S0-BCO-877

TEXTBOOK OF pediatric emergency medicine

TEXTBOOK OF pediatric emergency medicine

EDITORS **GARY R. FLEISHER, M.D., F.A.C.E.P.**
Assistant Director, Emergency Medicine
Children's Hospital, Philadelphia, Pennsylvania
Assistant Professor of Pediatrics
University of Pennsylvania School of Medicine

STEPHEN LUDWIG, M.D.
Director, Emergency Medicine
Children's Hospital, Philadelphia, Pennsylvania
Associate Professor of Pediatrics
University of Pennsylvania School of Medicine

ASSOCIATE EDITORS **FRED M. HENRETIG, M.D.**
RICHARD M. RUDDY, M.D.
JOHN M. TEMPLETON, JR., M.D.

CONSULTING EDITOR **BENJAMIN K. SILVERMAN, M.D.**
The Staff of the
Children's Hospital of Philadelphia

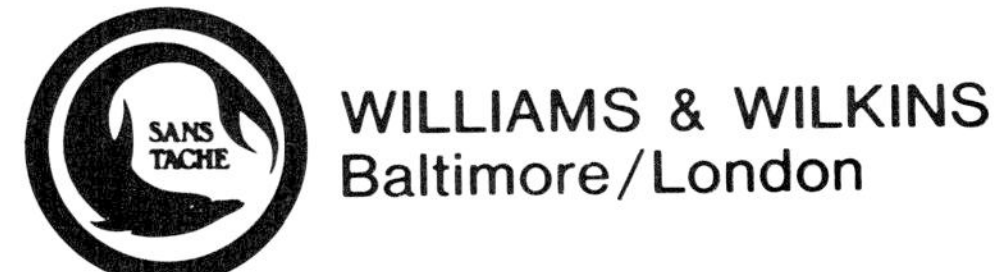

WILLIAMS & WILKINS
Baltimore/London

Accurate indications, adverse reactions, and dosage schedules for drugs are provided in this book, but it is possible that they may change. The reader is urged to review the package information data of the manufacturers of the medications mentioned.

Made in the United States of America

Reprinted 1984

Library of Congress Cataloging in Publication Data
Main entry under title:

Textbook of pediatric emergency medicine.

Includes index.
1. Pediatric emergencies. I. Fleisher, Gary. II. Ludwig, Stephen. [DNLM: 1. Emergencies—In infancy and childhood. WS 200 T355]
RJ370.T48 618.92′0025 82-7069
ISBN 0-683-03253-4 AACR2

Composed and printed at the
Waverly Press, Inc.
Mt. Royal and Guilford Aves.
Baltimore, MD 21202, U.S.A.

Dedication

For Their Love And Support
We Dedicate This Book To
Our Wives
Our Children
And Our Parents

Preface

For more than a decade, the editors have been caring for children in hospital emergency departments. Out of this chaotic milieu has arisen a concept of Pediatric Emergency Care which stems from the experiences of the editors in all aspects of the field, particularly clinical care and teaching.

As the editors groped with the vast array of clinical problems encountered among children in the emergency department and attempted to codify an organized approach for the housestaff and students, the lack of an appropriate source of information stood out sharply. Textbooks of Emergency Medicine relegated pediatrics to a single chapter, as if to suggest that small children had only a small number of problems. While references in pediatrics addressed all of the clinical issues at length, they did not speak to the needs of the emergency department physician nor to those more urgent and practical needs of the office pediatrician. All too often they dwelled on the intricate diseases at the expense of the common problems. Use of these textbooks has required making a diagnosis first, thereby limiting their usefulness in the evaluation of the sick child with a specific complaint or an unknown illness. They paid scant attention to cardiopulmonary resuscitation, surgical problems, and psychosocial emergencies and procedures. Although the multitude of manuals available came closest to providing an answer, they fell short in terms of the breadth and depth of their coverage.

While training residents from both emergency medicine and pediatric programs, the editors realized that neither group acquired the necessary knowledge and skills to adequately diagnose and treat the diversity of disease seen in the emergency department. The emergency medicine houseofficers often had only brief contact with children. In a survey encompassing 85% of all the Emergency Medicine Residency Programs in the United States in 1980, the directors indicated that an average of 4 months was dedicated to pediatrics. Residents trained in such programs often have difficulty in distinguishing the child with meningitis from one with a high fever due to otitis media.

While pediatric residents received a sufficient exposure to children, the editors noted deficiencies in several aspects of their education. Often, their experience with surgical problems and procedures was quite limited. The third year resident who could expound at length on systemic lupus erythematosus needed consultants to handle a child with a subungual splinter.

This book addresses both of the problems identified in the preceding discussion: (1) the lack of a single source of information on the emergency care of children and (2) the failure of existing references to treat material on pediatric illnesses in a fashion suitable for the emergency physician. It is designed as a resource for all physicians caring for children in the emergency department, regardless of their initial training—pediatrics, emergency medicine, family practice, surgery, or internal medicine.

This textbook is divided into seven major sections. More than anything else, the ability to deal with a multitude of life-threatening diseases separates the physician in emergency medicine from his colleagues in other specialties. Thus, pediatric resuscitation is covered in the *first section.*

The *second section* is problem-oriented and is organized on the basis of the chief complaints or primary concerns of children seen in the emergency department. Each brief chapter outlines an approach to the differential diagnosis of the symptom or sign, delineating both the potentially fatal and the less serious but common diseases. Often, the stated frequency of various illnesses in a given clinical situation derives from the experience of the contributors and the editors in the emergency department, rather than the tables available in specialty publications. These chapters offer a reasonable approach to evaluating children with various complaints and touch on management only briefly. Once a likely diagnosis has been reached by following the approach outlined, these chapters will guide the reader to a more detailed discussion elsewhere in the textbook.

The *third, fourth, and fifth sections* provide an in-depth analysis of diseases encountered in pediatric emergency medicine. Since each chapter could easily be expanded to its own textbook if it were to be all-inclusive, three compromises were necessary to make the book optimally compact and useful: (1) not every disease receives an individual discussion. Less common entities are grouped together or dealt with only in differential diagnosis, while a few very rare illnesses may not even be mentioned; (2) for some diseases, the discussion covers only those aspects that will bring the child to the emergency department. The text does not attempt to deal with emergencies originating within the hospital, such as in the delivery room, nursery, or operating room; and (3) clinical manifestations and management are stressed at the expense of etiology and epidemiology. An effort is made to give both sufficient background information to provide a perspective on the diseases and enough pathophysiology to enable the reader to understand the basis of the clinical manifestations and the therapeutic decisions.

The *sixth section* deals with the administration of a pediatric emergency facility. Children have unique administrative as well as medical problems. To cite just a few, there are the areas of child abuse, emancipated minors, and informed consent. Since children come to the emergency department with different diseases than adults, the level of staffing and the facilities are not the same as those in an emergency department serving primarily adults. While this section is geared to institutions limited to children, the principles will often apply equally to the care of children within the emergency departments of general hospitals.

The *last section* of the book gives a detailed account of the technical procedures used in caring for children in the emergency department. While it is appropriate for the physician trained in Pediatric Emergency Medicine to perform any of these procedures, their application in clinical situations should be tempered by the experience of the physician and the urgency of the situation. The section will serve as a guide to individuals learning these techniques under supervision and will be a resource in life-threatening emergencies. However, the inexperienced physician must keep in mind that many procedures are more difficult to successfully complete in children because of their smaller anatomic structures, making the incidence of complications greater. Thus, when the clinical situation allows for a delay, the novice should defer to others with more experience.

Acknowledgments

Those dedicated individuals who contributed to this book did so while simultaneously fulfilling many clinical, teaching, and research responsibilities. During the preparation of the book, more than 70,000 patients sought treatment in the Emergency Department of The Children's Hospital of Philadelphia. Each of the authors spent significant amounts of time in helping us to provide pediatric emergency care for our patients. For finding the additional time and using their literary skill to share their clinical experience and insight with us, they have our gratitude.

Preparing the manuscripts, facilitating communicating, and keeping track of the unending flow of paper required innumerable hours. Rose Beato served as the overall project secretary. Pat Marker and Ruth Davenport were also essential to our efforts, and many other individual secretaries provided invaluable assistance in times of crises. For the many nights and weekends, and for their never failing encouragement, they have our thanks.

By our departmental and administrative chiefs, we were given the freedom to work on this book and the guidance, trust, and support needed to complete the task. We greatly appreciate the professional milieu created by David Cornfeld, M.D., Chief of the Division of General Pediatrics, Mary Ames, M.D., Associate Vice-President of Ambulatory Services, James O'Neill, M.D., Surgeon in Chief of The Children's Hospital of Philadelphia, and Jean Cortner, M.D., Physician in Chief of The Children's Hospital of Philadelphia and Chairman of The Department of Pediatrics at The University of Pennsylvania School of Medicine.

Christine Young served as a medical illustrator and more. She was a visual editor. She provided us not only with masterful artwork, but also with sound advice and constant motivation. For this assistance, we are indebted to her. We thank also the staff of Williams & Wilkins, particularly our editors, Susan Vitale and Maureen Vardoulakis, for bridging the gap between the medical and publishing worlds.

Our final acknowledgment goes to the housestaff and the nursing staff of the Emergency Department of The Children's Hospital of Philadelphia. The dedication of these professionals in providing sensitive pediatric emergency care in our department provided the incentive for us to codify their skills into a textbook for practitioners everywhere. We hope that our effort will aid others in sharing in the joy of helping children.

Gary R. Fleisher, M.D.
Stephen Ludwig, M.D.

Contributors

Balu H. Athreya, M.D.
Senior Physician and Chief, Rheumatology Section
Children's Hospital of Philadelphia
Associate Professor Pediatrics
University of Pennsylvania School of Medicine
Clinical Director, Children's Seashore House

Lester Baker, M.D.
Senior Physician and Director, Division of Endocrinology/Diabetes
Director, Clinical Research Center
Children's Hospital of Philadelphia
Professor of Pediatrics
University of Pennsylvania School of Medicine

John W. Bender, M.D.
Research Fellow in Pediatric Hematology
Children's Hospital of Philadelphia
Instructor of Pediatrics
University of Pennsylvania School of Pennsylvania

Christopher C. Bergen
Former Associate Vice President
Children's Hospital of Philadelphia

Peter H. Berman, M.D.
Senior Physician and Director, Division of Neurology
Children's Hospital of Philadelphia
Professor, Departments of Neurology & Pediatrics
University of Pennsylvania School of Medicine

Harry C. Bishop, M.D.
Senior Surgeon
Children's Hospital of Philadelphia
Professor of Pediatric Surgery
University of Pennsylvania School of Medicine

John T. Boyle, M.D.
Assistant Physician, Division of Gastroenterology and Nutrition
Children's Hospital of Philadelphia
Assistant Professor of Pediatrics
University of Pennsylvania School of Medicine

A. Michael Broennle, M.D.
Senior Anesthesiologist
Children's Hospital of Philadelphia
Associate Professor of Anesthesiology
University of Pennsylvania School of Medicine

Derek A. Bruce, M.B., Ch.B.
Associate Neurosurgeon
Children's Hospital of Philadelphia
Associate Professor Neurosurgery & Pediatrics
University of Pennsylvania School of Medicine

Anthony A. Caldamone, M.D.
Fellow in Pediatric Urology Surgery
Children's Hospital of Philadelphia
Instructor in Urology Surgery
University of Pennsylvania School of Medicine

Edward B. Charney, M.D.
Associate Physician, Division of General Pediatrics, Child Development & Rehabilitation
Children's Hospital of Philadelphia
Assistant Professor of Pediatrics
University of Pennsylvania School of Medicine

Alan R. Cohen, M.D.
Assistant Physician, Division of Hematology
Director of Hematology, Coagulation and Hemoglobin Laboratories
Children's Hospital of Philadelphia
Assistant Professor of Pediatrics
University of Pennsylvania School of Medicine

MarJeanne Collins, M.D.
Associate Physician, Division of General Pediatrics, Adolescent Medicine Section
Children's Hospital of Philadelphia
Assistant Director, Student Health Service
University of Pennsylvania
Assistant Professor of Pediatrics
University of Pennsylvania School of Medicine

Gary Cupit, Pharm. D.
Adjunct Assistant Professor
University of Pennsylvania School of Medicine

Gary R. Diamond, M.D.
Associate Ophthalmologist
Children's Hospital of Philadelphia
Assistant Professor of Ophthalmology
University of Pennsylvania School of Medicine

Robert A. Doughty, M.D.
Associate Physician, Assistant Physician-in-Chief
Children's Hospital of Philadelphia
Assistant Professor of Pediatrics, Assistant Chairman
University of Pennsylvania School of Medicine

John W. Duckett, M.D.
Senior Urologist and Director of Pediatric Urology Surgery
Children's Hospital of Philadelphia
Professor of Urology Surgery
University of Pennsylvania School of Medicine

Gary R. Fleisher, M.D.
Associate Physician, Divisions of Infectious Diseases and General Pediatrics,
Pediatric Emergency Care Section
Assistant Director of Emergency Department
Children's Hospital of Philadelphia
Assistant Professor of Pediatrics
University of Pennsylvania School of Medicine

Joel E. Frader, M.D.
Ambulatory Care Center
Children's Hospital of Pittsburgh
Assistant Professor of Pediatrics
University of Pittsburgh School of Medicine

Michael H. Gewitz, M.D.
Assistant Cardiologist
Director, Pediatric Echocardiography Laboratory
Children's Hospital of Philadelphia
Assistant Professor of Pediatrics
University of Pennsylvania School of Medicine

Aron Goldman, B.A., M. Arch., M.D.
University of Pennsylvania School of Medicine

Daniel Hale, M.D.
Fellow, Division of Endocrinology
Children's Hospital of Philadelphia
Instructor of Pediatrics
University of Pennsylvania School of Medicine

Steven Halpern, M.D.
Fellow, Division of Oncology
Children's Hospital of Philadelphia
Instructor of Pediatrics
University of Pennsylvania School of Medicine

Steven D. Handler, M.D.
Associate Director, Department of Otorhinolaryngology & Human Communication
Children's Hospital of Philadelphia
Assistant Professor, Department of Otorhinolaryngology & Human Communication
University of Pennsylvania School of Medicine

Fred M. Henretig, M.D.
Assistant Physician, Division of General Pediatrics, Pediatric Emergency Care Section
Children's Hospital of Philadelphia
Assistant Professor of Pediatrics
University of Pennsylvania School of Medicine

Gordon R. Hodas, M.D.
Staff Psychiatrist
Philadelphia Child Guidance Clinic and Children's Hospital of Philadelphia
Assistant Professor of Child Psychiatry
University of Pennsylvania School of Medicine

Paul J. Honig, M.D.
Senior Physician and Chief—Dermatology Section, Division of General Pediatrics
Children's Hospital of Philadelphia
Associate Professor of Pediatrics in Dermatology
University of Pennsylvania School of Medicine

Charles G. Howell, M.D.
Assistant Surgeon
Chief Surgical Resident
Children's Hospital of Phildelphia
Instructor of Pediatric Surgery
University of Pennsylvania School of Medicine

David Jaffe, M.D.
Fellow, Emergency Pediatrics, Division of General Pediatrics
Children's Hospital of Philadelphia
Instructor of Pediatrics
University of Pennsylvania School of Medicine

Robert G. Kettrick, M.D.
Senior Anesthesiologist
Associate Director, Pediatric Intensive Care Unit
Children's Hospital of Philadelphia
Assistant Professor of Anesthesiology
University of Pennsylvania School of Medicine

Gerald B. Kolski, M.D., Ph.D.
Clinical Director, Allergy Section
Division of Allergy, Immunology, and Pulmonology
Children's Hospital of Philadelphia
Assistant Professor of Pediatrics
University of Pennsylvania School of Medicine

Jane B. Kuniewicz, B.S.N.
Associate Director, Ambulatory Services
Children's Hospital of Philadelphia

Beverly J. Lange, M.D.
Assistant Physician, Division of Oncology
Children's Hospital of Philadelphia
Assistant Professor of Pediatrics
University of Pennsylvania School of Medicine

Leo C. Lefebvre, Jr.
Director, Fiscal Affairs-Department of Pediatrics
University of Pennsylvania School of Medicine

Stephen Ludwig, M.D.
Associate Physician, Division of General Pediatrics, Pediatric Emergency Care Section
Director of Emergency Department
Educational Coordinator, Supportive Child Adult Network
Children's Hospital of Philadelphia
Associate Professor of Pediatrics
University of Pennsylvania School of Medicine

Kenneth R. Lyen, M.R.C.P.
Fellow, Division of Endocrinology
Children's Hospital of Philadelphia
Instructor of Pediatrics
University of Pennsylvania School of Medicine

Jack H. Neff, D.D.S.
Division of Dentistry
Children's Hospital of Philadelphia
Clinical Associate Professor of Dentistry
University of Pennsylvania School of Dental Medicine

Linda P. Nelson, D.M.D., M.Sc.D.
Acting Director of the Division of Dentistry
Children's Hospital of Philadelphia
Assistant Professor of Orthodontics and Pedodontics
University of Pennsylvania School of Dental Medicine

Michael E. Norman, M.D.
Senior Physician and Director, Division of Nephrology
Children's Hospital of Philadelphia
Associate Professor of Pediatrics
University of Pennsylvania School of Medicine

Roger J. Packer, M.D.
Assistant Physician, Division of Neurology
Children's Hospital of Philadelphia
Assistant Professor of Neurology and Pediatrics
University of Pennsylvania School of Medicine

Jan E. Paradise, M.D.
Assistant Physician, Division of General Pediatrics
Children's Hospital of Philadelphia
Clinical Assistant Professor of Pediatrics
University of Pennsylvania School of Medicine

George J. Peckham, M.D.
Senior Physician, Associate Department Chairman—Finance
Chief, Division of Neonatology
Children's Hospital of Philadelphia
Associate Professor of Pediatrics
University of Pennsylvania School of Medicine

William P. Potsic, M.D.
Director, Division of Otolaryngology & Human Communication
Children's Hospital of Philadelphia
Assistant Professor of Otorhinolaryngology & Human Communication
University of Pennsylvania School of Medicine

Russell C. Raphaely, M.D.
Senior Anesthesiologist
Associate Director, Department of Anesthesiology
Director of Pediatric Intensive Care
Children's Hospital of Philadelphia
Associate Professor of Anesthesiology
University of Pennsylvania School of Medicine

Kathleen R. Rosenberry, Pharm.D.
Clinical Pharmacist
Children's Hospital of Philadelphia
Clinical Assistant Professor of Pharmacology and Pediatrics
University of Pennsylvania School of Medicine

Richard M. Ruddy, M.D.
Assistant Physician, Division of General Pediatrics, Pediatric Emergency Care
Children's Hospital of Philadelphia
Assistant Professor of Pediatrics
University of Pennsylvania School of Medicine

John Sargent, M.D.
Staff Psychiatrist & Pediatrician
Philadelphia Child Guidance Clinic and Children's Hospital of Philadelphia
Clinical Assistant Professor of Pediatrics and Psychiatry
University of Pennsylvania School of Medicine

Thomas F. Scanlin, M.D.
Director, Cystic Fibrosis Center
Division of Allergy, Immunology and Pulmonology
Children's Hospital of Philadelphia
Assistant Professor of Pediatrics
University of Pennsylvania School of Medicine

Louise Schnaufer, M.D.
Associate Surgeon
Children's Hospital of Philadelphia
Associate Professor of Pediatric Surgery
University of Pennsylvania School of Medicine

Luis Schut, M.D.
Senior Surgeon and Chief of Neurosurgical Services
Children's Hospital of Philadelphia
Professor of Neurosurgery & Pediatrics
University of Pennsylvania School of Medicine

William Schwartz, M.D.
Senior Physician, Division of Nephrology and General Pediatrics
Children's Hospital of Philadelphia
Associate Professor of Pediatrics
University of Pennsylvania School of Medicine

Henry H. Sherk, M.D.
Assistant Orthopedic Surgeon
Children's Hospital of Philadelphia
Clinical Assistant Professor of Orthopedic Surgery
University of Pennsylvania School of Medicine

Benjamin K. Silverman, M.D.
Medical Editorial Consultant
Pediatric Practitioner
Clinical Affiliate
Children's Hospital of Philadelphia
Clinical Associate Professor
University of Pennsylvania School of Medicine

Howard McC. Snyder III, M.D.
Assistant Surgeon, Division of Urology Surgery
Children's Hospital of Philadelphia
Assistant Professor of Urology in Surgery
University of Pennsylvania School of Medicine

Leslie M. Sutton, M.D.
Assistant Neurosurgeon
Children's Hospital of Philadelphia
Assistant Professor of Neurosurgery
University of Pennsylvania School of Medicine

Anthony R. Temple, M.D.
Assistant Physician
Children's Hospital of Philadelphia
Adjunct Associate Professor
University of Pennsylvania School of Medicine

John M. Templeton, Jr., M.D.
Assistant Surgeon
Children's Hospital of Philadelphia
Assistant Professor of Pediatric Surgery
University of Pennsylvania School of Medicine

Josephine J. Templeton, M.D.
Assistant Anesthesiologist
Children's Hospital of Philadelphia
Assistant Professor of Anesthesiology
University of Pennsylvania School of Medicine

Ann E. Thompson, M.D.
Director, Pediatric Intensive Care
Children's Hospital of Pittsburgh
Assistant Professor of Anesthesia and Pediatrics
University of Pittsburgh School of Medicine

William J. Vasileff, M.D.
Provisional Staff, Department of Plastic Surgery
Children's Hospital of Michigan
Associate Staff, Department of Plastic Surgery
William Beaumont Hospital
Royal Oak, Michigan

Victoria L. Vetter, M.D.
Assistant Cardiologist
Children's Hospital of Philadelphia
Assistant Professor of Pediatrics
University of Pennsylvania School of Medicine

John B. Watkins, M.D.
Senior Physician and Chief, Division of Gastroenterology & Nutrition
Children's Hospital of Philadelphia
Associate Professor of Pediatrics
University of Pennsylvania School of Medicine

Linton A. Whitaker, M.D.
Senior Surgeon and Chief of Plastic Surgery
Children's Hospital of Philadelphia
Professor of Surgery
University of Pennsylvania School of Medicine

Carolyn L. Yancey, M.D.
Assistant Physician, Division of Rheumatology
Children's Hospital of Philadelphia
Assistant Professor of Pediatrics
University of Pennsylvania School of Medicine

Christine D. Young, M.A., A.M.I.
Medical Illustrator
Baltimore, Maryland

Moritz M. Ziegler, M.D.
Assistant Surgeon
Children's Hospital of Philadelphia
Assistant Professor of Pediatric Surgery
University of Pennsylvania School of Medicine

Contents

SECTION I

Life Support Emergencies

Stephen Ludwig, M.D., Section Editor

SECTION II

Signs and Symptoms

Fred M. Henretig, M.D., Section Editor

SECTION III

Medical Emergencies

Gary R. Fleisher, M.D., Section Editor

SECTION IV

Surgical Emergencies

John M. Templeton, Jr., M.D., Section Editor

SECTION VII

Procedures

Richard M. Ruddy, M.D., Section Editor

A. Michael Broennle, M.D., Michael H. Gewitz, M.D., Steven D. Handler, M.D., Charles G. Howell, M.D., David Jaffe, M.D., Robert G. Kettrick, M.D., William P. Potsic, M.D., John M. Templeton, Jr., M.D., and Josephine J. Templeton, M.D.

Introduction

UNDERSTANDING THE UNIQUE NEEDS OF CHILDREN

I. INTRODUCTION

The performance of a rapid, accurate clinical assessment of the child requires a familiarity with the elements of normal growth and development processes. The developmental level of the child guides the approach to the interview and examination, and the range of normal for various physical measurements and the significance of many clinical signs varies with age. In this introduction, we offer the reader a basic understanding of this growth process in order to facilitate the evaluation and treatment of the child. Familiarity with these principles will enhance the interpretation of the clinical findings and the application of the therapeutic techniques that are discussed in subsequent chapters.

When dealing with the usual adult patient, the demeanor of the physician has only a limited influence on the amount of information obtained; one who brusquely applies a cold stethoscope to the chest of an adult will detect just as many murmurs as one who takes a gentle approach with a warm instrument. However, physician interactions with children require special skills. The approach of the physician plays a crucial role in determining the amount and quality of information gathered during the clinical assessment. The key element to a successful approach is the ability to empathize and to understand things from the child's perspective. "Is there blood in your urine?" is less likely to be understood and to elicit an affirmative answer from a 5-year-old child with hematuria than, "Is your pee red?" Similarly, the cries of a hungry infant may well obscure the findings of localized rales whereas the child whose hunger has been sated by a bottle of formula will remain quiet, allowing for an adequate examination of the chest.

Only by experience can the physician ultimately learn to routinely perform a skillful history and physical examination of children of various ages. However, certain principles, based on a knowledge of growth and development, serve to guide those who are still acquiring new skills. By understanding the fears, intellectual abilities and needs of children, the physician can temper the desire for immediate information with age-appropriate techniques to gain cooperation from the child. Time spent in such an effort pays many dividends in all patient encounters, but particularly in the Emergency Department where the physician is often a stranger, the child has been stressed, and the diseases are potentially life-threatening.

After the physician has maximized cooperation on the part of the child and performed a thorough assessment, he or she must interpret the findings within the framework of growth and development. Abundant lymphatic tissue may raise the specter of cancer in an adult but signals only the normal maturation of the reticuloendothelial system in a 5-year-old. Similarly, a swelling above the eye of an adult might be an indication of frontal sinusitis, while such a disease could not possibly occur in a 1-year-old who had not yet aerated his frontal sinus.

II. GROWTH AND DEVELOPMENT

Every encounter with a child should begin with an assessment of the growth and development of that individual, both to decide upon an approach to the examination and to establish whether underlying disease has hindered these processes. Such an assessment may be hurried in the critically ill child and more leisurely in the absence of significant distress, but it must always be performed. Even in the child who has suffered a cardiopulmonary arrest, an accurate estimate

Table I.1
Formulas for Estimating Growth

Age	Weight (kg)	Height (cm)	Head Circumference (cm)
Birth	3.5	50	35
1 yr	10	75	47
2 yr	13	88	49
More than 2 yr	Add ~2 kg/yr	Add ~6 cm/yr	Not applicable

needs to be made for size and weight if resuscitation is to proceed adequately.

Experience and the use of certain established formulas provide quick estimates of growth (Table I.1) but they should never substitute for the use of standardized charts when time allows. Children should be weighed at each emergency visit. The physician should strive for precision

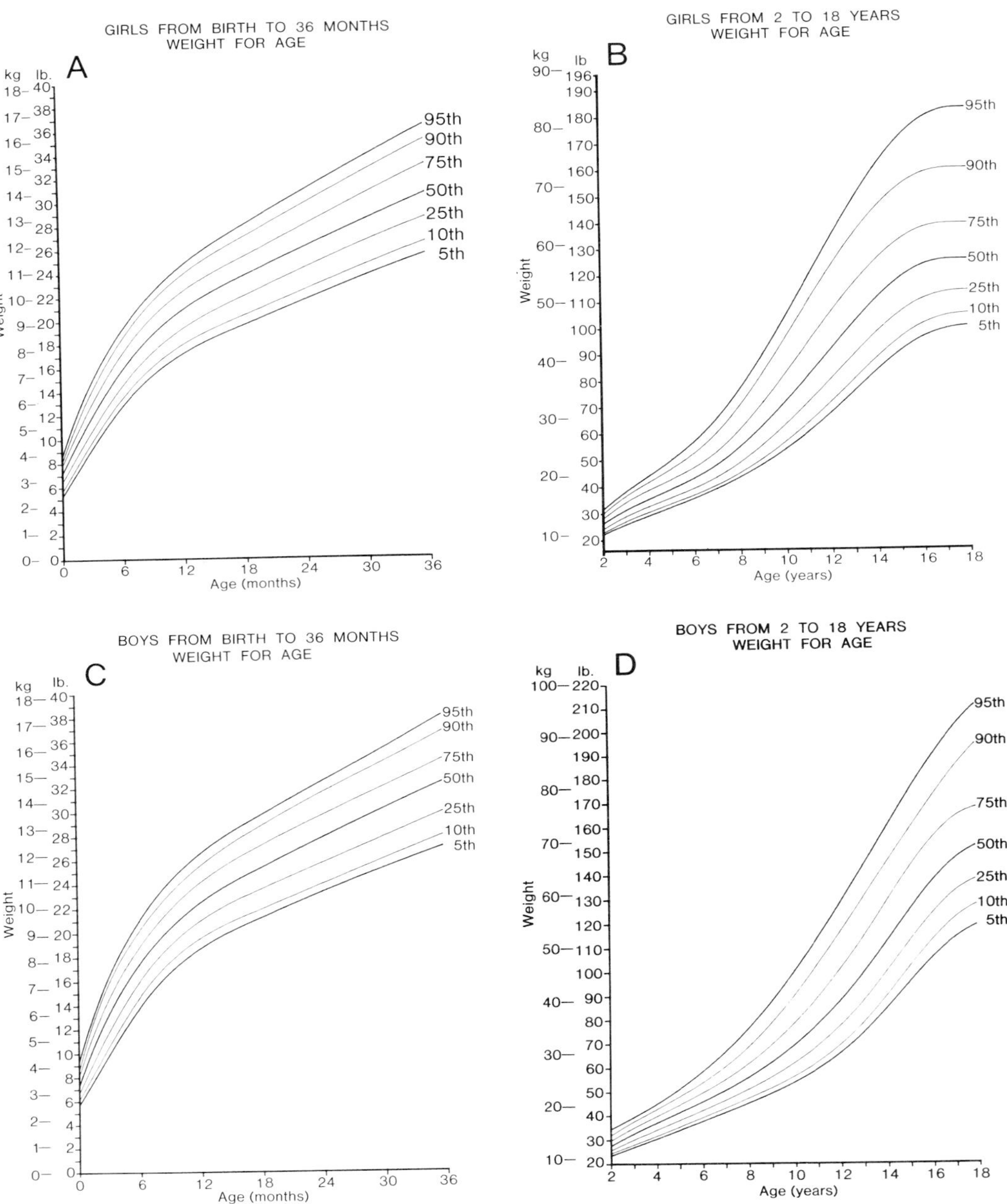

Figure I.1 Weight for age, birth to 36 months: (*A*) girls, (*C*) boys; 2 to 18 years: (*B*) girls, (*D*) boys. (Adapted from Health Resources Administration, National Center for Health Statistics, and Center for Disease Control.)

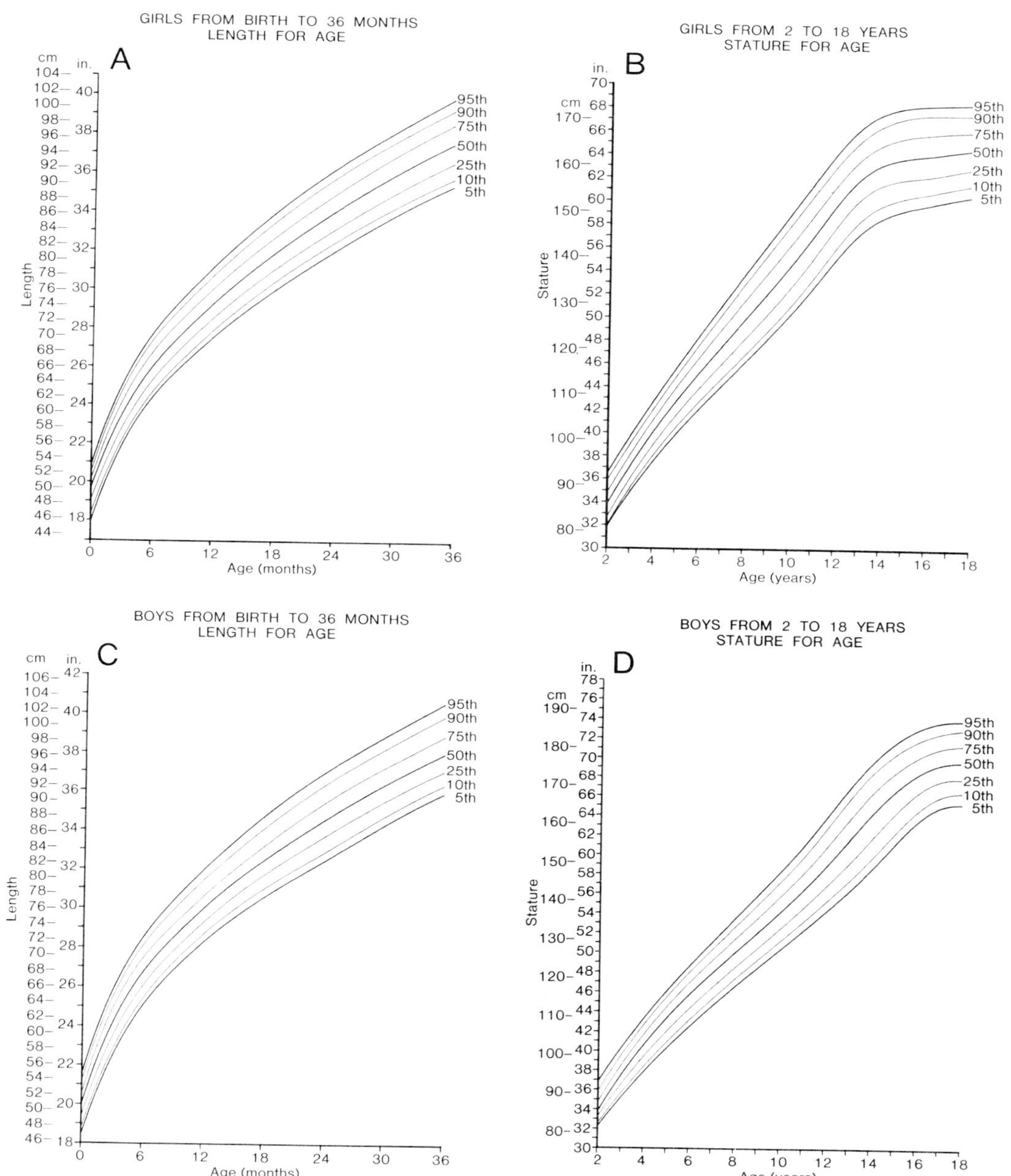

Figure I.2 Length for age, birth to 36 months: (*A*) girls, (*C*) boys; stature at 2 to 18 years: (*B*) girls, (*D*) boys. (Adapted from Health Resources Administration, National Center for Health Statistics, and Center for Disease Control.)

in obtaining and recording all measurements (Figs. I.1–I.3). The charts that are used should be appropriate for the age and sex of the child.

In assessing growth and development, measurements at different points in time are helpful if available. Children vary in all aspects of growth about a mean, but each individual child usually establishes and maintains a relatively

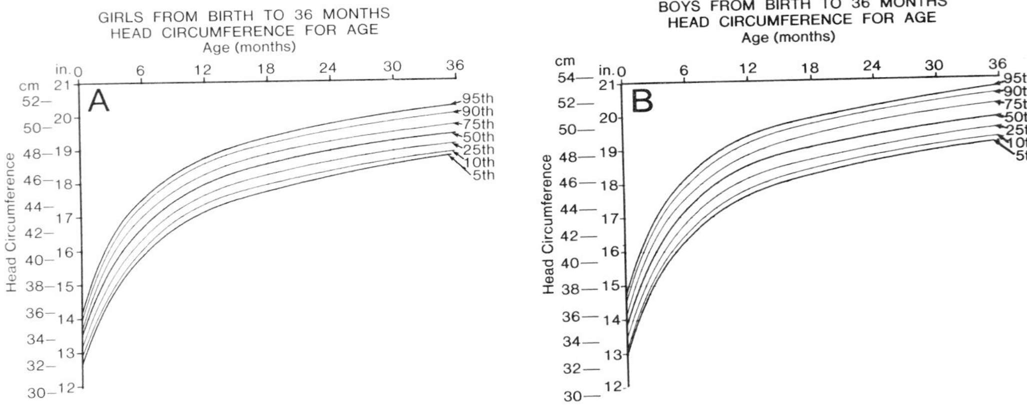

Figure I.3 Head circumference for age: (*A*) girls, (*B*) boys. (Adapted from Health Resources Administration, National Center for Health Statistics, and Center for Disease Control.)

constant rate of growth after birth. Thus, a child whose weight has fallen from the 90th percentile to the 3rd percentile over a period of 6 months should arouse more concern than the youngster who has been growing steadily along the 3rd percentile since infancy.

Expressions such as "Big is better" and "Small is beautiful" abound, but neither has any application to the process of growth and development. Rather, each child must be helped to achieve his maximal genetic potential, unimpeded by noxious environmental factors. Both deficient and excessive growth may indicate or result from underlying disease.

PHYSICAL GROWTH

The length of the term newborn infant usually varies between 45 and 55 cm (average 50 cm). The rate of increment for length is very rapid during the first few years of life but then declines until puberty. Growth may be altered by normal growth spurts as well as by a number of physical and environmental factors. The average child achieves a length of 75 cm by 1 year of age and a height of 100 cm by 4 years. Thereafter, the height increases by about 5 to 6 cm annually until puberty. During the pubertal growth spurt, boys grow about 20 cm and girls 18 cm.

WEIGHT

The change in a child's weight follows a pattern similar to that of length. During the first year of life, the average infant's weight triples so that the 3.5-kg term newborn develops into a 10-kg 1-year old. Prematures may even quadruple this birth weight in the first year. Subsequently, the rate of increment slows down; the older child gains 2 to 2.5 kg yearly.

The head is relatively large in proportion to the body at birth, having a circumference of about 35 cm. Compared to the height and weight, growth occurs very rapidly during the first 12 months of life and then slows down. The head circumference is about 46 to 47 cm at 1 year of age, 50 cm at 4 years, and 55 to 56 cm in the adolescent.

Different organ systems grow at different rates. While the central nervous system increases rapidly during the first 2 or 3 years of life, the genitals remain relatively dormant until puberty. The lymphatic system displays yet another pattern of growth; this tissue reaches a maximum size at 5 or 6 years of age and then declines. Primary teeth appear initially at 6 months of age and reach a full complement by 3 years. However, new secondary teeth do not erupt until 6 years of age.

DEVELOPMENT

A newborn can lift his or her head but is unable to move about. By 6 months of age most infants can sit, and by 1 year, walk. A 2- to 3-year-old child can run, jump, and pedal a tricycle. Gross motor abilities become increasingly sophisticated during the preschool years as the child develops the ability to skip and hop on one foot.

The 3- to 4-month-old infant can grab a toy, and the child of 6 to 7 months transfer objects from hand to hand. Before a year of age, pincer grasp usually develops sufficiently so that the child can pick up a small object such as a raisin. Toddlers develop the ability to copy geometric forms, and preschool age children can draw a human figure with 3 to 6 parts. Motor activities become increasingly specialized as they are applied to games and athletics at school.

During the latter part of the first year, the infant understands simple spoken phrases, but expression consists of only a few repetitive consonant sounds, such as "mama" or "dada." A few words appear at 1 year of age, and the 2-year-old knows several hundred words and utters brief sentences. The preschool age child forms longer sentences, knows his or her name, and can tell a story. During the elementary school period, children learn to express abstract concepts.

As the infant matures, different relationships evolve with adults in the environment. An infant less than 6 months of age usually does not distinguish between strangers and parents. However, the child between 1/2 and 3 years of age usually is shy of strangers; separation anxiety plays a major role during this period of development. After the third birthday, most children will allow strangers to approach if their manner is gentle and appropriate. Older children are more receptive to conversation and explanations.

III. APPROACH TO THE CHILD

Children needing emergency medical care find themselves in a strange and often threatening environment. The sights, sounds, and smells of the emergency department are alien to most children. The emergency department staff have the responsibility to do everything possible to minimize the trauma that may accompany a hospital visit. Every physical injury or illness has a concomitant psychological effect on the child. Many children will recount the story of their emergency department visit for weeks or months afterward. Some may retain vivid memories even into adulthood. Particularly stressful medical situations may become the foci of fears, phobias, or new symptoms. Thus, pediatric emergency care must be directed both to the child's body and to the psychological reactions to the illness or its treatment.

Beyond concern for the child's needs, having an effective approach to children makes pediatric emergency care more pleasurable for the emergency physician. A well planned and carried out approach to the child eliminates making every pediatric encounter a wrestling match between a screaming child and a frustrated physician witnessed by an audience of anxious and upset parents.

The approach to the child should be based on the child's developmental level. A recurring theme throughout this volume is that children are in a dynamic state of growth and development which makes them a unique patient population. By considering a few general principles, and then assessing and applying several developmentally appropriate principles, the emergency physician can lessen both the noise level in the department and, more importantly, the trauma left by the pediatric patient.

GENERAL PRINCIPLES

Several general principles should be applied to any endeavor with a pediatric patient. These guidelines should be followed regardless of the age or developmental level of the child. Adherence to these principles is more easily done if the physician attempts to view the situation through the child's eyes.

Environmental Considerations—The physician must be cognizant of the optimal environment for the child. Chapter 76 covers child oriented emergency department design and stresses structural and decor considerations. Most emergency departments were neither designed nor constructed with the pediatric patient in mind. Nonetheless, the emergency physician may compensate for this. Children should be segregated from acutely ill adult patients. The child who witnesses the treatment given to a seriously ill adult may be emotionally traumatized. Adults with psychiatric, drug or alcohol problems may be loud, abusive in their tone and apt to use foul language. Similarly, children with relatively minor illnesses should be sheltered from other children who are seriously ill. A calm, quiet environment is best for the child. The sound of a crying child will cause other children to succumb to their own fears.

If there are a few toys or books available, these will be effective in making the child feel more comfortable. Many physicians will carry a small toy or hand puppet in their black bag in order to gain the child's confidence. Wall posters, graphics, or mobiles can be used to attract the child's attention and make the physical examination easier.

An often overlooked aspect of the environment is room temperature. Small infants will be particularly sensitive to a cold environment and consequently will begin crying as soon as undressed. Older children who are febrile will also be affected by a low ambient temperature.

Parental Involvement—Parents should always be allowed to accompany their children during the emergency visit. Separation of the child and parent during a time when the child (and often the parents) is most anxious is counterproductive. Departmental policy should include regulations that allow maximal parent-child contact. In the case of a critically ill child, the clerk should gather billing and administrative information at the bedside rather than at the registration desk. On the other hand, parents who cannot tolerate the sight of a laceration repair should be positioned away from the surgical field but in physical contact with the child.

Children will often relax when witnessing a calm interchange between their parents and the doctor. Parents should be used constructively to gain history from the child, to help in the physical examination, and to soothe and support the child. Involving parents also lessens their anxiety and makes them feel comfortable in not losing their parental role even in the midst of a highly technical medical environment.

Communicate with the Child—Many physicians unaccustomed to working with children will overlook the value and the fun of communicating with the child. Even the infant will enjoy face to face contact with the physician and the sound of a friendly voice. Some children by the age of 2 or 3 years can give a history which is complete and accurate. Other children will enjoy playful banter, conversation about school, a sibling, or a friend, or discussion of an upcoming holiday or birthday. Children will be calmed to learn something about their doctor. An introduction by name is helpful. If the physician tells the child about himself or herself, the child will relate to the doctor as a person. This may diminish any threat perceived by the child.

Be Honest—Children are constantly being reminded about the value of honesty. Most children regard this virtue highly. Physicians must be honest with their pediatric patients in order to maintain credibility and build trust. Saying "this won't hurt a bit" before doing a venipuncture is dishonest. All rapport with the child will be lost. Children can handle most difficult situations if they are presented with the truth and allowed to express themselves. If a procedure must be done, they must be told so. This message can be softened by saying "It's all right to cry" or "I would not like it either" or "I am sorry but this is something that must be done." The days of preparing children for tonsillectomy by telling them that they are going to get some ice cream are gone.

Respect Modesty—Children of all ages should be respected for feelings of bashfulness or modesty. In particular, school-aged children and adolescents may have serious concerns about exposing their bodies to a stranger. All children should be offered hospital gowns. Although all parts of the body must be examined, including genitalia, this may be done in a stepwise fashion which demonstrates the physician's respect for the child.

AGE-SPECIFIC APPROACHES

Each child encountered in the emergency department is an individual. As such, each has unique characteristics which must be appreciated and understood in order to interact in the most positive way. As in-depth knowledge of the patient is a rare occurrence in the emergency department, the physician will be aided by relying on some age and developmental characteristic. Table I.2 summarizes the essential issues in this process including (1) the age of children; (2) their state of language, motor, and social development; (3) their fears; and (4) the techniques that may prove helpful.

Infancy (0–1 year)—Infants are in some ways the easiest to examine but in other ways the most difficult. Infants have little or no useful language development. Thus, there is no chance for the physician to discuss or reason with the patient. The child's world is very much the world for his/her parents, and the infant may feel most insecure when the parents are absent from the environment. Many infants even go through a stage of profound stranger anxiety. This is a period (5 to 9 months) when anyone but a parent will elicit a tearful reaction simply by approaching the child. At times even grandparents may be perceived as strangers. Comforting techniques at this age should involve careful use of

Table I.2
Developmental Approach to Pediatric Emergency Care Patients

Age (yr)	Important Development Issues	Fears	Useful Techniques
Infancy: 0–1	Minimal language Feel an extension of parents Sensitive to physical environment	Stranger anxiety	Keep parents in sight Avoid hunger Use warm hands Keep room warm
Toddler: 1–3	Receptive language more advanced than expressive See themselves as individuals Assertive will	Brief separation Pain	Maintain verbal communication Examine in parent's lap Allow some choices when possible
Preschool: 3–5	Excellent expressive skills for thoughts and feelings Rich fantasy life Magical thinking Strong concept of self	Long separation Pain Disfigurement	Allow expression Encourage fantasy and play Encourage participation in care
School age: 5–10	Fully developed language Understanding of body structure and function Able to reason and compromise Experience with self-control Incomplete understanding of death	Disfigurement Loss of function Death	Explain procedures Explain pathophysiology and treatment Project positive outcome Stress child's ability to master situation Respect physical modesty
Adolescence: 10–19	Self-determination Decision making Peer group important Realistic view of death	Loss of autonomy Loss of peer acceptance Death	Allow choices and control Stress acceptance by peers Respect autonomy

the parent. The parent should be close by. The child may need to be examined while in the parent's lap or held against the parent's shoulder. The sight, sound, touch and smell of the parent will be a comfort. A sudden separation, palpation with a cold hand or stethoscope, or the child's perception of the physician as a stranger may be all a source of patient distress.

Toddler (1–3 years)—The child of toddler age will have developed significant language skills. Language development is more advanced for receptive language than for expressive language. Thus, the toddler will understand more than he can express. The toddler will also have a more developed sense of self. The child sees a self-entity separate from the parents. This leads to the practice of self-assertion or what some refer to as the "terrible twos." The word "no" is the most frequently used.

Despite the apparent desire for individuation, the toddler is most fearful of separation from parents. This is characterized by the child's play in which he wanders or runs away from the parent but always returns to make sure that the parent is still there. Toddlers have also experienced a number of immunizations and may regard the physician as "needle giver."

Maintaining verbal communication with the child can be helpful. The child will understand a great deal of what is explained, although he may use a limited number of vocabulary words. Keeping the parents close by and allowing them to assist with the physical examination will be helpful. If one knows in advance that no venipuncture or intramuscular injection needs to be given, it may be helpful to reassure the child of this as early in the encounter as possible. Sometimes a statement such as "isn't it great that you are *not* going to have a needle today!" will smooth the way for a relaxed and quiet physical examination.

Preschool (3–5 years)—Preschool aged children have made many developmental gains. These children have developed a great deal of expressive language. They can express thoughts and feelings. They are clear about rules and regulations particularly if they have been in a structured preschool setting. Preschoolers have a well formed self concept and understand their position within the family and neighborhood. Preschoolers also have vivid imaginations and what some developmentalists have called "magical thinking." This is the age of imitation when children imitate what their parents do and what the latest "super hero" may be doing.

Preschool aged children have a well defined fear of pain. With a well formed self concept and body sense comes the concept that the body can be harmed or disformed. Children may be fearful that their leg has been removed when it has been placed in a plaster cast and cannot be seen.

The approach to the preschooler can be aided by having the child express his fears and fantasies. Fantasy can work in favor of the physician in two ways. First, some children may use their fantasies as a source of relaxation. The child who is undergoing a procedure such as laceration repair may become absorbed in a conversation about some fantasy. "Let's talk about all the things you are going to get for Christmas while I fix your cut. Tell me all the presents you want." Second, the child can be made the assistant doctor or nurse. The child can hold the stethoscope on his own chest. It is the fantasy of being like the paramedics seen on television. The child may be comforted by holding or manipulating the medical instruments, even trying them out on a doll. Play is a great vehicle for expression.

School Aged (5–10 years)—Children who are in school are easy to approach in that they have fully developed language skills. Many children have a beginning understanding of how the body works. Their sense of fantasy has been tempered by a more realistic view of the world. Children of school age have become used to reason and compromise.

The school aged child may not have a well formed concept of death. This may result in an exaggerated response to symptoms. For example, the child knows that blood is important for body function but may not know that the amount lost in a single episode of epistaxis is not life threatening. Many school aged children are still struggling with the fears of pain, body distortion, and separation from parents.

In approaching these children, language is the physician's most effective tool. The physician may wish to explain basics of pathophysiology and emphasize the body's mechanisms of repair. Children will want to know how things work. The physician can place the illness or injury in perspective. Project a positive outcome. Some children may express the fear of death or disfigurement and may need reassurance in these matters.

Adolescence (10–19 years)—The adolescent period is marked by a diverse array of developmental stages. It becomes more difficult to characterize an orderly sequence of skill aquisition. Adolescents seem to set and strive for their own developmental milestones, and it is this quality of self-determination that is the hallmark for the period. Chapter 71 covers the many problems which may be encountered during adolescence and offers some specific management techniques.

In striving to become an adult and in exercising self-determination, the adolescent most fears the loss of decision making power. Being treated like a child is intolerable. Self-esteem is often a tenuous quality and is also fiercely protected. The adolescent's body is undergoing radical change, so body image is another area of concern. Peer relationships become as important, perhaps even more important, than family relationships. For the adolescent, illness may mean returning to complete parental control and supervision, loss of freedom, distortion of body image, weakening self-esteem, and perhaps separation from or rejection by the peer group.

Using this cursory understanding of adolescence, the emergency physician must approach the child as if he were an adult. Taking the history from the parent without involving the patient will doom the physician to a difficult visit and perhaps noncompliance. Adolescents need explanations which appeal to their sense of control over their bodies. The adolescent must be reassured as far as body deformity, loss of function, or death. Relating this illness or injury to the experience of other teenagers may be helpful. At all costs, respect the adolescents' autonomy while letting them know that you are in control of the medical situation.

Gary R. Fleisher, M.D.
Stephen Ludwig, M.D.

SECTION I Life Support Emergencies

CHAPTER 1

Resuscitation—Pediatric Basic and Advanced Life Support

ROBERT G. KETTRICK, M.D., AND STEPHEN LUDWIG, M.D.

INTRODUCTION

Cardiopulmonary resuscitation (CPR) is a series of interventions aimed at restoring and supporting vital function after apparent death.

The urgent and immediate goal of resuscitation is to reestablish substrate delivery to meet the metabolic needs of the myocardium and brain. The overall goal is to return the patient to society without morbidity related to the resuscitation process.

Pediatric CPR has been largely based on the adult model of resuscitation. There is an orderly progression through the assessment and management of the ABC's—Airway, Breathing, and Circulation. Like the adult counterpart, pediatric CPR is best performed by a well-coordinated team of physicians, nurses, respiratory therapists, and other support personnel. Unfortunately, many experienced emergency physicians approach pediatric life support with uncertainty, anxiety, and confusion. This situation is usually related to a lack of familiarity with the distinctive knowledge and performance skills needed for supporting the pediatric patient. This chapter will emphasize those important differences between pediatric and adult CPR.

BACKGROUND

Incidence

There is no incidence data for pediatric resuscitations performed annually in the United States. We reviewed 130 resuscita-

Table 1.1
Leading "Causes" of Deaths of Children in the United States, 1975

Causes of Death	Age in Years			
	<1	1–4	5–9	10–14
Birth injury:				
Difficult labor, (hypoxia, anoxia)	26,585	10	6	2
Unintentional injuries	1,307	3,611	3,033	3,785
Motor vehicle injuries	(225)	(1,321)	(1,576)	(1,710)
Drowning	(40)	(743)	(501)	(690)
Fire	(135)	(617)	(360)	(220)
Firearms (unintentional)	(3)	(71)	(120)	(304)
Poisoning	(31)	(121)	(37)	(93)
Other	(873)	(738)	(439)	(768)
Congenital abnormalities	8,582	1,141	424	318
Malignant neoplasms	129	711	929	878
Influenza and pneumonia	2,201	527	177	185
Homicide	178	317	136	249
Cardiovascular diseases	814	338	232	344
Suicide	0	0	0	170
All others	10,699	2,405	1,248	1,363
Total	50,525	9,060	6,185	7,294

tion efforts which occurred between 1976 and 1980 at The Children's Hospital of Philadelphia. These resuscitations were those to which a Code Blue team (Resuscitation Team) was summoned. While other resuscitations were conducted in the operating rooms, cardiac catheterization laboratory, and intensive care unit, they were not included, as they did not involve the Code Blue team. This number therefore gives an approximation of the minimal number of resuscitations performed in a large children's hospital in which there are 6,000 admissions and 140,000 outpatient visits per annum.

We can estimate the incidence of potential resuscitations by examining the data on infant and childhood mortality. Table 1.1 shows the mortality rates and the leading causes of death for children in the United States in 1975. The death rate for children 1 to 4 years old in 1970 was 84.5 per 100,000 children. In the group 5 to 14 years old, the rate was 41.3 per 100,000 children. Note that there is a relatively higher mortality rate for young children.

Patient Characteristics

Age. In our series of 130 patients we found that the majority of children were at the younger end of the pediatric age range (Fig. 1.1). The mean age was 1.98 years and the median 5 months. The age range was between 2 weeks and 16 years. Although pediatric CPR education should generally be tailored to the anatomic and physiologic characteristics of the young child, emergency department staff must be prepared to cope with the full spectrum of age and size.

Etiology. The most common primary diagnoses of hospitalized pediatric patients requiring resuscitation involve the respiratory system (Table 1.2). Conditions such as pneumonia, bronchiolitis, asthma, aspiration, epiglottitis, and respiratory distress syndrome account for the largest group of diagnoses. Cardiac diagnoses and central nervous system disorders occur in roughly equal frequency, but half as often as respiratory diagnoses. Common cardiovascular diagnoses include congenital heart disease, septic shock, and severe dehydration. Central nervous system diagnoses include hydrocephalus (ventricular shunt failure), meningitis, seizure, and tumor.

In the emergency department the physician is more likely to encounter children whose cardiac arrest is due to sudden infant death syndrome (SIDS), trauma, or un-

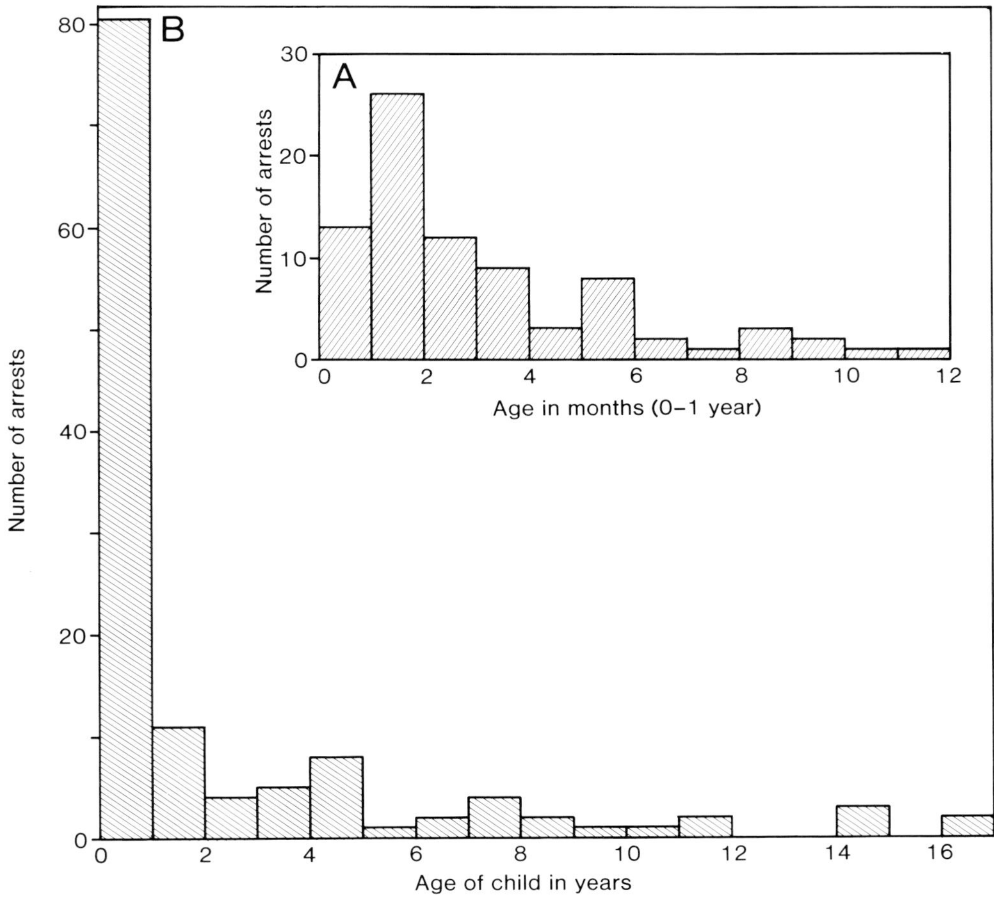

Figure 1.1 Histogram showing frequency of cardiac arrest as related to age in (*A*) months and (*B*) years from the Children's Hospital of Philadelphia survey.

known causes. Children with congenital anomalies, sequelae of prematurity, and birth trauma are also seen in the emergency department, as increasing numbers of children have survived the neonatal period and have been discharged from the hospital. The broad range of diagnoses encountered in our review of resuscitation is noted in Table 1.2. This clearly differs from the adult circumstance of resuscitation, where most arrests are related to coronary artery disease.

Demographics. There are no demographic studies to identify socioeconomic, racial, familial, or community characteristics of the pediatric patient who requires life support interventions. Such studies would be important for developing profiles of the high risk patient populations for subsequent development of surveillance or prevention programs.

Treatment Characteristics

Pediatric CPR presents the emergency department physician with several complexities and frustrations. The first difficulty often encountered is that the patient has received only minimal prehospital care. Pediatric patients are likely to be brought to the emergency department without the same field treatment that adult patients routinely receive. In many locales, paramedics are trained and equipped primarily to provide adult life support. Yet, they may be forced to initiate pediatric life support at the most basic level. In other areas, para-

Table 1.2
Diagnoses of Children Requiring Life Support By Body System, THE CHILDREN'S HOSPITAL OF PHILADELPHIA 1976–1980

Respiratory
Pneumonia
Aspiration
Asthma
Epiglottitis
Laryngotracheobronchitis
Respiratory failure/chronic lung disease
Bronchiolitis
Botulism
Primary apnea
Bronchopulmonary dysplasia
Cardiovascular
Congenital heart disease
Septic shock
Dehydration
Pericarditis
Congestive heart failure
Myocarditis
Central Nervous System
Acute hydrocephalus
Head Trauma
Seizure
Tumor
Meningitis
Hemorrhage
Gastrointestinal
Trauma
Enterocolitis
Bowel perforation
Bowel obstruction
Tracheoesophageal fistula
Miscellaneous/Multisystem
Sudden infant death syndrome
Drug ingestion
Tumors (non-CNS)
Multiple trauma

medics are limited by laws, regulations, or negative attitudes. Absent or inadequate prehospital care leads to longer periods of hypoxia and hypoperfusion which, in turn, directly affects prognosis and central nervous system morbidity.

The wide spectrum of age and diagnoses add additional complexity. The resuscitation team must provide an array of technical skills, drugs, and equipment. Without delay, the team must have the flexibility to adjust to the correct sizes and drug dosages for children.

Our experience shows that careful management of airway and breathing is extremely important. Because the cause of the arrest is often related to respiratory gas exchange and the child's myocardium is relatively resilient to hypoxemia, the rapid correction of hypoxemia may be all that is necessary to effect resuscitation. In one-third of the resuscitations we reviewed, resuscitation was effected with only oxygen and positive pressure ventilation.

For those patients who do not respond to airway and breathing management alone, life support will be significantly more difficult. In the emergency department, the lack of an immediate patient response usually predicts a need for multiple drug interventions. Our patients received a mean number of 4.5 drugs per patient.

One of the common frustrations to administering drugs is the establishment of an intravenous line. This technical skill continues to be the most frequent obstacle toward effecting successful CPR.

Dysrhythmia management is generally not a problem in pediatric life support. The absence of atherosclerotic vascular disease makes the child's myocardium less susceptible to dysrhythmia. As a result, antiarrhythmic medications and defibrillation are used infrequently. The most frequent cardiac rhythms to be recognized and managed are sinus bradycardia and asystole. The exceptions to this are those children with congenital heart disease and those who have sustained direct myocardial trauma (see Chapter 43). These children may present with unusual and difficult dysrhythmias which require esoteric management to effect a successful outcome.

Perhaps the greatest difficulty comes not with specific knowledge or technical skill, but with attitude. Many emergency departments are unaccustomed to resuscitating children and will become paralyzed when faced with the task. There is a fear that the child is somehow more fragile. In other circumstances there is over compensation to the point that the resuscitation of a child is prolonged beyond an optimal point for either the child or the family.

The emergency department team should review the effectiveness of each individual resuscitation effort. When the team recognizes that their efficiency and effectiveness with children is less than it is with adults, specific remedial education should be undertaken until this circumstance no longer exists.

Prognosis

The outlook for survival following CPR is very good for the pediatric patient. In our experience, if the arrest is rapidly recognized and skillfully managed, immediate survival may be as high as 90% and the survival to discharge rate 60%. These figures are based on a hospitalized population of children requiring resuscitation. For the emergency department patients the outcome is not as good but is still considerably better than the prognosis for adult arrest victims. In the emergency department the immediate survival may be as high as 60% while the survival to discharge rate is 40%. The poorer prognosis for emergency department patients may be attributed to delayed recognition of the arrest and to limited prehospital care.

CLINICAL MANIFESTATIONS

Infants and children who have experienced disruption of oxygen or glucose delivery to the brain may benefit from the various elements of basic or advanced cardiac life support. The clinical manifestations of those requiring immediate life support are most often related to failure of oxygen delivery to the skin, brain, and cardiovascular system. Cutaneous manifestations of oxygen deprivation include cyanosis, grayish hue, diaphoresis, and mottling. Manifestations of CNS hypoxia include confusion, delirium, seizures, and unresponsiveness. Cardiovascular manifestations include tachycardia, bradycardia, hypotension, and diaphoresis.

Glucose is the second essential substrate necessary for maintenance of central nervous system integrity. Severe hypoglycemia may be just as devastating as severe hypoxemia. Clinical manifestations are often similar to hypoxemia, as the primary effect on the central nervous system is coma. In addition, the effect of hypoglycemia on the cardiovascular system may lead to a secondary failure of oxygen delivery because of hypotension and related hypoperfusion.

A patient who has experienced a failure of substrate delivery to the central circulation must be resuscitated or supported until more specific diagnosis and management can be effected. Additionally, it is essential to identify those patients who are *at risk* for failure of substrate delivery. This can be accomplished by a physical examination with emphasis on evaluation for airway patency, gas exchange, and cardiovascular integrity. The laboratory may be helpful, as those with a low partial pressure of arterial oxygen (PaO_2), pH, glucose, hemoglobin, hemoglobin saturation, high $PaCO_2$ are at risk. Also, recognition of certain disease entities allows early intervention and prevention of cardiovascular collapse. Examples include epiglottitis, croup, and foreign body in the airway.

MANAGEMENT

Management Sequence

Once a child has been identified as requiring life support, a sequence of evaluations and interventions should be accomplished. Figure 1.2 shows the sequence of interventions for a patient requiring life support. Initially, central nervous system integrity is evaluated by the shake and shout maneuver. Vigorously shake the victim by the shoulders and at the same time shout at him and observe for response to these stimuli. If there is no response, the rescuer assumes that the brain is no longer receiving an adequate amount of oxygen and the three basic sequences of evaluation and management are initiated.

First, the airway is maneuvered so as to move the mandibular block of tissue up and off the posterior pharyngeal wall. The rescuer places his cheek next to the mouth and nose while he listens and feels for movement of air. At the same time the rescuer is watching the chest for any evidence of chest wall movement. If the patient is moving air independently, the rescuer simply continues to support the airway and looks to

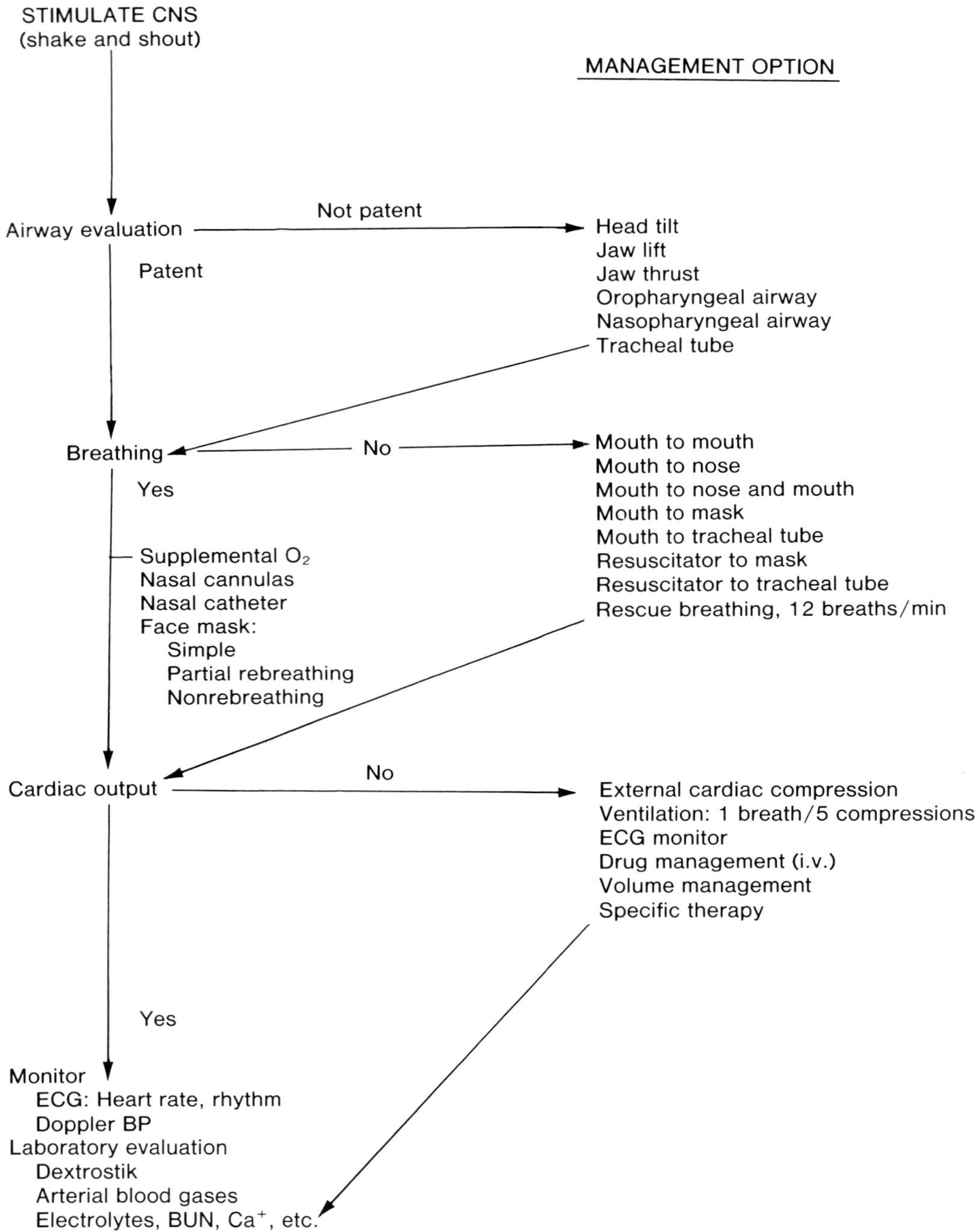

Figure 1.2 Management sequence for pediatric life support.

provide a mechanism for delivering supplemental oxygen. If the patient is not breathing spontaneously the rescuer must breathe for the victim, using an expired air technique. If advanced life support breathing technology is available, this may be employed. With the recognition that the airway is open and ventilation is occurring, the third phase of oxygen delivery is evaluated by feeling for arterial pulsations. Palpate the brachial, carotid, or femoral arteries. If palpable pulses are not present following a 15-sec evaluation, closed chest cardiac massage is initiated to provide a circulation. The adequacy of closed chest massage is initially determined by feeling for pulses. In determining whether or not the oxygen delivery system has been reestablished, look for improvement in the level of consciousness or a return to spontaneous breathing or an inherent cardiac rhythm.

Airway

EVALUATION

The first priority in the sequential evaluation and management paradigm of basic and advanced life support is evaluation and treatment of the airway. Look, listen and feel for evidence of gas exchange. *Look* at the chest to see if there is chest wall or abdominal movement suggestive of breathing effort. *Listen* over the mouth and nose for the sound of air movement. If a stethoscope is available, listen over the trachea. *Feel* with your cheek for evidence of air movement. If there is evidence of spontaneous breathing and no evidence of gas movement through the central airway, the presumptive diagnosis is that of airway obstruction.

MANAGEMENT

The most traditional noninvasive mechanism for handling an obstructed airway involves gentle flexion of the cervical spine on the thoracic spine and gentle extension of the occiput on the cervical spine (Fig. 1.3). The most effective manuver involves tilting the head back and lifting the chin forward by pulling or pushing the mandibular block of tissue forward (Fig. 1.3).

Most airway obstruction is related to the mandibular block of tissue falling posteriorly and lying against the posterior wall of the hypopharynx. This can be relieved by physically grasping the mandibular block and pulling it forward so that the lower anterior central incisors are anterior to the maxillary central incisors. The same result can be obtained by pushing the mandibular block of tissue forward. Place the fingers behind the angle of the jaw and push the jaw forward so that the lower central incisors are anterior to the upper central incisors (Fig. 1.3). These noninvasive maneuvers should be attempted before any of the more invasive airway adjuncts are utilized. Table 1.3 lists airway equipment which should be available for pediatric life support.

Artificial Airways

Oropharyngeal Airways. Oropharyngeal airways are used when manual manipulation of the airway is ineffective in maintaining airway patency. The purpose of the oropharyngeal airway is to stent or support the mandibular block of tissue off of the posterior pharyngeal wall. There are three basic parts to this airway (Fig. 1.4). The flange is used to prevent the airway from falling back into the mouth. It also serves as a point of fixation for adhesive tape. The bite block portion is designed to prevent approximation of the central incisors. A forceful bite may produce obstruction of an oral tracheal tube. The stent of the oropharyngeal airway is designed specifically to hold the tongue away from the posterior pharyngeal wall. Secondarily, the stent may provide an air channel or suction conduit through the mouth. The proper size oropharyngeal airway can be estimated by placing the airway along side the face so that the flange is at the level of the central incisors and the bite block portion is parallel to the palate. The tip of the airway should just approximate the angle of the mandible.

The airway should be placed by using a wooden spatula or tongue depressor to press the tongue into the floor of the mouth. The airway is then passed so that the stent conforms to the contour of the tongue. If the oropharyngeal airway is not inserted properly it may push the tongue backward into the posterior pharynx, aggravating or creating upper airway obstruction. If the airway is too long, it may touch the larynx and stimulate vomiting or laryngospasm.

Nasopharyngeal Airways. The purpose of this airway is to stent the tongue from the posterior pharyngeal wall (Fig. 1.3). It may also be used to facilitate nasotracheal suctioning. The length of the nasopharyngeal airway is estimated by measuring the distance from the nares to the

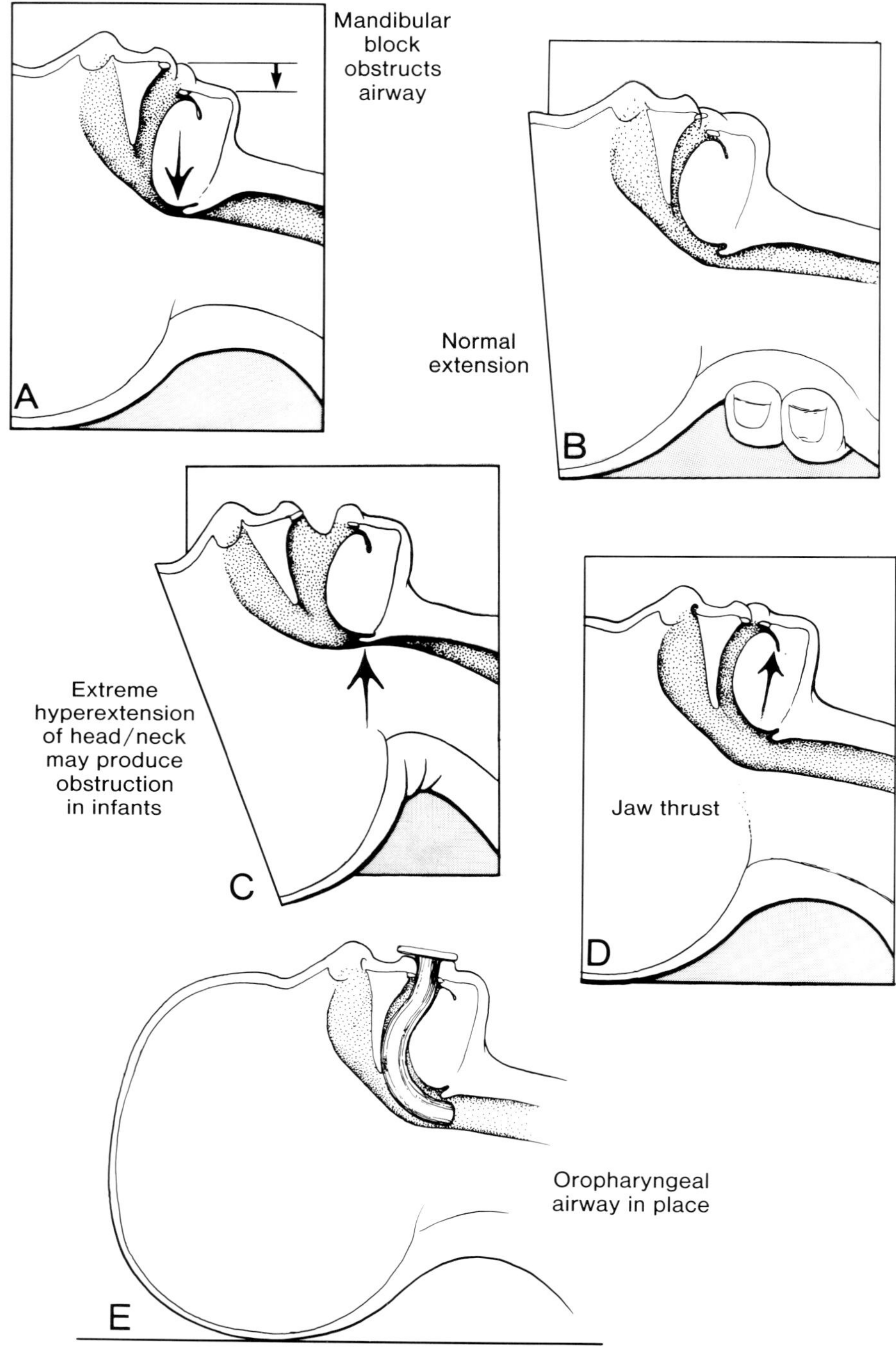

Figure 1.3 (*A*) Upper airway obstruction related to hypotonia. (*B*) Partial relief of airway obstruction by means of head extension. (*C*) Extreme hyperextension causing upper airway obstruction. (*D*) Fully open airway through use of jaw thrust and neck extension. (*E*) Oropharyngeal airway stenting mandibular block off of posterior pharyngeal wall.

Table 1.3
Airway Equipment Kit for Pediatric Resuscitation

1. Laryngoscope handle with knurled finish
2. Laryngoscope blades:
   Miller 0, 1, 2, 3
   MacIntosh 2, 3, 4
   Wis-Hipple 1.5
3. Oropharyngeal airways: Guedel sizes 00, 0, 1, 2, 3, 4
4. Nasopharyngeal airways: French sizes 12, 16, 20, 24, 28
5. Endotracheal tubes: I.D. sizes
   Uncuffed—2.5, 3.5, 4.5, 5.5, 6.5, 7.5
   Cuffed—5.5, 6.5, 7.5, 8.5
6. Stylet: infant, adult
7. Magill forceps: child, adult
8. Extra batteries and laryngoscope lamps
9. Suction catheters: French sizes 6, 8, 10, 12, 14

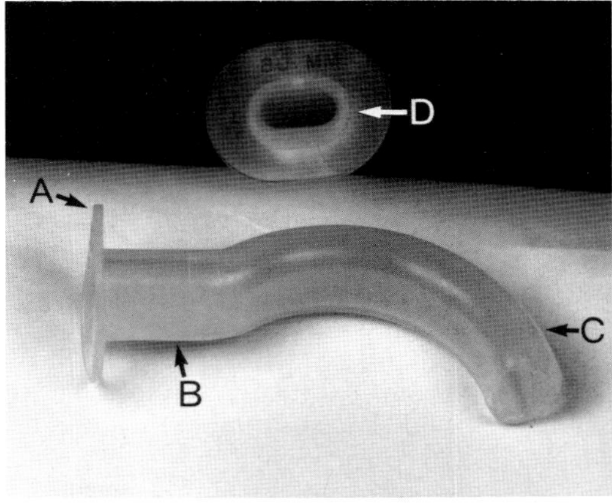

Figure 1.4 Oropharyngeal airway: (*A*) flange, (*B*) bite block, (*C*) stent, and (*D*) gas exchange or suction conduit.

tragus of the ear. The outside diameter of the airway should not be so large as to produce sustained blanching of the skin of the ala nasae. The nasopharyngeal airway is inserted through the nares and passed along the floor of the nostril into the nasopharynx and oropharynx so that it rests between the tongue and the posterior pharyngeal wall. Nasopharyngeal airways may lacerate the vascular adenoidal tissue found in the nasopharynx of children. Therefore adenoidal hypertrophy and bleeding diatheses are relative contraindications to the use of these airways.

Endotracheal Tubes. The purpose of the endotracheal tube (Fig. 1.5) is to supply a stable alternate airway. They are used to: (1) overcome upper airway obstruction, (2) isolate the larynx from the pharynx, (3) allow mechanical aspiration of secretions from the tracheal bronchial tree, and (4) facilitate mechanical ventilation or end expiratory pressure. The correct tube size can be approximated by using a simple formula based on the patient's age:

$$\text{Inside diameter (ID in millimeters)} = \frac{16 + \text{age in years}}{4}$$

Since this is an estimation, it is prudent to have the next smaller and larger size endotracheal tube available. In the pediatric patient, uncuffed tubes are used and are compatible with positive pressure ventilation. This is because in children there is a normal narrowing of the trachea at the level of the cricoid ring (Fig. 1.6). With proper tube selection this narrowing serves as a functional seal.

There are a variety of endotracheal tubes available. Tracheal tubes (Fig. 1.5) should be translucent to facilitate inspection of internal debris or occlusion, have a radiopaque tip marker, have the internal diameter noted proximally so that it is visible after intubation, have a distal vocal cord marker so that when the marker is placed at the level of the vocal cords the tip of the tube is in a midtracheal position, have centimeter markings along the course of the tube to be used as reference points for detecting tube movement, and meet the American National Standard Institute Z-79 guidelines for tracheal tubes and cuffs.

Laryngoscopy and Intubation (see procedure in Section VII). The purpose of laryngoscopy is to create a spatial plane through the mouth to the larynx through which an endotracheal tube can be passed into the trachea. The laryngoscope consists of a blade and a handle. It is used to identify the glottis and to compress the intervening soft tissue structures into the floor of the mouth. The three components of the laryn-

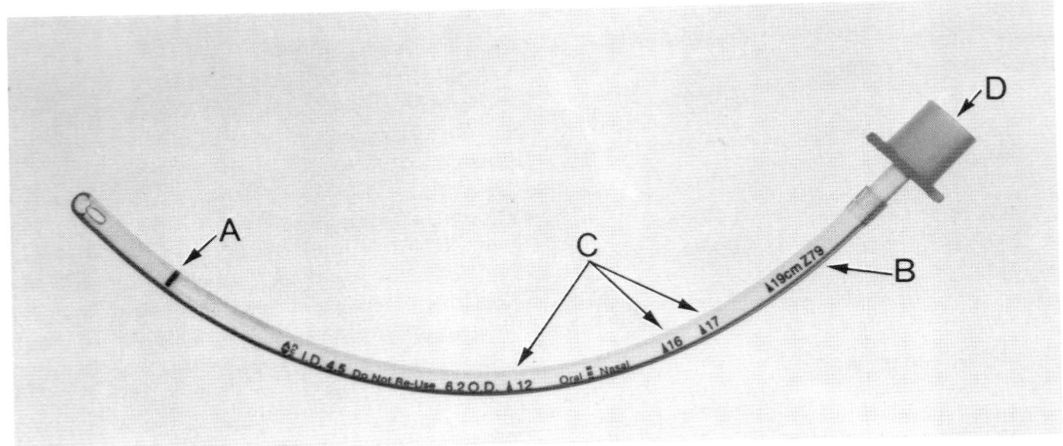

Figure 1.5 Oral tracheal tube: (*A*) vocal cord marker, (*B*) manufacturer indicating that tube meets ANSI-Z79 subcommittee standards, (*C*) distance in centimeters from tip of tube, and (*D*) standard 15-mm connector.

goscope blade are the spatula, the tip, and the flange. The spatula may be curved or straight and is used to compress tissue. The tip of the blade is used for positioning the spatula so that an optimal compression of the mandibular block or soft tissue can be effected. The purpose of the flange is to keep the tongue out of the way of the intubating channel. The laryngoscope is introduced into the mouth so that the tip of the blade slides down the right side of the tongue. As the tip of the blade follows the tongue posteriorly, it bumps into the anterior pillars of the tonsils. The tip is moved around the pillars of the tonsils until it bumps into the epiglottis. The tip is then positioned with respect to the epiglottis. When using a curved spatula, the tip is placed in the space between the tongue and epiglottis—the vallecula. When using a straight spatula, the tip is placed under the epiglottis with the leading edge resting on the aryepiglottic folds. Once the tip is properly placed, the spatula is shifted from the right side of the mouth to the middle of the mouth. This left lateral movement of the spatula allows the flange to push the tongue ahead of it, so that the tongue eventually occupies the left lateral one-third of the mouth while the blade occupies the middle third of the mouth. The right one-third of the mouth is then available as a channel through which the tracheal tube can pass. Once the tip of the blade is properly positioned and the flange has moved the tongue into the left corner of the mouth, the full surface of the spatula is used to compress the tongue into the floor of the mouth. With compression of the soft tissue of the mouth, exposure of the glottis should be effected and the tracheal tube can be passed. The tracheal tube should be fitted with a stylet. The purpose of the stylet is to provide some degree of curvature to the tube for those circumstances where a totally straight channel cannot be effected. The tracheal tube is passed through the glottis so that the ring marker near the tip of the tube is aligned with the vocal cords (Fig. 1.5). If the tube selected is of proper size and the ring marker is placed directly at the vocal cords, the tip of the tube should be at a midtracheal position.

Proper positioning of the tube is confirmed by ausculatating for breath sounds and observing for symmetrical chest movement. If breath sounds are not equal, the tube should be withdrawn slightly and the breath sounds and chest movement reevaluated. When circumstances allow, tube position should be confirmed with an anteroposterior (AP) chest roentgenogram. On the AP film the tip of the tracheal tube should be at a T2 to T3 vertebral level or

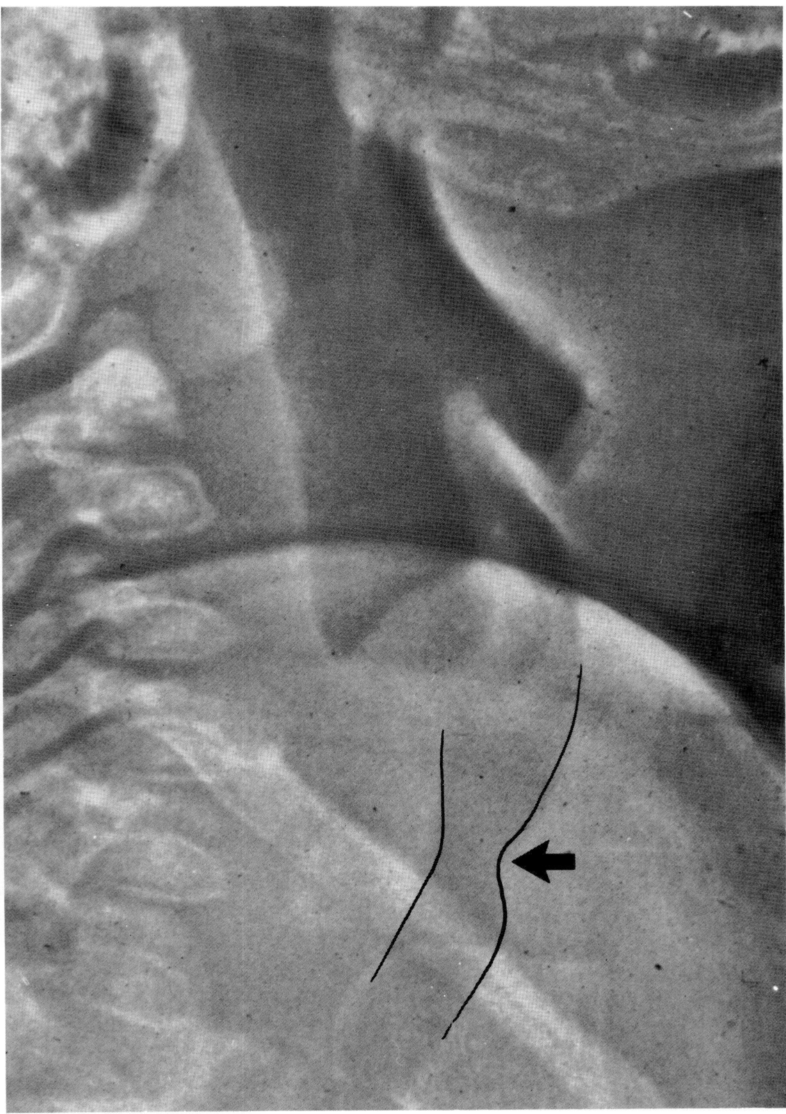

Figure 1.6 Lateral neck xeroradiograph showing narrowing at level of cricoid ring.

directly between the lower edges of the medial aspect of the clavicles.

Loss of an established airway is an unnecessary complication. The tracheal tube should be thoroughly secured with adhesive tape. The skin to which the adhesive tape is affixed should be cleansed, dried, and painted with tincture of benzoin.

The management of airway obstruction is detailed in a separate section at the end of this chapter.

Breathing

EVALUATION

When a clear and stable airway has been established, the patient should be reassessed. Look, listen, and feel for evidence of gas exchange. In infants, adequacy of ventilation is asessed by observing free uniform expansion of the lower chest and upper abdomen. This is in contrast to older children and adolescents where one looks for uniform upper chest expansion as a sign of adequate ventilation. Gas exchange should be confirmed by auscultation. First listen over the trachea to quickly establish that gas exchange is occurring through the central airway. Then listen to breath sounds bilaterally to assess for peripheral aeration and symmetrical lung expansion.

MANAGEMENT

Spontaneous Ventilation

If the airway has been established and the patient is breathing spontaneously, supplemental oxygen should be administered. While elimination of carbon dioxide is important, it is not nearly as important as delivery of oxygen. Children are quite resistant to the effects of severe hypercarbia and respiratory acidosis. They are not tolerant of even short periods of oxygen deprivation.

Oxygen Delivery Devices

A variety of oxygen delivery devices are available for use in patients who have stable airways without endotracheal tubes.

Nasal Cannulas. Two hollow plastic prongs arise from a flexible hollow face piece. Humidified oxygen delivered through the hollow tubing is directed to the nostrils. One hundred percent oxygen is run through a bubbler into the cannula system at a flow of 4 to 6 liters/min. Because of oropharyngeal and nasopharyngeal entrainment of air, the final oxygen delivery is usually 30 to 40%. The advantages of cannulas are that they are easy to apply, lightweight, economical, and disposable. Inefficiency of the bubbler humidifier is compensated for by the fact that the normal humidification and warming systems of the upper airway are not bypassd. The use of this device presumes that the patient's oxygen needs can be met with substantially less than 100% oxygen.

Nasal Catheters. These are flexible hollow tubes of about 30 cm in length which have holes in the terminal 2 cm of the catheter. The key to successful use involves proper placement. The catheter should be tested with low flow oxygen to ensure patency. After lubricating the catheter with a water-soluble lubricant, the catheter is passed along the floor of the nasal passage. The catheter should be observed in the mouth and pulled back until it sits just above or behind the uvula.

Catheter placement may precipitate a posterior pharyngeal hemorrhage in children with enlarged vascular adenoids. Use of oxygen catheters has been associated with gastric distention and rupture. If the catheter is not changed frequently with alternation of nostril placement, removal of the catheter can be quite painful. Catheter placement is somewhat uncomfortable and is poorly tolerated by most pediatric patients.

Oxygen Hoods. Oxygen hoods are clear plastic cylinders with removable lids (Fig. 1.7). They are used for delivery of oxygen to infants and come in a variety of sizes. They usually have a gas inlet system for wide bore tubing and a port for positioning the cylinder across the neck. Their purpose is to maintain a controlled environment for oxygen, humidity, and temperature. This can be done without producing a seal at the infant's neck. One can, without difficulty, deliver oxygen concentrations in the 80 to 90% range simply by increasing the O_2 flow to flood the canister. Because of their potential for delivering concentrations of oxygen which may be toxic to the eyes or lung of the infant, it is imperative to monitor both the fraction of inspired oxygen (FIO_2) and the PaO_2.

Oxygen Tent. The basic purpose of the tent is to provide a controlled and stable environment for humidity, temperature, and oxygen. They are useful for delivery of oxygen between 21 and 50%. Oxygen concentration may be variable because of a poor seal and frequent entry. Therefore, a tight fit and only necessary entry should be allowed. Tents impede access to the patient, and, if mist is used, the patient may be hidden in a cloud which makes skin color difficult to evaluate.

Oxygen Masks. Several types of oxygen masks can be used to offer the patient a wide range of inspired oxygen concentra-

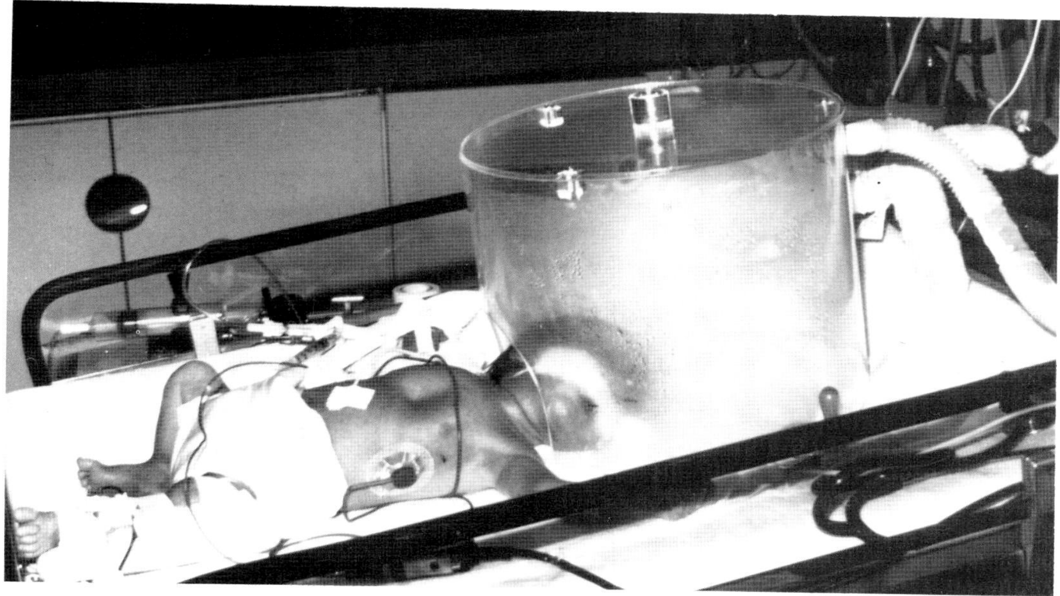

Figure 1.7 Infant oxygen hood.

tions. Masks are a hazard in patients prone to vomit. The mask can block the flow of vomitus and increase the risk of aspiration. Masks are contraindicated in patients who are obtunded or who have a vomiting diathesis.

Simple Masks. The purpose of the simple face mask is to deliver a moderate concentration of oxygen. These masks are lightweight and inexpensive. They can be used in a loose fitting fashion and are relatively comfortable. If the flow of oxygen is disrupted, the child can breathe through side ports. A minimal flow of oxygen is necessary to flush potential dead space. This type of oxygen delivery device does not bypass the upper airway mechanisms for warming and humidification of inspired gas. The disadvantages of the simple mask lie in the fact that it is difficult to provide a known and stable FIO_2. The FIO_2 will vary with the inspiratory flow rate of the patient and with the oxygen flow into the system. The actual pharyngeal FIO_2 may be difficult to predict or measure.

Partial Rebreathing Mask. These masks allow delivery of a higher oxygen concentration than a simple mask. They are also helpful in conserving oxygen. This system is a combined face mask and reservoir bag. When the flow rate into the bag is greater than the patient's minute ventilation and when the oxygen is adjusted so that the bag does not collapse during inhalation, there is negligible CO_2 rebreathing. They are usually used for midrange oxygen delivery. We use a partial rebreathing mask when we are trying to maintain an FIO_2 between 35 and 60%.

Nonrebreathing Masks. These are combined face mask and reservoir bag devices that have non-rebreathing valves incorporated into the face mask. They are useful for giving oxygen concentrations up to 100%

If the airway has been established and the child is not breathing spontaneously or gas exchange is not adequate, artificial ventilation should be started. The recommended rates for rescue breathing in infants and children are shown in Table 1.4.

Assisted Ventilation

If adjuncts for mechanical ventilatory support are not available, an expired air technique may be used. Patient size, type of available airway, and trial will determine which type should be used. The choices include: mouth to nose and mouth; mouth to mouth; mouth to nose; mouth to trache-

Table 1.4
Rate of Respiration

Infant:	20–24 breaths/min
Child:	16–20 breaths/min
Adolescent:	12–16 breaths/min

ostomy; mouth to mask; or mouth to endotracheal tube (Fig. 1.8).

Expired Air Techniques

Hand Squeezed, Self-inflating Resuscitators. These are the most commonly used resuscitators for infants and children. The elasticity of a self-inflating bag allows the bag to refill independently of gas flow. This feature makes the self-inflating bag easy to use for the inexperienced operator. Many of the self-inflating bags are equipped with a pressure limiting pop-off valve which is usually preset at 30 to 35 cm of water to prevent delivery of high pressures. Self-inflating bags which are not pressure limited should have a manometer in line. These resuscitators should be adapted to deliver 100% oxygen. In most cases this involves use of an oxygen reservoir adaptation to the unit (Fig. 1.9). Units without oxygen reservoir adaptations often deliver low concentrations of supplemental oxygen and therefore should be avoided.

The resuscitator may be used with a mask. When selecting a family of mask sizes, you should select a mask type which seals a variety of facial contours. Also the body of the mask should be sufficiently transparent so that vomitus can be easily recognized through the mask. We prefer the Rendall Baker Soucek type for infants and Ambu types for children and adolescents. Resuscitators, masks, and endotracheal tubes should be standardized so that any resuscitator can connect with any mask or endotracheal tube.

Anesthesia Bag. These resuscitators depend on an adequate gas flow to maintain a compressable unit which propels gas towards the patient (Fig. 1.10). An exit port must also be present so that the bag does not become a carbon dioxide reservoir. When used with an oxygen blender, any desired concentration of oxygen may be provided for the patient, because this system directly delivers the gas flowing into it. The major disadvantage of this type of bag is that it takes considerable experience to use effectively. One must be able to judge accurately the rate of gas flow into the bag and the rate of gas escape from the exit port so that under filling or over filling does not occur. If the bag is removed from a leak-tight patient application, it promptly deflates and one must wait for the reservoir to refill. Over filling the bag is dangerous, because high pressures can be transmitted to the lung and stomach.

Circulation

As with the other components of CPR, the circulation must be first assessed and then managed.

EVALUATION

Once the airway has been opened and gas exchange assured, the physician must evaluate the effectiveness of circulation by: (1) observing skin and mucous membrane color and (2) palpating a peripheral pulse. If the patient's color is ashen or cyanotic, the circulation may need to be enhanced.

The palpation of a peripheral pulse is mandatory. Often ineffective cardiac activity can be palpated over the child's thin chest wall. Thus the presence of an apical pulse may not be meaningful. The palpation of a strong femoral or brachial pulse (Fig. 1.11) will indicate presumptively that the cardiac output is adequate.

The resuscitation team will find it most helpful to have continuous blood pressure monitoring. Blood pressure measurements will help to quantify the effectiveness of cardiac function. An ultrasound or Doppler device may be necessary to detect systolic pressure at low levels in small infants.

As soon as possible, the team will also require continuous electrocardiogram monitoring in order to assess the development of dysrhythmia.

MANAGEMENT

Management may be divided into five phases: (1) external cardiac compression, (2) establishment of an intravascular route, (3) use of essential drugs, (4) use of secondary drugs, and (5) defibrillation.

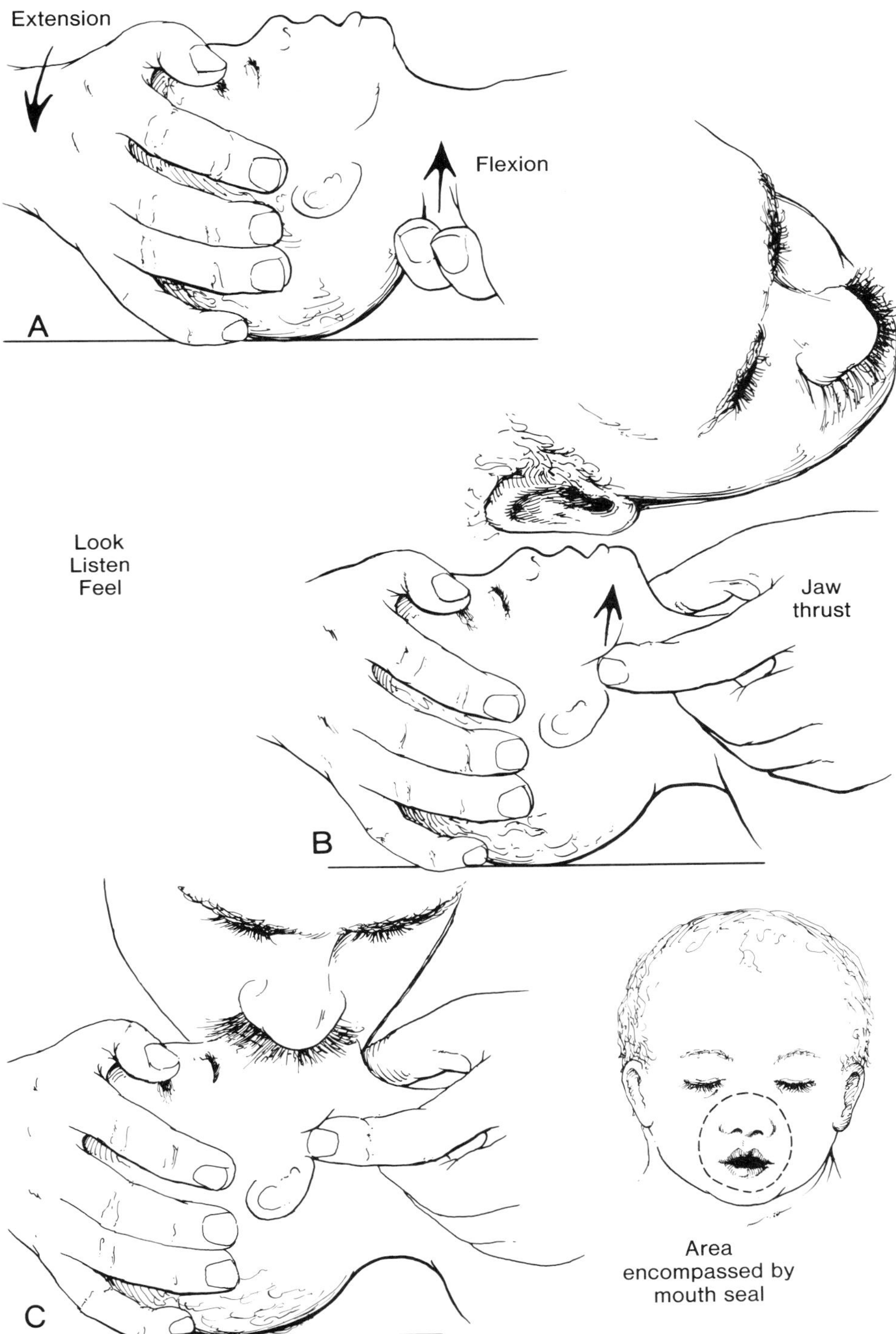

Figure 1.8 Basic life support—airway and breathing. (*A*) Positioning of head to open airway. (*B*) Evaluation for spontaneous ventilation. (*C*) Expired air (mouth-to-nose and mouth) ventilation.

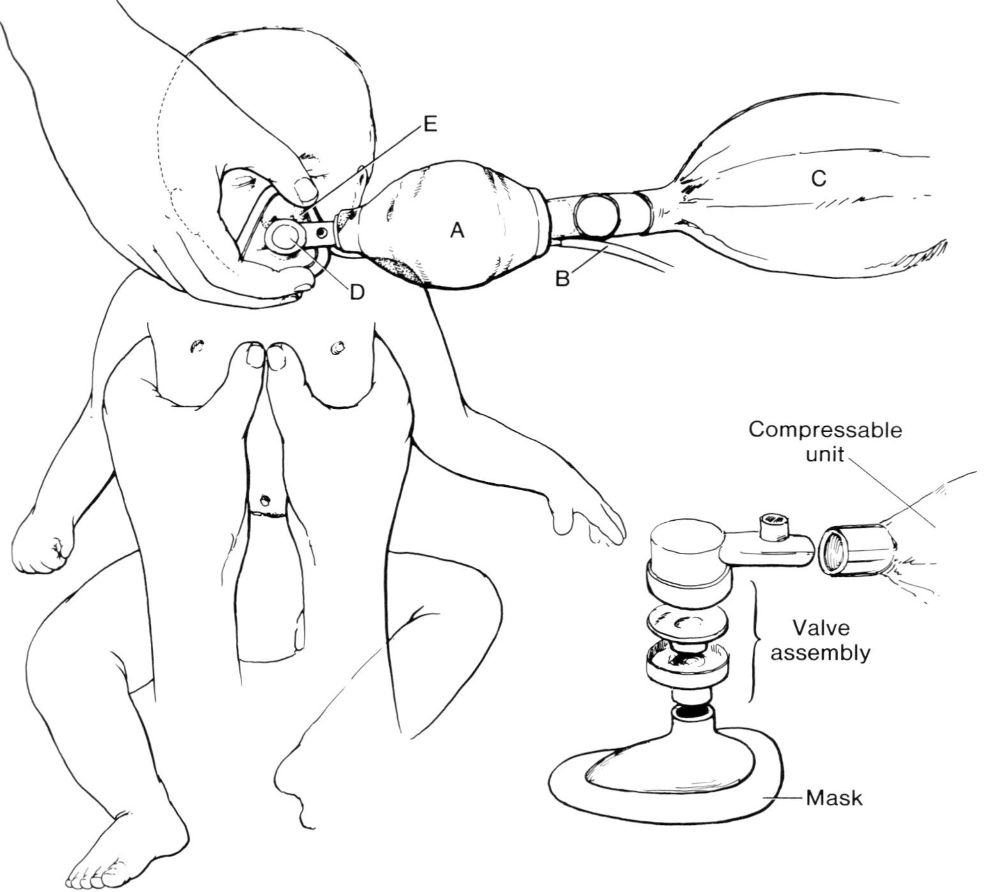

Figure 1.9 Self-inflating hand powered resuscitator: (*A*) compressible unit, (*B*) oxygen source, (*C*) oxygen reservoir, (*D*) one-way valve assembly, and (*E*) mask with transparent body.

External Cardiac Compression (ECC)

Absence of a peripheral pulse requires immediate institution of external cardiac compression (ECC) in order to establish at least a minimum circulation to the brain.

The mechanism by which blood moves during ECC compression has been the subject of recent investigation. The traditional view assumes that chest compression moves blood by direct cardiac compression. Therefore it was felt to be important to compress directly over the ventricles which were felt to be located under the middle one-third of a child's sternum. However, new information suggests that the movement of blood is caused by an increased intrathoracic pressure and expulsion of blood from the lungs through the left heart with simultaneous openings of both the mitral and aortic valves. Therefore, alternative mechanisms for producing blood flow during resuscitation are being investigated.

We recommend that compression should be applied evenly over the midsternum of the child. This standard technique has proven effectiveness. Compression over the lower one-third of the sternum should be avoided because of an increased risk of liver trauma.

The midsternal location for ECC can be found by spanning the sternum between the thumb and fifth finger and then measuring or judging the midpoint. Another method used in locating the midsternum is to find the point where the transnipple line intersects the sternum.

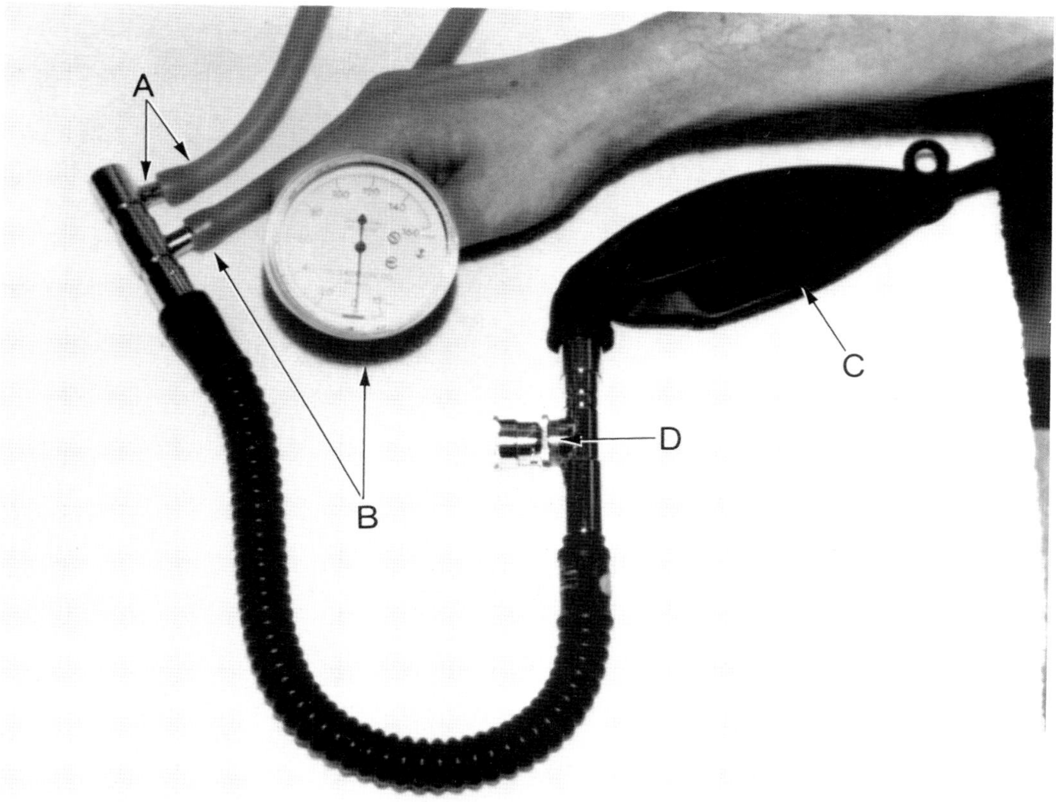

Figure 1.10 Anesthesia bag: (*A*) oxygen delivery port and tubing, (*B*) pressure monitoring line and gauge, (*C*) anesthesia reservoir bag, and (*D*) pressure pop-off valve.

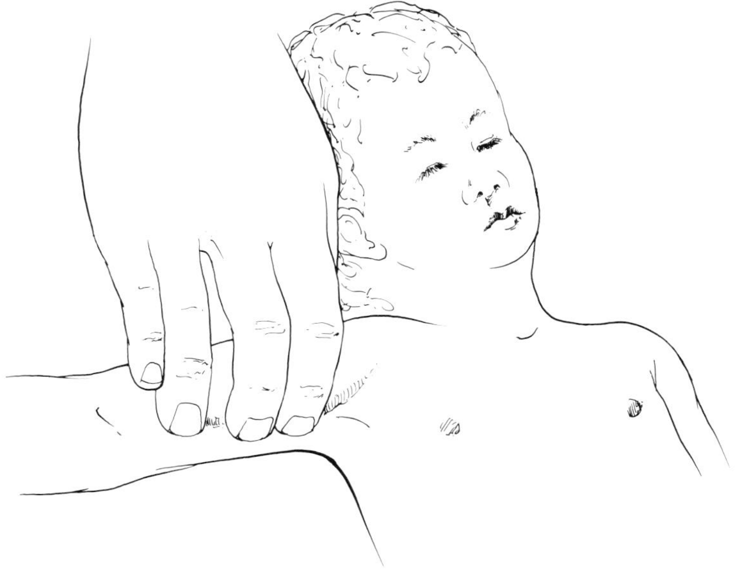

Figure 1.11 Palpation of brachial pulse on medial aspect of forearm.

Table 1.5
Ventilation/Compression Schedule for Pediatric Resuscitation

	Infant	Child	Adult[a]
Compression (rate/min)	100	80	60
Depth of compression (inches)	½–1	1–1½	1½–2
Ventilation (rate/min)	20	16	12

[a] Two person rescue.

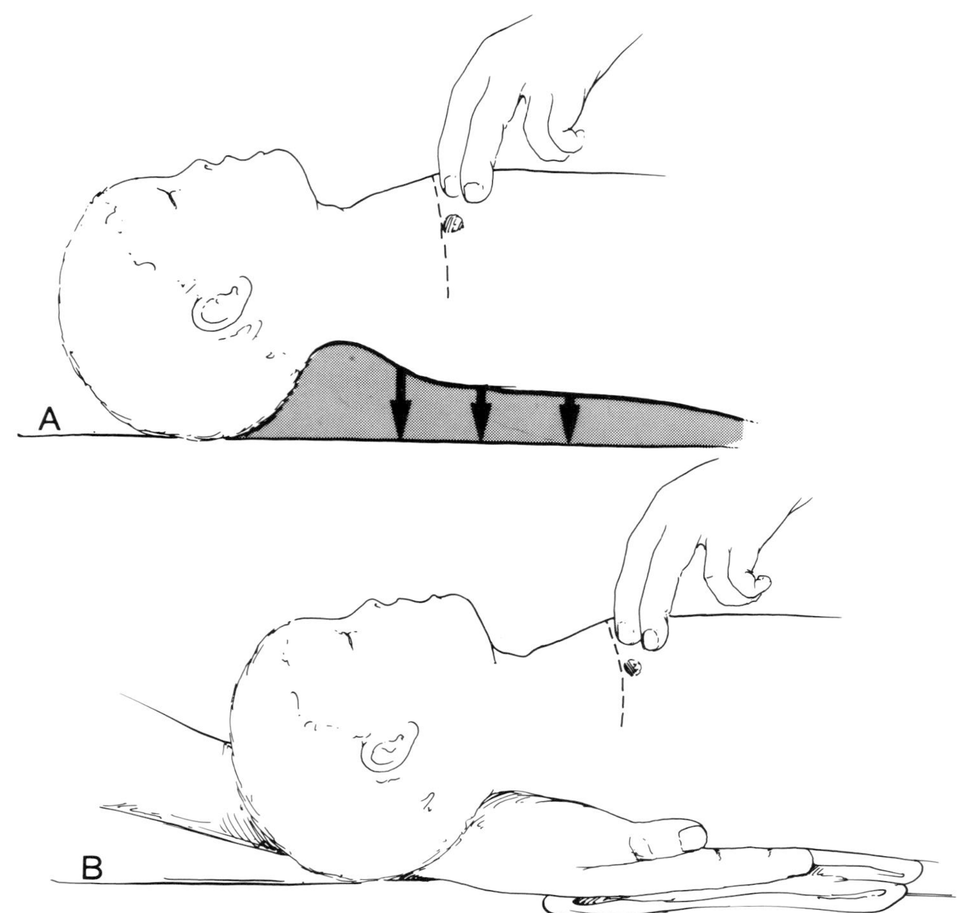

Figure 1.12 Thoracic cage support for external cardiac compression. (*A*) Dead space created by prominent occiput. (*B*) Hand providing thoracic support.

The depth and rate of compression is based on the child's age. Suggested rates and depths are shown in Table 1.5. Compression should be smooth, continuous, and uninterrupted. The compression phase should consume 60% of the time for the compression-release cycle. Jabby, jerky, brief compression may produce pressure pulses of adequate amplitude on a monitor, but blood flow will be inadequate for cerebral perfusion.

Because the child has a relatively large occiput, neck extension may elevate the shoulders and upper thorax off of the firm resuscitation surface. The resultant wedge-shaped dead space beneath the upper thorax may absorb the force of compression (Fig. 1.12*A*). The dead space must be filled with a firm substance so that the work of compression will not be lost. Place a firm towel or the rescuers hand beneath the upper thoracic spine (Fig. 1.12*B*). Compressions may then be applied with one or two fingers or with one hand in the older child. When using the technique developed by Thaler, the rescuer links his fingers beneath the thoracic spine and compresses with his thumbs (Fig. 1.13). This method is quite comfortable when using external cardiac compression on a newborn patient. With older children, try not to allow the encircling hands to limit the respiratory movements of the thorax.

Mechanical chest compressors should not be used for children. There is insufficient information about their effectiveness or safety for this patient population.

Intravenous Lines

The placement of an intravenous line is often the most difficult and time-consuming aspect of pediatric life support. Whenever possible, a central intravenous site should be obtained. Peripheral sites, although readily available, may be inadequate in getting drugs into the central circulation. Intracardiac administration of drugs is dangerous and should be avoided. However, when vascular access is inordinately delayed the technique may be used (Fig. 1.14). Intracardiac injection of drugs may injure an otherwise healthy myocardium. In the circumstance of CPR the cannulation of the subclavian vessel is difficult and is frequently associated with pneumothorax and hemothorax.

Two vessels that are easily cannulated and give access to the central circulation are the femoral and external jugular veins. Our vein of first choice is the femoral as its cannulation does not interfere with ongoing CPR. The femoral vein is located by palpating the femoral artery pulsation and moving just medially to it. If good external cardiac compression is being accomplished the pulsation should be present. When the pulse is not palpable, the physician should find the midpoint between the symphysis pubis and the anterior superior iliac spine on the plane of the inguinal ligament. The vein should be approached at a 45° angle to the skin 2 to 3 cm below the inguinal

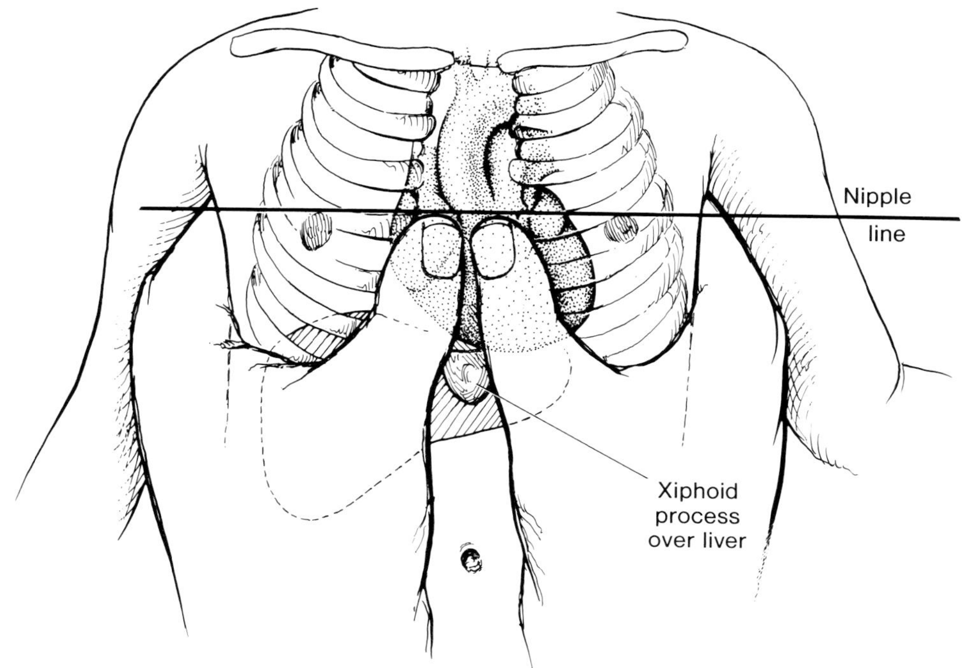

Figure 1.13 External cardiac compression—Thaler technique for infants.

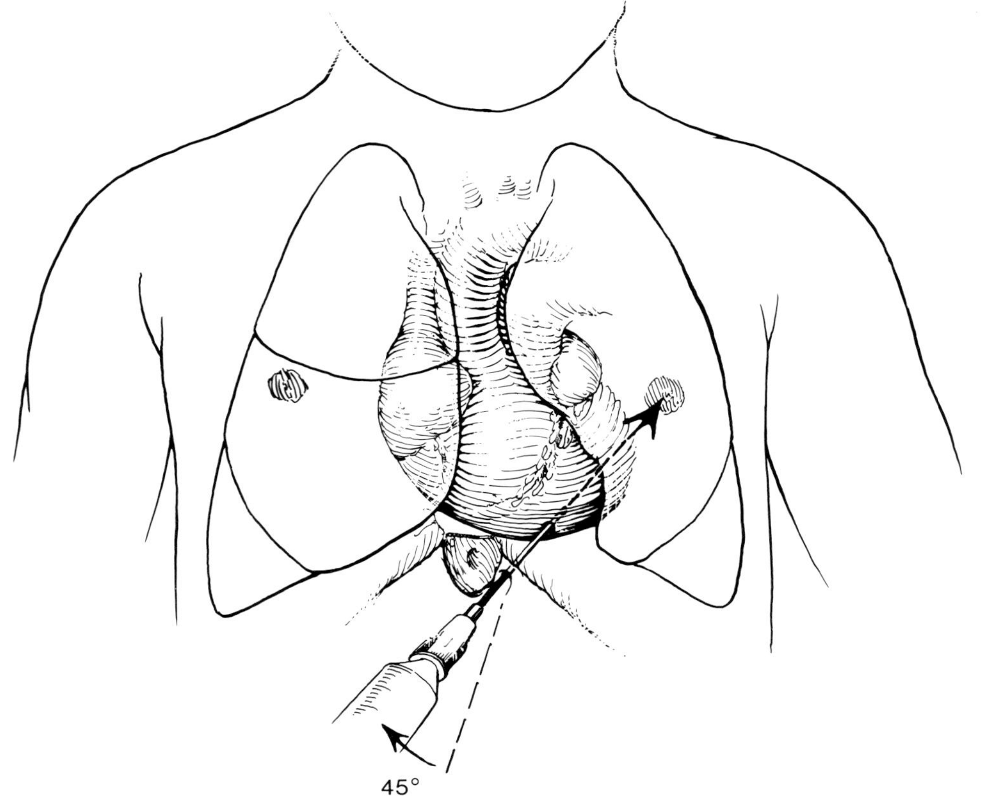

Figure 1.14 Needle position and landmarks for intracardiac injection.

ligament at the defined midpoint. The needle must not pass cephalad to the inguinal ligament as it may enter the peritoneal cavity and pierce bowel.

The external jugular is located by placing the child in a 20° head-down position. With the patient at this angle, the vein will fill and be seen as it courses over the midportion of the sternocleidomastoid muscle (see procedure in Section VII).

In cannulating either the femoral or external jugular vein the Seldinger technique is recommended (see procedure Section VII). The method employs a 22-guage, short beveled, thin walled needle. The needle is attached to a syringe and the vein is punctured and aspirated so that free blood flow into the syringe is seen. The syringe is then removed and blood sent for appropriate laboratory studies. A braided wire is introduced through the needle and positioned in the lumen of the vein. The needle is withdrawn over the free end of the wire. Next, a flexible Teflon catheter is passed over the wire and into the vein. Finally, the wire is removed from the lumen of the catheter, and the catheter is secured with suture. Although this technique requires several steps, it represents a safe and effective way to secure an intravenous line. It is particularly useful for the femoral and internal jugular veins.

If the Seldinger technique is not successful, an acceptable alternative is to cut down over the lesser saphenous vein just above the anterior and the medial malleolus (see procedure in Section VII). While well-known and commonly used, this method requires more extensive training to master. Also, it may require time to execute, even in experienced hands.

While waiting for the intravenous line to

be secured, the physician can administer certain drugs through the tracheal tube. It has been shown that epinephrine, atropine, and lidocaine can be given safely and effectively by the tracheal route. These drugs are absorbed at all levels of the respiratory tract. Some studies even show enhanced pharmacokinetics of drugs delivered by the tracheal route, including more rapid onset and longer duration of drug effect. It is recommended that the drugs be delivered deep into the lungs followed by a short period of hyperinflation. The drug doses are the same as those recommended in subsequent sections.

Essential Drugs

The essential drugs for advanced life support are oxygen, sodium bicarbonate, epinephrine, atropine, calcium and glucose (Table 1.6). Each agent has specific actions, indications, dosage, and untoward effects. Our recommended drug doses are based on kilograms of body weight. The resuscitation team must be able to estimate the weight of the child. If estimates prove too difficult, a standardized growth curve should be posted in the resuscitation area so that 50th percentile weight for the child's age may be used. If the pediatric drug dosage schedule is not used often, it is advisable to prominently display the schedule on the emergency department wall. Table 1.6 details the essential drugs.

Oxygen. In the cardiac arrest patient there are many factors which contribute to the pathophysiologic disruption of oxygen delivery, i.e., hypoxemia. A fundamental goal of basic and advanced life support is to correct cerebral and myocardial hypoxia before irreversible injury occurs.

Oxygen is indicated for any patient who is having decreased oxygen delivery to the tissues whether this is due to (1) pulmonary abnormality such as decreased air exchange, intrapulmonary shunting, or ventilation perfusion abnormality; (2) cardiac dysfunction such as decreased stroke volume or dysrhythmia; and (3) oxygen-carrying abnormalities such as low hemoglobin states or carbon monoxide poisoning. Any patient who is suspected to be hypoxemic should be given oxygen.

Table 1.6
Essential Life Support Drugs

Sodium bicarbonate	1 meq/kg i.v.
Epinephrine	10 μg/kg i.v. or i.t.
Atropine	0.01 mg/kg i.v. or i.t. (min 0.2 mg)
Calcium chloride	10 mg/kg i.v.
Calcium gluconate	30 mg/kg i.v.
Glucose	1.0 g/kg i.v.

The initial dosage of oxygen for the patient needing oxygen is 100%. The potential negative effects of high oxygen concentration are not a consideration in the life or death setting of CPR.

The physician should be familiar with the different oxygen delivery systems mentioned in the sections on airway and breathing. Oxygen concentrations delivered by mouth-to-mouth breathing vary from 17 to 21%. Bag valve mask devices deliver 21%. When an oxygen source is attached, they may deliver 30 to 60% and, when a reservoir is added, 100% may be achieved. Oxygen should be ordered like other drugs. The order should clearly specify the dose, mechanism, and duration of treatment.

Sodium Bicarbonate. With the onset of respiratory failure, the patient develops a respiratory acidosis. Rising levels of carbon dioxide in the blood produce a fall in pH. The immediate treatment for this type of acidosis is adequate ventilation. As the patient's circulation begins to fail, there is production of lactic acid and a metabolic acidosis. Sodium bicarbonate corrects the metabolic acidosis by combining with hydrogen to form carbon dioxide and water. This additional production of carbon dioxide must also be eliminated through ventilation.

Metabolic acidosis is a harmful by-product of the arrest, as acidosis further impairs cardiac and circulatory function. Acidosis depresses spontaneous cardiac activity, decreases the contractile force of the ventricle, and predisposes to ventricular fibrillation. Additionally, catecholamines such as epinephrine will be less effective in a patient whose metabolic acidosis is uncorrected.

It is not necessary to prove a diagnosis of

metabolic acidosis prior to treatment. Sodium bicarbonate is also indicated for the correction of suspected metabolic acidosis. This includes any patient who has arrested for more than a few minutes.

The initial dose of sodium bicarbonate is 1 meq/kg i.v. This should be given as full strength bicarbonate (1.0 meq/ml) for children over 6 months. For infants less than 6 months of age we recommend that the same dose be given, but in the form of half strength bicarbonate (0.5 meq/ml) in order to lessen the osmotic load of the drug.

Following the initial dose of bicarbonate, subsequent doses are best determined by measuring an arterial pH and calculating the dosage using the base deficit.

$$\text{Meq bicarbonate} = \frac{\text{base deficit} \times \text{weight (kg)} \times 0.4}{2}$$

The factor of 0.4 represents the bicarbonate distribution space which is 40% of the total body weight. The formula divides the dose by 2 in order not to overcorrect with bicarbonate and produce alkalemia. If an arterial blood gas determination cannot be made, subsequent doses of 0.5 meq/kg i.v. may be given every 10 to 15 min.

Untoward effects of bicarbonate include hypernatremia, alkalosis, and hyperosmolar states. Each of these effects are significant and can in themselves lessen survival. Hypernatremia and hyperosmolar states are most easily produced in the young infant. Alkalosis is poorly tolerated by the body. Thus, it is important to determine the exact need for bicarbonate as quickly as possible. Bicarbonate administration must always be secondary to the establishment of an airway and ventilations which are important for correcting the acidosis of respiratory origin.

There are other potential untoward effects of bicarbonate: the precipitation of bicarbonate and calcium in the intravenous line and the inactivation of catecholamines. To avoid these two problems we discourage the addition of bicarbonate to intravenous fluid reservoirs during the resuscitation. Bicarbonate should be given by direct intravenous administration and followed with a saline flush solution prior to giving subsequent medication, such as calcium or epinephrine. Intratracheal administration of bicarbonate can be hazardous. Bicarbonate is irritating to the airways, destroys lung surfactant, and can produce massive atelectasis. Also the large volume of bicarbonate usually required will virtually drown the patient.

Epinephrine. Despite the development of many new exogenous catecholamines, epinephrine remains the essential cardiac stimulant. Epinephrine actions include α- and β-adrenergic stimulation. The primary α effect is vasoconstriction and a resultant increase in systolic and diastolic blood pressure. The β-adrenergic action of the drug produces an increased inotropic (contractile force) and chronotropic (cardiac rate) effect. Additionally the β effect produces vasodilation of the coronary and cerebral vasculature. All of these actions are beneficial to the resuscitative effort.

Indications for the use of epinpephrine include asystole, electromechanical dissociation, and hypotension. It is also used to try to change a fine fibrillation pattern to a coarse one prior to defibrillation attempt. There is belief that a coarse fibrillation pattern is more easily converted.

The initial dose of epinephrine for asystole or electromechanical dissociation is 10 μg/kg i.v. Subsequent doses are given by a dose response method of titration. With this method the second dose is doubled to 20 μg/kg i.v., and the physician observes the patient for the desired response. If an inadequate response occurs, the dose should be doubled again. In the absence of underlying cardiovascular disease, this is a safe and effective approach. The dose of epinephrine for hypotension is 1 μg/kg i.v. An epinephrine infusion may be prepared by adding 6 mg of epinephrine to 100 ml of 5% dextrose in water (D5W). This creates a solution that has 60 μg/ml. By infusing this solution at 1 ml/kg/hour, the patient receives a dose of 1 μg/kg/min. If an intravenous line has not been established, epinephrine can be given intratracheally. The dose and concentration of the drug (1:10,000) should be the same. The drug is instilled into the tracheal tube and is followed by several positive pressure ventilations.

Epinephrine is a relatively safe drug and few untoward effects are seen in pediatric patients. Ischemia of the myocardium rarely occurs. There is the hazard of producing supraventricular or ventricular tachycardias, premature ventricular contractions, or ventricular fibrillation. Whenever possible the physician should avoid intracardiac injection of epinephrine, as this route is associated with greater risk and complications. As previously noted, mixing bicarbonate with epinephrine inactivates the epinephrine.

Atropine. The actions of atropine are parasympatholytic. Atropine has both peripheral and central effects. The peripheral effect is vagolytic and thus increases heart rate by increasing the rate of discharge from the sinoatrial node, while increasing conduction through the atrioventricular node. The central effect of atropine stimulates the medullary vagal nucleus and is produced with low dosage of the drug. The actions are opposite to those desired for resuscitation therapy.

The indication for atropine is bradycardia associated with: hypotension, premature ventricular ectopic beats, or symptoms of poor central nervous system or myocardial perfusion. Atropine may be used for second or third degree heart block although its actions may be only temporary for these dysrhythmias.

The dose of atropine is 0.01 mg/kg i.v. There is a minimum dose of 0.20 mg repeated every 5 to 10 min to a maximum total dose of 2.0 mg. Atropine may be given intratracheally if an intravenous route is not available.

The untoward reactions associated with atropine include: (1) paradoxical bradycardia, (2) atrial and ventricular tachyarrhythmias, and (3) myocardial ischemia. Paradoxical bradycardia is caused by the central action of atropine. This side effect can be avoided by using at least 0.2 mg for any patient being treated with atropine. Tachyarrhythmias occur but are not usually hemodynamically significant in the pediatric patient. Myocardial ischemia is rare in the absence of existing cardiac disease.

Calcium. The actions of calcium are to increase myocardial contractibility, increase ventricular excitability, and increase conduction velocity through the ventricular muscle. There is currently controversy about the use of calcium in CPR, but for the pediatric patient the positive cardiac stimulant effects require that it be maintained in the list of essential drugs.

The indications for calcium include asystole and electromechanical dissociation. Further, any situation in which there is a need for an increased inotropic effect is an indication for calcium.

The dose of calcium depends on the form of calcium used. Calcium chloride should be given as 10 mg/kg i.v. In the chloride form, calcium should be given only through a central venous line. Calcium gluconate has properties which make the calcium ion less available. Thus, the dose is 30 mg/kg i.v. Calcium gluconate may be given through a peripheral vein. When giving either form of calcium, the physician should infuse it slowly while watching the cardiac monitor for the appearance of bradycardia. The initial dose of calcium may be repeated once. However, subsequent doses should be guided by a serum ionized calcium level.

The untoward effects of calcium are significant. The patient who is made hypercalcemic may experience an arrest in systole. This is an untreatable situation in which even external cardiac compression will not be beneficial. Calcium must always be given slowly, particularly to the digitalized patient who is more prone to develop dysrhythmias.

Dembo and others have questioned the use of calcium in the asystolic adult patient. The measured serum calcium levels 5 min after infusion of a standard adult dose ranged between 12.9 and 18.2 mg/dl. Other studies show that calcium antagonist drugs appear to be protective against ventricular fibrillation in the ischemic myocardium. However, in our experience, fibrillation is not a common dysrhythmia.

Glucose. The action of glucose is to correct hypoglycemia. Glucose should be considered an essential drug. Infants have minimal glycogen stores for rapid conversion to glucose. Moreover many infants may have

Table 1.7
Useful Life Support Drugs

	Initial	Subsequent
Lidocaine	1 mg/kg i.v. or i.t.	10–20 μg/kg/min i.v.
Bretylium	5 mg/kg i.v.	10 mg/kg i.v.
Dopamine	10 μg/kg/min i.v.	
Isoproterenol	0.1 μg/kg/min i.v.	
Furosemide	1 mg/kg i.v.	2 mg/kg i.v.
Naloxone	0.01 mg/kg i.v.	Repeat
Methylprednisilone	30 mg/kg i.v.	
Dexamethasone	1 mg/kg i.v.	
Difibrillation current	2 watt-sec/kg	4 watt-sec/kg

had decreased caloric intake and excessive losses (diarrhea and vomiting) in the days prior to the arrest.

The dose of glucose is 1.0 g/kg i.v. A 25% solution should be used. Subsequent doses of glucose should be based on the serum glucose level.

Untoward effects include hyperglycemia and hyperosmolality, but these do not occur with the initial dose. There are no other adverse effects.

Useful Drugs

There are a number of useful or second line drugs which should be available for resuscitations. These secondary drugs are listed in Table 1.7.

Lidocaine. Lidocaine works by reducing the automaticity of ventricular pacemakers. Thus, it increases the fibrillation threshold. Ventricular fibrillation is a relatively uncommon event in pediatric resuscitations. However, when it occurs, lidocaine is the drug of choice. The initial dose is 1 mg/kg i.v. This dose may be repeated 3 times at 5-min intervals. Once the initial bolus has been given, an infusion of lidocaine 10 to 20 μg/kg/min should be initiated. If an intravenous line cannot be established, the initial dose of lidocaine may be administered by the tracheal route.

The adverse reactions of lidocaine include nausea, vomiting, lethargy, parasthesias, tinnitus, disorientation, and seizures. Central nervous system symptoms may be the first to appear. Later, symptoms of cardiac toxicity may appear, including depression of myocardial contractility and ventricular irritability. Heart block and eventual drug-induced asystole may occur. The metabolism of lidocaine is dependent on normal liver function. Thus, the dose must be modified for children with chronic congestive heart failure, hepatitis, or cirrhosis.

Bretylium. A second line drug for ventricular tachycardia or ventricular fibrillation is bretylium. The mechanism of action of bretylium has not been fully elucidated. It has been noted to have a positive inotropic effect in addition to its antiarrhythmic action.

The initial dose of bretylium is 5 mg/kg i.v. given rapidly. Then defibrillation is attempted. If defibrillation is not successful, repeat bretylium at 10 mg/kg i.v. and repeat the defibrillation attempt.

The most common untoward effect of bretylium is hypotension. The patient should be placed in a Trendelenburg position and the physician should be prepared to support the blood pressure with the administration of fluids. Bretylium is contraindicated in patients with a digitalis-induced dysrhythmia. The resuscitation team should be prepared to deal with the side effect of drug-induced vomiting.

Dopamine. Dopamine is a precursor of epinephrine. It has action on both α- and β-adrenergic receptors. Dopamine has a unique "dopaminergic" effect which increases blood flow to renal and mesenteric blood vessels. The dopaminergic effect occurs over the low dose range, 2 to 10 μg/kg/min. The cardiac actions of dopamine are similar to those of epinephrine and include a positive inotropic and chronotropic effect. There is also an increase in peripheral vascular resistance which causes an increase in blood pressure at moderate doses, 5 to 20 μg/kg/min. At high doses, greater than 20 μg/kg/min, there is a more marked increase in peripheral vascular resistance and a decrease in the renal and mesenteric blood flow.

Dopamine is indicated for the patient with hypotension and inadequate renal perfusion. The dose of dopamine is 10 μg/kg/min which is within the range for desired cardiac action. The standard infusion may be made by mixing 60 mg of dopamine in 100 ml of D5W. This solution is infused at a rate in milliliters per hour equal to the patient's body weight, e.g., in a 20-kg patient the solution is infused at a rate of 20 ml/hour. This simple method is appropriate for emergency department use, as minimal calculation is required. When the patient reaches an inpatient critical care unit, an infusion more suited for precision drug titration can be prepared. Dopamine may produce tachyarrhythmias as an untoward reaction. Ectopic cardiac beats, nausea, and vomiting may occur. Myocardial ischemia is a rare event in children. The drug must be used with careful monitoring. Rapid increases or decreases in the dose must be avoided. At low doses the dopaminergic effect may result in hypotension which must be supported with intravascular volume expansion. Extravasation of the drug into subcutaneous tissue may cause tissue necrosis. Thus, it should be given through a central line whenever possible. As with other catecholamines, dopamine should not be mixed with bicarbonate as this will inactivate the drug.

Isoproterenol. Isoproterenol is a synthetic catecholamine. The action of this drug is almost entirely through β-adrenergic receptors. The effects on the cardiovascular system are due to an increase in heart rate, increased contractile force, and an increase in venous return to the heart. Unlike epinephrine, isoproterenol produces peripheral arterial dilatation. Despite the decrease in vascular resistance, the drug usually produces an increase in blood pressure due to increased cardiac output.

Isoproterenol can be used for bradyarrhythmias which are not responsive to atropine. Heart block, sinus bradycardia, or nodal bradycardia may be treated, while the more definitive therapy of electrical pacing is arranged.

The dose of isoproterenol is variable. A simple infusion can be prepared by adding 0.6 mg of isoproterenol to 100 ml of D5W. Infusing the solution at a milliliter per minute rate equal to the patient's body weight in kilograms will deliver 0.1 μg/kg/min.

The adverse reactions of isoproterenol include tachyarrhythmias and myocardial ischemia. It should be used with extreme caution in children on digitalis. In the dehydrated or hypovolemic patient, isoproterenol may produce or aggravate existing hypotension. Thus, the physician must be prepared to support a further drop in blood pressure with intravascular volume repletion.

Furosemide. This diuretic agent is rapidly acting and thus is the agent of choice for treating acute pulmonary edema and congestive heart failure. Furosemide works by inhibiting reabsorption of sodium in the proximal and distal tubules and in the loop of Henle. In addition to its action as a diuretic, furosemide also acts to increase blood flow to renal vasculature.

The initial dose of furosemide is 1 mg/kg i.v. If there is not urine output within 20 to 30 min, a repeat dose may be given or the dose may be doubled. If the patient is hypovolemic the administration of furosemide may result in worsening of hypotension. Other adverse reactions include hypokalemia and hyperosmolality. Hypokalemia in the patient on digitalis therapy may result in the development of life-threatening dysrhythmias.

Naloxone. Naloxone is a narcotic antagonist. It works to block the action of both synthetic and natural narcotics. Naloxone reverses the actions of codeine, morphine, heroin, hydromorphone, and methadone. Children who have overdosed on these drugs may present with signs and symptoms of respiratory or cardiorespiratory arrest. The details of management of these poisonings are discussed in Chapter 71, "Adolescent Emergencies."

If narcotic overdose is suspected as the cause of the arrest, naloxone should be administered at 0.01 mg/kg i.v. This drug has a rapid onset of action and a short half-life. If a positive reaction to the agent is noted, a repeat dose should be given as often as every 3 to 5 min. After 3 to 5 doses a sustained effect should be apparent. There are no significant adverse reactions noted with naloxone.

Corticosteroids. There continues to be great controversy over the specific indications for the use of corticosteroids. There is general belief that steroids exert a positive effect on the shock state by stabilizing lysosomal membranes and by preventing the release of histamine and bradykinin. The possible clinical indications for the use of steroids include: (1) noncardiac pulmonary edema, for example, "shock" lung, (2) cerebral edema, and (3) septic shock.

The dose of corticosteroids is also controversial. However, current recommendations include methylprednisolone, 30 mg/kg i.v., or dexamethasone, 1 mg/kg i.v. The adverse reactions with short term administration of corticosteroids are minimal. There may be worsening of hyperglycemia and retention of sodium and water. The worsening of a bacterial infection is a theoretical risk which should not inhibit the short term use of steriods in a life-threatening situation.

Defibrillation. Defibrillation is a relatively uncommon intervention in pediatric resuscitation. It is unusual for a child's heart to fibrillate and thus there should be careful confirmation of the rhythm prior to attempted defibrillation. Unmonitored defibrillation of a child is not recommended. However, if the onset of fibrillation was monitored and the defibrillator is at the bedside, direct defibrillation should be attempted. Precordial thump is not recommended for use in children.

Defibrillation works by producing a mass polarization of myocardial cells with the intent that a spontaneous sinus rhythm returns.

Once the diagnosis of ventricular fibrillation has been made, the patient should be prepared for defibrillation. Acidosis and hypoxemia should be corrected. If the patient was unobserved or if a long interval of poor perfusion has elapsed, 100% oxygen and sodium bicarbonate (1 meq/kg) should be administered. Coarse (high amplitude), fibrillation is more easily treated than fine fibrillation (low amplitude). Fibrillation can be coarsened with the administration of epinephrine or calcium.

There is controversy in the literature about the correct electrode paddle size. Standard adult paddles are 8 cm in diameter. Pediatric paddles which are 4.5 cm in diameter are also available for most defibrillators. The correct size paddle is that one which makes complete uniform contact with the chest wall. The electrodes should be prepared with electrode paste or saline soaked pads. Placement of the paste or pads must be meticulous. The small size of the child's chest wall predisposes to bridging of the electric current. Electrical bridging will result in ineffective defibrillation and possible burning of the skin surface.

Once the correct paddles are selected and the electrode skin interface carefully prepared, the electrodes are ready to be placed on the chest wall. Both electrodes may be placed on the anterior chest wall, one at the right of the sternum below the clavicle and the other at the level of the xyphoid along the left midclavicular line. An anteroposterior placement of the electrodes is also acceptable; however, this is cumbersome in the usual resuscitation situation. Using either electrode placement, firm pressure should hold the paddles in contact with the skin. Personnel should be cleared from contact with the patient and the bed.

A dose of current for the initial shock is 2 watt-sec/kg. If the first defibrillation is unsuccessful, CPR is continued for 3 to 5 min and then the dose of current is doubled to 4 watt-sec/kg. If a third defibrillation shock is needed, the dose is again doubled to 8 watt-sec/kg.

Adverse reactions from defibrillation include myocardial injury from excessive current or from multiple discharges delivered in rapid succession (less than 3-min intervals). Another adverse reaction is the damage to skin and subcutaneous tissue that occurs when the electrode skin interfaces are inadequate. Alcohol pads should never be used as an electrode interface because of their flammable property.

STABILIZATION AND TRANSPORT

Once resuscitation has achieved cardiorespiratory stability, the patient should be transported to an inpatient special care unit for the critically ill. This transport may be several hundred yards or several hundred miles to a regional tertiary care pediatric hospital. In either circumstance the patient should be transported with: (1) appropriate advanced life support technology in place, (2) appropriately qualified personnel in attendance, and (3) options for further treatment or intervention immediately available.

Waddel has reported on the direct and indirect effects of movement within the hospital. Direct effects include patient discomfort, pain, and the physical stimulation of movement. Indirect effects include lack of equipment and facilities and the limitations which occur by being in motion, for example the ability to provide continuous ventilation while maneuvering the stretcher into a small elevator. All the equipment needed for a complete resuscitation should be available. Table 1.8 lists the equipment which is required. Transport should never be rushed, as this may result in direct morbidity to the patient. Pediatric patients are particularly prone to hypothermia and should be warmed in order to avoid the adverse hemodynamic effects of cold stress. This is particularly important for any young infant who has not established temperature control or the older child whose central nervous system pathology has resulted in loss of temperature regulation. Pediatric patients are likely to become physically active once CNS perfusion is adequate. Intravenous lines, endotracheal tubes, and nasogastric tubes must be well secured. Extremities must be restrained. The transport team must include a sufficient number of individuals to fully resuscitate the patient. Responsibility for the patient still rests with the resuscitation team until discharge of that responsibility takes place at the inpatient critical care unit.

Table 1.8
Essential Equipment for Transport in Pediatric Resuscitation

1. Airway box—items noted in Table 1.3
2. Portable suction—compact, battery operated
3. Bag-valve-mask with O_2 reservoir
4. Oxygen tank with yoke and flow meter
5. Intravenous fluids
6. Essential cardiac medications
7. ECG monitor defibrillator
8. Infusion pump—battery operated
9. Blood pressure apparatus—battery operated, doppler or ultrasound

DISCONTINUATION OF LIFE SUPPORT

Termination of life support in the emergency department is usually determined by whether or not the cardiovascular system can be supported with other than closed chest massage. If the heart and that supporting technology applied to it cannot sustain brain function, resuscitative effort should be discontinued. Obviously time must be allowed to mobilize and implement the appropriate technology and therefore most unsuccessful resuscitations often go beyond one hour.

Respiratory functions are easily supported mechanically and therefore are not used as markers for continuation or discontinuation of effort.

Brain death is becoming widely accepted as the ultimate determinate of death. It is a clinical diagnosis that should be confirmed by observations over a period of time or by studies documenting absence of cerebral blood flow or cerebral metabolic activity. We have seen infant botulism and postictal depression misdiagnosed as brain death and are therefore extremely cautious of making this diagnosis in the emergency department.

Ultimately, the diagnosis of death and subsequent discontinuation of resuscitative effort is a judgment that should be made by the senior physician directly attending the child.

Brain death is discussed in further detail in Chapter 4.

UPPER AIRWAY OBSTRUCTION

Background

If acute upper airway obstruction is not relieved properly and expeditiously, the child is likely either to die or to sustain a hypoxemic central nervous system injury. The emergency department physician, pressured by time to move through a sequence of evaluation and management, knows that inefficiencies or mistakes place the child at increased risk. Unfortunately, this is a circumstance that often generates panic. Panic can be avoided and the child's life saved if calm prevails and an orderly sequence of evaluations and interventions occurs quickly and atraumatically.

Clinical Manifestations

If the clinical process predisposing to upper airway obstruction has not evolved to produce complete airway obstruction, the usual clinical manifestations are related to an increased work of breathing or compromised oxygen exchange. Intercostal retractions qualitatively reflect the increased work of breathing. If the negative intrapleural pressure required to produce gas exchange is increased, retractions will be evident in the intercostal spaces. As the work of breathing continues to increase, retractions will be transmitted beyond the thoracic cage and one may see subcostal or supraclavicular retractions. In the extreme situation the sternocleidomastoid muscles are outlined by the negative intrapleural pressure transmitted into the neck. Another important clinical marker of airway obstruction is a decrease in breath sounds. Breath sounds should be auscultated both over the trachea and the peripheral lung fields. By following the pattern of inspiratory breath sounds one can appreciate a gradual diminution during progression of the process of airway obstruction.

Upper airway noises such as stridor, croupy cough and "bark," may be useful signs to identify those at risk for upper airway obstruction. The general appearance of air hunger or gasping respirations may indicate airway obstruction. Additionally, the symptoms of dysphagia, dysarthria and dyspnea should trigger a thorough evaluation of the airway.

Management

A number of tasks must be accomplished as quickly as possible once the patient has been identified as being at high risk for total airway obstruction. The child should receive supplemental oxygen and have his heart rate and blood pressure monitored. Equipment for managing an obstructed airway should be immediately available (Table 1.3). The hospital's identified airway specialist should be notified of the child's condition, and these individuals should move as quickly as possible to the emergency department. Beyond the emergency physician, speciality groups commonly identified as having airway expertise include: anesthesiologists, otorhinolaryngologists, nurse anesthetists, general surgeons, respiratory therapists, and cardiothoracic surgeons. It is important to keep in mind that the two important elements for successful management are technical expertise and judgment. These attributes are not necessarily found in the same individual. What may be necessary is a cooperative effort between those with technical expertise and those with the clinical experience and judgment.

If obstruction is not imminent, there is usually time to obtain a history and to perform an abbreviated physical examination. Additionally, chest x-ray and lateral neck x-rays may help to define more specifically the pathophysiologic process. These evaluations should only occur if there is no obvious evolution of the airway obstruction and if the natural history of the disease under consideration suggests further diagnostic studies.

If the patient is obtunded, the team must initiate the formal sequence of evaluation and management as previously described. The airway should be opened by flexing the cervical spine on the thoracic spine and tilting the head backward so that the skull is extended on the cervical spine. In addition to this maneuver, the jaw thrust or jaw pull may be employed by pushing or pulling the mandibular block of tissue forward off of the posterior pharyngeal wall. At this time the examiner evaluates the respiratory effort by looking, listening, and feeling for air flow. If the patient is breathing and there is gas exchange, the patient should receive supplemental oxygen and the sequence should progress toward an evaluation of the cardiovascular system. If the patient is not breathing, the oropharynx should be suctioned and oropharyngeal or nasopharyngeal airway placed in an effort to open the airway. With the airway in place the physician should reevaluate for gas exchange. If there is now gas exchange, supplemental oxygen should be administered. If there is no gas exchange, proceed immediately to laryngoscopy.

The purpose of laryngoscopy is twofold: the first priority is placement of an endotracheal tube; secondarily, the laryngoscopy may provide diagnostic information. If a foreign body is evident, try to intubate before attempting removal.

If the tracheal tube can be placed, the child should be oxygenated and ventilated. Then the cause of the upper airway obstruction should be evaluated and treated. If the child cannot be intubated a transcricothyroid membrane catheter should be inserted for delivery of supplemental oxygen (see procedure in Section VII). Jet ventilation may be accomplished through the catheter oxygenation system. Once the catheter is in place and oxygen is being administered, it is appropriate to reexamine the upper airway; look for a cause of the obstruction; and to reattempt placement of an endotracheal tube. If the airway cannot be secured at this time, a surgical team should be mobilized to perform a tracheostomy. Effective needle oxygenation and ventilation may permit transfer of the child to the operating room for tracheostomy. If circumstances do not allow oxygenation and ventilation, a formal tracheostomy may need to be performed in the emergency department.

SUMMARY

In most circumstances resuscitation of the pediatric patient can be approached with a sense of optimism for reversing the process which acutely threatens the child's life. Well organized and well qualified personnel can effect a high rate of successful resuscitation. However, organization and qualification require advanced planning, training, and preparation. Inherent to this preparation is the development of personnel disciplined to follow the sequence of evaluation and management for airway, breathing, and circulation. In additon, personnel must be familiar with those nuances of resuscitation peculiar to the age and size ranges of the pediatric population. A complete list of pediatric resuscitation equipment may be found in the Appendix (p. 1290).

References

American Heart Association: Standards for CPR and ECC. *JAMA* 244 (Suppl): 453–509, 1980.

Anthony CJ, Crawford EW, Morgan BC: Management of cardiac and respiratory arrest in children. *Clin Pediatr* 8: 647–654, 1969.

Babbs CF: New versus old theories of blood flow during CPR. *Crit Care Med* 8: 191–195, 1980.

Bishop RL, Weisfeld ML: Sodium bicarbonate administration during cardiac arrest. *JAMA* 235: 506–509, 1976.

Budassi SA, Bander JJ, Kimmerle L, Eie KF: *Cardiac Arrest and CPR*, pp. 45–56. Aspen Publication, Rockville, Md., 1980.

Chameides L, Brown GI, Raye JR, et al.: Guidelines for defibrillation in infants and children: Report of the American Heart Association Target Activity Group: Cariopulmonary resuscitation in the young. *Circulation* 56 (Suppl): 502–503, 1977.

Cote CJ, Jobes DR, Schwartz AJ, Ellison N: Two approaches to cannulation of a child's internal jugular vein. *Anesthesiology* 50: 371–383, 1979.

Debard ML: Cardiopulmonary resuscitation: Analysis of six years experience and review of the literature. *Ann Emerg Med* 10: 408–416, 1981.

Dembo DH: Calcium in advanced life support. *Crit Care Med* 9: 358–359, 1981.

Ehrlich R, Emmett SM, Rodriquez-Torress R: Pediatric cardiac resuscitation team: A 6-year study. *Pediatrics* 81: 152–155, 1974.

Filston HE, Johnson DG: Percutaneous venous cannulation in neonates and infants: A method for catheter insertion without cutdown. *Pediatrics* 48: 896–901, 1971.

Forney J, Ornato JP: blood flow with ventilation alone in a child with cardiac arrest. *Ann Emerg Med* 9: 624–626, 1980.

Gutgesell HP, Tacker WA, et al.: Energy dose for ventricular defibrillation of children. *Pediatrics* 58: 898–901, 1976.

Holbrook PR, Mickell J, Pollack NM, et al.: Cardiovascular resuscitation drugs for children. *Crit Care Med* 8: 8: 588, 762, 1980.

Kettrick RG, Ludwig S: Resuscitation in infants and children. *Curr Top Emerg Med* 1: 4, 1981.

Lee Terry KW, Templeton JJ, Dougal RM, Downes JJ: Selection of endotracheal tubes in infants and children. Presented to American Academy Pediatrics, Annual Meeting, Las Vegas, April, 1980 (submitted for publication).

Ludwig S, Kettrick RG, Parker M: Pediatric cardiopulmonary resuscitation: A review of 130 cases (submitted for publication).

Melker R, Cavallaro D, Krischer J: A pediatric gastric tube airway. *Crit Care Med* 9: 426–427, 1981.

Orlowski JP: Cardiopulmonary resuscitation in chil-

dren. *Pediatr Clin North Am* 27: 495–511, 1980.
Rudikoff MT, Freund P, Weisfeldt ML: Mechanisms of blood during cardiopulmonary resuscitation. *Circulation* 56–57 (Suppl III): 97, 1977.
Seldinger SI: Catheter placement over the needle in percutaneous arteriography. *Acta Radiol* 39: 368–376, 1953.
Singer J: Cardiac arrests in children. *JACEP* 6: 198–205, 1977.
Tahernia AC: Managing cardiac arrest in infants and children. *Postgrad Med* 47: 204–209, 1970.
Thaler MM, Stobie HC: An improved technique of external cardiac compression in infants and young children. *N Engl J Med* 269: 606–610, 1963.
Waddel G: Movement of critically ill patients within hospitals. *Br Med J* 2: 417–419, 1975.

CHAPTER 2

Shock

RUSSELL C. RAPHAELY, M.D.

INTRODUCTION

Shock may be defined as an acute syndrome (collection of symptoms) of cardiovascular failure resulting in vital organ malnutrition. Shock differs from simple hypotension. Major pathological alterations in tissue oxygenation and cellular activity occur as a result of hypoperfusion in shock.

Shock is traditionally classified into three etiologic types, (1) hypovolemic, (2) cardiogenic, and (3) septic. Hypovolemic, sometimes called hemorrhagic, is caused by acute blood or extracellular volume loss which results in diminished oxygen delivery to the body tissues. In cardiogenic shock the defect is in the myocardium which results in pump failure. All of the mechanisms of septic shock are less well understood. However, a major component is loss of vascular tone and integrity. Septic shock may also have myocardial and hypovolemic components. The types of shock do not always occur in pure form.

Little data exist on the incidence of hypovolemic or cardiogenic shock in children. Dupont and Spinx reported on a series of patients with bacteremia in which 25% of children with Gram negative bacteremia developed hypotension. Of the children, 30 days to 16 years of age, from whom Gram-negative organisms were recovered from their blood and who developed hypotension, 98% died. Of the entire group of bacteremic children, Gram-negative bacteria accounted for two-thirds of the cases with *Escherichia coli, Klebsiella, Enterobactor, Serratia* and *Pseudomonas* isolated predominantly. Other causitive microorganisms included *Staphylococcus, Streptococcus, Pneumonococcus, Clostridia, Rickettsia*, malaria, and virus. Apparently children develop hypotension associated with Gram-negative bacteremia less often then adults; however, those who do are more likely to die.

A better understanding of the pathophysiology and advances in monitoring and treatment presumably have decreased the morbidity and mortality rate.

PATHOPHYSIOLOGY

The pathophysiology of shock has many facets as each body tissue is involved. Several of the most important pathophysiologic responses are discussed in the sections which follow.

Intravascular Volume

Absolute or functional hypovolemia commonly occurs in shock. Absolute hypovolemia exists when blood, plasma, or electrolyte solution is lost. Although we easily recognize losses caused by hemorrhage, burns, severe vomiting, or diarrhea, we find more difficulty appreciating losses associated with peritonitis, accidental or surgical trauma, or increased capillary permeability. In these conditions, fluid remains within the body sequestered in areas outside the vascular space. Functional hypovolemia exists when vascular capacity increases, as in

Table 2.1
Naturally Occurring Vasoconstrictor Agents Playing a Role in Shock[a]

Vasoconstrictor	Major Sources	Site of Action	Means of Controlling
Norepinephrine	Sympathetic NS and adrenal medullae	Systemic	α-Adrenergic, β-blockers, ganglionic blockers
Epinephrine	Adrenal medullae	Systemic	α-Adrenergic, β-blockers, ganglionic blockers
Angiotensin II	Kidneys, blood, brain	Systemic, mesenteric	Converting enzymme inhibitors, receptor antagonists
Antidiuretic hormone (ADH)	Posterior pituitary	Systemic	[1-Deaminopenacillamine 4 valine, 8-D-arginine], vasopressin
Thromboxane A_2	Platelets	Cardiac, pulmonary, others	Tx synthetase inhibitors, Tx antagonists
Myocardial depressant factor (MDF)	Pancreas	Systemic	Membrane stabilizers, protease inhibitors
Serotonin (5-HT)	Platelets	Systemic	Anti-serotonergic agents
Prostaglandin $F_{2\alpha}$ ($PGF_{2\alpha}$)	Platelets and smooth muscle	Local and systemic	Cyclo-oxygenase inhibitors

[a] From R. A. Cowley and B. F. Trump: *Pathophysiology of Shock, Anoxia and Ischemia*. Williams & Wilkins, Baltimore, 1982.

spinal cord injury, anaphylaxis, and barbiturate overdosage.

Microvasculature

In response to decreased circulating blood volume, smooth muscle contraction, most notable in precapillary sphincters but also in the remaining portion of the arteriole, results from local sympathetic, vasoconstrictor nerve activity. Circulating vasoactive substances also affect vascular tone. Differential tonic activity in the microvasculature distributes blood volume to organs which lack reserve for decreased oxygen and energy substrate delivery. Initially, decreased flow reduces capillary hydrostatic pressure, favoring fluid movement from the interstitium into the capillary, thus augmenting blood volume. However, the precapillary sphincter quickly loses its responsiveness to nerve stimulation and relaxes when subjected to hypoxia, which ultimately occurs when local blood flow decreases even further.

Constriction of the capacitance vessels containing 60% of the blood volume, shifts blood to the central circulation. Strong sympathetic innervation mediates venous tone. Metabolic regulatory factors such as acidosis and hypoxia influence venomotor tone minimally. Continued venoconstriction in the presence of arteriolar and precapillary sphincter relaxation results in increased capillary hydrostatic pressure. The balance of forces across the capillary wall then favor fluid movement from the vascular space into the interstitium. When the pathophysiologic response is considered in toto, an initial beneficial compensatory response becomes a detrimental one.

Cardiac Performance

Decreased venous return and decreased coronary flow combine to diminish cardiac output. Vasoconstriction increases impedance to ventricular ejection, further reducing the output of the heart. Myocardial Depressant Factor, a 500 molecular weight water-soluble peptide containing 3 to 4 amino acid residues, exerts a direct negative inotropic effect on cardiac muscle.

Vascular Mediators

Extremely potent peptides of lipids appear to play a role in the development of ischemia and shock. The mechanism by which these naturally occurring substances exert that effect include: severe vasoconstriction and vasospasm; induction of platelet aggregation and thrombus formation; increased capillary permeability; and redistribution of blood flow away from vital tissues (see Table 2.1).

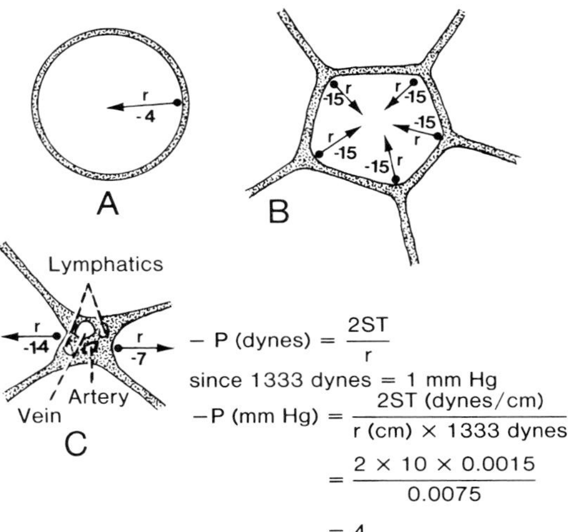

Figure 2.1. Effect of surface tension on the alveolar fluid and interstitial fluid pressure. (*A*) Assuming a spherical model of the alveolus with a radius of 75 μm and a surface tension of 10 dynes/cm, we calculate that the fluid lining the alveolus would be pulled away with a pressure of minus 4 mm Hg. (*B*) Assuming a polyhedral model, with the radius of curvature at the corners of 20 μm, the negative pressure in the corners would be minus 15 mm Hg. The pressure at the angles (not shown) where the alveolar air-liquid interface is cylindrical and where $-P = ST/r$ would be minus 7.5 mm Hg. (*C*) Dynamics at alveolar angles adjacent to interstitial space surrounding larger blood vessels and lymphatics; pressures of -7 to -14 mm Hg can be calculated, depending on the radius of curvature at the angles. (Redrawn from R. B. Mellins, and S. A. Stazcup: In *Disorders of the Respiratory Tract in Children*, p. 576, edited by E. L. Kendig and V. Chernick. W. B. Saunders, Philadelphia, 1977.)

Reticuloendothelial System

Dysfunction of this system occurs in experimental animals in shock partly due to a deficiency in circulating opsonic activity. Low levels of a humoral factor, plasma fibronectin, leads to diminished phagocytic activity. However, data on reticuloendothelial system dysfunction remain limited to animals, and its role in humans is uncertain.

Metabolic Alterations

Reduced aerobic and increased anaerobic glycolysis constitute the primary metabolic disturbances in shock. The shift to an inefficient energy production pathway results from decreased oxygen availability to the cells because of the hypoperfusion state. One mol of glucose yields 38 mol of ATP when aerobic glycolysis occurs. However, anerobic glycolysis generates only 2 mol of ATP from one mol of glucose. Cells consume the limited reserve of ATP very quickly. With exhaustion of the energy supply metabolic failure occurs.

Lactic acid accumulates within the cells, eventually spilling over into the blood and producing acidemia.

The cause of hyperglycemia observed in shock remains controversial. Increased circulating catecholamines contribute to the increased blood glucose. The source of the glucose appears to be hepatic glycogen acted upon by circulating epinephrine released from the adrenal medulla.

Lung

Recent experimental and clinical evidence implicates complement mediated polymorphonuclear granulocyte aggregation in the pulmonary capillary "leak" associated with shock. The complement fraction C5a, a 15,000 dalton cleavage product of C5 causes granulocytes to rapidly extrude membraneous veils and pseudopods which increase their tendency to adhere to each other as well as endothelial cells. Stimulated granulocytes produce the toxic oxygen species, superoxide and hydrogen peroxide, which damage the capillary endothelial cell and enhance injury caused by circulating endotoxin.

Damage to the capillary endothelium allows intravascular fluid to escape into the interstitium of the intraalveolar septum. Tight interdigitations of the epithelial cells resist fluid movement into the alveolar air spaces. The edema moves to the extraalveolar interstitium surrounding airways and blood and lymphatic vessels due to a pressure gradient created by nonuniform radii of curvature of juxtaposed alveolar air spaces. (Fig. 2.1). If lymphatic capacity for removal is exceeded, fluid accumulates initially in the interstitium of the bronchovascular pedicle, then in the intraalveolar interstitium. When interstitial hydrostatic pressure reaches 50 to 60 torr, the fluid breaks through into the alveolar air spaces. Presence of plasma, formed elements, and debris disrupt surfactant and prevent gas entry into the affected alveolus.

Additionally, neutrophils produce neutral and acid proteases which destroy structural proteins such as collagen, elastin, and fibronectin. The latter material, an adhesive glycoprotein, appears necessary for topographic order of interstitial cells and connective tissues. Furthermore, neutrophil proteases cleave fibrinogen, Hageman factor, complement, and other plasma proteins amplifying local lung injury by activating plasma factors which enhance further leukocyte aggregation and intravascular coagulation. Superoxide radicals permanently inactivate α_1-antitrypsin, which inhibits proteolysis. With this defense mechanism suppressed, proteolytic lung damage occurs.

The process damaging the alveolar epithelial cells eludes us. The injury appears reversible provided the basement membrane remains intact. Destruction of that structure apparently precludes restoration of normal alveolar architecture. Healing occurs by extensive fibroblastic proliferation with obliteration of the normal alveolar architecture.

Pulmonary artery hypertension, increased pulmonary vascular resistance and obliterated vascular beds burden the right ventricle with increased afterload. Thromboembolism, as well as extrinsic factors, appear operative in the rarefaction of the pulmonary vascular tree.

CLINICAL MANIFESTATIONS

While major pathophysiologic reactions occur immediately after the etiologic event, before the initial hypotensive episode, they for the most part go unrecognized unless we anticipate disaster and institute extensive monitoring. Decreased systemic arterial pressure most often identifies the patient in shock and signals the need for therapy. Tachycardia occurs as a compensation for diminished stroke volume. Vasoconstriction and diminished flow in the skin manifests as pallor, decreased skin temperature, mottling, and poor capillary refill. In the early stages of circulatory failure associated with infection one may observe oliguria with warm ruborus skin reflecting cutaneous vasodilatation in the hyperdynamic state.

Oliguria heralds diminished renal perfusion from decreased cardiac output and increased vascular resistance, as well as the kidney's attempt to restore intravascular volume by conserving salt and water.

The splanchnic vessels respond similarly to the renal vasculature. Vasoconstriction and decreased cardiac output deprive these viscera of oxygen and nutrients. Under the influence of ischemia, the bowel appears to be a source of undesirable vascular mediators or endotoxin. Additionally, decreased intestinal motility and distention may occur. Fluid accumulation in the energy-deprived cells and interstitium of the bowel may further aggravate hypovolemia.

Tachypnea leads to increased minute ventilation. Autonomic neuroactivity stimulates the respiratory center, resulting in increased alveolar ventilation (V_A). Nonrespiratory acidemia elicits a compensatory increase in V_A resulting in a fall in $PaCO_2$, thereby achieving more favorable acid base balance. Furthermore changes in pulmonary water content alter lung compliance. Finally, regional hypoperfusion increases wasted ventilation, requiring increased minute ventilation to maintain normal arterial carbon dioxide tension.

With advanced hypoperfusion, patients exhibit classical obtundation and stupor. However, in the early stages, particularly children who have no cerebrovascular disease, agitation and confusion occur more commonly. This altered mental status results from an inadequate attempt to maintain cerebral perfusion.

Monitoring

Measurement of several cardiopulmonary variables permits us to assess the complex clinical manifestations in the shock syndrome, and ultimately guides our therapy. Variables which reflect oxygen transport and oxygen consumption are most useful in predicting outcome, yet values outside the standard range of normal may be exhibited by patients who will survive. Therapy directed toward those values seen in eventual survivors may be defined as "preferred goals." If through therapy we achieve these "preferred goals" and ultimately realize improved outcome, we may consider these goals optimal.

Directly measured variables include: mean systemic arterial pressure; central venous pressure; hemoglobin; mean pulmonary artery pressure; pulmonary artery occluded pressure; blood volume; cardiac index; mean transit time; heart rate; body temperature; arterial pH, PCO_2, and hemoglobin saturation; mixed venous oxygen tensions.

To obtain these measurements we must insert peripheral systemic and pulmonary arterial catheters.

Systemic Arterial Catheters

Cannulation of a peripheral systemic arterial vessel has a very low cost/benefit ratio. Practice increases the success rate of cannulating the artery percutaneously, even in newborns. Trained personnel can insert a catheter into an artery exposed by a small skin incision, if percutaneous technique fails. Using teflon catheters of minimal and uniform diameter decreases the incidence of arterial occlusion by thrombosis. Continuous flushing with diluted heparin solutions of 1 unit of heparin per ml maintains patency of these catheters. Ischemia of tissue supplied by the artery which has been cannulated can be minimized by assuring adequate collateral flow. When the radial artery is used, a fiberoptic light source confirming the presence of the ulnar artery and the application of the modified Allen's test, confirms the presence of an effective alternate to the radial artery for blood flow to the hand.

We measure continuous systemic arterial pressure with transducer and amplifier equipped with auditory and visual alarms made to signal when preset limits are exceeded and occlusion or disconnection occurs. Arterial blood can be sampled frequently with minimal discomfort to the patient and analyzed for gas tensions, pH, and other important variables.

In children, arterial occlusion upon removal constitutes the most common complication of these catheters. Several factors influence the development of occlusion and recannulization. Catheters inserted by cutdown result in occlusion of the artery more frequently. Arteries cannulated for over 4 days occlude more often than those in which catheters remain in place for shorter periods. A greater catheter diameter to arterial diameter ratio will more frequently result in occlusion. Finally, recannulation usually occurs within 1 to 2 weeks and appears not to be influenced by the duration of cannulation.

Pulmonary Artery Catheterization

A balloon-tipped, flow-directed quadrilumen catheter made of extruded polyvinyl chloride is inserted into a peripheral vein and the tip carried by the blood flow through the heart into the pulmonary artery. When correctly positioned, the catheter lies in the center of the lumen of a distal pulmonary artery segment and measures pulmonary artery pressure. A latex balloon located at the tip of the catheter, when inflated, carries the catheter into a small branch of the vessel and prevents forward flow from the right ventricle from exerting its forces on the orifice distal to the balloon. A phased, delayed amplitude, dampened reflection of the left atrial pressure is then measured. A thermistor located 5 cm from the distal tip records blood temperature. Ten to 30 cm from the distal tip, depending on the user's specification, a second orifice exists to permit the introduction of chilled or room temperature dextrose and water into the blood for the measurement of cardiac output by the thermodilution technique. When the tip of the catheter is properly positioned in the pulmonary artery this orifice should lie within the right atrium, and pressures in that cardiac chamber can be measured.

Using 5 to 7 F catheters, we successfully catheterized the pulmonary artery 68 times in 49 children ranging in age from 1 month to 16 years, and weighing from 2.5 to 55 kg. We inserted all the catheters percutaneously using a Seldinger technique (see procedure in Section VII) with the femoral vein being the favored venous entry site. A fluoroscopic image intensifier facilitated placement in the majority of these insertions. We required an average of 50 min to properly place the catheter in the pulmonary artery.

Catheters remained in place for an average of just over 3 days with a range of between 10 min and 210 hours. Balloon rupture was the most common complication, calling for early removal of the catheter. Balloon life ranged from 10 min to 107 hours, and averaged 66 hours. No correlation between right atrial and pulmonary artery occluded pressure existed, suggesting that central venous pressure does not reliably reflect pressures on the left side of the heart in several diseases.

Two patients became hypotensive secondary to blood loss during catheter insertion. The wire was advanced too far into the femoral vein and venotomy was required for its removal. Postmortem examination revealed a thrombus in the inferior vena cava of these 2 patients. We recovered bacteria from 8 of 39 (20%) of the catheter tips upon removal and from the blood of 9 of 53 (17%) of the patients while the pulmonary artery catheters were in place. Table 2.2 shows the organisms cultured.

ECG and Heart Rate

ECG obtained from surface electrodes and displayed on a oscilloscope permits review of the electrical activity of the heart. A digital meter indicates heart rate and audio and visual alarms signal when preset limits are exceeded.

Table 2.2
Organisms Isolated from Systemic Catheter and Blood Cultures

	Catheter Tip	Blood
Enterobacter cloacae	1	3
Klebsiella pneumoniae	2	3
Pseudomonas aeruginosa	1	1
Pseudomonas fluorescens	2	1
Escherichia coli	—	1
Serratia marcescens	—	1
Klebsiella oxytoca	1	1
Acinetobacter anitratus	1	1
Staphylococcus epidermidis	2	1

Cardiac Output

Thermal technique for measuring cardiac output utilizes the principle of indicator dilution. When a solution (e.g. saline) of known temperature, different from the patient's blood temperature, and volume is injected, the average change in blood temperature recorded by a thermistor located downstream from the site of introduction of this fluid plotted against time entered into a modified Stuart-Hamilton equation yields cardiac output. Microprocessors facilitate the calculation and a digital meter displays the numerical value.

Thermal dilution technique compares favorably with more traditional methods for estimation of cardiac output. Determinations can be made rapidly and frequently. We inject a physiologic solution as the indicator and withdraw no blood from the patient. Small volumes of chilled indicator cause no significant change in blood temperature even in patients of less than 10 kg body weight.

Blood Volumes

Dilution of a known amount of radioisotope or dye in the plasma allows one to calculate the plasma volume. Introduction of labeled red blood cells and their dilution similarly permit determination of cellular volume. The sum, of course, equals the blood volume. In the absence of this assessment, we monitor filling pressures of the heart in response to infusions in order to judge the intravascular volume.

Gas Tensions, pH, Hemoglobin, Hematocrit, Total Proteins, and Colloid Osmotic Pressure

We analyze blood sampled from systemic artery and pulmonary artery (mixed venous blood) for oxygen and carbon dioxide tensions, hemoglobin, and hemoglobin saturation, hematocrit, pH, total proteins, and colloid osmotic pressure. Changes in oxygen content of right atrial blood parallel the pulmonary artery samples. Thus, right atrial blood (mixed venous blood) may be analyzed for oxygen and carbon dioxide tensions, hemoglobin and hemoglobin saturation, hematocrit, pH, total proteins, and colloid osmotic pressure.

Urinary Bladder Catheter

Perfusion and function of the kidneys may be estimated from urine output. Measurement is best done by urinary bladder catheter and a collection system. While urinary tract infection may occur from this indwelling device, in our opinion, the risk is justified when the patient's life is threatened by shock.

Computers

Numerouus variables may be measured and calculated. One system advocated by Shoemaker considers 35 cardiorespiratory variables in the evaluation of a patient's hemodynamic status. A programmed microprocessor automates calculation, organizes the data, and facilitates health care professional usage of the multitude of data which is acquired. The computer aids physicians, nurses, and others to recognize early and treat promptly deviations from desired goals. Furthermore, organization of the data into therapeutic and predictive indices allows caretakers to judge effectiveness of therapy as well as the likelihood of survival.

TREATMENT

Caretakers must institute orderly treatment immediately and gain inisight into etiology as therapy proceeds. Bodily compensation, generally inadequate, attempts to preserve flow to organs with little margin for interruption of oxygen and nutrients. Cells deprived of oxygen and energy substrate soon reach an irreversible state. Beyond this point, cell death proceeds, even if circulation is restored. The usual approach of diagnosis first, treatment later may not be appropriate and result in delay of much needed intervention. A plan directed at pathophysiology common to all types of shock allows caretakers to provide prompt treatment in this life-threatening condition. The plan includes first correcting hypoxia, then gaining vascular access for the administration of fluids and drugs (see Fig. 2.2).

Oxygenation

Oxygen delivery to tissues remains our primary focus in patients with shock. The

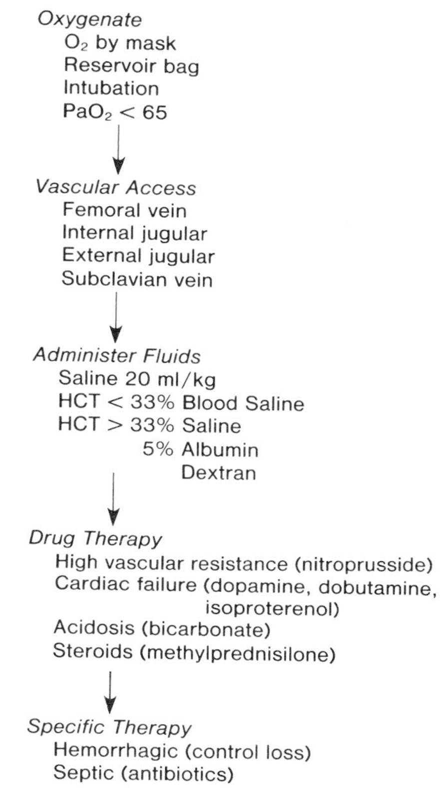

Figure 2.2. Management of shock—overview.

assurance of satisfactory oxygen content in the blood as it leaves the lungs a priori must be our immediate goal. We must eliminate airway obstruction. If we doubt the integrity of the natural airway, we insert an artificial airway (see Chapter 1). Oxygen administration by face mask and reservoir bag should precede laryngoscopy and tracheal tube placement to correct any hypoxia which exists, as well as to avoid further occurrence of hypoxia during tracheal intubation (see procedure in Section VII). We suggest the orotracheal intubation route initially. Nasotracheal intubation may follow once we achieve stability and correct abnormal arterial gas tensions. We administer one atmosphere of oxygen until arterial gas tension measurement indicates acceptable PaO_2. Subsequently we adjust FIO_2 to maintain arterial oxygen tension above 65 torr.

Early in the shock syndrome arterial hypoxia can be corrected by inspired oxygen concentrations below that generally accepted as toxic to the lung. Further interference with pulmonary gas exchange may require increases in transpulmonary distending pressure in order to avoid relying on toxic concentrations of oxygen. Since most of the gas exchange occurs during the exhalatory portion of the respiratory cycle, air containing lung volume decreases in that phase. As a result, in shock states most physicians favor end-expiratory pressure for correcting severe degrees of hypoxia.

Ventilatory failure occurs uncommonly in the early phase of shock. In fact, increased alveolar ventilation usually exists. However, as the syndrome progresses, severely deranged mechanics and fatigue may justify mechanical ventilation.

We must document the adequacy of gas exchange frequently and repeatedly. Often overlooked when caretakers focus on the failing circulation, we will not enhance cellular survival by achieving satisfactory blood flow unless oxygen content is adequate.

Vascular Access

We establish dependable vascular accesses by inserting large bore plastic catheters in peripheral veins if readily identifiable. However, often vasoconstriction precludes this. Alternately we seek central vein catheter placement. Favored entry sites for deep vein cannulation include: femoral, subclavian, internal and external jugular veins. We locate these vessels by their proximity to arteries. In seeking the lumen of these veins with a needle, the proximate artery may be accidentally entered. For this reason we favor small bore, thin walled, short beveled needles which make small holes in the artery easily sealed by brief compression. Once the needle tip enters the venous lumen, signified by blood aspirated into the attached syringe, we immobilize the needle, remove the syringe, and insert a flexible braided wire through the needle into the venous lumen. We then remove the needle and thread a catheter of appropriate diameter and length over the wire into the venous lumen, positioning the tip within the thorax, preferably in the right atrium (see procedure in Section VII). These catheters then serve a dual purpose of infusion devices as well as monitoring instruments.

Fluid Administration

Once we establish dependable venous access, we administer a fluid challenge of 20 ml/kg as rapidly as possible and assess systemic arterial pressure response to the fluid challenge. If systemic arterial pressure does not return to and remain at normal levels for patient's age following this fluid challenge, additional volumes are infused and titrated against central venous or right atrial pressures, since they correlate better with intravascular volume than does systemic arterial pressure. Initially we accept right heart filling pressures because of the greater ease in obtaining these measurements. However, if circulatory instability persists after achieving adequate right heart filling pressures, consider placement of a balloon-tipped flow-directed pulmonary artery catheter to obtain pulmonary artery occluded pressure, which more accurately reflects filling pressure of the heart.

A modification of Weil's "3.5 and 1.5 rule" (Fig. 2.3) helps us estimate volume deficits in pediatric patients. One observes the central venous pressure (CVP) for 10 min. If that pressure is less than 6 torr we infuse 4 ml/kg over 10 min, discontinuing the infusion if the central venous presssure rises at any time more than 3.5 torr. If, following the infusion, the central venous pressure has risen by less than 3.5 torr but more than 1.5 torr, we observe the patient for 10 min. If the central venous pressure remains above 1.5 torr of the starting value, we monitor the patient without administering additional fluid. If the central venous pressure declines to within 1.5 torr of the initial value, we again infuse 4 ml/kg over 10 min. We repeat these maneuvers until the systemic arterial pressure reaches a normal value, patient manifests other signs of restored circulation integrity, or the "3.5 and 1.5 rule" is violated. If the initial central venous pressure lies between 6 and 10 torr we administer 2 ml/kg over the 10 min period and look for the same central venous pressure changes. If the initial central venous pressure exceeds 10 torr, we infuse 1 ml/kg of fluid over 10 min and again observe the central venous pressure change.

Two points should be emphasized. First, we examine the change in central venous pressure measurement in response to the fluid infusion, rather than look for an absolute value. Secondly, because the veins are very distensible vessels and act as a reservoir for fluid, a three-fold increase in the volume of fluid contained in the venous system may be necessary before we see changes in the central venous pressure. When using the pulmonary artery occluded pressure (PAOP), substitute 7 and 3 torr for 3.5 and 1.5 torr central venous pressure measurements (Fig. 2.3).

Choice of Fluids

We maintain a hematocrit of 33%. We prefer to administer packed cells in combination with other blood component therapy, thereby more efficiently using this scarce resource. We employ fresh frozen plasma and platelets if clotting factors or thrombocytopenia exist.

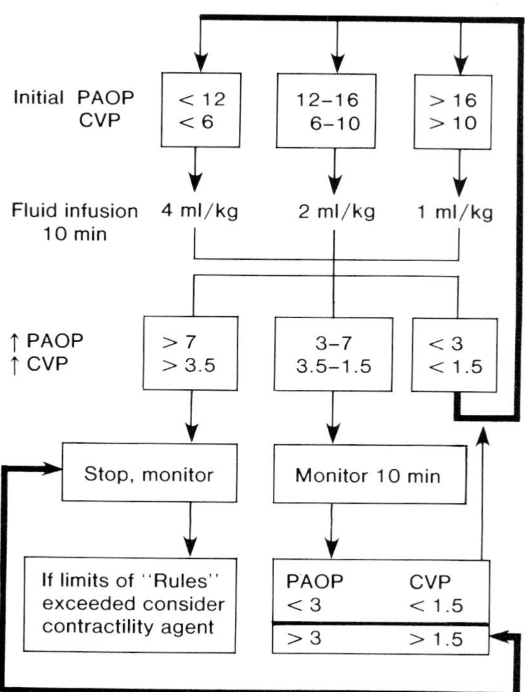

Figure 2.3. "7-3, 3.5–1.5 Rules" of Weil. (Adapted from M. H. Weil: *Journal of the American Medical Association*, 207: 337–340, 1969.) CVP = center venous pressure; PAOP = pulmonary artery occluded pressure.

If the hematocrit is greater than 30% or blood is not available, we use a 5% albumin in normal saline solution. Shoemaker examined the effect of colloid, crystalloid, and whole blood on several variables. Overall, he found that the synthetic plasma expander dextran, with molecular weight of 40,000 and 70,000, as well as albumin, produced the most favorable changes in the mean arterial pressure, cardiac index, left ventricular stroke work, pulmonary vascular resistance, and oxygen consumption. The dextrans are widely available and inexpensive, but cause decreased platelet adherence, thereby interfering with the clotting mechanism. This effect is seldom of clinical significance when less than 20 ml/kg/day of these solutions is administered. Crystalloids infused quickly leave the intravascular compartment and move into the interstitial water, which may already be increased in shock.

Vasodilator Therapy

If vascular resistance is high, vasodilator therapy may be helpful. Nutrient flow may be improved, left ventricular stroke work enhanced, and myocardial oxygen consumption decreased by lowering impedance to left ventricular ejection. We prefer a short-acting vasodilating drug such as sodium nitroprusside, beginning with 0.1 μg/kg/min. We increase the infusion rate exponentially until evidence of decreased peripheral vascular resistance exists, or the generally accepted safe dosage of between 8 and 10 μg/kg/min is reached. Toxic effects of sodium nitroprusside result from accumulation of cyanide, a metabolic product of the drug. Cyanide is cleared from the blood by conversion to thiocyanate, a reaction which is catalyzed by the liver enzyme rhodanese. Hypertension and metabolic acidosis are manifestations of toxicity from this drug. Treatment of the toxicity includes: sodium bicarbonate and intravenous hydroxocobalamin 0.1 ml/kg plus sodium nitrate 5 ml/kg, or amyl nitrite by

Table 2.3
Sympathomimetic Amines[a]

Acent	Dose Range	Peripheral Vascular Effect			Cardiac Effect	Comment
		Alpha	$Beta_2$	Delta	$Beta_1$	
Phenylephrine	0.1–0.5 μg/kg/min	4+	0	0	0	Increases systemic resistance without increasing inotropy; may cause renal ischemia
Isoproterenol	0.1–0.5 μg/kg/min	0	4+	0	4+	Strong inotropic and chronotropic agent: peripheral vasodilator; measure CVP—reduces preload; may "steal" renal blood flow
Norepinephrine	0.1–0.5 μg/kg/min	4+	0	0	2+	Increases systemic resistance; mildly inotropic; may cause renal ischemia
Epinephrine	0.1 μg/kg/min	2+	1–2+	0	2–3+	B_2 effect with lower doses; best for supporting blood pressure in anaphylaxis and drug toxicity
	0.2–0.5 μg/kg/min	4+	0	0	4+	
Dopamine	2–4 μg/kg/min	0	0	2+	0	Splanchnic and renal vasodilator; may be used with isoproterenol; increasing doses produce increasing alpha effect
	4–8 μg/kg/min	0	2+	2+	1–2+	
	>10 μg/kg/min	2–4+	0	0		

[a] From R. K. Crone: Acute circulatory failure in children. *Pediatric Clinics of North America*, 27: 534, 1980.

inhalation. The latter two drugs induce the formation of methemoglobin, which has a greater affinity for cyanide than the cytochrome oxidases. Toxicity from cyanide exists when serum concentrations exceed 200 μg/dl. Toxic levels of thiocyanate range from 5 to 10 ml/dl. Dillon and others have shown that infusion rates of up to 3.5 μg/kg/min of nitroprusside resulted in thiocyanate levels of 0.60 to 1.9 mg/dl with an average of just under 1 mg/dl an(1-2+ single patient a cyanide level of 64.1/dl.

Nitroglycerine affects predominantly the capacitance vessels. Venoconstriction in the postcapillary venule persists after ischemia. Hypoxia from ischemia overcomes the sympathetic neurally mediated arteriolar and precapillary sphincter constriction. Obstruction to flow leaving a capillary without reduction of inflow results in increased capillary hydrostatic pressure, favoring fluid movement out of the capillary into the interstitium. Recently, nitroglycerin has become available for intravenous administration. Perhaps this venodilator may prove to be more beneficial than those drugs which act predominantly on the arteriolar vasculature. We maintain systemic arterial pressure by prompt and adequate fluid infusion when vasodilators are administered and vascular capacity is increased.

Myocardial Contractility

Catecholamines are the drugs of choice for improving myocardial contractility in patients with shock because of their very short half-life and potency. The multiple effects upon the circulation are well documented and provide the basis for selection initially (Table 2.3). However, if optimal goals are not reached with one, the use of another or several in combination may achieve the desired goal. Currently, dopamine is our choice because of its specific effects on the splanchnic and renal circulation, in addition to its myocardial stimulating properties. We and others find the increase in heart rate to be an important part of the increased cardiac output caused by dopamine. In addition, Lange and others have found no significant increase in arterial resistance with dosages as high as 25 μg/kg/min.

Beginning with 2 μg/kg/min, we increase

the dose exponentially until we achieve a cardiac index of greater than 4.2 liters/sq m, an arterial mixed venous difference for oxygen of less than 5 ml/dl, or left ventricular stroke work of 60 gram meters or greater.

A feature ascribed to dobutamine, a new synthetic catecholamine, is direct β_1-adrenergic receptor stimulation resulting in increased myocardial contractility without marked tachycardia, or altered arterial resistance. In 21 infants and children ranging from 4 weeks to 14 years of age who demonstrated cardiogenic or septic shock, doses up to 10 mg/kg/min of dobutamine increased cardiac index between 23 and 30%. Unlike dopamine, the improvement was mainly due to an increase in stroke index, since no significant increases in heart rate occurred. Total systemic vascular resistance fell with doses of less than 7.5 mg/kg/min and authors observed no change in systemic or arterial blood pressure or total pulmonary vascular resistance. Infants less than 12 months of age demonstrated insignificant increases in cardiac index and stroke index. From this data, dobutamine appears to be useful in the management of infants and children with shock syndrome, particularly in patients older than 1 year.

Acid-Base Abnormalities

Our observations suggest that unless perfusion is adequate, infusion of sodium bicarbonate rarely maintains arterial pH. We therefore consider bicarbonate a temporary and immediate therapy to acutely alter arterial pH so that myocardial performance will be optimized. Ultimately, improved blood flow will result in a decrease in acid products of anaerobic metabolism and only then will H^+ concentration remain normal. We calculate the dose of sodium bicarbonate according to the following formula: bicarbonate administered in meq equals the body weight (kg) times base excess (BE) times 0.4. In the presence of acute hypercapnea, one-half of the calculated dose is administered and pH remeasured. If correction is not achieved, the remainder is infused. Suggested rate of administration should not exceed 2 meq/min.

Steroids

Shumer examined in adults the influence of steroids on mortality from septic shock. In a two-part study, one retrospective and the other prospective, he found improved survival in the steroid treated groups as compared to controls. He observed no difference in survival between those individuals treated with methylprednisolone sodium succinate or dexamethasone phosphate. Effects considered beneficial included: (1) reduction of granulocyte aggregation; (2) stabilization of lysosome membranes of white cells, thereby reducing release of enzymes which destroy the cell and when released into the blood stream activate vasotropic substances; (3) vasodilation; (4) improved capillary endothelial integrity and decreased intravascular fluid losses; (5) alleviation of the glucogenesis; (6) increased cardiac index; (7) increased oxygen transport; (8) increased oxygen consumption.

We administer 30 ml/kg of methylprednisolone as a bolus and repeat this dose one more time. Shumer believes steroids influence immunologic reactions by interfering with the complement activation cascade. Early use of steroids may prevent activation of complement. Once active complement components have been generated, the steroids exert little effect. Shumer also demonstrated that with repeated doses of glucocorticoids complications were more likely.

Other Specific Therapy

HEMORRHAGIC SHOCK

Obvious bleeding can be controlled initially with pressure and later with ligation, electrocautery, or repair of the open vessel. Gastrointestinal bleeding may respond to lavage with chilled saline or regional arterial vasoconstrictor infusion (Chapter 50).

SEPTIC SHOCK

We sample material from all possible sites of infection, immediately Gram stain the specimen, and choose antibiotic coverage accordingly. Organisms subsequently recovered by culture are tested for antibiotic sensitivity. We institute broad spectrum antibiotic coverage initially, followed by septic antimicrobial therapy when sensitivity studies are completed (see Chapter 45).

References

Bedford RF: Percutaneous radial artery cannulation—increased safety using teflon catheters. *Anesthesiology* 42: 219–222, 1975.

Bennett NR, Abbott TR: The use of sodium nitrate prusside in children. *Anesthesiology* 32: 456–463, 1977.

Carp H, Janoff A: Potential mediator of inflammation: Phagocyte-derived oxidants suppress the elastase-inhibitory capacity of alpha$_1$-proteinase inhibitor in vitro. *J Clin Invest* 66: 987–995, 1980.

Dillon TR, Janos GG, Meyer RA, et al.: Vasodilator therapy for congestive heart failure. *J Pediatr* 96: 623–629, 1980.

Dupont HL, Spinx WW: Infections due to gram-negative organisms: An analysis of 860 patients with bacteremia at the University of Minnesota Medical Center, 1958–1966. *Medicine* 48: 307–332.

Freed MD, Keane JF: Cardiac output measured by thermodilution in infants and children. *J Pediatr* 92: 39–42, 1978.

Hammerschmidt DE, Weaver LJ, Hudson LD, Craddock PR, Jacob HS: Association of complement activation and elevated plasma-C5a with adult respiratory distress syndrome: pathophysiological relevance and possible prognostic value. *Lancet* 1: 947–949, 1980.

Hosea S, Brown E, Hammer C, Frank M: Role of complement in a model of adult respiratory distress syndrome. *J Clin Invest* 66: 375–382, 1980.

Jacob HS: Damaging role of activated complement in myocardial infarction and shock lung: Ramifications for rational therapy. In *Critical Care—State of the Art*, pp I (L) 1–18, edited by WC Shoemaker, WL Thompson. Society of Critical Care Medicine, Fullerton, CA, 1980.

Janoff A, White R, Carp H, Harel S, Dearing R, Lee D: Lung injury induced by leukocytic proteases. *Am J Pathol* 97: 111–135, 1979.

Lang P, Williams RG, Norwood WI, Castaneda AR: The hemodynamic effects of dopamine in infants after corrective cardiac surgery. *J Pediatr* 96: 630–634, 1980.

Lefer AM: Blood borne humoral factors in the pathophysiology of circulatory shock. *Circ Res* 32: 129–139, 1973.

Lefer AM: Vascular mediators in ischemia and shock. In *Pathophysiology of Shock, Anoxia, and Ischemia*, pp 165–181, edited by RA Cowley, and BE Trump. Williams and Wilkins, Baltimore, 1982.

Mellins RB, Stalcup SA: Pulmonary edema in disorders of the respiratory tract in children, pp 573–592, edited by Kendig EI, and Chernick V. WB Saunders, Philadelphia, 1977.

Miyasaka K, Edmonds JF, Conn AW: Complications of radial artery lines in the pediatric patient. *Canad Anaesth Soc J* 23: 9–14, 1976.

Perkin RM, Levin DL, Reedy J, et al.: Hemodynamic effects of dobutamine in children with shock. *Crit Car Med* 9: 171, 1981.

Raphaely RC, Swedlow DB, Kettrick RG, et al.: Experience with pulmonary artery catheterization in critically ill children, Abstract. *Crit Care Med* 8: 265, 1980.

Seldinger SI: Catheter replacement of needle in percutaneous arterography: New technique. *Acta Radiol (Diagn) (Stockh)* 39: 368–376, 1953.

Shoemaker WC: Comparison of the relative effectiveness of whole blood transfusions and various types of fluid therapy in resuscitation. *Crit Care Med* 4: 71–78, 1976.

Shoemaker WC: Pathophysiology, monitoring and therapy of shock syndromes. In *Critical Care—State of the Art*, pp I (D) 1–63, edited by WC Shoemaker, WL Thompson. Society of Critical Care Medicine, Fullerton, CA, 1980.

Shumer W: Steroids in the treatment of clinical septic shock. *Ann Surg* 184(3): 334–341, 1976.

Stephenson LW, Edmunds Jr, LH, Raphaely RC, et al.: Effects of nitroprusside and dopamine on pulmonary arterial vasculature in children after cardiac surgery. Cardiovas Surg 1978, Suppl 1 *Circulation* 60: 104–110, 1979.

Weil MH, Shubin H: The "VIP" approach to the bedside management of shock. *JAMA* 207: 337–340, 1969.

Yamanda KM, Olden K: Fibronectins—adhesive glycoproteins of cell surface and blood. *Nature* 275: 179–184, 1978.

Zapol WM, Snider MT: Pulmonary hypertension in severe acute respiratory failure. *N Engl J Med* 296: 476–480, 1977.

CHAPTER 3

Emergency Department Anesthetic Management

JOSEPHINE J. TEMPLETON, M.D., and A. MICHAEL BROENNLE, M.D.

INTRODUCTION

Pediatric patients in the emergency department vary widely in requirements for analgesia, anesthesia, or life support. This chapter will review current and alternative principles and practices emphasizing those pertaining to the emergency department physician and indicating when specialists in anesthesiology should be consulted.

ANALGESIA AND SEDATION

Local Anesthetic Infiltration

Many pediatric patients require minor surgery to repair superficial lacerations and reduce simple fractures. Infiltration of a local anesthetic agent and restraint, using a "papoose" board, suffice for most simple lacerations. Intramuscular narcotics (morphine 0.1 mg/kg or meperidine 1 mg/kg) may provide adequate anesthesia in children over 1 year old for reduction of fractures. We discourage "cocktails" combining a sedative, narcotic, and tranquilizer, as they may oversedate and last for hours.

Ketamine was initially reported to be an agent safe for emergency department use but is now recognized to have all the hazards of other general anesthetics, including the potential for airway obstruction and aspiration. Ketamine should be used only by those fully trained in anesthesiology, working in properly staffed and equipped locations which, in most hospitals, means the operating suite.

Nitrous Oxide Analgesia

The use of nitrous oxide-oxygen inhalation analgesia has been reported recently in pediatric emergency department patients as young as 16 months old. In some children undergoing particularly painful procedures, local anesthetic infiltration still must be performed. Dentists have used nitrous oxide analgesia in office dental procedures for many years and appear to have the most thorough experience.

Currently we do not use nitrous oxide in the emergency department. To do so safely requires properly trained personnel with appropriately designed equipment. The individual administering the nitrous oxide must be skilled in airway management and cardiopulmonary resuscitation and cannot have any other responsibilities during the procedure. This person must maintain verbal contact with the patient, avoiding concentrations of nitrous oxide that render the patient unconscious. Most experience with nitrous oxide has been in elective patients following a planned interval since the last ingestion of food or liquid. The safety of nitrous oxide analgesia in the usual emergency situation (i.e., one assumes the patient has a "full stomach") has not been clearly defined.

Regional Anesthetic Blocks

Several regional anesthetic blocks may be useful in the emergency department. These require little technical skill but do necessitate the ability and equipment to manage adverse reactions. Intravenous access and resuscitative equipment must be readily available. Suggested doses of local anesthetic agents are indicated in Table 3.1.

As with all other forms of regional anesthesia, appropriate monitoring of cardiac rate, cardiac rhythm and blood pressure should be instituted before the block is performed. Airway equipment and emergency drugs should be readily available should the need arise.

Toxicity results from high serum levels of local anesthetic, which may result in convulsions and, less commonly, cardiovascular depression. Hypoxemia during the convulsion is the major threat; management consists of giving oxygen, supporting ventilation which requires a rapid sequence intubation in a patient with a full stomach, and stopping the convulsion with small doses of a barbiturate, such as thiopental, 1 mg/kg i.v.

To ensure the success of any regional method of anesthesia, there are several important factors which must be remembered. One must select the patient carefully. Some children will be emotionally unsuited for regional anesthesia. For example, past experiences with regional techniques will play an important part in the child's acceptance of the technique. The age and emotional state of the child at the time of the injury must be considered. Strategic placing of needles, syringes and other equipment away from the child's view is important in allaying the child's fears and pain.

Appropriate sedation of the child undergoing a regional technique is of paramount importance to assure the total success of the block. This can be accomplished either by a subanesthetic dose of ketamine (0.5 mg/kg) or diazepam (0.1 mg/kg) intravenously.

The procedure for simple digital nerve block is covered in the procedure described in Section VII.

Intravenous Regional Block (Bier Block)

The intravenous regional anesthetic block (Fig. 3.1) is appropriate for procedures on the arm that can be completed within the maximum tourniquet time, 90 min. By leaving the intravenous catheter in place, the duration of the procedure can be extended by allowing a period of circulation and then reinjecting the anesthetic agent. We do not use this technique for procedures involving the lower extremity because of the large amount of drug required. Typical procedures for which intravenous regional blocking is useful are reduction of forearm fractures and repair of moderately complex lacerations including tendon repairs.

A plastic intravenous catheter is placed in a hand vein with diluted heparinized saline (1 unit/ml) and plugged ("heparin lock"). A double tourniquet (e.g., Inflatomatic Dual Cuff Assembly, Zimmer USA, Warsaw, Indiana) or two narrow surgical tourniquets are placed over several wrapped layers of soft material (Webril) on

Table 3.1
Suggested Local Anesthetic Doses in Pediatric Patients

Anesthetic	Maximum Dose	Infiltration	Intravenous Regional	Brachial Plexus
Lidocaine (Xylocaine)	5–7 mg/kg	0.25–0.5%	0.5% 1.5–3 mg/kg	1%
Epinephrine 1:400,000 < 6 yr 1:200,000 > 6 yr		O.K.	No	O.K.
Bupivacaine (Marcaine; Sensorcaine)[a]	2 mg/kg	0.25%	0.25% 1.5 mg/kg	0.5%

[a] FDA. approved drug insert cautions: "Safety and effectiveness in children below the age of 12 have not been established."

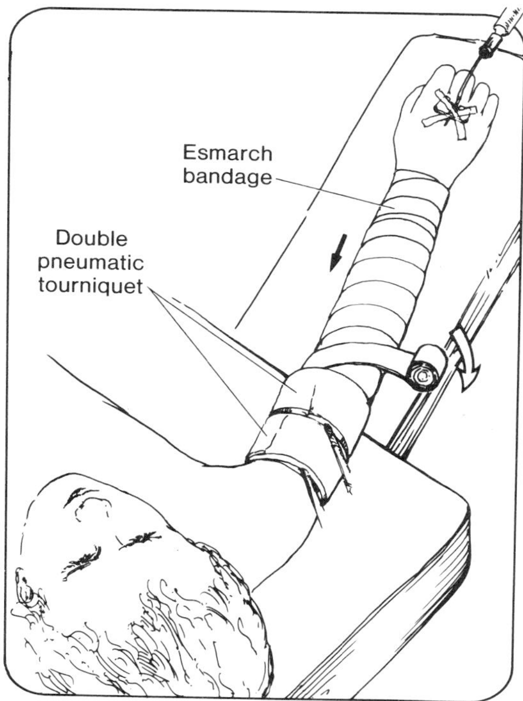

Figure 3.1. Intravenous regional block.

the arm. The arm is exsanguinated by raising it for 3 min, then wrapping the arm from the fingers centrally to the tourniquet with a snug elastic (Esmarch) roll. The proximal cuff is inflated to at least 150 torr over systolic pressure (maximum of 300 torr) and the elastic roll removed. An appropriate dose of local anesthetic is injected into the intravenous catheter. The catheter may then be removed, holding pressure over the puncture site. Onset of anesthesia is in approximately 5 min. If ischemic pain occurs under the proximal cuff, the distal cuff can be inflated over the now anesthetized arm allowing release of the proximal cuff. The tourniquet must remain fully inflated for at least 15 min to allow for "fixation" of the local anesthetic to the tissues, thus minimizing the possibility of systemic drug toxicity after tourniquet deflation. Blood level peaks are also minimized by alternately deflating/reinflating the tourniquet in 10 to 15-sec cycles for 3 to 4 min. Following a regional block using lidocaine, peak central venous blood levels occur in 4 to 6 min with equilibrium of venous and arterial concentrations at 30 min. Central venous and arterial levels equilibrate at 60 sec when 0.25% bupivacaine has been used. Surveillance of the patient should continue for at least 60 min following termination of a regional block. The anesthesic effect should only last about 10 min after tourniquet release if lidocaine 0.5% or bupivacaine 0.25% are used.

Axillary Block

The pediatric patient with a severely lacerated hand or fractured forearm is, in general, in need of prompt attention. The child is frightened, in pain, and for the most part will have a full stomach. Brachial plexus anesthesia is particularly indicated for the management of such lesions.

There are several approaches for anesthesia of the brachial plexus, the supraclavicular approach, the interscalene approach, and the axillary approach. We prefer the axillary approach in the child as it is better accepted. The axillary approach carries little or no risk of pneumothorax, injection in the subarachnoid space, or phrenic nerve block and it is relatively easy to perform.

For the performance of the axillary block (Fig. 3.2) the child is placed in a supine position with the head turned away from the operator while being distracted by an attendant. The arm is abducted 90° and the forearm is flexed at 45°, and externally rotated so that the dorsum of the hand lies on the table next to the patient's head in a "salute" position.

With the operator gowned and gloved, the axillary fossa is prepped in a sterile fashion. The axillary artery is then palpated and followed proximally to the insertion of the pectoralis major. Placing of the anesthetic solution at this level is more likely to reach the musculocutaneous and axillary nerves, which leave the axillary sheath at a very high level. At this point, a skin wheal is raised by means of a 25 gauge needle directly over the pulsation of the artery (Fig. 3.2*A*). The needle is then inserted at the level of the axillary pulse. The artery is approached by slowly advancing the needle until bright red blood is aspirated in the needle hub (Fig. 3.2*B*). The needle is then further advanced until blood is no longer

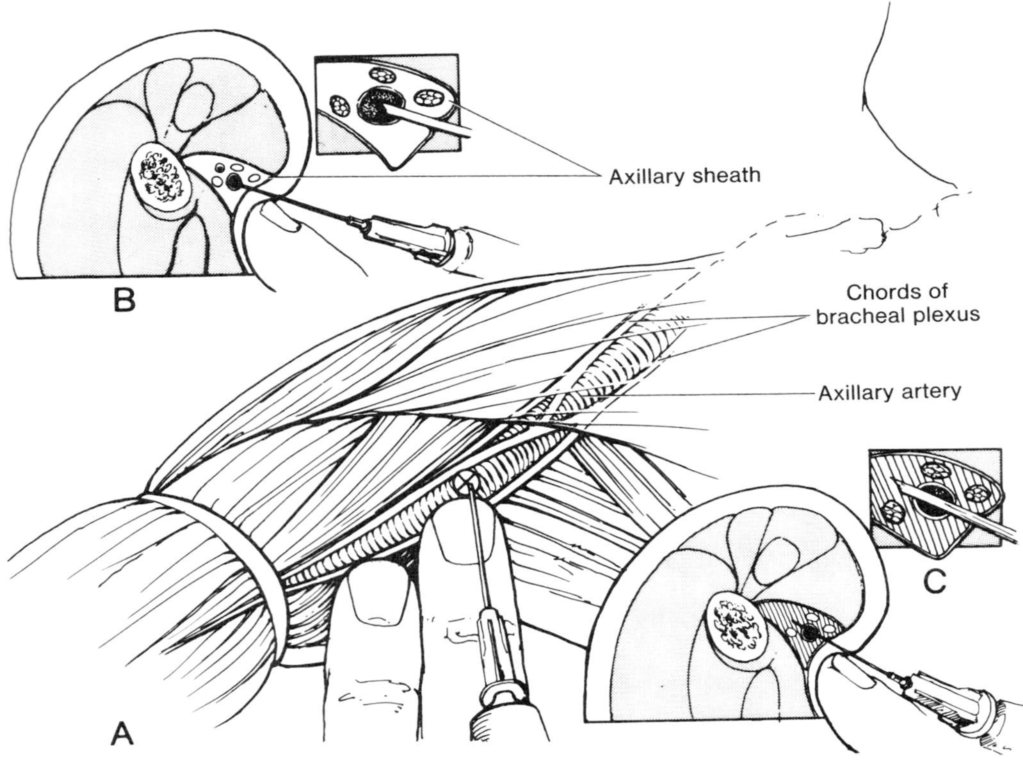

Figure 3.2 Axillary approach to brachial plexus block.

aspirated (Fig. 3.2*C*). Paresthesias need not be elicited with this approach. An appropriate amount of local anesthetic is then injected slowly while aspirating at frequent intervals to avoid inadvertant intraarterial injection. One or two milliliters of the anesthetic solution are retained (depending on the size of the patient) and injected subcutaneously over the artery in order to effectively block the intercostal nerve which runs superficial to the sheath on its course to innervate the upper inner aspect of the arm.

It takes 15 to 20 min (less in the young child) for the complete effect of the block to take place. The presence of vasodilatation and a blush is evidence that the block is effective. The child is then asked to touch his nose with the blocked arm; one sees that the child tries to follow the command but is not able, since the arm is now anesthetized.

GENERAL ANESTHESIA AND LIFE SUPPORT

The anesthesiologist should be notified as soon as a patient is identified as needing surgery in the operating suite, or general anesthesia to obtain diagnostic studies. Anesthesiologists may also provide life support during diagnostic studies such as computed tomography scanning.

Early involvement of anesthesiologists in the initial resuscitation and stabilization of the patient is desirable not only because the anesthesiologist can assist with technical procedures, but also to allow the anesthesiologist who will be managing the life support during surgery, to become familiar with the extent of the patient's injuries and treatment.

The initial consultation call to the anesthesiologist should include essential information such as the patient's *age*, estimated or actual *weight* and apparent *extent of injury*. This aids in organizing the appropriate anesthetic equipment. For the urgent situation of the severely injured patient it is ideal to have sufficient anesthesia personnel so that preparation of the anesthetizing location may proceed concurrently with the preanesthetic patient evaluation.

Preanesthetic Evaluation

The anesthesiologist should review the patient's acute and past medical history and perform an appropriate physical examination. Discussion with the parents should include reviewing prior anesthetic experiences, family history, and the current anesthetic plan allowing both patient, if mature enough, and parents an ample opportunity to ask questions. Only rarely will the immediate need for resuscitation or emergency surgery require that the discussion with the parents be deferred.

Premedication

Sedative drugs are rarely indicated prior to emergency surgery. Sedatives may be hazardous in causing depression in level of consciousness and loss of protective airway reflexes in patients who usually are assumed to have a "full stomach." In some circumstances narcotics may be indicated for pain, for example when the diagnostic evaluation is completed or when transport may be uncomfortable despite splinting of fractures. When indicated small incremental intravenous doses (morphine 0.05 to 0.1 mg/kg) with close monitoring should avoid obtundation. The drying effect of anticholinergics (atropine, 0.02 mg/kg; maximum 0.5 mg intramuscularly) is desirable at least 30 min prior to procedures such as bronchoscopy or esophagoscopy.

Intubation

Endotracheal anesthesia is indicated for all emergency general anesthetics. Most patients who require emergency anesthetics or urgent tracheal intubation are considered to have a "full stomach" and therefore are at risk of regurgitation and aspiration of acidic gastric contents into the airway. Aspiration may occur even if an interval as long as 6 hours or more has elapsed between the last oral intake and the induction. Injury, pain, anxiety, labor, and narcotics are all factors which may decrease gastric emptying in an unpredictable manner. Abdominal pathology such as appendicitis may cause an ileus. It is always prudent to assume that gastric contents are present. Endotracheal anesthesia is, therefore, indicated for almost all emergency anesthesia. An exception might be the child who has had a peaceful night's sleep with a splinted, relatively pain free fracture now coming for reduction.

A "*rapid sequence*" induction is the most desirable approach to emergency intubation of the patient with a "full stomach" unless the patient is already unconscious and flaccid. Essential equipment prepared beforehand should include: a functioning bag and mask or anesthetic circuit, tracheal tubes of appropriate sizes, a lubricated stylet, oxygen sources, two suction lines with "tonsil" or Yankauer suction tips capable of aspirating large volumes of gastric aspirate, and monitoring equipment including a precordial stethoscope, blood pressure monitoring devices, and electrocardioscope. Atropine, 0.01 to 0.02 mg/kg, is administered intravenously to block vagal reflexes. Patients over 5 years old are pretreated with a small dose of a competitive muscle relaxant, *d*-tubocurarine, 0.1 mg/kg i.v., or pancuronium, 0.01 mg/kg i.v., to decrease succinylcholine fasciculations which can cause a significant increase in intragastric pressure. Preoxygenation is performed for 3 min by applying high oxygen flow (5 to 10 liters/min) via a snug fitting mask/breathing circuit. Thiopental, 4 to 5 mg/kg i.v., is given immediately followed by succinylcholine, 2 mg/kg i.v., while an assistant applies pressure by firmly pushing the cricoid cartilage just below the thyroid cartilage, using the thumb and first two fingers in a fork configuration. This maneuver (Sellick's maneuver) occludes the esophagus against the vertebral body, effectively preventing retrograde passage of gastric contents. Without ventilating the patient, laryngoscopy and endotracheal intubation are performed as soon as the masseter muscles relax (15 to 20 sec in infants, 30 to 40 sec in older children). Once the tracheal tube is properly positioned, ventilation is begun. Following clinical confirmation of proper depth of placement and secure taping of the tracheal tube, the stomach should be aspirated by a large diameter (12 to 18 French) catheter. Specifics on endotracheal intubation are covered in Section VII.

Several cautions regarding "rapid sequence" intubation are necessary. Thiopental doses need to be reduced in frail or hypovolemic patients. Succinylcholine will cause paralysis with apnea for 5 min or more, and therefore is contraindicated when difficulty in intubating or ventilating with a mask is anticipated. Hyperkalemia sufficient to cause cardiac arrest may occur following succinylcholine administration to patients who have sustained burns, direct muscle trauma, or neurologic disorders resulting in motor deficits.

Pulmonary aspiration of gastric contents is common in obtunded or unconscious patients. Pulmonary dysfunction initially results from bronchospasm caused by the acid (pH 2.5 or less) and from atelectasis caused by aspirated particles. The immediate therapy is tracheal suctioning with consideration of bronchoscopy if the degree of atelectasis suggests the aspiration of larger particles. Respiratory care includes appropriate oxygen concentration and in some cases continuous positive airway pressure. Pulmonary lavage and steroids are not beneficial. Opinions vary on giving antibiotics immediately versus waiting for tracheal cultures to demonstrate significant bacterial flora.

Extubation criteria include satisfactory oxygenation and ventilation, restoration of muscle tone, adequate neurologic function including muscle tone, and pharyngeal protective reflexes. Equipment for reintubation must be available at the time of extubation.

Recovery

Patients who have had an anesthetic require a period of observation of at least 1 hour in a recovery room, intensive care unit, or similarly staffed area. Delivery of skilled close observation during the recovery period is difficult in the milieu of a regular nursing unit or emergency department.

DIAGNOSTIC STUDIES

An essential aspect of evaluating some pediatric emergency patients is obtaining sophisticated diagnostic studies, most commonly computed tomography (CT). Satisfactory studies are dependent on patients remaining completely still during the study, a requirement that may necessitate general anesthesia. Sedation produced by either intramuscular or intravenous medications is generally not recommended in the emergency patient because of the risks of airway obstruction and aspiration.

The patient with a head injury or multiple trauma needs close monitoring during transport to/from, and during the diagnostic procedure, in order to detect early signs of deterioration from increasing intracranial pressure or bleeding. Electrocardioscopes with pressure channels and suction apparatus can be battery powered and conveniently carried on a shelf constructed to fit securely over the patient's feet on a stretcher. Diagnostic study sites may be remotely located requiring advance planning to ensure the availability of an anesthetic machine with appropriate gases. We use a portable cart (Fig. 3.3) that is completely equipped with all the necessary equipment in addition to the anesthetic machine to safely conduct anesthesia in an isolated location. Sufficient personnel with requisite skills are required to transport the patient and aid the anesthetist in the induction of anesthesia. If adequate space is not available at the study site for induction of anesthesia, the induction should be done in the emergency department or operating room.

MANAGEMENT OF SPECIFIC CONDITIONS

General Trauma

To be effective, the anesthesiologist must discipline himself to follow an almost instinctive systematic approach. He must not be distracted by apparent injuries but must

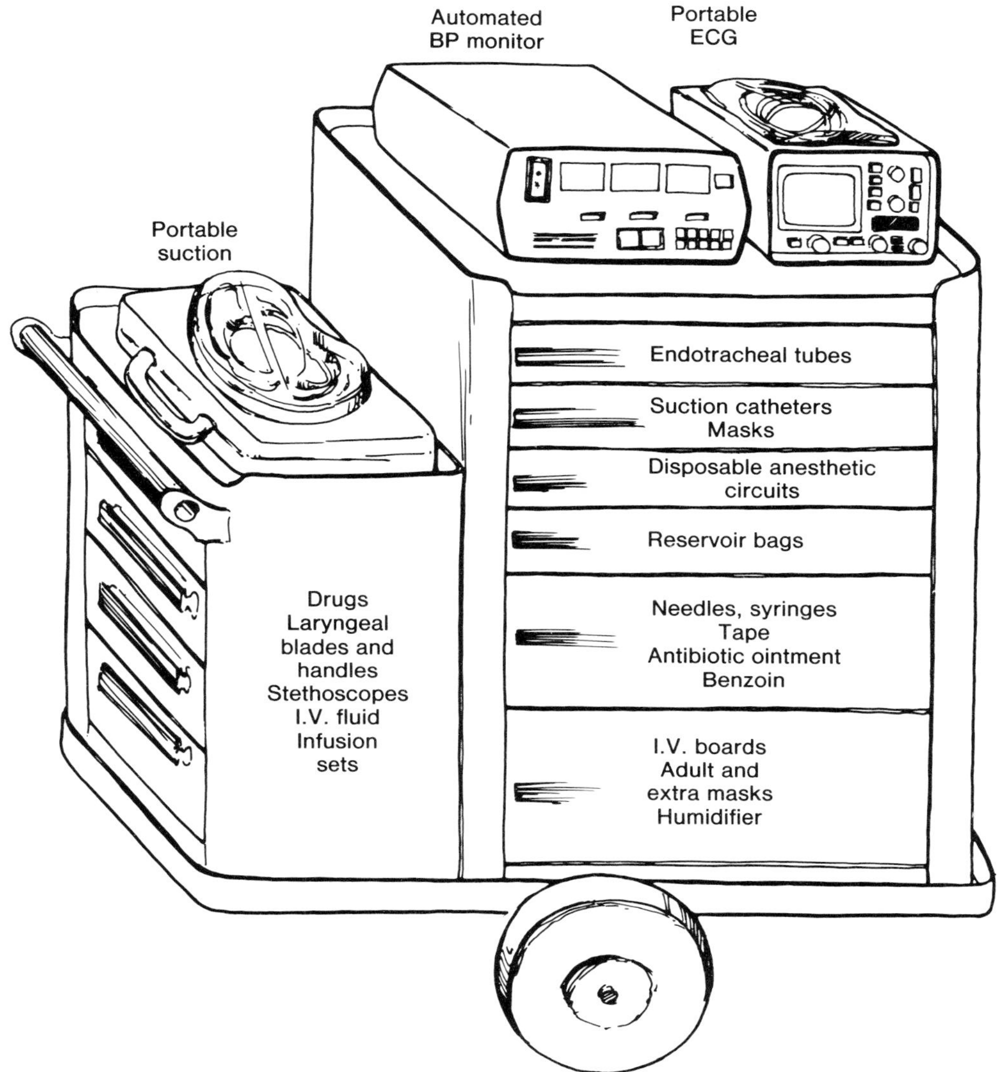

Figure 3.3 Transport cart for diagnostic studies.

sequentially assess airway patency, adequacy of oxygenation and ventilation, cardiac action, and peripheral perfusion. The anesthesiologist must then perform a brief assessment of the patient's neurologic status, specifically looking for signs of intracranial mass effect or increased intracranial pressure. This initial assessment can be easily performed in less than a minute, and it will direct where the initial resuscitative measures should be directed. There are two serious injuries which should be considered as they can be easily missed, particularly in the comatose patient. Injuries to the cervical spine can be silent and may be aggravated during movement of the patient or tracheal intubation. Traumatic diaphragmatic hernia is also a difficult condition to diagnose but should be suspected when there is evidence of trauma to the lower chest or upper abdomen.

Early diagnosis of shock is as important in the pediatric patient as it is in the adult. Unfortunately, the degree of shock is often underestimated in the pediatric patient. Pallor and poor capillary refill are strong evidence for hypovolemia. Tachycardia and hypotension are late signs of hypovolemic shock in small children whose peripheral vasculature is capable of marked vasoconstriction before decompensation occurs. A restless, anxious child with a thready pulse suggests inadequate cerebral perfusion. Shock, when not due to an obvious external hemorrhage, is usually due to intraabdominal or intrathoracic injuries. Therefore, in a hypovolemic patient, a bleeding site should be explored in the thoracic cavity by appropriate chest x-rays and tube thoracotomy, and in the abdomen by paracentesis (see Chapters 57, 59 and 60, and Section VII). Conversely head trauma rarely produces hypovolemia (unless there is such severe brainstem damage that the patient is terminal).

Respiratory noises such as gurgling and rattling may be indicative of partial respiratory obstruction and indicate a need for urgent attention to the airway. Repositioning of the patient or insertion of an artificial airway may be required. Early intubation is especially important in cases of facial injuries (including burns) before edema, blood, or debris distort the anatomy rendering endotracheal intubation more difficult or impossible.

A nasogastric tube should be inserted in all children who have sustained major trauma unless there is a definite contraindication. Gastric distention in the young child invariably accompanies major trauma. A distended tight abdomen can be a contributary factor to aspiration and interfere with ventilation.

Head Trauma

In children with head trauma and depressed sensorium, secondary morbidity may be related to unrecognized hypoxia resulting from airway obstruction. Therefore, the first management consideration should be the patency of the airway. If simple positioning does not correct the obstruction then oral tracheal intubation should be performed without delay.

Although the severely injured and flaccid child may require only atropine premedication for intubation, most patients with head injuries should be intubated with sedation and paralysis, in order to avoid the possibility of increasing intracranial pressure (ICP). Thiopental (4 to 5 mg/kg i.v.) is preferred as an induction agent because it decreases cerebral metabolism and reduces intracranial pressure. Pancuronium, 0.15 to 0.2 mg/kg i.v., has been suggested in place of succinylcholine because it is thought to be less likely to cause an increase in ICP. Paralysis is slower and less profound with pancuronium and will last over 1 hour. Lidocaine, 1 to 1.5 mg/kg i.v., prior to intubation, may be used to suppress the cough reflex and may exert a direct effect in lowering ICP. After intubation is accomplished, hyperventilation should be used to maintain a degree of hypocapnia with arterial carbon dioxide tension between 30 and 35 mm Hg, until the patient can be further evaluated. Continuous monitoring of the degree of hypocapnia can be measured with an end-tidal CO_2 monitor. Further measures to control intracranial pressure may be indicated, such as steroids, diuretics, and greater hypocapnia (partial pressure of arterial carbon dioxide ($PaCO_2$) = 25 mm Hg). These agents should not be used until a complete neurologic assessment has been made unless the status of the patient is rapidly deteriorating (see Chapter 67).

In patients with focal neurologic findings or signs of increased ICP, an intracranial subdural bolt should be placed, permitting monitoring and early specific treatment of increased ICP (see Chapter 67). Before the comatose patient is moved from the emergency department, cervical spine radiographs should be performed to rule out cervical spinal injury. Once stablized and monitored, the patient is ready for transport for further diagnostic studies, to the operating room, or to the Intensive Care Unit.

Thoracoabdominal Trauma

Thoracoabdominal injuries present particular anesthetic problems. Injury may directly involve the airway, making airway protection difficult. Additionally, impaired cardiorespiratory function may occur, especially in the case of a ruptured diaphragm, pneumothorax, or flail chest. During the assessment of the patient particular attention should be directed to the presence of pneumothorax especially where there are fractured ribs, causing respiratory and circulatory embarrassment. There may be severe hemorrhage secondary to major vessel injury requiring massive transfusion. Clinical evaluation of hypovolemic shock includes the possibility of hepatic or splenic rupture in abdominal trauma (Chapter 57).

When the patient has sustained severe abdominal injury, such as a hepatic injury, preparation for immediate and massive transfusion should be made with insertion of a large bore plastic cannula in an upper extremity vein. The importance of the location of intravenous cannula cannot be overstressed since the administration of intravenous fluids in the lower extremities may be lost. Once adequate circulation is improved, a central venous cannula should be inserted in the second upper limb or in the neck via the internal or external jugular vein. This will enable measurement of the central venous pressure and, at the same time, provides a second large route for volume infusion.

An attempt must be made to restore an optimal circulating blood volume and to maintain a hematocrit level which will ensure adequate oxygen transport to the tissues. Older children react to hypovolemia with pronounced vasoconstriction and near normal blood pressures even with losses up to 20% of their blood volume. Central venous pressure may initially be maintained, but will later fall as venous return to the heart becomes inadequate. Therefore, central venous pressure becomes a reasonable guide in judging adequate volume replacement. In infants and younger children, arterial blood pressure closely follows changes in intravascular volume, therefore, central venous pressure measurement does not appear as necessary as in older children (see Chapter 2).

Further information as to the adequacy of blood volume replacement and organ perfusion is obtained by the estimation of urine output. A urinary catheter should be inserted early. A urine flow of over 1 ml/kg/hour is an indication of adequate renal blood flow and, therefore, adequate organ perfusion. The general appearance of the patient should be constantly observed, particularly vasoconstriction of the skin vessels and capillary refill. This can be more objectively assessed by measuring skin temperature and core temperature. Core temperature can be measured by inserting a rectal probe in the rectum or inserting a probe in the nasopharyngeal or esophageal area. A rise in skin temperature with a constant core temperature would be indicative of improved perfusion due to an improved or expanded intravascular volume.

Attention should be paid to the temperature of the environment as radiant heat loss may be significant. This is especially important in the young child and infant. Fluids administered to the patient should be warmed to avoid a further drop in body temperature with possible stimulation of cardiac arrhythmias. Fluid and blood should be immersed in a controlled warm water bath whose temperature should not be higher than 40°C.

Fluid and Blood Therapy

All patients requiring anesthesia should be given regular maintenance intravenous fluids, 5% dextrose in 0.2 normal saline, according to the formula of Holliday and Seger:

The first 10 kg: 100 ml/kg/day
The second 10 kg: 50 ml/kg/day
Each kg over 20 kg: 20 ml/kg/day.

Trauma patients often require larger fluid volumes because of blood loss or sequestration of plasma-like fluid in the extravascular interstitial compartment known as the "third space." Third space fluid is found in sites of trauma where edema may be manifested; for example, after abdominal injuries, edema of the mesentery or bowel wall may occur, as well as accumulation of fluid in the bowel lumen.

Initial therapy of the clinically hypovolemic patient is based on the concept that otherwise healthy children will tolerate acute administration of 20 ml/kg of any volume expanding isotonic fluid (Ringer's lactate, normal saline, 5% albumin, plasma, or whole blood) without developing congestive heart failure or other sequelae. In the emergency department, Ringer's lactate or normal saline would be used initially. Heart rate, blood pressure, peripheral perfusion, and urine output are the parameters used to measure the patient's response to treatment. Following initial treatment, additional aliquots of 10 ml/kg may be repeatedly administered at rates determined by the apparent degree of volume deficit, until the deficit is corrected as reflected by a decrease in heart rate, increase in blood pressure and urine output, and improvement of peripheral perfusion.

Ringer's lactate must be given at a ratio of 2 to 3 ml/ml of blood loss since it equilibrates between the intravascular and extravascular interstitial fluid compartments. Third space requirements vary with the site and degree of trauma. Guidelines range from 2 to 3 ml/kg/hour for thoracotomies to 8 to 10 ml/kg/hour for extensive laparotomies. Although 40 ml/kg has been recommended as a maximum amount of intraoperative third space fluid replacement, personal experience suggests that individual cases must be evaluated on hemodynamic and peripheral perfusion parameters.

Transfusion of blood is based on the goal of maintaining a normal blood volume while allowing hemodilution by using nonblood replacement to a minimum hematocrit of 30% in children (40% in neonates). Depending on their initial hematocrit, children will usually tolerate non-blood replacement of 10 to 20% of their estimated blood volume (blood volume of infants, 80 ml/kg; children, 60 ml/kg). Blood loss in excess of this estimated allowable loss or serial hematocrits less than the minimum level, are treated by transfusion. We prefer whole blood over packed red blood cells to replace acute blood loss for several reasons. Whole blood: (1) can be administered faster, (2) most closely duplicates what is being lost, (3) eliminates need to decide on the appropriate diluting fluid, (4) maintains plasma protein levels, and (5) is less expensive than administering two components, i.e., packed cells plus plasma or 5% albumin. Although their efficacy is still not proven, we use 20 micron microfilters during the administration of all blood products except platelets.

Patients requiring massive transfusion, defined as blood replacement in excess of 1 blood volume, may develop specific deficiencies from banked blood. We serially determine ionized calcium levels as hypocalcemia may occur in rapidly transfused patients. Normal values for ionized calcium at Children's Hospital of Philadelphia are shown in Table 3.2 If low ionized serum calcium levels are measured or suspected by clinical impression, calcium gluconate, 30 mg/kg i.v., or calcium chloride, 10 mg/kg i.v., is slowly administered. Small infants may require 100 mg of calcium gluconate for every 100 ml of transfused blood. Calcium chloride should be given through a central venous line to avoid sclerosing peripheral veins. Fresh frozen plasma may be administered for labile clotting factors indicated by abnormal coagulation studies or empirically after 1 to 1.5 blood volumes have been transfused. Platelet concentrates may be necessary with a blood volume transfusion. Hyperkalemia and acidosis from large amounts of bank blood are problems not generally encountered if the patient has been successfully resuscitated, warmed, and adequately perfused. A metabolic alkalosis from metabolism of citrate preservative usually follows 12 to 36 hours after massive transfusion.

Ocular Trauma

Children with penetrating injuries of the eye are often quiet and they require little or no sedation. If the child appears anxious or uncomfortable preoperatively, then use of incremental doses of morphine, 0.1 mg/kg, will offer sedation and at the same time minimize depression of laryngeal reflexes.

Methods of induction of anesthesia and endotracheal intubation in these patients with full stomachs are controversial. The predominant view is that succinylcholine should be avoided since it increases intra-

Table 3.2
Serum Ionized Calcium

	Mean	Range + 2 S.D.
2–4 yr	2.58	2.24–2.74
5–17 yr	2.49	2.31–2.67
Adult	2.42	2.34–2.60

ocular pressure and may cause extrusion of the vitreous. We prefer a rapid sequence induction of anesthesia with thiopental, 5 to 6 mg/kg i.v., combined with pancuronium, 0.15 to 0.2 mg/kg i.v. Alternatively an inhalation induction with spontaneous ventilation and intubation facilitated by deep halothane is acceptable. For management of specific eye injuries, see Chapter 61.

Burns

Pediatric burn patients present six immediate problems for emergency department physicians and anesthesiologists. While initial focus tends to be on the extent of the injury and calculation of a fluid program according to one of the several burn formulas (see Chapter 64), reliable intravenous access and a site for blood pressure monitoring must be established. If the leg is uninvolved the posterior tibial artery may be used by placing a cuff, of the same diameter appropriate for the arm, above the ankle.

Heat loss through burned tissue is extraordinary, necessitating aggressive measures to preserve body temperature including high ambient temperatures in the emergency department and the operating room to prevent excessive cooling.

Respiratory function can be compromised from several causes including: a markedly increased metabolism with consequent increase in minute ventilation, a reduction in functional residual capacity, an increase in alveolar-arterial oxygen gradient, and decreases in both lung and chest wall compliance. These abnormalities are compounded in patients who have suffered "pulmonary burns" from heat or smoke inhalation. Facial or airway edema can develop rapidly in the initial hours after thermal injury. Patients with evidence or suggestion of airway edema should be intubated as soon as possible in anticipation of further swelling that may preclude intubation later. Intubation is strongly preferred over early tracheostomy because of the high mortality rate from infection following tracheostomy. Succinylcholine should not be used to intubate burn patients because massive potassium release may occur. Encephalopathy may occur early in the course from hypoxemia or hypovolemia and later from hyponatremia and septicemia.

Lastly, circumferential burns of the extremities or trunk can cause circulatory or respiratory embarrassment necessitating escharotomies within hours of an acute burn.

References

Aidinis SJ, Zimmerman RA, Shapiro HM, Bilanuick LT, Broennle AM: Anesthesia for brain computer tomography. *Anesthesiology* 44: 420–425, 1976.

Broennle, AM: Anesthesia for the pediatric patient. In *Surgical Pediatrics-Non-Operative Care*, pp. 83–98, edited by S Gans. Grune & Stratton, New York, 1979.

Crone RK: Nitrous oxide-oxygen sedation for minor surgery. *Pediatr Alert* 6: 57–58, 1981.

Dunbar BS, McGill WA, Epstein BS: Anesthesia for the injured child. In *The Injured Child*, pp. 107–125, edited by J Randolph. Year Book, Chicago, 1979.

Eather KF: Regional anesthesia for infants and children. *Int Anesthesiol Clin* 13: 19–48, 1975.

Feins NR: Multiple trauma. *Pediatr Clin North Am* 26: 759–771, 1979.

Goldberg AI: Anesthesia and intensive care. In *Pediatric Trauma*, pp. 105–136, edited by RJ Touloukian. John Wiley & Sons, New York, 1978.

Griffin CG, Campbell VD, Jones R: Nitrous oxide-oxygen sedation for minor surgery. *JAMA* 245: 2411–2413, 1981.

Moore DC, Crawford RD, Scurlock JE: Severe hypoxia and acidosis following local anesthetic-induced convulsions. *Anesthesiology* 53: 259–260, 1980.

Salem MR, Wong AY, Lin YH: The effect of suxamethonium on the intragastric pressure in infants and children. *Br J Anaesth* 44: 166–169, 1972.

Stark RA: A review of intravenous regional anesthesia. *Anesthesiol Rev* 9: 15–24, 1982.

Steward DJ, Creighton RE: Anesthetic management of the injured child. In *Care of the Injured Child*, pp 26–35. Williams & Wilkins, Baltimore, 1975.

Szyfelbein SK: Anesthetic considerations for major burn surgery. *ASA Refresher Courses in Anesthesiology* 8: 201–216, Lippincott, Philadelphia, 1980.

CHAPTER 4

Death

ROBERT G. KETTRICK, M.D.

INTRODUCTION AND DEFINITION

When a critically ill child comes to the emergency department the attending physician has a responsibility to provide those diagnostic, supportive, and management interventions necessary to reverse the processes which represent an immediate threat to life. On occasion, this goal is not achievable, and death occurs. In other circumstances a child is "DOA"—dead on arrival. Diagnosing and dealing with death in the emergency department requires a thorough knowledge of both medical and legal aspects of this event.

The common law definition of death generally consists of the permanent absence of respiration and circulation. However technological advances, organ replacement innovations, and life support systems have challenged the validity of this definition. We currently use a definition of death recommended by the President's Commission on the Study of Ethical Problems in Medicine, Biomedical and Behavioral Research, and approved by the Uniform Law Commissioners, the American Bar Association, the American Medical Association, the American Academy of Neurology, and the American Electroencephalographic Society. This commission defined death as either: (1) irreversible cessation of circulatory and respiratory functions; or (2) irreversible cessation of all functions of the entire brain, including the brain stem. The determination is to be made in accordance with "accepted medical standards."

PATIENT MANAGEMENT

Diagnosis of Death

When a child arrives in the emergency department with the presumptive diagnosis of death, the physician should confirm this diagnosis and record the appropriate physical examination. The statement of examination should reflect the following: the patient is apneic; there is no heart beat; there is no pulse; there is no motor activity; and the pupils are fixed and dilated. A statement of diagnosis is then written into the record and a time given to the pronouncement of death.

Resuscitative Efforts

Often patients present to the emergency department while receiving cardiopulmonary resuscitation by transport personnel. Emergency department personnel then assume the life support responsibilities from the transport team. Airway, breathing, and circulatory functions are assessed and supported in an effort to reestablish or maintain a cardiac output sufficient to provide vital organ (brain, heart, kidney) perfusion of oxygenated blood. When the circulatory system cannot be supported by other than external cardiac compression or direct massage after a reasonable period of resuscitative effort, the responsible physician should direct discontinuation of the resuscitative effort.

The resuscitative process may have provided cerebral perfusion adequate to sustain variable amounts of central nervous function—including a degree of consciousness. With discontinuation of resuscitative effort, a period of several minutes elapses before all evidence of brain activity disappears. It is appropriate to defer final examination until all motor activity is in abeyance. Thereafter, a physical examination is accomplished and recorded to provide documentary support of the diagnosis of death. Again, this examination should reflect: apnea; the absence of a heart beat, pulse and blood pressure; fixed dilated pupils; and the absence of motor activity. The details of resuscitation should be recorded along with the time noted for the pronouncement of death.

It is not uncommon with pediatric patients that the resuscitative effort reestablishes circulatory function. When this occurs, the appropriate life support interventions for respiratory and circulatory support should be maintained and refined, as appropriate. The physician then must reevaluate the central nervous system for evidence of dysfunction. If the clinical examination demonstrates an absence of both brain stem and cortical function, a diagnosis of brain death should be considered.

Brain Death

Brain death may be considered to have occurred when there is biologically irreversible cessation of brain function at both a cortical and brain stem level. The absence of cortical function is evidenced by the following: no spontaneous skeletal muscle activity greater than fasciculatory muscle movements; complete flaccidity of all muscles; and total unresponsiveness to painful stimuli either by withdrawal, facial grimacing, or assumption of postural movements. The presence of posturing (decerebrate, decorticate) suggests that both brain stem and higher functions may be intact. Posturing, therefore, is not consistent with the diagnosis of brain death.

Spinal segmental withdrawal reflexes may be preserved in the circumstance of brain death and must be discriminated from cerebral withdrawal response. In making this distinction, a painful afferent stimulus is provided to an extremity. The spinal reflex efferent response is confined to the same extremity as the stimulus. Also it is stereotyped, being similar in pattern with repeated stimulations. The cerebral withdrawal reflex is characterized by a variable response in the same extremity as well as a response in another extremity.

The absence of brain stem reflexes is evidenced by absence of: pupillary responsive to light, corneal reflexes; oculocephalic (Doll's eye) or oculovestibular (cold-caloric) reflexes, pharyngeal and carinal reflexes, and respiratory activity. The absence of respiratory activity is determined by the following process: (1) establish normocapnea; (2) administer 100% oxygen for at least 3 min; and (3) withdraw mechanical ventilation for 3 min and observe for respiratory effort. During the period of no mechanical ventilation, delivery of 100% oxygen through a Mapleson system should be continued.

When the patient has an intact circulation and a presumptive diagnosis of brain death, we generally admit the patient for a period of observation and support. After a 12-hour period of observation, the clinical examination is repeated and, if still consistent with brain death, an electroencephalogram is done. An isoelectric electroencephalographic tracing confirms the diagnosis of brain death. At that time the child is pronounced as dead. The support technology is then discontinued.

The interval between the presumptive diagnosis and final diagnosis is used to establish whether or not there are central nervous system depressants in the body in such quantities as to produce an appearance of brain death. If this is the case, the clinical examination and EEG must be repeated following the reversal or elimination of those drug effects.

Observation over time and the electroencephalographic examination allow discrimination between postictal depression with profound obtundation and brain death. Other circumstances which have produced erroneous diagnoses of brain death include severe infant botulism and overdose of neuromuscular blockers such as curare or pancuronium. Both represent circumstances of total motor paralysis. In each of these circumstances an EEG will confirm the presence of cortical function. In addition, the interval between the presumptive and final diagnosis can be utilized to establish a primary diagnosis or cause of death and to identify those resources appropriate to help the family cope with their loss.

If the process which has eventuated in a presumptive diagnosis of brain death is associated with elevations of intracranial pressure, an intracranial pressure monitoring bolt is inserted into the skull to measure and record the pressure. When the mean intracranial pressure is equal (±10 torr) to systemic mean arterial pressure for more than one hour, a four vessel cerebral arteriogram is done to confirm absence of cerebral blood flow. When an absence of cerebral blood flow is confirmed, along with a clinical examination compatible with brain death, the child is pronounced dead and life support technology is discontinued.

FAMILY INTERVENTIONS

Essential family members are allowed in the emergency department. Essential should be a definition of convenience. The nurse and physician determine what the family needs and what the emergency department environment can tolerate at that point in time. A rigid access policy will not allow the best possible care for the family. Guideliness, rather than policies, provide flexibility for individualizing your approach to the family (see Chapter 69).

The family should be allowed to "view" the child's body. A private area should be available for counseling or free expression of grief.

The extended family or mourners may come to the emergency department. The physician can be useful in insuring them that their loved one is being treated with dignity and that all appropriate efforts were made to save the child's life. Hospital personnel can often gain valuable information from these people as they work to insure that the family's needs are identified and met.

The emergency department physician often has to contend with crowds, other clinical responsibilities, and the pressure of other families who perceive that their child is in need of urgent evaluation and management. The press of other responsibilities does not relieve the physician from fulfilling his responsibility to the family of the dead child. When the physician cannot give the family his personal attention he should insure that this responsibility is delegated to those resources with proven value in helping families deal with death. The resources which we commonly draw upon include the chaplain, social worker, and certain experienced nurses.

Where a hospital chaplain is available, he or she can be invaluable in helping the family to begin to cope with their loss. Baptism or religious rites for the dying may be urgently requested or demanded. Whether or not a chaplain is immediately available, the emergency department should have a roster of clergy who are available at all hours to serve the immediate needs of those who desire religious services. The right person at the right time may do more to blunt the pain of the family than the more traditional members of the medical team. Where possible, representatives of the clergy should be formally integrated into that service effort which the hospital extends to the grieving family.

Social service should be contacted in order to ensure that follow-up is provided for those families whose innate resources appear inadequate to cope with the crisis of sudden death. Invaluable members of the hospital team, social workers are particularly effective in extending the medical community's ability to relieve suffering which occurs beyond the confines of the hospital.

The private physician should be notified as he is often in a position to provide direct counseling and reassurance. When the private physician knows the family dynamics, he may provide—in a sensitive and expeditious manner—those services that might otherwise come from the hospital chaplain or social worker.

SOCIETAL RESPONSIBILITIES

While there is a great sense of finality to the event of death, the physician and medical community responsibility does not end.

The emergency department physician's responsibilities extend beyond those of service to the child and his family. He must provide the mechanism for community review of the death. Pertinent history should be obtained from the family, and the patient should be examined to establish that the physical examination is compatible with the available history. Where there is discrepancy, that information should be passed on to the coroner or pathologist.

If no physician was in attendance during the last illness of the deceased or if the death was sudden, violent, suspicious, and not the result of natural causes, the death must be referred to the coroner.

When an autopsy is required, an explanation must be provided for the family. The family should know where the autopsy is to be performed in order to facilitate arrangements for subsequent disposition of the body. The mechanisms for obtaining information relative to the results of the autopsy should be made known to the family.

The emergency department chart must be completed and signed by the appropriate personnel. Thorough documentation of history, physical examination, and management should be accomplished. These records and their accuracy may be of great importance in any future civil or criminal review.

The tragedy and finality of a child's death may obfuscate our sense of responsibility to the child as an individual bonded into a family. As we go about fulfilling our limited medical responsibilities to the child, we must initiate the process of assessing the family needs. Ultimately, our major responsibility is to insure that those mechanisms which the family membership uses to cope with the loss are healthy rather than destructive.

References

Conference of Royal Colleges and Faculties of the United Kingdom: Diagnosis of brain death. Lancet November 13, 1976.

Gilder SS: 22nd World Medical Assembly—Death and the W.M.A. *Br Med J* 3: 493–494, 1968.

Harvard Medical School, Ad Hoc Committee of the Harvard Medical School to Examine the Definition of Brain Death: A definition of irreversible coma. *JAMA* 205: 337–340, 1968.

National Institute of Neurological and Communicative Disorders and Stroke: An appraisal of the criteria of cerebral death. *JAMA* 237: 982–986, 1977.

Report of the Ad Hoc Committee of the American Electroencephalographic Society on EEG Criteria for Determination of Cerebral Death: Cerebral Death and the Electroencephalogram. *JAMA* 209: 1505–1510, 1969.

Report of the Medical Consultants on the Diagnosis of Death to the President's Commission for the Study of Ethical Problems in Medicine and Biomedical and Behavioral Research: Guidelines for the determination of death. *JAMA* 246: 2184–2186, 1981.

SECTION II Signs and Symptoms

INTRODUCTION TO SECTION

In this section, the chapters focus on the problem-oriented approach to the rapid diagnosis and initial management of patients coming to the emergency department with specific signs or symptoms as chief complaints. The particular presenting complaints covered in the following chapters were chosen because they may result from serious diseases, requiring urgent diagnosis and therapy, or because they are quite commonly heard.

In each chapter, the sign or symptom is defined, and in most there will be a brief review of underlying pathophysiology. The chapter then concentrates on a realistic diagnostic approach that is applicable in the emergency department. These chapters will be supplemented in most cases by a table listing the common causes of each sign or symptom and an algorithm outlining the key steps in sorting out the differential diagnosis.

The chapters in this section mesh closely with those in the medical, surgical and psychosocial sections which are organized around specific diseases. Thus, there will be many cross-references in Chapter 21, "Fever," to specific topics in Chapter 45, "Infectious Diseases." These cross-references will guide the reader to text discussing details of the evaluation for and treatment of specific infectious diseases, once the likely diagnosis has been established. Brief comments on symptomatic therapy will be included only if specific treatments are not discussed elsewhere in the text.

Entire textbooks have been devoted to the differential diagnosis of pediatric signs and symptoms; the spectrum of childhood disease demands such lengthy works. However, the few rapidly progressive, life-threatening causes of each complaint may sometimes become obscured in an all-inclusive detailed discussion by the information presented on less urgent conditions. Thus, the chapters in this section emphasize the serious conditions of greatest concern to the emergency physician or the pediatrician in an emergency department. Readers interested in pursuing broader coverage of particular pediatric signs and symptoms are referred to the invaluable works of Illingworth and Green.

References

Green, M: *Pediatric Diagnosis.* W. B. Saunders, Philadelphia, 1980.

Illingworth, RS: *Common Symptoms of Disease in Children.* Blackwell, Oxford, 1979.

CHAPTER 5

Abdominal Pain

RICHARD RUDDY, M.D.

INTRODUCTION

Abdominal pain is a frequent complaint of children who come to the emergency department. Children with abdominal pain have a sensation of discomfort, varying from mild to agonizing, localized to the abdomen. The onset of abdominal pain frequently heralds a life-threatening emergency, calling on the clinician's talents to uncover the cause. The diverse etiologies include acute surgical diseases (i.e., appendicitis, strangulated hernia, trauma to a viscus); intraabdominal medical ailments (i.e., gastroenteritis, food poisoning, ulcer disease, urinary infections); extraabdominal conditions (i.e., pneumonia, tonsillitis, contusions of muscle and bone); systemic illnesses (i.e., "viral syndrome," leukemia, diabetes mellitus, sickle cell anemia); and functional abdominal pain.

PATHOPHYSIOLOGY

Abdominal pain can originate in at least three neural pathways: (1) visceral, (2) somatic, and (3) referred. (1) *Visceral* pain is generally a dull, aching sensation primarily in the midabdominal, epigastric, or lower abdominal region. Distension of a viscus stimulates nerves locally, initiating an impulse that travels through autonomic afferent fibers to the spinal tract and central nervous system. The nerve fibers from different abdominal organs overlap and are bilateral, accounting for the lack of specificity to the discomfort. (2) *Somatic* pain is usually well localized and intense in character. It is carried by somatic nerves in the parietal peritoneum, muscle, or skin unilaterally to the spinal cord level from T6 to L1. (3) *Referred* pain is felt at a location that is distant from the diseased organ as either a sharp, localized sensation or a vague ache. Afferent nerves from different sites, such as the parietal pleura of the lung and the abdominal wall, share pathways centrally. All three types of pain may be modified by the child's ability to tolerate pain. Psychogenic and environmental factors augment or inhibit the sensation to varying degrees in different individuals.

Certain illnesses are associated with abdominal pain that cannot be explained neurophysiologically. These include conditions such as tonsillitis with high fever and viral syndromes, though there may be tender intraabdominal lymphadenopathy as in the syndrome of mesenteric lymphadenitis. Thus, examination of the entire patient is always essential. The principle causes of abdominal pain in children are summarized in Table 5.1.

EVALUATION AND DECISION

The evaluation of the child with abdominal pain is an important and often difficult task. The assessment must focus on any history of trauma, the age of the patient, the onset and chronicity of the pain, the related symptoms and pertinent past history, and the physical findings (Fig. 5.1).

Table 5.1
Causes of Acute Abdominal Pain[a]

Infancy (<2 yr)	Preschool Age (2–5 yr)	School Age (>5 yr)
	Common	
Colic (age <3 months) Acute gastroenteritis "Viral syndromes"	Acute gastroenteritis Urinary tract infection Trauma Appendicitis Pneumonia, asthma Sickling syndromes "Viral syndromes" Constipation	Acute gastroenteritis Trauma Appendicitis Urinary tract infection Pelvic inflammatory disease Functional abdominal pain Sickling syndromes Constipation "Viral syndromes"
	Relatively Infrequent	
Trauma (possible child abuse) Intussusception Intestinal anomalies Incarcerated hernia Sickling syndromes	Meckel's diverticulum Henoch-Schönlein purpura (anaphylactoid purpura) Toxin Cystic fibrosis Intussusception Nephrotic syndrome	Pneumonia, asthma, cystic fibrosis Inflammatory bowel disease Peptic ulcer disease Cholecystitis, pancreatic disease Diabetes mellitus Pregnancy (ectopic and intrauterine), ovarian cyst Collagen disease Mittelschmerz
	Rare	
Appendicitis Volvulus Milk allergy Tumors (e.g., Wilms') Cystic fibrosis Toxin (heavy metal) Disaccharidase deficiency	Incarcerated hernia Neoplasm Hemolytic uremic syndrome Rheumatic fever, myocarditis, pericarditis Hepatitis Inflammatory bowel disease Choledochal cyst Hemolytic anemia Diabetes mellitus Porphyria	Rheumatic fever Toxin Renal calculi Tumor Testicular torsion Ovarian torsion

[a] Modified from W. Liebman and M. Thaler: In *Gastrointestinal Diseases*, Vol. 1, p. 411, edited by M. Sleisenger and J. Fortran. W. B. Saunders, Philadelphia, 1978.

Abdominal Pain with Trauma

Abdominal pain associated with trauma is covered in detail in the surgical section (Chapter 57, "Major Trauma," and Chapter 59, "Abdominal Emergencies"). The emergency physician first assesses the cardiovascular status (vital signs and clinical peripheral vascular perfusion) and the extent of visible injuries while simultaneously establishing intravenous access. He or she should perform a rapid, gentle, physical examination to separate superficial injury (i.e., muscle contusion) from significant intraabdominal trauma (i.e., splenic rupture or hepatic hematoma). Passage of a large bore nasogastric tube avoids gastric distension. Radiographs (e.g., chest and abdo-

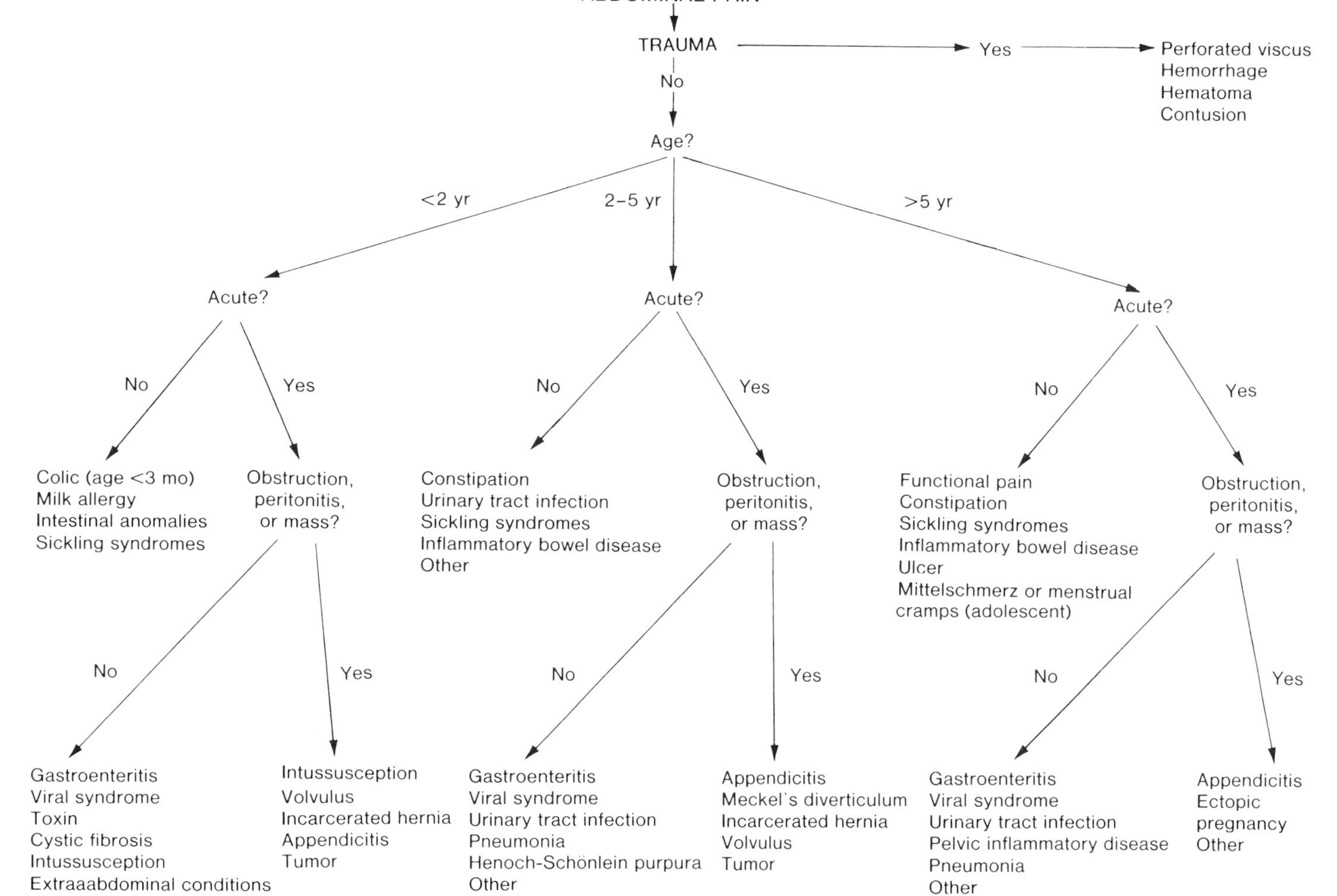

Figure 5.1 Evaluation of the child with abdominal pain.

men) and laboratory tests (e.g., CBC, urinalysis, and amylase) are indicated except in trivial injuries.

Abdominal Pain without Trauma

In assessing the child who develops abdominal pain without a history of trauma, the first responsibility of the emergency physician, after stabilization of the seriously ill patient, is to recognize the group of children requiring immediate surgical intervention, whether for appendicitis, intussusception, or other congenital or acquired lesions. Next, an effort should be made to diagnose any of the medical illnesses from among a large group of acute and chronic, abdominal and extraabdominal inflammatory disorders that require emergency nonsurgical management. Finally, the physician must deal with a host of self-limiting causes of abdominal pain and be able to manage the patient with a non-organic complaint.

INFANTS LESS THAN 2 YEARS OF AGE

The infant less than 2 years of age with abdominal pain is the most difficult to evaluate in the emergency department because the child cannot describe or localize the complaint. To the parent, the pain may consist of "crying out," of constantly drawing the legs up with sudden movements or jerks, of being inconsolable, or of irritability accentuated with fondling or rocking.

Acute Pain. In evaluating the uncomfortable infant, as described in the algorithm, look first at the onset of "pain," separating acute from recurrent. Then evaluate additional symptoms chronologically. Inquire about the presence of diarrhea, fever, and vomiting and their onset; this constellation of findings occurs most frequently with gastroenteritis. Cough may suggest pneumonia, broncholitis or asthma as the etiology of colicky pain. The story of episodic colicky pain with interposed quiet intervals, even in the absence of a "currant jelly" stool, makes one suspicious of intussusception or, occasionally, midgut volvulus.

The physical examination usually determines which diagnoses should be aggressively pursued. An ileus, manifest clinically by distension and absent bowel sounds, often accompanies surgical conditions, sepsis, and infectious enterocolitis, and may be seen with pneumonia or urinary tract infection. If an abdominal mass is palpable, intussusception, abscess, or neoplasm (usually of renal origin) are likely. Signs of partial or complete obstruction with peritonitis are indicative of a perforated viscus from intussusception, volvulus, or, occasionally, appendicitis or Hirschsprung's disease.

On auscultation of the chest, decreased breath sounds and rales may point to pneumonia. Abdominal pain and pallor can occur in neoplasia, as with bleeding into an abdominal Wilms' tumor, hepatoma, or neuroblastoma. The presence of pallor and pain also raises the possibility of sickling hemoglobinopathies with the development of either a vaso-occlusive crisis or a splenic sequestration. Rapid hemolysis from other causes where the spleen is enlarged acutely usually has associated jaundice. If bruising is noted, the physician must look for hemophilia or leukemia as the cause of abdominal pain.

Chronic Pain. When the abdominal pain is recurrent or chronic in infants under 3 months of age, and not accompanied by other findings or symptoms, the physician may make a diagnosis of "colic" (described at length in Chapter 13). There are, however, several serious uncommon causes of recurrent abdominal pain in infancy which must be considered. These include recurrent intussusception, malrotation with intermittent volvulus, milk allergy syndrome, and various malabsorptive diseases such as cystic fibrosis, celiac disease, and rarely, lactase deficiencies.

Laboratory Testing. In general, the history and physical examination will lead the emergency physician to the diagnosis. When there is obstruction, peritonitis, or a mass, a CBC and urinalysis are always indicated. Serum electrolytes and BUN are rarely useful unless dehydration and/or renal diseases are suspected. Abdominal x-rays may be helpful in confirming obstruction or the presence of a mass; a barium enema is indicated immediately in the case of suspected, uncomplicated intussusception. An upper gastrointestinal series may help to delineate malrotation, and an intravenous pyelogram, renal scan or ultrasound may be necessary if abnormalities of the kidney are felt to be likely.

CHILD 2 TO 5 YEARS OLD

Similar to the infant, the child 2 to 5 years of age usually has an organic etiology of his or her abdominal pain. The most common causes of abdominal pain are inflammatory processes, such as gastroenteritis and urinary tract infection.

As with the younger child, the emergency physician must first ascertain whether the abdominal pain is acute or chronic in onset. Those children with pain of recent onset are more likely to have surgical conditions. In every case, the physician must search for signs of obstruction or peritonitis, before attributing the etiology to a nonsurgical disease.

Acute Pain. The preschool child can often verbally describe pain and other symptoms, but such history may not be fully reliable, especially with regard to the true chronological order of events. Symptoms such as anorexia and vomiting suggest distension of an intraabdominal viscus; rectal bleeding points to early inflammatory bowel disease, infectious enterocolitis, intussusception, or a Meckel's diverticulum. Extraabdominal complaints are commonly present, such as cough, sore throat, headache; they are often indicative of a viral syndrome, pharyngitis, or pneumonia. Urinary symptoms may precede pyelonephritis, and polydipsia with polyuria may herald the onset of diabetes mellitus with abdominal pain from ketoacidosis.

The physical examination helps to separate the acute surgical abdomen with peritonitis or obstruction from less emergent conditions. The most important surgical causes of abdominal pain are acute appendicitis, and, occasionally, intussusception or malrotation. The presence of guarding and persistent abdominal tenderness with gentle palpation warns the emergency physician of a serious abdominal emergency. Usually, during a quiet relaxed examination, the pain from gastroenteritis abates; other "referred" abdominal pains (i.e., from pneumonia or tonsillitis) often seem to disappear when the child is reassessed in a calm fashion. Ill children with abdominal pain will occasionally have unusual diseases as listed in Table 5.1. The physical examination of such patients may show jaundice (hepatitis, hemolytic anemia), rash or arthritis (Henoch-Schönlein purpura), cardiac murmurs (rheumatic fever), friction rubs (pericarditis), or "acetone" on the breath (diabetes mellitus).

Chronic Pain. A history of recurrent abdominal pain suggests conditions such as sickle cell anemia, inflammatory bowel disease, cystic fibrosis, or asthma. Chronic constipation occurs not infrequently in children between 2 and 5 years of age, but psychogenic abdominal pain is unusual.

Laboratory Testing. The use of the laboratory parallels its role in young infants. Complete blood count and urinalysis are useful in this age range, either to point toward or away from appendicitis; if the appendix has not ruptured, the WBC count is usually normal or minimally elevated. WBC counts greater than 16,000 to 18,000/mm^3 suggest an acute bacterial infection or an intraabdominal abscess. A grossly abnormal urinary sediment points to urinary tract infection or occasionally glomerulonephritis, but does not exclude an inflamed appendix that is lying anteriorly near the bladder. Occasionally a hemoglobin electrophoresis is needed to make the diagnosis of sickling syndromes.

Radiographs may or may not be abnormal in children with gastrointestinal infections or appendicitis. Radiographic signs of appendicitis include localized bowel obstruction (a sentinel loop), an appendicolith, or obliteration of the psoas shadow. An abnormally thickened intestinal mucosa from inflammatory bowel disease or ascites from nephrotic syndrome favors the diagnosis of these nonsurgical emergencies. The chest x-ray often detects asthma with atelectasis or lower lobe pneumonia.

CHILD GREATER THAN 5 YEARS OLD

The school age child adds a new dimension to the spectrum of abdominal pain, that of psychosomatic illness. The leading organic causes of abdominal pain are inflammatory: gastroenteritis, appendicitis, and urinary tract infections. The child may also be the victim of chronic disease, as listed in Table 5.1. Colicky abdominal pain may rarely be associated with intussusception when there is a "lead" point for an intussusceptum (i.e., mesenteric adenitis, lymphoma, cystic fibrosis, anaphylactoid purpura). Abdominal pain with other symptoms may herald the presentation of inflammatory bowel, collagen, ulcer, gallbladder, pancreatic or liver disease. Abdominal pain in the menstruating, sexually active female may result from pelvic inflammatory disease, complications of pregnancy, or ovarian cyst, or dysmenorrhea.

Acute Pain. The history of abdominal pain is usually reliable in the older child. The presence of fever, cough, vomiting, and/or sore throat suggests an infectious cause. Associated diarrhea may be from infectious colitis, inflammatory bowel disease, or uncommonly, an appendiceal abscess irritating the bowel. A history of sexual activity increases the likelihood of pelvic inflammatory disease or an ectopic pregnancy, but this history may be denied by the adolescent female, particularly if she has been sexually abused. With urinary tract infections, urinary frequency and dysuria usually occur. Finally, pain that begins periumbilically and migrates to the right lower quadrant after 12 to 24 hours suggests appendicitis.

The findings on physical examination, including the rectal and pelvic (in the adolescent female), are again of paramount importance in this age group. Localized tenderness in the right lower quadrant or diffuse tenderness with involuntary guarding raise the suspicion of appendicitis or other diseases causing peritonitis.

Chronic Pain. Chronic abdominal pain may occur as a result of many of the conditions listed in Table 5.1. However, when the history and physical examination suggest a mild, self-limited disease or a nonorganic basis for the abdominal pain, emergency physicians should refrain from overutilizing the laboratory or x-ray department to allay the parents' fear of organicity. It is often a difficult task to provide reassurance and counseling in the busy emergency department to the enmeshed family and their child with abdominal pain; however, the time spent in this endeavor is well worth the effort. Counseling needs to be tailored to the level of sophistication of the family. Sometimes revisits to the emergency department should be scheduled for reappraisal, if referral to a primary physician cannot be arranged.

Functional abdominal pain precipitates more than 80% of physician visits by children for abdominal pain. It is generally episodic, radiates from the umbilicus and, by definition, has no organic etiology. The pain rarely occurs during sleep and has no particular associations with eating, exercise, or other activities. There may be a positive family history of gastrointestinal symptoms or migraine. The child's growth and development are normal, and the abdominal examination is unremarkable; occasionally, mild midabdominal tenderness, without involuntary guarding, is elicited. If performed, screening tests, such as complete blood count, sedimentation rate, and urinalysis are all normal.

The emergency physician's task is to allay any fears of serious organic disease while supporting the child who is truly feeling pain. As the long term solution to a functional complaint is not in the realm of the emergency department, one can only suggest a nonorganic cause of the pain and provide an avenue for continued supportive follow-up.

Laboratory Testing. In the majority of children with abdominal pain over the age of 5 years, laboratory tests are needed only to confirm a diagnosis that is suspected clinically. If appendicitis is being considered, a CBC and urinalysis should be obtained. Prior to rupture, the WBC count is usually minimally elevated and the urinalysis is normal. With perforation, the WBC count usually rises above 16,000 to 18,000/mm^3 and pyuria occurs occasionally. Again, radiographic findings with appendicitis may include a sentinel loop, an appendicolith, or obliteration of the psoas shadow. When inflammatory bowel disease is suspected in the child with abdominal pain, a sedimentation rate may prove useful, as it is almost invariably elevated with this group of disorders.

SUMMARY

Abdominal pain is one of the most frequent complaints of children who make emergency department visits. The history and physical examination should distinguish most cases requiring surgery or admission to the hospital; laboratory tests are indicated only to confirm diagnoses suspected clinically.

Inflammation, usually in the form of gastroenteritis, is the most frequent organic cause at all ages for abdominal pain; however, acute surgical conditions which are not always easy to diagnose must be excluded. Re-examinations on the same visit or the next day, as well as surgical consultation, are often necessary to decide on the need for hospitalization or surgery.

Nonabdominal causes of abdominal pain should receive consideration in children of all ages. A particularly common cause of abdominal discomfort in the older child is recurrent, functional pain.

References

Apley J: *The Child with Abdominal Pains.* F. A. Davis, Philadelphia, 1959.

Liebman, W, Thaler M: Pediatric considerations of abdominal pain and the acute abdomen. In *Gastrointestinal Disease*, Vol. 1, p. 411, edited by M Sleisenger and J Fortran. W. B. Saunders, Philadelphia, 1978.

Wolf SG: *Abdominal Diagnosis.* Lea & Febiger, Philadelphia, 1979.

CHAPTER 6

Arthritis and Arthralgia

ROBERT DOUGHTY, M.D.

INTRODUCTION

Arthritis is defined as "swelling of a joint or limitation of motion of a joint with heat or pain or tenderness." Pain or tenderness alone is not sufficient for the diagnosis of arthritis, since many conditions without true arthritis may be associated with joint pain, e.g., psychogenic arthralgia, tendonitis, myositis, and referred pain. In determining whether there is swelling of a joint it is important to consider the relation of the joint to surrounding bone and muscle tissue. Muscle wasting may make an adjacent joint appear swollen, and bony metaphyseal hypertrophy may mimic joint swelling. Joints on opposite sides of the body should be compared visually and by measurement whenever possible. This chapter will discuss the approach to the swollen, painful joint by discussing the approach to arthritis in general. This approach may also be used for cases without swelling when there is limitation of motion with heat, pain or tenderness.

Table 6.1 presents a differential diagnosis of conditions presenting with a swollen, painful joint, categorized by etiology. This broad differential diagnosis requires an organized approach in order to reach the correct diagnosis without excessive laboratory investigation and to lessen morbidity which may result from delay in diagnosis.

EVALUATION AND DECISION

Figure 6.1 presents an algorithm for evaluating children with a swollen, painful joint. Three major points to consider in approaching such children are: presence of fever, history of trauma, and duration of symptoms.

If there is a history of significant trauma there is a high likelihood that a hemarthrosis or traumatic effusion is the cause of a swollen painful joint. However, one must keep in mind that trauma may be incidental to a preexisting problem. Especially in a febrile child, one must be wary of accepting a traumatic etiology for arthritis without first excluding infectious arthritis by appropriate studies, including arthrocentesis and culture of joint fluid. If arthritis is recurrent and associated with fever and trauma, it is likely to be due to hemophilia, although chronic infection with fungus or tuberculosis must be excluded by culture of joint fluid. In the afebrile child, recurrent or chronic arthritis may result from internal derangements of the joint or from osteochondritis dissecans, which should be referred to orthopaedists, or from a rheumatic disorder.

History is quite important in narrowing the differential diagnosis of a child with arthritis. Involvement of multiple joints makes infection, internal derangement, or osteochondritis dissecans less likely and increases the likelihood of rheumatic fever and rheumatoid diseases. Morning stiffness is strongly suggestive of rheumatoid disorders, whereas afternoon pain more commonly occurs in traumatic arthritis, internal derangement, myositis (without true arthritis), and in functional conditions. A

Table 6.1
Swollen Joint—Differential Diagnosis by Etiology

Infection
- Acute bacterial
- Chronic fungal
- Mycobacterial

Trauma
- Simple
- Internal derangement
- Osteochondritis
- Hemophilia
- Ehlers-Danlos syndrome

Rheumatic Diseases and Inflammatory Conditions
- Juvenile rheumatoid arthritis
- Systemic lupus erythematosus
- Scleroderma
- Dermatomyositis
- Ankylosing spondylitis
- Reiter's syndrome
- Polyarteritis nodosa
- Anahylactoid purpura (Henoch-Schönlein)
- Stevens-Johnson syndrome
- Erythema multiforma
- Mucocutanous lymph node syndrome (Kawasaki disease)

Postinfectious Arthritis
- Viral infection—rubella, hepatitis B, EB virus
- Bacterial—streptococcus, gonococcus
- Cystic fibrosis

Hematologic Disorders
- Hemophilia
- Sickle cell disease
- Thalassemia

Tumor
- Leukemia
- Neuroblastoma

history of "locking of a joint" strongly suggests mechanical cartilage or ligament injury. Migratory arthritis is found in rheumatic fever, gonococcal arthritis, and Ehlers-Danlos syndrome. Severity of pain can suggest a diagnosis. Severe pain is characteristic of septic arthritis, acute traumatic arthritis, internal derangement, sickle cell disease, and gonococcal synovitis. The pain of rheumatic diseases like juvenile rheumatoid arthritis or systemic lupus erythematosus is generally more subacute and insidious.

There are certain key points on physical examination. A thorough joint examination must be performed on all patients with suspected arthritis. All joints (including cervical and lumbosacral spine, temperomandibular, and sternoclavicular joints) should be tested for swelling, warmth, tenderness, and range of motion. Relation of joint size to surrounding muscle mass should be considered. Adjacent muscle wasting can make a joint appear large or swollen. Objective measurement of circumference of pertinent joints and adjacent muscles should be recorded. Presence of muscle wasting or fixed joint contractures suggests chronicity of the process. Warmth of a joint establishes inflammation, even in the absence of fever, and may help direct the differential diagnosis.

The remainder of the physical examination should be thorough, to uncover associated systemic abnormalities which may point to the etiology of the arthritis. The patient should be specifically examined for alopecia (systemic lupus erythematosus—SLE); psoriasis (psoriatic arthritis); uveitis (juvenile rheumatoid arthritis—JRA, sarcoidosis, Reiter's syndrome); nasal or oral ulceration (SLE, Behçet's disease, Wegener's granulomatosis); lymphadenopathy (tumor, infection, rheumatoid disease); pneumonitis (SLE, systemic JRA); heart murmurs (acute rheumatic fever, subacute bacterial endocarditis with embolic septic arthritis); abdominal signs (inflammatory bowel disease); genital ulceration (Reiter's syndrome); peripheral cyanosis or ulceration (SLE, scleroderma); nail bed pitting (psoriatic arthritis); bruises (hemophilia); other rashes (SLE, JRA, gonococcal arthritis); and joint hypermobility (Ehlers-Danlos syndrome).

Laboratory studies should be performed only after initial narrowing of the differential diagnosis, based on presence of fever or trauma and duration of joint symptoms. Most commonly, a complete blood count (CBC), erythrocyte sedimentation rate (ESR) and radiographs of the affected joint(s) will have the highest yield in further defining the differential diagnosis. The CBC is especially helpful in evaluating malignancy, infection and sickle cell disease. The sedimentation rate usually differentiates inflammatory from noninflammatory

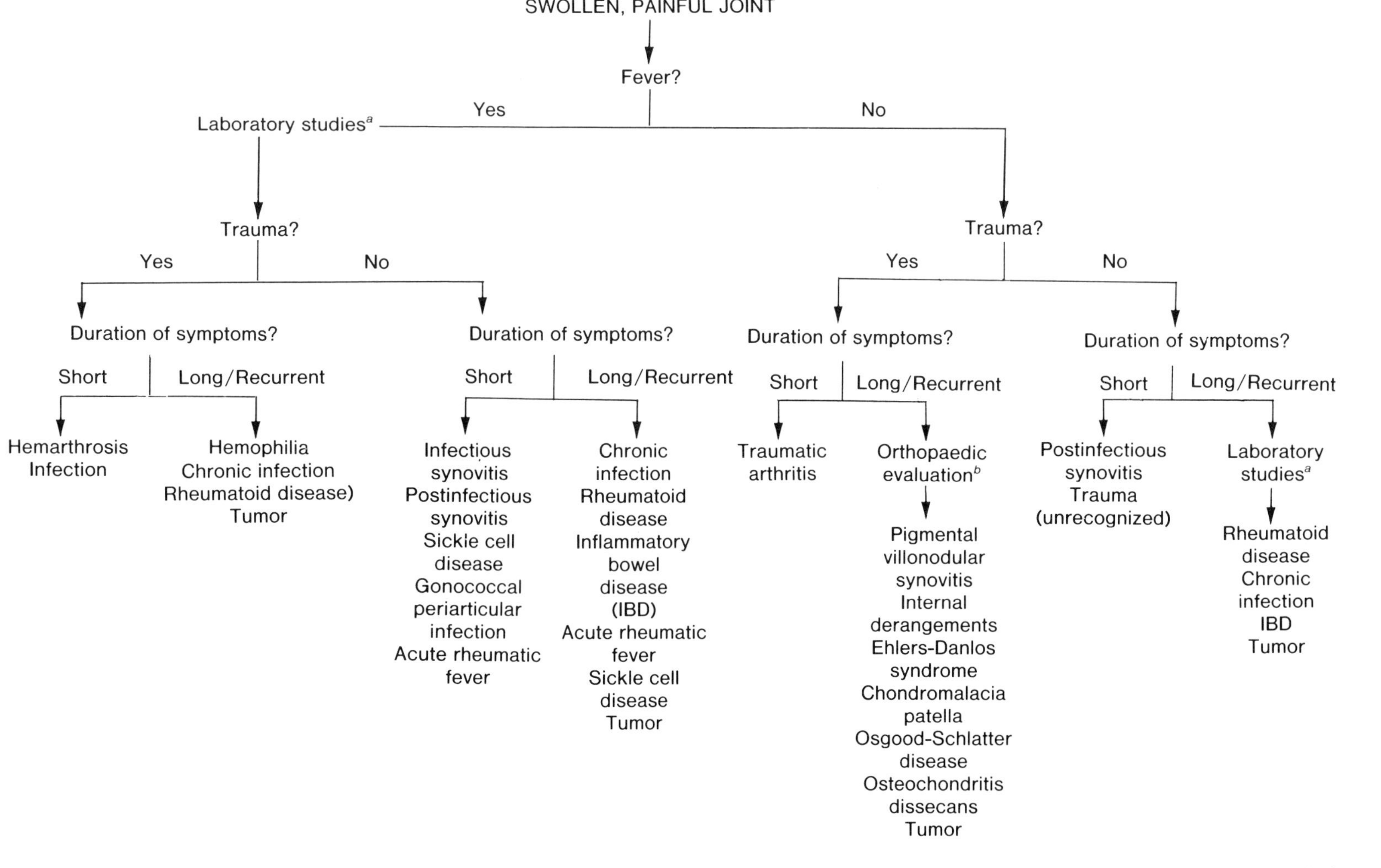

Figure 6.1 Diagnostic approach to the swollen, painful joint. (*a*) Laboratory studies: CBC, ESR, sickle preparation, x-ray, synovial fluid analysis, antinuclear antibody and rheumatoid factor. For febrile patients, consider chest x-ray and ECG. (*b*) Orthopaedic evaluation: arthroscopy, arthrogram,

Table 6.2
Characteristics of Common Pediatric Synovial Effusions[a]

Condition	Color	Clarity	Leukocyte Count (per mm^3)	Percent PMN	Glucose (serum-synovial fluid) (mg/dl)	Mucin Clot or String Test
Normal	Clear or straw-color	Transparent	200	10–20	0–10	Good
Traumatic arthritis	Straw-color or bloody	Opaque	2000	10–30	0–10	Good
Aseptic inflammatory arthritis (JRA, acute); rheumatic fever; postinfectious arthritis)	Cloudy, yellowish	Translucent	10–50,000	50–80	0–20	Fair to poor
Septic arthritis	Cloudy, yellow, gray or greenish	Opaque	50,000	90	20–50	Poor

[a] Abbreviations: PMN, polymorphonuclear leukocytes; JRA, juvenile rheumatoid arthritis.

Table 6.3
Revised Jones Criteria[a]
(Requires two major or one major + two minor and evidence of antecedent streptococcal infection (positive culture, ASO titer, history of recent scarlet fever) for diagnosis of rheumatic fever)

Major	Minor
Carditis	Fever
Migratory polyarthritis	Arthralgia
Chorea	Previous rheumatic fever or rheumatic heart disease
Erythema marginatum	Elevated ESR or positive CRP
Subcutaneous nodules	Prolonged PR interval

[a] From G. H. Stollerman, et al.: Jones criteria (revised) for guidance in the diagnosis of rheumatic fever. *Circulation*, *32*: 664, 1965.

causes of arthritis; however, it is important to remember that it may be normal in up to one third of children with JRA, especially the pauciarticular form. Radiographs should be carefully evaluated to look for effusions, leukemic lines, lytic lesions, periostitis, fractures, osteoporosis, growth arrest-recovery lines, and erosions.

If infection is suspected, arthrocentesis is necessary for definitive diagnosis. Arthrocentesis may also distinguish traumatic from inflammatory arthritis. Table 6.2 gives a summary of characteristics of synovial effusion in common causes of pediatric arthritis.

Other laboratory studies may be helpful. Presence of autoantibodies (e.g., antinuclear antibody, rheumatoid factor, or positive Coombs' test) or hypocomplementemia is strongly suggestive of rheumatoid conditions.

Elevated serum complement is seen in a variety of infectious, postinfectious, and rheumatoid inflammatory conditions.

A technetium bone scan can help establish whether inflammation is localized to a joint and periarticular space or whether the primary focus of inflammation is within the bone cortex. Disseminated asymptomatic lesions may also be detected by bone scan. The gallium scan may be helpful in documenting a pyogenic focus within a joint (although this may be done more easily by arthrocentesis) and in searching for occult sites of inflammation. If a gallium or bone scan is anticipated, arthrocentesis should be deferred, when possible, until after the scan, since the trauma of the arthrocentesis may affect results of the scan. In cases where the diagnosis of a chronic or recurrent effusion remains obscure, arthroscopy and/or synovial biopsy may be necessary to directly observe the joint anatomy, to obtain cultures (including those for fungi and mycobacteria), and to obtain material for histologic examination.

In many cases, careful observation and benign neglect are the most important diagnostic and therapeutic modalities. The primary exception to this is a case where bacterial infection is highly suspect. In such cases arthrocentesis must be performed promptly and, if results suggest infection, appropriate antibiotic therapy should be initiated pending culture results. An especially important example of this is septic arthritis of the hip. The vascular supply of the femoral head can be interrupted by the increased pressure of relatively small effusions, with catastrophic consequences. Consequently, if there is fever and limitation of hip motion suggestive of infection, orthopaedic consultation should be obtained promptly for arthrocentesis to permit the diagnosis of a septic hip.

Another potential emergency is migratory polyarticular arthritis in the presence of cardiac murmur. This raises a strong possibility of acute rheumatic fever. A chest radiograph and electrocardiogram may be helpful in evaluating the murmur. If there is evidence of carditis the patient should be admitted for the management of rheumatic fever since such a patient meets two major diagnostic criteria (Table 6.3).

In general, rheumatic disorders do not present as pediatric emergencies, but certain complications may become emergent as described in Chapter 56. Careful medical follow-up will assure that one does not miss a case of chronic rheumatic disease. The extent of evaluation should reflect the degree of patient disability and duration of symptoms.

CHAPTER 7

Ataxia

PETER H. BERMAN, M.D., AND ROGER J. PACKER, M.D.

INTRODUCTION

Ataxia may be defined as an impairment of the coordination of movement without loss of muscle strength. The coordination of movement is mediated by the cerebellum, which modifies muscle tone and contractions so that movements are performed smoothly and accurately.

The anatomy of the cerebellum and its afferent and efferent systems is intricate and complex, and a detailed description is beyond the scope of this chapter. Certain anatomic features, however, have particular clinical pertinence and merit comment.

The cerebellum is located in the dorsal portion of the posterior fossa of the cranial vault, and its ventral borders form the roof of the fourth ventricle. This anatomic relationship accounts for the fact that space-occupying mass lesions within the cerebellum frequently impede cerebrospinal fluid flow, leading to hydrocephalus and its associated signs of increased intracranial pressure.

The cerebellum is connected to the brainstem by paired superior, middle and inferior cerebellar peduncles which provide for passage of afferent and efferent connections to the rest of the central nervous system. Afferent connections originating from proprioceptive end organs in muscles, tendons, and joints reach cerebellar cortical neurons by way of the inferior cerebellar peduncles, after ascending through the spinal cord in the posterior columns and the spinocerebellar tracts. Extensive afferent connections originating from the labyrinths also pass through this peduncle. Afferent connections originating from the frontal motor cortex reach the cerebellar cortex through the middle cerebellum peduncles. These divergent afferent systems account for the fact that ataxia may result not only from intrinsic cerebellar dysfunction (cerebellar ataxia) but also from pathology involving the peripheral nerves and spinal cord tracts (sensory ataxia), labyrinths and vestibular pathways (labyrinthine ataxia), and the frontal lobes and cerebral pathways (frontal lobe ataxia).

The cerebellum consists of two lateral masses, the cerebellar hemispheres, which fuse medially into an elongated, narrow structure, the vermis. The cerebellar hemispheres are divided into lobes and lobules by fissures and sulci. The most inferior-ventral of these lobes, the flocculonodular lobes, fuse medially with the caudal portion of the vermis, the nodule, and receive the bulk of the vestibular afferent system. The cerebellar hemispheres are predominantly involved in the regulation of movement of the limbs; the rostral and caudal portions near the midline controlling the lower limbs, and the lateral midportion of the hemispheres controlling the upper limbs. The main afferent and efferent systems of the cerebellum either do not decussate or decussate and then redecussate, so that unilateral lesions of the cerebellum affect the function of ipsilateral limbs. The vermis and flocculonodular lobes are involved with the regulation of movement required for the maintenance of equilibrium when standing or walking.

This anatomical distribution leads to the two syndromes of cerebellar dysfunction that are seen clinically: the syndrome of the cerebellar hemispheres and the syndrome of the vermis or midline syndrome. In the syndrome of the cerebellar hemispheres, there is a gross disturbance of skilled movements of the ipsilateral limbs; the right cerebellar hemispheres controlling the coordination of the right limbs, and the left hemisphere, the left sided limbs. Distal movements tend to be more affected than proximal movements. In the midline syndrome, axial structures are predominantly involved, and swaying of the trunk when sitting, standing and walking is the most prominent clinical abnormality.

DIFFERENTIAL DIAGNOSIS

Ataxia may be an early, prominent sign of a wide variety of disorders. For the purposes of differential diagnosis, it is helpful to differentiate between acute, acute remitting and chronic ataxia. Chronic ataxias may be further differentiated into progressive and nonprogressive. Table 7.1. lists some of the more common conditions in which ataxia is an early or prominent sign.

Drug ingestion and other forms of intoxication are among the most common causes of acute ataxia. Although frequently associated with lethargy, stupor and other changes in mental function, ataxia may be the most prominent manifestation of toxicity (phenytoin, alcohol, lead, carbamazepine). Another common cause of acute ataxia is the syndrome of "acute cerebellar ataxia," a usually transient parainfectious illness of uncertain cause.

Ataxia may also be a prominent early sign of posterior fossa tumors, especially medulloblastoma, and other conditions associated with increased intracranial pressure, including nonneoplastic hydrocephalus, supratentorial tumors, and pseudotumor cerebri. Less commonly, acute ataxia may result from postinfectious encephalomyelitis, brainsteam encephalitis, head trauma, infectious polyneuritis (Guillain-Barré syndrome), or tick paralysis.

Table 7.1
Selected Etiologies of Ataxia in Childhood

Acute Ataxia
- Drug intoxication
- Acute cerebellar ataxia
- Head trauma
- "Brainstem" encephalitis
- Postinfectious encephalomyelitis
- Posterior fossa tumor
- Hydrocephalus
- Guillian-Barré syndrome
- Labyrinthitis
- Lead encephalopathy
- Hysteria

Acute Remitting Ataxia
- Hartnup disease
- Pyruvate decarboxylase deficiency

Chronic Ataxia
- Congenital anomalies of the cerebellum
- Ataxia-telangiectasia
- Friedreich's ataxia
- Hydrocephalus
- Posterior fossa tumor
- Leigh's syndrome (subacute necrotizing encephalopathy)

Acute remitting ataxia is seen as a manifestation of several rare metabolic diseases, including Hartnup disease and pyruvate decarboxylase complex deficiency states.

Chronic nonprogressive ataxia occurs as a consequence of congenital cerebellar anomalies, kernicterus, or perinatal hypoxic/ischemic injuries. Chronic progressive ataxia is usually a manifestation of herdofamilial disease (ataxia-telangiectasia, Freidreich's ataxia), although posterior fossa tumors, nonneoplastic hydrocephalus and congenital anomalies (Arnold-Chiari syndrome, Dandy-Walker syndrome) must also be considered.

CLINICAL APPROACH TO THE PATIENT WITH ATAXIA

History

The history will differentiate acute, acute remitting, chronic progressive, and chronic nonprogressive ataxia (Fig. 7.1). In acute ataxia, a history of recent ingestion of drugs or other toxic substances, infection or head

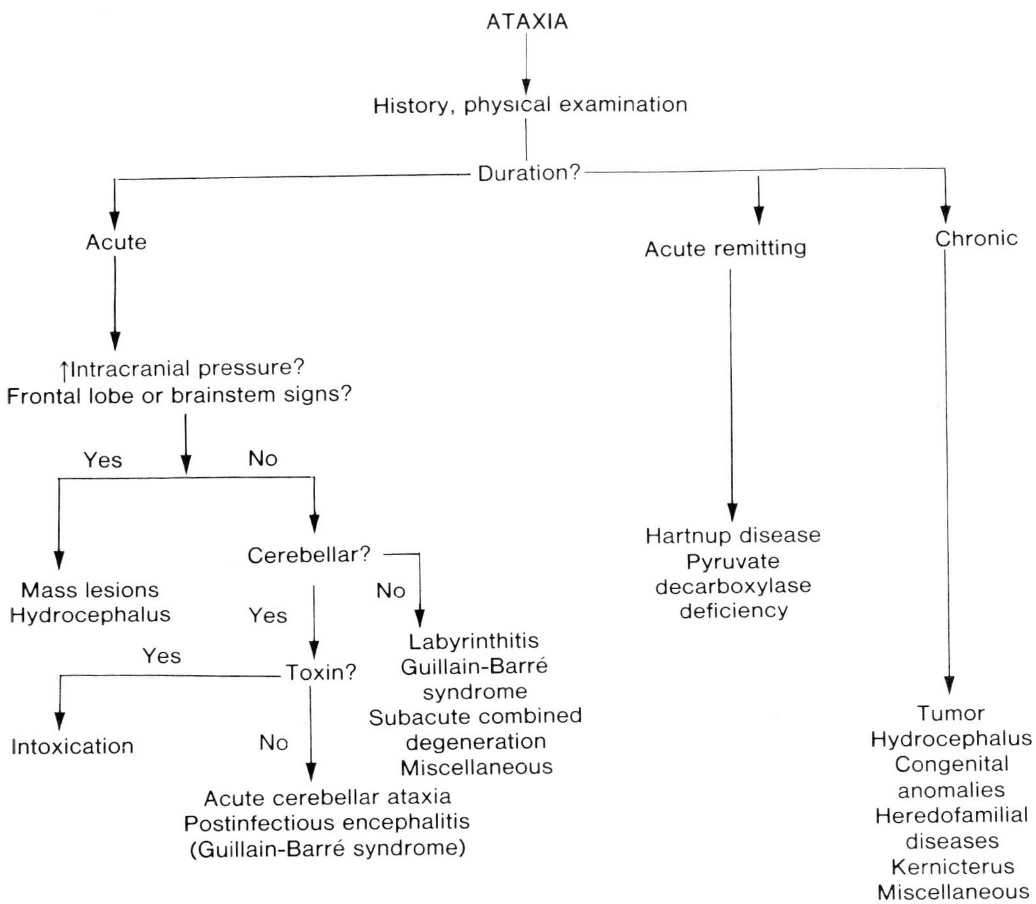

Figure 7.1 Approach to the diagnosis of ataxia.

trauma should be sought. When other etiologies are not apparent, it is often helpful to investigate the possibility of ingestion by specifically questioning parents about the availability of ataxia-producing agents in the home. A history of headache or changes in mental function or behavior may be seen in the child with posterior fossa tumors or frontal lobe ataxia. Vertigo frequently accompanies the ataxia of labyrinthine disease, and dysethesias or paresthesias may be reported in sensory ataxia.

Examination

The neurologic examination is not only helpful in distinguishing between cerebellar, laryrinthine, sensory and frontal ataxia, but may also determine the location of an abnormality within the cerebellum in instances of cerebellar dysfunction.

In young infants, most of the examination of motor coordination can be performed by observation of the child's spontaneous activity while sitting, standing, walking, and playing. Children old enough to cooperate are asked to stand erect with their feet as close together as possible, to walk in tandem fashion, and to turn quickly while walking. The finger-to-nose test and the heel-to-knee test are commonly used to assess coordination of the limbs, and the coordination of rapid alternating movements is assessed by asking the patient to tap his feet and his hands as quickly as possible.

Pure cerebellar ataxia is not associated with changes in mental function, weakness, or abnormality of sensation. Although nystagmus may be present if deep cerebellar structures are involved, there are no other signs indicating cranial nerve dysfunction unless brainstem function is disturbed from pressure or extension of a mass lesion.

Midline cerebellar disease leads to an equilibratory ataxia. With severe disease, there is a swaying or titubation of the head and trunk when sitting or standing, making the maintenance of an erect posture difficult. In milder involvement, the patient is able to stand erect but only with the feet apart (wide-based stance), and walking in tandem leads to swaying and lurching.

Disease of the cerebellar hemispheres leads to ataxia of the ipsilateral limbs, the lower limbs being predominantly affected by disease of the rostral and caudal poles near the midline, and the upper limbs with disease of the lateral midportions of each hemisphere. Several special terms describe nonequilibratory coordination deficits. Asynergy is the loss of coordinated action between muscle groups. Dysmetria is the loss of ability to gauge the distance, speed or power of a movement. Dysdiadochokinesia is a disturbance in the coordination of reciprocal agonist and antagonist muscles, leading to an inability to stop one set of movements and immediately follow it by the opposite set. These characteristic coordination deficits can readily be noted by observing the patient during spontaneous activity, or in the older, cooperative patient by asking him to perform the finger to nose or nose-finger-nose test with each upper limb and the heel to shin or toe to finger test with each lower limb. Dysdiadochokinesia is usually detected by having the patient alternately pronate and supinate his hands, either outstretched or with the elbows flexed and the shoulders adducted. Other movements involving reciprocal muscle groups, like opening and closing a fist or alternating dorsiflexing and plantar flexing the feet by tapping on the floor, may also be used.

Sensory ataxia is associated with other signs of peripheral sensory loss. Position and vibratory sense loss are the most frequent associated findings, but anesthesia to touch, hypesthesia to pain, and loss of temperature sensation may also be seen. Hyporeflexia is commonly found in cerebellar disease, but areflexia suggests sensory ataxia. In sensory ataxia, both equilibratory and nonequilibratory coordination deficits are more pronounced if the eyes are closed than if visual cues are permitted. This phenomenon explains the positive Romberg sign seen in disease of the proprioceptive pathways in which the patient is able to maintain an erect posture with the eyes open, but sways or falls when they are closed.

In labyrinthine ataxia, nystagmus is usually a prominent feature, and hearing deficits may be found.

Frontal lobe ataxia is the most difficult to differentiate clinically, unless other signs of frontal lobe disease, such as behavior, personality, or mental changes, snout reflex or palmomental reflex, are seen.

Laboratory Evaluation

The direction of laboratory assessment is dependent on the findings of the history and examination. Symptoms or signs of increased intracranial pressure such as headache, vomiting, or papilledema, or the presence of findings indicating brainstem involvement require a CT scan to rule out posterior fossa tumors and/or hydrocephalus.

Cerebrospinal fluid abnormalities may be present in child with some ataxia-producing diseases, such as acute cerebellar ataxia or Guillain-Barré syndrome; however, the presence of such abnormalities rarely necessitates a change in the direction of management, so lumbar puncture can be delayed until those conditions associated with increased intracranial pressure are completely excluded. Toxic screens of blood and urine are indicated in all instances of pure cerebellar ataxia. Vestibular function tests (electronystagnography, Nylen-Bárány maneuver) described in Chapter 16 (vertigo) may be helpful in differentiating labyrinthic ataxia. Electromyography and motor and sensory nerve conduction measurements may be helpful in differentiating sensory ataxias.

THERAPY AND MANAGEMENT

There is no therapy specific for ataxia. Fortunately, most conditions causing acute ataxia are self-limiting, and complete resolution of deficits will occur. During the period of acute ataxia, care must be taken to avoid injury. Sedatives should be avoided since they invariably exacerbate signs out of proportion to the amount given.

Reference

Swaiman KF: *Abnormalities of Gait in the Practice of Pediatric Neurology*, ed. 2, pp. 272–275, edited by KF Swaiman and FS Wright. C. V. Mosby, St. Louis, 1982.

CHAPTER **8**

Breast Lesions in Children and Adolescents

JOHN M. TEMPLETON, JR., M.D.

INTRODUCTION

Compared to many entities such as acute appendicitis which are much the same in children as they are in adults, the evaluation and management of breast lesions in children is a separate and almost unique field. For this reason most such problems should be evaluated by an experienced pediatrician or a pediatric surgeon who has an interest in the physiology of secondary sexual development and an understanding of the disorders which can occur in this development. The presence, for example, of a mass in the breast does not necessarily mean that a biopsy is required. Yet, someone with an adult orientation might be concerned about the possibility of cancer and recommend a biopsy. Unfortunately, the result, in a girl, of such a procedure might be the near total removal of the embryonic breast bud.

It is reassuring to know that the vast majority of breast lesions in children and adolescents are (1) benign and (2) relatively self-limited. When surgery is required, especially in a female, every effort is made to restore or preserve normalcy in the affected breast. Table 8.1 lists the principle causes of breast lesions in children and adolscents.

EVALUATION AND DECISION

Evaluation of a specific breast lesion in a pediatric patient is based first on whether or not there is inflammation; in the absence of inflammation, the key features are the patient's age and sex and the presence of a discrete mass or discharge. These latter features help to distinguish between the various physiologic, endocrinologic, neoplastic, and rare miscellaneous causes of pediatric breast disorders. The diagnostic evaluation is outlined in Figure 8.1.

Infection

Patients at any age may have the development of a localized or generalized cellulitis involving the breast tissue. This can be particularly a problem in neonates in whom the breast tissue is somewhat hypertrophied and in whom the ducts are temporarily open. As a result, bacteria tend to invade through the ducts and into the breast tissue itself. Following the newborn period, cellulitis and abscesses are not much of a problem in children until the onset of adolescence. Then with the hypertrophy of the underlying breast tissue, this tissue again becomes susceptible to cellulitis and/or abscess formation.

The most frequent organisms associated with such breast infections are streptococci or staphylococci. Streptococcal infections tend to produce a diffuse cellulitis. When severe, this cellulitis can develop into erysipelas of the breast with systemic toxic signs and symptoms. By contrast, infections due to staphylococci suppurate as they invade deeply into the tissue. As a result, the infection dissects between the fibrous septa leading to abscess formation and poten-

Table 8.1
Breast Lesions and Masses

- *I. Inflammatory Mass*
  - A. Cellulitis
  - B. Abscess
- *II. Noninflammatory Mass*
  - A. Infant
    - 1. Physiological hypertrophy
    - 2. Tumor (rare)
  - B. Childhood
    - 1. Premature thelarche
    - 2. Precocious puberty
    - 3. Prepubertal gynecomastia
    - 4. Carcinoma (rare)
  - C. Adolescence
    - 1. Male
      - a. Postpubertal gynecomastia
      - b. Exogenous stimulation
      - c. Endocrinopathy
      - d. Tumor (cancer, rare)
    - 2. Female
      - a. Fibrocystic disease
      - b. Fibroadenoma
      - c. Vaginal hypertrophy
      - d. Giant fibroadenoma
      - e. Fat necrosis
      - f. Cystosarcoma phylloides
      - g. Cancer (rare)
      - h. Papillomatosis

tially serious destruction of the breast tissue.

For the most part, these infections are the only breast disorders in children that require urgent treatment. In the earliest phases of these infections most patients should be treated with frequent hot soaks and antistaphylococcal antibiotics. If under this therapy the lesion becomes fluctuant, the patient should then undergo a formal surgical incision and drainage with culturing of the purulent material. In performing this drainage it is important to break up the multilocular pockets which are usually present. Based on the subsequent culture reports, the antibiotic coverage may be altered.

In the adolescent, the same treatment guidelines pertain as for the neonate. However, because of the greater mass of breast tissue involved, these infections more readily evolve into abscesses. One should, therefore, anticipate the need in most cases for surgical drainage and biopsy. In the older child if the infection appears to be unusually virulent, or if the patient has had recurrent infections, it is important to rule out the possibility of an unrecognized systemic illness such as diabetes mellitus.

Evaluation of a Breast Mass and/or Discharge in Prepubertal Children

Many children of either sex will have a prominence to the breast tissue bilaterally in the first few weeks of life. At birth there is no acinar development within the breast tissue. Yet, within a few days of life, a visible swelling may take place. This swelling is often associated with the secretion of a colostrum-like material, popularly known as "witches milk." Histologically such breast tissue has undergone hypertrophy with the development of acini in the duct system plus an increased vascularity of the stroma.

This breast hypertrophy in the neonate may correlate with a corresponding enlargement of the labia and the clitoris and occasionally a bloody vaginal discharge. This condition is thought by many to be the result of stimulation of the baby's hypophyseal system in the face of a progressive fall in the level of the maternal estrogens in the baby's circulation. It is generally self-limited and usually disappears entirely. Occasionally an overzealous mother may massage the breast in order to "get rid of all the milk." The result in such situations is an enhancement of the breast hypertrophy and the "milk" production. For any baby with persistence of such physiological hypertrophy one should apply cool compresses several times a day and be sure to terminate any manual stimulation.

Consultation with an experienced pediatric surgeon should be obtained if the abovementioned breast "hypertrophy" does not abate in the face of cold compresses and conservative management, or if a discharge or discrete mass develops. Such patients need to be followed closely although in most cases actual surgery will not be required. There may occur, for example, occasional cystlike obstructions to one of the ducts, or bleeding from the nipple due to a mild papillomatosis within one of the ducts. Some solid lesions such as a heman-

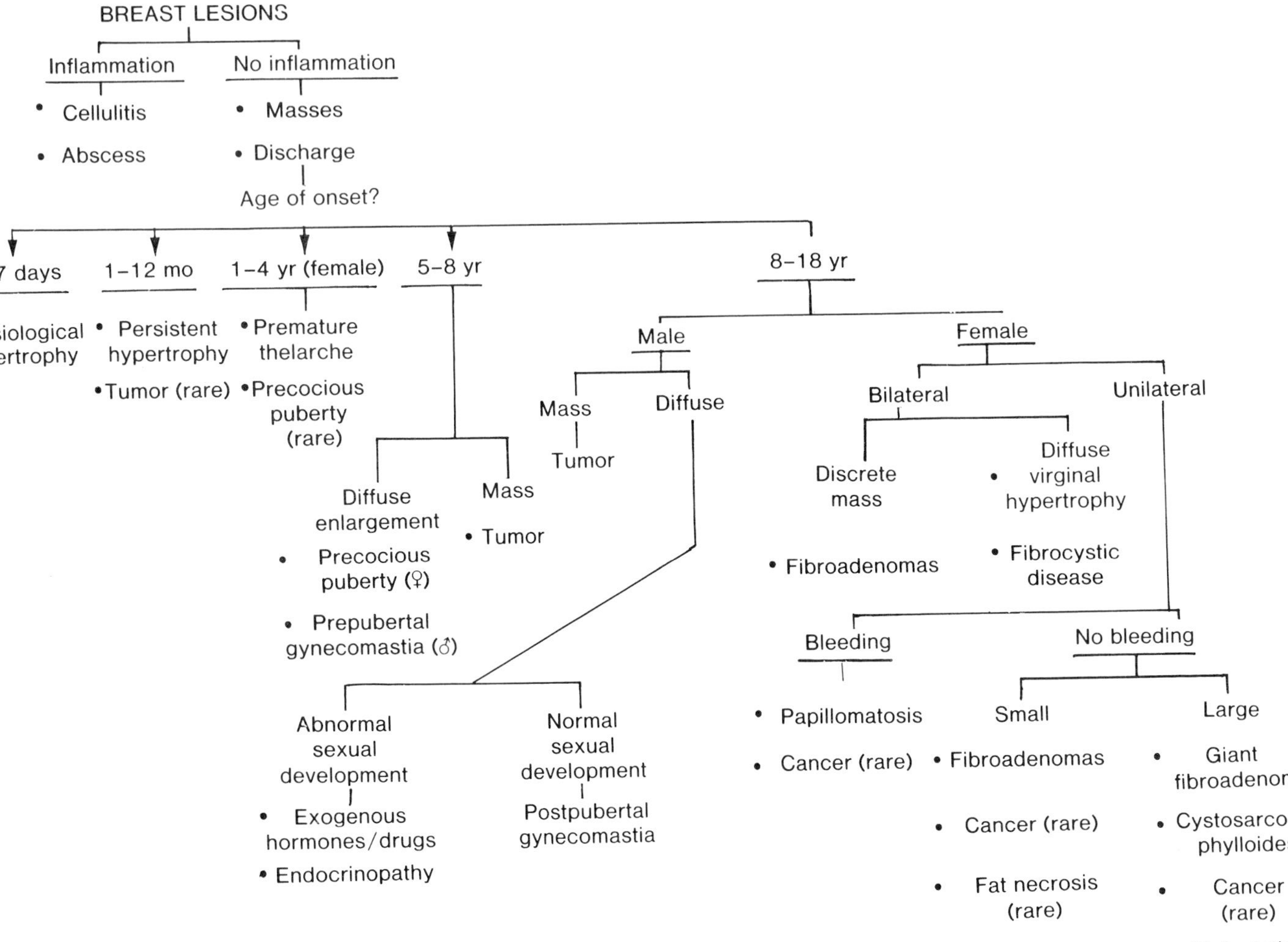

Figure 8.1 Evaluation of breast lesions in children and adolescents.

gioma may also involve the breast. If these lesions become worse, then on occasion one may need to consider surgery. Whereas, for the male, an excisional biopsy may be acceptable, only the most limited possible incisional biopsy should be performed in a female.

In females from the age of 1 to 4 years, one may encounter a unilateral, or occasionally a bilateral, enlargement of the underlying breast bud. This condition usually represents *premature thelarache* in which there occurs early development of the breast tissue only. There are no other manifestations of simultaneous sexual maturity such as genital enlargement, pubic hair development, an abnormal growth spurt, or menstruation. In general, true precocious puberty in this age is extremely rare.

The natural history of premature thelarache is that the enlargement of the breast bud is usually mild and self-limited. In time, the enlargement, in fact, resolves and the mass effect often abates. In such children one would rarely find it necessary to perform a biopsy. Follow-up by a pediatrician or pediatric surgeon is essential.

In male or female children, between the age of 5 and 8 years, one may encounter two abnormalities involving the size of the breast. One is a diffuse enlargement and the other is the presence of a specific mass. With diffuse enlargement, usually the entire breast is involved. Often both breasts increase in size. The physical examination of such breasts show a typical normal female pubertal breast development. Also there may be evidence of secondary sexual development and a growth acceleration. In the female such a condition represents precocious puberty. In the male it is referred to as prepubertal gynecomastia.

For the most part these lesions are idiopathic. Some of these patients may even be able to conceive, as in the case of a 5-year-old Peruvian girl who became pregnant and subsequently gave birth. There are, however, some specific etiologies which might produce precocious puberty, especially of a neurologic or endocrinologic nature. For that reason it is important to embark on a very thorough examination by an experienced pediatrician or endocrinologist.

In boys, the presence of breast development in this age group should be pursued with the same diligence as one would do for a young girl with precocious puberty. In both males and females, if a specific primary lesion is identified, then surgery may be required.

Also in the age range of 5 to 8 years one may encounter the development of a discrete breast mass in females and males. Such a mass is often eccentric in relation to the nipple and may, at first, not involve the entire breast tissue. These lesions are usually unilateral and may be associated with skin changes and occasional bleeding from the nipple. Such a situation suggests the possibility of a primary tumor. In a male, it would be appropriate to perform an excisional biopsy; for a female it is worth observing the lesion for several weeks to see if it will abate. This is particularly true if there is some bleeding in association with the lesion, as the underlying cause is most likely a benign papillomatosis which may, if mild, abate spontaneously. If the lesion does not abate, then one should consider a small incisional biopsy for histological determination.

Evaluation of the Postpubertal Child

Breast lesions in the postpubertal child from 8 to 18 years should be managed based upon the sex of the patient. In females, normal physiological thelarche may begin as early as 8 years of age. Initially, only one breast may enlarge. With observation one would expect the opposite breast to soon catch up in development.

When faced with an abnormal breast enlargement or mass in females, one needs to distinguish between unilateral lesions and bilateral lesions. In dealing with unilateral lesions the presence of bleeding is an important sign. If there is bleeding from the nipple, the usual diagnosis is papillomatosis. Rarely this may be a harbinger of carcinoma. If the bleeding persists one should plan for a limited biopsy based on the size and location of the lesion and the overall state of the breast development.

When there is no bleeding in the unilateral lesion, the possible etiologies depend on whether the lesion is small or large. Most small lesions measure 1 to 4 cm in size. The vast majority of these are fibroadenomas or foci of fibrocystic disease with one or more cysts. In a rare patient one might encounter fat necrosis or carcinoma. When the lesion is suggestive of fibrocystic disease with a cyst it is appropriate to aspirate the lesion if it persists. If fluid is obtained, the mass may shrink and no longer be an issue. If the aspiration is not successful, then a limited excisional biopsy would be appropriate.

For large lesions, the mass may range from 4 to 10 cm in size. The possible diagnoses include giant fibroadenoma, or, less commonly, cystosarcoma phylloides. Rare lesions include carcinoma or metastatic sarcoma. For these patients, an initial excisional biopsy is also indicated.

Some adolescent females may demonstrate bilateral lesions. Those lesions which are discrete may even be associated with more than one mass in the same breast. These lesions almost always represent fibroadenomas. In such cases it is not necessary to remove all of the masses. One may, instead, remove one or two of the largest lesions for histological confirmation and simply observe the other lesions over time.

When there is significant but diffuse enlargement of both breasts, the two leading possibilities are virginal hypertrophy or diffuse fibrocystic disease. If the enlargement is massive an eventual mammoplasty will be required.

In dealing with adolescent males, one must distinguish between two types of breast problems. One is an atypical mass that is usually eccentric and discrete. Most of the time these will represent a primary tumor necessitating an excisional biopsy.

Most other forms of adolescent male breast abnormalities are associated with diffuse enlargement of the entire breast. Such an enlargement is often bilateral. Many of these males will be overweight or quite heavy set. When the sexual and physical development is normal, the most likely diagnosis is postpubertal gynecomastia. This entity is often self-limited and will begin to abate after 1 to 2 years and largely disappear by the 3rd year. The unpleasant physical appearance of such breasts may be improved by placing the patient on a rigorous weight reduction program. During this period one needs to follow these patients closely and to provide assurance that there is no serious underlying abnormality. If at the end of 2 to 3 years the underlying breast enlargement has not begun to abate and if psychological factors begin to be a problem, then one can proceed with a subcutaneous mastectomy through a circumareolar incision.

An occasional adolescent male with diffuse and often bilateral breast enlargement will have other abnormalities in his physical and sexual development. Such a patient may demonstrate a paucity of pubic hair, small testes, and/or an immature pudgy appearance inconsistent with his age. In this situation, the physician must rule out an underlying endocrinopathy or the possibility of any exogenous hormones or drugs which can be associated with breast enlargement. Often a chromosomal analysis is also indicated. Such a careful evaluation is usually best handled by an experienced pediatric endocrinologist.

CHAPTER 9

Chest Pain

RICHARD M. RUDDY, M.D.

INTRODUCTION

The complaint of chest pain rarely represents an emergency in children, in contrast to the same complaint in adults. Although heart disease is not a common source of chest pain in children, the fear of a cardiac origin for the pain may evoke great anxiety in the child or the parents. Thus, a careful approach to the patient is still imperative in the pediatric patient. This section will first briefly review the pathophysiology of chest pain, then outline the differential diagnosis in childhood, and finally discuss the evaluation, as appropriate in the emergency department.

PATHOPHYSIOLOGY

In order to understand the possible origins of chest pain or discomfort, it is important to review how this sensation is transmitted. *Musculoskeletal pain* is produced by irritation of these tissues and is transmitted via the sensory nerves. The stimulus is carried through the nerve in the dermatomal or intercostal distribution to the dorsal root ganglia, up the spinal afferents, and into the central nervous system. This local, peripheral, sharp pain can also be produced by primary dorsal root irritation in the spine. Because of overlap of nerve distribution, pain may be sensed in locations distal to the irritation. For example, the third and fourth cervical nerves evoke pain as far caudally as the nipple line of the chest. *Tracheobronchial pain* is transmitted by vagal afferents in the large bronchi and trachea to fibers in the cervical spinal column. Dull, aching or sharp pain is felt in the anterior chest or neck. The irritation or sensation of cough is transmitted in a similar fashion. *Pleural pain* arises in the pain-sensitive parietal pleura and then travels through the intercostal nerves in the chest wall, giving rise to sharp, well localized pain. The visceral pleura is pain-insensitive. *Diaphragmatic pain* is transmitted by the intercostal or phrenic nerves. Peripheral diaphragmatic irritation may cause local chest wall pain because of the intercostal innervation. Central diaphragmatic stimulation travels by the phrenic nerve, with the distribution of pain referred to the shoulder of the affected side. The *esophagus* appears to be more pain sensitive in its proximal portion. Pain is transmitted by afferents to corresponding spinal segments, with resultant anterior chest or neck pain. The *pericardium* is innervated by portions of the phrenic, vagal, and recurrent laryngeal nerves as well as the esophageal plexus. This appears to give rise to a variety of sensations including chest or abdominal pain, dull pressure and even referred angina-like pain. Other mediastinal structures, such as the *aorta*, have pain fibers in the adventitia of the vessel wall. They transmit pain via the thoracic sympathetic chain to the spinal dorsal roots, giving rise to sharp, variably localized chest pain. Last, *cardiac* pain is probably transmitted via a number of routes, including the thoracic sympathetic chain and the cardiac nerves through the cervical and stellate ganglia. It has been proposed recently that pain arises from abnormal ventricular wall movement and stimulation of the pericardial pain fibers. These routes account for the sensation of cardiac chest pain as pressure or crushing pain substernally, or sharp pain in the shoulder, neck or arm.

DIFFERENTIAL DIAGNOSIS

A differential diagnosis of chest pain in children is included in Table 9.1. Most chest pain in children is due to acute respiratory disease, musculoskeletal injury, or anxiety. Chest pain in association with cardiorespiratory distress, however, demands immediate attention. In the case of trauma, cardiac or pulmonary compromise may arise from direct injury to heart, great vessels, or lung (see Chapter 60). Chest pain in the nontraumatized, yet dyspneic or cyanotic patient, most often stems from a respiratory problem, such as acute pneumonitis, asthma or pneumothorax (spontaneous or associated with cystic fibrosis or asthma). Rarely, severe chest pain in an acutely ill child may be due to a myocardial infarction resulting from aberrant coronary vessels, other underlying cardiac diseases (aortic stenosis), an acute arrhythmia, pericardial disease, or pulmonary embolus. Nonorganic chest pain may appear to cause respiratory distress in the hyperventilating teenager (see Chapter 72), but close examination should distinguish this syndrome from serious problems.

Chest pain in children usually occurs without associated cardiorespiratory signs of symptoms, often as a chronic problem. Mild to moderate strain or injury from ex-

Table 9.1
Causes of Chest Pain

I. Musculoskeletal/Neural
- A. Muscle
  - 1. Trauma—contusions, lacerations
  - 2. Infection—myositis
  - 3. Texidor's twinge
- B. Breast
  - 1. Physiological (fullness during menses or pregnancy)
  - 2. Mastitis
  - 3. Fibrocystic disease
  - 4. Tumor
- C. Bone
  - 1. Trauma—contusions, rib fractures
  - 2. Osteitis, osteomyelitis
  - 3. Costochondritis
- D. Intercostal nerve
  - 1. Neuritis—zoster, trauma
  - 2. Toxin
- E. Dorsal root
  - 1. Trauma
  - 2. Radiculitis—viral, postviral
  - 3. Spinal disease—scoliosis

II. Tracehobronchial (Proximal Bronchi)
- A. Foreign body
- B. Infection
  - 1. Tracheitis
  - 2. Bronchitis
  - 3. Pneumonia
  - 4. Cystic fibrosis
- C. Asthma

III. Pleural (Parietopleura and Diaphragm)
- A. Trauma—penetrating
- B. Pleurisy—viral, mycobacterial
- C. Pneumonia
- D. Cystic fibrosis
- E. Pneumothorax, hemothorax, chylothorax
- F. Empyema
- G. Subphrenic abscess
- H. Malignancy
- I. Postpericardotomy syndrome
- J. Pulmonary embolus/infarction
- K. Vaso-occlusive crisis (sickle cell anemia)

IV. Esophageal
- A. Foreign body
- B. Caustic ingestion
- C. Chalasia (esophagitis)
- D. Infection—Candida

V. Cardiac (Angina, Pericardial, Aortic)
- A. Angina—coronary insufficiency, anomalous vessels, pulmonary hypertension
- B. Obstructive heart disease
  - 1. Aortic stenosis, pulmonary stenosis
  - 2. Asymmetric septal hypertrophy (IHSS)
- C. Pericardial defects and effusions, pericarditis
- D. Acute arrhythmias
- E. Myocarditis
- F. Aortic aneurysm—idiopathic, syphilitic, Marfan's syndrome

VI. Central
- A. Anxiety—hyperventilation
- B. Idiopathic

ercise or trauma may produce a contusion or rib fracture. Inflammation of nerves, muscles, bones, costochrondral junctions, the esophagus, or the lower respiratory tract frequently causes organic chest pain. Both respiratory infection (pneumonia or bronchitis) and allergic respiratory disease (asthma) are important causes to consider. The toddler may aspirate a foreign body into the trachea or esophagus, with no adult being aware. Cardiac disease rarely causes chest pain in a child who appears generally well, but attention should be paid to diagnosing the rare patient with progresive obstructive heart disease, angina, mitral valve prolapse, or early pericardial or myocardial inflammation. A large group of children will be left whose pain fits best into an anxiety-induced or idiopathic category; however, beginning every evaluation with a broad differential diagnosis in mind can only help in the diagnosis and management of the child with chest pain.

EVALUATION AND DECISION

Child with Thoracic Trauma

The first step in evaluation of the child with chest pain is to perform a thorough history and physical examination. If there is any evidence of trauma to the chest, the patient requires rapid evaluation and resuscitation, as necessary (Fig. 9.1). Correction of myocardial or respiratory insufficiency may both diagnose and treat the cause of chest pain. Alveolar ventilation should be assessed for adequacy and bilateral symmetry to distinguish acute respiratory failure from hemothorax or pneumothorax. An insufficient cardiac output, as reflected by abnormalities of the pulse and/or blood pressure, suggests either a rhythm disturbance or tamponade, which causes muffling of the heart sounds and pulsus paradoxus. A discrepancy of the pulse or blood pressure between the extremities points to aortic diseases, such as traumatic avulsion or aneurysm, as the cause of chest pain. Many children with thoracic injuries but no respiratory distress will also complain of chest pain. Although a careful examination is mandatory in an effort to exclude significant intrathoracic trauma, the cause of the pain usually resides in the chest wall: contusions of the soft tissues or rib fractures. A history of significant trauma in the presence of cardiovascular abnormalities dictates that x-rays and an ECG be obtained. Radiographs also are indicated whenever rib fracture is suspected.

Child with No Thoracic Trauma

After initial stabilization, the physician should inquire as to a history suggestive of prior cardiorespiratory disease (Fig. 9.1). Children with respiratory illnesses, such as asthma or cystic fibrosis, are at risk for pneumothorax, acute respiratory failure from mucus plugging or pneumonitis, and acute pulmonary hypertension. Severe hypoxemia may accompany their chest pain. Auscultatory findings, such as rales or wheezing, may be minimal when obstructive pulmonary disease is moderately severe. In the child with a history of cardiac arrhythmias, congenital heart disease, cardiac surgery, or pericardial effusions, chest pain may signal an exacerbation of the underlying problem.

In the absence of prior cardiopulmonary disease or trauma, the approach must be directed toward unmasking evidence for any of the serious cardiorespiratory illness as listed in Table 9.1. However, most children with chest pain will be found to have less severe acute inflammatory processes of the respiratory tract or musculoskeletal system or a psychosomatic disturbance.

Infectious diseases of the respiratory tract cause fever, malaise, cough, and coryza and often involve several family members simultaneously. A first asthmatic attack should be suspected when an associated night cough, history of wheezing, or family history of atopy is present. The physical examination in asthma shows a prolonged expiratory phase of respiration and wheezing accentuated by a forced expiratory effort. In musculoskeletal inflammation, one should be able to elicit tenderness of the chest wall and a "trigger point," where palpation reproduces the pain. Pain following a dermatome unilaterally suggests intercostal neuritis; children with zoster (shingles) may have pain preceding the development of rash.

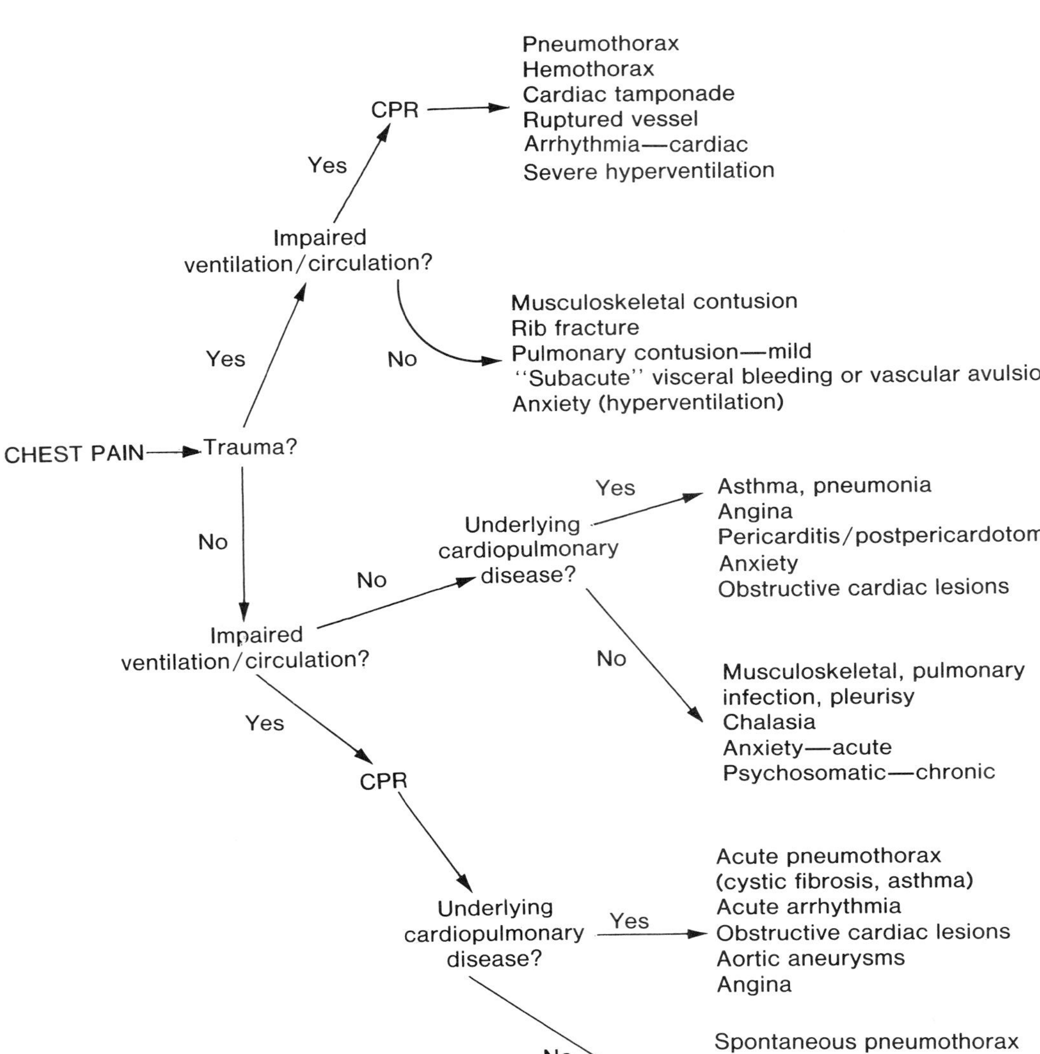

Figure 9.1 Diagnostic approach to chest pain in children.

When focal, peripheral pain is found without a "trigger point," the physician should consider pain referred from areas of sensory nerve overlap. A relationship of the pain to eating or swallowing suggests esophageal disease and often the physical examination is normal. "Texidor's twinge," or pericardial "catch," is a frequent cause of short duration, sharp pain in healthy teenagers and young adults, often related to exercise and located in the left substernal region. It may be caused by stretching of the supporting ligaments of the heart and is easily distinguishable from angina by its sudden, stabbing onset, a duration of less than 60 sec, and the absence of referral to other areas.

A thorough examination will usually uncover evidence of the cardiac and respiratory causes of chest pain listed in the table. Extrathoracic abnormalities, such as rashes or arthritis, may provide a clue to collagen disorders (Chapter 56) or other systemic illness. During examination of the heart and lungs, it is useful to relate normal findings to the child and family, as this reassurance often serves as the major "treatment" of self-limiting or functional problems.

Laboratory studies are sometimes indicated to help confirm a diagnosis or to relieve the anxiety of the child or family. Chest x-ray may show asthma, pneumonitis, pleurisy or spontaneous pneumothorax. The wide mediastinum of aortic aneurysm, abnormal cardiac silhouette due to a pericardial effusion or cardiomegaly, rib fractures, or metabolic bone derangements all produce characteristic radiographic changes. The presence of atelectasis may suggest mucus plugging or subtle evidence of pulmonary infarction from an embolus or a vaso-occlusive crisis of sickle cell anemia.

An electrocardiogram should be performed if cardiac disease is suspected. Although the ECG will often be normal, it may show signs of cardiac strain or ischemia with valvular heart disease, diseases of outflow obstruction, or angina. A decreased QRS voltage and electrical alternans confirms the presence of a pericardial effusion in the child with muffled heart sounds. Arrhythmias, such as atrial fibrillation and supraventricular tachycardia, may be identified by careful evaluation of a rhythm strip.

Studies other than a chest x-ray and ECG are infrequently necessary. An elevated leukocyte count with a shift to the left may point toward infection as the cause of pain. Examination of peripheral smear and a hemoglobin electrophoresis are indicated in the child suspected of having sickle cell disease as the etiology of chest pain. If an intraabdominal source for chest pain from diaphragmatic irritation is under consideration, an amylase should be obtained, as this is often elevated with pancreatitis. Esophageal causes of chest pain may often be diagnosed clinically, but a barium study or endoscopy may be required to confirm the findings. Pulmonary embolus, present occasionally in the older teenager or infirmed patient, requires the performance of nuclear scans or angiography for diagnosis.

A large group of children with chest pain will have no evidence of organic disease and no history of underlying cardiorespiratory disease or trauma. However, they may have a family history of chest pain. Often, there will be a stressful situation that has precipitated the chest pain. Complaints of chest pain and other somatic aches are often chronic, but no abnormalities are noted on the physical examination. Such children have psychogenic chest pain. To elicit the predisposing factors, the physician should interview the child and family away from the chaos of the emergency department, if possible. Occasionally, obtaining a chest x-ray and ECG is helpful in allaying parental fears of cardiac disease. However, definitive management requires referral to a primary care physician.

SUMMARY

Chest pain in children is a relatively infrequent sign of serious disease, but often has great importance to the patient or family. The majority of cases can be diagnosed by the emergency physician from the history and physical examination alone, although at times a chest x-ray and occasionally an ECG are helpful. Psychogenic chest pain is the most common occurrence and may be either chronic or related to an acute stressful event. The possibility of cardiac disease needs to be addressed directly by the examining physician in order to fully alleviate the patient's (or family's) anxiety. The most frequent causes of organic chest pain are musculoskeletal (traumatic or inflammatory) and infectious disorders, usually self-limited or easily treated diseases. Occasionally, serious abdominal, pulmonary or cardiac problems will require immediate attention.

References

Asnes R, Santulli R, Bemborad J: Psychogenic chest pain in children. *Clin Pediatr* 20: 788, 1981.

Driscoll D, Glicklich L, Gallen N: Chest pain in children: A prospective study. *Pediatrics* 57: 648, 1976.

Editorial: Texidor's twinge. *Lancet* 2: 133, 1979.

Green M: Chest pain. In *Pediatric Diagnosis*, Ed 3, p. 573. W. B. Saunders, Philadelphia, 1980.

MacBryde CM, Blacklow RS: Thoracic pain. In *Signs and Symptoms*. J. B. Lippincott, Philadelphia, 1970.

CHAPTER **10**

Coma

ROGER J. PACKER, M.D. AND PETER M. BERMAN, M.D.

INTRODUCTION

Stupor, coma, and other aberrations of consciousness are among the most common life-threatening emergencies faced by the emergency department physician. The final outcome, although usually not immediately determinable, is often influenced by the rapidity with which the physician makes appropriate assessments and decisions regarding the need for evaluative procedures and the institution of specific therapy. The primary objective of the care of the patient with an altered level of consciousness is the prevention of further brain damage. In addition to the prompt stabilization of the patient's vital functions, this requires the rapid determination of existing brain function and an organized approach to the search for reversible and treatable etiologies.

The various terms used to describe consciousness are ambiguous and for purposes of this discussion, the following simplistic definitions will be used. Consciousness is an awareness of one's self and environment. Alterations in consciousness represent a spectrum of abnormalities ranging from confusion to complete inability to be aroused (or unconsciousness). Confusion is thought of as a state of reduced awareness manifested by slowed, impaired cognitive abilities. In delirium the subject becomes increasingly unaware of his environment, often suffering from delusions, and may be agitated and violent. Stupor is a state of unawareness from which the patient can only be aroused by repeated, vigorous stimuli. The comatose patient is unresponsive and cannot purposefully respond to even the most vigorous stimuli. Coma has been further subdivided into categories such as semicoma, light, and deep coma, whose boundaries are quite indistinct and of questionable usefulness. Recently, more objective scales of unconsciousness, such as the Glascow coma scale, have been employed. However, these seem to have more usefulness in predicting outcome than in detecting signs of neurologic deterioration. A rare state of altered consciousness is akinetic mutism in which there is a silent, alert looking immobility with little evidence of mental activity. This occurs primarily in subacute and chronic state of unconsciousness and should be differentiated from the locked-in state (deafferent state or ventral pontine state). In the latter condition, the patient is aware of his environment but, due to bilateral supranuclear paralysis of all four extremities and cranial nerves, can only communicate with eye blinking and vertical eye movements.

These descriptive terms are not precise enough to describe subtle changes in the patient's level of consciousness and must be supplemented by detailed objective measures of neurologic function. These observations are necessary to identify early neurologic deterioration that may be potentially reversible.

PATHOPHYSIOLOGY

The state of full awareness is dependent on the integrity of the cerebral hemispheres and the ascending reticular activating system (ARAS). The ARAS, a polysynaptic neuronal network lying in the central core of the brainstem, thalamus, and hypothalamus receives inputs from and projects to the spinal cord, brainstem, and cerebral cortex. Transection or destruction of this region results in prolonged unresponsiveness. Central nervous system lesions produce coma by extensively bilaterally depressing or damaging the cerebral cortex, subcortical white matter, or upper thalamus, or by causing localized damage to the ARAS. The selective destruction of the ARAS, however, may result from focal mass lesions in the cerebral hemispheres which can displace or compress the brainstem (see Fig. 10.1).

The contents of the cranial cavity consist predominantly of three components, brain tissue, cerebral spinal fluid, and blood. An increase in the volume of one component is

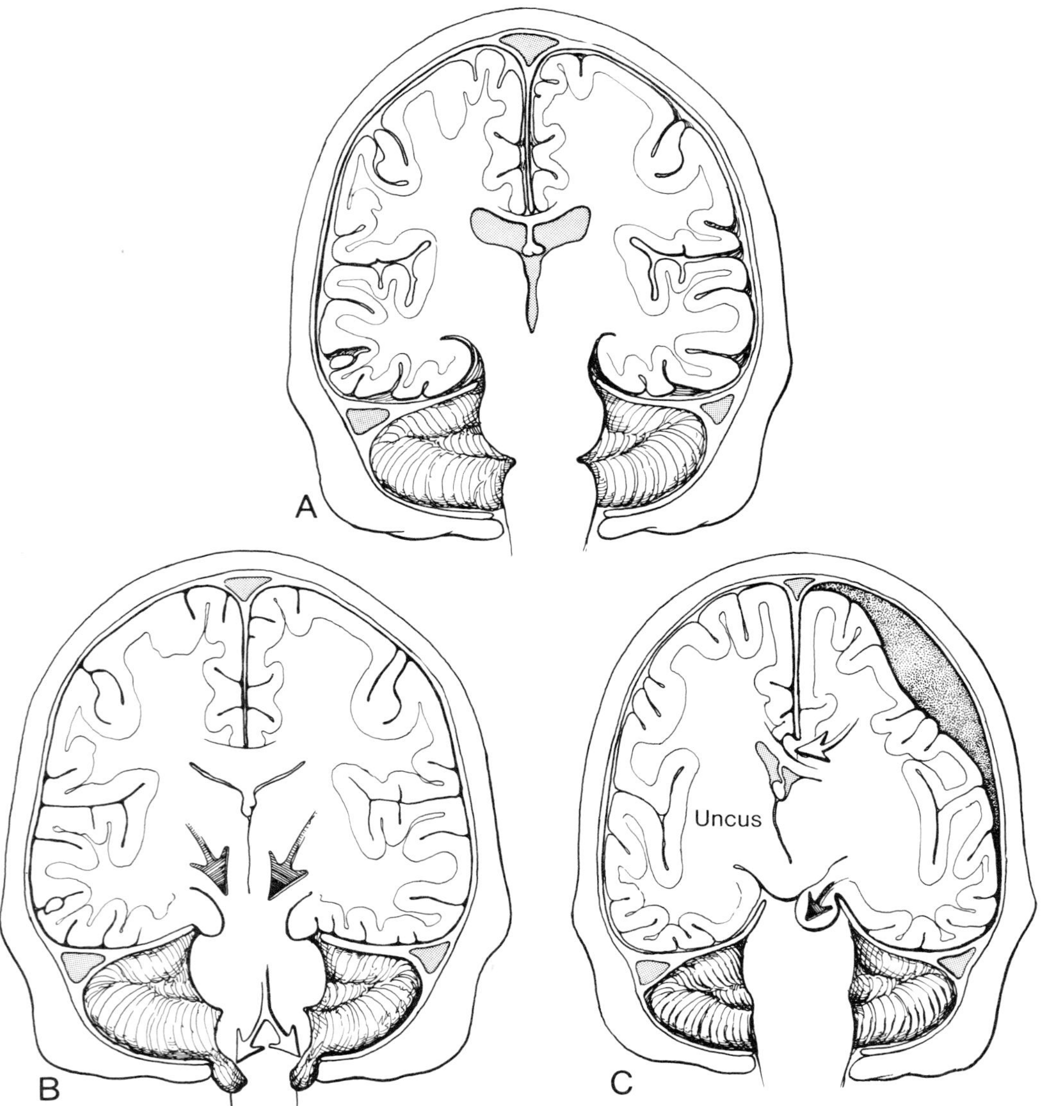

Figure 10.1 Intracranial contents. (*A*) Normal relationships. (*B*) Central herniation. (*C*) Uncal herniation.

compensated for by an enlargement of the cavity or the reduction or displacement of another component. Although the cranial cavity of a young child is somewhat more elastic than that of an adult (due to unfused sutures and anatomically open fontanelles), it can acutely tolerate only a limited increase in mass without rapidly increasing intracranial pressure. If the increase in mass cannot be compensated, the brain will be compressed against the rigid dural folds which support it. Clinically, the tentorium cerebelli is the most important septum, dividing the cranium into the anterior and posterior fossa. In the center of the tentorium there is a semioval opening through which the midbrain passes. In front of the midbrain lies the basilar artery (which supplies blood to the midbrain and pons) and the oculomotor nerve controlling eye movements and pupillary reactions. On top of the tentorium lie the temporal lobes with their most medial portions, the unci, bulging anteriorly into the tentorial notch in close proximity to the oculomotor nerve.

Displacement of brain through or against the tentorium causes injury to the brain, converting reversible central nervous system dysfunction into irreversible damage. Midbrain destruction may occur by direct compression of tissue against the tentorium. More frequently the basilar artery, which is tethered to the other intracranial vessels superiorly, is stretched and distorted, resulting in disruption of perforating vessels and secondary ischemia of the brainstem. In addition, compression of the cerebral aqueduct or the subarachnoid space around the brainstem may occur, hindering another means for cerebral compensation, displacement of cerebral ventricular fluid, and resulting in further increase in intracranial pressure. Less commonly, in the child with a subtentorial mass lesion, pressure is relieved by displacement of the brain up through the tentorial notch, causing similar distortion and vascular compromise.

As the brain is displaced, further damage occurs as it is compressed against another dural septum, the midline falx, which separates the cortex into halves. Shift laterally across the intracranial cavity causes compression of the medial hemispheres of the brain, resulting in vascular compromise, ischemia, swelling of tissues, and further build-up in intracranial pressure. Herniation of brainstem and parts of the cerebellum downward through the foramen magnum can also cause brainstem destruction, blockage of the flow of subarachnoid cerebral fluid, and vascular distortion. This distortion may cause severe respiratory and circulatory abnormalities and is often the ultimate cause of death.

With the recent widespread utilization in intracranial monitoring, decreased cerebral perfusion is an increasingly recognized sequela of increased intracranial pressure. Cerebral blood flow is dependent on a gradient between systemic arterial pressure and intracranial pressure. If this gradient, termed cerebral perfusion pressure (defined as mean arterial pressure minus mean intracranial pressure), falls below a critical level, blood flow to the cerebral cortex ceases, and irreversible brain damage results.

CLINICAL ASSESSMENT

The patient with an altered state of consciousness characteristically arrives at the emergency department at one point of what may be a rapidly evolving process. Although, as in all instances in medical practice, a thorough history and physical examination must eventually be done, the urgency of this situation demands a rapid, organized approach to determine the presence of worsening states and to identify rapidly remediable conditions before all the historical and physical information is available.

The questions which must be addressed immediately are:

1. Are the vital signs (pulse, respiration, blood pressure) of the child normal? If not, any respiratory or circulatory disturbances must be treated immediately.
2. Does the child have evidence for cerebral herniation? If so, immediate therapy must be instituted to reverse this process and the further destruction of brain.
3. Does the child have evidence for increased intracranial pressure? If so,

the child is at risk for cerebral herniation and steps must be taken to lower intracranial pressure.

4. Does the child have evidence for focal neurological disease?

The evaluation for increased intracranial pressure in the comatose child is based on the examination of the child's respiratory pattern, pupillary size and reactivity, extraocular movements, and motor posture and motor responses to stimuli. After these factors are assessed, the results must be analyzed to deduce the severity of neurologic dysfunction, the presence of increased intracranial pressure, or the occurrence of cerebral herniation. Two patterns of cerebral herniation often occur: (1) central (or rostrocaudal) herniation, resulting in a usually orderly progression of brainstem failure (see Table 10.1); or (2) uncal herniation, resulting in a somewhat less orderly progression of dysfunction (see Table 10.2). The clinical picture of uncal herniation is especially worrisome since deterioration may be unpredictable and extremely rapid soon after the appearance of the first clinical signs. However, the clinical picture and the etiologies of the two types of herniation often overlap.

Metabolic disturbances may result in increased intracranial pressure and signs of rostrocaudal dysfunction, but more frequently cause early changes in mentation. As the metabolic coma deepens, brainstem dysfunction occurs, but in a less stereotyped pattern, with sparing of certain brainstem functions, especially pupillary responses, despite compromise of other functions controlled at the same brainstem level (see "Differential Diagnosis").

Respiratory Patterns

Respiratory patterns may not only signal specific abnormalities in metabolic causes of coma, but also are useful in determining the level of the rostrocaudal cerebral dysfunction.

Hyperventilation in the stuporous or comatose patient signifies either compensation for metabolic acidosis (diabetes, uremia, lactic acidosis, drug ingestion) or primary respiratory alkalosis (salicylate poi-

Table 10.1
Central Syndrome of Rostro-Caudal Deterioration[a]

Stage	Respiratory Pattern	Pupillary Size and Reactivity	Oculocephalic-Oculovestibular	Motor Response to Noxious Stimuli
Early diencephallic	Cheyne-Stokes	Small pupils, reactive	Full dolls eye; full ipsilateral[b] tonic deviation	Appropriate (fends off stimuli) rigidity
Late diencephallic	Cheyne-Stokes	Small pupils, reactive	Full dolls eye (easy to obtain); full ipsilateral tonic deviation (easy to obtain)	Decorticate posture
Midbrain, upper pons	Central hyperventilation	Midposition, ± irregular pupils, unreactive	Impaired, dysconjugate	Decerebrate posture
Lower pons, upper medulla	Shallow or ataxic	Pinpoint, unreactive	Absent	No response

[a] From F. Plum and J.B. Posner: *Diagnosis of Stupor & Coma*, F.A. Davis, Philadelphia, 1980.
[b] Toward side of ice water irrigation.

Table 10.2
Syndrome of Uncal Herniation[a]

Pattern	Respiratory Pattern	Pupillary Size/Reactivity	Oculocephalic/Oculovestibular Response	Motor Response to Noxious Stimuli
Early third nerve	Normal	Unilateral,[b] moderately dilated pupil; dilated pupil reacts sluggishly	Full or dysconjugate[c]	Appropriate (fends off) or unilateral hemiparesis[b]
Late third nerve	Central hyperventilation or Cheyne-Stokes	Unilateral, widely[b] dilated pupil, unreactive	Dysconjugate (absent, late)[c]	Decortiate or decerebrate (may be assymetric)
Midbrain, upper pons	Central hyperventilation	Bilateral midposition pupils, unreactive	Impaired or absent	Bilateral, decerebrate

[a] From F. Plum and J.B. Posner: *Diagnosis of Stupor & Coma*, F.A. Davis, Philadelphia, 1980.
[b] Usually ipsilateral to side of lesion.
[c] Eye with dilated pupil does not move.

soning, hepatic coma, pulmonary disease, or psychogenic hyperventilation).

Hypoventilation in metabolic coma indicates either compensation for metabolic alkalosis (ingestion of alkali or loss of acid through the gastrointestinal tract or kidney) or respiratory acidosis (severe pulmonary or neuromuscular disease or central respiratory failure).

Abnormal respiratory patterns are also seen with rostrocaudal regression of coma due to mass lesions or other causes of increased intracranial pressure. The pattern associated with the mildest disturbance, *posthyperventilation apnea*, is characterized by 10 to 30 sec periods of apnea following a voluntary period of deep breathing (5 to 10 breaths). *Cheyne-Stokes respiration* is characterized by periods of hyperpnea alternating with apnea, the hyperpnea usually lasting longer than the apnea. Each cycle begins with a crescendo of deepening breaths followed by a decrescendo of smaller breaths until an apneic phase ensues. Cheyne-Stokes respirations imply bilateral hemispheric dysfunction with intact brain stem function. *Central neurogenic hyperventilation*, manifested by sustained, regular, rapid and deep respirations, points to midbrain dysfunction. *Apneustic breathing*, characterized by end inspiratory and/or end expiratory pauses lasting several seconds, and *ataxic* breathing, an irregular, sporadic respiratory pattern of varying amplitude, imply pontine and medullary dysfunction.

Pupillary Size and Responses

An evaluation of the size and the reactivity of the pupils to light is important in determining the level and location of lesions affecting the brain stem. In pathologic states confined to the cerebral hemispheres, subcortical white matter and posterior thalamic nuclei, the pupils function normally. With diencephalic involvement, the pupils are small (myotic), but their reaction to light is preserved.

With involvement of the midbrain, the pupils may be in midposition, slightly widened or irregular, or widely dilated (mydriatic). If the oculomotor nerves are involved, the light reflex is lost. With intrinsic midbrain involvement, the pupils are invariably involved bilaterally, although their size and reactions may be asymmetrical. Pontine lesions lead to constricted (myotic) pupils.

A unilaterally dilated pupil is a common early sign in the *uncal syndrome*, as the oculomotor nerve is compressed against the posterior cerebral artery by the medially displaced uncus of the temporal lobe. In the early stages, the ipsilateral pupil is only mildly dilated and the light reflex is retained. In clinical situations, it is important to differentiate this cause of asymmetric pupils from the Horner's syndrome (unilateral miosis, ptosis, and anhydrosis) which can occur from hypothalamic dysfunction.

Certain drugs that alter the state of consciousness also have fairly specific effects on the pupils (see Table 10.3).

Extraocular Movements

The position of the eyes at rest, the presence of spontaneous abnormal eye movements, and the ocular response to labyrinthine stimulation often provide important clues in the clinical assessment of patients in stupor and coma.

Conjugate deviation of the eyes at rest may occur with either cerebral hemispheric, usually frontal lobe, or pontine lesions. With cerebral lesions, the eyes are deviated to the side of the lesion, and labyrinthine responses (see below) are usually intact. With unilateral pontine lesions, the eyes are deviated away from the lesion, and labyrinthine responses are defective.

In the absence of lesions in the cerebral eye fields, the eyes in the comatose patient with intact brainstem function may be directed straight ahead or may be slightly divergent. Roving, conjugate, or slightly dysconjugate eye movements may also be seen. Midbrain lesions involving the oculomotor nucleus or nerve may cause the ipsilateral eye to be abducted, as may lesions involving the abducens nucleus or nerve in the pons. The *setting sun sign*, downward deviation of the eyes, is associated with paralysis of upward gaze and is due to an upper dorsal midbrain lesion. *Skew deviation*, in which one eye looks up while the other looks down, may occur with pontine lesions, but is usually of nonlocalizing significance.

Several types of spontaneous nystagmus may occur with brainstem pathology. *Convergent nystagmus*, characterized by a drifting divergent movement followed by a quick convergent component, indicates midbrain dysfunction in the tectal region. *Ocular bobbing*, episodes of intermittent downward displacement of the eyes, indicates pontine dysfunction. Unilateral vertical, horizontal, or rotary nystagmus may also occur in pontine lesions.

The ocular response to vestibular stimu-

Table 10.3
Drugs Resulting in Delerium/Coma

Drug	Physical Findings
Barbiturates	Small, reactive pupils, hypothermia, flaccidity (dolls eye may be absent)
Opiates	Pinpoint, reactive pupils, hypothermia, hypotension, hypoventilation, bradycardia
Psychodelics	Small, reactive pupils, hypertension, hyperventilation, dystonic posturing
Amphetamines	Dilated pupils, hyperthermia, hypertension, tachycardia, arrhythmia
Cocaine	Dilated pupils, hyperthermia, tachycardia
Atropine-Scopolamine	Dilated pupils, hyperthermia, flushing, hot, dry skin, supraventricular tachycardia
Glutethimide	Midposition, irregular fixed pupils, hypothermia, flaccidity
Tricyclic antidepressants	Hyperthermia, hypotension, supraventricular tachycardia
Phenothiazines	Hypotension, arrhythmia, dystonia
Methaqualone	As barbiturates, if severe tachycardia, dystonia

lation provides a means of assessing the integrity of cerebral nervous system function in the comatose patient. The caloric test, performed by flexing the patient's head to 30° and slowly injecting 50 ml of ice water through a catheter placed in the external auditory canal, is a standard technique for producing vestibular stimulation. In the normal patient, such stimulation will lead to conjugate, horizontal deviation of the eyes to the side of the injection with a compensating horizontal, rapid nystagmus to the opposite side. The nystagmus is under cortical influence, and, therefore, in coma from supratentorial lesions with intact brain stem function, the response may be limited to tonic conjugate deviation of the eyes. The integrity of this reflex is dependent on the function of the labyrinths, vestibular nerves and nuclei, abducens nuclei and nerves, medial longitudinal fasciculi, and oculomotor nuclei and nerves, structures that encompass dorsal lateral medulla, and lateral, medial, dorsal, and ventral parts of the pons and midbrain. Thus, an appropriate reflex indicates that much of the brainstem is intact. Partial abnormalities can be used to localize lesions within the brainstem, and absent reflexes suggest severe brainstem dysfunction.

The oculocephalic (doll's eye) reflex provides another means of producing vestibular stimulation, although the degree of stimulation is considerably less than in caloric testing. The oculocephalic response is produced by briskly rotating the patient's head from side to side. Its performance is contraindicated when a cervical spine injury is suspected. In a positive response, there is conjugate, horizontal deviation of the eyes opposite to the direction of the head rotation.

Motor Function

The motor system is initially evaluated by observation of the child's spontaneous movements and posture. Then, the tone of the muscles should be ascertained. Finally, noxious stimuli are applied, and the patient's response is observed. Asmmetry of function suggests hemiparesis which may signify midbrain compression due to uncal herniation. Two major stereotyped patterns of posturing should be recognized. The first is decorticate posturing which consists of some degree of opisthotonos, flexion of the arms, wrists and fingers with adducted upper extremities, and extension, internal rotation and plantar flexion of the lower extremities. This signifies diffuse damage to the cerebral cortex and subcortical white matter or basal ganglia. Decerebrate rigidity differs in that the opisthotonos is somewhat more marked, and the arms and hands are extended; it signifies more extensive damage involving the midbrain. With further depression of the brainstem, the patient becomes completely flaccid and unresponsive to stimuli.

Later Evaluation

After the patient is stable and the emergency evaluation outlined above is performed, a concise history must be obtained. Special concern should be placed on events just preceding the coma. However, questions about chronic mental status and personality changes should not be forgotten. A history for the presence of drugs in the home should be elicited. The general physical examination should likewise be succinct but complete. Special attention should be paid to the circulatory and respiratory systems. The patient's state of hydration must be evaluated. The patient's skin should be closely examined for signs of trauma or the presence of petechiae or rashes. The child should always undergo a complete neurologic examination searching for evidence of a focal deficit.

DIFFERENTIAL DIAGNOSIS

The etiologies of coma can be separated into three major categories: supratentorial, subtentorial, and metabolic (see Table 10.4). More important is the separation between comas due to raised intracranial pressure and all other causes.

Cerebral trauma is the most common etiology for supratentorial mass lesions that secondarily compromise consciousness. In children, epidural hematomas may follow minor blows to the head and occur without superficial signs of injury. The initiating event may be unseen or dismissed as trivial. The classic symptom complex of unconsciousness followed by a lucid interval and succeeded by deepening coma is rare. Ex-

Table 10.4
Commoner Etiologies of Unconsciousness

Supratentorial
- Trauma
  - Mass lesion (epidural, subdural, intracerebral hematoma)
  - Diffuse cerebral swelling
- Cerebral vascular accident
- Cerebral venous thrombosis
- Subdural empyema
- Intracerebral tumor (often with hemorrhage)

Subtentorial
- Tumors (often with hemorrhage)
- Trauma (epidural)
- Primary hemorrhage

Metabolic
- Anoxia
- Hypoglycemia
- Diabetic ketoacidosis
- Electrolyte abnormalities (sodium, potassium, calcium, magnesium)
- Exogenous poisonings
- Meningitis
- Encephalitis
- Reye's syndrome
- Hepatic encephalopathy
- Uremic encephalopathy
- Inborn errors of metabolism
- Hormonal abnormalities (thyroid, adrenal)
- Hypohyperthermia

tradural hemorrhage in childhood is usually venous, and thus the loss of consciousness may be gradual. The earliest neurologic sign may be pupillary dilatation on the side of the lesion.

Subdural hematoma is a common complication of recognized head injury; it is usually associated with external signs of trauma and immediate loss of consciousness. In these patients, the hematoma is often only one component of a diffuse injury that includes brain damage and edema. Chronic subdural hematomas rarely occur in children except in abused infants between the ages of 2 and 6 months. A history of recurrent vomiting, seizures, the presence of retinal or subhyloid hemorrhages, and a tense fontanelle suggest this diagnosis. Diffuse, severe head trauma may also result in diffuse swelling of the brain, increased intracranial pressure, and loss of consciousness without associated extracerebral or intracerebral collections of blood. Intracerebral hemorrhage may also occur after head trauma.

Nontraumatic supratentorial mass lesions may present with coma. Cerebrovascular accidents, though uncommon in childhood, may cause focal neurologic deficits, rapidly followed by status epilepticus and supervening unconsciousness. Subdural empyemas, also rare, occur primarily as a complication of previously undetected basilar skull fractures or chronic otorhinologic disease. Children with intracerebral tumors, which commonly produce focal neurologic dysfunction, may develop coma, especially after intratumor hemorrhage.

Subtentorial (posterior fossa) lesions may cause coma by either destroying the ARAS or compressing the brainstem from without and interfering with the blood supply of the area. They can be differentiated from supratentorial lesions only if localizing brainstem signs precede the onset of coma. Tumors may cause coma by direct compression or infiltration of the brainstem or by blockage of the ventricular system and secondary hydrocephalus. Though tumors more frequently cause chronic symptoms referable to the posterior fossa, in a recent review of posterior fossa tumors seen at The Children's Hospital of Philadelphia, nearly 20% of the children with these lesions presented with coma; this often occurred after hemorrhage into the tumor. In childhood, falls on the occipital region may result in massive posterior fossa venous sinus hemorrhage and unconsciousness. In approximately one-half of the cases, this occurs without specific symptoms referable to the area involved; however, x-rays of the skull usually show a fracture in the occipital area. Extremely rare causes of coma due to subtentorial lesions include hemorrhage into the brainstem and cerebellum due to arteriovenous malformations and demyelinating lesions of the brainstem.

Metabolic diseases causing coma are numerous. Changes in mental status are the earliest signs of metabolic encephalopathy. Respiratory function is involved relatively early, and abnormalities are often nonspecific secondary to changes in acid-base balance. Pupillary and ocular motility functions are spared initially with certain important exceptions. Motor abnormalities are often difficult to explain in metabolic disease; focal transient signs are surprisingly common. Other signs such as tremor, asterixis, and multifocal myoclonus may suggest a metabolic disturbance. Electroencephalogram changes may be very helpful in differentiating structural from metabolic diseases. The primary distinction is that metabolic diseases often cause partial dysfunction at many levels of the CNS rather than following clear anatomical boundaries.

Table 10.5
Metabolic Alterations Producing Coma

Acidosis
- Metabolic ($\downarrow$ph, $\downarrow CO_2$, $\downarrow HCO_3$)
  - Diabetic ketoacidosis
  - Reye's syndrome (uncommon)
  - Salicylism
  - Lactic (primary or secondary to anoxia, shock, seizures, etc.)
  - Exogenous poisons (ethylene glycol, methyl alcohol, paraldehyde)
  - Diarrhea
  - Uremia
- *Respiratory* ($\downarrow$pH, $\uparrow CO_2$, $\ddagger\uparrow HCO_3^-$)
  - Exogenous sedatives
  - Chest injury
  - Pulmonary dysfunction (intrinsic)
  - Brainstem dysfunction
  - Neuromuscular disease (myasthenia gravis, Werdnig-Hoffmann, botulism, etc.)
- Mixed ($\downarrow$pH, $\uparrow PCO_2$, $\downarrow HCO_3$)
  - Salicylism
  - Sepsis

Alkalosis
- Metabolic ($\uparrow$pH, $\uparrow PCO_2$, $\uparrow HCO_3$)
  - Vomiting
  - Bartter's syndrome
- Respiratory ($\uparrow$pH, $\downarrow PCO_2$, normal to $\downarrow HCO_3$)
  - Reye's syndrome (common)
  - Salicylism
  - Sepsis
  - Pneumonia
  - Hepatic coma

Arterial blood gases are often extremely helpful in categorizing the various causes of metabolic dysfunction (see Table 10.5). A decrease of oxygen delivery to the brain, causing either ischemia or anoxia, is the most common metabolic disturbance resulting in coma. This may be secondary to multiple systemic causes. Hypoglycemia is an important cause of coma since it is so readily treated. It is often secondary to excessive exogenous insulin, but also occurs with esidioblastosis or pancreatic adenomas. Transient focal neurologic symptoms occur frequently in hypoglycemia and may be misleading. Diabetic keto-acidosis with concomitant hyperosmolarity and lactic acidosis is another common metabolic cause of unconsciousness. Hyponatremia may occur as a primary cause of unconsciousness, but more frequently is secondary to CNS damage or infection, leading to the inappropriate secretion of antidiuretic hormone. Hypernatremia may complicate vomiting and dehydration and result in coma. Calcium excess or lack rarely may result in altered states of consciousness.

Hepatic and uremic encephalopathy are less frequent causes of coma in childhood. An altered mental state develops gradually in these conditions and often is associated with motor abnormalities such as multifocal myoclonus. One important common exception is Reye's syndrome (see p. 567). This syndrome is manifested by a history of recurrent vomiting and alterations in mental status rapidly leading to delirium. Although the diagnosis can only be made with certainty by liver biopsy, elevation of the serum ammonia level associated with this symptom complex suggests Reye's syndrome. This disease is not purely an hepatic encephalopathy, but is often complicated by diffuse brain swelling, raised intracranial pressure, and signs of central herniation. Urea cycle abnormalities have been described which are clinically indistinguishable from Reye's syndrome.

Intake of exogenous poisons is a frequent cause of coma, and correct diagnosis requires a high level of suspicion, an accurate history of accessible poisons around the home, and knowledge of the peculiar systemic and neurologic damage poisons can cause. A partial list of toxins is given in Table 10.3. Once again, arterial blood gases can be very helpful, especially in the case of drugs that cause severe metabolic acidosis, including methyl alcohol, ethylene glycol, and paraldehyde.

Meningitis and encephalitis may cause coma. The diagnosis and treatment of meningitis requires lumbar puncture even in the face of increased intracranial pressure. Among the encephalitidies, the diagnosis of herpes encephalitis (see p. 340) is of prime importance, since specific treatment is available. In the setting of a patient with a history of fever and headaches, who acutely or subacutely progresses to delirium and loss of consciousness, especially with focal neurologic findings, the physician should suspect a herpetic infection and perform appropriate studies.

Generalized seizures are another cause of prolonged unresponsiveness. This unresponsiveness usually lasts less than 30 min, but can be quite prolonged with severe repeated seizures. A rare cause of coma is petit mal status. In this instance, electroencephalography is diagnostic and allows for specific intervention.

Table 10.6
Emergency Management of Comatose Child

1. Assure ventilation and circulatory status; control body temperature
2. Draw baseline chemistries
3. Give glucose, naloxone
4. Evaluate for increased intracranial pressure. If increased:
   a. Hyperventilate
   b. Intravenous mannitol
   c. Intravenous corticosteroids
   d. Emergency computerized tomography
5. Evaluate for focal neurologic deficit (if present, emergency computerized tomography)
6. Evaluate for meningitis (if likely, lumbar puncture)
7. Draw arterial blood gas (if not already done)
8. Place indwelling urinary catheter
9. Evaluate for intoxications
   a. Urine and blood toxicology screen
   b. Urine FeCl
   c. Appropriate treatment (antidotes if possible)
10. Draw NH_4, liver and renal function studies
11. Transfer to intensive care unit (? intracranial monitoring)
12. Further laboratory evaluation

EVALUATION AND MANAGEMENT

Management of the comatose patient is directed at preventing further brain damage (see Table 10.6). Immediately upon arrival, the patient's respiratory rate, heart rate, blood pressure, and temperature should be obtained. The patient's airway is cleared and, if spontaneous ventilation is inadequate, immediate ventilation with a bag-valve-mask device should be begun. If oxygen cannot be adequately delivered by this means, endotracheal intubation is then performed. Supplemental oxygen should be delivered until adequate arterial oxygenation is documented. Arterial blood gases should be obtained rapidly. The patient's neck is manipulated minimally if there is any possibility of cervical spine injury, and portable lateral cervical spine films should be immediately obtained. Simultaneously, the patient's circulation is evaluated, and shock is immediately treated by volume expansion. A large bore secure intravenous line should be placed.

Once any cardiorespiratory disturbances have been treated, attention can be directed at making a diagnosis (Fig. 10.2). If the patient has sustained head trauma, he or she will require a CT scan to look for lesions amenable to surgical therapy. Signs of meningeal irritation point to the urgent need for a lumbar puncture. Even if there is concomitant evidence for increased intracranial pressure, the lumbar puncture should be performed since the need for specific bacteriologic information outweighs the risk of cerebral herniation. To lower the risk of herniation, such a child can be pretreated with hyperventilation and Mannitol, and the lumbar puncture should be performed with a small (22 gauge) needle. After withdrawal of blood for laboratory studies, the child with unexplained coma should receive 4 ml/kg of 25% dextrose in water intravenously while the physician observes the patient for any response. If the patient improves dramatically, a continuous infusion of 10% dextrose is begun. A failure to awaken after glucose administration makes the diagnosis of hypoglycemia unlikely. These patients should receive naloxone (0.01 mg/kg). The initial blood sample which was drawn should be sent for evaluation of serum sodium, potassium, chloride, CO_2, glucose, and calcium and a toxicology screen. After applying an electrocardiographic monitor, a twelve lead electrocardiogram should be performed as soon as possible. A Foley catheter should be placed and the initial urine sample analyzed. A portion of this urine should be sent for toxicology screening and another portion saved for ferric chloride determination.

After treatment of respiratory and circulatory disturbances, a thorough sys-

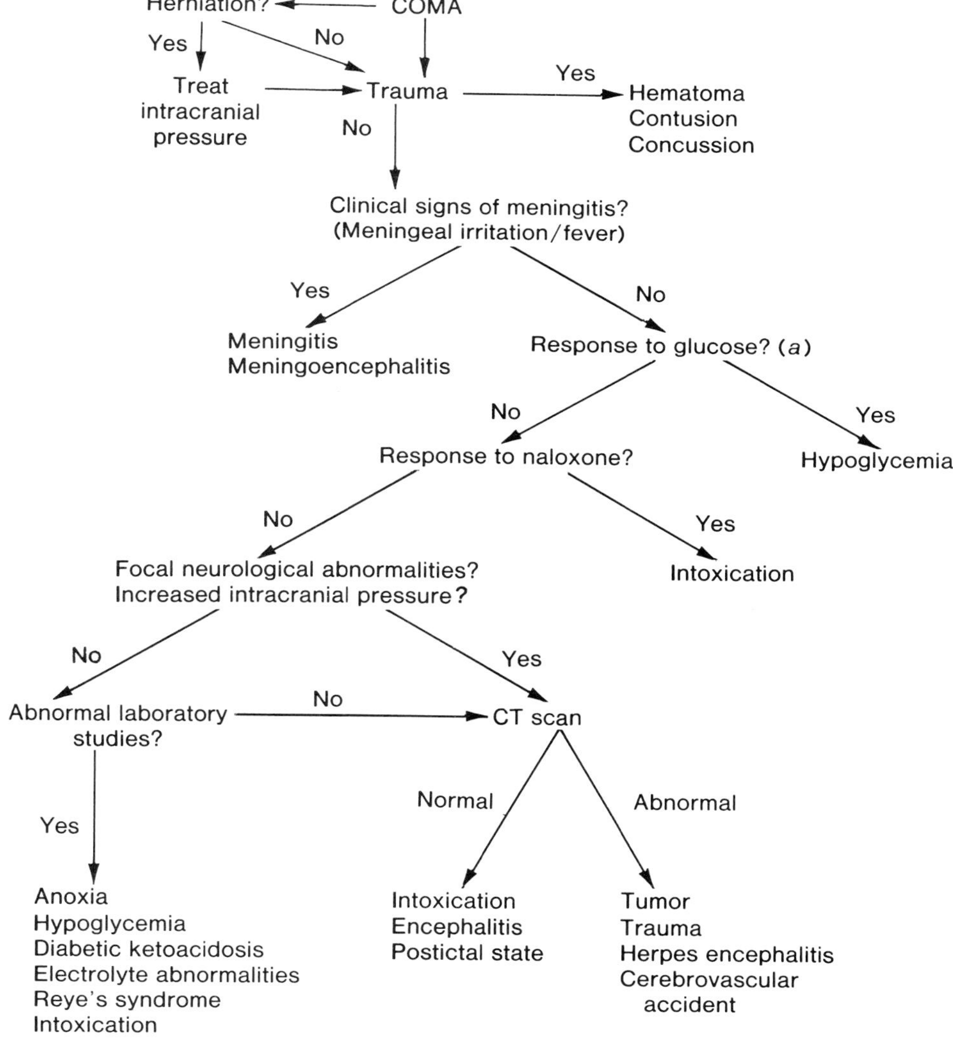

Figure 10.2 Evaluation of the child in coma with no apparent cause. This diagnostic approach assumes psychogenic "coma" has been ruled out. (*a*) If the glucose has been shown to be normal using any of the reagents for rapid measurement, proceed to the next step.

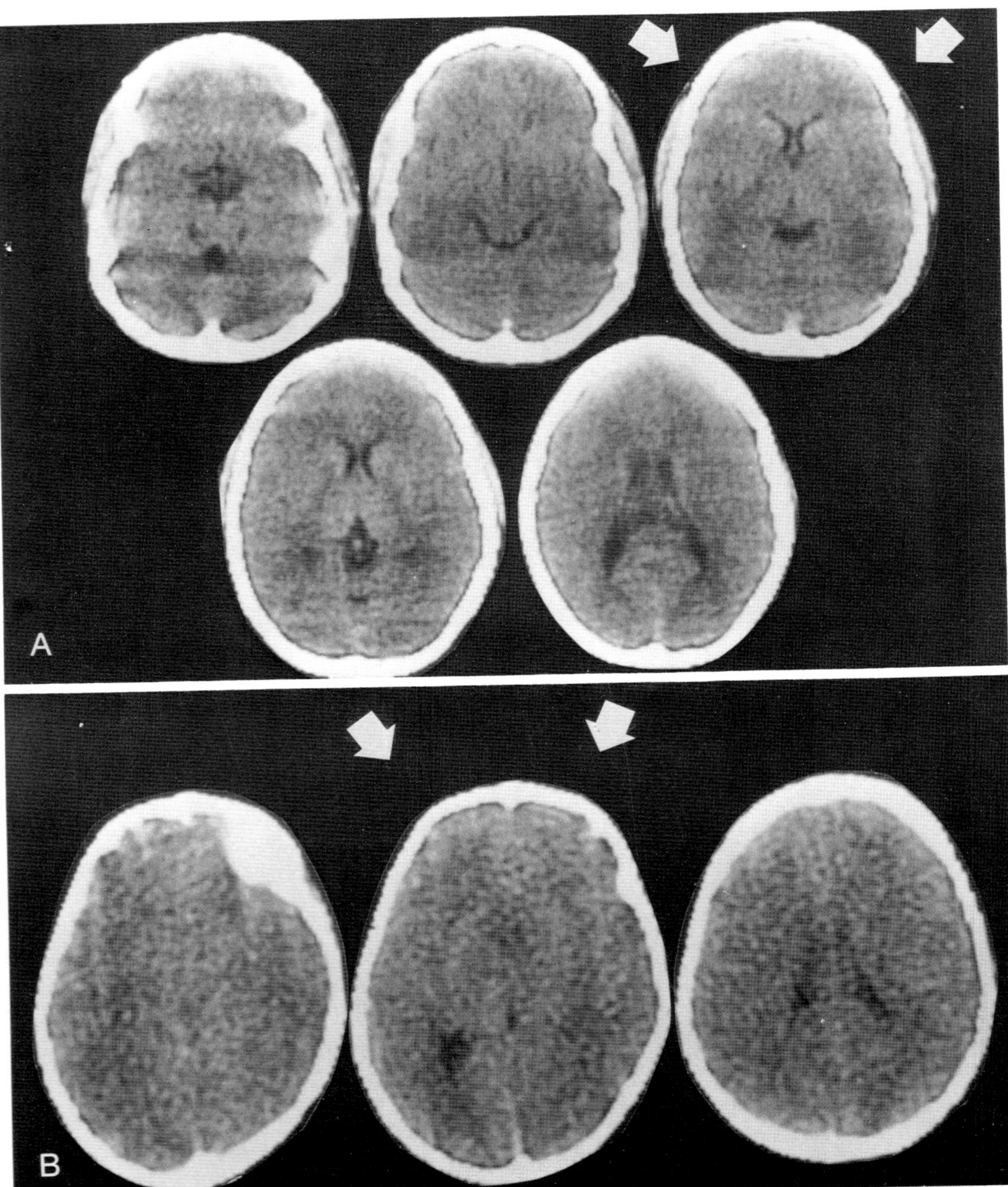

Figure 10.3 Computed tomography (CT) in acutely comatose children (*A*) normal CT (unenhanced) in child with drug intoxication, displaying normal size cisterns and ventricles; (*B*) abnormal CT (unenhanced) showing obliterated cisterns and small ventricles, in a child with increased intracranial pressure secondary to presumed "viral" encephalitis (a similar CT can be seen in diffuse brain swelling from multiple etiologies, hypoxia etc.); (*C*) abnormal CT (unenhanced) showing hypodensity of right cerebral cortex with obliteration of right lateral ventricle and shift of brain from right to left, in child with a right internal carotid stroke; (*D*) abnormal CT (unenhanced), displaying hyperdence mass in left epidural region of middle cranial fossa, with compression of brain and shift of ventricular system from left to right, in a child with a left epidural hematoma; (*E*) abnormal CT (unenhanced) showing hyperdence mass (blood) in the right frontal area with intraventricular and subarachnoid extension and resultant shift of brain from right to left, in a child with a posttraumatic intracerebral hematoma; (*F*) abnormal CT (enhanced) showing a contrasting enhancing mass in the fourth ventricle with obstruction and dilitation of the third and lateral ventricles, in a child with an ependymoma. (Computed tomograms courtesy of Robert A. Zimmerman, M.D., University of Pennsylvania.)

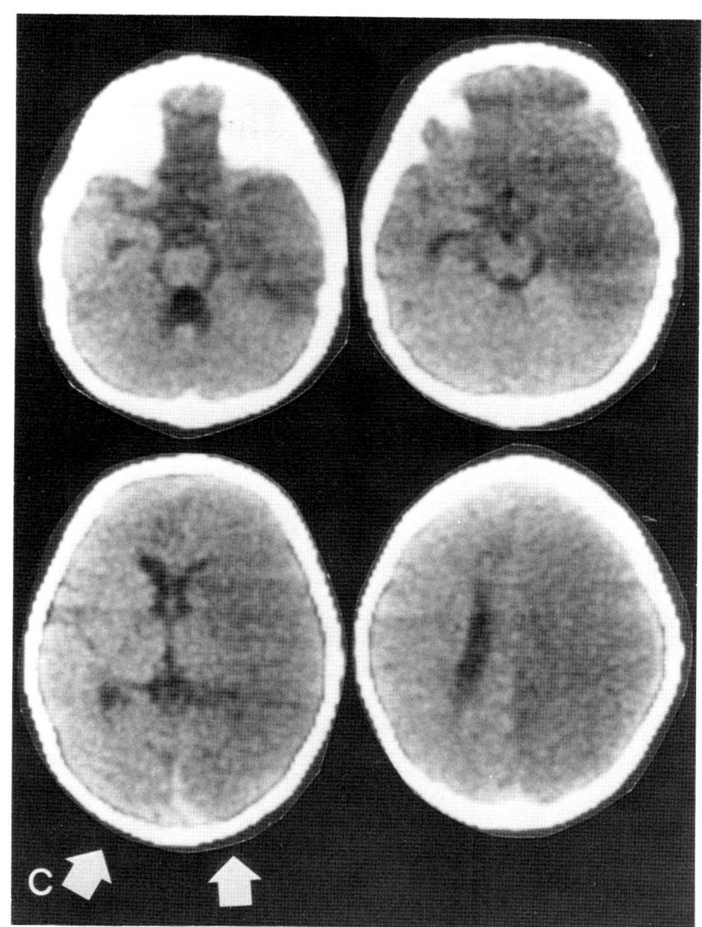
C

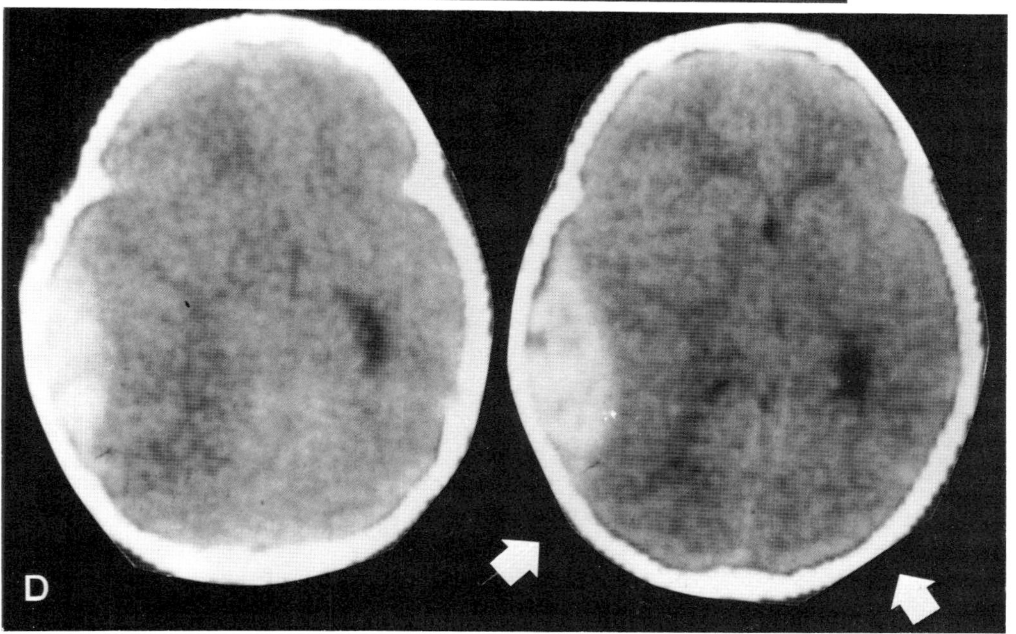
D

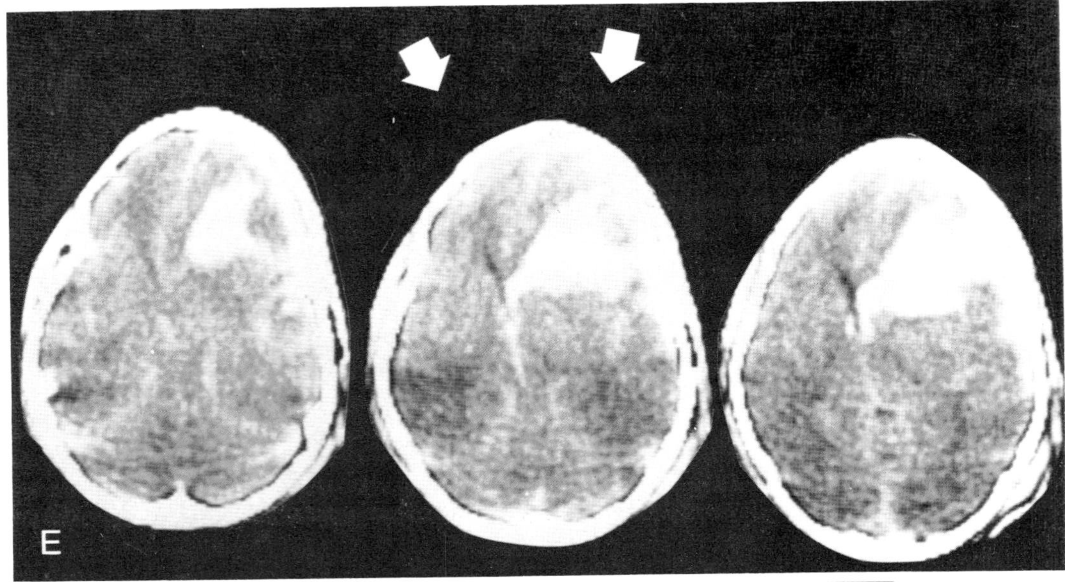

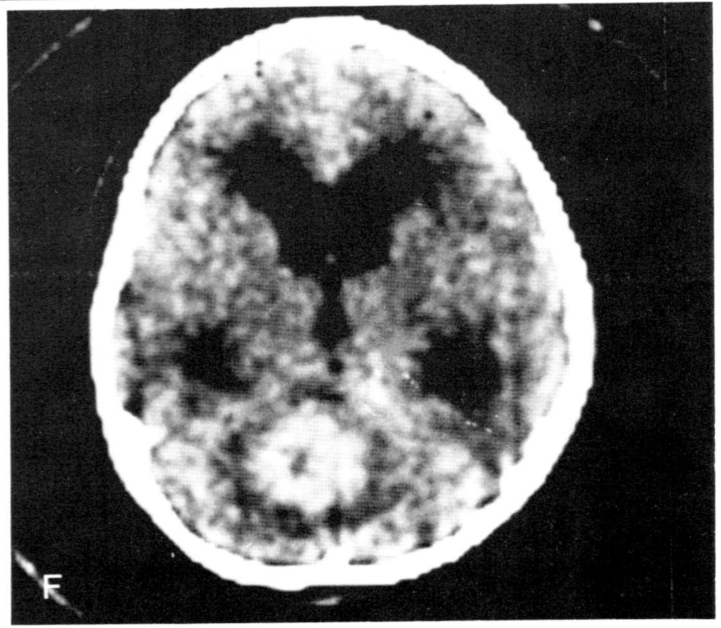

Figure 10.3 E–F

tematic neurologic evaluation of respiratory pattern, pupillary function, oculovestibular function, and skeletal motor function should be performed (as outlined above), looking for signs of increased intracranial pressure. If there is evidence for raised intracranial pressure, it must be immediately treated by (1) hyperventilation, and (2) drug therapy. The patient is hyperventilated in an attempt to decrease the partial pressure of CO_2 in the blood to a range of 20 to 25 Torr. A decrease in partial pressure of CO_2 lowers intracranial pressure by lessening cerebral blood flow; however, excessive hyperventilation may result in too drastic a decrease in blood flow and relative ischemia to the brain. Mannitol, an osmotic agent used to draw excess fluid from the brain, is infused intravenously in a 20% solution at 1.25 to 2 g/kg. Although somewhat controversial, if there is evidence for increased intracranial pressure, dexamethesone should be given at 1 to 2 mg/kg intravenously. After any circulatory insufficiency has been corrected, fluid (5% dextrose and 0.25 N saline solution) should be infused at 75% of the daily maintenance rate (see Chapters 44 and 67).

At this point, patients likely to have an intracranial lesion should undergo emergency CT scanning. In the acute situation, computerized tomography readily demonstrates the presence of mass lesions such as epidural, subdural, and intracerebral hematomas (see Fig. 10.3). It can also show the size of the ventricular system and the role of hydrocephalus in the etiology of the patient's unconsciousness. Diffuse brain swelling is well visualized in computerized tomography, and evidence for tentorial herniation can be seen. If the patient tolerates the CT scan, further information about the extent of damage may be obtained with the intravenous injection of contrast material. This is especially useful in outlining subacute subdural hematomas which may be isodense with brain or disturbances of the blood/brain barrier such as herpes encephalitis. If CT scanning is not available, brain scanning or arteriography should be performed if there is a high index of suspicion of a mass lesion. Skull x-rays are of little use in the care of the critically ill comatose patient. Rarely, if intracranial pressure cannot be reduced by the means outlined and there is evidence for severe head trauma, placement of burr holes may be life-saving.

If a metabolic etiology is strongly suggested at this point, an ammonia level, liver enzymes, BUN, and creatinine should be obtained. Arterial blood gases should be obtained if not done earlier. Ferric chloride testing of the urine may provide a clue as to the likelihood of poisoning. If there is a strong impression of intoxication, appropriate treatment should be carried out (see p. 491). An opiate ingestion is treated with naloxone (0.01 mg/kg), and an overdose of tricyclic antidepressant drugs with physostigmine (0.5–2 mg), both given intravenously.

While awaiting results of the laboratory studies, an electroencephalogram may be quite helpful. In the case of petit mal status, it shows a pathognomonic pattern. Other tests which may be obtained, depending on clinical impression at this point, include thyroid functions and serum cortisol levels. During this time care should be taken to protect the patient's eyes by patching them. The patient should be transferred to an intensive care unit for continued close observation. The emergency department physician should defer the institution of other modalities for controlling intracranial pressure, such as high-dose barbiturates. This treatment requires constant evaluation of central venous and arterial pressure as well as intracranial pressure monitoring, which are not adequately performed in the emergency department setting.

Throughout the initial period of treatment, the concerns of the patient's family should not be forgotten, and a member of the emergency department staff should make a point of keeping the family members informed of the patient's condition.

References

Lockman LA: Coma. In *The Practice of Pediatric Neurology*, pp. 92–105, edited by KF Swaiman and FS Wright, C. V. Mosby, St. Louis, 1975.

Plum F, Poser JB: *The Diagnosis of Stupor and Coma*, Ed. 3, F. A. Davis, Philadelphia, 1980.

CHAPTER 11

Constipation

STEPHEN LUDWIG, M.D.

INTRODUCTION

Although constipation rarely causes a life-threatening emergency, it is a common symptom in the emergency department. The bowel habits of children are watched closely by their parents and a great deal of folklore surrounds bowel functions. Many home remedies and over the counter preparations are used to alleviate presumed constipation. Despite frivolity of what some consider a societal preoccupation with bowel regularity, constipation may be the symptom of several serious health concerns. Constipation is defined by a combination of three factors: (1) stool consistency, (2) stool frequency, and (3) physical examination. Stool consistency describes the firmness or softness of the stool. The quality relates to the amount of water in the feces. Stool consistency varies with age and diet. For example, infants usually do not have formed stool. Stool frequency describes the time interval between bowel movements and also varies with age and diet. Moreover, there are individual differences in stool frequency. In diagnosing acute constipation it is important to note a decrease in stool frequency for that individual patient, not a specific numbered decrease. Both of the aforementioned factors must be considered in making the diagnosis of constipation.

There must also be a physical examination which is confirmatory. For example, a child who is being breast fed may have infrequent stools, perhaps once per week. Physical examination will show soft stool in the rectum and no abdominal fullness or mass in the left lower quadrant. Despite the infrequency of stool, this is *not* constipation. The child with severe functional constipation may pass frequent soft or liquid stools and may even be encopretic, yet on physical examination the physician may palpate a large fecal mass.

The pathophysiology of constipation is complex. A number of factors are important, including: diet, composition of the stool, gastrointestinal motility, and mechanical obstruction. Also, in order that normal defecation occur the child must perceive the stool in the rectum and then be able to contract the diaphragm and abdominal muscle. The anal sphincter must be relaxed against the force of stool bolus. A problem with any of the components of normal defecation may lead to constipation. At times more than one factor may be operative. Table 11.1 shows etiologies of constipation according to pathophysiology. It is the purpose of Figure 11.1 and the accompanying text to help the emergency department physician consider all the important diagnostic possibilities.

EVALUATION AND DECISION

The first step in the management of a child presumed to have constipation is to rule out pseudoconstipation. Pseudoconstipation refers to a parental complaint about constipation when in fact the condition does not exist. The history should include questions about stool consistency and stool frequency. The physical examination must

Table 11.1
Etiology of Constipation

- *I. Functional*
  - A. Fecal retention
  - B. Depression
  - C. Harsh toilet training
  - D. Toilet phobia
  - E. Avoidance of school bathrooms
  - F. Fecal soiling
- *II. Pain on Defecation*
  - A. Anal fissure
  - B. Foreign body
  - C. Sexual abuse
  - D. Laxative overuse
  - E. Proctitis
  - F. Rectal prolapse
- *III. Mechanical Obstruction*
  - A. Hirschsprung's disease
  - B. Pelvic tumor
  - C. Upper bowel obstruction
  - D. Rectal stenosis
- *IV. Decreased Sensation/Motility*
  - A. Drug-induced
  - B. Viral "ileus"
  - C. Neuromuscular diseases
    - 1. Hypotonia
    - 2. Werdnig-Hoffman disease
    - 3. Cerebral palsy
  - D. Endocrine abnormalities
    - 1. Hypothyroidism
    - 2. Hyperparathyroidism
    - 3. Hypercalcemia
  - E. Infant botulism
  - F. Spinal cord tumor
- *V. Stool Abnormalities*
  - A. Dietary
  - B. Dehydration
  - C. Malnutrition
- *VI. Pseudoconstipation*
  - A. Breast fed infant
  - B. Normal variation in stool frequency

include careful palpation of the abdomen and a rectal examination. Many parents will give a history that their infant grunts, turns red, and seems to strain to pass stool. The infant may even cry during defecation. All of these complaints are normal and are *not* in themselves diagnostic of constipation. If the child's stool is soft and physical examination is negative, constipation does not exist regardless of the stool frequency. Parents may feel that their child has a problem if a bowel movement has been missed for 1 day. Before considering any further diagnosis it is important to identify cases of pseudoconstipation and apply the appropriate parent/patient education.

Onset and Duration

If indeed constipation exists, the next differentiation is based on duration: acute versus chronic constipation. Acute constipation includes cases in which the onset has been 1 to 4 weeks prior to the emergency department visit. Chronic constipation has a duration greater than 1 month. Another important "break point" in the differential diagnosis has to do with the child's age at the symptom onset. Some parents will state that the child has been constipated since birth. This history is significant, as it raises the possibility of an anatomic problem such as Hirschsprung's disease. When the onset of constipation is at the age of toilet training it is most likely functional. The specific causes of constipation both chronic and acute are described in the sections which follow.

Chronic Constipation

HIRSCHSPRUNG'S DISEASE (CONGENITAL MEGACOLON)

Of all the causes of chronic constipation perhaps the most important diagnosis to be made is Hirschsprung's disease or congenital megacolon (see Chapter 59, "Abdominal Emergencies"). This is a congenital problem in which a portion of the colon, usually the rectosigmoid, is without ganglion cells. The normal propulsion of stool is unable to traverse the segment of colon which is not innervated. The term congential megacolon derives from the dilated segment of bowel proximal to the aganglionic segment.

Hirschsprung's disease may present in the newborn period with a failure to pass meconium, intestinal obstruction or as necrotizing enterocolitis. However, the majority of cases are recognized later in the first year of life in children presenting with constipation. A small percentage of cases are not recognized until later childhood. This latter group is unfortunately subjected to a variety of unsuccessful treatments and even

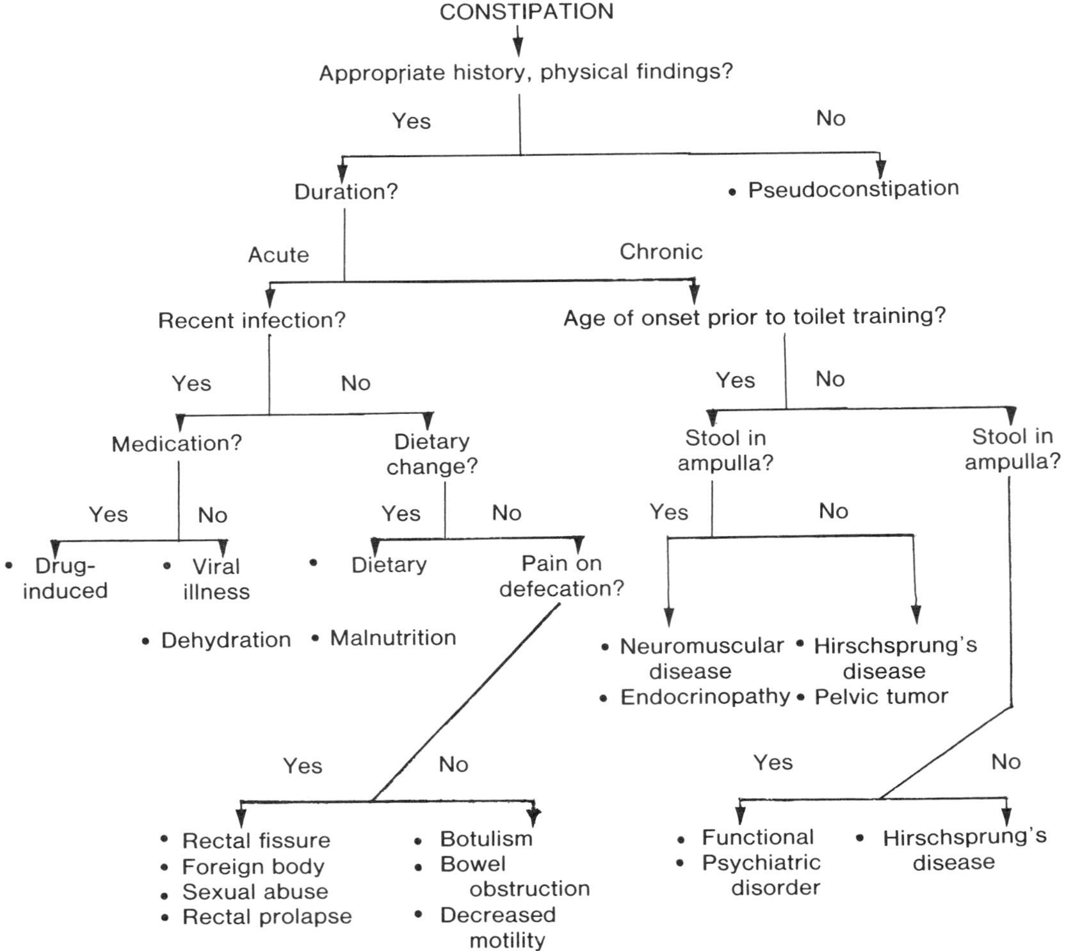

Figure 11.1 Approach to constipation.

psychotherapy. A subgroup of children has been defined as having ultrashort segment Hirschsprung's disease. In these children the aganglionic segment may be so short that clinical differentiation from functional constipation is difficult.

The diagnosis of Hirschsprung's disease is suspected when the history is one of chronic constipation with onset during the first year of life. There may be a history of increasing difficulty in passing stools; rarely has soiling occurred. The physical examination may indicate growth failure. The abdomen may be distended and a fecal mass will be palpable in the lower left quadrant. The key to making the diagnosis is the rectal examination in that there is an absence of feces in the ampulla. The diagnosis can be strengthened by the barium finding of an abrupt change in the bowel size between the ganglionic and aganglionic segments. Other barium enema findings are suggestive. Manometric studies of the bowel can also provide useful information in most cases. The definitive diagnosis can be made by rectal biopsy demonstrating absent ganglion cells.

If Hirschsprung's disease is suspected the child must be referred to a pediatric surgeon in order to establish the diagnosis and institute the appropriate surgical treatment (Chapter 59).

FUNCTIONAL CONSTIPATION

The most common cause of chronic constipation is functional. The cause of the condition is unknown. There seems to be a familial tendency and a higher concordance rate for monozygotic twins than for dizygotic twins. Some theorists suggest that harsh, early training may be a factor. Others implicate a tendency toward excessive reabsorption of colonic water that results in dry inspissated stool. Still other investigators have found abnormalities of bowel motility.

The child with functional constipation usually develops significant symptoms after the toilet training ages. Never is there an onset of constipation from birth, but at times there is a history of hard or dry stools in the first year of age. Encopresis or fecal soiling may occur. The child may report the passage of a huge stool. At times the stools may be hard and even blood streaked. Some parents have noted unusual behavior which has been called "retentive posturing." With such posturing the child forces stools in a retrograde direction in order to avoid defecation. The symptoms may include those of obstruction, anorexia, abdominal pain, irritability, decreased activity, or fecal soiling (paradoxical diarrhea).

On physical examination a left lower quadrant mass is noted and feces are easily palpable in the rectum. Rarely is there evidence of malnutrition or growth failure. The findings of the barium enema, manometrics, and biopsy are contrary to those in Hirschsprung's disease.

The management of functional constipation is difficult. The treatment can be initiated in the emergency department but must be continued in follow-up care. The child should be given cleansing phosphate enemas, in pairs, 1 hour apart. The dose is 1 oz per 10 kg body weight up to a maximum of 4 oz. The enema pairs may be repeated at 12-hour intervals until clearing is achieved. Both tap water and soap suds enemas are hazardous. The child is also given a lubricant such as mineral oil or Condremul at a dose of 1 to 2 oz per day. The oil should be administered twice a day, at bedtime and upon awakening. A multiple vitamin is given at midday. It is also possible to initiate important dietary therapy by increasing whole fresh fruit, cooked fruit, wheat or whole bran, raw vegetables, and juices. Cow's milk and processed sugars should be decreased.

Beyond these beginning treatment steps, the emergency physician must rely on the primary care provider or a referral source to continue the therapy. The ongoing management must be very structured and comprehensive. Frequent visits and educational intervention are required. Often, other psychosocial problems may require treatment. The duration of therapy may be months to years.

ENDOCRINE ABNORMALITIES

A number of endocrine abnormalities may cause chronic constipation. The most important of these is hypothyroidism. It is very important to recognize this during the first 6 months of life as it may herald a treatable cause of mental retardation. Besides constipation, the hypothyroid infant will also manifest feeding problems, sluggishness, somnolence, hypotonia, weak cry, hypothermia, and peripheral edema. Prompt recognition and treatment may spare neurologic sequelae. The reader is referred to Chapter 53, "Endocrine Emergencies," for a more complete discussion of hypothyroidism.

Other endocrine abnormalities which produce constipation include hyperparathyroidism and other hypercalcemic endocrinopathies.

NEUROMUSCULAR PROBLEMS

Constipation may also be a feature of conditions which cause muscular weakness. Children with hypotonia due to Werdnig-Hoffmann disease, myasthenia gravis, congential muscular dystrophy, or diffuse nonprogressive encephalopathy may suffer from constipation. Usually these children will be easily recognized by a careful physical and developmental examination.

PELVIC TUMORS

Rarely, children with pelvic tumors may have chronic constipation as a presenting complaint. It is important to perform a careful examination in all abdominal quadrants. Also the physician must examine the rectum after the stool has been evacuated, lest palpation of a pelvic tumor be missed. In female children the genitalia must be examined in order to document a perforated hymenal membrane. Hydrometrocolpos is often associated with constipation and urinary frequency. Intrauterine pregnancy is a cause of constipation in the adolescent. Chapter 52, "Gynecologic Emergencies," details the common pelvic mass lesions.

PSYCHIATRIC DISORDERS

Children with psychiatric disorders may complain of chronic constipation. In particular, depressed children on psychotropic drugs will be constipated. Other factors which may be contributory are lack of regular diet, lassitude, decreased activity and exercise, and general slowing of bodily function.

Acute Constipation

VIRAL ILLNESS

The most common etiology of acute constipation is a viral illness. Viral illness produces a nonspecific ileus and frequently a decrease in stool frequency. Additionally the child may have decreased intake and in some instances increased water losses through the respiratory tract or from fever.

DRUG-INDUCED

Children taking a medication may be prone to constipation. Those drugs which have been implicated include: antacids, anticholinergics, anticonvulsants, antidepressants, diuretics, iron, muscle relaxants, narcotics, and psychotropic agents. When prescribing any of these drugs the physician may anticipate constipation as a side effect. Children exposed to chronic laxatives may in fact become tolerant to them. Chronic laxative use may create a paradoxical constipation in which the laxative actually induces constipation. Heavy metals such as lead, mercury, arsenic, and phosphorus also produce constipation. Although these metals are generally not ingested as drugs, lead is ingested as pain chips and produces constipation, vomiting, and crampy abdominal pain. The paint chips may be visualized as radiodense particles on an abdominal radiograph.

DIETARY

When children change their diet they may experience an episode of acute constipation. This occurs when the family is experiencing a change in life-style; for example, around holidays, during a move, or on vacation. When the diet has increased carbohydrates (candy), increased milk, or decreased fruit, raw vegetables, whole grains or roughage, constipation is more likely to be dietary in etiology. Management consists of reversal of dietary habits. Dietary change should be attempted prior to the use of laxatives or chemical "stool softeners."

RECTAL PAIN

Rectal pain may be a cause for constipation. Pain is most commonly produced by an anal fissure. The passage of one hard stool may produce the fissure. The child then becomes reluctant to pass additional stools through the fissured area. The surface of the stool, when passed, is usually blood streaked. The diagnosis and management of rectal fissure is covered in Chapter 59, "Abdominal Emergencies."

Pain may be experienced as a child tries to pass a foreign body per rectum. Swollowed objects which have transversed the entire bowel without problem may become painful as rectal muscles squeeze down on them. Other objects are placed in the rectum by the child or a playmate. Rectal foreign bodies can usually be diagnosed either by palpation or abdominal radiograph.

Children may experience rectal pain and constipation following sexual abuse. Sexual abuse must be considered, especially if the child shows any other physical or behavioral changes (see Chapter 68).

DECREASED MOTILITY SYNDROMES

The final category of causes of acute constipation has to do with decreased motility syndromes. In recent years the most important entity has become infantile botulism. The reader is referred to Chapter 45, "Infectious Diseases," for the details of this infection. Constipation has been a very prominent early symptom. Since botulism has life-threatening potential it deserves special consideration in the differential diagnosis of constipation in the 1- to 8-month-old infant.

Other acute causes of decreased gastrointestinal motility are more obvious on physical examination. The child may have other neurologic abnormalities or findings of intestinal obstruction.

References

Davidson M, Kugler MM, Bauer CH: Diagnosis and management in children with severe and protracted constipation and obstruction. *J Pediatr* 62: 261, 1963.

Fitzgerald JF: Difficulties with defecation and elimination in children. *Am Gastroentiol* 6: 283, 1977.

Fleisher DR: Diagnosis and treatment of disorders of defecation in children. *Pediatr Ann* 5: 700, 1976.

Hope JW, Borns PF, Berg PK: Roentgenologic manifestations of Hirschsprung's disease in infancy. *AJR* 91: 217, 1965.

Levine MD: The school child with encopresis. *Pediatr Rev* 2: 285, 1981.

Roy CC, Silverman A, Cozzetto FJ: *Pediatric Clinical Gastroenterology*. C. V. Mosby, St. Louis, 1975.

Schnaufer L, et al.: Differentiation and management of incontinence and constipation problems in children. *Surg Clin North Am* 50: 895, 1970.

CHAPTER **12**

Cough

GERALD B. KOLSKI, M.D., PHD.

INTRODUCTION

Cough is often the initial symptom of a diverse group of diseases. The underlying mechanisms for the initiation of cough should be understood, before launching a discussion of causative conditions.

Coughing can be initiated either voluntarily or by reflexes. Cough receptors within the airway respond to a variety of stimuli by the initiation of cough. With stimulation, a deep inspiration occurs. Glottic closure, diaphragmatic relaxation, and muscle contraction against the closed glottis follow. This produces maximal intrathoracic pressure which allows rapid expulsion of air with glottic opening, causing significant shearing forces that help to clear mucus or foreign particles. Cough receptors in the airway respond to mechanical, thermal, inflammatory, and chemical stimuli. There are receptors in the nose, sinuses, ears, larynx, trachea, and major bronchi.

Mechanical stimuli include the inhalation of particulate matter, such as dust, or the compression of the airway, such as by a vascular ring or tumor. Thermal stimuli initiate coughing by acting through heat receptors in the airway. These receptors are stimulated by loss of heat from the airway and cause coughing with the inhalation of cold, dry air. Inflammatory stimuli produce coughing secondary to increased mucus production, irritation of the airway, and interstitial edema. These may occur secondary to an infectious or immune process. Chemical stimuli may also cause coughing by affecting irritant receptors. Cigarette smoke, air pollutants, and industrial occupational exposures all may produce coughing.

DIFFERENTIAL DIAGNOSIS

As is shown in Figure 12.1, the stimulus for the cough may originate in the upper or lower airway. In addition to the discussion of the airway, it is important to assess whether other systems may be involved in initiation of cough. The principal etiologies for cough are listed in Table 12.1

Nasal, Sinus, and Adenoid Disease

Some controversy surrounds the relationship of coughing to postnasal drip, whether from infection or inflammation in the nose, sinuses, or adenoids, but clinical experience suggests that there is a role for this association. The cough in these circumstances usually sounds loose and is often worse at bedtime when other mechanisms for clearing the mucus from the nasopharynx are not utilized. Nasal and sinus diseases are usually associated with significant congestion, discharge or nasal obstruction. Pale, boggy nasal turbinates, with a clear watery discharge suggest an allergic etiology for nasal or sinus disease. Since significant enlargement of the turbinates predisposes to sinus disease, x-rays may be indicated to assess whether there is involvement of the sinuses. Enlargement of the adenoids may also lead to postnasal drip

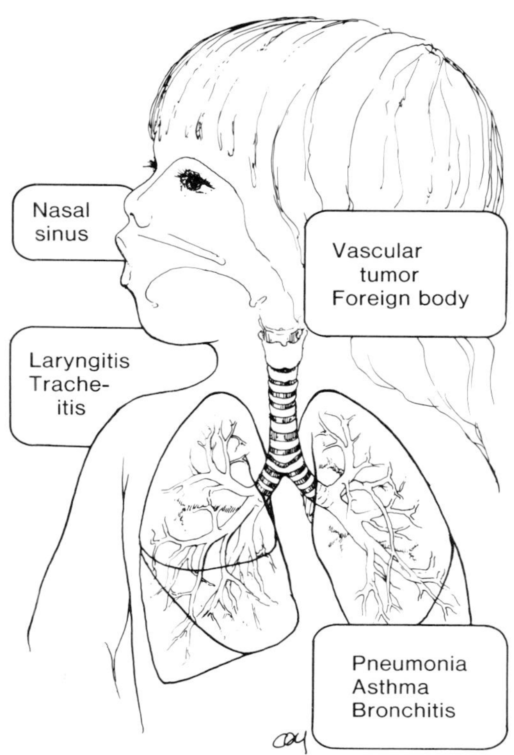

Figure 12.1 Cough stimulus origin.

and discharge with infection, causing an increase in coughing.

Hypopharynx and Larynx

A problem in swallowing coordination, congenital defects of the larynx, or enlargement of the tongue may predispose the child to difficulty with feeding. Such conditions may cause repeated aspiration of food, leading to recurrent coughing, especially with meals. Upper airway congenital defects should also be considered in the very small infant who develops coughing shortly after birth.

Trachea

Anomalies or disease processes of the trachea may cause a cough. Congenital defects, vascular rings, or tracheomalacia may all impair inspiration, thus producing a cough. A narrowing of the airway impedes the clearance of mucus and can thus result in cough. If there is also evidence of aspiration, other anomalies such as a tracheoesophageal fistula have to be considered. The acute onset of cough with fever suggests an infectious process. A dry, hacking cough associated (see Chapter 45) with inspiratory stridor points to laryngeotracheitis (croup). In addition to croup, however, the acute onset of coughing with evidence of inspiratory stridor may also be indicative of a foreign body in the larynx or extrathoracic trachea, especially in those infants who are beginning to crawl and put objects into their mouths.

Lower Airways

Neoplasms may cause lower airway obstruction and cough if they impinge on the airway. A Hodgkin's or non-Hodgkin's lymphoma with enlarged lymph nodes paratracheally can compromise the airway. Nonspecific inflammation of the airway as occurs with asthma, cystic fibrosis, bronchitis, or bronchiectasis leads to increased mucus production and cough. The association of cough with wheezing may help differentiate asthma from other diseases, but any condition in which there is significant obstruction may cause wheezing. In addition to the diseases that produce obstruction of the airway, other inflammatory conditions such as sarcoid may cause cough.

There are numerous infectious diseases which present with coughing, and these are discussed in detail in Chapter 45. However, it is important to review here some of the key characteristics that may help the examiner distinguish between the various classes of infectious agents associated with cough. The characteristic paroxysmal cough followed by a whoop that occurs with pertussis should be recognizable. Pneumonia due to certain viruses (especially adenovirus) and chlamydia may also have paroxysmal cough, though without the whoop. Most viral pneumonia is characterized by a dry, nonproductive cough. In contrast, bacterial pneumonia usually causes a cough producing purulent sputum.

Gastrointestinal Tract

In addition to pathology in the chest, several other systems may be involved in

Table 12.1
Etiologies for Cough in Children

I. Nasal, Sinus, Adenoid, and Ear Disease
- A. Infection
  - 1. Rhinitis—upper respiratory infection
  - 2. Sinusitis
  - 3. Adenoiditis
- B. Irritation: foreign body in ear, nose
- C. Tumor
  - 1. Nasal Polyps
  - 2. Neoplasm
- D. Inflammation
  - 1. Allergic rhinitis/sinusitis
  - 2. Nonallergic rhinitis

II. Hypopharynx and Larynx
- A. Infection
  - 1. Tonsillitis
  - 2. Laryngitis
- B. Congenital anomalies
  - 1. Cleft palate—predisposes to aspiration and nasal sinus disease
  - 2. Laryngotracheomalacia
  - 3. Laryngotracheal cleft
  - 4. Laryngeal web
- C. Tumors
  - 1. Vascular—hemangiomas
  - 2. Benign—papillomas
  - 3. Malignant
- D. Inflammation: allergic—laryngeal edema
- E. Neuromuscular diseases: swallowing dysfunction

III. Large Airways
- A. Infection: tracheitis
- B. Congenital anomalies
  - 1. Vascular ring
  - 2. Tracheal web
  - 3. Tracheoesophageal fistula
- C. Tumors
  - 1. External or internal compression of trachea
  - 2. Mediastinal tumors
- D. Irritation
  - 1. Noxious fumes
  - 2. Cigarette or marijuana smoking
  - 3. Inhaled particulates

IV. Small Airways/Lungs
- A. Infection
  - 1. Pneumonia
  - 2. Bronchiectasis
  - 3. Bronchiolitis
  - 4. Pleuritis
- B. Congenital anomalies
  - 1. Sequestered lung
  - 2. Congenital heart disease (with congestive failure)
- C. Inflammation
  - 1. Asthma
  - 2. Cystic fibrosis
  - 3. Chronic bronchitis
  - 4. Immotile cilia syndrome
  - 5. Sarcoidosis
- D. Tumors—with airway compression
  - 1. Lymphomas
  - 2. Mediastinal masses

V. Associated Systems
- A. CNS
  - 1. Psychogenic cough
  - 2. Phenic vagal irritation
- B. Gastrointestinal tract
  - 1. Gastroesophageal reflux
  - 2. Achalasia

initiating cough, most commonly the gastrointestinal tract. A direct connection between the GI tract and the airway, as in tracheoesophageal fistula may cause cough in the neonate. Gastroesophageal reflux has also been found to be a significant cause of pulmonary pathology and may be the etiology for recurrent pneumonia or asthma.

Central Nervous System

The central nervous system may be involved in initiating cough. Neurologic dysfunction may lead to incoordination of swallowing, absence of gag reflex, or a combination of these. Additionally the coughing mechanism itself may interact with the CNS as in the syndrome designated as cough syncope. In this situation, increases in intrathoracic pressure associated with cough decrease blood flow to the CNS and causes the patient to faint.

EVALUATION AND DECISION

In trying to establish a differential diagnosis for cough, it is helpful to separate

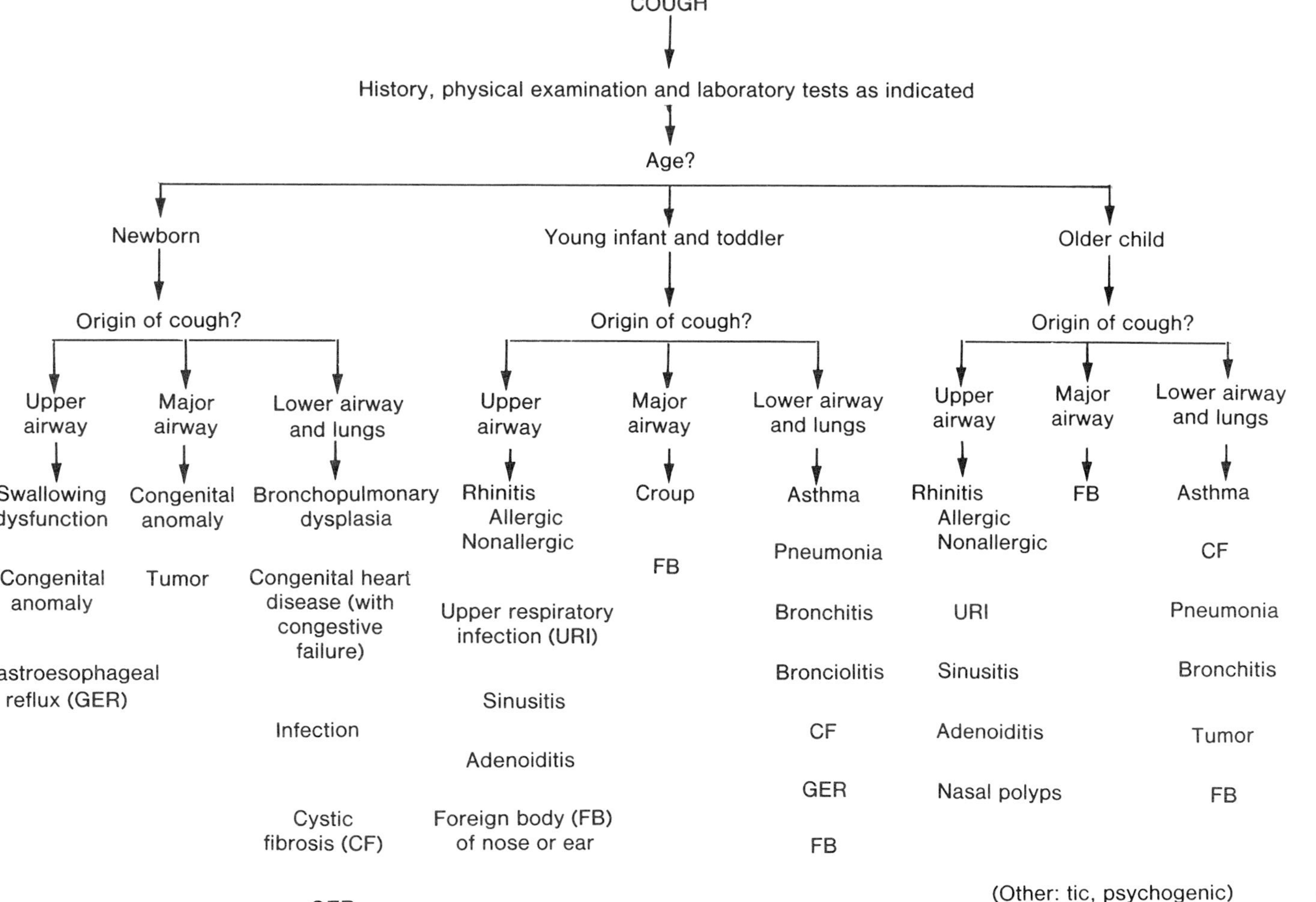

Figure 12.2 Diagnostic approach to cough.

children by age. Patients who present very early in life with coughing, especially in the neonatal period, are more likely to have congenital anomalies. A child who does well in the newborn period but develops a cough later is less likely to have a congenital anomaly of the airway. Above the age of 6 months, the acute onset of a cough should lead the physician to suspect foreign body aspiration. In the older age group, the common etiologies for cough can be divided into infectious causes (viral and bacterial), asthma, bronchitis, cystic fibrosis or nasal and sinus disease. However, an atypical clinical picture may suggest an unusual etiology, and it then becomes very important to attempt to ascertain where the cough is originating anatomically and what is its character. The diagnostic approach to cough is outlined in Figure 12.2.

In addition to the patient's age, the most important factor in making a specific diagnosis is the ascertainment of the anatomic origin of the cough. The characteristics of the cough itself, such as its timing, quality, and productivity, and associated features all can give valuable information as to the level in the respiratory tract at which the cough arises.

Timing

The time of day and the relationship to meals, environment, exercise, or position, are important in assessing the cause of the cough. Coughing which occurs after eating and at nighttime may be an indication that there is significant gastroesophageal reflux. In asthmatic children, coughing increases after exercise and at nighttime; such a cough may be the initial manifestation of a hyperactive airway.

Quality

The quality of the cough may be helpful in pinpointing the anatomic origin. A dry barking type of cough indicates upper airway inflammation as is seen with croup. If there is a change in voice along with the dry cough, laryngeal involvement is likely. A paroxysmal cough, associated with a whoop, suggests pertussis, whereas without the whoop it may indicate a tracheal or bronchial foreign body. A "brassy" cough accompanies tracheal irritation.

Productivity

The sputum associated with a cough may provide a clue to the diagnosis. An acute productive cough has a different significance than a dry perennial cough. The color, viscosity (thin or thick), and amount of sputum should always be assessed. In children it is often important to try to determine whether the patient is producing sputum but swallowing it. Parents may have an idea of whether the cough appears to be productive. Younger children often will vomit after swallowing a significant amount of mucus, and the nature of the vomitus may indicate how much sputum is being produced. A productive cough usually comes from an inflammatory response, such as a bacterial pneumonia, but may also be seen in patients with bronchospasm, after the spasm has been relieved.

Associated Features

In trying to assess the etiology for a cough, it is also very important to be aware of the circumstances surrounding the cough. The examination of organ systems not directly associated with the chest may shed light on the underlying cause of the cough. Fever, rash, rhinorrhea, headache, or sinus tenderness may all suggest specific etiologies for cough. The cough associated with hives and angioedema is likely to be of an allergic nature and to be associated with bronchospasm. The cough which comes on with high fever and shaking chills is more likely to be due to an infection.

In addition to ascertaining the patient's age and the particular manifestations of the cough, the diagnostic evaluation must include a particularly thorough physical examination of the airway and chest. If the patient is having difficulty on inspiration, the etiology of the cough is probably in the upper airway. If, however, the difficulty appears to be on expiration, the level of obstruction is probably within the chest. The child with a toxic general appearance often has an acute infection. The association of a rash may point to either an allergic or infectious process. On speculum examination of the nose, swollen turbinates, significant discharge, or drainage from the ostia of the sinuses may localize the cause of the cough to the upper airway. An examination of the throat should search for anatomical abnormalities and evidence of significant postnasal discharge. Auscultation of the chest indicates whether there is inspiratory or expiratory difficulty, equal aeration of the chest, or any significant localizing findings.

After the physical examination, the appropriate radiologic tests may be performed. The radiologic tests that may be helpful depend upon the likely site of pathology and include: sinus films, a lateral neck x-ray, fluoroscopy of the upper airway, chest x-ray, and barium swallow. Occasionally more sophisticated tests are necessary such as: tomograms of the chest and airway, or forced expiratory films (or lateral decubitus films in the preschool child) when looking for a foreign body. Where appropriate, some blood tests may be useful such as arterial blood gases, a complete blood count with differential, total eosinophil count, and erythrocyte sedimentation rate. Where an infectious etiology is felt to be likely, appropriate cultures may include: nasopharyngeal cultures for virus or bacteria, blood cultures, fluorescent antibody staining of secretions for virus or *Bordetella pertussis* and Gram stain and culture of sputum. Pulmonary functions in a cooperative patient can be especially helpful in determining the level and degree of obstruction. Evidence of obstruction in a patient with chronic cough can establish a diagnosis of asthma.

TREATMENT

The treatment for cough should always first focus on assessing the etiology for the cough. If a foreign body is lodged in the ear, nose, or airway, removal will be curative. If there is evidence of a bacterial infection, appropriate antibiotics should be used. Where there is underlying bronchospasm or a hyperreactive airway, bronchodilators are effective. Antihistamines and decongestants may be helpful to control the increased secretions in the allergic child. The most important step is to first determine the etiology for the cough which then allows for appropriate therapy.

CHAPTER **13**

Crying and Colic in Early Infancy

FRED M. HENRETIG, M.D.

INTRODUCTION

Crying is the means by which an infant may express discomfort, ranging from normal hunger and desire for company to severe, life-threatening illness. Many common minor irritations or illnesses need to be excluded by careful history and physical examination. Often, however, a normal thriving baby will develop a chronic pattern of daily paroxysms of irritability and crying known as colic. The attacks usually have their onset in the second to third week of life and may last for several hours, more commonly in the late afternoon or evening. The typical episode is described as paroxysmal crying that develops into a piercing scream as if the baby were in pain. The child may draw up his legs, the abdomen may appear distended, and flatus may be passed, leading the parents to conclude that the child is experiencing severe abdominal distress. The emergency physician may be confronted with such a patient and his worried, occasionally hostile parents (usually no earlier than 12 midnight!). Colic cannot be cured in the emergency department. Establishing an orderly approach to the infant with unexplained crying is important, however, in order to rule out the occasional physical illness and to provide preliminary guidance to the family.

Any unpleasant sensation can cause an infant to cry. There are numerous unproven theories about the etiology of colic. Cow's

Table 13.1
Conditions Associated with Abrupt Onset of Unconsolable Crying in Young Infants

I. Discomfort Due to Identifiable Illness

- A. Head and neck
  1. Meningitis
  2. Skull fracture/subdural hematoma
  3. Glaucoma
  4. Foreign body (especially eyelash) in eye
  5. Corneal abrasion
  6. Otitis media
  7. Caffey's disease
  8. Battered child syndrome
- B. Gastrointestinal
  1. Excess air due to improper feeding or burping technique
  2. Gastroenteritis
  3. Intussusception
  4. Anal fissure
  5. Milk intolerance
- C. Genitourinary
  1. Torsion of testis
  2. Incarcerated hernia
  3. Urinary tract infections
- D. Integument
  1. Open diaper pin
  2. Burn
  3. Strangulated finger, toe, penis (often due to an encircling hair)
- E. Musculoskeletal
  1. Battered child syndrome
  2. Extremity fracture (following a fall)

II. Colic—Recurrent Paroxysmal Attacks of Crying

milk allergy, immaturity of gastrointestinal tract or central nervous system, parental anxiety, poor feeding technique, and/or individual temperament characteristics have all been invoked. No one theory (or concomitant therapy) has gained uniform acceptance. Colic may be a syndrome that represents the manifestations of some or all of the above factors in varying degrees, in a normal population of babies whose tendency to cry varies along a normal distribution. Brazelton studied 50 normal infants prospectively from birth and found their average total crying time per day varied from approximately 1 hour at 2 weeks of age, to 3 hours at 6 weeks, and then decreased to 1 hour at 12 weeks. The range of crying spanned from about 1 hour/day in the "light fussers" to about 4 hours/day in the "heavy fussers" at 6 weeks of age. These estimates of crying time were made in a middleclass, private practice population whose mothers were advised to address any obvious needs the baby might have by offering food, burping, rocking, changing the diaper if necessary, etc. Thus, these estimates of crying time over the first 12 weeks of life seem to reflect a certain degree of unconsolable crying behavior which normal infants are destined to exhibit in the first 3 months of life (Table 13.1). The most persistent cryers in such a group would be diagnosed by most pediatricians as having "colic."

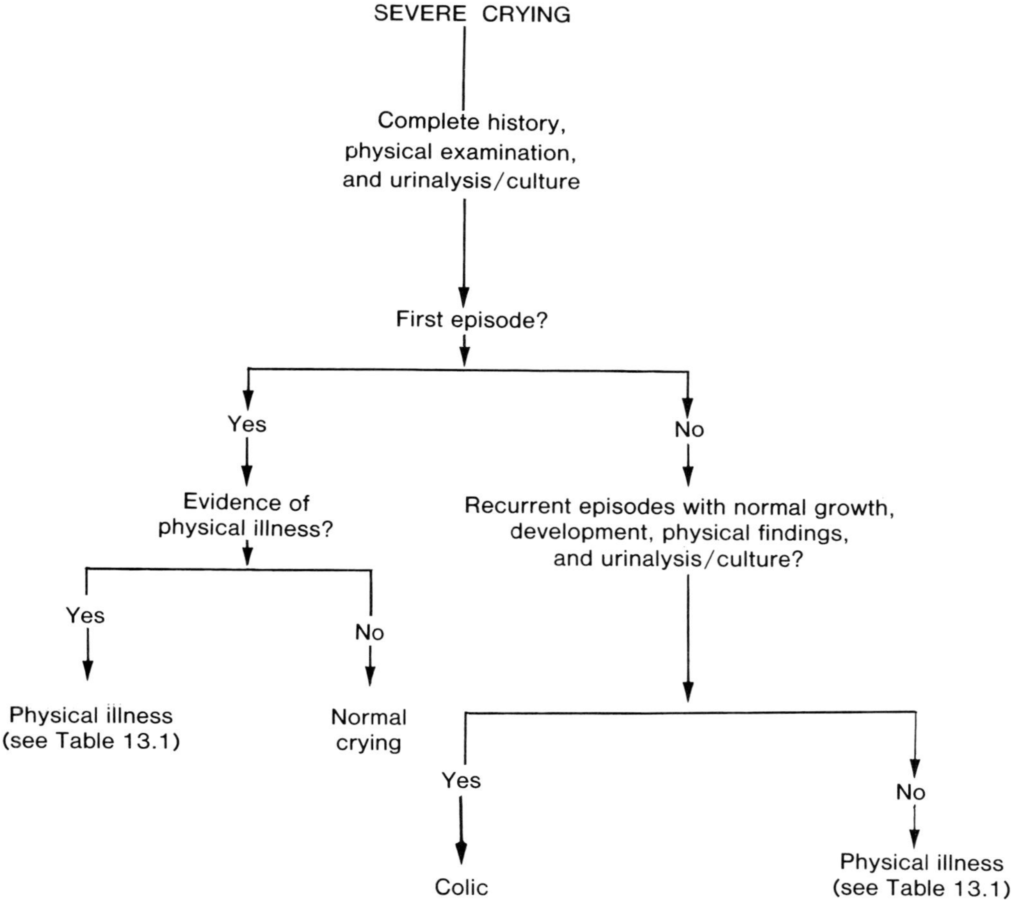

Figure 13.1 Approach to abrupt onset of severe crying in infancy.

EVALUATION AND DECISION

A careful history and physical examination with emphasis on head, eyes, ears, skin, abdomen, genitalia and extremities, plus analysis and culture of a urine specimen will usually enable the physician to diagnose identifiable illnesses or injuries causing severe paroxysms of crying (see Table 13.1). Over the time during which the crying attacks recur, the infant must demonstrate adequate weight gain (average 5 to 7 oz/week in the first months of life) and absence of physical disorders on several examinations, before underlying illnesses can be excluded and colic confidently diagnosed (Fig. 13.1). When it becomes clear that a given infant is experiencing colic, the practitioner faces a vexing problem. No dramatic cure is currently available, but the symptoms almost invariably resolve within 3 months of onset. In a treatment study by O'Donovan and Bradstock, blindly comparing homatropine/phenobarbital in alcohol, phenobarbital in alcohol, alcohol alone, and placebo, improvement in symptoms occurred over a 2-week period in 70% of babies regardless of modality. The physician can reassure the parents that their baby is thriving and will outgrow his colic.

The emergency department physician needs to be aware of colic as an entity, to initiate the evaluation described above, to rule out acute treatable illness, and to refer the family to a pediatrician for follow-up. They must understand that colic is not serious and does not last forever but will probably be a nuisance for several weeks to come. For immediate amelioration of crying at the time of the emergency department visit, no drug therapy or feeding change is recommended. Rather, most colicky babies derive some temporary relief from rhythmical motion, such as rocking, being carried or riding in a car, and continual monotonous sounds like those from a washing machine or electric fan. A purposefully chosen circuitous route for the car ride home (which combines motion and sound) should suffice as therapy for the first visit.

References

Brazelton TB: Crying in infancy. *Pediatrics* 29: 579–588, 1962.

Du JNH: Colic as the sole symptom of urinary tract infection in infants. *Can Med Assoc J* 115: 334–339, 1976.

Farron L, Farron D: The screaming baby blues. *Parents Magazine* 56–60, July 1981. (An excellent reference for parents)

O'Donovan JC, Bradstock AS: The failure of conventional drug therapy in the management of infantile colic. *Am J Dis Child* 133: 999–1001, 1979.

Wessel MA, et al.: Paroxysmal fussing in infancy, sometimes called "colic." *Pediatrics* 14: 421–435, 1975.

CHAPTER 14

Diarrhea

GARY R. FLEISHER, M.D.

INTRODUCTION

Diarrhea refers to an increase in the number of stools and/or a softening in their consistency. Because of the variability in the frequency and type of stools among children, absolute limits of normalcy are difficult to define. Rather, any deviation from the usual pattern established by an individual should arouse concern regardless of the actual number or water content. Some infants, particularly those who are breast fed, often have 5 or 6 loose stools daily as their normal routine; other healthy infants may produce only one formed stool every other day.

DIFFERENTIAL DIAGNOSIS

Diarrhea, with or without vomiting, frequently prompts a visit to the emergency department. Although most bouts of diarrhea seen in emergency departments in the United States are the result of infections that are self-limited, the potential for complications warrants a cautious approach. All children with diarrhea risk the development of dehydration, and those with bacterial infections may become bacteremic. Additionally, diarrhea may be the presenting sign of serious gastrointestinal disorders, such as an intussusception, Hirschsprung's disease, or malabsorptive syndromes. Table 14.1 presents the differential diagnosis of diarrhea.

EVALUATION AND DECISION

A diagnostic approach to the pediatric patient with diarrhea is outlined in Figure 14.1. The initial evaluation of the child with diarrhea should serve the dual purpose of exploring the possible etiologies and assessing the degree of illness. Pre-existing conditions in the child may account for the diarrhea or predispose to unusual causes; in particular, the emergency department physician should search for a history of previous gastrointestinal surgery or other ailments such as ulcerative colitis or regional enteritis. Immunodeficiency syndromes, neoplasms, and immunosuppressive therapy all lead to an increased susceptibility to infection. Institutionalized children and those recently returning from underdeveloped countries are more likely to harbor a bacterial or parasitic pathogen.

With the initial interview the physician should attempt to historically reconstruct the child's intake and output during the course of the illness. Detailed questions as to the number and size of stools, the frequency of emesis, and the amount of liquid taken orally allow for an estimate of fluid balance. Decreases in the frequency or volume of urination (or the number of diaper changes in the infant) suggest an inadequate output reflecting the development of dehydration.

The general physical examination can provide a clue to an underlying illness in the child who appears malnourished or small for his age. The weight of the child should always be measured carefully and compared to those previously recorded in the chart. If fever is present, infectious etiologies are most likely. The pulse and blood pressure, together with the turgor of the skin and mucous membranes, are useful

Table 14.1
Causes of Diarrhea

I. Infections
A. Enteral
1. Viruses: rotavirus, Norwalk agent, enteroviruses
2. Bacteria: *Salmonella, Shigella, Yersinia, Campylobacter,* pathogenic *Escherichia coli, Vibrio* spp., tuberculosis
3. Parasites: *Giardia, Entamoeba*
B. Nongastrointestinal (parenteral diarrhea)
II. Dietary Disturbances
Overfeeding, food allergy, starvation stools
III. Anatomic Abnormalities
Intussusception, Hirschsprung's disease, partial obstruction, blind loop syndrome, intestinal lymphangiectasis, short bowel syndrome
IV. Inflammatory Bowel Disease
Ulcerative colitis, Crohn's disease
V. Malabsorption or Increased Secretion
Cystic fibrosis, celiac disease, dissacharidase deficiency, acrodermatitis enteropathica, secretory neoplasms
VI. Systemic Illnesses
A. Immunodeficiency
B. Endocrinopathy: hyperthyroidism, hypoparathyroidism, congenital adrenal hyperplasia
VII. Psychogenic Disturbances (Irritable Colon Syndrome)
VIII. Miscellaneous
Antibiotic-associated, secondary lactase deficiency, neonatal drug withdrawal, toxins, HUS

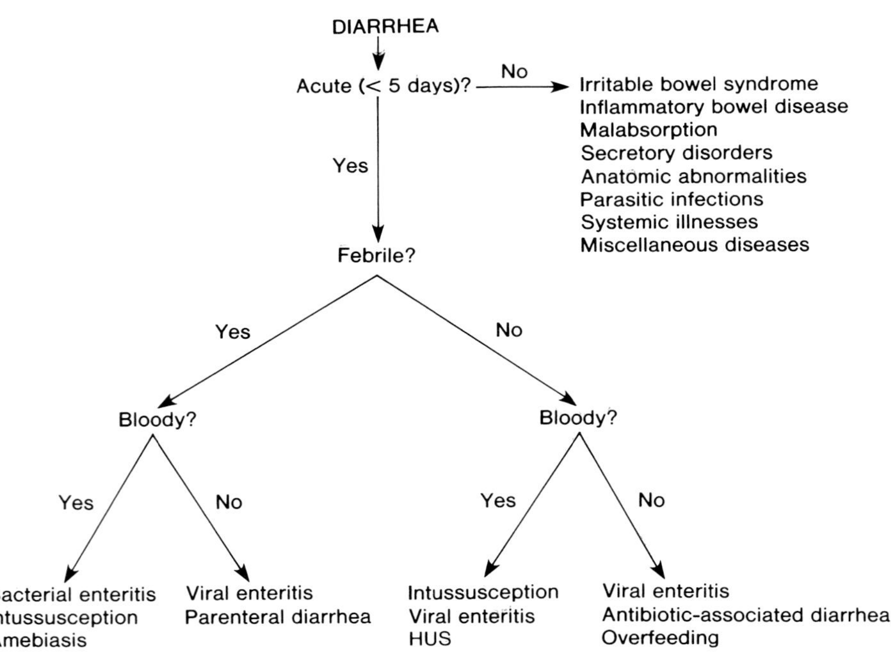

Figure 14.1 Algorithm for the evaluation of the child with diarrhea.

Table 14.2
Clinical Findings in Dehydration

Degree of Dehydration (%)	Skin	Mucosa	Pulse	Blood Pressure
0	Good turgor	Moist	Normal	Normal
5	Dry	Dry	Orthostatic increase	Orthostatic decrease
10	Tenting present	Very dry	Mildly increased	Mildly decreased
15	Poorly perfused	Parched	Markedly increased	Markedly decreased

in assessing the degree of dehydration (Table 14.2), except in the child who has hypernatremia. On abdominal examination, the finding of a mass (regional enteritis, intussusception) or evidence of obstruction is important.

A rectal examination should be performed in the child with chronic diarrhea. In the child with overflow diarrhea secondary to chronic constipation, the rectal ampulla contains a large amount of hard stool, but it is often empty in the patient with Hirschsprung's disease.

Acute Diarrhea

Most children coming to the emergency department with diarrhea have an acute illness of less than 5 days duration. In the majority of these patients, infections are the cause of their distress. Both infections of the gastrointestinal tract and those of other structures (otitis media, pyelonephritis) produce diarrhea in the child. An increase in stools due to an infection at a site remote from the gastrointestinal tract is referred to as parenteral diarrhea.

The child with acute diarrhea and a fever almost invariably has an infectious etiology for the gastrointestinal disturbance (p. 388). Although children with viral gastroenteritis may have a small amount of bright red blood on their stools or diaper from local irritation, the complaint of bloody diarrhea points more to a bacterial pathogen. Additional explanations for bloody diarrhea in the febrile child include inflammatory bowel disease, amebiasis, and intussusception.

In evaluating any child with a bloody diarrheal stool, the emergency department physician must consider the possibility of intussusception (Chapter 59). The associated signs and symptoms of vomiting, abdominal pain, and an abdominal mass may be absent. A barium enema under the supervision of a surgeon is needed if intussusception is suspected.

In the afebrile child with the acute onset of diarrhea, a viral infection remains the most common cause. If the child is taking an antibiotic, alterations in the bacterial flora of the bowel secondary to the medication should be suspected as the etiology of the diarrhea. Blood in the stools, particularly in association with vomiting and abdominal pain, warrants consideration of intussusception. Other possibilities include giardiasis, overfeeding in the infant, and, rarely, toxins.

Most children with the acute onset of diarrhea will be judged to have viral infections of the gastrointestinal tract or parenteral diarrhea and will not require any laboratory tests. However, several findings point to a bacterial enteritis and the need for a stool culture, including: (1) blood in the stools, (2) toxicity on examination, (3) travel in underdeveloped countries, (4) exposure to individuals living in institutional settings or known to have bacterial gastroenteritis, and (5) persistence after the initiation of dietary therapy. If bacterial enteritis is a consideration in the infant under 6 months of age, the physician should examine a stool smear for the presence of polymorphonuclear leukocytes after staining with methylene blue. The finding of large numbers of inflammatory cells indicates a bacterial infection and influences further management (see Chapter 45). When dehydration is clinically apparent (2 to 3%), the electrolytes, BUN, and urine specific gravity should be studied to help in the assessment of fluid loss and dehydration.

Chronic Diarrhea

Chronic diarrhea precipitates an emergency department visit by a child less frequently than does acute gastroenteritis. However, an apparent worsening of a longstanding disease may be a final frustration on the part of the parents, particularly on a weekend when the family's usual physician may be unavailable. The evaluation of chronic diarrhea usually requires a period of observation and laboratory evaluation beyond the scope of the emergency department. In the management of these children, the role of the emergency department physician is to select out those few children with emergent conditions and refer the remainder to their regular source of care. Particularly in the infant, consideration must be given to Hirschsprung's disease. A history of delayed passage of meconium, constipation since birth, and abdominal distension are compatible with this disease. A stool culture serves to diagnose the bacterial infections of the gastrointestinal tract and gives a head start on the evaluation to the physician who sees the child subsequently.

The child who returns to the emergency department with the persistence of an acute diarrhea illness, presumed to be viral in origin and with no evidence of malnutrition or dehydration, may often be managed without an extensive evaluation. Three causes are frequent: (1) bacterial infections, (2) secondary lactase deficiency from mucosal sloughing, and (3) starvation stools in the child who has inadvertently been continued on a clear liquid diet for several days. A stool culture should always be obtained. If the child has remained on a clear liquid diet, gradual refeeding is recommended. Milk and all milk products should be proscribed when secondary lactase deficiency is suspected.

TREATMENT

The treatments for the myriad causes of diarrhea are covered in the medical and surgical sections. However, the therapy for viral gastroenteritis or parenteral diarrhea merits a brief summary. Children with these conditions who are not dehydrated almost invariably respond to the institution of a diet limited to clear liquids for 24 hours, and then gradual refeeding. Antibiotics are contraindicated unless a specific treatable bacterial infection is identified. Antidiarrheal agents have no demonstrated effectiveness in childhood, and the combination of dephenoxylate and atropine (Lomotil), in particular, carries a grave risk of toxicity.

References

Blacklow NR, Cukor G: Viral gastroenteritis. *N Engl J Med* 304: 397, 1981.

Blair J, Fitzgerald JF: Treatment of nonspecific diarrhea in infants. *Clin Pediatr* 13: 333, 1974.

Gurwith MS, Williams TW: Gastroenteritis in children: A two-year review in Manitoba I. Etiology *J Infect Dis* 136: 239, 1977.

Pickering LK, Evans EJ, Munoz O, et al.: Prospective study of enteropathogens in children with diarrhea in Houston and Mexico. *J Pediatr* 93: 383, 1978.

Roy CC, Silverman A, Cozetto FJ: Diarrhea disorders. In *Pediatric Clinical Gastroenterology*, p. 173. C.V. Mosby, St. Louis, 1975.

CHAPTER **15**

Disturbed Child

JOHN SARGENT, M.D., AND GORDON R. HODAS, M.D.

INTRODUCTION

In this chapter an approach is presented for the diagnosis of the acutely disturbed child manifesting agitation and aggression or withdrawal. Further details of management of the conditions discussed below may be found in Chapter 70, "Psychiatric Emergencies."

Human beings generally respond to stress or personal threats by developing a fight or flight response. They either become aggressive in an attempt to confront the threat, or withdraw to maintain safety. Throughout development, regardless of age or developmental stage, children respond to threats either through fight (agitation and aggression) or flight (withdrawal). Although these behaviors may differ in their manifestations at different ages, the underlying responses are essentially similar throughout childhood.

At times the child's ways of responding to external events and changes in the environment are inadequate. In other situations a previously supportive environment no longer provides security and protection. As a result, the child may no longer be in control of his social and emotional responses. It is at this point of crisis that the emergency physician meets both the child and his caretakers.

Although agitation and withdrawal are distinctly different behaviors, it is important to recognize that a child in crisis can easily fluctuate from one to the other. For example, a sullen, withdrawn, and uncooperative adolescent may become agitated, angry, and disruptive in the face of additional stress. In addition, both agitation and withdrawal can result from the same underlying physical and psychological causes. Thus, both agitation and withdrawal as presenting symptoms in children in crisis are signs of significant emotional stress which the emergency physician should recognize and be prepared to treat.

The agitated child typically is anxious, upset, and unresponsive to attempts at support. The child may pace back and forth and may threaten staff or family. Speech is usually loud and may be abusive. Some, but not all, children may also be disoriented and out of contact with reality. Younger children when agitated may be behaviorally out of control, running about the examining room and having a severe temper tantrum. They may cry or strike out at the parent or physician. Older children or adolescents may be distraught, sullen, and angry as they meet the examiner. It is important for the emergency physician to be aware of his own responses to agitated children; feelings of anger and frustration in the physician often reflect the amount of stress that the child is experiencing. On the other hand, some children or adolescents may appear to be calm and under control when seen in the emergency department; however, information from the parents reveals significant destructiveness at home prior to coming to the hospital. In many cases, the improvement in the child's behavior in the emergency department is a response to the structure provided and the child's sense that help with the crisis will be forthcoming.

The withdrawn child primarily demonstrates significant unresponsiveness to the demands of his situation. He is inappropriately quiet and does not attempt to develop any relationship with the emergency physician. For younger children this withdrawal may be demonstrated by clinging behavior, whining, and crying. The child may be unresponsive to parents as well as the physician, instead responding to internal stimuli and demonstrating inappropriate affect. Older children may be sullen, unresponsive, or apathetic when asked about the precipitant of the current emergency department visit. It is important to distinguish emotional withdrawal from shyness, which is a temperamental quality, within the range of normal behavior.

DIFFERENTIAL DIAGNOSIS

A wide variety of both medical and psychiatric conditions can lead to a child developing significant agitation and withdrawal. These disorders are listed in Table 15.1 and include severe psychiatric disturbances, life-threatening medical conditions, and minor aberrations in the child's ability to respond to stressful events. Regardless of the underlying cause, an emotional state develops which disrupts the child's daily routine and the family's usual ways of coping with stress. Resumption of normal growth and development for the child requires that the underlying cause of the presenting behavior is appreciated and addressed.

Table 15.1
Differential Diagnosis of Agitation and Withdrawal in Childhood

- *I.* *Psychosis,* caused by:
  - A. Medical illness
  - B. Ingestion of toxic substance
  - C. Pervasive developmental disorder, i.e., autism
  - D. Adult type schizophrenia
  - E. Manic depressive illness
- *II.* *Depression*
- *III.* *Conduct Disorder*
- *IV.* *Adjustment Reaction of Childhood or Adolescence*
- *V.* *Attention Deficit Disorder*
- *VI.* *Medical Illness in the Absence of Psychosis*, i.e., thyrotoxicosis, temporal lobe epilepsy
- *VII.* *Sensory Deficit:* blindness, deafness
- *VIII.* *Severe Communication Disorder*, e.g., childhood aphasia

Psychosis

An acutely psychotic child may present to the emergency department as either anxious and agitated or as preoccupied and withdrawn. Psychosis refers to a mental state in which major disturbances in thinking, relating, and reality testing occur. Psychotic patients do not express themselves clearly and have difficulty answering direct questions. They may also be extremely suspicious and hostile.

Psychosis may be the result of a psychiatric disorder or a physical cause. Psychiatric causes of psychosis include early childhood autism, childhood schizophrenia, adolescent onset schizophrenia, and manic depressive disorder. Physical or organic causes of psychosis include either an ongoing medical illness or an acute intoxication with an exogenous substance. It is important that the emergency physician be able to determine the etiology of psychosis in a child, since treatment presupposes proper diagnosis.

Certain aspects of the child's mental status help to distinguish between psychiatrically based and organic psychosis. These differentiating features are outlined in Table 15.2. The child or adolescent who has developed an organic psychosis is likely to be disoriented, particularly with regard to time and place. The child's recent memory is also typically impaired in organic psychoses, and the child may be unable to describe the onset of his problems coherently. In addition, hallucinations when present are usually visual or tactile rather than auditory (though the latter may also be present). In contrast, the child with a psychiatrically based psychosis is likely to be oriented to person, place, and time, and should be able to report recent events accurately. Other intellectual and cognitive functions usually remain intact. Hallucinations, when present, tend to be auditory in nature, and a greater sense of suspiciousness is common. The rate of onset of psychosis is also revealing. Organic psychosis is more likely to be acute in onset or the result of acute deterioration in an ongoing chronic condition. A psychiatrically based psychosis is more likely to be gradual in onset, following a prolonged period of progressive social and emotional withdrawal.

Table 15.3 lists medical conditions in childhood which may induce, at some point in their course, acute psychosis with either agitation or withdrawal. As can be noted from the table, many of these illnesses are chronic conditions which may have been present for some time and under treatment. Therefore, it is extremely important with all psychotic children to obtain an accurate history of current and previous medical problems. Other medical conditions causing psychosis such as head injury and Reye's syndrome may develop acutely and may progress rapidly to unconsciousness and death unless identified and treated.

Table 15.4 lists drugs which may lead to psychosis characterized by either agitation or withdrawal. Some of these drugs are used illicitly and others are prescription drugs that are ingested either accidently or on purpose. In obtaining a history, a frequent important clue in intoxications is the acute onset of disordered thinking in the presence of visual hallucinations. Previous history of drug abuse and the availability of toxic substances are other important historical clues to the diagnosis of acute drug intoxication. Intoxications with alcohol, sedatives, antidepressants, anticholinergic agents and heavy metals can all be life-threatening if enough of the agent has been ingested and absorbed. Appropriate medical therapy must be instituted as rapidly as possible.

Psychiatric conditions leading to psychosis in the child or adolescent are frequently extremely distressing and may also be life-threatening. This threat to life can occur when the child's hallucinations are so disturbing that suicide is sought for desired relief. Further, as a part of psychosis, a

Table 15.3
Medical Conditions Which May Lead to Psychosis

I. Central Nervous System Lesions
- A. Tumor
- B. Brain abscess
- C. Cerebral hemorrhage
- D. Meningitis or encephalitis
- E. Temporal lobe epilepsy
- F. Closed head trauma

II. Cerebral Hypoxia
- A. Pulmonary insufficiency
- B. Severe anemia
- C. Cardiac failure
- D. Carbon monoxide poisoning

III. Metabolic and Endocrine Disorders
- A. Electrolyte imbalance
- B. Hypoglycemia
- C. Hypocalcemia
- D. Thyroid disease (hyper- and hypo-)
- E. Adrenal disease (hyper- and hypo-)
- F. Uremia
- G. Hepatic failure
- H. Diabetes mellitus
- I. Porphyria
- J. Reye's syndrome

IV. Collagen-Vascular Diseases
- A. Systemic lupus erythematosus
- B. Polyarteritis nodosa

V. Infections
- A. Malaria
- B. Typhoid fever
- C. Subacute bacterial endocarditis

Table 15.2
Differentiating Features of Organic and Psychiatrically Induced Psychosis[a]

Evaluation Feature	Organic Psychosis	Psychiatrically Based Psychosis
Onset	Acute	Gradual
Pathologic autonomic signs	May be present	Absent
Vital signs	May be abnormal	Normal
Orientation	Impaired	Intact
Recent memory	Impaired	Intact
Intellectual ability	May be impaired	Intact
Hallucinations	Visual	Auditory

[a] Children with both functional and organic psychoses will have impaired reality testing, inappropriate affect, thought disorder, poor behavior control, and disturbed relating ability.

Table 15.4
Exogenous Substances Causing Psychosis Following Ingestion of Significant Quantity

Alcohol
Barbiturates
Antipsychotics (e.g. phenothiazines)
Amphetamines
Hallucinogens—LSD, peyote, mescaline
Marihuana
Phencyclidene (PCP)
Quaalude
Anticholinergic compounds
Heavy metals
Cocaine
Corticosteroids
Reserpine
Opioids (e.g., heroin, methadone)

child may develop a delusional system such that he attacks another person who is seen as threatening. The psychotic child or adolescent may neglect his physical well-being through sleep deprivation and malnutrition. These deprivations themselves may intensify the child's vulnerability and exacerbate the psychosis. Thus, when dealing with the psychotic child or adolescent, it is imperative that the emergency physician evaluate the suicidal and homicidal potential of the patient as well as his overall physical condition and his ability to maintain himself.

Depression

Other children who may be brought to the emergency room for agitated or withdrawn behavior are those who are severely depressed. These children are more likely to be oriented, coherent in their thinking and able to discern reality from fantasy. However, there may be a history of deterioration in social and intellectual performance over the preceding months and evidence of withdrawal from important activities and relationships. The child may be described by his parents as being apathetic and may be extremely sad. The child may present as withdrawn and hopeless and may be quite difficult for the emergency physician to engage in conversation. Other depressed children may present as primarily anxious and angry, with minor concerns causing preoccupation and outbursts. Precipitants of depression and a sense of helplessness may include parental divorce or separation, loss of a parent through death, or a recent devaluation of personal abilities through poor academic performance, peer rejection, or the onset of significant physical illness. Once depression is identified as the cause of the child's agitation or withdrawal, it is extremely important for the emergency physician to inquire about the presence and nature of suicidal ideation. The physician should also ask about disturbances in appetite and sleep.

Other Conditions

Other psychiatric conditions, such as conduct disorders with severe behavioral disruption, adjustment reactions with interruption of normal coping mechanisms, and attention deficit disorder may also lead a child to present in the emergency department with significant agitation or withdrawal. With each of these problems, the emergency physician's first task is to screen for suicidal or homicidal ideation and intent. Then, after evaluating the problem, he can consider and pursue alternatives for further treatment and referral. The child or adolescent with a conduct disorder will often have a history of significant behavioral disruption, such as aggressiveness, stealing, fire-setting, truancy, and other forms of delinquency. The child presents as oriented and responsive, but may also be quite angry and resentful about being brought to the emergency department. The child's behavior may improve in the emergency department when it is clear to him that misbehavior or temper tantrums will not be tolerated.

A child with emotional disturbance due to an adjustment reaction will generally become calm as he recognizes the physician's concern and desire to understand his situation. An adjustment reaction is characterized by a deterioration of functioning from a previously higher level, in the presence of some precipitating event or situation. The child with an adjustment reaction is oriented and can usually explain his problems quite well. At times the precipitant may be a developmental event such as beginning a new school, increased peer pressure, or the emergence of secondary sexual characteristics during puberty. The precipitant may also be an acute event such as the loss of a parent through death or divorce.

A child with an attention deficit disorder is likely to have a history of impulsivity with associated distractibility, and a history of learning difficulties at school. Acute agitation or withdrawal requiring an emergency department visit is likely to be due to some consequence of the child's difficulties at school or at home.

Certain medical conditions, such as temporal lobe epilepsy and thyrotoxicosis, can also cause agitation and withdrawal without psychosis. The child with thyrotoxicosis will have tachycardia, appetite and sleep disturbances, weight loss, and possibly exopthalmos in association with the disordered behavior. The child with temporal lobe epilepsy may be identified through the history of seizures and auras and the possible presence of abnormal neurologic findings on physical examination. Differentiation between temporal lobe epilepsy and psychiatrically based behavioral disturbances may at times be difficult and may require neurologic and psychiatric consultation. Children with sensory dificits, such as blindness, deafness, or severe communication difficulties including developmental aphasia, may occasionally present in the emergency department with concomitant agitation or withdrawal and it is important for the physician to bear these possibilities in mind.

EVALUATION AND DECISION

The emergency assessment of the agitated or withdrawn child or adolescent involves three complementary areas. In actual practice the physician gathers data from all three areas at the same time, but for conceptual clarity we will discuss them separately. The first area involves determining if the problematic behavior is due to some *medical condition or organic state* and, if so, to make a diagnosis. To achieve this, the physician gathers information about the acute events leading to the emergency department visit, about any possible drug ingestions or drug use, and about the child's medical history. This is followed later by a complete physical examination. Potential life-threatening effects of the medical condition must be recognized and treated. Second, the *psychiatric manifestations* of the presenting condition, whether organic or psychiatrically based, are assessed. To do this, the physician performs a thorough mental status examination. Of particular concern is determining whether or not suicidal or homicidal intent is present. To complete the psychiatric evaluation of the child, the previous adjustment and the psychiatric history of the child are determined. These data should facilitate the diagnosis of psychiatrically based presenting problems. Third, the *family system and social support* for the child are assessed. This is done by observing the family's responses to the child during the emergency room visit and by assessing previous family functioning. Once these three areas have been evaluated, the physician can make an appropriate decision regarding disposition and further treatment.

Medical Conditions

First, in order to determine if the child's agitation or withdrawal is organically based, the physician should bear in mind the differential diagnosis of these behaviors, which include psychiatric as well as organic etiologies (Table 15.1). A complete history of the acute events leading up to the emergency department visit, including any changes in behavior or functioning of the child, should be obtained. This information will help the psychiatric as well as medical assessment of the child. The possibility of drug use or drug ingestions should be explored with the parents as well as the child. The child's past medical history should be carefully documented, and any previous episodes of the current behavior reviewed. In general, organically based problems are acute in onset, the result of an ingestion, an injury, or the worsening of a medical condition. At times the child's age may be helpful in suggesting certain diagnoses. For example, with children 12 years and over, intoxications with drugs of abuse are most common, while with younger children acute ingestions of medication or other toxic substances are more common.

The differentiating features of organic psychoses and psychiatrically based psychoses have been discussed and are listed in Table 15.2. Important information will come from the history (acuteness of onset of psychosis, presence of drug ingestion); the mental status examination (orientation, memory, intellectual function, nature of hallucinations); and the physical examination (presence of pathologic autonomic signs, abnormal vital signs, physical findings on medical and neurologic examinations). With an organic psychosis, the physician will consider the possible medical causes of psychosis (Table 15.3) as well as those due to ingestion (Table 15.4).

The medical evaluation of agitation and withdrawal requires that every child who presents with these behaviors in the emergency department receives a complete physical examination, including full neurologic evaluation. This will enable most significant ongoing organic illnesses as well as neurologic disease of traumatic, infectious, or structural origin to be detected. Pupillary abnormalities, when found in conjunction with abnormalities of pulse, temperature, and blood pressure, are suggestive of an acute intoxication. Abnormal reflexes suggest central nervous system disease and may warrant further diagnostic study. Mild incoordination, abnormalities of rapid alternating movements, and impaired tandem gait may be present in children with an attention deficit disorder. In situations where an acute intoxication is being considered, blood, urine and gastric aspirate should be obtained and sent for specific drug determinations and/or toxic screening as appropriate. Additional laboratory studies should be pursued in accordance with the findings of the physical examination, and may include a complete blood count, sedimentation rate, urinalysis, electrolytes, blood glucose, calcium, blood urea nitrogen, ammonia, and liver function tests. Thyroid studies are indicated when ongoing thyroid disease is suspected. With this information in hand, medical conditions when present can be diagnosed and appropriate treatment initiated.

Psychiatric Evaluation

The second major area in the emergency department approach to an agitated or withdrawn child involves assessing the psychiatric manifestations of the presenting condition. This is achieved through the mental status examination in conjunction with an evaluation of the child's previous level of adjustment and the past psychiatric history. The emergency department mental status examination is the important mechanism for determining the behavior and emotional condition of the child, including the possible presence of suicidal or homicidal intent. The child's mental status can be determined through direct interaction with the child, in the presence of the parents. It is important for the physician to approach the mental status examination systematically. With the various categories in mind, the physician can obtain much of the data during the history and physical examination. Other areas will require direct questioning of the child by the physician.

The categories of the mental status examination, as described in Chapter 70, "Psychiatric Emergencies" (see p. 1078) will be summarized here. The child's *appearance* will have already been noted by the physician. *Orientation* to person, place, time, and situation should be determined. Recent and long term *memory* should be tested, as should *cognitive functions*, which include intelligence, fund of knowledge, and the ability to reason and think (much of this information can be determined from the flow of the interview). The child's *behavior* should be assessed for activity level and age-appropriateness. The child's capacity for *relating* to the physician can be determined by the physician's noting not only the child's behavior with him but also his own internal responses to the child's behavior. Of particular importance in the emergency assessment of the child are affect and thinking. *Affect* refers to the predominant feelings displayed by the child. The examiner should observe the nature of the affect (happy, sad, angry, flat), its degree of appropriateness to the situation, and how it changes as various subjects are discussed. *Thinking* includes both thought processes and thought content. The coherence and goal directedness of verbal communication are assessed, and loose associations and speech lacking internal consistency are noted when present. Evaluation of thought content involves identifying the child's major themes and concerns. Preoccupations, such as hallucinations, delusions, and ideas of reference (present in psychosis) or sadness, hopelessness, and feelings of depression (present in depression), should also be sought. The child's strengths can be assessed from his spontaneous statements as well as his forthrightness in answering specific questions. The child's insight into the current problem should be noted, and his capacity to suggest a plan to deal with the present crisis evaluated.

Determining the presence or absence of suicidal or homicidal ideation and intent is an essential part of the mental status examination, and provides an opportunity to also ask about past attempts. The circumstances and intent of any previous suicidal or homicidal attempts should be thoroughly explored. The most effective way of determining such intent is by asking the child directly. Such an approach opens the subject in a way that is often reassuring to the child, thereby enabling the discussion to proceed.

As he proceeds with the mental status examination, the physician will develop a picture of the child that will lead to certain diagnostic possibilities. For example, the psychotic child will have bizarre or inappropriate affect, speech which is not goal directed, and may have hallucinations or delusions. Such a child typically relates poorly to the physician, avoiding eye contact, failing to respond to the physician's attempts to empathize with him, and perhaps engendering in the physician feelings of confusion and uneasiness. If the psychotic child is oriented with intact memory and cognitive functions, it is likely that the psychosis is psychiatrically based. If the child's orientation, memory, and cognitive functions are significantly impaired, it is probable that the psychosis is organic in nature. When the child's thinking is coherent and the affect is not bizarre or inappropriate, then it is likely that psychosis is not present. With depressed children, themes of sadness occur, and the physician may find himself attracted to the child and feeling sorry for him. This same reaction by the physician may also occur with children with an adjustment reaction. With a conduct disorder the history usually is quite informative, and the child's manner of relating may be distant or manipulative. The physician may find himself feeling angry at such children. The child with an attention deficit disorder may at times show distractability and impulsivity in the emergency department, but often these behaviors do not occur in one-to-one settings and will be revealed only by the history. The child who has some insight into his problem is more likely to have depression or an adjustment reaction rather than psychosis or a conduct disorder.

The child's previous level of adjustment offers important information needed for a complete profile of the child. The physician can ask about the child's family relations, peer relations, and school performance prior to the onset of the crisis. The child's major areas of interest and special competences should be appreciated. A child in an age-appropriate grade in a regular classroom who has had satisfactory involvement with friends and social activities in general has a good prognosis. The child from a chaotic family who is a loner and who attends school sporadically has a poorer prognosis. In all instances, however, it is important that the physician uncover some areas of strength of child and family, since this will serve as the basis for resolving the current crisis and pursuing further treatment.

Previous psychiatric hospitalization or outpatient treatment should be determined as well as any past incidents of suicidal or homicidal behavior. Knowledge of past and current medication use is also crucial. Family history of psychiatric disorder can easily be obtained at the same time that the child's history is taken.

Evaluation of Support Systems

Finally, emergency evaluation includes assessment of the family and social support system. To master a crisis, a child needs consistency and support within his environment. Information about who lives at home with the child, the nature of their relationships with each other, and any recent changes in family composition or in the child's living situation will help in understanding the current problem and in determining treatment.

The physician can gain information about the family through observation and direct questioning. In so doing, information about family relationships including the parents' level of concern and their ability to appreciate the child's current situation is obtained. Family structure is often revealed by noting which family members accompany the child to the emergency department. Typically, the family members with the child are more involved with him. The parents' description of the child during the history-taking offers insight into how the child is seen in the family. The extent to which the parents try to engage a withdrawn child or to calm and set limits with an agitated child should be noted, as well as the child's response to these efforts.

Parents' responses as the child is asked a question by the physician are also informative. Do the parents answer for him and interrupt when he tries to speak, or do they give their child an opportunity to form a relationship with the physician? The parental response suggests the degree to which the child's independent thinking and behavior are encouraged. If the child is not cooperating during the psychiatric or physical examinations, how effective are the parents in telling the child that he must cooperate? The parents' success in gaining the child's cooperation during the emergency department visit may offer a valuable clue as to their ability to effectively manage their child at home.

The physician can assess the degree of coping by the family in part by the way in which the family describes their problems. Responses suggesting that the parents are overwhelmed and disorganized should lead the physician to consider psychiatric consultation and possible hospitalization. The openness of the family in discussing recent difficulties is also important. Some families are extremely guarded and denying despite the presence of a major crisis that they are unable to manage. Other families offer a more balanced view of family functioning, instilling greater confidence in the physician.

The family should be asked about the adjustment of the child in the past and how earlier family difficulties were handled. Family history of emotional difficulties should also be obtained. The physician should be clear about who the major caretakers of the child have been through his life. In obtaining the family's perception of the crisis, it is best to begin by posing an open-ended question to each family member ("What do you think is going on with your son and in your family?"). After the family has responded, the physician can ask specific questions about recent significant events or changes that could be influencing the current situation.

In determining the disposition of a child in the emergency department with a psychiatric problem, the physician will be guided by the severity of the problem and by the ability of the family to manage the child on an outpatient basis. The physician should inquire as to what social supports are available to the parents. If extended family or close friends are available and the parents feel that their participation would be helpful, then the physician should encourage the parents to enlist such help. If other agencies are working with the family, their efforts should be coordinated with those of the hospital or mental health facility where the child receives treatment. Many families express a clear preference about whether or not their child should be hospitalized. The physician should keep this preference in mind, but should make his own decision based on the data about the child's physical and emotional well-being and his assessment of the family support system.

Disposition

As depicted in Figure 15.1, agitation and withdrawal can occur in the presence or absence of psychosis. When psychosis is present, the first task is to establish whether or not an organic cause is present.

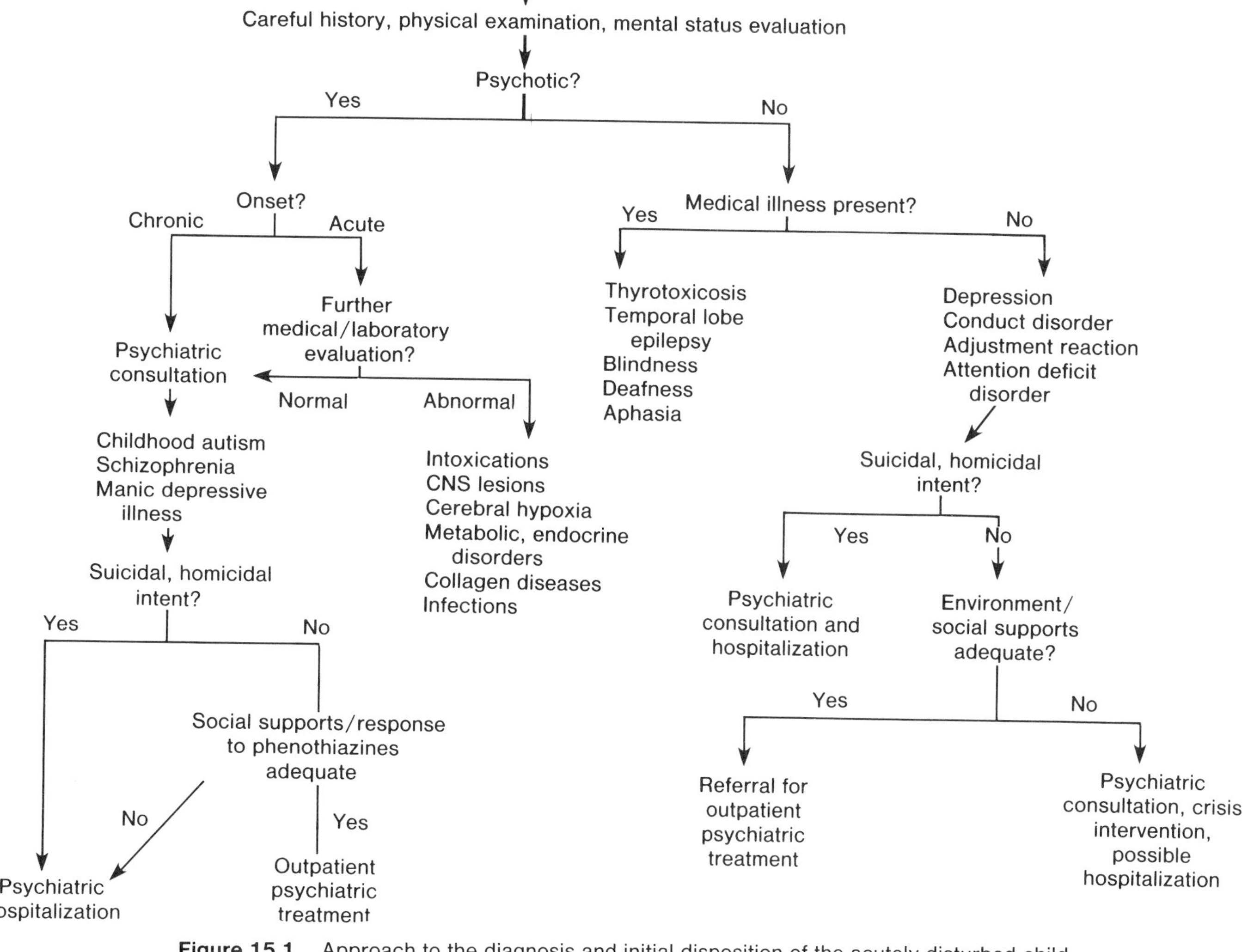

Figure 15.1 Approach to the diagnosis and initial disposition of the acutely disturbed child.

Organic psychosis always requires a full medical evaluation, observation, and treatment of the underlying condition, all of which are best accomplished through medical hospitalization. Psychiatric consultation is indicated in all cases of psychiatrically based psychosis. Psychotic patients, who are not suicidal or homicidal, may be referred for ongoing out-patient treatment following a positive response to antipsychotic medication (see Chapter 70, p. 1094). Psychotic patients who have suicidal or homicidal intent are usually hospitalized.

Psychiatric consultation is also indicated in the presence of active suicidal or homicidal ideation in the absence of psychosis. Persistent suicidal or homicidal intent is usually an indication for psychiatric hospitalization. When suicidal or homicidal thoughts are *absent*, the ability of the family and social support system to control the child's behavior and to prevent further emotional and physical harm should be assessed. If the support system is adequate, then referral to outpatient psychiatric treatment may be appropriate. The physician making a referral for outpatient psychiatric treatment should help the family to develop short-term measures to manage the child and relieve his distress until outpatient psychiatric treatment begins. When the support system is not deemed adequate, psychiatric hospitalization may be necessary, especially with such behavior as firesettings, repeated runaways, and persistent aggressiveness.

CHAPTER 16

Dizziness/Vertigo

ROGER J. PACKER, M.D. AND PETER H. BERMAN, M.D.

INTRODUCTION

Vertigo is a disturbance of the sensation of spatial orientation during which there is a feeling of whirling or rotation of either oneself or the environment. Subjective sensations of weakness and lightheadedness and objective disequilibrium are common associated findings. Vertigo may be transitory or persistent and difficult for the child to describe. The symptom of true vertigo implies dysfunction of the vestibular system. Its differentiation from similar sensations such as dizziness, faintness, lightheadedness, and transient clouding of consciousness, sometimes referred to as pseudovertigo, is the first step in diagnosis (Fig. 16.1). Despite a careful history such differentiation is often impossible, especially in children, and the documentation of the presence of true vertigo then depends on objective signs of vestibular function. Life-threatening causes of vertigo are rare and usually recognizable by associated audiologic or neurologic deficits.

PATHOPHYSIOLOGY

The awareness of one's position in space requires the integration of visual, vestibular and somatosensory stimuli. Disturbance in any of these inputs results in subjective and often objective imbalance, but vestibular dysfunction must occur to produce true vertigo. The inner ear or labyrinth, located in an osseous cavity within the petrous bone, consists of an inner membranous portion of interconnected sacs and ducts. The utricle, saccule, and three semicircular canals (the vestibular apparatus) contain specialized receptors supplying information concerning orientation and movement of the body. The organ of hearing, the cochlea, is also present in the labyrinth, and its integrity is important in the differential diagnosis of vertigo because of its anatomic relationship to the vestibular apparatus. Vestibular and auditory information are transmitted through the eighth cranial (auditory) nerve, which travels in close proximity to the fifth and seventh cranial nerves on its way to the vestibular nuclei in the lower pons and the upper medulla of the brainstem. Vertigo may be conceptualized as occurring on a *peripheral* basis, secondary to dysfunction of the vestibular apparatus, or on a *central* basis, following impairment of the vestibular nuclei or their brainstem connections. Temporal lobe dysfunction has also been described as a cause of vertigo.

DIFFERENTIAL DIAGNOSIS (see Table 16.1)

In childhood, peripheral vertigo is more common than central vertigo and may rarely occur as a complication of acute and chronic otitis media. Mastoiditis and associated suppurative labyrinthitis, with vertigo, fever and pain, is rare in the antibiotic era; but when present causes redness and warmth behind the ear. Variation of the mastoid pneumatization may make diagnosis somewhat difficult. Cholesteatomas, masses of desquamated epithelial cells occurring primarily or associated with chronic otitis media, invade bone and may result in

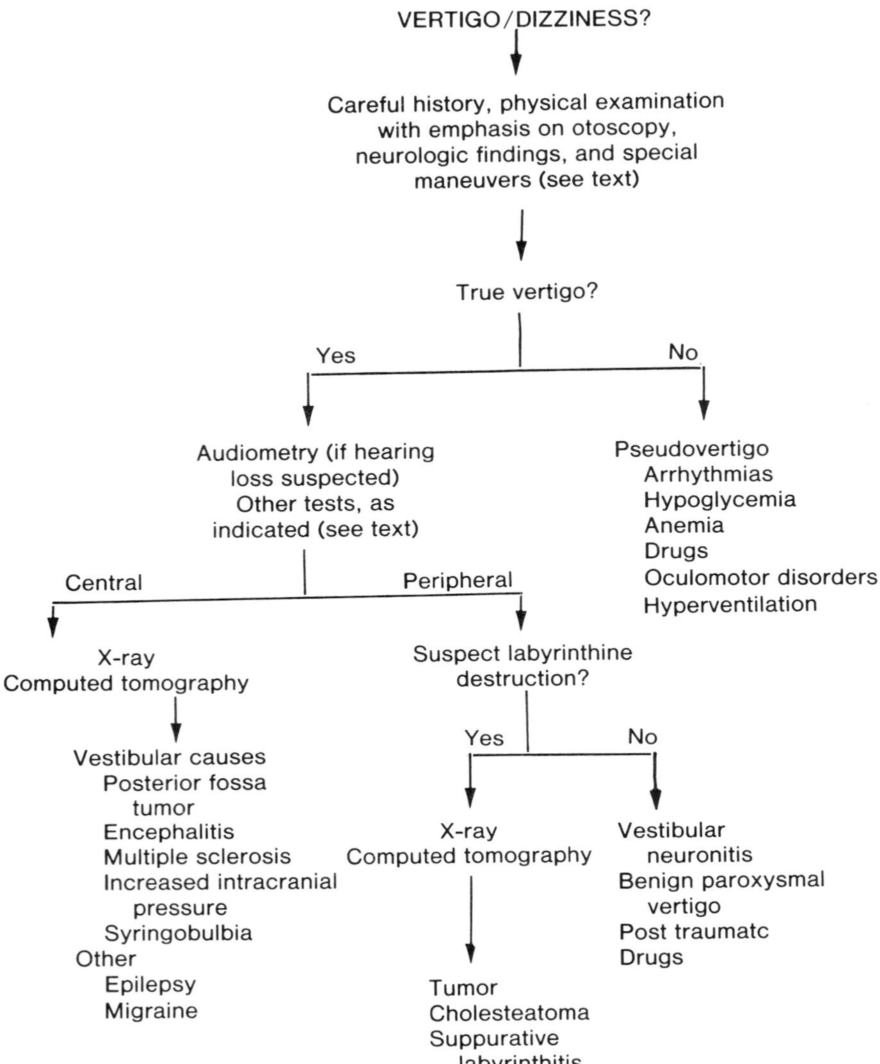

Figure 16.1 Diagnostic approach to the child with vertigo.

labyrinthitis and vertigo. Small bits of whitish debris in the middle ear is seen extruding from the perforated tympanic membrane. Radiologic studies disclose destruction of the temporal bone. Other rare mass lesions, such as rhabdomyosarcoma, may mimic cholesteatomas clinically.

Vertigo in the young child may be extremely difficult to diagnose. Benign paroxysmal vertigo, which occurs between the ages of 1 and 3 years, is heralded by acute episodes of imbalance. During the attack the child seems frightened, becomes pale and, if standing, either reaches for support or falls but does not lose consciousness. Subjective symptoms are difficult to ascertain. The attacks are usually brief, lasting seconds to minutes and may occur in clusters. Infrequently, these are associated with upper respiratory infection or middle ear infection. The cause of these attacks is unknown. Radiologic, audiographic, and electroencephalographic studies are normal. Tests of vestibular function are usually con-

Table 16.1
Vertigo in Childhood: Etiology

Peripheral Vestibular Dysfunction
Suppurative labyrinthitis (mastoiditis)
Labyrinth destruction, noninfectious (cholesteotoma, etc.)
Benign paroxysmal vertigo
Vestibular neuronitis
Drug related
Post-traumatic
Central Vestibular Dysfunction
Posterior fossa tumors
Increased intracranial pressure
Arnold-Chiari malformation
Syringobulbia
Multiple sclerosis
Other
Temporal lobe epilepsy
Migraine

sistent with peripheral vestibular dysfunction. This illness is most commonly confused with temporal lobe epilepsy. Vertiginous symptomatology may uncommonly be the sole clinical masnifestation of partial complex (temporal lobe) seizures and during these attacks vestibular function is said to be normal. However, usually the vertiginous symptoms are associated with other symptoms referable to the temporal lobe and also with abnormalities on electroencephalography. Vertiginous migraine may mimic temporal lobe epilepsy, but the history of associated headaches, occurring frequently, makes clinical differentiation possible.

An ill-defined entity of unknown etiology, vestibular-neuronitis (viral labyrinthitis), usually occurs in children over 10 years old but may occur at any age. It is often associated with intercurrent upper respiratory tract infection or middle ear infection. Viral labyrinthitis is not paroxysmal and is most symptomatic during the first 2 weeks of illness, slowly improving over the following 2 weeks. Vestibular function tests are abnormal during the disease, and spontaneous nystagmus is common. Audiologic tests are normal. Two frequently mentioned entities confused with vestibular-neuronitis, Ménière's disease and benign positional vertigo, are extremely rare in childhood. Ménière's disease results in recurrent paroxysmal vertigo, tinnitus, and hearing loss. Benign positional vertigo is manifest by intermittent vertiginous episodes associated with rapid changes of head position. Toxic labyrinthitis may occur following the administration of various drugs, most noteworthy the aminoglycosides. The onset of this illness is usually insidious, and the diagnosis may be missed if a careful history of drug intake is not performed. Other drugs which may rarely cause a similar toxic labyrinthitis include ethacrynic acid, salicylates, and quinine.

Vertigo may occur secondary to trauma. Sudden vestibular damage, occurring immediately after trauma, with resultant vertigo, nausea, vomiting, and spontaneous nystagmus poses little difficulty in the differential diagnosis. A more perplexing vertiginous syndrome, post-traumatic vertigo, occurs days and sometimes weeks following head trauma and is manifest upon sudden changes of head position. This is associated with abnormal vestibular function on testing. Primary differentiation is from dizziness as a component of the postconcussion syndrome. In the latter syndrome dizziness is rarely vertiginous and is associated with normal vestibular testing.

Vertigo on a central basis is extremely rare in childhood. When present secondary to tumors of the posterior fossa, such as brainstem gliomas, it tends to be overshadowed by associated neurologic deficits. Accoustic neuromas, tumors of the cerebellopontine angle, do present with vertigo but are rare until adulthood. Other rare reported etiologies of central vertigo are encephalitis, increased intracranial pressure, and syringobulbia. Multiple sclerosis can rarely present as vertigo in the adolescent.

No attempt will be made to discuss in detail all the nonvertiginous causes of dizziness (see Chapter 36). The importance of identifying cardiac abnormalities, such as arrhythmias and Stokes-Adams attacks, causing faintness or transient loss of consciousness, is clear. Hypoglycemia may also present similarly. Ingestion of drugs is a common cause of acute unsteadiness, subjective disequilibrium and nystagmus. As alluded to earlier, ocular motor dysfunctions, such as sixth nerve paresis, will result in double vision and subjective disequilibrium. Hyperventilation is probably the most common cause of lightheadedness in adolescence. These patients present with shortness of breath, paresthesias in their fingers and around their lips, and feelings of panic. Diagnosis can usually be made by history and by reproducing the complaint with hyperventilation in the emergency department (see Chapter 72). Psychiatric disorders and functional disorders with associated dizziness, though rare in early childhood, occur frequently in the adolescent years.

EVALUATION AND DECISION

Clinical differentiation between peripheral and central etiologies is often possible. Complaints of tinnitus, hearing loss, pain, or a sensation of fullness in the ear, as well as nausea and vomiting, are much more frequent with peripheral lesions. Paresthesia of the face, suggesting fifth cranial nerve involvement, indicates a central basis. The history of intermittent episodes of severe vertigo is much more consistent with peripheral disease, as central vertigo tends to be persistent and somewhat milder.

Important features on the physical examination include evidence of redness or warmth behind the ear, suggesting mastoiditis, serous labyrinthitis or bacterial labyrinthitis. Careful cranial nerve examination is mandatory for diagnosis. Involvement of the fifth or seventh cranial nerve implies central vertigo.

The fifth cranial nerve supplies sensation to the face and motor innervation to the muscles of mastication. Mass lesions in the pontocerebellar angle may result in abnormalities of pain, cold and touch sensation of the face and, less often, in deviation of the jaw to the side of the lesion. The seventh cranial nerve innervates the muscles of the face, and disruption of its fibers causes weakness of the upper and lower portions of the face. The corneal reflex tests for the integrity of both the fifth and seventh cranial nerves; its loss may suggest subtle asymmetries of cranial nerve function. A neural-sensory hearing loss, indicating eighth cranial nerve dysfunction, may be of cochlear or primary eighth nerve origin. Differentiation is often impossible at the bedside and requires further audiological evaluation. Spontaneous nystagmus may result from either central or peripheral vertigo. Nystagmus due to vestibular dysfunction is commonly a jerk nystagmus with a fast and slow component, the fast component being towards the side of impairment and increasing as one looks toward the lesion. It is primarily horizontal and decreased by fixation. A central basis for the nystagmus is likely if there are vertical or purely rotatory components to the nystagmus and if nystagmus changes direction when the direction of gaze is altered.

Extremely helpful in the diagnosis of vertigo are the inclusions of special tests which stimulate the symptom. These include hyperventilation; vasovagal maneuvers, such as Valsalva and carotid sinus stimulation; rapid changes of posture from lying to standing; rotation while standing (Bárány rotation) and the Nylen-Bárány maneuver. Not only should the patient's objective responses be evaluated during these procedures, but the child should be asked if these tests reproduce the subjective complaint. If they do not, the importance of the abnormality is questionable. The Nylen-Bárány maneuver is performed after seating the child on the edge of the examining table. The subject is then asked to quickly lie back and his head is tilted 45° backward and 45° to one side and maintained in this position for 60 sec. The eyes are observed for the onset, duration and direction of nystagmus. The child is then returned to the sitting position and the maneuver is repeated with the head turned to the opposite side. If nystagmus occurs, there is evidence for vestibular abnormality which can often be separated into central or peripheral categories (see Table 16.2).

Performance of additional tests after the initial evaluation is dependent on the clinical impression. These tests should not be done routinely but only if specifically indicated. Caloric testing, irrigation of the ear canals with both warm and cold water, may be used to confirm vestibular dysfunction. Electronystagnometry is a more sophisti-

Table 16.2
Nylen-Bárány Maneuver

Test	Central	Peripheral
Nystagmus	Yes	Yes
Latency	Immediate onset	Few seconds
Adaption	No	Yes
Fatigue	No	Yes (disappears on repetition)
Subjective vertigo	Usually absent	Present

cated means of monitoring caloric responses, and involves electro-recording the rate, direction, and amptitude of the nystagmus quantitatively with the eye open and closed. Audiometry should be performed if there is a suspicion for hearing loss. Other tests of auditory function, such as auditory recruitment, are useful in differentiating cochlear from eighth nerve dysfunction in the older child.

Radiographic studies are mandatory if one suspects central vestibular disease or labyrinth destruction. X-rays of the skull and mastoid area, including tomography of the auditory canal, are useful in the detection of infectious or destructive lesions. Computerized tomography with contrast enhancement is the procedure of choice if there is evidence of fifth or seventh nerve involvement. Electroencephalography should be performed only if there is a high index of suspicion that the vertigo is a seizure equivalent. For maximum yield it should be performed with the patient awake and asleep and with nasopharyngeal lead placement.

TREATMENT

The majority of causes of vertigo are benign, self-limited illnesses, and reassurance is the major aspect of therapy. In most cases, if the etiology is not readily apparent and there is no evidence of associated neurologic dysfunction or labyrinthine destruction, the child may be treated symptomatically and reevaluated before proceeding with more specific laboratory studies. In acute labyrinthitis, meclizine (12.5 mg b.i.d. to 25 mg b.i.d. for children over 12 years of age) results in symptomatic improvement of nausea and unsteadiness. Treatment of benign paroxysmal vertigo is hard to evaluate since the clinical course is unpredictable. There may be improvement with the use of diphenhydramine (5 mg/kg/day).

References

Brandt T, Daroff RB: The multisensory physiological and pathology vertigo syndromes. *Ann. Neurol* 7: 195–203, 1980.

Dix MR: Vertigo. *Practitioner* 211: 295, 1973.

Drachman DA, Hart CW: An approach to the dizzy patient. *Neurology* 22: 323–334, 1972.

Eviatar L, Eviatar A: Vertigo in children: comments on pathogenesis and management. *Clin Pediatr* 13: 940, 1974.

Fenichel GM: Migraine as a cause of benign paroxysmal vertigo of childhood. *J Pediatr* 71: 114, 1967.

Hart CW: Evaluation of post-traumatic vertigo. *Otolaryngol Clin North Am* 6: 157–168, 1973.

Koenigsberger MR, Chutorian AM, Gold AP, Shavey MS: Benign paroxysmal vertigo of childhood. *Neurology* 20: 1108–1113, 1970.

CHAPTER 17

Dysuria

WILLIAM SCHWARTZ, M.D.

INTRODUCTION

Dysuria, or the sensation of pain while voiding, stems from irritation of the bladder and urethra. While infection in the urinary tract is the most common cause of dysuria, chemicals, such as detergents or crystals, may produce the same symptoms (Table 17.1). The painful sensation is produced by the contraction of the bladder and the peristaltic activity of the urethra, which stimulate the pain fibers of the edematous and erythematous mucosa. Pain occurring at the end of micturition indicates that the trigone area of the bladder is involved. In general, there are few systemic symptoms with dysuria, but at times it is associated with pain in the lower abdomen or suprapubic area. Low grade fever may be present, and in a small number of cases there may be nausea or vomiting.

EVALUATION AND DECISION

When evaluating a child with dysuria, the physician should ask about trauma and about exposure to chemicals such as bubble bath, fabric softener, perfumed soap, or medications that may irritate the mucosal lining of the urethra or bladder. A negative history for injury may not be accurate, because most trauma is not remembered by the patient or, in the case of masturbation, is denied. The detection of gonococcal infections, a common cause of dysuria in adolescents, requires a sensitive historian to elicit an honest response to questions about sexual activity and exposures.

In addition to a routine physical examination, there should be special attention directed toward the genitourinary tract. A swollen or edematous urethra, a red vaginal mucosa, or a discharge from the urethra or vagina localize the source of the symptoms to the genitalia, obviating the need to look for other urinary tract diseases.

The most important task for the emergency physician is to diagnose or exclude an infection. Initially this is done on the basis of the history, physical findings, and

Table 17.1
Causes of Dysuria

- *I. Infection*
  - A. Urethritis
    1. *Neisseria gonorrhoeae*
    2. *Chlamydia* species
    3. Other
  - B. Cystitis
    1. Viral
    2. Bacterial (*Escherichia coli*, *Klebsiella pneumoniae*, *Pseudomonas aeruginosa*, others)
  - C. Pyelonephritis: bacterial (as above)
- *II. Chemical irritation*
  - A. Detergent
  - B. Fabric softener
  - C. Perfumed soaps
  - D. Bubble bath (?)
  - E. Spicy foods (?)
- *III. Trauma*
  - A. Local injury
  - B. Masturbation
  - C. Urinary stones

urinalysis; ultimately, cultures provide a definitive diagnosis (Fig. 17.1).

A urethral or vaginal discharge suggests an infection of the genitalia: urethritis in the male and either urethritis or vaginitis (see p. 618) in the female. *Neisseria gonorrhoeae* is the organism that most frequently causes disease in this area. A Gram stain will often provide a clue to the diagnosis. In the prepubertal female or the male of any age, the finding of Gram-negative intracellular diplococci confirms the diagnosis of gonorrhea; a culture should be obtained and treatment given (see p. 619). However, nonpathogenic organisms that colonize the vagina of the adolescent female have the same appearance as *N. gonorrhoeae* on Gram stain, necessitating confirmation of the diagnosis with a cervical culture before beginning treatment.

If no discharge is seen, the physician should obtain a urinalysis and urine culture from every child with the complaint of dysuria. The finding of pyuria (more than 5 to 10 WBCs per high power field) increases the likelihood of bacterial infection (urethritis, cystitis, or pyelonephritis) but does not prove the diagnosis. Inflammatory conditions, such as chemical urethritis, and nonbacterial infections may also evoke a

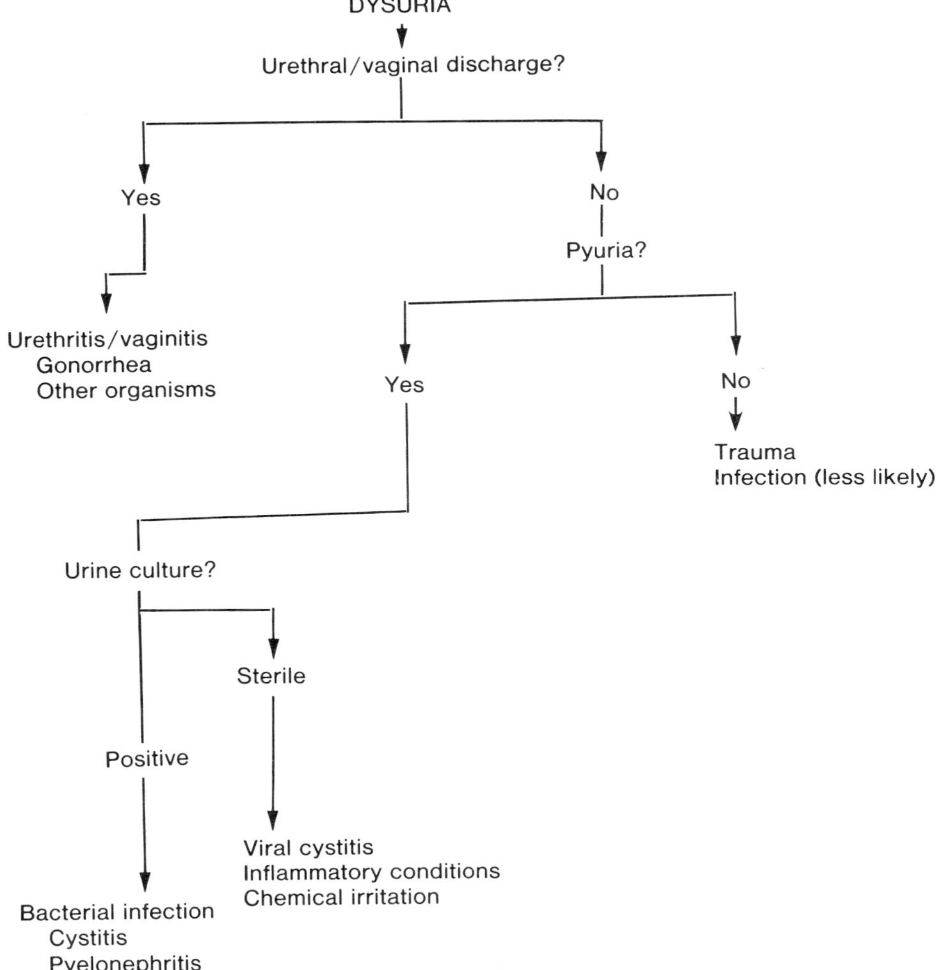

Figure 17.1 Approach to the diagnosis of dysuria.

leukocyte response. Thus, the physician should allow the results of the urine Gram stain and culture to guide the management of children with pyuria, rather than immediately beginning antibiotic therapy, unless fever and flank pain point to pyelonephritis.

In the child with dysuria in the absence of pyuria, local trauma or chemical irritation are the most likely etiologies for the pain. However, since as many as one-third of children with urinary tract infections do not have pyuria, a urine culture should be sent to the laboratory. Additionally, the adolescent requires cultures of the genital tract to diagnose mild gonococcal infections. Other noninfectious causes of dysuria, particularly urinary stones, occur infrequently in children.

The proper performance of the urinalysis requires meticulous attention to the details of the technique. Classically, if there is an infection, the urine will contain more than 5 WBCs per high power field after centrifugation at 3000 rpm for 5 min; there may be red cells, 0 to 2+ (100 mg/dl) protein, and bacteria on a Gram-stained smear. Factors that contribute to a decrease in the number of white cells include a very dilute urine and a delay of more than 6 hours before the sample is examined. There may be an increase in the number of white cells, unrelated to urinary infection, in a febrile patient or in a dehydrated patient. In these situations, it is best to hydrate the patient and repeat the urinalysis.

Culturing the urine is the most precise method of documenting an infection. The office screening techniques that rely on an agar coated plastic disk or Dipstick will accurately quantitate bacteruria. However, the products that contain a nitrite detector for rapid diagnosis require incubation of urine in the bladder for at least 4 hours, so they give a satisfactory result only if performed on the first urine of the morning. When two cultures are both positive, there is a 95% chance of accurately diagnosing a urinary tract infection. Too frequently in the emergency department, there is an unsterile collection of urine and institution of treatment before the outcome of the culture is known. If the patient is treated and the culture specimen lost or contaminated, it will be impossible to determine whether the patient was originally infected. Therefore, when the dysuria is mild and not associated with marked systemic symptoms, it is better to obtain a culture and postpone treatment for 24 hours when the culture can be examined for evidence of a significant infection (see Chapter 45).

Prior to obtaining the results of the urine culture, therapy directed at the symptom of dysuria can provide some relief from the pain. Generally, a dilute urine causes less irritation than a concentrated one, so a generous fluid intake should be recommended. For the child over 6 years of age, phenazopyridine (pyridium) at a dosage of 100 mg given 3 times per day may be helpful as a urinary tract anesthetic.

References

Paradise JE, Campos JM, Friedman HM, et al.: Vulvovaginitis in premenarcheal girl; clinical features and diagnostic evaluation. *Pediatrics* 70: 193, 1982.

Pryles CV, Eliot CR: Pyuria and bacteriuria in infants and children. *Am J Dis Child* 110: 628, 1965.

CHAPTER 18

Earache

WILLIAM P. POTSIC, M.D.

INTRODUCTION

"Earache" is pain interpreted by the patient to be in, on, or around the ear. The pain may vary like pain elsewhere in the body in its quality, intensity and duration. Children, depending upon their age and invidiual dispositions, tolerate pain to a different degree. Prelingual children are most often irritable, wake intermittently at night, or may appear lethargic. Older children can describe the pain more accurately. An experienced examiner can tell from facial expression if the child is experiencing pain. Young children often interpret a sensation of fullness as pain, but they do not have a painful expression on their faces.

Ear pain may be caused by a disease in the ear or may be nonotogenic in its origin. The etiology of otogenic ear pain is usually easily detected by otoscopic examination. Nonotogenic ear pain may be a neuralgia, psychogenic, referred from the head and neck area, or rarely referred from a site below the clavicles. Earache is only rarely associated with immediate life-threatening consequences. Table 18.1 lists the principal causes of earache.

EVALUATION AND DECISION

Ear pain is usually caused by an inflammatory process in the ear itself (Fig. 18.1). Acute suppurative otitis media and external otitis are the most common causes of earache seen in the emergency department. Acute otitis media produces a deep, boring, constant pain. There is often fever over 102°F (39°C) and the pain is not exacerbated by pulling on the ear. The diagnosis is easily made by otoscopy and this disorder should be treated with 10 days of appropriate antibiotics (see Chapter 45, p. 368). External otitis is caused by bacterial or fungal infection of the ear canal. It is a constant pain that is exacerbated by pulling or touching the ear or chewing. External otitis is usually associated with swelling of the ear canal and a foul-smelling aural discharge. It is easily diagnosed by otosocpy as well as visual examination of the external canal. It should be treated with 10 days of antibiotic-containing ear drops.

Viral acute otitis media and secretory otitis media are often associated with a sensation of fullness in the ear, which might be called earache by the patient. Otoscopic examination reveals *nearly* normal appearing landmarks with diffuse tympanic membrane inflammation. Herpes zoster oticus causes severe excruciating deep and superficial ear pain. It is associated with vesicular eruptions on the auricle, pharyngeal vesicles, facial paralysis and necrosis of the tympanic membrane on the same side. Viral ear infections can be treated only symptomatically.

Tumors of the middle ear or external canal are uncommon, but both benign and malignant tumors occur in these locations. Pain may be caused by the tumor itself or by secondary infection. Otoscopic examination will reveal abnormal tissue in the external meatus or middle ear.

Nonotogenic ear pain is the most frus-

Table 18.1
Causes of Earache

- *I. Otogenic*
  - A. Acute otitis media
  - B. Viral otitis
  - C. External otitis
  - D. Tumors
  - E. Herpes zoster oticus
- *II. Nonotogenic*
  - A. Mouth and pharynx
    1. Tooth abscess
    2. Impacted third molar
    3. Aphthous ulcer
    4. Pharyngitis/tonsillitis
    5. Peritonsillar abscess
    6. Pharyngeal tumor
  - B. Head and neck
    1. Sinusitis
    2. Parotitis
    3. Lymphadenitis
    4. Cervical spine disease
    5. Temporomandibular arthritis
  - C. Psychogenic

trating situation for the patient and examiner. The ear and surrounding tissues appear normal.

The sensory innervation of the ear is derived from four cranial and two cervical nerves. The regions supplied by these nerves may refer pain to the ear, and such pain is most often caused by an inflammatory process.

The most common source of referred ear pain is along the fifth cranial nerve and is of dental origin. Children or adolescents with erupting teeth may have ear pain. There may be as many as 32 potential tooth sources for referred pain. Invisible impacted third molars are a common cause of ear pain in adolescents. Oral mucosal ulceration from any cause, but most frequently aphthous ulcers, can result in earache. Sinusitis, sialadenitis, lymphadenitis and tumors of these regions may also cause pain. In the early phase of mumps, the patient may comlain of earache before parotid swelling is obvious.

The ninth cranial nerve supplies the oropharynx, nasopharynx and posterior third of the tongue. Inflammation is the most common cause of earache and is usually from pharyngitis and tonsillitis. Peritonsillar abscess or cellulitis causes unilateral earache. Earache is a common, but frequently unexpected, occurrence after an adenotonsillectomy. It usually occurs with swallowing and can occur at night, waking the child. Nasopharyngeal or oropharyngeal tumors such as lymphoma or rhabdomyosarcoma are also frequently associated with ear pain.

The tenth nerve supplies the base of the tongue, larynx, and trachea. Inflammatory or mass lesions in these areas may also cause pain. Seventh nerve pain is usually a precursor of Bells palsy or herpes zoster oticus. Cervical nerves C2 and C3 supply the mastoid and posterior pinna. Thus ear discomfort may result from cervical spine injuries, arthritis, or disk disease.

Neuralgia of any nerve supplying the head and neck may occur and cause atypical pain. However, when the otologic examination is normal, no lesion responsible for the pain can be found, and the pain does not fit the distribution of nerves V, VII, IX, X, C1, or C2, the pain may be psychogenic. Psychogenic pain is usually mild or moderate, occurring in a patient who suffers from either anxiety or depression.

Rarely thought of but potential sources of pain are the temporomandibular joint and the middle meningeal artery. With temporomandibular joint pain, the joint is usually tender to palpation. Middle meningeal pain is usually caused by tumors or meningitis and is associated with either generalized or focal neurologic signs. Ear pain from referred sources in the chest (myocardial infarctions) or abdomen (kidney infarct) is extremely rare.

The evaluation of ear pain should include a careful history. Constant pain is usually otogenic. Intermittent pain is usually referred or psychogenic. Severe pain is usually otogenic, but mild-to-moderate discomfort is often nonotogenic.

Otogenic causes of earache are easily diagnosed by otoscopy. A normal appearing ear should initiate a search for referred pain. If referred pain seems unlikely and does not fit the distribution of the cranial

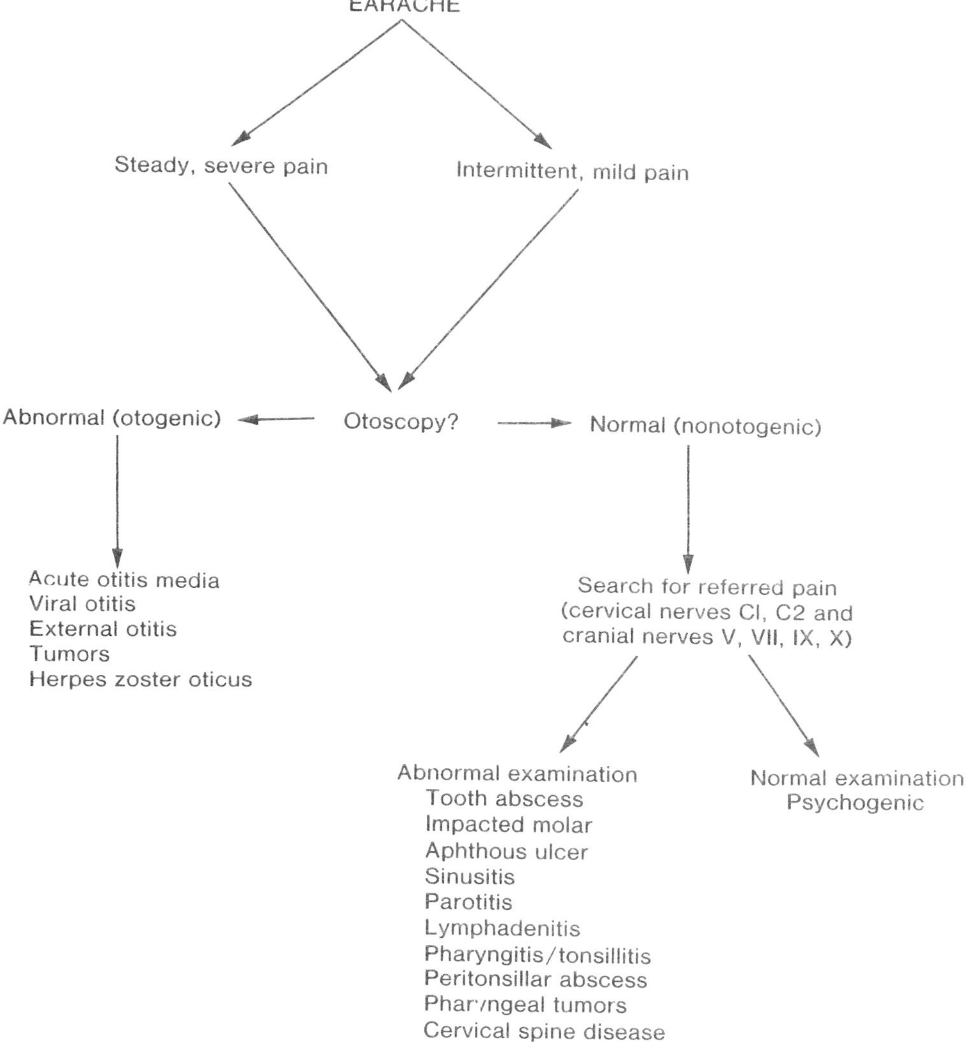

Figure 18.1 Approach to diagnosis earache.

or cervical nerves that refer pain to the ear, a psychogenic cause must be considered. Radiologic studies in the emergency department are rarely helpful to evaluate earache. Head and neck, as well as dental x-rays, are better obtained at a later time under optimal conditions. Any patient with persistent unexplained ear pain should be referred to an otolaryngologist for a complete head and neck examination including visualization of all mucosal surfaces that could refer pain to the ear. This includes nasopharyngoscopy, laryngoscopy, and hypopharyngoscopy.

CHAPTER 19

Edema

WILLIAM SCHWARTZ, M.D.

INTRODUCTION

Edema, the abnormal swelling of tissues from accumulation of fluid in the extravascular space, is a common emergency problem. This fluid characteristically appears either in the dependent portions of the extremities, distensible tissues such as the eyelids, scrotum, or labia, or in organs or extremities at the site of tissue damage. The major mechanisms that lead to this formation of edema are decreased intravascular oncotic pressure (clinically indicated by a decreased serum albumin), increased venous or lymphatic pressure, or vasculitis from an allergic reaction or hypersensitivity (Table 19.1).

PATHOPHYSIOLOGY

Hypoalbuminenia arises from decreased production of proteins due to hepatic disease or increased renal or gastrointestinal losses. When the albumin level is less than 2.5 g/dl, the oncotic activity in the vascular space is reduced enough for fluid to move into the soft tissues and eventually into the dependent extremities.

Edema formation without hypoalbuminemia requires an increased hydrostatic pressure that overcomes the oncotic pressure of intravascular protein and sodium, forcing fluid out of the vascular space. Hypervolemia from cardiac failure, salt retention, or estrogen-progesterone excess is the general mechanism responsible for increased hydrostatic pressure leading to edema. In the hypersensitive or allergic state, the formation of edema may be rapid and localized. This may be life-threatening

Table 19.1
Causes of Edema

Cardiovascular Disease
- Congestive heart failure
- Pericardial effusion (and tamponade)
- Infections
- Rheumatologic diseases
- Idiopathic
- Vasculitis or thrombosis

Hepatic Disease
- Liver failure
- Hepatitis
- Metabolic diseases
- Biliary atresia
- Congenital fibrosis

Renal Disease
- Nephrotic syndrome
- Glomerulonephritis
- Henoch-Schönlein purpura

Gastrointestinal Disease
- Chronic protein malnutrition
- Protein-losing enteropathy

Miscellaneous
- Urticarial reactions
- Local trauma or infections (cellulitis)
- Inappropriate secretion of antidiuretic hormone
- Drugs (oral contraceptives, lithium)
- Excess salt intake
- Premenstrual swelling
- Congenital anomalies

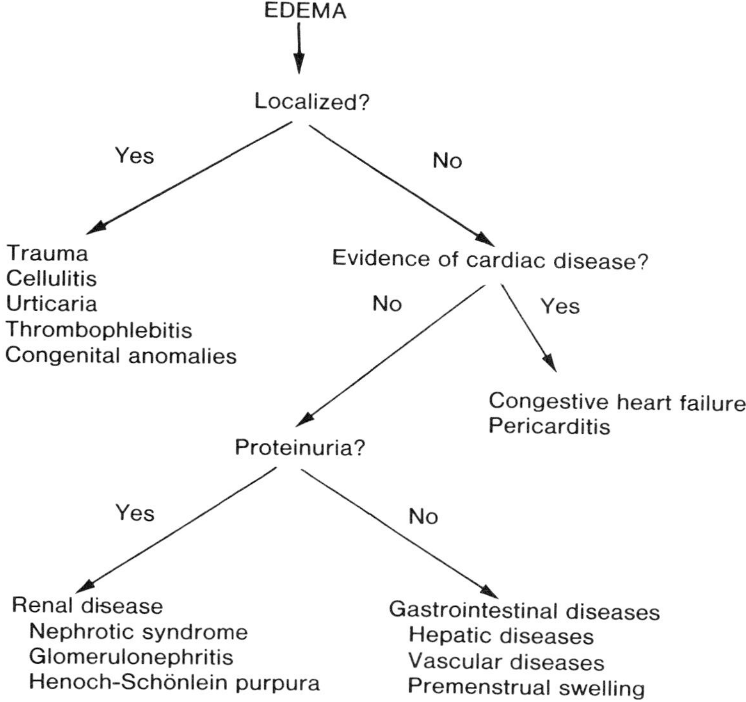

Figure 19.1 Approach to the diagnosis of edema.

if the edema is formed near the vocal cords or may be merely uncomfortable if restricted to the eyelids or ankles as seen with insect bites. If the basis of edema is decreased oncotic pressure or elevated hydrostatic pressure, the onset of symptoms is gradual and may exist for weeks or months before edema is appreciated by the patient or physician. Usually a 10 to 15% weight gain occurs before the patient comes to medical attention.

EVALUATION AND DECISION

Local Edema

Children come to the emergency department more often with local, rather than generalized, edema (Fig. 19.1). Most of these lesions result from minor trauma, infection of the subcutaneous tissues, or allergic (urticarial) reactions. Tenderness to palpation points to either trauma or infection, and fever often occurs with the latter. Particularly on the eyelids and around the lips, insect bites are likely to produce a very noticeable swelling. Whenever local edema occurs on the face, the physician should carefully evaluate the child for concurrent laryngeal involvement. Thrombophlebitis occurs rarely in the prepubertal child but may affect the adolescent; weight lifting and the use of oral contraceptive pills predispose teenagers to this condition. Rarely, lymphedema may result from congenital obstructions to lymphatic flow.

Generalized Edema

Generalized edema, usually an indication of significant underlying disease, occasionally occurs with less serious conditions. Certain drugs (oral contraceptive pills, lithium) may cause some individuals to become edematous during their administration; cessation of the drug produces a resolution of the swelling. Just prior to menstruation, adolescent females may complain of "bloating." The cyclical nature of this problem usually provides a clue to the diagnosis.

The evaluation of the edematous child demands requires careful attention to the cardiovascular examination. The clinical manifestations of congestive heart failure (CHF) or pericarditis are rarely subtle, if these conditions are sufficiently severe hemodynamically to produce edema. Tachycardia, tachypnea, adventitial pulmonary sounds, and hepatomegaly suggest CHF (see p. 000). In the child with a pericardial effusion, a pulsus paradoxus greater than 12 mm Hg, muffled heart tones, and jugular venous distension may accur (see p. 000). A chest x-ray will show an enlarged cardiac silhouette with both conditions.

Generalized edema that is not cardiovascular in origin most often arises secondary to diseases of the kidneys, particularly idiopathic nephrotic syndrome. Occasionally, other forms of the nephrotic syndrome, glomerulonephritis, or Henoch-Schönlein purpura (HSP) are responsible. The detection of significant proteinuria (3+ or 4+) confirms the diagnosis of nephrotic syndrome or nephritis, and such children require admission to the hospital for evaluation and treatment. In the child with HSP, the edema usually affects the lower extremities predominantly and is often accompanied by a purpuric eruption. If there is no involvement of the renal or gastrointestinal systems, the child with HSP may be treated as an outpatient.

Rarely, children with chronic hepatic or gastrointestinal diseases come to the emergency department with the recent appearance of edema. However, a careful history often uncovers a more insidious onset; the physician should question the child or parents about tight-fitting shoes or the need for a larger belt during the preceding months. Patients without an obvious explanation for their edema require hospitalization for their evaluation. If the finding of edema is questionable, a low serum albumin may confirm the diagnosis in some cases. Once the diagnosis is ascertained, the specific condition should guide further management.

CHAPTER **20**

Epistaxis

FRED M. HENRETIG, M.D.

INTRODUCTION

Epistaxis (nosebleeding) is a common symptom in young children and may be alarming to parents, who often overestimate the amount of blood loss. An orderly approach to history and physical examination is necessary to identify the small minority of patients requiring laboratory investigation or referral to an otorhinolaryngologist for specific treatment.

Two important factors contribute to the frequency of epistaxis in otherwise normal children. First, the nose is a favored site for recurrent minor trauma, especially habitual, often absent-minded, picking. Second, the small vessels supplying the nasal mucous membrane have little structural support, as the mucosa is closely applied to the perichondrium and periosteum of the nasal septum and lateral nasal walls. Further, the nasal mucosa is richly supplied with vessels forming plexiform networks. One such anastomosis of common etiologic significance is Kisselbach's plexus in Little's area of the anterior nasal septum, about 0.5 cm from the tip of the nose (see Fig. 62.6). Any factors which tend to cause congestion of the nasal vessels and/or drying of the mucosa will enhance the likelihood of epistaxis resulting from a given degree of trauma.

Local factors predominate in etiologic importance. In addition to minor accidental trauma and habitual picking, any cause of acute inflammation will predispose to bleeding. Acute upper respiratory infections, whether localized as in colds or whether secondary to more generalized infections such as measles, infectious mononucleosis, and influenzal illnesses, will contribute to the onset of epistaxis. Allergic rhinitis may also be a factor. Staphylococcal furuncles, foreign bodies, telangiectasias (Osler-Weber-Rendu disease), hemangiomas, or evidence of other uncommon tumors may be found on inspection. Juvenile nasopharyngeal angiofibroma is usually seen in adolescent males who may present with nasal obstruction, mucopurulent discharge and severe epistaxis. These tumors may bulge into the nasal cavity but often will require examination of the nasopharynx to be identified. Although benign, they can cause severe problems through local invasion of adjacent structures. A rare childhood malignant tumor, nasopharyngeal lymphoepithelioma, may cause a syndrome of epistaxis, torticollis, trismus and unilateral cervical lymphadenopathy. Rhinitis sicca refers to a condition common in northern altitudes during the winter, in which low ambient humidity, exacerbated by dry hot air heating systems, leads to dessication of the nasal mucosa with concurrent tendency to frequent bleeding. Other rare local causes of epistaxis include nasal diphtheria and Wegener's granulomatosis.

Systemic factors include hematologic diseases such as sickle cell anemia, leukemia, platelet disorders, hemophilia, and clotting disorders due to severe hepatic dysfunction.

Table 20.1
Differential Diagnosis of Epistaxis

I. Local Predisposing Factors
A. Trauma, picking
B. Local inflammation
1. Acute viral upper respiratory tract infection (common cold)
2. Bacterial rhinitis
a. Nasal diphtheria (rare)
b. Congenital syphilis
c. β-Hemolytic streptococcus
3. Foreign body
} Usually a blood-tinged purulent discharge
4. Acute systemic illnesses accompanied by nasal congestion: measles, infectious mononucleosis, acute rheumatic fever
5. Allergic rhinitis
6. Nasal polyps
7. Staphylococcal furuncle
C. Telangiectasias (Osler-Weber-Rendu disease)
D. Juvenile angiofibroma
E. Other tumors, granulomatosis (rare)
F. Rhinitis sicca

II. Systemic Predisposing Factors
A. Hematologic diseases
1. Primary hemorrhagic diatheses: leukemia, platelet disorders, hemophilias
2. Clotting disorders due to severe hepatic disease
3. Sickle cell anemia
B. Vicarious menstruation
C. Hypertension
1. Arterial (unusual cause of epistaxis in children)
2. Venous—as in paroxysmal coughing with diseases such as pertussis, cystic fibrosis.

Arterial hypertension is rarely a cause of epistaxis in children. Vicarious menstruation refers to a condition occasionally found in adolescent girls in which monthly epistaxis due to vascular congestion of the nasal mucosa occurs, concordant with menses and presumably related to cyclic changes in hormone levels (Table 20.1).

EVALUATION AND DECISION

As described above, epistaxis is a common event in normal children. It may be due to a combination of minor trauma and local predisposing factors, such as acute upper respiratory tract infection (URI) or nasal allergy, or to systemic conditions. It is usually first noted at about age 3 years and increases in frequency with age, until peaking prior to or in adolescence. Often parents will note hematemesis or melena, prompting them to seek urgent medical attention.

The evaluation of the child with epistaxis begins with a thorough history. Specific features to be sought include frequency of occurrence, difficulty in control (and adequacy of simple at-home first aid), history of trauma, nose-picking, frequent URI, allergic and chronic discharge, or obstructive symptoms. Specific questions regarding evidence for any systemic hemorrhagic disorder or family history of bleeding are asked. In adolescent girls, relation to menses is noted.

Physical examination must include a complete general examination with special attention paid to vital signs including blood pressure, evidence of hematologic disease (enlarged nodes, organomegaly, petechiae, or pallor) and, of course, inspection of the nasal cavity after reasonable efforts to stop the bleeding.

Since the vast majority of bleeding in children is from the anterior nasal septum, the simplest way to stop the hemorrhage is

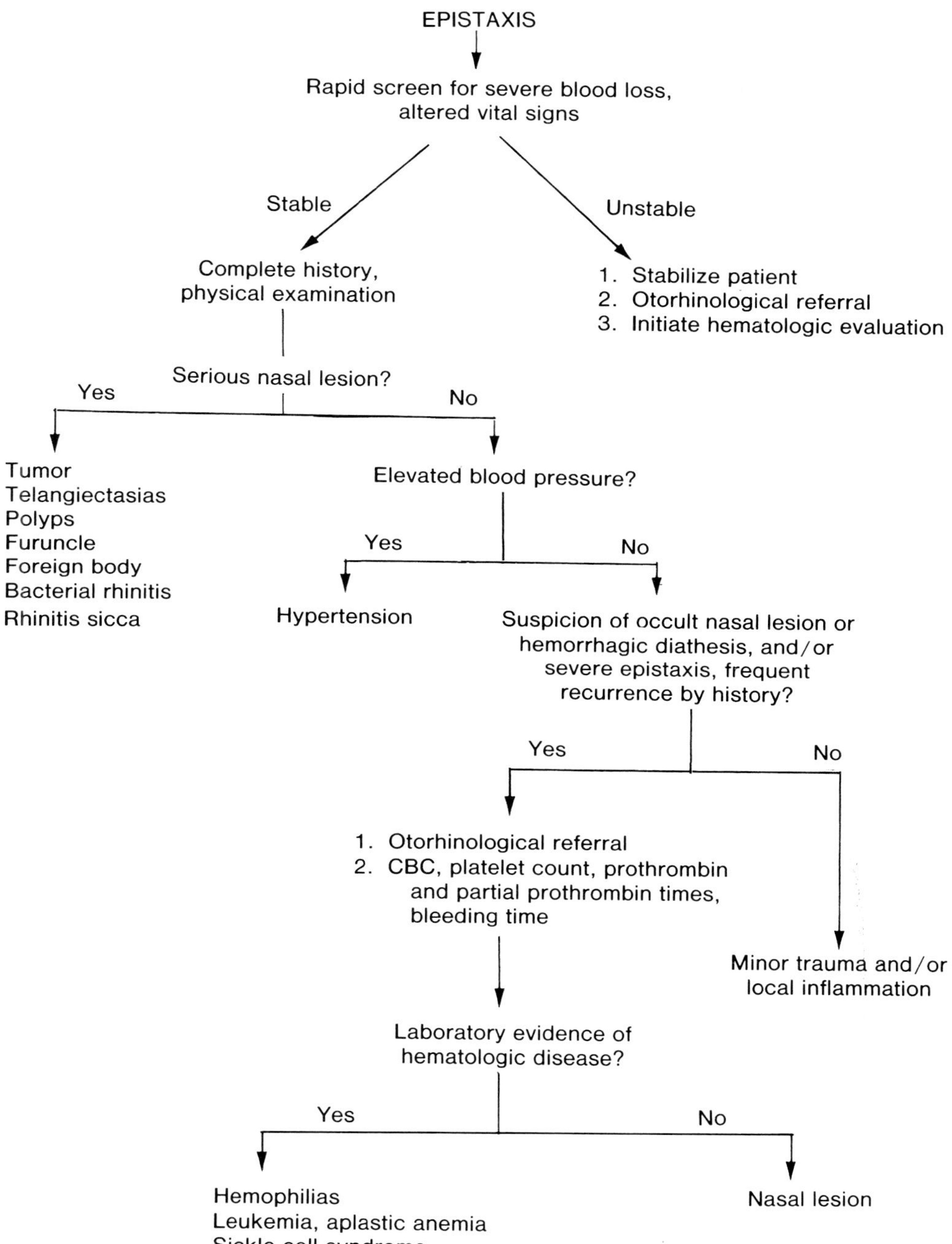

Figure 20.1 Approach to diagnosis of epistaxis.

by direct pressure on the bleeding site for 5 to 10 minutes by external compression of the nares between two fingers. In addition, a cotton (dental) roll may be placed under the upper lip to compress the labial artery. Occasionally, the addition of cotton-pledgets moistened with a few drops of epinephrine (1:1000) or cocaine (5%) solution or application of topical thrombin will help achieve hemostasis. The child should be sitting up with head tilted slightly forward during these procedures. If an anterior site of bleeding is identified, and particularly if bleeding has been recurrent, cautery with a silver nitrate stick may be warranted. For management of severe epistaxis not responsive to such measures, nasal packing and/or surgical ligation of vessels may be necessary.

In children without clinical evidence of severe blood loss, who have no suspicion of systemic factors, and for whom an anterior site of bleeding is identified and stopped readily with local pressure, no laboratory workup is indicated. Reassurance and education regarding appropriate at-home management need to be provided. Occasionally, recurrent epistaxis during an acute URI or flare-up of allergic rhinitis may be lessened with use of an antihistamine-decongestant preparation, although care must be taken not to dry the nose excessively causing epistaxis related to dry mucosa. During the winter, especially in the context of forced hot-air heating systems, a cool mist vaporizer may lessen crusting and drying of nasal mucosa with its subsequent predisposition to recurrent bleeding. Petroleum jelly, placed in the nostril twice daily, is also useful to maintain the normal moistness of the nasal mucosa.

All patients discharged from the emergency department after evaluation for significant epistaxis should be given specific instructions on nares compression and indications for repeat evaluation. For patients with specific local abnormalities, such as tumors, polyps, telangiectasias, etc., referral to an otorhinolaryngologist will, of course, be necessary. Such referral might also be considered, even with questionable findings on the emergency department nasal examination, if bleeding were severe, recurrent or suspected to be posterior in origin.

Finally, evaluation for hemorrhagic diathesis should be done in any child with pertinent positive findings on history, family history or physical exam. This would usually include prothrombin time, partial thromboplastin time, complete blood count, and bleeding time. Although the yield would be low in the absence of corroborative clinical features, some children whose epistaxis seems particularly severe or frequently recurrent might also deserve such screening. The above considerations are outlined in the epistaxis algorithm (Fig. 20.1).

References

Pimpinella PJ: The nasopharyngeal angiofibroma in the adolescent male. *J Pediatr* 64: 260, 1964.

Ritter FN: Vicarious menstruation. In *Differential Diagnosis in Pediatric Otolaryngology*, p. 216, edited by M Strome. Little, Brown, Boston, 1975.

CHAPTER 21

Fever

FRED M. HENRETIG, M.D.

INTRODUCTION

Fever, the abnormal elevation of body temperature, has been recognized for centuries by physicians as a sign of disease. Furthermore, the problem of the febrile child is one of the most frequently encountered in clinical pediatrics, accounting for as many as 20% of pediatric emergency department visits. Despite such considerable clinical experience, only in recent years has the pathogenesis of fever become somewhat clarified. The problem of appropriate clinical and laboratory evaluation of febrile children however, remains a major challenge to the pediatrician and emergency physician. The approach outlined below will enable the physician treating a febrile child in the emergency department to proceed systematically with the appropriate diagnostic steps and the institution of therapy. The principal causes of fever in children are listed in Table 21.1.

PATHOPHYSIOLOGY

Exogenous pyrogens (such as toxins, infectious agents, or antigen-antibody complexes) from many sources produce fever in man by inducing the production of a protein, endogenous pyrogen, by phagocytic leukocytes. This protein enters the circulation after its synthesis, interacts with specialized receptor neurons in the anterior hypothalamus, and leads to the production of prostaglandins, monoamines and probably cyclic AMP. These mediators in turn initiate signals via the posterior hypothalamus to the vasomotor center which results in peripheral vasoconstriction and conservation of heat, increased metabolic rate and concomitant heat production, and thus, ultimately, elevation of body temperature. Rarely, central nervous system dysfunction directly alters the hypothalamic set point.

It is difficult to pinpoint the lowest temperature elevation that is definitely abnormal for all children under all circumstances. Some children normally have rectal temperatures as low as 36.2°C (97°F) or as high as 38°C (100.4°F). Children, like adults, also normally have diurnal variation in temperature, with the peak usually occurring between 5:00 and 7:00 p.m. This variation is less pronounced in infants. In the 2- to 6-year age range, the temperature may vary by 0.9°C (1.6°F), and in children older than 6 years, diurnal variation may span 1.1°C (2°F). Factors such as excessive clothing, physical activity, hot weather, digestion of food, and ovulation can all raise temperature in the absence of disease. For the appropriately dressed child who has been at rest for 30 min, a rectal temperature greater than 38°C (100.4°F) will be defined as fever for this discussion. Oral and axillary temperatures are usually about 0.6°C (1°F) and 1.1°C (2°F) lower than rectal, respectively.

EVALUATION AND DECISION

The crucial importance of fever lies in its role as a sign of disease. Rarely, an extreme fever (temperature greater than 41.1°C

Table 21.1
Principal Conditions in Children Associated with Fever

- *I. Infections*
  - A. Central nervous system
    1. Meningitis
    2. Encephalitis
    3. Brain abscess
  - B. Ocular
    1. Periorbital (preseptal) cellulitis
    2. Orbital cellulitis/abscess
  - C. Airway and upper respiratory tract
    1. Common cold (''URI''—upper respiratory infection)
    2. Pharyngitis/tonsillitis
    3. Otitis media
    4. Acute cervical adenitis
    5. Acute sinusitis
    6. Peritonsillar, retropharyngeal, lateral pharyngeal wall abscess
    7. Croup
    8. Epiglottitis
  - D. Oral cavity and salivary glands
    1. Alveolar abscess
    2. Herpangina
    3. Herpetic gingivostomatitis
    4. Mumps
    5. Acute suppurative parotitis
  - E. Pulmonary
    1. Bronchitis
    2. Bronchiolitis
    3. Pneumonia
    4. Pulmonary tuberculosis
    5. Lung abscess
  - F. Cardiac
    1. Myocarditis
    2. Endocarditis
    3. Pericarditis
  - G. Gastrointestinal
    1. Acute gastroenteritis
    2. Hepatitis
    3. Cholangitis
    4. Appendicitis
    5. Peritonitis
    6. Pancreatitis
    7. Acute mesenteric adenitis
    8. Intraabdominal abscesses
  - H. Genitourinary
    1. Urinary tract infection
    2. Perinephric abscess
    3. Acute salpingitis
    4. Tubo-ovarian abscess
    5. Acute prostatitis
    6. Epididymitis
    7. Orchitis

Table 21.1—*Continued*

- I. Musculoskeletal
  - 1. Septic arthritis
  - 2. Osteomyelitis
  - 3. Myositis
- J. Cutaneous
  - 1. Cellulitis
  - 2. Exanthems (systemic infections usually associated with prominent rashes)
    - a. Roseola (presumed viral)
    - b. Rubeola
    - c. Rubella
    - d. Varicella
    - e. Hand-foot-mouth disease
    - f. Scarlet fever
    - g. Staphylococcal scalded skin syndromes (including toxic shock syndrome)
    - h. Syphillis, secondary
    - i. Meningococcemia (occasionally other primary septicemia)
    - j. Rocky Mountain spotted fever
- K. Systemic infections
  - 1. Bacterial sepsis (primary—especially meningococcemia)
  - 2. "Occult bacteremia" (especially pneumoccocal)
  - 3. Viruses
  - 4. Rickettsial, chlamydial, fungal, parasitic, and unusual bacterial infections
  - 5. Miliary tuberculosis

II. *Vasculitis Syndromes and Hypersensitivity Phenomena*
- A. Acute rheumatic fever
- B. Juvenile rheumatoid arthritis
- C. Systemic lupus erythematosis
- D. Polyarteritis nodosa
- E. Kawasaki's disease
- F. Dermatomyositis/polymyositis
- G. Mixed connective tissue disease
- H. Henoch-Schönlein purpura
- I. Serum sickness
- J. Stevens-Johnson syndrome
- K. Drug and immunization reactions

III. *Neoplasms*
- A. Leukemia
- B. Neuroblastoma
- C. Lymphoma
- D. Ewing's sarcoma

IV. *Poisonings*
- A. Atropine poisoning
- B. Salicylate poisoning
- C. Amphetamine poisoning
- D. LSD poisoning
- E. Miscellaneous drugs (e.g., phenothiazines, antidepressants and others with anticholinergic effect)

V. *Central Nervous System Disorders*
- A. CNS lesions in hypothalamus/brain stem
- B. Prolonged seizures
- C. Riley-Day syndrome

Table 21.1—*Continued*

VI. *Metabolic Diseases*
- A. Thyrotoxic crisis
- B. Etiocholanolone fever
- C. Acute intermittent porphyria

VII. *Miscellaneous Conditions*
- A. Dehydration
- B. Intravascular hemolysis
- C. Hemorrhage into an enclosed space
- D. Anhydrotic ectodermal dysplasia
- E. Extreme environmental heat excess
- F. Familial Mediterranean fever
- G. Sarcoidosis
- H. Chronic inflammatory bowel disease
- I. Factitious
- J. Major trauma (crush injuries)
- K. Other rare causes

(106°F) may pose a risk to a child in and of itself, and demand immediate management per se. However, in the vast majority of cases, the main task facing the physician is to make a diagnosis and treat the underlying disease causing the fever. If no specific treatment is necessary, the task becomes that of appropriate supportive care and follow-up.

Careful attention to history and physical examination will provide the most important clues to diagnosis, as well as help the physician gauge the overall toxicity of the child and thus the urgency of the situation. For young infants and toddlers especially, it is helpful to allow the child to sit on a parent's lap or be held in their arms while the history is obtained. Questions are asked concerning the onset and duration of the fever, the degree of temperature if taken, medications given (including antipyretics), associated signs and symptoms, and the presence of similar illnesses in sibs or playmates. Past medical history should focus on recurrent febrile illnesses, and particularly the presence of any diseases or drug regimens that would compromise normal host defenses, such as sickle cell disease, asplenia, malignancy, or immunosuppression. During the interview, the examiner notes the child's alertness, responsiveness to persons and objects (such as a proferred tongue blade or two), respiratory status, color, feeding activity, and age-related a propriateness of gross motor function. C ten, the observation that a young infa with an elevated temperature bangs h tongue blades together while eagerly drin ing from his bottle will convince the phys cian that a lumbar puncture is unnecessar On the other hand, the febrile infant wh appears irritable and/or inappropriately l thargic while being held by his parent b fore the examination, is one at high risk f a serious infection such as meningitis sepsis. The complaint or observation th the child's crying increases with parent attempts to comfort or fondle is critical note; such "paradoxical irritability" is a important sign of meningitis in infancy.

Other signs of severe, life-threatening in fections should be sought early in the eva uation of the febrile child (see Table 21.2 Altered sensorium, meningism or focal neu rologic findings are seen in central nervou system infections (though meningism is *no* commonly seen in infants less than 1 to years of age with meningitis). Strido drooling, retractions, and maintenance the head and neck in the "sniffing position (neck slightly flexed, head slightly extende on the neck and held quite still) are com mon presenting signs of upper airway ob structions such as acute epiglottitis or re tropharyngeal abscess. Dyspnea, cyanos or pallor, tachypnea, tachycardia, and hy

Table 21.2
Principal Life-threatening Acute Febrile Illnesses in Children

I. *Infection*
   A. Central nervous system
      1. Acute bacterial meningitis
      2. Encephalitis
   B. Upper Airway
      1. Acute epiglottitis
      2. Retropharyngeal abscess
      3. Laryngeal diphtheria (rare)
      4. Croup (severe)
   C. Pulmonary
      1. Pneumonia (severe)
      2. Tuberculosis, miliary
   D. Cardiac
      1. Myocarditis
      2. Bacterial endocarditis
      3. Suppurative pericarditis
   E. Gastrointestinal
      1. Acute gastroenteritis (fluid/electrolyte losses)
      2. Appendicitis
      3. Peritonitis (other causes)
   F. Musculoskeletal
      1. Necrotizing myositis (gas gangrene)
   G. Systemic
      1. Meningococcemia
      2. Other bacterial sepsis
      3. Rocky Mountain spotted fever
      4. Toxic shock syndrome

II. *Collagen-Vascular*
   A. Acute rheumatic fever
   B. Kawasaki's disease
   C. Stevens-Johnson syndrome

III. *Miscellaneous*
   A. Thyrotoxicosis
   B. Heat stroke
   C. Acute poisoning: atropine, aspirin, amphetamine
   D. Malignancy (rare): massive hemorrhage, hilar adenopathy compressing the trachea

potension reflect cardiorespiratory compromise as seen in infections such as severe pneumonia, pericarditis, bacterial endocarditis and septicemia. Hemorrhagic rashes occur in bacterial and rickettsial sepsis such as meningococcemia and Rocky Mountain spotted fever.

The remainder of the examination should focus on the likely sites of common infections in children: the ears, nose and throat; cervical lymph nodes; respiratory, gastrointestinal, and genitourinary tracts; integument; joints; and skeletal system. The tympanic membranes may show signs of acute otitis media such as redness, bulging, decreased motility, loss of landmarks and light reflex and drainage due to perforation. The nose, mouth or throat may have signs of inflammation pointing to acute upper respiratory infections (URI) including common colds, streptococcal pharyngitis, and herpetic gingivostomatitis. Cervical adenitis, a common complication of URI in children, may be apparent as a tender swelling on examination of the neck. An increase in the respiratory rate, presence of nasal flaring or retractions, and auscultatory abnormalities can suggest pneumonia and tracheobronchitis. The abdominal examination is usually unremarkable in common viral gastroenteritis, although ill-defined tenderness is often present. Suprapubic or flank tenderness would suggest urinary tract infection. Many febrile exanthems are so characteristic as to be diagnostic, examples including varicella, rubeola, and scarlet fever. Obvious joint inflammation in a febrile child points to septic arthritis; likewise, localized bony tenderness and inflammation suggest osteomyelitis.

Usually, a thorough history and physical examination will uncover the cause of an acute febrile illness (see Table 21.3). The most common diagnoses will be viral upper respiratory infections. Other viral illnesses such as gastroenteritis, stomatitis due to Coxsackie A (herpangina) or herpes simplex and exanthemata such as chickenpox and measles are readily identifiable sources of fever. However, some children with presumed viral illness have no definite focus of infection. Such patients are generally well-appearing despite their fever and, with the exceptions outlined below, should be managed symptomatically.

Common bacterial causes of acute febrile illnesses include otitis media, urinary tract infections, streptococcal pharyngitis, cervical adenitis, pneumonia and superficial skin infections, all of which usually give rise to

Table 21.3
Common Causes of Acute Febrile Illness in Children Seen in the Emergency Department

I. Infections
- A. Central nervous system
  1. Acute bacterial meningitis
  2. Viral meningoencephalitis
- B. Ocular
  1. Periorbital cellulitis
  2. Orbital cellulitis
- C. Upper respiratory tract
  1. Common cold
  2. Pharyngitis/tonsillitis
  3. Cervical adenitis
  4. Croup
  5. Epiglottitis
  6. Acute sinusitis
  7. Otitis media
- D. Oral cavity and salivary glands
  1. Alveolar abscess
  2. Herpangina
  3. Herpetic gingivostomatitis
  4. Mumps
- E. Pulmonary
  1. Acute tracheobronchitis
  2. Bronchiolitis
  3. Pneumonia
- F. Gastrointestinal
  1. Acute gastroenteritis
  2. Appendicitis
- G. Genitourinary
  1. Urinary tract infection
  2. Acute salpingitis
- H. Musculoskeletal
  1. Septic arthritis
  2. Osteomyelitis
- I. Cutaneous
  1. Cellulitis
  2. Viral exanthems
  3. Scarlet fever
  4. Miscellaneous systemic infections associated with prominent rash (e.g. meningococcemia and Rocky Mountain spotted fever)
- J. Systemic
  1. Primary septicemia—especially meningococcemia
  2. "Occult" bacteremia—especially pneumococcal
  3. Viral syndromes

II. Miscellaneous
- A. Drug and vaccine reactions including serum sickness
- B. Kawasaki's disease
- C. Salicylate poisoning

localizing signs and symptoms. However, these (particularly the urinary infections and pneumonia) as well as other localized infections (e.g., early osteomyelitis) can surprisingly silent at times. Additional recent investigations have shown that ba teremia occurs in 5% of young febrile ch dren who have minimal URI symptoms fever alone and who do not look clinical ill. The organisms recovered are *Strept coccus pneumoniae* in 60 to 70%, *Haem philus influenzae* type B in about 20%, a occasionally *Neisseria meningitidis* or *Sa monellae* as well. Almost all such bacte emic children are less than 24 months age, have a fever ≥39°C (102°F), and WBC count of ≥15,000/mm^3.

Given the above general consideratio an algorithmic approach to the child wi an acute febrile illness can be formulate using the following key features: overa degree of toxicity and presence of signs symptoms of life-threatening diseases, i munocompromized host status, age, degr of fever, and presence of other localizi features on history or physical exam (Fi 21.1). Laboratory studies are indicated on for selected situations as defined by th above clinical features. The vast majori of febrile children seen in an emergen department will need no laboratory testin

All children with fever require an imm diate rapid assessment upon arrival in th emergency department by a person qual fied to recognize neurologic signs such extreme impaired sensorium, irritability ongoing seizure activity, evidence of seve airway obstruction and/or inadequate ve tilation, circulatory insufficiency, hemo rhagic rash, and extreme hyperpyrexi (temperature ≥41.1°C (106°F)). If any these findings are present, or if the patie is immunocompromised by virtue of unde lying disease, asplenia or drug treatmen certain obvious management decisions an actions need immediate institution, ofte prior to establishment of definitive diagno sis (see algorithm in Fig. 21.1 and chapte on meningitis (45), septic shock (2), epiglo titis (62), pneumonia (45), and heat stroke hyperpyrexia (33). The febrile child comin to the emergency department with a histor of having had a seizure is a somewhat spe cial case.

A history of convulsions with fever ma portend serious central nervous system in fection. However, often a young child wit

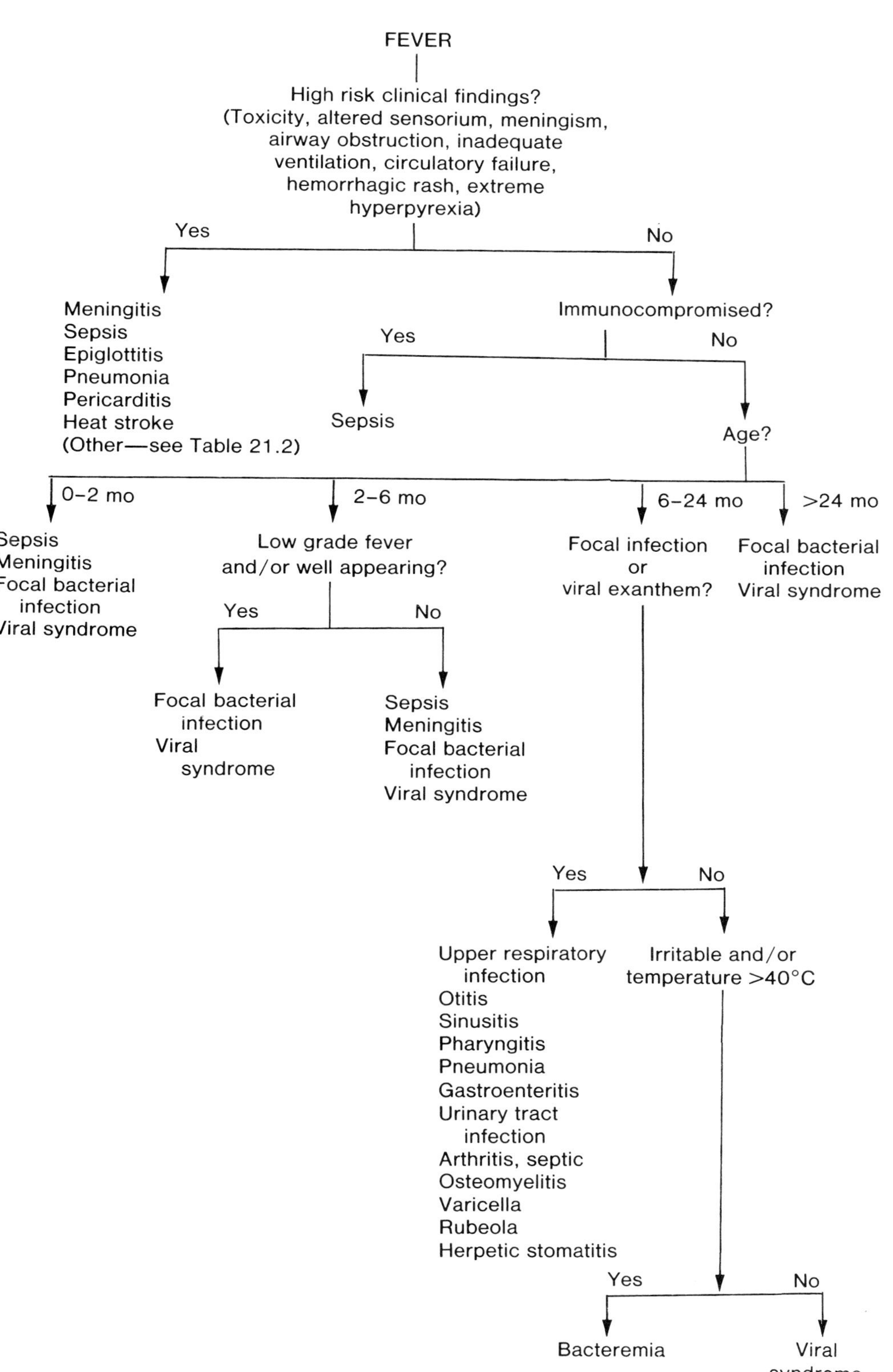

Figure 21.1 Approach to evaluation of the febrile child.

high fever will have had a single, brief, generalized seizure at home, or even in the emergency department waiting area, and still look very well at the time of examination. Simple febrile seizures are a common pediatric problem occurring in 3% of all children. They are defined as occurring only once per febrile illness, in children 6 months to 5 years of age. Furthermore the seizure must be brief (less than 15 min in duration), generalized, unaccompanied by neurologic findings, altered sensorium, or clinical signs of meningitis, and occur within 12 hours of onset of the fever (>38.5°C (101.3°F)).

The dilemma facing the emergency physician is to decide if such a child requires a lumbar puncture to rule out meningitis. Recent studies by several groups of investigators have shown that experienced pediatricians can diagnose on clinical grounds alone those children likely to have bacterial meningitis among a group with febrile seizures. However, because the clinical assessment of infants is fraught with uncertainty, it has been our usual practice to perform lumbar puncture in children less than 18 months of age with a first febrile seizure. Older children who show no clinical evidence of meningitis do not receive *routine* lumbar puncture. It is to be emphasized that: (1) this recommendation applies only to those children with *simple febrile seizures* as defined above and (2) children prone to recurrent simple febrile seizures may also contract meningitis and must be evaluated for this possibility, as any other child of similar age and clinical appearance.

Following the ascertainment that none of the above immediate threats to life, nor obviously recognizable signs of meningitis, are present, and with the above considerations regarding febrile seizures in mind, the careful history and examination outlined previously are undertaken. All children with fever (temperature ≥38°C (100.4°F)) who are less than 2 months of age receive a full laboratory investigation for serious infection, including CBC, chest x-ray, and urine, CSF and blood cultures ("septic work-up"). They are admitted to the hospital for observation with consideration given to starting presumptive antibiotic therapy (Chapter 45). Children between 2 months and 6 months are evaluated for degree of fever and degree of irritability. An occasional infant at this age may truly "look great" despite significant fever and be judged as requiring symptomatic treatment only without aggressive laboratory investigation or hospitalization. Those with high fever (temperature ≥39.5°C (103°F)), especially if they demonstrate even mild to moderate irritability and/or full anterior fontanel or meningism (the latter a rare sign in young infants) also deserve a septic workup. If all laboratory results are normal, such a child may be discharged on symptomatic treatment and/or antibiotics if an appropriate focus (i.e., otitis media) is found. However, even with normal laboratory parameters, these patients are at risk of bacteremia and subsequent focal infection, including meningitis. Thus, it has been our tendency to admit those who are 2 to 6 months with fever and *marked* irritability even when CBC and CSF are initially normal.

The febrile child 6 to 24 months of age with moderate irritability and/or meningeal signs also needs an evaluation including CBC, chest x-ray, and cultures of CSF, blood, and urine. If all results are normal, and the child looks better after antipyresis and a period of observation, he or she may be managed as an outpatient, again with appropriate symptomatic therapy and/or antibiotics for focal bacterial infections. For these children, as well as those who are clearly not ill enough to require lumbar puncture but still do not "look great," and/or have a temperature >40°C (104°F), we recommend the use of the total WBC as a guide to the risk of the "occult" bacteremia syndrome described previously. If the WBC is >15,000/mm^3, a blood culture is obtained, and oral antibiotics (usually amoxicillin, 50 mg/kg/day) begun. Follow-up is planned for 24 to 48 hours at which time clinical status and culture reports are reviewed (see bacteremia in Chapter 45). A chest x-ray is also helpful in children with high fever, especially if the WBC is >15,000/mm^3, since many times lobar pneumonia will be discovered despite a paucity of physical findings. Young infants, less than 12 months, especially if even moderately ill-appearing, are usually admitted to the hospital if diagnosed as having bacterial pneumonia or urinary tract infection.

The child older than 24 months can usually be managed on the basis of degree of irritability, evidence of meningeal signs, and/or other foci of infection found on history and physical. He or she need not be routinely screened for occult bacteremia. After excluding meningitis, there are several important infections which may be present in ill-appearing febrile children, without obvious initial focus, in this age group. These include meningococcemia, Rocky Mountain spotted fever, salmonellosis or shigellosis, and pyelonephritis. Early institution of presumptive therapy may be life-saving in some of these entities, so their possibility must be borne in mind with the toxic, febrile child at any age. Obviously, if certain very high risk features are missed during the initial triage (or evolved after triage) and are encountered early during the physician's careful clinical assessment (i.e., a significant purpuric rash), the child is managed with extreme urgency as befits his reclassification into the high risk category.

To reiterate, "occult" bacteremia, lobar pneumonia, and urinary tract infections in children often present as fever alone without localizing signs early in their course. Other relatively frequent causes of acute febrile illness syndrome to be kept in mind include intoxications (especially due to aspirin, atropinics, amphetamines, and antihistamines) and immunization reactions. With diphtheria-pertussis-tetanus (DPT) onset of fever is usually within 12 to 24 hours and may last 24 to 48 hours; with live measles or MMR vaccine onset of fever, if it occurs at all, is usually at 7 to 10 days, and sometimes a faint rash is seen.

SYMPTOMATIC TREATMENT

Over the years there has been considerable debate about the theoretical benefits of fever in the mechanism of host defense, but few definite benefits have been demonstrated in man. Most clinicians find that febrile children, especially those with high fever (temperature ≥39.5°C (103°F)), feel much better if temperature is brought down with antipyretic medication. Furthermore, antipyresis may allow the physician to see the child at "his best," and in particular can help in the decision to perform a lumbar puncture. However, such antipyresis may actually hamper accurate assessment of children with occult bacteremia, since such patients generally show at least mild to moderate irritability before antipyresis but often look quite well afterward (Henretig et al.). Thus, the ideal assessment of such patients would include observations of overall clinical appearance before and after antipyresis.

In general, antipyretic therapy should parallel the pathophysiologic basis of the fever. When due to altered hypothalamic set point, as in infection, antigen-antibody reactions and malignancy, attempts to reset the "thermostat" with aspirin or acetaminophen are most likely to enhance patient comfort. If fever is due to imbalance of heat production and heat loss mechanisms, such as in heat stroke, then rapid cooling by physical removal of heat is necessary and antipyretics will not help. Rarely, a patient with infection will have extreme hyperpyrexia (temperature ≥41.1°C (106°F)) and require urgent temperature reduction with both antipyretics and physical removal of heat, such as ice-water bath.

Current dosage recommendations for both aspirin and acetaminophen are 15 mg/kg given every 4 hours with usual maximum dose for both in the range of 650 mg every 4 hours. It is important to remember that many parents have great fear about even moderately high fever in their children and require reassurance that the fever itself, in its usual range of severity, does not cause damage. They need education regarding appropriate indications and dosing for antipyretic treatment, the lack of urgency in treating fever (unless temperature ≥41.0°C or there are prolonged febrile seizures), and most importantly the concept that the overall well-being of the child, in context with age, is usually far more important than the temperature per se.

References

Feder HM, Jr: Occult pneumococcal bacteremia and the febrile infant and young child. *Clin Pediatr* 19: 457–462, 1980.

Henretig FM, et al.: Clinical assessment of febrile infants at risk for occult bacteremia (abstract), Ambulatory Pediatric Association, San Francisco, 1981.

Jaffe M: Fever and convulsions—indications for laboratory investigations. *Pediatrics* 67: 729, 1981.

Lorber J, Sunderland R: Lumbar puncture in children with convulsions associated with fever. *Lancet*, 785, Apr 12, 1980.

McCarthy PL: Controversies in pediatrics: what tests are indicated for the child under 2 with fever. *Pediatr Rev* 1: 51–56, 1979.

McCarthy PL et al.: History and observation variables in assessing febrile children. *Pediatrics* 65: 1090–1095, 1980.

Schmitt BD: Fever phobia: misconceptions of parents about fevers. *Am J Dis Child* 134: 176–181, 1980.

HAPTER 22

Gastrointestinal Bleeding

JOHN T. BOYLE, M.D.

INTRODUCTION

In emergency department practice, the diatric patient is more likely than the ult to have acute rather than chronic strointestinal (GI) bleeding. The vast marity of patients who come to the emerncy department with "GI bleeding" have st small amounts of blood and are hemonamically stable. In such patients, two portant questions must be asked: (1) is e patient really bleeding? and (2) is the ood coming from the GI tract? Children th known or suspected causes of vomiting diarrhea in whom one or two drops or cks of blood are noted in the vomitus or ool should not be considered "GI bleeds" if their history or physical examination e otherwise unremarkable. Parents ould be reassured that the blood reprents merely local irritation, and the sympm treated. Likewise, a number of subances may simulate GI bleeding. Food loring, beets, Jello, Kool-Aid, antibiotic rups, and pyrinium pamoate may resemle red blood. Bismuth and iron preparaons, spinach, blueberries, grapes, and licrice may all be mistaken for melena. A areful history for recent epistaxis, dental ork, tonsillectomy, adenoidectomy and ore throat is also important. Chemical sts (Hematest or Hemoccult) to docuent intestinal blood loss should be rounely performed on material (vomitus, ool) which parents may bring to the emerency department.

The following discussion will deal with the approach to documented intestinal blood loss which, because of amount or clinical presentation, is felt to be pathological. The clinical presentation may be bright red or coffee ground hematemesis, or bright red, dark red, or tarry bowel movements.

EVALUATION AND DECISION

The list of causes of GI bleeding is extensive. A systematic approach to all patients includes: (1) initial assessment of the severity of the bleeding and institution of appropriate resuscitative measures; (2) establishing the level of bleeding within the GI tract; (3) pertinent history, physical examination and laboratory tests based on a knowledge of the various age related etiologies; and (4) emergency treatment based on general groups of causes.

Initial Assessment of the Patient

The physician who concentrates too quickly upon diagnosis at the expense of emergency care may jeopardize the child's life. The urgency of the intitial resuscitation will depend both on an estimate of the amount of blood lost in the stool or through vomiting and the patient's clinical status.

Parents tend to exaggerate the volume of blood their child has lost. The physician should request the parent to state specifically whether it was a drop, a spoonful, a cupful, or a quart. The clinical presentation may also delineate the potential severity of the bleeding. Bright red rather than coffee ground hematemesis points to a rapid rate of bleeding. Coffee ground material has been acted upon by gastric acid and usually indicates a low rate of bleeding. The estimated volume of blood loss should be correlated with the clinical status of the patient. Low blood pressure, orthostatic changes, tachycardia, severe pallor, poor capillary and venous filling, sweating, restlessness, and mental confusion all suggest significant blood loss and demand immediate measures. A child is capable of intense vasoconstriction to maintain his blood pressure. Perhaps the best indicator of significant acute blood loss is postural changes in pulse and blood pressure. A drop in systolic pressure of 10 mm Hg or more or an increase in 20 beats/min in pulse on moving the patient from supine to sitting position, suggests significant blood loss.

Hemoglobin and hematocrit are unreliable indices of the severity of acute GI bleeding because of a delay in hemodilution after acute blood loss. Even in a patient with overt hemodynamic instability, the initial hematocrit may be normal or only slightly decreased.

The resuscitation of the patient with hemodynamic instability or suspected significant volume loss is discussed in Chapter 2.

Establishing the Level of Bleeding

There are two general categories of bleeding. Upper GI bleeding refers to ble ing above the ligament of Treitz; lower bleeding is bleeding that is distal to t ligament of Treitz. In the majority of cas the clinical presentation together with n sogastric lavage will delineate the level bleeding within the GI tract (Fig. 22.1).

Hematemesis strongly suggests a ble ing site above the ligament of Treitz. T absence of hematemesis, however, does n eliminate the upper gastrointestinal tra as the source of blood loss, as upper tra bleeding frequently leads to melena rarely, the passage of gross maroon color blood or clots per rectum. Melena usua means bleeding from a site above the eocecal valve and is related to the effects digestive enzymes or bacterial action intraluminal blood. In general, the dark the blood in the stool, the higher it orig nates in the GI tract. Nevertheless, th stasis of blood in the right colon, lesions that area may cause melena. Hematochez usually means bleeding distal to the lig ment of Treitz; bloody diarrhea usually r flects colonic bleeding. Bright red bloo which streaks the surface of the stool us ally originates from the anorectal area.

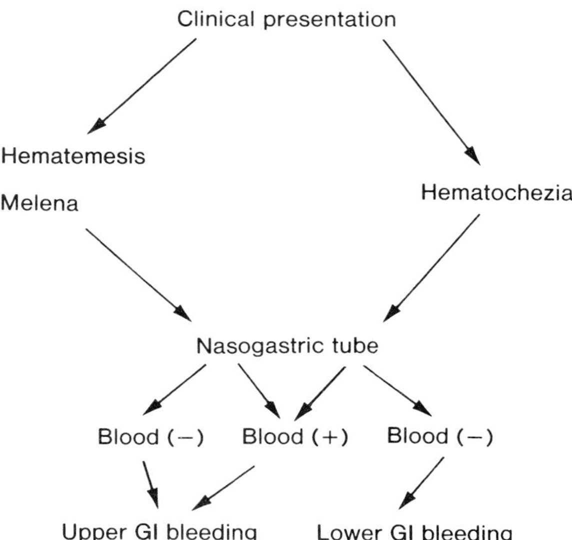

Figure 22.1 Establishing level of gastrointestinal (GI) bleeding.

All patients in whom the level of GI eeding is not obvious should have a na- gastric tube passed and their stomachs pirated. This is particularly important in .tients with no previous history of intes- ıal bleeding. Failure to document bleed- g from the upper GI tract early is often gretted several days later when initial agnostic studies are negative and the urce is still unclear. Not only is the pres- ıce of blood (bright red or coffee ground) the stomach diagnostic of an upper GI eed, but gastric lavage allows one to make ı estimate about the size of the bleed and hether the bleeding has stopped. It is im- ɔrtant to realize, however, that the ab- nce of blood by aspirate does not exclude .e possibility of upper tract bleeding, for eeding may have ceased or its source may › distal to a competent pylorus. Neverthe- ss, in one study of over 1000 patients, only % of those with upper GI bleeding had a ıstric aspirate negative for blood. On the her hand, a few blood streaks in the stom- :h contents may be secondary to trauma ıused by passage of the tube and should ɔt be taken as evidence of upper tract eed is historical data are not compatable.

Early Diagnostic Evaluation

In the emergency department, the phy- cian must seek information from the his- ɔry, the physical examination, and labo- ıtory tests which will narrow the range of iagnostic possibilities and help in deciding n appropriate strategies of intervention. pecific endoscopic and radiologic diagnostic techniques are rarely indicated in the early emergency evaluation of patients, but the clinical decision concerning the timing and sequence of subsequent special procedures is based on information obtained at the initial evaluation.

UPPER GI BLEEDING

Table 22.1 lists the age-related causes of upper GI bleeding. However 95% of cases of upper GI bleeding may be classified into two diagnostic categories: mucosal lesions and esophageal varices (Table 22.2). Mucosal lesions include esophagitis, gastritis, Mallory-Weiss gastroesophageal tears, stress ulcers, and peptic ulceration. While lesions in both categories may present with severe bleeding and hemodynamic instability, bleeding from mucosal lesions is usually self-limiting and will respond to conservative medical management. Bleeding from esophageal varices also usually stops spontaneously, but it carries a worse prognosis and requires a different mode of therapy. The object of the history, physical examination, and laboratory tests is primarily to distinguish between these two categories of upper GI bleeding. At the same time, clues to rare causes of upper GI hemorrhage should also be sought.

History

Suggestive of Mucosal Lesions. Is there a history of serious underlying GI disease, i.e., gastroesophageal reflux, peptic ulcer, inflammatory bowel disease? Is there a history of recent significant stress, i.e.,

able 22.1
tiology of Upper Gastrointestinal Bleeding Based on Age

Neonatal Period (<4 wk)	Infancy (<2 yr)	Preschool	School Age
. Bleeding diathesis	1. Stress ulcer	1. Stress ulcer	1. Chronic peptic ulcer
. Hemorrhagic gastritis	2. Esophagitis	2. Gastritis	2. Stress ulcer
. Stress ulcer	3. Gastritis	3. Mallory-Weiss tear	3. Gastritis
. Swallowed maternal blood	4. Mallory-Weiss tear	4. Esophageal varices	4. Mallory-Weiss tear
. Esophagitis	5. Pyloric stenosis	5. Esophagitis	5. Esophageal varices
. Foreign body irritation (nasogastric tube)	6. Vascular malformation	6. Foreign body	6. Esophagitis
. Vascular malformations	7. Duplication	7. Vascular malformation	7. Inflammatory bowel disease
. Duplication		8. Hemobilia	8. Vascular malformation
			9. Hemobilia

Table 22.2
Categories of Upper Gastrointestinal Bleeding

I. Mucosal Lesions (with common causes)
- A. Esophagitis: gastroesophageal reflux, moniliasis, herpes, corrosive, foreign body
- B. Mallory-Weiss tear
- C. Gastritis: drug induced (primarily aspirin), stress, alcohol, viral cytomegalovirus, herpes), bile reflux, foreign body or bezoar
- D. Stress ulcers: infection (sepsis, encephalitis, meningitis, hepatitis), dehydration, hypoglycemia, burns, head injury, postsurgical, difficult birth, aspirin therapy, steroid therapy
- E. Peptic ulcer

II. Esophageal Varices, Secondary Portal Hypertension
- A. Presinusoidal: cavernous portal vein transformation, acute portal vein thrombosis
- B. Sinusoidal: cirrhosis, hepatitis, infiltrative processes
- C. Postsinusoidal: Budd-Chiarri syndrome, right-sided congestive heart failure

infectious processes, dehydration, surgery, burns, head trauma, multiorgan trauma, difficult birth? Is there a history of toxic ingestion? What medications does the child take, specifically aspirin, nonsteroidal antiinflammatory drugs, steroids, reserpine, anticoagulants? Parents often consider taking aspirin so routine that they neglect to mention it. It is important to *specifically ask* about recent aspirin intake in all patients with upper GI bleeding. In addition, all adolescents should be questioned concerning alcohol ingestion.

A history of vomiting prior to the onset of bleeding episodes is important. Recurrent vomiting or regurgitation or unexplained pulmonary disease suggests gastroesophageal reflux or gastric outlet problems associated with esophagitis. Projectile vomiting in young infants points to pyloric stenosis, a condition which may result in secondary gastroesophageal reflux and esophagitis. Hematemesis following the acute onset of vomiting or retching at any age should suggest a Mallory-Weiss te Chronic peptic disease in the presch child is rare but often associated with f quent vomiting rather than pain.

Pain, particularly if increasing shortly b fore bleeding, suggests a GI lesion disru ing the mucosa. Dysphagia accompan esophageal lesions. On the other hand, M lory-Weiss tears and bleeding esophag varices rarely are preceded by pain. P and dysphagia, however, are hard sym toms to assess in young children and m be manifested only by irritability or a orexia. The absence of pain certainly do not exclude inflammatory mucosal lesion

Suggestive of Esophageal Varic The possibility of bleeding esophageal va ices is primarily suggested by the past me ical history. Variceal bleeding is rare infancy. A history of jaundice, hepatit and blood transfusion should be sought, should be a specific inquiry regarding liv disease in family members. Questio should be asked about neonatal conditio associated with portal vein thrombosis, i. sepsis, shock, exchange transfusions, o phalitis, and umbilical vein catherization

Suggestive of Other Conditions. In t well neonate, it is important to ask abo breast feeding and the possibility of regu gitation of maternal blood swallowed du ing feeding. Prompt diagnosis by means the Apt-Downey test for the absence fetal hemoglobin in the vomitus may ra idly allay fears and prevent costly and i vasive workup. Likewise, inquiries about family history of bleeding disorder or m ternal use of medications (such as aspiri anticoagulants or anticonvulsants) ma lead to the diagnosis.

Massive hemorrhage associated wi right upper quadrant pain and jaundice the post-trauma patient should arouse suspicion of hemobilia or bleeding into th bile tracts. A family history of polyposis also important.

Physical Examination

Suggestive of Mucosal Lesions. A no mal physical examination with the exce tion of mild to moderate epigastric or pe iumbilical tenderness is the hallmark most patients with mucosal bleeding. Mar exhibit the signs of a viral syndrome or other infectious processes. Oral thrush may lead one to suspect candida esophagitis, and lesions of the oral mucosa suggest the possibility of corrosive ingestion. A chest examination may show evidence of chronic aspiration or obstructive lung disease suggestive of gastroesophageal reflux.

Suggestive of Esophageal Varices. Jaundice, spider angiomas, palmar erythema, and abdominal distention point to chronic liver disease. Signs of intrahepatic portal hypertension include hepatomegaly, splenomegaly, and ascites. Isolated splenomegaly is suggestive of extrahepatic cavernous transformation of the portal vein.

Suggestive of Other Conditions. Petechiae or ecchymosis may suggest hemorrhagic diathesis or trauma. Melanotic pigmentation on the buccal mucosa occurs in patients with Peutz-Jegher syndrome. Hemangiomas or telangiectasia on the skin or oral mucosa often accompany angiodysplasia in the GI tract.

A careful ear, nose, and throat examination should be performed to rule out the possibility of swallowed blood from a nasopharyngeal source.

Laboratory Evaluation

Laboratory tests are not helpful in pinpointing the precise cause of upper GI bleeding. Mucosal lesions are more apt than esophageal varices to be associated with antecedent occult bleeding. Therefore, low mean corpuscular volume (MCV) and hypochromic, microcytic erythrocytes on initial blood count are more suggestive of a mucosal lesion. Initial low WBC and platelet counts may indicate hypersplenism from portal hypertension, but can also be caused by sepsis with associated stress mucosal ulceration. Abnormal liver studies including an elevation of the serum and bilirubin, transaminases, prothrombin time and a low serum albumin are suggestive of esophageal varices as an etiology for bleeding.

Further Diagnostic Evaluation

The major diagnostic alternatives in the further evaluation of upper GI bleeding include: fiberoptic endoscopy, barium contrast radiography, selective or superselective abdominal arteriography, and surgery (Fig. 22.2).

Fiberoptic endoscopy is clearly the most rapid and effective technique for detecting the exact source of upper GI bleeding. Five points have tempered our feelings about the need for emergency endoscopy in acute upper GI bleeding:

1. Eighty to 85% of upper GI bleeding stops spontaneously, and mucosal lesions can usually be distinguished from variceal bleeding by history, physical examination, and simple laboratory studies in most cases.
2. The diagnostic yield on endoscopy performed 12 to 24 hours after admission is as good as when it is performed immediately on admission. Therefore, if the patient responds quickly to resuscitation, one does not need to do emergency endoscopy in the middle of the night.
3. The improved diagnostic accuracy of double contrast barium radiography in detecting significant mucosal lesions capable of rebleeding make this test a valid alternative to endoscopy in evaluating stabilized patients.
4. Current studies have not confirmed that early diagnosis improves mortality and morbidity associated with bleeding. Transfusion requirements, need for emergency surgery, and duration of hospitalization seem to be no different whether early diagnosis is known or not. However, this may be simply a measure of the dangers of emergency surgical procedure on bleeding patients who are severely ill rather than of the usefulness of more accurate endoscopic detection of the bleeding source.
5. Despite numerous ongoing experimental studies evaluating endoscopic injection sclerotherapy, spraying of tissue adhesive, electrosurgery, cryosurgery, and laser photocoagulation, to date there are no practical endoscopic methods of controlling ongoing GI bleeding.

Therefore, we reserve emergency endoscopy for the patient who continues to bleed at a rate considered life-threatening (copius

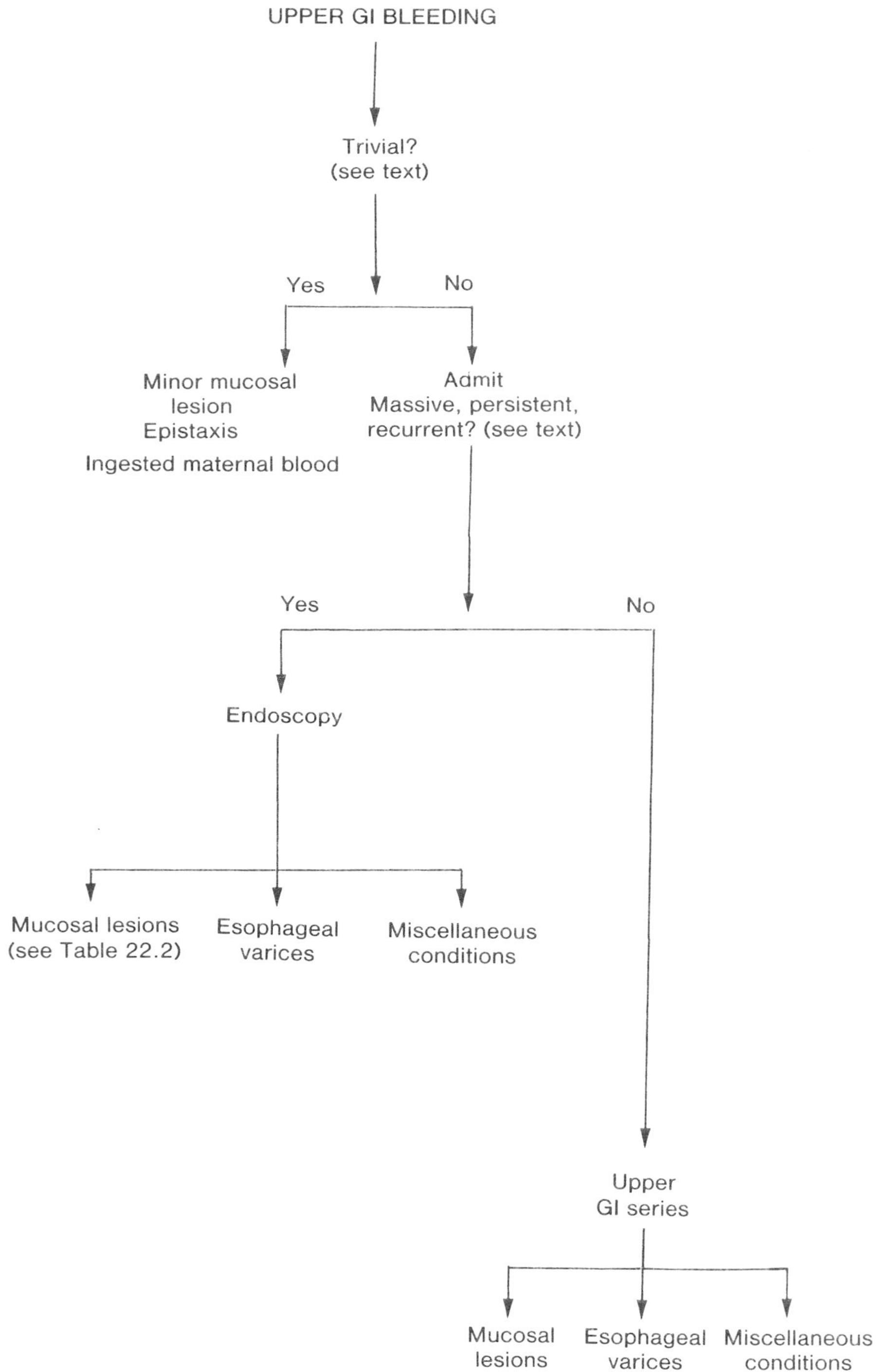

Figure 22.2 Diagnostic approach to upper gastrointestinal (GI) bleeding.

witnessed blood, continuing transfusion requirement, hemodynamic instability) despite initial medical therapy, and in whom a precise etiologic diagnosis will lead to specific medical or surgical therapy. Elective endoscopy is performed 12 to 24 hours following admission in patients who stop bleeding spontaneously but who (1) require transfusion or drop hematocrit below 30 or (2) have a history of previous unexplained upper GI bleeding episodes. All other patients, who have either stopped bleeding at the time of admission or soon after and who remain stable for 24 to 36 hours, are evaluated by air contrast barium contrast study.

It is now generally agreed that barium contrast radiography has little, if any, diagnostic usefulness in the presence of *active* GI bleeding. However, if the patient has a self-limited bleed, double air contrast x-ray performed 24 to 36 hours after admission will usually show lesions which are apt to re-bleed, particularly esophageal varices and peptic ulcer.

LOWER GI BLEEDING

The majority of GI bleeding in the pediatric age population, particularly over 1 year of age, originates distal to the ligament of Treitz. Furthermore, 70 to 80% of lower GI bleeding occurs in the anus, rectum, and colon. Unlike upper GI bleeding, specific diagnosis is more important in the management of lower GI bleeding. Table 22.3 lists the age-related causes of lower GI bleeding. Age is much more important diagnostic factor in lower GI bleeding than upper GI bleeding.

The approach to lower GI bleeding is based on three important points.

1. Severe lower GI bleeding leading to hemodynamic instability or requiring transfusion is rare in pediatrics. Nasogastric intubation is essential to rule out upper GI bleeding in any child with suspected significant lower GI bleeding. Meckel's diverticulum is the most common etiology of severe lower bleeding in all age groups, even given the fact that 50% of symptomatic Meckel's diverticula usually present before the age of 2 years. Inflammatory bowel disease and polyps are less frequent causes. Intestinal duplication can also contain ectopic gastric mucosa and produce bleeding by peptic ulceration of adjacent nongastric mu-

Table 22.3
Etiology of Lower Bleeding Based on Age

Neonatal Period	Infancy	Preschool	School Age
Well Infant			
1. Swallowed maternal blood	1. Anal fissure	1. Infectious colitis	1. Infectious colitis
2. Infectious colitis	2. Infectious colitis	2. Juvenile polyps	2. Inflammatory bowel
3. Milk allergy	3. Milk allergy	3. Anal fissure	3. Pseudomembranous enterocolitis
4. Hemorrhagic disease	4. Nonspecific colitis	4. Intussusception	4. Polyps
5. Duplication of bowel	5. Juvenile polyps	5. Meckel's diverticulum	5. Angiodysplasia
6. Meckel's diverticulum	6. Intussusception	6. Angiodysplasia	6. Hemolytic uremic syndrome
Sick Infant	7. Meckel's diverticulum	7. Henoch-Schönlein purpura	7. Hemorrhoids
1. Necrotizing enterocolitis	8. Duplication	8. Hemolytic uremic syndrome	8. Ischemic colitis
2. Infectious colitis	9. Hemolytic uremic syndrome	9. Inflammatory bowel disease	
3. Disseminated coagulopathy	10. Inflammatory bowel disease	10. Pseudomembranous enterocolitis	
4. Midgut volvulus	11. Pseudomembranous enterocolitis	11. Ischemic colitis	
5. Intussusception	12. Ischemic colitis		
6. Congestive heart failure			

cosa. Severe small and large bowel bleeding is also a complication of hemophilia. There have been only isolated reports of vascular lesions, lower bowel varices, ischemic colitis, and infectious diarrhea producing severe bleeding. GI bleeding in intestinal obstruction is a late finding and rarely is severe unless the problem goes undiagnosed for a prolonged period of time.
2. The main priority for the emergency physician is evaluating the patient with lower GI bleeding is to identify lower tract bleeding associated with intestinal obstruction. Intussusception and midgut volvulus secondary to malrotation are the major types of intestinal obstruction associated with lower GI bleeding. However, all causes of abdominal obstruction will eventually lead to GI bleeding if the vascular supply to the bowel is compromised. These include obstruction due to adhesions, incarcerated hernia, and other causes of volvulus such as Meckel's diverticulum, mesenteric cyst, and duplications. Forty percent of children with symptomatic Meckel's diverticula develop intestinal obstruction secondary to volvulus or intussusception (see Chapter 5).
3. In the vast majority of patients, rectal bleeding will be self-limiting, associated with diarrhea or constipation, and due primarily to inflammatory (bacterial colitis) or anorectal lesions (fissures and polyps).

In the emergency department, history, physical examination, and radiography are the primary means of distinguishing obstructive from nonobstructive causes of lower GI bleeding.

History

Suggestive for Obstructive Process. The age of the patient, type of abdominal pain, and color of the bleeding are important factors in the history of the patient with intestinal obstruction. One-half of the cases of intussusception occur in the first year of life; the majority of the rest during the second year. At any age, the acute onset of abdominal pain, vomiting, and distention associated with rectal bleeding is highly suggestive of intestinal obstruction. However, the occurrence of abdominal cramps accompanying rectal bleeding in an infant less than 2 should always be approached as intussusception until proven otherwise. Since bleeding in the obstructed patient is usually a late sign and indicates vascular compromise of the involved bowel, the blood is usually dark red (currant jelly).

Suggestive for Nonobstructive Processes. An infant with abdominal pain who passes a currant jelly stool is likely to have an obstructive lesion but, taken singly, youth, pain, and currant jelly stools are not specific for obstruction. Not uncommonly children with Meckel's diverticula, polyps, or angiodysplasia pass currant jelly stools, but these nonobstructive disorders cause painless rectal bleeding. Although pain is commonly associated with inflammatory lesions of the bowel, these are not obstructive processes. Inflammatory lesions are usually associated with diarrhea, tenesmus, and systemic symptoms such as fever, rash, arthritis, and arthralgia.

Age, again, is an important diagnostic factor in nonobstructive bleeding. Anal fissure is the most common cause of rectal bleeding in infancy and early childhood. Anal fissure is unusual in the adolescent, but, together with a history of diarrhea, should make one suspect Crohn's disease (see Chapter 50). Colitis secondary to milk allergy infrequently occurs after age 2 years. Juvenile polyps are rare before age 1 and after age 15 years. Inflammatory bowel disease is rare prior to 10 years of age. Hemorrhoids almost never occur during childhood.

The type of bleeding is also important. Bloody diarrhea and/or tenesmus point to inflammatory lesions, the most common etiology being bacterial infection. Nonspecific proctitis, in which no specific infectious etiology can be determined, is probably the second most common cause in infancy. Such patients are clinically well, but pass frequent small, loose, blood-streaked stools. Whether such patients have a viral-induced colitis or milk protein allergy is as yet unknown. Rotavirus has recently been implicated in bloody diarrhea. In any patient with bloody diarrhea, the emergency physician must maintain a high degree of suspicion for other causes of inflammatory bowel disease, i.e., pseudomembranous colitis, hemolytic-uremic syndrome, Henoch-Schönlein purpura, nonobstructive ischemic colitis, and ulcerative colitis or Crohn's colitis. In the neonate, necrotizing enterocolitis also has to be considered. In patients with a history of chronic diarrhea, especially adolescents who may not divulge a history of chronic rectal bleeding because of fear, special questioning regarding weight loss, fever, abdominal pain, rash, mouth sores, arthritis, and arthralgia may suggest a need for urgent further evaluation to look for ulcerative or Crohn's colitis. Chronic ischemic colitis is often overlooked in the historically evaluation of lower GI bleeding. Specific causes of nonobstructive ischemic colitis include: (1) postoperative after general anesthesia, (2) collagen vascular disease, (3) cardiac failure, (4) shock, (5) trauma, (6) intermittent volvulus or intussusception, (7) thrombotic thrombocytopenia purpura, (8) uremia, (9) digitalis toxicity, and (10) the use of oral contraceptive pills. One must also consider radiation enterocolitis in oncologic patients.

Constipation, or the passage of either large or hard stools, is commonly associated with the presence of anal fissure. Pain on defecation is suggestive of anal fissure, cryptitis or proctitis. A history of longstanding constipation with sudden onset of bloody diarrhea should suggest enterocolitis associated with Hirschsrpung's disease.

Drug history is again important, particularly recent antibiotic therapy which may be associated with pseudomembranous colitis. Enteric coated anti-inflammatory preparations, i.e. aspirin and nonsteroid anti-inflammatory agents, may produce ulceration in the small bowel.

Travel history, animal exposure, and sources of drinking water may all provide clues to the diagnosis. A family history of bleeding diathesis, polyps, or inflammatory bowel disease should be sought.

Physical Examination

Suggestive of Obstructive Processes. Abdominal distention, tenderness, a palpable mass, peritoneal signs, and hyperactive bowel sounds suggest obstruction. Hyperactive bowel sounds, however, may follow bleeding into the small bowel without obstruction.

Suggestive of Nonobstructive Processes. A relatively benign physical examination with the possible exception of mild to moderate periumbilical or lower quadrant tenderness is the hallmark of most patients with inflammatory lesions. Right lower quadrant fullness and tenderness suggest Crohn's disease. Growth retardation, fever, and swollen joints may all occur in children with inflammatory bowel disease.

Visual inspection of the anus by spreading the buttocks may show an anal fissure, cryptitis, or a severe diaper rash that oozes blood. Digital rectal examination is mandatory as 30 to 40% of rectal polyps are within reach of the examining finger. Significant pain on rectal examination suggests inflammatory colitis or proctitis.

As with upper GI bleeding, examination of the skin is important as findings may suggest bleeding diathesis, Peutz-Jeghers syndrome, or angiodysplasia (see p. 000). Ecchmyosis of the buttocks and lower extremities is a common manifestation of Henoch-Schönlein purpura. Eczema may be associated with milk allergy. Soft tissue tumors (osteoma, lipoma) suggest another polyposis syndrome, Gardner's syndrome. Erythema nodosum is the most common skin manifestation of inflammatory bowel disease. Café au lait spots are indicators of neurofibromatosis which is rarely associated with intramural neurofibromas of the bowel that can ulcerate, producing bleeding.

Radiologic Evaluation

A flat and upright abdominal x-ray should be obtained when the history and physical examination suggest an obstructive process. These may show obvious signs of obstruction; absence of rectal air, dilated proximal loops of bowel, air fluid levels, or

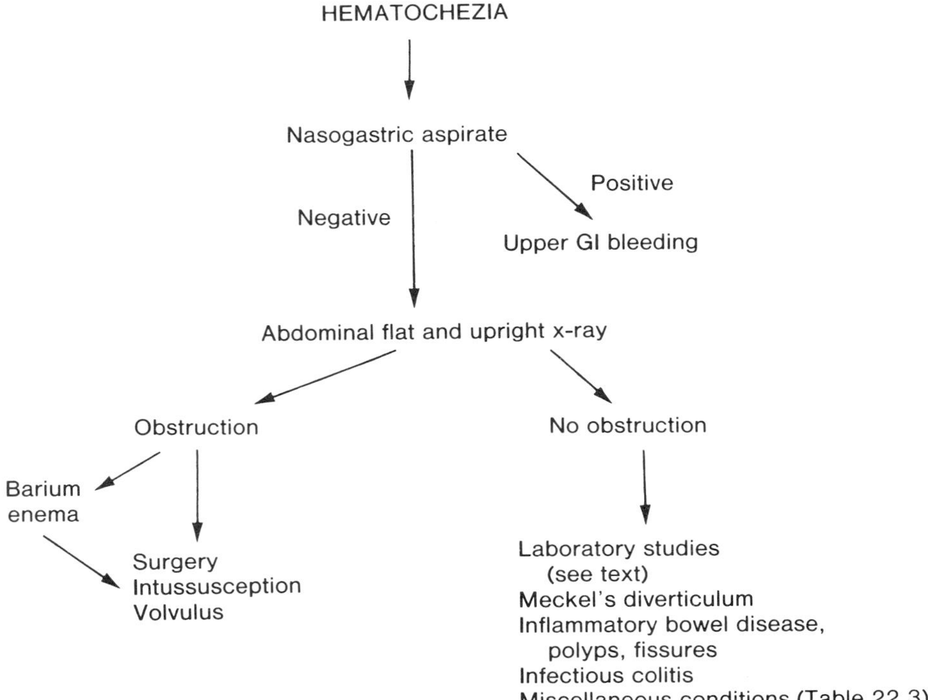

Figure 22.3 Diagnostic approach to lower gastrointestinal (GI) bleeding.

mass effect. However, the absence of definite obstructive signs in the face of a suggestive history or physical examination should not disuade further aggressive evaluation.

Further Diagnostic Evaluation

Having rule out obstructive processes by history, physical examination and abdominal x-ray, subsequent diagnostic evaluation of lower GI bleeding involves a logical sequential diagnostic plan which terminates at any point at which the cause for bleeding is found (Fig. 22.3). Since in most cases the bleeding is self-limiting, the urgency and extent of the evaluation is determined by the amount of bleeding, age of patient, associated clinical symptoms, and physical findings. It is not unreasonable to simply culture the stool and observe the well infant who has a few blood streaks in the stool and normal physical examination, or the child with the clinical signs of acute viral syndrome who presents with a scant amount of blood in a diarrheal stool.

In all cases, the evaluation should always begin in the emergency department. CBC, including red cell indices and smear, may give an indication of the chronicity of the bleeding. An elevated sedimentation rate points to inflammatory process. If bacterial colitis is strongly suspected, a Wright-stained smear of stool may be helpful; the presence of many neutrophils supports the diagnosis of infection. Some feel eosinophils in stool smear are suggestive of milk allergy, but they may also be seen infectious colitis. Stool cultures should be obtained not only for *Salmonella* and *Shigella*, but also *Campylobacter*, *Yersinia enterocolitica*, and *Clostridium difficile*. Culture of the latter three organisms requires special techniques and must be specifically requested. If available, stool should be assayed for enterotoxin produced by *C. difficile*. To exclude bacterial colitis, it is important to have at least three negative stool cultures. In the adolescent, an anorectal culture should be plated on Thayer-Martin media in order to exclude gonococcal proctitis. Stool should be collected for ova and parasites; but in addition, serological tests for amoeba should be drawn. Amoeba serology is positive in 90% of active cases.

Upon obtaining the above tests, the patient should be scheduled sequentially for proctosigmoidoscopy, Meckel's scan, air contrast barium enema, and upper GI series with small bowel follow through. Proctosigmoidoscopy confirms the presence of inflammatory colitis, and should always precede radiologic evaluation. Barium enema is performed only when known infectious etiologies of colitis have been rules out. As in the case of upper intestinal bleeding, double air contrast study of the large bowel is far superior to single contrast studies.

In the rare patient with unremitting lower intestinal bleeding requiring resuscitation and/or transfusion, exploratory laparotomy remains a reasonable approach since the likelihood of finding a remedial lesion is high, i.e. Meckel's diverticulum, polyp, and duplication. Nevertheless, there remains a significant number of patients in whom no bleeding site can be found. This number has been reported to be as high as 50%, but more likely is less than 20%. The development of new innovative diagnostic and therapeutic techniques over the past several years has enabled a more systematic approach to severe lower GI bleeding, providing the patient can be adequately stabilized by appropriate resuscitative measures. This sequential approach includes: (1) Meckel's scan; (2) technetium bleeding scan; (3) colonoscopy; and (4) angiography. Once again, it is important to emphasize that in massive rectal bleeding, one must always consider a duodenal bleeding site associated with a competent pylorus, leading to a negative nasogastric aspirate.

EMERGENCY TREATMENT

Upper GI Bleeding

Treatment of upper GI bleeding in the emergency department involves: resuscitation of the patient with hemodynamic instability, maintenance of intravascular volume and oxygen carrying capacity in the patient with active bleeding, control of bleeding by nasogastric lavage and other specific measures based on suspected etiology, and institution of preventive measures to prevent re-bleeding in patients who have stopped bleeding. The specifics of management are discussed in Chapter 50. Managing the problem of acute upper GI bleeding requires a team approach including the emergency physician, surgeon and gastroenterologist.

All pediatric patients with upper GI bleeding should be admitted to the hospital for observation and further evaluation even if they are hemodynamically stable, and the bleeding has stopped. Upper GI bleeding is associated with significant morbidity and mortality in the pediatric age group. Early recurrence of bleeding is common enough no matter what the cause to justify a period of close observation. The only exceptions are (1) children with known or suspected causes of vomiting, who bring up flecks of bright red blood in vomits and who have normal vital signs and physical exam, and negative nasogastric aspirate and (2) infants who vomit ingested maternal blood.

Lower GI Bleeding

Specific treatment techniques for lower GI bleeding must be predicated on accurate diagnosis. History and/or physical examination suggestive of intestinal obstruction should lead to urgent surgical consultation. Treatment for specific medical conditions is discussed in Chapters 50 and 59.

References

Katz LA: Advances in the approach to gastrointestinal bleeding in childhood. In *Digestive Disease in Children*, edited by E Lebenthal. Grune & Stratton, New York, 1978.

Law DH, Watts HD: Gastrointestinal bleeding. In *Gastrointestinal Disease: Pathophysiology; Diagnosis. Management*, Vol. 2, edited by MH Sleisenger and JS Fordtran. W. B. Saunders, Philadelphia, 1978.

Ostrow JD, Mulvancy CA, Hansell JR, Rhodes RS: Sensitivity and reproducibility of clinical tests for fecal occult blood with an emphasis on false-positive reactions. *Am J Dig Dis* 18: 930, 1973.

Roy CC, Morin CL, Weber AM: Gastrointestinal emergency problems in pediatric practice. *Clin Gastroenterol* 10: 225, 1981.

Roy CC, Silverman A, Cozzetto FJ: Symptoms; hematemesis; rectal bleeding. In *Pediatric Clinical Gastroenterology*, Ed. 2. C. V. Mosby, St. Louis, 1975.

Spencer R: Gastrointestinal hemorrhage in infancy and childhood: 476 cases. *Surgery* 55: 718, 1964.

CHAPTER **23**

Headache

EDWARD B. CHARNEY, M.D.

INTRODUCTION

Headache is a common complaint of childhood and adolescence. The numerous conditions associated with this symptom often result in a diagnostic challenge for the emergency department physician. Recognition of the pain sensitive structures of the head often assists in this initial evaluation process by localizing the anatomic origin of the headache.

Pain sensitive structures are either extracranial (i.e., paranasal and mastoid sinuses, ocular orbits, teeth, scalp and neck muscles) or intracranial (i.e., large intracranial venous sinuses and their tributaries, dura mater at the base of the skull, and the dural arteries including the anterior and middle meningeal and large arteries at the base of the brain). The brain parenchyma and much of the meningeal surface and ependymal linings of the ventricles are all relatively insensitive to pain. Headache localized to the anterior portion of the cranium through the fifth cranial nerve generally results from stimulation of pain structures on or above the tentorium, whereas headache posteriorly is generally transmitted from structures below the tentorium by the ninth, tenth, and upper three cervical nerves. Major pathophysiologic mechanisms operating upon these pain sensitive structures include: inflammation, traction, vasodilatation, and muscle contraction. The common causes of headache are listed by pathophysiologic classification in Table 23.1.

Inflammation

Acute purulent *meningitis* and viral *encephalomyelitis* frequently have headache as an early symptom, with inflammation of pain sensitive structures at the base of the brain and over the convexity. Localization depends on distribution of the meningeal irritation. The headache is often associated with neck stiffness, fever, and change in mental status. *Dental disease* may refer pain to distant points with either frontal, temporal, retroauricular or global headaches. These headaches are commonly aggravated by rinsing of the mouth with hot or cold water and are accompanied by dental abnormalities on either oral examination or dental radiographs.

Headaches may also be associated with inflammation of the *sinuses*. Inflammation and swelling of the sinus ostia, the most pain sensitive areas of nasal and paranasal structures, are the prime causes of such headaches. These headaches are usually characterized by localized pain and/or tenderness over the sinuses and rhinitis with nasal mucosa congestion. Maxillary antrums and ethmoid cells are present at birth and are usually of sufficient size to house infection, with resultant inflammation and headache. The pain originating from ethmoid sinusitis may be referred behind the eyes to the temporal or occipital areas. Frontal sinuses usually are not sufficiently developed and pneumatized until 6 to 10 years of age and therefore are unlikely to be the source of infection in preschool

Table 23.1
Pathophysiologic Classification of Headaches

- *I. Inflammatory*
  - A. Intracranial infections
    - 1. Meningitis
    - 2. Encephalitis
  - B. Dental infections
  - C. Sinus infections
- *II. Traction*
  - A. Increased intracranial pressure
    - 1. Cerebral edema
    - 2. Hydrocephalus
    - 3. Intracranial hemorrhage or hematoma
    - 4. Brain abscess
  - B. Neoplasm
  - C. Lumbar puncture
- *III. Vascular*
  - A. Febrile illness
  - B. Migraine
  - C. Systemic hypertension
  - D. Vascular anomalies
  - E. Seizures
  - F. Hypoxia
- *IV. Muscle Contraction*
  - A. Tension
  - B. Fatigue
- *V. Others*
  - A. Post-traumatic
  - B. Psychogenic
  - C. Ocular

children. In older children, frontal sinusitis usually causes pain just above the inner canthus of the inner eye on the affected side. Radiographic evidence of sinus involvement supports the clinical suspicion of sinusitis.

Traction

Displacement of the intracranial contents with traction on neighboring pain sensitive vessels and dura may result from increased intracranial pressure or an intracranial mass lesion (see Chapter 67). Increased intracranial pressure has several possible etiologies including the multiple causes of cerebral edema (i.e., pseudotumor cerebri, vasculitis, infection); obstructive hydrocephalus; epidural, subdural or intracerebral hematoma; brain abscess; ruptured intracranial aneurysm; and neoplasm. All of these diagnostic entities might be considered in the child who has severe headaches with clinical evidence of increased intracranial pressure with drowsiness, vomiting, diplopia, and papilledema.

Headaches following lumbar puncture are thought to be secondary to continued leakage of CSF through a dural hole, producing spinal fluid hypovolemia with traction on the base of the brain resulting from decreased reservoir volume. These headaches usually appear several hours after the procedure, persist for variable lengths of time (days to weeks), and tend to be exacerbated by the upright position and relieved with recumbency.

Vasodilatation

The major vascular headaches result from fever, systemic hypertension, migraine, or seizures. *Fever* associated with systemic illness (i.e., pharyngitis and viral syndrome) is the most common cause of all headaches in children. Febrile headaches resulting from increased intracranial vasodilation tend to be felt across the frontal and/or bitemporal regions, or occasionally in the retro-orbital area. They are constant or throbbing, intensified by body or head movement, and usually relieved by the combined antipyretic and analgesic effects of drugs such as acetylsalicylic acid or acetaminophen.

Systemic hypertension, often associated with acute glomerulonephritis or other renal diseases in children, may produce cranial arterial dilatation and headache. Coarctation of the aorta, pheochromocytoma, excessive steroid therapy and congential adrenal hyperplasia are less common sources of hypertension. Arterial dilation and headache may also result from the cerebral hypoxia associated with compromised cerebral circulation in congestive heart failure, vascular-occlusive events of sickle cell disease, or severe anemia.

Migraine is a common cause of recurrent headaches in childhood. Although the exact underlying pathophysiology is unknown, there are three recognized stages including: vasoconstriction of cerebral arteries, vasodilatation, and edema. There is usually a rather sharply defined clinical prodrome associated with the vasoconstrictive phase consisting of transient visual disturbances such as scintillating scotoma. Sensory modalities other than vision may be affected (i.e., paraesthesias, nausea, photophobia), and transient motor deficits (i.e., speech difficulties, hemiparesis) may occur. The pain of the vasodilatation stage in classic migraine headache is unilateral at the onset but often becomes generalized after 1 or 2 hours. It may last anywhere from 1 to 2 hours to 1 or 2 days. During the attack the child tries to avoid noises and bright lights and often finds relief through prolonged sleep. Children with complicated migraine will have transient hemiplegia or ophthalmoplegia as a manifestation of ischemia during the vasoconstrictive phase. The last stage of edema is often marked by a steady and dull headache accompanied by nausea. Family history is usually positive for similar migraine headaches. (For further discussion, see Chapter 44, p. 341.)

Headache may be the presenting manifestation of a *seizure disorder* in a child. The headache can occur either as an aura of a major motor seizure, during the postictal stage, or as the only manifestation of a seizure. There is no specific characteristic pattern or location; however, a significantly epileptiform electroencephalogram, presence of motor seizures, or dramatic response to anticonvulsants support the diagnosis (see Chapter 44).

Muscle Contraction

Sustained contraction of the skeletal musculature of the head and neck results in tension headaches. They are frequently precipitated by either emotional stress or fatigue, located usually in the back of the head and neck but occasionally generalized and described as a feeling of "tightness," "pressure," or a "band tightly around the head." Tension headaches are more commonly seen in adolescents than in young children.

Other

Headaches following *head trauma* frequently occur soon after return of consciousness and probably result from irritation of extracranial and intracranial pain-sensitive structures by small hemorrhages, edema, or vascular changes. There are no specific characteristics of post-traumatic headaches; however, persistence long after initial injury may be associated with a history of numerous psychogenic somatic complaints.

Controversy continues as to whether *ocular* abnormalities (i.e., refractive errors, astigmatism, strabismus, impaired convergence) can cause headaches. These ocular headaches should be relieved with proper corrective lenses. *Psychogenic* headaches are not uncommon in childhood and may be a symptom of depression or function for secondary gain, as in school avoidance.

EVALUATION AND DECISION

A complete history, physical examination, and neurologic examination are of paramount importance in evaluating the child complaining of headache. Emphasis is placed on eliciting the presence or absence of a history of head trauma, and the findings of fever, meningeal signs, other neurologic abnormalities, and hypertension. An approach to the differential diagnosis of headache utilizing these key clinical features is discussed below and outlined in Figure 23.1.

The presence of fever is helpful in initially guiding the diagnostic workup toward conditions with an infectious etiology. Both viral and bacterial meningitis may have headache as an initial symptom. Lumbar puncture should be performed in the child with signs of meningeal irritation (nuchal rigidity, Kernig and/or Brudzinski sign) on examination. Occurrence of other neurologic abnormalities, such as cranial nerve palsies, decreased sensorium or focal motor weakness, associated with fever and headache suggests a brain abscess which can be documented by computerized axial tomography. If the child with headache and fever has a completely normal neurologic examination, then attention should be directed to the sinuses and dentition. Localized tenderness over the sinuses or evidence of dental abnormalities on examination war-

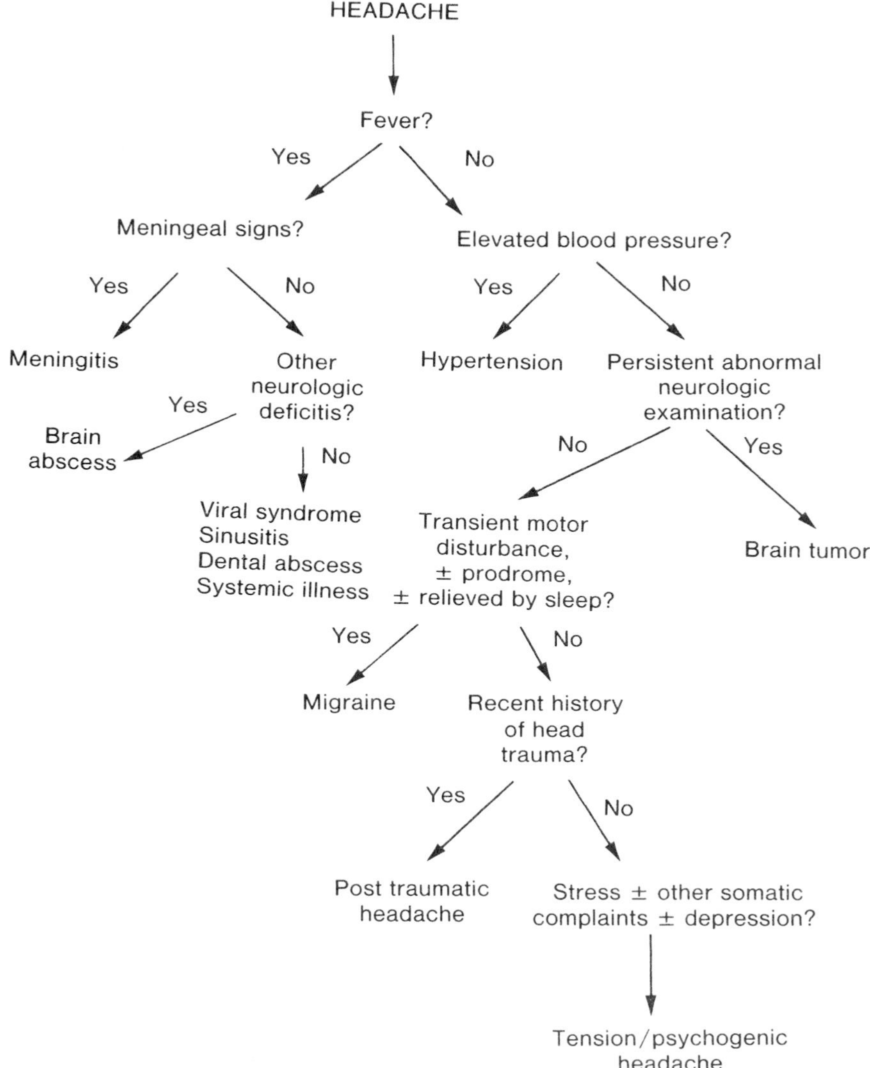

Figure 23.1 Approach to the diagnosis of headache.

rant radiographs of the sinuses or dentition, respectively. Headaches are commonly a symptom of the febrile response to a systemic illness and therefore the diagnostic workup should be limited in the child with a normal neurologic, sinus, and dental examination.

In the absence of fever, the evaluation for a child with a headache should begin with an accurate blood pressure recording. Diastolic pressures of greater than 100 to 110 mm Hg may be associated with headache. Children with hypertension should be assessed for evidence of renal disease by urinalysis, with specific attention for the cellular casts, proteinuria and/or hematuria of glomerulonephritis. Blood pressure recordings in both upper and lower extremities, along with cardiac auscultation, should be performed in the evaluation for aortic coarctation and associated hypertension. A detailed history regarding medications, particularly steroids, is essential in the diagnostic workup for hypertension, especially in the child on therapy for collagen vascular disease, malignancy, or asthma (see Chapter 46).

Complete neurologic and ophthalmologic examination is as crucial in the afebrile child complaining of headache as in the febrile child. Persistent abnormalities of either neurologic (i.e., ataxia and hemiparesis) or ocular systems (i.e., squint, papilledema, and recent onset of decreased visual acuity) are often associated with an intracranial mass producing increased intracranial pressure and headache. Intracranial hemorrhages or vascular anomalies frequently are associated with severe headaches that are sudden in onset, accompanied by stiff neck, not recurrent in nature, and usually followed by a decrease in the level of consciousness. Vascular abnormalities may also be associated with a cranial bruit.

Although brain tumor headaches often are characterized by their association with vomiting, are exacerbated by positional changes, and awaken the child from sleep, the most reliable evidence for such headache is the presence of abnormalities on neurologic and ocular examination. These abnormalities (i.e., ataxia, papilledema, and squint) are usually present within 2 months after the onset of headaches. Children with headaches that have been present for periods greater than 2 months and have a normal neurologic and ocular examination should be screened for the linear growth failure and/or diabetes insipidus, seen with the slow growing brain tumor, craniopharyngioma. Plotting several length measurements over time on standard growth curves, seeking a history for polydipsia or polyuria and testing urine specific gravity serve to screen the child with recurrent headaches over several months. The presence of persistent neurologic and/or ocular abnormalities or the development of linear growth deceleration warrants computerized tomographic scanning to investigate the possibility of brain tumor.

It is important to establish in the diagnostic workup whether the neurologic abnormalities are permanent or transient. Migraine headaches may have transient motor disturbances; however, there is often a positive family history for migraine and an associated prodrome. Electroencephalogram recordings vary considerably among children with migraine headaches. Therefore an accurate complete clinical history can often better establish the diagnosis. Accurate history taking may also reveal the occurrence of recent head injury that may be responsible for the headache in an otherwise healthy appearing child.

Tension or psychogenic headache should be a diagnosis of exclusion only after the aforementioned diagnostic scheme has been considered. Often these headaches occur in children where there is a positive family history of stress and/or multiple somatic complaints. School avoidance headaches are commonly characterized by prolonged school absenteeism and occurrence on week day mornings with relief during other periods of the day and weekends.

THERAPY

The majority of children presenting to the emergency department complaining of headache will have an associated febrile illness and will have considerable relief with rest and simple analgesic/antipyretic agents such as aspirin or acetaminophen. The child with suspected psychogenic or tension headache must receive the same critical historical, general physical and neurologic examination as the child with suspected "organic" headache. Reassurance and symptomatic relief with simple analgesia is often sufficient, until further in-depth assessment and management of these headaches can take place in a more appropriate medical setting than the emergency department. The treatment of headaches due to the various organic causes is discussed in appropriate chapters within this text.

References

Ad Hoc Committee on Classification of Headache: *JAMA* 179: 717, 1962.

Bachman DS, Hodges FJ, Friedman JM: Computerized axial tomography in neurologic disorders in children. *Pediatrics* 59: 352–363, 1977.

Berman P: Management of headache in children. *Pediatric Portfolio*, Vol. 1, No. 2, March 7, 1971.

Gass H, Goldstein AS, Ruskin R, Leopold NA: Chronic post-myelogram headache; isotopic demonstration of dural leak and surgical care. *Arch Neurol* 25: 168, 1971.

Hedges TR: An ophthalmological view of headache. *Headache* 11: 31, 1971.

Honig P, Charney E: Children with brain tumor headaches; distinguishing features. *Am J Dis Child* 136: 121, 1982.

Kriel RL: Headache. In *The Practice of Pediatric Neurology*, p. 154, edited by KW Swaiman and FS Wright. C. V. Mosby, St. Louis, 1975.

Livingston S, Whitehous D: Treatment of headaches in children. *Mod Treatment* 1: 1391, 1964.

McGovern JP, et al.: Headaches in children, part 1. *Headache* 1: 11, 1961.

Rothner AD: Headaches in children. *Headache* 19: 156–162, 1979.

CHAPTER 24

Hematuria

WILLIAM SCHWARTZ, M.D.

INTRODUCTION

Hematuria, the presence of red blood cells in the urine, is a common presenting complaint in the emergency department. A random red cell in the urine may be normal, but the appearance of 5 to 10 or more is abnormal and needs further investigation. It should be noted that many substances may color the urine red; further, both hemoglobinuria and myoglobinuria may cause the urine dipstick to be positive in the absence of red cells on microscopy (see Fig. 24.1). This discussion will be limited to the diagnostic approach to true hematuria.

PATHOPHYSIOLOGY

Red cells can be added to the urine at any point along the urinary tract from the glomerulus, through the tubule, collecting system, ureter, bladder and urethra. The presence of protein or tubular casts may help localize the source of the red cells. Although a small amount of protein may come from the tubules, the majority of the protein is derived from leakage through the basement membrane of the glomerulus. Red cells may become emmeshed in the protein matrix to form casts; thus, the presence of red cell casts point to bleeding in the glomeruli. Furthermore, glomerular bleeding that results in gross hematuria is usually manifested by "smokey" reddish brown urine (color of Coca-Cola or tea).

Common sites of nonglomerular bleeding are the renal papillae which are susceptible to necrosis from microthrombi and anoxia in patients with sickle cell hemoglobinopathies (especially AS and SC disease) or in those who have ingested toxins such as phenacetin. Severe bleeding from sites in the urinary tract below the glomerulus usually results in red urine that may contain clots but not red cell casts. Trauma to the kidney or bladder may cause hematuria either from contusions, hematomata or lacerations of the genitourinary tract. Increased vascularity from infection or chemical irritation will also lead to leakage of red cells into the urine. Bleeding may also occur rarely from tumors and cysts in the urinary tract. Most casts of hematuria are benign and idiopathic; since the amount of blood lost in the idiopathic cases is small, the bleeding is most likely secondary to a minimal leakage of red cells from a superficial blood vessel.

DIFFERENTIAL DIAGNOSIS

The differential diagnosis of hematuria is vast due to the long course of the urinary tract and the complicated steps in the formation of urine. The most common of the potentially serious renal causes of hematuria is acute post-streptococcal glomerulonephritis; infrequently, chronic nephritides are seen, either as primary renal diseases or in association with a systemic vasculitis as in lupus erythematosus, polyarteritis nodosa, or Henoch-Schönlein purpura. Other

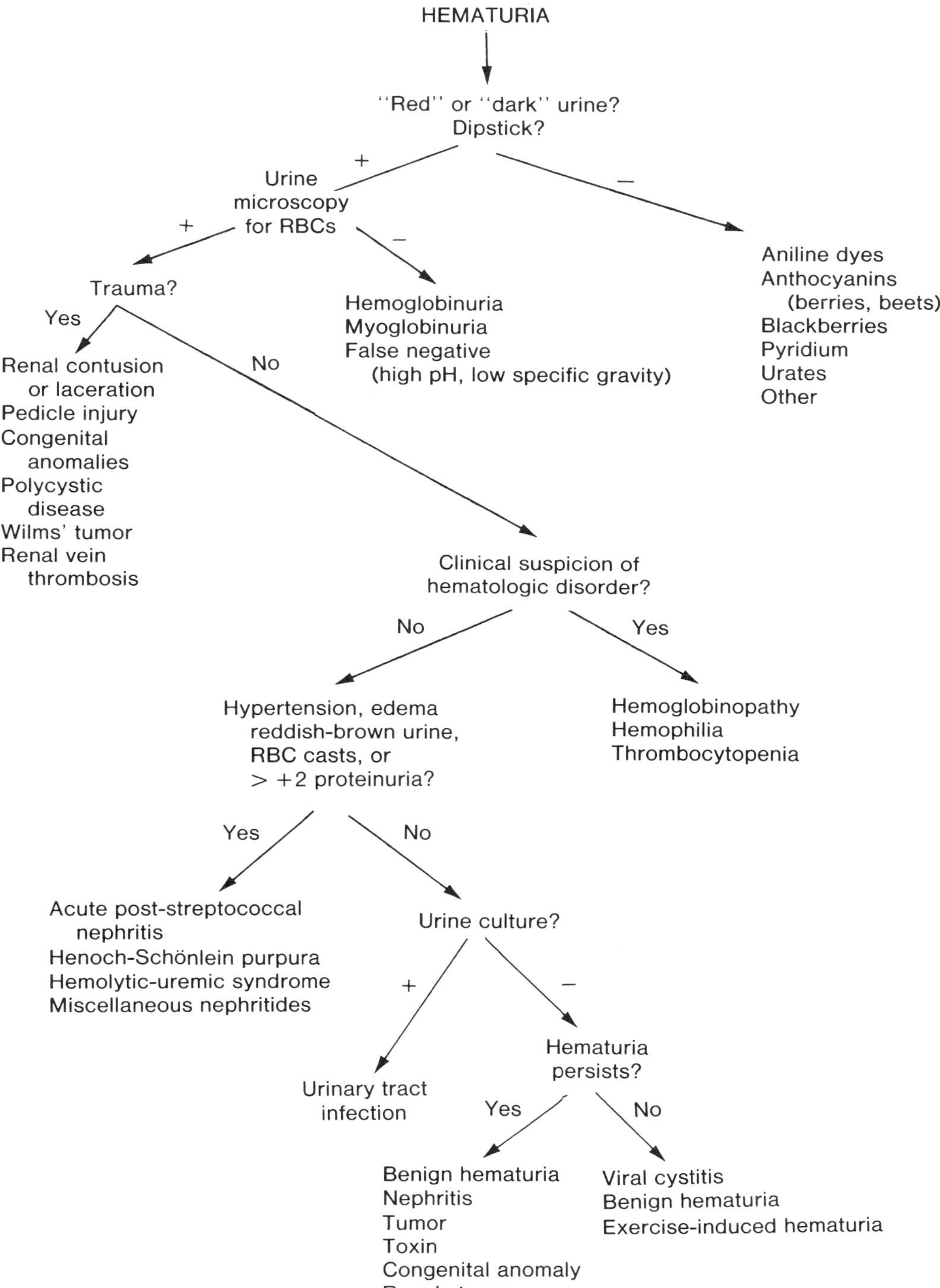

Figure 24.1 Approach to hematuria in the emergency department.

relatively common causes of hematuria that are usually readily identifiable after a thorough history and physical examination include trauma, urinary tract infection, and sickle cell hemoglobinopathies. When the child with hematuria is otherwise asymptomatic, most often no cause is found. This condition is usually referred to as benign (or benign recurrent) hematuria.

Hematuria may also be caused by congenital anomalies, including diverticula of the urethra and bladder, cysts of the kidney as in polycystic or multicystic kidney, and obstruction of the ureteropelvic junction. Wilms' tumor is associated with hematuria in about 15% of the cases. Although renal stones are not common in children, they should be considered if there is a family history of nephrolithiasis or a predisposing condition such as recurrent infection or bladder dysfunction as seen in myelomeningocele. Hypercalcuria and cystinuria are metabolic diseases that also predispose to renal stones and hematuria. The principal causes of hematuria are outlined in Table 24.1.

Table 24.1
Principal Causes of Hematuria in Children

- *I. Kidney*
  - A. Acute post-streptococcal glomerulonephritis
  - B. Other causes
    - 1. Pyelonephritis
    - 2. Trauma
    - 3. Tumor
      - a. Wilms' tumor
      - b. Leukemia
    - 4. Polycystic disease
    - 5. Collagen vascular disease
      - a. Systemic lupus erythematosus
      - b. Polyarteritis nodosa
      - c. Henoch-Schönlein purpura
    - 6. Hemolytic-uremic syndromes
    - 7. Hematologic disorders
      - a. Sickle cell hemoglobinopathies
      - b. Hemophilias
      - c. Thrombocytopenias
    - 8. Toxins
      - a. Phenacetin
      - b. Penicillins
      - c. Cephalosporins
      - d. Cyclophosphamide
    - 9. Hypercalcuria
    - 10. Cystinuria
    - 11. Renal stones
    - 12. Benign hematuria
- *II. Bladder*
  - A. Cystitis, infectious and chemical
  - B. Trauma
  - C. Toxins
  - D. Foreign bodies
- *III. Urethra*
  - A. Urethritis
  - B. Trauma
  - C. Diverticula
  - D. Foreign bodies

EVALUATION AND DECISION

The major task in evaluating a patient with hematuria in the Emergency Department is to identify the problems that need treatment or may be dangerous to the patient in the acute phase, such as renal trauma, malignancy, infection, or hypertension associated with acute nephritis (see Fig. 24.1). Historical information suggesting trauma, sickle cell disease, bladder irritation and any evidence of chronic or systemic disease should be sought. Family history regarding nephritis, deafness, renal stones, sickle cell disease or hemophilias, and renal anomalies is also important to elicit.

Physical findings of trauma or a mass in the abdomen or flank demand urgent intravenous pyelography. Often a hematologic disorder (leukemia, idiopathic thrombocytopenic purpura, hemophilia) may be suspected on the basis of findings such as petechiae, purpura, joint or mucous membrane bleeding, pallor, enlarged lymph nodes or splenomegaly. All black children with hematuria should have hemoglobin screening done. Evidence of nephritis on examination would include findings such as hypertension and edema. It is essential to measure the blood pressure in patients with hematuria; hypertension is seen in acute and chronic glomerulonephritis, in Wilms' tumor and in polycystic kidneys.

The laboratory investigation begins with a critical look at the urinalysis. Proteinuria may be present in any cause of bleeding but will not usually exceed 2^+ (100 mg/dl) if the only source of protein is from the blood. If there is more than 2^+ protein, the investigation should be directed towards glomerulonephritis. Tests for renal function, streptococcal antibodies, complement and electrolytes are indicated if the protein is $> 2^+$ and/or red cell casts are present on the initial urinalysis. However, since random protein tests are not reliable because they also reflect the state of the patient's hydration, a 24-hour collection of urine for protein would be preferable to determine if the proteinuria is significant. Further, the best time to detect casts is in the first urine specimen of the morning, since the urine will then be more concentrated than is likely on a random specimen taken after the patient has ingested liquids. Patients suspected of having glomerulonephritis should have throat and urine cultures, and all patients who are suspected of having urinary infection, or who are asymptomatic, should have a urine culture.

There is some controversy about the need for ordering an intravenous pyelogram (IVP) on all patients with hematuria. Since this is a reliable means to detect cysts, diverticula, tumors or obstruction, many physicians will use an IVP or ultrasound as part of their *initial* evaluation of hematuria, even in the absence of trauma or flank mass. Certainly if the hematuria does not seem to be due to an acute glomerulonephritis, and is persistent beyond a few days, an IVP would be considered necessary by most authors.

In the majority of patients, hematuria is chronic and asymptomatic, and there are no abnormal laboratory findings beyond the hematuria itself. These patients have benign hematuria. This diagnosis is one of exclusion and the patients should be followed for new signs or symptoms or the appearance of proteinuria. Benign hematuria may be associated with minor glomerular abnormalities but these patients do not need a renal biopsy since this invasion test is usually not helpful in making this diagnosis.

CHAPTER 25

Jaundice

JOHN B. WATKINS, M.D.

INTRODUCTION

Jaundice, recognized since antiquity as a cardinal sign of hepatic dysfunction, may have multiple etiologies. The excess bilirubin in the skin reflects an imbalance between rates of bilirubin formation and elimination of the pigment. Since bilirubin is derived from the breakdown of heme and must be largely conjugated in the liver before excretion can occur, accumulation of unconjugated bilirubin is due to excessive pigment formation from active hemolysis or an isolated deficiency of the hepatic conjugating mechanism. Conjugated hyperbilirubinemia, in contrast, is reflective of hepatobiliary dysfunction due to parenchymal disease or obstruction of the bile flow from an intra- or extrahepatic cause. These simple considerations provide the foundation for a practical approach to the diagnosis and management of extremely diverse conditions potentially responsible for hyperbilirubinemia and jaundice in all age groups (see Table 25.1).

EVALUATION AND DECISION

The first step in evaluating a jaundiced infant or child is to determine both the severity and type of the hyperbilirubinemia. This may be simply accomplished by performing both a total and direct serum bilirubin determination. Unconjugated hyperbilirubinemia is present when less than 15% of the total pigment reacts directly, and conjugated hyperbilirubinemia exists when the direct-reacting fraction exceeds 30% of the total. Additional testing may occasionally be necessary to classify the type of jaundice when the direct-reacting fraction is between 15 to 30% of the total.

Occasionally, the serum bilirubin level may be normal in a child who appears jaundiced. In this case the yellow cutaneous hue may be due to normal variation in the skin pigmentation or to carotenemia.

UNCONJUGATED HYPERBILIRUBINEMIA

The most important considerations in the evaluation of a child with unconjugated hyperbilirubinemia are the patient's age and the presence of anemia (see Fig. 25.1). Because some common disorders occur only during limited age ranges, division by age provides a useful basis for differential diagnosis.

The First Week of Life

Increased Hemolysis. Jaundice, clinically evident in the first 24 hours of life, is most often due to active hemolysis. In a large majority of newborns, maternal fetal blood group incompatibility (Rh or ABO) accounts for severe unconjugated hyperbilirubinemias. A direct Coombs' test is the standard procedure used to detect this type of hemolytic process. Red cell enzyme disorders, including deficiency of glucose-6 phosphate dehydrogenase and the rarer disorders such as pyruvate-kinase deficiency, must be diagnosed by specific enzyme as-

Table 25.1
Causes of Hyperbilirubinemia

- *I. Unconjugated Hyperbilirubinemia*
  - A. First 8 weeks of life
    - 1. Hemolytic disorders
      - a. Blood group incompatibility
      - b. Sepsis
      - c. Congenital spherocytosis
      - d. Red cell enzymopathies
      - e. Pyknocytosis
      - f. Congenital hypoplastic anemia
    - 2. Hepatic disorders
      - a. Crigler-Najjar syndrome
    - 3. Other
      - a. Physiologic jaundice
      - b. "Breast milk jaundice"
      - c. Congenital hypothyroidism
      - d. Upper gastrointestinal obstruction
      - e. Transient familial hyperbilirubinemia
  - B. Childhood
    - 1. Hemolytic disorders
      - a. Sickle cell anemia
      - b. Autoimmune hemolytic anemia
      - c. Other
    - 2. Hepatic disorders
      - a. Crigler-Najjar syndrome
      - b. Gilbert's syndrome
- *II. Conjugated Hyperbilirubinemia*
  - A. First 8 weeks of life
    - 1. Hepatic disorders
      - a. Biliary atresia
      - b. Neonatal hepatitis
    - 2. Congenital infections
      - a. Cytomegalovirus
      - b. Rubella
      - c. Syphilis
      - d. Other
    - 3. Metabolic disorders
      - a. Galactosemia
      - b. α_1-Antitrypsin deficiency
      - c. Tyrosinosis
      - d. Cystic fibrosis
      - e. Hereditary fructose intolerance
      - f. Other
    - 4. Extrahepatic biliary obstruction
      - a. Choledochal cyst
  - B. Childhood
    - 1. Hepatic disorders
      - a. Hepatitis
      - b. Drug-associated cholestasis
      - c. Dubin-Johnson syndrome
      - d. Rotor syndrome
    - 2. Metabolic disorders
    - 3. Congenital infections
    - 4. Extrahepatic biliary obstruction
      - a. Gallstones
      - b. Pancreatic disease

says in the red cells. Congenital spherocytosis can be determined on the basis of family history and characteristic appearance of the blood smears, and may occasionally present in the first days of life.

After the first day of life, jaundice is usually "physiologic" and due to immaturity of hepatic excretory function. However, "physiologic jaundice" is a diagnosis of exclusion. Other conditions must always be considered, particularly sepsis and causes of increased bilirubin formation due to red cell destruction.

Hemolytic conditions acquired during the first week of life may be due to reabsorption of a cephalohematoma, hemolysis due to vitamin K injections, and most importantly, neonatal sepsis. Inherited deficiency of bilirubin uridine 5′-diphosphate (UDP) glucuronyltransferase (Crigler-Najjar syndrome) is a rare disorder characterized by a rapid linear increase in the unconjugated serum bilirubin continuing after the fifth day in full-term newborns without any evidence of active hemolysis. In this condition, the serum bilirubin level may rise to as high as 30 mg/dl, all indirect-reacting, and only be temporarily lowered by exchange transfusions.

The Infant from 1 to 8 Weeks After Birth

The appearance of jaundice due to hemolytic and nonhemolytic conditions may be delayed in a number of infants until the second postnatal week or later. The most common cause, however, of an increase in unconjugated hyperbilirubinemia during this period is breast feeding. "Breast milk jaundice" is often reported to be familial and is generally not associated with other problems. The cause(s) of this unusual type of jaundice are not clearly defined. It may

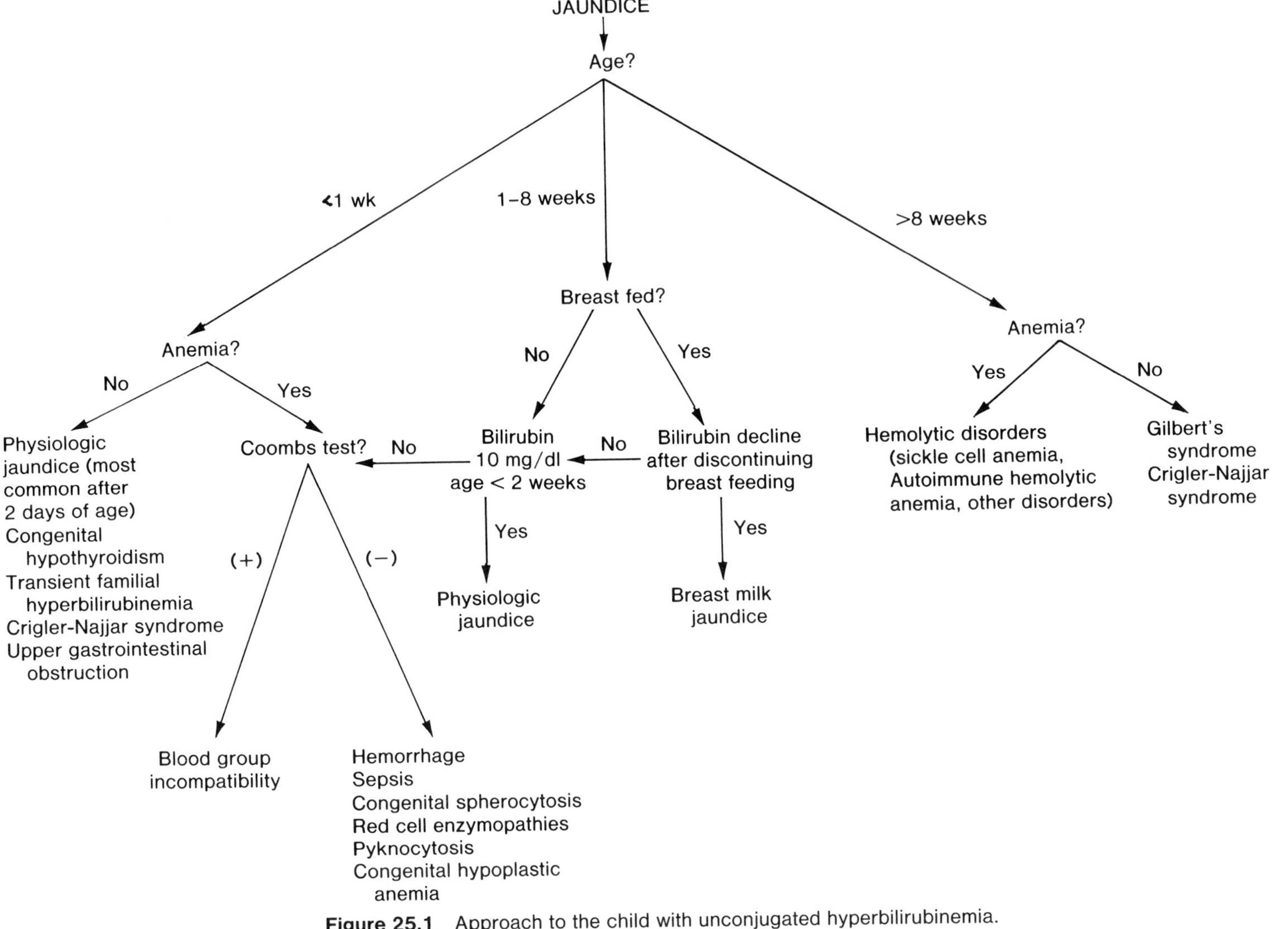

Figure 25.1 Approach to the child with unconjugated hyperbilirubinemia.

be due to the presence of abnormal female steroid hormone derivatives in the milk. Recent reports suggest that high concentrations of saturated free fatty acids secondary to human breast milk lipase activity promote the decrease in conjugation of bilirubin. The diagnosis of "breast milk jaundice" can be made when a rapid decrease in serum bilirubin follows the interruption of breast feeding for a few days. The resumption of breast feeding is usually not accompanied by a secondary rise in serum bilirubin, and the breast feeding may then be safely continued.

If an infant in this age range is not breast fed, or if the hyperbilirubinemia persists after the cessation of breast feeding, other conditions must be considered. Physiologic jaundice often accounts for a mild elevation of the serum bilirubin, but levels of more than 10 mg/dl merit further investigation. As for the infant in the first week of life (Fig. 25.1), a CBC and Coombs' test should be performed. Sepsis, urinary tract infection, and upper gastrointestinal obstruction are particularly serious conditions which must always be excluded before making a diagnosis of physiologic jaundice.

The Child Over 8 Weeks of Age

Jaundice occurs less frequently in children than in neonates. The most common disorders causing unconjugated hyperbilirubinemia after the first 2 months of life are the hemolytic anemias. Not infrequently, the child with previously undiagnosed sickle cell anemia develops jaundice with an acute infection.

Unconjugated hyperbilirubinemia without anemia is not often seen in children. Disorders such as Gilbert's syndrome or Crigler-Najjar syndrome may cause this clinical picture.

Conjugated Hyperbilirubinemia

The Infant Less than 8 Weeks of Age

Conjugated hyperbilirubinemia is always abnormal in early infancy. Multiple causes are listed in the table; however, infection, idiopathic liver disease ("neonatal hepatitis"), or biliary tract disease account for nearly 60 to 80% of cases in infants who develop conjugated hyperbilirubinemia during the first month of life. Therefore, as soon as conjugated hyperbilirubinemia is confirmed with the total and direct serum bilirubin reaction, the initial screening tests for infection and metabolic disease should be undertaken in the hospital in order to rule out potentially treatable causes of hepatic dysfunction. A relatively straightforward diagnostic approach is then available to the physician to further delineate between intrahepatic and extrahepatic biliary tract disease. In the emergency department, the serum glucose and a urine for reducing substances should always be obtained as certain metabolic disorders require urgent treatment.

The Child over 8 Weeks of Age

In the child over 8 weeks of age, conjugated hyperbilirubinemia may still be caused by some of the metabolic, infectious, and acquired lesions listed in Table 25.1. However, it is important to differentiate between an intrahepatic disorder and disease causing obstruction of the biliary tree. Viral hepatitis as the cause of jaundice, although common, should not be assumed. Drug related cholestasis always merits consideration and may require admission to the hospital or follow-up for proper evaluation. The physician should always inquire about previous episodes of jaundice, alcoholic stools, and/or abdominal pain. These symptoms suggest a more chronic condition or an underlying disorder leading to obstruction of the intra- or extrahepatic biliary tree. A thorough physical examination should be performed to search for an abdominal mass. Signs of peritoneal irritation, as seen in cholecystitis and pancreatitis, are often difficult to differentiate from the tender liver of hepatitis. Additionally, cutaneous and other physical findings (spider hemangiomas, ascites, splenomegaly, and growth failure) may point to chronic liver disease.

The use of the newer noninvasive diagnostic modalities such as ultrasound, computerized axial tomography, and endoscopic visualization of the extrahepatic biliary tree have improved the diagnostic accuracy in many patients. However, hospitalization in order to obtain a liver biopsy to confirm the diagnosis or to complete the necessary investigations is often required unless the clinical and laboratory findings suggest acute infectious hepatitis or drug-related cholestasis.

References

Allagille D, Odievre M: *Liver and Biliary Tract Disease in Children.* John Wiley & Sons, 1979.

Andres RK, Walker WA: Liver disease in infants. *J Pediatr* 90: 864, 1977.

Watkins JB, Katz A, Grand RJ: Neonatal hepatitis: A diagnostic approach. *Adv Pediatr* 24: 399, 1977.

HAPTER 26

Limp

ROBERT A. DOUGHTY, M.D.

INTRODUCTION

Limp is defined as an uneven, jerky, or)orious gait. Limp is easily recognized as departure from normal ambulation by th physician and parents; however, as-ssment of the etiology may be more dif-ult. The two phases of gait are the stance d swing phase. The former begins with e heel striking the floor and ends with eing off. The swing phase consists of nding the knee to about 70°, flexing the), and then extending the knee with dor-lexion of the foot to allow heel contact the next stance phase. Loss of rhythm-ty, weakness, or pain can cause alteration the coordinated process and produce a np.

Certain limps are characteristic of spe-ic abnormalities. The antalgic gait results m a short stance phase due to pain by ight-bearing on that extremity. The endelenberg gait is characterized by a wnward pelvic tilt during the swing phase e to weakness or pain of the contralateral iteus (medius) muscle. Marked difficulty mbing stairs frequently results from in-lvement of the quadriceps femoris or glu-is muscle groups. Careful observation of e gait may help pinpoint the weak or inful area.

It is difficult to outline a complete differ-tial diagnosis for limp since its causes iy be so varied. Table 26.1 lists many of e more common conditions associated th limp. The key to approach is to carefully observe the gait and localize the source of pain or weakness leading to the abnormality, as outlined in Figure 26.1.

EVALUATION AND DECISION

In the absence of obvious trauma, the critical conditions which must be excluded are joint and bone infections. Other serious disorders causing limp include tumor and hemoglobinopathy.

A careful history must be obtained. Presence of significant trauma reduces the likely differential, and radiographic studies will frequently make the diagnosis of fracture or hemarthrosis. With trauma, a normal radiograph, and presence of muscle or soft tissue tenderness to explain the limp, symptomatic treatment and observation is indicated. If the symptoms persist or worsen, repeat radiograph, bone scan, and hematologic studies may be necessary to rule out aseptic necrosis, infection, or other processes.

Other important historical features are presence of fever, anemia, malaise, or other evidence of systemic illness. These increase the likelihood of infection, connective tissue disease, or malignancy as the cause of limp.

Additional historical factors include: the degree of pain (severe with infection or fracture, milder with osteochondritis or rheumatoid disease, and even absent in Legg-Perthes disease, slipped capital femoral epiphysis or congenital dislocation of the hip); recent immunization in the lower

Table 26.1
Principal Causes of Limp by Major Cite of Pathology and Mode of Presentation[a]

	Long Bone	Any Joint: Includes Hip, Knee, Ankle[b]	Lumbosacral spine, Sacroiliac Joint, Pelvis	Hip[c]	Knee[c]	Ankle[c]	Foot	Skin/Soft Tissue	Neuromuscular System
Usual presentation:									
A. With trauma	Fracture Periostitis	Hemarthosis Sprain Dislocation	Intervertebral disc herniation	Slipped capital femoral epiphysis Aseptic necrosis	Referred hip pain Fractured patella Collateral/cruciate ligament tear	Sprain Epiphysial fractures of tibia, fibula		Tendonitis Bursitis Contusion Laceration	Muscle strain Muscle hematoma Nerve injury
B. With fever, systemic illness	Osteomyelitis Osteogenic sarcoma Leukemia Neuroblastoma Hemoglobin-opathy	Septic arthritis JRA Collagen disease Hemoglobinopathy Leukemia Neuroblastoma Osteomyelitis	Anklyosing spondylitis Discitis Sacral abscess	Transient synovitis	Referred hip pain		Ankylosing spondylitis (heel pain)	Thrombophlebitis Abscess Cellulitis Lymphadenitis	Viral myositis Trichinosis Dermatomyositis/Polymyositis Rhabdomyosarcoma Rhabdomyolysis
C. Without trauma, fever, systemic illness	Leg length discrepancy Osteoidosteoma	Tumor Postinfectious arthritis/synovitis Villonodular synovitis Aseptic necrosis	Scoliosis Scheuermann's disease	Transient synovitis Congenital dislocation Legg-Perthes disease Slipped capital femoral epiphysis	Referred hip pain Chondromalacia patella Osgood-Schlatter disease Osteochondritis dissecans		Flat feet New shoes Foreign body Paronychia Calcaneal spur Freiberg's disease Köhler's disease Plantar warts Bunions	Insect bite	Muscular dystrophy Postinfectious myositis Myasthenia gravis Spinal cord tumor Sacral tumor Diastometamyelia
Helpful diagnostic tests	X-ray CBC ESR Hgb elect. Bone scan	X-ray CBC ESR Hgb elect. Arthrocentesis RF ANA	X-ray CBC ESR HLA B27	X-ray	X-ray (include hips)	X-ray	X-ray CBC ESR HLA B27	CBC ESR Gallium scan	CBC ESR CPK Adolase Muscle biopsy Nerve conduction velocity Electromyography Myelography

[a] Abbreviations: JRA, juvenile rheumatoid arthritis; CBC, complete blood count with differential; ESR, erythrocyte sedimentation rate; Hgb elect., hemoglobin electrophoresis; Tech., technetium; RF, rheumatoid factor; ANA, antinuclear antibodies; HLA, histocompatability—antigen; CPK, creatine phosphokinase.

[b] See also tables and figure in Chapter 6.

[c] The disorders listed for any joint apply to hip, knee, and ankle. In addition, conditions particularly important to each joint are listed here.

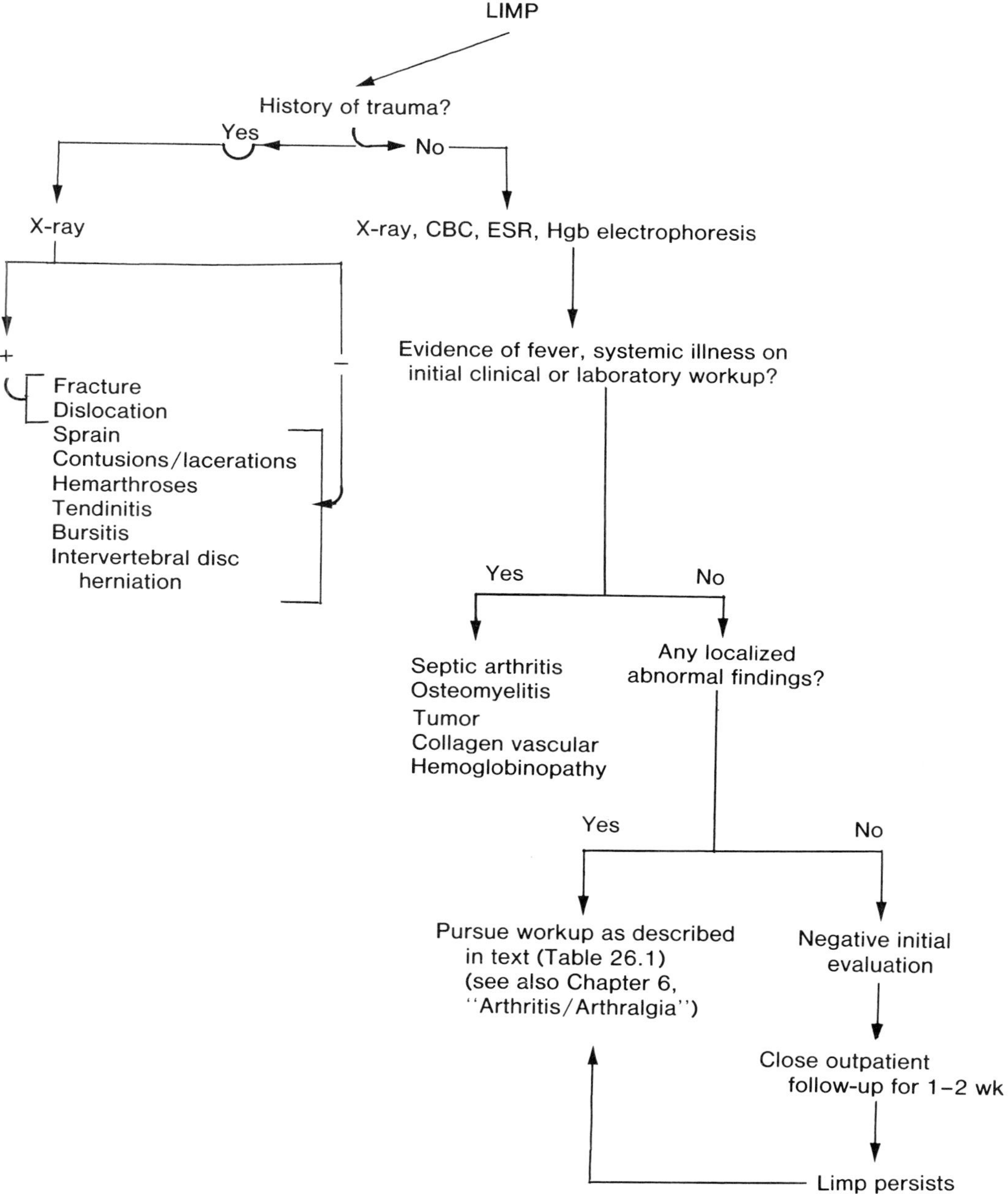

Figure 26.1 Approach to the child with a limp. *CBC*, complete blood count; *ESR*, erythrocyte sedimentation rate; *Hgb*, hemoglobin.

extremity; pattern of pain (relation to exercise, morning stiffness, absence on weekends); recent purchase of new shoes; and age of patient (1 to 3 years suggests trauma, transient synovitis, new shoes, or congenital dislocation of hip; 5 to 7 years suggests Legg-Perthes disease in males; adolescents frequently develop slipped capital femoral epiphysis, Osgood-Schlatter disease, or chondromalacia patella).

After a careful history, a complete physical examination should be obtained with the patient fully undressed. Careful attention should be paid to muscle strength testing, joint examination for warmth, swelling, tenderness and range-of-motion and a complete neurologic examination. Gait should be observed both with shoes off and on and the patient should be asked to climb up steps. Leg lengths should be checked (anterior superior iliac crest to medial malleolus) and thigh, knee, and calf circumferences should be measured. If pain is present, positions exacerbating and relieving the symptom should be sought to determine the exact source of pain. Finally, a rectal examination should be performed in the child with normal hips, legs and feet to rule out a rare sacral mass lesion causing limp.

The most useful laboratory studies for evaluating limp are: (1) the radiograph to rule out fractures, joint effusion (if not evident on physical examination) or lytic bone lesions; if the focus of pain is not apparent it may be necessary to obtain radiographs of the entire lower extremity, especially in young children who localize pain poorly; (2) complete blood count (CBC) as an indicator of infection, inflammation, malignancy or hemoglobinopathy; and (3) erythrocyte sedimentation rate (ESR) to help differentiate infectious and inflammatory processes from other causes of limp. Other potentially useful tests include technetium bone scan (especially for suspected aseptic necrosis, osteomyelitis, Legg-Perthes disease, septic arthritis, discitis, and osteoid osteoma); arthrocentesis (to differentiate septic arthritis from traumatic or rheumatoid arthritis); arthroscopy (for culture, synovial biopsy and to view internal derangements); and gallium scan (to localize occult infection or tumor).

Further discussion of major causes of limp can be found in Chapter 6, "Arthritis, Arthralgia," and in the chapters on orthopaedic, rheumatic, hematologic, neurologic and infectious disease emergencies.

When the initial history, physical examination and CBC, ESR and x-rays localize the site and etiology of pathology, the emergency physician can begin specific management. However, it is not uncommon for children with recent onset limp to remain undiagnosed despite a thorough initial evaluation. Such children may be managed as outpatients without further laboratory workup as long as close follow-up is assured. These patients should be re-evaluated every few days until the limp subsides (such patients usually having had minor trauma or mild transient synovitis), or until evidence of localization of pathology evolves. Limp lasting more than 1 to 2 weeks requires more extensive workup to rule out occult infection, tumor or collagen-vascular disease.

CHAPTER 27

Neck Mass

RICHARD M. RUDDY, M.D.

INTRODUCTION

Neck masses in children are common and represent a wide range of disorders. By definition, neck masses include any visible swelling that disturbs the normal contour of the neck between the shoulder to the angle of the jaw. Since the number of causes is extensive, this discussion will first emphasize recognition of those masses representing true medical emergencies. Then, the approach to nonemergent, but commonly seen, lesions will be described. Table 27.1 lists the important causes of neck masses of children.

Neck masses may arise from cellular hypertrophy, local infiltration, or cellular multiplication. Such changes occur secondary to inflammation, trauma, or antigenic or mitotic stimulation and often affect structures normally present, such as lymph nodes. By far the most common causes of neck mass in childhood are reactive adenopathy and adenitis. Congenital anatomic defects of the neck predispose children to develop masses, especially when infected or traumatized. Neoplasms may arise locally or from metastases.

True medical emergencies arise if neck masses compromise adjacent vital structures including the airway, carotid blood vessels, or cervical spinal cord. In rare cases, the principal threat to life is from systemic toxicity, such as infection leading to septicemia or the effects of excess hormone secretion in thyroid storm. Many large neck masses do not encroach on vital structures because their growth points outward. However, embarrassment about personal appearance or a concern of malignancy may be factors in the initiation of the emergency department visit.

EVALUATION AND DECISION

The first task in evaluating neck masses is to consider those disorders constituting true medical emergencies due either to local pressure on vital structures or systemic toxicity (Fig. 27.1). The initial history and physical exmination must rapidly screen for airway or cervical vessel compromise and cervical spine abnormality. One must specifically look for stridor, hoarseness, dysphagia, and drooling. The level of consciousness and breathing should be noted. Neck masses causing respiratory distress usually arise from trauma, infection, allergy, or neoplasm.

Child with a Neck Mass and Respiratory Distress or Systemic Toxicity

Trauma, from vehicular accidents or contact sports, may cause bleeding and hematoma formation near vital structures, such as the carotid artery or trachea. If the trauma involves the cervical spine, a hematoma may occur over fractured vertebrae. Even mild injuries may lead to severe hemorrhage and compression of vital structures of the neck in children with clotting

Table 27.1
Differential Diagnosis of Neck Mass by Etiology

- I. *Congenital*
  - A. Cystic hygroma (lymphangioma)
  - B. Hemangioma
  - C. Branchial cleft cyst
  - D. Thyroglossal duct cyst
  - E. Laryngocele
  - F. Dermoid cyst
  - G. Cervical rib
- II. *Inflammatory*
  - A. Infection
    1. Cervical adenitis—streptococcal, staphylococcal, fungal, mycobacterial; cat scratch disease
    2. Adenopathy—secondary to local head and neck infection
    3. Secondary to systemic "infection"—infectious mononucleosis, cytomegalovirus, toxoplasmosis, others
  - B. "Antigen"-mediated
    1. Local hypersensitivity reaction (sting/bite)
    2. Serum sickness, autoimmune disease
    3. Pseudolymphoma (secondary to phenytoin)
    4. Mucocutaneous lymph node syndrome
    5. Sarcoidosis
    6. Caffey-Silverman syndrome
- III. *Trauma*
  - A. Hematoma
    1. Sternocleidomastoid tumor of infancy
    2. Subcutaneous emphysema
    3. Arteriovenous fistulas
    4. Foreign bodies
  - B. Cervical fractures
- IV. *Neoplasms*
  - A. Benign
    1. Epidermoid
    2. Lipoma, fibroma, neurofibroma
    3. Keloid
    4. Goiter (with or without thyroid hormone disturbance)
    5. "Normal" anatomy or variant
  - B. Malignant
    1. Lymphoma—Hodgkin's disease, non-Hodgkin's lymphoma
    2. Leukemia
    3. Other—Rhabdomyosarcoma, neuroblastoma, nasopharyngeal squamous cell carcinoma, thyroid or salivary gland tumor

factor disorders (i.e., hemophilia) or platelet disorders (i.e., idiopathic thrombocytopenic purpura). Symptomatic arteriovenous fistulas may appear weeks after cervical trauma.

In children with obstructive lung diseases, such as asthma and cystic fibrosis, barotrauma may produce a pneumomediastinum which dissects into the neck. The high transpulmonary pressure generated in these diseases forces air through small alveolar leaks into the mediastinum or pleural space. The progression of a pneumomediastinum to pneumothorax may be

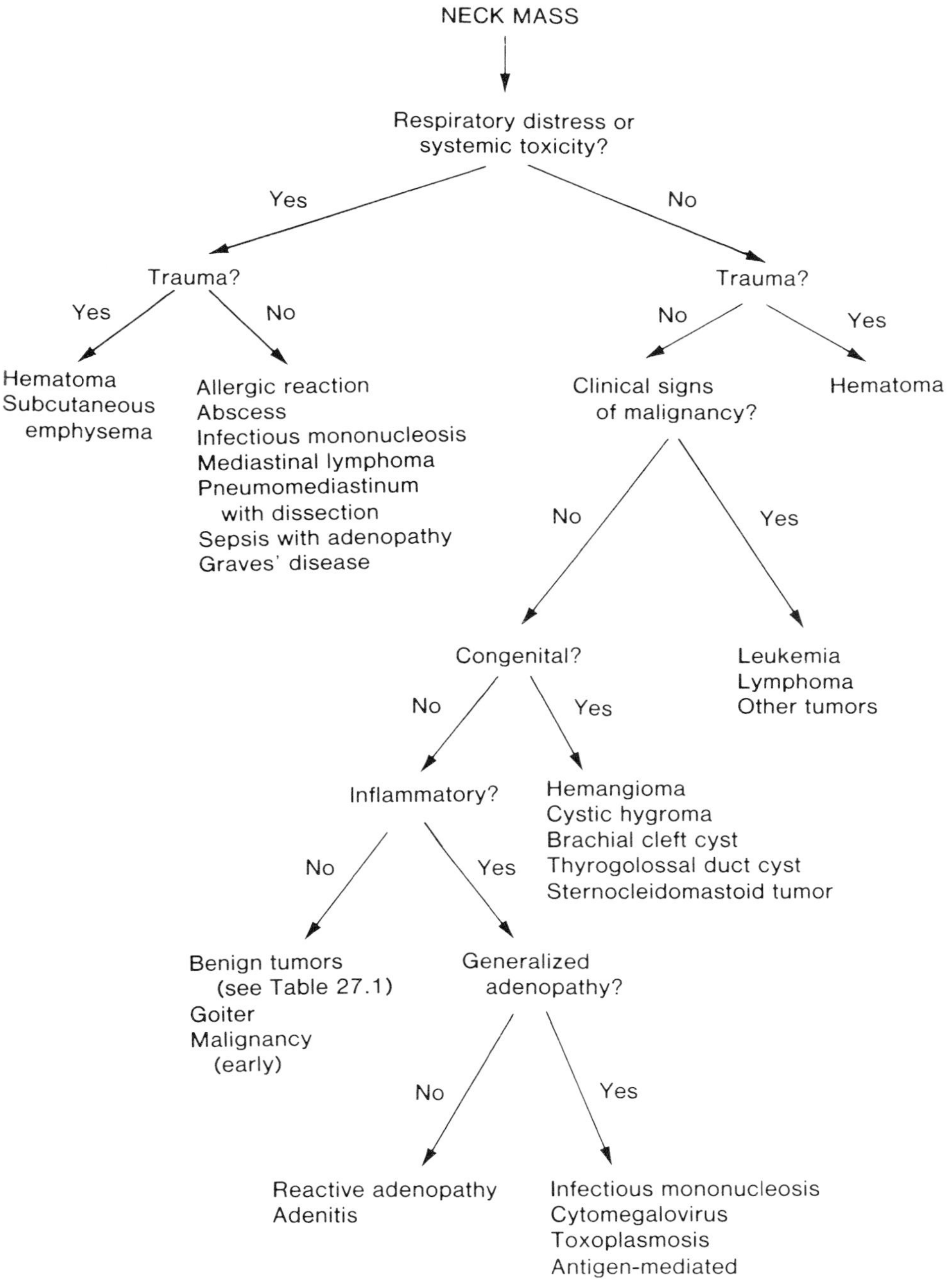

Figure 27.1 Evaluation of the child with a neck mass.

pid and requires the emergency physician be wary of the tachypneic child with a crepitant" neck mass.

Infections commonly cause neck masses, ut they usually do not constitute true emergencies. Exceptions include retropharyngeal, lateral pharyngeal, and peritonsillar abscesses; these may present with cervical adenitis and concomitant dysphagia, drooling, and stridor. Both airway compromise and carotid artery erosion may occur. In rare instances, patients with epiglottitis have been known to first complain of a neck mass. Occasionally, branchial cleft cysts become infected and progress to mediastinitis, or laryngoceles may become acutely infected and obstruct airflow. Massive tonsillar hypertrophy with infectious mononucleosis or dental infection spreading to the floor of the mouth and neck (Ludwig's angina), may cause both neck masses and airway compression.

Tumors of the neck in childhood may become large enough to encroach on vital structures. Cystic hygromas and hemangiomas occasionally enlarge sufficiently to interfere with feeding or obstruct the airway. Lymphoma, an important cause of neck mass, is suggested especially by painless enlargement occurring over several weeks to months; if mediastinal nodes are involved, the patient may rapidly develop a blockage of the intrathoracic trachea.

Last, *antigen*-mediated neck masses may precipitate an acute emergency if the swelling compromises the airway. Severe, local reactions to bee stings or other sensitizing allergens may cause enough tissue edema to obstruct the trachea.

When satisfied that vital structures are not critically involved, a thorough evaluation may proceed.

Child with a Neck Mass and No Distress

Once it is clear that the vital structures of the neck are not involved by a neck mass, a thorough evaluation is indicated. The physician should elicit details about trauma, the age of onset, duration, progression, presence of pain or discharge, and symptoms of systemic inflammation. Specifically, ascertain whether the mass changes with respiration, swallowing, or speech, as these findings point to an anatomic connection to muscle groups or internal structures of the neck. Recurrent unilateral masses, especially in young infants, should lead one to consider a cyst of congenital origin. Birth trauma, with bleeding into the sternomastoid muscle, may cause torticollis which presents at several weeks of age with a neck mass.

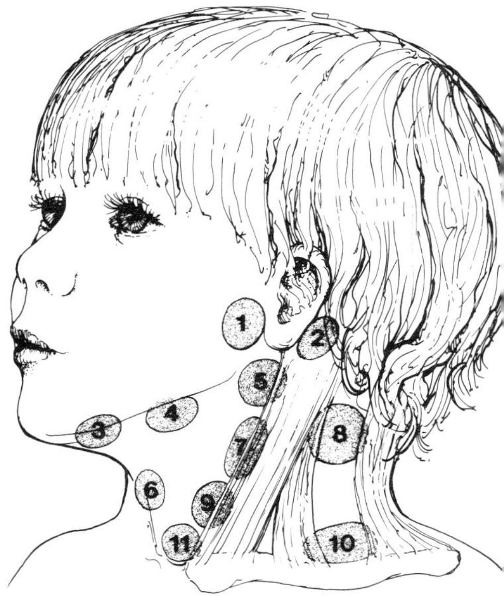

Figure 27.2 Differential diagnosis of ne mass by location.

Area 1. Parotid: Cystic hygroma, hem gioma, lymphadenitis, parotitis, Sjögren's a Caffey-Silverman syndrome, lymphoma

Area 2. Postauricular: Lymphadenitis, br chial cleft cyst (1st)

Area 3. Submental: Lymphadenitis, cys hygroma, thyroglossal duct cyst, dermoid

Area 4. Submandibular: Lymphadenitis, c tic hygroma, sialadenitis, tumor, cystic fibros

Area 5. Jugulodiagastic: Lymphadeni branchial cleft cyst (1st), parotid tumor, *n mal*—transverse, process C2, styloid proces

Area 6. Midline neck: Lymphadenitis, thy glossal duct cyst, dermoid, laryngocele, *n mal*—hyoid, thyroid

Area 7. Sternomastoid (anterior): Lymph enitis, branchial cleft cyst (2nd, 3rd), rare mors

Area 8. Spinal accessory: Lymphadenit lymphoma, metastasis (from nasopharynx)

Area 9. Paritracheal: Thyroid, parathyro esophageal diverticulum

Area 10. Supraclavicular: Cystic hygron lipoma, lymphoma, metastasis, *normal*— pad, pneumatocele of upper lobe

Area 11. Suprasternal; Thyroid, lipoma, d moid, thymus, mediastinal mass

(Modified from M. May: *Clinical Pediatrics*, 17, 1976.)

Details of chronicity, size, and progres- on and evidence of inflammation help dis- nguish between infection and neoplasm. asses that are greater than 3 cm in di- neter, nonpainful, enlarging, and of sev- al weeks duration suggest a malignancy, though some will be inflammatory in na- re.

The physical examination focuses on the termination of the location, size, shape, ntour, tenderness, attachment to under- ing tissue, crepitance, and fluctuance of e mass (Fig. 27.2). The surrounding area ould be palpated for additional lesions as ell as the normal structures of the neck, ch as the thyroid gland, sternomastoid uscles, trachea, and cervical spine. While scultating the chest for air entry and eath sounds, special attention should be ven to inspiration, as extra-thoracic air- ay obstruction from tracheal compression ill primarily affect that part of respiration. he examination of the head should be eticulous, including the scalp; local infec- ons of the middle ear, sinuses, tonsils, sopharynx, oral mucosa, dentition, pa- tid, or scalp represent the most common urces of neck masses in children.

Complete the rest of the physical exami- tion looking for systemic illness as the use of neck mass. The ill, pale, or bruised ild, especially with hepatosplenomegaly, ay have underlying leukemia or lym- oma. Signs of thyroid hormone excess or sence may be associated with goiter. Sys- mic infections, such as mucocutaneous mph node syndrome, causing cervical mphadenopathy may have associated fe- r, malaise, rash, or generalized lymphad- opathy. Systemic antigenic reactions oducing lymphadenopathy, such as se- m sickness or pseudolymphoma from enytoin, are possible, but uncommon, uses of neck masses.

The initial clinical impression determines e need for laboratory studies and x-rays. t times radiographs may be necessary: lateral neck films to look for causes of airway obstruction; cervical spine films to pinpoint fractures or dislocation; or chest films to view the mediastinum, pleura and lung for infection, tumor, pneumothorax or pneumomediastinum. Arterial blood gases may help determine the degree of airway obstruction in the child with respiratory distress. Compete white blood count and differential is often helpful in patients suspected of having an inflammatory mass and is essential when an oncologic cause is suspected. When bleeding due to trivial trauma is suspected as a cause of neck mass, platelet count, prothrombin time, and partial thromboplastin time should be done. Other studies are useful only if a specific disease is suspected, such as serum thyroid hormone levels in the case of a goiter or a heterophil antibody titer to diagnose infectious mononucleosis. Aspiration of a cystic neck mass may be both diagnostic and therapeutic. Anatomic defects with infection (i.e., branchial cleft or thyroglossal duct cysts) require special radiological and surgical studies, and neck masses suspicious of malignancy mandate a biopsy.

The use of diagnostic tests, therapy, and follow-up for children with neck masses will vary according to the initial impression. The majority of lesions are inflammatory and self-limited, requiring antimicrobial drugs, local care, and a repeat evaluation in 1 to 2 weeks. When a tumor is highly suspect, immediate referral to a surgeon or an oncologist is necessary. Hospitalization is indicated for patients with neck masses who have severe local disease or systemic toxicity.

References

Conn H, Conn R: Lymphadenopathy. In *Current Diagnosis*, pp. 25–29. W. B. Saunders, Philadelphia, 1974.

Green M: *Pediatric Diagnosis*, Ch. 14, p. 69. W. B. Saunders, Philadelphia, 1980.

May M: Neck masses in children; diagnosis and treatment. *Pediatr Ann* 5: 17, 1976.

CHAPTER **28**

Stiff Neck

ROBERT A. DOUGHTY, M.D.

INTRODUCTION

Stiff neck is caused acutely by discomfort resulting from cervical spine motion. Chronically this leads to wry neck or torticollis (derived from Latin *tortus* meaning "twisted" and *collum* meaning "neck").

Multiple congenital and acquired conditions may lead to stiff neck and/or torticollis. Muscular, neurogenic and osseous abnormalities may result in congenital torticollis. Causes of acquired stiff neck and torticollis include trauma, infection, neoplasia, inflammatory processes, neuromuscular lesions, phenothiazine reactions, hysteria, and a variety of syndromes. A differential diagnosis of causes of acute and chronic stiff neck is presented in Table 28.1. Although the most common causes of torticollis seen by the pediatrician are congenital muscular torticollis and torticollis associated with cervical spine or muscle trauma, an appreciation of the broader potential differential diagnosis is important in obtaining the correct diagnosis and management.

EVALUATION AND DECISION

In approaching the child with a stiff neck, important clinical features are: (1) presence or absence of fever, (2) presence of an abnormal cervical mass, (3) history of cervical trauma, and (4) duration of the symptom. An algorithm for approaching the child with a stiff neck is presented in Figure 28.1. The most important diagnosis to exclude with fever and a stiff neck is, obvious meningitis. In the child presenting with ver and torticollis one may neglect to ca fully test for meningism (including perfor ing Kernig and Brudzinski maneuvers); th should be done in all such cases since lu bar puncture is essential to accurately agnose the cause of meningism. With fev and tender cervical adenopathy, cervic adenitis is the likely diagnosis; successf treatment with antibiotics confirms the agnosis without extensive laboratory inve tigation. In chronic cases without a go response to antibiotic therapy, biopsy m be necessary to exclude tumor or establi the precise infectious agent. In the chi with fever and without a cervical mass meningism, a blood count and sedimen tion rate may be indicative of infection a lead to further studies such as a technetiu bone scan or gallium scan to establish t presence of focal infection such as verteb osteomyelitis or discitis. If bacterial infe tion or tumor involving cervical structur can be excluded, then other causes of st neck and fever are generally self-limit processes which will resolve with sympt matic therapy. If symptoms do not subsi within 1 or 2 weeks, further diagnostic stu ies are indicated.

In the patient with a stiff neck and fever, the presence of a mass suggests eith a chronic infectious process, tumor, or ste nocleidomastoid muscle inflammation. congenital torticollis the "tumor" or ma within the sternocleidomastoid muscle

Table 28.1
Stiff Neck

I. Acute Stiff Neck
- A. Trauma (cervical subluxation, muscle injury, hematoma, fracture of clavicle or cervical spine)
- B. Inflammation or infection (meningitis, cervical adenitis, vertebral osteomyelitis, viral myositis, arthropathy associated with pharyngitis, retropharyngeal abscess)
- C. Tumor (nerve, muscle, or bone tumor with swelling or nerve compression causing pain)
- D. Oculogyric crisis (usually painless)
- E. Hysteria
- F. Down's syndrome and acute atlantooccipital subluxation

II. Chronic or Recurrent Stiff Neck
- A. Congenital causes:
  1. Transient spasmodic torticollis of infancy
  2. Congenital muscular torticollis with sternocleidomastoid "tumor"
  3. Congenital hemivertebrae
  4. Klippel-Feil syndrome
  5. Ocular torticollis
  6. Congenital neuromuscular torticollis
- B. Acquired causes:
  1. Traumatic (cervical subluxation, rotary atlantoaxial subluxation, fractured clavicle, sternocleidomastoid injury)
  2. Infection (focal nerve, muscle, or bone infection; arthropathy associated with pharyngitis; cervical adenitis; retropharyngeal abscess; vertebral or rib osteomyelitis; discitis; viral or postinfectious myositis/neuritis)
  3. Tumor (midbrain or posterior fossa, cervical spinal cord, osseous tumor of cervical spine, lymphoma, rhabdomyosarcoma)
  4. Torticollis associated with vestibular disturbance (infection, postinfectious inflammation, tumor)
  5. Torticollis associated with ocular disturbance (midbrain or posterior fossa tumor, orbital tumor, strabismus)
  6. Miscellaneous causes/associations:
     - a. Osteoid osteoma of cervical spine
     - b. Associated with hyperthyroidism (usually adults)
     - c. Segmental dystonia
     - d. Cervical arthritis in juvenile rheumatoid arthritis
     - e. Torticollis with migraine headache
     - f. Torticollis with hiatal hernia and gastroesophageal reflux (Sandifer syndrome)
     - g. Atypical periodic paralysis
     - h. Myasthenia gravis
     - i. Syringomyelia
     - j. Mucopolysaccharidosis with atlantooccipital subluxation
     - k. Down's syndrome with atlantooccipital subluxation

generally not present at birth, but develops in the neonatal period and disappears spontaneously in 4 to 8 months. The chin of the patient points away from the affected side due to shortening of the sternocleidomastoid muscle. A facial asymmetry may occur with the unaffected side being more prominent and the cranium flattened on the contralateral occiput.

In other cases of sternocleidomastoid "tumor" or spasm, trauma is a common cause and cervical spine radiographs may be indicated even without a clear history of injury to establish a diagnosis of rotary subluxation or dislocation of the atlantoaxial articulation.

Another, less well-defined etiology of subluxation is the arthropathy due to ad-

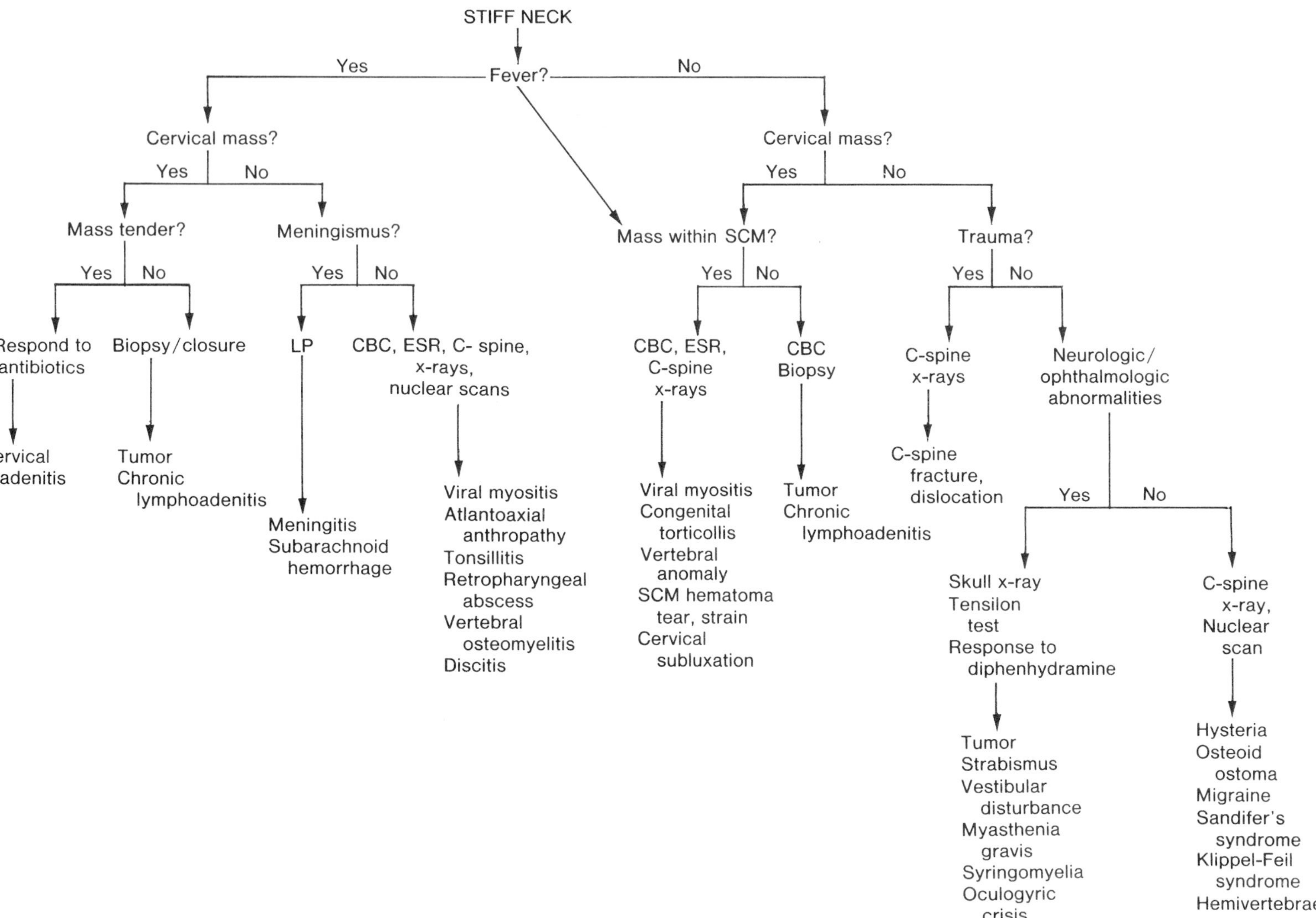
STIFF NECK
Fever?
Yes
No
Cervical mass?
Yes
No
Mass tender?
Yes
No
Respond to antibiotics
Cervical adenitis
Biopsy/closure
Tumor
Chronic lymphoadenitis
Meningismus?
Yes
No
LP
Meningitis
Subarachnoid hemorrhage
CBC, ESR, C- spine, x-rays, nuclear scans
Viral myositis
Atlantoaxial anthropathy
Tonsillitis
Retropharyngeal abscess
Vertebral osteomyelitis
Discitis
Cervical mass?
Yes
No
Mass within SCM?
Yes
No
CBC, ESR, C-spine x-rays
Viral myositis
Congenital torticollis
Vertebral anomaly
SCM hematoma tear, strain
Cervical subluxation
CBC
Biopsy
Tumor
Chronic lymphoadenitis
Trauma?
Yes
No
C-spine x-rays
C-spine fracture, dislocation
Neurologic/ ophthalmologic abnormalities
Yes
No
Skull x-ray
Tensilon test
Response to diphenhydramine
Tumor
Strabismus
Vestibular disturbance
Myasthenia gravis
Syringomyelia
Oculogyric crisis
C-spine x-ray, Nuclear scan
Hysteria
Osteoid ostoma
Migraine
Sandifer's syndrome
Klippel-Feil syndrome
Hemivertebrae

jacent inflammation in which mild subluxation may be associated with pharyngitis, tonsillitis, and other inflammatory processes adjacent to the cervical spine. This process is presumed to result from ligamentous weakening secondary to the local inflammatory process and is generally self-limited and without series complication other than local discomfort. Routine radiographic studies are frequently normal and do not exclude subluxation.

If a discrete mass is palpable and separate from the sternocleidomastoid then the physical character of the mass, its behavior with time (i.e., enlargement or regression) and presence of systemic symptoms will dictate whether biopsy need be performed to rule out a chronic infectious or malignant process.

In cases with a clear history of trauma where subluxation or fracture is suspected, cervical spine radiographs, including the important open-mouth odontoid view, are essential. A key clinical point in both rotary subluxation and atlantoaxial subluxation is that pain is localized to the long side of the neck—that is, the side to which the head is turned. This is in contrast to many of the inflammatory conditions with torticollis in which tenderness is localized in the region of the spastic sternocleidomastoid.

Neurologic, ophthalmologic, or vestibular dysfunction may lead to torticollis as a compensation for muscular or vestibular imbalance. Careful clinical examination with emphasis on cerebellar, extraocular muscle and vestibular function must be performed to exclude this possibility.

In patients with neck stiffness in whom all of the above diagnoses have been excluded, a number of possibilities remain. Sandifer syndrome, the association of hiatus hernia, torticollis, and gastroesophageal reflux must be considered in the child with recurrent vomiting or failure-to-thrive. Migraine has been reported to be associated with torticollis. Anatomic spinal abnormalities (congenital hemivertebrae, Klippel-Feil syndrome) may result in torticollis. Osteoid osteoma of the cervical spine may cause nocturnal cervical pain and is diagnosed by a positive radiograph or bone scan. Hysterical patients may also present with torticollis. Finally, children may present with torticollis and oculogyric crisis after taking phenothiazines, either as an accidental ingestion or when prescribed. A trial of intravenous diphenhydramine (1 mg/kg) may be both diagnostic and therapeutic.

In summary, although the potential differential diagnosis of a stiff neck is quite broad, traumatic and infectious causes (in particular, meningitis) require most prompt recognition. Other diagnoses may be established dependent upon duration and severity of symptoms and response to symptomatic therapy. For the majority of patients without clinical evidence of meningitis or trauma who present with acute symptomatology, no routine laboratory or radiologic workup is necessary.

References

Clark RN: Diagnosis and management of torticollis. *Pediatr Ann* 6: 231–239, 1976.

Kiesewitter WB, Nelson PK, Palladino US, Koop CE: Neonatal torticollis. *JAMA* 157: 1281–1285, 1955.

Lippman RK: Arthropathy due to adjacent inflammation. *J Bone Joint Surg* 35A: 967–979, 1953.

Shapiro R, Youngberg AS, Rothman SL: The differential diagnosis of traumatic lesions of the occipito-atlanti-axial segment. *Radiol Clin North Am* 11: 505–526, 1973.

Sullivan AW: Subluxation of the atlanti-axial joint; sequel to inflammatory processes in the neck. *J Pediatr* 35: 451–462, 1949.

CHAPTER 29

Oligomenorrhea

JAN E. PARADISE, M.D.

INTRODUCTION

In this chapter, possible etiologies for patients with oligomenorrhea and secondary amenorrhea are reviewed. Oligomenorrhea means infrequent menstruation and can be defined for the pediatric emergency physician as an interval of more than 6 weeks between two menstrual periods. If menstrual cycles do not resume within an arbitrarily chosen time span—3, 6, or 12 months according to various authorities—the term secondary amenorrhea is applied. In this chapter, we will use a single diagnostic approach for both oligomenorrhea and secondary amenorrhea. Some patients with anovulatory menstrual cycles have oligomenorrhea punctuated by episodes of excessive bleeding. An approach to the evaluation of abnormal vaginal bleeding is presented in Chapter 38.

Oligomenorrhea should be distinguished from hypomenorrhea, a pattern of light but regular menstrual periods that is not pathological. Although this section does not include a separate consideration of primary amenorrhea (failure to menstruate by a specified age, often 18 years), some of the disorders discussed below can produce primary rather than secondary amenorrhea as part of an overall delay in pubertal development.

The differential diagnosis of oligomenorrhea is given in Table 29.1.

EVALUATION AND DECISION

Diagnosis of Pregnancy

"Is she pregnant"? is always the first question to answer in evaluating an adolescent with one or several missed menstrual periods (Fig. 29.1). If the patient is not pregnant, her problem warrants methodical evaluation (see below). On the other hand, if she is pregnant, prompt diagnosis and referral are important both for the teenager who plans to continue her pregnancy and for the one who decides to seek a therapeutic abortion. Early and regular prenatal care is associated with reduced morbidity and mortality among pregnant teenagers and their offspring. Early diagnosis also allows the pregnant adolescent more time to decide on and arrange for a therapeutic abortion, if that is her choice. Presently, teenagers are twice as likely as older women to delay their abortions until the second trimester, when admission to hospital, with its greater morbidity and expense, is required.

Early pregnancy is not always easy to recognize. Symptoms of fatigue, nausea, vomiting (not necessarily in the morning), urinary frequency, and breast growth or tenderness are common, but by no means universal or specific. On pelvic examination, the first indication of pregnancy is softening of the lower uterine segment (Hegar's sign) and of the cervix (Goodell's sign)

Table 29.1
Differential Diagnosis of Oligomenorrhea

- *I. Hypothalamic-Pituitary Axis*
  - A. Delayed maturation
  - B. Psychological stress
  - C. Weight-related disorders
    - 1. Weight loss
    - 2. Marked thinness
    - 3. Anorexia nervosa
    - 4. Strenuous exercise
  - D. Chronic illness
  - E. CNS tumors
- *II. Ovary*
  - A. Ovarian failure
    - 1. Gonadal dysgenesis
    - 2. Cyclophosphamide
    - 3. Pelvic irradiation
  - B. Hormone-secreting tumors
- *III. Uterus*
  - A. Endometrial Destruction (rare)
    - 1. Surgical
    - 2. Tuberculous
- *IV. Hyperprolactinemic States*
  - A. Birth control pills
  - B. Phenothiazines
  - C. Other drugs
  - D. Pituitary adenoma
  - E. Lactation
- *V. Miscellaneous*
  - A. Pregnancy
  - B. Birth control pills
  - C. Polycystic ovary syndrome
  - D. Adrenal disease

at 4 to 6 weeks after the last menstrual period. By 6 weeks of gestation, the uterus changes from pear-shaped to globular, and between 6 and 8 weeks the vagina and cervix start to look bluish (Chadwick's sign). These changes occur in both ectopic and intrauterine pregnancies. A serviceable rule is that the pregnant uterus grows to about the size of a tennis ball at 8 weeks after the last menstrual period, becomes baseball-sized at 10 weeks, and softball-sized at 12 weeks. When the uterus is retroflexed, its size is more difficult to assess and rectovaginal palpation should be done. After 12 weeks, the uterine fundus is palpable above the symphysis pubis on abdominal examination. Fetal movement can be discerned after about 16 weeks. The fundus reaches the level of the umbilicus at 20 weeks of gestation.

The commercially available urine pregnancy tests will reliably give a positive result 6 weeks after the last menstrual period, when human chorionic gonadotropin (HCG) levels in serum reach several thousand international units per liter. A test may turn positive as early as 4 weeks after the last menstrual period, but a negative result at that time is not conclusive. A negative test performed 6 weeks or less after the last period should be repeated after an appropriate delay if the physician suspects pregnancy clinically. First-voided morning urine specimens are more concentrated and therefore more likely to yield positive tests. Blood or protein in the urine, and some drugs, principally phenothiazines and methadone, can produce falsely positive tests.

The recognition of an unruptured ectopic pregnancy is potentially life-saving. Fewer than 10% of ectopic pregnancies occur in young women under 20 years of age, but lower abdominal pain, abnormal vaginal bleeding, or a unilateral adnexal mass in any patient with a scanty or delayed menstrual period should alert the clinician to this possibility. Previous pelvic inflammatory disease is a predisposing factor. Patients using intrauterine devices for contraception also have a higher risk of ectopic pregnancy (3 to 5% of all pregnancies, compared to about 1% for non-IUD users), since nearly all intrauterine pregnancies are prevented. Because ectopic pregnancies result in relatively low hormone levels, urine pregnancy tests are negative in 50% or more of cases, and therefore not helpful for differentiating ectopic pregnancy from other disorders such as appendicitis, salpingitis, or ovarian cysts. One of the qualitative "serum pregnancy tests" will be much more reliable in this situation. The radioimmunoassay for the β-subunit of HCG in serum is highly sensitive and specific. The radioreceptor assay measures both HCG and luteinizing hormone. It might therefore be falsely positive at midcycle in a nonpregnant patient, but this is not a frequent problem in practice. Both of these serum assays are regu-

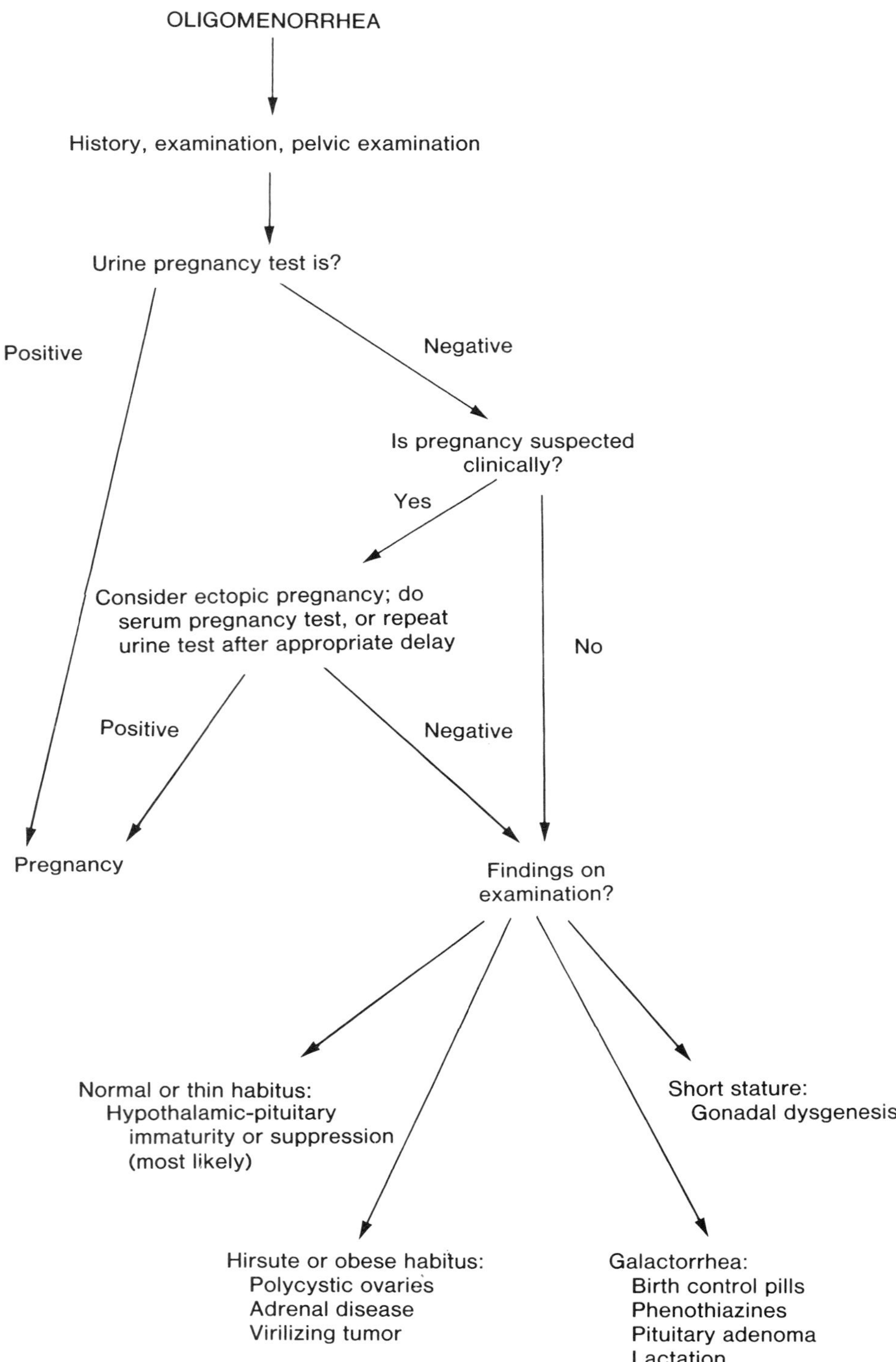

Figure 29.1 Approach to the diagnosis of oligomenorrhea.

larly positive 10 to 12 days after conception, before an anticipated menstrual period is even missed, and have been positive in about 95% of cases of ectopic pregnancy.

Evaluation of Nonpregnant Patients

If the physician can answer "No" to our original question—"Is she pregnant?"—the evaluation of an adolescent with oligomenorrhea can proceed at a more leisurely pace. During the first 2 years after menarche, irregular menstrual cycles are very common. The average girl requires about 15 months to complete her first 10 cycles, and some girls take much longer. As a rule, if an adolescent who complains of oligomenorrhea is fewer than 2 years past menarche, is not sexually active, and appears generally healthy, further investigation is not warranted. Of course, she should be reassured and followed.

Adolescents with a pattern of oligomenorrhea that has continued for more than 2 years after menarche, or that began after a regular menstrual pattern had already been established, need further evaluation. In the interview, historical details about the patient's menstrual pattern, growth, endocrine and central nervous systems, psychological status, and medications should be sought specifically. On physical examination, the patient's height and weight, visual fields, breasts, and pelvis should be checked carefully. The examination will separate the majority of patients from a minority with the important findings of (1) hirsutism, (2) obesity, (3) galactorrhea, and (4) unexplained short stature.

NORMAL AND THIN PATIENTS

Among adolescents who do not have hirsutism, obesity, galactorrhea, or short stature, suppression of the hypothalamic-pituitary axis is by far the commonest cause of oligomenorrhea. Psychological stress and abnormalities of body weight are the most frequent sources of this central disturbance. Accordingly, one should inquire about potential sources of emotional upset (family, friends, school, moving), recent weight loss, chronic illness or other causes of poor weight gain, behavior characteristic of anorexia nervosa, and strenuous exercise or participation in competitive sports.

Other diagnostic possibilities for oligomenorrheic patients include a wide variety of uncommon conditions. The history will provide a potential explanation in patients with ovarian damage or failure as a result of treatment with pelvic irradiation or cyclophosphamide. Endometrial destruction due to overvigorous curettage or pelvic tuberculosis is a rare cause of oligomenorrhea. Amenorrhea occurs in about 2% of menstrual cycles among patients who take birth control pills containing 50 μg or less of estrogen. "Post-pill amenorrhea" is diagnosed if spontaneous menstrual cycles do not resume within 6 months after the discontinuation of birth control pills. It can be attributed to an unrelated underlying condition (e.g., pregnancy, polycystic ovary syndrome, pituitary adenoma) in about two-thirds of cases; the remaining patients appear to have prolonged hypothalamic-pituitary axis suppression. Many patients with hyperprolactinemia and oligomenorrhea do not have concomitant galactorrhea to prompt a medical evaluation. Similarly, a substantial minority of patients with oligomenorrhea and laboratory features of the polycystic ovary syndrome lack either hirsutism or obesity or both. These patients with few characteristic symptoms or signs of disease will go unrecognized unless laboratory evaluation is undertaken.

HIRSUTE, OBESE, GALACTORRHEIC, AND SHORT PATIENTS

Ovarian enlargement, hirsutism, obesity, and amenorrhea constitute the classic clinical features of the polycystic ovary syndrome. Among women with this syndrome, about 70% are hirsute, 50% have amenorrhea, and 40% are obese. The ovaries can be normal in size, particularly during adolescence. If a patient's hirsutism is accompanied by other signs of virilization (clitoromegaly, deepening of the voice, temporal balding, marked acne), the possibility of adrenal disease or a virilizing tumor must be considered. Oligomenorrhea with galactorrhea and hyperprolactinemia occurs rarely during adolescence. It can be produced by drugs (most commonly birth control pills and phenothiazines), pituitary adenomas, and other central nervous system lesions. Of course, breast-feeding is regularly associated with oligomenorrhea. Unexplained short stature with oligomenorrhea is a clue to the diagnosis of gonadal dysgenesis. About 20% of the recognized patients with streak gonads and sex chromosome abnormalities have mosaic karyotypes (45X/46XX, for example). These patients are usually short (under 160 cm); some develop secondary sexual characteristics and spontaneous menstruation. Patients with classic Turner syndrome (45X karyotype) will instead have sexual infantilism and primary amenorrhea.

DIAGNOSTIC PROCEDURES

To differentiate among these many potential etiologies for oligomenorrhea after pregnancy has been excluded, determinations of serum levels of luteinizing hormone (LH), follicle-stimulating hormone (FSH), and prolactin can help either to corroborate an already suspected diagnosis or to categorize the patient whose history and physical examination have not provided many diagnostic clues. (Other laboratory tests should of course be performed whenever they seem appropriate.) Prepubertal levels of LH and FSH indicate hypothalamic-pituitary suppression in a postmenarchial patient; this pattern is the one most commonly found. An elevated LH level and a normal to low FSH are found in normal patients at the time of ovulation and in patients with the polycystic ovary syndrome. High FSH values occur in patients with ovarian failure. Elevated prolactin levels are uncommon, but must prompt an active search for pituitary disease in patients who are not using any of the drugs known to cause hyperprolactinemia and galactorrhea.

The administration of medroxyprogesterone acetate (10 mg orally daily for 5 to 7 days) provides an *in vivo* test of ovarian and endometrial function. If the hypothalamic-pituitary axis is producing some gonadotropin, the ovaries are responding with some estradiol production, and the uterine endometrium grows appropriately, the addition of exogenous progestin should produce at least scanty menstrual bleeding within 7 days after the drug regimen is completed. If menstrual flow appears, it provides both the patient and her physician with tangible evidence of the basic integrity of these organs. However, the procedure does not pinpoint a specific etiology for the oligomenorrhea.

References

Dale E, Gerlach DH, Wilhite AL: Menstrual dysfunction in distance runners. *Obstet Gynecol* 54: 47, 1979.

Dewhurst J: Secondary amenorrhea. *Pediatr Ann* 10: 496, 1981.

Emans SJ, Grace E, Goldstein DP: Oligomenorrhea in adolescent girls. *J Pediatr* 97: 815, 1980.

Kaufman ED, Mosman J, Sutton M, et al.: Characterization of basal estrogen and androgen levels and gonadotropin release patterns in the obese adolescent female. *J Pediatr* 98: 990, 1981.

Kleinberg DL, Noel GL, Frantz AG: Galactorrhea: a study of 235 cases, including 48 with pituitary tumors. *N Engl J Med* 296: 589, 1977.

Saxena BB: New methods of pregnancy testing in adolescent girls. *Pediatr Clin North Am* 28: 437, 1981.

CHAPTER 30

Pallor

JOHN W. BENDER, M.D., AND ALAN R. COHEN, M.D.

INTRODUCTION

Rosy cheeks in children have always been highly valued by their grandmothers and other trend setters in American life. Unfortunately, the loss or absence of this pleasing pink color is a relatively common problem in childhood. The development of pallor can be acute and associated with a life-threatening illness or it can be chronic and subtle, occasionally first noted by someone who sees the child less often than the parents. The onset of pallor can provoke anxiety for parents who are familiar with descriptions of the presentation of leukemia in childhood. In some instances, only reassurance may be needed as in the case of a light-complexioned or fair-skinned, nonanemic child. Even if there is a hematologic cause for the pallor, it is often a temporary condition readily amenable to therapy. However, pallor can portend a severe disease, and, when acute in onset, can herald a true pediatric emergency for which rapid diagnosis and treatment are needed.

The degree of pallor is dependent on the concentration of hemoglobin in the blood and the distribution of blood in the blood vessels of the skin. Any condition which decreases the concentration of hemoglobin or alters the distribution of blood away from the body's surface may present as pallor. Clinically, pallor due to anemia can usually be appreciated when the hemoglobin concentration is below 8 to 9 g/dl, although the complexion of the child and the rapidity of onset may influence this value. The hematologic causes for pallor in childhood are discussed below and further details regarding their management may be found in Chapter 47, "Hematologic Emergencies." Nonhematologic causes of pallor are briefly outlined in Table 30.1.

DIFFERENTIAL DIAGNOSIS

The differential diagnosis of the major hematologic causes of pallor in childhood is outlined in Table 30.2. The concentration of hemoglobin in the blood can be lowered by three basic mechanisms: decreased erythrocyte or hemoglobin production, increased erythrocyte destruction, or blood loss.

Decreased Production of Hemoglobin and Red Cells

NUTRITIONAL ANEMIAS

In childhood, the most common cause of decreased hemoglobin production is nutritional iron deficiency. This condition is usually seen in the first 2 years of life at which time the dietary iron content is often insufficient to meet the demands of the rapidly increasing red cell mass. Premature infants are particularly likely to develop iron deficiency anemia since iron stores at birth are less than those found in term infants while the growth (and, therefore, expansion of the red cell mass) of the premature infant is often faster than that of term infants.

Table 30.1
Pallor Without Anemia

Physiologic ("fair-skinned")
Shock: septic, hypovolemic, neurogenic, cardiogenic, anaphylactoid
Hypoglycemia
Respiratory distress
Skin edema
Pheochromocytoma

The early exhaustion of iron stores in premature babies may result in pallor by 6 months of age; in normal infants, signs of iron deficiency anemia are uncommon before 10 to 12 months.

The infant with severe iron deficiency is usually irritable and very pale. The lack of iron in the diet may be readily apparent or may be recognized only after careful questioning, particularly regarding the daily consumption of cow's milk. The hemoglobin concentration may be as low as 2 g/dl at the time of diagnosis. Conditions which increase cardiac output such as fever may provoke the development of congestive heart failure when anemia is severe.

The red cells are markedly microcytic and hypochromic in severe iron deficiency anemia. Variation in red cell size and shape is usually present and elongated, pencil-like cells are particularly common. The percentage of reticulocytes may be moderately elevated, but the absolute reticulocyte count is low. Treatment is usually instituted before confirmatory laboratory studies are available, but this rarely poses a problem since the diagnosis can be made on the basis of the history alone. The rapidity of the assay for free erythrocyte protoporphyrin, which is increased in iron deficiency anemia, makes this test particularly useful in the evaluation of the severely anemic child. Serum iron and ferritin levels have too long a turnaround time to be of much value in the emergency management of anemia.

Other nutritional anemias, such as vitamin B_{12} or folic acid deficiency, are uncommon in children in the United States and rarely develop in the absence of a grossly altered diet, extended hyperalimentation, intestinal resection, or chronic diarrhea. Unusual alterations of B_{12} and folic acid absorption and metabolism may cause symptoms similar to those of the nutritional megaloblastic anemias. Megaloblastic anemia is rarely severe enough to be life-threatening. The condition is characterized by normochromic, macrocytic red blood cells and hypersegmented neutrophils. The diagnosis of nutritional disorders is confirmed by the finding of low serum levels of folic acid or vitamin B_{12} and the response to folic acid or vitamin B_{12} replacement therapy.

HYPOPLASTIC AND APLASTIC ANEMIA

Pallor is usually the first sign of aplastic or hypoplastic anemia. Diamond-Blackfan syndrome is a congenital hypoplastic anemia that is usually detected in the first few months of life. The anemia can be severe at the time of diagnosis. The red cells are normocytic or macrocytic. The reticulocyte count is low. The white cell count is low in approximately 10% of affected patients, but thrombocytopenia occurs only rarely. The diagnosis is made by examination of a bone marrow aspirate which shows markedly reduced or absent erythrocyte precursors. The second major congenital hypoplastic anemia is Fanconi's anemia, a syndrome characterized by pancytopenia and associated abnormalities including microcephaly, strabismus, small stature, café au lait spots, mental retardation, and abnormalities of the thumbs and radii. Unlike Diamond-Blackfan syndrome, all three cell lines of the bone marrow are affected, and the hematologic abnormalities rarely develop before 4 years of age. The anemia is normochromic and macrocytic.

Acquired aplastic anemia can also present with severe pallor in children. The anemia is usually associated at diagnosis with granulocytopenia and thrombocytopenia. The condition is often idiopathic but has been associated with exposure to certain drugs and chemicals (chloramphenicol, benzene, pesticides), radiation, and viral infections (especially hepatitis). The diagnosis is made by an examination of the bone marrow.

Transient erythroblastopenia of childhood (TEC) is a condition often associated with a recent viral illness and characterized by moderate to severe anemia due to di-

Table 30.2
Pallor With Anemia

I. Decreased Erythrocyte Production
- A. Nutritional deficiencies
  1. Iron deficiency[a]
  2. Folic acid and vitamin B_{12} deficiency or associated metabolic abnormalities[a]
  3. Copper deficiency
- B. Aplastic or hypoplastic anemias
  1. Diamond-Blackfan syndrome
  2. Fanconi's syndrome
  3. Aplastic anemia[a]
  4. Malignancy: leukemia, lymphoma, neuroblastoma[a]
- C. Anemia of chronic disease: renal disease, inflammatory bowel disease, collagen-vascular disease, thyroid deficiency or thyrotoxicosis, malignancy
- D. Abnormal heme and hemoglobin synthesis
  1. Lead poisoning[a]
  2. Sideroblastic anemias
  3. Thalassemias

II. Increased Erythrocyte Destruction
- A. Erythrocyte membrane defects: hereditary spherocytosis, elliptocytosis, stomatocytosis, pyknocytosis, paroxysmal nocturnal hemoglobinuria
- B. Erythrocyte enzyme defects
  1. Defects of hexose monophosphate shunt: G6PD deficiency most common
  2. Defects of Embden-Meyerhof pathway: pyruvate kinase deficiency most common
- C. Hemoglobinopathies
  1. Sickle cell syndromes[a]
  2. Unstable hemoglobins
- D. Immune hemolytic anemia
  1. Autoimmune hemolytic anemia[a]
  2. Isoimmune hemolytic anemia[a]
  3. Infection
     - a. Viral: mononucleosis, influenzas, coxsackie, measles, varicella, cytomegalovirus
     - b. Bacterial: *Escherichia coli*, *Pneumococcus*, *Streptococcus*, typhoid fever, *Mycoplasma*
  4. Drugs: antibiotics, alpha methyl dopa
  5. Inflammatory and collagen vascular disease
  6. Malignancy[a]

III. Blood Loss
- A. Severe trauma[a]
- B. Anatomic lesions
  1. Meckel's diverticulum
  2. Peptic ulcer
  3. Idiopathic pulmonary hemosiderosis[a]

[a] Conditions that are known to present with acute, life-threatening anemia or are associated with other serious abnormalities.

minished red cell production. The mean corpuscular volume is usually normal at the time of diagnosis. The platelet and white blood cell counts are normal. The reticulocyte count is decreased and the Coombs test is negative. Bone marrow examination shows reduction or absence of erythrocytic precursors initially, followed by erythroid hyperplasia during recovery.

A hypoplastic anemia can be the presenting symptom of childhood malignancies. The pallor can be severe and, while all three cell lines of the bone marrow are usually affected, anemia may be the only hematologic abnormality. The diagnosis can be suspected from the presence of other symptoms or findings such as lymphadenopathy, bruising, limb pain, gum bleeding or an abdominal mass.

DISORDERS OF HEME AND GLOBIN PRODUCTION

Pallor may be the presenting sign of nonnutritional disorders of hemoglobin synthesis including the sideroblastic anemias and thalassemia syndromes. These disorders are characterized by a microcytic, hypochromic anemia. The sideroblastic anemia may be inherited (sex-linked) or acquired. Iron utilization within the developing red cell is abnormal, accounting for the presence of diagnostic ringed sideroblasts in the bone marrow. The serum iron and ferritin levels are usually markedly elevated. In the thalassemias, production of the globin portion of the hemoglobin molecule is defective. Cooley's anemia (β-thalassemia major) presents with severe pallor between 6 and 12 months of age, as the fetal hemoglobin level declines but the normal rise in hemoglobin A production fails to occur due to reduced or absent β globin production. While β-thalassemia is usually found in children of Mediterranean ancestry, this disease and associated disorders (e.g., E-β-thalassemia) are being seen with increasing frequency due to the recent influx of Southeast Asian refugees. The presence of hepatosplenomegaly and characteristic red cell morphology makes this diagnosis readily apparent.

Lead poisoning affects heme synthesis but significant anemia is unusual unless blood lead levels are markedly elevated. Iron deficiency is common in children with increased lead levels and usually accounts for the microcytic anemia found in these patients. If a concomitant hematologic disorder cannot be found in the anemic patient with plumbism, particular care should be given to the possibility of severe lead intoxication.

SYSTEMIC DISEASE

Numerous disorders which are not primarily hematologic may be associated with pallor and anemia. Occasionally pallor is the only presenting finding of a serious systemic disorder. Chronic inflammatory diseases such as juvenile rheumatoid arthritis and ulcerative colitis are often accompanied by a normocytic or microcytic anemia due to impaired iron utilization. The serum iron is reduced. The low iron binding capacity distinguishes the anemia of chronic inflammation from the anemia of iron deficiency. Similar clinical and laboratory findings may be associated with chronic infections such as subacute bacterial endocarditis. Other diseases in which anemia may be a prominent component include chronic renal disease, hyperthyroidism, and hypothyroidism. The anemia in these disorders is not severe enough to be considered a hematologic emergency unless complicated by other hematologic abnormalities. However, the anemia may be the first clue to an underlying disease in which early treatment may substantially improve the outcome.

Increased Red Cell Destruction

The numerous conditions associated with shortened red cell survival can be congenital, as in the case of the hemoglobinopathies and membrane and enzyme defects or acquired, as in the case of autoimmune hemolytic anemia and drug-associated hemolytic anemias. The hemoglobin levels in these disorders can be normal, slightly depressed or so low as to be life-threatening. This level is determined by the severity of the defect and the patient's ability to respond to the presence of a shortened red cell survival. Compensation is achieved by an increase in erythrocyte production as is evident from the elevated reticulocyte count that is usually found in these conditions.

An alteration in the patient's ability to compensate for increased red cell destruction may result in a severe, life-threatening exacerbation of the underlying anemia. This aplastic crisis, the result of a transient decrease in erythrocyte production in the presence of shortened red cell survival should be suspected in a patient with a known hemolytic anemia who develops increasing pallor and anemia associated with a reticulocyte count which is much lower than usual. Unfortunately, when the hemolytic anemia has not been previously diagnosed, the recognition of an aplastic crisis can be difficult since the findings are similar to those of transient erythroblastopenia of childhood or congenital erythrocyte hypoplasia (i.e., anemia with low or absent reticulocytes). Examination of the bone marrow may be helpful in distinguishing these disorders, since production of early red cell precursors has often resumed shortly after detection of an aplastic crisis. Frequently, the diagnosis of an aplastic crisis is made only after the underlying disorder has been recognized. Conversely, after resolution of a suspected aplastic crisis, every effort should be made to uncover an underlying condition that might cause shortened red cell survival. The differential diagnosis of such conditions is presented below.

MEMBRANE DISORDERS

The degree of pallor associated with anemia due to erythrocyte membrane abnormalities depends upon the hemoglobin level. In rare instances patients with hereditary spherocytosis, the most common of the membrane disorders, may develop significant anemia and pallor in the newborn period. Moderate or severe anemia is less common in the other membrane disorders, such as hereditary elliptocytosis and hereditary stomatocytosis. The anemia of the erythrocyte membrane disorders is accompanied by reticulocytosis. The red cell morphology frequently permits the diagnosis to be made from the peripheral smear. Since these disorders are usually inherited in an autosomal dominant fashion, a family history of anemia, splenomegaly, splenectomy or cholecystectomy may be helpful.

Infantile pyknocytosis is a hemolytic anemia which is seen during the first few months of life and is characterized by distorted and contracted erythrocytes and burr cells. The disorder may be associated with pallor and hyperbilrubinemia.

ENZYME DISORDERS

Erythrocyte enzymatic defects, such as pyruvate kinase deficiency and certain variants of glucose 6-phosphate dehydrogenase (G6PD) deficiency may be associated with pallor due to increased red blood cell destruction. In the latter disorder, pallor may be accentuated by acute hemolytic crises following exposure to oxidant stress (e.g., drugs, acidosis). Although alterations in red cell morphology are sometimes found in these enzyme disorders, assays of specific enzymes or substrates are required for diagnosis.

HEMOGLOBINOPATHIES

Pallor may result from the low hemoglobin level that is found in patients with sickle cell anemia and related hemoglobinopathies. Acute accentuation of pallor can result from an aplastic crisis, a complication of hemolytic disorders which is particularly common in sickle cell anemia. During an aplastic crisis, the normally elevated reticulocyte count may fall to zero, and the hemoglobin level may fall as low as 1 to 2 g/dl, resulting in severe pallor and signs of high output cardiac failure.

The sequestration crisis of sickle cell anemia and related hemoglobin disorders (SC disease, S-β thalassemia) results from acute pooling of red cells and plasma in the spleen. The sudden and severe anemia and the hypovolemia associated with this complication constitute a true hematologic emergency and, if untreated, may rapidly lead to death. The presence of increased pallor and acute enlargement of the spleen in a patient with a sickling disorder should prompt immediate investigation of a possible sequestration crisis. Although this complication rarely occurs in children with homozygous sickle cell disease after the age of 5 years, sequestration crises may occur much later in children with sickling disorders such as SC disease or S-β thalassemia in which early splenic infarction is less common.

IMMUNE HEMOLYTIC ANEMIA

Pallor due to autoimmune hemolytic anemia is usually acute in onset and may be associated with severe anemia. The presence of only moderate anemia (6 to 8 g/dl) at diagnosis should not detract from consideration of this disease as a hematologic emergency since brisk hemolysis may result in a sudden fall in hemoglobin level. Autoimmune hemolytic anemia is usually, but not always, characterized by a positive Coombs test and an increased reticulocyte count. Spherocytes are commonly seen in the peripheral smear. Other causes of immune hemolytic anemia include infections, drugs, inflammatory diseases, and malignancies.

Blood Loss

Although sudden, massive hemorrhage is usually accompanied by signs of hypovolemic shock, the repeated loss of smaller amounts of blood may be associated with few findings other than pallor. The finding of iron deficiency anemia despite normal dietary iron intake or iron supplementation may be a clue to the presence of chronic blood loss. For example, idiopathic pulmonary hemosiderosis is frequently confused with recurrent pneumonia until the hematologic findings of iron deficiency are appreciated. Gastrointestinal bleeding may also escape detection until pallor and anemia are pronounced.

EVALUATION AND DECISION

The initial assessment of the child with pallor should include an immediate determination of the degree of illness. Rapid treatment may be imperative for the severely ill child. In the presence of hypovolemic shock, immediate support of vascular volume is required. When high output cardiac failure due to severe anemia occurs, transfusion with small aliquots of packed red cells is necessary. Only after these initial therapeutic efforts have been completed can a thorough evaluation of the anemia proceed.

The need for immediate therapy may alter the usual approach to the investigation of pallor. For example, iron deficiency may be the most likely explanation for anemia in a 1-year-old black child with newly diagnosed meningitis. However, if the anemia is due to sickle cell disease, the management of the patient may require modification. Therefore, specific studies for sickling disorders should be performed in the initial stages of the evaluation of the anemia.

If the child with pallor is not acutely ill, a deliberate search for the cause of pallor should be undertaken (Fig. 30.1). While the history is being obtained, a spun hematocrit should be measured in the emergency department to ascertain the presence and severity of the anemia. The plasma layer in the hematocrit tube should be examined for the presence of a pink color indicative of free hemoglobin due to acute hemolysis.

A thorough yet relevant history should be obtained with particular attention to the type of onset of pallor. The slow development of pallor, often noticed only by a family member or friend who sees the child infrequently, suggests diminished red cell production as is found in bone marrow aplasia or iron deficiency. On the other hand, the acute onset of pallor is consistent with the brisk hemolysis found in autoimmune hemolytic anemia and is frequently accompanied by jaundice, dark urine, and cardiovascular changes.

After establishing the type of onset of the anemia, the history can be directed toward narrower categories of anemia or specific diseases. A detailed dietary history, with particular attention to milk intake, is important in young children with suspected iron deficiency; excessive consumption of cow's milk often results in iron deficiency. Vitamin B_{12} deficiency may accompany strict vegetarian diets and may occur in breast fed infants of vegetarian mothers. Nutritional folic acid deficiency is rare and can be readily deduced from the presence of severe dietary alterations and evidence of other vitamin deficiencies.

Sources of internal or external blood loss should be carefully sought. Chronic gastrointestinal bleeding may escape detection until iron deficiency anemia develops. Similarly, small pulmonary hemorrhages associated with idiopathic pulmonary hemosiderosis are often mistaken for other pulmonic processes until several recurrences of iron deficiency anemia suggest a hidden site of blood loss.

If fever, petechiae or increased bruising has occurred, multiple blood elements are probably affected. The circulation time of platelets and white cells is short in comparison with red cells. Therefore, clinical findings of thrombocytopenia and neutropenia are frequently present by the time pallor develops in patients with acquired aplastic anemia, Fanconi's anemia, and acute leukemia.

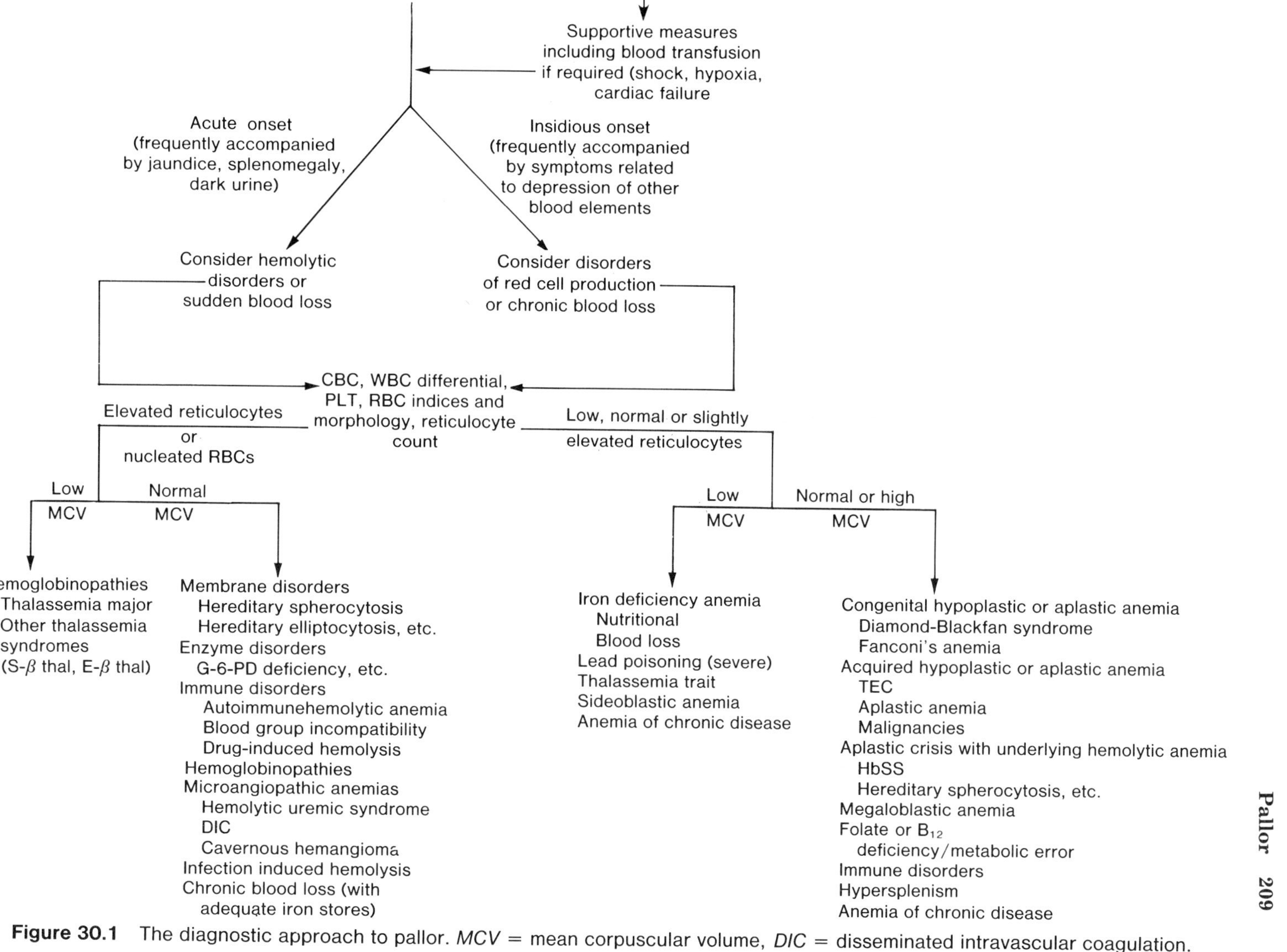

Figure 30.1 The diagnostic approach to pallor. *MCV* = mean corpuscular volume, *DIC* = disseminated intravascular coagulation.

The family history will be of assistance in the diagnosis of hemoglobinopathies and inherited disorders of red cell membranes and enzymes. Since results of previous hemoglobin testing may have been inadequately explained or inaccurately recalled, the family history should not preclude evaluation of the patient's hemoglobin phenotype if a sickling disorder is suspected. The presence of a microcytic anemia unresponsive to iron in the parents suggests a thalassemic disorder. A history of splenomegaly, splenectomy, or cholecystectomy in family members may help identify a hemolytic disorder such as hereditary spherocytosis or pyruvate kinase deficiency. Finally, a well-directed review of systems is essential in looking for systemic disorders such as chronic renal disease, hypothyroidism, or juvenile rheumatoid arthritis. Pallor may be the presenting complaint in these and other disorders.

In the examination of the severely anemic patient, pallor of the skin and mucous membranes is usually readily apparent. When anemia is less severe or when the skin color is dark, pallor only may be appreciated in the nailbeds and palpebral conjunctivae. The blood pressure and pulse should be measured to be sure that hypovolemic shock or high output cardiac failure are neither present nor imminent. If anemia or volume loss is mild, tachycardia may be present but normal blood pressure is preserved. A systolic flow murmur is usually heard if the hemoglobin level is below 8 g/dl. Lymphadenopathy and splenomegaly may suggest a malignancy or an infectious disease such as mononucleosis. However, when splenomegaly occurs without lymphadenopathy, attention is drawn to hemolytic disorders such as hereditary spherocytosis and autoimmune hemolytic anemia or hemoglobinopathies such as sickling disorders or Cooley's anemia. Scleral icterus may also be present in these disorders of shortened red cell survival. The finding of an unusually large and firm spleen in the absence of increasing scleral icterus suggests that red cells are being sequestered (splenic sequestration crisis of sickle cell disease, hypersplenism).

The skin should be examined for the presence of hemangiomas which might cause microangiopathic anemia. When this diagnosis is strongly suspected, careful auscultation of the abdomen and head may detect hemangiomas of the viscera. Bony abnormalities associated with red cell disorders include frontal bossing due to compensatory expansion of the bone marrow in hemolytic diseases and radial and thumb anomalies found in some patients with Fanconi's anemia.

Numerous classifications of anemia have been used to assist the physician in the laboratory investigation of pallor. Historically the reticulocyte count and the mean corpuscular volume (MCV) have been very helpful measurements in categorizing causes of anemia. The reticulocyte count can be performed rapidly and as shown in Figure 30.1 will distinguish anemias due to impaired red cell production (iron deficiency, hypoplastic anemia, etc.) from those due to shortened red cell survival (hemoglobinopathies, membrane disorders, etc.). With the use of electronic cell counters in most hospitals, the determination of the MCV provides a quick, accurate and readily available method of distinguishing the microcytic anemias (iron deficiency, thalassemia syndromes) from the normochromic (membrane disorders, enzyme deficiencies, autoimmune hemolytic anemia, most hemoglobinopathies) or macrocytic (bone marrow/stem cell failure, disorders of B_{12} and folic acid absorption or metabolism) anemias.

Nonetheless, the reticulocyte count and the MCV should be interpreted with caution. As shown in Figure 30.1, disorders of shortened red cell survival are not always characterized by an increased reticulocyte count. For example, reticulocytopenia may occur in autoimmune hemolytic anemia despite active hemolysis and increased erythropoiesis in the bone marrow. Chronic hemolytic disorders such as sickle cell anemia or hereditary spherocytosis may first be detected during an aplastic crisis when the reticulocyte count is low. Unless the underlying disorder is recognized, the physician may be misled by this finding. Furthermore, since the reticulocyte count is expressed as a percentage of total red cells, it must often be corrected for the degree of anemia. For example, a reticulocyte count of 4% in a

Table 30.3
Age-related Values for Mean Corpuscular Volume (MCV)

Age (yr)	MCV (fl)	
	Median	Lower limit[a]
0.5–2	77	70
2–5	79	73
5–9	81	75
9–12	83	76
1 2–14:		
Female	85	77
Male	84	76
1 4–18:		
Female	87	78
Male	86	77

[a] Third percentile. fl = femtoliters.

child with severe iron deficiency anemia (Hb 2 g/dl, RBC 1,000,000/cumm) is inappropriately low when expressed as an absolute number of reticulocytes (4% × 1,-000,000/cumm = 40,000/cumm).

The MCV varies with age, necessitating the use of age-adjusted normal values (Table 30.3). In addition, the measured MCV represents an average value. If microcytic and macrocytic red cells are present in the peripheral blood as, for example, in a patient with combined nutritional deficiency, the MCV may remain normal. Therefore, the peripheral smear should be carefully examined to determine whether the MCV reflects a single population of red cells of uniform size or two or more populations of distinctly different size.

As shown in Figure 30.1, the reticulocyte count and MCV help in the initial classification of anemia but leave the physician with broad categories of disease, rather than specific diagnoses. In many instances, the history and physical examination, when coupled with these laboratory measurements, will permit identification of a particular disorder. However, additional laboratory studies and careful examination of the peripheral smear are often required and can be readily performed while the patient is in the emergency department. The application of these procedures to diseases which are encountered frequently or are associated with unusually severe anemia is discussed below.

Increased Reticulocytes and Low MCV

The thalassemia syndromes associated with moderate or severe anemia can be recognized by the distinctive abnormalities of red cell morphology. In Cooley's anemia (thalassemia major), the red cells are generally small but vary markedly in size and shape. Many cells appear to contain little or no hemoglobin; the central pallor extends to the cell membrane. Nucleated red cells, basophilic stipling and polychromasia reflect active erythropoiesis. The parents of an affected child will usually have a low MCV characteristic of thalassemia trait.

Children with HbS-β thalassemia often have microcytic red cells, although the alterations in red cell morphology are not as dramatic as in Cooley's anemia. Sickled forms are often, but not always, present. Target cells are present. The solubility tests are positive due to the presence of HbS. Hemoglobin electrophoresis reveals HbS and reduced (less than 50%) or absent HbA.

Increased Reticulocytes and Normal MCV

Most membrane disorders can be readily identified by the characteristic changes in red cell shape which lend their name to the disease (e.g., spherocytosis, elliptocytosis, stomatocytosis). When the diagnosis of a membrane disorder is uncertain, examination of the parents' peripheral smears may be helpful since, in most cases, the inheritance pattern is autosomal dominant.

Abnormalities of red cell morphology are less striking in erythrocyte enzymatic defects. However, spherocytes and fragments may be found during episodes of active hemolysis in G6PD deficiency. If transfusion should be necessary, a pre-transfusion sample should be saved for assay of specific enzyme.

The reticulocyte count is usually markedly elevated in autoimmune hemolytic anemia but may be normal or only slightly elevated during the first days of the disease. In rare instances, reticulocytopenia persists. Spherocytes are usually present on the peripheral smear. Clumping of red cells due to agglutination may be seen. This agglutination sometimes causes a falsely elevated MCV as the electronic counter measures the volume of red cell couplets or triplets. The direct Coombs' test is positive in 90% of cases. Patients with a negative Coombs' test present a challenging diagnostic problem since the initial findings may be similar to those of an acute exacerbation of hemolysis in hereditary spherocytosis.

The recognition of homozygous sickle cell disease is usually accomplished by the finding of sickled red cells on the peripheral smear. Rarely, however, such cells may be absent, even during an acute illness. Target cells are commonly found in sickle cell disease but are more prominent in HbSC. Solubility tests are positive. Hemoglobin electrophoresis reveals the presence of the abnormal hemoglobin(s) and the absence of HbA. This confirmatory test takes less than 30 min to complete and should be performed whenever important therapeutic decisions depend on the result.

Red cell fragments are found in those diseases characterized by microangiopathic anemia. In hemolytic uremic syndrome, thrombocytopenia is present and renal function is impaired. The platelet count is also low in disseminated intravascular coagulation and clotting studies are abnormal. If intravascular hemolysis is severe, as in anemia associated with certain artifical cardiac valves, hemosiderin may be detected in the urinary sediment.

Low, Normal, or Slightly Elevated Reticulocytes and Low MCV

In severe iron deficiency anemia, red cells are markedly microcytic and show moderate variation in size and shape. Elongated red cells (pencil forms) are common. Platelets are frequently increased. As discussed previously, the erythrocyte protoporphyrin concentration is usually increased in iron deficiency, although values are lower than those found in severe lead poisoning.

Anemia is uncommon in lead poisoning but, when present, resembles the anemia of iron deficiency in its red cell morphology. Basophilic stipling is found in a small percentage of cases. The erythrocyte protoporphyrin is markedly elevated and the rapid measurement of this compound enables the physician in the emergency department to distinguish severe lead poisoning, which requires hospitalization and intensive chelation, from iron deficiency which can usually be treated on an outpatient basis (see Chapter 48, p. 521).

Low, Normal, or Slightly Elevated Reticulocytes and Normal or Elevated MCV

With the exception of mild macrocytosis, red cell morphology is usually normal in childhood disorders of bone marrow or stem cell failure. Thrombocytopenia and neutropenia are present in aplastic anemia and Fanconi's anemia. Although the platelet count and white count may occasionally be low in patients with Diamond-Blackfan syndrome, the red cells are most severely affected. Erythropoiesis alone is abnormal in transient erythroblastopenia of childhood and acquired pure red cell aplasia.

The clinical features at the onset of acute leukemia may closely resemble those of aplastic anemia. Examination of a bone marrow aspirate is required to distinguish these disorders. This procedure is rarely performed in the emergency department; therapy, such as corticosteroids, which might interfere in the interpretation of the bone marrow aspirate should be withheld until a definitive diagnosis has been made.

As discussed previously, children with hemolytic disorders may escape detection until pallor is noted during an aplastic crisis. The reticulocyte count and MCV are similar to those found in primary disorders of red cell production. An underlying hemolytic disease such as sickle cell anemia or hereditary spherocytosis can usually be recognized by finding characteristic red cells on the peripheral smear. In the autosomal dominant disorders of the red cell membrane, the presence of abnormal erythrocytes in the peripheral blood of one of the parents may further support the diagnosis. Solubility tests for HbS or hemoglobin electrophoresis should be performed to detect sickling disorders.

The MCV is usually increased in megaloblastic anemias unless other nutritional disorders are present. Hypersegmentation of the polymorphonuclear leukocytes is characteristic. In severe or long-standing megaloblastic anemia, neutropenia and thrombocytopenia may also be found. In such cases, the findings in the peripheral blood may be similar to those of aplastic anemia or even acute leukemia; examination of the bone marrow and measurement of specific nutrients (B_{12}, folic acid) are necessary to distinguish these disorders.

References

Alter BP: Bone marrow failure in children. *Pediatr Ann* 8: 53–70, 1979.

Buchanan GR, Boxer LA, Nathan DG: The acute and transient nature of idiopathic immune hemolytic anemia in childhood. *J Pediatr* 88: 780–783, 1976.

Cohen AR, Trotzky MS, Pincus D: Reassessment of the microcytic anemia of lead poisoning. *Pediatrics* 67: 904–906, 1981.

Dallman PR, Siimes MA, Stekel A: Iron deficiency in infancy and childhood. *Am J Clin Nutrition* 33: 86–118, 1980.

Pearson HA, Diamond LK: The critically ill child; sickle cell disease crises and their management. *Pediatrics* 48: 629–635, 1971.

Wang WC, Mentzer WC: Differentiation of transient erythroblastopenia of childhood from congenital hypoplastic anemia. *J Pediatr* 88: 784–789, 1976.

CHAPTER 31

Purpura

JOHN W. BENDER, M.D., AND ALAN R. COHEN, M.D.

INTRODUCTION

Blood in the skin or mucosal membranes is referred to as purpura. The unexplained appearance of purpura in a child is a finding which is disturbing to parents and may prompt a quick visit to the local emergency department or physician. This finding is also particularly disturbing to physicians since it may be the presenting sign of a myriad of diseases, some benign and others life-threatening, some treated easily and others requiring complex therapy.

When the onset of purpura is accompanied by massive hemorrhage or by bleeding in a critical site such as the central nervous system, the patient is easily recognized as being dangerously ill and appropriate measures are taken rapidly. However, when purpura is the only presenting complaint, the patient should still be considered as having the potential for life-threatening sequelae of disordered hemostasis. The cause of purpura should be established as rapidly as possible since early treatment may lead to a more favorable outcome. Fortunately, an understanding of the pathophysiology of purpura, a careful history and physical examination, and an appropriate laboratory evaluation will usually establish the cause of the bruising. This chapter will discuss the initial assessment and differential diagnosis of children with purpura. The management of emergency situations associated with these symptoms is discussed in Chapter 47, "Hematologic Emergencies."

PATHOPHYSIOLOGY

Purpura can be subdivided on the basis of its appearance into petechiae and ecchymoses. Petechiae are small (less than 3 mm diameter), reddish-purple, macular lesions. Ecchymoses are larger lesions which are frequently tender and, when severe, may be reaised above the level of the skin surface. Purpuric lesions do not blanch, a characteristic that distinguishes them from vascular dilatation or vascular anomalies. Under normal conditions, a purpuric lesion resolves in a predictable manner. The purple color gradually fades to golden brown as hemosiderin is formed. The golden brown color may then take as long as 6 weeks to resolve. This progressive and characteristic resolution of purpura is often helpful in determining the time and cause of an injury which resulted in purpura. For example, ecchymoses in various stages of resolution may be the major diagnostic finding in cases of child abuse with repeated assaults.

Complex mechanisms maintain vascular integrity and stop the flow of blood when a blood vessel is damaged. Any condition causing a loss of vascular integrity, a decrease in platelet number or function, or an abnormality of the numerous coagulation factors can result in purpura. Factors such as vitamin C which affect collagen synthesis are required for normal formation of connective tissue within the vessel walls. Platelets as well as pituitary and adrenal hormones contribute to the maintenance of the endothelial lining. When a blood vessel is injured, vasoconstriction and retraction usually occur immediately and decrease the flow of blood to the affected area. Platelets adhere to the damaged wall and, in response to the exposed subendothelial collagen, release adenosine diphosphate (ADP). This release reaction causes platelet aggregation at the site of injury and the formation of a platelet plug which is responsible for primary hemostasis. A decrease in the number of circulating platelets or an intrinsic or secondary alteration in platelet metabolism and aggregation may disrupt this early phase of hemostasis and result in localized or disseminated purpura.

The intrinsic pathway of coagulation is also activated by the exposed collagen (Fig. 31.1). A sequence of enzymatic reactions leads to the formation of a fibrin clot at the site of the injury. A related pathway (extrinsic pathway) is activated by tissue thromboplastin and contributes to the development of the fibrin clot. Factors XII, XI, IX, and VIII contribute exclusively to

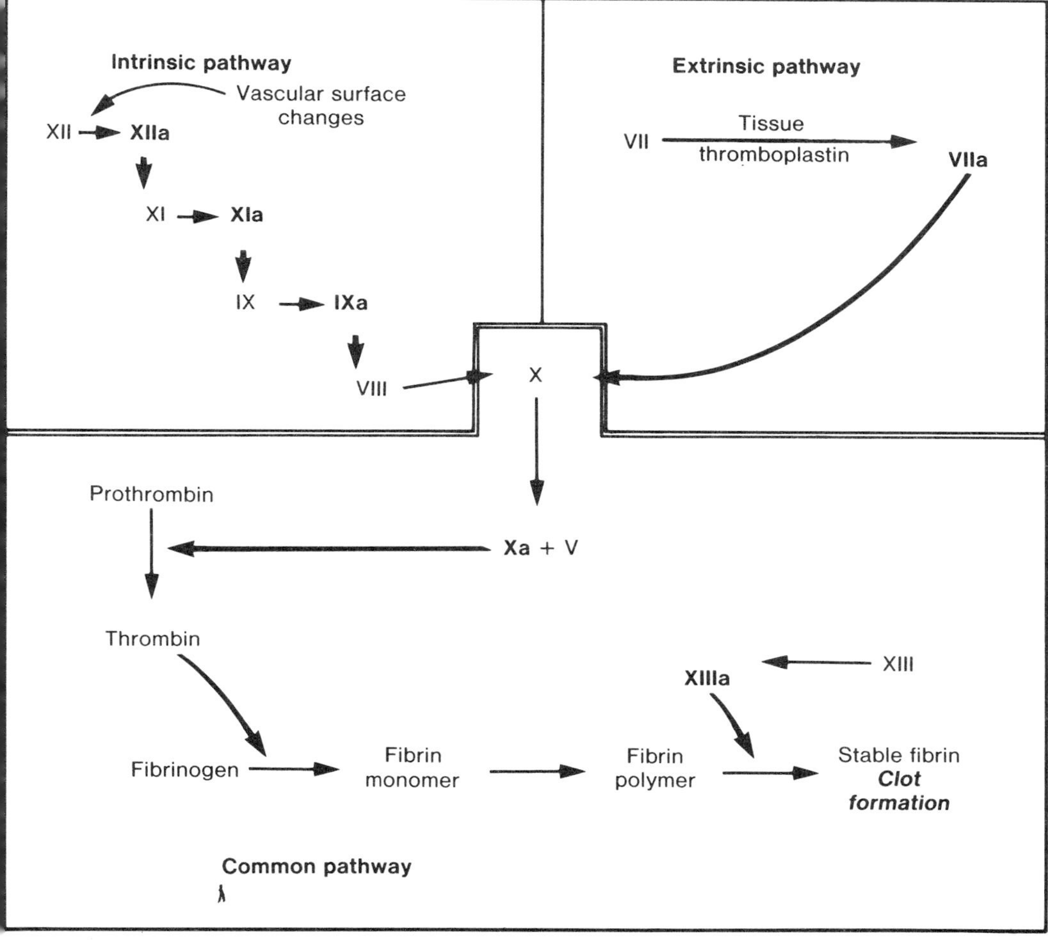

Figure 31.1 A simplified version of the coagulation "cascade." An abnormality in the extrinsic pathway results in a prolonged prothrombin time (PT). An abnormality in the intrinsic pathway results in a prolonged partial thromboplastin time (PTT). An abnormality in the common pathway results in prolongation of both the PT and the PTT.

the intrinsic pathway while factor VII is involved only in the extrinsic pathway. Factors X, V, II (prothrombin) and I (fibrinogen) are shared by both pathways. Defects in the clotting sequence interfere with the formation of a normal clot behind the platelet plug (secondary hemostasis). As is the case in platelet disorders, alterations in the coagulation pathway may be due to intrinsic abnormalities of the clotting factors or to abnormalities resulting from systemic diseases.

Disruption of the normal hemostatic mechanism at any point may result in purpura. Although the pathophysiology is complex and foreboding to most physicians when presented in detail, a basic understanding of altered hemostasis will enable the physician to categorize the wide variety of purpuric disorders and, therefore, to obtain a history, to perform a physical examination, and to select appropriate laboratory tests efficiently.

DIFFERENTIAL DIAGNOSIS

Loss of Vascular Integrity

Purpura may be due to numerous disorders which disrupt vascular integrity (Table 31.1). The most common cause of purpura due to vascular injury in children is trauma. The majority of active children have bruises, particularly on the anterior aspect of the lower extremities. However, it is not uncommon for a parent to bring a child to a physician with the complaint that the child bruises unusually easily. A thorough history and physical examination are often sufficient to distinguish the patient requiring further evaluation from the patient who requires only reassurance about normal childhood bruising from trauma. The child's level of activity should be correlated with the degree of bruising. Ecchymoses which might be acceptable in a child who enjoys climbing trees would be most surprising in a child who spends most of his leisure time reading. In addition, bruising which is on an area of the body infrequently exposed to trauma (e.g., chest, abdomen, back) or bruising which is out of proportion to the degree of trauma should be evaluated. Large, raised ecchymoses are rarely seen in the absence of significant trauma which is easily recalled. A history of sudden onset of excessive bruising without an associated change in activity also suggests an underlying disorder. Finally, even if the ecchymoses can be attributed to repeated episodes of minor trauma, the finding of excessive bruising may be due to the presence of a neurologic disorder in the child who seems unusually clumsy or uncoordinated.

Table 31.1
Causes of Purpura in Children Secondary to Disruption of Vascular Integrity

I. *Trauma:* accidental; child abuse
II. *Infection:* viral exanthems, infectious mononucleosis, bacterial endocarditis, rickettsial disease, streptococcal infection
III. *Drugs and Toxins*
IV. *Henoch-Schönlein Purpura*
V. *Vitamin C Deficiency*
VI. *Letterer-Siwe Disease*
VII. *Ehlers-Danlos Syndrome*
VIII. *Miscellaneous:* acute glomerulonephritis, rheumatic fever, collagen vascular diseases

Foremost in the mind of a physician caring for children must be the consideration that bruising is due to child abuse. Suspicion should be raised if the child has presented in the past with unexplained bruising or suspicious injuries, if explanations of the bruises are inconsistent, if they are confined to the buttocks, back or face, if they conform to the shape of a belt or cord, or if they are in various stages of resolution (see also Chapter 68).

Purpura can be the initial manifestation of numerous infectious processes. The purpura can be due to a disruption of the vascular integrity by the infecting agent or the body's reaction to the agent, an infection-induced thrombocytopenia, or disseminated intravascular coagulation (DIC) initiated by the septic process. The latter two disorders are discussed below. Capillary damage resulting in petechiae or ecchymoses can occur with the viral exanthems and is especially common with rubeola. The child with infectious mononucleosis, bacterial endocarditis, a rickettsial infection or streptococcal infection can present with urpura in the absence of coagulation or latelet abnormalities. Rocky Mountain potted fever should be strongly considered when the patient is from an area in which he disease is endemic or when there is a istory of tick exposure, especially in the nonths of April through October (see Chapter 45, p. 407).

The most serious infection that can cause urpura is meningococcemia, and this disrder must always be considered in a child resenting with purpuric lesions (Chapter 5, p. 358). The rapidity with which meingococcemia can progress may warrant he institution of antibiotic therapy in any moderately ill child with purpura until reults of cultures are available. Purpura fulminans is a particularly severe form of bleeding due in part to loss of vascular ntegrity and may accompany meningococemia as well as septicemia due to other organisms, scarlet fever, varicella, and rubeola. This disorder is frequently found in association with DIC and is characterized by the sudden onset of large ecchymoses and rapid development of gangrene of the extremities.

Numerous drugs and toxins can cause purpura as a result of increased capillary ragility or vasculitis. The parents of a child presenting with purpura should be quesioned closely regarding the recent use of any medications, including over-the-counter drugs and "home remedies." Drugs hat have been implicated include the sulfonamides, iodides, belladona, bismuth, mercurial compounds, the penicillins, phenacetin, and chloral hydrate. Corticosteroid treatment can cause the appearance of benign purpura, especially striated purpuric lesions just above the buttocks. The lesions resolve with discontinuation of corticosteroid therapy. The appearance of these lesions in a child not on corticosteroid therapy should initiate a search for endogenous corticosteroid production as in Cushing's disease. Vitamin C deficiency can also present with purpura ranging from scattered petechiae to substantial ecchymoses, particularly on the lower extremities. Scurvy is rare in the United States but can be seen in patients receiving hyperalimentation with inadequate vitamin C supplementation or in patients with iron overload. The purpuric lesions of scurvy heal rapidly after the administration of vitamin C.

Purpura resulting from an aseptic vasculitis within the corium may be the presenting symptom of Henoch-Schönlein purpura (HSP). The purpuric lesions are often accompanied by pink or brownish-pink macules or maculopapules which may later develop central areas of hemorrhage. They tend to coalesce and are usually located on the lower extremities, buttocks, and lower back. The platelet count is normal in uncomplicated HSP as are the prothrombin and partial thromboplastin times. Anaphylactoid purpura resembling HSP can also accompany acute streptococcal infections, rheumatic fever, acute glomerulonephritis, or collagen vascular disorders.

Rare disorders of childhood which may be associated with purpura due to loss of vascular integrity include Letterer-Siwe disease and Ehlers-Danlos syndrome. Letterer-Siwe disease is a histiocytic disorder with brown, crusted vesiculopapular skin lesions which are often purpuric. Petechiae may also be present. The pathogenesis of purpura in this disorder is uncertain but may be related to the widespread histiocytic infiltration. Ehlers-Danlos syndrome is an unusual defect in collagen synthesis. The altered blood vessel architecture causes capillary hemorrhage; rupture of major blood vessels may occur.

Platelet Disorders

THROMBOCYTOPENIA

Thrombocytopenia in childhood may be due to shortened platelet survival, decreased platelet production, or platelet sequestration (Table 31.2). However, certain illnesses and drugs may cause thrombocytopenia by more than one mechanism. For example, thrombocytopenia accompanying viral or bacterial infections may be due to decreased platelet production, antiplatelet antibody formation, or the presence of DIC. Similarly, thrombocytopenia associated with sulfonamide therapy may be due to diminished platelet production or immune-mediated platelet destruction. Conse-

Table 31.2
Causes of Childhood Purpura Secondary to Abnormalities of Intravascular Coagulation Function

I. Platelet Disorders
- A. Thrombocytopenia
  - 1. Decreased platelet survival
    - a. Immune mediated
      - i. Idiopathic thrombocytopenic purpura
      - ii. Collagen vascular diseases
      - iii. Drug-induced
      - iv. Sepsis
    - b. Disseminated intravascular coagulation
    - c. Hemolytic uremic syndrome
    - d. Thrombotic thrombocytopenic purpura
    - e. Wiskott-Aldrich syndrome
  - 2. Decreased platelet production
    - a. Malignancies (leukemia, neuroblastoma)
    - b. Sepsis: viral and bacterial
    - c. Drugs (bone marrow suppression)
    - d. Aplastic anemia, Fanconi's anemia
    - e. Storage disease (Niemann-Pick disease, Gaucher's disease)
    - f. Megaloblastic anemias
    - g. Osteopetrosis
    - h. Histiocytosis
  - 3. Platelet sequestration
    - a. Congestive splenomegaly
    - b. Large hemangiomas
- B. Qualitative platelet disorders
  - 1. Congenital
    - a. Glanzmann's thrombasthenia
    - b. Storage pool diseases; Bernard-Soulier syndrome, others
  - 2. Acquired. Drug-induced: aspirin, antihistamines, phenothiazines, glycerol, guaifenesin, carbenicillin

II. Factor Deficiencies
- A. Congenital: Deficiencies or alterations of every coagulation factor have been reported. Von Willebrand's disease, factor VIII deficiency (hemophilia A) and factor IX deficiency (hemophilia B) are most common
- B. Acquired: Disseminated intravascular coagulation, vitamin K deficiency, warfarin therapy, liver disease, renal disease, congenital heart disease, circulating anticoagulants (associated with malignancies and collagen vascular disease)

quently, further investigation may be required to determine the mechanism of thrombocytopenia and the appropriate treatment.

Increased Platelet Destruction

The most common form of thrombocytopenia in childhood is idiopathic thrombocytopenic purpura (ITP). This immunologic disorder is usually characterized by the acute onset of petechiae and ecchymoses, although symptoms occasionally occur more gradually. Epistaxis occurs in 30% of cases. Other bleeding manifestations are much less common. Although ITP occurs in children of all ages, most cases are seen between the ages of 2 and 6 years.

The onset of ITP usually follows a mild viral illness by 2 to 6 weeks and may be associated with infectious mononucleosis, cytomegalovirus infection, hepatitis, rubeola, mumps, and varicella. A similar relationship between ITP and rubeola and rubella immunization has been observed. ITP may be the first manifestation of systemic immunologic disorders such as systemic lupus erythematosus. A careful search for this association is particularly important in older children. The association of ITP with autoimmune hemolytic anemia is known as Evans' syndrome. Occasionally immune neutropenia may also be present.

The physical examination of the child with ITP reveals few abnormalities other than purpura. Enlargement of the spleen occurs infrequently. At the onset of purpura, the platelet count is usually below $20,000/mm^3$. In the absence of prolonged bleeding or antibodies to other hematologic elements, the hemoglobin concentration and white blood cell count are normal. A bone marrow aspirate is commonly performed to assess megakaryocyte production since the clinical presentation of aplastic anemia or acute leukemia rarely may be indistinguishable from ITP. A bone marrow aspirate is particularly important if treatment with corticosteroids is contemplated since this therapy may obscure the diagnosis of acute leukemia, thereby delaying appropriate therapy. Other laboratory studies which should be performed include an antinuclear antibody titer as a screening test for collagen vascular disorders and a reticulocyte count and direct Coombs test to detect immune hemolytic anemia.

Thrombocytopenia due to shortened platelet survival may be caused by fibrin deposition and platelet consumption as found in DIC (discussed below) and hemolytic-uremic syndrome (HUS). HUS is characterized by a microangiopathic anemia and uremia. Pallor, purpura, and signs of renal failure usually follow a prodrome of abdominal pain and diarrhea. Thrombotic thrombocytopenic purpura (TTP) is a disorder resembling HUS in its hematologic aspects but usually found in adults rather than children. However, this disorder has been described in the pediatric age group and may be particularly difficult to distinguish from HUS, although neurologic rather than renal symptoms are more prominent in TTP.

Infants with Wiskott-Aldrich syndrome, an X-linked recessive immunodeficiency disorder, may develop thrombocytopenic purpura beginning in the newborn period. Shortened platelet survival in this disease is due to an intrinsic platelet abnormality. The survival of transfused donor platelets is normal in children with Wiskott-Aldrich syndrome while survival of autologous platelets is shortened.

Numerous drugs have been reported to cause thrombocytopenia by the formation of platelet antibodies with resultant increased platelet destruction. The drugs causing thrombocytopenia which are most commonly used in children include sulfa compounds (including trimethoprim-sulfamethoxazole), digitoxin, phenytoin, acetazolamide, carbamazepine, and quinidine.

Decreased Platelet Production

Diseases associated with decreased amounts of functional bone marrow may also present with thrombocytopenia and purpura. Most notable in this group are the leukemias, neuroblastoma, histiocytosis, osteopetrosis, and storage diseases such as Gaucher's disease and Niemann-Pick disease. Decreased platelet production may also be due to abnormalities of development of the hematopoietic stem cell (aplastic anemia, Fanconi's anemia), ineffective megakaryocyte development (megaloblastic anemias) or, rarely, absence of a humoral factor (presumed thrombopoietin deficiency). Although pancytopenia may be present at the time of diagnosis of bone marrow disorders such as leukemia and aplastic anemia, thrombocytopenia may precede notable alterations in other elements in the peripheral blood.

Numerous drugs have been associated with thrombocytopenia due to decreased platelet production. Any drug capable of causing general bone marrow suppression can produce thrombocytopenia (most antibiotics, anticonvulsants, thiazide diuretics, etc). Drugs that specifically inhibit megakaryocyte production include the chlorothiazides, estrogenic hormones, ethanol, and tolbutamide.

The circulating platelets in disorders of platelet production are usually older and metabolically less active than those found in most diseases of shortened platelet survival. Consequently spontaneous purpura often appears at a platelet count of 25,000 to 40,000/mm^3 in leukemia or aplastic anemia but is infrequent in ITP except during the first week of illness.

Platelet Sequestration

Splenomegaly due to numerous causes (e.g., portal hypertension, storage diseases, primary splenomegaly) can result in sequestration of platelets and thrombocytopenia. The spleen is markedly enlarged and very firm in these disorders. Purpura due to platelet sequestration alone is rare but may result from associated liver disease. Platelet sequestration and consumption can also occur in large hemangiomas (Kasabach-Merritt syndrome).

QUALITATIVE DISORDERS OF PLATELETS

A clinical picture similar to that seen with thrombocytopenia can occur with a normal platelet count in the presence of a qualitative or functional platelet abnormality. These disorders can be congenital or acquired, and when congenital can present in infancy with prolonged oozing from venipuncture sites or the umbilical cord, ecchymoses, and petechiae. Glanzmann's thrombasthenia is an autosomal recessive disorder in which the platelet count is normal but the bleeding time is prolonged, clot retraction is poor, and platelet aggregation and adhesion are absent. Other inherited abnormalities of platelet metabolism (storage pool disease, aspirin-like defect, Bernard-Soulier syndrome) may be associated with purpura although bleeding is generally not as severe as it is in Glanzmann's thrombasthenia. Platelet dysfunction in addition to shortened platelet survival is found in Wiskott-Aldrich syndrome.

Acquired platelet dysfunction with purpura can occur in the presence of uremia or liver dysfunction and can also be caused by certain medications. Aspirin is the best known of the drugs that cause platelet dysfunction; a single dose of aspirin can alter platelet function for as long as 9 or 10 days. Platelet dysfunction has also been associated with antihistamines, propranolol, phenothiazines, glycerol, guaifenesin, and carbenicillin. These drugs interfere with the release of endogenous ADP and inhibit platelet aggregation and adhesion.

Factor Deficiencies

Purpura can be the presenting symptom of a congenital or acquired deficiency of coagulation factors. The most commonly encountered congenital deficiencies are hemophilia A (factor VIII deficiency) and hemophilia B (factor IX deficiency, Christmas disease). Although these disorders have an X-linked recessive mode of inheritance, the de novo appearance of the coagulopathy is not uncommon, particularly in children with severe hemophilia A (factor VIII activity $< 1\%$). Therefore, a family history of affected males may be helpful in establishing the diagnosis of hemophilia, but the absence of such a history does not eliminate this diagnostic possibility.

CONGENITAL DEFICIENCIES

Children with hemophilia frequently are detected when they develop purpura either spontaneously or after mild trauma. The diagnosis of hemophilia should also be entertained in newborns who develop excessive bleeding following circumcision and in infants with prolonged bleeding from lacerations of the lip, tongue, or frenulum. Prompt recognition of the disorder at this early age allows appropriate treatment, careful surveillance, and early genetic counseling for parents.

Coagulation tests in children with hemophilia A and B reveal a prolonged partial thromboplastin time and normal prothrombin time. The bleeding time is usually, but not always, normal. Specific factor assays will define the particular abnormality. Special care should be taken in establishing the diagnosis of factor IX deficiency in the young infant since the low factor IX levels found in normal infants in the first few days of life may overlap with the factor IX levels found in mild hemophilia B.

Less common congenital factor deficiencies which may cause purpura in childhood include fibrinogen and factors II (prothrombin), V, VII, X, and XI. As in hemophilia, clotting assays using plasma deficient in a specific factor will identify the particular abnormality. Alterations in fibrinogen function (dysfibrinogenemias) are also associated with purpura. Fibrinogen levels determined by clotting assay will usually be moderately reduced in these disorders.

Von Willebrand's disease is an often encountered bleeding disorder due to an alteration of the factor VIII molecule which adversely affects platelet function as well as clotting. The severity of this autosomal dominant disorder is extremely variable among affected individuals. While some patients may have spontaneous purpura, others remain asymptomatic and are only discovered after the diagnosis of von Willebrand's disease in a close relative leads to laboratory investigation of other family members. Occasionally, von Willebrand's disease is uncovered when an acquired alteration of hemostasis is superimposed upon the inherited abnormality. For example, bruising occurs very easily after aspirin ingestion in many patients with von Willebrand's disease. As in other disorders affecting platelet function, bleeding from mucosal surfaces (epistaxis, menorrhagia) is prominent in von Willebrand's disease. The laboratory abnormalities in von Willebrand's disease are variable and may fluctuate from week to week in the same patient. In its classical form, the disease is characterized by prolongation of the bleeding time, increased partial thromboplastin time, decreased levels of factor VIII coagulant activity and factor VIII related antigen, and diminished platelet aggregation in response to ristocetin (von Willebrand's factor). In practice, however, only one or two of the laboratory abnormalities may be found. Indeed, several determinations may be required to detect an abnormality or to confirm the diagnosis of von Willebrand's disease.

ACQUIRED DEFICIENCIES

Causes of acquired deficiencies of clotting factors include DIC, liver disease, vitamin K deficiency, circulating anticoagulants, uremia, and cyanotic congenital heart disease. DIC is a potential complication of infection (bacterial, viral, or rickettsial), extensive burns, severe trauma, malignancies (especially acute promyelocytic leukemia), snake and insect bites, shock and heat stroke. In DIC, the intravascular consumption of clotting factors may cause purpura due to factor depletion and, in severe cases, may lead to widespread, rapidly progressing purpuric lesions (purpura fulminans) associated with thrombosis or emboli. While other signs of serious illness are usually present in the child with purpura due to DIC, fever and purpura may be the only significant findings in the early stages of severe bacterial infections such as meningococcemia. Further investigations and appropriate therapy should proceed rapidly in such instances.

Laboratory abnormalities in DIC include one or more of the following: a decreased platelet count, prolonged prothrombin and partial thromboplastin times, decreased fibrinogen level and elevated fibrin split products. A microangiopathic anemia with red cell fragmentation may also be present.

Coagulopathies due to severe hepatocellular disease or vitamin K deficiency can present with clinical and laboratory findings which are very similar to those in DIC. A comparison of the laboratory values in these three disorders is shown in Table 31.3. Hepatocellular disorders which may cause purpura include Reye's syndrome, Wilson's disease, and toxic or infectious hepatitis. Vitamin K deficiency may be associated with malabsorption and chronic diarrhea. Purpura due to warfarin (Coumadin) therapy or ingestion can clinically resemble vitamin K deficiency. Hemorrhagic disease of the newborn due to decreased vitamin K stores at birth can be prevented by the administration of vitamin K routinely following delivery. However, this important step in normal newborn care may be overlooked when other problems develop in the delivery room, and a careful review of the records may be necessary to ensure that the young infant with purpura actually received vitamin K.

Circulating anticoagulants are rare in children but may be associated with malignancies or collagen vascular disorders. Numerous coagulation abnormalities have been demonstrated in vitro in patients with

Table 31.3
Comparison of Laboratory Values in Disseminated Intravascular Coagulation (*DIC*), Liver Disease, and Vitamin K Deficiency[a]

	PT	PTT	Fibrinogen	FSP	Platelet Count	Factor		
						V	VII	VIII
DIC	↑	↑	↓	↑	↓	↓	↓	↓
Vitamin K deficiency	↑	↑	N	N	N	N	↓	N
Liver disease	↑	↑	N to ↓	N to ↑	N to ↓	↓	↓	N to ↑

[a] PT, prothrombin time; PTT, partial thromboplastin time; FSP, fibrin split products. ↑ = increased or prolonged, ↓ = decreased, N = normal.

renal disease. However, bleeding is most commonly related to altered platelet function rather than defects in the fluid phase of coagulation. Abnormalities resembling those found in DIC have been associated with cyanotic congenital heart disease. Although the coagulopathy seems to be related to the degree of polycythemia, the underlying mechanisms remains unidentified.

EVALUATION AND DECISION

The evaluation of a child with purpura must combine speed and skill. The diagnostic approach is outlined in Figure 31.2. Purpura can be the initial sign of a life-threatening meningococcal infection requiring immediate treatment or the first sign of a complex social situation resulting in child abuse and requiring patient, thorough investigation. The initial approach should be dictated by the general appearance of the child and the presenting vital signs. A well appearing child with purpura and normal vital signs can be approached with less urgency than a febrile, lethargic child with purpura or a child with hemophilia, purpura of the neck, and respiratory compromise.

If the child with purpura appears well or if the more seriously ill child has been given appropriate emergency care, the evaluation of the purpura can proceed in an orderly fashion. The recent and past medical history should be carefully reviewed with the parents and child. The acute onset of purpura after a recent viral illness or immunization is consistent with an acquired disorder such as ITP. On the other hand, recurrent purpura since infancy suggests an inherited abnormality of platelets or clotting factors. Specific inquiries regarding past surgery, dental extractions or significant trauma should be made, since the absence of bleeding under these conditions would be unusual in most inherited disorders of even moderate severity. When previous bleeding has occurred, the site of bleeding may be helpful in establishing the alteration in the hemostatic mechanisms. Hemarthroses, a common problem in severe hemophilia, are rarely associated with platelet abnormalities. Conversely, petechiae and subconjunctival hemorrhages are frequently found in children with platelet disorders but occur rarely in hemophilia.

The family history should be reviewed for purpura or bleeding disorders. A positive family history in male relatives on the maternal side suggests factor VIII or factor IX deficiency. A history of bleeding or bruising in family members of both sexes suggests a condition with dominant inheritance such as von Willebrand's disease. However, as noted earlier, a negative family history does not preclude the diagnosis of von Willebrand's disease or hemophilia. A careful review of systems should also be obtained to evaluate underlying conditions such as uremia, hepatic disease, congenital heart disease, or malabsorption that might be associated with a coagulopathy.

The child should be examined carefully to assist in the diagnosis of the specific bleeding disorder and to evaluate hidden areas of hemorrhage. Particular attention should be paid to the skin. The distribution of purpura should be noted. Purpura on the lower extremities and buttocks suggests

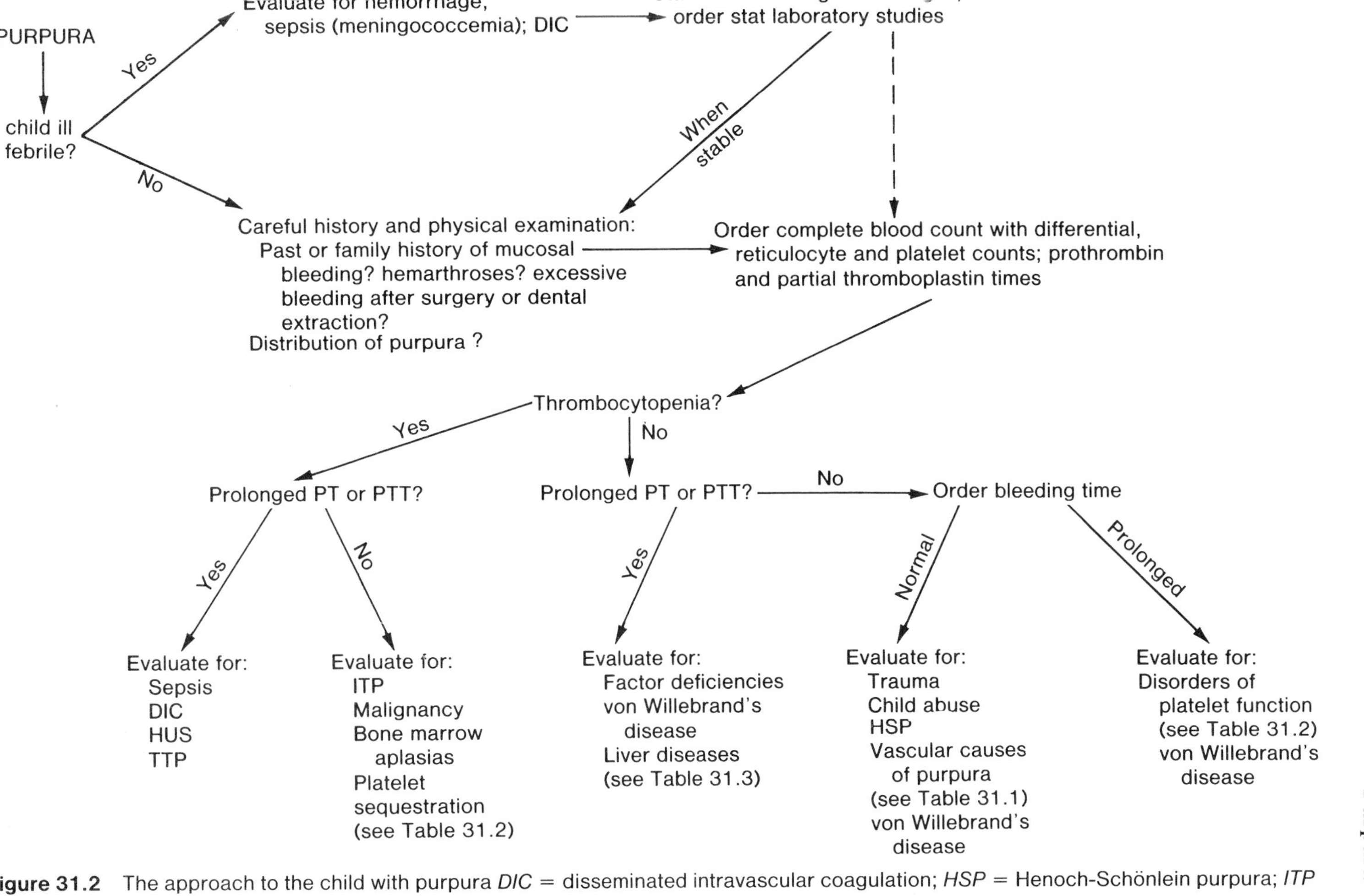

Figure 31.2 The approach to the child with purpura *DIC* = disseminated intravascular coagulation; *HSP* = Henoch-Schönlein purpura; *ITP* = idiopathic thrombocytopenic purpura; *TTP* = thrombotic thrombocytopenic purpura; *PT* = prothrombin time; *PTT* = partial thromboplastin time; *HUS* = hemolytic-uremic syndrome.

Henoch-Schönlein purpura and purpuric lesions on the palms and soles are often seen with rickettsial infections. When the purpuric lesion has an unusual shape such as a folded cord, child abuse should be suspected. Complete neurological assessment is mandatory when there is suspicion of head trauma in the face of a bleeding diathesis. The eyes should be examined for the presence of conjunctival, scleral or retinal hemorrage. The presence of lymphadenopathy or hepatosplenomegaly should be sought. Lymphadenopathy may be present in certain malignancies (leukemias) or viral infections (infectious mononucleosis, cytomegalovirus) that can present with purpura. Hepatomegaly may signal an underlying hepatic disorder causing a coagulopathy. Splenomegaly can be seen in infectious mononucleosis, leukemia, hepatic disease or the storage diseases. Inflammation or synovial thickening of the large joints is consistent with the hemarthroses seen in hemophilia or severe von Willebrand's disease.

The laboratory approach to a child with purpura is also influenced by the initial presentation and history. Every child pr senting with purpura should have a co plete blood count with a differential a platelet count, a prothrombin time and partial thromboplastin time. In most h pitals these tests can be done very quick so that therapy can be chosen or modifi on the basis of the results. A decreas hematocrit or hemoglobin concentrati may be indicative of past or present blo loss or bone marrow failure or replaceme The white blood cell count can give info mation regarding the possibility of sepsis leukemia. If sepsis is suspected the sme should be examined for the presence toxic granulation, vacuolization or Döh bodies. Atypical lymphocytes are seen wi many viral infections, especially monon cleosis.

Causes of abnormal screening coagul tion studies (platelet count, prothromb time, partial thromboplastin time, bleedi time) are outlined in Table 31.4. Dependi on the results of these initial tests and t clinical impression derived from the histo and physical examination, a more sophis cated laboratory evaluation can be unde

Table 31.4
Tests Frequently Employed in Evaluation of Purpura or Suspected Bleeding Disorders

I. Platelet Count (normal 150,000 to 500,000/mm^3)
Decreased: Increased platelet destruction, decreased platelet production, platelet seque tration (see Table 31.2)

II. Prothrombin Time (normal range may vary between laboratories)
Prolonged: Disseminated intravascular coagulation; vitamin K deficiency; warfarin ingestio deficiencies of factors II, V, VII, X (acquired or congenital), abnormalities of fibrinogen; liv disease; renal disease; congenital heart disease

III. Activated Partial Thromboplastin Time (normal range may vary between laboratories)
Prolonged: Disseminated intravascular coagulation; von Willebrand's disease; deficienci of factors V, VIII, IX, X, XI, XII, prothrombin and fibrinogen; vitamin K deficiency; hepa therapy or sample contamination; liver disease; renal disease; congenital heart disease

IV. Fibrinogen (normal > 150 mg/100 ml)
Decreased: Disseminated intravascular coagulation, liver disease, L-aspariginase therap dysfibrinogenemia, afibrinogenemia

V. Fibrin Split Products (normal < 1:20)
Increased: Disseminated intravascular coagulation, liver disease

VI. Bleeding Time (modified Ivy): (normal < 8 min, 30 sec)
Prolonged: Idiopathic thrombocytopenic purpura (early) and other thrombocytopenias, vo Willebrand's disease, platelet function disorders

VII. Rumpel-Leede Test (normal: 15 petechiae in 5-cm diameter area on forearm)
Abnormal: Conditions with increased capillary fragility (see Table 31.1), quantitative ar qualitiative platelet disorders (see Table 31.2)

aken. If emergency therapy is required before the cause of purpura is known, pretreatment plasma should be saved for later nvestigation of disorders such as von Willebrand's disease or other inherited factor leficiencies.

The emergency management of children with purpura is discussed in detail in Chapter 47. The general principles, however, are ather straightforward. When purpura is associated with a serious underlying disorder such as meningococcemia, treatment of hat disorder is usually the first priority. Treatment of the coagulopathy is based on he degree and site of bleeding and the actual hemostatic defects. In primary disorders of hemostasis, appropriate replacement therapy is used when the specific alteration is known. When the disease has not been fully defined, broad treatment with one or more blood products may be required while further laboratory studies are performed. In all instances, the standard measures for general emergency care should be fully employed during the evaluation and treatment of the purpuric disorders.

References

Bachman F: Diagnostic approach to mild bleeding disorders. *Semin Hematol* 17: 292–305, 1980.

Baugh RF, Hougie C: The chemistry of blood coagulation. *Clin Haematol* 8: 3–30, 1979.

Bloom AL: The von Willebrand syndrome. *Semin Hematol* 17: 215–227, 1980.

Brick RL: Disseminated intravascular coagulation and related syndromes; etiology, pathophysiology, diagnosis and management. *Am J Hematol* 5: 265–282, 1978.

McLure PD: Idiopathic thrombocytopenic purpura in children; diagnosis and management. *Pediatrics* 55: 68–74, 1975.

McLure PD: Idiopathic thrombocytopenic purpura in children; should corticosteroids be given? *Am J Dis Child* 131: 357–359, 1977.

Strauss HS: Diagnosis and treatment of hemophilia, a practical guide. Albany Medical College Publication, 1972.

Zuelzer WW, Lusher JM: Childhood idiopathic thrombocytopenic purpura; to treat or not to treat. *Am J Dis Child* 131: 360–362, 1977.

CHAPTER **32**

Red Eye

GARY R. DIAMOND, M.D.

INTRODUCTION

The outlines for differential diagnosis and initial management of the "red eye" will be described for the physician in an emergency environment. In order to develop an adequate differential diagnosis, it is necessary to take a sufficient history and be a good observer. A strong hand light, preferably with rheostat control, and fluorescein solution are essential. Access to a laboratory and a supply of culture transport materials are also necessary. The techniques involved with use of a slitlamp biomicroscope are of inestimable value, though few general emergency departments are so equipped. A few days under the direction of an ophthalmologist learning the essentials of slitlamp use will repay themselves many times during one's professional career. Table 61.2 in the chapter on ophthalmologic trauma lists necessary equipment for an initial comprehensive ophthalmologic examination in an emergency department.

The eye has only limited ways of responding to a given pathogen, the final common pathway involving vascular dilatation, pain, and reflex tear secretion. Thus, the clinician must use all data derived from thorough history taking and physical examination to arrive at a correct diagnosis.

EVALUATION AND DECISION

Classic differential diagnosis of the red eye includes uveitis, corneal foreign body, corneal abrasion, conjunctivitis, and acute glaucoma (Fig. 32.1 and Table 32.1). Acu glaucoma is quite rare in children, ar much iritis in children, especially that a sociated with pauciarticular juvenile rhe matoid arthritis, commonly presents wi a white eye. The overwhelming majority children with a red eye will have conjun tivitis or corneal abrasion. However, unre ognized glaucoma or uveitis can rapidly d stroy useful vision, and it is essential th the emergency department physician b able to distinguish these from the mo benign and common conjunctivitides.

For simplicity of organization, specifi of differential diagnosis and evaluation d cision in this chapter will be discussed u der the heading of each of the above ent ties.

Glaucoma

Acute glaucoma is the most immediatel vision threatening cause of red eye, as in traocular pressure can reach staggerin levels very rapidly and central retinal arter occlusion can quickly follow. This entity i fortunately quite rare in the pediatric pop ulation, but it does occur.

Examination will disclose a diffusely red tearing, tender eye. The cornea may b cloudly, and microcyst formation may b noted on the corneal surface. Hand light o slitlamp examination may disclose a shal low or nonexistant anterior chamber with iris close to or against the back surface o the cornea. Visual acuity testing should b attempted in each eye and the noninvolved eye examined to the best of one's ability

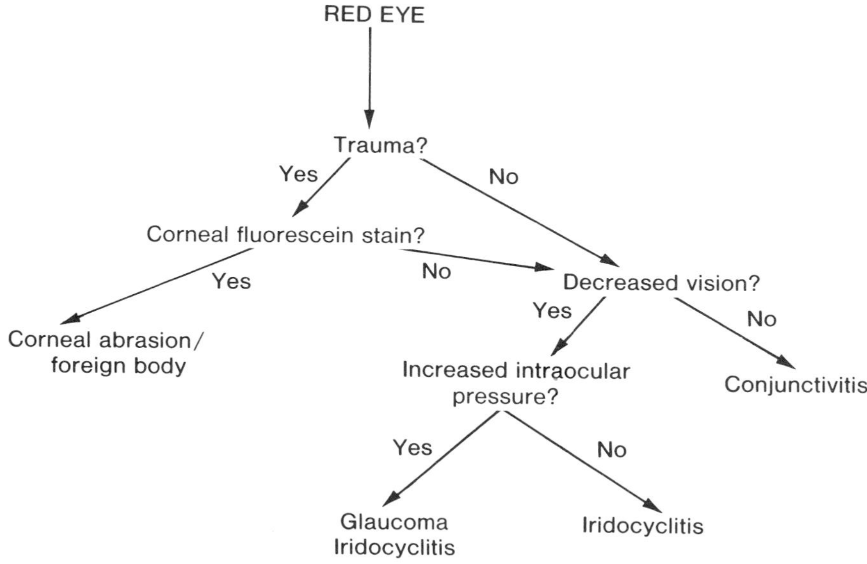

Figure 32.1 Diagnostic approach to red eye.

Table 32.1
Differential Diagnosis of Red Eye[a]

	Glaucoma	Abrasion	Uveitis	Conjunctivitis
History	Prematurity, oxygen, Marfan, homocystinuria	Trauma, contact lens	JRA, sarcoid, trauma	URI, contact lens
Symptoms	Pain, photophobia	Same	Same	Irritation, photophobia
Vision	Decreased	Nl or decreased	Nl or decreased	Usually Nl
Examination:				
Ext:	Watery discharge	Same	Same	Watery or purulent, lid swelling
IOP:	Increased	Nl	Increased, Nl, decreased	Nl
Cornea:	Cloudy, staining	Staining	Nl or band keratopathy	Staining (if keratitis is associated)
AC:	Nl or shallow	Nl	Cells, flare, hypopyon, hyphema	Nl
Pupil:	Fixed, mid-dilated	Nl or small	Small	Any size
ER diagnostic tests	IOP if possible	Fluorescein staining of cornea	Slitlamp, IOP if possible, complete physical exam, chest x-ray (unless obvious trauma)	Culture and Gram stain if purulent, add Giemsa stain if newborn (special handling if GC suspect)

[a] Abbreviations: IOP, Intraocular pressure; JRA, juvenile rheumatoid arthritis; GC, *Neisseria gonorrheae*; URI, upper respiratory infection; Ext, external examination; AC, anterior chamber; Nl, normal.

searching for early evidence of a similar process and therefore a clue to the diagnosis. Asymmetry of corneal diameter size or corneal diameter larger than 12 mm may suggest the presence of congenital or early onset glaucoma. Presence of hyphema or evidence of trauma should be sought. Measurement of intraocular pressure may be deferred to the ophthalmologist, but palpation with gentle tactile pressure will usually disclose the "rock-hard" eye and support the diagnosis of glaucoma.

Corneal Abrasions

Corneal abrasions are quite common and present frequently as red eyes, usually with pain and photophobia. History, as in traumatic iritis, may be helpful in the older child, but many abrasions are accidentally self-inflicted. The child may present with a foreign body sensation and the eye may be red with tearing and photophobia. It is safe to place one drop of topical anesthetic solution in the eye for the child's comfort and to permit further examination. Consider the possibility of corneal abrasion in any young infant who appears "colicky" without other explanation.

Topical fluorescein-impregnated papers are neater and less likely to be contaminated with microorganisms than bottled fluorescein solutions. One drop per eye is sufficient and will highlight abraded areas as dark green under fluorescent light.

Uveitis

The uveal tract consists of the choroid, ciliary body, and iris. Inflammation of any cause within this system will disturb the blood-aqueous barrier and liberate inflammatory cells and protein into the aqueous and/or vitreous. The term uveitis is a nonspecific one, which can be divided into iritis, cyclitis, or choroiditis. Iridocyclitis is a nearly equivalent term for uveitis.

Uveitis presents with pain, photophobia, tearing and a red eye which may be indistinguishable from the presentation of conjunctivitis or corneal foregin body. The absence of purulent discharge may help to distinguish uveitis from conjunctivitis, as may the absence of cervical or preauricular nodes and history of contacts. Absence of corneal staining with topical fluorescein will distinguish iritis from corneal abrasion, although trauma may cause either.

Helpful, if present, is a circumlimbal flush associated with uveitis, reflecting inflammation in the ciliary body which sits in this location inside the eye. As a rule the pupil in iritis is small, reflecting spasm of the sphincter muscle which lies in the uveal tract.

Three common causes of uveitis in children are juvenile rheumatoid arthritis, sarcoid, and trauma. Each of these will be discussed briefly.

Although the uveitis associated with pauciarticular rheumatoid disease in children is often detected in a white eye during routine or "protocol" directed slitlamp examination, some of these children will develop complications which can direct them to emergency care with a red eye. Band keratopathy secondary to calcium phosphate deposition in Bowman membrane of the cornea is often associated with recurrent epithelial erosions and signs and symptoms of corneal abrasion. Posterior synechia between iris and lens and peripheral anterior synechia between iris and cornea may lead to glaucoma and red eye. In end-stage disease, the shrunken, inflamed, painful eye may present a problem in differential diagnosis.

Sarcoid may present in the pediatric population with conjunctival and iris nodules as well as uveitis. Slitlamp examination may disclose greasy "mutton-fat" precipitates on the back of the cornea with cells and flare in the anterior chamber. The latter reflect a breakdown in the blood-aqueous barrier with an increase of protein and inflammatory cells into the eye. Cataract may develop and vitreous inflammation is common. The retina may manifest a vasculitis with perivascular hemorrhage and exudate development. Both posterior and peripheral anterior synechia may form, leading to glaucoma.

Traumatic iritis is the most common cause of uveitis in this age group, and history is helpful but may be circumspect. A high incidence of suspicion in the presence of mysterious circumstances may uncover the true etiology of the intraocular inflammation. Besides a red eye, circumlimbal flush and miotic pupil, severe trauma may cause lid edema, hyphema, layered white blood cells in the anterior chamber ("hypopyon"), iridodialysis, subluxated lens, retinal detachment, choroidal rupture, and macular hole formation. The initially consulted physician should recall the possibility of serious underlying ophthalmic damage.

Conjunctivitis

A history of upper respiratory infection or contact with conjunctivitis and an examination revealing a red, watery eye with preauricular and/or submandibular nodes and grainy appearance to the conjunctiva are highly suspicious for conjunctivitis. The older child may complain of an itchy-scratchy irritation. Symptoms may be worse early in the day, with lids stuck together in the morning upon arising. Viral or allergic conjunctivitis is more common in the older child, while gonococcal or chlamydial (inclusion) conjunctivitis are diseases of the newborn (see Table 32.2).

Laboratory tests can be helpful. Any conjunctivitis in the newborn requires culture, Gram and Giemsa staining and treatment as directed by the history, clinical presentation, stain results and culture.

Special care should be taken to culture the fragile gonococcal organism through standard microbiological techniques (chocolate agar, 5 to 10% CO_2 atmosphere, 35 to 37°C). A preliminary diagnosis of gonococcal conjunctivitis may be made if Gram-negative intracellular diplococci are seen on Gram stain. Other bacteria and sheets of polymorphonuclear neutrophils are occasionally found, common offenders being *Staphylococcus aureus*, *Streptococcus*, *Escherichia coli*, and *Pseudomonas*. Lack of bacteria and a mononuclear or polymorphonuclear infiltrate with watery discharge suggest viral conjunctivitis. Viral cultures are rarely indicated. Cytoplasmic inclusions in epithelial cells on Giemsa stain are indicative of chlamydia infection. Eosinophils are suggestive of an allergic etiology.

A high suspicion should exist for the possibility of herpes simplex conjunctivitis and keratitis in children with evidence of systemic herpes, past corneal infection, or red eye with watery discharge and absent organisms on Gram stain. The ophthalmologist will look for dendrite formation of the corneal ephithelial cells under slitlamp examination, reflecting infection with live herpes virus in the corneal ephithelium. Specific antiviral drops and ointments are available for herpes simplex.

Allergic conjunctivitis may be seasonal, with pale edematous swelling of the lid and conjunctiva, and symptomatology disproportionate to the presentation.

Any corneal opacity should be examined as soon as possible by an ophthalmologist to rule out a corneal ulcer, the management of which must be under ophthalmologic supervision.

Table 32.2
Etiologies of Conjunctivitis by Age (Listed in Approximate Order of Frequency of Presentation)

Less than 2 days	Chemical (silver nitrate)
2 days to 2 weeks	*Chlamydia trachomatis* (''inclusion blennorrhea'')
	Neisseria gonorrheae
	Escherichia coli and other Gram-negative bacilli
2 weeks to 3 months	*C. trachomatis*
	Viral
	N. gonorrheae
	Staphyloccocus aureus
	Streptococcus species
	E. coli and other Gram-negative bacilli
Greater than 3 months	Viral
	Allergy
	Bacterial, any above

CHAPTER **33**

Respiratory Distress

ANN E. THOMPSON, M.D.

INTRODUCTION

Respiratory disease accounts for a very large fraction of pediatric deaths each year in the United States. Trauma (including motor vehicle accidents, near drowning, and smoke inhalation), poisoning, and congenital anomalies represent a large part of the remainder, and respiratory failure frequently complicates these episodes.

If one surveys the population in a busy pediatric emergency department, symptoms of respiratory distress are exceedingly common. They range from trivial to life-threatening, demanding the physician's thorough understanding of the implications of a particular presentation in a child of a particular age. The principle causes of respiratory distress in children are listed by age in Table 33.1.

The primary role of the respiratory system is to meet the metabolic demands of the body; i.e. to provide oxygen and to eliminate carbon dioxide. Respiratory distress occurs whenever difficulty (whether perceived or actual) in meeting those requirements arises. Evidence of distress may be noted by the patient or by an observer (parent, teacher, or physician). Frank respiratory failure occurs when metabolic demands cannot be met. A number of definitions have been used, all somewhat arbitrary. Table 33.2 contains one set of useful criteria.

PATHOPHYSIOLOGY

Normal ventilation is the end result of the interaction of many elements in a complex system. Information from peripheral tissues, lungs, blood, and CSF, as well as from cortical centers, converges on the respiratory centers in the pons and medulla. Efferent impulses carried by the vagus, phrenic, and intercostal nerves cross neuromuscular junctions to the muscles of the chest wall, neck and abdomen effecting the bellows function of the system. Gases are conducted via the large and small airways to and from the alveolar-capillary membrane where actual gas exchange occurs. Flow through these conduits is also affected by autonomic innervation. Supporting structures, including ribs and spine, and elastic fibers of the pulmonary interstitium maintain the configuration of the system. Cardiovascular and lymphatic drainage maintain the fluid balance of the lung which in turn affects gas exchange and mechanical properties of the system.

Respiratory distress or dysfunction may occur as a result of increased metabolic demand or disruption at any point along the ventilatory pathway. A variety of factors predispose the *normal* infant or child to problems. The child with underlying structural or functional abnormalities may be especially vulnerable.

Premature and term infants have extremely active reflexes inhibiting respiration, including juxta-alveolar, Hering-Breuer, and intercostal stretch receptor output. Central nervous system processing of afferent information is markedly affected by sleep state, cold, drugs secreted into breast milk, and other metabolic derangements.

Table 33.1
Common Causes of Respiratory Distress in Children

Young Infant	Older Infant and Child
Pneumonia	*Pneumonia*
Bacterial	Bacterial
Viral	Viral
Aspiration	Other
Chlamydial	*Asthma*
Bronchiolitis	*Upper Airway Obstruction*
Septicemia	Croup
Upper Airway Obstruction	Epiglottitis
(especially congenital anomalies)	Peritonsillar abscess
Congenital Heart Disease	*Foreign Body Aspiration*
Intrathoracic Anomalies	*Congenital and Acquired Heart Diseases*
Diaphragmatic Lesions	*Near Drowning*
Vascular rings	*Smoke Inhalation*
Lobar emphsema	*Central Nervous System Dysfunction*
Cystic fibrosis	Trauma
Infantile Botulism	Infection
Metabolic Acidosis	Seizures
Gastroenteritis and dehydration	*Thoracic Trauma*
Salicylism	*Septicemia*
Miscellaneous causes	*Cystic Fibrosis*
	Neuromuscular Disease
	Guillain-Barré syndrome
	Spinal cord injury
	Metabolic Acidosis
	Diabetes mellitus
	Salicylism, other toxins
	Miscellaneous causes

The infant's chest wall is far more compliant and less stable than that of the older child or adult. The sternum is soft, the ribs are more horizontally placed, and the intercostal muscles are poorly developed. Most of the work of respiration is done by the diaphragm and a fraction of that work is lost in distortion of the rib cage. The loss increases dramatically in normal rapid eye movement sleep when diaphragm and intercostal muscles may not function synchronously, as well as in any situation where increased negative intrapleural pressure is necessary to provide an adequate inspired volume. The more negative the inspiratory pressure generated the greater the tendency to collapse of the rib cage with descent of the diaphragm, thereby limiting the flow of gases into the lung. (Apneic episodes may be precipitated by the increased stimulation of muscle stretch receptors that occurs in this situation.) Additional limitation of ventilatory capacity may arise from the greater fatiguability of the infant diaphragm and from any mechanical limitation of its function, including flattening of the normal curvature by hyperaeration of the lungs or external compression by abdominal distension.

The infant and young child are especially vulnerable to changes in the diameter of the airways. In the infant less than four months old, who is an obligate nose-breather, an upper respiratory infection may cause significant respiratory compromise. Hypertrophied tonsils and adenoids may occlude the upper airway, especially in the child with neuromuscular weakness or depression of the central nervous system. Although at birth the diameter of the trachea is one-third, and that of the bronchi one-half, that of the adult, a small increase in mucosal thickness in the infant will cause a much greater increase in resistance to air flow than in the adult, because resistance varies inversely with the fourth power of the radius of the airway. The situation is exaggerated even further when the diameter of the bronchioles is decreased. Elastic fibers maintaining alveolar and small airway patency are less well developed in early life, predisposing to airway closure and poor matching of ventilation and perfusion. The functional residual capacity of the lung is lower than in the older child, and any interruption in the supply of oxygen will result in a precipitous fall in the partial pressure of arterial oxygen (PaO_2).

In summary, the young infant and, to an important extent, the child under 5 years of age, has a central respiratory control apparatus that is not entirely adaptive, airways which are especially vulnerable to life-threatening obstruction, a bellows apparatus ill-equipped to perform the additional work required by alterations of respiratory function, and a reservoir of oxygen too small to provide even limited protection when ventilation is interrupted.

Table 33.2
Criteria for Respiratory Failure

Clinical
- Decreased or absent breath sounds
- Severe retractions and use of acessory muscles
- Cyanosis in 40% oxygen (excluding cyanotic congenital heart disease)
- Depressed level of consciousness and response to pain
- Poor muscle tone
- Expiratory grunting
- Weak to absent cough or gag reflex

Physiologic
- $PaO_2 < 60$ mm Hg in 60% oxygen (excluding cyanotic congenital heart disease)
- $PaCO_2 > 60$ mm Hg and rising
- Vital capacity < 15 cc/kg

Maximum inspiratory force (pressure) > −20 cm H_2O

Respiratory Failure Likely if Patient Exhibits 2 Clinical Findings and 1 Physiologic Parameter

EVALUATION AND DECISION

Triage and Stabilization

A patient developing respiratory distress may be in danger of imminent collapse of all vital function. Each child should be approached appropriately to the severity of the illness but with the possibility of catastrophe clearly in mind. In the first moments after arrival in the emergency department, the child's safety is addressed. The fascinating details of diagnosis and specific treatment follow later.

The child who is apneic on arrival in an emergency facility is, at most, only minutes away from cessation of cardiovascular function and irreparable central nervous system damage. It is obvious that resuscitation according to principles outlined elsewhere in the book should be begun at once. Once stability is achieved, the specific diagnosis can be pursued.

Children with signs of respiratory distress who are alert should be allowed to remain with their parents and be approached as gently as possible. Anxiety will increase minute ventilation and add substantially to the child's oxygen consumption. Gently, however, does not imply slowly or with disregard for the patient's safety. Any child perceived to have compromised ventilation should be immediately provided with humidified oxygen at the highest concentration available. Diagnostic and other therapeutic efforts can always be delayed for the few seconds needed, and supplemental oxygen provides a small but crucial margin of safety, increasing the likelihood of adequate cerebral and myocardial oxygenation.

Airway patency must be assured. No amount of supplemental oxygen will be effective if it does not reach the alveoli. Merely observing the respiratory efforts of the child is not an adequate assessment of ventilation; in fact, the most extreme efforts may be observed when airway obstruction exists in the presence of normal respiratory drive. One must be able to hear (with or without a stethoscope) and feel air movement. The patient with a depressed sensorium or one with neuromuscular disease may experience airway obstruction because of inability to maintain pharyngeal soft-tissue tone. Correct positioning of the head and neck and the jaw-thrust maneuver will often alleviate obstruction; a nasal or oropharyngeal airway may further improve air passage. These maneuvers are generally not appropriate for alert patients with normal muscle strength who will find an optimal position on their own.

Once supplemental humidified oxygen has been provided, additional basic assessment and therapy can begin. In the first moments, a brief history and physical examination are adequate for rapid localization of disease, assessment of its severity and rate of change, and selection of early measures to stop, control, or reverse the process. One can view therapeutic maneuvers as support for specific problems; e.g., controlled ventilation for the depressed central nervous system, mechanical support for a weakened chest wall, an artificial airway for an obstructed passage, supplemental oxygen for damaged alveoli, and so on.

Differential Diagnosis

Initially, the physician should attempt to separate respiratory dysfunction originating in the airways and pulmonary parenchyma from that caused by disruption of the ventilatory pathway at some other point. Although most children who develop respiratory distress have problems related to their lungs or airways, others may have disturbances of their central nervous system, musculature, chest wall, or metabolism. A careful physical examination serves as the first step in localizing the source of any respiratory difficulty. The diagnostic approach to the child in respiratory distress is outlined below and summarized in Figure 33.1.

Metabolic Disorders. The child with severe metabolic acidosis as a consequence of diabetes mellitus, marked dehydration, liver or renal disease, drug ingestions, or septicemia may be brought to medical attention because of deep rapid breathing. Attention must be directed to correcting the underlying condition and supporting ventilation. Failure to maintain compensatory ventilation may result in cardiovascular collapse.

Central Nervous System Disorders. The child with an altered sensorium produced by accidental ingestion, trauma, central nervous system infection, seizures, or intracranial mass lesions may demonstrate hypo- or hyperventilation, loss of pharyngeal tone with subsequent upper airway obstruction, or loss of protective airway reflexes. Arterial blood gas analysis, assessing effectiveness of ventilation, and physical examination, for stertorous or frankly obstructed breathing, and presence of a cough and gag will determine the need for intubation and mechanical ventilation. In the absence of a history or physical examination pointing to primary central nervous system disease, one must bear in mind that signs of restlessness, agitation, confusion, headache, seizures and coma may be a *consequence* of hypoxemia or hypercarbia.

Neuromuscular Disease. Respiratory inadequacy may also result from peripheral neuromuscular disease such as infantile botulism, spinal cord injury or Guillain-Barré syndrome. Spinal trauma or progressive weakness, hypotonia, hyporeflexia, a weak voice or cry, and a shallow or rocking respiratory pattern alert the physician to the likelihood of inadequate function of the chest wall as well as to the child's inability to maintain airway patency. Simple bedside pulmonary functions provide a quantitative assessment of the child's weakness: maximum inspiratory force (actually pressure) less negative than -20 cm H_2O and a crying vital capacity less than 15 cc/kg reflect weakness severe enough to prevent the child from expelling aspirated secretions or adjusting head position to maintain airway patency. In the absence of these measures, weakened cough and gag reflexes and inability to lift the head or legs from the bed reflect similar weakness. Arterial blood gas changes occur very late and may not be noted until the time of respiratory arrest.

Structural Disorders. In addition to neuromuscular weakness, structural abnormality of the chest wall may impair bellows function. Congenital or developmental skeletal deformity may restrict lung expansion severely enough to prevent the child from increasing ventilation enough to compensate for fever, increased secretions, or minimal parenchymal disease. Abdominal distension may seriously impair diaphrag-

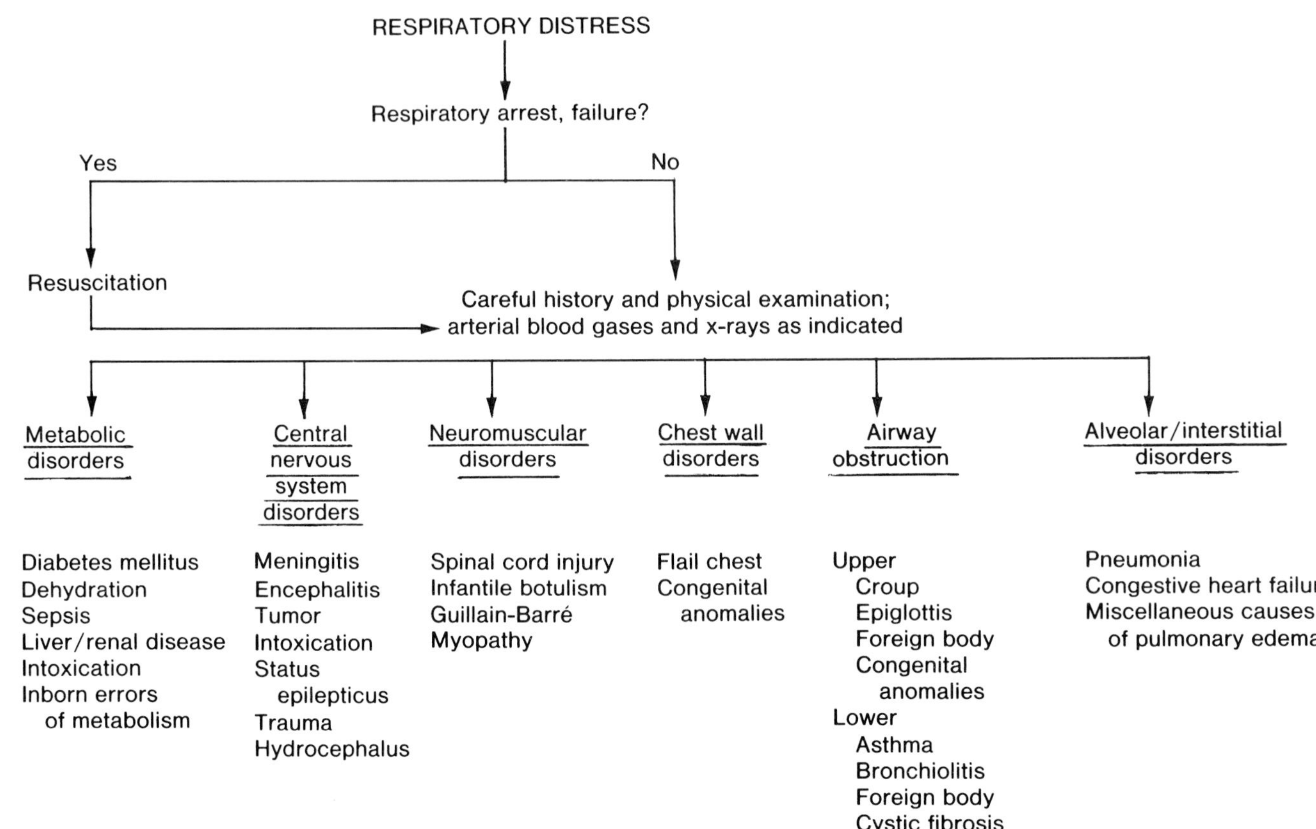

Figure 33.1 Diagnostic approach to the child in respiratory distress.

matic excursion and should be relieved if possible.

Upper Airway Obstruction. Obstructive disease is common in childhood, in part because of the vulnerability of small caliber airways described earlier. An effort should be made to localize the obstruction. The presence of snoring, stertorous breathing, or stridor indicates obstruction at or above the trachea, while wheezing is a consequence of lower airway disease (see also Chapter 35).

The child with stridor of abrupt onset, associated with high fever, sore throat, and drooling is likely to have epiglottitis. Similar symptoms but with a more gradual onset are attributable to other oropharyngeal infections, including peritonsillar and retropharyngeal abscesses. Stridor associated with low-grade fever or normal temperature and gradual worsening over hours or even days is typical of laryngotracheobronchitis (croup), although occasionally a previously well child awakens abruptly with stridor, barking cough, and severe respiratory distress. Identical complaints may arise as a result of foreign body aspiration if it then remains lodged in the upper airway. Infants under 6 months of age with stridor should be assumed to have some underlying structural basis for their distress, either as the primary problem or exacerbated by a viral respiratory illness.

Anteroposterior and lateral neck radiographs will provide conclusive diagnostic information in many cases. Examination of the oropharynx should be avoided or limited to inspection without instrumentation until epiglottitis can be excluded. Physical examination assessing the work of breathing is far more sensitive in this setting than arterial blood gas analysis, which may only serve to exacerbate the child's distress.

Any child with moderate to severe upper airway obstruction should be accompanied at all times by a physician prepared to intervene if complete airway occlusion occurs. If life-threatening asphyxia appears imminent, endotracheal intubation should be performed. Otherwise the child with epiglottitis or foreign body aspiration should be taken to the operating room where laryngoscopy, bronchoscopy, and/or intubation can be performed under controlled conditions. The child with croup should be carefully observed to assess the progression of disease. Aerosolyzed racemic epinephrine may relieve severe distress, but its effect is transient, and children requiring it should be admitted and observed in the hospital (see also Chapter 45, p. 374).

Lower Airway Obstruction. Lower airway obstruction producing wheezing may occur in many disease states. In infants under a year old, viral respiratory infection is most common, especially bronchiolitis and viral pneumonitis. Other causes relatively common in infancy include pertussis, bacterial pneumonia, cystic fibrosis, and congestive heart failure, especially in children with large left-to-right shunts. Many develop tachypnea alone, but additional signs typical of obstruction occur as the work of breathing increases, and apnea and cyanosis may supervene. The younger the infant, the more serious the problem of increased work, for the reasons described above.

A chest radiograph will show hyperaeration and diffuse interstitial markings or patchy atelectasis in bronchiolitis. Cardiomegaly and vascular engorgement seen radiographically combined with a physical examination revealing a murmur and hepatosplenomegaly point toward heart disease as the cause. The infant with cystic fibrosis may have similar symptoms, but the diagnosis of an underlying pulmonary disease is readily suspected with recurrent episodes, chronic cough, or failure to thrive.

Babies who are wheezing with bronchiolitis, but who are smiling, playful, pink in room air, able to feed well and exchange air freely, require little specific therapy. Those with rapid respiratory rates (>60/min), severe retractions, poor color in room air, or marked irritability or lethargy should be evaluated further. Arterial blood gases may reveal hypoxemia or hypercarbia. Infants in severe distress should be admitted, hydrated intravenously, and monitored closely for heart and respiratory rate.

Wheezing in older infants and children can generally be divided into acute and chronic or recurrent events. Acute episodes are often associated with foreign body aspiration, especially in the afebrile child after a paroxysm of coughing. Although parental observation of the child with a small object in his mouth makes the diagnosis obvious, such history is often not available. Differential air entry or wheezing and differential aeration on expiratory or decubitus chest radiographs support the diagnosis. The child with urticaria, mucosal edema and other signs of histamine release is likely suffering an acute allergic reaction.

Children with intermittent recurrent wheezing are frequently suffering from asthma which may be triggered by specific environmental stimuli, exercise, infection, or emotional stress. Similar symptoms may occur in the child with cystic fibrosis. Further discussion of these problems is found in Chapter 49. Occasionally intrathoracic masses may cause bronchial compression with progressively severe airway obstruction.

Alveolar and Interstitial Disorder. Evidence of airway obstruction (especially wheezing and retractions) is also present in many children whose primary problem is interstitial and alveolar disease, when terminal airways are edematous or filled with debris. The child of any age with cough, fever, rales or decreased breath sounds, and localized infiltrate or effusion on chest radiograph is likely to have bacterial infection. More diffuse infiltrates, frequently associated with upper respiratory tract symptoms, fever, and clear lungs, are typical of viral pneumonitis. Similar findings are noted in other atypical pneumonias (including pneumocystis, chlamydia, mycoplasma, etc). Congestive heart failure is likely in the child (most commonly an infant) with a murmur, hepatosplenomegaly, diffuse rales, and cardiomegaly and pulmonary vascular congestion or pulmonary edema on x-ray. Fever is usually absent but may complicate the diagnosis if failure is precipitated by the added stress of an infectious disease. Heart failure causing respiratory distress must also be considered in the child with a tachyarrhythmia or faint, muffled heart sounds.

If bacterial disease is likely, cultures should be obtained and antibiotics begun. If viral disease or aspiration is most likely, general supportive care is all that is necessary. Diuretic therapy may relieve symptoms of congestive heart failure. Digitalization, cardioversion of dysrhythmias, and other measures, should be considered in consultation with a cardiologist. Massive pleural effusion or pneumothorax should be decompressed with thoracentesis, and any fluid obtained should be examined and cultured.

The obviously cyanotic child should receive supplemental oxygen immediately and close attention until he or she is clearly well-oxygenated. Arterial blood gas analysis then guides further respiratory support: $PaO_2 < 60$ mm Hg on 60% oxygen merits intubation for more effective oxygen delivery and initiation of positive airway pressure if necessary; $PaCO > 60$ mm Hg indicates the need for mechanical ventilation. Because the ability to detect arterial hypoxemia clinically is notoriously poor, any child in significant distress with parenchymal disease should be evaluated with an arterial blood gas. Metabolic acidosis should be carefully corrected to decrease respiratory demands.

SUMMARY

In the evaluation and management of each child, one must keep in mind that many nonspecific symptoms alert the physician to respiratory compromise. Conversely, respiratory symptoms may originate outside of the airways and lungs, and assessment of the child's neurologic and cardiovascular status must be thorough. Children with respiratory dysfunction may change quickly. As a result, they require frequent reassessment with attention to heart rate, respiratory rate and pattern, blood pressure, adequacy of oxygenation, ventilation and perfusion. Because of the complexity of many of these illnesses and the risk of rapid change, assistance from physicians experienced in the management of critically ill children should be obtained promptly.

CHAPTER **34**

Scrotal Pain/Swelling

HOWARD McC. SNYDER III, M.D., ANTHONY A. CALDAMONE, M.D., AND JOHN W. DUCKETT, JR., M.D.

INTRODUCTION

Acute scrotal swelling in a child should be considered a surgical emergency. While some causes of acute scrotal swelling may be benign and require no more than observation, other causes of acute scrotal swelling may lead to the rapid loss of a testis if a delay in diagnosis and treatment occurs. The patient with such a chief complaint should be taken immediately to the emergency department with instructions to give the child nothing by mouth. In the emergency department, it is incumbent on the emergency physician to urgently consult a pediatric surgeon or a urologist familiar with the evaluation of acute scrotal swelling whenever testicular torsion is a possibility. Even for the most experienced clinician, certain diagnosis may be difficult and urgent scrotal exploration may be essential. Table 34.1 lists the principal causes of acute scrotal swelling.

EVALUATION AND DECISION

The evaluation of acute scrotal swelling is discussed here by consideration of the important entities causing *painful* versus *painless* scrotal swelling. This approach is outlined in Figure 34.1.

Causes of Painful Scrotal Swelling

Torsion of Testicular Appendage. There are several vestigial embryologic remnants which are commonly attached to the testis or epididymis and which may twist around their base producing venous engorgement, enlargement, and subsequent infarction. Typically, this occurs in boys in the prepubertal age group and has about an equal frequency as testicular torsion, the most important differential diagnosis. Scrotal pain is the usual presenting feature. While there may be associated nausea, vomiting, and diaphoresis, these symptoms are less common than with torsion of the testis. If the child is seen early after the onset of pain, scrotal tenderness and swelling may be localized to the area of the twisted appendage. Typically, this is on the superior lateral aspect of the testis. It may be possible to gently hold the testis and have the patient point to the specific point of pain. If this site is indicated to be the upper pole of the testis with the remainder of the testis being nontender, the diagnosis of a torsion of a testicular appendage is very likely. While the classic "blue dot" sign of an infarcted appendage may be visible, often this cannot be seen because of overlying edema.

In some cases, the degree of scrotal tenderness and edema increases to the point where differentiation from torsion of the testis becomes very difficult. Surgical exploration may be urgently required to be certain that a torsion of the testis is not present.

If the examiner is confident in the diagnosis of a torsion of an appendix testis, surgical exploration is not needed. These children should be sent home with analge-

Table 34.1
Causes of Acute Scrotal Swelling

Painful Scrotal Swelling
Torsion appendage testis
Torsion testis
Trauma—hematocele
Epididymitis—orchitis
Hernia—incarcerated
Painless Scrotal Swelling
Hydrocele and hydrocele of cord
Hernia—incarcerated
Idiopathic scrotal edema
Henoch-Schönlein purpura
Testis tumor
Antenatal torsion testis (newborn)
Generalized edematous states

sics and instructions to rest quietly. The child should return in 48 hours, having had nothing to eat or drink on the morning of the return visit. In the majority of cases, the child's pain will be improving and nothing further is indicated. There will occasionally, however, be a child who seems to have a disproportionate degree of discomfort from the torsion of these tiny appendages. For these children, removal of the appendage may shorten their morbidity. In the older cooperative child, this may be carried out under a spermatic cord block; but in the majority, a general anesthetic is required. We do not recommend contralateral scrotal exploration.

Torsion of the Testis. This represents the most common cause of acute painful scrotal swelling in children. As with torsion of an appendix testis, it occurs most frequently in the prepubertal age group. It results from an inadequate fixation of the testis to the intrascrotal subcutaneous tissue (Fig. 34.2), resulting in the so-called "bell-clapper" deformity. The testis in this deformity may rotate, producing torsion of the spermatic cord, venous engorgement of the testis, and subsequent arterial infarction.

The sudden onset of severe scrotal pain often with radiation to the abdomen and associated nausea and vomiting is typical. Often these episodes have their onset in the early morning. Other times, they may be associated with sports activity or mild testicular trauma which may be perceived by

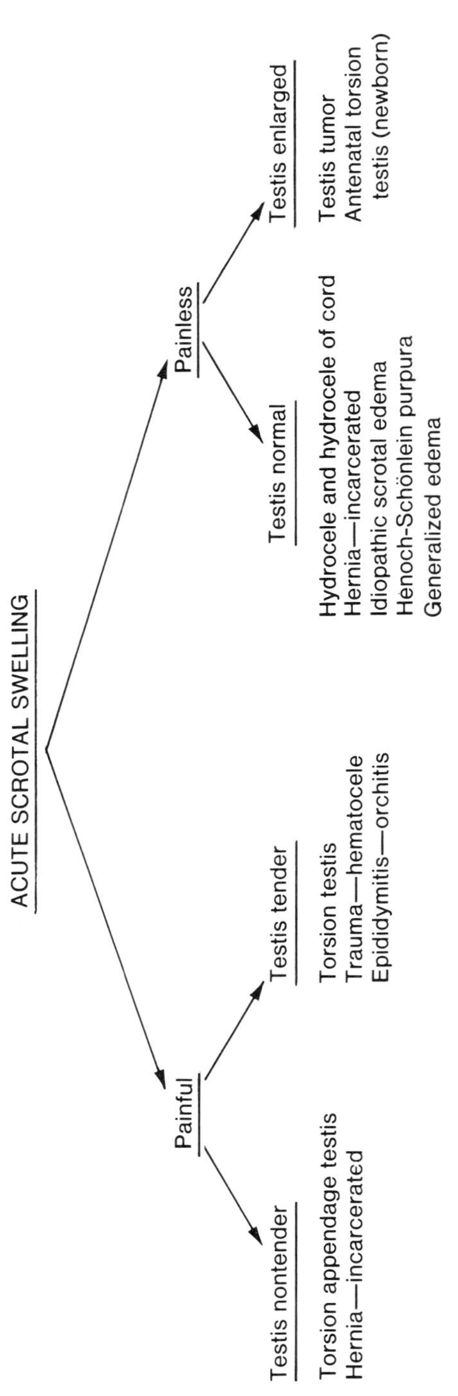

Figure 34.1 Diagnostic approach to acute scrotal swelling.

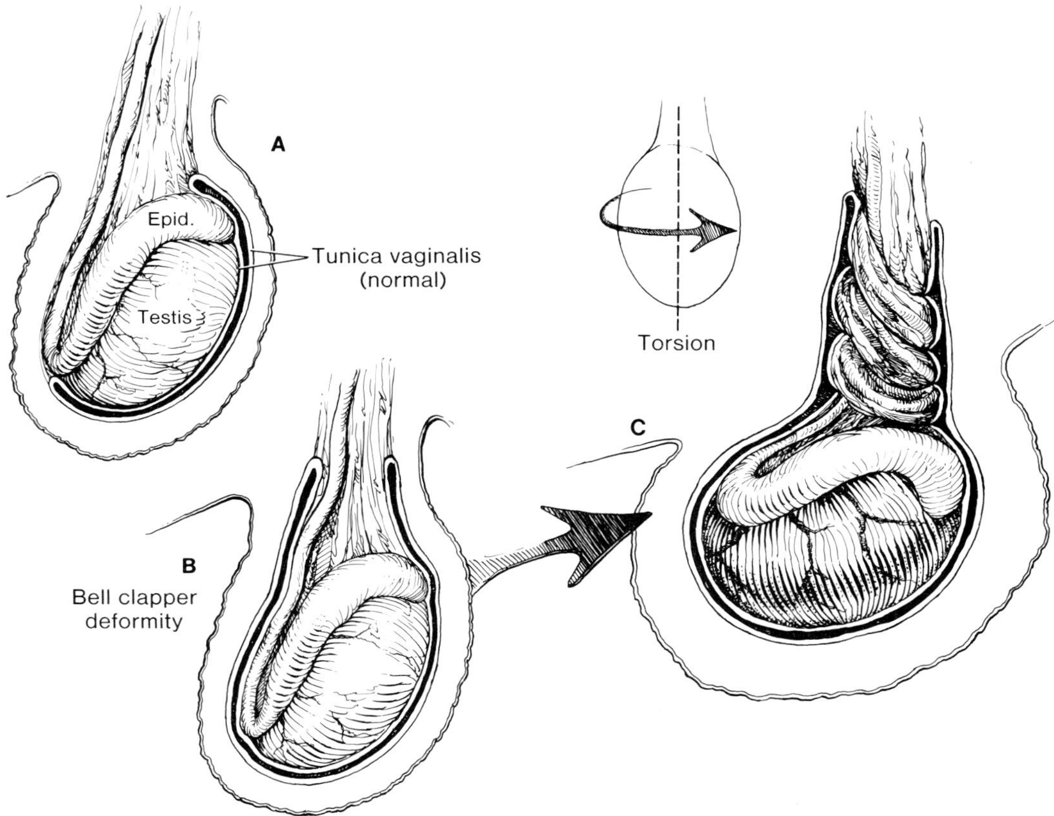

Figure 34.2 Torsion testis: abnormality of testicular fixation—bell-clapper deformity—permits torsion of spermatic vessels with subsequent infarction of the gonad. *Epid.* = epididymis.

the patient as cause of the pain. *The history of trauma is often misleading in patients with testicular torsion.*

As the pain may be referred to the abdomen, it is essential to be certain that the genitalia are carefully examined in every child who complains of abdominal pain. With torsion of the testis, there is typically found an acutely swollen and diffusely tender testis usually lying higher in the scrotum than its contralateral mate.

Time is of the essence in establishing the diagnosis of torsion of the testis. If a testis has been completely twisted sufficiently to fully obstruct its blood supply for greater than 6 hours, surgical detorsion is unlikely to salvage the gonad. However, clinically, it is impossible to determine whether the torsion has been partial or total. Therefore, it is an oversimplification to assume that if symptoms have been present for greater than 6 hours, an irreversible situation has developed that would preclude any attempt at testicular salvage. *The duration of symptoms does not always determine functional recoverability.*

While the diagnosis continues to be most reliably established by a skilled examiner familiar with acute scrotal lesions in children, in recent years diagnostic adjunctive studies have become available which may be of assistance. It must be stressed that if any appreciable time would be lost in arranging these studies, a preferred course is to proceed with surgical exploration.

The testicular nuclear perfusion scan with technetium-99 pertechnetate is helpful, but can have pitfalls in its interpretation. For example, the presence of a hydrocele or scrotal hernia may result in decreased counts on that side of the scrotum and may be confused with a torsion of the testis. Also, a severe degree of overlying scrotal edema may be associated with sufficient increased vascularity to obscure the underlying ischemic testis. The emergency physician seeing patients with scrotal swelling should *not* obtain a scrotal scan prior to seeking experienced advice. The scan should generally be reserved for confirmation in those cases in which the clinical impression is *against* torsion of the testis.

If a child is seen within a few hours of the onset of his torsion, before severe scrotal swelling has ensued, it may be possible to accomplish detorsion of the spermatic cord manually and thus restore blood supply to the testis. In a 1-year period at the Children's Hospital of Philadelphia, physicians in the Division of Urology carried this our in seven of nine patients with torsion of the testis. The Doppler ultrasound stethoscope provides a noninvasive evaluation of testicular blood flow and is a useful adjunct in manual detorsion of the testis. Initial examination will reveal decreased arterial flow to the affected testis when compared to the contralateral one. Intravenous morphine (0.1 mg/kg) is administered just before attempting detorsion. As torsion typically occurs in a medial direction, the detorsion should be carried out by rotating the testis outward toward the thigh. Relief of pain and reposition of the testis in a lower position in the scrotum suggests a successful outcome. This can be confirmed with the Doppler stethoscope by noting a return of normal arterial pulsations to the testis. While successful completion of manual detorsion may avoid the necessity of an emergency anesthetic for surgical reduction, it does not remove the necessity for a fixation of the testis to prevent the recurrence of this condition. An orchiopexy of the affected testis, as well as the contralateral one which is malfixed in more than 50% of cases, is recommended during the same hospitalization.

Trauma/hematocele. Scrotal trauma presents a spectrum of injuries ranging from minimal scrotal swelling to rupture of the testis with a tense blood-filled scrotum. Unless the testis can clearly be felt to be normal and without significant tenderness, urgent surgical evaluation and exploration should be undertaken. This approach is based upon two facts: (1) a ruptured testis has the best salvage rate when surgically repaired and (2) testicular torsion may present with a spurious history of trauma.

Epididymitis-Orchitis. Epididymital orchitis is rare in the prepubertal male. In this age group, it is safer to accept this diagnosis only after surgical exploration has ruled out the presence of torsion of the testis which is much more common. In the prepubertal boy, epididymital orchitis may indicate the presence of an anatomical abnormality of the urinary tract. Associated urinary tract infection is often present and anal-rectal anomalies may be present. In this age group, an appropriate evaluation requires urinalysis, urine culture, intravenous pyelogram, and voiding cystourethrogram.

In the postpubertal male, epididymital orchitis resembles the entity seen in adulthood. Rarely is there an underlying anatomical abnormality. The onset of swelling and tenderness is typically more gradual than with torsion of the testis or a testicular appendage. Early on, the epididymis may be selectively enlarged and tender, readily distinguished from the testis. However, shortly thereafter, the inflammation spreads to the testis and surrounding scrotal wall, making localization impossible. While elevation of the scrotum is said to relieve pain in epididymital orchitis (Prehn's sign), this has not been found to be useful in children, in separating this problem from torsion where elevation allegedly increases pain.

While white cells in the urinary sediment are seen more frequently in epididymitis than torsion, they are not consistently present. In a series of 18 cases of epididymitis in children, only 7 demonstrated microscopic pyuria and/or hematuria, and only 2 had a positive urine culture. In the older boy, as in the adult, *Chlamydia trachomatis* may account for many cases. Other organisms include those bacteria usually responsible for urinary tract infection.

Treatment consists of analgesic, sitz baths, elevation of the scrotum, and antibiotics. Trimethoprim sulfamethoxazole (40 mg/kg/day of sulfamethoxazole) and tetracycline (20 mg/kg/day) achieve best levels in epididymal tissue; however, their use is debatable in the patient with a negative urine culture. The patient should be warned that this process is frustratingly slow to resolve and that he may have 3 to 4 weeks of gradually subsiding discomfort and scrotal swelling.

Mumps Orchitis. Orchitis occurs in approximately 18% of postpubertal males with mumps parotitis. It is rare before puberty. In 70% of cases, it is unilateral and results in testicular atrophy in 50% of affected testes. The onset of mumps orchitis occurs from 4 to 6 days after parotitis is manifest. Although rare, orchitis has been reported in the absence of parotitis. ACTH and corticosteroids in adults may produce some degree of local relief of symptoms, but the course of mumps orchitis is not altered.

Causes of Painless Scrotal Swelling

Hydrocele. An accumulation of fluid within the tunica vaginalis surrounding the testis, i.e., a hydrocele, may be seen with torsion of the testis, epididymitis, trauma, or tumor. In these cases, the underlying testis is abnormal. If the testis can be felt to be normal and the hydrocele is not associated with any abnormality of the overlying scrotal soft tissues, then it is much more likely to be a simple hydrocele. In the infant, this is the result of fluid being left in this position after the processus vaginalis has closed. When there is no history of waxing or waning in the size of the hydrocele, it may be simply observed. Usually the fluid will be reabsorbed in the first 12 to 18 months of life.

If the hydrocele has a clear-cut history of changing in size, particularly if it is associated with thickening of the cord structures (the silk glove sign), then the diagnosis is that of a communicating hydrocele. Here the patent processus vaginalis does not generally close spontaneously and may enlarge to permit the development of hernia. Surgical exploration and high ligation of the processus vaginalis with removal of a portion of the tunica vaginalis to complete the decompression of the hydrocele is appropriate treatment. As a scrotal hernia may be confused with a hydrocele, aspiration should never be carried out in children.

Occasionally, a hydrocele of the cord will present as a scrotal swelling just above the testis. Differentiation from an incarcerated hernia may be difficult and may occasionally require surgical exploration. Surgical treatment as for a hydrocele of the testis is appropriate.

Hernia. While most inguinal hernias present in children with a mass in the groin, occasionally the hernia may extend and present as a scrotal swelling. An incarcerated hernia may produce pain in some patients. The diagnosis and treatment of hernia and incarcerated hernias is treated in Chapter 59, "Abdominal Emergencies" (p. 829).

Idiopathic Scrotal Edema. This is a rare entity comprising only 2 to 5% of acute scrotal swellings in otherwise normal children. The child usually is pain-free and has notable edema of the scrotal wall which may be bilateral and may extend up onto the abdominal wall. The skin of the scrotum may be erythematous. Through the edematous scrotum, the testes can be felt to be normal in size and nontender. This edema of the scrotal wall is of unknown etiology, although it is felt to probably represent a form of angioneurotic edema. No specific therapy has been demonstrated to be effective. The children spontaneously begin to improve within 48 hours regardless of treatment. Occasionally, scrotal edema is seen secondary to diseases causing generalized edema and/or ascites, such as nephrosis and cirrhosis.

Henoch-Schönlein Purpura. Occasionally, a child may be seen with a petechial rash on the scrotum as the initial presentation of this nonthrombocytopenic purpura. More typically, the rash begins on the lower extremities or buttocks and later may involve the scrotum. If the associated swelling is not great, the cord structures and testes can be felt to be uninvolved and normal. In a series of 59 boys seen with Henoch-Schönlein purpura, 9 had scrotal swelling, 4 of whom to such a degree that torsion of the testis was suggested. In such cases, surgical exploration may be necessary as the two entities have been rarely noted to coexist. Therapy is usually directed at the underlying vasculitic abnormality and is discussed in Chapter 47.

Testis Tumor. Testicular or peritesticular tumors are rare in children. They present as a usually painless, firm-to-hard scrotal swelling. There may be an associated hydrocele. Under age 2, the tumor is usually a yolk sac carcinoma. After puberty, germinal cell tumors, as found in the adult population, are seen. Evaluation of a solid testicular mass requires surgical exploration through a groin incision to permit control of the spermatic vessels and a possible radical inguinal orchiectomy.

Antenatal Torsion Testis (Newborn). A newborn boy may present with a painless, smooth, testicular enlargement which is usually dark in color. There may or may not be edema of the overlying scrotum. This is extravaginal torsion of the testis and probably occurs during the late period of embryonic development, as the testis descends into the scrotum. At this time, the testicular tunics are not yet attached to the scrotal tissue, and torsion of the entire testis with its tunics can occur. While the conventional course of action in the past has been surgical exploration, salvage of the testis has been extremely rarely, if ever, proven. As a result, simple observation of these cases is now felt to be sufficient.

References

Dresner ML: Torsed appendage: diagnosis and management; blue dot sign. *Urology* 1: 63, 1973.

Kaplan GW, King LR: Acute scrotal swelling in children. *J Urol* 104: 219, 1970.

CHAPTER 35

Stridor

STEVEN D. HANDLER, M.D.

INTRODUCTION

While stridor, or noisy breathing, is a relatively common symptom in children, its occurrence can often be very frightening to both the child and his parents. The presence of stridor in a child requires a complete and careful evaluation of the child by the emergency department physician in order to determine the etiology of the worrisome and, occasionally, life-threatening symptom. This chapter will discuss the causes of stridor or noisy breathing and will attempt to provide the emergency department practitioner with guidelines for the evaluation and management of the child presenting with stridor.

Normal respiratory efforts are usually not accompanied by any audible sounds. If there is some point of obstruction in the airway so that the normal respiratory volume of air must move faster to bypass the obstruction, turbulent air flow results, leading to noisy breathing. The stridor may originate from obstruction anywhere in the airway from the level of the anterior nares to the bronchi. Table 35.1 lists possible causes of stridor according to anatomical site.

The level of obstruction accounts for specific characteristics of the stridor that help to localize the site of airway blockage. Obstruction of the nose (foreign body, polyp) or nasopharynx (enlarged adenoids, tumor) causes snoring or snorting sounds. This type of stridor is often termed stertor. Because the passage of saliva and the flow of air are both impeded in pharyngeal obstruction, these patients often exhibit a "gurgling" type of noisy breathing. Laryngeal and subglottic obstruction is usually evidenced by high-pitched inspiratory stridor, while bronchial obstruction has characteristic expiratory wheezes. Tracheal obstruction usually presents with both inspiratory and expiratory stridor.

Esophageal foreign bodies will often present with stridor. The nature of the stridor depends on the location of the foreign body and the degree of blockage that it is causing. Foreign bodies in the middle or distal portions of the esophagus can cause compression of the anteriorly placed trachea, and thus present with the highpitched inspiratory and expiratory stridor characteristic of tracheal obstruction. If the foreign body is blocking the esophageal lumen and causing a back-up of saliva to the level of the pharynx, gurgling stridor characteristic of pharyngeal obstruction may result.

EVALUATION AND DECISION

The most common cause of stridor in the infant and young child is laryngomalacia. Once this diagnosis is made, treatment usually consists of close observation and parental reassurance that the condition will improve. Frequent causes of stridor in the older child include nasal obstruction related to an acute upper respiratory infection, adenotonsillar hypertrophy, croup, epiglottis, and foreign body of the upper aero-digestive tract. Depending upon the degree of

Table 35.1
Causes of Stridor in Children According to Site of Obstruction

I. Nose and Pharynx
- A. Congenital anomalies
  1. Lingual thyroid
  2. Choanal atresia
  3. Craniofacial anomalies (Apert's, Down's, Pierre Robin)
  4. Cysts (dermoid, thyroglossal)
  5. Macroglossia (Beckwith's syndrome)
  6. Encephalocele
- B. Inflammatory
  1. Abscess (parapharyngeal, retropharyngeal, peritonsillar)
  2. Allergic polyps
  3. Adenotonsillar enlargement (acute infection, infectious mononucleosis)
- C. Neoplasm (benign and malignant)
- D. Adenotonsillar hyperplasia
- E. Foreign body
- F. Neurologic syndromes with poor tongue/pharyngeal muscle tone

II. Larynx
- A. Congenital anomalies
  1. Laryngomalacia
  2. Web, cyst, laryngocele
  3. Cartilage dystrophy
  4. Subglottic stenosis
  5. Cleft larynx
- B. Inflammatory
  1. Croup
  2. Epiglottitis
  3. Angioneurotic edema
  4. Miscellaneous: tuberculosis, fungal, diphtheria, sarcoidosis
- C. Vocal cord paralysis (multiple etiologies)
- D. Trauma
  1. Intubation (laryngeal or subglottic edema, subglottic stenosis)
  2. Neck trauma
  3. Foreign body
- E. Neoplasm
  1. Subglottic hemangioma
  2. Laryngeal papilloma
  3. Cystic hygroma (neck)
  4. Malignant (rhabdomyosarcoma, etc.)
- F. Laryngospasm (hypocalcemic tetany)

III. Trachea and Bronchi
- A. Congenital
  1. Vascular anomalies
  2. Webs, cysts
  3. Tracheal stenosis
  4. Tracheoesophageal fistula
- B. Foreign body (tracheal or esophageal)
- C. Neoplasm (benign and malignant)
  1. Tracheal
  2. Compression by neoplasm of adjacent structure (thyroid, thymus, esophagus)
- D. Trauma: tracheal stenosis secondary to intubation or tracheostomy
- E. Inflammatory: bronchitis
- F. Immunological: asthma

airway obstruction, these problems, when identified, can be managed by the emergency department physician, or may require otolaryngic consultation and/or hospitalization (see Chapter 62).

In the evaluation of a child presenting to the emergency department with stridor, the first task is to assess the degree of airway obstruction. If the stridor is severe, emergency resuscitative efforts (laryngoscopy, intubation, tracheostomy) may be required. If the stridor is only mild or moderate, a more orderly evaluation process can be undertaken. The first step in this process is to obtain a complete and accurate history. The time of onset of the stridor together with any associated symptoms must be determined. Did the stridor of an infant become clinically apparent when the child was 4 to 6 weeks old (laryngomalacia) or was it present immediately after birth (vocal cord paralysis, subglottic stenosis, laryngeal web or cyst, choanal atresia)? Does the stridor worsen with straining or crying (laryngomalacia, subglottic hemangioma)? Is the stridor associated with a barky cough (croup) or is drooling present (epiglottis, foreign body of the esophagus)? Has there been an antecedent upper respiratory infection (croup, epiglottitis), history of neck trauma (laryngeal fracture, vocal cord hematoma) or possible foreign body ingestion? Is the stridor associated with feeding difficulties (tracheoesophageal fistula, cleft larynx, vascular ring/sling, neurologic disorder)? What are the characteristics of the voice/cry? Aphonic (laryngeal obstruction with foreign body)? Weak (neuromuscular disorder)? Hoarse (vocal cord paralysis, vocal cord nodules, granuloma, papilloma)?

The age of the child will often assist the physician in determining the source of the stridor. The young infant with stridor is most likely to have laryngomalacia, choanal atresia/stenosis, or subglottic stenosis. Croup and epiglottitis are more common in children between the age of 1 and 4 years. Adenotonsillar hypertrophy usually manifests itself between the ages of 2 and 8 years. While foreign bodies are most common in the toddler (1 to 3 years), they can present in any age group.

There is a great deal of information that can be obtained from a careful physical examination of the child presenting with stridor. The position that the child assumes can often help one to identify the level of obstruction. Children with airway obstruction at the level of the larynx or above (epiglottitis, adenotonsillar hypertrophy) will usually hyperextend their necks ("sniffing position") in an effort to straighten their upper airway and maximize air entry. This type of posturing does not help to relieve obstruction at the tracheal or bronchial level.

The quality of the stridor is important to assess in order to determine the level of the obstruction (see Fig. 35.1). Is the stridor snoring or snorting (nasal, nasopharyngeal obstruction) or gurgling (pharyngeal blockage)? If the stridor is high pitched, is it inspiratory (laryngeal, subglottic) or expiratory (bronchial)? Is it both inspiratory and expiratory (tracheal)? The relative lengths of the phases of respiration are also useful in identifying the source of the stridor. In children with laryngeal obstruction, the time of inspiration is greatly increased, while expiration tends to be prolonged in bronchial obstruction. Inspiration and expiration times are both increased in patients with tracheal obstruction.

Certain maneuvers can be performed during the physical examination of the child with stridor to assess the functional anatomy of the upper airway and to determine the cause of the stridor. These actions may have both diagnostic and therapeutic implications in the management of the child. The first maneuver should be to open the child's mouth and pull his mandible and tongue forward. If the stridor lessens, the obstruction is at the level of the larynx or higher. Nasal catheters should be passed to determine the patency of the nasopharyngeal airway. In patients with choanal atresia, the placement of an oral airway will help to make the diagnosis and to relieve the obstruction. Pulling the mandible and tongue forward will often relieve the obstruction in Pierre Robin syndrome. A nasopharyngeal airway will also relieve the stridor in a child with this syndrome as well as in one with adenotonsillar hypertrophy. Placing the child in the prone position can often lessen the stridor of laryngomalacia. The introduction of a laryngoscope can also

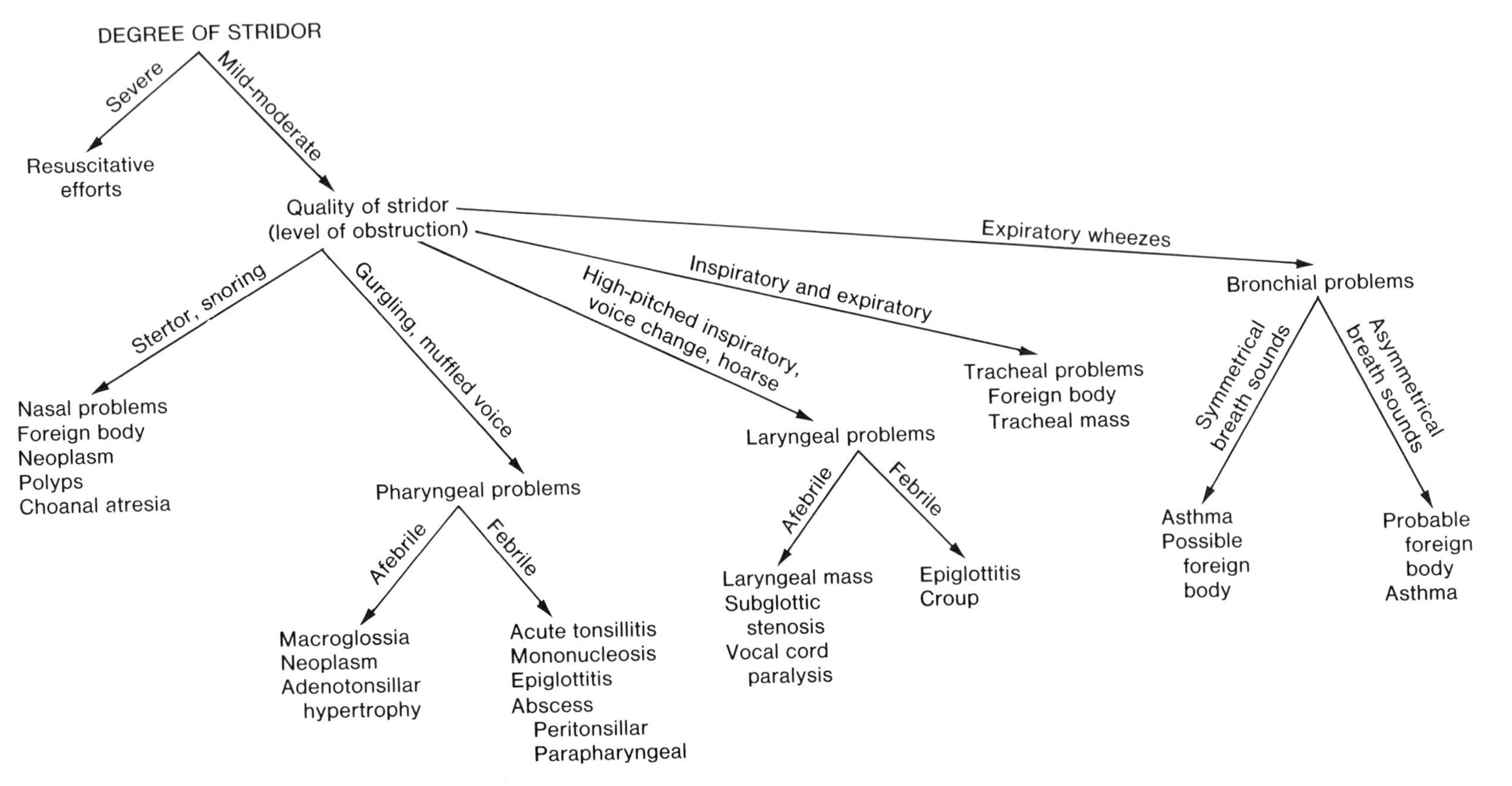

Figure 35.1 Diagnostic approach to stridor.

be useful in evaluating the stridor of laryngeal origin. The laryngoscope will support the laryngeal structures and decrease the stridor of laryngomalacia, but will not relieve the obstruction of vocal cord paralysis or subglottic stenosis. The child with likely epiglottitis represents a special case regarding examination (see Chapter 45, p. 376). Efforts to visualize the pharynx or epiglottis with a tongue blade may precipitate complete airway obstruction in such children.

Indirect laryngoscopy, while not applicable to all patients, is an important part of the examination of the child with stridor, especially of laryngeal origin. The otolaryngologist should be consulted to perform the indirect laryngoscopy. Information concerning the structure and function of the vocal cords can be obtained from this examination.

Radiographic studies are invaluable in the evaluation of the child with stridor. Anteroposterior and lateral views of the neck and chest are the first views obtained to look for mass lesions and extrinsic compression of the airway. Computed tomograms (CT), while not feasible for all patients, can often provide additional diagnostic information concerning the child with stridor. A barium swallow is useful in identifying vascular rings, tracheoesophageal fistulas, and neuromuscular disorders with aspiration and swallowing dysfunction. Fluoroscopy of the larynx can often help to determine vocal cord function. If any of the above studies point toward a vascular origin of the stridor, angiography is indicated.

Emergency management of the child with stridor will depend, of course, upon the cause of the noisy breathing and its severity. In some instances, the child is referred to a specialist (usually otolaryngologist) for further evaluation as an outpatient. In the more severe cases, immediate intervention is required in the emergency department. Oxygen, humidified air, nebulized racemic epinephrine, corticosteroids, laryngoscopy, intubation, and even emergency tracheostomy all have specific roles in the emergency department management of stridor depending upon its etiology (see Chapter 62).

Figure 35.1 presents an algorithm summarizing the emergency department diagnostic approach to the child with stridor.

Reference

Quinn-Bogard AL, Potsic WP: Stridor in the first year of life. *Clin Pediatr* 16: 913, 1977.

CHAPTER **36**

Syncope

EDWARD CHARNEY, M.D.

INTRODUCTION

Syncope or fainting is characterized by a brief, usually sudden, loss of consciousness and muscle tone due to cerebral ischemia. There is frequently a precipitating event. The child is almost always in either a standing or seated position at the time of the syncopal episode. Unconsciousness usually lasts for only several seconds; during this time, the child is often limp, unresponsive and diaphoretic with decreased blood pressure, diminished deep tendon reflexes, slow pulse, and dilated pupils. Only with a prolonged period of unconsciousness are there tonic clonic movements of the extremities. Mental alertness is usually present upon awakening (Fig. 36.1).

The principal causes of syncope may be divided into five major pathophysiologic categories: vasovagal, orthostatic or postural hypotension, cardiac, respiratory and metabolic (see Table 36.1). Occasionally, syncope may also occur as a manifestation of hysteria.

Vasovagal syncope, the most common form, is the fainting that results from a sudden loss of resistance in the peripheral circulation. Obvious emotional upsets are often responsible for these attacks which may be precipitated by feelings of fear, pain, anger, apprehension, and fatigue. The emotional trauma of procedures such as venipuncture or dental treatment may often be associated with this form of syncope. A formal religious service marked by prolonged erect posture in a warm and poorly ventilated environment is also a common setting for vasovagal syncopal attacks.

Orthostatic hypotensive syncope is infrequently encountered in children and adolescents, and is associated with an excessive and prolonged fall in blood pressure upon assuming the erect posture from a recumbent position. An unusual and uncommon form of this is micturition syncope which follows rapid bladder decompression, and in which there is reduced cardiac return associated with both postural hypotension and splanchnic vascular stasis.

Cardiac disease may on occasion be associated with syncope. Severe aortic or pulmonic stenosis, tetralogy of Fallot (in association with hypoxemic attacks), or pulmonary hypertension without shunting may result in syncope, particularly during or just after physical exertion (see also Chapter 43). Acute obstruction of the mitral valve orifice by a mobile left atrial myxoma is also a rare cause of syncope. Several unusual cardiac arrhythmias are commonly associated with syncope including: congenital complete AV block with Stokes-Adams attacks, sick sinus syndrome with sudden bouts of bradycardia or tachycardia, and paroxysmal ventricular tachycardia and prolonged Q-T interval associated either with autosomal recessive deafness or an autosomal dominant trait in families with normal hearing.

Respiratory causes of syncope include coughing or tussive episodes, hyperventilation, and breathholding. Tussive syncope often associated with asthma or pertussis

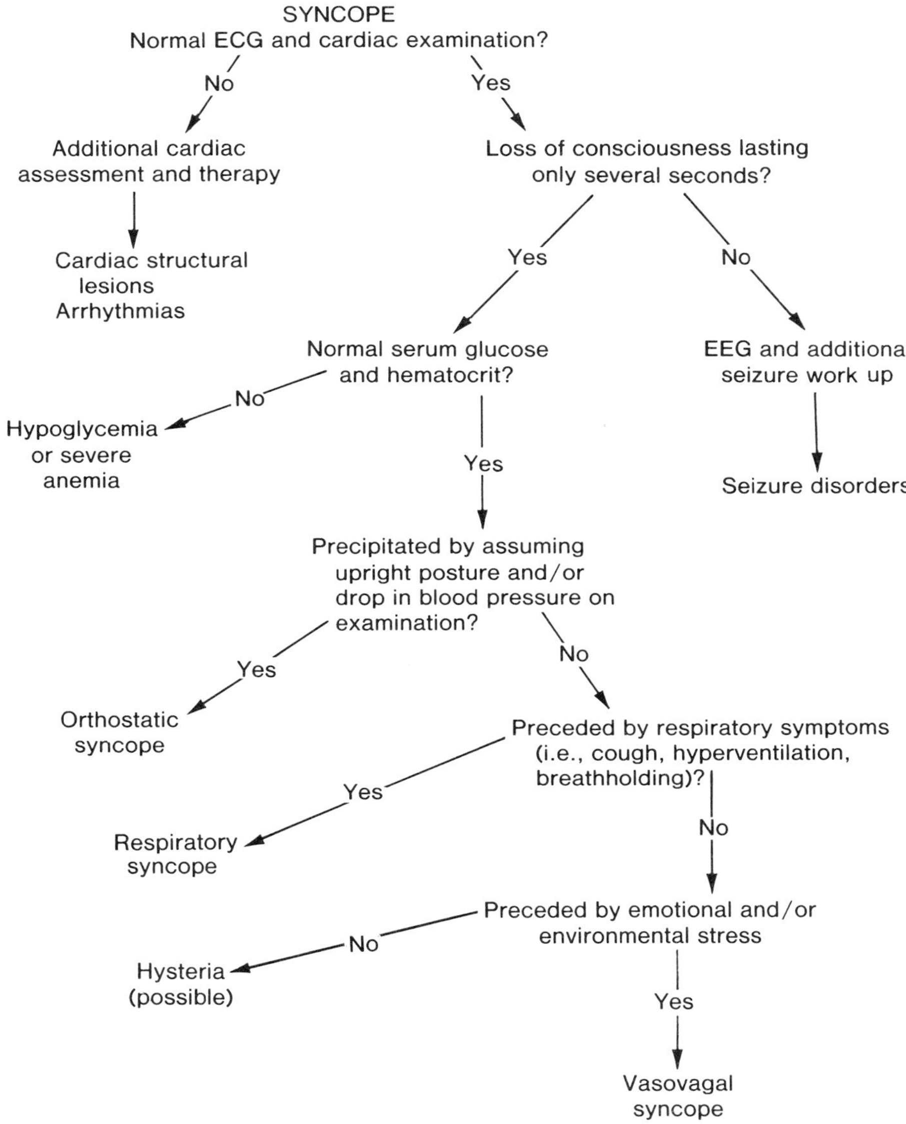

Figure 36.1 The diagnostic approach to syncope.

s probably a result of the hypoxia and educed cardiac return from the Valsalva naneuver or respiratory spasm after completion of coughing. Hyperventilation, with ts hypocapnia and cerebral ischemia, may e precipitated by anxiety or may be consciously induced while coupled with a Valsalva maneuver performed not uncomnonly in school grounds during recess time. Breathholding spells occurring in infants and toddlers are frequently precipitated by emotional upset and are either of the cyanotic or pallid nature (see Chapter 72).

Metabolic causes of syncope include anemia and hypoglycemia. Syncopal attacks from anemia are usually preceded by lightheadedness or giddiness, whereas those attacks associated with hypoglycemia are frequently preceded by pallor and sweating prior to the loss of consciousness.

EVALUATION AND DECISION

The emergency department physician must initially assess the cardiac status of all children presenting with a history of a syncopal episode. Observation is made for clinical cyanosis. Cardiac auscultation should be particularly directed at determining the presence of the systolic murmurs of aortic or pulmonary stenosis or diastolic murmur of a left atrial myxoma. An electrocardiographic rhythm strip should be obtained to assess the presence of any arrhythmias such as: AV block, sick sinus syndrome, or prolonged Q-T interval. Acute management and further diagnostic measures for these cardiac complications ar discussed in Chapter 43.

If the cardiac status of the child is deter mined to be normal, the physician mus then decide whether the period of loss c consciousness was syncopal in nature o part of a seizure. Differentiation betwee these two may be difficult; however, de tailed history, with a focus on circum stances of the event, possible precipitatin factors, and most importantly, duration c unconsciousness usually establishes the di agnosis. Distinguishing characteristics of seizure and syncope are outlined in Tabl 36.2. The neurologic examination will ofte separate the child in a post-ictal state wit prolonged unconsciousness and eventu confusion upon awakening from the mor alert and oriented child recovering from th brief syncopal attack.

An occasional adolescent may suffer at tacks of hysterical syncope. Such episode may be difficult to distinguish from bot vasovagal syncope and seizures. In gener such children manage to fall repeatedly be fore an audience, without hurting them selves, and the attacks may be accompanie by dramatic moaning. A careful histor may reveal significant psychosocial stres in the patient's home and family.

Additional history, with particular atter tion to the events preceding the syncop attack, will often be diagnostic in the chil who has a normal cardiac and neurologi examination. Orthostatic syncope will char acteristically be associated with a history c loss of consciousness occurring soon afte suddenly assuming an upright posture an may be further characterized by a pro longed drop in systolic pressure when aris ing from recumbent to erect posture o

Table 36.1
Causes of Syncope

- *I. Vasovagal*
- *II. Orthostatic*
- *III. Cardiac*
  - A. Structural lesions
    1. Aortic stenosis
    2. Pulmonic stenosis
    3. Tetralogy of Fallot
    4. Pulmonary hypertension
    5. Atrial myxomia
  - B. Arrhythmias
    1. AV block
    2. Sick sinus syndrome
    3. Prolonged Q-T interval
- *IV. Respiratory*
  - A. Cough
  - B. Hyperventilation
  - C. Breathholding
- *V. Metabolic*
  - A. Anemia
  - B. Hypoglycemia
- *VI.* Hysteria

Table 36.2
Differentiating Syncope from Seizure

	Syncope	Seizure
Period of unconsciousness	Usually seconds	Frequently 5 min or longer
Incontinence	Absent	May be present
Confusion upon awakening	Absent or mild	Marked
Tonic clonic movements	Occasionally present if unconsciousness is prolonged	Frequently present
EEG	Normal	Frequently abnormal

examination. Emotional and environmental stresses preceding the syncopal event suggest vasovagal syncope. Specific questions should be asked of both the child and observers of the attacks as to whether there were any antecedent periods of prolonged coughing, hyperventilation, or breathholding in order to establish the diagnosis of respiratory syncope. Even though there may not be the typical history of giddiness and light-headedness of anemic syncope or the pallor, sweating and fasting of hypoglycemic syncope, children with syncopal attacks should have hematocrits and measurements of the serum glucose as part of the initial diagnostic testing. If anemia or hypoglycemia are demonstrated, such patients are worked up as described elsewhere (Chapters 47 and 53).

THERAPY

Once the syncopal event has been distinguished from a seizure, and the child has had a normal cardiac examination, hematocrit and blood sugar, then the child and family should be counseled as to the benign ramifications of orthostatic, respiratory, or vasovagal syncope. Suggestions should be offered for avoidance of precipitating factors. Referral for appropriate counseling may be indicated if the syncope is felt to be on an hysterical basis.

References

Engel GL: *Fainting*, Ed. 2, Charles C Thomas, Springfield, Ill, 1962.

Enzer AB, Walker PA: Hyperventilation syndrome in childhood. *J Pediatr* 70: 521, 1967.

Jewell A, Lange-Nielson F: Congenital deaf-mutism, functional heart disease with prolongation of the Q-T interval, and sudden death. *Am Heart J* 54: 59, 1957.

Katz RM: Cough syncope in children with asthma. *J Pediatr* 77: 48, 1970.

Lombroso CT, Lerman P: Breathhold spells (cyanotic and pallid infantile syncope). *Pediatrics* 39: 563, 1967.

Lyll CB, Monroe JT, Flinn DE, Lamb LF: Micturtion syncope: Report of 24 cases. *N Engl J Med* 265: 982, 1961.

Wennevold A, Kungelbach J: Prolonged Q-T interval with cardiac syncopes. *Acta Paediatr Scand* 60: 239, 1971.

Wright FS: Recurrent paroxysmal nonepileptic disorders. In *The Practice of Pediatric Neurology*, edited by KF Swainman and FS Wright. C.V. Mosby, St. Louis, 1975.

CHAPTER **37**

Urinary Frequency

WILLIAM SCHWARTZ, M.D.

INTRODUCTION

Increased frequency of urination may represent multiple voidings of small amounts of urine or frequent production of large volumes. In the first situation, the problem is in the bladder; in the latter the etiology is the water balance of the body or dysfunction of the renal tubules' ability to concentrate urine (Table 37.1).

In the normal bladder, there are stretch fibers which sense the volume of urine in the bladder. When the bladder reaches a volume of 250 to 400 ml, it institutes voiding via the sacral nerves 2, 3, and 4, with relaxation of the external sphincter and a contraction of the bladder.

The mucosa is inflamed in infections and there is pain when the bladder contracts or urine passes through the urethra. Initially, the patient will not void and the bladder capacity increases. A painful sensation occurs when the volume of urine exceeds the capacity of the bladder. The passage of a small amount of urine will end the pain from the bladder distention but will also cause pain from the bladder contraction and irritation of the urethra. Because the bladder does not empty and urine continues to enter into the bladder from the kidneys, there is a cycle of frequent passages of small amounts of urine.

The cord bladder, where the sacral nerves are interrupted, is another situation where frequency occurs. There are two subgroups—the irritable bladder and the atonic bladder. In the former, the bladder is irritable, small, and sensitive to the presence of urine. Therefore, when urine enters the bladder, it contracts and a small amount of urine exits. In the other situation, the bladder is large and hypotonic so that there is a large urine volume, and small contractions occur when the volume exceeds the bladder capacity resulting in small frequent voidings.

The most common cause of frequency is anxiety. Many people will respond to feelings of anxiety by developing the urge to void. They usually pass small amounts of normal urine.

With normal bladder function, urinary frequency of large volumes of urine occurs secondary to the kidneys' response to a volume overload, or osmotic diuresis, or from the tubules' inability to concentrate. If large volumes of liquids are ingested, the intravascular volume expands and the osmolarity of the blood is lowered. The tubules respond by the production of a large amount of dilute urine. In diabetes mellitus, the serum glucose exceeds the capacity of the tubules to reabsorb glucose so that an osmotic diuresis and frequency occurs.

In chronic renal disease the tubules lose their ability to concentrate the urine so that large amounts of dilute urine are produced. In response to the thirst mechanisms, the patient drinks large volumes and then produces large amounts of dilute urine. This situation is similar to diabetes insipidus where the kidney cannot concentrate urine, and large volumes of dilute urine are produced.

EVALUATION AND DECISION

The first effort in investigating a patient with frequency is to further expand the description of the problem (Fig. 37.1). Are there small or large volumes? Are there pain, fever, or other symptoms that accompany the frequency? These questions are important because the primary task is to diagnose or exclude a urinary tract infection. Specific questions about symptoms of diabetes should also be included. As noted above, if there is a history of large volumes of urine that are passed frequently, the source of the problem is most likely in the kidney, while if there are small volumes the bladder should be investigated.

In addition to a complete physical examination, special attention should be directed toward the functioning of the sacral nerves 2 to 4. The presence of an anal wink and normal rectal tone is good evidence of functioning of these three nerves, and therefore the nerve supply of the bladder will also be intact. In a rare patient, a sacral dimple may indicate that there is a tract that may interrupt the sacral nerves or that there is a lipomeningocele which may compress the nerves.

The laboratory evaluation is relatively simple. A urinalysis and culture should be performed first to identify those patients whose frequency is associated with an infection. Likewise the presence of glycosuria

Table 37.1
Causes of Urinary Frequency

Bladder
Infection
Chemical cystitis
Cord bladder (injury to sacral nerves 2–4)
Anxiety
Kidney
Volume overload
Water intoxication
Increased intake
Osmotic diuresis
Diabetes mellitus
Diuretic ingestion
Tubular dysfunction
Chronic renal failure
Diabetes insipidus
Nephrogenic
Central

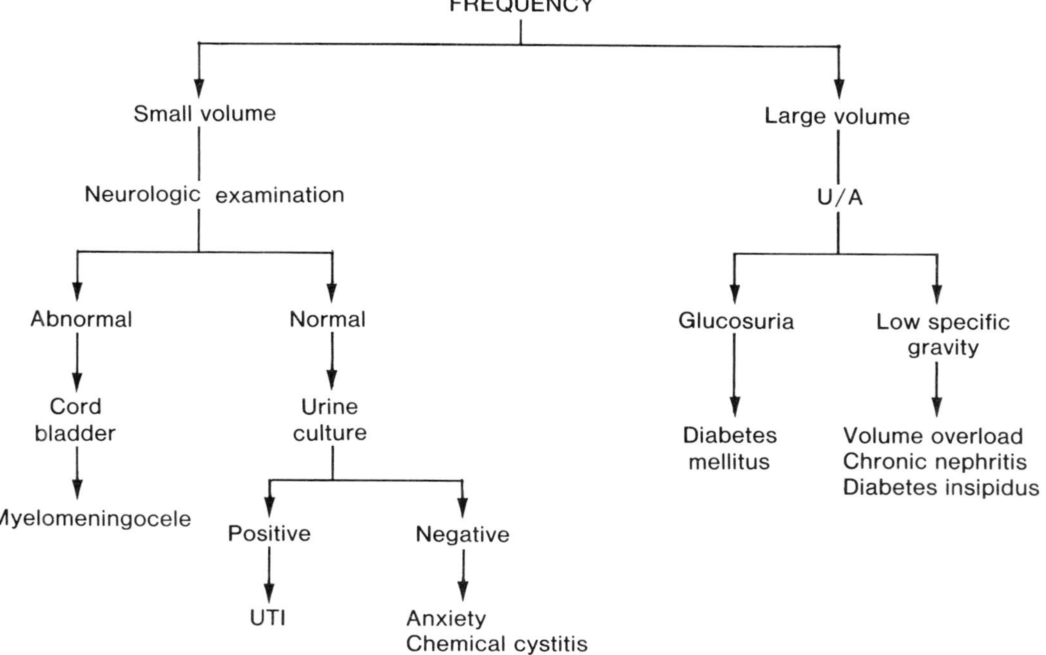

Figure 37.1 Differential diagnosis of urinary frequency. UTI = urinary tract infection; U/A = urinalysis.

will direct the evaluation toward diabetes. The combination of low specific gravity, proteinuria, and casts are seen in chronic renal failure, although not all of them need to be present at the same time. These patients need further studies of renal function, such as serum urea and creatinine and possibly a renal scan, IVP, or ultrasound. Patients with low specific gravity on a consistent basis may have compulsive water drinking leading to fluid overload or, on rare occasions, diabetes insipidus. If diabetes insipidus is suspected, the patient should be admitted for renal function tests including a water deprivation test. This test is dangerous and should not be performed as an outpatient or in a routine inpatient unit where the supervision is not adequate (see Chapter 46).

If infection and renal diseases are ruled out, the evaluation is then directed toward bladder dysfunction. A better description of the anatomy should be obtained through a voiding cystourethrogram. This may be followed by urodynamic studies if there is still a question about bladder capacity, tone, and contractions.

In many cases of urinary frequency, the workup may not be diagnostic. There are some instances where anxiety from a change in family or school can lead to frequency. In other cases, covert excessive drinking of water may be the cause of polyuria.

CHAPTER 38

Vaginal Bleeding

JAN E. PARADISE, M.D.

INTRODUCTION

Vaginal bleeding can be either a normal event or a sign of disease, and when pathologic, can indicate variously a local genital tract disorder, endocrinologic or hematologic disease, or a complication of pregnancy. During childhood, vaginal bleeding is abnormal after the first week or so of life and before menarche. After menarche, abnormal vaginal bleeding must be differentiated from menstruation, and in turn, menstrual bleeding must be categorized as either normal or excessive. Menstruation is defined as the spontaneous, periodic shedding of endometrial tissue and blood.

Menstrual patterns during the first 2 years after menarche vary widely, but it is possible to set outside limits. Ninety-five percent of young adolescents' menstrual periods are between 2 and 8 days long. A duration of 10 days or more is abnormal. An occasional interval of less than 21 days from the first day of one menstrual period to the first day of the next is normal for teenagers, but several very short cycles in a row are abnormal. Whether the quantity of a patient's menstrual bleeding is normal can be difficult to determine historically. However, it is uncommon for adolescents to soak more than 6 to 8 perineal pads or tampons a day. Normal menstrual bleeding *never* produces an acute fall in hemoglobin or hematocrit.

Because some disorders only produce vaginal bleeding in children or in postmenarchial adolescents, the diagnostic approach outlined in this chapter is divided into two age-related sections. However, since menarche can occur normally at any age between 10 and 16 years, the two sections cannot be separated at any single age (Table 38.1).

EVALUATION AND DECISION

Examination of Children

During the patient's general physical examination, the emergency department physician should be particularly alert for signs of hormonal stimulation—breast development, pubic hair growth, a dull pink vaginal mucosa, or physiologic leukorrhea. For the initial examination of the genitalia, an infant or child should be placed in a frog-leg position either on the parent's lap or on the examining table. The physician then gently separates the child's labia majora and inspects the introitus for a bleeding site. A vaginal speculum should not be used. If the vulva is normal, the child should next be placed in the knee-chest position to allow examination of her vagina. In this position, the girl is encouraged to relax her abdominal muscles while the examiner gently separates her labia and buttocks. The vagina will often fall open, and the physician can look for a foreign body, using an otoscope without a speculum as a light source (see Fig. 52.1B, p. 604). If no foreign body is seen, the child is returned to the supine position, and a vaginal specimen for culture is obtained, using either a soft plastic medicine dropper or a cotton-tipped swab moistened with nonbacteriostatic saline so-

Table 38.1
Differential Diagnosis of Vaginal Bleeding

- *I. At Any Time*
  - A. Trauma
  - B. Tumor
- *II. Before Normal Menarche*
  - A. Hormonal
    1. Neonatal bleeding
    2. Exogenous estrogen
    3. Precocious puberty
  - B. Nonhormonal
    1. Urethral prolapse
    2. Vaginitis
    3. Foreign body
- *III. After Menarche*
  - A. Dysfunctional uterine bleeding
  - B. Bleeding diathesis
  - C. Gonorrhea
  - D. Birth control pills
  - E. Intrauterine device
  - F. Ectopic pregnancy
  - G. Spontaneous abortion
  - H. Placenta previa
  - I. Abruptio placentae

lution. Finally, if the interior of the vagina could not be seen well, but the examiner suspects a foreign body or trauma, a rectal examination should be done to palpate the vagina indirectly and to check for lacerations.

VULVAR BLEEDING (*A* in Fig. 38.1)

Injuries of the vulva can produce lacerations, ecchymoses, or both. Any vulvar injury should alert the emergency department physician to the possibility of concurrent, potentially serious vaginal or rectal injuries (see below). Vulvar lacerations do not usually bleed excessively, but hematomas can extend widely through the tissue planes, forming large painful masses that occasionally produce enough pressure to rupture through the overlying vulvar skin. Since even minor periurethral injuries can produce urethral spasm that leads to acute urinary retention, the injured child's ability to void should be checked routinely. The possibility of sexual assault must be considered in the management of every child with a genital injury.

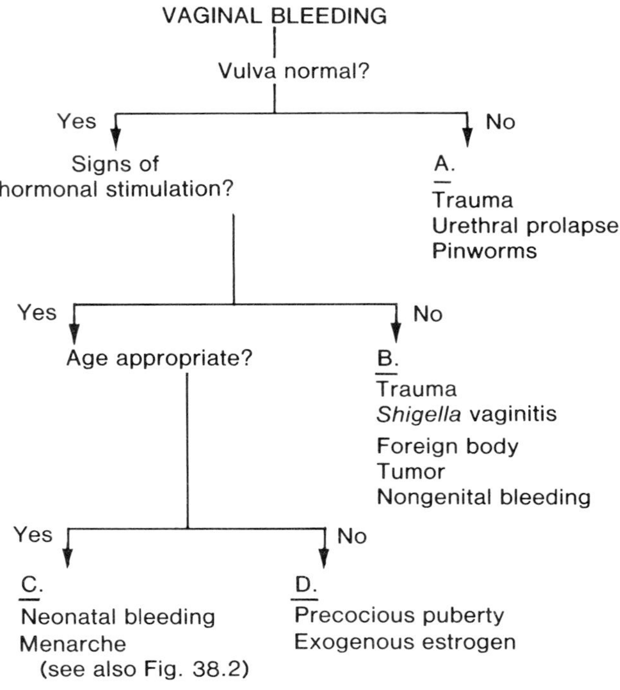

Figure 38.1 Vaginal bleeding before normal menarche.

Urethral prolapse is probably the com-
ıonest cause of apparent vaginal bleeding uring childhood (see Chapter 52). Some atients with urethral prolapse complain of ysuria or urinary frequency, but most are symptomatic. A prolapse is diagnosed by s characteristic doughnut shape (Fig. 52.6, . 671). The ring of protruding urethral ıucosa above the introitus is swollen and ark red with a central dimple that indiates the meatus. Often the prolapse is large nough to cover the vaginal introitus when ıe child is supine, and appears to protrude om the vagina. Bleeding comes from the chemic mucosa. If the diagnosis is in oubt, one may safely catheterize the blader through the prolapse to obtain urine. In ıost cases, surgical excision of the prolapse an be performed electively within a few ays of diagnosis.

If perineal excoriations are the source of leeding, the emergency department phycian should suspect rectal *Enterobius vericularis* infection. Pinworms characteriscally produce perirectal itching that is orse at night. Pinworm ova can often be een on low-power microscopic examinaon of perianal material that has been colcted with clear cellophane tape and then ttached to a glass slide.

AGINAL BLEEDING WITHOUT SIGNS F HORMONAL STIMULATION (*B* in Fig. 8.1)

Trauma, infection, and foreign bodies are he most common causes of vaginal bleedıg during childhood.

Vaginal bleeding after trauma indicates potential emergency. A penetrating narow object can damage the rectum, bladder, r abdominal viscera without producing ıuch external evidence of injury. Because aginal lacerations do not always produce great deal of bleeding or pain, the emerency physician cannot rely on the severity f the patient's symptoms to indicate the eriousness of the injury. Whenever a child ustains a genital injury, the physician must onsider the possibility that it was inflicted uring a sexual assault.

If trauma is suspected, the girl's abdomen hould be evaluated carefully. Lower quadant tenderness may provide a clue to intrabdominal injury. The vulva is inspected for bruises, and a rectal examination is performed to identify any lacerations. A general principle of management is that patients with vulvar, perianal, or vaginal injuries, even apparently minor ones, should undergo careful vaginal examination. This may require surgical consultation and sedation or general anesthesia, particularly in young children. Laboratory evaluation of the child with vaginal trauma should include a baseline hemoglobin determination and a urinalysis to screen for hematuria that might indicate urethral or bladder injury.

About half of all patients with shigella vaginitis have bleeding that may be more noticeable than the associated discharge. Most patients do not have concurrent diarrhea. A vaginal culture is needed for diagnosis and to check the organism's antibiotic sensitivity.

Although a chronic, foul-smelling discharge is generally considered the hallmark of a vaginal foreign body, some girls have intermittent scanty vaginal bleeding alone or with an unimpressive discharge. If a foreign body is strongly suspected but the vagina cannot be visualized and rectal palpation is normal, the patient should receive either gentle vaginal lavage (using saline solution, a 50 cc syringe with the plunger discarded, a red rubber catheter, and gravity), or an examination under anesthesia. Since the commonest foreign body, toilet paper, is not radiopaque, pelvic roentgenography is not likely to be helpful and should be avoided.

Genital tumors are a rare cause of vaginal bleeding. Adenocarcinoma of the vagina or cervix occurs in about 0.2% of daughters whose mothers took diethylstilbestrol or other estrogen-containing drugs during pregnancy. Vaginal bleeding may be the first symptom of this cancer or of sarcoma botryoides, but neoplasms are very uncommon. Urethral prolapse is sometimes mistaken for a malignant tumor, and should be considered in the differential diagnosis.

Occasionally, a patient with a history of bleeding has no abnormalities and no bleeding at the time of the examination. In this case, the history should be taken seriously since most parents are good observers, but the patient's urine and stool should be checked for blood. Vaginal foreign body and inapparent genital trauma are also in the differential diagnosis.

VAGINAL BLEEDING WITH SIGNS OF HORMONAL STIMULATION (*C* and *D* in Fig. 38.1)

During the first 2 to 3 weeks of life, and late in puberty, hormonal fluctuations produce physiologic vaginal bleeding of uterine origin. Before birth, full-term infants are exposed to high levels of circulating maternal estrogen that stimulates growth of the uterine endometrium as well as breast tissue in females. As this hormonal support wanes after birth, some infants have an endometrial slough that results in a few days of light vaginal bleeding. The bleeding will stop spontaneously, and requires no treatment except reassurance for the parents. Occasionally, a girl is brought to the emergency department by her family to confirm their belief that she is having her first menstrual period. In this case, if the adolescent's age and degree of pubertal development are appropriate for menarche (see Table 38.2), no further evaluation is necessary. Hormonal stimulation that produces vaginal bleeding in an older infant or child is a cause for concern. If the bleeding is cyclic, or associated with breast development (thelarche) or pubic hair growth (adrenarche) in a girl less than 8 years of age, she should be referred to an endocrinologist for evaluation of precocious puberty. The sequence of pubertal events is more likely to be abnormal in patients with precocious puberty. Rarely, a child is treated chronically with estrogen-containing medication (for example, for labial adhesions) that produces breast growth and eventual menstruation. The possibility that a girl with vaginal bleeding early in puberty simply has a nonendocrinologic disorder (foreign body, trauma, etc) must also be considered.

Vaginal Bleeding After Menarche (Fig. 38.2)

GENERAL CONSIDERATIONS

In the evaluation of postmenarchial adolescents with vaginal bleeding, a comprehensive history is important, and can sometimes lead directly to the likely diagnosis. The emergency department physician should ask specifically about the patient's menstrual chronology, including her age at menarche, her usual menstrual pattern, and the date of onset of her most recent menstrual period. Every patient who has been sexually active, regardless of age, should be asked whether she has ever been pregnant and if she has, about the pregnancy's outcome. Her current method of contraception should also be ascertained. The patient's mother, if she is present, should be asked whether her daughter was exposed to estrogen in utero.

Table 38.2
Chronology of Pubertal Development in Normal Girls

Tanner Stage	Breast	Pubic Hair	Average Age (yr)[a] Breast/Pubic hair	Cumulative % of Girls Reaching Menarche by Staging
1	None	None	—	
2	Breast buds; areolar enlargement	Long, downy, along labia	11.2/11.7	0
3	More growth; no separation on contours	Curly, coarse, along labia	12.2/12.4	25
4	Areola projects beyond breast contour	Covers mons pubis	13.1/13.0	90
5	Mature breast	Adult pattern, extends to thighs	15.3/14.4	100

[a] One standard deviation at each stage is approximately 1 year. Thus, it is uncommon for girls to begin breast growth before 9 years or after 13 years of age.

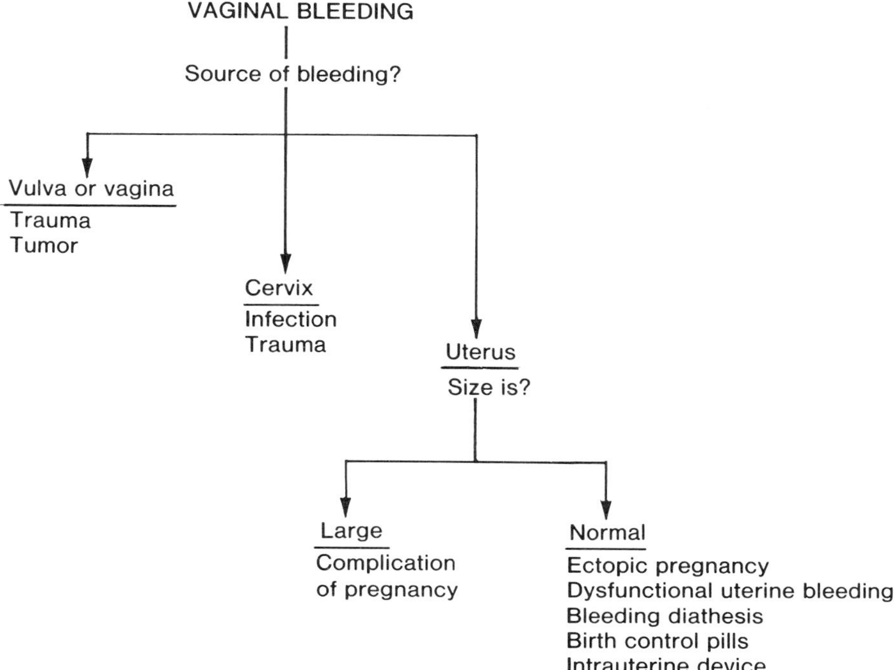

Figure 38.2 Vaginal bleeding after menarche.

During the physical examination, the patient's pulse and blood pressure are noted carefully. If she has been injured or is sexually active, a complete pelvic examination is performed. A speculum examination is not necessary for virginal adolescent patients who have not been injured, but a bimanual examination should be carried out routinely, since teenagers are not always candid about their sexual activity. If it is more comfortable, bimanual rectoabdominal palpation while the patient is in the lithotomy position can be substituted, or the examiner can place one finger intravaginally instead of two. In every case, a hemoglobin or hematocrit determination should be obtained to coroborate the patient's estimate of her blood loss. The examiner should not hesitate to order a urine or serum pregnancy test if there is any uncertainty about the diagnosis of pregnancy.

VULVAR OR VAGINAL BLEEDING

A minority of patients will prove to have vulvar or vaginal bleeding. Patients with bleeding from significant vulvar or vaginal lacerations should be referred to a gynecologist or surgeon. The evaluation and management of victims of sexual assault are discussed in detail in Chapter 68. Hymeneal tears produced by coitus require no treatment except reassurance for the patient. Bleeding genital warts should not be treated with topical podophyllin because toxic amounts of the resin can be absorbed systemically (see Chapter 52). Malignant tumors are a rare cause of vaginal bleeding during adolescence.

CERVICAL BLEEDING

Patients are very unlikely to be aware of cervical friability or bleeding caused by infection, since it is scanty. On examination, however, punctate cervical hemorrhages (a strawberry cervix) can be seen in about 3% of women with trichomonal vaginitis. Cervical lesions of *Herpes simplex* may also cause a small amount of bleeding. Patients with bleeding from cervical lacerations should be managed by a gynecologist.

UTERINE BLEEDING

The uterus is the source of the abnormal bleeding in most adolescents. In this situation, the patient's management will depend on whether or not she is pregnant. The diagnosis of early pregnancy is discussed on p. 198. Uterine bleeding during the first 20 weeks of pregnancy indicates either spontaneous abortion or ectopic pregnancy.

Threatened abortion is diagnosed if the patient has uterine bleeding, but the internal cervical os is closed, and tissue has not been expelled. The bleeding is usually light, and some patients have uterine cramps. An abortion is considered inevitable if the internal cervical os is open, and incomplete if tissue fragments have already been expelled from the uterus. The bleeding is usually heavier, and the patient reports painful uterine contractions. Urine pregnancy tests often remain positive for several days during spontaneous abortions prompted by death of an embryo, and should not be used to predict the outcome of a threatened abortion.

Septic abortion is diagnosed at any stage if signs of infection—usually fever, disproportionately severe pelvic pain, and leukocytosis—are present during spontaneous or induced abortion. In a missed abortion, the embryo is not expelled from the uterus within 4 weeks of its death. Dark bleeding is often seen. The patient's symptoms of pregnancy may have regressed, the uterus is smaller than it should be according to her menstrual history, and disseminated intravascular coagulation may occur. Although the emergency physician needs to be able to recognize these complications of pregnancy, every patient with a spontaneous abortion should be referred to an obstetrician for management and follow-up.

Bleeding during the second trimester of pregnancy is not common; the patient should be referred for obstetrical care. Third trimester bleeding is an obstetrical emergency because it can indicate placenta previa or an abruption. Pelvic examination is *not* performed, and the patient should be evaluated by an obstetrician without delay.

Vaginal bleeding occurs in 60 to 80% of patients who have ectopic pregnancies. The bleeding is usually light and is almost always accompanied by abdominal pain or tenderness. The timing of the bleeding sometimes leads the patient to consider it a normal menstrual flow, but most patients with ectopic pregnancy report having missed between one and three menstrual periods. The patient who uses an intrauterine device (IUD) for contraception and who complains of spotting and lower abdominal pain should be evaluated particularly carefully. Although these symptoms are common side-effects of the IUD itself, IUD-users are at a five-fold higher risk of an ectopically located pregnancy than are women who use other methods of contraception. On examination, the uterus is normal or only slightly enlarged, since it does not contain the gestational sac. In contrast to urine pregnancy tests which are often falsely negative, radioimmunoassays for the beta-subunit of human chorionic gonadotropin in serum are positive in about 95% of cases. Although it must always be considered, ectopic pregnancy is uncommon during adolescence; fewer than 10% of affected patients are under 20 years of age.

Most nonpregnant adolescents with abnormal vaginal bleeding have dysfunctional uterine bleeding (DUB), a result of anovulation. But, since there are no clinical or laboratory findings that can pinpoint this diagnosis, other possible etiologies must be excluded. The diagnosis and management of DUB are detailed in Chapter 52. Qualitative and quantitative platelet abnormalities are by far the commonest coagulation defects responsible for excessive menstrual bleeding. Females with von Willebrand's disease and idiopathic thrombocytopenic purpura are among those at risk. Patients whose menorrhagia occurs during the very first menstrual period warrant particularly close attention. Gonorrhea has been implicated as a cause of otherwise unexplained abnormal uterine bleeding; cervical cultures should therefore be taken routinely from sexually active adolescents. Patients taking birth control pills may have intermittent vaginal spotting or bleeding if they do not take their pills daily. Five to ten percent of woman whose pills contain 35 μg or less of estrogen will have spotting or bleeding even if they do take the pills properly. This breakthrough bleeding is most common during the first three months' use of such low-dose pills. Progestin-only contraceptive pills often produce menstrual irregularities. Oligomenorrhea, spotting, and breakthrough bleeding are all common among users of these "mini-pills." Adolescents who are not using hormonal contraception rarely have some spotting at the time of ovulation when estrogen levels fall transiently. Intrauterine devices do not affect the cyclicity of menstrual bleeding but produce intermenstrual spotting or a longer or heavier flow in about 40% of patients using them. Such variations in menstrual pattern are most prevalent during the first few months after an IUD is inserted.

References

Booher D, Little B: Vaginal hemorrhage in pregnancy. *N Engl J Med* 290: 611, 1974.

Breen JL: A 21 year survey of 654 ectopic pregnancies. *Am J Obstet Gynecol* 106: 1004, 1970.

Claessens EA, Cowell CA: Acute adolescent menorrhagia. *Am J Obstet Gynecol* 139: 277, 1981.

Dewhurst CJ, et al.: The regularity of early menstrual cycles. *J Obstet Gynaecol Br Commonw* 78: 1093, 1971.

Heller ME, et al.: Vaginal bleeding in childhood: A review of 51 patients. *Br J Obstet Gynaecol* 85: 721, 1978.

Huffman JW: Injuries to the genitalia during childhood. In *The Gynecology of Childhood and Adolescence*, Ed. 2, p. 213, WB Saunders, Philadelphia, 1981.

Robboy SJ, et al.: Prenatal diethylstilbestrol (DES) exposure: Recommendations of the diethylstilbestrol-adenosis (DESAD) project for the identification and management of exposed individuals. U.S. Dept. of Health and Human Services, NIH Publication No. 81-2049, 1981.

CHAPTER 39

Vaginal Discharge

JAN E. PARADISE, M.D.

INTRODUCTION

Normal infants, over 1 month of age, and prepubertal girls do not have liquid vaginal secretions. Consequently, any vaginal discharge in a female child is abnormal. However, vaginal discharges in neonates and girls who are pubertal may be either normal or abnormal, because during these time periods estrogen, either maternal or endogenous, stimulates growth of the vaginal epithelium and secretion of mucus by the paracervical glands. The resulting vaginal discharge consists of desquamated epithelial cells and mucus, is not irritating, and requires no treatment. It is known as physiologic leukorrhea. Vaginal discharges that persist beyond the neonatal period, that occur during childhood, or that are accompanied by discomfort in pubertal patients are abnormal and need to be investigated.

EVALUATION AND DECISION

General Considerations

Although the complaint of vaginal discharge is common among both children and adolescents, it is important for the emergency physician to recognize from the outset that this symptom is not necessarily either a sensitive or a specific indicator of actual lower genital tract disease. On the one hand, as noted in the definition above, an asymptomatic vaginal discharge during the first several weeks of life or after the onset of puberty is a normal occurrence, but is nevertheless likely to prompt an emergency department visit by the young pubertal girl concerned about this unexpected change in her body's function. Among prepubertal girls, on the other hand, complaints of vaginal discharge, irritation, itching, and dysuria can indicate urinary or gastrointestinal tract disease (cystitis or pinworms, for example), so the emergency physician cannot assume that the problem is specific to or limited to the genital tract. Thus, evaluation of children with the complaint of vaginal discharge must include historical information not only about genital symptoms, but also about urinary and gastrointestinal function. In addition, every child with genital complaints (and her parent) should be asked directly whether there is a possibility that she has had any sexual contact. Although physicians are often reluctant to raise this question, many parents will have considered it already, and some will have asked their daughters before the visit to the doctor. Parents who respond to a question about the possibility of sexual abuse with outrage or anger are more suspect for having abused their child than those who acknowledge its reasonableness. If the patient's history provides few diagnostic clues, then the physical examination and cultures will be the emergency physician's best guides to her proper management.

For examination of the external genitalia, infants and children should be placed in a frog-leg position either on the parent's lap or on an examining table. The genital mucosa of infants and children is normally reddish, not dull pink, since the epithelium

Table 39.1
Differential diagnosis of vaginal discharge[a]

- *I. During Infancy*
  - A. Physiologic leukorrhea
  - B. *Trichomonas vaginalis*
  - C. Ectopic ureter
  - D. Smegma
- *II. During Childhood*
  - A. Infections
    1. *Neisseria gonorrhoeae*
    2. *Shigella* species
    3. *Streptococcus pyogenes*
    4. *Candida albicans*
    5. *Chlamydia trachomatis*
  - B. Foreign body
  - C. Nonspecific vaginitis
  - D. Smegma
  - E. Sexual abuse
- *III. After Onset of Puberty*
  - A. Physiologic leukorrhea
  - B. Infections
    1. *Candida albicans*
    2. *Trichomonas vaginalis*
    3. *Gardnerella vaginalis*
    4. *Neisseria gonorrhoeae*
  - C. Foreign body

[a] This list includes only relatively likely entities in each age group and should not be considered exhaustive.

is relatively thin in the absence of estrogenic stimulation. This appearance of the introitus should not be mistaken for inflammation. Children should next be examined in the knee-chest position to check for the presence of a foreign body (see Figure 52.1B, p. 604). If the examiner sees a vaginal discharge when the child is in either position, a specimen should then be collected for culture. Soft plastic medicine droppers are convenient and comfortable to use for aspirating vaginal secretions. If a girl's secretions are minimal, the dropper can be used instead to instill and then withdraw nonbacteriostatic saline washings for culture. Alternatively, the physician can obtain secretions with a cotton-tipped swab moistened with nonbacteriostatic saline solution, but this method is usually less comfortable for the patient. If the volume of secretions allows it, a Gram stain and wet mounts with saline solution and 10% potassium hydroxide should also be prepared and examined microscopically. However, culture should be the first priority because positive identification of *Neisseria gonorrhoeae* can help to document cases of sexual abuse, and because microscopy cannot be used to identify infections caused by *Shigella* or *Streptococcus*.

A complete pelvic examination is rarely needed to evaluate the pubertal but premenarchial girl with lower genital tract complaints. The frog-leg position or the standard lithotomy position should be used for inspection of the girl's external genitalia, but speculum and bimanual examinations are not likely to be useful. On the other hand, standard speculum and bimanual pelvic examinations are indispensable for the evaluation of sexually active adolescents. Because these patients have high rates of both sexually transmitted infection and unsuspected pregnancy, the examiner should routinely obtain vaginal specimens for microscopy and cervical cultures for *N. gonorrhoeae* and should be alert for signs of pelvic inflammatory disease and pregnancy.

The patient's age and hormonal status should be considered first in the differential diagnosis of vaginal discharge (see Fig. 39.1). For a more detailed discussion of the specific vaginal infections to be mentioned in this section, the reader is referred to Chapter 52 (Vaginitis).

Infancy and Childhood

Physiologic leukorrhea is a normal, common vaginal discharge among female infants during the first 2 to 3 weeks of life. It is clear or white, slippery when fresh, and sticky when dried. Some neonates have associated withdrawal bleeding when maternal estrogen stimulation of the uterine endometrium wanes. Trichomonal vaginitis should be suspected if an infant's discharge persists beyond the neonatal period. An occasional baby whose mother has trichomonal vaginitis will acquire this infection during delivery. Infected infants may be irritable, and have a whitish or yellowish thin discharge. Uncommonly, infants have purulent discharge from an ectopically located ureter. This should be suspected more strongly if an infant's discharge is accompanied by signs of systemic infection (fever, vomiting, or poor appetite), or if a

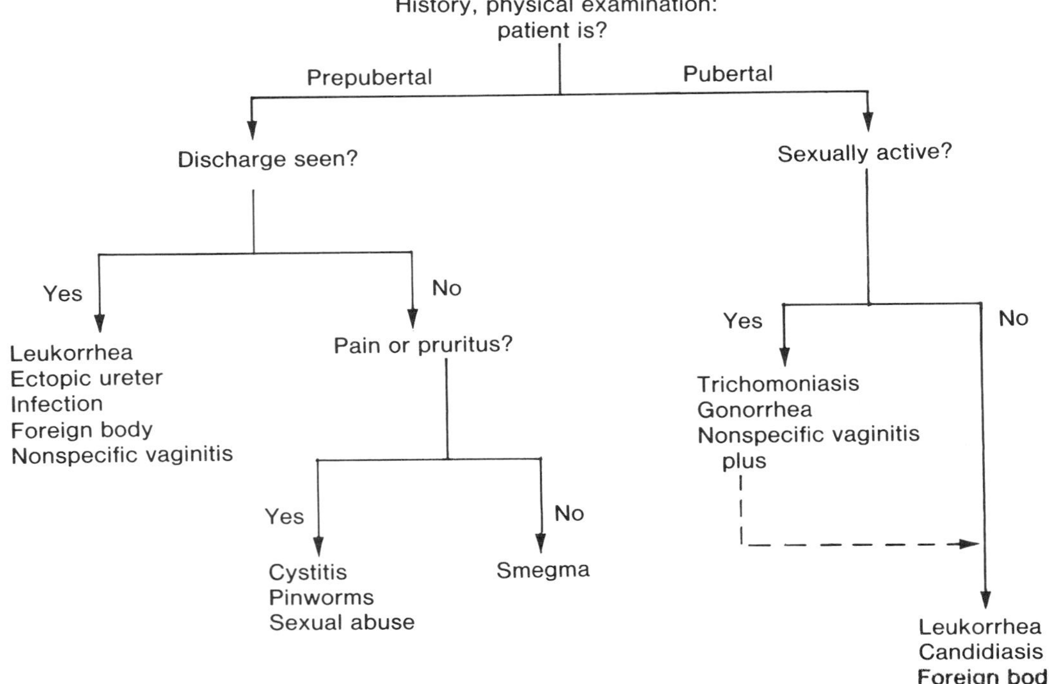

Figure 39.1 Decision tree for vaginal discharge.

child with a chronic discharge also has a history of recurrent urinary tract infections.

Among older infants and children, a visible vaginal discharge is most likely to indicate bacterial infection. Cultures for *N. gonorrhoeae* as well as other pathogens should be performed routinely, because in many cases neither the character of the discharge itself nor microscopy is diagnostic. Gonococcal infection produces a whitish to greenish purulent discharge. Bloody discharge occurs in half the cases of *Shigella* vaginitis. Vaginal infections with *Trichomonas vaginalis* are more likely to occur in infants under 6 months of age than in older children. Symptomatic chlamydial infections are rare except in children with concurrent or previous gonococcal vaginitis. It is therefore reasonable to reserve cultures for these latter two organisms for children whose bacterial cultures have already proved to be negative. As in adults, diabetes mellitus, broad spectrum antibiotic drugs, and immunodeficiency are risk factors for the development of candidal vaginitis in children.

An intermittently bloody, foul-smelling vaginal discharge is the classic complaint of the patient with a vaginal foreign body. However, since foreign bodies can produce either discharge or spotty bleeding alone, the diagnosis should be considered in every child with a complaint of discharge. Small wads of toilet paper are the commonest foreign bodies. The emergency physician must have a high index of suspicion if the child's vagina cannot be inspected satisfactorily while she is in the knee-chest position, because intravaginal toilet paper cannot often be palpated rectally. Less common foreign bodies—pencil erasers, pins, beads, nuts—are more likely to be palpable during rectal examination. Gentle vaginal lavage with saline solution can be used to flush out bits of toilet paper. Small round objects can sometimes be removed if the examiner places his finger in the rectum and then applies gently outward pressure. However, if the object is large or sharp, or simpler maneuvers fail, the patient may require examination and removal of the foreign body under general anesthesia.

Children with vaginal discharge that cannot be ascribed to any of the conditions just discussed are generally considered to have nonspecific vaginitis. This condition has been attributed to poor perineal hygiene and local irritation. Accordingly, frequent sitz baths, careful wiping anteroposteriorly after defecation, and the avoidance of presumed irritants (ballet tights, bubble bath, sand) are recommended for its treatment. These measures will produce improvement in a majority of patients with nonspecific vaginitis, but should not be used unless the appropriate diagnostic examinations and cultures have also been carried out.

Some girls with the complaint of vaginal discharge or irritation will have only vulvitis or no abnormality on examination of the genitalia. Genital smegma occurs in girls as well as in boys, and is sometimes mistaken by parents for a pathologic discharge. It consists of desquamated epithelial cells, is thick, yellow or white, and sticky, and is characteristically located in the labial folds and around the clitoral prepuce. However, if no discharge is seen, but the child has genital pain or pruritis, diagnostic possibilities include urinary tract infection and intestinal parasites (usually pinworms). Somatic genital discomfort is the presenting complaint of a small number of children who have been sexually abused, but are not injured or infected. The examiner must have a high index of suspicion to bring such cases to light.

Adolescence

With the onset of puberty, rising estrogen levels again promote the discharge of vaginal mucus and cells. This physiologic leukorrhea persists throughout the reproductive years, but for obvious reasons is most likely to arouse the concern of girls who are early in puberty. On microscopic examination, the discharge shows only abundant epithelial cells. Culture of a specimen is not necessary. Pubertal but premenarchial girls with genital itching are very likely to have candidal vaginitis, even in the absence of any predisposing factor. The associated cheesy discharge may be so scanty that it goes unmentioned or unnoticed. Among postmenarchial patients, birth control pills, broad spectrum antibiotics, diabetes mellitus, and pregnancy are all associated with an increased risk of acquiring vaginal candidiasis. Trichomonal infection is probably the commonest cause of abnormal vaginal discharge among sexually active adolescents who visit urban emergency departments. Associated pruritis, if present, is usually mild, and the discharge is frothy in only about 25% of cases. Cervical gonorrhea can produce a noticeable vaginal discharge, but the majority of infected adolescent girls have no lower genital tract symptoms. Nonspecific vaginitis, generally ascribed to infection with *Gardnerella vaginalis*, is characterized clinically by a fishy odor and the absence of visible vaginal inflammation. It is probably a sexually transmitted infection. On microscopic examination there are few polymorphonuclear leukocytes, but "clue cells" (vaginal epithelial cells studded with small Gram-negative rods) are seen. Microscopic examination of suspensions of vaginal discharge in 10% potassium hydroxide and saline solution will provide a diagnosis for half to three-quarters of patients with candidal and trichomonal infections documented by culture. Cervical Papanicolaou smears should not be used to diagnose vaginal infections since they yield falsely negative results in about 20% of patients with trichomoniasis and in 50% of patients with candidiasis. Similarly, Gram stains of cervical secretions are not sufficiently sensitive to be reliable for excluding the diagnosis of gonorrhea. A forgotten tampon is the commonest intravaginal foreign body. All foreign bodies will eventually give rise to foul-smelling discharge, but in general, they are an uncommon cause of vaginitis among adolescents.

References

Emans SJ, Goldstein DP: The gynecologic examination of the prepubertal child with vulvovaginitis: Use of the knee-chest position. *Pediatrics* 65: 758, 1980.

Henderson PA, Scott RB: Foreign body vaginitis caused by toilet tissue. *Am J Dis Child* 111: 529, 1966.

McLennan MT, Smith JM, McLennan CE: Diagnosis of vaginal mycosis and Trichomoniasis: Reliability of cytologic smear, wet smear and culture. *Obstet Gynecol* 40: 231, 1972.

CHAPTER 40

Vesicobullous Lesions

PAUL J. HONIG, M.D.

INTRODUCTION

The diagnosis of vesicobullous lesions in children over 1 month of age will be discussed in this section. The approach to such patients may be directed by certain key clinical features: a characteristic clinical appearance; chronicity, and/or presence at birth; associated fever or systemic illness; distribution of lesions; and age of the child. Such an approach is outlined in Figure 40.1.

CHARACTERISTIC CLINICAL APPEARANCE

Many times the appearance of a rash is so characteristic that a diagnosis becomes obvious. Such is the case with the entities listed in Table 40.1.

Linear or geometric areas of vesiculation are the best clues to the presence of allergic contact dermatitis. The shape of the dermatitis provides the information which helps identify the offending agent. The history of playing in a shrubbed area, camping, hiking, or being near burning leaves is helpful. Because children brush against poison ivy leaves, vesicles are often in a line. A round group of vesicles on the back of the wrist would point to contact sensitivity to nickel contained in the metal case of a wristwatch.

Dermatomal distribution of vesicles or bullae usually indicate the presence of herpes zoster. On rare occasions, as was described in infants, the same appearance may represent infection with herpes simplex. A positive Tzanck smear will indicate the presence of the herpes virus. Viral cultures are necessary to differentiate simplex and zoster.

Target or iris lesions are pathognomonic of erythema multiforme. The lesion has a dusky center that may blister and have successive bright red bordering rings. At times a doughnut-shaped blister occurs.

Pigmented lesions that blister after stroking or trauma (Darier's sign) indicate the release of histamine from a mast cell collection. This collection may be isolated (mastocytoma of the wrist) or generalized (urticaria pigmentosa). Blistering of such lesions generally only occurs until 2 years of age. After this time only urtication occurs.

DURATION

If there is no characteristic clinical appearance one must consider the duration of the rash. If it has been present for 4 weeks or more, it should be considered chronic. Rashes that come and go but take 4 weeks to disappear completely will not be considered chronic.

Chronic Rash (Duration 4 Weeks or More)

If the blistering disease has been present since birth (congenital) consider the diagnosis listed in Table 40.2.

Epidermolysis Bullosa Syndromes

Blisters usually occur in areas predisposed to trauma or friction. See Table 40.3 for differentiation of the various types.

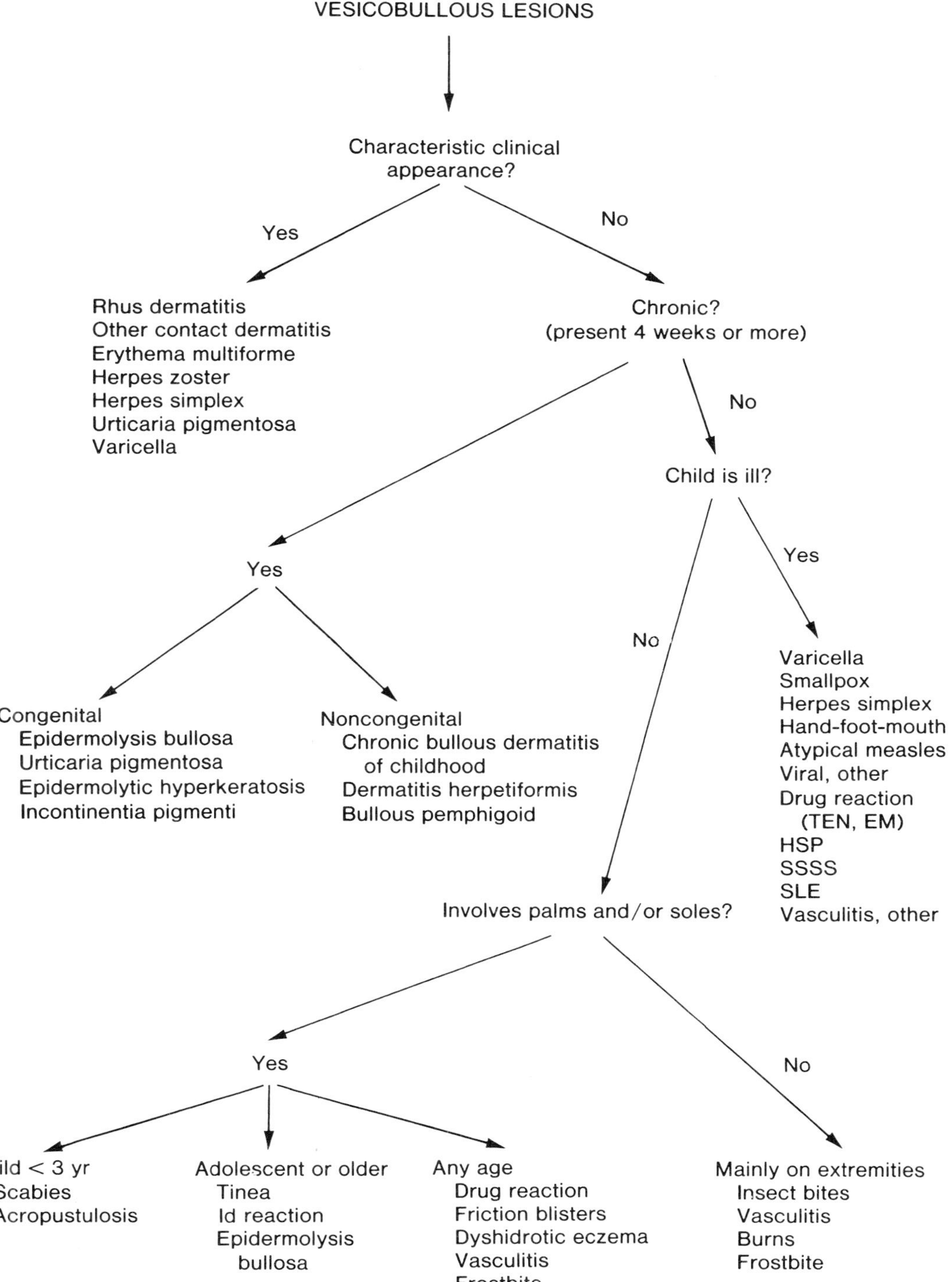

Figure 40.1 The diagnostic approach to the child with vesicobullous lesions. *HSP* = Henoch-Schönlein purpura; *SSSS* = staphylococcal scalded skin syndrome; *SLE* = systemic lupus erythematosis; *TEN* = toxic epidermal necrolysis; *EM* = erythema multiforme.

Table 40.1
Vesicobullous Rashes with Characteristic Clinical Appearance

Rhus dermatitis
Other contact dermatitis
Erythema multiforme
Herpes zoster
Urticaria pigmentosa
Herpes simplex
Varicella

Table 40.2
Congenital Blistering Diseases

Epidermolysis bullosa
Urticaria pigmentosa
Epidermolytic hyperkeratosis
Incontinentia pigmenti

Urticaria Pigmentosa

Mast cell disease (mastocytoma or urticaria pigmentosa) may cause blistering until 2 years of age. The pigmented solitary lesion most frequently occurs on the arm near the wrist. Lesions may be generalized. When a pigmented lesion feels infiltrated, think of this cause. Gentle mechanical irritation of such lesions causes urtication or blistering (Darier's sign).

Epidermolytic Hyperkeratosis (Congenital Bullous Ichthyosiform Erythroderma)

This autosomal dominant trait is categorized under the ichthyotic syndromes. Children with this problem have recurrent bullous lesions during infancy and childhood. The skin has a background of erythema, scales, and peels. The flexures are always affected, as are the palms and soles.

Incontinentia Pigmenti

This rare entity occurs almost exclusively in females. Inflammatory bullae erupt in crops in a linear distribution for the first several weeks to months of life. These affected areas then go on to a warty stage. Finally, swirl-like pigmentation occurs, but not necessarily in the areas previously involved with warty or blistering lesions. During the vesicobullous stage a high degree of peripheral eosinophilia occurs (18 to 50%).

If the blistering is noncongenital, one should think of the following conditions: chronic bullous dermatosis of childhood, dermatitis herpetiformis, and bullous pemphigoid. These conditions can be differentiated as outlined in Table 40.4.

Varicella (Chickenpox)

A delicate "tear drop" vesicle is characteristic of varicella. Lesions usually begin on the trunk. A progression through papules, vesicles, and crusts occurs rapidly (6 to 24 hours). All stages are present in an area at any given time. Mucous membranes are involved. Fever and malaise are usually present but are variable.

III Child

When the blistering lesions occur acutely one must determine if the child is febrile or ill. Conditions causing such systemic findings with associated blisters include those listed in Table 40.5.

Varicella (Chickenpox)

See previous section.

Hand-Foot-Mouth Disease

Caused by coxsackievirus A16, this infection is fairly characteristic. Vesicles are present on the palms, soles, and in the mouth. Other parts of the body may be involved. Fever, malaise, and abdominal pain may be present.

Viral (Nonspecific) and Other

Vesicles have been described in association with other coxsackievirus types (A4, 5, B1, 4), echo, reovirus, and *Mycoplasma pneumoniae* infections. These children are usually ill.

Drug Reactions

The presence of vesicles or bullae may indicate a drug reaction. Involvement of palms, soles, mucous membranes, or the presence of target lesions are other possible clues that this problem exists. Therefore, one must question about intake of prescribed and over-the-counter preparations.

Drug induced toxic epidermal necrolysis (TEN) may be associated with blisters. Histology which shows separation of dermis from epidermis *excludes* the staphylococcal induced problem. Also the staphylococcal scaled skin syndrome (SSSS) rarely occurs in children over 6 years of age. Think of a

Table 40.3
Epidermolysis Bullosa Syndromes

	Type	Inheritance	Clinical Features	Electron Microscope
Nonscarring	Epidermolysis bullosa simplex	Autosomal dominant	Bullae present at birth or early infancy; in areas of trauma; improves in adolescence; no mucous membrane involvement; nail involvement (20%)	Cleavage through basal cell layer above the basement membrane
	Recurrent bullous eruption of hands and feet (Weber-Cockayne disease)	Autosomal dominant	May present in first 2 years of life, but usually not before adolescence or early adulthood	Epidermal cleavage may be anywhere from the suprabasal to lower granular cell layer
	Junctional epidermolysis bullosa (Herlitz disease)	Autosomal recessive	Usually at birth; spontaneous bullae and large areas of erosion	Cleavage at junction of dermis and epidermis (above the basement membrane)
Scarring	Dominant dystrophic epidermolysis bullosa (dominant dermolytic bullous dermatosis)	Autosomal dominant	Early infancy and later; little or no involvement of hair and teeth; mucous membrane lesions and nail dystrophy	Dermal-epidermal separation beneath basement membrane
	Recessive dystrophic epidermolysis bullosa (recessive dermolytic bullous dermatosis)	Autosomal recessive	Present at birth; widespread scarring and deformity; severe involvement of mucous membranes and nails	Separation at dermal-epidermal junction (beneath the basal lamina)

Table 40.4
Noncongenital Chronic Blistering Disease

	Bullous Disease of Childhood	Bullous Pemphigoid	Dermatitis Herpetiformis
Type of lesions	Large, tense, clear bullae; annular plaques with active vesicular borders	Large, tense bullae	*Grouped* papulovesicles, bullae or urticarial lesions
Distribution	Scalp, lower trunk, genitals, buttocks, inner thighs	Trunk and flexor surfaces of extremities	Back, buttocks, scalp, extensor surface of extremities, often symmetric
Pruritus	None to severe	Mild	Intense
Mucous membrane involvement	No	Yes	No
Duration	Months to years	Months to years	Months to years
Immunofluorescence	+ or −	+	+
	Linear IgA on basement membrane (+ circulating IgA)	Linear IgG on basement membrane (+ circulating IgG)	Granular IgA at tips of dermal papilla of uninvolved perilesional skin
Treatment	Sulfapyridine or dapsone	Corticosteroids	Sulfapyridine or dapsone

Table 40.5
Blistering Diseases Associated with Fever and/or Systemic Illness

Chickenpox
Hand-foot-mouth
Viral (nonspecific) + other
Drug reaction (TEN, EM)[a]
Henoch-Schönlein purpura
Nonspecific vasculitis
Herpes simplex
Staphylococcal scalded skin syndrome
Systemic lupus
Atypical measles
Smallpox

[a] TEN, toxic epidermal necrolysis; EM, erythrema multiforme.

drug problem in children over six. The histology of SSSS demonstrates separation just below the stratum corneum.

Children with severe drug reactions may be very toxic. High fevers, malaise, joint problems, etc. can occur.

Henoch-Schönlein (HS) Purpura

Children with this syndrome may have blisters, due to severe involvement of blood vessels (vasculitis), in the typical distribution that occurs in this entity. Associated systemic problems include arthritis, abdominal pain, kidney disease (hematuria and/or proteinuria), and seizures.

Nonspecific Vasculitis

Children with vasculitic blisters, at times hemorrhagic, may be sick with fever, malaise, and other symptoms. Some go on to well-defined collagen vascular disease, others smolder, with no diagnosis ever being made.

Herpes Simplex

Primary infection with this virus may cause fever and regional lymphadenopathy. The first encounter for young children is usually herpetic gingivostomatitis. Vesicles involve the lips and rest of the mouth. These children are very uncomfortable and frequently refuse to eat or drink.

Herpes progenitalis may produce fever and local lymphadenopathy as well. Characteristic clusters of vesicles on an erythematous base occur. Frequently erosions or ulcerations evolve on the vulva or penis.

Diagnosis can be confirmed by a Tzanck smear showing aggregates of multinucleated giant cells.

Systemic Lupus Erythematosus (SLE)

Although not characteristic, bullous lesions can occur in SLE. Multisystem involvement suggests the diagnosis. Laboratory confirmation, which may include a skin biopsy and lupus band test, in conjunction with the complete clinical picture, are necessary for diagnosis.

Atypical Measles

An unusual macular, vesicular, or petechial rash occurs principally on the hands and feet. The children are very ill, with high fever, cough, and frequently a giant cell pneumonia. Children who received the killed measles vaccine are predisposed to this syndrome upon exposure to the wild virus. Therefore, careful questioning about measles vaccination is important. Killed measles vaccine was no longer recommended following the introduction of the live attenuated virus vaccine during the period of 1963 to 1965.

Smallpox

Unlike chickenpox, smallpox begins peripherally and extends to the trunk. The prodrome is long and severe (3 to 4 days). Lesions concentrate in areas of pressure or tightness of the skin and are all in the same stage in one area of the skin.

Otherwise Well Child

If the child is not ill search for blisters on the palms and soles.

Table 40.6
Acute Vesicobullous Diseases Involving Palms and Soles

Child < 3 years old
Scabies
Acropustulosis of infancy
Adolescent or older
Tinea pedis or manus
"Id" reaction
Epidermolysis bullosa of hands and feet
Any age
Drug reaction
Friction blisters or burns
Dyshidrotic eczema
Vasculitis (e.g., Henoch-Schönlein purpura)
Frostbite

Involves Palms and/or Soles

The age of the child will then help differentiate some of the disorders (see Table 40.6).

Child Less Than 3 Years Old

Scabies

Infants and very young children can have vesicobullous lesions on the palms, soles, head, and face. Don't be misled by this distribution and appearance. Generally, mother will be infested as well and exhibit the typical appearance of this disorder.

Acropustulosis of Infancy

The appearance of pruritic vesicopustules between 2 to 10 months of age on the palms and soles in black children should suggest this diagnosis. Vesicles frequently involve the lateral aspects of the fingers, palms, and soles. The entity was frequently diagnosed as dyshidrotic eczema in the past. Cyclic eruptions occur every 2 to 3 weeks lasting 7 to 10 days. Spontaneous disappearance occurs at 2 to 3 years of age.

Adolescent or Older

Tinea Pedis or Manus

Certain of the organisms causing tinea pedis or manus (e.g., *Trichophyton mentagrophytes*) induce a severe inflammatory reaction on the hands and feet. Vesicobullous lesions erupt on the palms, instep, or medial aspect of the foot. A KOH preparation confirms the presence of hyphae in either location.

"Id" Reaction

If the palms of an adolescent have blisters, look at their feet. Individuals with tinea pedis may have an allergic reaction to dissemination of antigen. A KOH preparation of the lesions on the palms will be negative for fungus.

Epidermolysis Bullosa of the Hands and Feet

See **Epidermolysis bullosae syndromes** in this chapter (Table 40.3).

Any Age

Drug Reaction

See **Ill Child** in this chapter.

Friction Blisters or Burns

Blisters appear on the palms and soles following trauma to the skin. The trauma is frequently due to a new activity (golfing, rowing, football) or new, possibly poorly fitted shoes.

Occasionally one sees accidental burns or burns secondary to child abuse. Abused children may have had cigarette burns or had their feet dipped in scalding water.

Dyshidrotic Eczema (Pompholyx)

Recurrent episodes of vesicles involving the palms, soles, and lateral aspects of the fingers is termed dyshidrotic eczema. On occasion large bullae occur. The problem is generally bilateral. There is frequently a personal or family history of atopy. KOH preparations of scrapings from the palms or soles are negative.

Vasculitis (HS purpura)

This entity may involve the palms and/or soles. See **Ill Child** in this chapter.

Frostbite

Fingers, toes, feet, nose, cheeks, and ears are affected. After exposed areas are damaged by the cold temperature, symptoms will occur on rewarming. Erythema, swelling and burning pain occur at first followed by vesicles and bullae (at times hemorrhagic) within 24 to 48 hours.

Extremities

If there is no involvement or minimal involvement of the palms and soles and the rash is concentrated on the extremities, one should consider insect bites, vasculitis, burns, and frostbite.

Insect Bites

Insects generally bite exposed skin surfaces. Therefore, heaviest involvement occurs on the head, face, and extremities. Mosquito bites occur in the warm weather months, while flea bites will occur any time of the year. Historical information to ask includes: contact with pets, camping trips, or other outdoor activities. When blisters are present, the more characteristic urticarial papules are usually present in other locations. If not, confusion with bullous impetigo is easily ruled out with a Gram stain (negative for bacteria).

Vasculitis (HS purpura)

Concentration of hemorrhagic bullae on the extremities and buttocks indicate HS purpura. The lower extremities are an area that is frequently involved due to settling of immune-complexes, cryoglobulins, etc. in that location.

Burns

Exposed areas are frequently involved. Children accidentally rub against hot objects causing burns and blistering.

In child abuse, children are intentionally burned with cigarettes (frequently mistaken for lesions of impetigo) or other heated objects. Children, at times, are submerged in scalding hot water. Usually both lower extremities are involved.

LABORATORY EVALUATION

If you don't have any idea what the blister is due to, these laboratory tests can be helpful.

Gram Stain

The Gram stain of fluid from an intact blister will be positive in impetigo and a secondarily infected lesion. However, it will be negative in all other conditions.

Tzanck Smear

Multinucleated giant cells will be present on Tzanck smear of material scraped from the base of an intact freshly opened vesicle caused by herpes simplex, herpes zoster, and varicella.

Bacterial or Viral Cultures

Occasionally cultures will help to confirm an etiologic diagnosis when Gram stain and Tzanck smear are negative or indeterminate.

Skin Biopsy

For perplexing cases undiagnosed by clinical and/or simple laboratory evaluation, dermatologic consultation and skin biopsy are required.

Many characteristic changes can be

Table 40.7
Pathologic Diagnosis of Vesicobullous Eruptions

Type of Blister	Site of Formation	Disease[a]
1. Subcorneal blister	Subcorneal	Impetigo SSSS
2. Blister due to intracellular degeneration	Upper epidermis	Bullous congenital icthyosiform erythroderma Epidermolysis bullosa of hands and feet Friction blisters
3. Spongiotic blister	Intraepidermal	Incontinentia pigmenti
4. Viral blister	Intraepidermal	Variola Herpes simplex Varicella-herpes zoster
5. Blister due to degeneration of basal cell	Subepidermal	Epidermolysis bullosa simplex Lichen planus Lupus erythematosus
6. Blister due to degeneration of basement zone	Subepidermal	Epidermolysis bullosa, dystrophic type Urticaria pigementosa Bullous pemphigoid Dermatitis herpetiformis Erythema multiforme, dermal type Drug induced TEN

[a] SSSS, staphylococcal scaled skin syndrome; TEN, toxic epidermal necrolysis.

found on histologic examination which lead to a definitive diagnosis (see Table 40.7). Lichen planus, SLE, TEN, SSSS, and vasculitis are some of the disease entities that can be identified by histologic studies.

If the picture on histology is compatible with erythema multiforme one should consider *direct immunofluorescence*. This will be negative in erythema multiforme but will be positive in bullous pemphigoid (linear IgG on basement membrane), dermatitis herpetiformis (granular IgA at tips of dermal papillae of uninvolved perilesional skin), and chronic bullous disease of childhood (linear IgA on basement membrane). Direct immunofluorescence can be negative in chronic bullous disease of childhood (CBDC).

Indirect immunofluorescence can be done to test for circulating antibodies. Circulating IgG is found in bullous pemphigoid; circulating IgA in CBDC.

CHAPTER 41

Vomiting

FRED M. HENRETIG, M.D.

INTRODUCTION

Vomiting, defined as the forceful, coordinated act of expelling gastric contents through the mouth, is a common symptom in children. Vomiting may be caused by a number of problems in diverse organ systems. While it often represents a transient response to a self-limited infectious, chemical or psychologic insult, it may also portend serious infections, metabolic disturbances, or diseases in the gastrointestinal, neurologic, or other major organ systems. Thus, an orderly approach to diagnosis is crucial.

Vomiting is a highly coordinated act, involving closure of gastric pylorus and glottis, relaxation of stomach, cardioesophageal junction and esophagus, and vigorous diaphragmatic and abdominal wall muscular contraction. A medullary vomiting center coordinates this action. Afferent stimuli to this center, which may trigger vomiting, arise from diverse areas of the body including the pelvic and abdominal viscera and peritoneum, genitourinary system, pharynx, labyrinth, and heart. A separate medullary site on the floor of the fourth ventricle, the chemoreceptor trigger zone, is responsive to various drugs or metabolic aberrations and may also serve as a source of afferent impulses to the vomiting center.

A related complaint, also often heard in the emergency department, is that of young infants who "spit up." This refers to the nonforceful reflux of milk into the mouth which often accompanies eructation. Such nonforceful regurgitation of gastric or esophageal contents is most often physiologic and of little consequence, although occasionally it represents a marked disturbance in esophageal function.

It is convenient to attempt to organize the many diverse causes of regurgitation and vomiting into age-related categories (Table 41.1). While there is considerable overlap, the most common and serious entities tend to fall into such groupings.

EVALUATION AND DECISION

General Approach

A brief perusal of the long list of causes for vomiting in Table 41.1 will serve to emphasize the need for an orderly approach to the differential diagnosis of this symptom. The approach advocated here will focus on three key clinical features: *age* of the child, evidence for *obstruction,* and signs or symptoms of *extra-abdominal* organ system *disease.* Other important points to consider include *appearance* of the vomitus, overall *degree of illness,* and *associated gastrointestinal symptoms.*

HISTORY

The history should focus on the key elements listed above. The patient's age is often critical, as certain important entities (especially those causing intestinal obstruction) are seen exclusively in neonates, older

Table 41.1
Vomiting and Regurgitation: Principal Causes by Usual Age of Onset and Etiology

I. *Newborn (Birth to 2 Weeks)*
   A. Normal variations
   B. Gastroesophageal reflux (± hiatal hernia)
   C. Esophageal stenosis, atresia
   D. Infantile achalasia
   E. Obstructive intestinal anomalies
      1. Intestinal stenosis, atresia
      2. Malrotation of bowel (± midgut volvulus)
      3. Meconium ileus (cystic fibrosis)
      4. Meconium plug
      5. Hirschsprung's disease
      6. Imperforate anus
      7. Enteric duplications
   F. Other gastrointestinal causes
      1. Necrotizing enterocolitis
      2. Cow's milk allergy
      3. Lactobezoar
      4. Gastrointestinal perforation with secondary peritonitis
   G. Neurologic
      1. Subdural hematoma
      2. Hydrocephalus
      3. Cerebral edema
      4. Kernicterus
   H. Renal
      1. Obstructive uropathy
      2. Renal insufficiency
   I. Infectious
      1. Meningitis
      2. Sepsis
   J. Metabolic
      1. Inborn errors of urea cycle, aminoacid, organic acid and carbohydrate metabolism (phenylketonuria, galactosemia)
      2. Congenital adrenal hyperplasia

II. *Older Infant (2 Weeks to 12 Months)*
   A. Normal variations
   B. Gastroesophageal reflux
   C. Acquired esophageal disorders (corrosive esophagitis ± stricture, foreign bodies, retroesophageal abscess)
   D. Rumination
   E. Gastrointestinal obstruction
      1. Bezoars, foreign bodies
      2. Pyloric stenosis
      3. Malrotation (with or without volvulus)
      4. Enteric duplications
      5. Meckel diverticulum (complications of)
      6. Intussusception
      7. Ascariasis
      8. Incarcerated hernia
      9. Hirschsprung's disease

Table 41.1—*Continued*

- F. Other gastrointestinal causes
  1. Gastroenteritis
  2. Celiac disease
  3. Peritonitis
  4. Paralytic ileus
- G. Neurologic
  1. Brain tumors
  2. Other intracranial mass lesions
  3. Cerebral edema
  4. Hydrocephalus
- H. Renal
  1. Obstructive uropathy
  2. Renal insufficiency
- I. Infectious
  1. Meningitis
  2. Sepsis
  3. Urinary tract infection
  4. Otitis media
  5. Pertussis
  6. Hepatitis
- J. Metabolic
  1. Metabolic acidosis (inborn errors of aminoacid and organic acid metabolism, renal tubular acidosis)
  2. Galactosemia
  3. Fructose intolerance
  4. Adrenal insufficiency
- K. Drug overdose
  1. Aspirin
  2. Theophylline
  3. Digoxin

III. Older Child (Over 12 Months)

- A. Gastrointestinal obstruction
  1. Acquired esophageal strictures
  2. Foreign bodies, bezoars
  3. Peptic ulcer disease
  4. Post-traumatic intramural hematoma
  5. Malrotation (with or without volvulus)
  6. Meckel diverticulum (complications of)
  7. Meconium ileus equivalent (cystic fibrosis)
  8. Ascariasis
  9. Incarcerated hernia
  10. Adhesions (postsurgical, peritonitis)
  11. Intussusception
  12. Hirschsprung's disease
- B. Other gastrointestinal causes
  1. Gastroenteritis
  2. Gastroesophageal reflux
  3. Appendicitis
  4. Peptic ulcer disease
  5. Pancreatitis
  6. Peritonitis
  7. Paralytic ileus

Table 41.1—*Continued*

- C. Neurologic
  1. Brain tumors
  2. Other intracranial mass lesions
  3. Cerebral edema
  4. Migraine
  5. Motion sickness
- D. Renal
  1. Obstructive uropathy
  2. Renal insufficiency
- E. Infectious
  1. Meningitis
  2. Urinary tract infection
  3. Hepatitic
  4. Upper respiratory infection (postnasal mucous drip)
- F. Metabolic
  1. Diabetic ketoacidosis
  2. Reye's syndrome
  3. Adrenal insufficiency
- G. Toxins and drugs
  1. Aspirin
  2. Ipecac
  3. Theophylline
  4. Digoxin
  5. Iron
  6. Lead (chronic)
- H. Other
  1. Pregnancy
  2. Psychogenic

infants or children beyond the first year of life. Evidence of obstruction, including symptoms of abdominal pain, obstipation, nausea, and increasing abdominal girth in addition to vomiting are sought. Other associated gastrointestinal symptoms may also include diarrhea, anorexia, flatulence, or frequent eructation with reflux. The suspicion of significant extra-abdominal organ system disease would be raised by neurologic symptoms, such as severe headache, stiff neck, blurred vision or diplopia, clumsiness, personality or school performance change, or persistent lethargy or irritability; by genitourinary symptoms such as flank pain, dysuria, urgency and frequency or ammenorrhea; or by common infectious symptoms such as fever or respiratory complaints.

The appearance of the vomitus (by history and inspection when a specimen is available) is often helpful in establishing the site of pathology. Undigested food or milk should suggest reflux from the esophagous or stomach due to lesions such as esophageal atresia (in the neonate), gastroesophageal reflux, or pyloric stenosis. Bilious vomitus suggests obstruction distal to the ampulla of Vater, although it is occasionally seen with prolonged vomiting of any cause when there is relaxation of the pylorus. Fecal material in the vomitus is seen with obstruction of the lower bowel. Hematemesis usually reflects a bleeding site in the upper GI tract; its evaluation is detailed in Chapter 22 (p. 160).

PHYSICAL EXAMINATION

The physical examination is directed first toward evaluating the overall degree of toxicity. (Does the baby look septic? Is there the unconsolable irritability of meningitis? Does the child exhibit the bent-over posture, apprehensive look, and pained avoidance of unnecessary movement typical of peritoneal irritation in appendicitis?) Then attention is aimed at the abdomen. Are there signs of obstruction such as ill-defined tenderness, distension, high-pitched bowel sounds (or absent sounds in ileus), or visible peristalsis?

The diverse nature of etiologies for vomiting make a "routine" laboratory or radiologic screen impossible. The history and physical must guide the approach in individual patients. Some well-defined clinical pictures demand urgent radiologic workup (e.g., abdominal pain and bilious vomiting in a child requires supine and upright plain films and a limited upper gastrointestinal series for evaluation of congenital obstructive anomalies such as malrotation; or a child with paroxysms of colicky abdominal pain and grossly bloody, mucousy stools requires immediate flat and upright abdominal films and usually a barium enema for the likely diagnosis of intussusception). Other situations require no x-rays (e.g., a typical case of viral gastroenteritis, or a classic history for pyloric stenosis with definite palpation of the pyloric tumor). In many cases, body fluid cultures or serum chemical analyses will be essential for making a diagnosis (meningitis, aspirin toxicity, Reye's syndrome, pregnancy); for the majority of straightforward common illnesses (gastroenteritis, cold with postnasal mucous drip), laboratory investigation is unwarranted.

Approach to Children by Age Groups

With these introductory concepts in mind, we can approach the differential diagnosis of the principal causes of vomiting on an age-related basis. An algorithm for such an approach utilizing the key clinical features outlined above is illustrated in Figure 41.1.

NEONATES

A careful history should focus on the perinatal events, onset and duration of vomiting, nature of the vomitus, associated gastrointestinal symptoms and the presence of symptoms referable to other organ systems. Newborn babies with the onset of vomiting in the first days of life should always be suspect for one of the common *congenital gastrointestinal anomalies* which cause obstruction, such as intestinal atresia, malrotation, meconium ileus, or Hirschsprung's disease. If the vomiting is bilious, bright yellow or green, an urgent surgical consultation is required. In the vast majority of cases, a serious and possibly life-threatening mechanical obstruction will be the cause of bilious vomiting. All patients in whom the possibility of gastrointestinal obstruction is entertained must have immediate flat and upright abdominal films. Other clinical features, such as toxicity and lethargy, usually attest to the length of time of the obstruction and its severity. Most neonates with a congenital basis for their bowel obstruction will present during their initial nursery stay. It will be uncommon, therefore, to see such babies for the first time in the emergency department.

Other serious causes of neonatal vomiting which may present to the emergency department include: infection, such as meningitis, sepsis, pyelonephritis, or necrotizing enterocolitis (it should be noted that such serious infections are often not accompanied by fever in the neonate); increased intracranial pressure due to cerebral edema, subdural hematoma or hydrocephalus; metabolic acidosis or hyperammonemia due to the rare inborn errors of aminoacid and organic acid metabolism; and renal insufficiency or obstruction. Such infants usually appear ill, with associated lethargy and irritability; sometimes fever, a full fontanel, a diminished urinary stream, an abdominal mass, or respiratory signs will suggest the correct etiology. Obviously, any ill neonate with vomiting even in the absence of obstruction will also require hospitalization and prompt evaluation for sepsis, neurologic, renal, and metabolic disease.

Commonly, however, a young infant in the first 2 to 4 weeks of life who appears entirely well is brought to the emergency department with the complaint of persistent vomiting. The birth history and perinatal course are unremarkable. The baby has gained weight appropriately (usually 5 to 7 oz/week after the first week of life), is vigorous, and has an entirely normal physical examination. Usually a closer description of the "vomiting" (or even better, a

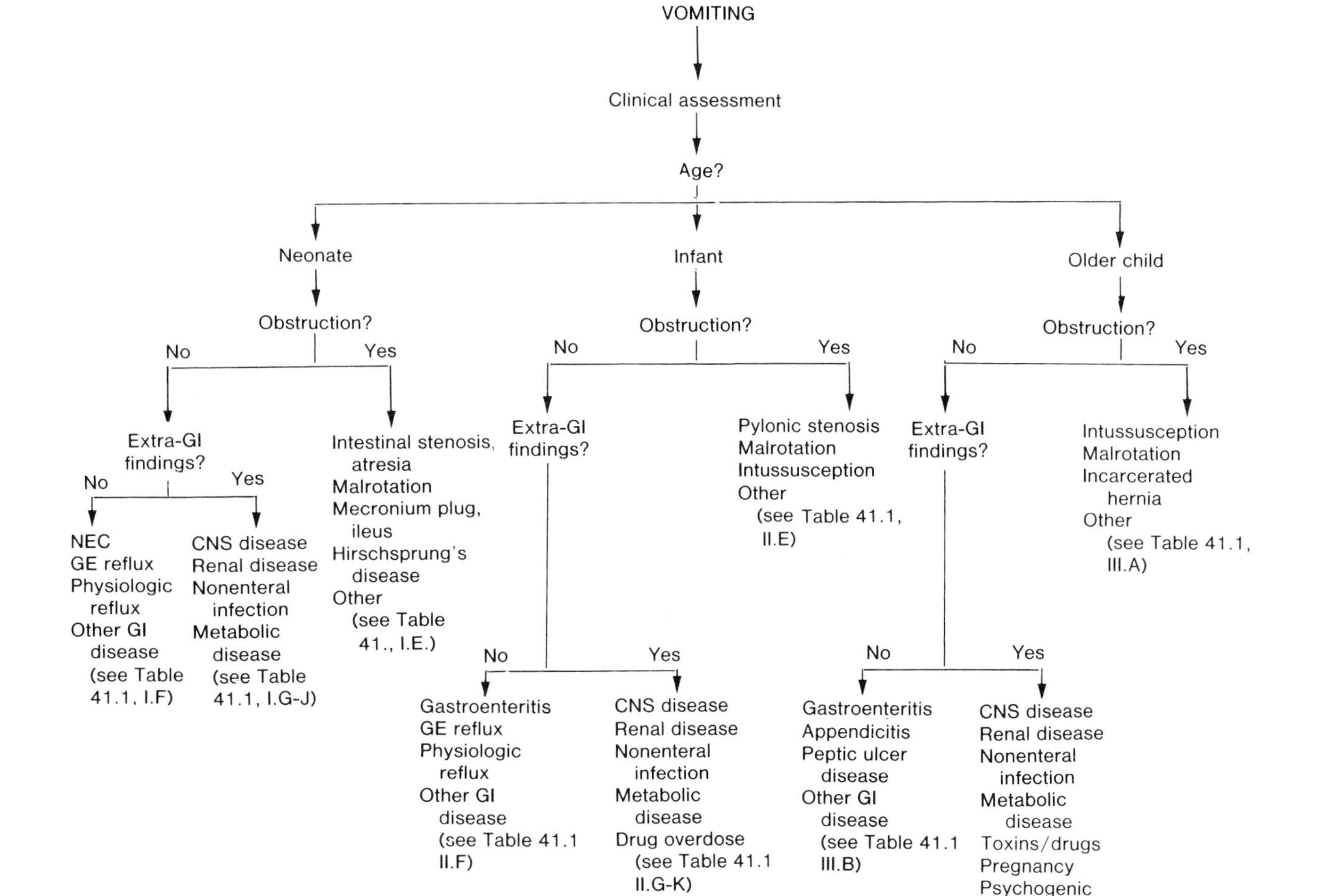

Figure 41.1 The diagnostic approach to vomiting. *GI* = gastrointestinal; *NEC* = necrotizing enterocolitis; *CNS* = central nervous system; *GE* = gastroesophageal.

trial feeding in the emergency department) reveals the problem to be *physiologic regurgitation,* or so-called "spitting up." This is a common and insignificant problem, probably representing some normal variation in maturation of cardioesophageal valve competence. These infants do not exhibit forceful abdominal contractions, but rather reflux milk into their mouths which dribbles out, usually when prone and often with a burp. The degree of reflux may be increased by improper feeding techniques such as failure to burp the baby, using nipples with holes that are too small, or bottle propping. Observation of a feeding trial and emphasis on good technique suffices for initial management of such babies. They should, like all newborns, be referred for ongoing pediatric care. Most babies outgrow such regurgitation by 6 to 9 months of age.

Other infants who regurgitate easily may not be so easily managed. Their course may be complicated by failure to thrive and recurrent aspiration pneumonia. Such infants are diagnosed as having the *gastroesophageal reflux syndrome (GE reflux)*, a more severe degree of cardioesophageal valve dysfunction. Barium swallow examination usually confirms the diagnosis and may reveal an associated hiatal hernia. Infants with GE reflux should be followed closely by a pediatrician. If they fail to improve on a vigorous medical regimen, they may require an antireflux surgical procedure.

OLDER INFANT

Infants presenting with vomiting after the first few weeks of life may still be manifesting intestinal obstruction, but the underlying etiologies are somewhat different than in the neonate. The important lesions responsible for mechanical obstruction in this age group include congenital hypertrophic pyloric stenosis, malrotation, intussusception, incarcerated hernia, enteric duplications, and complications of Meckel's diverticulum. Occasionally other anomalies that might be expected to present in the neonate, such as Hirschsprung's disease will appear only after several weeks or months of life. In all cases, these will have physical findings suggestive of intestinal obstruction and often specific for the level of obstruction. Having a high index of suspicion for both common and uncommon forms of intestinal obstruction is key to making a timely diagnosis.

The typical infant with *pyloric stenosis* (see Chapter 59, p 831) appears in the emergency department at 4 to 6 weeks of age with a chief complaint of projectile vomiting during or shortly after a feeding. Often a milder degree of vomiting will have been present for 1 to 2 weeks. The vomiting in pyloric stenosis is typically crescendo in nature, with increasing severity over days to weeks. By contrast, vomiting due to GE reflux tends to be relatively consistent over time; in malrotation, vomiting is sudden in onset or episodic. The vomitus is nonbilious, reflecting obstruction at the pylorus, and usually is voluminous, reflecting nearly the entire content of the feeding. The infant may become constipated if vomiting has been of sufficient duration. On examination an olive-sized mass can usually be palpated (most easily after vomiting has occurred) in the right upper quadrant to the right of the midline and just above the umbilicus. Peristaltic waves may be visualized moving from left upper to right upper quadrants again indicating obstruction at the pylorus. Unless the infant is significantly dehydrated, the child is usually vigorous and active although irritable due to hunger. The diagnosis of pyloric stenosis is a clinical one based on the typical history and palpation of the olive. Barium swallow x-ray, while helpful in atypical cases, is not necessary when the clinical findings are confirmed by surgical consultation.

Between 2 months and about 5 to 6 years of age, the most common cause of obstruction is *intussusception* (see Chapter 59, p 826). Most children develop this disorder between 3 months and 2 years of age. Early symptoms usually include paroxysms of colicky abdominal pain and vomiting, suggesting a gastrointestinal illness. Initially, the infant may appear relatively well between attacks, but some children will fall asleep or seem prostrate at these times. Initially, there may be a normal stool, but usually within 6 to 12 hours dark maroon blood is passed per rectum; this blood is often mixed with mucus earning the label of "currant jelly" stool. Some infants with intussusception, however, may present primarily with lethargy and decreased responsiveness, without striking gastrointestinal symptoms. Examination of the abdomen usually reveals a somewhat tender, sausage-shaped mass on the right side. The suspicion of intussusception mandates immediate surgical consultation and preparation of the patient for a possible laparotomy. Unless signs of peritonitis are present, a barium enema is usually indicated for diagnosis and often for therapy by hydrostatic reduction.

Other important causes of obstruction in the older infant include incarcerated inguinal hernia, volvulus, Hirschsprung's disease, or complications related to Meckel's diverticulum. The presence of an incarcerated hernia will be apparent on examination. Volvulus of the bowel will virtually always be associated with bilious vomiting. A good clue to diagnosis of Hirschsprung's disease is asking, "Has your child ever had a normal (unstimulated) bowel movement?" (see also Chapter 11, p. 103, and Chapter 59, p. 833). The obstructive complications of Meckel's diverticulum include intussusception and volvulus and have similar presentations to these types of obstruction due to other causes.

The principal nonobstructive causes of vomiting in the older infant include gastrointestinal, neurologic, renal, infectious, and metabolic disorders. Nonobstructive gastrointestinal disturbances are probably the most common cause for vomiting in this age group. *Viral gastroenteritis,* while usually manifesting predominantly as diarrhea associated with vomiting, will often begin with a prodromal phase of vomiting alone (Chapter 45, p. 388). Physical findings are usually limited to ill-defined and inconsistent abdominal pain and signs of a variable degree of dehydration. Vomiting in older infants will also be due at times to persistent GE reflux, as well as abdominal disorders uncommon in infancy, such as peptic ulcer disease or appendicitis. Occasionally vomiting is seen in paralytic ileus due to infection (pneumonia, peritonitis) or electrolyte disorders.

Neurologic causes of vomiting in infancy also include *mass lesions* such as tumor, abscess or intracranial hematoma (Chapter 44) as well as *meningitis* and *encephalitis.* There may be evidence of increased intracranial pressure: increasing head circumference, bulging fontanel, and split sutures before closure of the fontanel; papilledema is rarely noted during infancy. However, some brainstem tumors cause protracted vomiting by direct effect on the vomiting center without an accompanying increased pressure. Again, it is to be emphasized that meningism is rarely seen with meningitis in infancy, and that signs of increased intracranial pressure occur late (Chapter 45, p. 362). Early findings include fever, vomiting, lethargy and irritability, especially the paradoxic irritability of increased crying with parental fondling.

Infections outside the gastrointestinal and neurologic systems may cause vomiting in infants and occasionally in older children. The more important such infections are: otitis media, urinary tract infection, pertussis, and viral hepatitis. Positive physical findings on otoscopic examination are seen in otitis, along mild irritability, and often fever (Chapter 45, p. 368). Urinary infections may be surprisingly devoid of localizing signs and symptoms in preschool children (Chapter 63, p. 925); nonspecific gastrointestinal complaints including vomiting and abdominal pain, fever, irritability or anorexia may be the only presenting symptoms. Urinalysis and culture provide the specific diagnosis. Vomiting is also a common event after the paroxysms of coughing seen in infants with pertussis (Chapter 45, p. 386). It is a frequent symptom in the prodromal phase of infectious hepatitis, usually preceding the onset of jaundice (Chapter 50, p. 577). Abnormal liver function tests substantiate this latter diagnosis.

Renal and metabolic disorders also cause vomiting in the older infant. Renal failure (see p. 450), renal tubular acidosis (see p. 434) or rarely, diabetic ketoacidosis (see p. 632), may be seen in this age group. Hypoadrenalism (see p. 640), hepatic failure (see p. 578), Reye's syndrome (see p. 567), and inborn errors of metabolism such as galactosemia and fructose intolerance also may occur in infancy and have vomiting as a prominent symptom.

Occasionally parental overzealous use of over-the-counter or prescribed drugs in infants will lead to intoxication. Drugs which often produce vomiting in excessive doses include aspirin, theophylline, and digoxin; all of these intoxications are easily verified by associated signs and symptoms and specific drug levels. The problem of accidental ingestion is discussed below.

An additional rare cause of regurgitation or vomiting in infants, with onset usually at 6 to 12 months of age, is rumination (Chapter 72, p. 1145). This severe psychiatric disorder of infancy, though related to abnormal maternal-infant relationship, may progress to severe failure to thrive and death. These infants seem to self-induce the reflux, often by gagging themselves, and often appear to partially rechew and reswallow their vomitus.

OLDER CHILD

Many of the causes of intestinal obstruction and other important gastrointestinal diseases described in neonates and older infants may occasionally first appear in the older child (e.g. volvulus associated with malrotation and/or abnormal mesenteric attachments, Hirschsprung's disease, a meconium ileus "equivalent" in the child with cystic fibrosis, or an incarcerated hernia). Additionally, older children are often subject to blunt abdominal trauma; persistent vomiting after such injury may reflect obstruction due to a duodenal intramural hematoma or ileus secondary to pancreatitis. Gastroenteritis, as in infants, continues to be the most common cause of vomiting in the older child seen in the emergency department. Two entities that usually occur in older children, appendicitis and peptic ulcers, will be discussed here, although they also occur rarely in infancy.

Appendicitis (Chapter 59, p. 822) in a preadolescent child typically begins with periumbilical crampy abdominal pain, followed by vomiting within 1 to 2 hours. Then the pain shifts to the right lower quadrant, and fever develops. Younger children may deviate from this pattern by exhibiting less specific symptoms early in their illness and a more rapid progression to perforation and generalized peritonitis. As peritoneal irritation becomes well established, the child attempts to minimize any motion to his abdomen. Physical examination usually reveals localized involuntary right lower quadrant tenderness which may be easier to elicit by asking the child to cough, or hop on one foot. In addition, there may be rebound and referred rebound tenderness, and a tender fullness high on the right during rectal examination. Atypical positions of the appendix (e.g. retrocecal, retroilial, or pelvic) will be reflected in atypical areas of maximal tenderness, as well as confusing symptoms such as diarrhea or dysuria (due to appendiceal inflammation adjacent to colon or ureter/bladder). Pertinent laboratory findings include leukocytosis with a left shift in the differential count. The urinalysis is usually normal. Occasionally, in an atypical patient, abdominal x-rays may be helpful in showing a right lower quadrant fecalith, localized obstruction, and mass effect, as well as lumbar spine scoliosis.

Vomiting as a symptom of *peptic ulcer disease* in children is usually seen in association with abdominal pain (Chapter 50, p. 560). In young children, the pain is often nonspecific and not easily related to meals. In adolescents, the pattern becomes more classically related to food or antacids. There may be hematemesis and/or melena. The abdominal examination may be normal or reveal mild to moderate epigastric tenderness. A strong clinical suspicion of peptic ulcer disease should be confirmed with an upper gastrointestinal series and, at times, endoscopy.

Genitourinary causes of vomiting in the older child include urinary tract infection and obstructive urologic disease. An important additional concern in adolescent girls is early pregnancy (Chapter 29, p. 198). It is very common for such patients to visit the emergency department with the chief complaint of persistent vomiting (not necessarily only in the morning) for several weeks, and often there will be initial denial of sexual activity and/or amenorrhea. Physical findings at this stage of pregnancy may be subtle. Thus, prolonged vomiting in a postmenarchal girl should be pursued with the appropriate urine or serum gonadotropin assays (Chapter 29, p. 198).

The important extragastrointestinal infectious diseases of the older child causing vomiting have for the most part been discussed above under neonatal and infantile headings. Serious infections localize symptoms more readily in this older age group. Meningitis is usually accompanied by meningism after the age of 2 years, and urinary infections tend to present with dysuria, frequency and urgency as children approach school age. The toddler or school-age child may also vomit with pharyngeal irritation due to postnasal mucous drip from an upper respiratory infection.

Neurologic disease causing vomiting in the older child again represents primarily lesions causing increased intracranial pressure or direct irritation of the medullary vomiting center; they usually lead to papilledema and/or abnormal neurologic findings on examination. One important exception is childhood migraine (Chapter 44, p. 341). Preadolescent children do not usually manifest the classic migraine picture with aura, hemicranial headache, and scotomas. More often, they complain of relatively infrequent but quite severe, poorly localized headaches accompanied by nausea and vomiting and followed by sleep. The physical examination between attacks is usually normal. Another common but quite minor form of vomiting on a neurologic basis (due to labyrinthine stimulation) would be the propensity to motion sickness.

Metabolic aberrations, including hepatic, renal, and adrenal failure, all may cause vomiting in the older child as well as during infancy. Ketoacidosis presenting for the first time in an as yet undiagnosed diabetic occurs more commonly in older children, especially at school entrance age and later as adolescence begins (Chapter 53 p. 632). Vomiting may be the chief complaint of such children, although careful questioning usually uncovers a preceding 3- to 4-week history of polyuria, polyphagia, and polydipsia, and, at times, weight loss. A fruity breath odor, dehydration, hyperpnea, and varying degree of altered sensorium are typically present, and a urinalysis and serum glucose determination confirm the diagnosis of diabetic ketoacidosis.

The other important cause of vomiting to be emphasized here is *Reye's syndrome* (Chapter 50 p. 567). Although it may occur at any age, it tends to be seen more commonly in toddlers and school-age children. Typically, these children have had a preceding viral illness within the past 2 weeks (especially varicella and influenza) from which they have just recovered, or are recovering at the time of presentation. There is generally about 24 hours of severe, recurrent vomiting, followed immediately by progression through the varying stages of encephalopathy. Physical examination at the time of vomiting, prior to onset of encephalopathy, may be normal or show only hepatomegaly. Thus, it is crucial to pursue laboratory evidence of hepatic dysfunction in any child who raises the slightest suspicion of early Reye's syndrome, such as the patient with persistent vomiting in association with recent influenza-like syndromes or varicella, or persistent vomiting with even the mildest change in sensorium toward obtundation and/or delirium. Abnormal laboratory data in Reye's syndrome include elevated serum transaminase and ammonia, prolonged prothrombin time, and often hypoglycemia; however, bilirubin is usually normal, making other forms of severe liver disease very unlikely.

In the discussion regarding older infants, mention was made of occasional inadvertent drug overdosage by parents, causing intoxication-related vomiting. In children 1 to 3 years of age, accidental ingestion becomes a frequent problem. Acute poisonings that cause vomiting as a prominent symptom include aspirin, theophylline, digoxin, and iron sulfate (Chapter 48). Chronic lead poisoning also occurs in this pica prone age group. Early symptoms of lead intoxication are vomiting, colicky abdominal pain, anorexia, constipation, and irritability. Tragically, many such youngsters have been diagnosed as having nonspecific gastroenteritis syndromes initially, only to return days to weeks later with frank encephalopathy and ultimately severe neurologic sequelae. The history of pica and lead-paint exposure (peeling paint chips, especially in homes dating back to the 1940s and 1950s) should be sought in every toddler with persistent vomiting. The diagnosis of plumbism can be confirmed with elevated blood levels of lead and erythrocyte protoporphyrins.

Finally, the school-age child or adolescent may vomit on a psychologic basis. Acutely, brief episodes of vomiting may occur with any emotionally disturbing event. Children with school phobia or other significant psychiatric problem may vomit persistently. Before attributing the vomiting to a psychologic cause, a careful history, general examination, and complete neurologic examination will be necessary to minimize the likelihood of missing any organic etiology. An assessment of disturbed family dynamics, prior history of emotional disorders or evidence of depression and/or anxiety during the emergency department interview may corroborate the suspicion of vomiting on a psychologic basis and warrant a psychiatric referral.

References

Gryboski J: *Gastrointestinal Problems in the Infant*. W. B. Saunders, Philadelphia, 1975.

Roy CC, Silverman A, Cozzetto FJ: *Pediatric Clinical Gastroenterology*. C. V. Mosby, St. Louis, 1975.

(*Note:* See also Chapters 50 and 59 for references on specific disease entities.)

CHAPTER 42

Weakness

EDWARD CHARNEY, M.D.

INTRODUCTION

There are a large number of diagnostic considerations for the previously well child who presents to the emergency department complaining of recent onset of weakness or diminished muscle strength. One's initial diagnostic approach may vary considerably, depending upon specific clinical and historical features. This chapter will limit its discussion to the assessment of the child presenting with a sudden onset of severe weakness and associated flaccidity.

Flaccid paralysis marked by the inability to move one or several extremities voluntarily against gravity with absent or diminished deep tendon reflexes is characteristic of a lower motor neuron disease process affecting either the anterior horn cells, peripheral axons, neuromuscular junction, or muscle fibers. Upper motor disease affecting structures extending from the cerebral cortex to but not including the anterior horn cell, is characterized by increased tendon reflexes and spasticity; however, early in the clinical course there may be flaccid paralysis. Processes causing flaccid paralysis can be categorized into five general pathologic groups including: traumatic, infectious, toxic, metabolic and vascular (Table 42.1). Within each group there are several specific illnesses that may be identified in an emergency department after recognition of characteristic clinical courses, physical examinations, and laboratory results.

EVALUATION AND DECISION

Information most helpful in the critical assessment of the child with sudden paralysis can be discovered in a detailed history, with particular attention to trauma, toxic exposures, prodromal illness, and family history, and a physical examination, noting distribution of paralysis, associated cranial nerve weaknesses, and sensory changes. These clinical features guide the diagnostic approach as outlined in Figure 42.1.

Historical features pertinent to the acute onset of weakness include obvious trauma or toxin exposure, which direct the emergency physician immediately to the likely cause. A history of fever and/or viral prodromal illness is important in identifying the infectious and parainfectious etiologies. The past medical history is often notable for previous episodes of weakness in the metabolic and vascular disorders, and there may be a positive family history in some of these diseases (e.g., periodic paralyses, sickle cell disease).

Physical examination should concentrate on the neurologic findings. The distribution of paralysis will help to localize the site of pathology, as will any associated cranial nerve or sensory changes.

Laboratory workup must be individualized, as detailed below in the discussion of the important disorders causing acute onset of weakness. Patients with trauma will need x-rays of the spine, and those with hemi-

Table 42.1
Causes of Sudden Flaccid Paralysis

Traumatic
Vertebral fracture and/or dislocation with severe trauma
Mild trauma in patients with predisposing illness
Toxic
Tick paralysis
Botulism
Diphtheria
Infectious and Parainfectious
Guillain-Barré
Poliomyelitis
Transverse myelitis
Epidural abscess
Metabolic
Hypokalemia and hyperkalemia
Rhabdomyolysis
Acute intermittent porphyria
Vascular
Sickle cell disease
Congenital heart disease
Vascular malformations
Coagulopathy

paresis will usually require CT scanning. A lumbar puncture is indicated in the evaluation of the infectious and parainfectious disorders. Blood and urine for potassium, porphyrins or myoglobin determinations may occasionally be needed for the rare metabolic conditions discussed below.

Trauma

Traumatic fracture or dislocation of vertebrae may result in sudden paralysis, with either a complete or partial transection of the spinal cord. The trauma is often severe (i.e., motor vehicle accident, football injury); however, it may be mild, particularly in children with Down's syndrome or juvenile rheumatoid arthritis in whom there may be an associated cervical vertebral instability. Cord transections often result in both paralysis and sensory loss below the level of the lesion along with bladder and rectal incontinence. Radiographic studies demonstrating these vertebral changes should be done with care while immobilizing the child's neck.

Infectious

There are four major infectious or parainfectious diseases associated with acute flaccid paralysis. The most common of these is Guillain-Barré syndrome with its cellular infiltration and edema of the nerve roots, sensory ganglia, and peripheral nerves. Patients typically develop paralysis following either a nonspecific illness or a specific illness such as infectious mononucleosis. Flaccid paralysis is often acute in onset and symmetrical in distribution and ascends upward over a several hour to several day period. Sensory changes, if present, are generally less severe than the motor weakness. At a particular time in its clinical course, Guillain-Barré syndrome has the classic albumin-cytotologic dissociation with elevation of CSF protein (>60 mg/100 ml) without pleocytosis (<10 WBC/mm^3).

Poliomyelitis, one of the most common causes of acute flaccid paralysis in the preimmunization years, has an asymmetrical paralysis and associated signs of meningeal irritation such as nuchal rigidity and positive Kernig and Brudzinski signs. Sensory examination is normal and associated neurologic deficits follow the viral-induced pathologic processes in spinal cord gray matter, medulla, cerebrum, and cerebellum. There is CSF protein elevation and pleocytosis. In transverse myelitis, areas of inflammation and infarction in the spinal cord result in a clinical picture of flaccid paralysis in both legs along with rectal and bladder incontinence. There is also prominent sensory loss for pain and temperature. The exact relationship between antecedent viral illnesses and transverse myelitis is not well understood, even though there is frequently a several day history of fever, malaise, and myalgia prior to the onset of paralysis. There is often CSF protein elevation and pleocytosis.

Paralysis from an epidural abscess is generally not ascending in nature and frequently is associated with tenderness over adjacent vertebrae from pressure necrosis of the spinal cord. Hematogenous spread of staphylococci from an adjacent carbuncle or vertebral osteomyelitis may initiate development of the abscess. Lumbar puncture

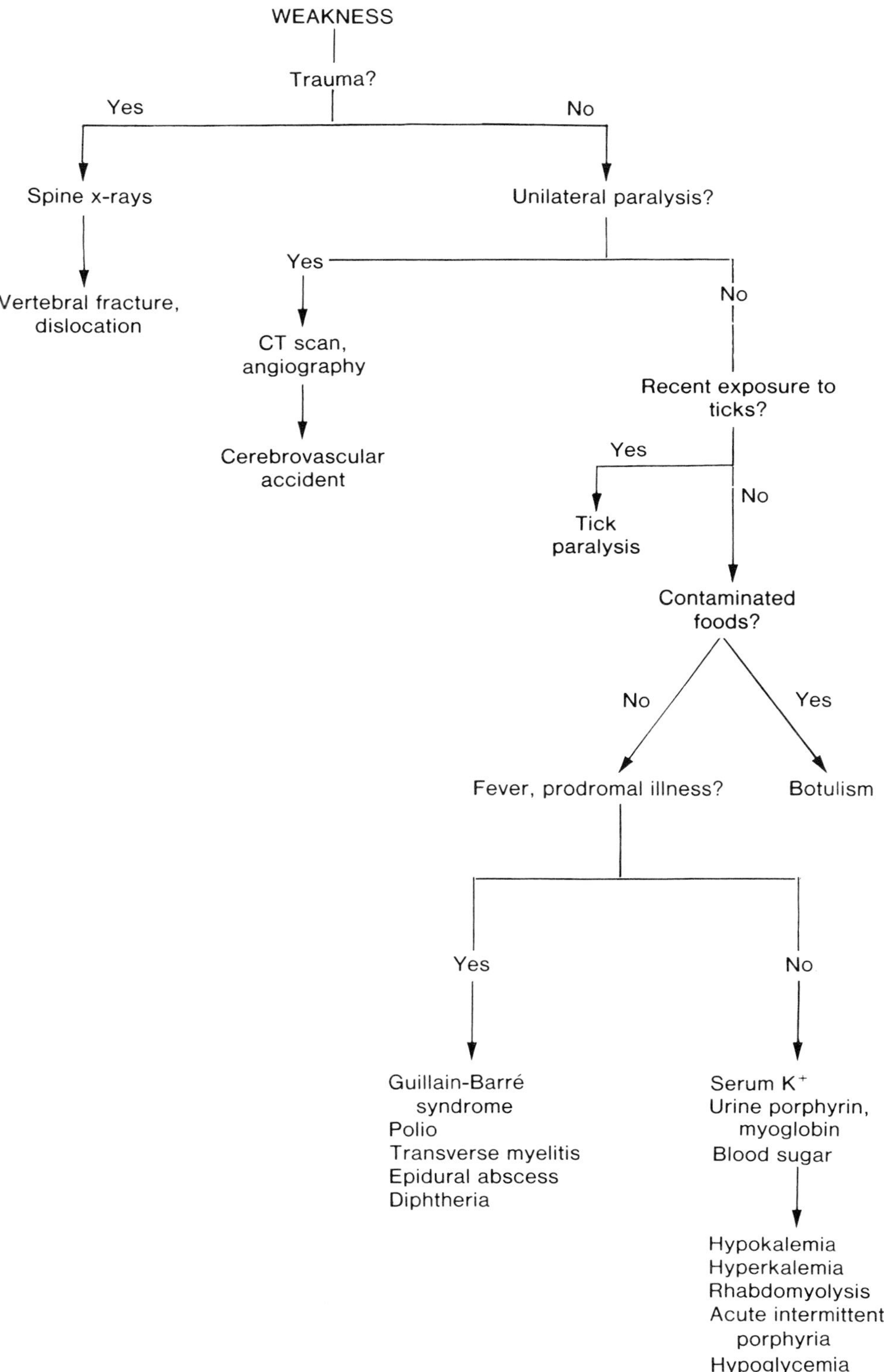

Figure 42.1 Diagnostic approach to acute onset of severe weakness.

in a child with an epidural abscess might reveal a complete subarachnoid block or CSF with marked pleocytosis and protein elevation.

Toxic

Toxins that can cause acute onset of flaccid paralysis include those derived from ticks, *Clostridium botulinum* and *Corynebacterium diphtheriae*. Both the dog tick (*Dermacentor variabilis*) and wood tick (*Dermacentor andersoni*) produce a toxin that results in an ascending flaccid paralysis similar to that observed in Guillain-Barré syndrome. *D. andersoni* is found primarily in the Rocky Mountain states and north into Canada, while *D. variabilis* is in the Southeastern United States. The toxin released prevents liberation of acetylcholine at nerve endings, and the paralysis occurs relatively rapidly with complete ascent to the bulbar area within 12 to 36 hours. Sensory changes tend to be minimal. Removal of the tick from the child's body results in dramatic and complete improvement. Tick paralysis, although not commonly encountered, should be considered in the differential diagnosis, particularly in spring and summer months of the endemic areas, when ticks are most active in their warm environment. Exposure to the tick often precedes the paralysis by 5 to 10 days, and therefore travel history is important.

C. botulinum toxin from contaminated food also produces paralysis by preventing release of acetylcholine at the myoneural junction. Accompanying symptoms of blurred vision, loss of accommodation, and diplopia usually occur within 24 to 48 hours after toxin exposure. A history of recently ingesting contaminated food and/or improperly canned food in a child with extremity paralysis accompanied by diplopia, dysphagia, and dysarthria is most suggestive of botulism from the *C. botulinum* toxin. If respiratory failure appears imminent on either clinical examination or pulmonary function tests, botulism antitoxin should be administered immediately. Definitive diagnosis of botulism may be made with EMG and stool culture. The toxin of *C. diphtheriae* frequently produces extraocular muscle weakness with squint and ptosis, and palatal paralysis with swallowing difficulties prior to the onset of limb paralysis. A latency period of 1 week to months exists between the exudative pharyngitis and paralysis. The toxic effects of *C. diphtheriae* should be suspected in a child with acute flaccid paralysis, stocking glove sensory loss, ptosis, and dysphagia who has not received adequate immunizations and has a history of exudative pharyngitis within the past 2 months. ECG in such a child might also document coexisting myocarditis.

Metabolic

Metabolic disturbances associated with acute onset of flaccid paralysis include: hypokalemia and hyperkalemia, rhabdomyolysis with myoglobinuria, and acute intermittent porphyria. Myopathic changes are present in the former two, whereas neuropathic changes exist in the latter one. Periodic attacks of paralysis caused by hypokalemia may be associated with: an autosomal dominant familial disorder, hyperthyroidism, hyperaldosteronism, chronic renal disease, ingestion of large amounts of licorice, or chronic vomiting or diarrhea. The familial form often presents in adolescence with sudden paralysis that may involve all the extremities after either a large carbohydrate meal or during rest following strenuous exercise. Sensory examination is normal. Autosomal dominant familial hyperkalemic paralysis is usually less severe. ECG is helpful for confirming both hypokalemia and hyperkalemia, and improvement of paralysis should ensue after intravenous correction of the potassium imbalance.

Myoglobinuria with sudden paralysis may result from excessive physical exertion, mild infection, or genetic disorders. If no specific etiologies are identified, then the clinical picture of acute paralysis with laboratory evidence of myoglobinuria is referred to as idiopathic rhabdomyolysis. Elevation of muscle enzymes in serum (creatine phosphokinase (CPK), serum glutamic-oxaloacetic transaminase (SGOT)) and evidence of myoglobinuria suggest abdomyolysis. Acute intermittent por-ıyria with abnormal excretion of por-ıyrin precursors is a rare autosomal dom-ant familial cause of flaccid paralysis. As-ciated abdominal pain and disturbances mentation and personality may be pres-ıt. Acute attacks can be precipitated by ugs such as barbiturates, sulfonamides, iseofulvin, estrogens, and alcohol.

Vascular

Sudden paralysis from infarction or hem-rrhage is unusual in childhood. These vents may occur with vascular anomalies f the spinal cord or brain, hemoglobinop-thies, coagulopathies, or cyanotic heart isease. Paralysis secondary to hemorrhage om a spinal cord vascular anomaly is often receded by pain in the back or abdomen ith sudden loss of all sensation and move-ıent. Cerebrovascular accidents associated ith sickle cell disease or cyanotic heart isease often result in hemiplegia, while pinal cord hemorrhage and paralysis in a hild with hemophilia may follow minor ack trauma. Unilateral paralysis of a child ithout the history of trauma is most con-istent with a cerebral vascular accident econdary either to CNS infection, sickle ell thrombotic crisis, embolic phenomena f congenital heart disease, AV malforma-ion, or idiopathic occlusive vascular dis-ase. The clinical suspicion of cerebrovascular accident can be confirmed by both CT scan and cerebral angiography.

In summary, the child with acute onset of flaccid paralysis should be evaluated for trauma, vascular accidents, infectious processes, toxin exposure or metabolic disturbances. Recognition of associated sensory disturbances and cranial nerve involvement are helpful in the diagnostic approach, along with a detailed history and emergency department procedures including lumbar puncture, spine x-rays, urinalysis, serum electrolytes, and ECG. Although dramatic recovery or improvement may result from emergency department management, the majority of children will require therapy in the hospital.

References

Ahmann P, et al.: Spinal infarctions due to minor trauma in children. *Neurology* 25: 301, 1975.

Fenichel GM, Swaiman KF, Wright FS, Spiro AJ: Neuromuscular disease. In *The Practice of Pediatric Neurology,* p. 927, edited by KW Swaiman and FS Wright. C. V. Mosby, St. Louis, 1975.

Gutman L, Pratt L: Pathophysiologic aspects of human botulism, *Arch Neurol* 33: 175, 1976.

Lagos, JC: *Differential Diagnosis in Pediatric Neurology.* Little, Brown, Boston, 1971

Markland LD, Riley HD Jr: The Guillain-Barré syndrome in childhood. *Clin Pediatr* 6: 162, 1967.

Paine RS, Byers RK: Transverse myelopathy in childhood. *Am J Dis Child* 85: 151, 1953.

Pearson CM, Kalyanaraman K: The periodic paralysis. In *The Metabolic Basis of Inherited Disease,* Ed. 3, edited by JB Stanbury, JB Wyngaard, DS Fredrickson. McGraw-Hill, New York, 1972.

SECTION III **Medical Emergencies**

CHAPTER 43

Cardiac Emergencies

MICHAEL H. GEWITZ, M.D., AND VICTORIA L. VETTER, M.D.

Congestive Heart Failure

BACKGROUND

Heart failure is best described as a syndrome in which the heart cannot maintain a level of tissue perfusion adequate to meet metabolic needs. In childhood, these needs also include growth and development. In this chapter we will outline the primary etiologic and physiologic factors which underlie the clinical presentation of the child in "congestive heart failure" and which influence management decisions.

Etiologic Considerations

Although the primary cause of congestive heart failure (CHF) in infancy and childhood is congenital heart disease, a panoply of conditions can be associated with the presentation of CHF in the presence of normal underlying cardiac structure. Table 43.1 lists the more common clinical entities associated with CHF, including both primary cardiac disease and conditions in which the heart is secondarily affected. In general, the principal physiologic problems which lead to impaired myocardial performance include: (1) excessive pressure loads such as with left heart obstruction; (2) excessive volume loads, such as with large left-to-right shunts, valvar regurgitation, or severe anemia; (3) primary inotropic depression such as with myocarditis, endocrinologic disorders, or coronary perfusion irregularities; and (4) rhythm abnormalities such as supraventricular tachycardia or severe forms of heart block.

In determining the cause of CHF, the history is critical and should not be glossed over in the rush to treat. Knowledge of preexisting cardiac disease is obviously important. A history of known hematologic disorders such as thalassemia or sickle cell anemia should also be elicited. Since heart failure can develop as a consequence of pressure overload of the right heart secondary to pulmonary vasoconstriction and hypoxia, a history of respiratory tract difficulties or breathing pattern irregularities should also be sought.

Table 43.1
Etiologic Considerations for Congestive Heart Failure

Congenital Heart Disease	Acquired Heart Disease	Endocrine/Metabolic	Other
1. Pressure overload: —Ventricular outflow obstruction (e.g., aortic stenosis; severe coarctation) —Left ventricular inflow obstruction (e.g., cor triatriatum) 2. Volume overload: —Left-to-right shunts (e.g., ventricular septal defect) —Anomalous pulmonary venous return —Valvar regurgitation (e.g., aortic insufficiency) —Arteriovenous fistulas 3. Other structural disease —Anomalous coronary artery —Traumatic injury 4. Rhythm disturbance —Supraventricular tachycardia —Complete heart block 5. Postoperative heart disease —Malfunctioning prosthetic valve	1. Myocarditis: —Viral infections —Kawasaki syndrome —Collegen vascular disease 2. Cardiomyopathy —Chronic anemia (e.g., thalassemia major) —Storage diseases 3. Pericardial disease 4. Rheumatic heart disease 5. Cor pulmonale —Acute (e.g., upper airway obstruction) —Cystic fibrosis —Neuropathies 6. Endocarditis	1. Hypoglycemia 2. Chronic anemia or acute blood loss 3. Sepsis 4. Calcium or magnesium disorders 5. Electrolyte disturbances	1. Ingestions —Cardiac toxins (e.g., digitalis) —Arrhythmogenics (e.g., tricyclic antidepressants)

With the appropriate physical findings and historical information, the diagnosis is usually evident in the older child. The principal problem of diagnosis centers on the infant in whom differentiation between CHF and primary respiratory tract disease can be difficult. Auscultation of cardiac murmurs is helpful, of course, but such murmurs may not always be audible, particularly in severe failure with low output. Parenchymal lung disease may result in systemic desaturation to the same degree as CHF with associated pulmonary congestion and ventilation-perfusion imbalance. Palpation of the liver edge below the costal margin in an infant may be related to hyperexpansion of the lungs and not to systemic venous congestion. Conversely, respiratory tract signs such as wheezing and retractions may be part of the clinical picture of heart failure in the absence of primary lung disease. The chest x-ray often fails to distinguish between cardiac and pulmonary disease since pulmonary markings often mimic infiltrative patterns. Generally, however, evidence of cardiac enlargement on the x-ray is a useful differential point. Other noninvasive methods, such as echocardiography, can also help to establish the diagnosis of cardiac disease

PATHOPHYSIOLOGY

There are four primary determinants of normal cardiac function, each of which may relate to the development of heart failure. (1) *Preload*, the volume at enddiastole which must be ejected by the left ventricle, closely reflects the intravascular volume status of the child in general and directly affects cardiac performance via the Frank-Starling relationship. (2) *Afterload*, the opposing force to ventricular ejection, relates to the tension that must be developed by the myocardium in order to eject a given preload. (3) *Contractility* can be viewed as an intrinsic property of cardiac muscle which permits the alterations in cardiac shape necessary for ejection and which is determined by fundamental properties of cardiac ultrastructure. (4) *Heart rate* (HR) is related both to intrinsic electrophysiologic capabilities of the specialized cardiac conduction system and to supervening neurologic input. It is directly related to cardiac output (CO) through the classic relationship: CO = HR × SV (stroke volume).

Compensatory Responses

In order to understand the basis for the clinical findings commonly associated with CHF, attention must be directed to the physiologic responses to inadequate cardiac function. These include *mechanical* effects, such as ventricular hypertrophy and ventricular dilatation; *neurohumoral* effects, principally involving the adrenergic nervous system; *biochemical effects* at the cardiac cellular level which alter myocardial energy metabolism and the excitation-contraction coupling process; and *hematologic* effects involving oxygen transport. Additionally, *pulmonary* responses including increased respiratory frequency and altered respiratory patterns also make up an important part of the clinical picture of CHF.

CLINICAL FINDINGS

The clinical manifestations of CHF are directly related to the above noted compensatory mechanisms:

1. *Cardiac enlargement* is usually the result of ventricular dilatation. While it may often be possible to detect cardiac enlargement by displacement of the cardiac impulse, the chest x-ray remains the most readily available method for assessing ventricular dilatation (Fig. 43.1). The other preeminent finding related to mechanical compensatory responses is ventricular hypertrophy which is easily distinguishable on the ECG (Fig. 43.2). As a compensatory mechanism, hypertrophy occurs before dilatation in pressure overload situations, whereas dilatation may occur first in volume overload of the heart. As a general rule, the cardiac size is a reliable guide to the overall fluid volume status of the infant or child.

2. *Tachycardia*, a heart rate of more than 160 in an infant or 100 in the older child, is easily detected clinically and confirmed by the ECG. This sign is a manifes-

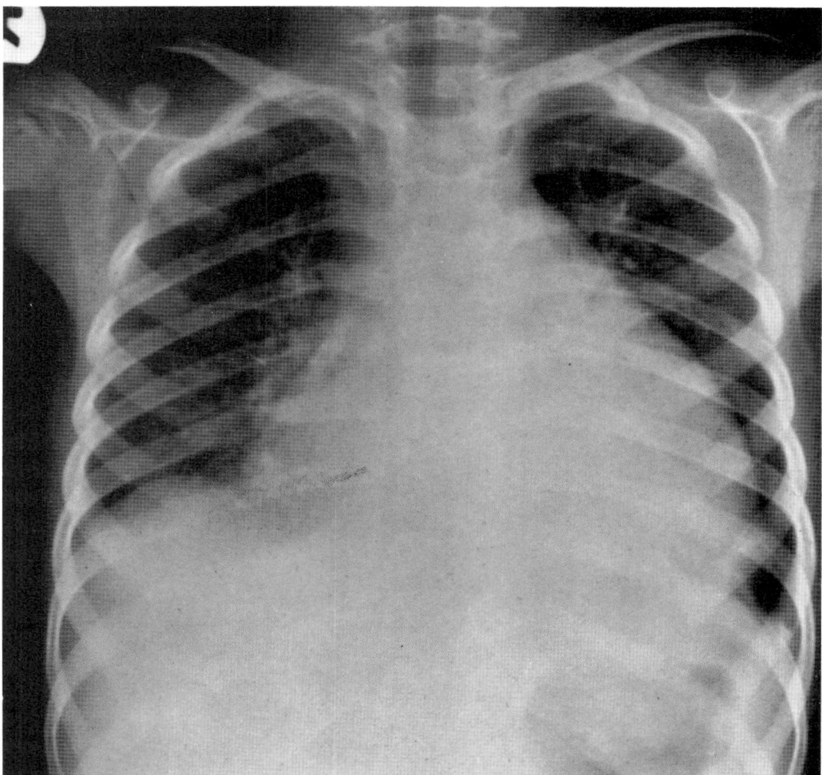

igure 43.1 Chest x-ray of child with congestive heart failure. Note cardiac enlargement and vidence of pulmonary venous congestion.

ation of increased adrenergic tone and :atecholamine release that is part of the ıeurohumoral response to diminished car- liac output.

3. Abnormalities of cardiac auscultation ıre also frequently present. The protodia- ;tolic *gallop*, or third heart sound (S_3), is ı manifestation of decreased ventricular :ompliance and increased resistance to fill- ng. Less frequently, the fourth heart sound, ›r atrial gallop (S_4), can be heard in chil- lren. It should be noted that these auscu- atory events can be normal findings in :hildhood, and thus the entire clinical pic- ure must be evaluated before defining their ;ignificance in any particular situation.

4. Respiratory responses, notably *tachy- nea*, are usually present as part of the ›icture of CHF. Frequently, rales, rhonchi ınd wheezing may be heard and should not ›e confused as signs of pulmonary paren- chymal disease rather than heart failure. In contrast, it is not unusual, particularly in infants, for rales to be absent despite the presence of tachypnea or wheezing, since experimental evidence indicates that considerable alveolar fluid accumulation is necessary for the development of rales. Thus, the presence of rales usually implies severe failure in an infant while pulmonary interstitial fluid collection, which occurs at an earlier stage, may be represented by tachypnea and wheezing alone. In older children, *dyspnea* with activity and *orthopnea* may also be present. A chronic *cough* also can be a sign of pulmonary congestion associated with CHF and not primary lung disease. Associated with these findings are chest *retractions*, reflecting the large negative intrathoracic pressures needed to ventilate stiff, fluid filled lungs.

5. *Growth failure and undernutrition*

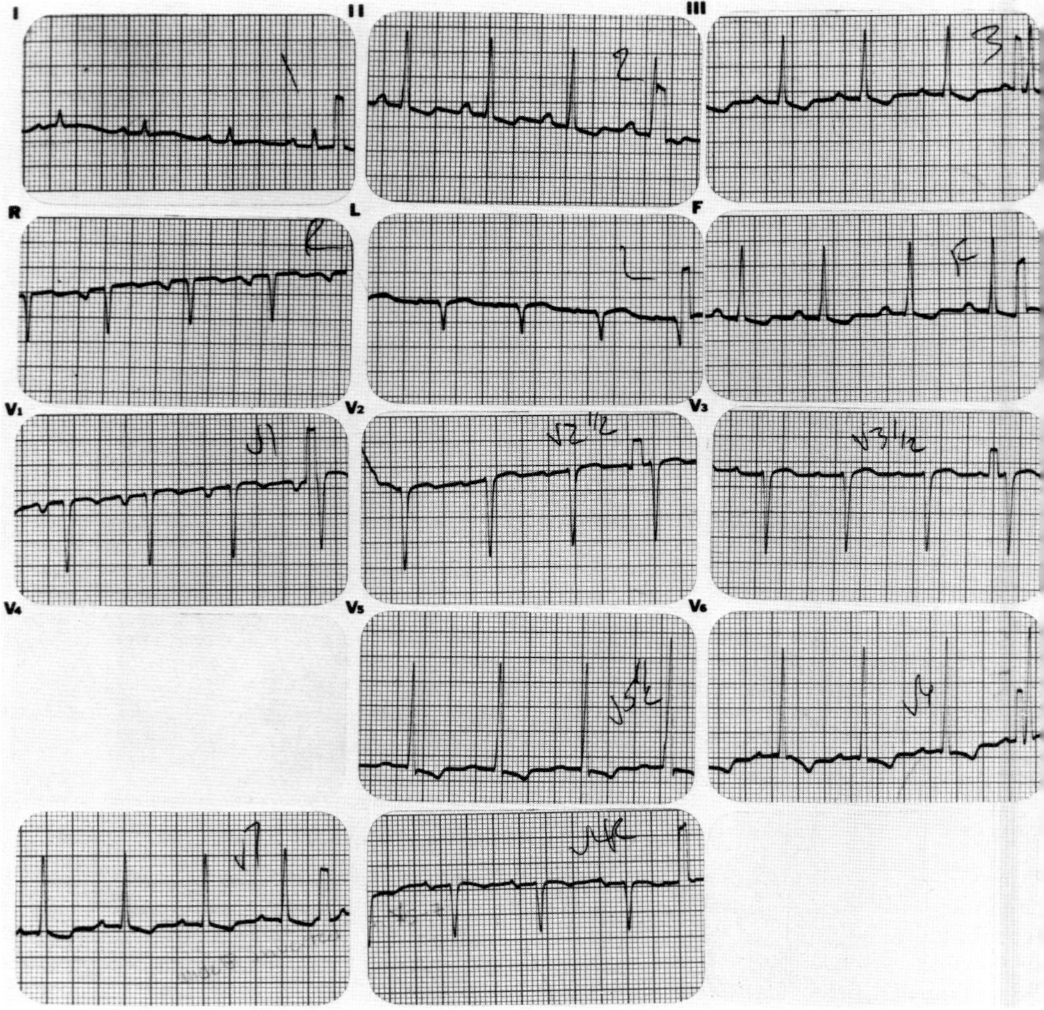

Figure 43.2 Electrocardiogram demonstrating left ventricular hypertrophy. Note increased R wave voltage in left precordial leads and abnormal T-wave changes.

may be important clinical correlates of chronic CHF. These reflect not only diminished cellular substrate availability as a result of inadequate tissue perfusion, but also increased caloric expenditure associated with heightened oxygen consumption and increased work of breathing. *Feeding difficulties*, which may be associated with the respiratory patterns noted above, aggravate caloric balance even further.

6. Cool, moist extremities and a generalized pallor may also be present and reflec peripheral vasoconstriction secondary t catecholamine release and the need t maintain blood pressure in the face of re duced cardiac output.

7. Central and peripheral fluid accumu lation with elevated systemic venous pres sure also accompanies CHF, reflecting im paired cardiac emptying and also impaire sodium and protein balance. *Hepatomeg aly, jugular venous distension*, and periph

eral edema represent the clinical manifestations of this aspect of the problem. *Pulsus alternans*, a beat-to-beat variability in the strength of the pulse, is also a clinical sign of cardiac mechanical decompensation.

The child with overt CHF who is seen in the emergency department may manifest nearly all of the above signs and symptoms. If severely ill, pallor will be evident, tachypnea prominent, and intercostal retractions visible. The liver is enlarged and palpable well below the right costal margin; a spleen tip may also be palpable. The pulses are weak and thready and the skin may be moist and cool to the touch. Auscultation of the chest reveals rales, rhonchi, and, sometimes, wheezes. Tachycardia is present, and auscultation of the heart sounds frequently elicits a gallop rhythm. Murmurs may be strikingly absent unless there is preexisting heart disease. A child with this spectrum of findings deserves immediate attention; acute heart failure in childhood usually implies an unstable situation with possible rapid deterioration.

Laboratory Findings

Usually a clinical diagnosis of CHF can be made without extensive use of x-rays or laboratory tests. Certain objective changes, however, may corroborate the clinical findings.

1. As noted, an x-ray of the chest shows an increased cardiothoracic ratio as well as pulmonary congestion. Kerley B lines or platelike atelectasis at the lung bases, reflecting dilated pulmonary lymphatics, may also be present. Pleural effusions occur commonly.

2. The ECG is a nonspecific indicator of cardiac decompensation. The precordial voltages decrease in certain conditions associated with CHF such as myocarditis, but may be normal or increased in other situations despite overt CHF. The ECG is helpful also for establishing an etiology such as in CHF secondary to a cardiac arrhythmia or to myocardial ischemia.

3. Echocardiography or radionuclide studies can be helpful in evaluating the child with CHF. The differentiation of an enlarged cardiac silhouette secondary to impaired cardiac performance with ventricular chamber enlargement rather than pericardial fluid accumulation can be best made by an ultrasound examination. Additionally, functional indices can be obtained as an objective measure of cardiac performance and of response to therapy.

4. Blood gas abnormalities may be present. Prolonged tissue hypoperfusion can result in metabolic acidosis of a significant degree, and the pulmonary abnormalities noted above may result in hypoxia.

5. Other abnormalities that may be present include electrolyte changes such as hyponatremia and hypochloremia and a reduction in hematocrit, based on dilutional factors. The sedimentation rate is usually lowered in active CHF. Additionally, in infants with CHF, serum glucose and calcium should be monitored, since deficiencies in either may be responsible in large measure for the impaired cardiac function. In situations of suspected perfusion abnormalities or inflammatory myocardial diseases, cardiac enzymes (creatine phosphokinase (CPK), in particular) may be elevated.

MANAGEMENT

For the patient requiring emergency treatment of CHF, initial medical therapy includes several therapeutic measures: (1) Supplemental oxygen should be supplied via a humidified system. In children, a tight-fitting mask or nasal cannulas may not be effective since excessive energy is expended fighting the use of such apparatuses. (2) Elevation of head and shoulders is helpful in the face of pulmonary edema, with maintenance of the lower extremities in a dependent position to increase peripheral pooling and, thus, diminish pulmonary blood volume. A "cardiac chair" or appropriate modification of an infant seat will establish this posture in the small baby. (3) Morphine sulfate (0.05 to 0.1 mg/kg subcutaneously) can be helpful in the face of agitation and air hunger associated with pulmonary edema. (4) Positive-pressure respiration via endotracheal intubation is sometimes indicated for severe situations,

Table 43.2
Digitalization with Digoxin

I. Usual Doses (i.m. or Oral)		
Age	Weight (g)	Dose (TDD)[a]
Premature infants	500–1000	20 μg/kg or 0.02 mg/kg
	1000–1500	20–30 μg/kg or 0.02–0.03 mg/kg
	1500–2000	30 μg/kg or 0.03 mg/kg
	2000–2500	30–40 μg/kg or 0.03–0.04 mg/kg
Full term to 1 month infants:		60 μg/kg or 0.06 mg/kg
1 month to 2 years		60–80 μg/kg or 0.06–0.08 mg/kg
2 years to 10–12 years		40–60 μg/kg or 0.04–0.06 mg/kg (no dose greater than 1.5 mg TDD)

II. Alterations in Usual Doses

1. Lower if renal function is impaired
2. Lower in presence of poor myocardial function (cardiomyopathy, myocarditis)
3. Lower in presence of metabolic imbalance (electrolyte abnormalities, hypoxia, acidosis)
4. *i.v. dose is 75% of oral or i.m. dose*

[a] TDD = total digitalizing doses.

particularly if arterial blood gas analysis shows respiratory decompensation ($PaCO_2$ $\geq$ 50 mm Hg). In infants, the use of controlled mechanical ventilation to improve respiratory status has greatly enhanced survival. (5) Bicarbonate therapy is rarely indicated to correct metabolic acidosis arising from diminished tissue perfusion. It should be remembered that administration of sodium bicarbonate in the face of respiratory decompensation is hazardous since further $PaCO_2$ elevation can occur. Additionally, bicarbonate given by rapid infusion can promote cerebral edema and rapidly affect serum osmolarity with deleterious effects. Also, an excessive sodium load can result from injudicious use of bicarbonate. Thus, only for severe acidosis (pH $<$ 7.2) should bicarbonate be considered and only then if respiratory function is satisfactory (see p. 21). (6) An intravenous infusion should be started to aid in both the administration of drugs and the strict monitoring and administration of fluids.

Blood products in the form of packed cells should be administered if the child is severely anemic. The use of antibiotics should be reserved for unequivocal evidence of infection or for situations in which circumstantial evidence is strongly suggestive and appropriate cultures have been drawn. The use of steroids may at times be indicated, particularly for heart failure precipitated by inflammatory myocardial disease. Decisions of this type, however should be made in concert with cardiac consultation. Treatment of arrhythmias resulting in CHF is discussed subsequently under "Cardiac Arrhythmias."

The mainstay of the medical management of CHF remains the use of digitalis (Table 43.2) to improve contractility, and diuretics to manipulate ventricular preload and intrapulmonary fluid. Recently, pharmacologic adjustments of afterload have also become an important part of treatment of CHF. Regardless of the specific modality of therapy, frequent reexamination and reevaluation is mandatory.

Digitalis

The drugs of choice for improving the inotropic condition of the heart are the digitalis glycosides; recent investigation have helped improve our understanding of the mechanisms of action of these agents and our adjusting their administration to specific clinical situations. Although the use of digitalis in infants was reported nearly 30 years ago, dosing regimens have been, until very recently, strictly empiric in their derivations. The use of a radioimmunoassay to determine serum digitalis levels has only modestly helped define a dosing format since in infants and children debate exists as to the true therapeutic concentration range. As noted in Table 43.2, the principal clinical value of digitalis pharmacokinetic studies thus far has been to verify that the same unit dose per kilogram of body weight is not necessarily best for children of all ages, and that premature infants in particular require close adjustment of dose based on body weight.

The mechanism of digitalis for improving cardiac performance centers on the regulation of the ionic movements which are part of the contractile process. In particular, inhibition by digitalis of ATPase interferes with the sodium pump mechanism allowing intracellular accumulation of sodium and consequently increasing the level of available calcium for contraction. The associated effect of intracellular potassium depletion may be related to the development of toxicity from digitalis preparations.

The result of digitalis administration for CHF is an increase in the force of cardiac contraction and, thus, an improvement in emptying of the ventricle. Intracardiac filling pressures are consequently reduced, cardiac output rises, cardiac size decreases, and heart rate slows. Eventually, use of the compensatory mechanisms noted above to maintain cardiac output is mitigated.

Several important points must be remembered when prescribing digitalis glycosides, regardless of the specific one selected or the route of administration. Diligent care must be used in relaying the prescribing information in order to avoid errors that may have fatal consequences. Calculations of the total digitalizing dose should be double-checked and clearly recorded. The microgram dosage should be unequivocally clear and the corresponding volume to be administered also written down. If possible, the prescription should be checked by other medical personnel. Decimal errors are inexcusable but all too frequent.

It must also be remembered that the route of administration has a significant bearing on the dosage prescribed. Parenteral digoxin preparations contain 100 μg/ml, and oral preparations contain 50 μg/ml. In the emergency setting, parenteral administration will frequently be the preferred route. If given intravenously, the child should be monitored for sudden changes in heart rate or rhythm, and the calculated oral dose reduced by 25%. Tissue perfusion levels should be assessed as satisfactory before intramuscular (i.m.) administration is contemplated since poor absorption from an i.m. dose (which can be painful) may undercut the therapeutic response.

Digoxin is administered in the dosages described in Table 43.2 (maximum, 1.5 mg). The total digitalizing dose is given over 24 hours; half initially, one-quarter in 8 hours, and one-quarter in another 8 hours. The daily maintenance dose is one-quarter of the total digitalizing dose divided into twice daily doses.

Poisoning from digitalis ingestion may itself be the precipitating cause for emergency evaluation. A variety of systemic manifestations may be associated with overdosage including nausea, vomiting, weakness, and worsening of preexisting heart failure. The ECG manifestations of digitalis excess are reviewed subsequently under "Irregular Heart Rates" and care should be taken to clarify the ECG distinctions between digitalis toxicity and more benign "digitalis" effect. In general, it is safest to assume that the appearance of a new major conduction disturbance in a child taking a digitalis preparation is related to the drug.

Treatment of *digitalis toxicity* involves cessation of the drug. Potassium supplementation may be helpful, specifically when potassium depletion has occurred because of dietary factors or diuretic therapy. Potassium should not be given to a patient with digitalis related AV block (see under "Cardiac Arrhythmias"). Diphenylhydantoin is particularly useful in disorders of impulse formation related to digitalis therapy (e.g., premature ventricular contractions). Some centers are experimentally assessing the efficacy of digitalis antibodies, but these are not generally available at this point. In instances of severe heart block, pacing may be required. The presence of digitalis is *not* an absolute contraindication for cardioversion and in certain instances cardioversion may be required to convert even a digitalis induced rhythm disturbance. On occasion, calcium EDTA (30 mg/kg intravenously slowly over 2 hours) may be used as an adjunct to the abovementioned forms of therapy. Careful monitoring is required, however, since hypocalcemia may be induced and since EDTA may negate the therapeutic effects of digoxin, resulting in worsening congestive heart failure.

Other Inotropic Agents

In situations of severely compromised cardiac output, isoproterenol or dopamine, both β-receptor agonists, have been successfully used in infants and children. Dobutamine, an analog of dopamine, has also recently been found to be useful in such circumstances.

Isoproterenol (Isuprel) has both vigorous inotropic effects and marked chronotropic effects. As noted under "Cardiac Arrhythmias," for persistent bradycardia, isoproterenol is the drug of choice. Cardiac rhythm effects may limit the use of isoproterenol, however, since induction of tachyarrhythmias is a known consequence of its administration. The starting dose is 0.1 μg/kg/min by continuous infusion (see Table 43.4).

Dopamine has achieved a wide degree of popularity because of its ability, at low doses ("dopaminergic effects"), to significantly augment renal blood flow directly, in addition to improving cardiac output. Furthermore, the chronotropic activity of the drug is somewhat less than isoproterenol, and there is less of a tendency to produce hypotension. Several recent studies have established the efficacy and safety of dopamine in infants and children. The drug is available in 5-ml ampules containing 200 mg of dopamine; this must be diluted in 250 to 500 ml of a neutral or acidic solution (usually 5 to 10% dextrose or saline). Dopamine must not be administered through the same intravenous solution as sodium bicarbonate since alkali will deactivate the drug. Initial doses in pediatrics range from 2 to 5 μg/kg/min given via continual infusion. For severe systemic hypotension 5 to 10 μg/kg/min may be used as the starting dose. The response should be relatively prompt, with an increase in heart rate and blood pressure followed by improvement in urine output. Increasing the infusion rate may be necessary, but at higher doses (15 μg/kg/min) the beneficial effects of dopamine on renal blood flow are mitigated, and at 20 μg/kg/min adrenergic effects predominate and renal blood flow may be reduced. Adverse effects from dopamine include nausea and vomiting and changes in cardiac rhythm, particularly in patients with preexisting arrhythmias and especially at higher infusion ranges (>10 μg/kg/min). Dopamine probably also elevates pulmonary vascular resistance and should be used with caution, if at all, in patients with pulmonary vascular obstructive disease. It should also be remembered that monoamine oxidase inhibitors may potentiate the effect of agents such as dopamine.

These agents should be administered under close supervision, with monitoring of arterial pressure, central venous and/or pulmonary wedge pressure, heart rate, and urinary output.

Diuretics

Alterations in renal perfusion and salt and water balance are well known correlates of CHF. Reduced renal blood flow can result in increased circulating volume and increased sodium and water reabsorption (through associated secondary hyperaldosteronism). Thus, diuretics have a critical role to play in the management of the child with congestive heart failure.

Currently, the so-called "loop diuretics" are used most commonly for the acute treatment of congestive heart failure. Furosemide (Lasix) is the most popular of these but ethacrynic acid (Edecrin) may also be used. Through effects on sodium and chloride transport in the loop of Henle, interference with urinary concentrating capability is achieved and diuresis is effected. An initial dose of 1 mg/kg intravenously will usually result in adequate urine flow within 1 to 2 hours of administration. If 3 to 5 ml/kg/hour urine flow is not achieved, a subsequent dose at an increment of 1 mg/kg can be given and repeated at hourly intervals to a maximum or 3 to 4 mg/kg. Close observation for changes in serum electrolytes, especially potassium, is important, particularly since intravenous digitalis may be concurrently given.

Thiazide diuretics are much less commonly used to treat acute congestive heart failure and are now reserved for more chronic situations, as oral agents. Nevertheless, agents such as hydrochlorothiazide or chlorothiazide, working at the tubular level, have good diuretic effects. Of recent interest is the thiazide-like compound, metalozone, which appears to be particularly useful when glomerular filtration rate is low. It is principally an oral agent, however, and to date pediatric experience with this drug is limited.

Spironolactone is considered as an adjunctive form of diuretic therapy in most situations and not as a first-line drug since its diuretic effect may not occur for 2 or 3 days. Aldosterone antagonism makes it suitable for use as an additional agent when potassium loss is a problem.

With the proper use of digitalis and diuretic therapy, improvement can be achieved in most children with CHF. Failure to improve requires scrutiny for any of the following: (1) persistent arrhythmia; (2) untreated or unrecognized infection; (3) anemia, especially in the infant with CHF; (4) inadequate or excessive digitalis dose, particularly in the patient with inflammatory myocardial disease; or (5) electrolyte disturbance, such as hypokalemia, which may be worsened with diuretics. If these entities can be ruled out, more intensive treatment is indicated to improve cardiac output.

Mention should be made in this context of the use of afterload reducing agents for CHF. This form of therapy, which has gained wide acceptance recently, should only be undertaken in selected circumstances after the treatments noted above have failed. The concept of afterload reduction is based on the physiologic principles defined earlier in this chapter. In heart failure, with reduced cardiac output, systemic vascular resistance is often elevated via compensatory mechanisms to maintain blood pressure. Preload reserve is utilized via cardiac dilatation to increase stroke volume, but at the expense of a decreased ability of the myocardium to shorten as needed to overcome the increased afterload. Thus, there is a mismatch of afterload and preload reserve in heart failure. For these reasons, attempts to reduce afterload by vasodilatation have been carried out. In several large adult series and in increasing numbers of pediatric cases, lowering of systemic vascular resistance with agents such as nitroprusside have been successful at significantly increasing cardiac output in the face of congestive heart failure. This form of treatment is highly specialized and requires extensive monitoring capabilities, since failure to maintain adequate cardiac filling can have disastrous results. At present, emergency use of afterload reduction to treat CHF should be limited to those well versed in cardiopulmonary physiology and carried out in an intensive care situation.

Cardiac Arrhythmias

GENERAL CONSIDERATION

BACKGROUND

Disturbances in cardiac rhythm are relatively common in infants, children and adolescents. An apparent increase in the incidence of cardiac arrhythmias in children can be explained by the extensive use of ECG monitoring equipment in children's hospitals, advances in cardiac surgery resulting in the survival of children with complex congenital heart disease, new techniques to investigate rhythm disturbances, and an increased awareness on the part of pediatricians and pediatric cardiologists of the manifestations of abnormal cardiac rhythms in children.

PATHOPHYSIOLOGY

The electrical impulse which initiates and coordinates the mechanical activity of the heart is propagated in an orderly manner through the normal heart. This electrical activity is initiated in the sinoatrial (sinus) node located at the junction of the superior vena cava and right atrium (Fig. 43.3). Activity then spreads through the atria to the AV node located in the lower part of the right atrium near the coronary sinus and just above the septal leaflet of the tricuspid valve. The impulse continues to the bundle of His which then divides into the right and left bundle branches in the ventricle. The bundle branches then divide into the Purkinje fibers of the ventricular myocardium and the entire ventricle is thus depolarized.

Arrhythmias in children are due to disturbances in impulse formation or conduction or both. In many children with rhythm disturbances, there is no recognizable cause. However, certain children have a propensity to develop arrhythmias. Some types of congenital heart disease have a relatively high incidence of associated cardiac arrhythmias. These include corrected transposition of the great vessels, Ebstein's anomaly of the tricuspid valve, congenital mitral stenosis, and asplenia-polysplenia syndromes. Other children may have congenital complete heart block or Wolff-Parkinson-White syndrome. Post surgical arrhythmias are commonly seen in children with transposition of the great vessels, tetralogy of Fallot, endocardial cushion defects and atrial septal defects. Acquired heart diseases with frequent rhythm disturbances include cardiomyopathies, rheumatic carditis or rheumatic heart disease, viral myocarditis, cardiac tumors and hemochromatosis.

Systemic diseases or abnormalities associated with cardiac arrhythmias include electrolyte disturbances, neuromuscular disorders (muscular dystrophy, Friedreich's ataxia), endocrine disorders (hyper- or hypothyroidism), inherited disorders of me-

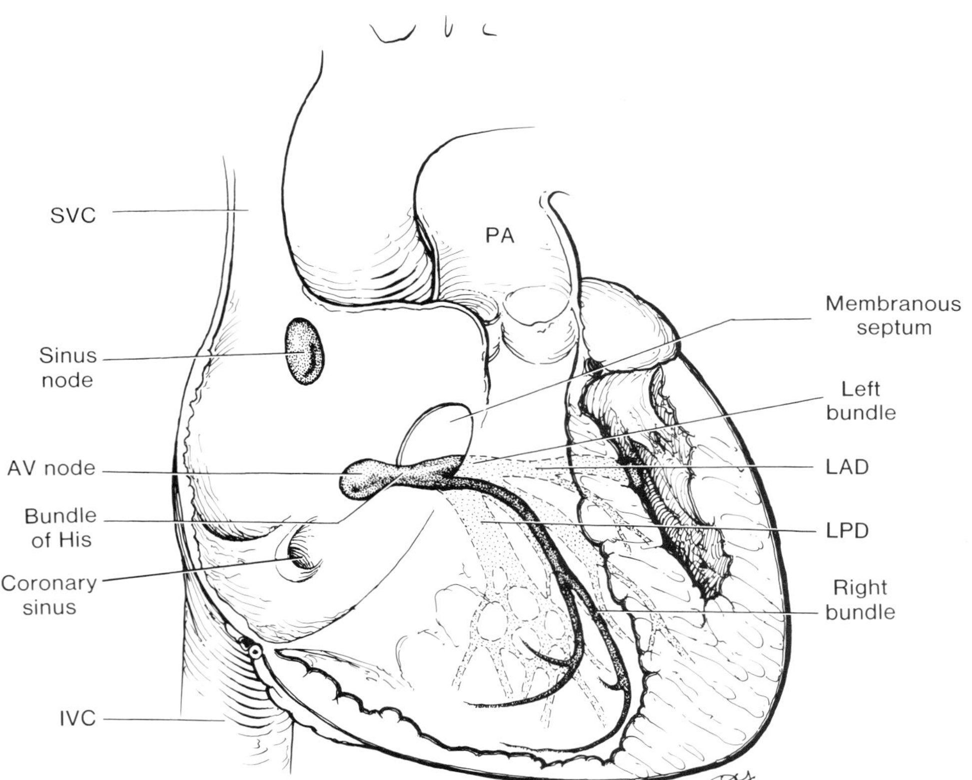

Figure 43.3 Schematic representation of the intracardiac conduction system. *SVC* = superior vena cava; *PA* = pulmonary artery; *LAD* = *left anterior division; LPD* = left posterior division; *IVC* = inferior vena cava.

tabolism (glycogen storage disease—Pompe's disease), collagen diseases (systemic lupus erythematosus), pulmonary disease (respiratory distress syndrome, cystic fibrosis), hematologic disorders (anemia, thalassemia major), neoplasms, renal diseases (uremia), infectious diseases, and central nervous system diseases (increased intracranial pressure, encephalitides). Drugs and toxic substances (digitalis, general anesthesia, aminophyllin, sympathomimetic drugs, epinephrine) can also lead to abnormalities of cardiac rhythm.

CLINICAL MANIFESTATIONS

Many children are not aware of or are unable to express their awareness of an abnormal cardiac rhythm. Thus, the physician must suspect the diagnosis from the secondary manifestations. Arrhythmias may surface in the following ways:

1. Symptoms of CHF (pallor, irritability, poor feeding, vomiting, dyspnea and diaphoresis);
2. Symptoms related to decreased cerebral blood flow (syncope, dizziness, inappropriate behavior);
3. Symptoms related to decreased coronary blood flow (anginal chest pain); and
4. Perception of the rhythm disturbance by the child (palpitations, skipped beats).

MANAGEMENT

Management of the child with a cardiac arrhythmia requires recognition of the manifestations of these disorders, diagnosis of the type of rhythm disturbance, understanding of the mechanism of the abnormality, knowledge of appropriate therapy (pharmacologic or other intervention), and judgment as to the appropriate timing and urgency of therapy. Once an abnormality in cardiac rhythm is suspected or found, the precise diagnosis must be made to institute appropriate treatment. This is generally dependent upon evaluation of the ECG. The resting ECG that is utilized to evaluate cardiac arrhythmias should include a long rhythm strip in addition to a complete 12 lead ECG. Lead 2 is frequently used for the rhythm strip, but a V_1 lead or another lead in which p waves are prominent may be more helpful. The rhythm on the ECG should be evaluated as to rate, regularity, mechanism, and origin of the disturbance.

Cardiac arrhythmias become emergencies when they produce hemodynamic alterations that result in a decreased cardiac output. To effectively treat cardiac arrhythmias, one must be able to identify specific arrhythmias, to recognize signs and symptoms of cardiac decompensation and to understand which arrhythmias are likely to rapidly produce cardiac decompensation. Most infants and children who have symptomatic arrhythmias will require cardiac consultation and admission to the hospital.

The cardiac arrhythmias to be discussed in this section will be classified according to their presentation to the physician: slow heart rates, rapid heart rates, and irregular heart rates. Slow heart rates that are most commonly seen in the emergency department include complete (or third degree) heart block, second degree heart block, sinus or junctional bradycardia, and the sick sinus syndrome. Supraventricular and ventricular tachycardias cause a rapid heart rate. Irregular rhythms are usually due to premature ventricular or atrial contractions and second degree heart block.

To determine whether a heart rate is abnormally fast or slow one must know the normal range of rates for children of various ages. Results of 24-hour continuous ECG monitoring are redefining the normal ranges. Table 43.3 illustrates ranges of rates accepted as normal.

SLOW HEART RATE

Complete Heart Block

Complete (third degree) atrioventricular (AV) heart block is the most common cause

Table 43.3
Normal Heart Rate Ranges

Age	Heart Rate (beats/min)
Newborn	80–180
1 week to 3 months	80–160
3 months to 2 years	80–150
2 years to 10 years	60–110
10 years to adult	50–90

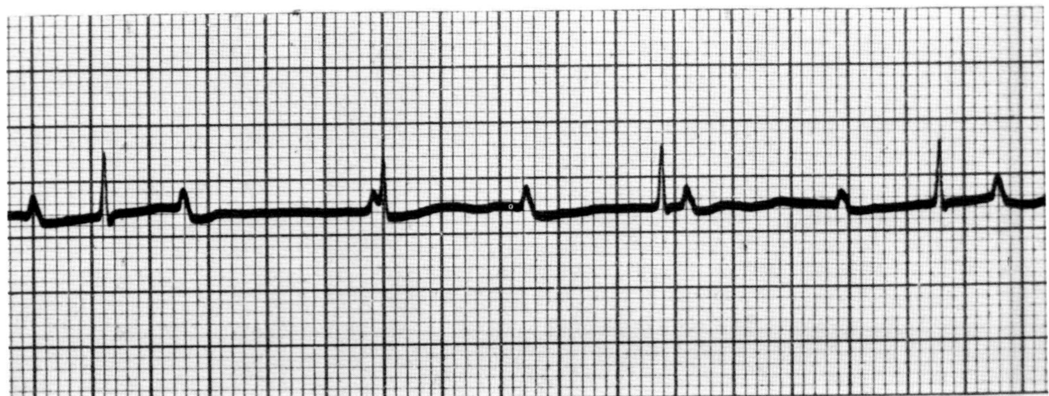

Figure 43.4 Example of complete heart block. Note absence of any regular P-R interval. Ventricular rate 62/min, atrial rate approximately 95 to 115.

Table 43.4
Treatment of Heart Block

Drug	Route	Dose
Epinephrine	i.v.	0.01 mg/kg (0.1 ml/kg of 1:10,000 solution or 0.01 ml/kg of 1:1000 solution)
	Infusion	0.2–0.4 μg/kg/min
Isoproterenol	Infusion	0.1–0.25 μg/kg/min
Ephedrine sulfate	i.v.	50 mg in 100 ml 5% dextrose in water in slow drip
	p.o. or i.m.	0.8–1.6 mg/kg/day in 4 doses

of significant bradycardia in infants and children. Complete heart block, which may be either congenital or acquired, results from a complete failure of conduction from atria to ventricles. The atrial rate is usually faster than the ventricular rate which is usually 40 to 80 beats per minute. A typical ECG is shown in Figure 43.4.

Congenital Heart Block

Congenital heart block may be idiopathic, associated with specific types of congenital heart defects such as corrected transposition of the great arteries or asplenia-polysplenia syndromes, or associated with collagen disease in the mother. Congenital heart block is being diagnosed more frequently in utero with the use of extensive fetal monitoring and sonography, but it may not be recognized for weeks or months after birth.

All infants with this disorder have bradycardia. Although some remain asymptomatic, others develop congestive heart failure and, occasionally, cardiovascular collapse. An ECG will differentiate sinus bradycardia from complete heart block. Sinus bradycardia should respond to the usual resuscitative measures: ventilation and oxygenation, treatment of acidosis, and catecholamine support of heart rate and blood pressure. The infant with complete heart block, who has severe congestive heart failure or is in shock, may also require intubation for adequate ventilation, oxygenation and treatment of acidosis. If there is no improvement with these measures, infusion of isoproterenol or epinephrine may increase the heart rate slightly allowing time for the placement of a temporary pacemaker (Table 43.4). A hydropic infant may require emergency phlebotomy as well as a potent diuretic such as furosemide (1 mg/kg, intravenously). Distressed infants with congenital heart block generally have rates below 50. If an infant is distressed with a rate greater than 50, one should suspect severe congenital heart disease in addition to the heart block. The infant in extremis from a slow heart rate may require immediate transthoracic cardiac pacing in the emergency department with special wires designed for this purpose. If time allows, placement of a temporary transvenous pacemaker either through the umbilical vein or femoral vein (see procedures in Section VII) under direct fluoroscopic observation in a cardiac catheterization laboratory is preferred. Temporary transvenous pacing is reserved for infants with signs of congestive heart failure, most commonly seen with rates less than 50 or in association with severe congenital heart defects. However, an infant with a rate of 45 should not be paced solely on the basis of heart rate, but should be observed for signs of congestive heart failure such as tachypnea, poor feeding, or hepatomegaly. The width of the QRS on the ECG does not always correlate with need for a pacemaker. Only a small percent of patients with congenital heart block require pacing and many of these escape the need for pacemakers until older.

Acquired Nonsurgical Heart Block

Acquired nonsurgical heart block may be idiopathic or associated with congenital heart defects, infectious diseases such as myocarditis or endocarditis, inflammatory processes (lupus, rheumatic fever), muscle diseases, cardiac tumors, or cardiac sclerosis. The emergency treatment of congenital and acquired nonsurgical heart block is similar. Subsequent implantation of a permanent pacemaker is based on symptomatology. A single typical Stokes-Adams or syncopal attack not related to neurologic or endocrinologic factors is considered to be an indication for pacemaker insertion, as these attacks may be fatal. The patient with acquired heart block who presents with a syncopal episode requires a temporary transvenous pacemaker. This should be left in place during induction of anesthesia for permanent pacemaker implantation, as serious arrhythmias have been noted to occur at this time.

Pharmacologic therapy plays a role if adequate ventilation, oxygenation, and the treatment of acidosis does not produce a normalization of the cardiac output as reflected by the blood pressure and peripheral perfusion. The initial drug to be used should be isoproterenol (Table 43.4) as it is most effective in increasing the heart rate. Epinephrine may be tried in place of, or in addition to, isoproterenol if bradycardia persists.

Temporary transvenous pacing may be required during the acute phase of an infectious process even when permanent pacing is not needed, as in a myocarditis. The presence of congestive heart failure is an additional indication for pacing.

Postsurgical Complete Heart Block

Postsurgical heart block is less common today than in the early days of surgery for congenital heart defects, with a current incidence of less than 2%. Improved knowledge of the location of the conduction system, as well as the implementation of intraoperative mapping techniques, has helped to decrease this serious postsurgical complication. Postsurgical complete heart block may be transient or permanent. Transient complete heart block generally resolves within 2 to 4 weeks. Permanent complete heart block generally presents immediately postoperatively but may occur many years after surgery. All patients with postsurgical permanent complete heart block should have implantation of permanent pacemakers. Emergency treatment of symptomatic postsurgical complete heart block includes pharmacologic support and temporary transvenous pacemaker placement until a permanent pacemaker can be placed.

Sinus Bradycardia

Sinus bradycardia is a heart rate below the normal range for age (Table 43.3). An ECG is necessary to rule out partial or complete heart block; P waves with a normal PR interval must preceed each QRS complex in sinus bradycardia. Sinus bradycardia is frequently associated with sinus arrhythmias. It often occurs in the athletic child or adolescent as a normal variant. Other causes of sinus bradycardia include hypothyroidism, increased intracranial pressure, and drugs such as propranolol or digoxin. Therapy of the underlying disorder is indicated.

Sick Sinus Syndrome

Sick sinus syndrome is a condition in which sinus node function is depressed and may present with a sinus bradycardia or slow junctional rhythm. Syncopal episodes may occur. This abnormal cardiac rhythm may be seen in children who have undergone atrial surgery for closure of an atrial septal defect, the Mustard procedure for correction of transposition of the great arteries, in association with a viral myocarditis, or as an idiopathic occurrence. Table 43.5 outlines the evaluation of the child with a suspected sick sinus syndrome. Evaluation will generally be performed by a pediatric cardiologist.

The urgency of the clinical picture determines the treatment of the child with sick sinus syndrome. The asymptomatic patient with a slow heart rate can be referred for consultation with a cardiologist. The child with congestive heart failure or inadequate perfusion from either a bradycardia or a tachycardia requires therapy directed at the specific arrhythmia and admission to the hospital. Isoproterenol or epinephrine infusions (Table 43.4) may temporarily increase the heart rate in a child with bradycardia but, in this situation, may precipitate tachyarrhythmias; thus, they should be administered cautiously. Symptomatic slow rhythms may require temporary or permanent cardiac pacing.

Table 43.5
Evaluation of Sick Sinus Syndrome

Test	Expected Normal Response[a]
Atropine (0.02–0.04 mg/kg)	HR > 90 beats/min >25–50% increase in HR
Isoproterenol (1–3 μg/min)	>25% increase in HR
Exercise	95% of expected normal rate
Electrophysiology study	Normal CSNRT (<550 msec) Normal SACT (45–105 msec)

[a] CSNRT = corrected sinus node recovery time, SACT = sinoatrial conduction time, HR = heart rate.

FAST HEART RATES

Supraventricular Tachycardia

BACKGROUND

Paroxysmal supraventricular tachycardia (SVT), also known as paroxysmal atrial tachycardia (PAT), is the most common significant arrhythmia seen in pediatric practice. Paroxysmal supraventricular tachycardia describes a group of arrythmias with similar ECG features but different mechanisms. These mechanisms have only recently been clarified by the use of specialized intracardiac pacing and recording techniques known as the electrophysiology mapping study and have been shown to originate in the sinus node, in the atrium, in the AV node, or in junctional conduction tissue.

A typical ECG seen in a pediatric patient with SVT is shown in Figure 43.5. Note the very rapid rate and the narrow QRS complex. P waves may be quite different from the usual sinus P wave with a prolonged PR interval. The rate of tachycardia in infants ranges from 220 to 320 beats/min. Older children have tachycardia rates that range from 150 to 250 beats/min. SVT with aberrancy has an ECG with a wide QRS complex and may resemble ventricular tachycardia.

The infant with SVT is most commonly less than 5 months of age and male (male:female = 3:2). Fifty percent of cases in infants are classified as idiopathic, 20% have associated conditions such as infection, fever, or drug exposure (most commonly cold medications containing sympathomimetic amines), 20% have congenital heart disease (Ebstein's anomaly or corrected transposition are most common), and 10% have Wolff-Parkinson-White syndrome (WPW). Older children with SVT are more likely to have WPW, concealed bypass tracts, or congenital heart disease.

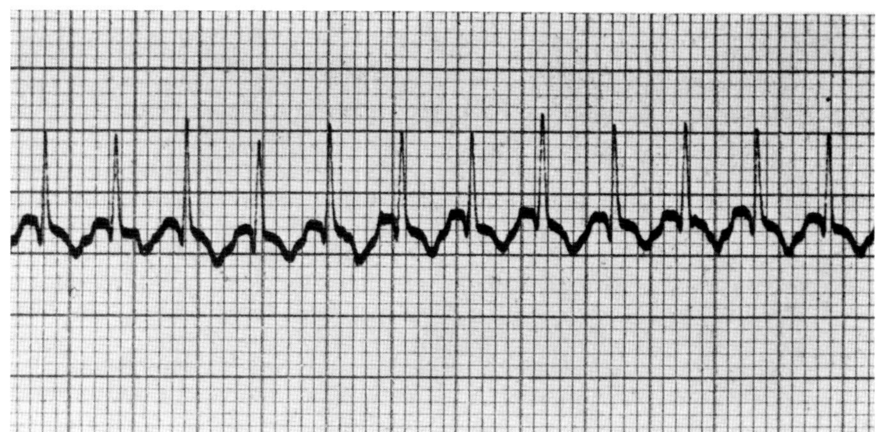

Figure 43.5 Supraventricular tachycardia, rate 300/min.

PATHOPHYSIOLOGY

New electrophysiologic catheterization techniques have provided much information about the mechanisms of SVT and have established that SVT is actually several arrhythmias including: (1) those due to reentry within the sinoatrial node, atrium, AV node and accessory pathways (Wolff-Parkinson-White syndrome) and (2) those caused by enhanced automaticity of specialized atrial fibers. The supraventricular arrhythmias most commonly seen in pediatric patients include AV nodal reentrant SVT, WPW with SVT, concealed bypass tracts with SVT, and atrial flutter or atrial fibrillation.

The concept of AV nodal reentry as a mechanism for SVT was first proposed by Mines in 1913, and the presence of dual pathways in the AV node was shown subsequently by Moe and colleagues. Recently, programmed stimulation has demonstrated the role of reentry in SVT. By convention, the dual pathways have been labeled alpha (α) and beta (β). The α pathway is slower conducting, but has a shorter refractory period than the faster conducting β pathway. The application of this concept to human SVT is shown in Figure 43.6. During sinus rhythm the atrial impulse traverses the faster conducting beta pathway to produce a single QRS complex. The impulse simultaneously travels down the α (slow) pathway, reaching the His bundle shortly after it has been depolarized and rendered refractory by the impulse that was conducted down the β pathway. In response to an atrial premature depolarization, the impulse is blocked in the β pathway due to its longer refractory period and proceeds slowly down the α pathway. If conduction down the α pathway is slow enough to allow the previously refractory β pathway time to recover, an atrial echo results. However, if the α pathway does not recover in time to permit subsequent antegrade conduction, only a single atrial echo results. An earlier atrial premature depolarization (Fig. 43.6) also blocks in the β pathway, but conducts more slowly down the α pathway and arrives later to exit retrogradely from the β pathway and produce an echo. However, because of the longer antegrade conduction time, the α pathway has had sufficient time to recover and a sustained AV nodal reentrant tachycardia results.

If conduction delay and refractoriness in both pathways are appropriate, a continuously circulating wavefront of electrical activity ensues, resulting in a reentrant tachycardia. The conditions for reentry may be found in the sinus node, atrium, AV node and accessory pathways, and the Purkinje fibers of the ventricles. The most common form of SVT in pediatrics is due to sustained reentry within the AV node or a bypass tract.

The rate of SVT appears to reflect the conducting properties of the AV node. Pa-

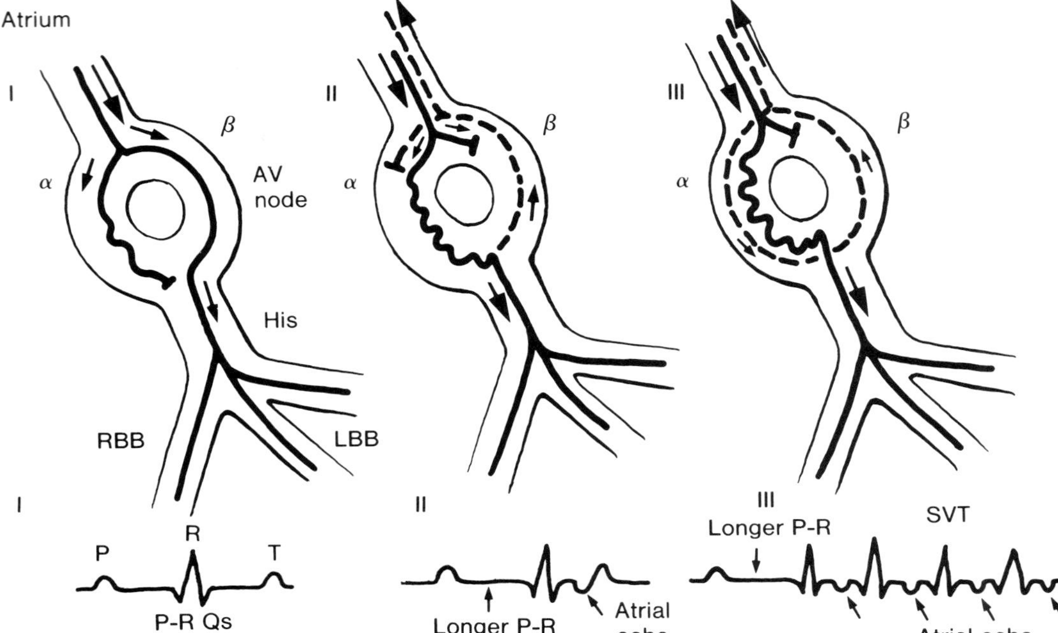

Figure 43.6 Schematic representation of conduction pathway and corresponding ECG in the development of AV nodal reentry. *RBB* = right bundle branch; *LBB* = left bundle branch. See tex for full discussion.

tients whose AV nodes conduct slowly, either spontaneously or due to the effects of drugs like digitalis or propranolol, have slower rates during SVT.

SVT is the usual clinical problem which affects patients with the Wolff-Parkinson-White syndrome. The arrhythmia has all the characteristics of reentry but the reentrant circuit involves an extra AV nodal accessory pathway. Wolff-Parkinson-White complexes, which consist of a short PR interval and a widened QRS complex with a slurred upstroke (delta (δ) wave), are generally not seen during the tachycardia, but only after conversion to normal sinus rhythm as shown in Figure 43.7. The WPW complex represents the presence of a bypass tract connecting atria and ventricles. The short PR interval and δ wave characteristic of WPW syndrome are produced by conduction over the accessory pathway which has different electrophysiological properties than the normal AV conduction system. The ventricular complex is a fusion beat with a variable contribution from the accessory pathway. The greater the contribution from the accessory pathway, th larger the δ wave and more bizarre th QRS.

Episodes of SVT in WPW syndrome ar usually initiated by a premature atrial de polarization which blocks antegrade con duction in the accessory pathway and trav els to the ventricles over the normal A conducting system. The impulse, upo reaching the ventricular insertion of th bypass tract, can travel retrograde up th bypass tract to the atrium and reenter th AV node to start a "circus movement" typ of tachycardia.

Thus, reentrant supraventricular tachy cardia in WPW syndrome is analogous t AV nodal reentrant SVT with the bypas tract functioning like a β pathway (fas conduction, long refractory period) and th AV nodal His Purkinje system functionin like an α pathway (slow conduction, shor refractory period). Since antegrade conduc tion during SVT occurs over the usual A conducting system, the QRS complexes wi be normal. In rare cases, the route of reen try may be reversed, and the bypass trac

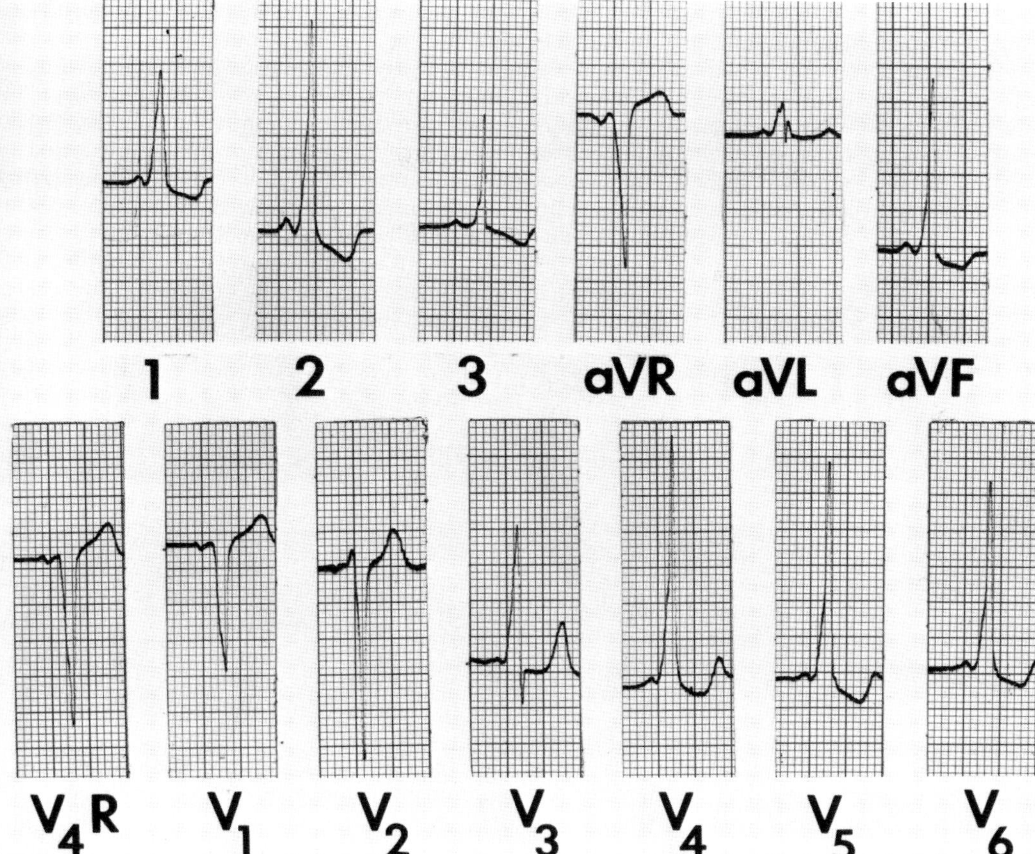

Figure 43.7 Electrocardiogram in Wolf-Parkinson-White syndrome. Note wide QRS, presence of delta wave (slurred upstroke of R), and short P-R interval.

forms the antegrade limb. In these cases, the QRS complexes will be wide and bizarre, and the arrhythmia may simulate ventricular tachycardia.

A concealed bypass tract indicates that the bypass tract is utilized only as the retrograde limb of the reentrant circuit during SVT but is not utilized during normal resting rhythm. Thus, the resting ECG appears normal.

Because the ventricle must be depolarized prior to retrograde conduction up the bypass tract, atrial activation must always follow ventricular activation; therefore, the P wave follows inscription of the QRS complex. The PR interval is usually less than 50% of the RR interval. In AV nodal reentrant SVT, the P wave may or may not be visible but, if visible, is generally closely related to the preceding QRS complex.

The identification of the mechanism of the tachycardia in SVT is helpful from a therapeutic point of view, so that a medication known to act specifically on the AV node, on the accessory pathway, or on the atrial tissue may be chosen. In addition, if the tachycardia can be reproducibly initiated in the electrophysiology laboratory, the efficacy of a specific drug can be tested in the laboratory rather than empirically chosen.

CLINICAL MANIFESTATIONS

The clinical findings in the patient with SVT depend on the duration of the arrhythmia and the presence or absence of an underlying heart defect. In the patient with no congenital heart defect or myocardial dysfunction, CHF will usually appear only after 24 hours of a rapid rate. However, when the patient is first seen in the emergency department, the precise onset of the SVT is rarely certain. Likewise, the presence of associated heart defects is generally unknown. Therefore, one must treat all patients with some degree of urgency.

The infant with SVT may present with only a fast rate or may have varying degrees of CHF (poor feeding, irritability, respiratory distress) or shock. The infant may be acidotic and appear to be septic.

The child over 5 or 6 years of age will usually complain of some symptom such as chest pain or a rapid heart beat. The child may also present with signs of CHF but is unlikely to be quite as ill when first seen as the infant or young child unless a congenital heart defect or primary myocardial disease is present.

MANAGEMENT

As the mechanisms of SVT are now identifiable, treatment can be chosen for the specific forms of SVT. However, the main principle of treatment in any cardiac arrhythmia is that the form of therapy is determined by the urgency of the situation. Thus, a different mode of treatment is chosen for the patient with tachycardia in shock than for the asymptomatic patient who has only a fast heart rate (Table 43.6).

When the SVT is due to AV nodal reentry, any intervention that interrupts the critical relationship of conduction and refractoriness in the AV node can interrupt the tachycardia. However, the patient's response to the drugs or maneuvers is not always predictable. The methods used most frequently are those that further slow AV nodal conduction. In adult patients, carotid sinus pressure or ocular pressure frequently can terminate the tachycardia by increasing vagal tone which slows conduction and prolongs refractoriness within the AV node. Although these maneuvers are often ineffective in children, the occasional successful attempt justifies their initial use. Ice water or ice bags applied to the face have been utilized, but this maneuver has been shown to produce asystole in the presence of an immature autonomic nervous system and should be reserved for older children who are monitored.

Any patient with SVT who presents in shock, with acidosis, or severely compromised should be treated immediately with DC cardioversion at a dosage of 1 to 2 watt-sec/kg. The dosage may be continually doubled until effective or a level of 10 watt-sec/kg is reached. Cardioversion synchronized to the QRS complex should be used, if available, to lessen the chance of ventricular fibrillation. If fibrillation should occur, repeat cardioversion will generally convert the patient to normal sinus rhythm. The older patient should be given a sedative or short acting anesthetic and preparations should be made for airway support and ventilation if needed. The presence of digoxin in the patient should not prevent the use of cardioversion when needed. Once the patient has converted, the chosen chronic treatment should be initiated immediately.

Children who have only mild to moderate failure may be treated medically, as many patients will convert rapidly after pharmacologic treatment. Agents, other than digitalis, useful for the treatment of SVT are reviewed in Table 43.7. The preferred medical treatment of AV nodal SVT in children is digoxin which works by prolonging AV nodal conduction and refractoriness in both the fast (β) and slow (α) pathways. When refractoriness of the fast pathway is prolonged greater than conduction down the slow pathway, inability to initiate SVT results.

Table 43.6
Treatment of Supraventricular Tachycardia[a]

Clinical Status	Treatment
↑ HR, asymptomatic	Digoxin, parenteral (i.m. or i.v.) in infant, parenteral or oral in older child
↑ HR, mild CHF	Digoxin, parenteral
↑ HR, moderate CHF	Digoxin, parenteral (i.v.) or DC cardioversion
↑ HR, severe CHF, shock	DC cardioversion

[a] CHR = congestive heart failure, HR = heart rate.

Table 43.7
Antiarrhythmic Agents for Supraventricular Tachycardia and Ventricular Tachycardia

Drug	Intravenous	Oral
Propranolol	0.1 mg/kg/dose q6h	1 mg/kg/dose q6h
Procainamide	5–15 mg/kg in 30 min	15–50 mg/kg/day in 6 doses
Quinidine sulfate		15–60 mg/kg/day in 4 doses
Phenylephrine	0.005–0.01 mg/kg/dose	
Lidocaine	1–2 mg/kg/dose Infusion 10–50 μg/kg/min	
Phenytoin	2–4 mg/kg over 5 min	1st day 20 mg/kg 2nd day 10 mg/kg 3rd day 10 mg/kg Maintenance—4–10 mg/kg/day

The usual digitalizing dose appropriate for age is used (Table 43.2). The route (intravenous or intramuscular) is dependent on the status of the patient. Intravenous digoxin should be used in the presence of congestive heart failure with decreased perfusion. As noted earlier, the intravenous dose should be calculated to be 75% of the oral or intramuscular dose. The interval of time preceding the second and third doses of the total digitalizing dose should again be determined by the patient's status. These additional doses may be required after only 2 to 4 hours. If the tachycardia persists after three doses, one to two additional doses may be given.

Propranolol, which also prolongs AV nodal conduction and refractoriness in both α and β pathways, may be used in the moderately ill child who does not respond to digoxin. The dosage is 0.1 mg/kg intravenously. Digoxin seems to be slightly more effective than propranolol in treating SVT. Raising the blood pressure with α-adrenergic agents such as phenylephrine can terminate the SVT by stimulating the vagus through the baroreceptor reflexes (Table 43.7). Termination of AV nodal reentrant SVT by these agents and by vagal maneuvers almost always occurs by gradual slowing and then antegrade block in the slow (α) pathway. Thus, in most instances, the tachycardia is terminated by a so-called nonconducted atrial echo.

Procainamide and quinidine in relatively high doses may be used under the guidance of a cardiologist to terminate AV nodal SVT by blocking retrograde conduction in the fast (β) pathway (Table 43.7). SVT can also be converted in the catheterization lab by rapid atrial pacing. An electrode catheter is placed in the high right atrium. Rapid pacing (faster than the SVT rate) will frequently interrupt the reentrant cycle and result in normal sinus rhythm. Even when normal sinus rhythm cannot be achieved, a slower rate may be obtained if 2:1 AV nodal block is produced by rapid atrial pacing.

The treatment of SVT in Wolff-Parkinson-White syndrome or in a concealed bypass tract is similar to the treatment of AV nodal reentrant SVT since the AV node participates in one limb of the reentrant circuit. Propranolol is an exceptionally effective drug since it markedly shows AV nodal conduction and prolongs refractoriness while having no significant effects on the accessory pathway. Digoxin, with similar effects on the AV node, must be used cautiously in WPW since it can shorten the refractory period of the bypass tract and enhance conduction in the accessory pathway. In a patient with an associated atrial tachyarrhythmia such as atrial flutter or atrial fibrillation, digoxin may lead to a rapid ventricular response or ventricular fibrillation secondary to rapid conduction of the atrial impulse down the bypass tract. A high percentage of adults with WPW and SVT also have atrial fibrillation, but the incidence of this association is unknown in children. Quinidine and procainamide are often very effective in this type of SVT as they act on the accessory pathway to slow conduction and prolong refractoriness and thus interrupt the retrograde limb of the reentrant circuit.

Intravenous verapamil may become an important drug for the emergency treatment of SVT in infants and children. European trials have shown verapamil to be rapidly effective in a dose of 0.075 to 0.15 mg/kg. This drug remains an investigational agent in children in the United States.

Infants with SVT should receive treatment for the first year of life even if there are no recurrences. Studies have shown that only 20% will recur if the medicines are continued for this period of time. We would also advise treatment of those infants who spontaneously convert from documented episodes of SVT as these children are predisposed to have recurrences. Older children or infants, who are difficult to control and have multiple recurrences, often requiring combinations of digoxin and propranolol or digoxin and procainamide, must be managed individually and should not routinely have their medicines discontinued after 1 year. Children with SVT should not be treated for upper respiratory tract infections with sympathomimetic amines. Instead, if needed, pure antihistamines, such as chlorpheniramine maleate or triprolidine HCl, may be utilized.

Atrial Flutter and Atrial Fibrillation

Atrial flutter and fibrillation occur uncommonly in children. Atrial flutter consists of rapid, regular atrial excitation at rates of 280 to 480 beats per minute (Fig. 43.8). The ventricular response depends on atrioventricular nodal conduction which may allow 1:1, 2:1, 3:1 or 4:1 conduction. The typical ECG reveals saw-toothed flutter waves best seen in leads 2 and V_1. Atrial flutter is most commonly seen in children with congenital heart disease, especially postoperatively after Mustard repair for transposition of the great arteries, but can also occur idiopathically or congenitally.

Atrial fibrillation consists of totally disorganized rapid atrial activity (at a rate of 400 to 700 beats/min) with a variable ventricular rate secondary to varying AV block. Atrial fibrillation is seen most commonly in adolescents with long standing rheumatic or congenital mitral disease or in patients with hyperthyroidism.

Children with atrial fibrillation or flutter raise the same therapeutic problems as those with SVT. If cardiac compromise does not necessitate immediate cardioversion, the initial treatment is digoxin. In the child who is stable, having a normal blood pressure and adequate perfusion, the physician should allow 24 hours for a response to digoxin before adding a second drug such as procainamide or quinidine. Failure to achieve a normal rhythm after an additional 24 to 48 hours calls for cardioversion at that time. Therapeutic drug levels for these agents, which should be obtained in a steady state of drug administration are listed in Table 43.8.

Automatic Atrial or Junctional Tachycardias

Automatic atrial or junctional tachycardias may be quite difficult to control and are often associated with inflammatory states such as myocarditis. Digoxin (in relatively low doses initially to avoid ventricular arrhythmias in a sensitive myocardium) and procainamide have been most effective. Once the abnormal rhythm has converted, chronic therapy must be initiated; otherwise, the arrhythmia is likely to recur.

Ventricular Tachycardia

Ventricular tachycardia is defined as three or more consecutive premature ventricular contractions (Fig. 43.9). The heart rate usually is 150 to 200 beats per minute but may be slower or more rapid. These contractions may be hemodynamically inefficient and result in syncope and death. The etiology may be electrolyte imbalance, metabolic disturbances, cardiac tumors, drugs, cardiac catheterization or surgery, congenital heart disease, cardiomyopathies, prolonged QT syndrome, or idiopathic.

Ventricular tachycardia is being seen more commonly in children who can be divided into three groups: (1) patients with

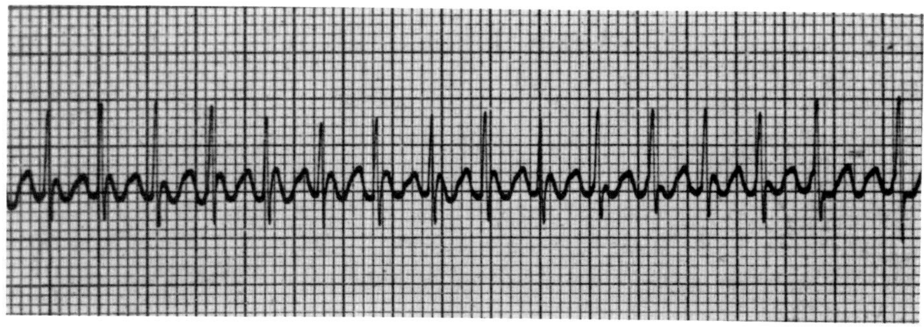

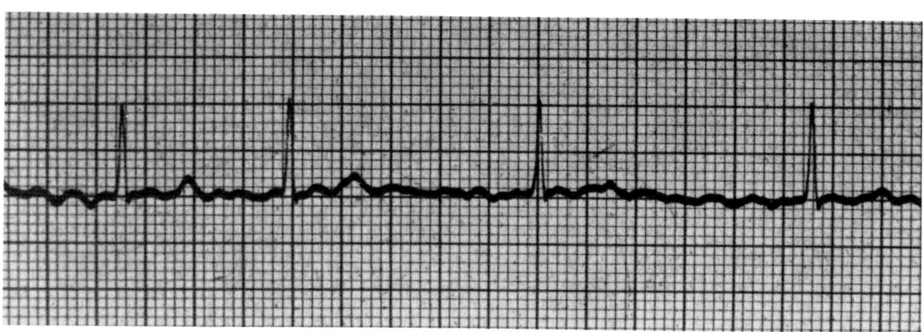

Figure 43.8 (*Top*) Atrial flutter. Sawtooth baseline is apparent. Regular QRS with ventricular rate of 250. (*Bottom*) Atrial fibrillation. Irregularly irregular QRS with course erratic baseline undulations representing fibrillatory waves.

Table 43.8
Serum Drug Levels in Treatment of Atrial Flutter and Atrial Fibrillation

Digoxin	1.5–3.5 ng/ml
Propranolol	20–150 ng/ml
Procainamide	3–10 μg/ml
Quinidine	2.5–6 μg/ml
Phenytoin	10–20 μg/ml
Lidocaine	1–5 μg/ml

indentifiable noncardiac causes (electrolyte imbalance, etc), (2) patients with no underlying heart disease and no extracardiac disturbances, and (3) patients with either congenital or acquired heart disease

In those children with identifiable extracardiac abnormalities (Group 1), the underlying disturbance is treated. Children with no known cardiac or extracardiac causes for ventricular tachycardia (Group 2) require treatment if they have a sustained, rapid arrhythmia. As with SVT patients, the urgency of treatment is dependent on the clinical status. In cases of shock, impending cardiac decompensation or cardiac failure, DC cardioversion at 2 to 5 watt-sec/kg should be used. Intravenous lidocaine at 1 to 2 mg/kg may also be effective (Table 43.7); a continuous infusion of lidocaine at 10 to 50 μg/kg/min may be required. Intravenous procainamide at 5 to 15 mg/kg over 30 min and intravenous phenytoin at 2 to 4 mg/kg over 15 to 20 min may help to control the arrhythmia.

Rapid atrial or ventricular pacing may be used for overdrive suppression or conversion to normal rhythm if pharmacologic therapy fails or is contraindicated. Chronic treatment with procainamide, quinidine, propranolol, or phenytoin has been effective for long-term control of this arrhythmia.

There is no data to determine whether

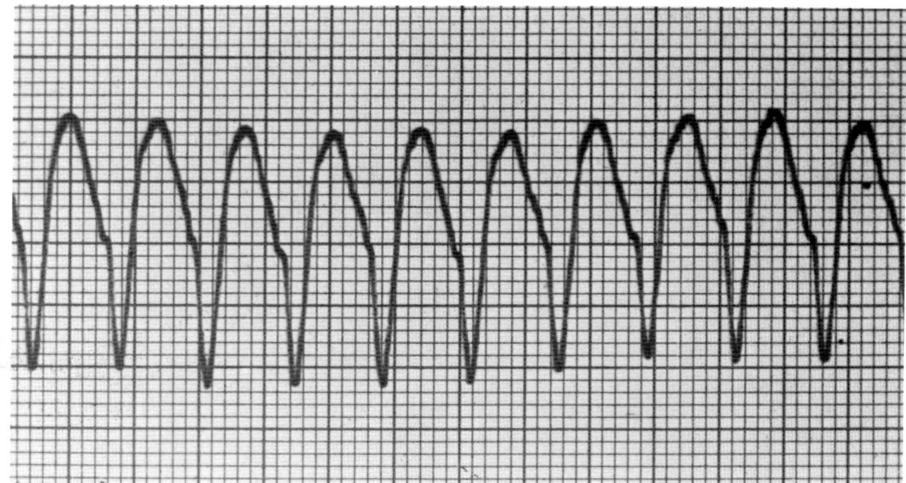

Figure 43.9 Ventricular tachycardia. Wide QRS with rate of approximately 250; sinusoidal pattern.

asymptomatic patients with idiopathic slow ventricular tachycardia should be treated with antiarrhythmic agents. Certainly, the patient should not be made more toxic by the therapy than by his arrhythmia.

Patients with congenital heart disease (Group 3) and ventricular tachycardia raise a different issue. Often these patients have some degree of hemodynamic compromise and do not tolerate the ventricular tachycardia at all. The emergent and chronic treatment is similar to that outlined above but may be required even more urgently. All patients with congenital heart disease and ventricular tachycardia require therapy, even if the rates are relatively slow or the patient is asymptomatic.

Ventricular Fibrillation

Ventricular fibrillation consists of chaotic irregular ventricular contractions with cessation of circulation. Electrical defibrillation with correction of precipitating factors (acidosis, electrolyte imbalance, hypoxia) may result in conversion to normal sinus rhythm. The treatment of cardiac arrest is discussed in Chapter 1.

IRREGULAR HEART RATES

Premature Depolarizations

BACKGROUND

The primary irregular rhythm which may require attention is the premature ventricular contraction. Premature ventricular contractions (PVC) are seen as premature, wide, bizarre-shaped QRS complexes. Generally the T wave is opposite in direction to the main deflection of the QRS. There is usually a compensatory pause following the premature beat. P waves may reveal AV dissociation, retrograde conduction, or be absent. When a rhythmic pattern of PVCs is established, the designation of bi-, tri-, or quadrigeminy is made depending on whether that beat follows every second, third, or fourth sinus beat.

PATHOPHYSIOLOGY

Ventricular premature contractions often occur without identifiable cause in children and have been considered benign. However, PVCs are seen in children with congenital heart disease and congestive heart failure, myocarditis, cardiomyopathies, cardiac tumors, hemochromatosis, or electrolyte imbalance. They are also seen in association with various forms of drug administration including general anesthesia, digoxin, sympathomimetic amines, and phenothiazine tranquilizers. However, especially if multiple or multifocal, PVCs may be precursors of ventricular tachycardia or fibrillation.

CLINICAL MANIFESTATIONS

Children who present with PVCs are frequently asymptomatic and unaware of their arrhythmia especially if they are under the age of 5 years. If the PVC is appreciated, the child may complain of a "skipped" or "hard" beat, a fluttering or pounding in the chest, difficulty breathing, or chest pain. If the PVCs are frequent and/or associated with heart disease (congenital or acquired), the child may note dizziness or a rapid heart beat. Frequent PVCs in the presence of compromised cardiac function may worsen the cardiac output and produce signs and symptoms of congestive heart failure.

MANAGEMENT

The only PVCs which require treatment are those that cause or are likely to cause hemodynamic compromise. This would generally be seen in the context of frequent PVCs in a patient with myocarditis, cardiomyopathy or a congenital heart defect (pre- or postoperative) and abnormal underlying cardiac function. The treatment may include lidocaine, procainamide, quinidine, propranolol or phenytoin as outlined in the section on ventricular tachycardia. Although digoxin is not generally considered for patients with PVCs or ventricular tachycardia, those patients with poor myocardial function, as evidenced by the clinical findings of CHF or ECG evidence of abnormal myocardial function, may benefit from digitalization.

Isolated multiform or coupled PVCs in an asymptomatic patient with a normal heart may not require treatment, but this decision must be individualized after consultation with a cardiologist. Rarely is emergency treatment of this type of patient required and investigations using 24-hour continuous ECG monitors, exercise stress testing, and electrophysiologic catheterization studies may be utilized to determine the appropriate management.

Premature atrial or premature junctional contractions generally do not require treatment. Other variations or normal rhythm in children which do not require treatment include sinus arrhythmia and wandering atrial pacemakers.

First and Second Degree Heart Block

First degree heart block reflects slowed conduction from the sinus node to the ventricle and is manifested by a prolonged PR interval. It is seen with digoxin intoxication, certain types of congenital heart disease (primum and secundum atrial septal defects), and in inflammatory diseases such as rheumatic or viral myocarditis.

Second degree heart block results in the failure of some impulses to traverse the AV node. The Wenckebach phenomenon, a form of second degree heart block, is a result of progressive slowing of AV conduction and is seen as a progressively prolonged PR interval and eventual dropped beat. Other forms of second degree heart block include 2:1, 3:1, and 4:1 block.

Children with first and second degree heart block are rarely symptomatic unless the associated heart rate is low enough to decrease the cardiac output. In such instances, signs and symptoms of congestive heart failure may be present.

Both first and second degree heart block may be associated with digitalis toxicity requiring that the digitalis dose be adjusted downward or temporarily held. Otherwise, first degree heart block does not need therapy. Second degree heart block is treated only if it produces a heart rate sufficiently slow to interfere with cardiac output. In this instance, the management is the same as that outlined for complete heart block (see p. 301).

Arrhythmias Associated with Electrolyte Abnormalities

Alterations in electrolyte concentrations may influence cardiac rate, rhythm, and automaticity and lead to arrhythmias. Potassium and calcium abnormalities are the most common electrolyte alterations that produce arrhythmias, but abnormalities in magnesium and acid-base balance are also important. A combination of ionic alterations is commonly responsible for arrhythmias. Any patient with a significant arrhythmia should be evaluated for an electrolyte disturbance. ECG changes may be characteristic and lead to suspicion of a specific electrolyte abnormality. Normal ECG intervals (P-R, QT) are listed in Table 43.9.

Hyperkalemia

Hyperkalemia is common in hospitalized children and produces recognizable ECG alterations (Fig. 43.10). Peaked T waves are

Table 43.9
P-R Interval, QRS Duration, and QT Interval Related to Rate and Age (and Upper Limits of Normal)[a]

I. P-R

Rate	0–1 Mo	1–6 Mo	6 Mo–1 Yr	1–3 Yr	3–8 Yr	8–12 Yr	12–16 Yr	Adult
<60						0.16(0.18)	0.16(0.19)	0.17(0.21)
60–80					0.15(0.17)	0.15(0.17)	0.15(0.18)	0.16(0.21)
80–100	0.10(0.12)				0.14(0.16)	0.15(0.16)	0.15(0.17)	0.15(0.20)
100–120	0.10(0.12)			(0.15)	0.13(0.16)	0.14(0.15)	0.15(0.16)	0.15(0.19)
120–140	0.10(0.11)	0.11(0.14)	0.11(0.14)	0.12(0.14)	0.13(0.15)	0.14(0.15)		0.15(0.18)
140–160	0.09(0.11)	0.10(0.13)	0.11(0.13)	0.11(0.14)	0.12(0.14)			(0.17)
160–180	0.10(0.11)	0.10(0.12)	0.10(0.12)	0.10(0.12)				
/180	0.09	0.09(0.11)	0.10(0.11)					

II. QRS

	0–6 Mo	1–6 Mo	6 Mo–1 Yr	1–3 Yr	3–8 Yr	8–12 Yr	12–16 Yr	Adult
Seconds	0.05(0.065)	0.05(0.07)	0.05(0.06)	0.06(0.07)	0.07(0.08)	0.07(0.09)	0.07(0.10)	0.08(0.10)

III. Q-T

Cycle Length (sec)	Heart Rate (per min)	Average Q-T (sec)	Cycle Length (sec)	Heart Rate (per min)	Average Q-T (sec)
1.50	40	0.45(0.49)	0.85	70	0.36(0.38)
1.40	43	0.44(0.48)	0.80	75	0.35(0.38)
1.30	46	0.43(0.47)	0.75	80	0.34(0.37)
1.25	48	0.42(0.46)	0.70	86	0.33(0.36)
1.20	50	0.41(0.45)	0.65	92	0.32(0.35)
1.15	52	0.41(0.45)	0.60	100	0.31(0.34)
1.10	55	0.40(0.44)	0.55	109	0.30(0.33)
1.05	57	0.39(0.43)	0.50	120	0.28(0.31)
1.00	60	0.39(0.42)	0.45	133	0.27(0.29)
0.95	63	0.38(0.41)	0.40	150	0.25(0.28)
0.90	67	0.37(0.40)	0.35	172	0.23(0.26)

[a] Modified with permission from W. G. L. Guntheroth: *Pediatric Electrocardiography*, W. B. Saunders, Philadelphia, 1965.

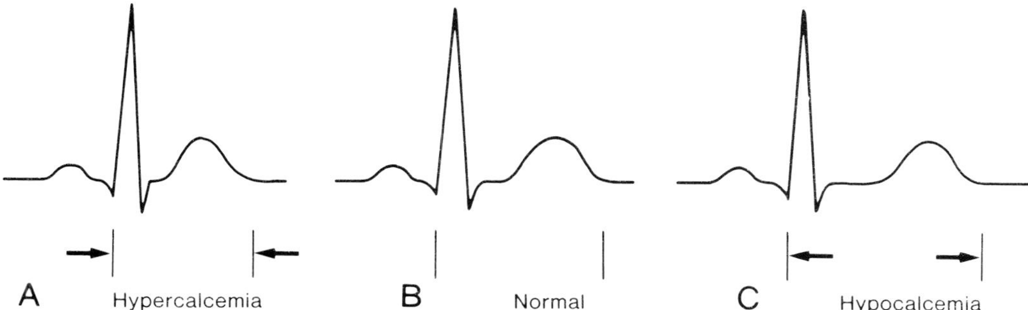

Figure 43.10 Electrolyte effects on ECG QT interval. Note prolongation with hypocalcemia, shortening with hypercalcemia.

seen at a serum concentration of 5 to 6 meq/liter, and the QRS widens with a concentration exceeding 6 meq/liter. The QT interval increases with the increasing QRS duration. P wave amplitude decreases, P wave duration increases, and the PR interval increases above 7 meq/liter. Above 8 to 9 meq/liter P waves disappear, the ventricular rate becomes irregular, and severe bradycardia with sinus arrest, block or idioventricular rhythms occurs, often with a sinusoidal wave pattern. Ventricular fibrillation or asystole occurs at serum concentrations greater than 12 to 14 meq/liter. Low serum calcium enhances the myocardial toxicity of hyperkalemia. Likewise, acidosis potentiates hyperkalemia by producing potassium ion efflux from cells. Potassium may potentiate the effect of digoxin to delay AV conduction and generally should not be given to patients with AV block secondary to digoxin toxicity.

Hypokalemia

Serum potassium concentrations of less than 2.7 meq/liter generally produce typical ECG changes in ventricular repolarization. These changes include a U wave amplitude greater than 1 mm, seen best in leads V_2 and V_3, and ST segment depression greater than 0.5 mm. The QT interval lengthens and the T wave flattens with progressive hypokalemia. The PR interval may be prolonged and intraventricular conduction delayed with widening of the QRS complex. With marked hypokalemia, P wave and QRS amplitude may increase. Other arrhythmias which have been associated with hypokalemia include ectopic atrial and ventricular complexes, ectopic atrial tachycardia with block, AV dissociation, second degree AV block, ventricular bigeminy, ventricular tachycardia and ventricular fibrillation.

Patients on digoxin who become hypokalemic are especially susceptible to arrhythmias because of the synergistic effects of digoxin and hypokalemia on automaticity and conduction.

Hypocalcemia

Hypocalcemia produces characteristic ECG changes which consist of QT interval prolongation secondary to ST segment prolongation and occasional reversal of the T wave. The ECG changes correlate with ionized calcium, as the degree of QT prolongation generally is proportional to the degree of hypocalcemia. Ectopic rhythms, though uncommon, have been reported and include supraventricular tachycardia, 2:1 AV block and complete heart block. The effects of calcium and potassium on myocardial cells are antagonistic.

Hypercalcemia

Hypercalcemia, with levels above 12 mg/dl, produce a shortened QT interval, a shortened ST segment, and normal or prominent U waves. Severe hypercalcemia causes PR interval prolongation, QRS prolongation, and occasionally second and third degree heart block. Elevated serum calcium decreases the effect of hyperkalemia and potentiates digoxin toxicity. Thus, calcium should be administrated to patients on digoxin cautiously, and with the heart rate being monitored.

Hypomagnesemia

Low magnesium levels are frequently associated with hypokalemia and hypocalcemia, and the ECG abnormalities seen may be those associated with any or all of these aberrations. Ectopic beats and T wave changes are commonly noted. Ventricular fibrillation has been reported.

Hypermagnesemia

Hypermagnesemia of 3 to 5 meq/liter or higher may be associated with a delay in atrioventricular and intraventricular conduction.

Treatment of these electrolyte abnormalities is discussed in Chapter 46.

PERICARDIAL DISEASE

BACKGROUND

There are few medical situations in which a simple, quickly performed medical procedure can result in immediate, life saving results. Among these is pericardiocentesis for cardiac tamponade. The technical aspects of periocardiocentesis are discussed (Procedure Section VII). This section will focus on etiologic concerns, clinical findings, and other initial management measures that must be taken to satisfactorily evaluate and treat the child with pericardial disease.

Three forms of illness can affect the pericardium. *Pericarditis,* usually not a true medical emergency, is a nonspecific term denoting inflammatory disease. *Pericardial effusion,* a condition requiring close evaluation but not necessarily requiring emergency treatment, implies fluid accumulation within the pericardial space. *Cardiac tamponade,* a true medical emergency requiring immediate attention, connotes a situation in which impairment of ventricular filling has resulted from either pericardial fluid accumulation or constriction of the heart by an abnormally thickened pericardium, resulting in impairment of cardiac output.

Table 43.10 reviews some of the principle cause of pericarditis in childhood. When considering the etiology of pericardial dis-

Table 43.10
Causes of Diseases of the Pericardium

Infectious	Noninfectious, Inflammatory	Traumatic	Oncologic	Chronic
Bacterial	Acute rheumatic fever	Postpericardiotomy syndrome	Leukemia	Constrictive pericarditis
Viral	Systemic lupus erythematosus	Chest wall injury	Lymphoma	Subacute effusion pericarditis
Fungal	Uremia	Foreign bodies with pericardial contact	Pericardial cyst	Blood dyscrasias
Parasitis	Radiation		Cardiac rhabdosarcoma	
Tuberculous	Juvenile rheumatoid arthritis			

ease and its clinical correlates, it is important to remember that the pericardium is in continuity with the surrounding intrathoracic structures. Thus, conditions affecting the pleura, the mediastinal structions, or the diaphragm may affect the pericardium as well.

Infectious diseases remain the most likely cause of pericarditis in childhood. While a viral etiology is frequently presumed to be causative, in only about 20 to 30% of the time is an actual viral pathogen confirmed. Coxsackie (group B) and ECHO viruses are paramount, but a host of other agents including rubella, Epstein-Barr virus, adenovirus, influenza virus and mumps virus have all been associated with pericardial inflammation and pericardial effusion. Rarely, viral disease results in cardiac tamponade.

Purulent pericarditis, on the other hand, is frequently a medical emergency because of associated cardiac tamponade and because of important sequelae which may be mitigated by early effective treatment. While it is a disease seen at all pediatric ages, approximately 30% of the cases involve children under the age of 6 years. *Staphylococcus aureus*, *Haemophilus influenzae*, *Neisseria meningiditis*, *Streptococcus pneumoniae*, and other streptococci are the principal bacterial agents responsible for childhood pyogenic pericarditis, although other pathogens have been recovered occasionally. Associated infections, such as respiratory tract disease, osteomyelitis or pyogenic arthritis may be present and clinically helpful for suspecting the specific organism involved. For example, a recent review noted that a preponderance of cases of staphylococcal peridarditis were associated with infections distant to the pericardium, such as osteomyelitis, while most cases of *H. influenzae* pericarditis were associated with respiratory tract infection.

PATHOPHYSIOLOGY

As noted earlier, pericardial inflammation itself is not usually a lifethreatening situation. Of concern for the physician evaluating a child in an emergency situation are the hemodynamic sequelae of either fluid accumulation in the pericardial space or scarring and thickening of the pericardium leading to restriction of cardiac filling. Usually, there is a small amount of intrapericardial fluid (under 30 to 50 ml) which exists in an equilibrium state between secretion into the pericardial space and reabsorption. With a sudden accumulation of fluid or with a more gradual increase of large amounts of fluid within the pericardial sac, interference with ventricular filling occurs, leading to decreased stroke volume and to falling blood pressure. Cardiac filling may be compromised through several interrelated mechanisms including increased ventricular enddiastolic pressure, a decreased gradient for venous return, premature atrioventricular valve closure, and shortened diastolic time. The clinical manifestation of these physiologic aberrations, known as cardiac tamponade, is directly related to the severity of these abnormalities and to compensatory mechanisms evoked to overcome them.

CLINICAL FINDINGS

A history of onset of respiratory difficulties after resolution of an upper respiratory illness may indicate pericardial disease in some instances. Chest pain, usually a benign symptom in childhood, is frequent with pericardial inflammation. This pain may be variable depending upon position. Not uncommonly, abdominal pain may be the presenting symptom.

The child with significant pericardial effusion may show clinical signs that are similar to several of those noted in the preceeding section on congestive heart failure. *Tachypnea*, secondary to raised pulmonary venous pressures and decreased pulmonary compliance, is usually present. This may be associated with intercostal retractions. Reduced cardiac output may result in peripheral *vasoconstriction*, manifested by cool extremities, pallor, or decreased systemic blood pressure. Elevated systemic venous pressures cause *neck vein distension*, *hepatomegaly*, and on occasion in more of a chronic picture, *protein loss* either via the gastrointestinal tract or the urine. *Tachycardia* is a universal finding and is representative of an effective compensatory mechanism, but only up to a point. This compensation is limited, as diastolic filling times become further shortened by the increased heart rate.

The cardiac auscultatory findings directly relate to the degree of pericardial fluid accumulation. A *friction rub*, the scratching, harsh sound frequently heard throughout the cardiac cycle, is often not audible with significant amounts of intrapericardial fluid and may become apparent only after pericardiocentesis. The heart sounds are usually distant, or muffled, and the apical impulse weak. In general, the presence of a quiet precordium in the face of the above noted respiratory and circulatory changes should alert the examiner to the possibility of pericardial disease with effusion.

The sine qua non of cardiac tamponade is *pulsus paradoxus*. The finding of a paradoxical pulse greater than 20 mm Hg is unequivocal evidence of circulatory compromise. Additionally, most investigators assume that as little as 10 mm Hg is suggestive of hemodynamic impairment.

The physiologic mechanisms underlying pulsus paradoxus can be viewed as exaggerated examples of the integrated functioning of the cardiopulmonary unit. Normally, a small fall (under 10 mm Hg) in systolic blood pressure is noted with inspiration as a result of several factors. As negative intrathoracic pressure is generated by the inspiratory effort, the gradient for systemic venous return increases favoring right heart filling. At the same time, diaphragmatic descent exerts a traction effect on the heart limiting both filling and ejection. Additionally, there may be some decrease in pulmonary venous return since the gradient from pulmonary veins to left atrium is probably reduced. Thus left heart output and systemic blood pressure are reduced. The pericardium itself is an additional variable factor. In general, since it envelops the heart, it tends to retard expansion of ventricular volume, normally only to a limited degree. Thus, in normal respiration, the pericardium exerts a further volume reducing effect on the left ventricle. In pericardial disease states, as the pericardium itself becomes more rigid or as fluid in the pericardial space increases and intrapericardial pressure rises, the restriction to left ventricular output becomes greater and the consequent decline in systemic blood pressure steeper.

The best method of detecting pulsus paradoxus is to first measure blood pressure in the usual method at expiration and then to inflate the cuff a second time to a few mm Hg above the systolic pressure and allow the cuff to slowly deflate. As the pressure falls, the Korotkoff sounds will disappear with each inspiration. At the point where they cease to disappear, becoming equal to that auscultated during expiration, the measured blood pressure is recorded. The difference between the initial maximum systolic pressure and the final measurement is the "pulsus paradoxus."

It should be noted that pulsus paradoxus is not a finding unique to cardiac tamponade. It is a frequent finding in respiratory tract disease such as asthma and may also be present in congestive heart failure without pericardial effusion.

LABORATORY FINDINGS

The laboratory findings will vary according to the underlying causes of pericardial disease. Although cardiac tamponade is a clinical diagnosis, certain laboratory tools can be extremely helpful in clarifying the situation.

The ECG will show diminished precordial voltage in most instances of significant intrapericardial fluid accumulation (Fig. 43.11). With pericarditis, an associated current of injury pattern reflecting myocardial involvement, seen as elevations in the S-T segments, may also be present. Diffuse T wave inversions are also a frequent finding. The heart size is increased on chest x-ray with pericardial effusion, but can be entirely normal if there is not a significant amount of intrapericardial fluid. The lung fields may be clear, but one should look for associated bronchopneumonia or pleural effusions which may be helpful for diagnostic considerations. In some situations, as with constrictive pericarditis, the heart size may be relatively small. If the patient has had previous chest x-rays, a sudden increase in heart size should always arouse

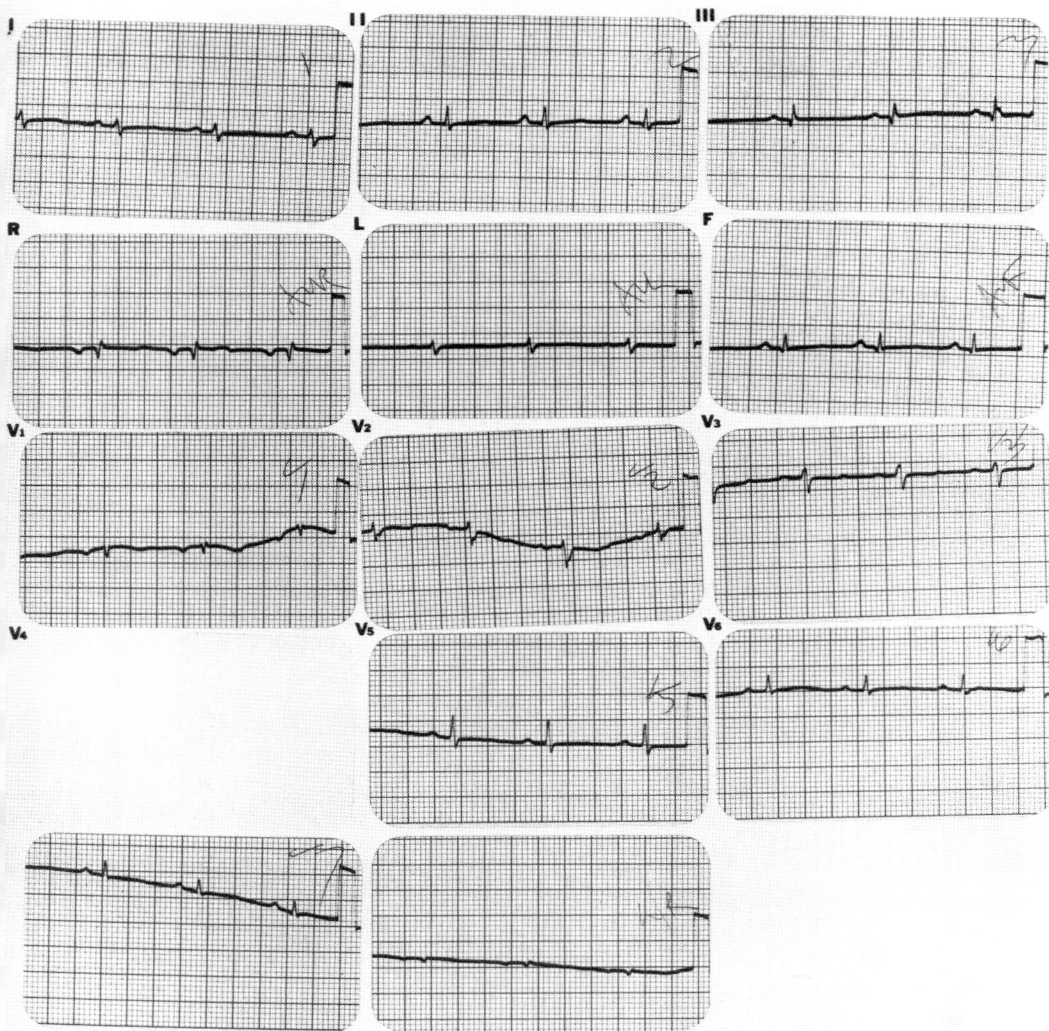

Figure 43.11 Electrocardiogram in pericardial effusion. Generalized low voltage present. ST-T wave flattening is present.

suspicion for the presence of pericardial effusion.

Echocardiography has become the diagnostic procedure of choice for determining the presence and amount of intrapericardial fluid. An echo-free space between the epicardium and the pericardium can be readily identified (Fig. 43.12) with a negligible incidence of false positive diagnoses in experienced hands. Quantitation is not exact, but evidence of both anterior and posterior fluid accumulation suggests a large collection. Either single crystal m-mode echocardioraphy or two dimensional real time echocardiographic studies can be used. Additionally, serial evaluation of the pericardial space is easily accomplished using echocardiography and is helpful for observing the effects of treatment and for evaluating indications for further therapeutic maneuvers after initial drainage measures.

When infectious pericardial disease is suspected, as with the evaluation of any other potentially life threatening infection,

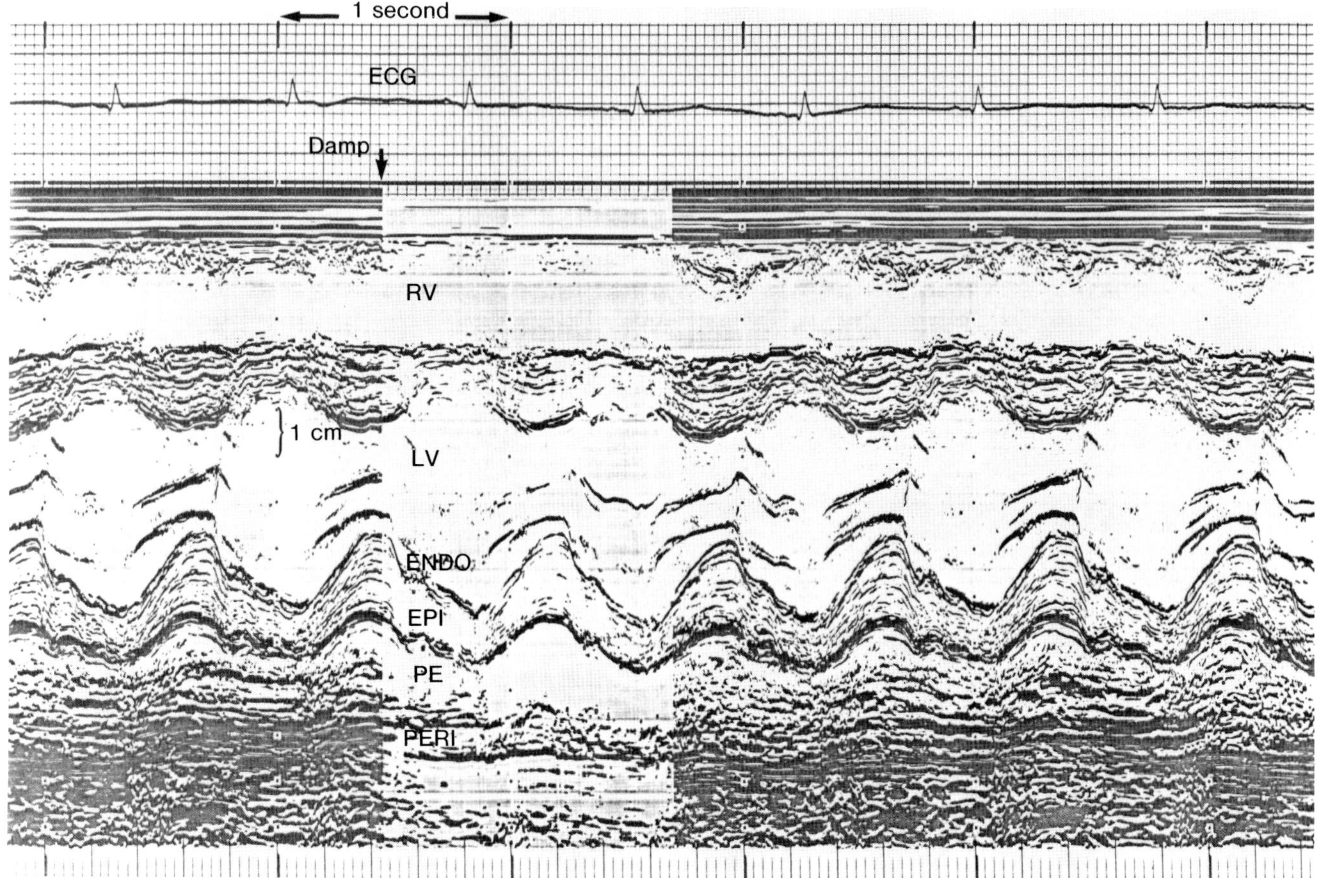

Figure 43.12 M-mode echocardiogram in pericardial effusion. Note absence of echos (clear area) between epicardium and pericardium, representing intrapericardial fluid. *RV* = right ventricle; *LV* = left ventricle; *ENDO* = endocardium; *EPI* = epicardium; *PE* = pericardial effusion; *ECG* = electrocardiogram; *PERI* = pericardium.

a complete bacteriologic evaluation should be initiated before commencing antibiotic therapy.

MANAGEMENT

For pericarditis without evidence of pericardial effusion, emergency invasive treatment is usually not mandated. Symptomatic therapy for pain should be prescribed and bed rest in the hospital is advisable. The patient should be followed closely for the development of complications such as myocarditis, pericardial effusion or cardiac tamponade. Diagnostic evaluation to identify the cause should be initiated.

For pericardial effusion, a more definitive approach is needed. Careful evaluation of vital signs and frequent attention to development of pulsus paradoxus are mandatory. Cardiology consultation should be obtained and the patient admitted for evaluation. Diagnostic pericardiocentesis will often be required in the *de novo* presentation, particularly without evidence of other forms of systemic disease; it is always required with the suspicion of a purulent pericardial process. Usually, in the presence of purulent pericarditis, an open drainage procedure is indicated. It is contingent upon the emergency department physician to ensure cardiovascular stability in the presence of pericardial effusion, since tamponade can develop rapidly once maximum pericardial distensibility has been reached.

The management of cardiac tamponade requires intense medical vigilance. While it may be possible in relatively mild or highly selected situations to manage the effusion conservatively, it is generally necessary to remove the fluid. A full discussion of the techniques employed for pericardiocentesis in the emergency situation is available on p. 000. This can be a lifesaving technique and, when successfully done, shows clearly the fruitful outcome of appropriate, decisive evaluation and treatment procedures.

INFECTIOUS ENDOCARDITIS

BACKGROUND

One of the persistently difficult problems of pediatric medicine has been the evaluation and management of the child with infectious endocarditis. While long term treatment issues generally are not within the province of emergency medical care, it is critically important for the emergency department physician to be aware of the clinical context in which bacterial endocarditis is a consideration. It may also be incumbent upon the emergency physician to initiate therapy in certain instances, and it is always crucial to avoid unnecessary clouding of the diagnosis.

Etiologic Factors

The most frequent setting for infectious endocarditis is the child with preexisting congenital heart disease, but marked variability exists in terms of the specific associated lesions (Fig. 43.13). It is disturbing to note, however, that 1 in 10 cases of endocarditis occurs in children with no preexisting history of cardiac abnormality. These children may be among the most ill, pre-

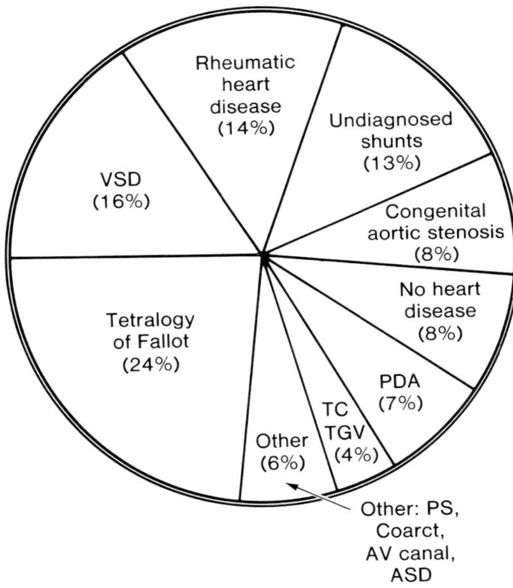

Figure 43.13 Distribution of cardiac lesions in 266 cases of bacterial endocarditis. *PDA* = patent ductus arteriosus; *ASD* = atrial septal defect; *PS* = pulmonary stenosis; TC = TGV = (Redrawn with permission from E. L. Kaplan: *Infective Endocarditis*, Monograph 52, American Heart Association, Inc., Dallas, 1977.)

senting with their illness as part of an acute bacterial endocarditis picture.

Certain factors predispose a child to the development of endocarditis. Well known among these are dental and surgical procedures. Dental procedures even without periodontal disease can yield significant bacteremia. Unfortunately, many types of ordinary daily events are associated with at least transient bacteremia (Table 43.11), and one wonders, in fact, why more cases of endocarditis are not evident. Of note, cardiac catheterization is rarely associated with the development of endocarditis.

The specific congenital heart lesions which are associated with endocarditis are numerous, but certain physiologic conditions appear to be most important. Diseases in which there is a highly turbulent stream of blood or a high velocity of flow are particularly prone to this complication. Such lesions include ventricular septal defect, aortic valve stenosis and mitral valve disease. Children with postoperative systemic-to-pulmonary shunts are also in this category. In contrast, atrial septal defect is a lesion associated with a low risk for endocarditis, as the shunt flow is of low velocity. Prosthetic valve endocarditis does occur, as has been noted in adult studies, and will probably become of increasing concern in children as more valve surgery is done.

Table 43.11
Transient Bacteremia and Various Procedures or Conditions[a]

Procedures	Bacteremia (%)
Tooth extractions (no gingivitis)	34
Tooth extractions (gingivitis)	70–75
Endontic procedures	4
Chewing mint candy	20
Brushing teeth	40
Oral irrigation device	27–50
Massage of infected tonsil	23
Urethral surgery	57
Massage of infected prostate	67
Barium enema	11
Bronchoscopy	15
Sigmoidoscopy	5–10

[a] Modified with permission from D. Kaye (Ed.): *Prophylaxis of Endocarditis*, pp. 245–265, University Park Press, Baltimore, 1976.

Microbiology. Causative organisms include both fungi and bacteria. While viridans streptococci remain the most frequent isolates, other pathogens have become increasingly prevalent in the recent past. In particular, staphylococci are now considered to be causative of more than 35% of the cases. Additionally, bacteria of relatively high incidence in childhood endocarditis include enterococci, *Haemophilus* sp., and pneumococci. The particular agent isolated is somewhat dependent upon the clinical context; for example, postoperative children with congenital heart disease appear to have a higher incidence of staphylococcal endocarditis. Age also appears to be a factor relating to type of organism.

CLINICAL FINDINGS

Of course, the sine qua non of a positive diagnosis is the recovery of organisms obtained by blood culture. In order to arrive at that point, however, a high degree of suspicion must be maintained. Frequently, early signs and symptoms can be subtle and persist for a considerable period of time before the diagnosis is made. With streptococcal endocarditis, this is a common situation. As a rule, persistence of fever in any child with congenital heart disease should prompt the clinician to carefully consider the possibility of endocarditis.

The classic findings of fever, a change in the cardiac examination, splenomegaly, and evidence of emboli are usually present in severe cases, but may require serial examinations to elucidate. Emboli may be discovered by careful funduscopic examination, by observation for conjunctival lesions, or by meticulous scrutiny of the nail beds, palms of the hands, soles of the feet, and other skin surfaces. Microscopic hematuria should be recognized as an important sign of endocarditis in the appropriate clinical context. Scrapings of cutaneous emboli may be helpful for rapid identification of infecting organisms.

Complications

The mortality from infective endocarditis has decreased considerably in recent years. Currently, most series cite a fatality rate of

15 to 20%. While this is still a high percentage, especially for pediatric illness, it should be remembered that over 50% mortality was the norm in the 1950s and that the disease was nearly always fatal in the preantibiotic era.

Other complications occur in as many as 50 to 60% of cases. Systemic or pulmonary emboli, depending on the intracardiac site of the vegetation, are a major source of concern and indication for prompt initiation of treatment. Major neurologic sequelae can arise from focal embolization to the central nervous system; thus, the presentation of a new neurologic deficit in a child with heart disease can be another clinical clue to the diagnosis of endocarditis. Myocarditis, myocardial abscesses, valvar obstructions associated with large vegetations, and ruptured sinus of Valsalva are other important complications.

Acute bacterial endocarditis, or the development of an acute situation such as new aortic insufficiency, should be considered a true medical emergency. Often, early reparative surgery will be required to save the child's life in this situation. These children are critically ill and *congestive heart failure is a grave sign in the context of suspected endocarditis.* Characteristic heart murmurs may be absent in this setting and their absence should not be taken as a cause for optimism. Other surgical indications include the development of a cardiac arrhythmia such as heart block, continued embolization, and continued positive blood cultures after initiation of therapy. Hemodynamic changes can transpire quickly, demanding frequent examinations even while the child is awaiting hospital admission or transfer from the emergency department area.

MANAGEMENT

Treatment of infective endocarditis should be started as early as possible after appropriate evaluation is completed. Blood cultures must be drawn regardless of the presence or absence of classic clinical findings. In order to facilitate the diagnosis, the physician, particularly one evaluating a child with heart disease with unexplained fever, must obtain blood for appropriate cultures at an early stage. In the majority of cases of endocarditis, the causative organism will be recovered from the initial two blood cultures. Particular emphasis should be placed on avoiding contamination of the sample site. Growth of spurious organisms can be misleading and dangerously time-consuming, since bacteria on the skin can themselves be implicated in endocarditis. It is not mandatory to obtain cultures at the time of fever spikes since bacteremia is fairly constant in the untreated patient. Early consultation should be sought from a cardiologist since, frequently, specialized procedures such as echocardiography can help pinpoint the diagnosis rapidly even in relatively difficult situations (Fig. 43.14).

In every instance, the diagnosis of infectious endocarditis implies long term antibiotic therapy and, thus, most management issues arise after the patient has left the emergency area. In general, antibiotic therapy should be instituted as soon as the diagnosis is made. If the patient is critically ill, it may be necessary to initiate therapy even before laboratory confirmation by cultures can be returned. Certainly, stabilization of the patient with heart failure, initiation of the diagnostic workup, and mobilization of the relevant medical personnel are the responsibilities of the emergency department physician in dealing with the child with suspected endocarditis. If the situation requires the initiation of therapy without definition of the microbial agent, many authors would recommend the combination of an aminoglycoside, such as gentamicin (5 to 7.5 mg/kg/day) and a penicillinase resistant penicillin such as oxacillin (150 mg/kg/day). Others advocate the use of ampicillin (200 mg/kg/day) and gentamycin as the initial drug therapy in this particular situation.

Much mention has been made of the value of antimicrobial prophylaxis in mitigating the development of infectious endocarditis. While it should be noted that the benefits of prophylaxis have never been fully substantiated, nevertheless, it remains incumbent upon the physician seeing a child with heart disease in the emergency department to make sure that prophylaxis

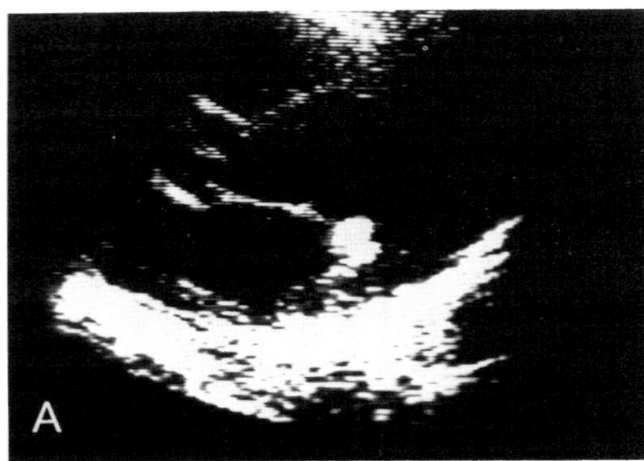

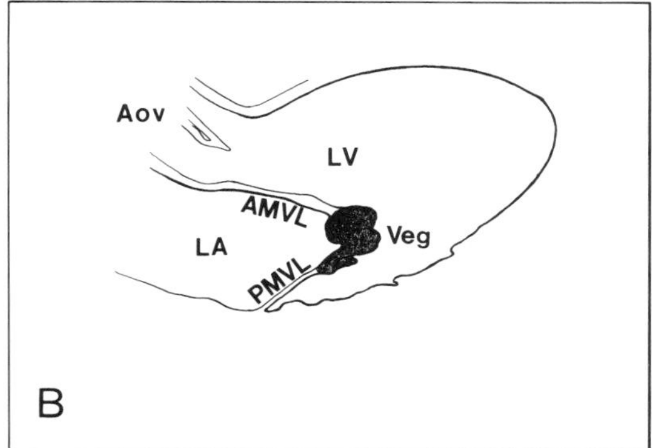

Figure 43.14 (*A*) Long axis parasternal two-dimensional echocardiogram in patient with mitral valve pneumococcal endocarditis. (*B*) *Aov* = aortic valve; *LV* = left ventricle; *AMVL* = anterior mitral valve leaflet; *PMVL* = posterior mitral valve leaflet; *Veg* = vegetation; *LA* = left atrium.

has been implemented if warranted. Guidelines have been established by the American Heart Association (Table 43.12). As a general rule, such measures are practical only in the face of a well-defined predisposing event. The usual child with heart disease who presents with a routine febrile illness does not require prophylactic antibiotics. Unnecessary hasty administration of antibiotics when not indicated can be harmful since obfuscation of the ultimate diagnosis may result in damaging delay.

If systemic antibiotics are contemplated for other infectious indications, a complete blood count and a blood culture should be drawn before initiation of therapy in most instances. In particular, these measures should be taken for the child with heart disease and a major infection, such as pneumonia or cellulitis, even if no clinical evidence of endocarditis is immediately apparent. It is not mandatory to admit the child with heart disease and an intercurrent febrile illness to the hospital on every occasion, and the above noted laboratory studies may be helpful in making such a decision. Clinical judgement, however, remains the best immediate guide as to the necessity for hospitalization. While a high degree of suspicion and alertness for the possibility of endocarditis is mandatory, the emergency physician should resist the temptation to indiscriminantly administer antibiotics to the child with heart disease.

HYPOXEMIC ATTACKS

BACKGROUND

Children with cyanotic congenital heart disease in which pulmonary blood flow is reduced, such as tetralogy of Fallot, may experience periodic episodes of intense hypoxemia. Emergency attention is usually sought for these episodes at the nearest convenient medical location. Thus, the emergency physician caring for children should have a good understanding of the associated physiologic and management principles.

PATHOPHYSIOLOGY

The reasons for the acute nature of these episodes have never been unequivocally defined. Initial thoughts that "cyanotic spells" were caused by spasmodic contraction of the portion of right ventricular outflow tract known as the "infundibulum" cannot provide the entire explanation since children with pulmonary atresia, in whom no subpulmonic infundibulum has developed, can also experience hypercyanotic attacks. Additional theoretical concerns have focused on (1) sudden changes in systemic vascular resistance and in venous return to the heart which consequently effect the intracardiac right-to-left shunt, (2) alterations in sensitivity of the respiratory center, (3) marked changes in heart rate, or (4) some combination of all of these. A sche-

Table 43.12
Pediatric Regimens for Prophylaxis of Bacterial Endocarditis[a]

I. Prophylaxis for Dental Procedures and Surgical Procedures of the Upper Respiratory Tract

	Most congenital heart disease (3); rheumatic or other acquired valvular heart disease; idiopathic hypertrophic subaortic stenosis; mitral valve (4) prolapse syndrome with mitral insufficiency	Prosthetic heart valves (5)
All dental procedures that are likely to result in gingival bleeding (1, 2)	Regimen A or B	Regiman B
Surgery or instrumentation of the respiratory tract (6)	Regimen A or B	Regimen B

(1) Does not include shedding of deciduous teeth.
(2) Does not include simple adjustment of orthodontic appliances.
(3) For example, ventricular septal defect, tetralogy of Fallot, aortic stenosis, pulmonic stenosis, complex cyanotic heart disease, patent ductus arteriosus, or systemic pulmonary artery shunts. Does not include uncomplicated secundum atrial septal defect.
(4) Although cases of infective endocarditis in patients with mitral valve prolapse syndrome have been documented, the incidence appears to be relatively low and the necessity for prophylaxis in all of these patients has not yet been established.
(5) Some patients with a prosthetic heart valve in whom a high level of oral health is being maintained may be offered oral antibiotic prophylaxis for routine dental procedures except for the following: parenteral antibiotics are recommended for patients with prosthetic valves who require extensive dental procedures, especially extractions, or oral and gingival surgical procedures.
(6) For example, tonsillectomy, adenodectomy, bronchoscopy, and other surgical procedures of the upper respiratory tract involving disruption of the respiratory mucosa.

Regimen A — Penicillin

1. *Parenteral-oral combined*: Aqueous crystalline penicillin G (30,000 units/kg i.m.) *mixed with* procaine penicillin G (600,000 units i.m.). Given 1 hr prior to the procedure and then penicillin V (500 mg orally) every 6 hr for 8 doses. For children under 60 lb (25 kg), the dose of penicillin V is 250 mg.
2. *Oral*: Penicillin V (2.0 g orally) 30 min to 1 hr prior to procedure and then 500 mg orally every 6 hr for 8 doses. For children less than 60 lb, use 1.0 g orally 30 min to 1 hr prior to the procedure and then 250 mg orally every 6 hr for 9 doses.

For patients allergic to penicillin: Use either vancomycin (see Regimen B) or use erythromycin (20 mg/kg) orally 1½–2 hr prior to the procedure and then 10 mg/kg every 6 hr for 8 doses.

Regimen B — Penicillin plus Streptomycin

Aqueous crystalline penicillin G (30,000 units/kg i.m. *mixed with* procaine penicillin G (600,000 units i.m.) *plus* streptomycin (20 mg/kg i.m.). Timing of doses for children is the same as for adults. For children less than 60 lb, the recommended oral dose of penicillin V is 250 mg every 6 hr for 8 doses.

For patients allergic to penicillin: Vancomycin (20 mg/kg i.v.) over 30 min to 1 hr. This should not exceed 44 mg/kg per 24 hr. Start initial infusion ½ to 1 hr prior to the procedure, then erythromycin (10 mg/kg) every 6 hr for 8 doses.

Table 43.12—*continued*

II. Prophylaxis for Gastrointestinal and Genitourinary Tract Surgery and Instrumentation

Aqueous crystalline penicillin G (30,000 units/kg i.m. or i.v.)
or
Ampicillin (50 mg/kg i.m. or i.v.)
plus
Gentamycin (2.0 mg/kg i.m. or i.v.)
or
Streptomycin (20 mg/kg i.m.)

Give initial doses 30 min to 1 hr prior to procedure. If gentamycin is used, then give a similar dose of gentamycin and penicillin (or ampicillin) every 8 hr for 2 additional doses. If streptomycin is used, then give a similar dose of streptomycin and penicillin (or ampicillin) every 12 hr for 2 additional doses. During prolonged procedures or in the case of delayed healing it may be necessary to provide additional antibiotics. For brief outpatient procedures such as uncomplicated bladder catheterization, one dose may be sufficient. In patients with compromised renal function it may be necessary to modify antibiotic doses.

For patients allergic to penicillin: Vancomycin (20 mg/kg given i.v. over 30 min to 1 hr) plus streptomycin (20 mg/kg i.m.). A single dose of these antibiotics begun 30 min to 1 hr prior to the procedure is probably sufficient, but may be repeated in 12 hr.

[a] Modified from: Statement by Committee on Rheumatic Fever and Bacterial Endocarditis of the Council on Cardiovascular Disease in the Young of the American Heart Association: Prevention of bacterial endocarditis. *Circulation*, *56:* 139A, 1977.

matic cycle of postulated mechanisms is noted in Figure 43.15.

Any number of precipitory events related to these physiologic factors can be associated with the development of cyanotic spells. Frequently, they are morning events, noted shortly after awakening. This may be related to the sudden changes in cardiac output that occur after arousal from a long sleep. Other times of likelihood for the appearance of hypercyanosis include periods of dehydration, invasive medical procedures, or other significant stresses.

CLINICAL FINDINGS

The diagnosis of a hypoxemic spell is usually self-evident. Aside from the obvious cyanosis and the history of heart disease, there may also be a preceding history of squatting with exertion or of other positional vagaries that the parents may recall. It is not necessary for the child to have been overtly cyanotic before the onset of a spell, as many such episodes can occur in children with little or no cyanosis otherwise. During a spell, the child may be irritable and crying or may be lethargic and even unconscious. Hyperpnea is a feature of the syndrome and should be distinguished from tachypnea or from other abnormal respiratory patterns which may signal other medical problems associated with cyanosis. During a spell, there may be a notable absence or lessening of a previously heard heart murmur since pulmonary blood flow through the stenotic right ventricular outflow tract is considerably reduced. Laboratory investigations, such as arterial blood gas analysis, should ordinarily be avoided in the initial evaluation. If the attack is prolonged and associated with deepening sensorium changes, assessment of acid-base balance and ventilatory status may be indicated.

MANAGEMENT

The child with a hypoxemic spell requires immediate attention. Appropriate positioning, oxygen, and administration of morphine are the standard initial therapeutic measures, and these usually result in prompt abatement of the attack.

Subcutaneous morphine has traditionally been used in the treatment of cyanotic

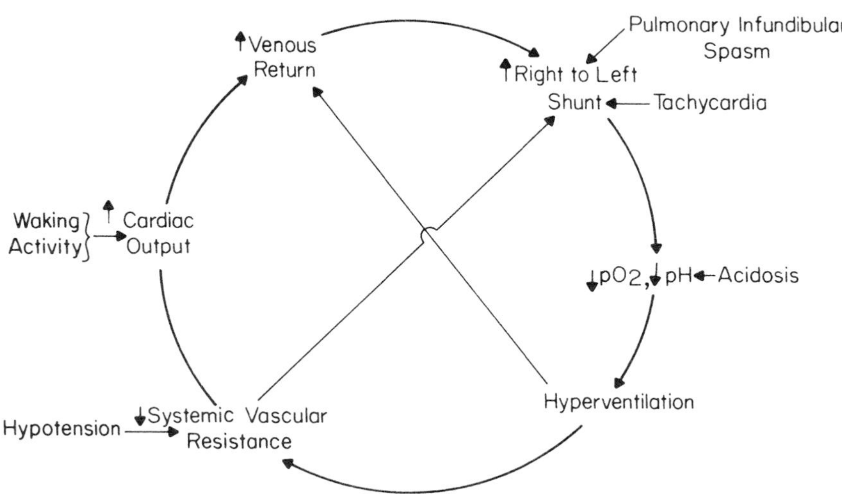

Figure 43.15 Schema of interrelated events in the genesis of hypoxemic spells. See text for discussion. (Reproduced with permission from C. L. Anthony et al.: *Pediatric Cardiology*, Medical Outline Series, p. 193, Medical Examination Publishing Co., Inc., Garden City, N. Y., 1979.)

spells. Relatively large doses are given (0.1 to 0.2 mg/kg) although the precise mechanism of action is not known. Morphine probably does not act to inhibit catecholamine action at the cardiac level but may abort the cycle of hyperpnea and vasomotor changes by depressing the respiratory center. A theoretical negative effect of morphine is its tendency to lower systemic vascular resistance.

Oxygen should be administered, since PaO_2 levels may be quite low and some benefit in terms of oxygen saturation may be obtained from even relatively small increments in dissolved oxygen. However, in the face of marked reduction of pulmonary blood flow, as occurs with a "spell," oxygen will not have a dramatic effect.

The child should be placed in a knee-chest position and calmed, if possible. If the attack persists, additional therapeutic steps are needed. Sodium bicarbonate may be indicated; the dosage dependent upon arterial pH. Propranolol has also come to be recognized as efficacious in this situation, and an intravenous dose of 0.2 mg/kg over 4 to 5 min may yield relatively prompt improvement. Whether the effect of propranolol is primarily upon infundibular contraction, upon the hyperpneic ventilatory response, or upon systemic vasomotor tone, or all of these, is not clear. It should be remembered that propranolol is not to be used if the patient has a coincident history of asthma.

Intravenous fluids should be administered in the severe spell in maintenance doses (see p. 415), at least, as pulmonary blood flow and right ventricular output are volume dependent. Functionally, right ventricular outflow obstruction may be heightened in the face of depleted intravascular volume.

Vasopressors have been advocated as alternative or adjunctive therapy for hypoxemic spells. Phenylephrine (Neo-Synephrine) can be given intravenously as a dilute solution of 10 mg/100 ml and infused at 10 μg/kg/min. Heart rate should be monitored and frequent blood pressure assessment carried out if this type of agent is used. Methoxamine (10 mg/100 ml) or metaraminol (50 mg/100 ml) may also be used. These drugs, by increasing systemic vascular resistance, favorably reduce intracardiac right-to-left shunting and, thus, improve systemic oxygenation. Digitalis, epinephrine, or norepinephrine, however, should not be used in this setting.

If any underlying condition exists, such

as a cardiac rhythm disturbance, prompt correction according to the principles noted under "Cardiac Arrhythmias" (p. 299) may quickly alleviate this situation.

Cardiac consultation is advisable as soon as feasible in order to make extended management decisions, even if the spell has abated with the above measures. In most situations, if the spell has required more than oxygen and positional adjustment to abate, hospitalization will be indicated. Usually, although relieved with therapy, the occurrence of spells is an indication to proceed with the appropriate surgery for the cardiac defect.

ACUTE RHEUMATIC FEVER

BACKGROUND

Although the large numbers of rheumatic fever patients seen in the past have greatly dissipated in the face of improved diagnosis and treatment of streptococcal infections, the disease does still occur within the pediatric population; thus, the emergency physician should be aware of its clinical manifestations. In general, care of the child with rheumatic fever is a chronic process often involving the use of extended care facilities. Nevertheless, proper initial therapy can greatly affect the long term outlook, and early diagnosis can be critically important.

PATHOPHYSIOLOGY

It has been clearly established that streptococcal infection is a necessary precedent for the development of rheumatic fever. In particular, a history of infection by this organism of the upper respiratory tract should be carefully sought in any suspected case. The precise mechanistic relationship between antecedent streptococcal infection and rheumatic fever, however, remains ill defined. Many serologic types of Group A streptococci can be associated with acute rheumatic fever so that the antigenic factors involved are common to various strains of the organism. The particular host factors which determine who succumbs to acute rheumatic fever and who does not, despite identical infections, are also poorly defined. A clear-cut familial pattern has never been identified. The more common theoretic considerations relating streptococcal infection and acute rheumatic fever are: (1) an immunologic (autoimmune) response involving host reaction to infection with a target organ being the heart, specifically, endocardial tissue; (2) a persistence of organism despite therapy, with localization to cardiac tissue; and (3) a direct reaction to the organism such as cardiotoxicity from streptolysin O produced by the organism. Thus far, no evidence of direct cardiac infection has developed, making experimental evaluation difficult.

CLINICAL FINDINGS

The diagnosis of rheumatic fever requires a high index of suspicion. The time-honored Jones criteria (Table 43.13), if unequivocally present, usually establish the diagnosis, but the situation may not always be entirely clear-cut.

A complete careful physical examination is the mandatory first procedure. Special attention should be given to eliciting joint pathology and cutaneous findings whose presence may facilitate the diagnosis in difficult cases. All of the major Jones criteria are derived through clinical examination, which usually needs to be repeated at frequent intervals. Among the major criteria, *carditis* can be easily overdiagnosed. Misinterpretation of functional ("innocent")

Table 43.13
Rheumatic Fever Manifestations[a]

Major:
- Carditis
- Arthritis
- Subcutaneous nodules
- Erythema marginatum
- Chorea

Minor:
- Fever
- Elevated erythrocyte sedimentation rate
- Prolonged PR interval
- Arthralgia
- Previous rheumatic fever

[a] Diagnostic criteris should also include evidence of a preceding β-hemolytic streptococcal infection. (After T. D. Jones: The diagnosis of rheumatic fever. *JAMA*, *126:* 481, 1944.)

murmurs, whose auscultation is heightened in the presence of fever or agitation, often causes undue concern. In the appropriate clinical setting, the presence of an apical systolic murmur, characteristic of mitral insufficiency, or of a basal diastolic decrescendo murmur, typical of aortic insufficiency, *are* important signs of carditis. The presence of a pericardial effusion, congestive heart failure, or pericarditis also strongly suggests the carditis component of acute rheumatic fever, even in the absence of valvar murmurs. Care must be taken to exclude other causes for cardiac findings, such as deteriorating congenital heart disease, which may result in cardiac decompensation not related to a rheumatic process. If at all possible, the examining physician should attempt to document a change in previous clinical findings in children with preexisting heart disease (or previous rheumatic fever episodes). While regurgitant lesions, such as aortic or mitral insufficiency, are common components of the acute manifestations of rheumatic fever, stenotic lesions, such as aortic or mitral stenosis, are not usually seen with a first attack of acute rheumatic fever.

Polyarthritis is the most frequently found major criterion. It should be remembered that this is true joint inflammation, not arthralgia. Tenderness, motion restriction, heat, redness, and swelling are the signs to be elicited. In contrast to other forms of collagen disease, joint involvement in rheumatic fever is usually migratory and multiple, and tends to localize to larger joints of the extremities. It may be necessary to avoid rapid use of anti-inflammatory agents in patients with suspected acute rheumatic fever in order to clarify the diagnosis of migratory polyarthritis.

The cutaneous criteria are *erythema marginatum* and *subcutaneous nodules*. These findings are not as frequent as arthritis and carditis and are rarely present as the only major criteria. Nodules usually occur in situations of recurrent rheumatic fever or chronicity. They are found over extensor surfaces of joints, such as elbows or knees, are firm and decidedly nontender, and are movable on palpation. Erythema marginatum characteristically appears on the trunk and proximal extremities and is an extremely evanescent finding. The application of heat may accentuate its appearance. This rash is notable for its fine, lacy appearance with central blanching and a serpiginous pattern. It is not pruritic and is usually easily distinguishable from drug rashes or other viral exanthems.

Chorea is the fifth of the major criteria defined by Jones. It is a relatively rare finding that is limited to children over the age of 3 years, and can occur quite some time after the initial streptococcal infection, making accurate diagnosis difficult. Chorea is typified by involuntary purposeless movement of the extremities and facial grimacing. Notable emotional lability is also a part of the picture. The emergency department diagnosis of acute rheumatic fever rarely depends upon the finding of chorea as the principal manifestation. The physician, however, should be aware of the possibility of the diagnosis in a child presenting with this finding and arrange for appropriate further evaluation of the etiologic basis for the chorea.

The "minor criteria" defined by Jones are nonspecific indices of inflammatory disease and, frequently, are sources of overdiagnosis of acute rheumatic fever. The fever associated with acute rheumatic fever is notable for its lack of associated chills or rigor. It is typically low grade, and fevers of greater than 104°F (40°C) or a history of a febrile seizure should point to other illnesses. The wildly fluctuating fever of juvenile rheumatoid arthritis ("quotidian" pattern) is usually not a part of the rheumatic fever picture. Elevation of the erythrocyte sedimentation rate (ESR) or C-reactive protein should be present in acute rheumatic fever, but severe congestive heart failure may lower the ESR. A prolonged P-R interval is a frequent occurrence in acute rheumatic fever but also an extremely nonspecific finding. It does not necessarily correlate with the presence of organic murmurs and can be found in other inflammatory cardiac diseases or as a result of certain drugs. Overemphasis of the significance of P-R prolongation is a frequent cause of improper diagnosis.

Emphasis needs to be placed upon the

inclusion with the modified Jones criteria of evidence of recent streptococcal infection. Culture documentation is helpful, but serologic evidence may be the most rewarding and diagnostic. The widespread use of the multiple antibody test (Streptozyme) has made serologic confirmation of recent streptococcal infection much easier. The antistreptolysin O test (ASO) remains a commonly used single serologic test and is well standardized. Levels greater than 250 Todd units in older children and greater than 333 in younger children are present in active rheumatic fever. As many as 20% of otherwise normal children can have elevated ASO titers and, depending upon the time course of the illness, other antibody determinations may be required.

The differential diagnosis of acute rheumatic fever includes many diseases which fall under the classification of "collagen-vascular" as well as other types of diseases. The Jones criteria themselves can include a spectrum of illnesses such as juvenile rheumatoid arthritis, serum sickness, systemic lupus, and even bacterial endocarditis or septic arthritis. Viral processes, such as myocarditis or pericarditis, need also be excluded, as well as intracardiac lesions such as left atrial myxoma.

In summary, careful application of the Jones criteria plus documentation of a streptococcal infection of recent onset should enable the physician to diagnose acute rheumatic fever most, but not all, of the time. Patience must be exercised in arriving at the diagnosis, since initiation of therapy may suppress findings critical for the diagnosis. Thus, decisions to treat must be tempered with the understanding that it is vital to collect as much definition of the disease process as possible.

As noted earlier, acute phase reactants such as the sedimentation rate and C-reactive protein are elevated in acute rheumatic fever. A CBC should be drawn in order to screen for anemia or an elevated white blood cell count. Leukocytosis is not only a manifestation of infection, but may be considered an "acute phase reactant" as well. Throat cultures (at least two) should be obtained before penicillin therapy is started. In addition, the streptococcal screen previously described should be obtained. Blood cultures will frequently be drawn, with appropriate concern, to rule out subacute bacterial endocarditis, a problem which can present in an identical fashion to acute rheumatic fever.

A chest x-ray to assess heart size can be helpful for gauging the severity of carditis, as well as objectivity verifying its presence. An ECG should be taken to ensure that a rapid pulse rate is the result of sinus tachycardia and to enable measurement of P-R interval. If pericardial disease or intracardiac myxoma need to be ruled out, an echocardiogram can provide highly sensitive information. These latter procedures, of course, will usually be completed after cardiac consultation has been requested. The appropriate laboratory procedures to help rule out other forms of collagen-vascular disease are described in Chapter 56.

MANAGEMENT

Acute rheumatic fever requires admission to the hospital and chronic management. That is, a prolonged treatment course is indicated once the diagnosis is made. Thus, most considerations in caring for a child with acute rheumatic fever will not be made in the emergency department setting. It should be restated that a rush to treat with anti-inflammatory drugs (aspirin or steroids) in a poorly documented case may obscure the ultimate diagnosis and delay further therapy, thereby compromising more than helping the patient.

Principles of management include: (1) treatment of the active streptococcal infection, (2) rest, (3) anti-inflammatory agents, and (4) treatment of chorea. *All* patients with acute rheumatic fever should receive a course of penicillin to eradicate any streptococci present. Intramuscular benzathine penicillin in appropriate dosage for age and weight (see Chapter 45) is preferable. Bed rest is indicated for as long as evidence of active inflammation is present. It should be initiated upon suspicion of the diagnosis and is best done during the initial period in a hospital setting. Anti-inflammatory drugs (salicylates or steroids) may be indicated, but the tendency to begin such therapy before confirmation of the diagnosis as outlined above should be resisted. If arthritis without carditis is present, aspirin is usually sufficient (see Chapter 56). Treatment of carditis may include steroids in selected cases, but that is a decision to be undertaken once the child is hospitalized and a cardiologist consulted. Treatment of chorea is also a long-term management issue with agents such as diazepam or haloperidol currently favored (see p. 350). Recent evidence also suggests a role for steroids in the treatment of chorea as well as for the presence of carditis.

On occasion the child with acute rheumatic fever may present with significant cardiac compromise involving either congestive heart failure associated with a large degree of valvar regurgitation or pericardial effusion resulting in cardiac tamponade. Initially, the heart failure or tamponade should be managed as outlined in the previous sections, and then consideration given of the rheumatic process.

One of the most important aspects of management of the patient with rheumatic fever is prevention of recurrent attacks. It has been clearly documented that penicillin can be effective in this setting, with minimal patient risk. The most reliable method of prophylaxis is intramuscular, with monthly injections of 1.2 million units of benzathine penicillin G being the preferred treatment. Oral penicillin, 200,000 units twice daily, is an alternative prophylactic regimen. Sulfonamides may be used, as well as erythromycin in patients sensitive to penicillin. Recommended dosages for the sulfonamides are 0.5 to 1.0 g daily, depending upon weight, and 250 mg twice daily for erythromycin. While recommendations as to the duration of prophylaxis are currently under scrutiny, most centers continue antibiotics for a minimum of 10 to 15 years after the initial diagnosis and some for life. Increasing age may lessen susceptibility to streptococcal disease, but reliable evidence is lacking to substantiate conclusively this impression. The physician who evaluates a child with known rheumatic heart disease for any reason should review the prophylaxis status of the child at every occasion.

References

Congestive Heart Failure

Chaterjee K, Parmley WW: The role of vasodilator therapy in heart failure. *Prog Cardiovasc Dis* 19: 301, 1977.

Driscoll DJ, Gillette PC, McNamara DG: The use of dopamine in children. *J Pediatr* 92: 309, 1978.

Engle MA: Treatment of the failing heart. *Pediatr Clin North Am* 11: 247, 1964.

Engle AM, Lewey JE, Lewey PR, et al.: The use of furosemide in the treatment of edema in infants and children. *Pediatrics* 62: 811, 1978.

Friedman WF: The intrinsic physiologic properties of the developing heart. In *Neonatal Heart Disease*, p. 21, edited by WF Friedman, M Lesch, EH Sonnenblick. Grune & Stratton, New York, 1973.

Kaplan S: New aspects of management of congestive heart failure. In *Pediatric Cardiovascular Disease*, edited by MA Engle, Cardiovascular Clinics 11/2. F. A. Davis, Philadelphia, 1981.

Neill CA: The use of digitalis in infants and children. *Prog Cardiovasc Dis* 7: 399, 1965.

Ross J, Jr: Afterload mismatch and preload reserve; a conceptual framework for the analysis of ventricular function. *Prog Cardiovasc Dis* 18: 225, 1976.

Rudolph AM: Cardiac failure in children; a hemodynamic overview. In *The Myocardium—Failure and Infarction*. p. 102, edited by E Braunwald. HP Publishing, New York, 1974.

Talner NS: Heart failure. In *Heart Disease in Infants, Children and Adolescents*, Ed. 2, p. 660, edited by AJ Moss, FH Adams, GC Emmanoulides. Williams & Wilkins, Baltimore, 1977.

Cardiac Arrhythmias

Anderson ED, Jacobsen JR, Sandoe E: Paroxysmal tachycardia in infancy and childhood. *Acta Paediatr Scand* 62: 341, 1973.

Garson A, Gilette PC, McNamara DG: Supraventricular tachycardia in children; clinical features, response to treatment, and long-term follow-up in 217 patients. *J Pediatr* 98: 875, 1981.

Gilette PC: Cardiac dysrhythmias in infants and children. In *Pediatric Cardiovascular Disease*, p. 79, edited by MA Engle, AN Brest. F. A. Davis, Philadelphia, 1981.

Hernandez A, Strauss A, Keliger RE, et al.: Idiopathic paroxysmal ventricular tachycardia in infants and children. *J Pediatr* 86: 182, 1975.

Lundeberg A: Paroxysmal tachycardia in infancy; follow-up study of 47 subjects ranging in age from 10 to 26 years. *Pediatrics* 51: 26, 1973.

Nadas AS, et al.: Paroxysmal tachycardia in infants and children. *Pediatrics* 9: 167, 1952.

Park MK, Guntheroth WG: *How to Read Pediatric ECG's*. Yearbook, Chicago, 1981.

Roberts N, Gelband H: Arrhythmias. In *Heart Disease in Infants, Children and Adolescents*, p. 676, edited by A. Moss, FH Adams, GC Emmanouilides. Williams & Wilkins, Baltimore, 1977.

Roberts ND, Gelband H. (eds): *Cardiac Arrhythmias in the Neonate, Infant, and Child*. Appleton-Century-Crofts, New York, 1977.

Surawicz B: Electrolytes and the electrocardiogram. *Postgrad Med* 66: 123–129, 1974.

Vetter VL, Josephson ME, Horowitz LN: Idiopathic recurrent sustained ventricular tachycardia in children and adolescents. *Am J Cardiol* 47: 315, 1981.

Videback J, Andersen ED, Jacobsen JR, Sandoe E, et

al.: Paroxysmal tachycardia in infancy and childhood. 11. Paroxysmal ventricular tachycardia and fibrillation. *Acta Paediatr Scand* 62: 349, 1973.

Pericardial Diseases

Echeverria P, Smith EWP, Ingram D, et al.: *Haemophilus influenzae* pericarditis in children. *Pediatrics* 56: 808, 1975.

Engle, MA, Zabriskie FB, Senterfit LB, et al.: Postpericardiotomy syndrome; a new look at an old condition: modern concepts. *Cardiovasc Dis* 44: 59, 1975.

Gersony WM, Hordof AJ: Infective endocarditis and diseases of the pericardium. *Pediatr Clin North Am* 25: 831, 1978.

Hirschmann JV: Pericardial constriction. *Am Heart J* 96: 110, 1978.

Shabetai R, Fowler ND, Guntheroth WG: The hemodynamics of cardiac tamponade and constrictive pericarditis. *Am J Cardiol* 26: 481, 1970.

Van Regen D, Strauss A, Hernandez A, et al.: Infectious pericarditis in children. *J Pediatr* 85: 165, 1974.

Infectious Endocarditis

Gersony WM, Hayes CT: Bacterial endocarditis in patients with pulmonary stenosis, aortic stenosis, or ventricular septal defect. *Circulation* 56 (Supp 1): 1, 1977.

Johnson DH, Rosenthal A, Nadas AS: A forty year review of bacterial endocarditis in infancy and childhood. *Circulation* 51: 581, 1975.

Kaplan FL, Taranta AV (eds.). *Infective Endocarditis—An American Heart Association Symposium*, Monograph No. 52. Am Heart Assn, Dallas, 1977.

Kaplan FL, Anthony BF, Bisno A, et al.: Prevention of bacterial endocarditis. AHA Committee report. *Circulation* 56: 135A, 1977.

Sande M, Scheld W: Combination antibiotic therapy of bacterial endocarditis. *Ann Intern Med* 92: 390, 1980.

Wann LS, Dillon JC, Weymann AE, et al.: Echocardiography in bacterial endocarditis. *N Engl J Med* 295: 135, 1976.

Hypoxemic Attacks

Boncheck LI, Starr A, Sunderland CO, et al.: Natural history of tetralogy of Fallot in infancy. *Circulation* 48: 392, 1973.

Honey M, Chamberlain DA, Howard J: The effective beta-sympathetic blockage on arterial saturation in Fallot's tetralogy. *Circulation* 30: 501, 1978.

Morgan BC, Guntheroth WG, Bloom RS, et al.: A clinical profile of paroxysmal hyperpnea in cyanotic congenital heart disease. *Circulation* 31: 66, 1965.

Nudel DB, Berman MA, Talner NS: Effects of acutely increasing systemic vascular resistance on oxygen tension in tetralogy of Fallot. *Pediatrics* 58: 248, 1976.

Acute Rheumatic Fever

Committee to Revise the Jones Criteria—American Heart Association: Jones criteria (revised) for guidance in the diagnosis of rheumatic fever. *Circulation* 32: 664, 1965.

Committee on Prevention of Rheumatic Fever and Bacterial Endocarditis of the American Heart Association: Prevention of rheumatic fever. *Circulation* 55: 1, 1977.

DiSciasco G, Taranta A: Rheumatic fever in children. *Am Heart J* 99: 635, 1980.

Kaplan EL: Acute rheumatic fever. *Pediatr Clin North Am* 25: 817, 1978.

Markowitz M, Gordis L: *Rheumatic Fever*, Ed. 2. W. B. Saunders, Philadelphia, 1972.

Siegel AC, Johnson EE, Stollerman GH: Controlled studies of streptococcal pharyngitis in a pediatric population. 1. Factors related to the attack of rheumatic fever. *N Engl J Med* 265: 559, 1961.

Wannamaker LW: The chain that links the heart to the throat. *Circulation* 48: 9, 1973.

CHAPTER 44

Neurologic Emergencies

ROGER J. PACKER, M.D., AND PETER H. BERMAN, M.D.

INTRODUCTION

Neurologic dysfunction, whether due to primary nervous system damage or secondary to systemic disease, often results in life-threatening conditions requiring immediate management. The care provided in the emergency department frequently determines the extent of ultimate neurologic damage. Neurologic assessment, at times difficult in the child with neurologic deficits, is the basis for proper management of the patient. Ancillary tests, such as lumbar puncture, computed tomography, myelography, and electroencephalography, although often indispensable, require an understanding of the nature and anatomic location of neurologic injury for appropriate utilization. If used indiscriminately, they may delay treatment and result in further damage to the child.

In this chapter, an attempt will be made to discuss the more common conditions which present with acute neurologic dysfunction and rarer diseases in which proper management is lifesaving. The illnesses will be classified by the symptomatology most frequently heralding their presence: seizures, encephalopathy, headaches, disorders of motor function, disorders of balance, and cranial nerve dysfunction.

SEIZURES

BACKGROUND

Seizures are among the more common symptoms leading to an emergency department visit. A number of epidemiologic studies indicate that from 4 to 6% of children will have at least one seizure in the first 16 years of life. Fortunately, recurrent seizures or other signs of neurologic dysfunction will only occur in a small number of these children. However, the first seizure is always a frightening, anxiety-producing event.

A seizure is defined as a transient involuntary alteration of consciousness, behavior, motor activity, sensation, and/or automatic function due to an excessive rate and hypersynchrony of discharges from a group of cerebral neurons. A convulsion is a seizure with prominent alterations of motor activity. Epilepsy is a condition of susceptibility to recurrent seizures. The term implies chronicity, but it is important to stress that epilepsy in childhood need not be a lifelong condition. Epilepsy and seizure disorder are synonomous terms. There are multiple causes for seizures as listed in Table 44.1.

Most seizures are brief, lasting less than 10 to 15 min. Prolonged seizures or convulsions are those which last more than 10 to 15 min. Status epilepticus occurs when seizures are continuous or repetitive for an hour or longer, and the patient does not regain consciousness during this time interval. Serial seizures are repetitive over a prolonged time period, but consciousness may be regained at intervening intervals.

Febrile Convulsions

The relatively common association of fever and seizures in infants and young chil-

Table 44.1
Etiologic Classification of Convulsive Disorders

- *I. Acute*
  - A. Infections
    1. Simple febrile seizures
    2. Intracranial infections (meningitis, encephalitis, cerebral abscess, sinus thrombophlebitis)
    3. Shigellosis
  - B. Toxic/metabolic disturbances
    1. Hypernatremia
    2. Hyponatremia
    3. Hypocalcemia
    4. Hypomagnesemia
    5. Hypoglycemia
    6. Pyridoxine deficiency
    7. Renal diseases
    8. Liver diseases
    9. Exogenous toxins
    10. Inherited metabolic disorders
  - C. Intracranial hemorrhage
  - D. Anoxia
  - E. Hypertension
  - F. Trauma
  - G. Brain tumors
  - H. Miscellaneous
- *II. Chronic*
  - A. Idiopathic
  - B. Postanoxic injury
  - C. Postinfectious injury
  - D. Posttraumatic injury
  - E. Posthemorrhagic injury
  - F. Posttoxic injury
  - G. Degenerative diseases
  - H. Congenital disorders

dren has been noted in the medical literature since the days of Hippocrates. In the adult and older child the association of fever and convulsions is relatively rare and connotes an underlying central nervous system infection. In the infant and young child, however, fever and convulsions are frequently associated, and the fever is usually of extracranial origin. CNS infections are found in less than 1% of children under 7 years of age presenting with a febrile convulsion.

Febrile convulsions are divided into "simple" and "complex" on the basis of the clinical characteristics of the seizures. "Simple" febrile convulsions are brief (lasting less than 10 to 15 min) and generalized (without any features suggesting focal CNS onset). "Complex" febrile seizures are prolonged and/or have focal features.

Several further clinical characteristics at the time of the seizure define a group of patient with the syndrome of Simple Febrile Convulsions. The syndrome is important not only because it represents the most common form of childhood epilepsy, but also because of several special associated prognostic and therapeutic implications. Simple febrile convulsions are characteristically brief (less than 15 min in duration), generalized, and occur at the onset (first 24 hours) of a febrile illness in children between 1 and 4 years of age with a normal neurologic examination, including normal psychomotor development. The interictal electroencephalogram in these children is normal except for possible transient postictal generalized background slowing. The family history frequently is positive for similar simple febrile seizures in childhood and negative for other types of seizure disorders. Children with one simple febrile seizure have a 30% chance of having a second simple febrile seizure, and the incidence of further simple febrile seizures remains at approximately 30% with each succeeding convulsion. The likelihood of developing recurrent febrile seizures is less than 1 to 2 in 100, and, in prospective studies, no deleterious educational or behavioral effects have been detected.

The 30% recurrence rate can be reduced to approximately 10% by phenobarbital therapy at therapeutic serum concentrations, but such therapy is associated with a high incidence of significant drug-related behavioral changes. Therapy with other anticonvulsants has thus far not been shown to be effective. Intermittent anticonvulsant therapy, at the time of fever, is not effective since the convulsions tend to occur early in the course of a febrile illness, and there is not sufficient time for the attainment of therapeutic blood levels.

PATHOPHYSIOLOGY

The basic pathophysiologic abnormality common to all seizures and convulsions is the hypersynchrony of neuronal discharges.

The exact mechanisms responsible for this abnormality have not yet been completely defined, but both genetic and constitutional factors play a role. During a seizure, cerebral blood flow, oxygen and glucose consumption, and carbon dioxide, lactic acid, and pyruvate production increase. If the patient remains well ventilated, the increase in cerebral blood flow is sufficient to meet the increased metabolic requirements of the brain. Brief seizures rarely produce lasting deleterious effects on the brain; however, prolonged and serial seizures, and especially status epilepticus, may be associated with permanent neuronal destruction. Several factors, including a local decrease in pH from pyruvate and lactic acid accumulation and hypoglycemia, may be responsible for this effect.

CLINICAL MANIFESTATIONS

Briefly, seizures can be classified according to seizure type. Generalized seizures include grand mal, petit mal and myoclonic seizures (infantile spasms). Partial (focal) seizures include motor, sensory, and psychomotor (complex partial, temporal lobe) seizures. Partial seizures frequently evolve into generalized convulsions, especially in patients not on anticonvulsant medication.

Grand Mal Seizures

The onset of grand mal seizures is usually abrupt, although 20 to 30% of children may experience a sensory or motor aura. If sitting or standing, the child falls to the ground. The face becomes pale, the pupils dilate, the eyes deviate upward or to one side, and the muscles contract. As the increased tone of the thoracic and abdominal muscles forces air through the glottis, a grunt or cry may be heard. Incontinence of urine or stool is frequent. After this brief tonic phase (10 to 30 sec), clonic movements occur. The child is unresponsive during the seizure and remains so, postictally, for a variable period of time.

Petit Mal Seizures

Petit mal seizures have an abrupt onset and cause a brief loss of consciousness, usually less than 30 sec in duration. The child does not fall, but may drop articles being carried. Commonly, there are motor manifestations such as eye blinking or rhythmic nodding. Although there is no postictal period, an occasional child with petit mal status may appear to be in such a state.

Myoclonic Seizures

Myoclonic seizures occur in the first 2 years of life and are characterized by a sudden dropping of the head and flexion of the arms ("jackknifing"). The episodes occur quickly, frequently, and often several hundred times daily.

Partial (Focal) Seizures

Focal seizures may be either motor or sensory. In childhood, motor manifestations occur more commonly, usually involving the face or hand. Spread occurs in a fixed pattern determined by the anatomic origin of the nerve fibers innervating the various muscle groups. If a seizure remains focal, the child maintains consciousness; however, focal seizures often become generalized.

Complex Partial (Psychomotor) Seizures

Psychomotor seizures in childhood usually manifest as purposeful but inappropriate, repetitive motor acts; fugue states or episodes of confusion are rarely seen. An aura is common, usually a cry or an attempt to run. This is followed by a loss of time, and a child who is standing or sitting generally falls to the ground. Postictal drowsiness almost always follows the seizure.

MANAGEMENT

A seizure must always be viewed as a symptom of an underlying pathologic process. The gravity of this process varies from a relatively benign genetic predisposition to the differential diagnosis of serious infectious, metabolic, structural, or degenerative diseases. In the care of the child with seizures (particularly grand mal), the attention of the physician must be focused first on stopping the seizure and providing supportive care; second, on establishing the underlying cause; third, on initiating appropriate prophylactic treatment; and finally, on assuring the availability of appropriate follow-up care.

Stopping the Seizures

It is unusual for the child with a brief seizure to arrive in the emergency department actively convulsing, since, by definition, such seizures last less than 15 min. Therefore, the actively convulsing child is usually already in a prolonged or serial seizure state. The administration of nasal oxygen and the insertion of an oropharyngeal airway are a vital part of the initial management of the unconscious, actively convulsing child. Except for the oropharyngeal airway, there is no benefit from inserting other objects, e.g., padded tongue blade, into the mouth. Trismus occurs frequently in generalized seizures but is transient. If the teeth are tightly clenched, even the placement of the airway should be deferred until it can be inserted without undue trauma during a phase of relaxation.

Following steps to ensure the adequacy of ventilation and circulation, anticonvulsant medication should be administered. If the convulsion is generalized, the intravenous route of administration is preferable, unless technical difficulties cause undue delay. Infants with a first seizure should receive 100 mg of pyridoxine initially. Three drugs, diazepam, phenytoin, and phenobarbital are available for intravenous use as anticonvulsants; only phenobarbital can be used intramuscularly. There is no unanimity of opinion concerning which of these drugs is the best initial agent. Each has its advantages and disadvantages. With the dose and rate of administration required for the treatment of the actively convulsing child, all have the potential to depress cardiorespiratory function.

Diazepam is especially useful as the first drug of choice in children known to be epileptic and on maintenance therapy with other anticonvulsant drugs. It is administered intravenously in an initial dose of 0.2 to 0.3 mg/kg (maximum 10 mg) at a rate of approximately 1 mg/min. The main advantage of its use is the rapidity of its action, the seizure stopping within minutes of its administration when it is effective. Its disadvantages include the relatively short duration of its action (another anticonvulsant medication must be administered within 15 to 20 min even when diazepam has been effective in stopping the seizures), and its prolonged sedative effects. The administration of repeated doses of diazepan in the emergency department should be avoided since the potential for severe respiratory depression and hypotension is increased. If phenobarbital has been used as the initial drug of choice, the use of diazepam is also contraindicated since its cardiorespiratory depressive effects are potentiated by high concentrations of barbiturates.

Phenobarbital is especially useful as the first drug of choice in children not previously treated with anticonvulsant medication. It is administered intravenously in a dose of 10 mg/kg (maximum 120 to 150 mg). The dose can be diluted in 30 to 50 ml of an intravenous dextrose or saline solution and administered slowly over a 5 to 10 min period of time, reducing the possibility of severe respiratory depression. If the seizure stops during the time of administration, the rate can be slowed further but the full dose should be administered to prevent recurrence. Following the administration of this initial dose, further administration of phenobarbital should be delayed for at least 1 to 2 hours. If the convulsions continue, however, phenytoin can be administered.

Phenytoin is especially useful as a second drug when the initial dose of phenobarbital or diazepam is ineffective. It must be administered directly into a vein or intravenous tubing since further dilution may lead to crystallization. Phenytoin should never be injected intramuscularly since its absorption from this site is slow and erratic. An appropriate initial dose is 10 mg/kg, administered slowly over a 10 min period with monitoring of the cardiac rate and rhythm. Its advantages include the absence of respiratory depression, even following the prior administration of diazepam, and minimal sedative effects. Its disadvantages include the necessity for slow, direct infusion, its potential for producing cardiac arrhythmia, and the delay between administration and full effect.

One approach is to administer phenobarbital (10 mg/kg) first to the child not on anticonvulsant medication, and diazepam

(0.2 to 0.3 mg/kg) to the child on anticonvulsants. If convulsions persist for 15 min, an initial dose of phenytoin (10 mg/kg) is administered. A second dose of phenobarbital (5 mg/kg) is administered 30 to 60 min after the administration of phenytoin, followed by a second dose of phenytoin (10 mg/kg) 30 min later, if convulsions persist.

Establishing an Underlying Cause

Seizures are always a symptom of an underlying abnormality of neuronal function. The exact cause of this abnormality may be identifiable (symptomatic seizures) or may remain obscure even after the most extensive evaluation (cryptogenic or idiopathic seizures). The latter, however, is a diagnosis of exclusion, and in the evaluation of a child with seizures a search for a specific etiology is always warranted. Seizures may be symptomatic of a wide variety of pathologic conditions (Table 44.1) and a full etiologic evaluation is beyond the scope of a simple emergency department visit. The evaluation should focus on the differentiation of those conditions which, although relatively rarely found, require, and at times are, amenable to specific therapy.

The first step in the evaluation is a thorough history and a physical examination with particular attention to the neurologic assessment. The results of the history and physical examination will be most helpful in determining the direction of the search for a specific cause. For instance: in the child with fever and seizures, the investigation should be directed toward finding the source and cause of the fever; in the child with seizures and signs of focal neurologic deficit and/or increased intracranial pressure, toward identifying the nature and extent of a possible intracranial structural lesion; and, in the child with seizures and developmental delay, toward determining the cause of the retardation.

Laboratory tests that have been recommended for the evaluation of patients with seizures include serum chemistries (glucose, calcium, magnesium, sodium, BUN, SGOT, SGPT, ammonia, and lead), urinalysis including amino acid and organic acid screens, lumbar puncture, electroencephalography, skull x-rays, computerized tomography of the head, and anticonvulsant serum levels. There is little to be gained by establishing a routine, "shotgun" approach to the laboratory investigation of the child with seizures. Some procedures are mandatory in certain situations and of little value in others. Factors playing a role in determining the extent and direction of laboratory assessment include the age of the child, the history (e.g., trauma, ingestion), and the presence or absence of abnormal findings on examination, e.g., fever, developmental delay, focal neurologic deficit, or increased intracranial pressure. All children with a first seizure should have metabolic studies performed including serum electrolytes, glucose, and calcium. Other laboratory tests, however, have particular pertinence to the evaluation of patients in whom a cause is not readily apparent after the results of the initial tests are available.

Lumbar Puncture. Although less than 1% of children with febrile seizures have CNS infection, seizures often occur in the course of acute bacterial meningitis, a condition that requires spinal fluid examination for diagnosis. Lumbar puncture is mandatory in the evaluation of all febrile seizures associated with signs of meningeal irritation. However, there is little consensus about the role of spinal fluid examination in the evaluation of patients with febrile seizures without signs of meningeal irritation. One approach is to perform a lumbar puncture if the febrile convulsions are prolonged or serial, if the fever had been present for more than 48 to 72 hours before the seizure, or if the child is less than 18 months of age. A lumbar puncture is rarely indicated for the evaluation of an afebrile child without meningeal signs in the emergency department.

Computerized Tomographic (CT) Scans of the Head. CT scanning of the head allows for detailed analysis of the gross anatomy of intracranial structures by a noninvasive technique. CT scans are especially helpful as an aid in the evaluation of patients with convulsions associated with signs of focal neurologic deficit, increased intracranial pressure, or more than transient changes in level of consciousness.

Electroencephalography. Electroencephalography is an important laboratory aid in the evaluation of seizure types, response to treatment, and prognosis. It is rarely of benefit in the acute management of a seizure disorder.

Skull X-rays. Skull x-rays are useful in the evaluation and management of traumatic seizures for determining the presence and extent of skull fractures. They may also show signs of chronic increased intracranial pressure or, on rare occasions, intracerebral calcifications in brain tumors or congenital infections. In these circumstances, however, a CT scan will yield much more definitive information. Skull x-rays have not been found to be valuable in the evaluation of febrile seizures.

Anticonvulsant Serum Concentrations. Poor compliance is one of the more common causes for recurring seizures in a previously well-controlled epileptic, and the availability of technology for the rapid and reliable assay of most anticonvulsants in a small amount of serum has had a dramatic beneficial effect on patient management. Anticonvulsant serum concentrations should always be performed when seizures occur in a known epileptic on such medication.

Initiating Anticonvulsant Medication

Anticonvulsant therapy should be initiated in all patients who have had one or more seizures unless:

1. The seizures were symptomatic of a readily reversible condition.
2. The circumstances of the seizures were such that a diagnosis of the syndrome of Simple Febrile Seizures can be established.
3. The seizure occurred in the last stages of a syncopal attack.
4. The description of events is such that it is unclear that a definite seizure occurred.

Phenobarbital, phenytoin, and carbamezapine (Tegretol) are the most commonly used anticonvulsant medications for the treatment of grand mal, focal, and complex-partial seizures.

Phenobarbital remains the most commonly used initial drug, primarily because of its low cost and low toxicity. The effective serum concentration ranges between 15 to 40 μg/ml. This serum level usually can be maintained with a dose of 3 to 6 mg/kg/day in children and 1 to 2 mg/kg/day in adolescents, administered in divided doses twice a day. Daily doses greater than 90 mg are hardly ever necessary. With the administration of such a maintenance dose in the previously untreated patient, effective serum concentrations will not be reached for 2 to 3 weeks. A loading dose of approximately twice the maintenance dose (6 to 10 mg/kg/day in children and 2 to 4 mg/kg/day in adolescents) for 2 to 3 days will bring the serum concentration to the therapeutic range within 48 to 72 hours. Such loading doses are usually associated with considerable transient drowsiness. There is a wide margin between the anticonvulsant and soporific effects of phenobarbital, and drowsiness rarely persists at the recommended doses. Decreased attention, hyperactivity, and alterations of mood occur in 30 to 50% of infants maintained on phenobarbital. These behavioral changes are the most frequently encountered side effects and often are sufficiently undersirable to force the change to another drug.

Phenytoin. The effective serum concentration of phenytoin is between 10 and 20 μg/ml. To achieve this level, maintenance doses of 7 to 10 mg/kg/day in children under 20 kg, 5 to 7 mg/kg/day in children between 20 and 40 kg, and 5 mg/kg/day in children above 40 kg are usually required. There is, however, considerable variation in the metabolism from individual to individual, and serum levels should be obtained after the initiation of this medication. Saturation of biotransforming enzyme systems frequently occurs between serum levels of 10 and 20 μg/ml so that small changes in dose in this range may lead to relatively large changes in serum levels.

With the administration of such maintenance doses, it will take from 1 to 2 weeks to achieve a plateau in the serum level. Loading doses of 4 times the daily dose (maximum 20 mg/kg/day) on the first day and 2 times the daily dose for the next 2 days will bring serum levels into the therapeutic range within 24 hours; side effects rarely occur with this loading dose. Gingival hyperplasia is a common side effect and may be seen with phenytoin concentrations in the therapeutic range. It can be minimized with good dental hygiene. Ataxia, the most common adverse reactions, rarely occurs unless serum levels are over 30 μg/ml.

Carbamazepine. The effective serum concentrations of carbamazepine range between 6 and 12 μg/ml, but with this drug there is little correlation between clinical efficacy, toxicity, and the serum concentration. Recommended maintenance doses range between 10 and 20 mg/kg/day, divided into 3 daily doses. The administration of a total maintenance dose to a previously untreated patient frequently results in drowziness, at times severe lethargy, so that this drug should be initiated by gradually increasing the dose to a full maintenance level over 7 to 10 days.

The ultimate goal of anticonvulsant therapy is the prevention of further attacks without the appearance of undesirable side effects. This goal can be accomplished in the majority of patients with the use of a single drug prescribed in appropriate amounts and taken faithfully. Compliance is most important in the treatment of seizures, and is often understandably difficult to obtain since medications must be taken regularly, for long periods of time, even when no obvious problem exists.

ENCEPHALOPATHY

Encephalopathy is an imprecise term implying diffuse brain dysfunction with or without alterations in the level of consciousness (see Chapter 10). The emergency department physician must often decide if the degree of irritability, uncooperativeness, and lethargy of a child is proportionate to the degree of systemic illness, if it is due to fear, or if it represents cortical dysfunction. Since cognitive functions, such as speech and reasoning, are often untestable in the child, this decision is dependent on a careful history and neurologic examination. Encephalopathy may be secondary to diffuse processes which interrupt the availability of substrates on which brain tissue is dependent, such as oxygen and glucose; which disturb the biochemical mechanisms necessary for brain cell function, as in hepatic or renal failure; or which compress, disrupt, or destroy neural tissue. The metabolic conditions that cause cortical dysfunction are covered in Chapters 46 and 50. This chapter will discuss only conditions causing primary brain dysfunction commonly seen in the emergency department.

Encephalitis (Non-herpetic)

BACKGROUND

Encephalitis is an inflammation of the brain parenchyma often with an associated lepto-meningeal involvement. CNS dysfunction is due to direct invasion of brain by a pathogen, most frequently a virus, or secondary to immunologic mechanisms. Viral encephalitis commonly follows a viremia, although spread can occur rarely via peripheral nerves or the nasal mucosa. Host factors, especially immunocompetence, modify the extent and duration of the disease.

Viral encephalitidies are caused by a wide variety of viruses which lead to clinically indistinguishable illnesses. In general, the incidence of sequelae is higher in children under 1 year of age. Mumps is the most common cause of meningoencephalitis, and up to 50% of patients with mumps parotitis will have cerebrospinal fluid pleocytosis. The illness classically occurs several days to 2 weeks after the onset of parotitis, but may precede the onset of systemic illness or occur without parotitis, and it tends to be mild. Measles encephalitis is less common since the advent of widespread live immunization. The onset usually occurs during the prodromal period, or after the rash has appeared. Ataxia is the most common neurologic abnormality, and sequelae occur in up to 30% of the cases. Varicella encephalitis occurs 2 to 9 days after the onset of the rash; severe infections are uncommon, except in the immunosuppressed host.

The arthropod/borne encephalitidies, including St. Louis, western equine, eastern equine, and Californina encephalitis, occur in sporadic and epidemic forms, frequently in late summer or early fall, and tend to cluster in localized geographic areas. Sequelae may be severe and mortality high, especially in Eastern Equine encephalitis. Outbreaks of enteroviral (Coxsackie, echovirus) encephalitis are common in the late summer and early fall and may be associated with a mild paralytic illness. Poliomyelitis, caused by another enterovirus, produces a paralytic or nonparalytic illness and results in significant morbidity and mortality. Although rare since the advent of live virus immunization, this disease still occurs in epidemics in nonimmunized communities. Cytomegalovirus, usually causing intrauterine infection, may result in encephalitis in the immunosuppressed child. Lymphocytic choriomeningitis is characterized by primarily meningeal symptoms, and marked CSF pleocytosis between 700 and 1,000 cells is common.

Postinfectious or postimmunization encephalitidies are arbitrarily separated from the viral encephalitidies. Considered "postviral" since virus cannot be isolated from or demonstrated in brain tissue, they are characterized histologically by perivenous demyelination, thought to be on an immunologic basis. They are more frequently complicated by concomitant acute transverse or ascending myelitis than acute viral infections. Acute hemorrhagic leukoencephalitis and acute dissemminated encephalomyelitis are probably more explosive variants of "postinfectious" encephalitis.

CLINICAL MANIFESTATIONS

The onset of encephalitis may be abrupt or insidious, and is characteristically associated with fever, headache, and signs of meningeal irritation. Neurologic deficits and the level of consciousness are dependent on the degree and location of cerebral involvement.

Laboratory assessment is often nonspecific. The blood count usually shows a mild polymorphonuclear or monocuclear leukocytosis. A cerebrospinal fluid pleocytosis is variable and, if present, is usually under 500 cells. These cells may be predominantly polymorphonuclear early in the course of the illness; however, a mononuclear predominance is common later. Spinal fluid protein and glucose are usually normal. Virus isolation from the cerebrospinal fluid may be difficult but should be attempted, as should viral isolation from other body sites including the nasopharynx, skin lesions, urine, and feces. Serologic evidence for viral infection, though useful later, is of little help in making an immediate diagnosis. Electroencephalography demonstrates diffuse focal slowing and may be helpful in the differential diagnosis, especially in herpes simplex encephalitis.

DIFFERENTIAL DIAGNOSIS

Brain abscesses, partially treated bacterial meningitis, tuberculous meningitis, rickettsial disease, and brain tumors may mimic viral encephalitis and have similar cerebrospinal fluid profiles. Brain abscesses and tumors are demonstrable by computerized tomography. Tuberculous meningitis, characterized by greater elevations in the spinal fluid protein than seen in viral encephalitis and a diminution in the spinal fluid glucose, is commonly associated with radiographic evidence of pulmonary tuberculosis. The TB skin test may be negative if the patient is anergic. If doubt persists after the initial evaluation, the patient should be treated with antituberculous drugs. Partially treated meningitis should be suspected when there is a history of recent antibiotic usage. Counterimmunoelectrophoresis of the cerebrospinal fluid and urine may disclose a bacterial infection even if Gram stains and cultures are negative. Rocky Mountain spotted fever, the most common rickettsial disease in the United States, occurs 2 days to 2 weeks following a tick bite. This illness is heralded by high fever followed by a petechial rash (see Chapter 45), but may occasionally cause an encephalitis prior to the cutaneous manifestations.

MANAGEMENT

At present, the treatment of non-herpes encephalitis is primarily supportive. Since these patients are at risk for the development of inappropriate ADH secretion, fluid restriction is necessary early in the course of the illness, and serum electrolytes must be monitored diligently throughout the course of the illness.

Herpes Encephalitis

Herpes simplex encephalitis causes death or neurological sequelae in over 70% of patients. It tends to present with high fevers, focal or generalized seizures, and focal neurologic findings with supervening coma. The cerebrospinal fluid profile is consistent with viral encephalitis, and in addition, red cells are present in 50% of cases. Electroencephalography may show focal slowing or periodic localized epileptiform discharges. CT or brain scanning discloses focal areas of parenchymal involvement in some patients. Unfortunately, since none of these findings are pathognomonic for herpes simplex encephalitis and the clinical picture may vary, a definitive diagnosis requires demonstration of the virus. Viral culture takes at least 2 days and serological assays for virus antibody or antigen, even in the cerebrospinal fluid, are unreliable. The only rapid reliable method of virus demonstration is brain biopsy.

Treatment of herpes simplex encephalitis with adenosine arabinoside has resulted in a decrease in mortality and some improvement in morbidity. However, the drug must be given at high fluid volumes in patients at risk for inappropriate ADH secretion and hyponatremia, and it potentially causes bone marrow depression. In addition, it must be used early in the disease, prior to the onset of coma, to be of maximum benefit. For these reasons, we recommend that all patients with possible herpes simplex encephalitis should undergo emergency electroencephalography, brain scan, or computerized tomography. If focal deficits are demonstrated, a brain biopsy should be performed. Pending results of the biopsy, treatment with adenosine arabinoside should be started.

Reye's Syndrome

Reye's syndrome, a common cause of acute encephalopathy, is characterized by recurrent vomiting and alterations in the state of conciousness, usually following a viral illness. This encephalopathy is associated with fatty infiltration of the liver, and the diagnosis can be made with certainty only by liver biopsy. However, a presumptive diagnosis can be made if an elevated blood ammonia level is present. Early diagnosis is mandatory, for aggressive control of increased intracranial pressure may be lifesaving. A complete discussion of pathogenesis, diagnosis, and treatment is given in Chapter 50.

HEADACHE

Headaches of varying character, severity, and etiologies affect patients of all ages. Much of the CNS, including the brain parenchyma, is devoid of pain sensors. Pain sensitive cranial structures include the proximal portions of the large cerebral arteries, the arteries of the dura and scalp, the intracranial venous sinuses, and the dura at the base of the skull. Compression or distortion of these structures, as well as involvement of the facial sinuses, orbits, teeth, scalp, muscles, and cervical roots of the spinal cord may result in headache. The presence of focal neurologic impairment or alteration in the level of consciousness requires a complete evaluation for intracranial causes of headache. Morning headache and projectile vomiting, said to be common symptoms of headaches secondary to increased intracranial pressure, can be found in headaches due to different etiologies and are variable in children with intracranial mass lesions. A full discussion of the differential diagnosis of the etiologies of headache is given in Chapter 23.

Migraine

BACKGROUND

Migraine, recurrent headaches separated by long symptom-free intervals, is probably the most frequent cause of episodic headaches in childhood. Migraine is considered "classic" when the headache is well-localized and preceded by an "aura," and "common" when it is not. The common form of migraine predominates in childhood. Basilar migraine is a migraine variant involving the posterior cerebral circulation in which brainstem symptoms, which may include transient loss of consciousness, predominate. Cluster headaches, which are unilateral, occur in runs and are associated with autonomic changes, are a rare migraine variant in childhood.

PATHOPHYSIOLOGY

The pathogenesis of migraine is not fully delineated, but the headache is thought to be secondary to paroxysmal vascular instability resulting in intracranial vasoconstriction followed by extracranial and possibly intracranial vasodilatation. These vascular changes often occur sequentially resulting in premonitory motor, visual, or sensory symptoms (the vasoconstrictive phase), and then headache (the vasodilation phase). The biochemical basis of this instability may be due to depression of sertonergic brainstem neurons, although many neuronal transmitter abnormalities have been described.

CLINICAL MANIFESTATIONS

In childhood, migraine is commonly associated with nausea, vomiting, abdominal pain, and the desire to go to sleep. The headaches may be pulsating and unilateral but less frequent than in adulthood. Auras occur in less than half of migrainous children. A family history of migraine is helpful in diagnosis, and a disproportionate number of migrainous children have episodes of motion sickness, dizziness, vertigo, or frank paroxysmal events. Approximately 60% of migrainous children are male. During the headaches, analgesics are relatively ineffective, and children seek a quiet, dimly lit area to rest or sleep. Occasionally, the attacks awaken the children from sleep. Common trigger factors in childhood include emotional stress, lighting changes, and minor head trauma. Foods, such as lunch meats, which contain nitrates, and cheeses, which contain tyramine, are less frequent but important triggers. The physical examination usually shows no focal neurological deficits.

MANAGEMENT

The diagnosis of migraine is almost exclusively based on the history and is supported by the absence of abnormalities on examination. Given an accurate history, differentiation from tension headaches, sinusitis, and headaches secondary to intracranial lesions is usually possible; studies such as skull x-rays, electroencephalography and computerized tomography are rarely indicated. From 20 to 90% of migrainous children have been reported to have nonspecific electroencephalographic abnormalities, but the EEG is usually not helpful in diagnosis.

"Complicated" migraine, in which sensory or motor abnormalities persist throughout and after the headache, are somewhat more common in children than in adults. At times, there is a history of similar events in other family members. These abnormalities may take any form, but most commonly hemiplegic or ophthalmoplegic deficits are noted. Unless these episodes have occurred previously, their presence warrants further neurologic evaluation.

The acute migrainous attack should be treated with mild analgesics such as aspirin and bed rest. Stronger analgesics should be avoided, but may be used if the headache prevents sleep. If nausea and vomiting are marked, rectal or intramuscular administration may be necessary. Sedatives, such as chloral hydrate (25 to 50 mg/kg, up to maximum of 1 g by mouth) are more useful than analagesics to promote sleep.

Ergot preparations such as ergotamine tartrate (1 to 2 mg sublingually at onset of attack, repeated at 30 min intervals; not more than 3 tablets in 24 hours or 10 tablets in 1 week), acting primarily as vasoconstrictors, are more effective than placebo in aborting acute attacks; but, they must be utilized early in the headache to be effective, preferably at the outset of the prodrome. Since most young children cannot identify an aura, their use is limited before adolescence. Common side effects of ergot preparations include nausea, vomiting, cramps, and distal paresthesias, all which may intensify the symptoms of migraine. Sensitivity to ergots may vary and this makes proper dosage difficult. A reasonable approach is to begin with 1 mg sublingually in the adolescent. Preparations of ergot with additional drugs such as phenobarbital and caffeine are available; however, there is little evidence that they are more efficacious. Oxygen delivered at a concentration of 100% via mask has a mild vasoconstrictive effect, and it is reported to be useful in aborting severe attacks. If migraines are frequent and severe, prophylactic treatment is possible.

ISORDERS OF MOTOR FUNCTION

Every level of the neural axis is involved the performance of motor tasks. Dys-unction of the cerebral cortex, diencepha-n, cerebellum, brainstem, spinal cord de-ending tracts, anterior horn cells, periph-al nerves, neuromuscular junction, or uscle can result in disruption of motor unction. Anatomic localization is usually ossible after evaluation of the distribution nd character of the deficit (see Table 44.2).

Acute Hemiplegia of Childhood

ACKGROUND

Acute hemiplegia of childhood is not a isease but a syndrome resulting from com-romise of the vascular supply of the brain, ccurring primarily in children under 3 ears of age.

LINICAL FINDINGS

Classically, a previously well infant de-elops a focal clonic seizure associated with fever ranging from 38.5 to 39.5°C. This eizure later becomes generalized, the child ses consiousness, and flaccid hemiparesis ecomes apparent upon cessation of seizure ctivity. Initially, deep tendon reflexes are bsent, and the Babinski response is exten-or on the side of involvement. Generally, he face and upper extremity are involved o a greater extent than the lower extrem-ty, and there may be associated aphasia or emianopsia.

Hemiplegia in older children tends to ccur without major alterations in the state f consciousness or seizure activity. The nset of hemiplegia may be subacute or arely stuttering.

In the acutely hemiplegic child, the cere-rospinal fluid is usually normal but may how a mild pleocytosis and slightly in-reased protein. The EEG classically re-eals unilateral slowing.

ANAGEMENT

An initial evaluation should be per-ormed to identify potentially treatable auses of acute hemiplegia including epi-

Table 44.2
Neurologic Motor Paresis: Localization

	Upper Motor Neuron	Anterior Horn Cell	Neuromuscular Junction	Peripheral Nerve	Muscle
Tone	Increased (may be decreased acutely)	Decreased	Normal, variable	Decreased	Decreased
Distribution	Pattern (hemiparesis, paraparesis, etc.) Distal ≫ proximal	Variable, asymmetric	Fluctuating, cranial nerve involvement	Nerve distribution	Proximal ≫ distal
Reflexes	Increased (may be decreased early)	Decreased to absent	Normal (unless severely involved)	Decreased to absent	Decreased
Babinski	Extensor	Flexor	Flexor	Flexor	Flexor
Other	Cognitive dysfunction, atrophy only very late	Fasciculations, atrophy, no sensory involvement	Fluctuating course	Sensory nerve involvement, atrophy, rare fasciculations	No sensory deficits, tenderness, signs of inflammation

dural, subdural, or intracerebral hematoma, brain abscess, bacterial meningitis, viral encephalitits, (particularly due to herpes simplex), brain tumors with sudden intraparenchymal hemorrhage, hemoglobinopathies, and vasculitis. The laboratory evaluation should include a complete hematologic evaluation and sedimentation rate. If there is evidence for a mass lesion, emergency computerized tomography is indicated. Lumbar puncture can usually be delayed until after computerized tomography unless there is a strong suspicion of bacterial meningitis. EEG is important in distinguishing acute hemiplegia of childhood from mass lesions. Cardiac evaluation, including echocardiography, is necessary in all children, since treatment for cardiac embolization is lifesaving. Hemoglobin electrophoresis should also be performed to exclude sickling disorders.

After the inital evaluation, the patient should be observed for the next 24 to 48 hours. Management is initially aimed at preventing further neurologic damage. Anticonvulsants are given to control seizures, if present, and to prevent further seizure activity. Postictal paralysis, or Todd's palsy, usually clears within 24 hours but occasionally lasts longer. Arteriography should be performed on all children in whom an etiology is not evident at this point, since at times an unsuspected arteriovenous malformation of the brain or other abnormalities may be found.

Transverse Myelitis

BACKGROUND

Transverse myelitis is a destructive process of the spinal cord with resultant insidious or acute weakness and sensory dysfunction. Transverse myelitis is not a disease per se, but rather the result of any number of destructive processes affecting the spinal cord. In childhood, it most commonly occurs on a presumed autoimmune basis following viral illnesses such as measles or mumps, or, less commonly, after vaccination. If there is evidence for cerebral dysfunction, the term encephalomyelitis is appropriate. In later childhood or adolescence, it may be the initial symptom c multiple sclerosis, a condition that can b diagnosed only in retrospect when evidenc of neurologic impairment occurs at a diffe ent level of the neuro-axis at a later dat When the illness is temporally related to bout of optic neuritis, the term Devic's di ease is sometimes used, but is just a syr onym for another form of multiple sclerosi Transverse myelitis may sometimes occu as a component of adrenoleukodystroph Vasculitis, such as systemic lupus, ma rarely involve the spinal cord and caus transverse myelopathy.

PATHOPHYSIOLOGY

During the course of the illness, the in tial area or areas of spinal cord inflamma tion may extend rostrally and caudally t involve an extensive area of the spinal cor Since segments of the body supplied by th spinal cord below the level of highest cor involvement already demonstrate dysfunc tion, the rostral extension of the proces results in ascending symptoms.

CLINICAL MANIFESTATIONS

Initial symptoms include lower extremit paresthesia, local back pain, unilateral o bilateral lower extremity weakness, and ur nary retention. A preceding history of a upper respiratory, gastrointestinal, or ex anthematous infection occurs in approx mately 50% of patients. At the time of d agnosis, fever and meningismus are com mon in childhood. Characteristically, th insidious onset of paresthesia or weaknes of the lower extremities progresses ove days, or rarely, weeks, and then is replace by the abrupt occurrence of static paraple gia or quadraplegia and, in the cooperativ child, a detectable sensory level. In othe children, the course of progression may b less than 12 hours. The sensory loss gener ally involves all modalities, although spinothalamic deficit (pain) may occu without posterior column dysfunction (vi bration). The weakness is usually symmet ric, but may be asymmetric. Initial flaccid ity may be replaced by spasticity after variable interval as "spinal shock" wear ff. Sphincter disturbance of both the bowel nd bladder occurs in most patients, blad-er distention being the most common ini-ial sign of damage.

Both the peripheral leukocyte count and edimentation rate are normal. Lumbar uncture shows a normal or slightly ele-ated opening pressure and a mild pleocy-osis in the cerebrospinal fluid in nearly alf of patients at the time presentation. 'he cerebrospinal fluid protein may be el-vated, but the glucose is usually normal.

IFFERENTIAL DIAGNOSIS

Transverse myelitis is a diagnosis of ex-lusion and every patient with signs of cord ysfunction should undergo myelography o rule out potentially treatable processes ompressing, invading, or interfering with he blood supply of the spinal cord. These sions include epidural or subdural abscess r hematomas; extradural or intradural tu-iors; inflammatory or carcinomatous pro-esses of the leptomeninges; spinal arterio-enous malformations; and vertebral or in-ravertebral disc disease. In transverse iyelitis, the myelogram is usually normal, lthough in a minority of cases the cord is iildly widened. Early in the course of ill-ess, prior to the onset of upper motor euron signs, it may be difficult to differ-ntiate between acute polyneuritis (Guil-ain-Barré syndrome) and transverse mye-tis; however, in Guillain-Barré syndrome, owel and bladder function is commonly pared until later in the disease, and a dis-inct sensory level is not present.

IANAGEMENT

Treatment of transverse myelitis is sup-ortive and some degree of recovery occurs i approximately 80% of cases. All children ith this syndrome should be hospitalized. 'reatment with systemic and intraspinal orticosteroids and emergency laminec-omy has not improved outcome. High dose orticosteroids (Decadron 1 to 2 mg/kg, up o 100 mg i.v., followed by 0.5 mg/kg every hours i.v. or p.o.) should be begun until ord compression by a mass lesion is ruled ut.

Acute Polyneuritis

BACKGROUND AND PATHOPHYSIOLOGY

Acute polyneuritis, also known as the Guillain-Barré syndrome, is characterized by symmetric ascending paralysis. The hallmark of this disease, pathologically, is primary demyelination of motor and sensory nerves, believed secondary to auto-immune mechanisms. It occurs in children in all age groups, but is uncommon before 3 years of age. An antecedent respiratory or gastrointestinal infection precedes the onset of illness by 1 to 2 weeks in over 75% of childhood cases.

CLINICAL MANIFESTATIONS

The onset of weakness is commonly insidious, and paraesthesias or other sensory abnormalities are prominent in 50% of cases. The paraesthesias and paralysis are usually symmetric and ascending, although variation may occur. Early in the course of illness, distal weakness is more prominent than proximal weakness. Deep tendon reflexes are depressed or absent at the time of diagnosis. Cranial nerve abnormalities occur during the illness in over half the cases and may be the predominant finding, especially in the "Fisher variant" of this syndrome, which is characterized by oculomotor palsies, ataxia, and areflexia. The most common cranial nerve deficit is seventh (facial) nerve palsy followed in decreasing frequency by impairment of the ninth, tenth, and eleventh cranial nerves and oculomotor abnormalities. Internal ophthalmoplegia and papilledema have been described rarely. Autonomic dysfunction occurs frequently and results in blood pressure lability and cardiac abnormalities; it is a disproportionate cause of morbidity and mortality. Urinary retention may occur but is more common late in the illness.

The primary aid in diagnosis is lumbar puncture, which demonstrates an elevated protein, normal glucose, and less than 10 white blood cells per cu mm—the so called albumino-cytologic disassociation. The protein elevation occurs in almost all cases but may be delayed for weeks, usually peaking in the second or third week of illness. Electrophysiologic evidence for Guillain-Barre syndrome is the presence of nerve conduction velocity delay and is usually not demonstrable until the second or third week of illness. Emergency electromyography and nerve conduction velocity testing is not indicated.

DIFFERENTIAL DIAGNOSIS

The differential diagnosis includes the various neuromuscular causes of weakness: poisoning with neurotoxins such as lead, thallium, and arsenic; acute intermittent porphyria; and tic paralysis. The most difficult distinction is between Guillain-Barré syndrome and poliomyelitis. In polio, paralysis tends to be asymmetric; the tendon reflexes are variably depressed; the prodromal phase is more explosive; and high fever and meningismus tend to be more prominent.

MANAGEMENT

Management is based on the premise that the illness is progressive, somewhat unpredictable in tempo, ascending, and potentially life-threatening. The patient must be hospitalized and closely observed for respiratory compromise. Impending respiratory distress must be anticipated, and routine respiratory monitoring should be aided by specific measures of respiratory function. Arterial blood gases and pulmonary function studies should be obtained immediately. Since autonomic dysfunction is common, blood pressure must be closely monitored and abnormalities vigorously treated. Intravenous access should be obtained at the first sign of vascular instability. Other treatments such as corticosteroids and plasmapheresis are of unproven benefit in the acute form of illness.

Myasthenia Gravis

BACKGROUND AND PATHOPHYSIOLOGY

Myasthenia gravis manifests by fluctuating weakness of cranial and skeletal musculature, exacerbated by exertion. More commonly a disease of adulthood, myasthenia gravis occurs in childhood in thre major forms: transient neonatal, infantil and juvenile.

In myasthenia, antibodies directe against acetylcholine receptor protein the postsynaptic neuromuscular junctio cause intermittent failure of neuromuscula transmission and fluctuating weakness.

CLINICAL MANIFESTATIONS

The juvenile form, accounting for almos 25% of all cases of myasthenia gravis, clir ically mimics the adult disease. The mea age of onset is 8 years, with a female pre dominance of approximately 4 to 1. Th onset of symptoms may be insidious c acute. The majority of cases affect the cra nial nerves, and any cranial nerve can b involved in combination or isolation. Bila eral ptosis is the most frequent crani nerve deficit, followed in incidence by ocu lomotor impairment. Generalized trunca and limb weakness is present at onset in u to 40% of cases. The diagnosis should b suspected if there is a history of worsenin weakness during continual activity or if fa tigability of muscle strength is demonstra ble. Illnesses confused with myasthenia in clude the muscular dystrophies, congenita myopathies, inflammatory myopathie acute and chronic polyneuropathies, an in the infant, botulism.

The tensilon test is the backbone of di agnosis. In this procedure, an anticholines terase drug edrophonium (Tensilon), whic has a 30 sec onset and an approximately min duration of action, is slowly given in travenously at a dose of 0.2 mg/kg up to maximum dose of 10 mg. Initially, one tenth of the total dose is given and, if n hypersensitivity or severe cholinergic reac tions (such as bradycardia) are noted, th remainder of the dose is administere Since Tensilon is short-lived, interpretatio of the response requires close monitoring o a muscle or muscle group in which improve ment can be clearly seen, such as the eyeli elevators. In small children, this is ofte impossible and longer acting anticholines terases such as neostigmine (0.125 mg in a infant, and 0.04 mg/kg in an older child can be used. Electromyography provide electrophysiologic evidence for myasthenia gravis, but may be negative when the disease is confined to the cranial nerves.

MANAGEMENT

Although myasthenia gravis is a potentially life-threatening illness, specific management can usually be delayed until after diagnosis is assured. Obviously, if there is evidence for respiratory compromise, ventilatory support is mandatory. Treatment is begun with the use of anticholinesterases to prolong the availability of acetylcholine at the neuromuscular junction. Presently, the anticholinesterase of choice is Pyridostigmine (Mestinon), at a starting dose of 1 mg/kg by mouth every 4 hours, adjusted according to the clinical response. Other agents, such as corticosteroids or antimetabolites, may be of benefit in selected cases but must be used cautiously and only after anticholinesterases have failed to control symptoms. If there is any concern of respiratory compromise or if severe weakness is present, the child should be immediately hospitalized.

Myasthenia has a fluctuating, unpredictable course which can be exacerbated by intercurrent illness and by certain drugs, particularly the aminoglycoside antibiotics. In a known myasthenic, rapid worsening and respiratory compromise (myasthenia crises) may be difficult to differentiate from deterioration secondary to overdose of anticholinesterases (cholinergic crises) because the muscarinic side effects of the anticholinesterases, such as nausea, vomiting, cramps or muscle fasciculations, may be absent. Differentiation can at times be made by giving 1 to 2 mg of edrophonium intravenously, after assuring respiratory sufficiency. This should result in rapid improvement in the patient with a myasthenic crisis. However, this procedure may be falsely positive, and, if the diagnosis is unclear, the patient should be withdrawn from all anticholinesterases and, if necessary, maintained on mechanical respiration for 48 to 72 hours. Cholinergic crises require the immediate withdrawal of all anticholinesterases. Myasthenic crises respond variably to additional anticholinesterases, and plasmapheresis may be particularly useful in this situation. Both myasthenic and cholinergic crises mandate admission to the hospital.

Botulism

BACKGROUND AND PATHOPHYSIOLOGY

Botulism is an increasingly recognized cause of acute weakness in previously well infants under 6 months of age. The illness is secondary to intestinal colonization by *Clostridium botulinum*, which produces a toxin, impairing acetylocholine release from the nerve terminal. Spores of *C. botulinum* are of ubiquitous origin and the various host factor predisposing to intestinal colonization are poorly understood. Honey has been found to be a particularly contaminated food.

CLINICAL MANIFESTATIONS

The initial symptom is usually constipation followed insidiously by lethargy and feeding difficulties. Physical findings at the time of presentation, in decreasing incidence, are hypoactive deep tendon reflexes, decreased suck and gag, poorly reactive pupils, bilateral ptosis, oculomotor palsies, and facial dyplegia. Differential diagnosis includes all the potential causes of lethargy and poor feeding in infancy, and the majority of infants are initially misdiagnosed. Laboratory studies, including the leukocyte count and lumbar puncture, are normal. The diagnosis is established by identification of *C. botulinum* toxin in the feces; the toxin has not been isolated from the serum in any infantile cases to date. Electromyography, however, may supply immediate information. In a recent study of 11 children with bacteriologically confirmed botulism at the Children's Hospital of Philadelphia, electromyographic examination showed the presence of BSAPS (brief small action potential) in all cases, and 82% demonstrated incremental responses to repetitive motor nerve stimulation. Although nonspecific, in the proper clinical setting these findings are highly suggestive of botulism.

MANAGEMENT

Management requires hospitalization for observation for respiratory compromise. The use of cathartics or other laxatives to reduce the amount of *C. botulinum* present in the intestine has not been of proven benefit. Botulism antitoxin has resulted in anaphylactic reaction in infants and is not recommended. Antibiotics such as pencillin, although widely utilized, have not been shown to eradicate the organism from the bowel or result in clinical improvement.

Myositis

BACKGROUND

Myositis is an acute inflammatory muscle disease, most commonly secondary to viral infection. Myalgias are frequently associated with viral illness, but severe inflammation causing muscle weakness is uncommon. The illness tends to strike school-age children; it usually follows epidemics of influenza virus, but also is caused by Coxsackie A and B viruses.

CLINICAL MANIFESTATIONS

Viral myositis is characterized by 2 to 4 days of flu-like symptoms, followed by the acute onset of severe muscle pain, especially in the gastrocnemius and soleus muscles, that often causes the child to refuse to walk. Strength may be difficult to assess due to discomfort, and weakness is variable. The neurologic examination is otherwise normal. Elevated serum muscle enzymes are the rule; the creatinine phosphokinase (CPK) may be 10 times normal. The peripheral white blood cell count may be reduced, with a mean of approximately 5000/cu mm in most series.

DIFFERENTIAL DIAGNOSIS

Myositis may rarely occur secondary to multiple abscesses with *Staphylococcus aureus* and after trichinosis infection. The latter is characterized by mild muscle tenderness, weakness, and eosinophilia. The muscular dystrophies may cause diagnostic confusion, but can be differentiated by their insidious onset, distribution of weakness, and inheritance pattern. Distinction between dermatomyositis and viral myositis is often difficult early in the illness. Dermatomyositis is usually heralded by insidious, progressive muscle weakness and tenderness, a characteristic purplish discoloration over the upper eyelid; erythematous eruptions over the malar region of the face, metacarpal, phalangeal, and interphalangeal joints of the fingers, and extensor surfaces of the elbows and knees (see page 56). However, in some cases the onset is more explosive, and, early in the disease, the rash may be less prominent. The serum muscle enzymes are usually elevated and the sedimentation rate is occasionally high. Later in the illness, the distinction is easier since dermatomyositis runs a chronic, often remitting course.

MANAGEMENT

Since viral myositis usually has a benign course, with the vast majority of children improving over a 1-week period without sequelae, treatment is supportive. Bed rest is all that is usually needed.

Periodic Paralysis

Periodic paralysis is a rare illness, inherited in an autosomal dominant fashion which results in episodes of severe weakness. The major forms of illness include hyperkalemic, normokalemic, and hypokalemic periodic paralysis. Thyrotoxicosis may also be associated with episodic paralysis, and treatment results in the cessation of attacks. Serum potassium abnormalities are thought to be epiphenomenons of yet undelineated muscle membrane abnormalities. Histologic examination of muscle during the attack may disclose a vacuolar myopathy. Characteristically, a previously well patient develops a flaccid weakness in his trunk and upper thighs which gradually involves the remainder of the skeletal muscles. The attacks last hours to days, and, between the attacks, the muscular strength is usually normal, although a minority of patients have residual muscular weakness.

The hyperkalemic form begins in infancy and childhood, and attacks occur predominantly during the period of rest after vigorous exercise. The episodes may affect extraocular movements and commonly last only a few hours. Myotonia is usually associated with the illness. During the attack, plasma potassium is elevated, as is urine potassium secretion. In severe attacks, intravenous glucose, calcium, and insulin infusions may be helpful. Daily acetazolamide or hydrochlorthiazide may prevent attacks, although proven dosage in childhood is unclear and should only be begun after diagnosis is confirmed.

Hypokalemic periodic paralysis occurs primarily in young adults. Trigger factors include vigorous exercise, heavy carbohydrate meals, and the cold. During an attack, potassium levels are usually 2 to 2.5 meq/liter, and electrophysiologic examination demonstrates unstimulatable muscles. Treatment includes oral, or rarely intravenous, potassium. The avoidance of trigger factors, the utilization of slow released potassium preparations and diuretics, as used for the hyperkalemic form of illness, may prevent episodes.

Normokalemic periodic paralysis causes severe and prolonged attacks. Paralysis is worsened by potassium administration but may be improved by careful infusion of sodium chloride. Preventive treatment with acetazolamide or 9-α-fluorodihydrocortisone may be useful.

DISORDERS OF BALANCE

Disturbances of motor function in which there is an impairment of control of coordinated movement may result from dysfunction of various portions of the neuroaxis, including the peripheral nerves, posterior columns of the spinal cord, brainstem, vestibular apparatus, cerebellum and cerebral cortex (especially with acute hydrocephalus) in childhood. Differentiation is challenging and dependent on careful evaluation for associated symptoms and neurologic deficits (see Chapters 7, 67).

Acute Cerebellar Ataxia

Acute cerebellar ataxia is characterized by the acute onset of unsteadiness in a previously well child. It is seen primarily between the ages of 1 and 4 years, but can occur at any time during childhood. The cause of the illness is unknown; however, since antecedent viral infections occur in over half of patients 2 to 3 weeks prior to illness, it is considered para- or postinfectious.

The child develops acute truncal unsteadiness with a variable degree of distal motor difficulty, such as tremor and dysmetria. Cerebellar scanning speech and eye coordination deficits, such as nystagmus, are also variable. Resolution of symptoms is complete in most children within 2 weeks of onset, but mild residual neurologic deficits have been reported in up to 30% of the cases. Differentiation is difficult from the other causes of acute ataxia (see Chapter 7) when the ataxia occurs in isolation.

MANAGEMENT

Care should be taken to exclude a posterior fossa tumor, especially in children with a insidious or chronic course. Any child with associated neurologic deficits should undergo computed tomography. Cerebrospinal fluid analysis, disclosing a mild pleocytosis in over 50% of patients, may be reassuring to the physician but is nonspecific. Lumbar puncture is not necessary in most children but should be performed in any child with an uncharacteristic clinical course. The child should be hospitalized, unless symptoms are very mild and daily follow-up can be assumed.

Viral Labyrinthitis

Viral labyrinthitis is an ill-defined entity usually occurring in children over 10 years of age. It is characterized by the acute onset of vestibular dysfunction, often associated with an intercurrent upper respiratory tract infection. The illness tends to peak over a 2-week period and slowly improves. Symptomatic treatment is of some benefit. A further discussion of this entity and differential diagnosis and management is given in Chapter 62.

Benign Paroxysmal Vertigo

Benign paroxysmal vertigo is an illness affecting children primarily under the age of 4 years. It is manifest by acute episodes of imbalance, lasting seconds to minutes, between which the child is asymptomatic.

During the spell, the child characteristically becomes frightened and pale, but does not lose consciousness. Vestibular functions tests are abnormal and suggest peripheral vestibular disease. The etiology of this illness is unknown, the course self-limited and benign, and treatment supportive. For a further discussion of differential diagnoses and management see Chapter 7.

MOVEMENT DISORDERS

Involuntary movements are a component of many disorders of the CNS. The movements tend to be complex. A rigid classification into specific subtypes, based on the character, predominant anatomic localization, rhythmicity, and frequency is arbitrary, but useful in deducing the cause of the disorder (Table 44.3). Movements such as chorea, athetosis, dystonia, ballismus, and certain types of tremors suggest dysfunction of the extrapyramidal nervous system, a collection of nuclei (including the caudate, putamen, globus pallidus, and substantia nigra) and tracts which have multiple connections to the other portions of the CNS regulating movement. A multiplicity of neurotransmitters, including dopamine, acetylcholine, norepinephrine, serotonin, and γ-aminobutyric acid, control the extrapyramidial system. Recent localization and understanding of their function has allowed for symptomatic, at times dramatically successful, treatment of involuntary movements. Involuntary movements are also caused by damage to the cerebellum or its outflow tract, especially sustention (on maintaining fixed position) and intention tremors. Myoclonus may occur secondary to cerebral cortex, brainstem, or spinal cord disease, and is best thought of as a subtype of seizure. It, as other forms of seizures, may occur during sleep. Tics, another form of involuntary movements, may be extremely difficult to distinguish from chorea and are best differentiated by their stereotypic character. They are probably the most common involuntary movement disorder, but are not true neurologic emergencies. Many illnesses may present with involuntary movements and are diagnosed by associated neurologic findings. Cerebellar disease is discussed on page 349.

Sydenham's Chorea

BACKGROUND

Sydenham's chorea, the most common form of acquired chorea in childhood, occurs primarily between the ages of 3 and 13 years. Manifest by involuntary movements, coordination difficulties and emotional lability, its onset may be abrupt or insidious. Sydenham's chorea is thought to be a poststreptococcal disease and may occur months after the primary bacterial infection. The pathophysiology of the illness is

Table 44.3
Movement Disorders

Movement	Character	Location	Speed	Rythmicity	Stereotyped
Chorea	Jerky	Anywhere, may be unilateral	Rapid	Irregular	No
Athetosis	Writhing	Primarily distal	Slow	Irregular	At times
Dystonia	Writhing	Primarily proximal	Slow	Irregular	At times
Ballismus	Flailing	Proximal (involve entire limb)	Rapid	Irregular	No
Tremor	May be resting, sustention or intention	Most marked distal	Variable	Regular	Yes (may be variable, dependent on action, stress)
Myoclonus	Jerky	Anywhere	Rapid	Irregular	Variable
Tic	Jerky	Anywhere, more common face, neck	Rapid	Variable	Yes

nknown. Serologic evidence for preceding rep infection is absent in up to a quarter ' cases, and only one-third of patients have ssociated manifestations of rheumatic feer at the time of diagnosis.

LINICAL MANIFESTATIONS

The involuntary movements may be sube at first and exacerbated by stress. Inially, the movements classically affect the ce and distal portion of the upper extremies and consist of rapid, involuntary ranom jerks. This results in the milk-maid and in which the child's hand can not aintain a uniform strength while grasping e examiner's hand. The involuntary ovements disappear during sleep. There usually associated muscular hypotonia id marked coordination difficulties, and eech is often quite jerky. Hemichorea, in hich the abnormal movements are preominately unilateral, occurs in some of the ses. The deep tendon reflexes are normal, though occasionally the patellar reflex is id to be "hung up." There is no evidence r upper motor neuron disease.

IFFERENTIAL DIAGNOSIS

Due to the frequent lack of associated anifestations of poststreptococcal disease id at times absence of serologic evidence r streptococcal infection, diagnosis can be fficult. Chorea must be distinguished om other movement disorders (See Table .3). Damage secondary to perinatal asyxia may also cause chorea; this tends to come apparent in the first 3 years of life id to possess an athetoid component. untington's chorea, inherited in an automal dominant fashion, is rare in childod and frequently associated with rigidy, ataxia, and mental deterioration. Failial paroxysmal choreoathetosis is differitiated by the paroxysmal nature of the tacks and lack of associated hypotonia id emotional lability. A vasculits, such as stemic lupus erythematosus, may rarely esent with choreiform movements as the st manifestation. Children with learning sabilities may have associated choreiform ovements that mimic mild cases of Synham's chorea. Drug ingestion may cause jerky movements indistinguishable clinically from chorea. Many degenerative diseases, such as Lesch-Nyhan syndrome and Wilson's disease may have choreiform features, but should be distinguishable by associated findings.

MANAGEMENT

Initially, all patients should have a hematological profile, sedimentation rate, and streptozyme drawn. Electrocardiograms should also be performed. If there is a question concerning diagnosis, further tests such as computed tomography, lumbar puncture, and serological evaluation for collagen vascular disease might be helpful, but they are not usually necessary on an urgent basis.

The success of any treatment is hard to evaluate since the course is so unpredictable. Drugs employed to treat this disease have included phenobarbital, phenothiazines, and nordiazepam—all have had questionable efficacy. Haloperidol 0.5 to 1 mg twice daily has been reported to result in improvement within 2 to 3 days. Since patients with Sydenham's chorea have an increased incidence of rheumatic carditis, prophylactic penicillin should be employed, unless other specific etiology is determined for the chorea.

CRANIAL NERVE DYSFUNCTION

The cranial nerve nuclei are closely packed in the brainstem, and their peripheral axons are integrally related to many vital portions of the CNS, cerebral vasculature, and cranial cavity. Due to these anatomic interrelationships, multiple cranial nerve involvement and associated neurologic dysfunction is common with diseases of the brainstem. Characteristic of brainstem disease is crossed symptomatology, with cranial nerve deficits ipsilateral to the lesion and motor and sensory deficits of more caudal neurologic structures contralateral to the lesion. The combinations and etiologies of such lesions and the multiple eponyms used to describe such deficits are legion. Radiographic analysis of the base of the skull and sellar region, coupled with computerized tomographic analysis of the intracranial structures, is often necessary for diagnosis.

Optic Neuritis

BACKGROUND

Optic neuritis is an acute inflammation of the optic nerve characterized by an impairment of vision, progressing over hours or days, and associated with tenderness of the eyeball exacerbated by eye movement. The disease is primarily unilateral, but an increased incidence of bilateral involvement is found in childhood. Optic neuritis in childhood is most commonly presumed to be on an auto-immune basis following a viral disease, including the childhood exanthems. At times, a contiguous sinusitis may cause the illness. Twenty percent of patients with unilateral optic neuritis will develop multiple sclerosis at a later date, but there is little benefit in making this diagnosis prior to the development of other symptoms of neurologic dysfunction.

CLINICAL MANIFESTATIONS

On examination, decreased visual acuity and decreased color vision are associated with a relative afferent pupillary deficit to light and a central scotoma in the affected eye. The relative afferent pupil defect is demonstrated by the swinging flashlight manuever, during which the pupil of the affected eye constricts briskly when light is shown into the contralateral eye (the consensual light reflex) and dilates when light is then immediately shown into the affected eye. Fundoscopic examination discloses a swollen optic disc and often flame hemmorhages; in the rare cases of retrobulbar optic neuritis, fundoscopic examination is normal.

MANAGEMENT

Before beginning any treatment for optic neuritis, the diagnosis must be firmly established. The primary distinction is between optic neuritis and papilledema secondary to increased intracranial pressure. Papilledema is almost always bilateral and associated with normal vision and normal pupil reactivity until late in the disease. In cases of bilateral optic neuritis, differentiation may be impossible since fundoscopic findings are identical in the two illnesses. If any doubt persists of increased intracranial pressure, the patient should undergo evaluation by computerized tomography of the brain and, if the CT scan is normal, cerebrospinal fluid analysis.

In the uncomplicated, unilateral case of optic neuritis evaluation should include a complete blood count, sedimentation rate and x-rays of the skull with special attention to the paranasal sinuses. The course of the illness is variable, with most patients recovering to normal or near-normal vision over 4 or 5 weeks. Treatment with high dose systemic corticosteroids, such as prednisone 2 mg/kg/day orally for 7 to 10 days or retrobulbar injections of corticosteroids has not been shown to improve the ultimate prognosis, but may result is a slightly faster resolution of symptoms.

Oculomotor Palsy

Dysfunction of the third cranial nerve may result from lesions anywhere between the third nerve nuclei in the midbrain and the passage of the nerve through the superior orbital fissure of the orbit. The nerve innervates the pupil, the upper eyelid, and the muscles of the eye responsible for upward and inward movement. The pupillomotor fibers lie superficially in the nerve and, because of their location, compression of the nerve may result initially in pupillary dilatation without other signs of oculomotor dysfunction. More anterior lesions, involving the cavernous sinus, and generalized peripheral nervous system illness, such as myasthenia gravis and acute polyneuritis, tend to spare pupillary function.

A completely isolated paresis of the third nerve will result in a ptotic lid, a semidilated nonreactive pupil, and an eye which is deviated outward and downward. Isolated third nerve lesions are rare in childhood and require a careful evaluation for associated findings, suggesting more extensive brainstem disease.

Etiologies of third nerve dysfunction include compressive or infiltrative lesions of the midbrain, demyelination, meningeal sease, and masses in the cavernous sinus ıd orbit. Proper evaluation includes radio- 'aphic studies of the orbit and sella, com- ıterized tomography of the brain and cra- al cavity, cerebrospinal fluid analysis, ıd, in selected cases, arteriography of cer- ›ral vasculature. Postviral third nerve ılsy probably occurs, but is rare. Ophthal- oplegic migraine is a disease of childhood ıat is frequently overlooked. Typically an ›isode of severe headache, associated with ıusea and vomiting, occurs, and, as it re- lves, a painless ophthalmoplegia becomes 'ident. In a young child with this charac- ristic presentation, especially with a pos- ıve family history for migraine or compli- ıted migraine, arteriography should not performed. These episodes may recur ıd paresis usually resolves within 1 month. ny child with a pupil-sparing third nerve ıresis should undergo Tensilon testing to ıle out myasthenia gravis.

Abducens Palsy

The sixth cranial nerve runs a long course om its nucleus in the caudal pons to the teral rectus muscle, which it innervates. linically, the involved eye turns inward ıd cannot fully abduct. Isolated acute pa- sis results in diplopia which is most severe ›on lateral gaze ipsilateral to the side of volvement. Due to its intimate anatomic lationship with the ipsilateral horizontal ıze center, a nuclear lesion always pro- ıces an ipsilateral gaze palsy.

The etiologies of abducens paresis are gion, and differential diagnosis is made ore difficult since an isolated sixth nerve ılsy is commonly a nonspecific sign of creased intracranial pressure. When there concommitant involvement of other cra- al nerves, a full evaluation including com- ıterized tomography and cerebrospinal ıid analysis is indicated. A well-recog- zed syndrome of inflammation of the pet- us bone secondary to middle ear infection ;radenigo's syndrome), is characterized facial weakness, pain in the face, and teral rectus weakness. Sixth nerve palsies e common following closed-head trauma, pecially with associated basilar skull frac- re. Involvement of the third or fourth cranial nerves suggests cavernous sinus or orbital disease.

The evaluation of isolated, nonnuclear sixth nerve paresis in childhood is controversial. In one study, done at a tertiary referral center, one-third of such cases were secondary to intracranial tumors. However, cases of abducens palsy secondary to increased intracranial pressure, without other evidence for increased pressure such as papilledema, are rare, if they occur at all. The otherwise well child with an isolated nonnuclear sixth nerve paresis should be carefully examined and middle ear infection should be ruled out. Other than a peripheral blood count and skull films for the evaluation of sinus disease, no further laboratory tests are indicated at the time of presentation. The child should be carefully followed; if, after a period of 2 to 3 months, no improvement is noted, further evaluation including computerized tomography and cerebrospinal fluid evaluation is indicated.

Bell's Palsy

Bell's palsy is an acute, idiopathic unilateral paralysis of the upper and lower musculature of the face. It is believed to be secondary to edema of the facial nerve as it passes through the facial canal within the temporal bone. Further localization within the facial canal is possible after evaluation of the function of the branches of the facial nerve which supply taste to the anterior two-thirds of the tongue and innervate the lacrimal and salivary glands and the stapedius muscle. However, the major differentiation is between paralysis on a central (or upper motor neruon basis), which spares the upper half of the face; and peripheral involvement, which involves the entire face. The latter is most commonly due to Bell's palsy. Prior to the onset of paralysis there is a history of upper respiratory infection in over half of the subjects.

Pain localized to the ear is a common first manifestation of illness, followed rapidly by paralysis which reaches its maximum extent over the next few hours. The face is pulled to the unaffected side and there is difficulty closing the eyes, drinking, and controlling salivation. The diagnosis is based on exclusion of other causes of acute cranial nerve dysfunction such as Guillain-Barré syndrome, Herpesvirus infection, mastoiditis, brainstem tumor, and diabetes. Baseline studies which should be obtained on all patients include a blood count, leukocyte count, sedimentation rate, and fasting blood sugar. Any associated neurologic abnormality, specifically in the other cranial nerves, necessitates further evaluation, including computed tomography.

Treatment is somewhat controversial. Corticosteroids are of possible value. They must be used early in the disease and at high doses (prednisone, 2 mg/kg/day), for 7 to 10 days to be of benefit. Electrodiagnostic evaluation with the measurement of nerve threshold to electrical stimulation is of prognostic value after the first 72 hours of illness, but supplies no useful information at the onset of illness. Recovery is more common with incomplete paralysis and with electrophysiologic evidence for incomplete denervation. Complete recovery is seen in 60 to 80% of children beginning during the second to third week of illness. During the period of recovery, special care should be taken to protect the cornea by the installation of bland ointments and patching of the involved eye. The child should be referred for reexamination to assure a recovery during the expected time period.

References

Seizures

Dodson, WE, Prensky, AL, DeVivo, DC: Management of seizure disorders: Selected aspects Part 1. *J Pediatr* 89:527, 1976.

Encephalitis

Barza M, Paulker SG: The decision to biopsy, treat or wait in suspected herpes encephalitis. *Arch Intern Med* 92: 641, 1980.

Johnson RT, Mims CA: Pathogenesis of viral infection of the nervous system. *N Engl J Med* 278: 23, 1968.

Sells CJ, Carpenter RL, Ray C: Sequelae of central-nervous system entervirus infection. *N Engl J Med* 293: 1, 1975.

Whitley RJ, Soong S, Dolen R, et al.: Adenine arabinoside therapy of biopsy-proved herpes simplex encephalitis. *N Engl J Med* 297: 289, 1977.

Ziegler DK: Acute disseminated encephalitis. *Arch Neurol* 14: 476, 1966.

Headache

Ad Hoc Committee on Classification of Headach *JAMA* 179: 717, 1962.

Raskin NH, Appenzeller O: *Headache*. Volume XI Major problems in internal medicine, W. B. Sau ders, Philadelphia, 1980.

Migraine

Golden S, French JH: Basilar migraine in young ch dren. *Pediatrics* 56: 722, 1975.

Millichap J: Recurrent headaches in 100 childre *Childs Brain* 4: 95, 1978.

Prensky AL: Migraine and migrainous variant in p diatric patients. *Pediatr Clin North Am* 23: 46 1976.

Prensky AL, Sommer D: Diagnosis and treatment migraine in children. *Neurology* 29: 506, 1979.

Hemiplegia

Gold AP, Carter S: Acute hemiplegia of infancy a childhood. *Pediatr Clin North Am* 23: 413, 1976.

Gold AP, Challenor YB, Gilles FH et al.: Strokes Children. *Stroke* 4: 835(Part I), 1007(Part II), 197

Transverse Myelitis

McAlpine D, Lumsden CE, Acheson ED; *Multip sclerosis. A reappraisal.* E. & S. Livingston, Edi borough, Scotland, 1968.

Paine RS, Byers RK: Transverse myelopathy in chil hood *Arch Dis Child* 85: 151, 1953.

Ropper AH, Proshanzer DC: The prognosis of acu and subacute transverse myelopathy based on ear signs and symptoms. *Ann Neurol* 4: 51, 1978.

Acute Polyneuritis

Evan B: Polyneuropathy in childhood. *Pediatrics* 6 96, 1979.

Low L, Schneider J, Carter S: Polyneuritis in childre *Pediatrics* 63: 76, 1978.

Marks HH, Augustyn P, Allen RJ: Fisher's syndron in children. *Pediatrics* 60: 726, 1977.

Myasthenia Gravis

Drachmen DB: Myasthenia Gravis. *N Engl J M* 298: 136, 1978.

Millichap, JG: Diagnosis and treatment of myasthen gravis in infancy, childhood, and adolescence. *Ne rology* 1007, 1960.

Patten M: Myasthenia Gravis: Review of diagnos and management. *Muscle Nerve* 1: 190, 1978.

Botulism

Berg BO: Syndrome of infant botulism. *Pediatrics* 5 321, 1977.

Johnson RO, Clay SA, Arnon SB: Diagnosis and ma agement of infant botulism. *Amer J Dis Child* 13 586, 1979.

Myositis

Antony JH, Procopis PG, Ooiriev RA: Benign acu childhood myositis. *Neurology* 29: 1068, 1979.

Banker BO, Victor M: Dermatomyositis (systemic a

giopathy) of childhood. *Medicine* 45: 261, 1966.
Dietzmann DE, Schaller JG, Ray GC, et al.: Acute myositis associated with influenza B infection. *Pediatrics* 57: 255, 1976.
Dubowitz V: Treatment of dermatomyositis in childhood. *Arch Dis Child* 51: 494, 1976.
Jacob JC: Methotrexate and azathioprine treatment of childhood dermatomyositis. *Pediatrics* 59: 212, 1977.

Acute Cerebellar Ataxia

Cottom DG: Acute cerebellar ataxia. *Arch Dis Child* 32: 181, 1957.
Weiss S, Carter S: Course and progress of acute cerebellar ataxia in children. *Neurology* 9: 711, 1959.

Viral Labyrinthitis

Dix MR: Vertigo. *Practitioner* 211: 295, 1973.

Benign Paroxysmal Vertigo

Koenignsberber MR, Chutorian AM, Gold AP, et al.: Benign paroxysmal vertigo of childhood. *Neurology* 20: 1108, 1970.

Movement Disorders

Fahn S: Differential diagnosis of tremors. *Med Clin NA* 56: 1363, 1972.
Lockman LA: Movement disorders. In *The Practice of Pediatric Neurology*, p 218, C.V. Mosby, St. Louis, 1975.
Puvoisen R: Clinical diagnosis of the dyskinesia. *Med Clin North Am* 56: 1321, 1972.

Sydenham's Chorea

Aron AM, Freeman JM, Carter S: The national history of Sydenham's Chorea. *Am J Med* 38: 83, 1965.
Shenkar DM, Grossman MJ, Klawans NL: Treatment of Sydenham's Chorea with haloperidol, *Dev Med Child Neurol* 15: 19, 1973.

Optic Neuritis

Arnason BGW: Optic neuritis and multiple sclerosis. *N Engl J Med* 289: 1140, 1973.
Bradley WA, Whitty WD: Acute optic neuritis: Prognosis for development of multiple sclerosis. *J Neurol Neurosurg Psychiatry* 31: 10, 1968.
Glaser TS: *Optic Neuritides in Neuro-opthalmology* p 104. Harper & Row, New York, 1978.

Oculomotor Palsy

Friedman AP, Harter DH, Merritt HM: Opthalmoplegic migraine. *Arch Neurol* 7: 320, 1962.
Smith A: Oculomotor disorders. In *Textbook of Neurology*, edited by AB Johnson, BK Jones, p 255. Harper & Rowe, New York, 1978.

Abducens Palsy

Robertson DM, Hines JD, Rucher CW: Acquired 6th nerve paresis in children. *Arch Opthalmol* 83: 574, 1970.

Bell's Palsy

Adour KK: Diagnosis and management of facial paralysis. *N Engl J Med* 307: 348, 1982.

CHAPTER 45

Infectious Disease Emergencies

GARY R. FLEISHER, M.D.

INTRODUCTION

Although not as dramatic as multiple trauma or cardiac arrythmias, infection precipitates more emergency department encounters than either of the above conditions. Fever is the single most common chief complaint among children seen in the emergency department at The Children's Hospital of Philadelphia. Though only a small fraction of patients with infections die, such diseases, being so much more common than noninfectious conditions with a high fatality rate, account for a large percentage of deaths in the emergency department. Russo and colleagues reviewed the charts of children dead on arrival in Newark, NJ, and found that infection ranked second only to trauma as a cause of death.

The approach to the febrile child is outlined in Chapter 21. In this chapter infections are divided anatomically as follows: generalized (bacterial), central nervous system, upper respiratory, lower respiratory, gastrointestinal, bone and soft tissue, and genital. Infections of the urinary tract are discussed in Chapters 17 and 63 and of the heart in Chapter 43. Systemic nonbacterial illnesses, including the childhood exanthems, and several miscellaneous syndromes are dealt with as a group at the end of the chapter.

For each anatomic area, the realtive frequency of disease due to various pathogens is discussed and an approach is given for establishing a specific etiology. I have then provided a more extensive description of the serious and/or treatable conditions, often clustering similar or less significant pathogens. The recommendations for management are derived from published literature. In certain areas, particularly as regards the indications for admission, scant information exists. Thus, it has been necessary at times to offer as guidelines the management protocols we have found successful in the emergency department at The Children's Hospital of Philadelphia, even though they may not have been subjected to vigorous clinical trials.

BACTEREMIA AND SEPSIS

In both bacteremia and sepsis, a bacterial pathogen has invaded the bloodstream. The presence or absence of toxicity differentiates these two entities: bacteremia is relatively asymptomatic, while sepsis is accompanied by signs of serious systemic illness. Since these infections represent a continuum whereby some children with bacteremia proceed to develop the manifestations of sepsis, a separation into distinct diagnostic categories is not always possible. Bacterial infection in the bloodstream may occur in isolation (primary) or in association with focal disease (secondary). This section will be limited to primary infections.

Bacteremia

BACKGROUND

In bacteremia, viable organisms proliferate in the bloodstream but produce no evidence of serious infection other than fever. *Streptococcus pneumoniae* causes 50 to

Table 45.1
Organisms Recovered from the Blood of Children with Unsuspected Bacteremia

Authors	Year	No. of Positive Cultures	Pathogen (% of total isolates)				
			Streptococcus pneumoniae	*Haemophilus influenzae*	*Neisseria meningitidis*	*Salmonella* spp.	Other
Henretig et al.	1982	22	82	9	0	9	0
Waskerwitz et al.	1981	17	53	29	6	6	6
Baron et al.	1980	8	88	12	0	0	0
Hamrick et al.	1978	28	61	29	7	3	0
McCarthy et al.	1977	24	63	21	8	8	0
McCarthy et al.	1976	47[a]	66	13	2	6	13
Teele et al.	1975	19	79	11	0	0	10
McGowan et al.	1973	31	61	20	3	3	13

[a] Analysis limited to children with an initial diagnosis of fever of unknown origin, upper respiratory infection, otitis media, or pneumonia.

60% of primary bacteremias and *Haemophilus influenzae*, 20 to 30%. Less frequently encountered pathogens include salmonellae, *Neisseria meningiditis*, the Group A *Streptococcus*, and rarely others. Table 45.1 summarizes the bacteria isolated in prospective studies of bacteremia.

Bacteremia occurs frequently among febrile children seen in the emergency department, but is unusual in the first 6 months of life. McGowan and colleagues recovered pathogens from 22 of 551 (4%) of children with an elevated temperature treated as outpatients. In this series, blood cultures were positive in 1 of 74 (1%) of infants ≦ 6 months of age, 11 of 116 (9.5%) of children 7 to 12 months old, 5 of 131 (3.8%) of those 13 to 24 months, and 5 of 225 (2.2%) over 24 months of age. McCarthy et al. identified bacteremia in 117 of 1,783 (6.5%) of children with a temperature ≥ 37.7°C. Again, the incidence was highest between 6 and 24 months of age.

PATHOPHYSIOLOGY

There appears to be a continuum of disease, starting with colonization and progressing through bacteremia, which may have three outcomes: (1) spontaneous resolution; (2) sepsis; or (3) focal infection. The factors have not yet been completely defined that determine which children become colonized, which colonized children become bacteremic, and which bacteremic children improve without therapy. Clearly, exposure to carriers plays a role, accounting for the increased incidence of asymptomatic carriage and disease among household contacts of patients with infections due to *N. meningiditis* or *H. influenzae*.

Bactericidal antibody in the serum has been shown to protect against meningococcal disease; however, some individuals without such antibodies do not progress beyond colonization. Among 492 military recruits studied by Goldschneider and colleagues, 54 lacked bactericidal antibody to meningococcus group C. Twenty four of these 54 men acquired the organism in the nasopharynx and 11 showed a bactericidal antibody response. Five of those without such a response developed meningococcal meningitis. A concurrent viral infection may increase the likelihood of bacteremia in a colonized individual by disrupting the normal mucosal barrier.

CLINICAL MANIFESTATIONS

By definition, primary bacteremia presents with a paucity of symptoms and signs. The complaints are usually those of malaise or an upper respiratory infection. Fever, without evidence of a source, is the only physical finding.

McCarthy and colleagues attempted to define the history and observation variables useful in assessing febrile children. Observation of behavior (playfulness, alertness, and consolability) had the strongest correlation with the overall assessment; however, 9 of 21 children subsequently shown to have serious illnesses were not initially categorized as being moderately or severely ill.

Henretig and colleagues tested whether the initial overall assessment of the response to an antipyretic drug administered in the emergency department could distinguish febrile children with bacteremia from those with viral infections. Neither the initial assessment nor the magnitude of the decrease in temperature was predictive for the presence or absence of organisms in the bloodstream.

The WBC count exceeds 15,000/cu mm in 75% of children with bacteremia due to *S. pneumoniae* and 50% due to *H. influenzae.* Although both the erythrocyte sedimentation rate and the C-reactive protein are usually elevated in patients with bacteremia, these tests provide only minimal additional information.

MANAGEMENT

A discussion on the management of bacteremia must address three issues: (1) the evaluation for bacteremia in the febrile child with a seemingly trivial illness, (2) the treatment of the child with suspected bacteremia but no signs of sepsis or focal disease, and (3) the therapy of proven bacteremia. Although controversy plagues all these areas, the information accumulated over the last decade clearly shows some limitations to clinical judgement and points to the not infrequent occurrence of serious complications from bacteremia.

The likelihood of bacteremia in the child between 3 and 24 months of age with a fever ≧ 40°C, coupled with the difficulties of clinical assessment in these youngsters, makes obtaining a WBC count mandatory. With lower fevers in these young children or with temperatures ≧ 40°C in children > 24 months of age, the physician can rely more firmly on clinical judgement. In the child who is felt to be particularly irritable or toxic, but not so ill as to require an admission to the hospital, a WBC count should be drawn. Blood cultures are sent to the laboratory from any of these children who have a WBC count ≧ 15,000/cu mm. Additionally, patients who have a lumbar puncture performed in the emergency department, as part of an evaluation for febrile seizures or suspected meninigitis, should have cultures of their blood.

Although not definitive, several studies have suggested that bacteremic children less frequently continue to be bacteremic or develop focal infections if they have received oral antibiotic therapy that is effective against the organism isolated from their bloodstream. Thus, the child identified on the basis of age, fever, clinical assessment, and WBC count as a likely candidate for bacteremia should receive an oral antibiotic and return for a reexamination in 48 hours. Amoxicillin, 50 mg/kg/day, appears to be the most reasonable choice in terms of its antibacterial spectrum and low toxicity.

The management of the patient with proven bacteremia hinges on the identity of the pathogen. All patients from whom *H. influenzae* is recovered should enter the hospital for intravenous antibiotic therapy. If *S. pneumoniae* is isolated, the clinical findings at the repeat examination determine the subsequent treatment. Children without fever or evidence of a serious infection (meningitis, pneumonia, cellulitis) should receive oral penicillin, 50,000 units/kg/day for 10 days; all others require hospitalization.

Sepsis

BACKGROUND

In sepsis, bacteremia exists in association with signs of serious systemic illness. The etiology of sepsis varies with age in the otherwise healthy child.

During the first 2 months of life, the Group B *Streptococcus* has recently replaced *Escherichia coli* as the commonest cause of sepsis. There are over 10,000 cases of neonatal disease due to this organism yearly in the United States. Eickoff and colleagues reported in 1964 that the group B *Streptococcus* was the commonest isolate in neonatal sepsis, accounting for 25% of the infections. In 1964, 11 of 22 neonates with sepsis at their hospital had Group B *Streptococci* and 7 had *E. coli.* Seigel and colleagues in 1979 described an incidence of neonatal sepsis with the Group B *Streptococcus* of 2.5 per 1,000 live births and with *E. coli* of 0.6 per 1,000 live births.

N. meningiditis, *H. influenzae*, and *S. pneumoniae* infect the newborn only occasionally, but then emerge as the most frequent causes of sepsis in childhood. The Group A *Streptococcus*, *Staphylococcus aureus*, and salmonellae are relatively rare.

Sepsis occurs less frequently than bacteremia; however, large numbers of children with meningococcemia are occasionally seen in epidemics. Over 1,500 cases of meningococcal sepsis are reported yearly in the United States, most affecting children. The usual annual incidence has been estimated at 1 per 100,000 population, although in one epidemic the attack rate was 838 per 100,000 children.

Certain conditions impose on children án increased susceptibility to sepsis. These include neoplasia, immunodeficiency syndromes, immunosuppresive therapy, asplenia, and sickle cell disease. The hemoglobinopathies pose a particularly urgent problem for the physician in the emergency department because of their relative frequency and the fact that overwhelming sepsis may occur in the young prior to the initial clinical manifestation of the underlying hematologic disease. Among 326 consecutive children with sickle cell hemoglobinopathies seen at the Children's Hospital of Philadelphia in a single year, the temperature was $\geqq$ 38.0°C in 154, and 4 of those with fever had positive blood cultures. Two of the 4 were septic and the other 2 were bacteremic, but the immediate institution of antibiotic therapy may have prevented the rapid appearance of systemic toxicity.

PATHOPHYSIOLOGY

As discussed under bacteremia, the first step toward sepsis occurs with colonization of the host by a potentially pathogenic bacteria. The site of colonization is usually the pharynx in older children, but may be the umbilicus or bowel in the neonate. Among immunosuppressed children, organisms residing in the gastrointestinal tract often invade the bloodstream.

Not every child with bacteremia develops the clinical manifestations of sepsis. The intrinsic virulence of the pathogen determines, in part, whether the bacteremia will resolve spontaneously. *H. influenzae* bacteremia results in sepsis or a focal infection in 50 to 80% of children, while salmonellae almost always remain asymptomatic. Host factors also assume an important role in clearing circulating bacteria. The young child, particularly under 2 years of age, has a greater tendency to become seriously ill.

CLINICAL MANIFESTATIONS

The duration of the history in a child with sepsis is variable. While some children are febrile for several days during a preceding bacteremia, others develop a sudden dramatic illness. The interval between the initial fever and death may be less than 12 hours in fulminant meningococcemia. The child progresses with continued sepsis from malaise to profound lethargy and finally obtundation. Although fever is the cardinal sign of infection, children under 3 months of age often remain afebrile with sepsis; hypothermia is common in the first month of life.

A marked tachycardia occurs early in the course of the disease, often exceeding 200/min in the first 3 months of life, 175 between 4 months and 2 years of age, and 150 in the older child. Hypotension and tachypnea are present. The skin is cold and poorly perfused; additionally, petechiae and purpura may appear.

The hemoglobin and hematocrit are usually normal, falling occasionally from hemolysis as seen with disseminated intravascular coagulation (DIC). Although leukocytosis usually accompanies sepsis, an overwhelming infection occasionally produces neutropenia. The WBC count is rarely normal, and the differential is almost always shifted to the left; metamyelocytes and band forms often make their way into the peripheral blood. As the infection progresses, the platelet count decreases. It is distinctly unusual to have evidence of cutaneous hemorrhage from sepsis without thrombocytopenia. Similarly, the prothrombin time (PT), partial thromboplastin time (PTT), and fibrin degradation products rise with the ongoing comsumption of the clotting factors. The electrolytes reflect a metabolic acidosis, and occasionally mild hyponatremia occurs; the BUN is normal. A Gram stain of a petechial scraping shows the etiologic agent in one-third of the cases. In the infant, hypoglycemia may occur.

MANAGEMENT

Although the initial therapy for sepsis is directed at the preservation of vital functions, every effort must be made to obtain the appropriate diagnostic studies. Blood should be drawn for culture, CBC, platelet count, PT, PTT, electrolytes, BUN, arterial blood gas analysis, SGOT, and SGPT as the initial intravenous line is inserted.

During the first hour, normal saline with 5% dextrose is given at 20 ml/kg/hour. The unstable patient requires central venous, arterial, and urinary catheters. The initial laboratory studies, the response to the bolus of saline, and the measurements of the intravascular status determine the type and quantity of the subsequent fluids and the need for vasopressors (see Chapter 2).

Under 2 months of age, ampicillin, 200 mg/kg/day, and gentamicin, 7.5/kg/day, are administered. Chloramphenicol, 100 mg/kg/day, replaces gentamicin in the older child and also in the young infant when bloody diarrhea, suggestive of salmonellosis, is present. The benefit of corticosteroids remains uncertain; however, data from animal models and retrospective studies in humans point to a salutory effect. We administer methylprednisolone, 120 mg/kg/day divided into 4 doses, during the first 24 hours.

Blood components are given as indicated by the results of the initial hematologic studies. If the hemoglobin is < 10 g/dl, packed red cells are administered at 10 ml/kg. Thrombocytopenia (< 50,000/cu mm) is corrected with platelet concentrates at 0.2 units/kg and decreased clotting factors with fresh frozen plasma, 10 ml/kg. For the child with hypoglycemia (glucose < 50 mg/dl), glucose should be given at a dose of 1 g/kg in the form of a 25% solution. Heparin plays no role in the emergency department care of the child with sepsis but may be useful subsequently to treat severe thrombotic episodes.

CENTRAL NERVOUS SYSTEM INFECTIONS

Three important infectious syndromes involve the CNS: meningitis, encephalitis, and brain abscess. Since encephalitis and brain abscess usually confront the emergency department physician as problems in the differential diagnosis of various neurologic manifestations, they are discussed as neurologic emergencies in Chapter 44.

Meningitis, an inflammation of the membranes lining the CNS, results from an infection or irritation on a noninfectious basis. Inflammation of the meninges produces a pleocytosis in the cerebrospinal fluid (CSF) allowing, in most cases, for the diagnosis of meningitis by examination of this readily accessible material. However, organisms may occasionally infect the meninges without eliciting a cellular reaction, either because sufficient time has not elapsed for a leukocyte response or the pathogen is of low virulence.

In the emergency department setting, the vast majority of the cases of meningitis result from infection of the CNS. Table 45.2 lists those organisms which are the more frequent invaders of the meninges. The most important initial task confronting the emergency department physician is the identification of children with bacterial meningitis. This is a common, life-threatening pediatric infection amenable to therapy

Table 45.2
Organisms Causing Meningitis

Viruses
Enteroviruses
Herpes simplex
Lymphocytic choriomeningitis
Mumps
Other
Mycoplasma
Bacteria
Haemophilus influenzae
Streptococcus pneumoniae
Neisseria meningitidis
Escherichia coli
Group B *Streptococcus*
Salmonella
Listeria monocytogenes
Mycobacterium tuberculosis
Fungi
Candida albicans
Cryptococcus neoformans
Parasites
Cystercercosis
Amoebae

Table 45.3
Usual Ranges for CSF WBC count, Protein and Glucose in Normal Infants and Children and in Those with Viral or Bacterial Meningitis

	Neonate	Child	Bacterial Meningitis	Viral Meningitis
WBC (per cu mm)	<30	<10	200–20,000	10–1000
Protein (mg/dl)	<170	<40	>100	40–100
Glucose (mg/dl)	>30	>40	<30	>30

if diagnosed early in the course. The sine qua non for the diagnosis of meningitis is examination of the CSF. Routine studies performed on this fluid should include cell count with differential, glucose, protein, Gram stain, and bacterial culture. Appropriate media for inoculation of the specimen would include a combination such as blood, chocolate, and MacConkey agar. In selected cases, additional studies are indicated, such as counterimmunoelectrophoresis, lactate level, acid fast stain, India ink preparation, serologic test for syphilis, cryptococcal antigen, and cultures for anaerobic bacteria, mycoplasma, mycobacteria, and fungi. Values of various parameters of the CSF are presented for healthy individuals and those with viral and bacterial meningitis (see Table 45.3).

The spinal fluid ordinarily contains no red blood cells. The presence of blood indicates either contamination from a traumatic lumbar puncture or hemorrhage in the CNS. If the density of the red cells is constant from the first to the third tube and the cells are crenated, the likelihood of CNS hemorrhage is greater. Certain infectious agents, such as herpes simplex virus, may produce a hemorrhagic meningoencephalitis.

More than nine white blood cells in the CSF from a child and 29 from a neonate indicates inflammation of the meninges. However, a specimen is sometimes obtained early in the course of meningitis before an inflammatory reaction has been invoked. Thus, an occasional child with fewer than 10 cells in the CSF will later develop the physical and laboratory manifestations of meningitis.

In viral infections of the CNS, the white blood count in the spinal fluid usually ranges from 10 to 1000/cu mm. Occasionally, a WBC as high as 2500/cu mm may be seen. There is usually a predominance of mononuclear cells. Bacterial meningitis, on the other hand, evokes an intense infiltration of leukocytes, with a predominance of neutrophils. The cell count is usually in the range of 1000 to 20,000/cu mm, but may be even higher.

The cerebrospinal fluid glucose is normally one-half to two-thirds of the serum glucose. Equilibration between the serum and CSF glucose levels has been estimated to require at least 30 min. Thus, a rapid decrease in the serum glucose may obscure a wide variance from the CSF level, while a sudden elevation may lead to a falsely large discrepancy. Since the stress of a lumbar puncture produces hyperglycemia, a serum glucose for comparison with the CSF level should be obtained before attempting this procedure. In viral meningitis, the CSF glucose, which is usually in the normal range, may be as low as 30 mg/dl. The glucose in bacterial meningitis frequently falls below 30 mg/dl. Hypoglycorrhachia accompanying mild mononuclear pleocytosis should arouse a suspicion of tuberculous meningitis.

A normal CSF protein is less than 40 mg/dl in the child and 170 mg/dl in a neonate. While there is minimal elevation of the protein in viral meningitis, the level in bacterial meningitis is generally in the range of 100 mg/dl or greater.

Additional studies, such as counterimmunoelectrophoresis and CSF lactate, may be helpful in distinguishing bacterial from viral meningitis. However, these more sophisticated tests seldom play a role in the emergency department.

Bacterial Meningitis

BACKGROUND

Although almost any bacteria can cause meningitis, over 90% of the cases in children result from infections with five organisms: *H. influenzae*, *S. pneumoniae*, *N. meningitidis*, *E. coli*, and the Group B *Streptococcus*. The most common organism varies with the age of the child (see Figure 45.1). In the first month of life, *E. coli* and, more recently, Group B *Streptococcus* are usually isolated. Between 30 and 60 days of age, *H. influenzae* has been shown to be the commonest cause of meningitis (71% in the series of Friedman and Fleisher) with the Group B *Streptococcus* second in frequency during this interval. After the first 2 months of life, *H. influenzae* causes the majority of meningeal infections. The reported frequency has been as high as 66%. Also common are *S. pneumoniae* and *N. meningitidis*. *Salmonella*, an infrequent etiologic agent in the United States, should be suspected in the first year of life if meningitis occurs in association with gastroenteritis.

Meningitis occurs frequently in children; it has been estimated that there are 30,000 cases of bacterial CNS infection yearly, leading to over 3,000 deaths and 2 to 3 times as many permanent sequelae. Approximately 1 in every 2,000 children develops bacterial meningitis per year. At the Children's Hospital of Philadelphia, which has 10,000 admissions and 70,000 acute ambulatory visits annually, there are 50 to 60 children hospitalized in each 12-month period with bacterial meningitis. Bacterial meningitis may occur at any age, but one-quarter of the cases are reported in the first year, two-thirds before 5 years, and three-quarters prior to adulthood.

PATHOPHYSIOLOGY

Microorganisms gain access to the CNS via two potential pathways. Most commonly in children, a preceding septicemia leads to hematogenous seeding of the meninges. Alternatively, direct extension may occur from a purulent parameningeal focus.

Colonization of the nasopharynx sets the stage for the subsequent development of meningitis in the majority of bacterial CNS infections in the older child. In the infant, who is susceptible to infection with gram-negative enteric organisms, the bowel is often the source of the pathogen. This is also the case beyond the neonatal period

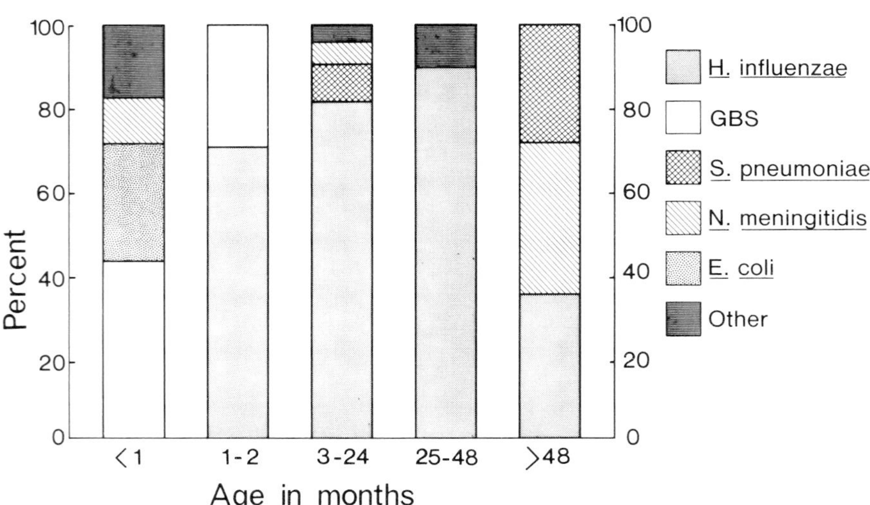

Figure 45.1 The frequency of the bacteria causing purulent meningitis over a 2-year period at the Children's Hospital of Philadelphia is shown by age.

Table 45.4
Signs and Symptoms of Meningitis

Age	Symptoms	Signs	
		Early	Late
0–3 months	Irritability	Lethargy	Bulging fontanelle
	Altered sleep pattern	Irritability	
	Vomiting	Fever (±)	
	Lethargy		
4–24 months	Irritability	Fever	Nuchal rigidity
	Altered sleep pattern	Irritability	Lethargy
	Lethargy		
>24 months	Headache	Fever	Brudzinski sign
	Stiff neck	Nuchal rigidity	Kernig sign
	Lethargy	Irritability	Lethargy

with less common bacteria such as *Salmonella*. A small percentage of the children colonized with a potential pathogen will develop bacteremia, but most will spontaneously terminate this event; over 80% of the cases of bacteremia with *S. pneumoniae* resolve without leading to local infection. While meningitis is more common following the recovery of *H. influenzae* from the blood, the majority of such children also escape CNS infection. Splenectomized individuals, or those who have infarcted spleens on the basis of inherited hemoglobinopathies, cannot limit the spread of bacteremia as successfully as those who are immunologically intact.

Although a less common predecessor to meningitis, purulent collections contiguous to the CNS do also frequently produce such infections. Sinusitis is the most frequent offender. Organisms may also occasionally invade the meninges directly from the middle ear. However, meningitis following otitis media usually results from bacteremia, unless a congenital or posttraumatic fistula in the temporal bone provides access to the CSF.

CLINICAL MANIFESTATIONS

The signs and symptoms of meningitis vary with the age of the child (see Table 45.4). Particularly in the first 3 months of life, the clinician must maintain a high index of suspicion for this disease.

Before 3 months of age, the history is that of irritability, an altered sleep pattern, vomiting, and decreased oral intake. In particular, paradoxical irritability points to the diagnosis of meningitis. Irritability in the infant without inflammation of the meninges is generally alleviated by maternal fondling; however, in the child with meningitis, any handling, even directed toward soothing the infant, may increase irritability by its effect on the inflamed meninges. The amount of time spent sleeping may either increase due to obtundation or decrease from irritability. Bulging of the fontanelle, an almost certain sign of meningitis in the febrile ill-appearing infant, is a late finding.

As the child passes beyond the age of 3 months, the symptomatology gradually becomes more specific for involvement of the CNS. There is a marked change in the level of activity. However, it is only in the child more than 2 years old that meningitis manifests with complaints of headache and neck stiffness.

The physical examination in the young infant rarely provides specific corroboration, even when the history suggests meningitis. Fever is often absent in these children, despite the presence of bacterial infection. On the other hand, any child less than 2 to 3 months old, presenting to the emergency department with a documented temperature $\geqq 38.5°C$, should be assumed to have meningitis unless disproven by the spinal fluid findings. The physical signs are sufficiently elusive that one cannot rely on the examination to definitively rule out meningeal infection. In several studies, 10 to 20% of these young infants had meningitis despite being judged clinically well by experienced pediatric houseofficers.

After 3 months of age, increasing, but not absolute, reliance can be placed on the physical findings; fever is almost invariably noted. Specific evidence of meningeal irritation will often be present including nuchal rigidity and, less frequently, Kernig and Brudzinski signs. In those instances where a lumbar puncture fails to confirm the diagnosis of meningitis despite the presence of meningeal signs, one must pursue other conditions which can mimic the findings on physical examination. Conditions capable of producing meningismus (irritation of the meninges without pleocytosis in the CSF) include severe pharyngitis, retropharyngeal abscess, cervical adenitis, arthritis or osteomyelitis of the cervical spine, upper lobe pneumonia, subarachnoid hemorrhage, pyelonephritis, and tetanus.

At times, meningitis manifests initially as a convulsion. In the infant under 6 months of age with a seizure, a lumbar puncture is mandatory to discern the presence of CNS infection. However, the occurrence of a seizure in a febrile child over 6 months of age presents a dilemma for the clinician. Febrile seizures are very common, affecting 5% of children, and will underlie most of these episodes. However, it may be difficult to distinguish a simple febrile seizure in an ill-appearing child with a high fever from early meningitis due to the vague symptomatology and lack of definitive physical findings in the first 2 years of life. Additionally, the occurence of a convulsion may obscure such meningeal signs as nuchal rigidity which may be masked by the hypotonia of the postictal period. Opinion varies as to whether a febrile seizure can be distinguished clinically from a seizure secondary to meningitis. In one study, 20% of children thought to have a first febrile seizure on the basis of the history and physical examination eventually were determined to have meningitis. However, other investigators have reported more success in making such a clinical differentiation. Because of the difficulty of establishing a clinical diagnosis in the young child, we recommend a lumbar puncture in every child under 18 months of age with a first febrile seizure. In the older child or in the case of a recurrent febrile seizure, the experienced clinician may choose to be guided by the physical findings and the evolution of the illness over the ensuing 12 to 24 hours.

The child with meningitis often has a complicated course beginning in the emergency department or even preceding arrival at the hospital (see Table 45.5). Shock, seizures, and hyponatremia strike at any age, while apnea and hypoglycemia affect predominantly infants less than 3 months of age. Although sterile subdural effusions and empyemas usually occur later in the disease, they merit consideration in the infant with signs of herniation and a bulging fontanelle.

MANAGEMENT

Bacterial meningitis is a medical emergency that requires the immediate institution of therapy. If the disease is diagnosed and treated promptly, mortality dwindles to less than 5%. Antibiotics should be given intravenously at the completion of the lumbar puncture. If meningitis is suspected, but attempts to obtain CSF are unsuccessful, this failure should not delay the drug therapy. It is safer to presumptively treat a child with a sterile pleocytosis than to handle the complications of progressive CNS infection. Similarly, inability to achieve venous access should not retard the administration of antibiotics. The intramuscular route provides a suitable, temporary alternative.

The age of the child determines the spectrum of microorganisms causing meningitis and the selection of antibiotic therapy (see Table 45.6). In the first 30 days of life the most likely organisms include the Gram-negative enteric rods and the Group B *Streptococcus*. The enteric pathogens are

Table 45.5
Complications of Meningitis

Early	Late
Apnea	Hyponatremia
Shock	Subdural empyema
Hypoglycemia	Seizures
Hyponatremia	
Seizures	

Table 45.6
Initial Antibiotic Therapy of Meningitis[a]

	Drug	Dose
0–30 days	Ampicillin and	300 mg/kg/day
	Moxalactam or	200 mg/kg/day
	Gentamicin	7.5 mg/kg/day
31–60 days	Ampicillin and	300 mg/kg/day
	Chloramphenicol	100 mg/kg/day
>60 days	Ampicillin and	300 mg/kg/day
	Chloramphenicol	100 mg/kg/day

[a] See appendix for age-adjusted and maximal dosages.

almost always sensitive to the aminoglycoside antibiotics; however, recent studies have suggested that moxalactam, a third generation cephalosporin, may be more effective. Penicillin or ampicillin, but not the antistaphylococcal penicillins, effectively treats the Group B *Streptococcus*. Ampicillin and an aminoglycoside or moxalactam thus provide coverage for the most frequent pathogens in the first month of life. The spectrum of these antibiotics also includes less common organisms in the neonate, such as *S. pneumoniae*, *N. meningitidis*, and *Listeria monocytogenes*. *Salmonella* is a somewhat unusual cause of meningitis in the United States, but may be isolated in 1 to 2% of such infections. Increasingly, this organism is resistant to ampicillin. Thus, the isolation or strongly suspected presence of *Salmonella* from the gastrointestinal tract dictates the inclusion of chloramphenicol.

Between 30 and 60 days of age, *H. influenzae* emerges as a major pathogen, and the Gram-negative enteric bacilli decrease in frequency. The Group B *Streptococcus* remains a common isolate, and *S. pneumoniae* and *N. meningitidis* occur sporadically. National surveillance indicates that 15 to 20% of *H. influenzae*, type B, isolated in the United States, show resistance to ampicillin. However, less than 1% of the organisms are resistant to chloramphenicol. Thus, ampicillin and chloramphenicol are chosen.

After the first 2 months, *H. influenzae* is clearly the predominant pathogen causing meningitis. It is followed in frequency by *S. pneumoniae* and *N. meningitidis*. This group of organisms responds to initial therapy with the combination of ampicillin and chloramphenicol. Again, chloramphenicol is an essential partner to ampicillin because of the increasing percentage of *H. influenzae* strains resistant to the latter antibiotic. Since *H. influenzae* remains common throughout childhood, despite a decrease in the frequency with advancing age, the initial therapy is the same in the adolescent.

In addition to the antibiotic administration aimed at the eradication of the offending organism, supportive therapy for complications (see Table 45.5) is an essential ingredient in the care of the child with meningitis. Laboratory studies on every patient should include a CBC, electrolytes, BUN, prothrombin and partial thromboplastin time, glucose, and blood culture. A rapid assessment should be made as to the adequacy of ventilation. The CNS edema which accompanies inflammation of the meninges may produce obtundation and hypoventilation. In the infant, apneic episodes are not uncommon. Thus oxygen, intubation, and assisted ventilation may all be required. Bacteremia, which usually accompanies meningitis, may lead to septic shock. This condition demands vigorous fluid resuscitation with normal saline. The response to an initial bolus of 20 ml/kg of saline determines the need for further therapy such as the use of cardiotonic agents (Chapter 2). The urgency to provide adequate perfusion to the vital organs by expanding the intravascular volume takes precedence over concerns about edema in the CNS.

Hyponatremia often accompanies meningitis, resulting from water retention due to the inappropriate secretion of antidiuretic hormone (SIADH). Occasionally, the oral administration of hypotonic solutions by the parents during the preceding prodromal illness may produce fluid overload and a low serum Na. If the child is felt to have seizures on the basis of hyponatremia, the physician should give 3% NaCl (see Chapter 46).

After the correction of dehydration or shock, the rate of fluid administration to the child with meningitis should be at 75% maintenance (see Chapter 46). Generally 0.2% NaCl is used for this purpose. Failure of the serum Na to rise in the hyponatremic child mandates further restriction on hydration.

Hypoglycemia occurs as a reaction to septicemia and stress. It is a more common concomitant of meningitis in the first 3 months of life. If the blood glucose is below 50 mg%, 25% glucose should be given at a dosage of 1 g/kg. This must be followed by an infusion of 5% glucose and monitoring of the response. Occasionally, 10% glucose will be necessary to maintain an acceptable serum level.

Seizures occur in 25% of children with bacterial meningitis and occasionally in those with viral infections. One should always be suspicious of derangement of the glucose or sodium as a cause of convulsive activity. However, most seizures are caused by irritation of the brain from the infectious process. They are controlled in the usual fashion with valium, phenobarbital, and dilantin (see Chapter 44).

Subdural effusion and, less often, empyema occur in 20 to 40% of children with meningitis, but usually appear later in the course and remain asymptomatic. In the rare infant with herniation due to a subdural collection, percutaneous drainage relieves the pressure on the brain and produces marked improvement (see Chapter 67).

Aseptic Meningitis

BACKGROUND

The aseptic meningitis syndrome is defined here as an inflammation of the meninges occurring in the absence of bacterial growth on routine culture media. A child whose initial spinal fluid findings suggest an aseptic meningitis may occasionally turn out to have a purulent infection since bacteria do not always elicit a marked polymorphonuclear leukocytosis early in the course. Additionally, bacteria with unusual growth requirements, inhibited by subtherapeutic concentrations of antibiotics, or sequestered in pockets adjacent to but not directly communicating with the CSF, may all produce an aseptic meningitis syndrome.

Both infectious and noninfectious diseases cause the aseptic meningitis syndrome (see Table 45.7). By far the most common etiology is viral meningitis. Despite underreporting, the Centers for Disease Control in the United States collected 9,000 cases in 1979.

Aseptic meningitis occurs throughout the year. However, the incidence of enteroviral infections, which are responsible for a large number of the cases, peaks in the summer in temperate regions. Thus, outbreaks of aseptic meningitis are more often seen in the warm months.

PATHOPHYSIOLOGY

The multiple causes of the aseptic meningitis syndrome produce inflammation of the meninges by different mechanisms. Even among the viral infections, the patho-

Table 45.7
Aseptic Meningitis Syndrome

Infectious
Viruses
Early or partially treated bacterial meningitis
Parameningeal infection
Unusual bacteria
Leptospirosis
Syphilis
Tuberculosis
Fungal
Cryptococcous
Parasitic
Trichinosis
Toxoplasmosis
Noninfectious
Neoplasm
Hemorrhage
Hypersensitivity reactions

genesis varies considerably. Some viruses lead to an immune reaction in the CNS while others directly invade the neural tissue. Access to the meninges is usually hematogenous but may be achieved by ascension along peripheral nerves.

CLINICAL MANIFESTATIONS

The signs and symptoms of aseptic meningitis resemble those of bacterial infections of the CNS but are not usually as severe. The infant shows only lethargy and irritability while the older child complains of a headache and stiff neck. Vomiting may occur and this may be persistent. There is often a history of a concommitant upper respiratory or gastrointestinal viral illness.

Fever usually occurs but not infrequently hovers around 38.5°C. The infant appears toxic, but the older child may remain remarkably well. Nuchal rigidity in a patient who is alert and conversant suggests aseptic, rather than bacterial, meningitis. Shining a flashlight in the eyes often elicits photophobia. The fontanelle of the infant usually maintains a normal configuration but occasionally bulges. Aside from positive Kernig and Brudzinski signs, the neurologic examination often shows no abnormalities. The presence of an altered level of consciousness or focal neurologic deficits points to meningoencephalitis rather than aseptic meningitis (see Chapter 44).

MANAGEMENT

All children with aseptic meningitis should have, in addition to the usual CSF studies, a CBC, electrolytes, and a BUN. Therapy does not extend beyond supportive care. Dehydration from prolonged emesis may necessitate intravenous fluid administration. After any deficit has been corrected, the rate should be set to provide three-quarters of the daily maintenance requirement to avoid overhydration and the possible aggravation of cerebral edema in the child who develops an encephalitic component.

Because the CSF findings in aseptic meningitis occasionally overlap those in bacterial infections, hospital admission is usually warranted until the spinal fluid culture results are available. However, the experienced clinician may choose to follow the older child as an outpatient if the family is reliable.

UPPER RESPIRATORY TRACT INFECTIONS

Infections in children involve the upper respiratory tract more frequently than any other area of the body. Included in this category are nasopharyngitis (common cold), stomatitis, pharyngitis, sinusitis, otitis, peritonsillar abscess, retropharyngeal abscess, laryngotracheobronchitis (croup), and epiglottitis. Because the most common causative organism varies between sites, infection in this area demands a specific anatomic diagnosis if the physician is to proceed with the appropriate diagnostic evaluation and therapy.

Nasopharyngitis (URI)

Nasopharyngitis, or the common cold, is a viral illness of the upper respiratory tract in children. The most frequently isolated organisms are the rhinoviruses and coronoviruses. Prospective family studies have shown that five or six episodes occur yearly during childhood. The illness is characterized by fever of less than 39°C and coryza. There may be a mild conjunctivitis and injection of the pharynx. Although the tympanic membranes may show a slightly dull appearance and decreased mobility, the characteristic features of acute purulent otitis media (erythema, loss of the landmarks, and bulging) are absent. Therapy is limited to a recommendation for rest, adequate hydration, saline nose drops, and antipyretic agents. Neither antibiotics nor antihistamine decongestant combinations prevent secondary bacterial infections, such as acute purulent otitis media.

Stomatitis

Stomatitis, an infection of the mouth, is caused by herpes simplex and the Coxsackie viruses at any age, and by *Candida albicans* ("thrush") in the infant (see Chapters 62 and 66). Viral infections cause vesicular lesions initially and ulcerations and plaques subsequently. Treatment is limited to systemic antipyretic and analgesic drugs, and the local application of topical analgesics, dosed by weight, such as 2% viscous xylocaine. *C. albicans* produces white plaques on the mucosa that bleed if scraped. Nystatin, 200,000 units q.i.d., leads to a prompt resolution of this condition.

Pharyngitis

Pharyngitis is an infection of the throat including the tonsils. In the immunocompetent child, several viruses, *Mycoplasma pneumoniae*, and only a few bacteria cause pharyngitis. Common viral isolates include the adenoviruses, influenza viruses, enteroviruses, parainfluenza viruses, and the Epstein-Barr virus (EBV). Although many bacteria have been reported as possible causes of pharyngitis, only three organisms have a well defined role: the Group A *Streptococcus*, *Corynebacterium diphtheriae*, and *N. gonorrhoeae*.

Pharyngitis is a common infection in children. Moffet and colleagues reported that 128 of 230 visits to an infirmary by youngsters of school age at a children's home were due to pharyngeal infections. The group A *Streptococcus* causes almost half of such infections between 5 and 15 years of age, but is uncommon in the first 3 years of life. In one study of 50 children less than 3 years old with exudative pharyngitis, only 7 had illness due to streptococci.

For practical purposes, pharyngitis can be considered as streptococcal (bacterial) or nonstreptococcal (viral). Since the symptomatology of the two types overlap, the physician can reliably distinguish the more important streptococcal infections only with the aid of a throat culture. Certain clinical features, however, favor a bacterial etiology. Such infections more often have an abrupt onset with fever and sore throat; cough and coryza are uncommon. Examination of the pharynx shows an erythematous mucosa, often with exudate and petechiae on the posterior palate. Additionally, the cervical lymph nodes often become enlarged and tender.

Although unusual, complications may occur with bacterial pharyngitis; both suppurative and nonsuppurative sequelae can result from streptococcal infections. The latter category includes acute rheumatic fever and glomerulonephritis. Viral pharyngitis resolves spontaneously in 2 to 5 days with the exception of EBV, as discussed under *Infectious Mononucleosis* (see page 406).

In the emergency department, a throat culture should be obtained from all children with pharyngeal inflammation and those complaining of a sore throat. Culture-proven infections due to the Group A *Streptococcus* are treated with penicillin. While a single injection of benzathine penicillin, 30,000 units/kg, obviates all problems with compliance, oral phenoxymethyl penicillin, 50 mg/kg/day, provides an acceptable alternative if prescribed for 10 days. Erythromycin, 40 mg/kg/day, is used for penicillin-allergic children. Antipyretic agents, fluids, and adequate rest should be recommended. Since there are studies which indicate that antibiotics shorten the course of streptococcal pharyngitis minimally if at all, there is no reason to hastily give these drugs before confirming a bacterial etiology by culture.

Otitis Media

BACKGROUND

Otitis media (OM) refers to inflammation within the middle ear. There are several classifications for the various types of OM; for the purpose of management in the emergency department, the disease can be divided into four categories on the basis of duration and the presence or absence of pathogenic bacteria. Table 45.8 provides the schema for classification according to the duration, the physical findings, and the bacteriology (see also Fig. 45.2). Acute purulent otitis media (APOM) has a sudden onset and is due to a bacterial infection. Chronic purulent otitis media (CPOM) denotes a bacterial infection persisting for more than 2 weeks. Acute serous otitis media (ASOM) is characterized by a sterile effusion in the middle ear for less than 2 weeks. In chronic serous otitis media (CSOM) the effusion persists for more than 2 weeks. If the fluid in the middle ear be-

Table 45.8
Classification of Otitis Media

Type	Duration	Bacteria[a]	Typanum	Signs and Symptoms
APOM[b]	<2 weeks	Yes	Red, bulging	Fever (50%), earache
CPOM	≧2 weeks	Yes	Perforated	Draining ear
ASOM	<2 weeks	No	Dull, retracted, ± fluid	None, decreased hearing, fullness
CSOM	≧2 weeks	No	Retracted, fluid	None, decreased hearing, fullness

[a] *Streptococcus pneumoniae*, *Hemophilus influenzae*, or *Streptococcus pyogenes*.
[b] APOM = acute purulent otitis media; CPOM = chronic purulent otitis media; ASOM = acute serous otitis media; CSOM = chronic serous otitis media.

comes viscous, mucoid otitis media (MOM) may be substituted for CSOM.

The bacterial flora of middle ear infections varies somewhat with age. Although gram-negative enteric bacilli and *S. aureus* cause 15 to 20% of OM during the first month of life, *S. pneumoniae* and *H. influenzae* predominate at all ages, even in the neonate. *S. pneumoniae* can be recovered from about 40%, and *H. influenzae* from 20%, of children with OM between 1 month and 10 years of age. Among older children and adolescents, *H. influenzae* decreases in frequency but remains a significant pathogen. Over 90% of the *H. influenzae* causing OM are nontypable, and most of the remainder are type B. The incidence of ampicillin resistance among *H. influenzae* has increased, climbing as high as 30% in Washington, DC. At the Children's Hospital of Philadelphia, 15% of OM in children between 1 month and 12 years of age was due to *H. influenzae* in a survey in 1981; 15% of all *H. influenzae* isolates showed resistance to ampicillin.

APOM concerns the emergency department physician to a far greater extent than the other varieties of ear disease. This is the most common bacterial infection in childhood. Howie and Ploussard found at least one episode of OM in two-thirds of the children in their practice by their second birthday, and 1 in 7 children had more than 6 episodes.

OM is more common in the winter in temperate climates. This is presumably related to the higher incidence of upper respiratory infections during the colder months.

PATHOPHYSIOLOGY

Any discussion of the pathophysiology of OM provokes great controversy among both pediatricians and otolaryngologists. However, it appears that abnormal function of the eustachian tube contributes to the development of OM in most cases. Possible mechanisms for obstruction of the eustachian tube include hypertrophied nasopharyngeal lymphoid tissue or intrinsic abnormalities of the various components of this structure. Whatever the cause, blockage impairs ventilation of the middle ear leading to an accumulation of fluid behind the tympanic membrane. This effusion then provides a fertile environment for the proliferation of bacteria from the heavily colonized nasopharynx.

CLINICAL MANIFESTATIONS

Studies by Howie, Paradise, Klein and others have shown the variable spectrum of OM. An infection in the middle ear may produce no symptoms, being detected only on examination, or cause obvious localizing pain. In the young child, the initial manifestation is often fever, irritability, or diarrhea. Children beyond the age of 3 years generally, but not invariably, complain of pain in the ear. Less frequent symptoms include vertigo and hearing impairment.

Fever, occurring in 25 to 50% of children with APOM, serves only to arouse suspicion of infection in the middle ear. The diagnosis rests in the usual clinical settings on the accurate interpretation of the otoscopic findings, a skill gained only by experience with the pneumatic otoscope. If cerumen obscures the tympanic membrane, a sufficient quantity must be cleared to allow adequate visualization. Either a blunt currette or an apparatus for irrigation (ear syringe or Water-Pik) will adequately remove such material in most cases.

The tympanic membrane in APOM bulges out at the examiner as a result of the positive pressure generated by the production of purulent material in the middle ear cavity. Although the drum is sometimes red, it more often appears yellow due to the exudate behind it. A convex contour of the drum in the child suspected of having APOM is sufficient to make this diagnosis, regardless of the color of the tympanum. The diffuse injection of the normal tympanum, which is often exaggerated by crying, should not be confused with the intense erythema of infection.

Difficulty arises in differentiating serous otitis media (SOM) from APOM and in diagnosing "early" APOM, particularly in the child with a preexisting middle ear effusion. The tympanic membrane has decreased mobility in both APOM and SOM; however, it is usually retracted in the latter condition.

The WBC count, if obtained, usually falls within the normal range or shows a mild leukocytosis. An occasional young child may have a count of 20,000 to 30,000/cu mm. Tympanocentesis yields an organism in 60 to 70% of the cases, but blood cultures are usually sterile.

Acute complications occur infrequently in OM since the advent of effective antibiotics. Local suppuration may involve the mastoids and rarely leads to meningitis or brain abscess. Perforations will generally heal spontaneously (see Chapter 67). A child with OM in the first year or two of life may develop dehydration from vomiting and diarrhea associated with the infection.

MANAGEMENT

Uncomplicated OM in the child over the age of 1 month should be treated with oral antibiotic therapy on an outpatient basis. Amoxicillin, 50 mg/kg/day in 3 divided doses, remains the drug of choice in most areas of the United States. If the local resistance patterns dictate the use of an antibiotic effective against ampicillin-resistant *H. influenzae*, either cefaclor, 50 mg/kg/day in 3 divided doses, or the combination of erythromycin and sulfasoxazole, 40 mg/kg/day of erythromycin in 3 divided doses, serve as alternatives. Both of these drugs can be used in children with a history of penicillin allergy.

If APOM persists during therapy with amoxicillin or recurs within 2 days of its discontinuance, ampicillin-resistant *H. influenzae* emerges as a likely cause of the infection. Cefaclor, erythromycin/sulfasoxazole, and trimethoprim/sulfamethoxazole (40 mg/kg/day of sulfamethoxazole in 2 divided doses) are all effective in this situation. Failure of such a second course of antibiotics to eradicate the infection mandates a tympanocentesis for culture.

The management of OM in the first month of life has provoked controversy due to: (1) the occurrence of gram-negative enteric bacilli and *S. aureus* in middle ear infections in these children; and (2) the decreased ability of the neonate to resist infection. If a child under 1 month of age presents with fever or irritability and is found to have OM, we admit the child for intravenous antibiotic therapy pending the outcome of cultures of the blood, urine, and spinal fluid.

Infants between 4 and 12 weeks of age with OM can be managed as outpatients, since *S. pneumoniae* and *H. influenzae* are the predominant organisms. However, other sources of infection, including meningitis, must be excluded in the febrile child before attributing the source of a temperature elevation to OM alone.

Otitis Externa

Otitis externa (OE), or swimmer's ear, indicates an infection affecting the auditory canal and external surface of the tympanic membrane but sparing the middle ear. Multiple organisms, particularly *P. aeruginosa*, play a role in this disease. There is usually a history of recent swimming, but occasional cases are seen in children whose only submersion occurs during normal bathing. The child complains of an earache that may be unilateral or bilateral, and purulent ma-

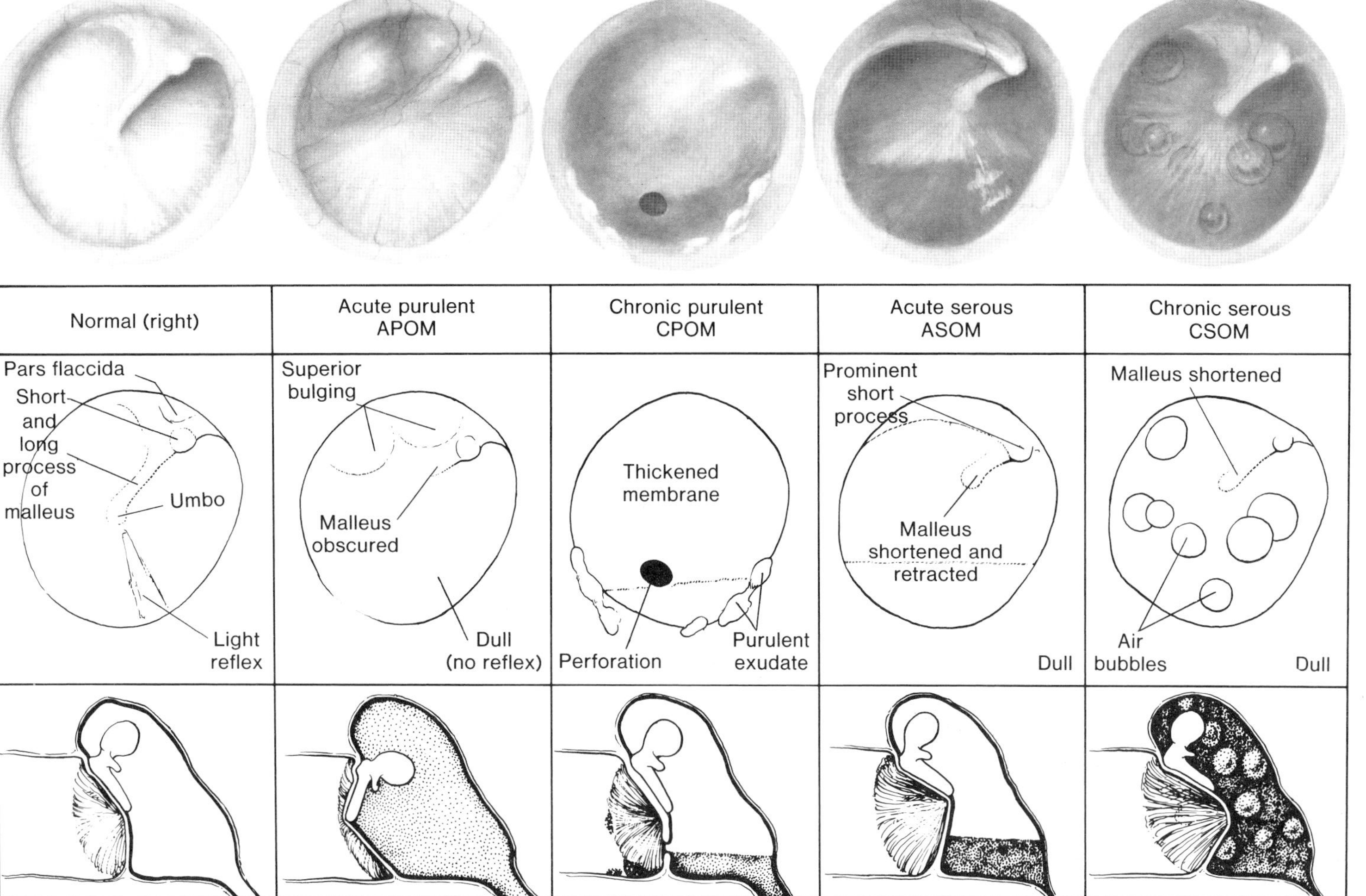

Figure 45.2 Appearance of the tympanic membrane in different types of otitis media.

terial often drains from the ear. Fever is never present unless there is an associated illness. Unlike OM, pulling on the ear lobe to straighten the canal in preparation for otoscopic examination elicits marked tenderness. A cheesy white exudate fills the canal, often obscuring the TM. If the ear is shielded from exposure to water, otic solutions containing antibiotics and corticosteroids (Cortisporin, Lidosporin) provide a rapid cure. They are given in a dosage of 4 drops 4 times/day for 1 week. Should a local cellulitis develop, systemic antibiotics are indicated (see page 395).

Sinusitis

BACKGROUND

Sinusitis is an inflammation of the paranasal sinuses: maxillary ethmoid, frontal, or sphenoid. The ethmoid and maxillary sinuses are present at birth, but the frontal and sphenoid do not become aerated until 6 or 7 years of age. Either an acute or a chronic infection may occur, each characterized by a different, but overlapping, group of symptoms. Sinusitis is not a common illness in children. Among 2,613 patients seen in an office practice, Breese et al. made this diagnosis in only 6 (0.23%).

Wald and colleagues studied the bacteriology of sinusitis in children using cultures of material obtained by antral puncture. They recovered 47 organisms from 30 children: 17 *S. pneumoniae*; 11 nontypable *H. influenzae*; 9 *Branhamella catarrhalis*; 2 *Streptococcus viridans*; 7 group A *Streptococcus*; and 1 *Moraxella*. Hamory and colleagues found a similar spectrum of pathogens in adults with maxillary sinusitis. Although anaerobic organisms and *S. aureus* have been reported occasionally, they do not play a role in most of these infections in childhood. *H. influenzae*, type B, frequently causes ethmoiditis and periorbital cellulitis.

PATHOPHYSIOLOGY

Infection of the sinuses arises in a fashion similar to that described for APOM. Organisms ascend from the nasopharynx and cause disease if the mucosal barrier of the sinus or the normal pattern of drainage has been altered.

CLINICAL MANIFESTATIONS

The presentation of acute sinusitis varies in some respects with the age of the child. Usually, the infection follows a viral upper respiratory illness. Cough occurs in 75% of the patients. Unlike adolescents, young children do not often complain of a headache or facial pain. A fever is noted in about half of the children with sinusitis. Nasal discharge occurs in almost all of these infections and is often the symptom that brings the child to the emergency department. The area of the face overlying the sinus swells in 10 to 20% of the patients with maxillary disease, and periorbital or orbital edema and cellulitis even more commonly accompany ethmoiditis.

The child with chronic sinusitis complains only of chronic cough and rhinorrhea. Fever, headache, and facial pain are unusual. Often abnormal findings are not seen on examination.

The WBC count is normal in 60 to 80% of children with sinusitis. In 10 to 30% of these infections, transillumination of the sinuses shows a discrepancy between the two sides. The sinus x-ray is abnormal in almost every child with sinusitis; there may be an air-fluid level, complete opacification, or mucosal thickening. Of 60 sinuses in 30 children evaluated radiographically by Wald and colleagues, 4 were normal, 38 showed complete opacification, 15 showed mucosal thickening, and 3 showed an air-fluid level. Hamory et al. obtained x-rays on 43 patients with 58 episodes of sinusitis. Eighteen had an air-fluid level, 18 opacification, 12 mucosal thickening, and 10 no abnormalities.

Although sinusitis usually responds to oral antibiotic therapy, serious complications occasionally result from the local spread of the suppuration. These include orbital infection, brain abscess, epidural or subdural empyema, and cavernous sinus thrombosis. Proptosis and paralysis of the extraocular muscles point to the accumulation of purulent material within the orbit. Following intracranial extension, the child appears toxic and usually has a detectable neurologic deficit.

MANAGEMENT

All children suspected of sinusitis should have an x-ray evaluation of their sinuses. Among this group of patients clinically felt to be at risk for an infection, any abnormality (air-fluid level, opacification, or mucosal thickening) suffices to confirm the diagnosis. Amoxicillin, 50 mg/kg/day, effectively treats the common pathogens, *S. pneumoniae* and *H. influenzae*. Children with sinusitis require admission if they are less than 2 years old, have facial swelling and tenderness, or develop any complications.

Peritonsillar Abscess

A peritonsillar abscess, or "quinsy," results from the accumulation of purulent material within the tonsillar fossa. The group A *Streptococcus*, various anaerobic organisms, and occasionally *S. aureus* are isolated from these lesions, which are rare in children.

The complaints of trismus and difficulty speaking separate a peritonsillar abscess from the far more common pharyngitis. The voice sounds muffled, and the child drools profusely. Both tonsils may swell, but the enlargement of one is more pronounced. Usually the abscessed tonsil becomes sufficiently large so as to push the uvula to the opposite side of the pharynx, and the examiner can palpate a fluctuant mass intraorally. The WBC count is elevated.

All children with a peritonsillar abscess should be hospitalized and treated with antibiotics and drainage. Penicillin, 100,000 units/kg/day, is usually sufficient, but the results of the culture and Gram stain of material from the infected tonsil will determine the final choice of therapy, since *S. aureus* is occasionally recovered. In the unusual child with respiratory compromise, aspiration of the abscess can be life-saving in the emergency department. This is accomplished using an 18-gauge 3 ½-inch spinal needle mounted on a 10 ml syringe (see Chapter 62).

Cervical Lymphadenitis

BACKGROUND

Cervical lymphadenitis is a bacterial infection of the lymph nodes in the neck. This condition must be distinguished from lymphadenopathy, an enlargement of one or more lymph nodes that occurs with viral infections or as a reaction to bacterial disease in structures draining to the nodes.

S. aureus causes lymphadenitis in the majority of those children with an identifiable pathogen. Barton and Feigin isolated *S. aureus* from 27 (36%) and the group A *Streptococcus* from 19 (26%) of 74 children with this condition. Other organisms that rarely play a role include anaerobic bacteria, *H. influenzae*, *Yersinia pestis*, gram-negative bacilli, *Francisella tularensis*, *Actinomyces*, and *Mycobacteria*.

PATHOPHYSIOLOGY

The causative organisms in cervical adenitis initially colonize the nares or pharynx. Dental abscesses may also be a source of pathogens. Whether or not they produce a local infection, the bacteria can spread to the lymph nodes in the neck. If not contained by the child's immune system, they proliferate within the node and evoke an inflammatory response.

CLINICAL MANIFESTATIONS

Children with cervical lymphadenitis present with a swelling in the neck. If sufficiently old, the child will usually complain of pain. Fever occurs only occasionally, more often in children under a year of age. The infected node varies in size from 2 to 8 cm. Initially it has a firm consistency, but fluctuance develops in about 25%. The skin overlying the node becomes erythematous, and edema may surround it.

The WBC count is usually normal but may be elevated in the younger, febrile child. Aspiration of the node often identifies the organism by both Gram stain and culture, even if fluctuance is not appreciated. The children with infections due to *M. tuberculosis* usually react to the PPD-S skin test and have changes compatible with tuberculosis seen on x-ray of the chest.

Complications of bacterial adenitis are unusual. Organisms such as *S. aureus* and the group A *Streptococcus* can spread locally if unchecked. A sinus tract develops in some children infected with *Mycobacteria*. Recurrence of the infection occurs in conditions such as chronic granulomatous disease.

MANAGEMENT

Children with cervical adenitis who are otherwise healthy should receive an antibiotic effective against *S. aureus* and the Group A *Streptococcus*. Agents such as dicloxacillin, 50 mg/kg/day, or cephalexin, 50 mg/kg/day, have activity against both of these organisms. If the node is fluctuant, aspiration provides useful etiologic information and speeds the rate of resolution. All children with lymphadenitis should have a PPD-S skin test and be followed until the infection subsides.

Children under 3 months of age and those who appear toxic or have developed a draining sinus are best managed in the hospital. A failure to improve while on oral antibiotic therapy or a positive skin test with PPD-S necessitate subsequent hospitalization.

Retropharyngeal Abscess

A retropharyngeal abscess fills the potential space between the anterior border of the cervical vertebrae and the posterior wall of the esophagus. The usual pathogens are the group A *Streptococcus*, anaerobic organisms, and, occasionally, *S. aureus*. These infrequent infections occur most often in young children.

The child with a retropharyngeal abscess presents with a clinical picture similar to that seen with epiglottitis (see page 376), but the onset is less abrupt. Fever and a toxic appearance are common. As purulent material collects, the fluctuant mass obstructs the larynx and esophagus leading to stridor and drooling. The abscess may cause meningismus; thus, this diagnosis should be considered in the child with nuchal rigidity but no pleocytosis in the cerebrospinal fluid.

Although a retropharyngeal infection can rarely be seen as a midline swelling on examination of the pharynx, it is usually difficult to observe this finding in the uncooperative child. If the diagnosis is suspected, a lateral neck x-ray should be obtained. The radiograph shows an increase in the width of the soft tissues anterior to the vertebrae. Ordinarily, the width of this space is less than half of that of the adjacent vertebral body if the examination is done with the neck properly extended.

A retropharyngeal abscess poses a risk to the patency of the airway. All children with this infection should be hospitalized under the care of an otolaryngologist. In the emergency department, intravenous access should be secured, penicillin given in a dosage of 100,000 units/kg/day, and cardiorespiratory monitoring instituted. In the event of respiratory arrest, intubation, or less commonly tracheotomy, becomes necessary.

Laryngotracheobronchitis (Croup)

BACKGROUND

Croup, or laryngotracheobronchitis, is a viral infection which involves the larynx and may extend into the trachea and bronchi. It is a common infection, with at least 10 cases of croup to every one of epiglottitis among children presenting to the emergency department. Though most children with croup are treated as outpatients, Rapkin reported there were 32 admissions for croup in 1971 at the Children's Hospital of Newark. During the winter of 1969–1970, there were 30 admissions for croup to the Children's Hospital of Philadelphia. Hoekelman reported that 3 (1.2%) of 246 healthy term infants in a pediatric practice developed croup during their first year of life. This infection is the commonest etiology for stridor in the febrile child (see Chapter 62).

Parainfluenza virus can be recovered from about 60% of children with croup. Additional causes of the disease are influenza, adenoviruses, measles, and respiratory syncytial virus. Bacteria play no role.

Croup occurs more commonly in the winter months. Children between the ages of 6 months and 3 years are affected most frequently. The diagnosis of croup in a child ıore than 3 years old should arouse the uspicion of an underlying anatomic abnorıality.

ATHOPHYSIOLOGY

The viral pathogens that eventually prouce croup invade the epithelium of the harynx initially. Spread occurs downward) the larynx and occasionally further along ıe respiratory tract. The infection causes ndothelial damage, mucus production, loss f ciliary function, and edema. There is rythema and swelling of the vocal cords nd the subglottic larynx. A fibrinous exuate partially occludes the lumen of the ·achea.

LINICAL MANIFESTATIONS

Croup begins insidiously with the onset f fever and coryza. During the next 1 to 2 ays, the infection spreads further along ıe airway, producing signs of upper respiatory obstruction. Inspiratory stridor deelops at this stage of the illness, and a arking cough is heard. The child may be nable to maintain adequate oral intake.

Although the severity of croup varies, the ıajority of children appear mildly to modrately ill in contrast to the toxic patients ith epiglottitis. The fever usually ranges om 38° to 39°C. There is tachycardia and ıchypnea, but the respirations rarely exeed 40 breaths/min. Suprasternal and subostal retractions frequently accompany roup. On auscultation of the chest, the xaminer may hear either stridor alone in ıild disease or rhonchi and wheezes with ıore extensive involvement of the respiraory epithelium. Cyanosis occurs only in ıe minority of children with severe croup.

The WBC count is generally normal; mphocytosis may occur as with other iral infections. The lateral neck x-ray ıows subglottic narrowing from soft tissue dema in severe disease. However, the maority of the radiographic studies of the irway are normal or disclose only balloonıg of the hypopharynx. Rather than conrm the diagnosis of croup, X-ray examiation more often excludes other illness ıch as epiglottitis or retropharyngeal abcess. The arterial blood gas shows neither hypoxia nor hypercarbia unless respiratory fatigue ensues.

Both dehydration and upper airway obstruction may complicate croup. Because of the respiratory distress and the toxicity associated with a febrile illness, the ability to maintain normal hydration will decrease in some children. Dehydration then occurs in the face of increased fluid losses via the pulmonary and cutaneous routes.

An occasional child with croup develops marked upper airway obstruction. Signs suggestive of impending respiratory failure include: (1) hypotonicity; (2) marked retractions; (3) decreased or absent inspiratory breath sounds; (4) depressed level of consciousness; (5) tachycardia out of proportion to the fever; and (6) cyanosis. Although an arterial blood gas is not needed in the evaluation of children with mild croup, this study plays a role in deciding on the therapy in more severe cases. Respiratory failure is defined as a $PaCO_2 \geqq 60$ mmHg or a $PaO_2 < 100$ mmHg in 100% oxygen. However, significant respiratory compromise is present in croup when the $PaCO_2$ rises over 45 mmHg and the PaO_2 falls below 70 mmHg in room air.

MANAGEMENT

Many children with croup never seek medical attention. Of those who present to the emergency department, the majority can be managed as outpatients. The indications for admission are dehydration and/or significant respiratory compromise. If any of the signs of respiratory failure are noted, hospitalization becomes necessary. A lateral neck x-ray is needed only if the diagnosis is uncertain clinically, and an arterial blood gas should be obtained in those cases where the clinical picture is not decisive. In addition, the physician should consider the social milieu of the family. Hospitalization provides the safest course for the child when the parents are unreliable caretakers or transportation to the emergency department for a reevaluation proves an obstacle to further treatment.

Antibiotic administration has no place in the treatment of croup, as the viral etiology of this illness has been well established. In a retrospective review of children with croup, Rapkin found no difference in the outcome among children who did or did not receive antibiotics.

Mist therapy lessens the severity of croup. Water droplets penetrate to the area of inflammation in the larynx and provide moisture to the mucosa.

Corticosteroids have long been mentioned as potential aids in the treatment of croup, but the initial controlled studies on these agents failed to substantiate the early anecdotal successes. However, Leipzig et al. found dexamethasone effective in a controlled study in 1979. Methodologic flaws plague all the published investigations, making their interpretation difficult as discussed by Tunneson and Fienstein. Until sufficient data becomes available, the decision to prescribe corticosteroids will remain arbitrary. It is not our policy to use these agents routinely in the emergency department.

Racemic epinephrine, delivered either by positive pressure or nebulization, has also been tried in the management of croup. Adair et al. described significant improvement among children with this disease in their initial study. However, Gardner et al. did not confirm the benefit of racemic epinephrine. Subsequent investigations have also noted a rebound phenomena with this form of therapy; some children show rapid improvement but deteriorate over the next 1 to 2 hours. Thus, we do not advocate the administration of racemic epinephrine to children in the emergency department who are not being hospitalized. However, this mode of therapy is useful for the child with significant airway obstruction awaiting admission to the intensive care unit.

Epiglottitis

BACKGROUND

Epiglottitis is a life-threatening bacterial infection of the epiglottis and the surrounding structures. Recent authors have suggested that supraglottitis would be a more appropriate appellation.

Epiglottitis occurs with regularity in children, accounting for 1 of every 1,000 pediatric admissions. Recent reviews indicate an incidence of 4 cases per year at Denver Children's Hospital, 5 at Buffalo Children's Hospital, and 6 at the Children's Hospital of Philadelphia. Epiglottitis ranks second in frequency to croup as an infectious cause of stridor. It occurs more often than retropharyngeal abscess or diphtheria.

H. influenzae causes over 90% of the cases of epiglottitis. *S. pneumoniae* and the group A *Streptococcus* are also occasionally etiologic agents in this illness. However, *S. aureus* has not been shown to be a pathogen in epiglottitis, with the exception of a single atypical neonatal case.

Although more common in the winter months, epiglottitis occurs through the year. This disease usually strikes children between the ages of 3 and 7 years; however, infants and adults with epiglottitis have been well described.

PATHOPHYSIOLOGY

The pharynx of normal children is often colonized with potentially pathogenic microorganisms such as *H. influenzae* and *S. pneumoniae*. Occasionally, these bacteria penetrate the mucosal barrier and invade the bloodstream. During the course of bacteremia, focal infection may occur at several sites including the epiglottis and surrounding structures. Infection causes inflammatory edema beginning on the lingual surface of the epiglottis where the submucosa is loosely attached. The swelling progresses rapidly to involve the aryepiglottic folds, the arytenoids, and finally the entire supraglottic larynx. Tightly bound epithelium on the vocal cords halts the spread at this level. The tremendous reduction in the caliber of the airway results in turbulent air flow on inspiration, manifest clinically as stridor.

There are two possible mechanisms to explain the sudden respiratory arrest which not infrequently complicates this disease. The swollen epiglottis may be drawn into the glottis, acting like a plug to obstruct the flow of air, but this seems unlikely because the edematous, inflamed tissues of the supraglottic region become relatively tense. More likely, aspiration of oropharyngeal ecretions occludes an already narrowed ryngeal inlet.

LINICAL MANIFESTATIONS

Epiglottitis has an abrupt onset. The du- tion of illness prior to presentation is ten as short as 6 hours and rarely exceeds hours. Among the 21 children reported y Greenberg and Schisgall, an average of 7 hours elapsed between the first symptom nd hospital admission. Faden found a ean duration of symptoms related to air- ay obstruction of 0.9 days. The parents rst note the onset of fever. Shortly there- ter, the child develops stridor and labored spirations. As the disease progresses, the upraglottic edema interferes with the abil- y to swallow secretions; thus, drooling is complaint in 60 to 70% of cases. One-half the children with epiglottitis will com- ain of a sore throat. Aphonia, hoarseness, nd cough are infrequent. Although both oup and epiglottitis manifest with stridor a febrile child, the examiner can usually fferentiate these two illnesses on the basis the clinical features (see Table 45.9).

The anxious appearance of the child with piglottitis strikes the examiner immedi- ely. In order to maximize air entry, these ildren assume a sitting position with their ws thrust forward. Cyanosis may occur in e later stages of the illness. The temper- ure, almost always elevated, often reaches level of 40°C. Tachycardia is a constant ature. While the patients are universally chypneic, the respiratory rate infre- uently exceeds 40 breaths/min. Stridor n be heard without a stethoscope, but auscultation of the lungs reveals no other adventitious sounds. Marked retractions are seen, predominantly involving the suprasternal and subcostal musculature.

As will be discussed under *Management*, attempts to visualize the epiglottis are hazardous and should be avoided in the child with suspected epiglottitis. However, the examiner can view the pharynx without the use of a tongue depressor. The mucosa is seen to be erythematous and pooled secretions are present in about half of the children. Occasionally, a swollen cherry red epiglottis protrudes above the base of the tongue and is visible without instrumentation.

The WBC count is usually elevated in children with epiglottitis. As in other diseases resulting from bacteremia with *H. influenzae*, a leukocytosis in the range of 15,000 to 25,000/cu mm and a shift to the left occur in response to the infection. Culture of the blood yields a pathogen in 80 to 90% of the cases, and of the epiglottis, following the placement of an airway, in about half.

A lateral neck x-ray is pathognomonic of epiglottitis. There are three characteristic features: (1) a swollen epiglottis; (2) thickened aryepiglottic folds; and (3) obliteration of the vallecula (Fig. 45.3). The normal epiglottis has a thin, curved silhouette that has been likened to a bent finger, convex on one side and concave on the other. As a result of inflammatory edema from infection, it swells and assumes a configuration that is convex on both sides. This has been called the "thumb sign." The airway below

able 45.9
piglottitis and Croup: A Comparison

	Epiglottitis	Croup
natomy	Supraglottic	Subglottic
tiology	Bacterial: *Haemophilus influenzae*	Viral: Parainfluenza
ge range	3 to 7 yr	½ to 3 yr
nset	6 to 24 hr	24 to 72 hr
oxicity	Marked	Mild to moderate
rooling	Frequent	Absent
ough	Unusual	Frequent
oarseness	Unusual	Frequent
/BC	Leukocytosis	Normal

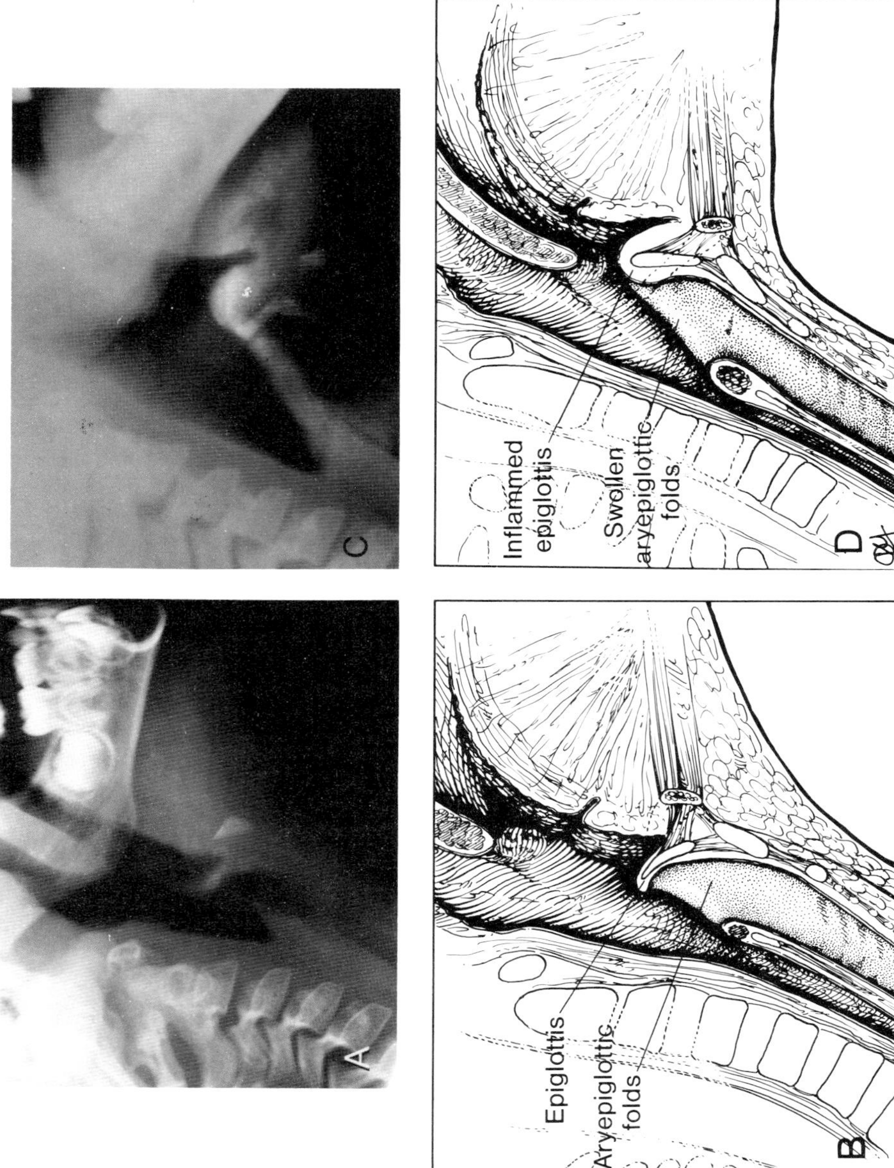

Figure 45.3 Appearance of the lateral neck region in the normal child (A and B) and the child with epiglottitis (C and D).

he level of the vocal cords appears normal n the lateral neck x-ray of a child with piglottitis.

The most serious complication of epiglottitis is sudden respiratory obstruction. This ay occur unpredictably at any point in he illness, prior to seeking medical attention, in the emergency department, or after ospitalization. Although a child with minimal respiratory distress may occasionally ave a total obstruction, marked retractions and labored breathing should serve as warning of an impending airway catastrophe.

An additional complication of this illness s extraepiglottic spread of the infection. During the course of the bacteremia, seeding may involve the meninges, lungs, pericardium, synovial membranes, and soft tissues. Thus, the initial examination should ttempt to elicit signs of infection at these dditional sites. Among 72 children reviewed by Molteni, chest x-rays showed neumonia in 18 (25%). Although no cases f meningitis were seen in this series, infection of the CNS has been described in association with epiglottitis.

MANAGEMENT

When a child is suspected of having epiglottitis, the thrust of the management plan s to make a definitive diagnosis and institute therapy prior to the onset of airway obstruction. The major pitfall in this process is the vigorous examination of the posterior pharynx without having considered he possibility of supraglottic infection. Such manipulation initiates laryngeal obstruction in a large number of children with epiglottitis.

The initial steps in management are based on the degree of respiratory distress and the likelihood of epiglottitis as judged from the clinical features (Fig. 45.4). Some children with epiglottitis will have total or nearly total airway obstruction as the initial presentation of their disease. In this situation, treatment precedes any diagnostic evaluation—steps are taken to maintain an adequate exchange of air.

The majority of children, however, manifest lesser degrees of stridor and respiratory compromise with fever. The clinician must decide whether the constellation of historical and physical features point to croup or epiglottitis. When the findings weigh in favor of epiglottitis, immediate preparation should be made for the insertion of an artificial airway; this includes collecting the necessary equipment and summoning the proper personnel. At our institution, both the anesthesiologist and otorhinolaryngologist are involved in the care of these children, in addition to the pediatrician in the emergency department. Following the appropriate preparations, a physician should accompany the child to the radiology department for a lateral neck radiograph. An intravenous infusion using a plastic cannula should be started in the cooperative patient. However, if the child becomes agitated or the procedure lengthy, the x-ray must be obtained immediately rather than persisting with attempts to gain

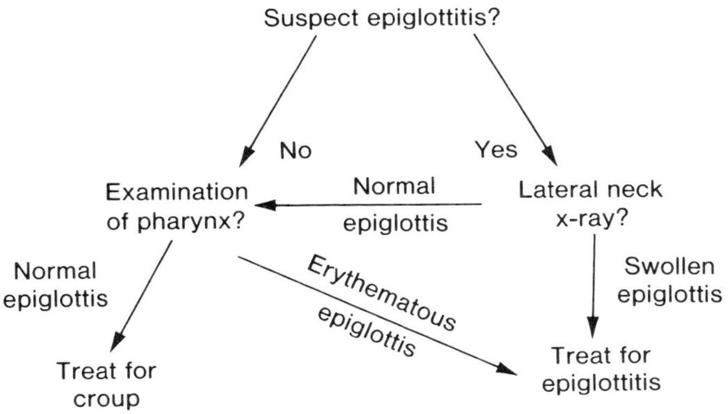

Figure 45.4 Approach to the febrile child with stridor.

intravenous access. The lateral neck x-ray either confirms or disproves the clinical diagnosis. If epiglottitis is verified radiographically, the anesthesiologist next performs endotracheal intubation in the operating suite or the otolaryngologist proceeds with a tracheostomy. On the other hand, the emergency physician can examine the pharynx if the radiograph shows a normal supraglottic area.

In most children with stridor, the history will favor croup, which is more common than epiglottitis. The child will not appear toxic or show signs of air hunger. In such situations, a lateral neck x-ray is not indicated. Rather, the pharynx can be directly visualized with a tongue depressor to confirm the absence of a swollen, inflammed epiglottis.

A review of the mortality statistics in epiglottitis emphasizes the importance of an artificial airway in the management of this illness. Rapkin described a fatal outcome in 20% of the children treated with antibiotics and observation alone. In 1978, Cantrell et al. summarized 749 cases of epiglottitis. The mortality varied with the method of airway management as follows: tracheostomy, 3 deaths among 348 children (0.86%); endotracheal intubation, 2 in 216 (0.92%); no artificial airway, 13 in 214 (6.1%).

Antibiotics play an essential part in the treatment of epiglottitis by eradicating the local infection and limiting the spread to other sites. Both ampicillin, 200 mg/kg/day, and chloramphenicol, 100 mg/kg/day, are administered in 4 divided doses. Steroids have not been shown to be useful in epiglottitis.

LOWER RESPIRATORY TRACT INFECTIONS

The most frequent lower respiratory tract infections in childhood include bronchiolitis and pneumonia. Occasional episodes of pertussis and pulmonary tuberculosis are also seen.

Pneumonia is an inflammation of the lung tissue that may follow either a noninfectious or an infectious insult. In the emergency department, the febrile child with an acute onset of pneumonia almost alway has an infection. The causative organism in pneumonia vary according to the age c the child (see Table 45.10). While vir agents account for 60 to 90% of pneumoni bacteria, particularly *S. pneumoniae*, pla a major role. *M. pneumoniae* increases i frequency after puberty. Unusual causes c pneumonia in the immunocompetent chil include *M. tuberculosis*, Rickettsia, Fung and Protozoa.

Bacterial Pneumonia

BACKGROUND

Bacterial pneumonia is an inflammatio of the pulmonary parenchyma due to bacterial pathogen. In the first weeks of lif group B *Streptococci* and gram-negativ bacilli cause the majority of such infection (see Table 45.10). Between 2 weeks and months of age, viruses and chlamydia ar most frequent, and viruses remain the com monest isolates throughout childhoo Among the bacteria, *S. pneumoniae* pre dominates at every age beyond the new born period. *H. influenzae* ranks second t

Table 45.10
Lower Respiratory Tract Infections

Age	Infecting Organism
2 wk	Bacteria
	Group B Streptococcus
	Gram negative bacilli
	Viruses
2 wk to 2 mo	Chlamydia
	Viruses
	Bacteria
	Streptococcus pneumonia
	Staphylococcus aureus
	Haemophilus influenzae
2 mo to 3 yr	Viruses
	Bacteria
	S. pneumoniae
	H. influenzae
	S. aureus
3 yr to 12 yr	Viruses
	Bacteria
	S. pneumoniae
	Mycoplasma pneumoniae
13 yr to 19 yr	*M. pneumoniae*
	Viruses
	Bacteria
	S. pneumoniae

he pneumococcus, usually occurring in the rst 3 years of life. *S. aureus* causes a severe ut infrequent pneumonia in young chil-ren; 60% of these infections occur in the rst year of life. Other less common isolates nclude the Group A *Streptococcus*, *N. eningiditis*, and anaerobic bacteria.

Definitive studies on the relative fre-uency of the various pathogens have not een performed in a randomly selected out-atient population of children. Since an rganism is not usually recovered from the lood, establishing an etiologic diagnosis equires recovery of the pathogen from ither pleural fluid or the pulmonary paren-hyma. However, pleural effusion accom-anies only a minority of bacterial pneu-ionias, and a direct aspiration of the lung, lthough quite safe, cannot be justified on hildren who are sufficiently well to be ianaged as outpatients. Thus, one must xtrapolate the data collected on hospital-zed children or those with more severe ifections to estimate the spectrum of path-gens in uncomplicated bacterial pneu-ionia.

ATHOPHYSIOLOGY

In the majority of pneumonias, the athophysiology remains unknown. Patho-ens reach the lung, either by hematoge-ous dissemination or by aspiration. In *H. ifluenzae* pneumonia, the organism can be ecovered from the bloodstream in 90% of ne children, often 1 to 2 days before the ppearance of the infiltrate. This suggests hat bacteremia precedes the pulmonary ifection. However, bacteremia is found in nly 10% of the pulmonary infections with *. pneumoniae* at the time of diagnosis. 'hus, aspiration must play a greater role in he pathogenesis of infections with this or-anism, or else the preceeding bacteremia esolves prior to the development of pneu-ionia.

Following invasion of the pulmonary tis-ue by bacteria, an acute inflammatory re-ction ensues. There is an exudation of both uid and polymorphonuclear leukocytes, ollowed by the deposition of fibrin. Several ays later, macrophages appear in the al-eoli. The accumulation of fluid in a lobe of the lung leads to the characteristic lobar consolidation seen on the chest x-ray.

CLINICAL MANIFESTATIONS

Bacterial pneumonia generally has an ab-rupt onset with fever, often accompanied by chills. A cough is a common but nonspe-cific complaint. The young child reacts to bacterial infection in the chest with leth-argy and/or a decreased appetite. Occasion-ally, pleuritic involvement produces pain with respiratory effort.

The observation of the child at rest prior to the examination often provides the key to the diagnosis of pneumonia. Tachypnea out of proportion to the fever is frequently the only sign, particularly in the first year of life. On the other hand, the child breath-ing at a normal rate seldom has a bacterial infection of the lung. A hasty effort at aus-culation that disturbs the quiet infant ob-scures this finding.

Fever is almost universally present, rang-ing from 38.5°C to 41°C. Grunting respira-tions in a young child should arouse a strong suspicion of pneumonia. Localized findings, more often seen in the child over a year of age, include inspiratory rales, de-creased breath sounds (often the only ab-normality), and less frequently dullness to percussion. Gastric dilatation may accom-pany pneumonia; occasionally, the abdom-inal findings in pulmonary infections mimic appendicitis. With upper lobe pneumonia, the pain may radiate to the neck causing meningismus; the diagnosis of pneumonia must therefore be explored in the child with nuchal rigidity and normal cerebrospinal fluid.

In the emergency department, every child suspected of pneumonia should have an x-ray of the chest. Although an occa-sional child who is dehydrated may have a clear x-ray, the radiographic evaluation confirms or denies the diagnosis of bacterial pneumonia in most cases. This is important in a clinical setting not conducive to conti-nuity of care. Additionally, the x-ray may provide information on the disease process. A lobar consolidation is assumed to be a bacterial disease needing treatment with antibiotics, while a diffuse interstitial infil-trate suggests a viral infection that can be managed with symptomatic therapy. Bilateral involvement, pleural effusion, and pneumatoceles point to more severe disease.

Further laboratory studies are obtained only on specific indications. A WBC may be helpful in differentiating viral from bacterial disease or in assessing the likelihood of bacteremia in the young child. The WBC is usually over 15,000/cu mm and not infrequently exceeds 30,000/cu mm. McCarthy et al. reported that the C-reactive protein correlated with the bacteremia and lobar infiltrates more closely than the WBC; however, this test is less readily available than the WBC.

The most common complication of pneumonia is dehydration occurring in young children. Electrolytes and a BUN are useful in assessing the degree of fluid loss. Rarely, extensive pulmonary involvement compromises ventilation leading to respiratory failure. Arterial blood gases are indicated to confirm this diagnosis. A pleural effusion accumulates in the majority of infections due to *S. aureus* and *H. influenzae* and less often with *S. pneumoniae*. Bacteremia may result in additional foci of infection including meningitis, pericarditis, epiglottitis, and septic arthritis.

MANAGEMENT

The majority of children with pneumonia respond to outpatient antibiotic therapy. Since most of the infections are due to *S. pneumoniae*, penicillin is our drug of choice. A single dose of procaine penicillin, 50,000 units/kg, is administered intramuscularly followed by oral penicillin V, 30 mg/kg/day for 10 days. Alternatively, either ampicillin or erythromycin may be used. Supportive therapy includes antipyretics and adequate hydration. Antitussives have no place in the treatment of pneumonia. Every child should return within 24 hours for a second evaluation.

Any child should be hospitalized who appears to be toxic on the basis of the physician's clinical judgment. Firmer, but not unarguable, indications for admission are listed in Table 45.11. The child under a year of age does not tolerate bacterial pneumonia as well as those who are older. Ad-

Table 45.11
Indications for Admission

I	Age < 1 year
II	Respiratory compromise
III	Pleural effusion
IV	Pneumatocele
V	Failure to respond to penicillin within 2 hours
VI	Dehydration

ditionally, potentially serious infection with *S. aureus* and *H. influenzae* occu more often in the first year of life. Th radiographic detection of a pleural effusio or pneumatocele also suggests a pathoge other than *S. pneumoniae*. Effusion should be cultured by thoracentesis whic requires subsequent observation of th child in the hospital. Although a persister elevation of the temperature is well de scribed in children with pneumococca pneumonia that subsequently respond t penicillin, failure of the fever to defervesc after the administration of procaine pen cillin suggests a greater likelihood of mor virulent pathogens.

Viral Pneumonia

BACKGROUND

Several viruses are able to infect th lungs of children and adolescents. Respira tory syncytial and parainfluenza virus ar the commonest isolates, particularly in th first year of life. Other viruses can caus pneumonia including influenza, adenovi ruses, enteroviruses, rhinoviruses, measles varicella, rubella, herpes simplex, cytomeg alovirus, and Epstein-Barr virus. Pulmo nary disease complicates upper airway in fections with influenza, varicella, and th Epstein-Barr virus more frequently in th adolescent. The annual incidence of vira pneumonia peaks in the first 5 years of lif at 40 per 1,000, and then declines wit advancing age.

PATHOPHYSIOLOGY

The majority of viruses causing pneu monia initially invade the epithelium of th upper respiratory tract and spread locall to the lungs. The infection evokes an in ammatory response that consists primar- y of mononuclear cells. Following infec- on, the epithelial cells slough into the rway, and obstruct the bronchi producing e hyperinflation characteristically seen the chest x-ray.

A few viruses may reach the lungs via ematogenous dissemination. These in- ude measles, varicella, rubella, cytomeg- ovirus, herpes simplex, and Epstein-Barr rus.

LINICAL MANIFESTATIONS

Viral pneumonia has its onset over a 2 to day period, being more gradual than with cterial infection. Cough, coryza, and a w grade fever occur frequently. Particu- rly with RSV infections in the first 3 onths of life, an apneic spell may be the st sign to draw attention to the illness.

The fever in viral pneumonia is usually ss than 39°C. As with bacterial infections, chypnea in the undisturbed child may be e only physical finding. Rales are fre- ently audible diffusely throughout the est and wheezing may also be present. ith more severe disease, the child shows gns of respiratory failure: grunting, cy- osis, and changes in mental status.

The WBC count varies widely in viral eumonia. Although leukocytosis over ,000/cu mm may occur in some cases, ch elevated counts should arouse a sus- cion of bacterial disease.

The radiographic examination provides eful clues to the type of pathogen causing pneumonia, but can never confirm a viral fection nor rule out a bacterial etiology. ost typically, the x-ray in a child with ral pneumonia shows bilateral air trap- ng and peribronchial thickening. A diffuse crease in the interstitial markings is also mmonly seen. However, the findings can ry from barely detectable increases in lume to segmental infiltrates. Decubitus ms occasionally detect small effusions. ue to the limitations in obtaining reliable ltures for bacteria, it is safest to presume bacterial etiology in the child with a lobar filtrate, a pleural effusion, a temperature er 39°C or signs of clinical toxicity. Par- ularly in a dehydrated child, the chest x- y may fail to show a lobar consolidation early in the course of a bacterial pneu- monia.

Most viral pneumonias resolve without specific therapy. Potential complications include dehydration, apnea, and local pro- gression of the infection. Apnea is frequent in the first 3 months of life.

MANAGEMENT

The physician must attempt to make an etiologic diagnosis in pneumonia on the basis of the clinical and radiographic find- ings without the benefit of pathognomonic laboratory tests. A WBC count should be obtained if there is uncertainty as to the likely etiology. In such cases, a leukocytosis over 15,000/cu mm would weigh against a viral infection.

If a viral pneumonia is strongly sus- pected, no specific therapy need be given. An example of such a situation would be a well-hydrated 5 year old child with a grad- ual onset of cough, a temperature of 38.0°C, scattered bilateral rales, WBC < 15,000/cu mm, and the finding of hyperaeration on chest x-ray. Treatment in this case would be limited to antipyresis and hydration with a follow-up visit in 24 hours. Because the infant under 3 months of age may become apneic during the course of viral pneu- monia, these young children need observa- tion in the hospital.

Mycoplasmal Pneumonia

BACKGROUND

M. pneumoniae is one of the commonest causes of pneumonia among children more than 5 years old. In younger children, infec- tions with this organism are often limited to the upper respiratory tract or, occasion- ally, the bronchial tree. By the end of ado- lescence, 90% of the population has anti- bodies to *M. pneumoniae.*

PATHOPHYSIOLOGY

The initial infection with *M. pneumoniae* occurs on the surface of the respiratory epithelium. Destruction of these cells causes them to slough into the lumen of the bronchi. The infection evokes an inflam- matory response, primarily by mononuclear leukocytes.

CLINICAL MANIFESTATIONS

Pneumonia due to *M. pneumoniae* begins insidiously with fever and malaise. After 3 to 5 days, the child develops a nonproductive cough, hoarseness, sore throat, and in one-quarter of the cases, chest pain. Fever is almost invariably present and may reach a level of 40°C. Children seldom develop much respiratory distress, with the exception of those who are less than 5 years old or also have sickle cell anemia or an immunodeficiency. Rales are heard in 75% of these infections, often bilaterally. The pharynx may appear inflamed, and some investigators have noted ear infections, particularly bullous myringitis, in association with pneumonia due to *M. pneumoniae*. In 10% of patients, a maculopapular or, less often, a vesicular rash occurs; rarely, erythema multiforme, urticaria, or petechiae are seen.

The WBC count is usually normal in infections due to this pathogen. A cold agglutinin titer ≧ 1:32 is found in the majority of patients with lobar infiltrates from an *M. pneumoniae* infection, but may also occur, though less frequently, with viral and bacterial illnesses. The organism may be recovered by culture; however, this procedure requires more than a week and is not readily available. The radiographic findings show considerable variation. Between 10 and 25% of children will have lobar consolidation. Scattered segmental infiltrates, interstitial disease, and combinations of all the above patterns may be seen. Pleural effusions occur in 5% of the cases.

Numerous complications are described in association with *M. pneumoniae* infections, but they occur infrequently. These include hemolytic anemia, arthritis, encephalitis, meningitis, and neuropathy.

MANAGEMENT

The diagnosis of Mycoplasmal pneumonia is presumptively based on the clinical and x-ray findings and the cold agglutinin titer. An older child or adolescent with the gradual onset of a mild bilateral pneumonia should be treated for this infection. On the other hand, a lobar infiltrate in a 5-year old will usually be assumed to be of bacterial etiology regardless of the level the cold agglutinins. The results of cultur and specific serologic assays entail too gre a delay to be useful to the clinician in t emergency department. Erythromycin, mg/kg/day, provides effective therapy f *M. pneumoniae* infections. The response more pronounced in the older child wi lobar disease than in the younger child wi a diffuse infiltrate.

Chlamydial Pneumonia

BACKGROUND

Two species of *Chlamydia* cause pne monia: *Chlamydia psittaci* and *Chlamyd trachomatis*. Psittacosis, a severe pne monia due to *C. psittaci*, is quite rare; ho ever, recent reports have shown that *trachomatis* is the most frequently r covered pathogen from children with af brile pneumonias between 4 and 12 wee of age.

PATHOPHYSIOLOGY

Among infants born to pregnant wom with vaginal colonization by *C. trachom tis*, one-third to one-half will acquire t organism. These infants are at risk for t subsequent development of pneumonit Arth et al. described the pathologic exam nation in a culture-proven chlamydi pneumonitis as showing a mononucle consolidation with occasional eosinoph and neutrophils and marked necro changes in the bronchioles.

CLINICAL MANIFESTATIONS

Infants with chlamydial pneumonia us ally have a stacatto cough that may reser ble the paroxysms seen in pertussis. In ha of the cases, conjunctivitis precedes t onset of respiratory symptoms. Pneumon with this organism only rarely produces fever. Mild retractions, hyperresonanc and diffuse rales are noted on examinati of the chest. Hyperaeration of the lun depresses the liver, allowing the edge to b palpated 1 to 2 mm below the right cost margin.

Although the WBC count is usually the normal range, the total number of e sinophils rises slightly (400/cu mm) in 75 these patients. Elevated immunoglobulin vels, though nonspecific, occur frequently ith chlamydial infections, but seldom with ral. Mild hypoxemia is common. The est x-ray shows hyperaeration of the ngs and a diffuse increase in the intersti- l markings. Lobar consolidations and eural diffusions are not seen.

Although usually a mild illness, chlamyd- pneumonia may be complicated by the currence of mucus plugging of the bron- i, apnea, and severe impairment of oxy- nation. It is not possible to predict which fants with an initially mild course will ve a stormy one.

ANAGEMENT

Because of the difficulty in making a finitive etiologic diagnosis and the poten- l for life-threatening complications, chil- en with presumed chlamydial pneumon- s should be admitted to the hospital. ythromycin, 40 mg/kg/day, may shorten e course and should be given. As more owledge accumulates about the course of is disease and the effect of antimicrobial erapy, it may be possible to define a oup of infants who can be treated on an tpatient basis.

Bronchiolitis

ACKGROUND

Bronchiolitis is a pulmonary infection of ung children characterized by wheezing. espiratory syncytial virus causes the ma- rity of these illnesses, but other viruses, rticularly parainfluenza, are isolated oc- sionally. Additionally, *M. pneumoniae* is so an occasional cause of bronchiolitis.

The epidemiology of bronchiolitis pri- arily follows the pattern of its principle thogen, the respiratory syncytial virus. ost of these infections occur in the winter, d the majority of the children are be- een 2 and 8 months of age. Although me authorities do not accept the diagno- s of bronchiolitis after the age of 1 year, hers believe that the disease occurs until e 2 years. Hoekelman noted 3 episodes of onchiolitis in his pediatric practice nong 246 infants being cared for during eir first year of life.

PATHOPHYSIOLOGY

Respiratory syncytial virus, the most frequent cause of bronchiolitis, invades the epithelial cells of the nasopharynx and spreads to the mucosa of the lower respiratory tract by cell-to-cell transfer. The infection causes death of the cells lining the bronchi which then slough into the lumen. The production of mucus increases, and mononuclear cells infiltrate the area. Clumps of necrotic epithelium and mucus initially decrease the diameter of the bronchi causing turbulent air flow, particularly on expiration when the luminal diameter normally decreases. Eventually, plugging of the bronchi produces hyperinflation and atelectasis.

CLINICAL MANIFESTATIONS

Bronchiolitis begins as an upper respiratory illness with cough and coryza. Over a period of 2 to 5 days, signs of respiratory distress appear. The parents will often be able to hear the child wheezing.

Fever occurs in two-thirds of children with bronchiolitis. They often appear ill on overall assessment. The respiratory rate climbs to at least 40/min, and may reach 80 to 100/min. Nasal flaring and retractions of the intercostal and supraclavicular muscles are noted and increase as the disease progresses. In bronchiolitis and other lower respiratory tract infections, the intercostal retractions are more pronounced than the supraclavicular, the opposite of the findings in croup and epiglottitis. Wheezes and a prolonged expiratory phase are heard in all children with bronchiolitis, often without a stethoscope; rales are minimal. As the ventilatory muscles fatigue, the child will have grunting respirations; only in the most severe cases does cyanosis occur.

The WBC count in bronchiolitis is normal. Usually the chest x-ray shows only a hyperaerated chest, but there may occasionally be areas of atelectasis. If respiratory failure supervenes, the PaO_2 decreases and carbon dioxide is retained.

The complications of bronchiolitis include dehydration, respiratory failure, and bacterial superinfection. Pneumothorax and pneumomediastinum are rarely seen.

The increased respiratory effort in bronchiolitis not uncommonly prevents an infant from maintaining an adequate oral intake. Careful attention should be paid to the details of fluid balance when taking a history. Ten percent to 20% of infants with bronchiolitis develop significant respiratory compromise. Cyanosis, decreased inspiratory breath sounds, and lethargy on examination point to ventilatory failure. Bacterial superinfection is uncommon in the early stages of the illness, occurring more commonly in hospitalized infants. However, pulmonary consolidation seen on the chest x-ray suggests a potential bacterial pneumonia.

MANAGEMENT

Every child in the emergency department suspected of having bronchiolitis should have a chest x-ray taken, both to look for findings compatible with this diagnosis and to help exclude other entities such as pneumonia or a foreign body. A WBC count, arterial blood gas, electrolytes, and BUN are obtained only if the diagnosis is uncertain or the clinical picture suggests that complications have occurred.

Although not often successful, an injection of epinephrine 0.01 ml/kg (1:1000) may at times diminish the wheezing and improve the aeration in the child with moderate to severe disease. When this maneuver meets with success, further therapy with susphrine, 0.005 ml/kg, and theophylline, 24 mg/kg/day, is indicated. Presumably, these children have either underlying asthma or bronchiolitis with a significant amount of bronchospasm.

If the child does not respond to epinephrine or has only mild distress, bronchodilators should not be given. Therapy is limited to antipyretics and the encouragement of adequate oral intake, and the infant should be examined again after 24 hours. Dehydration, secondary bacterial infection, and marked respiratory distress necessitate admission to the hospital. Although not validated in infants with bronchiolitis, a score of 4 or more on the asthma scale (Chapter 49) suggests significant respiratory compromise. An arterial PaO_2 below 70 tor in room air also suggests a need for hospitalization.

Pertussis

BACKGROUND

Pertussis, or whooping cough, is an infe tion of the respiratory tract caused by *Bo detella pertussis*. Occasionally, a simil clinical syndrome is caused by *Bordetel parapertussis*, the adenoviruses, or chl mydia. Young children most frequent contract pertussis, but the incidence in a olescents has increased recently. Althoug vaccination has contributed to the mark decrease in the frequency of this diseas several thousand cases occur yearly in th United States.

PATHOPHYSIOLOGY

Following inhalation, *B. pertussis* org nisms attach to the epithelial cells of th respiratory tract. Multiplication of the ba teria leads to infiltration of the mucosa wi polymorphonuclear leukocytes and lym phocytes. Inflammatory debris in the l men of the bronchi and peribronchial lym phoid hyperplasia obstruct the smaller ai ways, causing atelectasis.

CLINICAL MANIFESTATIONS

Although pertussis can be divided in three stages for discussion, a clinically di tinct syndrome does not evolve until th disease has progressed to the second stag Initially, the symptoms mimic a viral upp respiratory infection. This first stage (c tarrhal), characterized by a mild coug conjunctivitis, and coryza lasts for 1 to weeks. An increasingly severe cough he alds the onset of the second stage (paro ysmal) which continues for 2 to 4 week Following a prolonged spasm of coughin the sudden inflow of air produces the cha acteristic whoops. Vomiting often occu after such an episode. When not coughin the child has a remarkably normal physic examination, except for an occasional su conjunctival hemorrhage. During the thi stage (convalescent), the intensity of th cough wanes.

The WBC count in children usual reaches a level of 20,000 to 50,000/cu m with a marked lymphocytosis, but su changes are not often seen in infants le than 6 months of age. While a chest x-r occasionally shows the characterist haggy right heart border, more often the ıng fields appear clear. *B. pertussis* can be lentified by fluorescent antibody staining f mucus obtained from the nasopharynx r, less frequently, recovered by culture of ıis material.

Complications frequently occur during a out of pertussis. Most immediately life ıreatening is complete obstruction of the irway by a mucus plug leading to respira- ›ry arrest. While secondary bacterial neumonia has a more insidious onset, it ccounts for 90% of the fatalities from per- ıssis. Encephalitis may manifest with sei- ıres or coma; sudden increases in intratho- ıcic pressure can cause intracranial hem- rrhages, rupture of the diaphragm, and ectal prolapse.

ANAGEMENT

Except for occasional situations in which ıorescent antibody testing is immediately ailable, the diagnosis of pertussis rests on inical grounds. Children with an unmis- kable paroxysmal cough followed by a hoop should be assumed to have the dis- ıse. When the clinical picture is cloudy, a BC count and chest x-ray should be ob- ıined. The x-ray helps to eliminate other ıuses of a severe cough (foreign body, acterial pneumonia, cystic fibrosis, tuber- ılosis), and the WBC count provides con- rmatory evidence if a marked lymphocy- ›sis is found. Because of the grave risk of ›mplications, all children under 1 year of ge diagnosed as pertussis should be ob- rved in the hospital. Older children who ıow signs of respiratory compromise, such s cyanosis during paroxysms of coughing, r develop complications also require ad- ıission. Treatment includes erythromycin,)/mg/kg/day, maintenance of adequate ydration, and a level of respiratory sup- ort appropriate to the severity of the dis- ase.

Tuberculosis

ACKGROUND

In the United States, tuberculosis is aused almost exclusively by *M. tubercu- ›sis* and occurs in childhood in several inical forms. Although currently an un- sual infection, it should be kept in mind as an occasional, treatable cause of morbidity and mortality.

PATHOPHYSIOLOGY

Tubercle bacilli enter the body via the respiratory tract, producing an initial focus in the lungs. This lesion usually remains subclinical but may progress locally, resulting in a primary tuberculous pneumonia. During the primary infection, the organisms can disseminate hematogenously. Such spread may remain quiescent or, in a young child, lead to miliary tuberculosis. Seeding of various organs occurs and may produce focal infections, a particularly serious concern with meningeal involvement.

Usually, the immune system limits the initial infection. However, reactivation of these foci may cause disease years later at any site involved during dissemination. Pulmonary lesions reactivate to produce tuberculous pneumonia in adults and adolescents much more often than children.

CLINICAL MANIFESTATIONS

Most infections by *M. tuberculosis* in children never cause any significant symptoms. Among the myriad of possible clinical presentations, three stand out as particular concerns to the emergency physician: primary pneumonia, miliary tuberculosis, and meningitis.

The onset of primary tuberculosis pneumonia resembles that of bacterial infections of the lungs. It begins with fever and tachypnea; rales and an area of dullness are found on examination of the chest. The WBC may be elevated with a shift to the left, and the chest x-ray shows a lobar consolidation, accompanied frequently by hilar adenopathy and less often by pleural effusion or cavitation. Although the primary pneumonia often resolves spontaneously, the child occasionally follows a downhill course due to local progression. Clinical findings that should arouse a suspicion of tuberculous pneumonia in the child otherwise thought to have a bacterial infection of the lung include: (1) pleural effusion; (2) cavitation; (3) toxicity; and (4) a failure to respond to antibiotic therapy.

Miliary tuberculosis begins with an abrupt rise in temperature but a paucity of other physical findings. Subsequently, respiratory symptoms and enlargement of the liver, spleen, and superficial lymph nodes occur. The WBC is usually in the range of 15,000/cu mm. Although the chest x-ray initially shows no lesions, a diffuse mottling appears 1 to 3 weeks after the fever. Miliary tuberculosis is a consideration in a child with a persistent fever and hepatosplenomegaly.

Tuberculous meningitis comes on insidiously with a low-grade fever, apathy, and, in 50% of patients, vomiting. After 1 to 2 weeks of nonspecific illness, neurologic signs appear, including drowsiness and nuchal rigidity; untreated, the child lapses into coma. The CSF shows a mononuclear pleocytosis and an elevated protein concentration.

MANAGEMENT

A child suspected of having pneumonic, meningeal, or miliary tuberculosis should be admitted to the hospital for evaluation and possible chemotherapy. Among inner city populations where the risk of tuberculosis is greatest, the routine placement of a tine or Mantoux test in children with lobar pneumonia should be considered.

GASTROINTESTINAL INFECTIONS

Gastroenteritis is an inflammation of the alimentary tract that, in its acute form, is overwhelmingly infectious in origin. Viruses are the organisms most commonly found in children with diarrhea in the United States and can be isolated from 30 to 40% of children with acute gastroenteritis. In 10 to 25%, bacteria are recovered including salmonellae, *Shigella*, *Campylobacter*, *Yersinia*, and pathogenic *E. coli*. Occasionally *Vibrio* species and parasitic infestations cause diarrheal diseases, but current diagnostic techniques are unable to identify an etiologic agent in most of the remaining episodes.

Viral hepatitis is covered in Chapter 50 under *Gastrointestinal Emergencies*. Bacterial infections of the liver, almost exclusively abscesses, are quite rare in otherwise healthy children; more commonly, they complicate an immunosuppressive disease, or therapy, or affect the neonate.

Because calculi in the bile ducts rarel occur during childhood, cholecystitis occu much less frequently than in the adul Occasionally episodes are seen in adole cents or children predisposed to stone fo mation as in the chronic hemolytic an mias. Less commonly, salmonellosis or le tospirosis produces acalculous cholecystiti

In childhood, peritonitis almost invar ably reflects an intraabdominal catastroph requiring surgical intervention. Howeve the accumulation of ascitic fluid in a chil with disease such as nephrosis and cirrhos allows for the development of a primar infection of the peritoneum.

Viral Gastroenteritis

BACKGROUND

Viral gastroenteritis occurs primarily i two forms caused by different pathogen The Norwalk virus produces an illnes characterized by an explosive onset an vomiting, more severe than diarrhea; th symptoms are self-limited, resolving in 2 c 3 days. It occurs in epidemics most often i the winter and affects predominantl school-age children.

Rotavirus, on the other hand, produce a severe, prolonged diarrheal illness. It oc curs more frequently in young children a though family members may be affecte Other viruses may play a role in gastroer teritis. These include enteroviruses, coror aviruses, and adenoviruses.

Viral gastroenteritis is a common illnes Among United States families, it trails onl the common cold in frequency. Rotaviru are the most frequently isolated pathogen particularly among children who develo dehydration. While most episodes term nate spontaneously, viral infections of th gastrointestinal tract cause considerabl loss of time from school and occasionall require treatment in the hospital.

PATHOPHYSIOLOGY

Rotaviruses invade the intestinal epithe lial cells where they can be visualized b electron microscopy. The histology of th mucosal layer is disturbed during the activ infection and for 3 to 8 weeks afterwarc Functional abnormalities accompany th morphologic changes including depressions of disaccharidase levels. Although Norwalk virus may invade the mucosal lining of the intestine, it has not been detected intracellularly. Histologic changes occur and persist for 2 weeks, and disaccharidase levels decline during the infection.

CLINICAL MANIFESTATIONS

Children with viral gastroenteritis are usually brought to the emergency department with a complaint of diarrhea and/or vomiting. The numbers of stools may vary from 2 or 3 to 15 or 20 daily. Most commonly there are 6 to 8 bowel movements per 24 hour period; the stools range from semisolid in consistency to watery. While hematochezia may occasionally occur in viral infections, the presence of blood in the stool should suggest a bacterial gastroenteritis. Vomiting may either accompany diarrhea or be the sole manifestation of a viral gastroenteritis. The daily frequency of emesis varies in the same range as for diarrhea. After forceful emesis, streaks of blood may be present in the vomitus. Most children with viral gastroenteritis beyond the age of 2 or 3 years complain of crampy abdominal pain. In more severe illnesses, the parent may relate a history of decreased oral intake and oliguria.

Children with viral gastroenteritis are usually febrile. However, in the child more than 3 years of age, a temperature over 39°C suggests a bacterial enteritis. Tachycardia and hypotension reflect dehydration in severe episodes. While the respiratory rate is usually normal, tachypnea occurs when acidosis is present. The abdomen is soft and nondistended. While the child may perceive palpation as being uncomfortable, this maneuver does not elicit localized or rebound tenderness. Auscultation reveals hyperactive bowel sounds. The skin turgor is decreased and the mucous membranes dry only in severe gastroenteritis with dehydration (see Chapter 14).

No laboratory studies are indicated in the uncomplicated case of gastroenteritis. The CBC, electrolytes, and BUN are all within the normal range. If oral intake fails to keep pace with the efflux of fluids from the alimentary tract, dehydration occurs. The sodium, usually normal, may drop to 110 meq/liter to rise to 170 meq/liter, and the bicarbonate is invariably low. With mild dehydration, the serum bicarbonate hovers just below the normal level at 18 to 20 meq/liter; however, values of 10 to 12 meq/liter are usually found in the face of prolonged diarrhea. The BUN reflects both the state of hydration and the adequacy at the recent intake of protein. It may climb as high as 100 mg/dl in children who lose over 10% of their body weight. However, in a child who has been maintained on clear liquids, the BUN will not accurately indicate the degree of dehydration since urea arises as a breakdown product during protein metabolism. Although the hemoglobin and WBC count are usually normal in the child with viral gastroenteritis, hemoconcentration may occur with dehydration.

MANAGEMENT

Uncomplicated viral gastroenteritis usually remits in 2 to 5 days and does not require treatment in the hospital. All children should be carefully weighed in the emergency department prior to discharge to provide a baseline for follow-up. Both the vomiting and diarrhea will generally respond to a brief cessation of oral intake. After 4 hours of abstinence, the diet should be resumed gradually and restricted to clear liquids. While juices will suffice for 1 to 2 days in the child over 6 months of age, commercially prepared solutions of known composition (Pedialyte, Lytren) provide more reliable hydration in the young child or for longer periods of time. Preparation of salt-containing fluids at home by the family notoriously leads to errors, and this procedure is to be condemned. Similarly, the physician should avoid the use of boiled skim milk, a hypertonic solution which may produce hypernatremia.

Antiemetics and antidiarrheal medications provide minimal, if any, relief to the child. Additionally, many of these medications carry significant risks. Kaopectate has been shown to increase stool losses of water and electrolytes. Although the combination of diphenoxlate and atropine (Lomotil) may be successful in adults, toxic reactions in children limit its usefulness. Trimethobenzomide (Tigan) is ineffective as an antemetic in children, and the phenothiazine compounds frequently produce adverse side effects, such as extrapyramidal reactions or oculogyric crises.

Dehydration is the only significant complication of viral gastroenteritis. Whenever the physician suspects that a child has lost more than 2 to 3% of body weight, electrolytes and a BUN should be obtained. These tests will establish the degree of acidosis and the presence of hyponatremia or hypernatremia.

The child with dehydration can be managed on an outpatient basis with oral fluids if the decrease in body weight is less than 5%, the sodium is normal, and the BUN less than 25 mg/dl. Additionally, the child must demonstrate the ability to take fluids orally before leaving the Emergency Department. A bolus of intravenous fluids, such as 10 ml/kg of normal saline, may be administered when the degree of dehydration is judged to be 5% but the gastroenteritis is waning.

Children who are more than 5% dehydrated or have alterations in the serum sodium (less than 130 meq/liter or more than 145 meq/liter) require hospitalization. Intravenous therapy should be started in the emergency department, particularly if there is evidence of vascular instability (see Chapter 14).

Bacterial Gastroenteritis

BACKGROUND

Five pathogens commonly produce gastroenteritis: *Salmonella*, *Shigella*, *Yersinia*, *Campylobacter*, and pathogenic *E. coli*. Together these organisms cause 10 to 25% of the diarrheal illnesses seen in children coming to the emergency department. In underdeveloped countries and occasionally in the United States, *Vibrio* species must also be considered.

Salmonella, *Shigella*, and *Yersinia*, gram-negative bacilli in the Enterobacteriaceae family, do not normally inhabit the alimentary tract. Thus, recovery of one of these organisms suffices for the diagnosis of the etiology of gastroenteritis. *E. coli*, however, is part of the normal bowel flora, only occasionally assuming a pathogenic role. Unfortunately, identification of disease-producing strains is not readily available to the clinician. *Campylobacter* are mobile comma-shaped gram-negative rods in the *Vibrio* species. They are not considered normal bowel flora.

PATHOPHYSIOLOGY

Salmonellae gain access to the small intestine following ingestion. Gastric acid is usually lethal to the organism, but large numbers of bacteria may overcome this defense mechanism. Studies have shown that 10^5 virulent organisms will induce disease in 30% of healthy adults and 10^9 in 95%. Patients with gastrectomies are more susceptible to *Salmonella* infection than those with an intact stomach. Salmonellae can penetrate the epithelial layer to the level of the lamina propria and evoke a leukocyte response. Generally the infection extends no further, but bacteremia may occur, especially in young children. Several species, notably *S. choleraesuis* and *S. typhi* readily enter the circulation via the lymphatics. Salmonellae produce diarrhea by multiple mechanisms. Several toxins have been identified; additionally, prostaglandins may be released which stimulate the active secretion of fluids and electrolytes.

Certain shigellae attach to binding sites on the surface of the intestinal mucosal cells. The organisms penetrate the cells and proliferate within them. Intraepithelial multiplication destroys the cell and produces mucosal ulcerations. Invasion of the epithelium evokes an intense inflammatory response. At the base of the ulcerated lesions, erosion of blood vessels may lead to bleeding. Other shigellae elaborate exotoxins that can produce diarrhea. These toxins result in increased secretion of fluid and electrolytes by the intestinal mucosa.

Although the pathophysiology of infection due to *Y. enterocolitica* has not been completely elucidated, clues are available from animal models and occasional pathologic specimens. The organisms are thought to produce terminal ileitis; inflammatory changes and ulcerations have been visualized at endoscopy. The infection elicits a neutrophilic response, particularly around the Peyer's patches. It then extends to the mesenteric lymph nodes which are destroyed by microabscess formation and may enlarge considerably. Occasionally, further dissemination occurs with involvement of the liver and spleen. Although an enterotoxin has been identified in cultures of *Y. enterocolitica* maintained at 26° to 30°, production *in vivo* has not been established.

The pathogenesis of *Campylobacter* enteritis remains unknown. Attempts to demonstrate toxin production have not met with success, and the organism has been shown to lack invasive properties. At autopsy, extensive hemorrhagic ulcerations of the bowel have been described.

CLINICAL MANIFESTATIONS

Signs and Symptoms

A careful epidemiologic history often provides a clue to the diagnosis of *Salmonella* infections. Foodborne outbreaks occur frequently in the summer. After an incubation period of 8 to 48 hours, the child experiences crampy abdominal pain and nausea. The stools are watery and may contain blood, but this is not the rule. Fever is noted in the majority of children. Unless protracted diarrhea has led to clinically apparent dehydration, the physical examination is unremarkable. Abdominal tenderness or distension are unusual findings. The leukocyte count is usually 10,000 to 15,000/cu mm. Methylene blue staining of the stool shows the presence of polymorphonuclear leukocytes, but not in sheets as seen with *Shigella*. A single rectal swab leads to isolation of salmonellae from over 90% of children with this infection.

Shigellae may cause an asymptomatic infection, mild gastroenteritis, or bacillary dysentery. Mild illnesses are more common. Children so affected will complain of frequent watery stools but few constitutional symptoms. The temperature remains normal in most cases, and the physical examination is unremarkable.

Bacillary dysentery begins suddenly with fever and abdominal pain. Diarrhea commences shortly thereafter. The stools, which number 10 to 12 daily, contain mucus and blood, and tenesmus is common. Children with this form of shigellosis have a fever, often in the range of 39° to 40°C. Palpation of the abdomen frequently elicits diffuse tenderness but no evidence of peritoneal irritation.

An occasional *Shigella* infection may produce irritation of the CNS because of the release of toxin prior to the onset of diarrhea. Thus, shigellosis must be considered in the differential diagnosis of meningismus in the absence of a pleocytosis in the CSF. A seizure may actually be the first manifestation of the illness.

While there are no pathognomonic laboratory findings in shigellosis, two abnormalities strongly suggest this organism as the cause of gastroenteritis. The leukocyte count often shows many band forms which exceed the mature neutrophils in number. Poh described this phenomenon in 85% of 123 children with shigellosis between the ages of 2 months and 8 years. The total WBC may show a leukopenia or a leukocytosis, but most commonly hovers in the normal range. Because shigellae invade the intestinal mucosa, they elicit a profound inflammatory response. This exudation of white cells leads to the finding of sheets of neutrophils in the stool after methylene blue staining. A single rectal swab suffices for the isolation of shigellae from the majority of children with this illness.

Children with gastroenteritis due to *Y. enterocolitica* usually have an abrupt onset of diarrhea. The stools are frequently watery and may contain blood, but vomiting generally remains inconsequential. Patients with this illness often complain of severe abdominal pain, sometimes prior to the onset of diarrhea. Delorme et al. noted this symptom in 6 of the 35 children, half of whom were 1 to 5 years of age. In an epidemic in a school in New York State, 37 of 38 patients had abdominal pain. The potential severity of the abdominal pain in this disease is illustrated by the fact that 16 patients in this outbreak mistakenly underwent an appendectomy.

Gastrointestinal infection with *Y. enterocolitica* usually elicits a febrile response. The mean temperature in the young adolescents reported by Black et al. was 38.7°C with a range of 37.2°C to 40.0°C; it exceeded

37.8°C in over 95% of the patients. Younger children appear to develop a fever less frequently. The abdominal examination is usually benign, but palpation produces marked tenderness in the subset of patients with mesenteric adenitis. Arthritis and skin rashes occur in 5 to 10% of patients with this disease.

The mean WBC in children with yersiniosis is usually normal, although leukocytosis with a shift to the left occurs occasionally. The electrolytes and BUN are normal. Examination of stool stained with methylene blue reveals polymorphonuclear neutrophils. The organism can be recovered from stool culture but requires enrichment techniques. Although a single specimen is diagnostic in 70 to 80% of illnesses, a second sample should be obtained in the face of a previous negative culture when the clinical suspicion of disease remains strong.

Campylobacter enteritis is characterized by the abrupt onset of fever and abdominal pain, followed shortly by diarrhea. The temperature frequently remains normal in children less than 3 months of age, but ranges up to 40°C in the older child. Vomiting occurs uncommonly and rapidly resolves. Two-thirds of children complain of abdominal pain which may be severe. The number of stools varies from 2 to 20 daily; they are watery and contain blood in at least 50% of the cases. Karmali and Fleming found frank blood in the stools of 95% of their patients. The physical examination is generally unremarkable. Although the abdominal pain occasionally simulates appendicitis, palpation of the abdomen elicits minimal tenderness. Signs of dehydration are found only rarely.

The WBC in *Campylobacter* enteritis usually remains less than 12,000/cu mm, the highest being 22,500/cu mm in one study; on occasion, there may be a shift to the left. The electrolytes and BUN are usually normal. Maki et al. found fecal leukocytes in 4 of 5 patients with enteritis due to *Campylobacter*. The organism is not frequently isolated from the blood but can be easily recovered from the stool using appropriate media. When available, phase contrast microscopy can demonstrate the organism in fresh stool specimens.

In general, features of the history and physical examination suggestive of a bacterial rather than a viral gastroenteritis include: (1) diarrhea of greater than 4 days duration; (2) blood in the stool; (3) fever ≧ 39.5°C; and (4) toxicity. While a viral gastroenteritis may produce all of the above findings, their presence enhances the likelihood that a bacterial pathogen is involved.

Complications

The complications of *Salmonella* gastroenteritis include dehydration and spread of the infection beyond the confines of the gastrointestinal tract. During a bacteremia focal infections may develop including meningitis, osteomyelitis, endocarditis, and pneumonia. However, most episodes of bacteremia terminate spontaneously. Dehydration is diagnosed on the basis of the clinical findings: dry mucous membranes decreased skin turgor, tachycardia, and hypotension. The BUN will climb to levels above 20 mg/dl depending on the amount of fluid loss and the protein intake during the illness. While the electrolytes are most often normal, both hyponatremia and hypernatremia may occur.

Bacteremia is most common in young children. In a study by Hyams et al., 25% of hospitalized patients with *Salmonella* gastroenteritis had the organism recovered from their blood. Although a high fever usually accompanies spread to the circulation, the physical examination is often devoid of any signs of serious illness. The WBC is greater than 15,000/cu mm in most cases, and culture of the blood leads to recovery of the organism.

Enteric fever also occurs from the dissemination of certain serotypes of *Salmonella*. The disease is characterized by chills and fever, often rising in a steplike pattern to 40°C. Diarrhea does not necessarily precede or coexist with the systemic illness. A relative bradycardia in relation to the height of the temperature is a hallmark of enteric fever. Splenomegaly and a macular rash, or rose spots, are detectable in 20 to 30% of patients. Leukopenia characterizes the hematologic picture. Both blood and stool cultures may be negative. The diagosis may rest on a fourfold rise in the gglutinin titers.

Invasion of the bloodstream may lead to arious focal disease. Meningitis most commonly affects the youngest children. The eatures are identical to those observed in CNS infections with other purulent organisms (see page 363). Bone and joint involvement has a peculiar predilection for children with sickle cell hemoglobinopathies. Endocarditis and pneumonia are less requently seen.

The complications of shigellosis include lehydration, bacteremia, seizures, and colonic perforation. Dehydration frequently ccompanies dysenteric infections and is liagnosed on the basis of the usual clinical indings. Bacteremia and perforation are oth rare, occurring in less than 1% of gasrointestinal infections.

Most episodes of gastroenteritis with *Yersinia* are self-limited, resolving before lehydration develops. Appendicitis occasionally results from obstruction of the appendiceal lumen by swollen lymphoid tissue. The incidence is unknown, but 5 of 38 patients in the New York State epidemic underwent removal of appendices that were suppurative. Bacteremia and focal infection ollow gastroenteritis almost exclusively in he compromised host, particularly in association with thalassemia.

Campylobacter infections occasionally ead to dehydration, but less frequently han is seen with the other bacterial pathogens in the gastrointestinal tract. Rarely, bacteremic or focal infections occur.

MANAGEMENT

Salmonella gastroenteritis is usually a self-limited illness. In the majority of cases, he disease is not sufficiently distinct or severe to suggest to the clinician the need or a diagnostic evaluation. However, life-threatening complications occur with predictable regularity in certain susceptible hosts: infants under 6 months of age and children with sickle cell hemoglobinopathies.

The treatment of *Salmonella* gastroenteritis should be directed towards the maintenance of adequate hydration. As with viral infections, limitation of the diet to clear liquids suffices in most children. Antibiotic therapy neither ameliorates the course of the gastroenteritis nor eradicates the organism from the intestinal tract. In fact, several studies have suggested prolonged carriage following the administration of antibiotics. The indications for admission of a child with diarrhea suspected or proven to be due to salmonellae are: (1) dehydration; (2) focal infection; (3) age less than 6 months; and (4) sickle cell anemia. If bacteremia is suspected, intravenous therapy with both ampicillin, 200 mg/kg/day, and chloramphenicol, 100 mg/kg/day, is given immediately. Up to 20% of salmonellae show resistance to ampicillin, depending on the geographic area.

Shigellosis stands alone as the only form of bacterial gastroenteritis for which antibiotics have been proven efficacious. Antimicrobial therapy shortens both the course of the illness and the duration of excretion of the organisms in the stool. Treatment alleviates the symptoms and signs of the gastroenteritis and limits transmission of the disease. Ampicillin, 200 mg/kg/day, and trimethoprim-sulamethoxazole (10 mg trimethoprim and 50 mg sulfamethoxazole kg/day) are useful for sensitive organisms. The increasing resistance of shigellae to ampicillin dictates the choice of TMP-SMX as the initial agent prior to isolation of the organism and identification of the sensitivity pattern.

Supportive therapy is an important aspect of the management of shigellosis. The initial oral intake should be limited to solutions with physiologic concentrations of glucose and electrolytes. As the diarrhea begins to abate, solid foods can be added. Dietary manipulation will lead to resolution of the disease in some children prior to the isolation of the organism. Antibiotic therapy may be omitted in such cases, unless there is a particular concern about spread in a closed population.

As with other varieties of infectious gastroenteritis, medications designed to provide symptomatic relief from diarrhea have no demonstrated efficacy. In particular, paregoric or combinations of diphenoxylate and atropine (Lomotil) are contraindicated. Dupont et al. showed that diarrhea persisted longer in infected volunteers treated with antibiotics and diphenoxylate/atropine than those receiving only antibiotics.

Most episodes of shigellosis can be handled on an outpatient basis. Indications for admission include: (1) age ≦ 6 months; (2) dehydration; and (3) bacteremia (rare). Prior to the definitive diagnosis of shigellosis, particularly with significant bleeding, hospitalization may be required because of a concern about noninfectious entities such as a Meckel's diverticulum.

The majority of children with yersiniosis can be treated as outpatients. Initially the diet should be limited to clear liquids. Although *Y. enterocolitica* is usually sensitive *in vitro* to tetracycline, chloramphenicol, colistin, gentamicin, and kanamycin, current studies have demonstrated no benefit from antibiotic therapy of uncomplicated gastroenteritis. Persistent diarrhea may, however, respond to antimicrobial treatment. Suspected or proven sepsis merits intravenous administration of antibiotics such as gentamicin. The indications for admission include: (1) dehydration; (2) severe abdominal pain suggesting appendicitis; and (3) underlying diseases such as thalassemia.

Campylobacter enteritis is a self-limited but prolonged illness; diarrhea persists for more than a week in one-third of children. These organisms exhibit almost universal sensitivity to erythromycin which can be given orally at a dosage of 40 mg/kg/day. However, antimicrobial therapy has not been proven to decrease the duration of diarrhea.

SKIN, SOFT TISSUE, AND BONE INFECTIONS

Infections of the skin, soft tissues, and bones include the following: impetigo, cutaneous abscesses, lymphadenitis, cellulitis, pyomyositis, septic arthritis, and osteomyelitis. Chapter 58 on minor surgical problems deals with cutaneous abscesses. Among the others, impetigo and cellulitis are both common complaints in the emergency department. While children with bone and joint infections are seen only occasionally, the differential diagnosis of several common complaints (fever, limp) often includes these conditions. Thus, the emergency physician dealing with children should be familiar with such infections, particularly since a delay in the institution of therapy can result in appreciable morbidity. Pyomyositis is rare in the United States, occurring more commonly in tropical regions.

Impetigo

BACKGROUND

Impetigo is a bacterial infection of the skin confined to the epidermis. A deeper variety of impetigo, ecthyma, involves the dermis as well. Bullous impetigo, a different disease, is characterized by pustules greater than 1 cm in diameter. Impetigo is a frequent infection in children, particularly during the summer months. It occurs in epidemics during the warm weather in confined populations of children.

Any strain of the Group A *Streptococcus* can infect the skin, including nephritogenic varieties. In bullous impetigo, *S. aureus* invades the integument; bacterial toxins produced by this organism lead to the accumulation of purulent material and the evolution of bullae.

PATHOPHYSIOLOGY

The intact epidermis forms a relatively impervious barrier to bacteria. However, a breach in the integument, even if too small to be noticed by the patient, allows for the entry of pathogens and the development of impetigo. In streptococcal infections, toxins, such as streptolysins, elaborated by the organism promote local spread of the process.

CLINICAL MANIFESTATIONS

Impetigo is more common in young children, particularly under the age of 6 years. Typically, a parent will bring a child to the emergency department complaining of sores of the body. There are no associated systemic ailments such as fever or malaise. Physical examination shows a healthy child with a normal temperature. The lesions usually ooze serous fluid, but may be crusted as well. Surrounding erythema is minimal, and the regional lymph nodes often do not enlarge noticeably.

Laboratory studies are not routinely obtained in children with impetigo. The

Group A *Streptococcus* can be recovered from the lesions in about 80% of the cases if there is any doubt as to the diagnosis. The WBC count is normal.

The complications of impetigo include spread of the infection locally and remote nonsuppurative disease. Occasionally, impetigo may progress to cellulitis. If the lesions are caused by nephritogenic streptococci, glomerulonephritis may develop. The attack rate for glomerulonephritis has been as high as 1% in certain epidemics; however, the incidence is far less in the usual clinical setting.

MANAGEMENT

Outpatient antibiotic therapy cures impetigo in 95% of children. Penicillin is the drug of choice and can be administered either orally or intramuscularly. Intramuscular benzathine penicillin, 50,000 units/kg, provides a highly effective single dose treatment. Alternatively, penicillin V can be given orally at a dose of 30 mg/kg/day for 10 days. Erythromycin is the drug of choice for the child allergic to penicillin. Local therapy is not helpful.

S. aureus, an organism resistant to penicillin, causes bullous impetigo. For this disease, antistaphylococcal penicillins are recommended. Dicloxacillin can be given at a dose of 50 mg/kg/day for 10 days or erythromycin at 40 mg/kg/day.

Lymphadenitis

Lymph nodes in any region of the body may become infected. Regardless of the site of involvement, the same considerations apply as discussed under cervical lymphadenitis (see page 373). *S. aureus* and the Group A *Streptococcus* are the most frequent pathogens. The finding of inguinal or axillary adenitis should prompt a meticulous search for a portal of entry for bacteria on the extremities. Locating an impetiginous lesion or other breech in the integument provides reassurance that the lymph node enlargement is due to infection rather than neoplasm. Particularly in the adolescent, inguinal adenitis suggests a need to look for sexually transmitted pathogens (see page 400). The child with lymphadenitis should be treated with antibiotic therapy and drainage if fluctuation occurs. Dicloxacillin, 50 mg/kg/day, or cephalexin, 50 mg/kg/day, are both effective against the usual pathogens.

Cellulitis

BACKGROUND

Cellulitis is an infection of the skin and subcutaneous tissues. Any anatomic area may be involved, but the body can be divided, for etiologic considerations, into two regions: (1) the face; and (2) the scalp, neck, trunk, and extremities.

Facial cellulitis includes buccal, periorbital, and less frequently orbital lesions. *H. influenzae* causes 50% of these infections; the remainder are due to *S. aureus*, Group A *Streptococcus*, *S. pneumoniae*, and rarely other organisms. Bacteremia is present in 90% of the cases of *H. influenzae* disease.

On the other hand, *S. aureus* causes the majority of nonfacial cellulitis. Fleisher and colleagues recovered this organism from 70% of extremity lesions with an identifiable etiology, either as the sole pathogen or in combination with Group A *Streptococcus*. Only 2 to 5% of nonfacial cellulitis results from infection with *H. influenzae* and, as with facial lesions, the organism usually invades the bloodstream.

Cellulitis is a frequent infection that is more common in temperate climates when the weather is warm. Precise statistics on the incidence of cellulitis are not available; however, during the summer months this infection accounts for approximately 1 of every 500 visits to the emergency department of the Children's Hospital of Philadelphia.

PATHOGENESIS

Cellulitis follows either hematogenous dissemination of a pathogenic organism or local invasion. Surgical or traumatic wounds may serve as a portal of entry for bacteria. This is the route by which *S. aureus* and Group A *Streptococcus* usually gain access to the subcutaneous tissue. Toxins produced by the organisms allow for local spread. Alternatively, invasion of the bloodstream may precede the appearance of cellulitis. The lesions seen with *H. influ-*

enzae follow a bacteremia, and the organism is recovered from the blood in 90% of children. *S. aureus* and Group A *Streptococcus* are less frequently spread by this mechanism.

CLINICAL MANIFESTATIONS

The child with cellulitis develops a local inflammatory response at the site of infection with erythema, edema, warmth, pain, and limitation of motion. There may be a history of a prior wound or insect bite. Facial infections are more common during the first 5 years of life. Fever is unusual unless the etiology of the infection is *H. influenzae*. Only 10 to 20% of children with cellulitis due to other organisms become febrile. The lesion itself is erythematous and tender but not fluctuant; red streaks may radiate proximally along the course of the lymphatic drainage. The regional lymph nodes usually enlarge in response to the infection.

With cellulitis due to *S. aureus* or Group A *Streptococcus*, the WBC is normal in most children. More extensive lesions or bacteremia, seen only occasionally, evoke a leukocytosis. A culture obtained from the leading edge of the cellulitis will yield a pathogen in half of the cases, but cultures of the blood usually remain sterile.

On the other hand, bacteremia accompanies *H. influenzae* cellulitis; this organism is isolated from the blood in 90% of the patients. The WBC is greater than 15,000/cu mm as a rule, usually with a shift to the left.

The complications of cellulitis, though infrequent, include both local and metastatic spread of infection. The organisms may invade deeper tissues, producing septic arthritis or osteomyelitis. During the course of bacteremia, a frequent occurrence in *H. influenzae* infections, there may be involvement of the meninges, pericardium, epiglottis, or synovial membranes. Multifocal areas of cellulitis should arouse a suspicion of hematogenous dissemination. Occasionally, cellulitis provides a clue to an infection originating in deeper anatomic structures. Thus, a lesion on the abdomen may be a sign of peritonitis.

MANAGEMENT

The majority of children with nonfacial cellulitis can receive antibiotic therapy as outpatients, but the physician must first exclude the presence of *H. influenzae* (Fig. 45.5). Since *S. aureus* and Group A *Streptococcus* are most frequently isolated, treatment should be directed at these organisms. Acceptable alternatives include a semisynthetic penicillin such as dicloxacillin (50 mg/kg/day) or cephalexin (50 mg/kg/day); *S. aureus* are generally resistant to penicillin and ampicillin. A CBC, blood culture, and aspirate culture are not necessary.

If a child with a nonfacial cellulitis has a fever, the likelihood of a bacteremic infection with *H. influenzae* increases. A WBC and cultures from the lesion and the blood should be obtained. In cases where the WBC is $<$ 15,000/cu mm, antibiotic therapy is given as above and the patient asked to return the following day. A leukocytosis in association with a temperature $\geqq$ 38.5°C mandates admission for intravenous treatment with oxacillin (150 mg/kg/day) and chloramphenicol (100 mg/kg/day).

Children with facial cellulitis are partic-

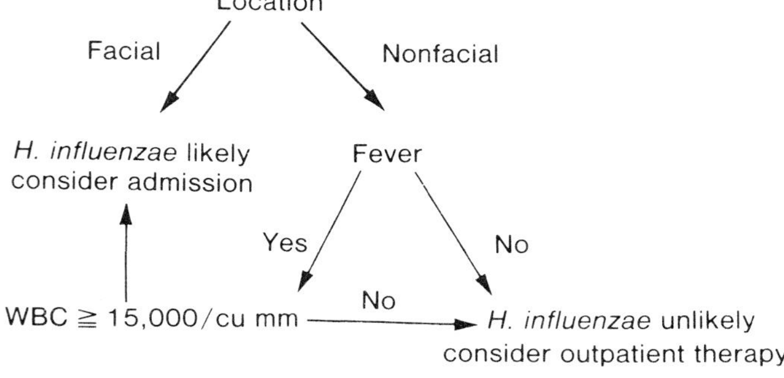

Figure 45.5 Approach to the child with cellulitis.

ılarly likely to be bacteremic with *H. influ-ɘnzae*. Thus, they should receive intrave-ıous therapy with oxacillin and chloram-ɔhenicol to treat this organism as well as *S. ɑureus* and Group A *Streptococcus*.

Septic Arthritis

ƷACKGROUND

Septic arthritis is an infection within a joint space. The incidence of this infection is unknown; however, Nelson reported that 20 children were admitted yearly between 1966 and 1970 to two large pediatric services in Dallas. As opposed to adults, children who develop septic arthritis are generally otherwise healthy. Males are affected twice as commonly as females.

The bacterial etiology of septic arthritis varies with age. During the first 2 months of life, the Group B *Streptococcus* and *S. auerus* predominate. Gram negative enteric bacilli, *Candida* species, and *N. gonorrheae* are seen sporadically.

Between 3 months and 3 years of age, *H. influenzae* emerges as the commonest pathogen, being isolated from 60 to 80% of children with septic arthritis. *S. aureus* is the second most frequent organism found. After 3 years of age and until puberty, *S. aureus* causes the majority of joint infections. The Group A *Streptococcus*, the pneumococcus, and *H. influenzae* are less commonly recovered.

The incidence of gonococcal arthritis in teenagers has varied in different reports depending on the frequency of sexual activity in the population studied. Among sexually active adolescents, *N. gonorrhoeae* is the most common cause of septic arthritis, trailed closely by *S. aureus*.

Many other organisms occasionally invade the joint space, some only in special circumstances. *P. aeruginosa* shows a peculiar predilection for septic arthritis of the foot following puncture wounds. In the child with sickle cell anemia, salmonellae frequently cause septic arthritis. The gram-negative bacilli are almost never recovered from previously healthy children, but are seen in immunosuppressed patients. *Mycobacterium tuberculosis* is rarely recovered at any age.

PATHOPHYSIOLOGY

Septic arthritis generally results from the hematogenous dissemination of an organism, either into the joint or the bony metaphysis. Rarely, a pathogen gains access to the joint by direct inoculation or spread from a contiguous site of infection. Although many children give a history of recent trauma, the role played by injury remains unknown. In gonococcal arthritis, the initial site of infection may be the genitals, pharynx, or rectum. Dissemination from the cervix follows menstruation when shedding of the organism is highest.

Bacteria in the joint space evoke an inflammatory response with an infiltration of neutrophilis. The accumulation of purulent material distends the joint capsule, producing the physical and radiographic findings.

CLINICAL FEATURES

Infection within a joint produces pain and limitation of motion of that joint. Thus, the site of the arthritis determines the initial complaint. Ninety percent of children have a monoarticular arthritis, involving the lower extremity (hip, knee, and ankle) in the majority. Thus, a limp is the commonest presenting symptom. If a joint in the arm is involved, there will be decreased mobility of the upper extremity.

With infections in deeper joints, the pain may radiate to contigious anatomic structures. Children with a septic hip often complain of an ache at the knee, and sacroiliac arthritis may mimic appendicitis, pelvic neoplasm, or urinary tract infections. Although the duration of symptoms in septic arthritis is less than 3 days in over half of the children with these conditions, the delay in diagnosis may reach 3 or 4 weeks with sacroiliac arthritis.

The findings are often vague in the first 6 months of life. Pyoarthritis may cause paradoxical irritability, an increase in crying on being fondled as is seen with meningitis. The infant with a septic hip usually lies quietly holding the leg abducted and externally rotated.

Sixty to 70% of children with septic arthritis have a temperature $\geqq$ 38.5°C. The absence of fever occurs most commonly in the adolescent with a gonococcal infection or the neonate. An erythematous swelling surrounds a superficial joint that is infected. Although a temperature difference exists between the affected and unaffected sites, it can be difficult to discern in the febrile child. Inflammation within the joint distends the capsule and produces pain with movement. If a child can put an extremity through a full range of motion, septic arthritis is unlikely.

The ESR is the most consistently abnormal laboratory study. Molteni observed an elevated ESR in 32 of 37 (86%) of children with septic arthritis; the median value was 50 mm. The WBC count varies from < 5000 to > 20,000/cu mm. Although a leukocytosis with a shift to the left occurs commonly, as many as 20% of children will have a WBC count < 10,000/cu mm. If septic arthritis is diagnosed early, an x-ray of the joint will not show any pathologic changes. The first radiographic alteration to be noted is edema of the adjacent soft tissues, which is not pathognomonic of inflammation in the joint. Later, distension of the capsule becomes visible and bony destruction may be seen late in the course of the infection.

The thickness of the tissues surrounding the hip joint makes the detection of an effusion difficult by physical examination. X-ray of the hip should always be obtained if there is a possible infection in this joint. Early in the course, the tendon of the obturator internis is displaced medially as the muscle passes over the distended hip capsule. Continued accumulation of an inflammatory exudate forces the femoral head laterally and upward, disrupting the arc formed by the femoral head and the pelvis (Shenton's line).

No constellation of laboratory and radiographic results can rule out the diagnosis of septic arthritis; an analysis of the joint fluid is mandatory if the index of suspicion is high. Infection causes an infiltration of polymorphonuclear leukocytes into the joint space. Although intraarticular WBC counts > 100,000/cu mm are traditionally associated with infection, a lesser cellular response is frequently noted. Nelson found a WBC count in the joint fluid < 25,000/cu mm in 9 of 31 (34%) children with proven bacterial arthritis. The joint fluid glucose is reduced to less than 40 mg% in only 25 to 50% of patients, but the Gram stain of the synovial fluid shows organisms in 75%. Because inflammatory exudates have bacteriostatic properties, cultures of joint fluid yield an organism in only 60% of cases. A pathogen is recovered from the bloodstream in 40% of children with septic arthritis, more frequently if *H. influenzae* is the cause of the disease.

The complications of septic arthritis include both local and distant spread of the infection. Osteomyelitis frequently accompanies joint infections in the first year of life due to the location of the metaphysis within the joint capsule. During the process of hematogenous dissemination, bacteria may invade sites other than the joint. Simultaneous infections may occur in the meninges, pericardium, or the soft tissues; these are particularly frequent with *H. influenzae*.

MANAGEMENT

Septic arthritis demands prompt management; in particular, infection in the hip joint should be considered an emergency. Pressure generated by purulent material within the joint space can compromise the vascular supply of the femoral head, leading to necrosis and eventual loss of normal ambulation.

The initial treatment is aimed at relieving the pressure within the joint and controlling the infection. At the time of the diagnostic aspiration, as much purulent fluid as possible should be removed. Immediate surgical intervention is needed for hip infections.

All children with septic arthritis require admission to the hospital for intravenous antibiotic therapy. The initial choice of antimicrobials depends on the age of the child and the Gram stain. If no organisms are apparent on examination of the joint fluid, presumptive antibiotic therapy is begun as follows: ≦2 months of age—penicillin 250,000 units/kg/day, oxacillin 150 mg/kg/day, and gentamicin 7.5 mg/kg/day; > 2 months to ≦3 years of age—oxacillin 150 mg/kg/day and chloramphenicol 100 mg/kg/day; >3 years of age—oxacillin 150 mg/kg/day up to a maximum of 6 g/day.

Osteomyelitis

BACKGROUND

Osteomyelitis is an infection of the bone; a variant, discitis, affects the intervertebral disc space. Bremmer and Neligman estimated that 1 in 5,000 children less than 13 years of age develop osteomyelitis. There were approximately 10 children with bone infections admitted yearly to the pediatric service at Parkland Memorial Hospital in Dallas between 1959 and 1973.

S. aureus causes osteomyelitis in the majority of children regardless of age. During the neonatal period, the Group B *Streptococcus* is the second most frequent isolate; *N. gonorrhoeae* and gram negative enteric bacilli are also found. *H. influenzae* has been recovered from about 2% of bone infections in children, generally from those less than 3 years of age. Granoff et al. described three children with *H. influenzae* osteomyelitis between the ages of 21 and 28 months; Dich et al. had 4 patients less than 2 years of age and a fifth between ages 2 and 5 years. The Group A *Streptococcus* causes 5 to 10% of osteomyelitis in childhood. Other pathogens are recovered infrequently, including *S. pneumoniae*, *Y. enterocolitica*, *Brucella* species, anaerobic organisms, *M. tuberculosis*, and *Actinomyces* species.

P. aeruginosa frequently infects the bones of the foot following a puncture wound. In children with sickle cell hemoglobinopathies, *Salmonella* species account for almost half of the cases of osteomyelitis.

PATHOPHYSIOLOGY

In the majority of children with osteomyelitis, organisms reach the bone via the bloodstream. Occasional infections follow the direct inoculation of pathogens or spread from a contiguous focus. During hemotagenous dissemination, organisms lodge in the sinusoidal vessels of the metaphysis at the site of sludging or thrombosis. Bacterial proliferation evokes an inflammatory exudate. Within the confined space of the bone, the pressure generated by the accumulation of purulent material can necrose the cortex and elevate or rupture the periosteum. If the metaphysis is contained within the joint capsule, septic arthritis may ensue.

CLINICAL FEATURES

Osteomyelitis causes bone pain as the infection progresses. The site of the osteomyelitis determines the presentation of the disease. In 90% of cases a single bone is involved. The femur and tibia are the most common bones infected, making limp a common presentation. In a study of 100 consecutive children with a limp seen at the emergency department of the Children's Hospital of Philadelphia, osteomyelitis was diagnosed in 2%.

Osteomyelitis affects the bones of the upper extremity in 25% of cases. These children complain of pain on motion of their upper extremities.

The multiplicity of bones that may be involved leads to a wide spectrum of chief complaints. Vertebral osteomyelitis manifests as backache, torticollis, or stiff neck, and involvement of the mandible causes painful mastication. Infection of the pelvis is particularly elusive and may masquerade as appendicitis, neoplasm, or urinary tract infection. Infants with osteomyelitis localize the symptoms less well than older children. Initially, irritability may be the only complaint.

Fever exceeds 38.5°C in 70 to 80% of children with osteomyelitis. The infant with a long bone infection often manifests pseudoparalysis, an unwillingness to move the extremity. Movement may also be decreased in the older child, but to a lesser degree. Point tenderness almost always is seen in osteomyelitis; however, it is found in other conditions such as trauma, may be difficult to discern in the struggling infant, and does not always occur early in the course of the infection. Percussion of a bone at a point remote from the site of an osteomyelitis elicits pain in the area of the infection.

When purulent material ruptures through the cortex, diffuse local erythema and edema appear. This finding occurs frequently in infants and is confined primarily to children in the first 3 years of life before the cortex thickens sufficiently to contain the inflammatory exudate. Weissburg et al. noted swelling of the extremity in 14 of 17 patients with osteomyelitis under 1 month of age.

The ESR provides a useful screening test for osteomyelitis, as bony infection almost always leads to an elevation. Nelson found an ESR < 15 mm/hr in only 4 of 88 children with osteomyelitis, and the mean value was 70 mm/hr. Although the WBC may reach a level of 20,000/cu mm, it falls within the normal range in two-thirds of the cases. Cultures from the blood yield an organism in 50%, and from the bone in 70%, of children with osteomyelitis.

X-rays of the affected area should always be obtained if osteomyelitis is suspected, even though they are often normal early in the course. The first change, noted after 3 to 4 days, is deep soft tissue swelling which is seen as a subtle shift of the lucent deep muscle plane away from the bone. Within 3 to 10 days, the muscles swell and obliterate the lucent planes which usually separate them radiographically. Visualization of osseous destruction requires the loss of 50% of the bony matrix in an area at least 1 cm in diameter. This amount of demineralization occurs only after 10 to 12 days of infection. At this stage, lytic lesions and periosteal elevation are apparent on the x-ray.

Recently, radionuclide scanning has provided another useful diagnostic tool for the clinician. Uptake of compounds such as technecium is seen at sites of increased metabolic activity which occurs in an infection before sufficient bony destruction has occurred to be seen on conventional x-rays. If scintigraphy is available, the patient with suspected osteomyelitis and a normal x-ray should have this study. However, the absence of increased uptake does not preclude bony infection. Some patients will have decreased uptake because the accumulation of purulent material decreases the blood flow to the site. Additionally, Fleisher et al. and others have shown that the scan may be entirely normal early in the course.

The complications of osteomyelitis include the spread of infection either locally or to remote sites, chronic infection, and irreparable bony destruction. The later two complications are determined by the length of the delay in the institution of therapy and the adequacy of treatment, whereas distant foci of infection pose an immediate problem.

MANAGEMENT

All children strongly suspected or known to have osteomyelitis require admission to the hospital for intravenous antibiotic therapy. The emergency department physician should withold antibiotics until the orthopaedic surgeon has evaluated the child and attempted to culture the bone at the site of infection.

GENITOURINARY INFECTION

Urinary track infections in the child are discussed in Chapters 17 and 63. Of the venereal infections, the three important diseases in the United States are gonorrhea, syphilis, and genital herpes. Although this section will provide a brief general background on these entities, it will primarily emphasize features unique to pediatrics.

Gonorrhea

BACKGROUND

The term gonorrhea will be used to describe a genital infection with *N. gonorrhoeae*, but the organism can also produce disease at other sites. The incidence of gonorrhea has increased recently, and there are 1,000,000 cases reported yearly in the United States. The highest rate of gonococcal infection is found in adolescents and young adults. When looked for, however, gonorrhea is not infrequent in prepubertal youngsters. Paradise et al. studied 38 consecutive prepubertal females with vaginitis from the emergency department at The Children's Hospital, recovering *N. gonorrhoeae* from 4. The age-specific rates for gonorrhea reported in one study were 6.1 of 100,000 from 0 to 9 years and 37.4 of 100,000 from 10 to 14 years. Gonococcal conjunctivitis occurs most frequently in the first month of life, although cases have been described in older children and adults. Other forms of gonococcal infection are rare in children.

PATHOPHYSIOLOGY

A child acquires gonorrhea by direct contact with infected secretions. The gonococci adhere to the surface of columnar epithelial cells and then penetrate through the intracellular spaces to the subepithelial tissues. They evoke an inflammatory response with polymorphonuclear leukocytes. Extension may occur via the lymphatics or the bloodstream.

CLINICAL MANIFESTATION

The most common form of infection with *N. gonorrhoeae* seen among children in the emergency department is infection of the genitals. Prepubertal girls develop a vaginitis, rather than a cervicitis as seen in adult women, due to differences in the vaginal mucosa. Vaginal irritation, dysuria, and a discharge are the most frequent complaints. Boys have a urethral discharge and, occasionally, swelling of the penile shaft. Henretig has described a boy with urinary retention due to gonorrhea. Fever, systemic signs and symptoms, and spread to the pelvic organs occur rarely.

A Gram stain shows gram-negative intracellular diplococci in the majority of children with gonorrhea. Cultures allow for a definitive identification of the organism, a crucial issue from the medicolegal standpoint. Pharyngeal and rectal cultures will each be positive in 5 to 10% of cases where the organism is not isolated from the genital tract.

Despite the widespread use of prophylactic silver nitrate in the eyes of newborns, gonococcal conjunctivitis continues to appear sporadically. A thick, purulent discharge quickly replaces the initial mild erythema from chemical irritation. A Gram stain of the exudate usually shows the organism, and cultures are almost always positive.

Disseminated gonorrhea and pelvic inflammatory disease emerge as problems in the sexually active adult. A complete discussion on these entities is found in Chapter 52.

MANAGEMENT

All children with suspected gonorrhea should have cultures of the genitals, pharynx, and rectum, and a serologic test for syphilis. Genital infection is treated with procaine penicillin, 100,000 units/kg intramuscularly, given 1 hour after an oral dose of probenecid, 25 mg/kg. Spectinomycin, 40 mg/kg, is administered intramuscularly if the child is allergic to penicillin. Because the usual mode of acquisition is venereal, a report must be made to the appropriate community department dealing with child abuse.

No infant under 1 month of age with conjunctivitis should leave the emergency department prior to the performance of a Gram stain and culture of the ocular exudate. The finding of gram-negative diplococci on the smear mandates admission to the hospital for intravenous penicillin therapy.

Syphilis

Syphilis is an infection due to *Treponema pallidum.* The rate of this disease has been increasing in the United States, but it is uncommonly encountered in children. However, scattered congenital infections are seen, and an incidence of 20 per 1,000,000 has been reported in older adolescents.

Congenital syphilis usually presents with the same clinical picture as other intrauterine infections such as rubella and cytomegalovirus. Characteristic features include jaundice and hepatosplenomegaly in an ill-appearing newborn. However, some infants have only a few stigmata, and the diagnosis is overlooked in the nursery. These children may turn up in the first months of life with skin lesions, a persistent nasal discharge, and painful extremities (pseudoparalysis of Parrot). Darkfield examination of the cutaneous lesions can identify the spirochetes, and the serologic test for syphilis is positive. Additionally, x-rays may show lesions of the long bones.

Acquired syphilis presents in the teenager, as in the adult, in the first stage with a chancre and in the second stage with cutaneous or mucosal manifestations. The rash of secondary syphilis may resemble pityriasis rosea, and all sexually active patients diagnosed with this disease, particularly with involvement of the palms or soles, should have a serologic test for syphilis. Other lesions include white patches on the mucous membranes and flat topped warts (condyloma lata) around moist areas. Such lesions shed spirochetes detectable by dark-field microscopy.

Congenital syphilis will be rarely diagnosed in the emergency department and the delay involved in confirmation will move the treatment out of the realm of the emergency physician. All such children require admission to the hospital. In acquired disease, benzathine penicillin, 2.4 million units, is given intramuscularly in a single dose for early syphilis and in three doses, each separated by a week, for syphilis of more than 1 year's duration.

Herpes Genitalis

Herpes simplex can infect the genitals, as well as other anatomic sites. Although the commonest cause of genital ulceration seen among adolescents and adults at venereal disease clinics, this entity is unusual in prepubertal children.

Genital pain is a frequent complaint with infections due to herpes simplex and may precede the appearance of the lesions. Characteristically, the virus produces grouped vesicles on an erythematous base; however, erosion of the overlying skin often leaves only ulcers at the time of the first visit. Particularly with a primary infection, the inguinal lymph nodes enlarge.

Visual inspection often suffices for the diagnosis in the adolescent. Either a Tzanck smear (see Chapter 54) or a viral culture can verify the clinical impression. In children, a culture should always be obtained, since the disease is rarely seen and needs medicolegal confirmation. A serologic test for syphilis and bacterial culture are needed to rule out coexisting veneral infections. Although occasionally spread by nonsexual contact, the physician must explore the possibility of sexual abuse when herpes genitales occurs prior to puberty.

NONBACTERIAL SYSTEMIC INFECTIONS

Viral Syndrome

The term viral syndrome is used to refer to a generalized illness presumed clinically to be due to a virus and characterized by malaise and usually fever. Numerous agents have been implicated, including influenza, enteroviruses, and others. Nonspecific viral syndromes and viral upper respiratory infections account for most of the febrile visits made by children to the emergency department.

A viral syndrome begins with malaise and fever. The temperature varies from 37°C to over 40°C, greater elevations occurring in children less than 2 years of age. Particularly with influenza, children who are able to verbalize their discomfort will complain of diffuse aching. There may be a cough or occasional bout of emesis. Signs of mild inflammation may be seen in the upper respiratory tract.

The physician arrives at a diagnosis of a nonspecific viral syndrome by excluding other diseases on the basis of the history and physical examination. At times, a WBC count will be needed to determine if the child with a high fever is at risk for occult bacteremia. Treatment is limited to antipyresis and the maintenance of an adequate oral intake. Antibiotics will not prevent secondary bacterial infections and should not be prescribed. The parents must be instructed to seek further care if the fever persists for more than 48 hours.

Measles

BACKGROUND

Measles is a disease caused by a specific myxovirus and characterized by fever, cough, coryza, conjunctivitis, and a rash. Since the introduction, on a large scale, of effective vaccines this disease has markedly decreased in incidence. Currently only 25,000 cases are reported yearly to the Centers for Disease Control, a tenfold decline from the level of the mid twentieth century.

PATHOPHYSIOLOGY

Measles virus enters the body via the upper respiratory tract where local replication is believed to occur. A transient viremia ensues, and virus spreads to the reticuloendothelial system. A secondary viremia then follows, producing the clinical disease.

CLINICAL MANIFESTATIONS

Fever and malaise herald the onset of measles. During the course of the illness, the temperature often rises to 40°C. Within 24 hours, coryza, conjunctivitis, and cough develop. Koplik's spots appear on the buccal mucosa by the third day of fever. These are seen as fine white spots on an erythematous background and have been likened to grains of sand. The rash erupts on the fourth or fifth day. The exanthem is maculopapular in appearance and begins on the face and neck. The lesions are heaviest on the upper portion of the body, often coalescing. As the rash advances down the trunk, the prodromal findings (cough, coryza, conjunctivitis) and the Koplik's spots resolve. The rash involves the extremities on its third day, but has already begun to fade on the face.

A leukopenia accompanies uncomplicated measles. Specific antibodies, initially absent from the serum, reach detectable levels 2 weeks after the onset of illness.

Complications, which are unusual, fall into two categories: (1) extension of the viral infection; and (2) secondary bacterial infection. The virus itself may produce inflammation of the lower respiratory mucosa leading to laryngotracheitis, bronchitis, and/or pneumonia. Encephalitis occurs in 1 of every 1,000 cases of measles; this is a debilitating illness with a mortality rate of 15%. Thrombocytopenia and corneal ulcerations are seen infrequently. Lymphoid hyperplasia in the bowel can occlude the lumen of the appendix leading to inflammation of this organ; histologic examination of surgically removed tissue confirms the diagnosis of measles on the basis of the characteristic giant cells. Acute purulent otitis media is the commonest bacterial complication of measles and cervical adenitis occasionally occurs. Pneumonia, although usually viral, may have a bacterial etiology.

MANAGEMENT

The clues gathered from the history and physical examination suffice for the diagnosis of measles by the experienced clinician. However, as the number of cases dwindles, the physician is less likely to be familiar with the disease. Often, serologic studies are required to confirm the etiology, particularly among the first few children seen in sporadic outbreaks.

Measles runs a self-limited course. Bed rest and antipyretic therapy help to keep the child comfortable. Antitussives, antihistamines, and topical ophthalmic preparations have no role. Prophylaxis against secondary bacterial infections with antibiotics is not warranted.

Children with uncomplicated measles or superficial secondary infections such as otitis and cervical adenitis can be treated as outpatients. Hospitalization is required when there is evidence of significantly severe laryngotracheobronchitis, as discussed earlier in this chapter. Lower respiratory tract or CNS involvement necessitate admission to the hospital.

Measles is a preventable disease. Susceptible contacts should receive immune serum globulin, 0.25 ml/kg, as a single dose.

Rubella

BACKGROUND

Rubella is a childhood infection due to a specific togavirus. Prior to the advent of vaccination, epidemics occurred every 6 to 9 years; 488,796 cases were reported to the Centers for Disease Control in the United States in 1964, the year of the last outbreak in this country. Presently, there are an estimated 25,000 to 50,000 cases per year. Rubella traditionally occurs in children 5 to 9 years of age, but the incidence among teenagers is increasing.

PATHOPHYSIOLOGY

The initial site of inoculation is the upper respiratory tract where local replication occurs. A viremia ensues, disseminating the virus to the skin.

CLINICAL MANIFESTATIONS

Only 10% of the children experience prodromal symptoms such as fever, malaise, cough, and mild conjunctivitis. However, such complaints are frequently voiced by the adolescent. The rash begins on the face and spreads downward, reaching the extremities by the end of the second day. The lesions are pink maculopapules that may coalesce. The lymph nodes in the postauricular, suboccipital, and posterior cervical chains enlarge and become somewhat tender. During the first 2 days of illness, the temperature usually rises, but remains under 39°C.

The WBC count often decreases in rubella and a few atypical lymphocytes may appear. A fourfold rise in specific antibodies occurs after 10 to 14 days.

Complications of rubella are rare in children but include encephalitis, thrombocytopenia, and arthritis or arthralgia. Painful and/or swollen joints occur frequently in adolescents. Encephalitis has an incidence of 1 in 6,000 cases of rubella and usually resolves spontaneously.

MANAGEMENT

Rubella is difficult to diagnosis clinically due to its infrequent occurrence and the plethora of exanthems with a similar appearance. Situations that require a definite etiologic diagnosis, such as the pregnant adolescent, demand serologic confirmation. Children with rubella can be managed as outpatients with antipyretic therapy. Only the rare child with encephalitis or thrombocytopenia requires admission to the hospital.

Varicella/Zoster

BACKGROUND

Herpesvirus varicellae causes two clinical illnesses, varicella (chickenpox) and zoster (shingles). Varicella occurs during a primary infection and zoster following a reactivation of latent virus.

Varicella is a frequent infection in children, usually between 2 and 8 years of age. Almost 90% of susceptible household contacts of an index case develop the disease. By adolescence, serologic surveys have shown a seropositivity rate of 70 to 80%. Zoster, on the other hand, affects adults predominantly. More than 60% of the cases are in individuals over 45 years of age.

PATHOPHYSIOLOGY

The virus enters the body via the oropharynx and replicates locally. Viremia presumably occurs after exposure and before the onset of the exanthem. During an episode of varicella, the virus invades sensory nerve endings and ascends to the dorsal root ganglion where it becomes latent. Zoster follows reactivation of the latent virus.

CLINICAL MANIFESTATIONS

Varicella

A mild prodrome, lasting 1 to 3 days frequently precedes the exanthem of varicella; however, the first sign of illness may be the rash. The child runs a fever, usually less than 39.5°C, and may complain of malaise. Lesions erupt initially on the upper trunk or face and spread centripetally. Pruritis is universal.

The abnormal findings on physical examination are limited to the elevated temperature and the skin and mucus membrane lesions. Initially, the exanthem consists of erythematous papules that evolve into vesicles and then pustules over 6 or 8 hours. The early vesicles have a diameter of 2 to 4 mm and a "dewdroplike" appearance. Since new lesions erupt in crops for 2 to 4 days, papules, vesicles, and pustules are usually seen together. An exanthem involves the mucosa of the oropharynx and, occasionally, the vagina. The severity of the cutaneous manifestations varies widely, and there may be from 1 to more than 1,000 lesions.

There are few laboratory derangements in varicella. The WBC occasionally shows a leukocytosis, and the SGOT and SGPT may be mildly elevated. In adolescents, the chest x-ray reveals an interstitial infiltrate in 5 to 10% of the patients even though there may be no respiratory symptoms.

Varicella runs a self-limited course in the majority of cases, but is occasionally a more serious illness. Fleisher et al. recently reviewed 96 children hospitalized with complications of this disease during a 5-year period at the Children's Hospital of Philadelphia. Of the group, 81 were immunocompetent children older than 1 month of age; they experienced complications including encephalitis (20), pneumonia (5), hepatitis (8), bacterial superinfection (22), Reye's syndrome (17), unusual cutaneous manifestations (5), medication overdoses (5), exacerbation of an underlying chronic disease (2), and dehydration (1).

Encephalitis takes two forms: a diffuse cerebritis with coma and seizures, and a cerebellitis with ataxia. Since bacterial meningitis can also complicate varicella, an analysis of the spinal fluid should be done even if viral encephalitis is suspected. There will often be a mild pleocytosis (10 to 300 cells) and a slight elevation of the protein (40 to 80 mg/dl). If the encephalopathy is felt to be due to Reye's syndrome, a serum ammonia should be obtained.

Zoster

Zoster appears suddenly in most children without any warning symptoms such as pain or pruritis. The lesions are grouped vesicles on an erythematous base in a dermatomal distribution. In 15 to 20% of cases, extradermatomal cutaneous dissemination occurs. However, spread to the viscera does not occur in the immunocompetent child. If the eruption occurs along the ophthalmic branch of the trigeminal nerve, the cornea may be involved. The appearance of vesicles on the tip of the nose should evoke a suspicion of ocular involvement that can be best seen after fluorescein staining of the eye.

MANAGEMENT

Visual inspection suffices for the diagnosis of varicella; no laboratory studies are indicated. Acetaminophen is given to control the fever, and antihistaminic drugs provide some relief from the pruritis. Benadryl, 5 mg/kg/day, or hydroxyzine, 2 mg/kg/day, can be used. The child cannot attend school for 1 week after the eruption of the first lesion.

Immunosuppressed children with varicella will require hospitalization in order to receive intravenous adenine arabinoside which has recently been shown to prevent visceral dissemination. Complications mandating admission to the hospital include Reye's syndrome, pneumonia, and encephalitis, except in the mildest cases. Superficial bacterial infections such as impetigo, cellulitis, and adenitis can be treated with oral antibiotic therapy such as dicloxacillin, 50 mg/kg/day. Children with deeper bacterial infections, i.e. septic arthritis, should receive antibiotics intravenously.

As with varicella, there is no specific therapy for zoster. Antipruritic and antipyretic agents provide symptomatic relief. Immunocompromised children should be admitted to the hospital. Ocular involvement merits consultation with an ophthalmologist.

Roseola

Roseola infantum, or exanthem subitum, is a common, self-limited, presumably viral infection of infants. The child, usually less than 3 years of age, presents with a high fever, ranging up to 40.5°C, and a paucity of physical findings. There may be mild irritability but no coryza, pharyngeal infection, or conjunctivitis. After 2 to 4 days of illness, the fever drops precipitously and a rash appears. The lesions are discrete, pink maculopapules, 2 to 3 mm in diameter. They fade with pressure and do not coalesce. The exanthem appears on the trunk initially and spreads outward. Roseola resolves without complications other than an occasional febrile convulsion. The diagnosis of roseola is made on the basis of the clinical course, often in retrospect. If a WBC count is obtained, leukopenia will be seen. Treatment is limited to antipyretic agents.

Erythema Infectiosum

Erythema infectiosum, or fifth disease, is an exanthematous illness of childhood thought to be due to a viral etiology. It occurs most commonly between 2 and 12 years of age. The appearance of a rash marks the onset of the disease; fever or other prodromal symptoms are infrequent. The rash involves the face initially, conferring on the child a "slapped cheek" appearance. Maculopopular lesions erupt 24 hours later, initially on the upper portion of the extremities and then spread both proximally and distally. Fading of the central portion of the lesions gives a lacelike appearance to the rash. Arthralgia, arthritis, and hemolytic anemia have been reported but are rare. There is no specific therapy.

Infectious Mononucleosis

BACKGROUND

Infectious mononucleosis (IM) is a disease characterized by malaise, fever, pharyngitis, lymphadenopathy, and splenomegaly. In 1968, Henle and Henle showed that the Epstein-Barr virus (EBV) causes this illness.

EBV infections are frequent, but usually asymptomatic, during the first years of life. In childhood, sporadic infections occur and infectious mononucleosis is occasionally diagnosed. By late adolescence, 50 to 90% of individuals are seropositive, a higher prevalence of antibodies being found in teenagers of lower socioeconomic status. EBV infections are again common between 15 and 25 years of age in more affluent individuals; half of the seroconversions are accompanied by the clinical manifestations of IM.

PATHOPHYSIOLOGY

Several studies have suggested that EBV is transmitted via intimate oral contact. The virus infects B lymphocytes which may spread to the various lymphoid tissues in the body. Sensitized T-cells destroy the infected B-cells and limit the production of virus; these cells are the atypical lymphocytes that appear in the circulation.

CLINICAL MANIFESTATIONS

IM begins insidiously with fever and malaise. Three-fourths of children with this illness will complain of a sore throat. Although a child may recover from IM in 7 to 10 days, the symptoms usually last for 2 to 4 weeks. This persistence of symptoms separates the patient with IM from those with pharyngitis due to the Group A *Streptococcus* or to other viruses. Occasionally, the onset resembles that of infectious hepatitis.

The child with infectious mononucleosis is febrile in 90% of cases at presentation. Enlarged lymph nodes are uniformly palpable. While the lymphadenopathy may be limited to the cervical region, involvement of the axillary and inguinal areas occurs commonly. Pharyngitis due to any pathogen produces an increase in the size of the anterior cervical nodes, but EBV characteristically affects the posterior cervical and submental glands as well. In 75% of cases, the pharynx is inflamed, often with an exudate. The spleen enlarges in 60% of children and the liver in 25%. Periorbital edema and a diffuse maculopapular rash are seen occasionally.

The hemoglobin and hematocrit are normal in the uncomplicated disease. Although the total WBC count does not often increase much beyond 15,000/cu mm, levels up to 30,000/cu mm are seen in 10 to 15% of children. A higher leukocyte count casts some doubt on the diagnosis of IM. There is an absolute lymphocytosis with many atypical mononuclear cells; however, 16% of children presenting with IM in one series had fewer than 10% atypical lymphocytes, and 58% had fewer than 20% of such cells. The mainstay for the diagnosis of IM in the adult is the heterophil antibody test, but these antibodies reach levels detectable by routine assays in only 50% of children. Confirmation of a heterophil negative case of IM requires Epstein-Barr virus-specific serologic assays. The SGOT and SGPT are elevated in the majority of children.

The most worrisome complications of IM for the emergency department physician are splenic rupture and airway obstruction. Even minor trauma can cause a rent in the capsule of the enlarged spleen seen in IM; these children manifest the usual signs of intraperitoneal hemorrhage. Occasionally, massive lymphoid hyperplasia of the tonsils occludes the upper airway leading to stridor and retractions. The site of narrowing is easily visualized on examination. Less common complications include encephalitis, pneumonia, myocarditis, hemolytic anemia, and thrombocytopenia.

MANAGEMENT

A WBC count and heterophil antibody titer usually suffice for the confirmation of the clinical diagnosis. Epstein-Barr virus-specific antibodies are indicated only for heterophil negative cases.

Specific therapy is not available. Adequate rest and nutrition should be maintained, and antipyretic agents will increase the comfort of the child. The treatment of a child with uncomplicated IM does not require the administration of corticosteroids.

If complications develop, the child should be admitted to the hospital. Corticosteroids almost always dramatically shrink the enlarged tonsils of the child with airway obstruction. Prednisone is given at 2.5 mg/kg for the first day and tapered over 5 days.

Rocky Mountain Spotted Fever

BACKGROUND

Rocky Mountain spotted fever (RMSF) is an infection caused by *Rickettsia rickettsii*; it is the most frequently occurring rickettsial disease in the United States. Ticks harbor the organism and transmit it to humans during blood sucking. Although named for the area of the country where the causative agent was discovered, most cases of RMSF occur in the states along the eastern coast of the United States. The incidence of the disease peaks during the warmer months. It affects individuals of all ages, but two-third of the victims are children and adolescents. Each year, over 1,000 cases are reported to the Centers for Disease Control.

PATHOPHYSIOLOGY

Rickettsiae are inoculated during blood sucking by a tick and replicate locally. In animal models, the organisms disseminate hematogenously and invade the endothelial lining of the small blood vessels. The infection induces an inflammatory reaction in these cells leading to swelling, necrosis, thrombosis, and finally occulsion of the vascular lumina. The diffuse vasculitis underlies the widespread clinical manifestations that may involve almost every organ.

CLINICAL MANIFESTATIONS

The incubation period of RMSF ranges from 2 to 10 days, but usually lasts one week. The initial symptoms of headache and malaise are followed by fever. The rash erupts on the third or fourth day of illness. In over half the cases reviewed by Vianna, the exanthem appeared first on the wrists and ankles and spread inward toward the trunk. The initial lesions are maculopopular but become hemorrhagic in the ensuing 24 to 48 hours if the disease remains unchecked.

The findings on examination vary with the duration of the disease. Early in the course of the illness, the child remains alert. Conjunctivitis and a rash may be the only signs. Edema begins in the periorbital regions and involves the extremities as the vasculitis progresses. Splenomegaly is found in one-third of the cases. Although the sensorium is clear initially, obtundation, and finally coma, develop after several days of illness.

The WBC count remains normal or rises slightly with RMSF. Thrombocytopenia occurs in 75% of patients during the first stages of the disease; later, disseminated intravascular coagulation may develop with a prolonged PT and PTT as well as elevated fibrin split products. Most patients have hyponatremia but no other electrolyte abnormalities. Bradford and Hawkins noted a decrease in the serum sodium among 88% of children. Recently, immunofluorescent staining has been used to identify rickettsiae in the endothelial cells of dermal vessels from skin biopsies. Even when myocarditis remains clinically silent, the electrocardiogram may show signs of myocardial dysfunction. The earliest changes consist of an elevation of the ST segment: later, the P-R interval may become prolonged and arrythmias may occur.

Complications of RMSF which demand immediate attention include shock and seizures. Vascular collapse occurs due to the combination of the endothelial damage and inadequate hydration in the obtunded patient. Tachycardia, hypotension, and an impaired peripheral perfusion point to a decrease in the intravascular volume. Convulsions occur not infrequently in the comatose child with RMSF. Either hyponatremia or a cerebral vasculitis may underlie the seizure activity. In some cases, mild increases in the CSF cell count and protein concentration are seen. Occasionally, the hemorrhagic diathesis needs immediate treatment in the emergency department. Myocarditis and nephritis are also seen.

MANAGEMENT

A CBC, platelet count, electrolytes, PT, PTT, and serologic titers should be obtained on the child with suspected RMSF. These studies will help to both pin down the diagnosis and influence the management. Since no routinely available test confirms the diagnosis of RMSF early in its course, treatment must be initiated presumptively. The mildly ill child with a fever, maculopopular exanthem, and a history of a tick bite can be treated as an outpatient. Chloramphenicol, 50 mg/kg/day, is the drug of choice under age 8 years and tetracycline, 50 mg/kg/day, in older youths.

Admission is indicated in several situations: (1) clinical evidence of toxicity; (2) encephalitis; (3) thrombocytopenia (platelet count < 150,000/cu mm) or derangements in the clotting studies; and (4) hyponatremia (Na < 130 meq/liter). In the emergency department, an intravenous infusion should be started and sufficient fluids administered to maintain an adequate blood pressure as discussed under septic shock. Chloramphenicol, 50 mg/kg/day, can be given alone if the illness is clearly felt to be RMSF; in practice, however, broader antibacterial coverage is often used because bacterial sepsis cannot be excluded.

MISCELLANEOUS INFECTIONS

Rabies

Rabies is a viral infection of the brain that is almost invariably fatal. Although the actual disease is extremely rare in the United States, potential exposure in the form of animal bites occur frequently. Dogs bite 1,000,000 to 2,000,000 people per year, and 75% of the victims are children.

The decision as to whether or not to give prophylaxis for rabies is influenced by the species of animal, the condition of the animal, the ability to study the animal, and the prevalence of rabies in the region (see Table 45.12). The incidence of rabies in the area should be available from the local health department. When the physician determines that prophylaxis is necessary, human rabies immune globulin (HRIG), 20 IU/kg, and human diploid cell vaccine (HDCV) are used. After cleaning the wound, half of the HRIG is given locally and the remainder at a distant site. Arrangements should be made for the child to receive HDCV from the health department in the community.

Tetanus

Clinical tetanus is caused by the toxin produced by *Clostridium tetani*. The disease is rare in the United States due to the widespread use of the vaccine. Neonatal tetanus from infections of the umbilicus by the organism continues to be reported occasionally. However, the more common problem for the emergency physician is the use of prophylaxis following traumatic wounds. Both tetanus toxoid, 0.5 ml, and human tetanus immune globulin, 250 units, may be indicated, depending on the type of wound and the prior immunization history (see Table 45.13). Tetanus-prone wounds include punctures, crush injuries, and injuries contaminated by animal excreta or left untreated for more than 24 hours.

Botulism

BACKGROUND

Botulism is a paralytic illness produced by neurotoxins elaborated by *Clostridum botulinum*. The disease may result from the ingestion of preformed toxin or from the

Table 45.12
Rabies: Postexposure prophylaxis

Species	Condition of Animal	Escaped (E) or Captured (C)	Treatment
Wild: bat, fox, skunk, coyote, racoon	Regard as rabid	C	None, pending brain examination
		E	HRIG and HDCV[a]
Wild: other	Not applicable	C or E	Varies by species and region
Domestic	Healthy	C	None, pending observation
		E	HRIG and HDCV
	Suspected rabid	C or E	HRIG and HDCV

[a] HRIG = human rabies immune globulin; HDCV = human diploid cell vaccine.

Table 45.13
Guidelines for Tetanus Prophylaxis

No. of Primary Immunizations	Years since Last Booster	Type of Wound	Recommendation
2	Irrelevant	Low risk	T[a]
		Tetanus prone	T+ TIG[b]
3	10	Low risk	T
		Tetanus prone	T
3	5–10	Low risk	No treatment
		Tetanus prone	T
3	5	Low risk	No treatment
		Tetanus prone	No treatment

[a] T = tetanus toxoid.
[b] TIG = human tetanus immune globulin.

elaboration of toxin by organisms in a wound or the gastrointestinal tract. Of particular concern to the physician caring for children is infantile botulism due to toxin formed in the intestines. Almost 200 cases of this disease in the United States were reported to the Centers for Disease Control in 1980.

PATHOPHYSIOLOGY

During growth, *C. botulinum* releases neurotoxins that are the most potent poisons known on a weight basis. They interfere with neurotransmission at peripheral cholinergic synapses by blocking the release of acetylcholine.

CLINICAL MANIFESTATIONS

Botulism from the ingestion of toxin causes vomiting in half of the cases. The patients complain of weakness and a dry mouth; constipation and urinary retention may occur. Paralysis is noted within 3 days, usually affecting first the cranial nerves and then the extremities. The patients are alert and febrile. Abnormalities of the neurologic examination include ptosis, extraocular palsies, fixed dilated pupils, symmetrical weakness, and hyporeflexia. Both the ileus and urinary retention seen in this disease may lead to abdominal distension.

Infantile botulism occurs in children in the first 6 months of life who are otherwise healthy. Constipation is the first symptom of the disease, but may not be sufficiently severe as to draw attention to any underlying illness. After several days, mild lethargy, weakness, and a decreased appetite are noted. Occasionally, the onset of lethargy and weakness may be so precipitous as to resemble bacterial sepsis or meningitis.

On examination, the infant is quiet, with little discernable movement, and has a weak cry. Fever is not a part of this syndrome. The child sucks on a nipple with difficulty and may be unable to swallow. The absence of a gag reflex, profound hypotonia, and hyporeflexia in infantile botulism help to distinguish this illness from bacterial sepsis.

The WBC count is normal in botulism. Organisms may be recovered by anaerobic culture techniques from the gastrointestinal tract in infantile or wound botulism, but identification of the toxins requires the specialized facilities of the Public Health Department. All children suspected of botulism should have an electromyogram which shows a characteristic pattern of brief duration, small amplitude, overly abundant, motor unit action potentials (BSAP).

Respiratory failure is a potentially life-threatening complication in botulism of any variety, and ventilatory support is often required. The profound bulbar weakness in infantile botulism often prevents an adequate fluid intake; dehydration occurs frequently.

MANAGEMENT

Since there is no immediately available test to diagnosis infantile botulism, the initial evaluation of these infants aims at excluding other causes of lethargy and weakness such as sepsis, poliomyelitis, myasthenia gravis, neuropathy, and drug ingestion. A lumbar puncture is often performed in the emergency department to rule out meningitis, and electrolytes and a BUN are useful to assess hydration.

The children all require admission to the hospital. Monitoring of the pulse and respiratory rate should be begun in the emergency department. An intravenous line should be started for the administration of fluids to correct dehydration and in anticipation of a possible respiratory arrest. Neither antibiotics nor antitoxin ameliorate the course of infantile botulism. Because they may potentiate the neuromuscular blockage, aminoglycoside antibiotics should be avoided when treating for possible sepsis.

Children with foodborne and wound botulism also require admission to the hospital. Antitoxin is available from the Centers for Disease Control and should be administered after consultation with the staff at this agency.

Toxic Shock Syndrome

BACKGROUND

The toxic shock syndrome (TSS) is characterized by severe prolonged shock and is probably caused by a toxin produced by *S. aureus*. Todd et al. initially described this syndrome in seven children, aged 8 to 17 years, but the majority of the subsequently reported episodes have occurred in postpubertal females, often after a menstrual period. Between October 1979 and May 1980, investigators at the Centers for Disease Control were able to collect information on 55 cases.

PATHOPHYSIOLOGY

Colonization by a phage-group-1 toxin producing staphylococcal strain sets the stage for the development of the TSS. The enterotoxins of these organisms are pyrogenic and enhance the susceptibility to shock from endotoxins.

CLINICAL MANIFESTATIONS

TSS begins suddenly with high fever, vomiting, and watery diarrhea. Pharyngitis, headache, and myalgias may also occur and oliguria rapidly develops. Within 48 hours the disease progresses to hypotensive shock. The patient has a fever, usually 39 to 41°C, a diffuse, erythematous maculopopular rash, and hyperemia of the mucus membranes. Often, marked disorientation evolves.

The WBC count is elevated with a shift to the left. Thrombocytopenia occurs frequently, being present in over 75% of the children reported by Todd. The majority of patients develop disseminated intravascular coagulation and have an elevated PT and PTT. Additional abnormalities in the laboratory studies may include an elevated SGOT, SGPT, BUN, creatinine, and creatinine phosphokinase. The serum calcium and phosphate may be decreased.

MANAGEMENT

The initial diagnosis of TSS rests on the constellation of clinical and laboratory findings. The following laboratory tests should be obtained from all children suspected of having this syndrome: CBC, platelet count, PT, PTT, fibrin split products, electrolytes, BUN, creatinine, SGOT, SGPT, and creatinine phosphokinase. Cultures of the blood, urine, stool, throat, and vagina serve both to isolate *S. aureus* and to rule out other infectious causes of shock. A lumbar puncture will often be required to exclude bacterial meningitis.

The management of TSS is the same as that for shock due to other organisms (Chapter 2). The physician should secure venous access with a plastic cannula and administer sufficient fluids to maintain an adequate blood pressure. Monitoring of the intravascular volume and urine output usually requires the placement of central venous and peripheral arterial lines and a urinary catheter.

References

Introduction

Russo RM, Gururaj VJ, Sheth KA, et al.: Pediatric DOA: Causes of death. *New York St J Med* 78: 1045 1978.

Bacteremia and Sepsis

Bratton L, Teele DW, Klein JO: Outcome of unsuspected pneumococcemia in children not initially admitted to the hospital. *J Pediatr* 90: 703, 1977.

Eickoff TC, Klein JO, Daly AK, et al.: Neonatal sepsis

and other infections due to group B beta hemolytic streptococci. *N Engl J Med* 271: 1221, 1964.

Feder HM: Occult pneumococcal bacteremia and the febrile infant and young child. *Clin Pediatr* 19: 457, 1980.

Goldschneider T, Gotschlich EC, Artenstein IM: Human immunity to the meningococcus. I. The role of humoral antibodies. *J Exp Med* 129: 130, 1969.

Hamrick HJ, Murphy TS: Bacteremia in 28 ambulatory children. *Clin Pediatr* 17:109, 1978.

Hänninen P, Terho P, Toivanen A: Septicemia in a pediatric unit. *Scand J Infect Dis* 3: 20, 1971.

Johnston RB, Sell SH: Septicemia in infants and children. *Pediatrics* 34: 473, 1964.

McCarthy PL, Grundy GW, Spiesel SZ, et al.: Bacteremia in children: An outpatient clinical review. *Pediatrics* 57: 861, 1976.

McCarthy PL, Jekel JF, Dolan TF: Comparison of acute phase reactants in pediatric patients with fever. *Pediatrics* 62: 716, 1978.

McCarthy PL, Jekel JF, Dolan TF: Temperature greater than or equal to 40°C in children less than 24 months of age: A prospective study. *Pediatrics* 59: 663, 1977.

McCarthy PL, Jekel JF, Staskwick CA, et al.: History and observation variables in assessing febrile children. *Pediatrics* 65: 1090, 1980.

Roberts KB, Borzy MS: Fever in the first eight weeks of life. *Johns Hopkins Med J* 141: 9, 1977.

Siegel JD, McCracken GH, Jr., Threlkeld N, et al.: Single dose penicillin prophlaxis against neonatal group B streptococcal infections. *N Engl J Med* 303: 669, 1980.

Stiehm ER, Damrosch DS: Factors in the prognosis of meningococcal infection. *J Pediatr* 68: 457, 1966.

Supure JS: Hyperpyrexia (temperature>40°C) in children *Ann Emerg Med* 8: 130, 1979.

Tiele DW, Pelton SI, Myles JAG, et al.: Bacteremia in febrile children under 2 years of age: Results of culture of blood of 600 consecutive children seen in a "walk-in" clinic. *J Pediatr* 87: 227, 1975.

Meningitis

Baker CJ, Barrett FF, Gordon RL, et al.: Suppurative meningitis due to streptococci of Lancefield group B: A study of 33 infants. *J Pediatr* 82: 724, 1973.

Feigin RD, Shackelford PG: Value of repeat lumbar puncture in the differential diagnosis of meningitis. *N Engl J Med* 289: 571, 1973.

Friedman A, Fleisher G: Meningitis: Update of recommendations for the neonate. *Clin Pediatr* 19: 395, 1980.

Laxer RM, Marks MI: Pneumococcal meningitis in children. *Am J Dis Child* 131: 850, 1977.

Lepow ML, Carver DH, Wright HT, Jr, et al.: A clinical, epidemiological, and laboratory investigation of aseptic meningitis during the four year period 1955–1958. Observations concerning etiology and epidemiology. *N Engl J Med* 266: 1181, 1962.

Moore CM, Ross M: Acute bacterial meningitis with absent or minimal cerebrospinal fluid abnormalities. *Clin Pediatr* 12: 117, 1973.

Silver TS, Todd JK: Hypoglycorrhachia in pediatric patients. *Pediatrics* 58: 67, 1978.

Swartz MN, Dodge PR: Bacterial meningitis—a review of selected aspects. *N Engl J Med* 272: 725; 779; 842; 898; 954; 1003, 1965.

Nasopharyngitis

Davis SD, Wedgewood RS: Antibiotic prophylaxis in acute viral respiratory disease. *Am J Dis Child* 109: 544, 1965.

Townsend EH, Jr., Radebaugh JE: Prevention of complications of respiratory illnesses in pediatrics practice. A double blind study. *N Engl J Med* 266: 683, 1962.

Pharyngitis

Breese BB, Disney FA: The accuracy of the diagnosis of beta streptococcal infections on clinical grounds. *J Pediatr* 44: 670, 1954.

Honikman LH, Massell BF: Guidelines for the selective use of throat cultures in the diagnosis of streptococcal respiratory infections. *Pediatrics* 48: 573, 1971.

Moffet HL, Cramblett HG, Smith A: Group A streptococcal infections in a children's home. II. Clinical and epidemiological patterns of illness. *Pediatrics* 33: 11, 1964.

Moffet HL, Siegel AC, Doyle HK: Nonstreptococcal pharyngitis. *J Pediatr* 73: 51, 1968.

Otitis Media and Externa

Brownlee RC, Jr., Deloach WR, Cowan CC, Jr., et al.: Otitis media in children: Incidence, treatment, and prognosis in a pediatric practice. *J Pediatr* 75: 636, 1969.

Feingold M, Klein JO, Harlan JE, et al.: Acute otitis media in children. *Am J Dis Child* 111: 361, 1966.

Howie VM, Ploussard JG, Slayer J: The "otitis-prone" condition. *Am J Dis Child* 129: 676, 1975.

Jenkins BH: Treatment of otitis externa and swimmer's ear. *JAMA* 175: 402, 1961.

Paradise JL: Otitis media in infants and children *Pediatrics* 65: 917, 1980.

Paradise JL, Smith CG, Bluestone CD: Tympanometric detection of middle ear effusion in infants and young children. *Pediatrics* 58: 198, 1976.

Schwartz R, Rodriquez WJ, Khan WN, et al.: Acute purulent otitis media in children older than five years: Incidence of *Haemophilus influenzae* as a causative organism. *JAMA* 238: 1032, 1977.

Shurin PA, Pelton SI, Donner A, et al.: Persistence of middle ear effusion after acute otitis media in children. *N Engl J Med* 300: 1121, 1979.

Tetzlatt TR, Ashworth C, Nelson JD: Otitis media in children less than twelve weeks of age. *Pediatrics* 59: 827, 1977.

Sinusitis

Brooks I, Friedman EM, Rodriques WJ, et al.: Complications of sinusitis in children. *Pediatrics* 66: 568, 1980.

Hamory BH, Sande MA, Sydnor A, et al.: Etiology and antimicrobial therapy of acute maxillary sinusitis. *J Infect Dis* 139: 197, 1979.

Shopfner CE, Rossi JO: Roentgen evaluation of paranasal sinuses in children. *Am J Radiol* 118: 176, 1973.

Wald ER, Milmoe GJ, Bowen A, et al.: Acute maxillary sinusitis in children. *N Engl J Med* 304: 749, 1981.

Peritonsillar and Retropharyngeal Abscesses

Flodstrom A, Hallander HO: Microbiological aspects of peritonsillar abscesses. *Scand J Infect Dis* 8: 157, 1976.
McCurdy JA, Jr: Peritonsillar abscess. *Arch Otolaryngol* 103: 414, 1977.
Sprinkle PM, Veltri RW, Kantor CM: Abscesses of the head and neck. *Laryngoscope* 84: 1142, 1974.

Lymphadenitis

Barton LL, Feigin RD: Childhood cervical lymphadenitis: A reappraisal. *J Pediatr* 84: 846, 1974.
Dajani AS, Garcia RE, Wolinsky E: Etiology of cervical lymphadenitis in children. *N Engl J Med* 268: 1379, 1963.

Laryngotracheobronchitis (Croup)

Adair JC: Ten year experience with IPPB in the treatment of acute laryngotracheobronchitis. *Anesth Analg* 50: 649, 1971.
Eden AN, Larkin VD: Corticosteroid treatment of croup. *Pediatrics* 33: 768, 1964.
Gardner HG, Powell KR, Roden VJ, et al.: The evaluation of racemic epinephrine in the treatment of infectious croup. *Pediatrics* 52: 52, 1973.
Hall CB, German JM, Breese BS, et al.: Parainfluenza viral infections in children: Correlation of shedding with clinical manifestations. *J Pediatr* 91: 194, 1977.
Hoekelman RA: Infectious illnesses during the first years of life. *Pediatrics* 59: 119, 1977.
Liepzig B, Oski FA, Cummings CW, et al.: A prospective randomized study to determine the efficacy of steroids in the treatment of croup. *J Pediatr* 94: 194, 1979.
Tercero-Talavera Fl, Rapkin RH: Antibiotic usage in the management of laryngotracheobronchitis. *Clin Pediatr* 13: 1074, 1974.
Tunnessen WW, Feinstein AR: The steroid croup controversy: An analytical review of methodological problems. *J Pediatr* 96: 751, 1980.

Epiglottitis

Berenberg W, Kevy S: Acute epiglottitis in childhood. *N Engl Med* 258: 870, 1958.
Faden HS: Treatment of *Haemophilus influenzae* type b epiglottitis. *Pediatrics* 63: 402, 1979.
Greenberg LW, Schisgall R: Acute eipglottitis in a community hospital. *AFP* 12: 123, 1979.
Johnson GK, Sullivan JF, Bishop LA: Acute epiglottitis—Review of 55 cases and suggested protocol. *Arch Otolaryngol* 100: 333, 1974.
Molteni RA: Epiglottitis: Incidence of extraepiglottic infection; Report of 72 cases and review of the literature. *Pediatrics* 58: 526, 1976.
Rapkin RH: The diagnosis of epiglottitis: Simplicity and reliability of radiographs of the neck in the differential diagnosis of the croup syndrome. *J Pediatr* 80: 96, 1972.
Rapkin RH: Tracheostomy in epiglottitis. *Pediatrics* 52: 426, 1973.
Wetmore RF, Handler SD: Epiglottitis: Evolution in management during the last decade. *Ann Otol Rhinol Laryngol* 88: 822, 1979.

Bacterial Pneumonia

Asmar BI, Slovis TL, Reed JO, et al.: *Haemophilus influenzae* type b pneumonia in 43 children. *J Pediatr* 93: 389, 1978.
Bechamps GJ, Lynn HB, Wenzl JE: Empyema in children: Review of the Mayo Clinic experience. *Mayo Clin Proc* 45: 43, 1970.
Forbes GB, Emerson GL: Staphylococcal pneumonia and empyema. *Pediatr Clin North Am* 4: 21, 1957.
Klein JO: Diagnostic lung puncture in the pneumonias of infants and children. *Pediatrics* 44: 486, 1969.
Marshall R, Teele DW, Klein JO: Unsuspected bacteremia due to *Haemophilus influenzae*: Outcome in children not initially admitted to hospital. *J Pediatr* 95: 690, 1979.
McCarthy PL, Frank Al, Ablow RC, et al.: Value of the C-reactive protein test in the differentiation of bacterial and viral pneumonia. *J Pediat* 92: 454, 1978.
Mimica L, Donoso E, Howard JE, et al.: Lung puncture in the etiologic diagnosis of pneumonia. *Am J Dis Child* 122: 278, 1971.
Shullteworth DB, Charney EL: Leukocyte count in pneumonia. *Am J Dis Child* 122: 393, 1971.

Nonbacterial Pneumonia

Arth C, Von Schmidt B, Grossman M, et al.: Chlamydial pneumonitis. *J Pediatr* 93: 447, 1978.
Beem M, Saxon E: Respiratory tract colonization and a distinctive pneumonia syndrome in infants with *Chlamydia trachomatis*. *N Engl J Med* 296: 396, 1977.
Beem MO, Saxon E, Tripple MA: Treatment of chlamydial pneumonia of infancy. *Pediatrics* 63: 198, 1979.
Brolin I, Wernstedt L: Radiologic appearance of mycoplasmal pneumonia. *Scand J Respir Dis* 59: 179, 1978.
Foy HM, Cooney MK, McMahon R, et al.: Viral and mycoplasmal pneumonia in a prepaid medical care group during an eight year period. *Am J Epidemiol* 97: 93, 1973.
Harrison HR, English MG, Lee CK, et al.: *Chlamydia trachomatis* infant pneumonitis. *N Engl J Med* 298: 702, 1978.

Bronchiolitis

Been M, Wright FH, Fasam DM, et al.: Observations on the etiology of acute bronchiolitis in infants. *J Pediatr* 61: 864, 1962.
Chanock RM, Kim HW, Vargoska HJ, et al.: Respiratory syncytial virus. Virus recovery and other observations during a 1960 outbreak of bronchiolitis, pneumonia, and minor respiratory disease in children. *JAMA* 176: 647, 1961.

Pertussis

Bass JW, Klenk EL, Korherine JB, et al.: Antimurobial treatment of pertusis. *J Pediatr* 75: 768, 1969.
Brooksaler F, Nelson JD: Pertussis: A reappraisal and report of 190 confirmed cases. *Am J Dis Child* 67: 56, 1967.

Whitaker JA, Donaldson P, Nelson JD: Diagnosis of pertussis by the fluorescent antibody method. *N Engl J Med* 263: 850, 1960.

Tuberculosis

Lincoln EM, Sewell EM: *Tuberculosis in Children.* McGraw Hill, New York, 1963.

Harris VJ, Scharf V, Duda F, et al.: Fatal tuberculosis in young children. *Pediatrics* 63: 912, 1977.

Gastroenteritis

Black RE, Jackson RJ, Tsac T, et al.: Epidemic *Yersinia enterocolitica* infection due to contaminated chocolate milk. *N Engl J Med* 298: 76, 1978.

Blackow NR, Cugor G: Viral gastroenteritis. *N Engl J Med* 304: 397, 1981.

Blair J, Fitzgerald SF: Treatment of nonspecific diarrhea in infants. *Clin Pediatr* 13: 333, 1974.

Butzler JP, Alexander M, Segers A, et al.: Enteritis, abscess, and septicemia due to *Yersinia enterocolitica* in a child with thalassemia. *J Pediatr* 93: 619, 1978.

Delorme J, Laverdiere M, Martinease B, et al: Yersiniosis in children. *Can Med Assoc J* 110: 281, 1974.

Dupont HL, Hornick RB: Adverse affect of Lomotil therapy in shigellosis. *JAMA* 226: 1525, 1973.

Evans RG, Dadsweli VJ: Human vibriosis. *Br Med J* 2: 240, 1967.

Guerrant RL, Moore RA, Kirschenfeld PM, et al.: Role of toxigenic and invasive bacteria in acute diarrhea of childhood. *N Eng J Med* 293: 567, 1975.

Gurwith MJ, Williams TW: Gastroenteritis in children. A two-year review in Manitoba. *J Infect Dis* 136: 239, 1973.

Jacobs JC: *Yersinia enterocolitica* arthritis. *Pediatrics* 55: 236, 1975.

Karmal MA, Fleming PC: Campylobacter enteritis in children. *J Pediatr* 94: 527, 1979.

Kohl S, Jacobson VA, Nahmias A: *Yersinia entercolitica* infections in children. *J Pediatr* 80: 77, 1976.

Kohl S: *Yersinia enterocolitica*: A significant new pathogen. *Hosp Pract* 131: 81, 1978.

Maki M, Maki R, Besikari T: Faecal leukocytes in campylobacter associated diarrhea in infants. *Acta Pediatr Scand* 68: 271, 1979.

Nelson J, Kusmiesz H, Jackson L, et al: Trimethoprim-sulfamethoxazole therapy for shigellosis. *JAMA* 235: 1239, 1976.

Pai CH, Sorger S, Lackman L, et al: Campylobacter gastroenteritis in children. *J Pediatr* 94: 589, 1979.

Rodriquez WJ, Kim HW, Arrobia JO, et al: Clinical features of acute gastroenteritis associated with human reovirus-like agents in infants and young children. *J Pediatr* 91: 188, 1977.

Rosenstein BH: Salmonellosis in infants and children. *J Pediatr* 70: 1, 1967.

Skirrow MB: Campylobacter enteritis: A new disease. *Br Med J* 2: 9, 1977.

Impetigo

Dajani, AS, Ferrieri P, Wanamaker LW: Natural history of impetigo. *J Clin Invest* 51: 2863, 1972.

Dillon HC: The treatment of streptococcal skin injections. *J Pediatr* 76: 676, 1970.

Cellulitis

Barkin RM, Todd JK, Amer J: Periorbital cellulitis in children. *Pediatrics* 62: 390, 1978.

Dajani AS, Barson AI, Thiramoorthi MC: Systemic *Haemophilus influenzae* disease: An overview. *J Pediatr* 94: 355, 1979.

Fleisher G, Ludwig, S, Campos J: Cellulitis: Bacterial etiology, clinical features, and laboratory findings. *J Pediatr* 94: 355, 1977.

Santos JI, Jacobson SA, Swensen P, et al: Cellulitis: Treatment with cefoxitin compared with multiple antibiotic therapy. *Pediatrics* 67: 887, 1981.

Varma BK: Cellulitis in children—A five year review. *Penn Med* 80: 43, 1977.

Uman SJ and Kunin CM: Needle aspiration in the diagnosis of soft tissue infections. *Arch Intern Med* 135: 959, 1975.

Septic Arthritis

Chusid MJ, Jacobs WM, Stay JR: Pseudomanas arthritis following puncture wounds of the foot. *J Pediatr* 94: 429, 1979.

Memon IA, Jacobs NM, Yeh TF, et al.: Group B streptococcal osteomyelitis and septic arthritis. *Am J Dis Child* 133: 921, 1979.

Molteni RA: The differential diagnosis of benign and septic joint disease in children. *Clin Pediatr* 17: 19, 1978.

Nelson, JD: The bacterial etiology and antibiotic management of septic arthritis in infants and children. *Pediatr* 50: 437, 1972.

Pittard WB, Thullen JD, Fanaroff AA: Neonatal septic arthritis. *J Pediatr* 88: 621, 1976.

Schaad UB, McCracken GH, Nelson JD: Pyogenic arthritis of the sacroiliac joint in pediatric patients. *Pediatrics* 66: 375, 1980.

Osteomyelitis

Bremmer A, Neligman G: Pyogenic Osteitis. *Recent Adv Pediatr* 2: 354, 1958.

Capitanio MA, Kirkpatrick JA: Early roentgen observations in acute osteomyelitis. *Am J Roentgenol* 108: 488, 1970.

Dich PQ, Nelson JD, Haltallin KC: Osteomyelitis in infants and children: A review of 163 cases. *Am J Dis Child* 129: 1273, 1975.

Edward MD, Baker CJ, Wagner ML, et al: An etiologic shift in infantile osteomyelitis: The emergence of the Group B streptococcus. *J Pediatr* 93: 578, 1978.

Fleisher GR, Paradise JE, Plotkin SA, et al.: Falsely normal radionuclide scans for osteomyelitis. *Am J Dis Child* 134: 499, 1980.

Granoff DM, Sargent E, Jolivette D: *Haemophilus influenzae* Type B osteomyelitis. *Am J Dis Child* 132: 488, 1978.

Minnefor AB, Olson MI, Carver DH: Pseudomonas osteomyelitis following puncture wounds of the foot. *Pediatrics* 47: 598, 1971.

Trevis S, Khettery J, Broker FH, et al.: Osteomyelitis: Early scintigraphic detection in children. *Pediatrics* 57: 173, 1976.

Waldvogel FA, Vasey H: Osteomyelitis: The past decade. *N Engl J Med* 303: 360, 1980.

Weissburg ED, Smith AL, Smith DH: Clinical features

of neonatal osteomyelitis. *Pediatrics* 33: 505, 1974.

Genitourinary Infections

Ackerman AB, Goldfaden G, Cosmides JC: Acquired syphilis in early childhood. *Arch Dermatol* 106: 92, 1972.

Branch G, Paxton R: A study of gonococcal infection among infants and children. *Public Health Rep* 80: 347, 1965.

Fleisher G, Hodge D, Cromie W: Penile edema in childhood gonorrhea. *Ann Emerg Med* 9: 314, 1980.

Hare M, Mowla A: Genital herpes virus infection in a prepubertal girl. *Br J Obstet Gynae Col* 84: 141, 1977.

Henretig FM: Acute urinary retention secondary to severe gonococcal balanoblennorrhea. *Pediatrics* 67: 734, 1981.

Tomeh MO, Wilfert CM: Venereal disease of infants and children at Duke University Medical Center. *North Car Med J* 34: 109, 1973.

Systemic Viral Infections

Barken RM: Measles Mortality: Analysis of the primary cause of death. *Am J Dis Child* 129: 307, 1975.

Fleisher G, Henle W, Henle G, et al.: Primary Epstein-Barr virus infections in American infants: Clinical and serological observation. *J Infect Dis* 139: 553, 1979.

Fleisher G, Henry W, McSorley M, Arbeter A, Plotkin S: Life-threatening complications of varicella. *Am J Dis Child* 135: 896, 1981.

Fleisher G, Lennete ET, Henele G, et al.: Incidence of heterophil antibody responses in children with infectious mononucleosis. *J Pediatr* 95: 63, 1979.

Fleisher G, Paradise J: Atypical lymphocytosis in children. *Ann Emerg Med* 10: 424, 1981.

Fleisher GR, Paradise JE, Lennette ET: The leukocyte response in childhood infectious mononucleosis. *Am J Dis Child* 135: 699, 1981.

Krugman S, Ward R, Katz S: *Infectious Disease of Children.* C. V. Mosby, St. Louis, 1981.

Weinstein L: Failure of chemotherapy to prevent the bacterial complications of measles. *N Engl J Med* 253: 679, 1955.

Rocky Mountain Spotted Fever

Bradford WD, Hawkins HK: Rocky Mountain spotted fever in children. *Am J Dis Child* 131: 1228, 1977.

Fleisher G, Lennette ET, Honig P: Diagnosis of Rocky Mountain spotted fever by immunfluorescent identification of Rickettsia ricketsii in skin biopsy tissue *J Pediatr* 95: 63, 1979.

Hattwick MAW, Retailliau H, O'Brien RJ: Fatal Rocky Mountain spotted fever. *JAMA* 240: 1499, 1979.

Vianna NJ, Hinman AR: Rocky Mountain spotted fever in Long Island. *Am J Med* 51: 725, 1971.

Woodward TE, Pederson CE, Oster CN, et al.: Prompt confirmation of Rocky Mountain spotted fever Identification of rickettsiae in skin tissues. *J Infect Dis* 134: 297, 1976.

Botulism

Grover W, Peckham G, Berman P: Recovery following cranial nerve dysfunction and muscle weakness in infancy. *Dev Med Child Neurol* 16: 163, 1979.

Johnson RO, Clay SA, Arnon SS: Diagnosis and management of infant botulism. *Am J Dis Child* 133: 586, 1979.

Pickett J, Berg B, Chaplin E, et al: Syndrome of botulism in infancy: Clinical and electrophysiologic study. *N Engl J Med* 295: 770, 1976.

Tetanus

Freelander FC: Tetanus neonatorum. *J Pediatr* 39: 448, 1951.

Turner TB, Velasco-Joven EA, Prudovsky S: Studies on the prophylaxis and treatment of tetanus. *Bull Johns Hopkins Hosp* 102: 71, 1958.

Weinstein L. Tetanus. *N Engl J Med* 289: 1293, 1973.

Rabies

Plotkin SA, Wiktor TJ, Koprowski H, et al.: Immunization schedules for the new human diploid cell vaccine. *Am J Epidemiol* 103: 75, 1976.

Toxic Shock Syndrome

Davis JP, Chesney PJ, Wand PJ, et al.: Toxic shock syndrome: Epidemiologic features, recurrence, risk factors, and prevention. *N Engl J Med* 303: 1429, 1980.

Todd J, Fishant M, Kapral F, et al.: Toxic-shock syndrome associated with phage-group-I staphylococci. *Lancet* 2: 1116, 1978.

CHAPTER 46

Renal and Electrolyte Emergencies

MICHAEL E. NORMAN, M.D.

ELECTROLYTE DISORDERS

Isotonic Dehydration

BACKGROUND

Isotonic dehydration reflects a loss of total body water coupled with a loss of Na* of an equal magnitude. Clinically, significant dehydration occurs commonly in childhood. Several factors predispose infants and children to dehydration including: (1) the frequent development of acute infections with high fevers, (2) their tendency to develop vomiting and diarrhea with nonenteral as well as enteral infections, and (3) the greater ratio of surface area to mass in the child.

Children may lose fluids through the gastrointestinal tract, the kidneys, and/or the skin. In the otherwise healthy child, gastrointestinal losses account for most instances of dehydration, the majority of these being due to either a viral or bacterial enteritis.

PATHOPHYSIOLOGY

An understanding of dehydration in the child requires a familiarity with fluid balance in the healthy individual as well as the pathophysiology of excessive fluid losses.

The daily maintenance fluid requirement is directly related to caloric expenditure. Since surface area correlates best with caloric expenditure, this parameter often serves as a guide to fluid therapy. However, the physician must either memorize estimated surface areas for children of various ages or calculate the area for each child using a nomogram based on the height and weight. Alternatively, the weight alone can rapidly provide a basis for establishing maintenance requirements. Since surface area increases at a slower rate than body mass (weight), the increment in maintenance fluids per kilogram decreases as the child grows in size. The maintenance requirement can be calculated from the following formulas:

Weight (kg)	*Fluid/24 hours*
<10	100 ml/kg
11–20	100 ml × 10 + 50 ml for each kg over 10
>21	100 ml × 10 + 50 ml × 10 + 20 ml for each kg over 20

The maintenance requirement for electrolytes directly relates to the caloric expenditure which also determines the requirement for water. For Na, this is 2 to 3 meq/100 ml and for K, 2 meq/100 ml. As an example, a 30-kg child would have a daily maintenance requirement for fluid of 1700 ml (100 ml/kg × 10 kg + 50 ml/kg × 10 kg + 20 ml/kg × 10 kg). The requirement for Na would be 34 to 51 meq and for K, 34 meq.

* Extreme hyperproteinemia and/or hyperlipidemia may result in an apparently low Na concentration in the extracellular fluid by decreasing the percentage of water contained in a unit volume of plasma (normally 93%). This displacement is given by the formula: ml H_2O per 100 ml plasma = 99.1 − [(1.03 × total lipid in g/dl) + (0.73 + total protein in g/dl)].

Isotonic dehydration is defined as a loss of total body water with the maintenance of a normal serum [Na] ranging from 135 to 145 meq/L. The final [Na] in the extracellular fluid (ECF) is a function not only of what is lost from the body but of the composition of replacement fluids administered at home and transcellular shifts of fluid as well. The initial loss of fluid from the body depletes the ECF; gradually, water shifts from the intracellular space to maintain the ECF and this fluid is lost if dehydration persists. If dehydration is acute (the duration of the illness is <3 days) approximately 80% of the fluid loss is from the ECF and 20% from the intracellular fluid (ICF). Additional fluid moves out of the ICF if the loss continues for 3 or more days. In such cases the proportion of fluid lost from the two compartments is 60% from the ECF and 40% from ICF. ECF contains predominately Na at a concentration of 140 meq/L and ICF, K at a concentration of 150 meq/L.

CLINICAL MANIFESTATIONS

A careful history taken from the parents of a child with isotonic dehydration helps both to establish the cause for the fluid loss and to estimate the degree of depletion. Specific inquiries must be made as to the volume of the child's intake and output, focusing on gastrointestinal and renal function. The physician should ask about the amount and duration of vomiting, diarrhea, and/or other abnormal losses as well as the adequacy of urine flow. In infants, the absence of tears with crying and a decrease in the number of wet diapers suggest the presence of dehydration.

The physical examination should begin with a careful weighing of the child since this is the most accurate clinical indicator of dehydration. The signs of dehydration become more apparent as the degree of dehydration increases (Table 14.2, Chapter 14, "Diarrhea"). With a 5% loss of body weight, the skin and mucous membranes feel dry, but there are no signs of vascular instability. Tachycardia and hypotension appear if the loss of fluid exceeds this mark, and the skin turgor shows a marked decrease. The development of acidosis leads to tachypnea and contributes to poor peripheral perfusion. If the child has lost more than 10% of body weight in a brief period of time, signs of shock may appear including a rapid, thready pulse, marked hypotension, and cold, clammy skin (see Chapter 2).

By definition, the [Na] falls within the normal range, 135 to 145 meq/L, in isotonic dehydration. In mild dehydration, the serum bicarbonate is usually 15 to 20 meq/L, but it may drop to 6 to 10 meq/L with more severe losses. The [K] is usually normal (3.5 to 5.0 meq/L), although transcellular shifts due to acidosis may elevate the serum level (see p. 427). The BUN rises proportionately to the degree of fluid loss, varying from 20 to 30 mg/dl in mild dehydration to 50 to 100 mg/dl in more severe cases. However, the BUN may show less of an increase than expected from the clinical estimate of dehydration if the child's protein intake has been markedly limited in the preceding 24 to 48 hours.

Urine flow is usually scant or absent, but an effort should be made to obtain a specimen. In older children with dehydration, the specific gravity rises above 1.020, often reaching 1.035. Infants, however, have a relative lack of renal concentrating ability. Even in the face of severe dehydration in the child in the first three months of life, the urine specific gravity may be only 1.020.

MANAGEMENT

In all children with significant dehydration ($\geqq$5%), an intravenous infusion should be started and blood sent to the laboratory for measurement of electrolytes and BUN. The child with shock demands immediate fluid resuscitation and monitoring as described in Chapter 1. With lesser degrees of dehydration, the optimal type and rate of fluid infusion is calculated on the basis of the child's estimated ideal weight and degree of dehydration. Sufficient fluids are administered in the first 24 hours to fulfill the maintenance requirement and correct the total deficit; half of the deficit is replaced in the first 8 hours.

Example. A 5-month-old infant has a 3-day history of diarrhea and a decreased oral intake. One week previously, she weighed

5.0 kg in the pediatrician's office. Now she weighs 4.5 kg and has a temperature of 37.0°C, pulse of 120/min, respiratory rate of 30/min, and blood pressure of 80/40. The child's skin and mucosa are dry, and the skin shows "tenting" if lifted. The urine specific gravity is 1.028, and the serum electrolytes are as follows: [Na] 135 meq/L; [K] 4.0 meq/L; [Cl], 90 meq/L; and [HCO_3], 9.0 meq/L. The BUN is 30 mg/dl.

This infant has lost 10% of its body weight. Since acute decreases in weight reflect fluid loss, the fluid deficit is 500 ml. Dehydration has occurred over a 3-day period indicating that 60% of the loss is from the ECF and 40% from the ICF. Thus, the Na and K deficits are calculated as follows:

$$\text{Na deficit} = 140 \text{ meq}/100 \text{ ml} \times 60\% \times 500 \text{ ml} = 42 \text{ meq}$$
$$\text{K deficit} = 150 \text{ meq}/1000 \text{ ml} \times 40\% \times 500 \text{ ml} = 30 \text{ meq}$$

The maintenance requirements for this infant are 500 ml of fluid (100 ml/kg × 5 kg), 15 meq of Na (3 meq/100 ml × 500 ml), and 10 meq of K (2 meq/100 ml × 500 ml) for each 24-hour period.

One half of the fluid and Na deficit is replaced during the first 8 hours of rehydration. Thus, the infant would receive 250 ml of deficit fluid with 21 meq of Na. In addition to this, one third of the maintenance requirement, or 175 ml of fluid with 5 meq of Na, would be given for a total of 425 ml of fluid with 25 meq of Na.

Only half of the K deficit is corrected during each of the first 2 days, and this is done at a constant rate. Since the maintenance K for this infant is 15 meq and the deficit is 30 meq, the amount of K administered would be 30 meq daily for the first 48 hours. The solution would also need to contain an appropriate amount of bicarbonate (see p. 435).

Disorders of Sodium (Na) Homeostasis

Hyponatremia

BACKGROUND

Hyponatremia is defined as a measured serum Na concentration of less than 135 meq/L in the ECF. No specific environmental or genetic factors are known to result in hyponatremia. The etiologies of hyponatremia are multiple and diverse, but can be grouped into four categories (Table 46.1).

PATHOPHYSIOLOGY

Basic Mechanisms. To understand hyponatremia, two fundamental principles regulating Na and water balance will be reviewed. First, total body Na determines ECF volume, because water moves freely throughout all body compartments to restore a disturbed osmotic equilibrium and Na is the predominant regulator of osmotic equilibrium in the ECF space. Hyponatremia may result after the restoration of osmotic equilibrium in response to an absolute or relative gain of water or an absolute or relative loss of salt from the body. Looked at in this way, it should be clear that total body Na can be normal, low, or even increased in the face of hyponatremia. Second, the kidney normally defends against hyponatremia by its ability to dilute

Table 46.1
Etiologies of Hyponatremia

I. *Normal Total Body Water and Na (Hyperosmolar Hyponatremia)*
   A. Hyperglycemia[a]
   B. Mannitol, glycerol therapy
II. *Increased Total Body Water and Na (Edema-forming States)*
   A. Congestive heart failure
   B. Nephrosis
   C. Cirrhosis
   D. Acute renal failure
III. *Decreased Total Body Water and Na (Hypovolemic States)*
   A. Gastrointestinal losses (vomiting, diarrhea, fistulas)
   B. Renal losses (diuretics, renal tubular acidosis, primary interstitial disease)
   C. Adrenal (mineralocorticoid) deficiencies
   D. Third space losses (ascites, burns)
IV. *Increased Total Body Water but Normal Total Body Na*
   A. Syndrome of inappropriate antidiuretic hormone
   B. Water intoxication

[a] For every 100 mg/dl rise in plasma glucose concentration above normal, there is a corresponding decrease in plasma sodium concentration of approximately 1.6 meq/liter.

the urine. Since urinary dilution depends on glomerular filtrate rate (GFR), proximal tubular reabsorption of Na, delivery of fluid to the distal tubular diluting segment and antidiuretic hormone (ADH), disturbances in any of these mechanisms could lead to hyponatremia.

Applications. The causes of hyponatremia are listed in Table 46.1 and grouped according to the net changes in total body water and total body Na. When glucose, mannitol or glycerol is present in plasma in high concentrations, water moves into the ECF, lowering Na concentration in the face of elevated osmolality (Table 46.1, *I*). In the edema forming states listed under *II* in Table 46.1, a decreased effective circulating plasma volume is sensed by the kidney as hypoperfusion. Sodium is maximally reabsorbed, the urine is concentrated because of maximum ADH secretion, and hyponatremia often ensues. Acute reduction in GFR, and decreased delivery of fluid to the distal tubular diluting site, often results in hyponatremia in acute renal failure, especially if the patient is ingesting hypotonic fluids. When extrarenal losses of Na and water lead to negative Na balance and a diminished ECF volume (Table 46.1, *III*), inhibitory signals from the osmoreceptors to block ADH release are overcome by stimulatory signals from the volume receptors. Water reabsorption is maximal, the urine is concentrated and hyponatremia results. In renal and adrenal Na wasting (Table 46.1, *III*), negative Na balance and ECF volume contraction occur in the face of inappropriately high urine Na concentrations. In the specific situations of diuretic abuse or adrenal insufficiency, hyponatremia results from a fall in GFR and an increased compensatory proximal Na reabsorption, leading to decreased delivery of fluid to distal diluting segments. ADH is also stimulated and renal water excretion falls. Structural renal disease also impairs Na and chloride reabsorption at the diluting site leading to hyponatremia. Finally, hyponatremia occurs in states of markedly increased water intake or inappropriate water reabsorption by the kidney under the influence of ADH (Table 46.1, *IV*). Although only one third of the increased total body water is distributed in the ECF, this modest volume expansion will lead to an inappropriately high urinary Na concentration and increased quantitative Na excretion. The most common causes of hyponatremia seen in the emergency department are gastrointestinal losses and water intoxication, the latter occurring particularly in infancy.

CLINICAL MANIFESTATIONS

Symptoms and signs of hyponatremia per se are directly related to both the absolute level and the rate of fall of serum Na from the normal range, but are in themselves somewhat nonspecific (Table 46.2). For example, one child may be dramatically symptomatic at a serum Na of 125 meq/L if the Na had fallen 15 meq/L in only 1 to 2 hours and equilibrium had not yet been restored, whereas a second child might be totally asymptomatic at a serum Na of 120 meq/L if the Na had fallen 20 meq/L in 2 to 3 days and osmotic equilibrium had been reestablished. Specific symptoms and signs do not correlate with specific levels of serum Na. The clinical examination can help in limiting the possible diagnoses to explain the hyponatremia. Thus, patients with obvious edema would fall into category *II* in Table 46.1, and those with obvious signs of a contracted ECF volume would fall into category *III*.

Complications requiring urgent diagnosis include Cheyne-Stokes respirations and seizures. However, a clouded sensorium and pathologic reflexes are often warning signs of seizures. The laboratory studies required to initiate the assessment of most children with symptomatic hyponatremia are given in Table 46.3.

Table 46.2
Symptoms and Signs of Hyponatremia

Symptoms	Signs
Anorexia	Clouded sensorium
Nausea	Decreased tendon reflexes
Muscle cramps	Pathologic reflexes
Lethargy	Cheyne-Stokes respiration
Apathy	Hypothermia
Disorientation	Pseudobulbar palsy
Agitation	Seizures

Table 46.3
Laboratory Evaluation of Hyponatremia

I. Blood
- A. Electrolytes (Na, K, Cl, HCO_3)
- B. BUN, creatinine
- C. Liver function tests
- D. Osmolality

II. Urine
- A. Urinalysis including specific gravity
- B. Urine Na
- C. Urine creatinine
- D. Urine osmolality

MANAGEMENT

Armed with a working knowledge of pathophysiology, the clinical history and examination, and the few simple laboratory tests as outlined in Table 46.3, the emergency physician should be able to rapidly diagnose the specific cause of hyponatremia in most cases. A specific diagnosis is necessary because therapies differ markedly, depending on the etiology of the hyponatremia. A working schema is outlined in Figure 46.1.

In the patient with hyponatremia in the face of obvious contraction of ECF volume, reexpansion with isotonic saline is the appropriate therapy. The volume and rate of infusion are dictated by estimates of fluid (i.e., weight) loss from the history and physical examination. In shock, 20 ml/kg of isotonic saline or 10% dextrose in isotonic saline can be administered rapidly over 1 hour and then repeated as necessary until the blood pressure and peripheral circulation return to normal. Underlying diseases, such as renal tubular acidosis and adrenal insufficiency, can be most effectively treated by specific replacement therapy. Diuretics, if previously given, should be promptly discontinued.

In water intoxication, restriction of daily free water administration by 25 to 50%, depending on the chronicity and severity of the hyponatremia, is the treatment of choice. In the acutely ill patient, temporary relief of symptoms may be accomplished by elevating the serum Na by 10 meq/L with the intravenous administration of 3% sodium chloride in the following manner: ml 3% NaCl (0.5 meq/ml) to give = 10 meq/L × body wt (kg) × 0.2 (ECF space). Alternatively, 10 to 12 ml/kg of 3% NaCl can be infused over 1 hour.

In simple water intoxication, the normal kidney responds with maximal urinary dilution which, when coupled with restriction of water intake, will rapidly restore Na concentration to normal. In the syndrome of inappropriate secretion of ADH (see p. 647), water restriction is the initial treatment of choice but is not always effective.

Finally, in the edema-forming states and acute renal failure, hyponatremia is usually mild and water restriction will usually suffice. In some patients, diuretics may be necessary to treat the underlying disease. In such situations, free water excretion is increased but at the risk of inducing ECF volume contraction through increased Na excretion.

Admission is recommended for any patient with symptomatic hyponatremia or severe hyponatremia per se (<130 meq/L) when the etiology is not obvious.

Hypernatremia

BACKGROUND

Hypernatremia is defined as a measured serum Na concentration of greater than 145 meq/L in the ECF. The frequency of hypernatremic dehydration as a cause of hypernatremia reflects different geographical patterns of feeding practices for children with vomiting and diarrheal illnesses. In some regions the use of hyperosmolar (especially hypernatremic) oral solutions contributes to the observed hypernatremia. Currently published recommendations for use of commercially prepared balanced electrolyte solutions in the oral therapy of diarrhea should counter this problem.

As with hyponatremia, the etiologies of hypernatremia can be grouped into four major categories (Table 46.4) on the basis of net changes in total body water and Na.

PATHOPHYSIOLOGY

The same general principles regulating Na and water balance must be applied to understand conditions of hyper- as well as hyponatremia. In hypernatremia, there is either an absolute or relative water deficit, which can occur in the face of normal,

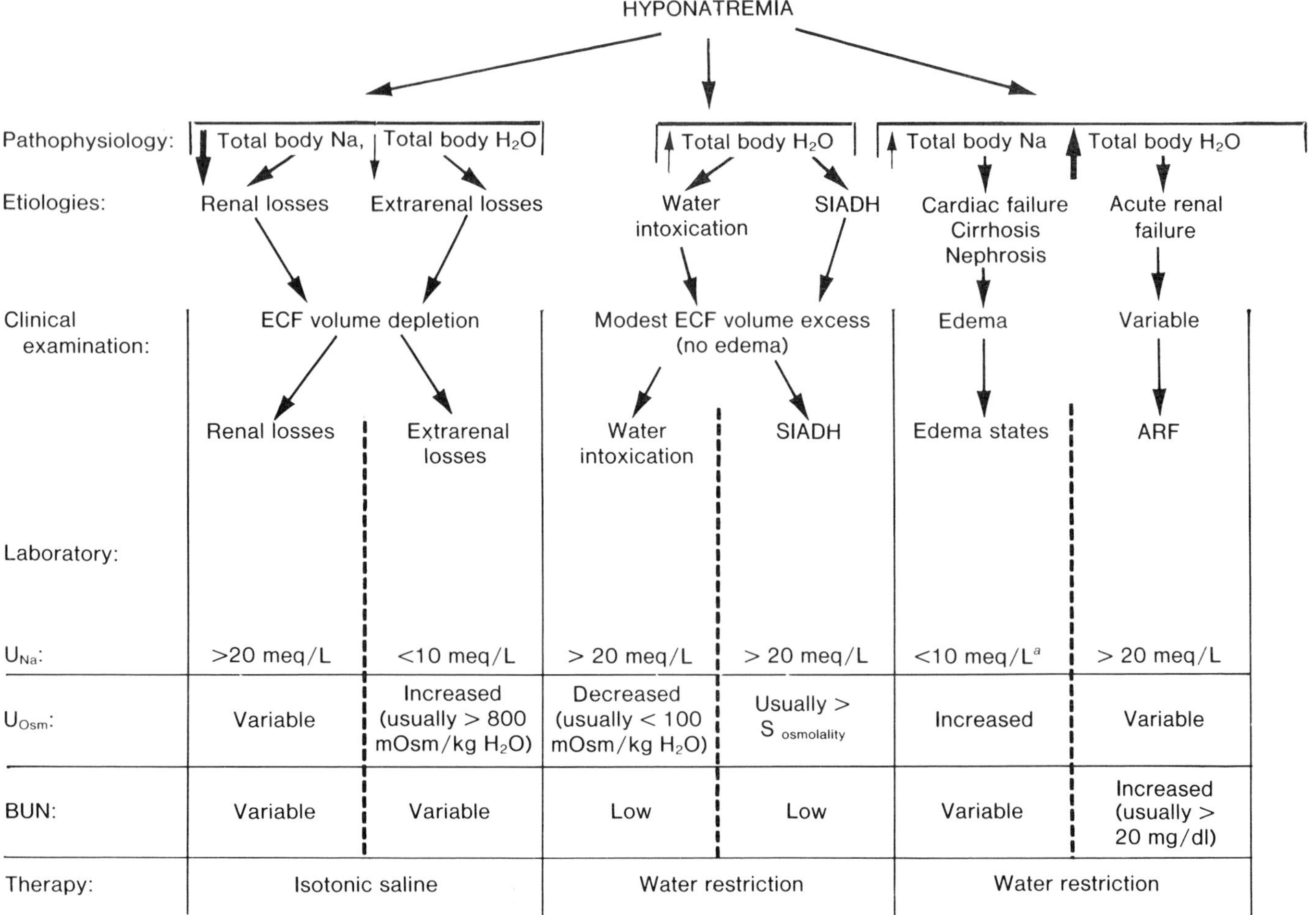

Figure 46.1 Approach to hyponatremia. U_{Na} = urinary sodium; U_{Osm} = urinary osmolality; SIDAH = syndrome of inappropriate antidiuretic hormone; *ECF* = extracellular fluid; (*a*) = in the absence of prior diuretic therapy.

increased or even decreased total body Na (Table 46.4).

In Na poisoning, water moves into the ECF in response to an increase in Na, and the initial physical findings are usually those of obvious expansion of the ECF (Table 46.4, *I*). Eventually, some of this "new" ECF water will be lost when the kidney excretes the extra Na.

An important cause of hypernatremia in pediatrics is the ADH-"deficiency" syndrome (Table 46.1, II.B), due to partial or complete central diabetes insipidus and partial or complete nephrogenic diabetes insipidus. The latter may be due to a variety of primary renal tubular disorders, hypokalemia, hypercalcemia and/or the rare familial form inherited usually as a sex-linked dominant trait. These patients with "pure" renal water losses manifest signs of neither ECF expansion nor depletion, unless of course they are denied free access to water or have an associated hypothalamic (e.g., thirst center) disturbance, in which case signs of ECF volume depletion supervene. Normally, the maximum stimulus for urinary concentration is a body weight loss of 3 to 5%; this response is blunted or absent in diabetes insipidus, and the urine is inappropriately hypotonic. Compulsive water drinking is sometimes confused with pituitary diabetes insipidus, but can be easily separated if the following facts are remembered: (1) in the former, polyuria is due to polydipsia, whereas in the latter the converse is true; (2) water intake is variable in compulsive water drinking, but consistent in diabetes insipidus; (3) the onset of polyuria is usually gradual in compulsive water drinking, but often abrupt in diabetes insipidus; and (4) serum Na concentration is usually normal to low in compulsive water drinking but elevated in diabetes insipidus! Occasionally a child will lose large quantities of water through hyperventilation or sweating in a hot, humid environment without adequate water replacement, leading to hyponatremia. Here, too, the normal renal response concentrates the urine, although the Na concentration may vary.

Table 46.4
Etiologies of Hypernatremia

I. Increased Total Body Na or Increased Total Body Na Greater than Increased Total Body Water
- A. Na poisoning (accidental; Na bicarbonate therapy)
- B. Hyperaldosteronism (rare in children)

II. Normal Total Body Na; "Pure" Water Loss
- A. Insensible losses—respiratory and skin
- B. Renal (central and nephrogenic diabetes insipidus)

III. Decreased Total Body Na Less than Decreased Total Body Water
- A. Extrarenal (gastrointestinal)[a]
- B. Renal (osmotic diuretics: glucose, mannitol, urea)

IV. Normal Total Body Na and Water with Abnormal Central Osmotic Regulation of Water Balance
- A. Essential hypernatremia

[a] In diarrheal states, hypernatremia usually results from a combination of relatively greater water than Na losses coupled with relatively greater Na than water replacement.

When total body Na is reduced due to abnormal gastrointestinal fluid losses, the physical signs are those of contraction of the ECF with recent weight loss, dry mucus membranes and, once fluid losses are very marked, poor skin turgor (Table 46.4, *III-A*). The renal response is directed toward restoring the ECF volume with maximum conservation of Na and water. Thus, the urine is concentrated and contains little Na. During an osmotic diuresis, more water than Na is lost in hypernatremia and volume depletion. Excessive solute, unreabsorbed in the proximal tubule, obligates water delivery distally and impairs free water generation. This leads to a reduced renal concentrating capacity, enhancing urinary Na and water losses (Table 46.4, III.B).

Finally, a few children have been described with primary central nervous system tumors or infection, leading to a resetting of the osmoreceptors governing water balance at a higher than normal level (Table 46.4, *IV-A*). When serum osmolality is then perturbed about that new setting, appropriate renal diluting or concentrating responses occur. The hypernatremia fluctuates but is usually mild.

This most common cause of hypernatremia in the emergency department is hypernatremic dehydration secondary to diarrhea.

CLINICAL MANIFESTATIONS

Most of the symptoms and signs of hypernatremia result from cellular dehydration as water moves into the ECF space to lower osmolality. Brain cells are the most vulnerable to water loss, especially if the loss is acute. Symptoms and signs range from lethargy and irritability to muscle weakness, convulsions and coma. If, on the other hand, hypernatremia develops more slowly, brain cells defend their volume by manufacturing additional intracellular solute (so-called idiogenic osmoles) which reduces water loss to the ECF. Therefore, symptoms and signs are related both to the level of serum Na concentration and its rate of rise. By the same token, therefore, rapid restoration of ECF osmolality to normal after the slow development of a hyperosmolar (e.g., hypernatremic) state does not permit brain cells to inactivate idiogenic osmoles, and cerebral edema may result! Finally, because ECF volume is defended early in the course of a dehydrating illness associated with hypernatremia, the classic physical sign of decreased skin turgor is absent until total fluid losses are severe (~10 to 15% of body weight).

The major complications of hypernatremia which require urgent diagnosis are seizures and coma.

The laboratory studies required to initiate the assessment of most children with symptomatic hypernatremia are the same as those given for hyponatremia in Table 46.3. In addition, hypernatremia is the initial manifestation of primary central nervous system disease in some children, and a formal neurologic evaluation may be indicated after treatment of the electrolyte disturbance.

MANAGEMENT

As in the hyponatremic states, the emergency physician should be able to reach a specific category of disease or diagnosis armed with a working knowledge of pathophysiology, clinical evaluation of the status of ECF volume, and a few simple serum and urine tests. Since emergency therapies vary considerably between the disorders noted in Table 46.4, accuracy of interpretation is important. Figure 46.2 provides a working schema.

In patients who are severely dehydrated and in shock, reexpansion with isotonic saline is the appropriate initial therapy (see under "Hyponatremia"). Osmotic diuretics, if previously given, must be stopped. Replacement of water and Na losses with hypotonic electrolyte solutions is appropriate but, in the case of diarrhea, serum Na should be lowered slowly (usually no more than 10 to 15 meq/L/24 hours) to guard against brain edema. In hypertonic dehydration, free water deficit of 4 ml/kg for every meq/L of serum Na greater than 145 meq/L should be replaced over 48 to 72 hours.

For example, a 5-month-old infant has a 3-day history of diarrhea. Last week she weighed 5.0 kg but now she weighs 4.5 kg. She has been receiving undiluted skim milk and "salt water" orally. Vital signs are normal. Electrolytes are: [Na] 160 meq/L; [Cl] 120 meq/L; [CO_2] 10 meq/L; and [K] 3.5 meq/L. This patient has lost 10% of her body weight, but is asymptomatic because of relative preservation of the ECF space in hypernatremia. That percentage of the total (i.e., 500 ml) fluid deficit that is to be replaced as solute-free water is calculated as follows:

$$\text{Free water (ml)} = [160\text{–}145 \text{ meq/L}] \times 4 \text{ ml/kg} \times 5 \text{ kg} = 300 \text{ ml}$$

This is given slowly over 2 days in order to lower serum Na by approximately 10 meq/L. The other 200 ml of the deficit are also given slowly over 2 days as solute-containing fluid. Calculation of the Na deficit (i.e., the amount of Na to put in the remaining 200 ml of volume deficit) can be made from any one of a number of general formulas that are based on certain fundamental assumptions about fluid and electrolyte physiology as discussed under Isotonic Dehydration. If one views the solute-containing fluid deficit as coming 40% from the ICF and 60% from the ECF, then deficits of Na and K are as follows:

1. ECF: 60% × 200 ml × 145 meq/L, [Na] = 17 meq
2. ICF: 40% × 200 ml × 150 meq/L, [K] = 12 meq

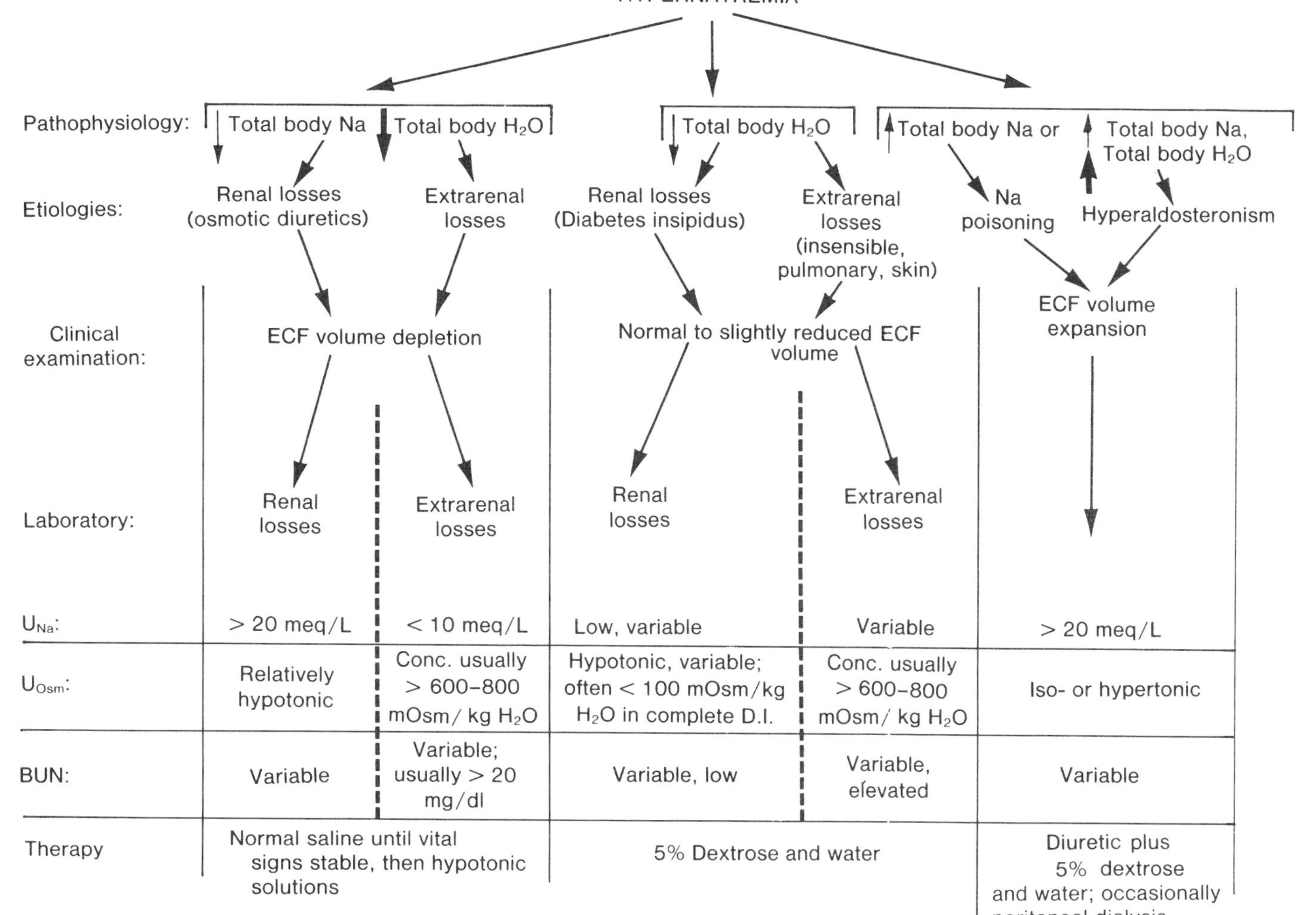

Figure 46.2 Approach to hypernatremia. U_{Na} = urinary sodium; U_{Osm} = urinary osmolality; *ECF* = extracellular fluid.

In practice, the usual tonicity of the total deficit plus maintenance fluid that is infused is usually ¼ to ½ normal tonicity for Na.

In patients with increased insensible water losses, simple free water replacement with glucose solutions is all that is required. Here, monitoring weight and serum Na concentrations are useful guides to the adequacy of therapy. Correction can usually be given over several days.

The emergency treatment of the diabetes insipidus syndromes is free water replacement, monitoring vital signs, clinical signs of dehydration and serum Na concentration as guides to the rate and volume of replacement. There is no place for the use of various antidiuretic agents that promote ADH release or mimic its actions in central diabetes insipidus, or for thiazide diuretics in nephrogenic diabetes insipidus as initial therapies.

Children who are victims of acute salt poisoning and severely symptomatic can safely have serum Na concentrations lowered rapidly either by a combination of loop diuretics (furosemide 0.5 to 2 mg/kg every 12 hours) and glucose water administration or, rarely, peritoneal dialysis against a Na-free dialysate. The latter procedure should only be carried out in consultation with a pediatric nephrologist. Admission is recommended for any patient with symptomatic hypernatremia or severe hypernatremia per se (greater than 160 meq/L) when the etiology is not obvious.

Disorders of Potassium (K) Homeostasis

Hypokalemia

BACKGROUND

Hypokalemia is defined as a measured serum K concentration of less than 3.5 meq/L. No specific environmental factors are known to result in hypokalemia. A rare genetic cause of hypokalemia which affects children is familial periodic paralysis. The etiologies of hypokalemia are varied. With the exception of transcellular shifts of K, most causes of hypokalemia result in increased renal K excretion either as a primary or secondary event. The four major categories of hypokalemia are shown in Table 46.5.

Table 46.5
Etiologies of Hypokalemia

I. *Apparent K Deficit (Transcellular Shifts)*
   A. Alkalosis
   B. Familial hypokalemic periodic paralysis
II. *Decreased Intake*
   A. Anorexia nervosa
   B. Unusual diets (rare in pediatrics)
III. *Extrarenal Losses*
   A. Protracted vomiting (e.g., pyloric stenosis or gastric suction)
   B. Protracted diarrhea
   C. Ureterosigmoidostomy
   D. Laxative abuse (rare in pediatrics)
   E. Increased sweating (cystic fibrosis)
IV. *Renal Losses*
   A. Diuretic abuse (naturetic, osmotic agents)
   B. Renal tubular acidosis
   C. Diabetic ketoacidosis
   D. Excessive mineralocorticoid effect
      1. Primary/secondary hyperaldosteronism
      2. Bartter's syndrome
      3. Licorice abuse (rare in pediatrics)
      4. Cushing's syndrome (rare in pediatrics)
   E. Excessive administration of "impermeant anions" (carbenicillin)

PATHOPHYSIOLOGY

Basic Mechanisms. When confronted with unexpected hypokalemia, the emergency physician is, for all practical purposes, dealing with one of two pathophysiologic situations: (1) K shifts into cells in exchange for H^+ ion, or (2) extrarenal or renal losses. K shifts into cells in response to alkalosis and out of cells in response to acidosis; for every 0.1 unit rise or fall in pH, there is a reciprocal change in ECF K concentration of approximately 0.6 meq/L. Insulin facilitates cellular uptake of K by a mechanism as yet unexplained but which is independent of glucose uptake. In view of these observations, and the knowledge that K is primarily an intracellular cation, it can be appreciated that ECF K concentration does not reflect the status of total body K. Therefore, when evaluating total body K in light of disturbances in ECF K concentrations, the plasma pH or H^+ ion concentration must be known.

The mechanisms governing renal K excretion are outlined in Table 46.6. Potassium is filtered at the glomerulus and virtually completely reabsorbed in the proximal tubule. That K which appears in the

Table 46.6
Factors Governing Renal K Excretion

Aldosterone
Na delivery to the distal tubule
H^+ ion secretion
Nonreabsorbable anion
Urine flow rate
K intake

urine is the result of distal tubular secretion. Hyperaldosteronism increases Na-K exchange in the distal tubule. Conditions which increase Na delivery to the distal tubule, such as volume expansion, also lead to increased K excretion.

Applications. Alkalosis increases distal tubular delivery of bicarbonate (i.e., luminal negativity) which in turn enhances K secretion; secretion is also enhanced by the high cellular K concentration in response to the elevated systemic pH. Increased urine flow rate enhances K excretion. Finally, increased K intake increases renal excretion. In familial hypokalemic periodic paralysis, an as yet undefined abnormality in muscle cell membranes leads to a movement of K into cells with a consequent fall in serum K.

Renal conservation of K in response to a reduced intake or extrarenal losses is slower than that for Na, and takes 1 to 2 weeks to occur. Potassium depletion and the resultant hypokalemia that occur with vomiting do not result primarily from the K lost in the vomitus itself! In fact, the gastric fluid concentration of K is only 5 to 10 meq/L. Rather, renal losses account for most of the K deficit seen with vomiting. ECF volume depletion leads to secondary hyperaldosteronism and alkalosis leads to increased bicarbonate delivery to the distal tubule. Both of these phenomena increase urinary losses of K. In addition, with continued volume depletion, alkalosis is maintained because the proximal tubule preferentially reabsorbs Na bicarbonate to restore ECF volume (filtered chloride is reduced and K shifts into cells). Early in the course of vomiting, hypokalemia can be corrected merely by restoring ECF volume with isotonic saline without K supplements, providing convincing evidence of the role of volume contraction in causing renal K wasting! Chronic diarrhea results in large K losses. Ureterosigmoidostomy can lead to K and bicarbonate secretion in exchange for Na and Cl reabsorption, resulting in a hyperchloremic, hypokalemic acidosis. In cystic fibrosis, volume contraction can result from excessive cutaneous losses of water, Na and Cl through increased sweating in the summer months. This may lead to renal K wasting and alkalosis.

One of the hallmarks of renal tubular acidosis is hypokalemia, which is paradoxical in view of the corresponding acidosis. Renal K wasting results from secondary hyperaldosteronism and bicarbonaturia. The marked glycosuria of diabetic ketoacidosis increases urine flow rate and distal Na delivery, thus enhancing K excretion. Bartter's syndrome is an uncommon, poorly understood cause of hypochloremic, hypokalemic metabolic alkalosis. Hypokalemia is frequently profound and resistant to replacement therapy. The mechanism is probably either a primary renal chloride or K leak. Impermeant anions such as phosphate, sulfate, and organic compounds enhance K excretion by increasing tubular luminal negativity, thus increasing K secretion.

CLINICAL MANIFESTATIONS

The cause of hypokalemia can usually be suspected as belonging to one particular diagnostic category after obtaining a careful history. For example, in familial periodic paralysis, the weakness comes on gradually over a few hours and may last 48 to 72 hours. It may be heralded by short episodes of weakness in one or more extremities. It usually occurs during periods of rest after vigorous exercise or a carbohydrate load.

Potassium depletion can result in widespread disturbances in cellular physiology and function, although symptoms are usually not seen at serum K concentrations above 3 meq/L. The major abnormalities and their clinical consequences are listed in Table 46.7. The most important clinical manifestations of hypokalemia relate to abnormal neuromuscular function. Impulse formation and propagation and the resultant muscle contraction are impaired in both striated and smooth muscle, leading to ileus, tetany, skeletal muscle weakness,

Table 46.7
Pathophysiological (Clinical) Consequences of Hypokalemia

Muscle cell dysfunction (rhabdomyolysis)
Cardiac cell dysfunction (myocardiopathy, arrhythmias)
Neuromuscular dysfunction (weakness-paralysis, ileus, tetany, encephalopathy with underlying liver disease)
Renal (polydipsia, polyuria, concentration defect)

Table 46.8
Laboratory Evaluation of Hypokalemia

I. Blood
- A. Electrolytes (Na, K, Cl, HCO_3)
- B. BUN
- C. Glucose
- D. Arterial blood gas
- E. Creatinine phosphokinase

II. Urine
- A. Urinalysis
- B. Urine Na, K, Cl
- C. Urine pH
- D. Urine osmolality

III. Other[a]
- A. ECG
- B. Plain abdominal x-ray
- C. Upper gastrointestinal series

[a] Selection of studies depends upon the suspected diagnosis.

and, if severe enough, paralysis and areflexia.

Hypokalemia may cause rhabdomyolysis with myoglobinuria. Alteration of the cardiac action potential by slowing the rate of repolarization leads to conduction abnormalities and arrhythmias. ECG changes include depression of ST segments, reduced T wave voltage and increased U wave voltage. However, while the signs and symptoms of hypokalemia generally parallel its rate of development and its severity, ECG changes frequently fail to correlate with serum K. They are helpful if present but not reassuring if absent! In the presence of digitalis, however, hypokalemia is much more likely to produce cardiac arrhythmias.

Complications requiring urgent diagnosis include acute respiratory failure from muscle paralysis, cardiac arrhythmias, and myoglobinuria which can lead to acute renal failure.

Laboratory and radiologic evaluations are outlined in Table 46.8. Generally, in situations of total body K depletion, a 1 meq/L fall in serum K concentration reflects a 100 to 200 meq K deficit. This figure may be somewhat lower in young children. The blood glucose rises in diabetes mellitus and creatinine phosphokinase with rhabdomyolysis. An increased BUN reflects contraction of ECF volume. If the electrolytes reveal a hyperchloremic hypokalemic metabolic acidosis with a normal anion gap and an alkaline urine pH, renal tubular acidosis should be suspected. When there is a hypochloremic metabolic alkalosis, the urine electrolytes are helpful. A urine chloride less than 10 meq/L suggests vomiting, cystic fibrosis or diuretic abuse as the cause of hypokalemia. A urine chloride of greater than 20 meq/L points to one of the disorders leading to mineralocorticoid excess. When the urinary K is less than 20 meq/L, several conclusions can be drawn. First, the K deficiency has probably been present for at least 2 weeks. Second, the kidney can be excluded as the route of K depletion. On the other hand, a urinary K concentration of greater than 20 meq/L suggests either K wasting of short duration or a primary renal loss. In similar fashion, a urinary concentrating defect which persists in the face of a stimulus to concentrate bespeaks chronic K depletion.

MANAGEMENT

When hypokalemia results from simple transcellular shifts in response to alkalosis without an accompanying K deficit, correction of the pH is all that is required. In periodic paralysis, K supplementation with 2 to 6 meq/kg/day is recommended with careful monitoring of serum K to avoid hyperkalemia as paralysis subsides. An important principle to remember when treating hypokalemia is that before K can move into cells, it must first traverse the relatively small intravascular compartment. Slight changes in serum K concentration can effect large changes in transmembrane electrical potential gradients and, by this, neuromuscular excitation. Therefore, in most circumstances K repletion should be slow (over days) and given by the oral route once urine flow is confirmed. Intravenous loading should be avoided except under very special conditions (see below). Despite the fact that ECF K concentration does not accurately reflect total body K deficits, serum K concentration is the only practical way of assessing adequacy of replacement and avoiding unwanted complications. This author generally estimates the K deficit from the degree of hypokalemia and the blood pH, and replaces it over 2 to 3 days (assuming no on-going losses). If i.v. fluids must be used, no more than 40 meq/L of K should be given by peripheral vein, and 80 meq/L by central vein. In terms of the quantitative rate of repair, this should be no more than 0.2 to 0.3 meq K/kg/hour. However, if potentially life-threatening cardiac arrhythmias or respiratory paralysis are evident, up to 1 meq/kg/hour can be given by infusion pump with continuous ECG monitoring in an intensive care unit. Finally, the selection of the specific K salt used in repairing deficits is important. Generally, potassium chloride should be used if there is alkalosis and potassium bicarbonate or its equivalent if there is acidosis. In states of ECF volume depletion from any cause, volume replacement with isotonic saline is as important as K replacement in normalizing serum K and turning off renal K wasting.

The child with symptomatic hypokalemia requires admission for therapy and monitoring (and possibly for diagnostic workup), as does any child with a serum K of less than 3.0 meq/L.

Hyperkalemia

BACKGROUND

Hyperkalemia is defined as a measured serum K concentration of greater than 5.0 meq/L. No specific environmental factors are known to result in hyperkalemia. The etiologies of hyperkalemia are varied. With the exception of transcellular shifts of K, most of the common causes of hyperkalemia result from impaired renal excretion due to decreased glomerular filtration, low urine flow, or decreased tubular secretion. Occasionally, exogenous or endogenous (i.e., from cell breakdown) K loading is responsible for the observed hyperkalemia. The categories of hyperkalemia are shown in Table 46.9.

PATHOPHYSIOLOGY

Pseudohyperkalemia is seen when blood is drawn after prolonged application of a tourniquet but is easily diagnosed by repeating the K measurement after drawing blood without a tourniquet. It may also occur with extreme leukocytosis or extreme thrombocytosis. In these situations, the diagnosis is made by measuring the WBC or platelet count or plasma K. Hyperkalemia resulting from transcellular K shifts in response to acidosis can be seen with normal or decreased total body K. In the former case, simple correction of the pH is all that is required. However, hyperkalemia from acidosis usually occurs in the face of total body K deficits such as diarrheal dehydration or diabetic ketoacidosis. Here it is vitally important to begin K replacement while the pH is being returned toward normal, thus avoiding a sudden fall in serum K concentration as it shifts back into cells.

The pathophysiology of hyperkalemia in cases of endogenous K release from cells is straightforward. Cellular catabolism occurs in the face of negative nitrogen balance from any cause; in pediatrics this usually results from dietary protein restriction. In-

Table 46.9
Etiologies of Hyperkalemia

I. *Pseudohyperkalemia (Hemolysis, Extreme Leukocytosis or Thrombocytosis)*
II. *Apparent K Excess (Transcellular Shifts)*
    A. Acidosis
III. *Increased Intake*
    A. Endogenous (rhabdomyolysis, massive hemolysis)
    B. Exogenous (suicide attempt with K salts)
IV. *Decreased Excretion*
    A. Acute or chronic renal failure (oliguria)
    B. Adrenal corticoid deficiency (acute adrenal insufficiency, hyporeninemic hypoaldosteronism)
    C. Use of K-sparing diuretics in renal failure or in conjunction with dietary K supplements.

jury from trauma or burns can accelerate K delivery into the ECF, but life-threatening hyperkalemia rarely ensures if renal function is intact. The commonest cause of hyperkalemia encountered in the emergency department is probably metabolic acidosis followed by reduced renal excretion. The latter occurs commonly in acute renal failure from any cause, especially when there is concomitant oliguria (see Table 46.6 for factors controlling urinary K excretion). In chronic renal failure, normal serum K levels are usually noted, provided that the glomerular filtration rate falls slowly, allowing the residual functioning nephrons to increase K excretion. Therefore, the development of hyperkalemia usually signals a sudden increased excretory burden or transcellular shifts. In adrenal corticoid deficiency states or in patients receiving K-sparing diuretics, distal tubular secretion of K is impaired. Although more commonly seen in adults, patients with diabetes mellitus and mild renal insufficiency may develop a syndrome of hyporeninemic hypoaldosteronism with hyperkalemia. Glucocorticoid production is normal, as is serum Na concentration, separating these patients from those with acute adrenal insufficiency.

CLINICAL MANIFESTATIONS

The predominant symptoms and signs are neuromuscular. Paresthesias are followed by weakness and even flaccid paralysis. Major toxicity is reflected in the ECG. The earliest change is symmetrical peaking of the T wave, then widening of the QRS complex and lengthening of the PR interval. First degree heart block, loss of the P wave, ventricular arrhythmias, and cardiac standstill may follow. Cardiac arrest is more commonly seen with hyper- than with hypokalemia. In general, the ECG changes parallel the degree of hyperkalemia when it has developed acutely. The presence of any ECG changes associated with hyperkalemia mandates urgent diagnosis and therapy.

The laboratory evaluation of hyperkalemia is outlined in Table 46.10. While hypokalemia may cause rhabdomyolysis, hyperkalemia is often an early and life-threatening consequence of rhabdomyolysis from other causes. An elevated BUN and creatinine point to acute renal failure. The urinary electrolyte pattern of the untreated patient can be quite helpful if one suspects adrenal corticoid deficiency. In acute adrenal insufficiency, urine Na concentration is inappropriately high, and urine K concentration inappropriately low for their respective serum concentrations.

Table 46.10
Laboratory Evaluation of Hyperkalemia

I. Blood
- A. Electrolytes (Na, K, Cl, HCO_3)
- B. BUN, Creatinine
- C. Glucose
- D. Arterial blood gas
- E. Creatinine phosphokinase

II. Urine
- A. Urinalysis
- B. Urine Na, K, Cl
- C. Urine pH
- D. Urine osmolality

III. Other
- A. ECG

MANAGEMENT

There are three general techniques employed in lowering serum K levels to normal: (1) reverse the membrane effects, (2) transfer K into cells, and (3) enhance renal excretion of K. If patients are asymptomatic, serum K is less than 6.5 meq/L, and the ECG is normal or reveals only peaked T waves, all that may be required is discontinuation of K intake, removal of K-sparing diuretics if they are being used, and treatment of acidosis. Exceptions to this occur in acute oliguric renal failure and rhabdomyolysis, where the serum K level may rise to much higher levels precipitously, and a more aggressive therapeutic approach is indicated.

When there are more widespread ECG changes and/or a serum K greater than 7.0 meq/L, several available therapies are designed to move K into cells acutely, including glucose and insulin, and Na bicarbonate. The latter agent has recently been shown to be effective even in the absence of acidosis.

With the onset of cardiac arrhythmias or a serum K level greater than 8.0 meq/L, urgent therapy is needed. Under continuous ECG monitoring, intravenous calcium is given first to reverse potentially life-threatening arrhythmias without altering serum K. Calcium accomplishes this by restoring a more normal differential between the threshold and resting transmembrane potentials. This may then be followed by glucose and insulin, and Na bicarbonate.

For more long-term control of hyperkalemia, the cation exchange resin Na polystyrene sulfonate (Kayexelate) can be administered. Finally, in patients with oliguric renal failure, peritoneal dialysis will remove potassium, although the immediate fall in serum levels may reflect redistribution due to the alkalinizing effect of dialysis and the glucose load in the dialysate itself. The doses of drugs used to treat hyperkalemia, the recommended rates of administration and onset of action are detailed in Table 46.11.

Any child with symptomatic hyperkalemia or a serum K level of greater than 6.5 meq/L deserves admission for therapy and additional work-up.

Disorders of Calcium (Ca) Homeostasis

Hypocalcemia

BACKGROUND

Hypocalcemia beyond the neonatal period is defined as a measured total serum Ca concentration of less than 9.0 mg/dl. In older infants and children, hypocalcemia may result from a variety of genetic as well as acquired disorders. In addition, vitamin D deficiency leading to hypocalcemia may result from unusual living styles such as the avoidance of sunlight and vitamin D-containing foods. There are four major categories of hypocalcemia in infants and children as denoted in Table 46.12.

PATHOPHYSIOLOGY

Basic Mechanisms. The skeleton contains 99% of total body Ca; the remaining 1% is distributed in intravascular, interstitial and intracellular fluids. Most of the skeletal Ca is in a nonexchangeable pool and is unavailable for moment-to-moment

Table 46.11
Emergency Treatment of Hyperkalemia

Technique	Agent	Dose	Rate of Administration	Onset/Duration of Action	Comments
Reversal of membrane effects	10% calcium gluconate	0.5 ml/kg	2–5 min i.v.	Min/30–60 min	ECG monitor; discontinue if pulse rate <100
Movement of K into cells	Na bicarbonate, 7.5% (1 meq ≈ 1 ml)	2–3 ml/kg	30–60 min	30 min/1–4 hr	May use in the absence of acidosis
	Glucose 50% plus insulin (regular)	1 unit for every 5–6 g glucose	Same	Same	Monitor blood glucose
Enhanced excretion of K	Kayexalate	1 g/kg	Can be given in 10% glucose (1 g in 4 ml) every 4–6 hr	Hours/variable	Can be given p.o. or by rectum

Table 46.12
Etiologies of Hypocalcemia

- *I. True Hypoparathyroidism*
  - A. Familial, with or without multiple endocrine abnormalities ("autoimmune")
  - B. DiGeorge syndrome
  - C. Postsurgical
  - D. Idiopathic
  - E. Magnesium deficiency
- *II. End-organ Resistance to Parathyroid Hormone*
  - A. Pseudohypoparathyroidism
  - B. Insensitivity to cyclic AMP
- *III. Abnormalities of Vitamin D Metabolites*
  - A. Primary D deficiency (dietary, sunlight)
  - B. Secondary D deficiency
    - 1. Malabsorption (coeliac disease, biliary atresia, etc.)
    - 2. Anticonvulsant therapy
    - 3. Chronic renal failure
  - C. Primary D resistance (familial hypophosphatemic rickets)
  - D. Secondary D resistance
    - 1. Fanconi syndromes (cystinosis, Lowe's syndrome, etc.)
    - 2. Renal tubular acidosis
  - E. Primary D dependence
    - 1. Type I (deficient 1, α-hydroxylase)
    - 2. Type II (end-organ resistance to 1,25[OH]$_2$D)
- *IV. Miscellaneous*
  - A. Hypoproteinemia
  - B. Hypernatremic dehydration with K deficiency
  - C. Postacidotic tetany
  - D. Diuretic abuse
  - E. Phosphate loading

regulation of Ca homeostasis which includes bone remodeling plus a wide range of metabolic activities. The Ca in the rapidly exchangeable pool is present in the body fluids described above, in the cell cytosol, and on the surfaces of recently mineralized bone. Preservation of normal total serum Ca within relatively narrow limits is regulated by dietary intake, gastrointestinal absorption, both gastrointestinal and renal excretion, and bone resorption. In addition, there is an as yet unclear but reciprocal relationship between serum Ca and serum inorganic phosphorus; factors raising phosphorus result in a lowering of serum Ca and vice versa. The active form of vitamin D [1,25(OH)$_2$D] promotes Ca and phosphorus absorption from the gut when present in physiologic concentrations. It also enhances the parathyroid hormone (PTH)-dependent mobilization of Ca from mineralized bone and has a small but important action on the renal conservation of Ca. Thus 1,25(OH)$_2$D is a Ca promoting hormone which serves to raise serum Ca in response to hypocalcemia and/or increased tissue demands for Ca. PTH secretion is enhanced by hypo- and suppressed by hypercalcemia. Serum Ca is raised in response to increased PTH by at least two mechanisms: (1) increased Ca resorption from bone, and (2) increased renal excretion of phosphorus. Calcitonin acts in response to hypercalcemia by inhibiting bone resorption and thus lowering Ca delivery into the ECF. The action of both 1,25(OH)$_2$D and PTH is through receptor binding and stimulation of mediators such as cyclic-AMP. Therefore, hypocalcemia could result from an absolute deficiency of one or both of these compounds, end-organ resistance due to a lack of receptors or abnormal receptor binding, or impaired formation or action of the mediators.

Applications. Examples of all of these potential abnormalities have now been described and are outlined in Table 46.12. The etiologies of hypocalcemia listed under 46.12, *I* and *II* are rarely encountered in the emergency department setting.

In simple or primary vitamin D deficiency, impaired Ca absorption and bone resorption cause the observed hypocalcemia, although 1,25(OH)$_2$D may be normal or even elevated in blood. The anticonvulsant agents diphenylhydantoin and phenobarbital probably induce hepatic microsomal enzymes which increase the conversion of 25(OH)D in the liver to inactive metabolites. Hypocalcemia is uncommon in children taking anticonvulsant agents unless they are also receiving a poor Ca intake and have little sunlight exposure. When chronic renal insufficiency is moderate to severe (i.e., glomerular filtration rate 50% of normal or lower), a decrease in renal mass leads to decreased production of 1,25(OH)$_2$D. In addition, decreased renal excretion of phosphorus causes hyperphosphatemia and a reciprocal fall in serum Ca. Secondary hyperparathyroidism then ensues. Dietary intake of Ca is often decreased in these patients. For all of these reasons, hypocalcemia is very common and often resistant in this condition. Occasionally, hypocalcemia is seen in acute renal failure, especially when acidosis is vigorously treated with alkali.

Hypocalcemia is not commonly seen but may occur in familial hypophosphatemic rickets. The mechanism is unclear. Hypophosphatemia rather than hypocalcemia is the hallmark of disturbed mineral homeostasis in Fanconi's syndrome. In renal tubular acidosis, the combination of hypercalciuria secondary to obligatory bicarbonaturia and acidosis, and probable impairment in $1{,}25(OH)_2D$ production may lead to hypocalcemia. Hypocalcemia is often profound and refractory to therapy in the various forms of vitamin D dependence. The characteristic blood profile in this and the other abnormalities of vitamin D metabolism are outlined in Table 46.13.

Hypocalcemia due to a lowered protein-bound fraction is commonly associated with the hypoproteinemia of nephrotic syndrome or protein-losing enteropathy, though ionized Ca is normal. The hypocalcemia is mild, usually in the range of 7.5 to 9.0 mg/dl, and rarely causes symptoms. Hypernatremic dehydration in association with a K deficit results in hypocalcemia for reasons that are unclear. Overvigorous correction of acidosis, especially in the dehydrated child, will drive Ca into bone, resulting in hypocalcemic tetany. Diuretic abuse with the potent loop blockers (ethacrynic acid, furosemide) may cause massive hypercalciuria and hypocalcemia, especially in the face of a hypochloremic alkalosis. Phosphate loading, either exogenous or endogenous (e.g., lysis of tumor cells) will result in hyperphosphatemia, with a corresponding fall in serum Ca until the extra phosphorus is excreted.

CLINICAL MANIFESTATIONS

The signs and symptoms of hypocalcemia per se are primarily neuromuscular in origin. Nonspecific findings such as vomiting, muscle weakness, and irritability are common. In addition to the characteristic tetany and positive Chvostek and Trousseau signs, there may be frank seizures or laryngospasm with upper airway obstruction. Rickets is characterized by thinning of the inner table of the skull (craniotabes), enlarged costochondral junctions (rachitic rosary), and thickening of the wrists and ankles. The ECG may reveal a prolonged Q-T interval.

Complications requiring urgent diagnosis include frank tetany, laryngospasm and seizures. Laboratory studies which should be included in the initial evaluation are listed in Table 46.14. If the diagnosis is not clear after these studies are completed, PTH should be measured, since it serves to differentiate most of the causes of hypocalcemia from primary hypoparathyroidism and hypomagnesemia. The diagnosis of primary hypoparathyroidism is established by finding hypocalcemia, hyperphosphatemia, undetectable PTH and a normal renal and skeletal (calcemic) response to exogenous PTH. Hypomagnesemia may also result in functional hypoparathyroidism. The characteristic laboratory profiles of the various vitamin D abnormalities are outlined in Table 46.13. In this latter group of diseases, symptomatic hypocalcemia is often preceded by poor linear growth and clinical rickets.

Table 46.13
Blood Profile in Disorders of Vitamin D Metabolism

Disorder	Ca (mg/dl)	Phosphorus (mg/dl)	25(OH)D (ng/ml)	$1{,}25(OH)_2D$ (pg/ml)	PTH (μl eq/ml)
Primary D deficiency	↓	↓	↓[a]	NL or ↑	↑
Secondary D deficiency					
Anticonvulsant therapy	NL or ↓	NL or ↓	↓[a]	NL or ↓	?
Renal failure	NL or ↓	NL or ↑	NL	NL or ↓	↑[a]
Primary D resistance	NL	↓[a]	NL	NL	NL or ↑
Primary D dependence	↓[a]	↓	NL	NL ↓ or ↑	↑

[a] Denotes the characteristic abnormal finding. NL = normal blood level.

Table 46.14
Laboratory Evaluation of Hypocalcemia

I. *Blood*
  A. Ca, phosphorus, alkaline phosphatase
  B. Magnesium
  C. Total protein, albumin
  D. BUN, creatinine
  E. PTH
  F. pH
II. *Urine*
  A. Ca, phosphorus
  B. Creatinine
III. *Other*[a]
  A. ECG
  B. Skull, chest x-ray
  C. Skeletal survey

[a] Selection of studies depends upon the suspected diagnosis.

MANAGEMENT

The emergency treatment of choice for hypocalcemia from any cause other than hypomagnesemia is intravenous calcium. It should be given under cardiac monitoring at a starting dose of 0.5 to 1.0 ml/kg as 10% Ca gluconate administered over 3 to 5 min. The infusion should stop if the heart rate falls below 60/min. Once symptoms are relieved, Ca gluconate can then be added to the i.v. solution (100 mg elemental Ca/kg/24 hours) or Ca may be administered orally. Oral preparations for chronic Ca supplementation include Ca lactate (13% calcium by weight), Ca gluconate (9% calcium by weight) or, if volume is a limiting factor, Ca chloride (21% calcium by weight). When magnesium deficiency is suspected or confirmed as the cause of hypocalcemia, magnesium should be administered, usually by the i.m. route. One gram of 50% magnesium sulfate contains 99 mg of magnesium or roughly 8 meq. The dose of magnesium is 0.5 meq/kg or 0.125 ml/kg of the 50% solution. Children with unanticipated hypocalcemic tetany, seizures or laryngospasm should be admitted for treatment and workup for the underlying cause of the hypocalcemia.

Hypercalcemia

BACKGROUND

Hypercalcemia is defined as a measured total serum Ca concentration of greater than 11.0 mg/dl. The discussion will exclude hypercalcemia in the newborn. The major etiologies of hypercalcemia in infants and children are outlined in Table 46.15. Hypercalcemia can result from increased Ca absorption from the gut or increased Ca resorption from bone. Hypercalcemia will occasionally result from a massive increase in dietary Ca intake or a reduction in the renal excretion of Ca.

PATHOPHYSIOLOGY

In hyperparathyroidism, increased bone reabsorption of Ca results in hypercalcemia, and decreased renal reabsorption of phosphorus results in hypophosphatemia. Because PTH stimulates bone turnover, alkaline phosphatase is elevated. PTH is inappropriately elevated for the level of serum Ca and confirms the diagnosis. Measurement of PTH, however, would not differentiate primary hyperparathyroidism from a malignancy producing ectopic PTH or a PTH-like material. Skeletal x-rays often support the diagnosis by revealing osteitis fibrosa, subperiosteal bone resorption and generalized demineralization. Although more commonly seen in adults, patients may present with or have associated Ca nephrolithiasis and renal colic.

Infantile hypercalcemia has an uncertain etiology. Hypersensitivity and in utero excessive exposure to vitamin D have been

Table 46.15
Etiologies of Hypercalcemia[a]

I. *Primary Hyperparathyroidism (Rare in Pediatrics)*
  A. Sporadic
  B. Familial (with or without associated endocrine abnormalities)
II. *Infantile Hypercalcemia*
III. *Vitamin D Intoxication*
IV. *Immobilization*
V. *Malignant Disease*
  A. Bony metastases (especially lymphoreticular)
  B. Ectopic production of parathyroid hormone or other bone-resorbing factors
VI. *Miscellaneous*
  A. Sarcoidosis (rare in pediatrics)
  B. Thiazide diuretics
  C. Hypervitaminosis A

[a] This list is not meant to be comprehensive, but includes the important etiologies in children.

raised as causative factors. The disorder is clinically recognized in early infancy by a characteristic facies (pug nose, fat nasal bridge, "cupid's bow" upper lip), failure to thrive, slow development and hypotonia. Hypercalcemia may disappear later in the first year of life, but mental retardation usually persists. Peripheral pulmonic and/or supravalvular aortic stenosis are characteristic associated findings.

The vitamin D toxicity syndromes can usually be suspected from the history; hypercalcemia is the result of increased Ca absorption. If the intoxicating compound was conventional vitamin D, the hypercalcemia may be prolonged because of the storage of this compound in adipose tissue.

Immobilization hypercalcemia occurs typically in the adolescent who is growing rapidly. Acute injury or illness requiring prolonged immobilization (especially in traction) leads first to hypercalciuria and then to hypercalcemia. The presumed etiology is increased bone resorption in the face of decreased or arrested bone mineralization.

Lymphoreticular malignancies in childhood may be associated with hypercalcemia from one of several mechanisms: (1) bony metastases with localized bone resorption; (2) rarely, the elaboration of a PTH-like peptide by tumor cells; and (3) release of other bone-resorption-promoting factors such as prostaglandin E or osteoclast activating factor. In sarcoidosis there is a heightened sensitivity to the Ca absorbing effects of vitamin D, but the precise mechanism is unclear. Thiazide diuretics reduce renal Ca excretion probably by two mechanisms: (1) ECF contraction leading to enhanced proximal tubular reabsorption of Ca with Na, and (2) increased renal tubular sensitivity to PTH-induced Ca reabsorption. Hypervitaminosis A can increase skeletal resorption of Ca leading to hypercalcemia. Associated and characteristic findings are failure to thrive, dry skin and rash, poor hair texture, papilledema and headache.

CLINICAL MANIFESTATIONS

Symptoms and signs of hypercalcemia are listed in Table 46.16 and are grouped by organ system. Mild hypercalcemia (Ca 11 to 13 mg/dl) usually produces headache, irritability and gastrointestinal upset. When serum Ca rises above 14 to 15 mg/dl abruptly, a life-threatening hypercalcemic crisis may occur consisting of severe vomiting, hypertension, polyuric dehydration, acute renal failure and coma. Laboratory studies which should be included in the initial evaluation are shown in Table 46.17. In any patient with unexplained hypercalcemia, an appropriate workup for hidden malignancy should be initiated once the hypercalcemia is controlled.

Table 46.16
Signs and Symptoms of Hypercalcemia

I. *Neurologic*
   A. Headache, irritability, lethargy, fatigue
   B. Weakness, seizures, coma
   C. Hyporeflexia, behavioral changes
II. *Gastrointestinal*
   A. Anorexia, nausea, vomiting, constipation
   B. Dehydration
III. *Cardiovascular*
   A. Bradycardia, hypertension, short Q-Tc interval (ECG)
IV. *Renal*
   A. Polydipsia, polyuria
   B. Hypokalemia, aminoaciduria, nephrocalcinosis, nephrolithiasis
V. *Dermatologic*
   A. Pruritus
   B. Band keratopathy, ectopic calcification

Table 46.17
Laboratory Evaluation of Hypercalcemia

I. *Blood*
   A. Ca, phosphorus, alkaline phosphatase
   B. Total protein, albumin
   C. BUN, creatinine
   D. Parathyroid hormone
   E. Vitamin D[a]
II. *Urine*
   A. Ca, phosphorus
   B. Creatinine
III. *Other*[b]
   A. ECG
   B. Skull, abdominal x-ray
   C. Skeletal survey
   D. Intravenous pyelogram

[a] If vitamin D intoxication is suspected, blood for 25(OH)D should be drawn acutely and sent to the appropriate reference laboratory.
[b] Selection of studies depends upon the suspected diagnosis.

MANAGEMENT

The choice of therapy depends on whether or not the kidneys are functioning normally. The initial emergency treatment for symptomatic hypercalcemia is designed to enhance Ca excretion by saline infusion at a rate of twice maintenance followed by bolus injections of furosemide, 1 to 2 mg/kg every 6 to 8 hours. The amount and rate of saline to be administered will depend on the state of hydration and presence or absence of hypertension or pre-existing cardiac disease. Treatment of a hypercalcemic crisis depends on the underlying etiology. It always requires hospitalization in an intensive care setting. If malignancy is suspected, mithramycin may be given (25 μg/kg, i.v.). Vitamin D intoxication may be treated with infusions of phosphate or sulfate salts followed by oral prednisone (1 to 2 mg/kg/day). In acute oliguric renal failure, peritoneal or hemodialysis against a low Ca dialysate is usually effective, albeit slowly over hours. Any child in hypercalcemic crisis or with a serum Ca over 13 mg/dl should be admitted for therapy and diagnostic evaluation.

Disorders of Acid-Base Homeostasis

Metabolic Acidosis

BACKGROUND

Definition. Of the four primary acid-base disorders, only metabolic acidosis will be discussed in this section because it is the most frequently encountered acid-base disturbance in pediatric emergencies. Metabolic acidosis is defined as a net gain in H^+ ions or a net loss of bicarbonate (HCO_3^-) ions in the ECF. Clinically, this is reflected by a fall in plasma or serum HCO_3^- (or in some laboratories total CO_2 or tCO_2 which is approximately 95% HCO_3^-). The lower limit of normal for infants and children is 20 meq/L.

Epidemiology. Most of the common causes of metabolic acidosis are acquired. However, certain inborn errors of metabolism may present clinically with severe metabolic acidosis in the first few months of life. An important epidemiologic consideration in all children with unexplained metabolic acidosis is accidental or intentional poisoning with any of a number of agents.

Etiology. The etiologies of metabolic acidosis are conveniently grouped into two major categories: those with a normal anion gap (also known as the "delta" or "R" fraction) and those with an increased anion gap. The anion gap is determined from the serum electrolytes by the following formula: serum electrolytes by the following formula:

$$\text{anion gap} = \text{serum [Na] meq/L} - [Cl^- + HCO_3^-] \text{ meq/L}$$

Potassium is not included in this formula because it is present in relatively low concentrations which vary slightly compared to the other ions. The anion gap represents the sum of anions unmeasured by routine electrolyte determinations, and normally is made up by phosphate, sulfate, organic anions such as lactate and negatively charged plasma proteins. In adults, the anion gap is 12 ± 4 meq/L; adequate normal values have not been published in children but may be 2 to 4 meq/L higher. This author uses 16 ± 4 meq/L as the normal range under 2 years of age. The etiologies of metabolic acidosis are outlined in Table 46.18.

PATHOPHYSIOLOGY

Basic Mechanisms. Metabolic acidosis results from one of three general patho-

Table 46.18
Etiologies of Metabolic Acidosis

I. *Elevated Anion Gap Acidosis*
   A. Diarrheal dehydration
   B. Diabetic ketoacidosis
   C. Renal failure (acute or chronic)
   D. Inborn errors of metabolism
   E. Poisons (e.g., salicylates, ethanol, ethylene glycol)
   F. Lactic acidosis (e.g., hypoxia, sepsis, idiopathic)
II. *Normal Anion Gap Acidosis*
   A. Hypernatremic dehydration (older children)
   B. Renal tubular acidosis
   C. Hyperalimentation
   D. Enteric fistulas (e.g., pancreatic) or enterostomies
   E. Ureterosigmoidostomy
   F. Drugs (e.g., Sulfamylon, ammonium chloride, amphotericin, acetazolamide)
   G. Early renal failure (chronic interstitial nephritis)

physiologic mechanisms: (1) increased H^+ ion delivery into the ECF, (2) increased HCO_3^- loss from the ECF (gastrointestinal or renal), and (3) decreased renal H^+ ion excretion. The end result is a fall in serum tCO_2 or HCO_3^-; the pH which is the negative logarithm of the $[H^+]$ is usually below normal (<7.37) unless there is a second acid-base disturbance driving the pH in the opposite direction.

ECF $[H^+]$ or pH is maintained within very narrow limits by a series of buffers, the most important of which is the bicarbonate buffer system. It operates in both the ECF (35% of total buffering) and ICF of red blood cells (18% of total buffering) and provides immediate defense against life-threatening acidemia. It is an excellent and versatile buffer system for two reasons: (1) the carbonic acid-bicarbonate system represents a weak acid-strong conjugate base system that readily accepts protons of H^+ ions from nonvolatile acids in the usual range of plasma pH, and (2) the product resulting from adding H^+ to this system is CO_2 which can be blown off by the lungs, thus blunting the net change in H^+ or pH.

The overall buffering mechanisms in response to metabolic acidosis are listed in Table 46.19. Of practical importance is the length of time it takes each of these mechanisms to operate in returning pH toward normal. Eventual full correction of metabolic acidosis requires renal excretion of excess H^+ ions, which takes several days to accomplish. Normally, children produce twice as much acid per day as adults (i.e. 2 to 3 meq/kg), which results from a combination of endogenous metabolism and ion exchange at the surface of growing bone.

Table 46.19
Buffering Mechanisms in Metabolic Acidosis

1. Extracellular buffering (instantaneous)
   $H^+ + Buf^- \rightarrow HBuf$
   $H^+ + HCO_3^- \rightarrow H_2CO_3$
2. Respiratory buffering (10–15 min)
   $H^+ + HCO_3^- \rightleftharpoons H_2CO_3 \rightleftharpoons H_2O + CO_2 \uparrow$
3. Intracellular buffering (2–4 hr)
   Diffusion of H^+ into cells
   H^+ + proteinate$^-$ $\rightarrow$ H protein
   H^+ + hemoglobinate$^-$ $\rightarrow$ H hemoglobin
   $H^+ + PO_4^- \rightarrow HPO_4^-$

Since the final pH resulting from metabolic acidosis is a reflection of the extent of the physiologic compensatory (i.e., adaptive) response as well as the magnitude of the initiating disturbance, we must briefly consider this adaptive response. The compensatory response to metabolic acidosis is hyperventilation. This process produces a respiratory alkalosis, defined as a PCO_2 lower than normal (e.g., 40 mm Hg) which returns the pH *toward*, but *not to* normal. This response is immediate and, for all practical purposes, is completed by the time the emergency physician sees the child with a metabolic acidosis (e.g. > 12 to 24 hours after the onset of the inciting illness). The stimuli to hyperventilation are probably: (1) via peripheral chemoreceptors immediately sensing the fall in plasma pH or rise in H^+, and, somewhat later, (2) the respiratory center sensing similar changes in CSF. These later changes do not occur immediately because PCO_2 diffuses across the blood-brain barrier faster than HCO_3^- and initially the CSF pH may actually rise! A useful formula which predicts the normal adaptive response to metabolic acidosis is:

$$PCO_2 = 1.5 \times [HCO_3^-] + 8 \pm 2$$

If the PCO_2 is greater than expected from the calculations, suspect a second acid-base disturbance, respiratory acidosis. In other words, the compensatory response is inadequate. If, on the other hand, there is an exaggerated compensatory response with a PCO_2 lower than expected from the calculations, suspect a primary respiratory alkalosis. Note that this formula probably does not apply to pH values less than 7.00.

Net renal acid excretion is accomplished by two mechanisms: (1) H^+ ion secretion by the renal tubule in exchange for HCO_3^- ion, and (2) H^+ ion binding to ammonia. Negligible H^+ ion is quantitatively excreted in the free state.

Applications. (1) *Elevated anion gap.* Let us first consider the causes of an elevated anion gap acidosis (Table 46.18). Diarrheal dehydration in infants and young children is the most common cause of metabolic acidosis. It tends to produce an elevated anion gap because of the early development of tissue catabolism and starvation ketosis. This results in increased H^+ ion production in association with release of increased amounts of organic anions into the ECF. Diabetic ketoacidosis results in the increased production of β-hydroxybutyric acid and acetoacetic acid which raise the anion gap. In severe renal failure, there is accumulation of normally occurring anions including phosphates, sulfates and creatinine. In addition, tissue catabolism ensues early in the face of oliguria and decreased caloric intake. The acidosis itself is also contributed to by decreased ammonia production by the damaged kidney.

A number of the rarely seen inborn errors of metabolism may present with severe metabolic acidosis after the institution of milk (protein) feeds. Various poisons, but especially salicylates, cause metabolic acidosis either by their metabolic conversion to acids which are fully ionized at body pH, or by liberating endogenous acids as a consequence of interfering with normal metabolic pathways. Lactic acidosis is probably a more common cause of metabolic acidosis than is currently recognized in pediatrics. It most typically develops in the setting of acute circulatory and/or respiratory failure with shock, hypoxia and poor tissue perfusion. A common predisposing event is sepsis with gram-negative organisms. Hepatic failure, drugs and toxins, Type I glycogen storage disease and pulmonary embolus are other causes seen in childhood. In a significant number of patients, the cause is unknown. Primary hyperventilation will produce moderate elevations in serum lactate but rarely leads to symptomatic acidosis.

(2) *Normal anion gap.* We can now turn to a consideration of the common causes of a normal anion gap acidosis (Table 46.18). In most cases, this results from a relative or absolute hyperchloremia. In hypernatremic dehydration secondary to diarrhea seen in adults and children, increased Cl^- reabsorption in the large bowel may account in part for the relative hyperchloremia. In addition, in extreme hypertonic states (i.e., serum Na greater than 165 meq/L), Na^+ may be underestimated relative to Cl^- if electrolytes are being measured by the autoanalyzer technique. The hyperchloremia seen in both the proximal and distal forms of renal tubular acidosis is thought to result from a renal loss of HCO_3^- without a corresponding loss of chloride. The Na^+ deficit occasioned by the loss of $NaHCO_3$ and other Na^+ salts in turn leads to volume contraction, stimulating the renal tubular reabsorption of NaCl. Effectively, $NaHCO_3$ is replaced by NaCl in the ECF. Another clue to the diagnosis is an inappropriately alkaline urine pH (> 5.5) in the face of systemic acidosis.

Other more rare causes of a normal anion gap acidosis include therapy with hyperalimentation solutions, amphotericin B and Sulfamylon.

Enteric fistulas and ureterosigmoidostomies probably produce a normal anion gap acidosis via enhanced Cl^--HCO_3^- exchange in the bowel.

Chronic interstitial nephritis with early renal failure (glomerular filtration rate 25 to 50% of normal) may result in a hyperchloremic acidosis. The pathophysiologic picture is one of renal tubular acidosis with renal bicarbonate wasting, but an additional component is reduced ammonia production and ammonium excretion.

CLINICAL MANIFESTATIONS

The clinical manifestations of metabolic acidosis usually reflect the predisposing illness and are not in themselves unique. Nonetheless, in some patients the presenting complaints appear to result primarily from the acid-base disturbance, in that they resolve after bicarbonate therapy. The signs and symptoms include tachypnea with or without hyperventilation, abdominal pain, vomiting, unexplained fever and lethargy. Tachypnea and hyperpnea are characteristic of severe lactic acidosis, and coma may ensue if the pH is markedly depressed. There is often an associated but unexplained leukocytosis.

The urgency to diagnose metabolic acidosis is linked to the clinical imperative of defending the blood pH within a life-sustaining range. Factors which mandate rapid diagnosis (therapy) include: (1) a severely depressed blood pH (<7.15 to 7.20) indicating marked acidemia, (2) a critically ill patient with multisystem disease, especially pulmonary and/or renal disease, (3) inability to effectively treat the underlying disease, and (4) the combination of hypoxia and acidemia which together can cause myocardial depression.

The laboratory studies required to diagnose and characterize metabolic acidosis are given in Table 46.20. A measurement of pH is needed to assess the potential urgency of alkali therapy, and the remainder of the arterial blood gas analysis is needed to assess the adequacy of respiratory compensation. The simultaneous measurement of blood and urine pH will provide a clue to the diagnosis of renal tubular acidosis; this diagnosis is also suspected in the patient who has hypokalemia rather than normo- or hyperkalemia.

MANAGEMENT

The choice of therapy is alkali, and the preferred agent is almost always $NaHCO_3$. Sodium lactate, given as lactated Ringer's solution, is an acceptable alternative, provided that liver function is normal and lactic acidosis is ruled out. Patients require treatment if the serum HCO_3 is less than 15 meq/L and/or the pH is less than 7.20, unless the underlying disorder is simple diarrheal dehydration. In that case, discontinuing oral intake and administering i.v. fluids are usually the only therapies required. The diarrhea usually stops and the kidney corrects the acidosis.

Of equal importance to the choice of alkali therapy is the amountof bicarbonate to use and the rate of repair. The bicarbonate or buffer deficit requires some estimate of the "bicarbonate space" which in health equals the ECF space or 20% of body weight in liters. Recent experimental studies in dogs, however, have suggested that the bicarbonate space is increased in severe metabolic acidosis to as much as 50% and, in lactic acidosis, even to 100%! The proposed reason for this is the movement of excess H^+ ions out of the ECF into other body compartments. Calculations of the HCO_3 deficit may therefore be as follows:

Mild/moderate acidosis (pH 7.20 to 7.37):

HCO_3^- deficit in meq = ("normal" serum [HCO_3^-] − "observed" serum [HCO_3^-]) × 20% of total body weight in liters

Table 46.20
Laboratory Evaluation of Metabolic Acidosis

I. Blood
- A. Electrolytes (Na, K, Cl, HCO_3)[a]
- B. Arterial blood gases
- C. BUN, creatinine
- D. Glucose
- E. Toxic screen[b]
- F. Lactate, pyruvate[c]

II. Urine
- A. Dipstick (pH, glucose, protein)

[a] Calculate the anion gap.
[b] Or measurements of specific drugs if suspected or causing the acidosis.
[c] If available.

Severe acidosis (pH less than 7.20):

HCO_3^- deficit in meq = ("normal" serum [HCO_3^-] − "observed" serum [HCO_3^-] × 50% of total body weight in liters

If the volume of infused solution must be limited, 7.5% $NaHCO_3$ (1 meq/ 1 ml) is used; otherwise, lesser concentrations should be employed. Full correction of serum HCO_3^- should never be attempted; a reasonable goal is to increase serum HCO_3^- in increments of 5 to 10 meq/L until a level of 15 to 18 meq/L is achieved. At this point, maintenance HCO_3^- therapy can be continued at roughly 2 meq/kg/day unless the underlying cause of the acidosis has been successfully treated.

Requirements for alkali can vary because acid production may continue and/or the distribution space for bicarbonate theoretically could change. Frequent checks of serum HCO_3^- must accompany therapy. Overzealous alkali therapy is risky and can lead to a variety of complications outlined in Table 46.21. In some patients, such as those with uremic acidosis, chronic bicarbonate therapy may not be indicated because stabilization occurs with only mildly positive H^+ ion balance (HCO_3^- greater than 15 meq/L) and the Na load occasioned by additional alkali therapy may aggravate preexisting hypertension or congestive heart failure. Any child requiring intravenous alkali therapy should be admitted to the hospital.

Table 46.21
Complications of Alkali Therapy in Metabolic Acidosis

- I. *Hypokalemia*
  - A. K^+ losses as part of the disease process (e.g., renal tubular acidosis, diabetic ketoacidosis)
  - B. K^+ shifts into cells
- II. *Alkalosis*
  - A. Overcorrection
  - B. Persistent hyperventilation
  - C. Endogenous manufacture of HCO_3^-
- III. *CSF Acidosis*
  - A. Delay in equilibration of HCO_3^- across the blood-brain barrier
- IV. *Sodium Overload*
- V. *Hypocalcemic Tetany*
  - A. Ca^{2+} binding to protein
  - B. Ca^{2+} incorporation into bone

Table 46.22
Nephrotic Syndrome

Syndrome and Histologic Pattern	Usual Response to Corticosteroids[a]
I. *Primary*	
A. Minimal change (also lipoid nephrosis, "nil" disease)	S
B. Focal segmental sclerosis	R
C. Membranoproliferative nephritis	R
D. Membranous nephropathy	±S
E. Proliferative nephritis	
1. Mesangial	S
2. Focal	R(?)
3. Diffuse	R(?)
II. *Secondary*	
A. Lupus nephritis	S
B. Sickle cell anemia	R
C. Henoch-Schönlein purpura	R
D. Hereditary nephritis	R
E. Drugs, toxins	R
F. Infections	R
G. Miscellaneous	R

[a] S = sensitive; R = resistant.

NEPHROTIC SYNDROME

BACKGROUND

Definition. Nephrotic syndrome is the clinical expression of a variety of primary and secondary glomerular disorders, the hallmarks of which are: (1) hypoproteinemia (serum albumin < 3.0 g/dl); (2) heavy proteinuria, initially or at some point in the illness (> 40 mg/sq m/hour in a 24-hour urine); (3) edema; and less consistently (4) hyperlipidemia (predominantly triglycerides and cholesterol). Primary nephrotic syndrome is the term applied to diseases limited to the kidney. They are further classified according to the response to corticosteroid therapy and histology on renal biopsy. Secondary nephrotic syndrome is the term applied to multisystem disease in which the kidney is involved. Occasionally, nephrotic syndrome will develop as a consequence of exposure to environmental agents including heavy metals and bee venom. Table 46.22 lists the most important disorders in each category.

Epidemiology. Nephrotic syndrome is worldwide in distribution. It tends to occur more commonly in boys than in girls. The mean age of onset tends to be earlier (< 6 years) in primary nephrotic syndrome than in secondary nephrotic syndrome (> 6 years). Incidence and prevalence figures show some geographic variation: in the United States, the figures are 1.3 to 2.8/100,000 and 14 to 16/100,000 children, respectively. Although the disease is usually sporadic, a familial incidence is clearly established with a polygenic inheritance pattern. The infantile or congenital form of nephrotic syndrome is particularly common in children of Finnish extraction and is inherited as an autosomal recessive trait.

Etiology. The etiologies of the primary and most of the secondary glomerular disorders associated with the nephrotic syndrome are largely unknown. By far the most common form of nephrotic syndrome is that associated with "nil disease" or minimal change on renal biopsy. It is also called idiopathic nephrosis of childhood and accounts for 80% of pediatric cases. There is no definite association with antecedent bacterial (e.g., streptococcal) or viral infections, although the presenting illness and episodes of clinical relapse are often associated with upper respiratory or gastrointestinal infections. An immunologic basis for nephrotic syndrome has been suggested from a number of studies which have reported: (1) persistently elevated serum IgM levels, (2) circulating immune complexes, (3) spontaneous relapses with natural measles infections (which are known to induce suppression of cell-mediated immunity), (4) suppression of lymphocyte proliferative responses in vitro by serum from patients with nephrotic syndrome, (5) hyperactivity of lymphocytes from patients when exposed to renal antigens in vitro, and (6) response of some patients to immunosuppressive agents. The strongest argument against an immunologic factor as a cause of nephrotic syndrome has been the failure to find immune reactants or inflammation in kidney biopsies, despite repeated studies of these patients.

The typical age of presentation of primary nephrotic syndrome is 18 months to 5 or 6 years. When nephrotic syndrome appears in the neonatal period, one is likely dealing with the congenital or Finnish-type nephrotic syndrome which is steroid-resistant and carries generally a fatal prognosis. Conversely, nephrotic syndrome presenting in a teenager is much more likely to be associated with a primary or secondary form of underlying nephritis, and renal biopsy is generally indicated.

PATHOPHYSIOLOGY

The hallmark of nephrotic syndrome is edema, signaling salt and water retention. Although the mechanisms of edema formation are incompletely understood, it is generally believed that the initiating factor is a large glomerular leak of proteins, predominantly albumin, leading to hypoalbuminemia. The leak is probably related to some noninflammatory immunologic or metabolic process which reduces the negative charges in the glomerular basement membrane. These charges are primarily represented by sialic acid residues which ordinarily repel albumin and other negatively charged plasma proteins. With loss of serum albumin and other plasma proteins, the intravascular oncotic pressure falls and fluid moves out of the vascular and into the interstitial spaces, in accordance with Starling's principles. Since the liver ordinarily has a large synthetic capacity for albumin, the persistent hypoalbuminemia noted in most nephrotics is probably not simply due to urinary losses. Other contributing factors suggested in the literature, but not proven, are: (1) decreased protein intake, (2) decreased synthesis, and (3) increased catabolism. Once plasma oncotic pressure falls, extracellular volume is reduced, which the kidney "reads" as a decreased effective circulating arterial volume. Proximal tubular sodium reabsorption is increased in response to this stimulus. The renin-angiotensin system is also stimulated, aldosterone secretion rises, and distal tubular sodium reabsorption intensifies. This secondary hyperaldosteronism serves to perpetuate the edema-forming state. The increased lipid turnover seen in nephrotic syndrome is characterized by elevations in serum triglycerides and cholesterol. The stimulus to this increased synthesis is unknown but is related to the degree of hypoproteinemia. Limited studies have pointed to a reduction in lipoprotein lipase and/or other circulating lipolytic factors and a selective retention of large molecular weight lipoproteins.

CLINICAL MANIFESTATIONS

Presentations. The major presenting complaint is edema, which may be localized or diffuse. A typical story is that of a 2- or 3-year-old with puffy eyes who was treated for allergies but did not improve. A rapidly changing belt, trouser or shoe size may be indicative of rapid weight gain before there is detectable edema. The rate and degree of edema formation varies from child to child and appears to be directly related to the degree of hypoalbuminemia. This, in turn, reflects both the degree of albuminuria and the dietary protein intake. The degree of edema is also dependent upon and varies inversely with the urine output which is typically reduced in the full-blown case. In fact, in some patients true oliguria ($<$ 300 ml/sq m/day) may be seen, although it almost never signifies acute renal failure. Rarely, there is abrupt and massive salt and water retention leading to respiratory distress because of a combination of hydrothorax and ascites with elevation of the diaphragm. Ascites may also be associated with various abdominal complaints such as anorexia, nausea and vomiting which are thought to be due to edema of the intestinal wall since they disappear with successful treatment of the edema.

Complications. The acute complications of nephrotic syndrome occur in two groups of patients: (1) those presenting de novo or in relapse but not on steroids, and (2) those presenting in relapse or remission while still receiving pharmacologic doses of steroids (Table 46.23). Bacterial infections are noted with increased frequency in both groups, though much more common in the steroid-treated children. The types of infections include cellulitis, peritonitis, sepsis, pneumonia, meningitis, and arthritis. More recently gram-negative organisms have been reported as frequently as gram-positive organisms, the most common of which is *Streptococcus pneumoniae.* The typical signs and symptoms of infection may be masked in the steroid-treated nephrotic child, especially when the dose of steroid is quite high (e.g., 2 mg/kg/day of prednisone). Even peritonitis may occur without local abdominal signs in the child with ascites because the accumulated fluid prevents painful contact between the inflamed visceral and parietal layers of the peritoneum.

Symptomatic hypovolemia, which can progress to shock despite the presence of edema, results from injudicious fluid restriction, excess diuretic administration, or a combination of both factors. This complication should never happen once the patient is under medical management. The problem is not total body water or salt depletion, but intravascular depletion due to the abnormal distribution of what amounts to excess total body salt and water in the interstitial spaces. The signs and symptoms are those common to any child with hypovolemic shock.

Table 46.23
Acute Complications of Nephrotic Syndrome

I. Without Steroid Therapy
- A. Bacterial infection
- B. Hypovolemia
- C. Hypercoagulability (thromboembolic phenomena)
- D. Respiratory embarrassment

II. With Steroid Therapy
- A. Bacterial Infection[a]
- B. Hypovolemia[a]
- C. Hypercoagulability[c]
- D. Respiratory embarrassment
- E. Hypertension
- F. Altered behavior
- G. Steroid withdrawal (benign intracranial hypertension)

[a] These complications occur more frequently after steroid therapy.

Hypercoagulability, the tendency to form venous thromboses and thromboemboli, stems from many factors in nephrotic syndrome including hyperlipidemia leading to hyperviscosity, thrombocytosis and increased levels of circulating fibrinolytic inhibitors. Renal vein, pulmonary artery, and peripheral pulmonary emboli are particularly devastating manifestations of hypercoagulability in nephrotic syndrome. The addition of steroid therapy enhances this risk by mechanisms that are unclear, though it is believed that prednisone exerts some anti-heparin effect in man. For these reasons, nephrotic children should never have femoral or other deep venipunctures unless no alternative vascular access exists.

As mentioned above, massive ascites may rarely lead to acute respiratory embarassment, the treatment for which includes emergency paracentesis.

In steroid-treated children, acute rises in blood pressure with symptoms of headache, blurred vision or frank encephalopathy may occur at any point in the clinical course. The diagnosis of hypertensive encephalopathy does not require a specific level of systolic and/or diastolic blood pressure. Rather, it is the degree of blood pressure change and rate of rise which causes symptoms (see p. 445). Acute mood changes, ranging from euphoria to depression, are associated with the introduction, sudden increase, or decrease of steroid therapy. Symptomatic complaints include irritability with a low frustration level, hyperwakefulness at night, and emotional lability with crying and withdrawal. Abrupt reductions in steroids may lead to benign intracranial hypertension characterized by headaches, vomiting, and occasional papilledema which are not associated with arterial hypertension.

Although hyponatremia and hypocalcemia are frequently noted in the laboratory (see "Laboratory and Radiologic Studies" below), they are rarely associated with acute symptoms.

Laboratory and Radiologic Studies. Laboratory studies can be grouped into three general categories: (1) those required to confirm nephrotic syndrome, (2) those designed to categorize nephrotic syndrome as primary or secondary, and (3) those designed as aids to medical management. These studies are outlined in Table 46.24.

Hypoalbuminemia, defined as a serum albumin less than 3.0 g/dl, occurs in virtually every child with nephrotic syndrome. The measurement of the urinary protein concentration varies somewhat with urinary volume, but is usually 3 to 4+ (300 to 1000 mg/dl) in the untreated patient. Heavy proteinuria is the most reliable indicator of nephrotic syndrome and is defined as a 24-hour urine protein excretion of greater than 40 mg/sq m/hour or approximately 1 g in a 30-kg child. The urinalysis occasionally shows red blood cells and casts, suggesting an underlying nephritis, although this will not distinguish between causes of primary versus secondary nephrotic syndrome. In most nephrotics, the urine specific gravity is high, generally over 1.020.

The child with nephrotic syndrome often has an elevated hematocrit due to intravascular dehydration. It is typical for nephrotic children to have depressed serum Na levels, usually in the range of 120 to 135 meq/L. This rarely causes symptoms and does not require specific treatment. Hypocalcemia is also frequent but usually asymptomatic; the fall in Ca usually parallels that of albumin. Although the baseline uric acid is normal, many of these children later receive diuretic agents that can cause hyperuricemia. An initial elevation of the BUN in the range of 20 to 40 mg/dl is not at all uncommon and may reflect a reduction in GFR due to low plasma volume. Persistent azotemia can result from persistent reduction in GFR (an ominous prognostic sign) or, more commonly, from any combination of injudicious fluid restriction, increased catabolism due to poor dietary intake and/or infection, and/or steroid therapy. Serum creatinine should serve to differentiate these two categories, and either confirm or deny a true impairment in renal function due to intrinsic renal damage.

Table 46.24
Laboratory Tests in Nephrotic Syndrome

I. Diagnostic Tests to Confirm Nephrotic Syndrome
- A. Serum proteins (albumin, globulin)
- B. Serum cholesterol
- C. Urine protein
  - 1. Qualitative (dipstick: albumin)
  - 2. Quantitative (24-hr collection)

II. Diagnostic Tests to Distinguish Primary from Secondary Nephrotic Syndrome
- A. Urinalysis (evidence of nephritis)[a]
- B. Screening test for sickle cell anemia
- C. Serum immunoglobulins
- D. Serum C3 complement
- E. Serum antinuclear antibody, DNA binding
- F. Hepatitis B surface antigen

III. Management Tests
- A. CBC, especially hematocrit
- B. Serum Na, K, CO_2, Cl, Ca, uric acid
- C. Serum creatinine, BUN

[a] Hematuria plus proteinuria generally indicates nephritis, especially if there are cellular (e.g., red blood cell) casts in the sediment.

Management. Acute management of the nephrotic syndrome can be divided into two categories: specific and supportive. In the emergency department, the primary goal is usually either to restore and preserve intravascular volume or to treat symptomatic edema.

Despite the presence of peripheral edema, shock is treated in the usual way with 20 ml/kg/hour of normal saline until circulation is restored (see Chapter 2). If the child is clinically dehydrated and hemoconcentrated (hematocrit greater than 50%) but not in shock, a trial of Na-poor fluids orally at twice maintenance is preferable to immediately starting hypotonic intravenous solutions (i.e., 5% dextrose in 0.25 N salt solution). Fluids should be given in small amounts (1 to 4 oz) at frequent intervals (1 to 4 hours) to avoid vomiting due to an edematous gut. While Na restriction is indicated for an edematous nephrotic child, water restriction is rarely indicated and will only further decrease a usually low urine output.

The on-going state of intravascular hydration can be assessed by serial hematocrit tests. If the patient is symptomatic from massive edema, a trial of diuretics is warranted. Symptoms include difficulty ambulating, abdominal discomfort, skin breakdown and respiratory distress. Furosemide, 1 to 2 mg/kg/day, in two divided oral doses can be used. If there is no response, additional diuretics may be added which act at other sides in the tubule, thus enhancing the diuretic effect. Commonly used agents are spironolactone and hydrochlorthiazide, both starting at 1 mg/kg/day in two doses. Diuretics will not usually work, however, if the serum albumin concentration is less than 1.5 g/dl. When it appears urgent to remove some edema fluid, a combination of albumin infusions followed 30 min later by i.v. furosemide is often effective. The dose of albumin is 1 g/kg given as 25% salt-poor albumin followed by 0.5 to 1.0 mg/kg of furosemide. Paracentesis is rarely indicated but may bring prompt relief of severe respiratory distress from massive ascites.

Prednisone is generally begun at a dose of 2 mg/kg/day in 2 to 3 divided doses after the workup is initiated and a tuberculin test is placed. If the patient has previously been prednisone-responsive and is on either no drug or a maintenance program, a return to full therapy is indicated, provided frank relapse is obvious. If not, a quantitative 24-hour urine test should be ordered. Concurrent administration of a low sodium antacid may reduce the risk of gastric irritation.

Antibiotics are not administered prophylactically, but are used when a bacterial infection is suspected and the physician is awaiting results of appropriate cultures. This is particularly true if the patient is receiving Cytoxan or chlorambucil as well as prednisone. Penicillin has been the appropriate first choice in the past to treat *S. pneumoniae*. However, in view of reports of increased gram-negative bacterial infections in nephrotic children, it may be necessary to broaden this coverage. In the presence of documented infection, high-dose steroid treatment should be reduced but not discontinued. Halving the daily or alternate day dose (if 2 mg/kg or more) is appropriate, but no lower than 10 to 15 mg/day. Finally, good hygiene and a balanced high-protein diet are important adjuncts to therapy.

Indications for emergency admission of a child with active nephrotic syndrome are listed in Table 46.25. As in diabetes mellitus, the admission of a newly diagnosed child is as much for patient and parental education as it is for further workup and treatment. If a patient is more than 10% dehydrated, has orthostatic hypotension, and/or has a hemoglobin over 16 g/dl or a hematocrit over 50%, admission is advised for fluid therapy with close observation of vital signs and urine output.

HYPERTENSION

BACKGROUND

Definition. For the purposes of this review, hypertension is defined as a systolic and/or diastolic blood pressure greater than two standard deviations above the mean for age and sex. This definition, however, implies that the blood pressures have been taken carefully several times during the course of evaluation, and that the child is not diagnosed as being hypertensive until the mean values from two or three such evaluations have been established over several weeks. The emergency department physician is not afforded this opportunity for continued surveillance and is often dealing with symptomatic children who are severely hypertensive. Nonetheless, as with all patients who are diagnosed as being hypertensive, strict attention must be paid to the technical details of the measurement. The apparatus must calibrate to "zero," the cuff should be ½ to ⅔ the width of the upper arm, the inflatable bladder should encircle the arm, and note should be taken of undue patient anxiety, pain or muscle contraction.

Table 46.25
Indications for Admission for Nephrotic Syndrome

Newly diagnosed patient
Severe dehydration (e.g., poor intake, persistent vomiting)
Unexplained fever (e.g., suspected bacterial infection)
Refractory edema (e.g., respiratory distress)
Peritonitis
Renal insufficiency (e.g., elevated serum creatinine)

all of which can elevate both the systolic and diastolic readings.

This author finds it useful to group children into four major age categories when defining upper limits of systolic and diastolic blood pressures (Table 46.26). Additionally, it is useful to think of hypertension in terms of its four different presentations, each of which will be discussed under "Clinical Manifestations": (1) asymptomatic or minimally symptomatic hypertension, (2) malignant hypertension, (3) accelerated hypertension, and (4) hypertensive encephalopathy.

Epidemiology. Hypertension is a major worldwide public health concern; in the United States alone it is estimated that 40 million adults are hypertensive or roughly twice the number reported in yearly surveys. It has only been in recent years that pediatricians have recognized hypertension as a widespread and frequent health problem in children. Hypertension occurs throughout childhood and shows no sexual preference. As with adults, it probably occurs more frequently in blacks than in whites. There appear to be certain predisposing factors in genetically susceptible children. These include: (1) dietary sodium intake, (2) physical inactivity, and (3) obesity. In addition, genetic studies have also shown "clustering" of hypertension in certain families with strongly positive histories. Finally, infants who have high-normal or frankly elevated blood pressures tend to "track" along the same blood pressure percentiles as they progress through childhood.

Etiology. Now that essential hypertension is acknowledged as a cause of hypertension in childhood, pediatric hypertension should be divided into primary and secondary causes (see Table 46.27). Generally, the endocrinologic, cardiac, neurologic and miscellaneous causes of hypertension produce relatively mild and asymptomatic increases in blood pressure and affect systolic more than diastolic readings. The one exception is pheochromocytoma, a very rare disease in children. Steroid-induced hypertension usually requires several weeks of pharmacologic doses to develop (e.g., 2 mg/kg/day of prednisone). Occasionally, primary (essential) hypertension will produce symptoms such as headaches, abdominal pain, and/or visual disturbances, but rarely leads to malignant hypertension with or without encephalopathy. Most children with severe elevations of diastolic blood pressure (e.g., greater than 100 mm Hg under 10 years; greater than 115 mm Hg over 10 years of age) and hypertensive crises have a secondary renal or renovascular cause for their hypertension. In several large surveys of severe diastolic hypertension reported from tertiary referral cen-

Table 46.26
Hypertension

Age (yr)	Upper Limit (mm Hg)	
	Systolic	Diastolic
0–2	110	65
3–6	120	70
7–10	130	75
11–15	140	80

Table 46.27
Etiologies of Hypertension

I. *Primary*
   A. Essential hypertension
II. *Secondary*
   A. Renal
      1. Acute or chronic glomerulonephritis
         a. Postinfectious
         b. Henoch-Schönlein purpura
         c. Systemic lupus erythematosus
         d. Membranoproliferative nephritis
      2. Hemolytic-uremic syndrome
      3. Pyelonephritis (reflux nephropathy)
      4. Obstructive uropathy (with or without urinary infection)
      5. Segmental hypoplasia (Ask-Upmark kidney)
      6. Renal vascular disease (renal artery stenosis, embolus)
      7. Hemodialysis or renal transplant patients
   B. Endocrine
      1. Pheochromocytoma
      2. Cushing's syndrome
      3. Treatment with adrenocortical steroids
      4. Hyperthyroidism
   C. Cardiac
      1. Coarctation of the aorta
      2. Congestive heart failure (multiple causes)
   D. Neurologic
      1. CNS infection, drugs, tumor
   E. Miscellaneous drugs or poisons

ters, the four most common etiologies in order of decreasing frequency were: (1) chronic glomerulonephritis, (2) chronic (primary or secondary) pyelonephritis, (3) coarctation of the aorta, and (4) renal artery stenosis. The younger the child and the higher the blood pressure, the more likely it is that an underlying cause for hypertension will be found.

PATHOPHYSIOLOGY

Measured blood pressure results from the interaction of physiologic mechanisms regulating vascular volume and cardiac output on the one hand, and peripheral vascular tone on the other hand. Since pressure equals flow times the resistance to flow, blood pressure (BP) equals cardiac output (CO) times total peripheral resistance (TPR) or:

$$BP = CO \times TPR$$

Factors which influence CO either directly or through changes in vascular volume include circulating aldosterone levels, the autonomic nervous system, renal regulation of sodium balance, and small vessel compliance (i.e., capacitance and resistance).

The distribution of the blood volume is as important as the total blood volume itself in affecting blood pressure. Normally, volume is distributed partly in "resistance" vessels on the arterial side of the circulation. When blood volume is increased primarily in the resistance vessels, CO and BP are much more likely to rise than when the increase is primarily in the capacitance vessels. Factors which influence TPR by inducing either vasoconstriction or vasodilitation include activity of the autonomic nervous system, levels of circulating catecholamines and levels of circulating angiotension II (see Fig. 46.3).

Obviously, hypertension occurs when an increase in CO is not matched by a physiologic and reciprocal fall in TPR, and vice versa. In clinical practice, however, hypertension is only rarely due to a *single* pathophysiologic abnormality, such as activation of the renin-angiotensin system leading to vasoconstriction and thereby to increased TPR, or excessive salt and water retention leading to increased blood volume and CO.

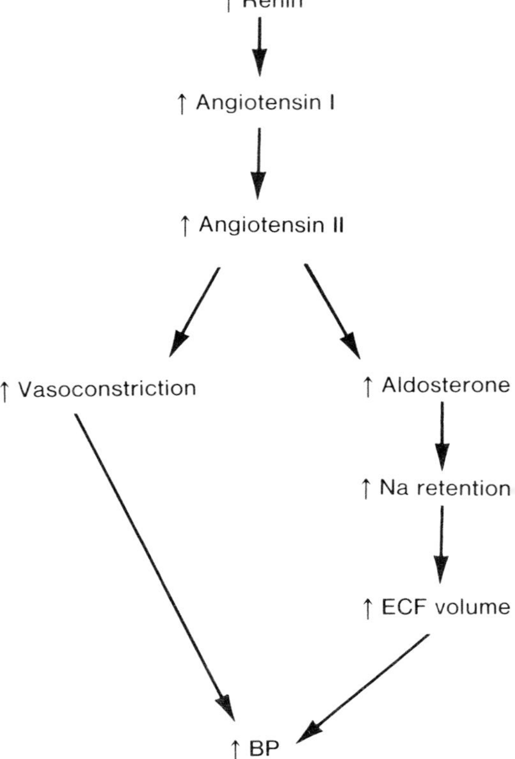

Figure 46.3. Mechanisms generating hypertension. *ECF* = extracellular fluid; *BP* = blood pressure.

Rather, one can think of hypertension as developing in two phases: (1) an initial or generating phase, which may be due primarily to increased CO or to vasoconstriction, and (2) a maintenance phase, which is almost always the result of increased CO from any one of a number of causes. Generally, the history and physical examination provide reliable guides in assessing the relative roles of CO and TPR in the acutely hypertensive child. Using this information, the emergency department physician can make a rational selection of initial antihypertensive drugs.

The pathophysiology of hypertensive encephalopathy is controversial. What is generally agreed upon is that autoregulation of cerebral blood flow is disrupted, leading either to over-regulation with exaggerated vasospasm and ischemic injury, or under-regulation with breakthrough of the circulation, increased cerebral flow and cerebral edema.

CLINICAL MANIFESTATIONS

As outlined above, hypertension usually presents in one of four ways (Table 46.28). First, there is the asymptomatic or mildly symptomatic child with mild to moderate elevations in blood pressure (130 to 160 mm Hg systolic; 80 to 110 diastolic). Acute symptoms are usually nonspecific and include headaches, abdominal pain, epistaxis and irritability. If the hypertension is chronic, failure to thrive and deteriorating school performance may be prominent complaints.

Malignant hypertension is characterized by marked elevations in systolic and/or diastolic blood pressure (e.g., 160 mm Hg or higher systolic under 10 years of age; 170 mm Hg or higher systolic over 10 years; 110 mm Hg or higher diastolic under 10 years; 115 mm Hg or higher diastolic over 10 years) and is often associated with spasm and tortuosity of the retinal arteries, papilledema, and hemorrhages and exudates on fundoscopic examination. This condition is much more commonly seen in adults than in children. Accelerated hypertension is defined as an acute rise in systolic and/or diastolic blood pressures superimposed upon previously existing hypertension. In both malignant hypertension and accelerated hypertension, the patient may present with dramatic symptoms and signs such as heart murmur, congestive heart failure, lower motor neuron facial palsy and hematuria.

Hypertensive encephalopathy is frequently seen in malignant hypertension and consists of a combination of symptoms and signs which often vary from patient to patient (Table 46.29). No single symptom or sign is diagnostic of this syndrome; the diagnosis is confirmed by demonstrating a rapid improvement in the symptoms and signs after the blood pressure is lowered. While there is no generally agreed-upon level of systolic and/or diastolic blood pressure at which encephalopathy occurs, most investigators believe that the rate of rise in the blood pressure is as important as the actual level itself. In this, as in all forms of severe hypertension (which are almost always secondary), the presenting complaints are usually attributable to the hypertension itself and not to the underlying disease.

Table 46.28
Clinical Presentations of Hypertension

Asymptomatic or mildly symptomatic
Malignant hypertension
Accelerated hypertension
Malignant hypertensive encephalopathy

Table 46.29
Malignant Hypertensive Encephalopathy

Nausea, vomiting
Headaches
Altered mental status (neuropsychiatric symptoms, confusion, stupor, coma)
Visual disturbances (blurry vision, decreased visual acuity, diplopia)
Seizures, stroke

Ascertaining the cause for increased blood pressure in the acutely hypertensive child with an abnormal neurologic examination presents a difficult challenge (Table 46.30). In general, when there is primary neurologic disease with secondary hypertension, the hypertension is usually mild and predominantly systolic. To determine whether the hypertension caused the neurologic abnormalities or vice versa, the physician must first observe the neurologic response to lowering the blood pressure. If signs and symptoms clear rapidly, then he is probably dealing with true hypertensive encephalopathy. In addition, primary neurologic disease can be screened for by a spinal tap (if a mass lesion is not suspected) or a CAT scan if a mass lesion or an intracranial bleed is suspected.

The urgency of prompt treatment of malignant hypertensive encephalopathy is attested to by the fact that fully one third of severely hypertensive children develop neurologic abnormalities which may be sudden in onset yet leave permanent deficits. These include cortical blindness, infarction of the optic nerve, and hemiplegia.

Finally, in patients with an acute exacerbation of long-standing hypertension,

Table 46.30
Differential Diagnoses of Hypertensive Encephalopathy

Head trauma
Cerebral hemorrhage or infarction
Meningitis, encephalitis
Brain tumor
Uremic encephalopathy

overzealous antihypertensive therapy can produce relative hypotension and paradoxically lead to some of the neurologic abnormalities cited above.

When confronted with newly diagnosed hypertension in the child, the physician should ask three important questions: (1) is the hypertension primary or secondary, (2) is there evidence of target organ injury, and (3) are there associated risk factors that would worsen the prognosis if the hypertension was not treated or treated unsuccessfully? The laboratory and radiologic workup can then be conveniently divided into three categories, as outlined in Table 46.31. The laboratory and radiology studies listed in the table are intended to be comprehensive, covering children with the full range of secondary causes of hypertension. Obviously, the emergency physician can usually establish a strong working diagnosis from the history and physical examination, and selected laboratory tests. A few examples should suffice to highlight this point.

Case 1. A 13-year-old obese black male has occasional bifrontal headaches and a blood pressure of 155/95 (mean of three readings). Fundoscopic and cardiovascular examinations are normal. The family history is positive for hypertension in an obese mother and maternal grandmother, and the diet contains excessive fried food.

Comment. This story is classical for essential hypertension and the only diagnostic studies that are required immediately are a urinalysis and urine culture, though many physicians would do a CBC, and tests for creatinine and electrolytes as well. Studies for target organ damage and associated risk factors should be done at a later time.

Case 2. An 11-year-old girl presents with the gradual onset of headaches and weight loss and the acute onset of abdominal pain

Table 46.31
Laboratory Tests in Hypertension

I. Diagnosis: Primary or Secondary
- A. Laboratory
  1. Urinalysis
  2. Urine culture
  3. Urinary catecholamines
  4. CBC with platelet count and blood smear
  5. Serum Na, K, Cl, CO_2, Ca, P_i
  6. Serum BUN, creatinine
  7. Serum C3 complement, antistreptolysin-O titer, antinuclear antibody
  8. Plasma renin
- B. Radiology
  1. Chest x-ray
  2. Intravenous pyelogram
  3. Voiding cystourethrogram
  4. Cardiac catheterization
  5. Renal ultrasound
  6. Renal scan
  7. Renal arteriogram
- C. Other
  1. ECG

II. Tests for Target Organ Injury
- A. Urinalysis
- B. Chest x-ray
- C. ECG

III. Tests for Associated Risk Factors
- A. Serum lipid profile (e.g., lipoprotein electrophoresis)
- B. Serum uric acid

with vomiting and blurry vision. She has a past history of three episodes of "cystitis" and cystoscopy with urethral dilitation. Examination reveals a thin girl in obvious pain with a blood pressure of 180/120 (mean of three readings) and arteriolar spasm and papilledema on fundoscopic examination. Urinalysis reveals clear urine with a specific gravity of 1.005 but otherwise is negative.

Comment. The likely diagnosis here is pyelonephritis-reflux nephropathy given the history of urinary infections, the parodoxically low urine specific gravity and the level of blood pressure. After stabilization of the blood pressure, the patient should be admitted. Urine cultures, intravenous pyelogram (IVP) and voiding cystourethrogram (VCUG) are the appropriate studies to order first. One might expect to see renal scarring with or without vesicoureteral reflux. Note that, in pyelonephritis, the level of glomerular filtration rate does not correlate with the elevation in blood pressure so the BUN and creatinine may be normal in this patient.

Case 3. A 10-year-old, previously well boy has a gradual onset of aggressive, sullen behavior followed by a severe headache, decreased visual acuity and a generalized seizure. Family and past medical histories are negative. Blood pressure is 220/150 (mean of three readings), there is florid papilledema with hemorrhages and exudates in the retina, cardiac enlargement and a bruit over the left flank.

Comment. The presumptive diagnosis is hypertensive encephalopathy due to renal artery stenosis which may present at any age. Once the blood pressure is stabilized, the patient is admitted for renal scan and arteriogram. A hypertensive IVP is no longer recommended in the evaluation of such patients because of the high rate of false negative studies.

Case 4. A 6-year-old boy presents with obvious symptoms and signs of congestive heart failure and red-brown urine. Urine output has been "low." He had a sore throat 10 days ago. The blood pressure is 160/110 (mean of three readings), there is obvious congestive heart failure with peripheral edema, and the urine reveals 3+ protein, large blood and 40 to 50 RBC, 10 to 20 WBC, 3 to 6 granular and 0 to 2 red blood cell casts per high power field.

Comment. This patient has acute glomerulonephritis (presumably poststreptococcal infection) with acute hypertension and oliguria leading to salt and water retention and congestive heart failure. His blood pressure needs immediate therapy and he must be admitted. The BUN and creatinine will probably be elevated and there may also be hyperkalemia. These studies are required immediately. Later serologic tests will confirm the diagnosis. The entrance point into the workup is the urinalysis which immediately points to some form of glomerulonephritis as the cause of secondary hypertension.

Patients with coarctation of the aorta are suspected by the presence of a heart murmur and diminished femoral pulses and blood pressures which are higher in the arms than in the legs. There is cardiomegaly on the chest x-ray. Those patients with hemolytic-uremic syndrome are anemic, thrombocytopenic and invariably develop red blood cell fragmentation on the blood smear. Finally, children with acute or chronic obstructive uropathy can be screened with renal ultrasound which is an excellent noninvasive technique for detecting hydronephrosis in the acutely ill child. Subsequent IVP and VCUG may then be needed to localize the site of the obstruction.

MANAGEMENT

Once hypertension is recognized and established, it should be treated. However, not all children appearing in the emergency department with hypertension require immediate treatment or admission. If hypertension is discovered by accident and is not the reason for the patient's complaints, medical follow-up for repeated measurements is indicated before therapy, especially if the elevation is mild (i.e., no more than 10 to 15 mm above the upper limits of normal for systolic and diastolic pressures given in Table 46.26). If the blood pressure is moderately elevated (see p. 445) but the patient is asymptomatic, two options exist. First, arrangements can be made for elective workup in an outpatient setting in the near future and either a thiazide diuretic or the β-blocker propranolol may be initiated at low dose (see Table 46.32). Alternatively, the patient may be admitted to begin an evaluation and therapy under hospital observation. Patients with severe hypertension (see p. 445) must always be admitted after initial parenteral antihypertensive therapy in the emergency department.

An overall management approach to the hypertensive child was formulated by the Special Task Force on Hypertension in Children and is outlined in Table 46.33. Turning to hypertensive emergencies, there are several "rules to live by":

1. Acute, de novo hypertension is more likely to cause symptoms and signs than chronic hypertension at any equivalent level of blood pressure and should be treated more aggressively;
2. In severe hypertension, always lower the blood pressure first before investigating the patient for an underlying cause;
3. Hypertensive encephalopathy is a bona fide

Table 46.32
Drugs Used in Hypertensive Crises

Drug	Initial Dose	Administration	Interval to Repeat or Increase Dose	Daily Maximum Dose		Onset of Action	Common Side Effects
				mg/kg	Total mg		
Nitroprusside	0.5 μg/kg/min	Infusion	30–60 min	8.0 μg/kg/min	?	Instantaneous	Hypotension, thiocyanate toxicity, salt and water retention
Diazoxide	3–5 mg/kg	Rapid i.v. push for 2–3 doses	15–30 min	10–15	?	Minutes	Tachycardia, salt and water retention, occasional delayed (>30 min) onset of action
Hydralazine	0.1–0.2 mg/kg	i.v. infusion over 15–30 min, every 4–6 hr	8–24 hr	1–2	100	15–30 min	Tachycardia, flushing, headache, vomiting, salt and water retention
Propranolol	1 mg/kg p.o., i.v.[a]	t.i.d. or q.i.d.	3–6 days	4–6	200–400	2–4 hr	Bradycardia, drowsiness, malaise; contraindicated in asthma
Reserpine	0.07 mg/kg, i.m.[b]	Every 12 hr	—	0.15	?	1–3 hr[b]	Nasal stuffiness, lethargy
Furosemide	1–2 mg/kg	i.v. push over 3–5 min	8–12 hr	10	?	Minutes	Extracellular fluid volume contraction, exacerbates hypertension in previously dehydrated patient; hypocalcemia, metabolic alkalosis, hearing loss if given too rapidly

[a] Consult pediatric nephrologist.
[b] When given with hydralazine 0.15 mg/kg as a single i.m. injection, this combination has proven effectiveness in acute poststreptococcal glomerulonephritis.

Table 46.33
Recommended Drug Regimen for Children with Hypertension by Age and Severity[a, b]

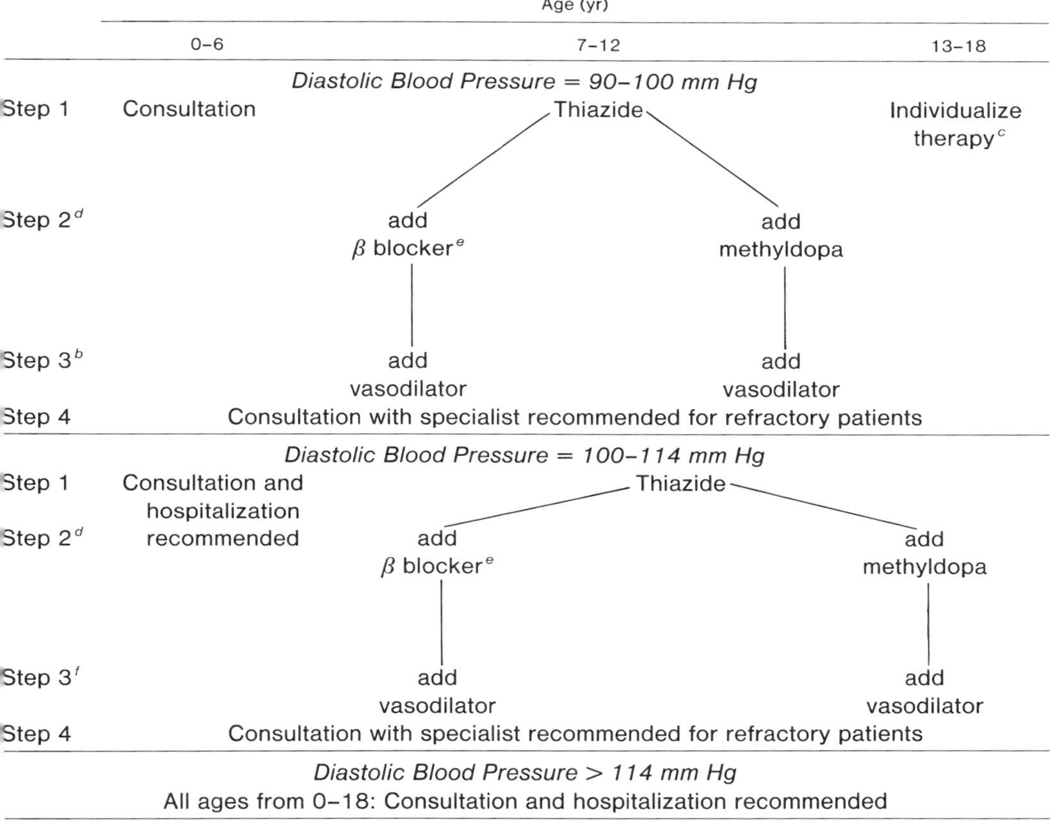

	Age (yr)		
	0–6	7–12	13–18
	Diastolic Blood Pressure = 90–100 mm Hg		
Step 1	Consultation	Thiazide	Individualize therapy[c]
Step 2[d]		add β blocker[e] — add methyldopa	
Step 3[b]		add vasodilator — add vasodilator	
Step 4	Consultation with specialist recommended for refractory patients		
	Diastolic Blood Pressure = 100–114 mm Hg		
Step 1	Consultation and hospitalization recommended	Thiazide	
Step 2[d]		add β blocker[e]	add methyldopa
Step 3[f]		add vasodilator	add vasodilator
Step 4	Consultation with specialist recommended for refractory patients		
	Diastolic Blood Pressure > 114 mm Hg		
	All ages from 0–18: Consultation and hospitalization recommended		

[a] Reproduced with permission from *Pediatrics*, *59* (suppl): 797, 1977.
[b] After appropriate evaluation and nondrug management, drug therapy may be considered indicated.
[c] Drug therapy not always required. Consider weight control and avoidance of salt abuse. Systematic follow-up. Recheck annually at minimum.
[d] Reserpine has been omitted from recommended drug regimens because of the many adverse effects it can produce in children, e.g., emotional depression and lability, sedation, stuffy nose.
[e] Propranolol is the β blocker of choice; it is not currently approved by the Food and Drug Administration for use in children.
[f] Clonidine and prazosin have not been evaluated in children and clinical data are not available. Guanethidine is most effective in the erect position and least effective in the supine position; consequently, its value in infants is limited.

medical emergency and must be treated as such to avoid sudden death or severe disability;

4. Short-acting parenterally administered antihypertensive agents are preferred in treating the newly diagnosed (and presumably recently hypertensive) patient;

5. Thiazides are the preferred diuretics of choice when renal function is normal or near normal; conversely, the loop blockers (furosemide, ethacrynic acid) are preferred in the patient with renal insufficiency; and

6. When given in combination, most antihypertensive drugs are synergistic in their combined effects.

Generally, most hypertensive crises in pediatric patients can be controlled, given the availability of new classes of potent antihypertensive agents and the expertise to use them. If the blood pressure is moderately to severely elevated but the patient is asymptomatic with normal fundi, hydralazine may be given by slow intravenous drip over 15 to 30 min (see Table 46.32). When there is malignant hypertension or hypertensive encephalopathy, diazoxide is the preferred agent of many because it acts almost immediately, can be repeated again in 15 to 30 min, may provide a surprisingly long duration of blood pressure control (8 to 12 hours with normal renal function and 12 to 24 hours in acute renal failure), and usually does not cause postural hypotension. However, it must be given by direct intravenous injection over 5 sec, as it is heavily protein-bound and does cause marked salt and water retention. Thus, if the patient is edematous (acute glomerulonephritis) or is in heart failure (e.g., acute glomerulonephritis, renal artery stenosis, pyelonephritis), diazoxide should be followed by a diuretic agent to provide for maximum effects. If, on the other hand, the patient has had significant vomiting and/or diarrhea and is ECF volume-contracted, immediate use of diuretics may exacerbate the hypertension, or at the very least blunt the antihypertensive action of the vasodilators. It is wise to begin a β-blocking agent such as propranolol in the extremely tachycardiac patient who is to receive a vasodilator. Generally speaking, the other sympatholytic agents used routinely as maintenance antihypertensive agents are not suited to treatment of acute hypertensive crises because of a slow onset of action.

In the occasional patient who is resistant to intravenous diazoxide, nitroprusside is the "court of last resort" and is invariably effective. However, its use mandates hospitalization and monitoring in an intensive care setting since it is administered by an infusion pump and can produce rapid hypotension. The duration of nitroprusside therapy is limited to 48 to 96 hours because of the accumulation and relative toxicity from thiocyanate, one of its principal metabolites.

The most promising of the newer generation of antihypertensive agents is the converting enzyme inhibitor, Captopril. Although pediatric doses and dose schedules remain to be established, preliminary reports have demonstrated remarkable effectiveness in children with difficult-to-control renal hypertension whose hypertension has entered an accelerated or malignant phase. The doses, dose intervals, onset of action and important side effects of the drugs used in hypertensive crisis are outlined in Table 46.32.

At this juncture, a brief comment about resistant hypertension is in order. When a previously diagnosed and treated hypertensive child appears in the emergency department with an exacerbation of symptomatic hypertension, several diagnostic considerations must be entertained:

1. The technique of blood pressure measurement is incorrect:
2. The patient is not taking one or all of the prescribed drugs in the prescribed fashion;
3. The physician has prescribed incorrect doses of drugs;
4. The patient has increased the salt content of his/her diet;
5. The patient is anxious or in pain; and/or
6. The disease or syndrome leading to hypertension has progressed.

The role of the emergency department physician is to rule out the first five considerations before increasing the doses of drugs or admitting the patient to the hospital, although this is not always easy to do!

Indications for hospitalization of the hypertensive child include malignant hypertension or hypertensive encephalopathy, accelerated hypertension with significant symptoms and signs, or severe hypertension regardless of clinical complaints, as outlined in Table 46.33.

ACUTE RENAL FAILURE

BACKGROUND

Definition. Acute renal failure (ARF) is an acute reduction in renal function as reflected by a decreased glomerular filtration rate (GFR). It may occur de novo or superimposed upon preexisting renal disease. Cardinal features are solute retention, demonstrated by a rise in serum BUN and/or creatinine concentrations (i.e., azotemia) and oliguria or, more rarely, anuria. Oli-

oliguria has been variably defined in the pediatric patient as: (1) a urine output ≤ 300 ml/sq m/day, (2) urine output ≤ 400 ml/day, (3) urine output ≤ 0.5 or ≤ 1 ml/kg/hour for an undefined period of time, and (4) urine output ≤ 0.5 or ≤ 1 ml/kg/hour for 12 to 24 hours. In the emergency department setting, precise measurements of previous urine output are rarely available, so it is most convenient to use the figure ≤ 1 ml/kg/hour for an unspecified period. True oliguria can then be confirmed later after 24 hours of hospital observation.

Although much less common in children than in adults, ARF can occur in the face of normal or near-normal urine output, particularly after burns or exposure to nephrotoxins. Finally, ARF can and should also be defined anatomically in terms of the localization of the insult. Thus, azotemia and oliguria may be due to prerenal, renal (i.e., parenchymal), or postrenal (i.e., obstructive) factors. There are important clinical distinctions to make, since if recognized promptly, prerenal and postrenal causes of ARF can frequently be reversed with appropriate therapy.

Epidemiology. ARF is generally sporadic in nature. There are no clearly defined environmental factors which play a role in the common causes of pediatric ARF, other than the variety of infectious agents which have been linked with hemolytic-uremic syndrome (HUS). Rarely, myoglobinuric ARF is secondary to a genetic abnormality in muscle metabolism. The incidence of ARF in hospitalized children beyond the neonatal period is not known. At the Children's Hospital of Philadelphia, approximately 5 to 10 children have ARF upon admission and another 30 to 40 are seen in consultation in the hospital each year.

Etiology. As suggested in the definition of ARF, an anatomic approach to considering various etiologies is useful (Table 46.34). Prerenal factors include: (1) decreased cardiac output resulting from various hemodynamic abnormalities which cause left ventricular failure or cardiogenic shock, (2) true hypovolemia resulting either from excessive salt and water losses or from hemorrhage, and (3) "relative" hypovolemia resulting from an altered distribution of salt and water out of the ECF space (i.e., "third-spacing") as seen in nephrotic syndrome, cirrhosis, pancreatitis and burns.

Table 46.34
Causes of Acute Renal Failure[a]

I. Prerenal
- A. Decreased cardiac output (cardiogenic shock)
- B. Decreased intravascular volume (hemorrhage, dehydration, "third-spacing")

II. Renal
- A. Primary renal parenchymal disease
  1. Vascular (acute glomerulonephritis, HUS[b])
  2. Interstitial (pyelonephritis, drug-induced)
- B. Acute tubular necrosis
  1. Ischemic injury (see I-B, above)
  2. Nephrotoxic injury (antibiotics, uric acid)
  3. Pigmenturia (myoglobinuria, hemoglobinuria)

III. Postrenal
- A. Obstructive uropathy
  1. Posterior urethral valves
  2. Intra-abdominal tumor
  3. Nephrolithiasis (rare)
- B. Renal vein thrombosis (rare outside of the neonatal period)

[a] Major pediatric causes of acute renal failure are listed in parentheses.
[b] Hemolytic-uremic syndrome.

Primary renal (parenchymal) causes of ARF can be divided into two general categories: (1) inflammatory diseases which are usually immunologic or infectious in nature such as acute poststreptococcal glomerulonephritis, methicillin-induced hypersensitivity interstitial nephritis or pyelonephritis, and (2) ischemic or nephrotoxic injuries which have been grouped under the general heading of acute tubular necrosis. Of increasing pediatric interest and perhaps importance are nephrotoxins that have long been known to play an important role in adult ARF. Most prominent in this regard are drugs, including several commonly used antibiotics (aminoglycosides and cephalosporins), heavy metals (mercury, lead, cisplatinum) and diuretics (thiazides and furosemide). When administered together, the antibiotics and diuretics appear to act synergistically in their nephrotoxic effect. Uric acid may also have a direct nephrotoxic effect as well as causing renal tubular (luminal) obstruction.

Postrenal or obstructive factors include, most commonly, posterior urethral valves and abdominal lymphomas or rhabdomyosarcomas causing extraureteral or extravesical compression. Rarely, a large kidney stone will obstruct the bladder outlet or the urethra.

The frequency of various etiologic factors in ARF differs markedly between adults and children, as seen in Table 46.35. Medical causes are much more common in children; postsurgical ARF is much more common in adults. Although the incidence of nephrotoxic ARF in children is very low (Table 46.35), it reflects the data from several older published series and focuses more on the newborn and younger infant than the older child. As stated previously, this author believes that the true incidence of nephrotoxic ARF is increasing, and it must be searched for aggressively in the initial evaluation.

PATHOPHYSIOLOGY

Early concepts of the pathophysiology of parenchymal ARF in man suggested that various predisposing factors led to a final common pathway of renal ischemia, which in turn resulted in tubular injury. This theory gave way to the theory of "vasomotor nephropathy" which suggested that ARF could be divided into an *initial phase*, mediated either by ischemia or nephrotoxic injury, and a *maintenance phase*, which resulted from increased intrarenal renin release and consequent intrarenal vasoconstriction. Recent studies, however, have thrown doubt on this model as satisfactory to explain oliguria and/or solute retention in all patients with ARF. In some animal models, vasoconstriction and renal ischemia may lead to a parallel decrease in renal blood flow and GRF in the *initial* phase of ARF, but renal blood flow spontaneously returns to normal (or is restored with vasodilators) despite a persistently low GRF with oliguria in the maintenance phase of ARF. It is more likely that parallel changes in renal blood flow and GRF explain the solute retention and oliguria of prerenal ARF rather than intrinsic ARF. What differentiates pre-renal from intrinsic ARF is: (1) preservation of tubular function in the former, especially maximum urinary concentration and sodium reabsorption (see "Clinical Manifestations"), and (2) response of azotemia and oliguria to volume replacement.

Table 46.35
Categories of Acute Renal Failure

Category	Approximate Incidence (%)[a]	
	Adults (N = 2476)	Children (N = 362)
Medical	24	85
Postsurgical	43	11
Toxin	10	<1
Trauma	14	?
Miscellaneous	9	4

[a] Adult data are based on two large series; pediatric data are based on six series, three of which focus on the newborn and infant less than 1 year of age.

Current theories about the pathogenesis of ARF in man are based on studies in several animal model systems which have led to an appreciation of four major factors that are probably operative singly or in combination in all forms of human intrinsic ARF. These are: (1) decreased renal blood flow; (2) decreased glomerular filtration (i.e., decreased glomerular permeability, K_f, and/or glomerular surface area); (3) tubular luminal obstruction; and (4) tubular backleak. A summary of one proposed schema for the pathogenesis of ARF in man is outlined in Figure 46.4. What is important to emphasize is that in most patients with ARF, more than one pathophysiologic abnormality is operating at any given time.

CLINICAL MANIFESTATIONS

Presentations. The presentation of ARF can be very variable and usually relates to the underlying disorder. Typical symptoms and signs are given in Table 46.36 together with the likely diagnosis. This list is by no means comprehensive but emphasizes those disorders likely to be encountered. Most children are oliguric or give a history of "decreased urination." If solute retention is severe, the clinical manifestations of uremia may ensue and obscure, for the moment, the underlying diagnosis (Table 46.37). One consideration that must always be raised in a patient with suspected ARF is whether or not it has occurred de novo or is superimposed upon

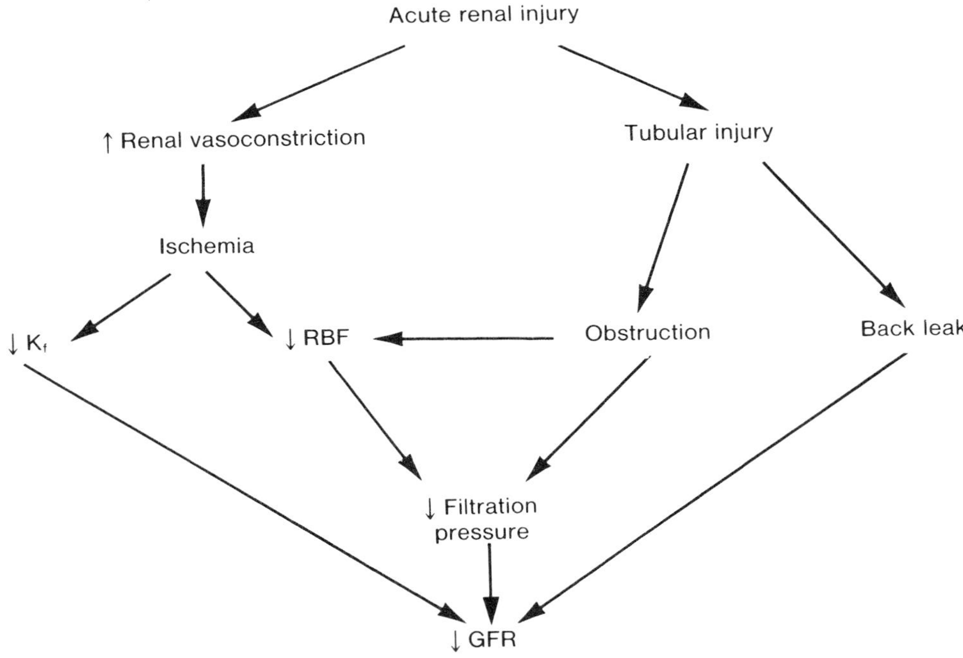

Figure 46.4 Acute renal failure pathogenesis. K_f = glomerular capillary ultrafiltration coefficient: K_f = glomerular permeability × filtering surface area; *RBF* = renal blood flow; *GFR* = glomerular filtration rate. (Adapted from J. H. Hostetter et al.: *Contemporary Issues in Neprhology, Acute Renal Failure*, Vol. 6, edited by B. M. Brenner and J. H. Stem. Churchill Livingstone, New York, 1981.)

Table 46.36
Acute Renal Failure Presenting Symptoms and Signs[a]

Syptoms	Signs	Likely Diagnosis
Nausea, vomiting	—	Gastroenteritis (ATN)
Diarrhea	Dehydration, shock	Gastroenteritis (ATN)
Hemorrhage	Shock	ATN
Fever	Petechiae, bleeding	Sepsis, DIC (ACN)
Melena	—	HUS
Sudden pallor	—	HUS
Grand mal seizures	—	HUS
Fever, chills	Flank tenderness	Pyelonephritis
Fever, skin rash	Erythema multiforme, purpura	AIN HSP nephritis
Sore throat	Hypertension	PSGN
Pyoderma	Edema	PSGN
Grand mal seizures	Congestive heart failure	PSGN
Trauma	Muscle tenderness	Myoglobinuria
Myalgia	Myoedema	Myoglobinuria
Antibiotics, diuretics	—	Nephrotoxic acute renal failure
Variable urine output	Suprapubic mass	OU

[a] ATN = acute tubular necrosis, DIC = disseminated intravascular coagulation, ACN = acute cortical necrosis, HUS = hemolytic-uremic syndrome, AIN = acute interstitial nephritis (''hypersensitivity nephritis''), HSP = Henoch-Schönlein purpura nephritis, PSGN = poststreptococcal glomerulonephritis, and OU = obstructive uropathy.

Table 46.37
Acute Renal Failure: Clinical Uremia

- *I. Gastrointestinal*
  - A. Nausea, vomiting, diarrhea
  - B. Hiccoughs, fetid odor
  - C. Hematemesis, melena
- *II. Cardiovascular*
  - A. Pericarditis
- *III. Dermatologic*
  - A. Pruritus
  - B. Uremic "frost"
- *IV. Neurologic*
  - A. Apathy, fatigue
  - B. Psychiatric disturbance
  - C. Seizures
  - D. Asterixis
  - E. Coma
  - F. Peripheral neuropathy

preexisting chronic renal failure. Clinical clues that may lead to the latter diagnosis are failure to thrive, a history of polyuria/polydipsia, continued good urine output despite historical and physical evidence of dehydration, and physical evidence of renal rickets. Relevant laboratory data supporting the diagnosis of chronic renal disease will be reviewed below.

Complications. It is the immediate or occasionally the delayed complications of ARF, not ARF itself, that confront the emergency department physician with the most important diagnostic and therapeutic challenges. The major complications in terms of frequency and threat to life are: (1) severe hyperkalemia with impending or actual cardiac arrhythmia, (2) congestive heart failure with pulmonary edema, usually secondary to hypertension, (3) malignant hypertensive encephalopathy with seizures, (4) urinary tract infection with associated urinary obstruction, and (5) metabolic seizures.

Hyperkalemia occurs after many causes of ARF, but particularly in association with myoglobinuria and after open heart surgery. It is aggravated by hemolysis, acidosis, infection and catabolic stress. Congestive heart failure and malignant hypertensive encephalopathy typically occur in many forms of acute glomerulonephritis, but especially in poststreptococcal glomerulonephritis. The risks of rapid destruction of renal parenchyma by bacterial organisms is dramatically increased in the face of obstructive uropathy. Such patients usually present with systemic symptoms and signs of infection including fever, chills, vomiting, abdominal pain and costovertebral angle tenderness. Metabolic seizures are most often due to uremia and not to hyponatremia and/or hypocalcemia, which are frequently present in ARF. Hyponatremia is mild and usually develops slowly. Hypocalcemia usually does not cause tetany in the untreated patient because of coexistent metabolic acidosis.

Laboratory and Radiologic Studies. Of particular importance in differentiating the three anatomic forms of ARF are the urinalysis and the so-called urinary indices. In the critically ill patient who has not passed urine, a sterile straight catheterization of the bladder is appropriate to obtain a sample. The urinalysis is most helpful in separating glomerulonephritis from the other causes of ARF. In the typical case of acute glomerulonephritis, the dipstick shows large amounts of blood and protein, and there are red blood cells, granular and cellular (i.e., red blood cell) casts in the spun sediment. Patients with prerenal ARF and those with acute tubular necrosis typically have little blood or protein by dipstick and an unremarkable sediment save for hyaline casts. Occasionally, the latter group will have prominent numbers of renal tubular epithelial cells and epithelial cell casts in the sediment, but the author has found this to be generally unhelpful.

The major differentiation of prerenal ARF from acute tubular necrosis is by urine concentration as measured by specific gravity. Typically, the patient with prerenal ARF has a concentrated urine (specific gravity greater than 1.025), whereas the patient with acute tubular necrosis tends to have an isosthenuric urine (specific gravity 1.005 to 1.015). Hematuria by dipstick examination without corresponding red blood cells in the sediment suggests hemoglobinuria or myoglobinuria as the cause of ARF, especially if pigmented granular casts are also seen. Renal tubular and bladder epithelial cells and epithelial cell casts are commonly seen in nephrotoxic ARF or drug induced (hypersensitivity) acute interstitial nephritis. Eosinophils on a Wright's stained urine sediment make the latter diagnosis much more likely. Marked pyuria, leukocyte casts and a positive Gram stain of the urine all support the diagnosis of acute pyelonephritis, with or without a coexistent obstruction.

Urinary indices refer to the ratios of the simultaneously measured solutes sodium, creatinine, and urea, and osmolality in "spot" samples of blood and urine. The primary purpose of these indices is to assist in differentiating prerenal ARF from acute tubular necrosis. These indices have generally replaced the BUN/creatinine ratio and "spot" urine sodium concentrations, which are too variable to reliably separate prerenal from renal ARF. They are outlined in Table 46.38.

Other diagnostic studies are outlined in Table 46.39. HUS is typically characterized by thrombocytopenia, microangiopathic hemolytic anemia with red blood cell fragmentation, and oliguria. However, early in the course of HUS the only abnormal findings may be a rising BUN and falling hemoglobin, or bloody diarrhea alone, suggesting inflammatory bowel disease. The coagulation profile is often abnormal in HUS and always so in disseminated intravascular coagulation. Low C3 complement is seen in 90% of children with poststreptococcal glomerulonephritis, and elevated streptococcal serologies occur in 85 to 95% of such children, depending on the number of antibodies measured. A typical patient with poststreptococcal glomerulonephritis is presented in the section on "Hypertension" (Case 4). Elevated antinuclear antibody titers are found in virtually all patients with lupus nephritis, albeit a rare cause of ARF. High IgE levels and absolute eosinophilia suggest acute interstitial nephritis. Elevated CPK is an invariable accompaniment of rhabdomyolysis and myoglobinuria. In patients with massive hemolysis, serum haptoglobin falls to undetectable levels and elevated plasma hemoglobin may impart a pink-red color to the serum. An elevated 24-hour urine excretion of uric acid supports the diagnosis of uric acid nephropathy as the primary cause of ARF. A potentially useful screening test is the urine uric acid to creatinine ratio on a "spot" urine specimen; if the ratio is ≥ 1.0, it supports this diagnosis. Most of the other causes of ARF result in a raised serum but not urine uric acid.

Renal ultrasound has replaced IVP as the initial x-ray study of choice to differentiate postrenal (obstructive) from intrinsic renal causes of ARF. This is particularly true in critically ill patients, since the ultrasound evaluation is a noninvasive procedure without the risk of intravenous injection of contrast. The ultrasound examination will not usually show the specific site

Table 46.38
Acute Renal Failure: Urinary Indices[a]

Indices	Acute Renal Failure	
	Prerenal	Intrinsic[b]
Older Children and Adults		
U/P urea nitrogen	> 8	< 3
U/P creatinine	> 40	< 20
U/P osmolality	> 500 mOsm/kg H_2O; > 1.5	< 350 mOsm/kg/H_2O; < 1.5
FE_{Na} (%)[c]	< 1.0	>1.0
Neonates and Infants		
U/P urea nitrogen	Variable	Variable
U/P creatinine	Variable	Variable
U/PO osmolality	> 1.0	< 1.0
FE_{Na} (%)[c]	> 2.5	< 2.5

[a] U_x/P_x refers to simultaneously measured urine and plasma concentrations of x.
[b] Refers to classical acute tubular necrosis from various causes.
[c] Fractional excretion of filtered sodium = (U/P)Na/(U/P) creatinine × 100.

Table 46.39
Acute Renal Failure Laboratory Tests for Diagnosis

Test	Diagnosis[a]
Blood	
Platelet count	HUS, DIC
Blood smear	HUS, DIC
Coagulation profile	HUS, DIC
Blood culture	DIC, acute pyelonephritis
Streptococcal serologies	PSGN
C3 complement	PSGN
Antinuclear antibody	Systemic lupus erythematosus-nephritis
IgE, eosinophil count	AIN
Aminoglycoside level	Nephrotoxicity
Creatinine phosphokinase (CPK)	Myoglobinuria
Haptoglobin, "pink" plasma	Hemoglobinuria
Urine	
Culture	Acute pyelonephritis
Protein (24 hr)	Acute nephritis
Uric acid (24 hr or $U_{uric}/U_{creatinine}$ ratio)	Uric acid nephropathy
Radiology	
Renal ultrasound	Obstructive uropathy
Intragenous pyelogram	Obstructive uropathy, pyelonephritis
Voiding cystourethrogram (VCUG)	Underlying chronic renal disease, obstructive uropathy
Renal flow scan	Acute tubular necrosis (cortical necrosis), renal vascular insult

[a] HUS = hemolytic-uremic syndrome, DIC = disseminated intravascular coagulation (bacterial sepsis), PSGN = poststreptococcal glomerulonephritis, and AIN = acute interstitial nephritis ("hypersensitivity"nephritis).

of obstruction, but the IVP should not be performed until the patient is cardiovascularly stable and well hydrated. The IVP subsequently provides data on renal size, position and, to some extent, function. Information gained may include: (1) evidence of obstruction, (2) pyelonephritic scarring, and (3) small, contracted kidney suggesting underlying chronic disease. An early but persistent nephrogram phase of the IVP, without normal concentration of the dye in the pelvocalyceal system, supports the diagnosis of acute tubular necrosis with tubular backleak. The VCUG is often underused in the initial evaluation of suspected causes of postrenal ARF. It is the best test to diagnose posterior urethral valves (the most common obstructive cause of ARF) and provides additional information about the presence or absence of coexistent vesicoureteral reflux. The renal scan is best used to assess blood flow to and within the kidneys. In experienced hands, the scan can also assess renal size and differentiate intrinsic renal from postrenal causes of ARF. It may be used in conjunction with ultrasound in the child whose clinical status rules out the immediate use of IVP dye. An additional advantage of the scan over IVP is that it does not require a minimal level of estimated glomerular filtration rate to be performed (i.e., serum creatinine $\leq$ 4.0 mg/dl).

MANAGEMENT

When confronted in the emergency department with a child who has ARF, the examining physician should always ask himself four questions about therapy: (1) Is this prerenal ARF and can parenchymal ARF be prevented by the appropriate fluid therapy? (2) Are there any life-threatening complications evident at this time which must be treated immediately? (3) Is there urinary tract infection with associated obstruction that must be relieved immediately? and (4) Are there indications for immediate peritoneal dialysis or hemodialysis? An initial set of laboratory tests provides a guide for subsequent management (Table 46.40).

1. If prerenal ARF is suspected from the clinical history, physical examination and urinary indices, fluid resuscitation should be employed. Confirmation of this diagnosis requires a resumption of normal urine flow and a decrease in solute retention following restoration of euvolemia. An approach to fluid resuscitation is outlined in Table 46.41. A single exception to this approach might be the patient who is euvolemic or even hypervolemic but in cardiogenic shock. In the critically ill, unconscious or uncooperative patient with an uncertain urine output, this author favors placement of an indwelling urinary catheter to accurately monitor urine output.

One clinical condition that demands the use of mannitol and furosemide is myoglobinuria or hemoglobinuria. Here the purpose of therapy is to prevent tubular obstruction by pigmented proteins after ECF volume is restored. The order of therapy in Table 46.41 is revised; 1 to 2 mg/kg of furosemide i.v. is given initially followed 5 to 10 min later by 0.5 mg/kg of mannitol. After urine flow is established, an infusion of 5% mannitol in one-quarter strength saline can be administered as ml for ml replacement of urine until the pigmenturia has resolved. Finally, as indicated in Table 46.41, failure to respond to a fluid challenge or a fluid plus diuretic challenge has one of three explanations: (1) volume losses have been underestimated, (2) there is coexistent urinary obstruction, or (3) the patient has already developed parenchymal ARF! The major risk of mannitol occurs in parenchymal ARF because if not excreted, it will recirculate and may cause ECF volume expansion.

Table 46.40
Acute Renal Failure: Laboratory Tests for Management

Blood:
Hemoglobin, hematocrit
BUN, creatinine
Electrolytes (Na, K, Cl, HCO_3)
Blood gas (optional)
Ca, Pi, Mg, uric acid
Other:
Chest x-ray
ECG
ECHO cardiogram

2. Regarding life-threatening complications of ARF, the therapy of malignant hypertension has previously been discussed. Hyponatremia is common but rarely symptomatic in ARF unless it is due to ECF volume depletion. In euvolemic or clinically edematous patients, the treatment is fluid restoration and not extra sodium. Hypocalcemia is also common but rarely symptomatic in ARF and should not be treated with supplemental calcium until and unless the serum phosphorus concentration is known. Failure to take this precaution may result in raising the $Ca \times P_i$ product and risk ectopic calcification or further renal damage! Metabolic acidosis does not need correction unless the serum bicarbonate is less than 15 meq/L, and only then with slow replacement with 1 meq/kg/day of bicarbonate and frequent monitoring. "Overshoot" alkalosis can easily occur in the face of a rapidly changing GRF and urine flow. Also, a sudden shift of the pH toward normal or an alkaline range can convert asymptomatic hypocalcemia into frank tetany. Treatment of hyperkalemia is often the most urgent goal in ARF. Specifics of therapy for varying levels of serum K are outlined in Table 46.42.

3. If the clinical picture, urinalysis and Gram stain suggest urinary tract infection, coexistent obstructive uropathy must be ruled out rapidly. It can be immediately suspected because acute pyelonephritis in the unobstructed patient rarely causes ARF. Absence of a history of difficulty voiding or failure to palpate an enlarged bladder does not rule out obstruction and a renal ultrasound should be obtained.

4. The indications for dialysis are outlined in Table 46.43. Generally, peritoneal dialysis is favored over hemodialysis, although the latter may be more efficient at removing certain nephrotoxins and potassium. The reasons for favoring peritoneal dialysis are: (1) its ready availability, (2) the relatively simple technique employed, and (3) its safety in terms of preserving cardiovascular stability or minimally dis-

Table 46.41
Acute Renal Failure (ARF): Immediate Therapy of Prerenal ARF

I. Dehydration with Shock
- A. 20 ml/kg/hr of 10% dextrose in one-half strength sodium bicarbonate (75 meq/L) until vital signs stable and urine flow re-established (6–10 ml/kg/hr)
- B. Repeat hourly if necessary for 1–2 doses
- C. After hour 2 or 3, if no urine flow, catheterize
- D. If no urine in bladder, give furosemide, 2 mg/kg i.v.[a]
- E. If no urine flow, treat as parenchymal ARF

II. Hemorrhage with Shock
- A. 20 ml/kg/hr of plasma, or if unavailable, crystalloid solution as listed in Ia
- B. Transfuse when blood available (whole fresh blood or packed red blood cells plus fresh frozen plasma)
- C. After hour 2 or 3, if no urine flow, catheterize
- D. If no urine in bladder, give furosemide, 2 mg/kg i.v.[a]
- E. If no urine flow, treat as parenchymal ARF

[a] Mannitol can be substituted for furosemide at a dose of 0.5 g/kg (2.5 ml/kg of a 20% solution) infused over 10–20 min.) A urine flow of 6–10 ml/kg/hr should be established in the first several hours.

Table 46.42
Acute Renal Failure: Emergency Treatment of Hyperkalemia

1. Serum [K] 5.5–7.0 meq/L (normal ECG):
   Kayexelate 1 g/kg p.o. or per rectum[a]
2. Serum [K] > 7.5 meq/L or > 7.0 meq/L with abnormal ECG[b]:
   Step 1. Calcium gluconate 0.5 ml/kg as 10% solution over 2–4 min with ECG monitoring. Stop when pulse rate falls 20/min or to < 100/min
   Step 2. Sodium bicarbonate 3.3 ml/kg of 7.5% solution
   Step 3. Glucose 1 ml/kg as 50% solution. If hyperkalemia persists, infuse a 20–30% glucose solution with 0.5 unit regular insulin/kg. Keep blood sugar < 300 mg/dl
3. Serum [K] persistently > 6.5 meq/L:
   Dialysis

[a] Kayexelate exchanges 1 meq K for 1 meq Na and lowers serum [K] by approximately 1 meq/L within 4 hr. It can be administered p.o. with food or beverage, by nasogastric tube or per rectum in 10% glucose/water (1 g in 4 ml) or in 20% sorbitol (50–100 ml). It must be retained for at least 30 min.
[b] Serum [K] > 7.0 with a normal ECG can be treated as outlined in 1.

Table 46.43
Acute Renal Failure: Indications for Peritoneal Dialysis

Uremic syndrome
BUN > 100 mg/dl
Persistent hyperkalemia (serum [K] > 6.5 meq/L)
Persistent metabolic acidosis (serum [HCO_3] < 10 meq/L)
Persistent congestive heart failure
Oliguric acute renal failure secondary to hemolytic-uremic syndrome or rhabdomyolysis with myoglobinuria

turbing cardiovascular instability! It is generally not recommended in patients with generalized vasculitis, heat stroke, or very recent abdominal surgery.

Any child with suspected or proven ARF from any cause deserves hospitalization.

References

FLUID AND ELECTROLYTE DISTURBANCES

Isotonic Dehydration, Hyponatremia, Hypernatremia

DeFronzo RA, Thier SO: Pathophysiologic approach to hyponatremia. *Arch Intern Med* 140: 897, 1980.
Editorial: Hyponatremia. *Lancet* 1: 1334, 1976.
Humes HD, Narins RG, Brenner BW: Disorders of water balance. *Hosp Pract* 14: 133, 1979.
Moses AM, Miller M: Drug-induced dilutional hyponatremia. *N Engl J Med* 291: 1234, 1974.
Norman ME: The physiology of fluid-electrolyte and acid-base balance in children, Part II. In *Clinical Diagnosis Quiz*, Vol. 5, No. 6, edited by PJ Honig, WW Tunnessen Jr. Creative Medical Publications, Syracuse, N.Y., 1980.
Schrier RW: Renal sodium excretion, edematous dis-

orders, and diuretic use. In *Renal and Electrolyte Disorders*, edited by RW Schrier. Little, Brown, Boston, 1976.

Schrier RW: New treatments for hyponatremia (Editorial). *N Engl J Med* 298: 214, 1978.

Schrier RW, Berl T: Disorders of water metabolism. In *Renal and Electrolyte Disorders*, edited by RW Schrier. Little, Brown, Boston, 1976.

Hypokalemia, Hyperkalemia

Cohen JJ: Disorders of potassium balance. *Hosp Prac* 14: 119, 1979.

Editorial: Familial hypokalemic periodic paralysis. *Lancet* 1: 1140, 1981.

Gabow P: Disorders of potassium metabolism. In *Renal and Electrolyte Disorders*, edited by RW Scrhier. Little, Brown, Boston, 1976.

Reineck HJ: The control of potassium homeostasis. *Kidney* 12: 13, 1979.

Hypocalcemia, Hypercalcemia

Root AW, Harrison HE: Recent advances in calcium metabolism; I. Mechanisms of calcium homeostasis. *J Pediatr* 88: 1, 1976.

Root AW, Harrison HE: Recent advances in calcium metabolism; II. Disorders of calcium homeostasis. *J Pediatr* 88: 177, 1976.

Metabolic Acidosis

Foreman JW: Metabolic acid-base disorders. In *Metabolic Disease, A Guide to Early Recognition*, edited by RW Cohn, K Roth, S Segal. W. B. Saunders, Philadelphia (in press).

Lyons H: Increased anion gap acidosis. In *Acid-Base and Electrolyte Balance*, edited by AB Schwartz, H Lyons. Grune & Stratton, New York, 1977.

Lyons H: Acidosis of kidney disease. In *Acid-Base and Electrolyte Balance*, edited by AB Schwartz, H Lyons. Grune & Stratton, New York, 1977.

Schwartz, AB: Differential diagnosis of metabolic acidosis using anion gap. In *Acid-Base and Electrolyte Balance*, edited by AB Schwartz, H Lyons. Grune & Stratton, New York, 1977.

Winters RW: Pathophysiology of acid-base disorders. In *The Body Fluids in Pediatrics*, edited by RW Winters. Little, Brown, Boston, 1973.

NEPHROTIC SYNDROME

Barnett HL, Schoeneman M, Bernstein J, et al.: The nephrotic syndrome. In *Pediatric Kidney Disease*, Vol. II, Chap. 53, edited by CM Edelmann Jr. Little, Brown, Boston, 1978.

Giangiacomo JG, Cleary TG, Cole BR, et al.: Serum immunoglobulins in the nephrotic syndrome. *N Engl J Med* 293: 8, 1975.

Habib R, Kleinknecht C: The primary nephrotic syndrome of childhood; classification and clinicopathologic study of 406 cases. In *Pathology Annual*, p. 165, edited by SC Somers. Appleton-Century-Crofts, New York, 1971.

Levinsky RJ, Malleson PN, Barratt TM, et al.: Circulating immune complexes in steroid-responsive nephrotic syndrome. *N Engl J Med* 298: 126, 1978.

Rubin MI: Nephrotic syndrome. In *Pediatric Nephrology*, Chap. 19, edited by MI Rubin, TM Barratt. Williams & Wilkins, Baltimore, 1975.

White RHR, Glasgow EF, Mills RJ: Clinicopathologic study of nephrotic syndrome in childhood. *Lancet* 1: 1353, 1970.

HYPERTENSION

Balfe JW, Rance CP: Recognition and management of hypertensive crises in childhood. *Pediatr Clin North Am* 25: 159, 1978.

Fleischmann LE: Management of hypertensive crises in children. *Pediatr Ann* 6: 72, 1977.

Gill DG, daCosta M, Cameron JS, et al.: Analysis of 100 children with severe and persistent hypertension. *Arch Dis Child* 51: 951, 1976.

Hulse JA, Taylor DSI, Dillon MJ: Blindness and paraplegia in severe childhood hypertension. *Lancet* 2: 553, 1979.

Lloyd-Still J, Cottom D: Severe hypertension in childhood. *Arch Dis Child* 42: 34, 1967.

Ram CVS: Hypertensive encephalopathy. *Arch Intern Med* 138: 1851, 1978.

Report of the Task Force on Blood Pressure Control in Children: *Pediatrics* 59 (suppl): 797, 1977.

Tarazi RC: Management of the patient with resistant hypertension. *Hosp Pract* 16: 49, 1981.

ACUTE RENAL FAILURE

Anderson RJ, Schrier RW: Clinical spectrum of oliguric and nonoliguric acute renal failure. In *Contemporary Issues in Nephrology, Acute Renal Failure*, Vol. 6, edited by BM Brenner, JH Stein. Churchill Livingstone, New York, 1981.

Bastl CP, Rudnick MR, Narins RG: Diagnostic approaches to acute renal failure. In *Contemporary Issues in Nephrology, Acute Renal Failure*, Vol. 6, edited by BM Brenner, JH Stem. Churchill Livingstone, New York, 1981.

Ellis D, Gartner JC, Galvis AG: Acute renal failure in infants and children; diagnosis, complications and treatment. *Crit Care Med* 9: 607, 1981.

Hostetter JH, Wilkes BM, Brenner BM: Mechanisms of impaired glomerular filtration in acute renal failure. In *Contemporary Issues in Nephrology, Acute Renal Failure*, Vol. 6, edited by BM Brenner, JH Stem. Churchill Livingstone, New York, 1981.

Lieberman E: Management of acute renal failure in infants and children. Nephrosis 11: 193, 1973.

Mathew OP, Jones AS, James E, et al.: Neonatal renal failure; usefulness of diagnostic indices. *Pediatrics* 65: 57, 1980.

Miller TR, Anderson RJ, Linas SL, et al.: Urinary diagnostic indices in acute renal failure. *Ann Intern Med* 89: 47, 1978.

Ng RCK, Suki W: Treatment of acute renal failure. In *Contemporary Issues in Nephrology, Acute Renal Failure*, Vol. 6, edited by BM Brenner, JH Stem. Churchill Livingstone, New York, 1981.

Schrier RW: Acute renal failure; pathogenesis, diagnosis and management. *Hosp Prac* 16: 93, 1981.

Smotens P, Stein JH: Pathophysiology of acute renal failure. *Am J Med* 70: 479, 1981.

Trainin EB, Spitzer A: Treatment of acute renal failure. In *Pediatric Kidney Disease*, edited by CM Edelmann Jr. Little, Brown, Boston, 1978.

CHAPTER 47

Hematologic Emergencies

JOHN W. BENDER, M.D., AND ALAN R. COHEN, M.D.

INTRODUCTION

Hematologic disorders arise in children who have been previously well, who have known blood diseases, or who have systemic diseases. While the particular setting in which a serious blood abnormality occurs may affect some facets of emergency care, the initial measures of support, diagnosis and treatment are based on general principles which frequently cross the boundaries between the usual categories of blood disorders. In the following discussion of hematologic emergencies, particular emphasis is placed on these principles as they apply to disorders of red cells, white cells, platelets and coagulation. The initial evaluation and treatment of life-threatening disorders are described in detail. Where controversy exists regarding specific management problems, alternative approaches are presented.

DISORDERS OF RED BLOOD CELLS

Severe anemia is a pediatric emergency which requires rapid evaluation and treatment to prevent hypoxia, congestive heart failure, and death. The classification of causes of anemia according to (1) blood loss, (2) increased red cell destruction and (3) decreased red cell production is familiar to most physicians and provides an excellent starting point for the evaluation of the anemic child. In Chapter 30, these categories are used for the differential diagnosis of hematologic causes of pallor and for the appropriate selection of initial laboratory studies. In the following section, the same classification is applied to the emergency management of specific hematologic disorders.

Blood Loss

Trauma is the leading cause of major hemorrhage in children. Every emergency physician must be prepared to act quickly and systematically when confronted with an actively bleeding child. The initial approach often requires the joint effort of a team of doctors and nurses in order to accomplish numerous tasks simultaneously. Within the first few minutes the nature of the accident, an estimate of blood loss and the presence of major current or chronic illnesses, including bleeding disorders, should be determined. The adequacy of the airway must be assured. Vital signs should be measured frequently in order to detect early signs of hypovolemic shock. All clothing should be removed, and the child should be examined for sites of bleeding other than those found upon initial inspection. Intravenous access should be established, preferably in a large vein, and blood samples should be drawn for a complete blood count (including platelet count), screening coagulation studies (prothrombin time and partial thromboplastin time), and the crossmatching of donor blood. A spun hematocrit should be measured immediately in the emergency department. If bleeding is brisk and sustained or if there is any suggestion of hypovolemic shock, volume expanders should be infused. Although colloid preparations such as 5% albumin are more efficient for the maintenance of intravascular volume than crystalloids such as saline or Ringer's lactate, the latter solutions may be more readily available and should be used until colloid is ready.

After immediate stabilization has been completed and external hemorrhage has been slowed or stopped, the child should be evaluated for internal hemorrhage. This evaluation is especially important when the nature of the trauma is unclear or when multiple areas of the body may have been involved as in automobile or bicycle accidents. The importance of locating internal hemorrhage is underscored by the too common occurrence of hypovolemic shock and death in the child whose skin lacerations were sutured but whose ruptured spleen went undetected. In many instances, the examination for internal hemorrhage should be performed in consultation with a surgeon who is experienced in the management of multiple trauma. Suspicion of internal bleeding should be raised in the presence of a continuously falling hematocrit or continuing signs of hypovolemic shock despite control of external bleeding and the replacement of seemingly adequate volume. Respiratory compromise, a protuberant abdomen, or changing sensorium may be further clues to the presence of internal hemorrhage. Further studies, including radiographs of the chest and abdomen, peritoneal lavage, and computerized axial tomography of the head, should be instituted when appropriate.

The approach to blood transfusion (Table 47.1) can be divided into three levels of intervention, depending upon the clinical findings and the laboratory data. (1) If bleeding has been controlled, vital signs are stable, the hematocrit remains above 20%, and further bleeding is considered unlikely, the initially crossmatched blood should be held for at least 24 hours and then released for other use if no longer required for this patient. (2) If bleeding has led to hypovolemic shock but tissue oxygenation is not critically affected, intravascular volume should be supported with crystalloid or colloid solutions until a crossmatch has been performed and compatible donor blood is available. A similar approach should be used if the hematocrit slowly falls to a level less than 15 to 20% or if the hematocrit remains stable at a low level but further bleeding is considered likely (e.g., esophageal varices). (3) Only when bleeding is accompanied by life-threatening hypoxia should uncrossmatched group O, Rh negative blood be administered. Transfusion of blood with minor blood group incompatibilities may result in immediate hemolysis and renal failure or, more commonly may result in sensitization of the recipient to red cell antigens, making future blood compatibility testing difficult. The determination of the patient's ABO or Rh blood group can be performed within a few minutes, so that selection of ABO and Rh compatible donor units is almost always feasible.

Increased Red Cell Destruction

Membrane Disorders

The anemia in disorders of the red cell membrane (hereditary spherocytosis, hereditary elliptocytosis, stomatocytosis, liver disease) is rarely severe enough to constitute a hematologic emergency. However, the hemoglobin level may fall even further when red cell destruction increases (hemolytic crisis) or red cell production slows (aplastic crisis). These complications usually are associated with acute infections and are self-limited. Hemolytic and aplastic crises are particularly common in young infants, perhaps as a result of their increased susceptibility to viral infections.

The hemolytic crisis is characterized by increasing jaundice, falling hemoglobin level and increasing reticulocyte count. In contrast, the aplastic crisis is associated with slowly increasing pallor, worsening anemia and low or absent reticulocytes. In those children with red cell membrane disorders associated with brisk hemolysis (hemoglobin level less than 8 to 9 g/dl and reticulocytes greater than 5 to 7%), these crises may produce acute symptoms of anemia and, in rare instances, red cell transfusions may be required. The hemoglobin level should be routinely checked in children with known disorders of the red cell membrane and increasing pallor or jaundice associated with an infectious illness.

Table 47.1
Guidelines to Transfusion Therapy

Blood Component	Indication	Dose
Whole blood	Immediate restoration of blood volume and red cell mass after trauma or surgery; exchange transfusion	—[a]
Packed red blood cells (PRBC)	For all nonemergency transfusions or emergency restoration of red cell mass (may be combined with saline or fresh frozen plasma for volume expansion or exchange transfusion)	—
Frozen red blood cells	Same indications as PRBC but contains no leukocytes or plasma; helpful in patients who have had febrile transfusion reactions	—
White blood cells	Recommended only for severely neutropenic patients with documented or strongly suspected sepsis	One unit daily (each unit contains approximately 10×10^8 granulocytes)
Platelets	For hemorrhagic complications due to thrombocytopenia or abnormal platelet function	0.2–0.4 unit/kg (maximum 10–20 units/dose)
Fresh frozen plasma	Volume expansion; to provide missing coagulation factors or immunoglobulins	10–20 ml/kg/dose

[a] Calculation of red blood cell transfusion requirements:

Ml of required packed RBC = (blood volume[b] × (desired hematocrit − present hematocrit)/hematocrit of packed RBC[c]).

[b] Blood volume (ml) = 0.08 × body weight (grams).
[c] Packed RBC usually have a hematocrit of 70–80 vol%.

The diagnosis of an aplastic crisis should only be considered in a child with a known hemolytic disorder. The red cell lifespan in normal individuals is sufficiently long so that anemia due to transient marrow aplasia is uncommon. If a child with no previous hematologic abnormality develops anemia and reticulocytopenia, examination of a bone marrow aspirate and further studies in consultation with a pediatric hematologist should be performed before transfusions are administered.

Older children and adolescents with red cell membrane disorders may develop gallstones due to increased red cell destruction and bilirubin release. Cholelithiasis or cholecystitis in affected patients should be managed the same way as it is in patients without underlying hematologic disease.

Metabolic Abnormalities

Like the red cell membrane disorders, erythrocyte metabolic abnormalities usually do not cause severe anemia. However, certain non-African variants of glucose 6-phosphate dehydrogenase (G6PD) deficiency are exceptions. These disorders are associated with chronic hemolysis and episodes of acute and sometimes life-threatening anemia usually after exposure to oxidant drugs or chemicals (Table 47.2). Acute intravascular hemolysis usually occurs within 1 to 3 days of oxidant exposure and is characterized by pallor, malaise, fever,

Table 47.2
Drugs and Substances Commonly Associated with Acute Hemolysis in Children with Glucose 6-Phosphate Dehydrogenase (G6PD) Deficiency

Antimalarials (primaquine and quinine most common)
Sulfonamides (including salicylazosulfapyridine and trimethoprim-sulfamethoxazale)
Acetanilid
Acetylphenylhydrozine
Nalidixic acid and nitrofurantoin
Naphthalene
Fava beans
Aspirin (does not cause acute hemolysis with G6PD deficiency when used in therapeutic doses)

scleral icterus, abdominal and back pain, and dark urine. Treatment should include removal of the offending agent and fluid administration to prevent renal tubular damage. When hemolysis is severe, red cell transfusions may be required. However, if the diagnosis is uncertain, a pretransfusion blood sample should be saved for further diagnostic studies.

Autoimmune Hemolytic Anemia

BACKGROUND

One of the most serious causes of severe anemia in children is autoimmune hemolytic anemia (AIHA). This antibody-mediated disorder occurs most commonly in young children. Affected erythrocytes are removed prematurely from the circulation by macrophages of the reticuloendothelial system. Although AIHA may be associated with infections, drugs, inflammatory diseases or malignancies, a specific cause can rarely be identified in pediatric patients.

CLINICAL MANIFESTATIONS

Although this disorder may occasionally be indolent and may go undetected for days or weeks, AIHA is usually associated with the sudden onset of pallor, jaundice, and dark urine. The hemoglobin level may be as low as 1 to 2 g/dl at the time of diagnosis. When the anemia is this severe, the child may appear moribund and desperately ill. Signs of congestive heart failure may be prominent.

The anemia is usually accompanied by reticulocytosis, although the reticulocyte count may be below 5% during the first few days of the illness. Occasional patients remain reticulocytopenic for prolonged periods. Spherocytes are frequently found on the peripheral smear and red cell fragments may also be present. Free hemoglobin in the urine produces a positive dipstick reaction for blood in the absence of red cells on microscopic urinalysis. When hemolysis is severe enough to exceed the renal clearance of hemoglobin, the plasma will be pink, and careful inspection of the plasma layer of a spun hematocrit may provide an early diagnostic clue. The direct Coombs' test using broad spectrum Coombs' serum (IgG, IgM and complement) is usually positive in childhood AIHA. Acute hemolysis is most commonly associated with positive reactions using IgG and/or complement specific Coombs' serum. Although the antibody may be shown to have specificity in vitro (usually in the Rh system), the shortened survival of "compatible" blood suggests the presence of wider activity of the identified antibody or the presence of additional undetected antibodies.

MANAGEMENT

The management of the child with AIHA should be aggressive since the hemoglobin level may fall precipitously. Hospitalization for careful observation and treatment is usually necessary. The immediate institution of corticosteroid therapy (prednisone 2 mg/kg/day or equivalent doses of parenteral preparations) may prevent or reduce the need for red cell transfusions. While steroid therapy is usually recommended for patients with warm-reacting antibodies (usually IgG or complement), occasional patients with cold-reacting antibodies seem to respond favorably, and thus a trial of steroids seems warranted, particularly in the severely anemic patient, regardless of the results of initial serologic studies. A response to steroids often occurs within the first few days of therapy.

Red cell transfusions are particularly

hazardous in patients with AIHA and should be reserved for children with severe anemia and signs of hypoxia or cardiac failure. The presence of a nonspecific antibody in the patient's serum makes it difficult to find a unit of donor blood that is compatible in the major crossmatch (donor cells and patient serum). The finding of an apparently compatible unit may pose even greater danger since the physician is lured into a false sense of confidence when, in fact, an undetected antibody may still cause a severe hemolytic transfusion reaction. The use of the "least incompatible" unit is a common practice although data supporting this approach are lacking. The best policy is to avoid transfusion whenever possible. If red cells are required and a compatible donor unit can be found, this unit should be used. Otherwise, ABO and, if possible, Rh compatible units should be administered despite the incompatibility in vitro. The recognition of the risks of transfusion in children with AIHA should not lead to the withholding of "incompatible" blood when transfusion therapy is required to prevent severe morbidity or death.

Whether the unit of red cells appears compatible or incompatible on the basis of serologic studies, special precautions should be taken during the actual transfusion. The first 5 ml should be administered in no less than 15 to 20 min, and the patient should be observed closely for malaise, back pain, fever and other signs of acute hemolysis. The plasma layer of the spun hematocrit should be carefully inspected for the pink color of free hemoglobin. If any of these findings is present, the transfusion should be stopped and normal saline should be administered until a new unit can be prepared. If the patient is asymptomatic and the plasma is clear, the remainder of the unit should be given with continuing close observation.

In rare instances, the hemoglobin level continues to fall despite steroids and red cell transfusion, necessitating alternative therapeutic attempts to sustain life. Exchange transfusion or plasmapheresis may remove sufficient antibody to allow improved survival of transfused red cells. If these measures fail, emergency splenectomy may be required.

Nonimmune Acquired Hemolytic Anemia

Acute hemolytic anemia in children may be caused by infections, chemicals or drugs that damage the red cell directly. These disorders resemble AIHA in their clinical presentation and should be considered in the child with acquired hemolytic anemia and a negative Coombs' test. Infectious agents that may induce hemolytic anemia include malaria (which is of particular importance in Southeast Asian refugees), protozoa, and a wide variety of gram-positive and gram-negative organisms. Chemicals and drugs that cause hemolysis include naphthalene, nitrofurantoin and salicyl sulfasalazine. Treatment is directed at elimination of the offending agent. Red cell transfusions are usually unnecessary unless anemia is severe (hematocrit $<15\%$) or accompanied by signs of congestive heart failure.

Erythrocyte Fragmentation Syndromes

Red cells will undergo fragmentation and lysis when subjected to excessive physical trauma within the cardiovascular system. Hemolytic anemias due to red cell fragmentation have been associated with abnormalities of the heart (valve homografts and synthetic prostheses, uncorrected valvular disease), great vessels (coarctation of the aorta) and small vessels (hemolytic uremic syndrome, thrombotic thrombocytopenic purpura, collagen vascular disease, hemangiomas). Physical findings are related to the underlying disorder. The presence of red cell fragments on the peripheral smear strongly suggests mechanical damage to the erythrocyte. When small vessels are involved, thrombocytopenia may also be present. Hemolytic anemia associated with valvular or great vessel disease rarely causes severe anemia. However, iron deficiency due to intravascular lysis and urinary excretion of hemosiderin in renal tubular epithelial cells may aggravate the hemolytic anemia. Oral iron supplementation may obviate the need for transfusions. When hemolysis is due to small vessel disease, treatment of the underlying disorder (collagen vascular disease) or primarily affected organs (renal failure in hemolytic uremic syndrome) is the first priority. Red cell transfusions should be reserved for the treatment of symptomatic anemia. Since the hemolysis is due to extracorpuscular factors, survival of transfused cells may be markedly shortened. The management of intravascular coagulation associated with several of these disorders is discussed later in this chapter (p. 486).

Decreased Red Cell Production

Disorders of red cell production, unless accompanied by shortened red cell survival, are characterized by a slowly progressive anemia. Consequently, the physician does not often encounter many of the difficulties associated with acute, life-threatening hemolysis. However, the insidious onset of anemia when erythropoiesis is impaired may delay recognition of the disorder, and severe anemia and cardiac failure may be present at the time of diagnosis. Tissue oxygenation may be inadequate because of the low hemoglobin level, and conditions that increase the cardiac rate or output (fever, exercise) may precipitate congestive heart failure in the previously compensated patient. In addition, anemia secondary to diminished red cell production may be associated with an underlying, severe illness such as leukemia, neuroblastoma or aplastic anemia in which other life-threatening hematologic abnormalities (severe neutropenia or thrombocytopenia) may be present. Thus, the patient with impaired production of erythrocytes may be equally as ill as the patient with acute hemolysis.

The important role of the history, physical examination and laboratory studies in the initial evaluation of the child with decreased red cell production is described in Chapter 30. Initial management should include basic support of cardiorespiratory function and identification and treatment of conditions such as fever which may be compounding the problems of severe anemia. The patient with hypoxia or cardiac failure requires red cell transfusions. As described earlier, the urgency of the clinical situation dictates the need to abbreviate the standard crossmatching procedures. A pretransfusion blood sample should always be saved for further diagnostic studies as well as determination of the patient's red cell antigen profile should chronic transfusion therapy be necessary. The initial transfusion should be given as a small aliquot of packed red cells. In many instances, the symptoms of severe anemia will be relieved after the hemoglobin level has risen only 1 or 2 g/dl. The administration of additional blood is rarely necessary in the early stages of therapy. Furthermore, the added volume may precipitate cardiac failure in the face of a preexisting high output state. A helpful rule of thumb is to administer a number of milliliters per kilogram of packed red cells equivalent to the hemoglobin level. For example, a child with aplastic anemia, a hemoglobin level of 3 g/dl and early signs of cardiovascular compromise would be given 3 ml/kg of packed red cells. Some physicians routinely administer diuretics (such as furosemide 1 mg/kg/dose) during the transfusion of a severely anemic patient. An alternative approach is to reserve diuretic therapy for those patients who develop signs of increasing cardiac compromise during the transfusion.

Aplastic and Hypoplastic Anemias

The differential diagnosis of aplastic and hypoplastic anemias is discussed in Chapter 30. Most of these disorders have a protracted course and, after initial stabilization of the patient, require intensive diagnostic evaluation and careful assessment of chronic therapy rather than emergency management. Transfusion should be used with particular caution in the initial management of patients with hypoplastic and aplastic anemias since exposure to HLA and other antigens may adversely affect engraftment of transplanted bone marrow in patients who might otherwise have benefited from this procedure. Washed or frozen thawed red cells will markedly reduce exposure to donor white cells and platelets.

When affected patients do not require immediate transfusion, a bone marrow aspirate may be helpful in predicting the course of the disease during the next few days and, in particular, the likelihood that red cell transfusions will be required. For example, a patient with transient erythroblastopenia of childhood has a hemoglobin level of 4.0 g/dl and absent reticulocytes at the time of diagnosis. If examination of the bone marrow reveals only an occasional pronormoblast, a further decrease of the hemoglobin concentration should be anticipated and red cell transfusions will almost certainly be required. If, on the other hand, the bone marrow aspirate shows numerous erythrocyte precursors progressing through all levels of red cell maturation, a peripheral reticulocytosis can be expected within 24 hours and red cell transfusions will be unnecessary (Fig. 47.1).

Nutritional Anemias

Nutritional anemias in childhood constitute more of a public health problem than a hematologic emergency. However, the hemoglobin level may, on occasion, be very low at the time of diagnosis. In certain instances such as vitamin B_{12} deficiency in an infant exclusively breast-fed by a vegetarian mother, nonhematologic symptoms such as coma may be more prominent than the anemia. Stabilization and improvement can usually be achieved with replacement of the deficient nutrient. Nucleated red cells or reticulocytes usually appear within 48 hours of replacement therapy in folic acid or vitamin B_{12} deficiency and within 72 hours of therapy in severe iron deficiency anemia. Because of this rapid response, red cell transfusions are rarely required unless symptoms associated with the anemia pose a serious threat. A response to replacement therapy should not preclude further investigation of the origin of the anemia, especially when the dietary history is inconclusive. For example, iron deficiency anemia may be due to repeated small pulmonary hemorrhages or chronic bleeding from an intestinal lesion rather than inadequate iron intake. Similarly, megaloblastic anemias may be caused by deficient intrinsic factor or abnormalities of folic acid transport rather than a seriously altered diet.

Iron replacement therapy consists of 3 to

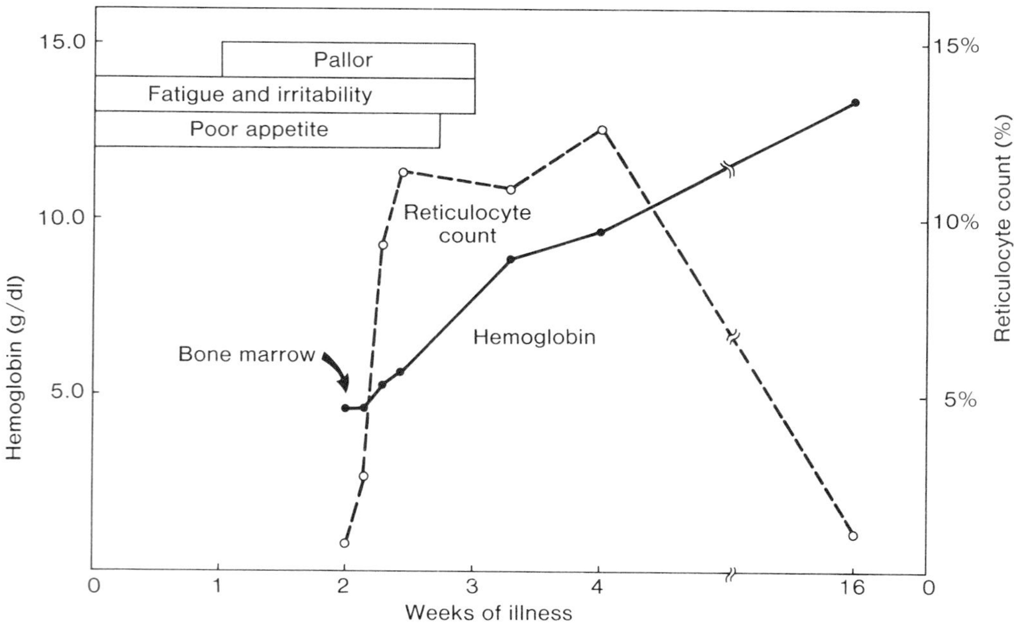

Figure 47.1 Clinical course of transient erythroblastopenia of childhood (TEC) in a 2-year-old girl. There was a 1- to 2-week history of pallor, fatigue, and decreased appetite. A bone marrow aspirate showed an active erythroid series which was reflected in the subsequent reticulocytosis and full hematologic recovery.

6 mg/kg/day of elemental iron given orally as ferrous sulfate in 2 or 3 divided doses. Parenteral iron is painful and dangerous. Moreover, the hematologic response to intramuscular or intravenous iron dextran is no faster than the response to oral iron. Replacement doses of 1 mg of folic acid and 100 μg of vitamin B_{12} daily are undoubtedly excessive, but their common usage reflects the safety and the concentrations of the available compounds.

The administration of supplemental iron, vitamin B_{12} or folic acid should not be considered a substitute for adequate dietary intake when nutritional deficiency is inadvertent. Unlike most hematologic emergencies, the rapid improvement after treatment of these disorders may reduce the likelihood of further visits despite attempts to assure adequate follow-up care. Therefore, a strong effort to restructure the diet should begin at the time of the initial contact.

DISORDERS OF HEMOGLOBIN STRUCTURE AND PRODUCTION

The disorders of hemoglobin structure and production which are most often encountered in a pediatric emergency room are the sickle hemoglobin syndromes (sickle cell anemia, hemoglobin SC disease, hemoglobin S-β thalassemia and others). While most physicians are familiar with these diseases, the frequency with which affected patients are seen may lead to a false sense of complacency, leaving subtle findings undetected. On the other hand, thalassemia major and methemoglobinemia occur much less commonly than the sickling disorders. Lack of familiarity with these diseases may delay recognition of serious illness, resulting in severe morbidity and even death. In the following section, particular attention will be paid to the recognition of unusual but serious diseases and the management of the many and diverse complications associated with the hemoglobinopathies.

Sickle Hemoglobin Disorders

BACKGROUND

The sickling disorders are responsible for a large percentage of hematologic emergencies and a major proportion of total visits for any reason in many pediatric emergency departments. Although the basic molecular lesion in these disorders is well defined, the mechanisms responsible for the numerous complications remain poorly understood and treatment is often unsatisfactory. Nonetheless, early recognition and aggressive management of specific problems may alleviate unnecessary suffering and prevent much of the morbidity and mortality associated with the sickling disorders. Optimal long-term care should be provided at a center with specialists familiar with sickle cell disease and all of its complications.

CLINICAL MANIFESTATIONS/ MANAGEMENT

Presentation. It is important to identify the ill child with a previously undiagnosed sickling disorder so that appropriate therapy is instituted. The diagnosis of sickle cell disease should be considered in black children with unexplained pain or swelling (especially of the hands or feet), pneumonia, meningitis, sepsis, neurologic abnormalities, splenomegaly or anemia. The hemoglobin level and reticulocyte count are inadequate screening tests for the sickle hemoglobinopathies since values in affected patients (especially those with hemoglobin SC disease and S-β thalassemia) may overlap with normal values. Similarly, the peripheral smear may be devoid of sickled cells. Definitive testing for sickling disorders can be accomplished in 30 min by hemoglobin electrophoresis on cellulose acetate at alkaline pH. If this test is not available, standard solubility tests can be used to identify the presence of sickle hemoglobin. However, solubility tests do not distinguish patients with sickle cell trait, hemoglobin SC disease or other sickle variants from patients with sickle cell anemia (hemoglobin SS). Therefore, the results of solubility screening tests must be considered in the context of the clinical presentation and other laboratory studies. In addition, whether the screening test is positive or negative, confirmatory testing by hemoglobin electrophoresis is mandatory in all patients with hematologic or nonhematologic emergencies which may be related to sickle cell anemia.

Sepsis. A combination of impaired immunologic functions, including early loss of normal splenic activity, contributes to the markedly increased frequency of sepsis in patients with sickle cell disease and the fulminant nature of this complication. The risk of bacterial sepsis in the patient with sickle cell disease is increased several hundred-fold in comparison with the normal population. *Streptococcus pneumoniae* and *Haemophilus influenzae* are the most common pathogens although enteric organisms also occur with increased frequency. The period of greatest risk is between the ages of 6 months and 3 years when development of protective antibodies is limited and splenic function is diminished or absent.

The common occurrence of fever with no obvious source in young children with sickle cell disease makes the distinction between serious bacterial infections and benign, self-limited viral disorders a particularly frustrating problem. Unfortunately, no single physical finding or laboratory test can accurately identify the septic patient. The physician consequently must choose between the safety of admitting most or all young, febrile patients with sickle cell disease and the risk of sending home a child who may later develop signs of overwhelming sepsis.

In many centers the first approach is used; young children with sickle cell disease and unexplained fever are admitted to the hospital and treated with antibiotics until results of blood cultures are available. In other centers, particular weight is given to certain findings in the physical examination or laboratory evaluation. Factors which may favor the presence of sepsis include age less than 3 years, high temperature, leukocytosis, increased absolute band count and presence of toxic granulations, vacuoles or Döhle bodies in neutrophils. The finding of Howell-Jolly bodies in the red cells reflects the loss of splenic function and emphasizes the vulnerability of the patient to fulminant sepsis. Since bacterial sepsis has a particularly strong association with young age and high fever in children with sickle cell disease, patients less than 3 years of age with temperatures in excess of 39°C should be hospitalized for therapy with antibiotics. However, many children with sickle cell anemia who are older than 3 years or who have fevers less than 39°C also require hospitalization for observation or therapy. Decisions regarding the appropriate management of these patients should be made after consideration of the clinical and laboratory findings discussed above.

Because unexplained fever is uncommon in older children in general, the diagnosis of bacterial sepsis should be strongly considered in the older child with sickle cell anemia and fever. A careful assessment of the child's clinical condition should take into account the factors noted earlier. If the child appears toxic, admission for antibiotic treatment is advisable even in the absence of high fever or leukocytosis. Perhaps most importantly, good follow-up care must be assured. When a child of any age with sickle cell disease and fever is managed as an outpatient, a second visit within 24 hours of the initial visit should be mandatory.

The treatment of sepsis in patients with sickle cell disease should include the rapid institution of antibiotic therapy and aggressive management of septic shock. As in other patients with no splenic function, clinical deterioration may be extremely rapid. The patient who is alert upon arrival in the emergency department may be moribund and hypotensive 30 min later. Antibiotic therapy should include ampicillin and chloramphenicol for appropriate coverage of *S. pneumoniae*, *H. influenzae* (including β-lactamase producers), salmonellae and other gram-negative organisms. Even if vital signs are normal, intravenous fluids should be administered at twice the maintenance rate unless specifically contraindicated (e.g. intrinsic heart disease, meningitis). Septic shock should be treated in the same way as in patients without hematologic disorders (see Chapter 2). Red cell transfusions or partial or total exchange transfusions may reduce the likelihood of secondary organ damage due to massive sickling in the presence of hypoxia, stasis and acidosis.

Other Infections. Children with sickle cell disease are affected more frequently with infections other than sepsis in comparison with their hematologically normal counterparts. Meningitis, pneumonia, septic arthritis and osteomyelitis may be responsible for substantial morbidity and mortality unless promptly recognized and appropriately treated. The level of suspicion for meningitis should be particularly high in the young, irritable child with sickle cell disease and unexplained fever. Antibiotic therapy of meningitis is similar to that recommended for hematologically normal children with this disorder. However, exchange transfusion, to lower the percentage of sickle hemoglobin, may theoretically reduce the risk of intracerebral sickling and infarction in areas of local swelling and possible red cell sludging. This procedure may also help resolve the conflict between the need for maintenance or greater fluid therapy to prevent vaso-occlusion and the need to restrict fluids in the face of cerebral swelling and possible inappropriate antidiuretic hormone secretion. If hemoglobin S is less than 30% of the total hemoglobin, sickling is unlikely and fluid management can be dictated by the central nervous system findings.

Pneumonia accounts for the majority of hospital admissions for infection in children with sickle cell anemia. The affected patient is usually tachypneic, even after antipyretic therapy. Rales, ronchi and physical findings of lobar consolidation may be present. However, in some children, particularly those who are somewhat dehydrated, physical findings may be far less striking. Rales may only be heard after several hours of rehydration. Because pneumonia may escape detection on physical examination, a chest radiograph should be obtained in children with sickle cell disease and unexplained fever.

The problem of identifying the responsible pathogen in patients with sickling disorders and pneumonia is similar to that encountered in hematologically normal children (see Chapter 45). Although pneumonia due to *S. pneumoniae*, gram-negative organisms and *Mycoplasma pneumoniae* is more common in sickle cell disease, a causative organism is rarely found in cultures of the blood or sputum. Consequently, therapy is usually begun with intravenously administered ampicillin and modified according to the clinical response. In the very ill child, the identification of the causative organism should be pursued more vigorously with aspiration of pleural fluid, when present, or aspiration of actual lung tissue. Oxygen should be administered to all children with sickle cell disease and pneumonia.

Septic arthritis and osteomyelitis present particularly difficult diagnostic problems in children with sickle cell disease since the clinical findings so closely resemble those found in infarctions of the bone. A careful physical examination and judicious use of laboratory tests will help the physician weigh the relative likelihood of infection and infarction. If symptoms are of recent onset (<3 days), a ^{99m}Tc-diphosphonate bone scan in conjunction with a ^{99m}Tc-sulfur colloid bone marrow scan may be helpful in distinguishing the two processes. In osteomyelitis, the bone scan shows increased uptake and the bone marrow scan is normal. In bone infarction, the bone scan is normal but the bone marrow scan shows decreased uptake. Closed or open bone aspiration should precede the institution of antibiotic therapy in the patient with suspected osteomyelitis. Similarly, aspiration of an affected joint should be performed if septic arthritis is suspected. In most instances, swollen, warm and tender joints are due to local infarction. The presence of other sites of concurrent infarction and the patient's description of the pain as typical "crisis pain" may be helpful in identifying the cause as vaso-occlusion. The total white cell count and differential count of the joint fluid may be similar in septic arthritis and sterile effusion secondary to infarction. Therefore, the Gram stain and culture are especially important. Septic arthritis of the hip deserves special mention since delayed intervention may result in necrosis of the femoral head. Children with this complication usually appear quite ill and hold the limb in a "frog leg" position. Confirmation of septic arthritis by joint aspirate should be followed as soon as possible by surgical decompression.

Vaso-occlusion. Infarction of bone, soft tissue and viscera may occur as a result of intravascular sickling and vessel occlusion. Children may have only pain or may have symptoms related to the affected organ (e.g., hematuria in papillary necrosis, jaundice in hepatic infarct, seizures or weakness in central nervous system ischemia, respiratory distress in pulmonary infarction). Initial management usually centers around control of pain, general supportive measures and differentiation of vaso-occlusion and disorders unrelated to the hematologic abnormality.

The treatment of the child with a painful crisis requires an objective assessment of the severity of the discomfort and an appropriate use of analgesic therapy. Once nonsickling disorders have been ruled out, hydration should be undertaken with 0.5 N saline at a rate of 1.5 to 2 times maintenance fluid requirements (see Chapter 46). The choice of analgesic is aided by familiarity with the patient's previous crises. Hesitancy in the use of parenteral narcotics may result in inadequate pain relief, mounting anxiety and a loss of trust between physician and patient. This is a particularly common occurrence when the patient has had repeated emergency room visits, and physicians are suspicious of the stated degree of discomfort. The use of the placebo saline injection is to be decried as an insensitive and potentially cruel test of the patient's pain level. Meperidine (1.5 to 2.0 mg/kg) or morphine sulfate (0.10 to 0.15 mg/kg) should be administered intramuscularly and further therapy should be based upon the degree and duration of pain control. Admission to the hospital is necessary if continuing parenteral analgesic therapy is required, if fluid intake is inadequate, or if the child has had several visits for the same problem. Repeated 4-hour stints in the emergency department will often leave the child and family exhausted and will infrequently prevent hospital admission.

Several specific areas of vaso-occlusion deserve special attention. Between 6 and 24 months of age, dactylitis is a common manifestation of sickle cell disease. Infarction of the metarcarpals and metatarsals results in swelling of the hands and feet. These episodes recur frequently. Pain usually resolves after several days, but swelling may persist for 1 or 2 weeks. Treatment is similar to that described above for a painful crisis.

Because it is difficult to distinguish pulmonary infarction from pneumonia on the basis of physical findings and noninvasive laboratory studies, these two disorders are classified together under the heading of "acute chest syndrome." Fortunately, pulmonary infarction is not associated with substantial morbidity in children with sickle cell disease and, therefore, specific therapy is rarely required.

Infarction of abdominal and retroperitoneal organs may produce clinical findings that closely resemble the findings in a variety of nonhematologic diseases. The distinction between occlusion of the mesenteric vessels and appendicitis or other causes of an acute abdomen is, at times, particularly difficult. Physical findings and laboratory studies are remarkably similar. The onset and quality of the pain may be familiar to the patient and readily recognized as typical "crisis pain." On the other hand, the patient may describe the symptoms as distinctly different from episodes of infarction, giving support to the diagnosis of an acute abdomen. Since painful crises occur far more frequently than appendicitis and other causes of acute abdomen, a period of careful observation is warranted unless the patient is severely ill (e.g., perforated appendix). Repeated assessment of the abdominal examination and the clinical response to fluid therapy will help identify the child with an acute abdomen and will reduce unnecessary and risky emergency surgical procedures in children with sickle cell disease. The hours required for exchange transfusion prior to surgery provide an additional period of observation, during which symptoms may abate.

Hepatic infarction may also create a diagnostic dilemma since the acute onset of jaundice and the abdominal pain which characterize this disorder are similar to the symptoms of hepatitis and cholecystitis. The distinction between infarction and cholecystitis is particularly important since recurrent gallbladder disease is an indication for cholecystectomy. Ultrasonography of the abdomen often shows a dilated common bile duct or the presence of stones in the duct in children with biliary tract disease when the study is performed shortly after the onset of symptoms. The initial management of these disorders is similar to that previously described for vaso-occlusive crises (i.e., fluids, analgesics). A nasogastric tube may relieve abdominal discomfort due to distention.

The major emergencies related to vaso-occlusion within the genitourinary tract are hematuria due to renal papillary necrosis and priapism. The hematuria of papillary necrosis is usually painless and frequently persistent. A history of recent trauma, streptococcal infection or recurrent urinary tract infection should alert the physician to other causes of hematuria. Similarly, the presence of hypertension suggests the presence of nephritis rather than simple vaso-occlusion. Microscopic examination of the urine shows numerous red cells with vaso-occlusion, but red cell casts are rarely seen. Pyuria and proteinuria in excess of what might be attributed to the blood in the urine are not found in papillary necrosis but may be indicative of nephritis. The hematocrit or hemoglobin level should be measured since the hematuria, if persistent or severe, may markedly worsen the chronic anemia. For the patient who is otherwise well, diagnostic studies can be accomplished on an outpatient basis and a trial of increased oral fluids (twice maintenance) should be undertaken. However, in many instances, admission to the hospital will be required for intravenous hydration. Alkalinization of the urine may reduce bleeding but is difficult to accomplish and usually unnecessary. When hematuria is severe, red cell transfusions are sometimes required for treatment of anemia. Transfusions or exchange transfusions may also be useful in shortening the coarse of hematuria.

Priapism is an unusually painful and frightening form of vaso-occlusion. The penis becomes swollen, edematous and very tender. Urination may be difficult. The initial treatment consists of fluid therapy and analgesics. Once again, red cell transfusions or exchange transfusions may promote resolution, but these forms of therapy should be reserved for patients with no response to the more conservative measures. Aspiration of the corpora and surgical shunting procedures have been recommended for adult patients to prevent impotency after an episode of priapism. However, this complication is extremely uncommon in children, and, therefore, such invasive treatment is rarely required.

Infarction of the central nervous system is a catastrophic form of vaso-occlusion. The initial presentation varies from the mild and fleeting symptoms of a transient ischemic attack to seizures, hemiparesis, coma and death. Physical findings usually define the area of cortical infarction. Supportive therapy should be instituted immediately. A one and one-half or two volume exchange transfusion should begin as soon as blood is ready. This procedure will reduce the likelihood of further intravascular sickling and may prevent extension of cortical damage.

Cerebral aneurysms occur with increased frequency in patients with sickle cell disease. The origin of this complication, which is usually detected in teenagers or adults, remains obscure but may be related to local vessel occlusion or ischemia. Unfortunately, the aneurysm escapes detection until after a major, and frequently fatal, subarachnoid or intracerebral bleed. The severe morbidity and high mortality associated with ruptured cerebral aneurysms require careful evaluation of the patient with sickle cell disease and headaches or neurologic findings. Immediate surgical intervention should follow radiologic confirmation of bleeding.

Less common areas of infarction which may be particularly confusing to the physician include the orbits and cervical spine. Vaso-occlusion involving the bones of the orbit may produce findings similar to those of orbital cellulitis. Tenderness and fever may be present in bony infarction but are usually less remarkable than when found in cellulitis. A bone marrow scan using ^{99m}Tc-sulfur colloid may demonstrate decreased uptake in the affected area, avoiding the need for prolonged antibiotic therapy.

Vaso-occlusion which presumably occurs in the cervical spine causes marked meningismus. A spinal tap may be necessary to rule out meningitis. As in other situations, the patient's evaluation of the pain may be very helpful in distinguishing vaso-occlusive processes from more serious disorders.

Splenic Sequestration Crisis. The sudden enlargement of the spleen with resulting sequestration of a substantial portion of the blood volume is a life-threatening complication of sickle cell disease. Because this crisis requires the presence of vascularized splenic tissue, it usually occurs before 5 years of age in patients with homozygous sickle cell disease but may occur much later in children with other sickling disorders such as SC disease or S-β thalassemia. The patient undergoing a severe sequestration crisis may first complain of left upper quadrant pain. Within hours, the patient becomes very pale, ill-appearing, lethargic and disoriented. The physical examination shows evidence of cardiovascular collapse; hypotension and tachycardia are often present. The level of consciousness falls. The hallmark of a severe sequestration crisis is a spleen which is markedly enlarged in comparison with previous examinations and unusually hard. The hematocrit or hemoglobin level is much lower than during routine visits and the reticulocyte count is usually increased (Fig. 47.2). Mild neutropenia or thrombocytopenia may be present.

Recognition of this complication should be immediate so that life-saving therapy begins without delay. The rapid infusion of large amounts of normal saline or albumin is necessary to restore intravascular volume. Although a sufficient number of red cells to relieve tissue hypoxia may be released by the spleen following initial resuscitation, transfusion with packed red cells (2 to 10 ml/kg) is often required in more severe cases. Whole blood transfusions may help relieve the dual problems of intravascular volume depletion and impaired tissue oxygenation. Reversal of shock and a rising

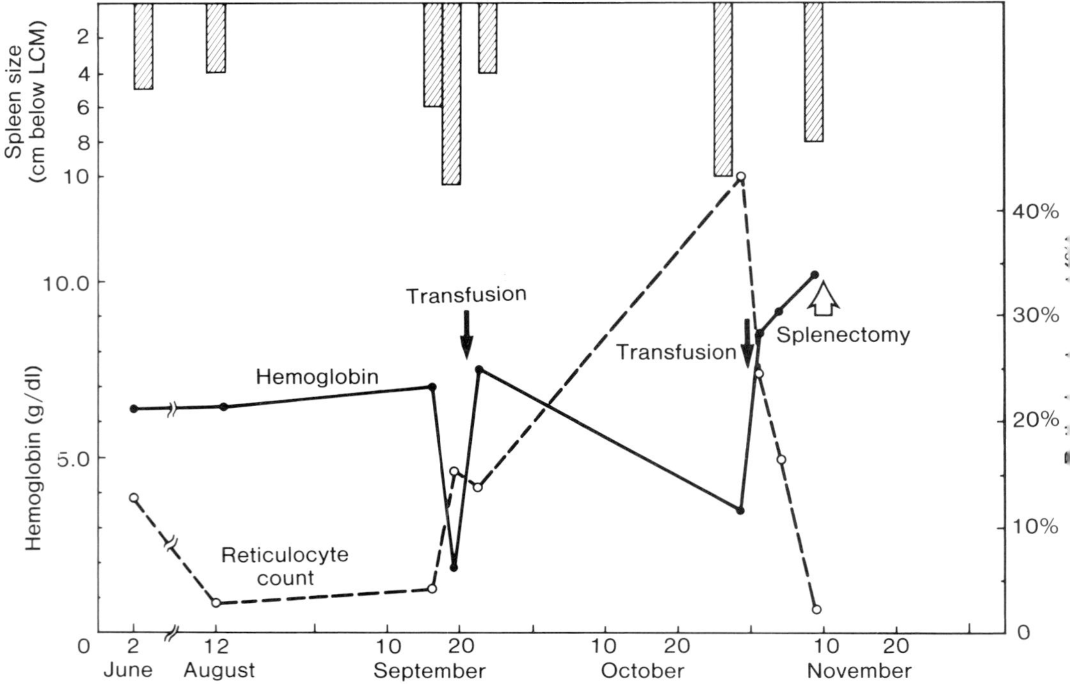

Figure 47.2 Clinical course of a 6-year-old black girl with hemoglobin S-β^0 thalassemia and two splenic sequestration crises which were characterized by abdominal pain, increased splenic size, and a rapid fall in hemoglobin concentration.

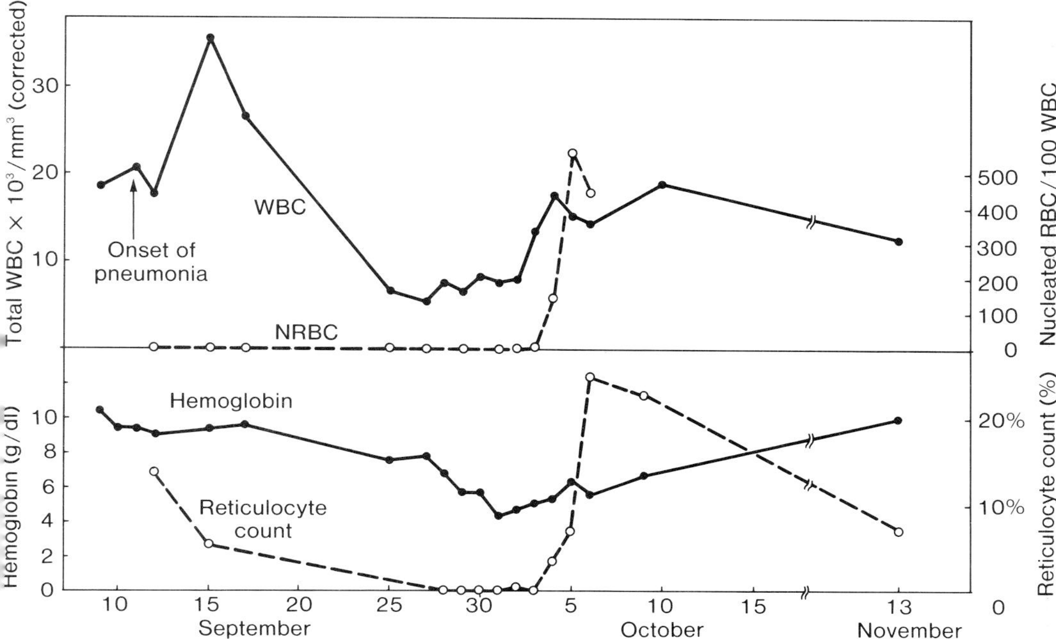

Figure 47.3 Aplastic crisis in a 5-year-old black girl with sickle cell anemia and *Mycoplasma pneumoniae* pneumonia. Her aplastic crisis was characterized by a low hemoglobin level and reticulocytopenia. The white blood cell count was also transiently decreased. Recovery was characterized by reticulocytosis, marked increase in the number of nucleated red blood cells and a rise in hemoglobin level.

hematocrit signal improvement of a sequestration crisis. The spleen gradually becomes less firm and smaller.

Aplastic Crisis. Increased bone marrow erythroid activity (as reflected by the elevated reticulocyte count and presence of nucleated red cells in the peripheral blood) partially compensates for the shortened red cell survival in sickle cell anemia and other hemolytic disorders. If erythropoiesis slows or ceases, this precarious balance is disturbed, and the hemoglobin level may fall rapidly. The event which most commonly causes erythroid aplasia is a current or recent viral or bacterial infection. Progressive pallor is unaccompanied by jaundice or other signs of hemolysis. Severe anemia may result in dyspnea and changes in level of consciousness. The hemoglobin level is unusually low and reticulocytes are decreased or absent (Fig. 47.3). During the early phase of an aplastic crisis the bone marrow has a paucity of erythroid activity. During the recovery stages, erythroid activity increases and the cells steadily mature. The level of red cell maturity can be used to predict the appearance of reticulocytosis in the peripheral blood and this information may be helpful in determining whether the patient needs a red cell transfusion or can await the recovery of the bone marrow without further compromising oxygen delivery. If a red cell transfusion is required, a small aliquot is usually sufficient to raise the hemoglobin concentration to a level which assures adequate oxygenation until red cell production recovers.

Hemolytic Crisis. Worsening anemia and increasing reticulocytosis may accompany viral and bacterial infections in children with sickle cell disease. Scleral icterus is more prominent than usual. The findings are consistent with an increasing degree of active hemolysis. The hemoglobin level rarely falls low enough to require specific therapy. Hematologic values return to the usual level as the infectious process resolves.

The long-term management of many of the complications of sickle cell disease is beyond the scope of this chapter but has been discussed in detail in review articles and textbooks. In most instances, a thorough understanding of the extended care is necessary for correct management of the initial stages of hematologic emergencies. The clinical course and previous laboratory data of the patient should be familiar to someone involved in the care of the acute problem. Therefore, the treatment of hematologic emergencies in children with sickle cell disease is accomplished best in a center which also provides comprehensive care to affected patients.

Thalassemia Major (Cooley's Anemia)

BACKGROUND

The thalassemias are a group of disorders characterized by an inability to synthesize sufficient amounts of the globin component of hemoglobin. In β thalassemia major, the most common of the homozygous thalassemia syndromes, the affected child produces little or no hemoglobin A and is usually transfusion dependent from early childhood. The β thalassemia gene occurs commonly in countries bordering the Mediterranean Sea as well as in the countries of Southeast Asia. Although most of the problems associated with these disorders are due to long term transfusion therapy, the severe anemia at the time of diagnosis may constitute a hematologic emergency.

CLINICAL MANIFESTATIONS

Children with β thalassemia major usually develop a sallow complexion and increasing fatigue between the ages of 6 and 24 months. Weight gain and linear growth may be retarded. Physical examination shows pallor and enlargement of the liver and spleen. The hemoglobin level may be as low as 3 or 4 g/dl, and the mean corpuscular volume (MCV) is below 65 fl. The red cells are hypochromic and microcytic with striking variation in size and shape; nucleated red cells are present in the peripheral smear. Thalassemia major is readily distinguishable from severe nutritional iron deficiency. In the latter disorder, the dietary history is grossly abnormal, organomegaly is uncommon, changes in red cell morphology are less impressive, and nucleated red cells are rarely seen in the peripheral smear. The diagnosis of thalassemia major should be considered in a child with severe microcytic anemia and an appropriate ethnic background. Although severe anemia is extremely rare in heterozygous thalassemia disorders, thalassemia trait and concomitant iron deficiency may be particularly difficult to distinguish from a homozygous thalassemia disorder.

MANAGEMENT

The moderate anemia which is usually present at the time of presentation allows sufficient time for a careful diagnostic evaluation and outpatient transfusion therapy. However, when anemia is severe and congestive heart failure is present or imminent, the need for red cell transfusion may be urgent. In such instances, pretransfusion blood should be saved for appropriate diagnostic studies (hemoglobin electrophoresis) and initial red cell antigen typing. If transfusion is necessary, small aliquots of red cells (2 to 3 ml/kg) should be given. The administration of a rapidly acting diuretic (furosemide 1 mg/kg/dose) may diminish the risk of fluid overload. Partial exchange transfusion has also been recommended for patients with severe anemia to prevent further increases in intravascular volume and myocardial stress. Since patients with thalassemia major and severe anemia invariably have a lifelong dependence on red cell transfusions, the use of uncrossmatched blood should be scrupulously avoided at the time of presentation in order to prevent sensitization to foreign red cell antigens.

Methemoglobinemia

BACKGROUND

Methemoglobinemia is an uncommon cause of cyanosis in infants and children but is capable of causing severe problems and even death. Cyanosis results from a disproportionate amount of heme iron being present in the ferric rather than ferrous state. Under these conditions, oxygen binding by hemoglobin is severely impaired. The diagnosis of methemoglobinemia should be considered whenever cyanosis occurs in the absence of demonstrable cardiac or pulmonary disease.

The disturbance in the usual balance between ferrous and ferric iron may be due to alterations of hemoglobin structure (hemoglobin M), abnormalities of red cell enzymes (methemoglobin reductase) or exposure to oxidant drugs or chemicals (Table 47.3). The inherited forms of methemoglobinemia may be characterized by chronic cyanosis. However, in the absence of a specific oxidant stress, further symptoms are uncommon and treatment is given primarily for cosmetic reasons. When acute methemoglobinemia results from an oxidant stress, oxygen delivery may be severely compromised and the patient becomes acutely ill. If the agent acts as a direct oxidant, the onset of symptoms is rapid. If, however, methemoglobin formation is due to a metabolite of the original compound or due to secondary alterations in red cell metabolism, symptoms may be delayed. For example, methemoglobinemia is seen 12 to 15 hours after exposure to nitrobenzene.

CLINICAL MANIFESTATIONS

Symptoms depend on the concentration of methemoglobin. When methemoglobin comprises 10 to 25% of total hemoglobin, only cyanosis occurs. As the level rises to 30 to 50%, dyspnea, tachycardia, dizziness, fatigue and headache may be noted. Severe lethargy and stupor are often present when the methemoglobin concentration exceeds 50%, and death may occur at concentrations above 70%. If anemia is present, oxygen delivery is further compromised and toxicity may be more severe at lower concentrations of methemoglobin.

Accurate diagnosis and rapid therapy will prevent serious damage. The diagnosis should be strongly suspected when oxygen administration fails to affect the cyanosis. To eliminate an anatomic abnormality as a cause of oxygen unresponsive cyanosis, an attempt should be made to oxygenate the patient's blood in vitro. As a rapid screening test, a drop of blood is placed on filter paper. After waving the filter paper in the air for 30 to 60 sec, normal blood will appear bright red, while blood from a patient with methemoglobinemia will remain reddish-brown. Spectrophotometric assays can be used for confirmation of methemoglobinemia as well as determination of the level of methemoglobin.

Table 47.3
Substances and Drugs Commonly Implicated in the Formation of Methemoglobin in Children

I. Drugs
- A. Silver nitrate
- B. Sulfonamide antibiotics
- C. Quinones
- D. Phenacetin
- E. Benzocaine

II. Domestic and Environmental Substances
- A. Foods containing nitrates or nitrites
- B. Well water containing nitrates
- C. Anilin dyes (certain marking inks, dyes for some clothing and shoes, some crayons)
- D. Naphthalene (moth balls)
- E. Soap enemas
- F. Certain industrial compounds (nitrobenzenes, nitrous gases, organic amines)

MANAGEMENT

The treatment of methemoglobinemia depends on the clinical severity. In all cases, an attempt should be made to identify an oxidant stress and, once identified, to remove the causative substance. If symptoms are mild after oxidant exposure, therapy is unnecessary. Red cells with normal metabolism will reduce the methemoglobin in several hours. If the symptoms are severe, 1 to 2 mg/kg of methylene blue as a 1% solution in saline should be infused intravenously over 5 min. A second dose can be given if symptoms are still present 1 hour later. Since methylene blue can act as an oxidant at high doses, the total dosage should not exceed 7 mg/kg. Failure of methylene blue to improve the course of methemoglobinemia may be due to concomitant G6PD deficiency since the therapeutic effect requires an intact hexose monophosphate shunt. Under these conditions, ascorbic acid may be of some value, but, if symptoms are severe, exchange transfusion may be required. Even if treatment with methylene blue or ascorbic acid in the emergency department is successful, any child with symptomatic methemoglobinemia should be admitted to the hospital for close observation and further evaluation of the underlying abnormality or causative agent.

DISORDERS OF WHITE CELLS

Infection is the most significant complication associated with either quantitative or qualitative white cell disorders. In some children, death may follow a single episode of acute, overwhelming sepsis. In others, repeated local infections may cause severe organ damage or may culminate in a fatal, disseminated fungal infection. The appropriate emergency management of the child with white cell abnormalities and fever or other signs of infection may have a profound impact on both the length and quality of the patient's life.

Neutropenia

The most common forms of neutropenia and abnormal neutrophil function are listed in Table 47.4. Neutropenia is usually defined as an absolute neutrophil count below 1000/cu mm. When the neutrophil count falls below 500/cu mm, the patient exhibits an increased susceptibility to infections caused by normal skin, respiratory or gastrointestinal flora. Between 500 and 1000/cu mm, susceptibility to infection is less

Table 47.4
Causes of Neutropenia and Disorders of Neutrophil Function in Children (See Hematology Text for Complete Listings)

I. *Congenital Neutropenia*
   A. Kostmann's syndrome (infantile genetic agranulocytosis)
   B. Familial benign neutropenia and severe neutropenia (autosomal dominant)
   C. Neutropenia associated with immunoglobulin disorders
   D. Reticular dysgenesis
   E. Neutropenias associated with phenotypic abnormalities (metaphyseal chondrodysplasia, cartilage-hair hypoplasia)
   F. Chronic neutropenia of childhood
   G. Cyclic neutropenia
II. *Acquired Neutropenias*
   A. Drugs and chemical toxins
   B. Infection (bacterial, viral, rickettsial and protozoal)
   C. Bone marrow infiltration (leukemia, neuroblastoma, lymphoma)
   D. Nutritional deficiencies (starvation; anorexia nervosa; vitamin B_{12}, folate and copper deficiencies)
   E. Immune neutropenias (collagen vascular diseases, Felty's syndrome, neonatal isoimmune neutropenia, autoimmune neutropenia, transfusion reactions)
III. *Disorders of Neutrophil Function*
   A. Cellular defects of chemotaxis (Job syndrome, "lazy leukocyte" syndrome, congenital icthyosis, chronic renal failure, diabetes, rheumatoid arthritis, bone marrow transplantation, malnutrition, infection)
   B. Secondary defects of chemotaxis (Chédiak-Higashi syndrome, hypogammoglobulinemia, chronic mucocutaneous candidiasis, Wiscott-Aldrich syndrome, chronic granulomatous disease)
   C. Complement abnormalities and congenital absence of opsonin system
   D. Disorders of defective degranulation (Chédiak-Higashi syndrome)
   E. Defective peroxidative killing of bacteria and fungi (chronic granulomatous disease, myeloperoxidase deficiency)
   F. Acquired disorders of phagocytic dysfunction (severe iron deficiency, malnutrition, malignancies, severe burns)

marked but the host's ability to combat more typical infections is impaired. However, management of the patient cannot be based on the absolute neutrophil count alone since other, often unknown factors contribute to the severity of the clinical course. For example, serious, recurrent bacterial infections are common in Kostmann's neutropenia and death frequently occurs in early childhood. In contrast, the clinical course of chronic benign neutropenia is much milder. Yet the absolute neutrophil counts in the two disorders frequently overlap. Similarly, serious infection is unusual in immune-mediated neutropenia, although the absolute neutrophil count may be less than 500/cu mm, a level at which severe morbidity and substantial mortality may be found in children with leukemia undergoing chemotherapy (see p. 699).

The management of localized infection or unexplained fever in the child with neutropenia depends in large part on the underlying disorder and the patient's previous history of infection. In neutropenic states associated with repeated, severe infections, an aggressive attempt to identify a causative organism should be undertaken. Blood cultures and appropriate cultures from identified areas of infection (e.g., skin abscess, cellulitis) should be obtained. When fever cannot be attributed to a specific site of infection, cultures of the blood and urine are necessary. The cerebrospinal fluid should be examined and cultured whenever central nervous system infection is suspected. If the child appears ill or toxic, broad spectrum intravenous antibiotic therapy should be instituted with modification of therapy when culture results are available. Initial treatment should include antibiotics effective against *Staphylococcus aureus* and other gram-positive organisms as well as enteric bacteria including *Pseudomonas aeruginosa*. If no source of fever is identified and the child appears well, observation in the hospital without antibiotic therapy may be considered.

Decisions regarding admission to the hospital and treatment are often more difficult in children with more benign neutropenic states. Although infections are usually mild and localized in these patients, severe infections rarely may occur. A white cell count and differential may be valuable since, in some children, the white count will rise to normal or near normal levels during acute infection. Further laboratory investigation and treatment once again depend on the physical examination of the child as well as the previous history of infection. In most instances, antibiotic therapy can be reserved for those children with a specific source of bacterial infection. Careful follow-up is required, however, for children in whom fever is unexplained or attributed to probable viral infection.

A particularly perplexing problem arises when a child is found to be neutropenic during an evaluation of fever. In most instances, both the fever and neutropenia are due to a viral illness. Under these circumstances, serious secondary bacterial infections are unlikely to occur, and admission to the hospital and antibiotic therapy are probably unnecessary. However, since the neutropenia usually cannot be attributed with certainty to a viral illness, other causes of neutropenia should be carefully sought. The patient or parents should be questioned regarding the use of drugs which are associated with neutropenia (e.g., penicillins, phenothiazines, phenytoin). The family history should be explored for recurrent infections or deaths in early childhood which might suggest a congenital neutropenia. Underlying disorders such as malignancies or nutritional disturbances should be considered. If the child appears even moderately ill, admission to the hospital for further evaluation is appropriate.

Disorders of Neutrophil Function

Numerous disorders of neutrophil function have been described. These disorders are associated with serious infections to a variable extent. Therefore, the evaluation and treatment of the patient with abnormal neutrophil function should be based on the specific etiology. Particular attention should be paid to those disorders such as chronic granulomatous disease in which the site of infection (liver, bones, gastrointestinal tract) and causative organisms are distinctly unusual.

DISORDERS OF PLATELETS

The clinical course and management of patients with platelet abnormalities are determined primarily by the etiology of the underlying disorder. For example, at the same level of thrombocytopenia, bleeding is more common in disorders of platelet production than in immune-mediated disorders of platelet survival. Consequently the treatment of suspected bleeding following trauma should be more aggressive in the former disorder. The numerous causes of thrombocytopenia and abnormal platelet function are discussed in Chapter 31 and form an important background to the following section in which emphasis is placed on the management of bleeding emergencies in accordance with the underlying causes. The approach to a child with purpura or bleeding and no prior history of a bleeding disorder can also be found in Chapter 31. Finally, a discussion of the management of the many problems of lesser urgency which are associated with chronic platelet disorders is provided by textbooks of pediatric hematology.

Idiopathic Thrombocytopenic Purpura (ITP)

BACKGROUND

ITP is the most frequently encountered platelet disorder of childhood. Serious bleeding is rare, occurring in only 2 to 4% of cases. This low incidence is particularly remarkable since the disease is most common between the ages of 1 and 4 years when children are particularly prone to trauma as they learn to walk, run and climb. The risk of serious bleeding decreases sharply after the first week of illness, reflecting the presence of newly formed platelets with greater hemostatic activity.

CLINICAL MANIFESTATIONS/ MANAGEMENT

Petechiae and ecchymoses are the most common findings at the time of diagnosis of ITP but present no danger to the patient. Nonetheless, in many centers newly diagnosed patients are begun on a limited course of 2 mg/kg/day of prednisone to raise the platelet count and possibly prevent the occurrence of serious bleeding, such as intracranial hemorrhage, during the initial stages of the disease. Although corticosteroid therapy is effective in increasing the platelet count above levels found in untreated patients during the second week of illness, the low incidence of hemorrhagic complications in ITP has made it impossible to ascertain the clinical benefits of such therapy. If steroids are used, a bone marrow aspirate should be obtained prior to therapy to be certain that the diagnosis is correct. Occasional patients with leukemia have been mistakenly diagnosed as having ITP. Therapy with prednisone in these patients delays accurate diagnosis and may adversely influence the long-term outcome.

Bleeding may be particularly prominent in some patients with ITP. Epistaxis, gum bleeding, hematuria and menstrual bleeding are particularly persistent and anemia and iron deficiency may follow prolonged oozing. Local therapeutic measures, such as pressure and topical phenylephrine, may be helpful in stopping nosebleeds. However, when bleeding occurs in sites where local therapy is impossible or when bleeding continues despite conservative measures, treatment with prednisone should be instituted A dose of 2 mg/kg/day should be continued for 2 weeks, then stopped or tapered during the third week. Excessive menstrual bleeding may require hormonal therapy. If serious bleeding does not stop despite these measures, a transfusion of 0.2 unit/kg (maximum 10 units) of random donor platelets should be administered (Table 47.1). Although these transfused platelets are susceptible to the same antibody-mediated destruction as autologous platelets, their survival may be sufficiently long to stop or retard active bleeding.

Life-threatening hemorrhage is a rare complication of ITP that requires immediate recognition and therapy. Intracranial hemorrhage is the major cause of death in ITP although fatal bleeding has occurred in other sites. As noted earlier, serious bleeding is more common in the first week of the illness but may occur at any time. The child with ITP who has sustained head trauma or who has developed signs of increased intracranial pressure (headache, vomiting, lethargy) or focal neurologic deficits should be evaluated immediately. The platelet count should be measured; since, in the absence of severe trauma, intracranial hemorrhage is very unusual in the child with ITP whose platelet count is above 50,000/cu mm. If there is any suspicion of intracranial bleeding based on either a history of moderate or severe head trauma or the presence of neurologic abnormalities, hydrocortisone, 8 to 10 mg/kg, should be administered intravenously and 0.4 unit/kg of random donor platelets (maximum 15 to 20 units) should be infused immediately thereafter. When necessary, the volume of plasma in the platelet preparation can be reduced by centrifuging the platelets, removing a portion of the plasma and resuspending the platelets.

If further investigation documents intracranial bleeding or if the patient's clinical course deteriorates due to continuing hemorrhage, the patient must undergo splenectomy and, if appropriate, neurosurgical exploration. If the spleen had been removed previously, exchange transfusion or plasmapheresis with subsequent platelet transfusion should follow the initial treatment with corticosteroids and platelets.

Although the management of patients with ITP and obvious signs of intracranial hemorrhage is straightforward, a much more common and perplexing problem is the treatment of the asymptomatic child who has sustained mild or moderate head trauma. While no firm rules are possible, management should be based on the duration of disease, tendency to bleed as demonstrated by the presence of petechiae or ecchymoses, platelet count and likelihood of careful followup.

Immune-Mediated Neonatal Purpura

Serious bleeding may occur in the newborn or young infant with isoimmune thrombocytopenia or in the infant born to a mother with ITP. A discussion of the pathophysiology and diagnosis of these disorders is beyond the scope of this section. However, since mortality may be high in these disorders, the management of actual or potential bleeding deserves special emphasis. The brain is the major site of serious bleeding perhaps because of trauma sustained during vaginal delivery. Consequently, in many centers all newborns with immune thrombocytopenia and platelet counts below 20,000 to 50,000/cu mm receive a platelet transfusion (0.2 unit/kg) following vaginal delivery. Further therapy depends on the clinical course and subsequent platelet counts. In isoimmune thrombocytopenia, random donor platelets are usually destroyed rapidly due to the presence of the same offending antigen as that found on the infant's platelets. However, maternal platelets will survive normally and should be used if the platelet count is low after transfusion of random donor platelets or if signs of bleeding are present. Treatment of the thrombocytopenic infant born to a mother with ITP is more difficult since survival of all donor platelets is markedly shortened. If signs of generalized bleeding are present or if vital organs are impaired by local hemorrhage, a two-volume exchange transfusion should be performed to remove a portion of the circulating antiplatelet antibody. A platelet transfusion should be administered immediately after completion of the exchange transfusion. While steroids have not been proved to be efficacious in these disorders, their use, particularly in neonatal thrombocytopenia due to maternal ITP, has been advocated by some physicians.

The recognition of immune-mediated neonatal thrombocytopenia is important for counseling of the parents and preparation for future deliveries as well as for the treatment of the affected child. In some instances, maternal ITP has been recognized only after delivery of a thrombocytopenic newborn. In isoimmune thrombocytopenia, accurate diagnosis allows appropriate counseling regarding the risk to infants born of subsequent pregnancies. In addition, maternal platelets can be prepared just prior to future deliveries so that they are available for immediate transfusion if needed. These factors make it imperative for the physician to obtain appropriate diagnostic studies in the thrombocytopenic infant.

Nonimmune Thrombocytopenia and Abnormalities of Platelet Function

Serious bleeding due to decreased platelet production or impaired platelet function usually responds rapidly to an infusion of random donor platelets (0.2 unit/kg, maximum 10 units). However, unless part of a program of prophylactic therapy, transfusions should be reserved for severe or persistent bleeding. Many affected patients have chronic disorders and require repeated transfusion. The excessive use of platelet transfusions, whether prepared from multiple, single or HLA matched donors, may contribute to the early formation of antiplatelet antibodies, making future transfusions more difficult and, in many instances, less effective.

DISORDERS OF COAGULATION

Coagulation abnormalities are responsible for a large proportion of hematologic emergencies. Indeed, children with hemophilia often use the emergency department as their primary source of acute care since bleeding episodes frequently occur at odd hours and require immediate treatment. This section places particular emphasis on the management of bleeding which poses a direct threat to life or to normal, long-term organ function in children with common inherited and acquired coagulopathies. The rarer inherited disorders of coagulation are not discussed in detail. Bleeding episodes are usually similar to those found in the more common disorders. Appropriate replacement products are listed in Table 47.5.

Inherited Disorders

BACKGROUND

The most common inherited bleeding disorders are factor VIII deficiency (hemophilia A), factor IX deficiency (hemophilia B) and von Willebrand's disease. The severity of bleeding in the hemophilias can usually be predicted from the level of factor coagulant activity. If less than 1% of the deficient factor is present (severe hemophilia), bleeding episodes occur frequently and are often unrelated to trauma. If the factor level is between 1 and 5% (moderate hemophilia), spontaneous hemorrhage is less common but bleeding occurs in response to minimal trauma. If the factor level is greater than 5% (mild hemophilia), significant trauma is usually required to induce bleeding. Although very low factor VIII coagulant activity is associated with severe bleeding in von Willebrand's disease, the relationship between laboratory findings and clinical course is less predictable than in hemophilia, and the severity of von Willebrand's disease in a particular child is best judged on the basis of the patient's own bleeding history.

The classification of inherited bleeding disorders according to severity is very important in assessing patients who have sustained trauma or who have signs of active bleeding. For example, after mild head

Table 47.5
Specific Factor Deficiencies and Replacement Therapy

Factor Deficiency	Replacement Therapy
Fibrinogen (I) (also dysfibrinogenemias)	Cryoprecipitate Fresh frozen plasma Fibrinogen concentrates
Prothrombin (II)	Fresh frozen plasma
Factor V	Fresh frozen plasma
Factor VII	Fresh frozen plasma
Factor VIII	Cryoprecipitate Factor VIII concentrates Fresh frozen plasma
Factor IX	Fresh frozen plasma Factor IX concentrates
Factor X	Fresh frozen plasma
Factor XI	Fresh frozen plasma
Factor XII	Fresh frozen plasma
Factor XIII	Fresh frozen plasma

trauma the patient with severe hemophilia is at greater risk of developing intracranial bleeding than the patient with mild hemophilia and therefore must be managed more aggressively. On the other hand, when extensive hemorrhage is seen in a child with mild hemophilia, significant trauma has probably occurred and injury to deeper organs should be suspected.

CLINICAL MANIFESTATIONS/ MANAGEMENT

Joint Bleeding. Hemarthroses are a common complication in hemophilia, frequently occurring in the absence of trauma in severe disease. The large joints such as the knees and elbows are commonly affected. Initial replacement therapy should be designed to raise the factor level to 25 to 30% (see below). Further treatment is usually unnecessary unless pain persists or swelling increases. When the involved joint has been the site of recurrent hemorrhages, several doses of replacement therapy may be required. Initial immobilization of the joint is often helpful and can be easily accomplished with a plaster splint that extends to the next joint distally. The pain associated with joint bleeding usually resolves within a few hours of treatment and, therefore, analgesics are often unnecessary. However, if pain is severe, analgesic therapy should be given orally. Aspirin must not be used since its inhibitory affect on platelet function may further aggravate the clotting disorder. Acetaminophen, either alone or in combination with codeine, is usually sufficient. The repeated use of outpatient therapy with narcotics should be carefully avoided since the risk of drug addiction in severe hemophilia is substantial.

Bleeding in the hip is a particularly serious problem. As the joint becomes distended, blood flow to the femoral head may be impeded, resulting in aseptic necrosis. The hip is also a difficult joint to immobilize. Consequently, re-bleeding is more likely in the hip than in other joints. Local tenderness is usually present and the child prefers to lie in the "frog leg" position. A radiograph of the hip shows widening of the joint space. Because of the importance of achieving and maintaining hemostasis in this joint, initial correction to 50% (see p. 485) is often followed by several days of continuing replacement therapy (30% correction every 12 hours). Hospitalization may be required for immobilization, using either strict bed rest or traction.

The role of arthrocentesis varies from center to center. Removal of the blood from the joint has been helpful in allowing early mobilization and maintaining normal range of motion. Other indications for arthrocentesis include relief of pain if the joint is severely distended and prevention of further synovial damage in the chronically affected joint. Although the physical examination and laboratory findings may be similar in septic arthritis and hemarthrosis, the history and the patient's description of the pain ("just like my other bleeds") are usually sufficient to distinguish these two disorders, making arthrocentesis for diagnostic purposes unnecessary. Furthermore, while joint bleeding is very common in hemophilia, septic arthritis is extremely rare. Correction to 30 to 50% should be achieved prior to tapping the joint. How prominent a role arthrocentesis plays in the emergency management of joint bleeds may ultimately depend on the availability of consistent, experienced orthopaedic care. Like most procedures, the risk-benefit ratio of a joint tap is greatly reduced if the physician has extensive experience with the procedure and its role in the care of the particular disease.

Muscle Bleeding. Most muscle bleeding is superficial and easily controlled with a single dose of replacement therapy to achieve 30% correction. However, emergencies may arise when substantial blood loss occurs or when nerve function is impaired. Extensive hemorrhage is most commonly found in retroperitoneal bleeds (e.g., ileal-psoas) or thigh bleeds. Retroperitoneal bleeds are frequently accompanied by lower abdominal pain. A mass is sometimes palpable deep in the abdomen and sensation in the distribution of the femoral nerve may be diminished. Loss of the psoas shadow may be seen on an abdominal radiograph and a hematoma may be demonstrated by ultrasonography. The hemoglobin level should be measured initially and, if bleeding persists, at regular intervals thereafter.

Treatment consists of hospitalization, bed rest, initial correction to 50 to 60% and maintenance of a 30% factor level until pain has resolved and ambulation has been successfully achieved.

Nerve paralysis and Volkmann's contracture are associated with bleeding into the volar compartment of the forearm. Consequently, hemorrhage in this area should be treated with an initial correction of 50 to 60% and, if abnormal muscle or nerve function is present or if swelling increases, maintenance of factor levels above 30% until resolution of symptoms. Patchy sensory loss is frequently associated with compression of superficial nerves and may persist for several months before normal sensation reappears.

Subcutaneous Bleeding. Hemorrhage under the skin may cause extensive discoloration but is rarely dangerous and usually requires no therapy unless compression of critical organs occurs. Pressure on the airway from a subcutaneous bleed of the neck may be life-threatening, requiring steps to assure airway patency such as an endotracheal tube in addition to correction of the factor level to at least 50%. Careful observation of children with bleeding in the muscles of the neck is mandatory since airway obstruction may be sudden.

Oral Bleeding. Mouth bleeds are particularly common in young children with hemophilia. The presence of fibrinolysins in saliva may lead to persistent oozing in the absence of aggressive management. The site of bleeding should be identified. If a weak clot is present it should be removed and dry topical thrombin placed on the site. Initial correction should be 30 to 50%. Frequently, one or more additional treatments is necessary to achieve adequate clot formation and prevent re-bleeding when the clot falls off. The antifibrinolytic agent, ϵ-aminocaproic acid (EACA), is a useful adjunct in the treatment of oral bleeding. The drug should be administered orally in a dose of 100 mg/kg every 6 hours with a maximum daily dose of 24 g. Since children may swallow a substantial amount of blood, actual blood loss may be underestimated by the patient or family, and measurement of the hemoglobin level is helpful, particularly if bleeding has persisted for more than 24 hours. As in bleeds of the neck muscles careful evaluation of airway patency is essential. Complete airway obstruction may result from extensive bleeding in the tongue.

Gastrointestinal Bleeding. Hemorrhage from the gastrointestinal tract is rarely severe in hemophilia unless an anatomic lesion such as a duodenal ulcer or diverticulum is present. Maintenance of the factor level above 30% for 2 or 3 days is usually sufficient. If bleeding persists, appropriate diagnostic studies are necessary.

Urinary Tract Bleeding. Atraumatic painless hematuria is the most common manifestation of renal bleeding in children with hemophilia. Specific lesions are rarely identified and intravenous pyelography can often be reserved for those patients who fail to respond to initial replacement therapy. Ultrasonography, on the other hand, carries no risk and may be helpful in identifying the occasional patient with a subcapsular or intrarenal hemorrhage. If bleeding is persistent, moderate to severe anemia may develop and the hemoglobin level should be carefully monitored. In the absence of trauma or a demonstrable lesion, several approaches to ensuring hemostasis seem equally effective. Bed rest without replacement therapy is often successful. In some centers, one or two initial doses of factor replacement (30 to 70%) are used in combination with bed rest for at least 24 hours after gross hematuria has ceased. A brief course of orally administered prednisone has also been effective.

While disagreement regarding the optimal method of treating painless hematuria persists, there is no difference of opinion regarding the potential hazard of EACA in affected patients. The strong, antifibrinolytic activity of this drug may cause formation of ureteral clots and outflow obstruction. Although EACA is an effective and seemingly safe agent in the treatment of hematuria associated with sickle cell anemia or sickle cell trait, its use in children with hemophilia has been accompanied by obstructive uropathy and should therefore be avoided.

When the child with hemophilia develops hematuria or flank tenderness after trauma a more aggressive approach to diagnosi and treatment is required. Ultrasonography or intravenous pyelography should be performed as soon as possible to look for subcapsular or intrarenal bleeding. In order to prevent parenchymal damage and deterioration of renal function, replacement therapy to achieve a level of 70 to 100% should be administered immediately. If a lesion is demonstrated using the techniques noted above, replacement therapy should be continued for 7 to 10 days. If no lesion has been identified, a shorter course of therapy is usually sufficient, using resolution of pain and hematuria as an endpoint. The hemoglobin level and renal function tests should be followed carefully.

Intracranial Hemorrhage. Bleeding within the cranial vault is a complication of hemophilia that fully justifies the concern, anxiety and urgency attached to it. In practical terms, however, head trauma in children with hemophilia is common while intracranial hemorrhage is comparatively rare. Thus, the physician must be able to recognize as well as treat the child at risk without exposing other patients to unnecessary hospitalization, diagnostic studies or therapy.

The management of the hemophiliac with head trauma but no neurologic signs requires careful attention to the severity of the bleeding disorder, type of trauma, previous history of intracranial bleeding and likelihood of close followup. Even with consideration of these factors, good fortune remains an important ingredient. Children with seemingly insignificant trauma may develop the first obvious signs of intracranial bleeding several days later when concern has diminished. To prevent such occurrences, every child with reported head trauma is treated with at least one dose of replacement therapy in some centers. However, this approach carries the risk and expense of frequent therapy. More importantly, in an effort to prevent yet another visit to the emergency department, the child or parent may fail to report a serious episode of trauma. Consequently, other centers use an approach which is still conservative although slightly less rigid. If the trauma is mild (e.g., a light bump on the forehead), the child is observed at home for the usual signs of intracranial hemorrhage or increased intracranial pressure. When the trauma is somewhat more substantial (e.g., falling down 2 or 3 carpeted stairs), the child is evaluated by the physician, given replacement therapy to achieve a level of 50 to 70%, observed for several hours in the office or emergency department and, if well, discharged. If, however, moderate or severe trauma has occurred (e.g. hitting the head on the dashboard; falling off a changing table onto a hard floor), hospital admission and repeated doses of replacement therapy are essential.

Unfortunately, the severity of trauma usually defies quantitative analysis and the physician is left with substantial uncertainty. When the child with head trauma is not hospitalized, parents should be well informed about signs of intracranial bleeding. In particular, parents (and physicians) must remember that bleeding may be slow and, therefore, neurologic symptoms and signs may be delayed. Repeated visits may be necessary to accurately monitor the child's neurologic examination in order to detect intracranial hemorrhage as early as possible. At the first suggestion of the complication (headache, vomiting, etc.), hospitalization and treatment are mandatory.

The management of the hemophiliac with neurologic findings in the presence or absence of head trauma begins with replacement therapy and those measures required for life support and treatment of increased intracranial pressure. Levels of the appropriate factor should be raised to 100%. Factor concentrates (see below) are generally used because the actual concentration of factor in this preparation has been measured, and, therefore, the post-treatment factor level can be predicted with reasonable accuracy. The indications for surgery are similar to those for children without coagulation disorders, provided an appropriate correction of clotting abnormalities has been achieved.

Preparation of the Hemophiliac for Emergency Surgery. The child with hemophilia is subject to the surgical emergencies that affect children with normal hemostasis (e.g., appendicitis, compound fractures) as well as those hemorrhagic complications requiring immediate operative intervention. In some instances, a bleeding episode may be confused with an acute abdomen. For example, retroperitoneal hemorrhage may mimic acute appendicitis. If time allows, a trial of replacement therapy may be helpful in distinguishing the two disorders. If, on the other hand, the child's clinical condition worsens or the need for surgery has been definitively established, correction up to 100% should be given and the partial thromboplastin time (PTT) measured to assure its normalization. Since the PTT is normal when the factor VIII or IX level is as low as 20%, measurement of factor coagulant level is needed to assess the adequacy of response to treatment when levels above 20% are desired. This test cannot always be performed prior to surgery but is essential in the postoperative management of the hemophiliac. Therefore, surgery in a child with hemophilia should rarely, if ever, be undertaken in a hospital without appropriate laboratory facilities.

REPLACEMENT PRODUCTS

The three blood products commonly employed for the treatment of children with hemophilia are fresh frozen plasma, cryoprecipitate and lyophilized factor concentrates. The correct use of these products is important not only to ensure adequate hemostasis but also to minimize risks associated with treatment and to reduce costs when possible.

Fresh Frozen Plasma. Fresh frozen plasma contains both factor VIII and factor IX activity, and, therefore, is particularly useful in the treatment of the newborn or young infant with an inherited, but undefined, disorder of coagulation. However, the relatively low concentration of these factors (1 unit/ml) restricts the use of fresh frozen plasma in older children. For example, at least 600 ml of fresh frozen plasma are required for the treatment of a minor joint bleed in a 50-kg boy with factor VIII deficiency. In contrast, only 150 ml of cryoprecipitate (see below) are needed to achieve the same level of factor replacement in this patient. In smaller children, the total volume of fresh frozen plasma required for treatment is less and its low risk of post-transfusion hepatitis in comparison with pooled concentrates makes it an excellent alternative to the latter product in the treatment of factor IX deficiency. The use of fresh frozen plasma rather than factor IX concentrates is especially important in children with mild factor IX deficiency since the limited need for therapy does not warrant the increased exposure to hepatitis viruses. As a general rule, fresh frozen plasma should be used for those patients with mild or moderate factor IX deficiency who have had little or no exposure to concentrates, unless the type of hemorrhage requires a high and precisely predicted level of correction. The role of fresh frozen plasma in children with severe factor IX deficiency is similar in many centers although factor IX concentrates are used from the time of diagnosis by other pediatric hematologists.

Cryoprecipitate. When plasma is frozen and then slowly thawed, the precipitate contains enriched factor VIII activity (100 units of factor VIII activity in 20 to 30 ml of plasma). Thus, factor VIII is concentrated 3- to 5-fold in comparison with fresh frozen plasma and the volume required for therapy is proportionately smaller. However, like fresh frozen plasma, the actual factor VIII activity in a given bag (or unit) depends on the level in the donor and therefore, may vary widely. Actual factor VIII activity in a particular bag of cryoprecipitate is rarely assayed although most blood banks know the average factor VIII recovery in their laboratory. If only one or two bags are being administered, the total administered factor VIII activity is unpredictable since the bags may be unusually high or low in factor VIII activity. When a larger number of bags are given, the total factor VIII content is more likely to reflect the average activity for units of cryoprecipitate prepared in that particular blood bank.

Since each bag of cryoprecipitate is made from a single donor, the risk of post-transfusion hepatitis is low in comparison with factor VIII concentrates. Because it carries such a low risk of hepatitis, cryoprecipitate remains the preferred replacement product for emergency treatment of children with factor VIII deficiency unless they are receiving regular therapy with concentrates or unless the type of hemorrhage requires knowledge of the precise concentration of factor in the replacement product. As an example of the latter situation, a 6-month-old boy weighing 8 kg would require approximately 300 units of factor VIII to achieve a correction of 100%. Although this level theoretically can be achieved with three bags of cryoprecipitate, the actual factor VIII content in each bag may range from 50 to 150 units and the total amount of factor VIII administered might be as low as 150 units. In contrast, each vial of factor VIII concentrate has been assayed for factor VIII coagulant activity, thus permitting administration of a known amount of factor.

Concentrates. The concentrations of factor VIII and factor IX in the lyophilized products are enriched 10- to 20-fold in comparison with fresh frozen plasma. The high factor concentration and the measured factor content in each vial make these products uniquely suitable for the treatment of major hemorrhage. In addition, most older children with hemophilia use factor concentrates for home therapy and, therefore, the product may be suitable for the emergency treatment of even minor bleeding episodes. However, as discussed earlier, the factor concentrates are associated with a substantially higher risk of post-transfusional hepatitis since the product is made from a large pool of donors. In addition, administration of factor IX concentrates (which also contain factors II, VII and X) has been followed by disseminated thrombosis, most commonly in patients with pre-existing liver disease. Therefore, the use of factor concentrates should be reserved primarily for those children with hemophilia who cannot be treated adequately with fresh frozen plasma or cryoprecipitate.

Calculation of Dosage. Two formulas are commonly used for determining the number of units of factor VIII or factor IX necessary to achieve a specific level:

Factor VIII:

a. Wt of patient (kg) × desired level of correction (%) × 0.4 = number of units

   or

b. One unit of factor VIII per kg raises the measured factor level by 2%. ((desired level/2) × wt of patient [kg] = number of units)

Factor IX:

a. Wt of patient (kg) × desired level of correction (%) × 0.6 = number of units

   or

b. 1 unit of factor IX per kg raises the measured factor IX level by 1.5%. ((desired level/1.5) × wt of patient [kg] = number of units)

The calculations for each factor yield similar, though not identical, results. In the treatment of minor bleeding episodes, a calculated correction of 30% usually provides a sufficient margin of safety to make small differences in calculated dosages insignificant. In the treatment of major hemorrhages, however, the achieved level of factor activity should be measured directly since the in vivo recovery varies widely among patients no matter which formula is used and since inadequate hemostasis may lead to severe morbidity or death.

For children with von Willebrand's disease, doses of factor VIII of 15 units/kg and 30 to 50 units/kg are commonly used for the treatment of minor and major hemorrhages, respectively. However, the response to treatment with fresh frozen plasma or cryoprecipitate is not as predictable in this disorder as it is in factor VIII deficiency. The clinical course and the bleeding time are the most useful measurements of the response to therapy and need for further treatment.

MANAGEMENT OF PATIENT WITH INHIBITORS

The treatment of bleeding episodes in the child with hemophilia and high levels of antibodies to the missing or diminished factor is difficult, controversial and frequently unsatisfying. For children with antibodies to factor VIII, the treatment of bleeding episodes with factor IX concentrates at a dose of 75 units/kg produces a favorable clinical response in comparison with placebo. The reason for this response remains unknown, and the failure of approximately 50% of treated patients to respond to this product adds further confusion to the understanding of the hemostatic mechanism. Factor IX concentrates with increased levels of activated factor or factor VIII inhibitor bypassing activity (FEIBA) are being evaluated at the present time but are not widely available for the treatment of children with inhibitors. In the absence of predictable response to treatment with factor IX concentrates, good local care, including splinting for joint bleeds and topical thrombin for accessible oral lacerations, remains a cornerstone of therapy.

Extensive resources, experience and ingenuity are necessary for the treatment of major hemorrhages in the patient with antibodies to factor VIII. Very large doses of factor VIII (>100 units/kg) may be sufficient to overwhelm low levels of circulating inhibitor and achieve measurable factor VIII activity and initial hemostasis. However, those patients who are "high responders" to the factor VIII antigen will develop rising titers of antibody within 3 to 5 days, making further therapy with factor VIII useless. Despite the predictable antibody rise, this brief period of factor VIII therapy may be sufficient to stop bleeding in a critical organ such as the brain. The concomitant use of immunosuppressive therapy has not inhibited antibody response in most patients although this approach has been advocated by some investigators.

If no response to factor VIII infusion occurs, or if initial antibody titers are too high to warrant such a trial, factor IX concentrate should be used. The success of such therapy must be judged by the clinical response of the patient, making careful, repeated evaluations mandatory. Should the patient's condition worsen, as, for example, deepening coma in the child with head trauma, a two-volume exchange transfusion may remove sufficent antibody to allow a response to factor VIII administration. However, since 50% of the IgG inhibitor is tissue bound and will rapidly return to the plasma, further infusions of factor VIII will be unsuccessful unless preceded by a similar exchange transfusion.

Some patients with low levels of factor VIII antibodies have no anamnestic response to factor VIII infusion and can be managed satisfactorily with this product alone. These patients have usually been identified by their response to previous therapy.

The treatment of patients with antibodies to factor IX has not been clearly defined. Factor IX concentrates containing increased levels of activated factor or factor VIII inhibitor bypassing activity have been beneficial in some cases. Exchange transfusion followed by infusion of factor IX concentrate may also be useful if the hemorrhage is severe or life-threatening. Fortunately, the incidence of factor IX deficiency is only 15% of the incidence of factor VIII deficiency. Therefore, despite the equivalent likelihood of developing inhibitors in the two disorders, few patients with factor IX deficiency and inhibitors will require therapy.

The recognition of a newly developed inhibitor may be equally as important as the treatment of a patient with a known inhibitor. With the development of an inhibitor, patients with severe hemophilia frequently experience no change in their already difficult clinical course. However, the response to therapy is usually noted to be less satisfactory. If an inhibitor is suspected at the time of emergency therapy, a PTT should be measured after therapy since, in the presence of a strong inhibitor, a level of factor activity adequate to normalize the PTT (20 to 30% factor VIII) is rarely achieved. An inhibitor screen can also be performed by mixing the patient's plasma with normal plasma and demonstrating a prolonged PTT in comparison with normal plasma mixed with saline. The level of inhibitor can be measured using more sophisticated techniques. Although the PTT need not be measured after routine treatment of minor hemorrhages, this study should always be used to demonstrate an elevation in factor activity in the treatment of major hemorrhage since a failure to respond to initial therapy may compromise organ function or life itself.

Disseminated Intravascular Coagulation

Disseminated intravascular coagulation (DIC) is an acquired disorder of hemostasis which may be due to numerous causes but in children most commonly accompanies septic shock. The clinical and laboratory findings of DIC are described in Chapter 31. The treatment of this disorder should be directed primarily toward correction of the underlying disorder. Although correction of the hemostatic abnormality may temporarily decrease bleeding or prevent formation or extension of thrombosis, mortality remains extremely high when shock is not reversed in the first several hours.

Abnormal coagulation studies are frequently found in the absence of actual bleeding in DIC. Attempts to correct these abnormalities are of little or no value in preventing later bleeding or altering the outcome of the underlying illness. If persistent or severe bleeding occurs, replacement of the consumed blood products may be helpful. Platelet transfusions (0.2 to 0.4 unit/kg) and fresh frozen plasma (15 ml/kg) should be used to correct severe thrombocytopenia or substantially prolonged tests of clotting function. Although the administration of platelets and clotting factors may theoretically provide the necessary ingredients for further pathologic clotting, there is little evidence to suggest that such therapy is, in practice, responsible for worsening organ damage. However, replacement therapy should be stopped if bleeding does not improve after one or two infusions of the appropriate product.

The role of therapy with heparin in DIC remains controversial. Although anticoagulation may slow the progression of disseminated thrombosis and resulting ischemia and hemorrhage, such therapy may itself lead to fatal bleeding complications. Furthermore, as noted earlier, anticoagulation does not appear to affect patient survival and therefore should not interfere with the primary goal of reversing shock. Nevertheless, administration of heparin is commonly recommended for patients with DIC and purpura fulminans (see Chapter 31) or severely compromised renal function due to thrombosis and ischemia. Heparin may be given by intermittent intravenous injection (50 to 100 units/kg every 4 hours) or continuous intravenous infusion (12.5 to 25 units/kg/hr) following an initial bolus injection of 50 to 100 units/kg). The dose should be adjusted to maintain the PTT at 1½ to 2 times the normal value. Once further consumption of coagulation factors has been slowed or halted, administration of plasma and platelets may restore normal components of clotting. However, the actual benefit of the seemingly paradoxical use of anticoagulants and coagulation factors is unproven.

OTHER HEMATOLOGIC EMERGENCIES

Postsplenectomy Sepsis

Splenectomy may cure or ameliorate several hematologic disorders. However, loss of the spleen is associated with a markedly increased risk of sepsis due to *Streptococcus pneumoniae, Neisseria meningiditis, Escherischia coli, Haemophilus influenzae,* and other bacteria, especially in young children. The frequency of pneumococcal sepsis is particularly high as this organism accounts for one-half of the episodes of postsplenectomy sepsis. If the hematologic disorder is immunologic in origin (autoimmune hemolytic anemia) or accompanied by other gaps in host defense (Wiskott-Aldrich syndrome), the incidence of sepsis is especially high. More important, the mortality due to sepsis in asplenic patients is markedly increased, averaging higher than 50% and rising to more than 80% in the presence of some immunologic abnormalities.

Although pneumococcal immunization and prophylactic antibiotics may reduce the occurrence of postsplenectomy sepsis, the most important facet of management is early detection and treatment. The presence of fever in an asplenic patient demands an immediate and careful evaluation to identify a source of infection. If the fever cannot be definitively attributed to a benign process such as an upper respiratory infection or if the patient appears unusually ill, the institution of parenteral antibiotic therapy pending results of cultures is usually indicated. The rapidity with which patients develop irreversible shock makes even a brief period of observation very risky and underscores the need for aggressive management of the symptomatic child.

Transfusion Reaction

BACKGROUND

Acute hemolytic transfusion reactions due to blood group incompatibility constitute a major hematologic emergency and may result in massive hemorrhage, renal failure and death. The uncommon occurrence of this problem is, in large part, a tribute to careful blood banking practices and close attention to the administration of the red cell product. Unfortunately, the rarity of acute hemolytic reactions may lead to a sense of complacency regarding transfusion and a loss of familiarity with the signs and symptoms of massive red cell destruction at a time when red cell transfusions are being administered with increasing frequency.

CLINICAL MANIFESTATIONS/ MANAGEMENT

The characteristic findings of an acute hemolytic transfusion reaction include apprehension, fever, chills, abdominal or flank pain, chest tightness and hypotension. If one or more of these findings develops, the transfusion should be stopped immediately since the severity of symptoms is related directly to the amount of hemolysis. Saline should be administered at 1½ to 2 times the maintenance rate (see Chapter 46). A spun hematocrit should be examined for the presence of hemoglobin which imparts a pink color to the plasma. The urine should also be examined for hemoglobin which causes a positive dipstick reaction for blood in the absence of red cells on microscopic analysis. The name, identification number and blood type of the patient should be compared with those on the unit of blood to ensure that the blood was given to the patient for whom it was intended. Finally, an aliquot of the unit should be returned to the blood bank for confirmation of the original compatibility testing.

Further management of an acute hemolytic transfusion reaction is directed toward maintenance of normal blood pressure and urine output and treatment of intravascular coagulation. Rapid intravenous hydration is mandatory to prevent renal shutdown. Diuretics, including mannitol (1 g/kg), may also be helpful. Intravascular coagulation should be treated with heparin, using doses similar to those described earlier for DIC from other causes.

Nonhemolytic transfusion reactions are more common and, in most instances, less severe than hemolytic reactions. Sensitization to plasma proteins may cause urticaria. Fever, chills and headache occur frequently in repeatedly transfused patients who have become sensitized to white cell and platelet antigens. While these reactions pose little danger to the patient, they may be difficult to distinguish from the more urgent hemolytic reaction. Before continuing the transfusion, urine and plasma should be checked for the presence of hemoglobin. If these studies are unrewarding, the physician must decide whether or not the clinical condition of the child warrants discarding the remainder of the unit or finishing the transfusion with supportive therapy such as antipyretics or antihistamines. Fortunately, the increasing use of frozen thawed red cells which contain neither plasma nor white cells has drastically reduced the incidence of nonhemolytic reactions in chronically transfused patients. As a corollary, a hemolytic reaction should be given particularly strong consideration when fever and chills occur in a child receiving frozen thawed red cells.

References

Alter BP, Rappaport JM, Parkman R: The bone marrow failure syndromes. In *Hematology of Infancy and Childhood*, Ed. 2, edited by Nathan DG and Oski FA. WB Saunders Co, Philadelphia, 1981.

Barrett-Connor E: Bacterial infection and sickle cell anemia: An analysis of 250 infections in 166 patients and a review of the literature. *Medicine* 50: 97, 1971

Buchanan GR, Boxer LA, Nathan DE: The acute and transient nature of idiopathic autoimmune hemolytic anemia in childhood. *J Pediatr* 88: 780, 1976.

Corrigan JJ, Jordan CM: Heparin therapy in septicemia with disseminated intravascular coagulation. *N Engl J Med* 283: 778, 1970.

Hathaway WE: The bleeding newborn. *Semin Hematol* 12: 175, 1975.

Heene DL: Disseminated intravascular coagulation: Evaluation of therapeutic approaches. *Semin Thromb Hemostas* 3: 291, 1977.

Lux SE and Wolfe LC: Inherited disorders of the red cell membrane skeleton. *Pediatr Clin North Am* 27: 463, 1980.

McClure PD: Idiopathic thrombocytopenic purpura in children: Diagnosis and management. *Pediatrics* 55: 68, 1975.

McIntosh S, Rooks Y, Ritchey AK, Pearson HA: Fever in young children with sickle cell disease. *J Pediatr* 96: 199, 1980.

Montgomery RR, Hathaway WE: Acute bleeding emergencies. *Pediatr Clin North Am* 27: 327, 1980.

Pearson HA, Diamond LK: The critically ill child: Sickle cell disease crises and their management. *Pediatrics* 48: 629, 1971.

Pincus SH, Boxer LA, Stossel T: Chronic neutropenia in childhood. *Am J Med* 61: 849, 1976.

Singer DB: Postsplenectomy sepsis. *Perspect Pediatr Pathol* 1: 285, 311, 1973.

CHAPTER 48

Toxicologic Emergencies

FRED M. HENRETIG, M.D., GARY C. CUPIT, PHARM.D., AND ANTHONY R. TEMPLE, M.D.

MEDICAL TOXICOLOGY

Medical toxicology as a science and as a clinical discipline has been of increasing interest and concern over the past two decades, particularly for primary care specialists, emergency physicians, and intensivists. Medical toxicology, which deals with toxic effects of overdose or excessive administration of drugs or other chemicals, also interfaces with, and to some degree overlaps, disciplines such as environmental toxicology, forensic or analytical toxicology, industrial medicine, and basic research toxicology, but its singular focus is the medical treatment of the poisoned patient.

The problem of poisoning in the emergency department is considerable. Estimates of poisoning episodes annually in the United States range in the millions. Poisonings may be either accidental or intentional. Accidental poisonings make up some 80 to 85% or more of all poisoning exposures, while intentional poisonings comprise the other 10 to 15%. Individuals in this latter group have a much higher rate of treatment in the emergency department, hospitalization, and intensive care. Among children age 5 and under, essentially all poisonings are accidents related to exploratory behavior. While less common, the physician must also consider, especially in urban areas, the possibility of both environmental exposures and suicide attempts in children.

The scope of toxic substances involved in poisonings is broad, requiring a wide range of knowledge. Table 48.1 presents the 25 categories of substances most frequently ingested by children under 5 years of age in the United States for the year 1978. Table 48.2 presents the 20 most common drugs involved in adolescent and adult emergency department poisoning visits for the year 1979. It is obvious from these data that the profile of pediatric poisonings differs from that of adult exposures. The most important differences between the pediatric and the adult profile, by type of agent, is in the higher percentage of cases in which psychopharmacologic drugs (sedatives, tranquilizers and antidepressants) were the cause of the poisoning in adults and the much higher frequency of exposures to household chemicals and plants in children.

There are five basic modes of exposure to poisoning: ingestion which accounts for the vast majority of occurrences, followed in decreasing frequency by ocular exposure, cutaneous or topical exposure, envenomation, and inhalation. Poisonings may be the result of both acute or chronic exposures. Most poisonings are acute, and the victims are typified by the child who surreptitiously invades the medicine cabinet or the storage area for household cleaners or the adolescent or adult who takes a massive number of pills in a fit of despair. Chronic poisoning refers to toxicity produced over some period

Table 48.1
Categories of Substances Most Frequently Ingested by Children under 5 Years of Age Reported to the National Clearinghouse for Poison Control Centers for 1978[a]

Type of Substance	1978	
	No.	Percent
1. Plants	11,010	11.7
2. Soaps, detergents, cleaners	5,836	6.2
3. Antihistamines, cold medications	4,003	4.3
4. Perfume, cologne, toilet water	3,748	4.0
5. Vitamins, minerals	3,677	3.9
6. Aspirin	3,557	3.8
Baby	2,557	0.4
Adult	380	0.4
Unspecified	640	0.7
7. Household disinfectants, deodorizers	2,752	2.9
8. Miscellaneous analgesics	2,752	2.9
9. Insecticides (excluding mothballs)	2,675	2.9
10. Miscellaneous internal medicines	2,303	2.5
11. Fingernail preparations	2,270	2.4
12. Miscellaneous external medicines	2,151	2.3
13. Liniments	2,016	2.2
14. Household bleach	1,863	2.0
15. Miscellaneous products	1,627	1.7
16. Cosmetic lotions, creams	1,625	1.7
17. Antiseptic medications	1,603	1.7
18. Psychopharmacologic agents	1,463	1.6
19. Cough medicines	1,443	1.5
20. Hormones	1,386	1.5
21. Glues, adhesives	1,384	1.5
22. Rodenticides	1,347	1.4
23. Internal antibiotics	1,246	1.3
24. Corrosive acids, alkalies	1,204	1.3
25. Paint	1,204	1.3

[a] Adapted from the National Clearinghouse for Poison Control Centers, 1978.

of time in which a toxic substance accumulates in the body producing toxic results; it is best exemplified by environmental exposure to lead or other heavy metals. In the drug category, chronic toxicity can also exist. Aspirin poisoning that occurs in infants and small children or in older adults as a result of salicylate accumulation following administration of too much drug for too long a period of time is typical of therapeutic toxicity. Chronic toxicity is a special problem for the clinician, because the source is not always obvious, the toxicity not always clear, and toxic process not often obvious until serious clinical derangements occur.

Responding to this need, health professionals have made a number of important strides. In the early 1950s, at the insistence of pediatricians and public health officials, the first poison control center was established. Shortly thereafter, the American Association of Poison Control Centers was organized. Recently, the American Board of Medical Toxicology was incorporated. Though few in number, the diplomates of this organization have taken the first steps in fulfilling an important specialty need in medicine. Other organizations have formed special poison prevention committees (American Academy of Pediatrics) or toxicology committees (American College of Emergency Physicians), and toxicology topics have become a substantive part of

Table 48.2
Twenty Most Common Drugs Involved in Emergency Room Poisoning Episodes Reported to Drug Abuse Warning Network for 1979[a]

Drug	Total No. of Mentions
Alcohol-in-combination	25,032
Diazepam	18,557
Heroin/Morphine	6,822
Aspirin	6,682
PCP[b]/PCP combinations	6,002
Flurazepam	4,666
Marijuana	4,555
d-Propoxyphene	3,585
Amitriptyline	3,297
Acetaminophen	3,296
Methaqualone	3,270
Chlordiazepoxide	2,869
Cocaine	2,846
Phenobarbital	2,799
Secobarbital/Amobarbital	2,516
Hydantoin	2,466
Methadone	2,415
Over-the-counter sleep aids	2,260
Chlorpromazine	2,170
Amphetamine	1,996

[a] Adapted from Project Dawn Annual Report-1979: DEA-NIDA, 1979.
[b] PCP = Phencyclidine.

many continuing education courses. Knowing how to manage a poisoning is an important part of clinical medicine.

GENERAL PRINCIPLES FOR MANAGING THE POISONED CHILD

Institution of Basic Life-Support Measures

As in all critically ill patients, the initial assessment and management should include establishment of an airway, artificial ventilation, and appropriate measures to restore circulation. Specific attention should be paid to the heart rate, blood pressure, central nervous system function (reflexes, response to verbal and painful stimuli, and pupil size and response to light), and hydration (see Chapter 2).

Historical Evaluation

Whenever the poisoned patient is first encountered, an assessment of the potential severity of the toxic exposure should be made as soon as possible. Basic historical information to obtain includes: (1) confirmation that a toxic exposure has occurred, (2) identification of the toxic agent(s), (3) the route and magnitude (dose) of the exposure, (4) the time of the exposure, and (5) the present condition of the victim, including signs, symptoms and recent changes in the patient's status. With an accurate history, it is often possible to make a judgment regarding the level of treatment required. Whenever serious poisoning is a possibility, the victim must be seen by appropriately trained personnel. It is crucial that management proceed rapidly and in a logical and organized manner.

Obtaining Specimens for Analytical Toxicologic Analysis

Once basic life-support measures have been instituted and while other management procedures are being performed, specimens should be collected for qualitative and quantitative toxicology screens. This requires the availability of sophisticated analytical toxicology support.

Termination or Minimization of Toxic Exposure

A number of methods may be utilized to terminate the patient's exposure to a toxic substance or mitigate its effects. For respiratory exposure, removal of the victim from the toxic environment is usually all that need be done, with careful observation for latent effects of exposures to pulmonary irritants. Involved eyes should be washed for at least 10 to 15 minutes with water. For dermal exposure the skin should be immediately flushed with water and then washed with copious amounts of water and soap if available; all contaminated clothing should be removed. For ingestions, the principal effort is focused on gastrointestinal decontamination including dilution, evacuation, binding, and catharsis.

Simple Dilution

Dilution is indicated only when the toxin produces local irritation or corrosion. Water or milk are acceptable diluents. On the other hand, for drug ingestions dilution alone should not be used since it may increase absorption by increasing dissolution rates of the tablets or capsules or promote more rapid transit into the lower gastrointestinal tract. However, administration of fluids during the induction of emesis is appropriate.

Gastric Decontamination

Gastric evacuation may be of value up to 24 hours postingestion, but is most effective if done within 2 to 4 hours. Emesis is preferred for the removal of ingested poisons in children and is indicated except when the patient has ingested caustics, or when the patient is comatose, experiencing seizures, or has lost the gag reflex. The drug of choice of inducing emesis under most circumstances is ipecac syrup (not fluid extract). A dosage of 30 ml for adolescents, 15 ml for children, and 10 ml for infants under 1 year of age, given with at least 8 oz of water or other liquid, will produce vomiting in nearly 100% of patients. If vomiting does not occur within 20 to 30 min, the dose should be repeated. Apomorphine also has been used, but is fraught with complications or discomfort. When apomorphine is used, naloxone (Narcan) may be necessary to stop protracted vomiting or to reverse sedative effect.

In the adolescent or adult, gastric lavage may be preferable to emesis. In order to carry out a satisfactory lavage, the largest nasogastric or orogastric lavage tube which can be reasonably passed should be used (ideally a French size 36 nasogastric or 50 orogastric). Gastric contents should be initially aspirated before any lavage fluid is introduced. The lavage fluid used can be either water or 0.45 N saline. Lavage should be continued until the return is clear, usually requiring a total volume of at least 2 liters.

Activated Charcoal

Activated charcoal minimizes absorption of toxins by adsorbing them on its surface. Its use should be considered in all cases of poisoning although a number of compounds are not well adsorbed (iron, cyanide), or in selected circumstances its use may interfere with other crucial therapy (orally administered antidotes). Activated charcoal is most effective if given during the first several hours after ingestion. Approximately 5 to 10 g of activated charcoal should be administered for each gram of drug or chemical ingested.

A minimum of 20 g of activated charcoal should be given to a child in situations where the amount of toxic substance ingested is unknown, and 50 to 100 g in adolescents. The activated charcoal should be mixed with a sufficient amount of water to make a slurry that can then be taken orally or administered by nasogastric tube. When used in conjunction with ipecac syrup, activated charcoal should not be given until vomiting has occurred, since it will otherwise inactivate the ipecac. It should also be noted that the once advocated "universal" antidote comprised of activated charcoal, magnesium oxide and tannic acid, is not recommended. Similarly, burnt toast is not effective. Repeated dosing of charcoal may be beneficial for children who have taken drugs undergoing enterophepatic recirculation or active excretion into gastric fluid; enhanced clearance of several drugs with repeated charcoal dosing has also recently been demonstrated by Berg and colleagues, even in the absence of such active excretion or recirculation.

Catharsis

After emesis or lavage, catharsis may be used to hasten the elimination of remaining ingested material. The agents usually recommended for this purpose are saline cathartics, such as sodium or magnesium sulfate in a dose of 250 mg/kg, administered as a 20% solution. The cathartic may be repeated every 1 or 2 hours as long as bowel sounds are present, up until there is passage of any administered charcoal. Mineral oil or stimulant cathartics, such as castor oil, are not recommended since they may increase absorption of some poisons or unnecessarily extend the cathartic effect.

Antidotal Therapy

The overall number of ingestions for which a specific antidote is necessary or available is small. Where a specific antidote can be used, it is vital that it be administered as early as possible and in an appropriately monitored dose. Those antidotes that should be available for immediate administration include: sodium nitrite/sodium thiosulfate (cyanide), atropine (cholinesterase inhibitors), methylene blue (methemoglobinemic agents), oxygen (carbon monoxide), and naloxone (narcotic respiratory arrest). Other antidotes usually do not require such urgent administration and may be given subsequent to initiation of other management modalities. Even when available, antidotes do not diminish the need for meticulous supportive care or other therapy. Indiscriminant use of antidotes without other forms of management should be discouraged. Table 48.3 summarizes a list of commonly used antidotes, suggested doses, and their indications for use.

Hastening the Elimination of an Absorbed Poison

The procedures available for enhancing the elimination of an absorbed poison that have the greatest value are diuresis, dialysis and hemoperfusion. Because some risk is involved, these measures are indicated only in those cases where the patient's recovery would be otherwise unlikely or where a specific significant benefit is expected.

Diuresis

Diuresis may be useful in cases of poisoning with agents that are excreted primarily by the renal route. Fluid diuresis may increase glomerular filtration, and, if accompanied by proportionally less tubular reabsorption of the toxic agent, may result in enhanced excretion. However, water diuresis, achieved simply by administering large fluid loads, has limited value. The addition of a diuretic drug such as furosemide (1 mg/kg/dose) is more likely to enhance excretion, but preferably one should use osmotic diuresis with mannitol or urea, which will prevent reabsorption of an ingested drug. Diuresis has been shown to be particularly effective with long-acting barbiturates and salicylates and is often combined with alkalinization.

Ionized diuresis takes advantage of the principle that excretion is favored when a drug is in its ionized state. Alkaline or acid diuresis involves selection on the basis of the pK_a of the toxic agent so that the ionized drug will be trapped within the tubular lumen and not reabsorbed. For drugs that are weak acids, alkalinization of the urine will be effective. Acid diuresis similarly may enhance the excretion of weak bases. As previously noted, the combination of alkaline and osmotic diuresis has been shown to be beneficial in barbiturate poisoning. This combination is efficacious in adult salicylate poisoning, but satisfactory alkalinization of the urine is difficult to achieve in children.

Criteria for initiating diuretic therapy include: (a) a systolic blood pressure of 90 mm Hg or higher, (b) clinical evidence of adequate renal function, (c) no evidence of cardiac failure, (d) no evidence of respiratory insufficiency, (e) duration of coma expected to be at least 72 hours, (f) drug blood level in the serious or potentially fatal range, and (g) the drug should be well excreted with the renal route.

Mannitol is given as a 25% solution in a loading dose of 0.5 g/kg. A satisfactory flow, once established, can be maintained using a 10% mannitol solution. Urea is given in a 50% solution at an initial rate of 1 ml/kg/hour over a period of 4 hours. A maintenance infusion is then administered at a rate of 0.25 ml/kg/hour. Urine output, fluid input, Na, K, Cl, CO_2, BUN, Ca, P, serum osmolality, urine osmolality and central venous pressure should be monitored during diuresis. Ideally, the initial diuretic load should produce a urine output of approximately 5 ml/kg/hour. Additional doses of diuretics should be adjusted to produce a urine output of 6 to 9 ml/kg/hour. Diuresis may be discontinued when the patient regains consciousness, serious toxic manifestations abate, or when drug blood levels are below the toxic range.

Urine alkalinization can be initiated with sodium bicarbonate at a dose of 1 to 2 meq/kg intravenously over a 1- to 2-hour period. Throughout this period, urine pH should be monitored. The infusion should be continued at the same rate or modified to maintain a urine pH of 8.0 or greater. Acidifica-

Table 48.3
Summary of Local and Systemic Antidotes

Poison	Local Antidote	Systemic Antidote
Acetaminophen	Activated charcoal (not to be used if *N*-acetylcysteine is to be given)	*N*-Acetylcysteine (Mucomyst) initial dose of 140 mg/kg orally in Coca-Cola, Pepsi, Fresca, grapefruit juice, or water; then, 70 mg/kg every 4 hr for 68 hr (17 doses)
Acids, corrosive	Dilute with water or milk	
Alkali, caustic	Dilute with water or milk, then give demulcent	
Alkaloids (coniine, quinine, strychnine, etc.)	Activated charcoal	
Amphetamines	Activated charcoal	Chlorpromazine, 1 mg/kg i.m. or i.v. (administer slowly if given i.v.); may repeat in 15 min; reduce to 0.5 mg/kg if other CNS depressants involved.
Anticholinergics	Activated charcoal	Physostigmine (adult: 2 mg; child: 0.5 mg) may be given i.v., i.m., or s.c.; may repeat in 15 min until desired effect is achieved; subsequent doses may be given every 2–3 hr p.r.n.
Anticholinesterases Organophosphates Neostigmine Physostigmine Pyridostigmine	Activated charcoal	Atropine, 1–2 mg (for children under 2 yr, 1 mg or 0.05–0.1 mg/kg) i.m. or i.v. repeated every 10–15 min until atropinization is evident; then give pralidoxime chloride 25–50 mg/kg (1 g in adults) i.v.; repeat in 8–12 hr p.r.n.
Carbamates		Atropine as above, but *do not* use pralidoxime
Antihistamines	(*see* Anticholinergics)	
Arsenic	(*see* Heavy metals)	
Atropine	(*see* Anticholinergics)	
Barium salts	Sodium sulfate, 300 mg/kg	Sodium or magnesium sulfate, 10 ml of 10% solution i.v. every 15 min until symptoms stop
Belladonna alkaloids	(*see* Anticholinergics)	
Bromides		Sodium or ammonium chloride, 6–12 g/day p.o., or the equivalent as normal saline, every 6 hr i.v.
Cadmium	(*see* Heavy metals)	
Carbon monoxide		100% oxygen inhalation for no more than 2 hr followed by inhalation of room air
Cholinergic compounds	(*see* Anticholinesterases)	
Copper	(*see* Heavy metals)	
Cyanide		*Adult:* Amyl nitrite inhalation (inhale for 15–30 sec every 60 sec) pending administration of 300 mg sodium nitrite (10 ml of a 3% solution) i.v. slowly (over 2–4 min); follow immediately with 12.5 g sodium thiosulfate (2.5–5 ml/min of 25% solution) i.v. slowly (over 10 min)

Table 48.3—*Continued*

Poison	Local Antidote	Systemic Antidote
		Children (Na nitrite should not exceed recommended dose as fatal methemoglobinemia may result):
	Hemoglobin / *Initial dose 3% Na nitrite i.v.*	*Initial dose 25% Na thiosulfate i.v.*
	8 g / 0.22 ml (6.6 mg)/kg	1.10 ml/kg
	10 g / 0.27 ml (8.7 mg)/kg	1.35 ml/kg
	12 g (nl) / 0.33 ml (10 mg)/kg	1.65 ml/kg
	14 g / 0.39 ml (11.6 mg)/kg	1.95 ml/kg
Detergents, cationic	Ordinary soap solution	
Ethylene glycol	(*see* Methanol)	
Fluoride	Calcium gluconate or lactate, 150 mg/kg, or milk	Calcium gluconate, 10 ml of 10% solution, given slowly i.v. until symptoms abate; may be repeated p.r.n.
Formaldehyde	Milk or egg whites; or 1% solution of ammonium acetate or carbonate, preferably with lavage	
Gold	(*see* Heavy metals)	
Heavy metals:	Milk or egg whites	BAL (dimercaprol): 3–5 mg/kg dose deep i.m. every 4 hr for 2 days, every 4–6 hr for an additional 2 days, then every 4–12 hr for up to 7 additional days
	Usual chelators used:	*EDTA:* 75 mg/kg 24 hr deep i.m. or slow i.v. infusion given in 3–6 divided doses for up to 5 days; may be repeated for a second course after a minimum of 2 days; each course should not exceed a total of 500 mg/kg body weight
Arsenic	BAL	
Cadmium	satisfactory use not demonstrated	
Copper	BAL, penicillamine	
Gold	BAL	
Lead	BAL, EDTA, penicillamine (*see* Table 48.8)	
Mercury	BAL, penicillamine	
Silver	Satisfactory use not demonstrated	*Penicillamine:* 100 mg/kg/day (max 1 g) p.o. in divided doses for up to 5 days; for long-term therapy do not exceed 40 mg/kg/day
Thallium	Satisfactory use not demonstrated	
Hypochlorites	(*see* Alkali, caustic)	
Iodine	Starch solution, 3–10%	
Iron	Sodium bicarbonate, 1–5% solution, preferably by lavage (Deferoxamine, 2 g/L in 1–2% bicarbonate lavage, and as post-lavage intragastric bolus, 10 g/50 ml—see text)	Deferoxamine, 20–40 mg/kg i.v. given as slow drip over 4-hr period not to exceed 15 mg/kg/hr; followed by 20 mg/kg every 4–8 hr until urine color normal or iron level normal (can give 20 mg/kg i.m. every 4–12 hr if no i.v. sites available)
Isoniazid	Activated charcoal	Pyridoxine (vitamine B_6) 1 g per g of INH ingested, 5–10% concentration in 5% dextrose in water, i.v. over 30–60 min
Lead	(*see* Heavy metals)	
Mercury	(*see* Heavy metals)	
Methanol		Ethanol, loading dose to achieve blood level of 100 mg/dl *Adult:* 0.6 g/kg body weight + 7–10 g to be infused i.v. over 1 hr *Child:* 0.6 g/kg body weight to be infused i.v. over/hr

Table 48.3—*Continued*

Poison	Local Antidote	Systemic Antidote
		Maintenance doses should approximate 10 g/hr in adults and 100 mg/kg/hr in children, to be adjusted according to measured blood ethanol levels
Methemoglobinemic agents: Nitrites, Chlorates, Nitrobenzene		Methylene blue, 1–2 mg (0.1–0.2 ml/kg) of a 1% solution i.v. slowly over 5–10 min if cyanosis is severe (or methemoglobin level is greater than 40%)
Narcotics	Activated charcoal	Naloxone, 0.005–0.01 mg/kg (adult 0.4 mg) i.v. every 2–3 min intervals p.r.n. (second choice of agents includes levallorphan, 0.2 mg/kg or nalorphine 0.1 mg/kg i.v. given as above)
Nitrites	(*see* Methemoglobinemic agents)	
Oxalate	Dilute with water or milk, then give calcium gluconate or lactate, 150 mg/kg	Calcium gluconate, 10 ml of 10% solution, given slowly i.v. until symptoms abate; may be repeated p.r.n.
Phenol	Dilute with water or milk, then give activated charcoal, castor oil, vegetable oil	
Phenothiazines (neuromuscular reaction only)		Diphenhydramine, 0.5–1.0 mg/kg i.m. or i.v.; or benztropine, 2 mg i.m. or i.v.
Phosgene		Methenamine, 20 ml of 20% solution (4 g) i.v. Probably ineffective after full development of pulmonary edema
	(*see* Anticholinesterases)	
Quaternary ammonium compounds	(*see* Detergents, cationic)	
Silver	(*see* Heavy metals) Normal saline (lavage)	
Thallium	(*see* Heavy metals) Activated charcoal; may be given continuously to remove metal excreted via enterohepatic circulation	
Tricyclic antidepressants	(*see Anticholinergics*)	
Warfarin		Vitamin K_1, 0.5–1.0 mg/kg i.m. or i.v. *Adults:* 10 mg i.m. or i.v. *Children:* 1–5 mg i.m. or i.v.

For Envenomation[a]

Animals	Antivenin[b]
Snake, Crotalidae (all North American rattlers and moccasins)	Antivenin (Crotalidae) Polyvalent (Wyeth)
Snake, coral	Antivenin (*Micrurus fulvius*), monovalent (Wyeth)
Spider, black widow	Antivenin, *Latrodectus mactans* (Merck, Sharp & Dohme)

[a] *Note:* All antisera should be tested for sensitivity to horse serum.
[b] See package insert for dosage and administration.

tion of the urine is usually initiated with ammonium chloride at a dose of 75 mg (2.75 meq/kg/dose) orally every 6 hours via a nasogastric tube until the urine pH is equal to or less than 5.0. The urine should be maintained at this pH. As an adjunct to this therapy, ascorbic acid in a dosage range of 0.5 to 2.0 g in 500 ml of fluid can be administered intravenously at a maintenance infusion rate every 6 hours.

Dialysis

Dialysis is indicated for selected cases of severe poisoning or when renal failure is present. Indications for dialysis depend both on patient-related and drug-related criteria. Patient-related criteria include: (a) anticipated prolonged coma with the high likelihood of attendant complications, (b) development of renal failure or impairment of normal excretory pathways, and (c) progressive clinical deterioration in spite of careful medical supervision. Drug-related criteria are: (a) satisfactory membrane permeability, (b) a correlation between plasma drug concentration and drug toxicity of the agent, (c) plasma levels in the potentially fatal range or the presence of a significant quantity of an agent which is normally metabolized to a toxic substance, and (d) significant enhancement of clearance during dialysis expected.

Hemodialysis is the most effective means of dialysis. Because it requires highly technical skills and both a physician and a technician, it is not always available, but is an essential consultative service for units managing severe poisoning cases. Peritoneal dialysis is considerably less efficient than hemodialysis, but is more readily available and is reasonably simple and safe. However, substances that are highly protein-bound are dialyzable only if protein is added to the dialysis fluid. The most convenient procedure is the use of 5% serum albumin (Albumisol) containing appropriate amounts of essential electrolytes. Gastric dialysis or continuous gastric lavage has been used to remove agents which are actively excreted into the stomach. Drugs in this category are generally weak bases, such as mepivacaine or the tricyclic compounds. This procedure has yet to be shown to remove significant amounts of drug.

Hemoperfusion

Hemoperfusion, the process of passing blood through an extracorporeal circuit and a cartridge containing an adsorbent after which the detoxified blood is returned to the patient, is also effective in drug removal. Although there are some reservations regarding the extent to which hemoperfusion can be utilized, it appears to be at least as effective and possibly more effective than hemodialysis for a number of agents. Indications for use are similar to those for hemodialysis.

APPROACH TO CHILD WITH INGESTION OF UNKNOWN POISON

Children who are poisoned do not always come to the emergency department with a clear history of exposure followed by the onset of symptoms. Often, they develop signs and symptoms of illnesses that mimic other diseases and give no history of a toxic exposure. Thus, the emergency department staff must always consider the possibility of an ingestion when treating young children.

General features that suggest the possibility of poisoning include: (1) acute onset; (2) age range of 1 to 5 years; (3) past history of pica or known, accidental ingestion; (4) substantial environmental stress, either acute (arrival of a new baby, serious illness in a parent) or chronic (marital conflict, parental inadequacy); (5) multiple organ system involvement; (6) significant alteration in level of consciousness; and (7) a clinical picture that seems especially puzzling. The findings on physical examination may also suggest an intoxication. Of particular interest are those clinical manifestations related to *altered vital signs*, *neuromuscular* dysfunction, *eye* findings, *skin* changes, and unusual *odors* on the breath. Some of the important poisons responsible for such clinical signs and symptoms are outlined in Table 48.4.

There are also specific combinations of toxic signs and symptoms that may suggest specific types of poisonings. These "toxidromes" (Mofenson and Greensher) are often so characteristic as to provide guidance for early therapeutic trials before laboratory confirmation of a specific diagnosis is available (see Table 48.5).

THE NONTOXIC INGESTION

Frequently the emergency department physician will be asked about a childhood ingestion of some common household products, many of which are nontoxic, unless

Table 48.4
Clinical Manifestations of Poisoning[a]

I. Vital Signs
- A. Pulse
  - 1. Bradycardia
    - a. Gasoline
    - b. Digoxin
    - c. Narcotics
    - d. Organophosphates
    - e. Cyanide
    - f. Carbon monoxide
    - g. Plants (lily of the valley, foxglove, oleander)
  - 2. Tachycardia
    - a. Alcohol
    - b. Amphetamines and sympathomimetics
    - c. Atropinics
    - d. Tricyclic antidepressants
    - e. Theophylline
    - f. Salicylates
    - g. Cocaine
- B. Respirations
  - 1. Slow, depressed
    - a. Alcohol
    - b. Barbiturates (late)
    - c. Narcotics
    - d. Sedative/hypnotics
  - 2. Tachypnea
    - a. Amphetamines
    - b. Barbiturates (early)
    - c. Methanol
    - d. Salicylates
    - e. Carbon monoxide
- C. Blood pressure
  - 1. Hypotension
    - a. Methemaglobinemia (nitrates, nitrites, phenacetin)
    - b. Cyanide
    - c. Carbon monoxide
    - d. Phenothiazines
    - e. Tricyclic antidepressants
    - f. Barbiturates
    - g. Narcotics
  - 2. Hypertension
    - a. Amphetamines/sympathomimetics (especially phenylpropanoloamine in over-the-counter (OTC) cold remedies, diet pills)
    - b. Tricyclic antidepressants
    - c. Phencyclidine
    - d. Phenothiazines
    - e. Antihistamines, atropinics
- D. Temperature
  - 1. Hypothermia
    - a. Ethanol
    - b. Barbiturates

[a] Adapted from H. C. Mofenson and J. Greensher: *Pediatrics, 54:* 336, 1974.

Table 48.4—*Continued*

- c. Sedative/hypnotics
- d. Narcotics
- e. Phenothiazines
- f. Antidepressants
- g. Clonidine

2. Hyperpyrexia
   - a. Atropinics
   - b. Quinine
   - c. Salicylates
   - d. Amphetamines
   - e. Phenothiazines
   - f. Tricyclics
   - g. Theophylline

II. Neuromuscular

A. Coma
1. Narcotic depresssants
2. Sedative/hypnotics
3. Anticholinergics (antihistamines, antidepressants, phenothiazines, atropinics, OTC sleep preparations)
4. Alcohols
5. Anticonvulsants
6. Carbon monoxide
7. Salicylates
8. Organophosphate insecticides

B. Delirium/Psychosis
1. Alcohol
2. Phenothiazines
3. Drugs of abuse—phencyclidine, LSD, peyote, mescaline, marijuana, cocaine, heroin, Methaqualone
4. Sympathomimetics and anticholinergics (including prescription and OTC cold remedies)
5. Steroids
6. Heavy metals

C. Convulsions
1. Alcohol
2. Amphetamines
3. Phenothiazines
4. Antidepressants
5. Antihistamines
6. Camphor
7. Boric acid
8. Lead
9. Organophosphates
10. Isoniazid
11. Salicylates
12. Plants: water hemlocks

D. Ataxia
1. Alcohol
2. Barbiturates
3. Carbon monoxide
4. Diphenylhydantoin
5. Heavy metals
6. Organic solvents
7. Sedative/hypnotics
8. Hydrocarbons

Table 48.4—*Continued*

- E. Paralysis
  - 1. Botulism
  - 2. Heavy metals
  - 3. Plants: poison hemlock
- *III. Eyes*
  - A. Pupils
    - 1. Miosis
      - a. Narcotics
      - b. Organophosphates
      - c. Plants: mushrooms (muscarinic type)
    - 2. Mydriasis
      - a. Amphetamines
      - b. Atropinics
      - c. Barbiturates (if comatose)
      - d. Cocaine
      - e. Methanol
      - f. Glutethamide
      - g. LSD
  - B. Nystagmus
    - 1. Diphenylhydantoin
    - 2. Sedative/hypnotics
    - 3. Carbamazepine
    - 4. Glutethimide
    - 5. Phencyclidine (both vertical and horizontal)
    - 6. Barbiturates
    - 7. Ethanol
- *IV. Skin*
  - A. Jaundice
    - 1. Carbon tetrachloride
    - 2. Acetaminophen
    - 3. Napthalene
    - 4. Phenothiazines
    - 5. Plants: mushrooms, Fava bean
    - 6. Heavy metals: iron, phosphorus, arsenic
  - B. Cyanosis (unresponsive to oxygen, due to methemoglobinemia)
    - 1. Aniline dyes
    - 2. Nitrites
    - 3. Benzocaine
    - 4. Phenacetin
    - 5. Nitrobenzene
  - C. Pinkness to redness
    - 1. Atropinics and antihistamines
    - 2. Alcohol
    - 3. Carbon monoxide
    - 4. Cyanide
    - 5. Boric acid
- *V. Odors*
  - A. Acetone: acetone, methyl and isopropyl alcohol, phenol and salicylates
  - B. Alcohol: ethanol
  - C. Bitter almond: cyanide
  - D. Garlic: heavy metal (arsenic, phosphorus and thallium), organophosphates
  - E. Oil of wintergreen: methyl salicylates
  - F. Hydrocarbons: hydrocarbons (gasoline, turpentine, etc.)

Table 48.5
Toxidromes

Anticholinergics (atropine, antidepressants (TCA), phenothiazines, antihistamines)	VS—Fever, Tachycardia, hypertension, (cardiac arrhythmias—TCA) CNS—Delirium/psychosis/convulsions/coma Eye—Mydriasis Skin—Flushed, hot dry skin
Amphetamines	VS—Fever, tachycardia, hypertension CNA—Hyperactive to delirious and tremor, myoclonus, psychosis convulsions Eye—Mydriasis Skin—Sweaty
Narcotics	VS—Bradycardia, bradypnea, hypotension, hypothermia CNS—Euphoria to coma, hyporeflexia Eye—Pinpoint pupils
Organophosphates (and muscarinic mushroom poisoning)	VS—Bradycardia, tachypnea (secondary to pulmonary manifestations) CNS—Confusion to drowsiness to coma, convulsions; muscle fasiculations, weakness to paralysis Eye—Miosis, blurry vision, lacrimation Skin—Sweating Odor—Garlic Misc.—Salivation; bronchorrhea, bronchospasm, and pulmonary edema; urinary frequency and diarrhea
Barbiturates, sedatives/hypnotics	VS—Hypothermia, hypotension, bradypnea CNS—Confusion to coma, ataxia Eye—Nystagmus, miosis or mydriasis Skin—Vesicles, bullae
Salicylates	VS—Fever, hyperpnea CNS—Lethargy to coma Odor—Oil of wintergreen (with methylsalicylate) Misc.—Vomiting
Phenothiazines	VS—Postural hypotension, hypothermia, tachycardia, tachypnea CNS—A. Lethargy to coma, tremor, convulsions B. Extrapyramidal syndromes: Ataxia Torticollis Back arching Oculogyric crisis Trismus Tongue protusion or heaviness **Eye—Miosis (majority of cases)**

VS = vital signs. (Adapted from H. C. Mofenson and J. Greensher: *Pediatrics, 54:* 336, 1974.

taken in huge amounts. The availability of a list of such nontoxic products often leads to immediate relief of parental anxiety and avoids the institution of unnecessary noxious interventions. Before using such a list, however, several precautions need to be borne in mind. The fact that an ingestion is nontoxic does not necessarily mean it has no medical significance. Ingestions often occur in the context of a suboptimal environment. There may be poor supervision or unusual family stresses surrounding the accident, or the ingestion may not have been accidental. Several criteria have been suggested by Mofenson and Greensher to qualify an ingestion as "nontoxic." These include the assurance that only *one identifiable product* is ingested in a well-approximated *amount*, that the product label includes *no cautionary signal word*, that the child is *symptom-free* and *less than 5 years old*, and that an appropriate mechanism is available for telephone *follow-up*. With these criteria in mind, Table 48.6 provides an updated list of nontoxic ingestions.

ACETAMINOPHEN POISONING

BACKGROUND

Acetaminophen (*N*-acetyl-*p*-aminophenol, APAP), has become a commonly used analgesic-antipyretic, being second in frequency of usage only to aspirin in the United States. It is now one of the 5 most common drugs accidentally ingested, and

Table 48.6
Products that Are Nontoxic when Ingested in Small Amounts[a]

Abrasives	Hand lotions and creams
Adhesives	Hydrogen peroxide (medicinal 3%)
Antacids	Incense
Antibiotics	Indelible markers
Baby-product comestics	Ink (black, blue)
Ballpoint pen inks	Laxatives
Bath oil	Lipstick
Bathtub floating toys	Lubricating oils
Battery (dry cell)	Lysol brand disinfectant (not toilet-bowl cleaner)
Bleach (less than 5% sodium hypochlorite)	Magic markers
Body conditioners	Matches
Bubble-bath soaps	Mineral oil
Calamine lotion	Newspaper
Candles (beeswax or paraffin)	Paint (indoor, latex)
Caps	Pencil (graphite)
Chalk	Perfumes
Cigarettes or cigars	Petroleum jelly
Clay (modeling)	Phenolphthalein laxatives (Ex-Lax)
Colognes	Porous-tip marking pens
Contraceptive pills	Putty (less than 2 oz)
Corticosteroids	Rubber cement
Cosmetics	Shampoos (liquid)
Crayons (marked AP, CP)	Shaving creams and lotions
Dehumidifying packets (silica or charcoal)	Soap and soap products
Detergents (phosphate)	Suntan preparations
Deodorants	Sweetening agents (saccharin, cyclamates)
Deodorizers (spray and refrigerator)	Teething rings (water sterility)
Elmer's glue	Thermometers (mercury)
Etch-A-Sketch	Thyroid tablets
Eye makeup	Toothpaste
Fabric softeners	Vitamins (without iron)
Fertilizer (if no insecticides or herbicides added)	Warfarin (rat poison)
Fish-bowl additives	Watercolors
Glues and pastes	Zinc oxide (Desitin)
Grease	Zirconium oxide
Hair products (dyes, sprays, tonics)	

[a] Adapted from H. C. Mofenson and J. Greensher: *Pediatrics, 54:* 336, 1974.

one of the 10 most common drugs used by adolescents and adults in intentional self-poisoning. Fortunately, accidental ingestion in young children has been associated with little morbidity, and only two deaths have been reported in this group.

PATHOPHYSIOLOGY

The major toxicity of APAP is severe hepatic damage. APAP is metabolized in three ways by the liver: (1) glucuronidation, (2) sulfation, and (3) metabolism via the cytochrome P450 pathway to form a potentially toxic intermediate, which in turn conjugates with glutathione. In a massive overdose, glutathione becomes depleted, thus allowing the undetoxified intermediate to bind to hepatocytes, leading to cellular necrosis. This damage is reflected by rising liver enzymes, hepatic dysfunction and, in severe poisonings, hepatic failure and death. The use of *N*-acetylcysteine as an antidote relates to this molecule's ability to act as a glutathione surrogate.

CLINICAL MANIFESTATIONS

Initially, the signs and symptoms of APAP ingestion are vague and nonspecific, including nausea and vomiting, anorexia, pallor and diaphoresis. These manifestations usually resolve within 12 to 24 hours, and the patient appears well for 1 to 4 days. During this latent period, liver enzymes may rise, and jaundice with liver tenderness may ensue. Most patients have a gradual resolution of their hepatic dysfunction, though without antidotal treatment about 2 to 4% of intoxications that develop toxic plasma levels will go on to hepatic failure and death. Such patients with severe toxicity develop further clinical evidence of hepatic disease at 3 to 5 days postingestion. Anorexia, malaise and abdominal pain may progress to signs of liver failure with hepatic coma.

The severity of an intoxication may be predicted by the amount ingested, if accurately known, the intensity of the initial symptoms, and the plasma level of APAP. Doses of APAP less than 150 mg/kg in children are likely to be harmless. Severe toxicity in adolescents or adults usually occurs with overdoses in the 10- to 15-g range. Initial gastrointestinal symptoms, though vague, are generally more pronounced when the overdose is large. However, the only reliable indication of the potential severity of the hepatic damage is the plasma APAP level, taken at least 4 hours postingestion. A nomogram (see Fig. 48.1) is available for using this value in the prediction of likely toxicity. We recommend use of the lower line of the nomogram, plotted 25% below the possible toxicity line, in order to err on the safe side in making therapeutic decisions.

MANAGEMENT

The basic toxicologic principles of preventing absorption apply to APAP overdoses, with one important exception. After emesis or lavage, routine use of activated charcoal is *not* recommended, since it may adsorb *N*-acetylcysteine (a specific antidote for APAP). If a multiple drug ingestion has occurred and it is felt that charcoal is vital, it should subsequently be removed by lavage prior to the administration of *N*-acetylcysteine. Cathartics, such as magnesium sulfate, facilitate the elimination of APAP from the bowel and also enhance its metabolism via the sulfation pathway.

N-Acetylcysteine, given orally, lessens the severity of hepatic damage if used within 16 hours of ingestion, and deaths due to APAP are preventable when it is used within 24 hours. This antidote can be mixed with fruit juice or soda to disguise its foul smell, or it can be administered by lavage tube. Only mild gastrointestinal side effects result from its usage. Since *N*-acetylcysteine remains an investigational antidote, to obtain permission for its use and to continue to gather data regarding its efficacy, the treating physician should call the Rocky Mountain Poison Control Center (800-525-6115). A protocol for the management of APAP overdose, adapted from Rumack and Peterson, is outlined in Table 48.7.

ALCOHOLS AND GLYCOLS

The alcohols and glycols are some of the most frequently found organic compounds

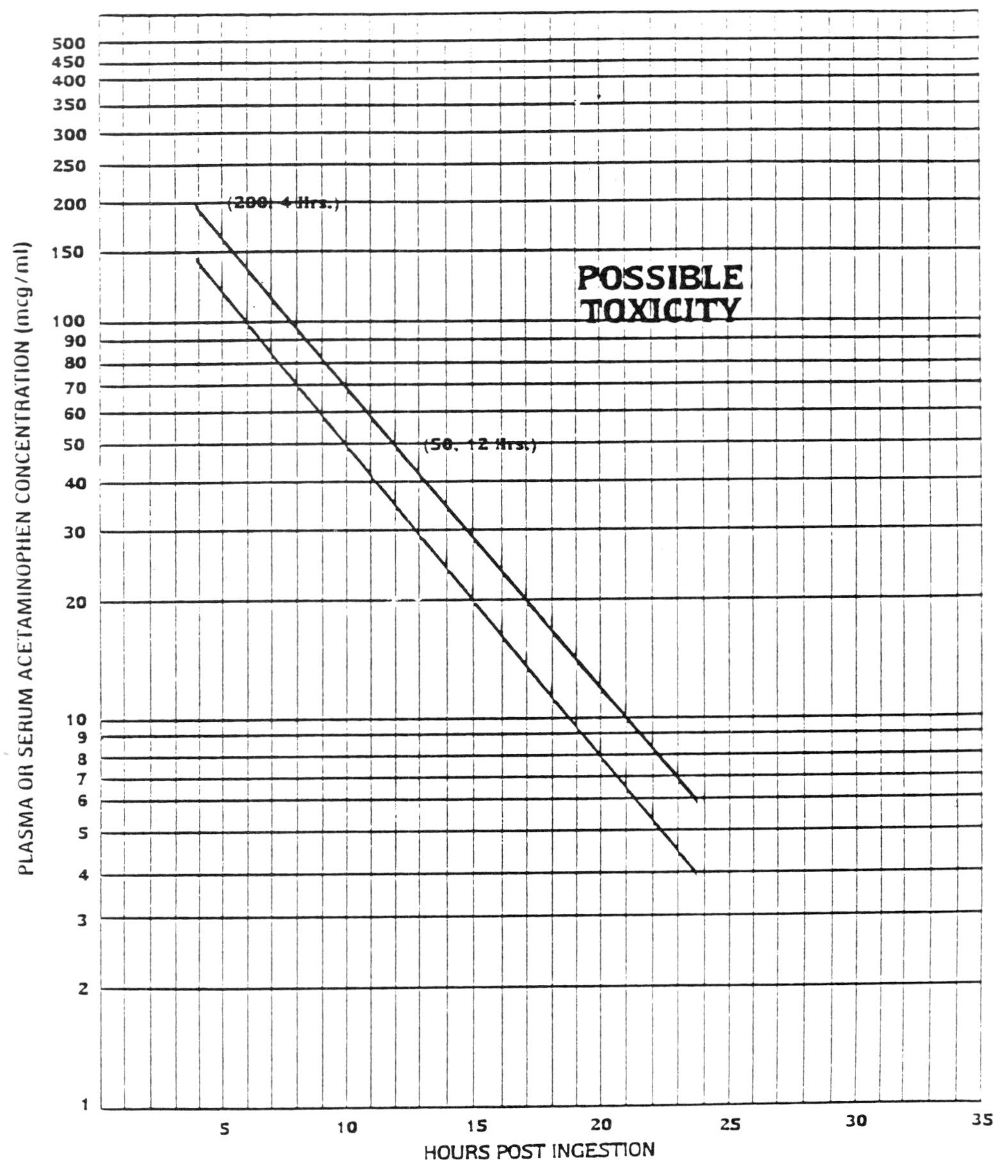

Figure 48.1 Nomogram for estimating severity of acute acetaminophen poisoning. (Adapted from B. H. Rumack and H. Matthew: *Pediatrics*, *55:* 871–876, 1975. Copyright, American Academy of Pediatrics, 1975.)

in the environment. Ethanol, or ethyl alcohol, is the most commonly encountered solvent and is used as a topical antiseptic, chemical intermediate, beverage and, in some instances, as a rubbing alcohol. Methanol, or methyl alcohol, functions as a solvent in many industrial and home products. Isopropyl alcohol finds use as a solvent, a fuel for alcohol lamps, or most commonly, as a rubbing alcohol. Paraldehyde, an alcohol, not normally encountered in the home environment, is frequently used in the treatment of many neurological disorders, including alcohol withdrawal. Ethylene glycol was originally discovered as a substitute for glycerin and has been used in

Table 48.7
Protocol for *N*-Acetylcysteine (NAC) Treatment in Acute Acetaminophen (*N*-Acetyl-*p*-aminophenol, APAP) Overdose[a]

1. Empty stomach by ipecac-induced emesis or lavage
2. Induce catharsis, preferably with sodium or magnesium sulfate
3. Omit the administration of charcoal unless another drug has been ingested
4. If the quantity ingested is thought to be less than 150 mg/kg, after inducing emesis and catharsis, obtain the 4-hr plasma level before proceeding with antidotal therapy or hospital admission. (This assume a rapid turn-around-time of the result of the plasma APAP level, so that treatment could be instituted within 16 hr of ingestion if the level was high)
5. If quantity ingested is estimated to be well in excess of 150 mg/kg, administer loading dose of NAC if within 24 hr of ingestion (140 mg/kg p.o.—repeat if vomiting occurs within 1 hr)
6. Obtain 4-hr (or later) plasma APAP level (and consider toxicology screen in adolescent suicide attempts)
7. Using nomogram (lower line), estimate risk of hepatic toxicity. If toxicity possible, admit and continue NAC at 70 mg/kg every 4 hr for a total of 17 doses. In this case, obtain also CBC and platelets, BUN, creatinine, liver function tests, glucose and electrolytes. Repeat liver function tests every 24 hr
8. If stat plasma APAP levels are unavailable, the patient should receive the entire course of treatment and laboratory monitoring
9. Avoid diuresis, dialysis and hemoperfusion, as they are not necessary and have not been shown effective

[a] Adapted from B. H. Rumback and R. G. Peterson: *Pediatrics*, *62* (Suppl.): 898, 1978.

commercial products, such as detergents, paints, lacquers, pharmaceuticals, polishes, and cosmetics. It is most frequently encountered as a de-icer or antifreeze.

Ethanol

The most frequently ingested alcohol is ethanol. After ingesting either an alcoholic beverage or cosmetics, such as perfumes, children may develop a staggering gait or nausea and vomiting. Since ethanol is a central nervous system depressant, they deteriorate to stupor, coma, and eventually death, if significant quantities are consumed. Blood concentrations <50 mg/dl rarely result in sensory or motor impairment. Values of 100 to 150 mg/dl are consistent with intoxication and cause mild neurological findings. Lethal blood alcohol concentrations range from 250 to 500 mg/dl in children. These concentrations may be lower if concomitant drugs are ingested, such as tranquilizers, sedatives or antihistamines. In patients who are found unconscious, hypoglycemia, which may lead to convulsions, may be a serious complication. Additionally, peripheral vasodilation and central nervous system depression may lead to hypothermia. The amount of liquid that is of concern when ingested by a child depends upon the concentration of alcohol. For a beverage such as beer (5% alcohol), approximately 30 ml/kg must be ingested before serious toxicity results. Similar estimates are 10 ml/kg for wine (14% alcohol) and 5 ml/kg for an 80 proof liquor (40% alcohol).

The management of an ethanol ingestion in children begins with emesis if the child is not comatose, convulsing or without a gag reflex. If any of these conditions are present, then gastric lavage should be performed. After evacuation, administer activated charcoal in the amount of 30 to 60 g for young children and 60 to 100 g for adolescents. Elimination from the gastrointestinal tract is particularly useful, since ethanol does not achieve a peak blood concentration until 30 min to 2 hours after ingestion. With food in the stomach, a delay of even greater time may occur. The rapid administration of activated charcoal has been shown to produce lower than expected ethanol blood concentrations. The additional administration of a cathartic, such as magnesium sulfate in a dose of 250 mg/kg, will aid in clearing the activated charcoal from the gastrointestinal tract. In a stuporous or comatose patient, the immediate institution of an intravenous drip infusion of 10% glucose prevents convulsions due to hypoglycemia.

Since alcohol is metabolized by the enzyme alcohol dehydrogenase in the liver, its elimination rate is dose dependent. This means that with higher blood alcohol concentrations, a slower elimination will occur, because the capacity of the body to produce alcohol dehydrogenase is limited. The rate of reduction in blood alcohol concentration varies from 10 to 25 mg/dl/hour. The institution of hemodialysis is rarely indicated in an alcoholic ingestion, but may be useful in those patients who have impaired liver function or a blood alcohol concentration greater than 300 to 350 mg/dl. Hemodialysis can eliminate alcohol at a rate of 3 to 4 times the metabolic capacity of the body; however, the risk of hemodialysis should always be weighed against the likely outcome with supportive care alone.

Isopropyl Alcohol

Poisoning with isopropyl alcohol may be particularly insidious since oral ingestion is not the only route of exposure. Children developing severe symptomatology, including coma, following topical application of isopropyl alcohol for the relief of fever have been reported. Since isopropyl alcohol is usually available in a 70% concentration by volume, the ingestion of 2 to 2.5 ml/kg of this solution may lead to symptoms. This compound causes many of the same features of ethanol ingestion with the additional complication of severe gastritis when ingested by the oral route. Some clinicians have observed a more severe acidosis than is seen with ethanol ingestion; in any patient with coma, a severe acidosis and an unexplained osmolar gap (the difference between calculated and observed osmolarity) the physician should consider alcohol as a likely toxic ingestion. Another difference between isopropyl alcohol and ethanol is that isopropyl alcohol is much more readily absorbed from the gastrointestinal tract, resulting in a peak blood concentration 1 hour after ingestion. Although metabolism of this compound is also hepatic, it results in the formation of acetone. Plasma concentrations remain higher for a longer time period than those of ethanol. Treatment for patients who ingest isopropyl alcohol or ethanol is similar.

Methanol

While methanol is used primarily as a solvent for industrial purposes, it is found in other compounds that are contained in the home. It may be contained in fuels for stoves, in jelled fuels for heating small dishes (e.g., Sterno), and in many paint removers. Of all the alcohols previously discussed, methanol causes the greatest concern; not only is methanol poisonous, but its metabolites, formaldehyde and formic acid, cause more harm than methanol itself. The metabolites are responsible for the severe metabolic acidosis and ocular symptoms frequently associated with methanol ingestion. The conversion of methanol to its toxic metabolites occurs very slowly at a rate of about 15 to 20% of the metabolic elimination of ethanol.

The clinical effects of a methanol ingestion usually occur after a latent period of 12 to 24 hours. This delay occurs as the result of the metabolic conversion of methanol to its toxic by-products. In large ingestions, acute methanol poisoning may cause severe CNS depression, metabolic acidosis, and a number of reversible or irreversible optic changes. In subacute ingestions, the nonspecific neurological symptoms of methanol intoxication resemble those of ethanol "hangover," including malaise, headache and dizziness. During recovery from a mild ingestion, occasional paresthesias of the extremities may develop.

The most significant clinical concern from a methanol ingestion is a severe acidosis. This acidosis is the result of the formation of formic acid and formaldehyde which are thought to be 5 and 50 times more toxic than methanol itself. An elevated amylase occurs in many patients who develop pancreatic necrosis. The ophthalmic abnormalities that develop during methanol intoxication may be either temporary or permanent in nature. These include blurred or double vision, changes in color perception, or sharply reduced visual acuity. Permanent abnormalities may include diminished pupillary light reaction, reduced visual acuity, and defects of optic nerve fiber bundles; blindness may ensue. The occurrence of permanent visual defects correlates directly with the degree of metabolic acidosis, the duration of the acidosis, and the quantity of methanol ingested. An interesting gastrointestinal finding in methanol poisoning is the occurrence of constipation and obstipation during recovery from methanol ingestion.

The treatment of methanol ingestion consists of removing, or causing the elimination of, methanol from the body and preventing the formation of its toxic metabolites. As with other alcohol ingestions, emesis or gastric lavage when indicated should be performed as soon as possible. Activated charcoal may be instilled into the gastrointestinal tract unless oral treatment of the methanol ingestion is attempted in the manner described below. In all instances where there is a history of methanol ingestion, a blood methanol concentration should be determined as rapidly as possible. Patients in whom the concentration exceeds 20 mg/dl require immediate therapy with ethanol. Patients who have a blood methanol concentration greater than 50 mg/dl need hemodialysis along with the administration of ethanol.

To prevent the formation of toxic metabolites from methanol, allowing it to be eliminated via the kidney in its unchanged form, ethanol has been advocated as an effective antidote. Ethanol has a greater affinity than methanol for alcohol dehydrogenase and blocks the conversion of methanol to its toxic metabolites by the enzyme in the liver. For ethanol to be effective in a methanol poisoning, a blood concentration of 100 mg/dl of ethanol must be maintained for 2 to 3 days or until methanol concentrations are less than 20 mg/dl and no acidosis is present. To achieve and maintain a blood ethanol concentration of 100 mg/dl, it is first necessary to administer a loading dose either intravenously or orally of 0.6 g/kg of absolute alcohol. A maintenance dose of 100 mg/kg/hour is then given, following the patient's blood concentration to assure a concentration of ethanol of 100 mg/dl. Individual monitoring has shown that some patients require as much as 125 to 150 mg/kg/hour to maintain an effective concentration. It is not necessary to only use absolute alcohol in the management of these patients. Alcoholic beverages may be utilized with the understanding that many of these compounds contain only 40 to 50% alcohol; however, this is advantageous, since the oral administration of absolute alcohol should not be in a concentration greater than 25 to 30%. It must be remembered that a proof designation of a beverage is twice the alcohol concentration expressed as a percentage, e.g. 80 proof equals 40% alcohol.

If hemodialysis is also utilized in the management of a methanol poisoning, there must be an increase in the amount of ethanol infused per hour to account for the dialyzability of ethanol as well as methanol. During hemodialysis, the maintenance dose of ethanol should be doubled for a total 200 to 250 mg/kg/hour.

In those situations where thrombophlebitis occurs from the intravenous route, or adequate supplies of absolute alcohol are not available, treatment with oral therapy is useful. However, if activated charcoal has been administered previously in the course of treatment, adequate blood concentrations of ethanol may not be obtained by this route. Therefore, these patients should receive intravenous therapy until the gastrointestinal tract is cleared of charcoal.

During therapy for methanol intoxication, the profound acidosis that develops must be treated with adequate ventilation and the concomitant administration of sodium bicarbonate as determined by analysis of blood gases.

Ethylene Glycol

The ingestions of ethylene glycol, while infrequent, causes significant morbidity and occasional mortality in adolescents and young adults.

The toxic effects of ethylene glycol are related to the metabolic products of the parent compound, such as oxalic acid. The metabolites are produced via the alcohol dehydrogenase pathway. Since this pathway is utilized also by alcohol, the same course of treatment applies to ethylene glycol as to methanol, with the addition of other antidotes.

The clinical syndrome of ethylene glycol intoxication manifests itself in three different stages. The first stage consists of predominately central nervous system manifestations and is accompanied by a profound metabolic acidosis. In this early stage, mild hypertension, tachycardia, and a low grade fever are often present. Nausea and vomiting commonly occur and, with larger doses, intoxication is followed by coma, convulsions and even death within a few hours. Another frequent finding is the presence of hypocalcemia. It is believed to be due to chelation of the calcium ion by oxalate arising from the metabolism of ethylene glycol; this forms relatively insoluble calcium oxalate crystals. Hypocalcemia has been reported to be severe enough to cause tetany and cardiac malfunction. Urinalysis usually reveals a low specific gravity, proteinuria, microscopic hematuria, and crystalluria. The second distinct state is ushered in by coma and cardiopulmonary failure; it is usually the result of complications of acidosis and hypocalcemia. With rapid correction and treatment, this stage may be avoided. The third stage usually occurs after 24 to 72 hours. Renal failure of varying severity emerges as the dominant problem. Usually a picture of acute tubular necrosis develops. With supportive therapy, return to normal or near normal renal function may be expected. A delayed finding also noted during recovery from the last stage is the presence of myalgia. This is usually found in conjunction with an elevated creatine phosphokinase level.

The diagnosis of ethylene glycol poisoning should be based either on the history, or when, in the absence of diabetic ketoacidosis, there is: (1) alcohol-like intoxication without the odor of alcohol, (2) coma with metabolic acidosis and a large anion gap, or (3) a urinalysis demonstrating massive calcium oxalate crystalluria. The initial therapy of ethylene glycol intoxication includes emesis or gastric lavage and the installation of activated charcoal. Plasma concentrations of ethylene glycol and oxalic acid are difficult to determine and may not be readily available; thus, they provide little help in the diagnosis or management of an acute intoxication. The treatment of metabolic acidosis alone significantly increases survival in patients. Correction of acidosis should, therefore, begin immediately with sodium bicarbonate and appropriate ventilation. The manifestations of hypocalcemia may be alleviated by the prompt institution of therapy with calcium gluconate or chloride. Thiamine and pyridoxine are both precursors to cofactors that are necessary for the degradation of ethylene glycol to byproducts less toxic than oxalic acid. Therefore, the administration of large doses of thiamine (0.25 to 0.5 mg/kg) and pyridoxine (1 to 2 mg/kg) in the first 24 hours is recommended. This will assist in avoiding depletion of reserves of these compounds, and thus avoids subsequent increased oxalate production. When blood ethylene glycol concentrations are unavailable or the history is incomplete, preparation must be made for the institution of hemodialysis in those patients who are severely symptomatic and/or comatose. The other form of therapy which must be instituted as rapidly as possible is the infusion of ethanol with the same considerations used in the management of methanol poisoning. With the institutions of these measures in a rapid and sequential fashion, it is possible to avoid many of the acute and long-term sequelae of ethylene glycol ingestion.

ANTIHISTAMINES

Antihistamines are used as a treatment for children with allergic diseases, as sedatives and antinauseants, and to prevent motion sickness. They are present in many cough syrups, available both over the counter and by prescription. Antihistamines may also be found in combination with analgesics, sympathomimetic amines, and caffeine for the symptomatic relief of the common cold. They are combined with analgesics, such as salicylamide, and an anticholinergic drug, such as scopolamine, for use as a non-prescription sleep medication.

Finally they are included in some liquid cough and cold preparations, which may also contain ethanol as the solvent.

Antihistamines may either depress or stimulate the central nervous system. Used therapeutically, central nervous system depression is most commonly seen, manifesting as drowsiness or dizziness. With increasing doses, stimulation results in insomnia, nervousness and restlessness. In antihistamine overdose, the central nervous system stimulatory effects of the drug predominate. In children, central nervous system stimulation causes excitement, tremors, hyperactivity, hallucinations, and with higher doses, tonic-clonic convulsions. Children are also more likely to have signs and symptoms of anticholinergic poisoning: flushed skin, fever, tachycardia and fixed dilated pupils. Death from antihistamine ingestion in children usually is the result of uncontrolled seizures progressing to coma and cardiorespiratory arrest.

The treatment of antihistamine poisoning requires an accurate history of the time of ingestion and the type and quantity of drug consumed. The antihistamines are rapidly absorbed, and gastric lavage may not return any ingested drug, unless gastric emptying has been delayed by either food or other drugs. Of particular importance is the type of drug ingested since numerous sustained-released antihistamine products are on the market. These sustained-release or time-released preparations should be eliminated from the gastrointestinal tract by either emesis or catharsis.

Patients with seizures require anticonvulsant therapy immediately. Preferably short term control may be gained using diazepam, in a dose of 0.05 to 0.2 mg/kg i.v. With a known history of antihistamine ingestion, it is possible to utilize physostigmine to reverse the anticholinergic effects of the antihistamine. This is usually administered in a dose of 0.5 mg slowly i.v. with a time period of 5 minutes between doses. When repeating the dose, the lowest effective dose should be utilized. If not effective, no more than 2 mg should be administered. It should be noted that if physostigmine is administered too rapidly or in too large a dose, seizures may result. Atropine should be available to reverse severe cholinergic effects that may occur with physostigmine use (see also p. 529 in section on tricyclic antidepressants).

Once seizures are controlled, or in the absence of seizures, the gastrointestinal tract should be evacuated. Syrup of ipecac may be administered or gastric lavage performed. Afterward, activated charcoal should be administered to prevent further absorption of the antihistamines. This is particularly important with the sustained-release preparations. The concomitant administration of a cathartic, such as magnesium sulfate, is extremely important. Other manifestations of anticholinergic poisoning may include hyperthermia, which should be managed with either tepid water sponging or cooling blankets.

ASPIRIN POISONING

BACKGROUND

Aspirin poisoning is a major problem for the emergency physician. Salicylate poisoning serious enough to require hospitalization is due to accidental ingestion in about 60% of cases, and due to therapeutic overdosing in about 40%. However, in recent years, more than 80% of fatal cases have occurred as the result of therapeutic overdose.

Several causative factors may work together to explain the seriousness of such chronic, therapeutic intoxication. The aspirin dose may be excessive (as in the use of 325 mg "adult" tablets, by mistake, instead of 80 mg "baby" tablets). Several salicylate containing medications may be given simultaneously, such as cold remedies and upset-stomach preparations. At times, intoxication might result from normal dosing in a dehydrated patient. Additionally, the diagnosis of chronic salicylism is often delayed, because its symptoms may resemble those of the disease for which it is being used (i.e., fever, vomiting and tachypnea in a child with viral respiratory infection and/or gastroenteritis syndrome).

PATHOPHYSIOLOGY

The direct effects of aspirin on metabolism are multiple. Aspirin stimulates the medullary respiratory center, gluconeogenesis, lipid metabolism and tissue glycolysis inhibits enzymes of the Krebs cycle and amino acid metabolism uncouples oxidative phosphorylation and interferes with the mechanisms of hemostasis. Secondary effects include fluid and electrolyte loss, respiratory alkalosis, metabolic acidosis and impaired glucose metabolism.

The initial effect of respiratory stimulation is independent of increased oxygen consumption or carbon dioxide production. It results in increases in both the rate and depth of respiration, leading to a decreased $PaCO_2$ and an increased blood pH. Simultaneously, several mechanisms are working to produce a metabolic acidosis, including Krebs cycle inhibition with resultant lactic acidosis and ketone body formation due to increased lipid metabolism.

The balance between these mechanisms may result in either a predominant alkalosis or acidosis. Children with mild to moderate salicylate intoxication usually have respiratory alkalosis, but in severe poisonings, metabolic acidosis tends to predominate in a mixed acid-base picture.

Glucose homeostasis is seriously altered in acute aspirin poisoning. Early in the course, hyperglycemia usually occurs due to decreased peripheral utilization. Later, hypoglycemia may supervene as glucose stores are depleted.

Fluid and electrolyte disturbances may be multifactorial, resulting in dehydration, hyponatremia or hypernatremia, and hypokalemia. Among the contributing factors are increased heat production and increased insensible water losses from the skin, emesis, increased renal water, sodium and potassium loss due to organic aciduria, and increased respirations with increased insensible losses through the lungs. The patient with severe salicylate poisoning may lose 4 to 6 liters of water/m^2. It should be noted that a patient with aspirin poisoning may manifest hyperglycemia, glucosuria, ketonuria, and metabolic acidosis; thus, this condition may mimic diabetic ketoacidosis. However, patients with salicylate poisoning rarely have blood sugars above 200 mg/dl.

Minor or unusual aspirin effects include: renal tubular shedding epithelial cells with protein in the urine; a syndrome that resembles inappropriate secretion of antidiuretic hormone in children with chronic therapeutic aspirin poisoning; and a reversible toxic hepatitis manifested by elevation of liver enzymes.

CLINICAL MANIFESTATIONS

The initial clinical signs and symptoms the estimate of dose ingested, and the measurement of salicylate levels all serve to gauge the severity of a given acute aspirin poisoning. However, in cases of chronic therapeutic salicylism, the clinical picture is the most useful guideline.

The estimated amount of drug ingested may be predictive of the severity of the clinical syndrome. Ingestions of less than 150 mg/kg are usually benign. In the range of 150 to 300 mg/kg, mild to moderate toxicity usually occurs. Ingestions of greater than 300 mg/kg generally show more severe symptomatology, and an overdose of more than 500 mg/kg may cause death. Such guidelines do not apply to chronic therapeutic poisoning, but it has been observed that toxicity results when doses of greater than 100 mg/kg/day have been taken for 2 or more days.

In the child with a mild overdose of salicylates, mild to moderate hyperpnea occurs, at times with some degree of lethargy. Moderate reactions cause severe hyperpnea and neurologic findings, including lethargy and/or hyperirritability. Severe aspirin toxicity is manifested by severe hyperpnea with coma, often complicated by convulsions.

The Done nomogram (Fig. 48.2) is a further aid in gauging the likely severity of a given acute overdose, though it is of no value in chronic salicylism. The earliest time to obtain a useful salicylate level is 6 hours after an acute ingestion, in order to allow for absorption and distribution of the drug. Serial determinations may help monitor the efficacy of treatment and/or clarify a patient's prognosis.

MANAGEMENT

The usual efforts to prevent absorption of any toxin, including ipecac-induced emesis or lavage, followed by charcoal administration and catharsis (as described on p.

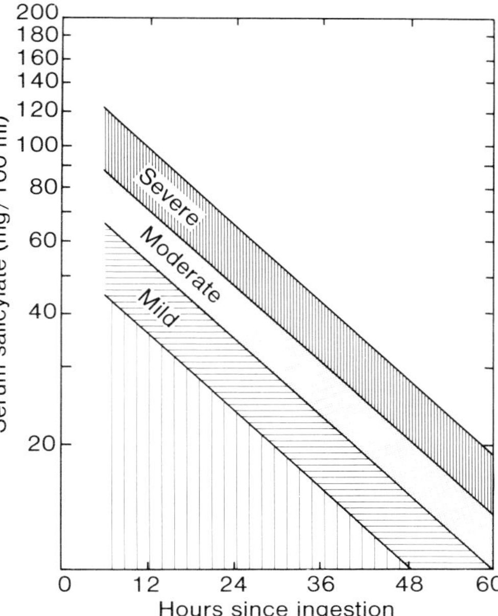

Figure 48.2. Done nomogram for estimating severity of acute salicylate poisoning. (Adapted from A. K. Done: *Pediatrics, 26:* 800, 1960. Copyright, American Academy of Pediatrics, 1960.)

492), should be initially employed. Specific therapeutic goals in salicylate intoxication include correction of fluid and electrolyte disturbances and the enhancement of salicylate excretion.

Fluid therapy should aim at restoring hydration and electrolyte balance, and promoting renal salicylate excretion. Since dehydration may be significant, the fluid infusion rate should be 10 to 15 ml/kg/hour for the first 2 hours. The initial fluid, in order to replace both Na and bicarbonate losses, should contain 5% dextrose with 75 meq of Na, 50 meq of Cl and 25 meq of HCO_3 per liter. If the patient has severe acidosis (pH < 7.15), additional bicarbonate will be necessary (usually 1 to 2 meq/kg every 1 to 2 hours). Subsequent hydration fluids may be given at a rate of 4 to 5 ml/kg/hour until the salicylate level falls to therapeutic values, which may take as long as several days. Fluid composition during this stage of treatment should approximate 5% dextrose with 40 meq of Na, 35 meq of K, 50 meq of Cl and 20 to 25 meq of HCO_3 per liter, although, again, additional HCO_3 may be necessary for persistent acidosis.

Alkalinization of the urine favors movement of salicylate from intracellular sites through plasma into urine. The urine may be alkalinized by giving additional HCO_3 at doses of 1 to 2 meq/kg every 1 to 2 hours until the urine pH reaches 8.0. However, achievement of such a high urine pH in acutely poisoned children may be difficult, due to the degree of organic aciduria present and to complicating potassium depletion.

Further salicylate elimination can be achieved with hemodialysis or hemoperfusion, although such invasive therapies should be reserved for seriously ill children. Our criteria currently include: (1) extremely elevated salicylate levels (> 160 mg/dl initially or > 130 mg/dl at 6 hours), (2) intractable acidosis (pH < 7.1), (3) evidence of renal failure, (4) persistent neurologic dysfunction, and/or (5) progressive clinical deterioration despite standard treatment.

HOUSEHOLD CLEANING PRODUCTS AND CAUSTICS

Household Cleaning Products

BACKGROUND

Until the early 1950s, cleaning products used for home laundry and maintenance and for personal hygiene were usually some form of soap. However, soap has the disadvantage of forming an insoluable precipitate that clings to surfaces such as skin, bathtubs, clothes, or dishes. Most products today use synthetic detergents which do not form troublesome precipitates. Soap is one type of surface active agent ("surfactant"). A "detergent" is any cleansing product. In common usage, though, the word "detergent" has come to mean a household cleaning product that is based on non-soap surfactants, used mainly for laundering and dishwashing. Other cleaning products include disinfectant cleaners; cleaners for drains, ovens, and toilet bowls; bleaches; and ammonia. These agents are of concern to the toxicologist because they are often involved in human ingestions, being used widely in the home in areas easily accessible to children. Furthermore, animal studies and clinical observations have shown some of these products to be injurious to human tissues following topical applications.

Each year about 6% of reported accidental ingestions involve "soap, detergents, or cleaners," 2 to 3% are due to "household bleaches," and 1 to 2% to "corrosive acids and alkalies" (e.g., ammonia, drain cleaners). Close to 90% of these cases involve children under 5 years of age. About 14% of cases involving detergents and cleaners become symptomatic, but fewer than 1% are hospitalized. For household bleaches, 24% are symptomatic and about 2% require hospitalization. Over 95% of household cleanser exposures occur inside the home, mainly in the kitchen and bathroom. An important statistic is the high frequency of exposures that occured while the products were in use (72.1% of cases) as opposed to the number of accidents (23.8%) which occurred while they were in storage. In less than 3% of cases had the product been discarded. Further, in 54% of cases, the products were in their original containers, while in 46% they were transferred to a different one.

Toxicology of Individual Products

Product Composition

Detergents are mixtures of both inorganic and organic ingredients. The primary organic component is a surface active agent (surfactant), a substance which lowers water surface tension enabling it to "wet" surfaces more effectively in order to remove dirt, soil, and grease.

Detergents also often contain "*builders*," inorganic salts, which inactivate minerals that interfere with detergency and which also maintain appropriate pH of the washing solution. Some common builders include phosphates, carbonates, silicates, and aluminosilicates. Detergents may also contain small amounts of other ingredients including soil-redeposition inhibitors, whitening agents, fabric softeners, agents to control sudsing, enzymes, bleaches, perfumes, and colorants.

Bleaches intended for household use contain sodium peroxide, sodium perborate, or sodium hypochlorite in variable concentrations. The most common such bleaches contain solutions of 3 to 6% sodium hypochlorite, but granular bleaches can have stronger concentrations. Commercial bleaches contain peroxides or perborates. *Household ammonias* usually contain weak solutions of ammonia, whereas industrial ammonias are often far more concentrated.

Product Toxicology

Since cleaning products present in the home are usually mixtures of ingredients, their biological effects are not always predictable by knowledge of the chemical properties of individual ingredients. Fortunately, the systemic toxicity of most ingredients and cleaning products themselves due to acute oral exposure is not high. However, the topical reactions range from mild irritation to corrosive effects.

Irritation or burns of the oral mucosa, esophagus, and stomach can result from the ingestion of many household cleansers. The eye is also susceptible to injury from exposure to cleaning products. The majority of household soaps and detergents do not cause substantial harm, and thus, differ from lye or similar corrosives. However, they can be irritants and cause erythema, erosion, and subsequent inflammation if left in contact with mucosa for a lengthy time. In most cases there are minimal sequelae, with recovery of the injured mucosa over a period of a few days. However, several specialty products such as selected laundry products, detergents for automatic dishwashers, cleaners for walls or hard surfaces, and particularly drain cleaners and oven cleaners, are strong enough to cause severe oral, esophageal, and gastric mucosal injury. As a rule, such products are identifiable by their very alkaline pH or by warnings on the label. Cleaning products shown to be capable of substantial injury after toxicologic testing are required by law to carry appropriate warning labels.

Many of these products induce vomiting after ingestion. Thus, it would be unusual for large amounts of most soaps or detergents to be accidentally ingested without the occurrence of spontaneous vomiting. This may explain the observed low incidence in one recent study of symptomatic exposures, especially those in which patients required medical care beyond a call to the local poison center. Symptoms, when reported, were all related to the irritating effects of the products on the gastrointestinal tract, and included nausea and/or vomiting, mouth irritation and uncommonly, abdominal pain. In this study, no patients manifested hematemesis, hematochezia, dysphagia, painful swallowing or other evidence of esophageal injury.

Soap. Soaps are generally only minimally toxic. As mild irritants, they may produce inflammation of the skin, eyes, mouth and gastrointestinal tract. Large amounts of soap may induce emesis or lead to mild diarrhea.

Surfactants. Surfactants are also usually of low toxicity, except for those products with a high degree of alkalinity. Of the various types of detergents, cationic formulations are more toxic than anionic or nonionic detergents. Cationic detergents are often found in disinfectant cleansers and fabric softeners. Concentrated solutions will have caustic qualities; more dilute solutions show marked irritant effects. Systemic absorption of cationic detergents may produce generalized toxic symptoms, including central nervous system disturbances, such as restlessness, confusion and muscle weakness, that may progress to cyanosis, respiratory paralysis and convulsions.

Builders. The addition of builders to detergents changes the final product's toxicity. Silicates and carbonates (found in "low phosphate" detergents) and certain phosphates (such as trisodium phosphate) may raise the pH of the detergent and make it much more corrosive. Highly alkaline detergents can produce severe eye irritation, burns of the mouth and esophagus, and hemorrhagic gastritis. Dishwasher detergents have a very high pH and some may cause toxic effects comparable to alkaline caustics (see below).

Bleaches. Household bleaches tend to be mild to moderate irritants and generally cause no tissue destruction. They may result in mild oral or esophageal burns, or irritation of the skin or eyes. Bleaches may induce emesis. One study of almost 400 patients demonstrated no esophageal strictures or perforations after chlorine bleach ingestion. Our experience also has been that burns and scarring are not caused by household hypochlorite bleaches. Other bleaches may contain sodium peroxide or sodium perborate. The former has low toxicity, but sodium perborate decomposes to peroxide and borate, which is more alkaline and irritating and may lead to the toxic systemic effects of boric acid. Solid-form bleaches are of potentially greater toxicity because they are far more concentrated.

Ammonia Compounds. Weak ammonia solutions are mildly irritating, but concentrated solutions may be caustic. Ingestion of household ammonia causes erythema and superficial erosion. The vapors irritate the eyes, respiratory tract and other mucous membranes. Fumes from concentrated ammonia solutions can cause severe irritation of the eyes with profuse tearing. Such fumes when inhaled may also cause severe respiratory tract irritation, which can produce a sensation of tightness of the chest and persistent cough, and may progress to a delayed onset pulmonary edema. Industrial strength ammonia acts as a caustic agent.

Mixing Chemicals. It is important to note the phenomenon that occurs with the mixing of hypochlorite bleaches with other household cleansers. Such mixing may result in the release of gases that are very irritating to the pulmonary tract; such exposure, when prolonged, may cause pulmonary edema. When hypochlorite is mixed with strong acids, chlorine gas is released. Hypochlorite mixed with ammonia will lead to the production of chloramine gas.

MANAGEMENT

Dilution with water or milk should be instituted immediately with all ingestions involving soaps, detergents, or household cleansers. In those cases where mucosal irritation is noted or might be expected, demulcents should be used. Emesis is rarely indicated. However, since delayed spontaneous emesis often occurs, the patient should be kept in an upright posture for at least 2 hours. With more alkaline products, the mucosa effected should be examined. Esophagoscopy is not indicated, except when the product is found to be caustic. Gastrointestinal discomfort may be alleviated with mild analgesics. If significant diarrhea or vomiting occurs, fluid and electrolyte deficits may require treatment. Figure 48.3 outlines the approach to emergency management of possible household cleaning product ingestions.

For eye contact, begin irrigation immediately, gently flushing the eye with water until the material is completely removed. This is best accomplished by tilting the head back and gently streaming copious amounts of cool or lukewarm water from a container onto the eye. The eye should be thus flushed continuously for 15 min, particularly if the package label indicates potential risk for ocular injury. When the product is identified as corrosive to the eye, ophthalmologic consultation should be sought as soon as possible for a complete eye examination.

In cases of skin contact, thorough rinsing with water prevents a prolonged exposure. Limited skin contact is not usually a problem.

When there is fume inhalation, the essential first aid measure is removal from contaminated air. For prolonged exposures, or if early symptoms occur, observation for delayed-onset, severe pulmonary manifestations is indicated.

Caustics

BACKGROUND AND PATHOPHYSIOLOGY

Strong alkalis and acids cause direct destruction of tissue. Acids produce coagulation necrosis which usually causes superficial damage, rather than deep, penetrating

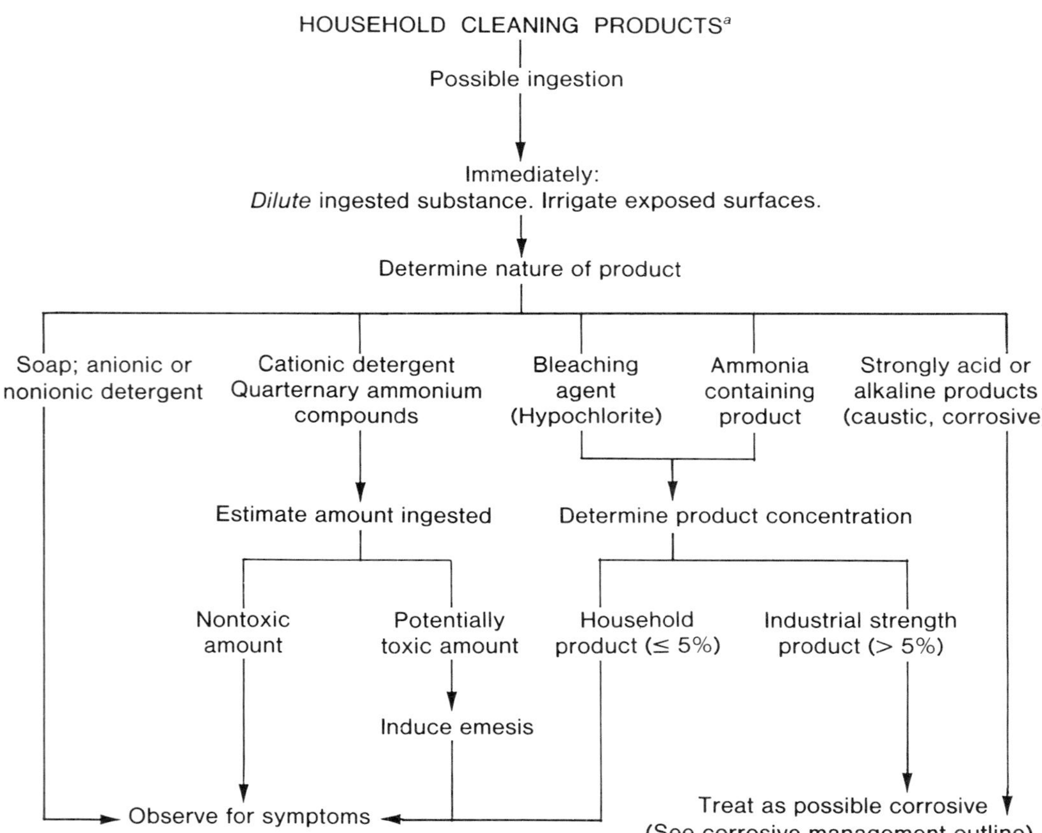

Figure 48.3 Algorithm for management of household cleaning product ingestion. [a] Adapted from: Temple AR and Lovejoy FH, Jr.: *Cleaning Products and Their Accidental Ingestion*, Soap and Detergent Assoc., NY, NY, 1980.

burns. Alkalis cause a deep and penetrating liquefaction necrosis, which often have severe consequences, such as esophageal perforation. Such deep burns are often associated with severe scarring, and ultimately, with stricture formation. A few household cleansers may contain alkalis or acids, but usually in concentrations below those necessary to cause caustic effects. Acid corrosives include the mineral acids such as hydrochloric, sulfuric and nitric, used in metal cleansers and other products. Hydrofluoric acid is used in etching glass and as a corrosive in many industries. Oxalic acid is found in some industrial bleaches and metal cleansers and in some household products such as metal polishers, anti-rust treatments and paint removers. Oxalic acid causes corrosive effects on mucous membranes; oxalates may also lead to systemic toxicity via combination with serum calcium, producing severe hypocalcemia and tetany, and by renal tubular damage due to the oxaluria. Common household products containing acid corrosives, such as toilet bowl and metal cleaners, are the most common source of acid caustic exposures. However, many home accidents involve acids brought home (often in unmarked food containers) by parents from the workplace.

Alkali caustics are also found in household products and thus may cause serious accidental poisonings in children. Lye (sodium hydroxide) in crystalline or liquid form is used as an oven cleaner or drain pipe cleaner (e.g., Drano, Pronto, Liquid Plum'r, and Easy-Off). Sodium hydroxide is a constituent of the tablets used to test for glycosuria (Clinitest). Although most homes contain corrosive alkalis such as oven cleaners and drain cleaners, the average parent recognizes the extreme danger of such products and usually makes an effort to keep them stored safely. However, other products such as some electric dishwasher detergents, are also highly alkaline, and thus, quite corrosive. These products tend to be less generally appreciated as hazardous and may be more available for accidental ingestion by a curious toddler.

CLINICAL MANIFESTATIONS

Ingestions of both acid and alkali caustic substances cause immediate severe burning of exposed surfaces usually with intensely painful swallowing that soon leads to complete inability to swallow (Fig. 48.4). Associated glottic edema may cause immediate airway obstruction and asphyxia. Severe acid ingestions often cause gastric necrosis and may be complicated by gastric perforation and peritonitis. With alkali, severe damage is more commonly found in the esophagus, and death from esophageal perforation, mediastinitis and pneumonia may occur. As noted above, alkalis also produce severe esophageal strictures in survivors of the acute toxicity.

MANAGEMENT

The approach to management of caustic ingestions, as outlined in Figure 48.4, begins with rapid clinical assessment of cardiorespiratory function, neurologic status, evidence of gastrointestinal hemorrhage, and the state of hydration. Basic life-support measures may need to be instituted, as in glottic edema causing upper airway compromise. As noted above, most patients with significant exposures develop symptoms early, and may appear critically ill. However, even patients with minimal symptoms and absence of mouth burns may have significant esophageal lesions; thus, all patients with convincing exposures to a caustic substance need esophagoscopy to evaluate fully for the presence of esophgeal burns.

Simple dilution instituted immediately after ingestion may be very beneficial. Four to twelve ounces of water or milk should be given. Swallowing may be difficult but should be attempted if possible. Afterward, the mouth should be rinsed as well. Caustic ingestions are a contraindication to induction of emesis or gastric lavage. Efforts to neutralize the caustic with mild acids or bases may possibly cause tissue damage due to exothermia and, thus, their use is controversial.

If the eyes are involved, irrigation as described previously should immediately be started, and carried out for at least 15 min, with longer periods for crystalline caustics. Alkali eye injuries require urgent ophthalmologic consultation. Skin contamination also deserves prolonged rinsing with water

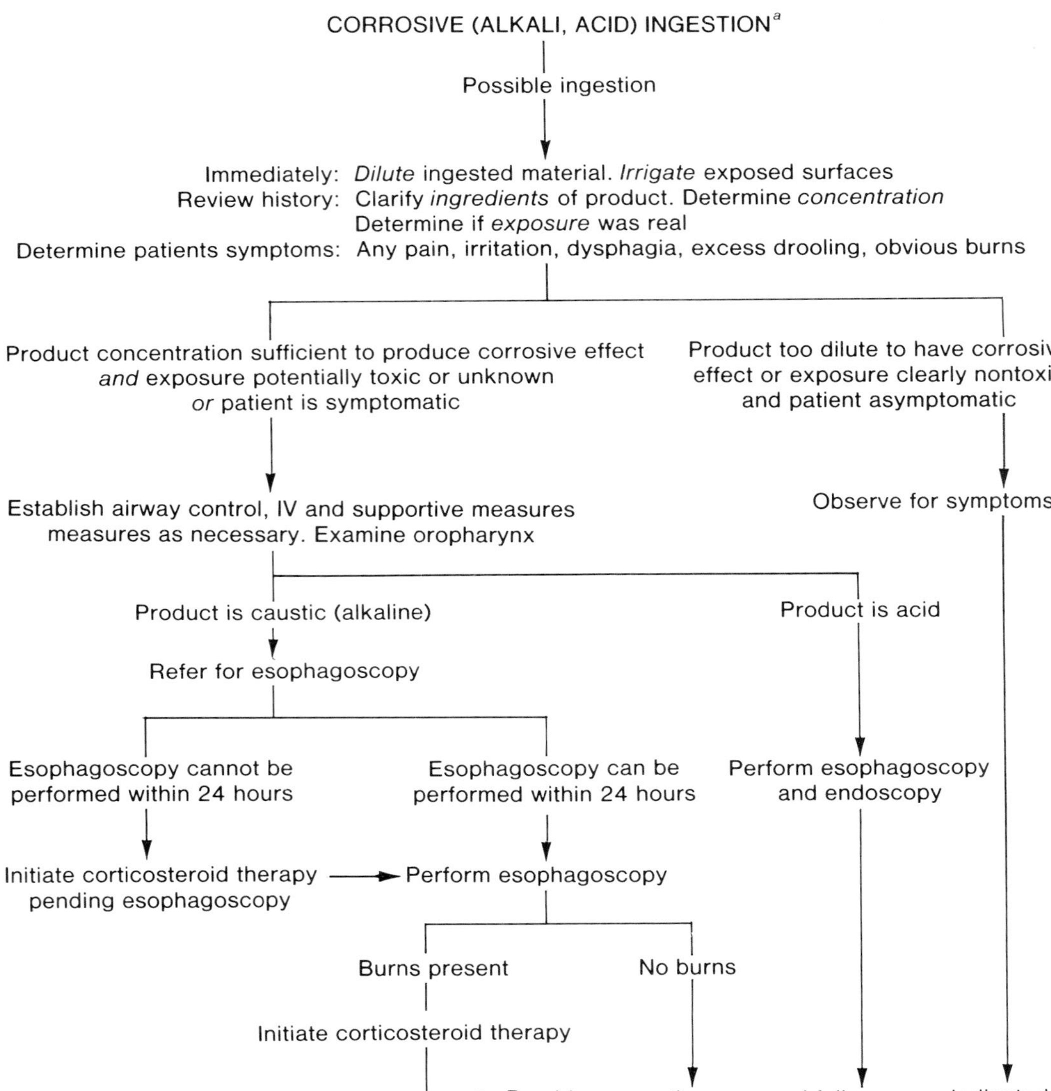

Figure 48.4 Algorithm for management of corrosive ingestion. [a] Adapted from: Temple AR an Lovejoy FH, Jr.: *Cleaning Products and Their Accidental Ingestion*, Soap and Detergent Assoc New York, 1980.

and removal of contaminated clothing. Irrigation should continue until the skin is free of alkali, as determined by disappearance of the soapy sensation.

The next phase of management calls for further evaluation. All exposed surfaces, especially the oropharynx, should be scrupulously examined. A CBC and chest x-ray should be obtained, the latter particularl if any respiratory signs or symptoms ar noted. Referral to an endoscopist must b done on an immediate basis.

Analgesic therapy may be necessary fo severe pain. The patient should not be al lowed any oral intake and requires the in stitution of a secure intravenous line, if nc previously necessary for basic life support. Most authorities currently feel that early corticosteroid treatment is beneficial; parenteral prednisolone (2 mg/kg/24 hours) or methylprednisolone (1.6 mg/kg/24 hours) may be used initially. If esophagoscopy can be performed within the first day post-ingestion, the consulting otolaryngologist may wish to defer steroid treatment until after endoscopy. All patients are admitted, and intensive supportive care with monitoring for acute complications such as mediastinitis, pneumonitis and peritonitis continued.

The long-term management of survivors with severe caustic esophageal burns and stricture formation is complex, involving many surgical, medical and psychologic stresses to the patient. Years of repeated bougienage may be necessary, and some patients will require esophagectomy with colonic interposition in an effort to replace the destroyed esophagus. The patient may not be capable of tolerating solid foods for prolonged periods of time.

HYDROCARBONS

Hydrocarbons are carbon compounds that are liquid at room temperature and are often found as solvents, fuels and additives in household cleaners and polishes. They contain a mixture of straight chain and branched aliphatic hydrocarbons. The major toxicity of these compounds stem from their low surface tension and vapor pressure, which allow them to spread over large surface areas, such as the lungs when aspirated, leading to a necrotizing chemical pneumonitis. Originally, it was believed that the aspiration of these substances into the lungs, secondary to the vomiting that acompanies their ingestion, was responsible for the major pulmonary toxicity. It has been shown, however, that the mere presence of the substance in the hypopharynx can cause chemical pneumonitis by spread to contiguous surfaces in the airway. In addition to the pulmonary findings, there may be associated central nervous system symptoms, secondary to systemic absorption of some of the hydrocarbons; rarely liver, kidney or myocardial injury occurs.

The amount of a hydrocarbon that has been ingested by a pediatric patient is often difficult to quantify. Less than 1 ml of some compounds, when aspirated directly into the trachea, may produce severe pneumonitis and eventual death. Other compounds are difficult to aspirate and are not well absorbed from the gastrointestinal tract. Generally, compounds such as asphalt or tar, lubricants (e.g., motor oil, household oil, heavy greases), and mineral oil or liquid petrolatum are not toxic when ingested. In a retrospective study of hydrocarbon ingestions in children, Anas et al. demonstrated that the vast majority of children (880 out of 950) developed no symptoms after the ingestion of a hydrocarbon compound.

The major toxicity associated with other hydrocarbons is related to their viscosity. Products with viscosity of 150 to 250 Saybolt Seconds Units (SSU), such as the oils mentioned above, have a very limited toxicity, but those with a viscosity in the range of 3 to 35 SSU or lower, such as furniture oils or polishes, have a high aspiration hazard. For this reason, induction of emesis is not recommended for compounds such as mineral seal oil (found in furniture polish) or signal oil. These compounds do not appear to be absorbed from the gastrointestinal tract, but they are clearly associated with a high risk of severe aspiration pneumonitis.

Induction of emesis is generally recommended for compounds that have inherent central nervous system toxicity or a potential for systemic toxic effects. These compounds include the halogenated hydrocarbons (e.g., trichloroethylene, carbon tetrachloride) and aromatic hydrocarbons (e.g., toluene, xylene, benzene, turpentine). Additionally, any petroleum distillates, regardless of their viscosity, should be evacuated from the gastrointestinal tract if they contain dangerous additives, such as heavy metals or insecticides.

Other hydrocarbon compounds including gasoline, kerosene, charcoal lighter fluid, turpentine, and mineral spirits are unlikely to produce systemic symptoms following accidental ingestion. Usual guidelines include the induction of emesis only when an amount greater than 1 to 2 ml/kg of body weight has been ingested of these compounds, and in the absence of spontaneous vomiting. Therefore, emesis is generally not recommended unless a large ingestion has occurred, usually as a suicide attempt.

Patients who ingest hydrocarbons may begin by choking, coughing and gagging as the product is swallowed and then vomit shortly following ingestion. Aspiration of the product at the time of the initial swallowing may cause aspiration pneumonitis. Generally, if the patient is coughing upon arrival at a treatment facility, aspiration has already occurred and admission is required. In this event, a chest x-ray should be obtained early in the course of the ingestion, and compared with another x-ray, repeated 24 hours after initial observation. General treatment calls for the induction of emesis where indicated above, followed by the administration of a cathartic; activated charcoal has not been useful in preventing the absorption of hydrocarbons. Asymptomatic children with a normal physical examination should be observed for 4 to 6 hours in the emergency department; if they remain well and have a normal chest x-ray after the period of observation, they may be discharged.

Treatment of hydrocarbon pneumonitis is basically that of supportive care. Antibiotics should be not used prophylactically, but reserved for specific infections, should they develop. The use of corticosteroids in the treatment of aspiration from hydrocarbons has been associated with increased morbidity, and is not recommended. In the event of hypotension or bronchospasm, epinephrine is contraindicated since hydrocarbons are known to cause ventricular irritability and predispose to fibrillation.

IRON POISONING

BACKGROUND

Iron poisoning is one of the most common potentially fatal intoxications in children. Most serious childhood poisonings result from ingestion of adult-intended ferrous sulfate tablets (which unfortunately look very much like candy). A common scenario is that the victim is a toddler whose mother has just had a new baby; the increased demands on mother's attention and almost universal prescription of iron to post-partum women combine to set the stage for this ingestion. Cases have also been reported of poisonings resulting from ingestion of iron-fortified children's vitamins.

Sufficient data to define a safe lower limit for toxic iron ingestions are not available. As little as 30 mg/kg of elemental iron has caused toxicity, while ingestions of > 50 mg/kg often produce toxic effects. Of course, it is often impossible to know the exact number of tablets ingested. As few as ten 300-mg $FeSO_4$ tables have been fatal to a young child. Furthermore, the elemental iron content of whole bottles of chewable vitamins is usually about 1200 mg. Legislation now demands child-proof caps for vitamin bottles containing more than 250 mg elemental iron.

PATHOPHYSIOLOGY

Iron toxicity is due to both a direct caustic effect on the gastrointestinal mucosa and the presence of free iron in the circulation. Pathologic changes include hemorrhagic necrosis of stomach and intestinal mucosa, and lesions in the liver ranging from cloudy swelling to areas of complete necrosis. Occasionally, pulmonary congestion and hemorrhage are noted. Excess free iron is believed to act as a mitochondrial poison, particularly in the liver, with resulting changes in cellular energy metabolism and the production of metabolic acidosis.

CLINICAL MANIFESTATIONS

The clinical effects of iron poisoning are classically divided into four phases. Phase I represents primarily the effects of direct mucosal injury and usually lasts 6 hours. Vomiting, diarrhea, and gastrointestinal blood loss are the prominent early signs; when severe, the patient may lapse into early coma and shock, due to volume loss and metabolic acidosis.

Phase II, which lasts from 6 to 24 hours after ingestion, is marked by dimunition of the gastrointestinal symptoms. With appropriate therapy to replace fluid and/or blood losses, the child may seem relatively well and often goes on to full recovery without any subsequent symptoms. However, this remission may be transient and be followed by Phase III, characterized by cyanosis and profound metabolic acidosis. The child may develop coma, seizures, and intractable shock. This phase is felt to represent the hepatocellular injury with consequent disturbed energy metabolism; elevated levels of lactic and citric acids are noted in experimental iron poisoning before cardiac or respiratory failure occurs. Jaundice and elevated transaminases are noted in this phase. A Phase IV has been described in survivors of severe iron poisoning, marked by pyloric stenosis, due to scarring, and consequent obstruction.

Laboratory abnormalities often associated with severe iron intoxication include leukocytosis, hyperglycemia, metabolic acidosis, hyperbilirubinemia and increased liver enzymes, and a prolonged prothrombin time. If fluid loss is marked, there will be hemoconcentration and elevated BUN. Abdominal films may show radio-opaque material in the stomach, but the absence of this finding does not indicate a trivial ingestion.

MANAGEMENT

All children alleged to have ingested iron are potentially at significant risk for life-threatening illness. However, severe iron poisoning is quite uncommon when compared to the number of children who develop only mild symptoms or remain entirely asymptomatic. Thus, the emergency department physician needs an approach that encompasses both the response to the severely poisoned child, as well as the majority who will remain well.

As noted earlier, the amount of iron ingested is often hard to quantify, and minimal "safe" amounts are not well established. Serum iron levels have been shown to correlate with the liklihood of developing symptoms (usually a reflection of the serum iron exceeding the iron-binding capacity and resulting in free circulating iron). Usually, iron levels below 350 mg/dl, when drawn 2 to 6 hours postingestion, predict an asymptomatic course. Patients with levels in the 350 to 500 mg/dl range often show mild Phase I symptoms but rarely develop serious complications. Levels greater than 500 mg/dl suggest significant risk for Phase III manifestations. However, the serum Fe determination is not always available on a "stat" basis.

Recently, Lacouture et al. demonstrated that early clinical assessment and several simple laboratory screening tests are quite predictive of patients whose iron levels are greater than 300 mg/dl, and thus at possible risk (conservatively) for serious intoxication. Vomiting, diarrhea, serum glucose greater than 150 mg/dl, WBC count greater than 15,000/mm^3 and the finding of radiopaque material on abdominal x-ray all showed a high correlation with an elevated serum iron; no patient who remained asymptomatic for six hours post ingestion went on to develop late onset symptoms. With these observations in mind, it is possible to construct a protocol for the triage and initial management of the patient who has ingested a possibly toxic amount of iron (Fig. 48.5).

Categorization

Patients arriving with severe early symptoms including vomiting, diarrhea, gastrointestinal bleeding, depressed sensorium, or circulatory compromise require urgent, intensive treatment in the emergency department. The first priority is obtaining venous access. Simultaneously blood is drawn for CBC, blood glucose, electrolytes, BUN, liver function tests, serum iron, total iron binding capacity, and type and crossmatch. Lavage should be started with as large a bore tube as possible. Blood pressure should be supported with normal saline or Ringer's lactate (see Chapter 2). Specific chelation therapy with intravenous deferoxamine (as described below) is begun immediately in all severely poisoned patients. An abdominal x-ray should be obtained as soon as possible after lavage to determine the efficacy of the gastric evacuation.

Patients with only mild vomiting and diarrhea in the early postingestion period still need urgent treatment but usually do quite well. Emesis is induced, followed with lavage, and then by a postlavage x-ray. Blood studies as noted above are drawn,

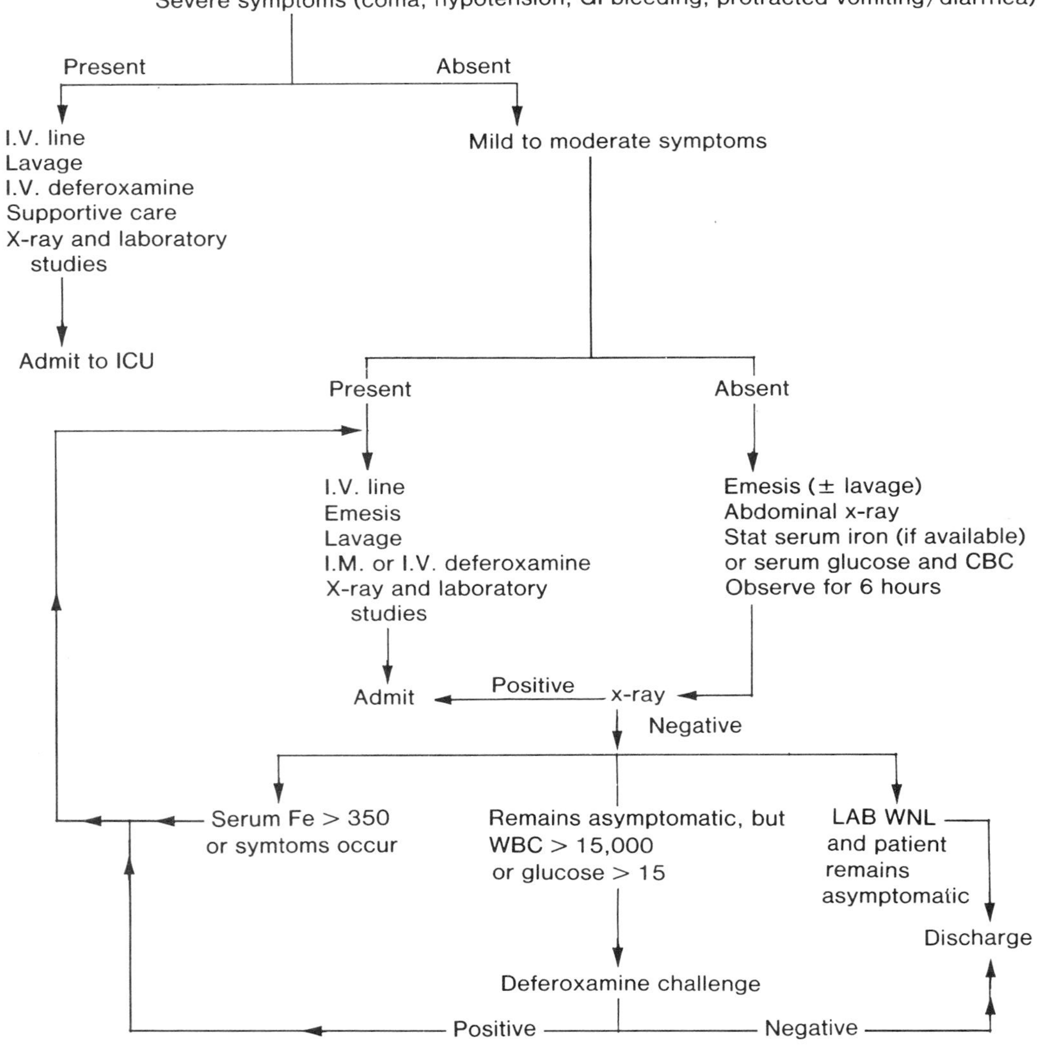

Figure 48.5 The initial approach to the patient ingesting a possibly toxic dose of iron. *ICU* = intensive care unit; *WNL* = within normal limits.

and parenteral deferoxamine therapy begun.

The asymptomatic patient who has presumably ingested iron also requires emesis. Some authorities would still recommend postemesis lavage, though in the authors' opinion this may at times be omitted. If serum iron levels are immediately available, blood should be sent for this study, an abdominal x-ray obtained, and the patient observed. An iron level taken 2 to 6 hours after ingestion of < 350 mg/dl in an asymptomatic patient with a normal x-ray would suggest that the patient is at minimal risk and may be discharged. Iron levels above 350 mg/dl, the development of any symptoms, or a "positive" x-ray should lead to admission and management as described above for the mild to moderately ill patient.

When serum iron levels are not available on an emergency basis, the WBC count and serum glucose may be used as screening laboratory tests, in addition to the abdominal x-ray. Patients are observed for 6 hours in the emergency department. Those who have normal screening tests and remain asymptomatic may be discharged. Patients with abnormal screening laboratory tests should have an iron level sent, for later reference, and be given a deferoxamine challenge (50 mg/kg intramuscularly up to a maximum of 1 g). The appearance of a pinkish-orange ("vin rose") color to the urine indicates the presence of iron-deferoxamine complex in the urine and correlates well with a significantly elevated serum iron level. A positive deferoxamine challenge thus also mandates admission and further treatment. Patients asymptomatic after 6 hours, with a negative challenge, may be discharged.

TREATMENT

The treatment for acute iron poisoning includes efforts to decrease absorption and hasten excretion as well as appropriate supportive care.

Ipecac-induced emesis is the first step in preventing absorption, if the patient has a normal level of consciousness and intact gag reflex. Activated charcoal is not effective in binding iron salts. For serious poisonings, it is also recommended that emesis be followed by gastric lavage, in the hopes of both minimizing any direct mucosal injury due to residual particulate matter and in effecting the precipitation of residual iron salts to a less absorbable form by using specific lavage fluids. This latter goal has led to considerable controversy in choosing the best solution. Currently most authors recommend a 1 to 1.5% bicarbonate solution, though Robotham and Leitman have recently argued strongly for lavaging with alkalinized deferoxamine, 2 g/L, as well as giving a postlavage intragastric bolus of 10 g of this agent in 50 ml of water. In the Emergency Department at Children's Hospital we have prepared our lavage solution by diluting stock deferoxamine to a concentration of 2 g/L in 1.5% bicarbonate. The previously recommended practice of lavaging with diluted Fleets enema solution is contraindicated because of the risk of severe hypertonic phosphate poisoning.

Chelation therapy with parenteral deferoxamine enhances the excretion of iron. For severe poisonings, especially those complicated by shock, the most efficacious route is a continuous intravenous infusion, the maximum recommended dose being 15 mg/kg/hour (maximum daily dose 360 mg/kg, up to 6 g total). A higher infusion rate may itself be associated with hypotension. For patients with mild symptoms, or those who are asymptomatic but require therapy on the basis of high serum iron or positive challenge test, treatment may be either by the intravenous (20 to 40 mg/kg infused over 4 hours) or intramuscular (20 mg/kg g4h to g8h) route. Chelation is continued until the urine color and/or serum iron level return to normal.

At times the post-lavage abdominal x-ray will demonstrate residual radiopaque material. If the quantity of material is deemed significant and the patient's condition so allows, consideration should be given to gastroscopy or even gastrotomy to effect its removal. Large clumps of coalesced iron tablets in the stomach or duodenum have led to severe hemorrhagic infarction of these viscera with subsequent perforation, peritonitis and death. As noted above, even in such patients who survive the acute phase there will be considerable risk of subsequent pyloric or bowel stenosis with obstruction, usually 4 to 6 weeks postingestion. In this regard, we also urge early pediatric surgical consultation for patients in the first few days postingestion with any evidence of peritoneal irritation.

Once the patient has been initially stabilized, further problems may include: hypotension, profound metabolic acidosis, hypo- or hyperglycemia, anemia and colloid loss due to gastrointestinal hemorrhage (after equilibration), renal shutdown due to shock, and hepatic failure with an associated bleeding diathesis. The maintenance of an adequate urine output is critical to prevent renal failure and to foster excretion of the iron-deferoxamine complex. If renal failure supervenes, chelation may be continued with concurrent dialysis, since the complex is dialyzable.

LEAD POISONING

BACKGROUND

Although lead poisoning is usually the result of chronic ingestion by pica prone children or occupational exposure in adults, patients with lead poisoning may come to the emergency department with varied complaints of recent onset that often mimic diverse acute illnesses. Fortunately, severe lead encephalopathy is now rare, due in large part to widespread screening programs and early treatment of asymptomatic or mildly ill children. However, the risk of lead intoxication is still significant, and the emergency physician and pediatrician must maintain a high index of suspicion in every community where children have ready access to lead, particularly in the summer when most cases occur.

Sources of Lead

The major source of excess lead absorption in children is lead-based paint, widely used in home interiors through the 1940s. The average lead intake for a normal 2-year-old child (due to general environmental contamination) is on the order of 100 mg/day. The lead content of one average sized lead-based paint chip is 8000 mg, which explains how the child with pica can rapidly accumulate an enormous total body lead burden. In addition to the ingestion of macroscopic-sized chips of paint, inner city children are often exposed to house dust, with a high lead content due to finely crumbled paint particles, which gets on their hands and toys. Repetitive mouthing can lead to increased lead exposure even in the absence of observable pica. Although classically a disease of poorer inner city residents, the recent phenomena of young, middle class families moving into older sections of large cities and renovating townhouses therein has led to an expanded population at risk. This is because the sanding, stripping and burning of lead based paint from woodwork in such houses has also been associated with lead intoxication in the occupants. Other unusual sources of lead exposure include the burning of battery casings for heat (a source that may be increasing due to the "energy crisis"), soft well water carried by out-dated lead pipes, improperly home-glazed ceramics, drinking glass glazed decals, and dust or dirt alongside heavily travelled roads due to auto emissions.

PATHOPHYSIOLOGY

Absorption of lead occurs through both gastrointestinal and pulmonary routes, although the former predominates in pediatric intoxications. Lead is then compartmentalized into three main areas: bone, soft tissues and blood. Excretion occurs slowly through urine, feces and sweat. Children are probably at double jeopardy compared to adults in that there is experimental evidence that younger animals have increased absorption and also a heavier distribution into soft tissues (including the brain). Concomitant nutritional deficiency, especially low dietary iron and calcium, may enhance intestinal lead absorption. Unfortunately, the same group of children at greatest risk for lead poisoning by virtue of age and residence are also likely to be at risk for dietary deficiency, especially of iron.

Lead exerts its toxic effect principally by enzyme inhibition, particularly on enzymes rich in sulfhydryl groups. In man, the most obvious effect is on the heme synthesis pathway, which is interrupted at several points resulting in abnormally high levels of porphyrins and their precursors. Other cellular systems known to be affected by lead include the cytochrome chain in hepatocytes and brain adenyl cyclase.

CLINICAL MANIFESTATIONS

Early signs and symptoms of plumbism are notably vague and nonspecific. Abdominal complaints including colicky pain, constipation, anorexia and intermittent vomiting are common; of course these same symptoms are often ascribed to relatively normal 2-year-olds by their parents. The child with early plumbism may also show listlessness and irritability. When encephalopathy begins, the child develops persistent vomiting and becomes drowsy, clumsy or frankly ataxic. As encephalopathy worsens, the level of consciousness deteriorates further, and seizures commonly occur. Pathological examination of brains of children who have died of lead encephalopathy shows severe cerebral edema with vascular damage; intracranial pressure is often, though not invariably, increased during the encephalopathy. When spinal fluid is examined, it often reveals a picture similar to that of aseptic meningitis with a mononuclear pleocytosis and elevated protein; however, lumbar puncture should be avoided if possible, due to the risk of subsequent herniation. Peripheral neuropathy often occurs in adults with lead poisoning but is rare in children, although it is seen occasionally in those with an underlying hemoglobinopathy. Other organs may be damaged by lead. The kidneys may develop disturbances ranging from slight aminoaciduria to a full Fanconi syndrome with glycosuria and phosphaturia in addition to aminoaciduria. Very high lead levels are also associated with a microcytic anemia, due to a defect in hemoglobin synthesis. However, most anemia seen in children with excess lead levels is actually due to concurrent iron deficiency. A sensitive laboratory measure of lead effect on heme synthesis is the evaluation of erythrocyte protoporphyrin (EP), a heme precursor. Moderately elevated EP levels are seen in iron deficiency, but levels above 250 to 300 mg/dl are almost always due to lead poisoning.

MANAGEMENT

The asymptomatic child discovered to have a lead level in the 30 to 69 μg/dl range, particulary if the EP is greater than 250 μg/dl, deserves immediate referral to a pediatrician or toxicologist. Such children will require environmental investigation, further evaluation, and possibly therapy. All symptomatic children, or those with lead levels higher than 70 μg/dl, need immediate hospitalization and treatment as outlined below, as well as pediatric consultation in order to ensure adequate postchelation follow-up.

The remainder of this discussion is addressed primarily to the early recognition and treatment of plumbism, including acute lead encephalopathy. We focus here on this single aspect of chronic childhood lead poisoning as it represents a true medical emergency.

Recognition

As stated above, to recognize mildly symptomatic patients with lead poisoning (or asymptomatic children with high lead levels at great risk to soon become symptomatic) requires a high index of suspicion. All children between 1 and 5 years of age are suspect if they have (1) persistent vomiting, listlessness or irritability, clumsiness, or loss of recently acquired developmental skills; (2) afebrile convulsions; (3) a strong tendency to pica, including a past history of, or current visit for, acute accidental ingestions; (4) a deteriorating pre-World War II house or a parent with industrial exposures; (5) a family history of lead poisoning; (6) iron-deficiency anemia; and (7) evidence of child abuse or neglect.

The child aged 1 to 5 years who comes to the emergency department with an acute encephalopathy presents the physician with a dilemma: lead intoxication requires urgent diagnosis, but confirmation with a blood lead level is usually not available on an immediate basis. A constellation of historical features of lead poisoning increases the likelihood of the diagnosis. These features include: (1) prodromal illness of several days to weeks duration suggestive of mild symptomatic plumbism, (2) occurrence in the summer months, and (3) a history of pica and source of exposure to lead. Several nonspecific laboratory findings make lead poisoning likely enough to warrant presumptive chelation therapy until confirmation by lead levels is available. These findings would include: (1) microcytic anemia; (2) elevated EP level, especially if greater than 250 μg/dl; (3) basophilic stippling of peripheral erythrocytes, or if feasible, of red cell precursors on bone marrow examination; (4) elevated urinary coproporphyrins*; (5) glycosuria; (6) aminoaciduria; (7) radiopaque flecks on abdominal x-rays; and (8) dense metaphyseal

* A test for urine coproporphyrins can be performed in the emergency department if the reagents are available. A fresh urine specimen is acidified to pH 4.0 with drops of glacial acetic acid. Coproporphyrin is then extracted from the urine with (freshly opened, peroxide-free) ether. The ether-coproporphyrin layer is pipetted into a test tube, to which 1.5 N HCl is added in a volume equal to the original urine volume. The coproporphyrin is then extracted into the HCl layer, which is viewed under a fluorescent light (i.e., Wood's lamp). If excess coproporphyrins are present, the acid layer will fluoresce a brillant orange-red color.

bands on x-rays of knees and wrists (lead lines).

Abnormalities on examination of CSF are also indicative of lead encephalopathy, including a lymphocytic pleocytosis, elevated protein and increased pressure. However, a lumbar puncture should not be performed if lead encephalopathy is strongly suspected, since there would be a considerable risk of herniation. If CSF must be examined in order to rule-out bacterial meningitis, the minimal amount (< 1 ml) necessary should be obtained. Alternatively, one might institute treatment for presumed meningitis, perform a determination of the lead level, and consider a delayed lumbar puncture after several days if lead level was normal.

Treatment

The treatment of lead poisoning involves relocation of the child to a lead-free environment, chelation therapy, and appropriate supportive care. Symptomatic patients are at great jeopardy of developing encephalopathy with subsequent death or neurologic sequelae. Additionally, asymptomatic patients with very high lead levels (especially greater than 70 to 80 μg/dl) are also at significant risk for developing CNS involvement and require urgent treatment.

The specific chelating drugs commonly used for lead intoxication are edathamil calcium disodium (Ca EDTA) and 2,4-dimercaptopropanol (British Anti-Lewisite or BAL). Side effects of Ca EDTA include local reactions at injection sites, fever, hypercalcemia and renal dysfunction manifested by rising BUN and abnormal urine sediment with proteinuria, hematuria and/or epithelial cells. The major side effects of BAL include nausea and vomiting, so that for the first day or two of BAL therapy it is prudent to maintain the patient on intravenous fluids, and clear liquids or nothing by mouth. BAL also induces hemolysis in patients with glucose 6-phosphate dehydrogenase (G6PD) deficiency. Its use is hazardous if the patient has severe hepatic dysfunction, and it forms a toxic complex if given concurrently with iron.

Asymptomatic children found to have lead levels > 70 μg/dl require immediate hospitalization and treatment for 5 days with Ca EDTA alone. If the lead level is > 100 μg/dl or there are mild symptoms, BAL is added for the first 2 days (Table 48.8). Supportive care includes adequate hydration to promote good urine output. Symptomatic children without frank encephalopathy should receive chelation therapy with a combination of Ca EDTA and BAL. Supportive care includes close monitoring for signs of encephalopathy and, again, maintenance of urine flow.

Patients with encephalopathy require more aggressive combination chelation therapy with Ca EDTA and BAL (Table 48.8), as well as intensive supportive care. Fluid therapy is critical and must be individualized. Adequate urine flow is needed to excrete the lead-chelate complexes; however, fluid overload must be avoided in order not to exacerbate cerebral edema. A reasonable goal is to supply basal water requirements, maintaining urine production at 0.35 to 0.5 ml/kcal/24 hours. Metabolic requirements in children may be calculated as 100 kcal/kg for 0 to 10 kg, plus 50 kcal/kg for 10 to 20 kg, plus 20 kcal/kg for each additional kg.

Seizures commonly occur in acute encephalopathy, and should be controlled with anticonvulsant drugs (see Chapter 44). Hypothetical precautions have been made about the use of phenobarbital in lead encephalopathy (i.e., synergistic disturbances in porphyrin metabolism), but its clinical use has not been associated with any noticeable deleterious effect.

Recent advances in the management of cerebral edema and increased intracranial pressure (see Chapter 44) have not been evaluated in a controlled fashion in the context of lead encephalopathy. However, it seems reasonable to expect that such measures as forced hyperventilation, mannitol or glycerol osmotic therapy, and steroids in high doses would have a salutory effect. Whether more aggressive measures such as continuous intracranial pressure monitoring, induced hypothermia, and barbiturate coma would further decrease mortality or morbidity is unknown at this time

Table 48.8
Chelation Treatment of Lead Poisoning[a]

Drug	Dose	Route
BAL and Ca EDTA combination	BAL[b]: 500 mg/m² per 24 hr, in divided doses, every 4 hr	i.m.
	Ca EDTA[c]: 1500 mg/m² per 24 hr, in divided doses, every 4 hr	i.m.
Ca EDTA[c, d] alone	1000 mg/m²/24 hr in divided doses every 8–12 hr for 3–5 days	i.m.

[a] Adapted from *Preventing Lead Poisoning in Young Children: A Statement by the Center for Disease Control*, p. 20, April 1, 1978.

[b] give BAL alone first, then give BAL and Ca EDTA 4 hr later and every 4 hr at separate deep i.m. sites. Usual course 5 days for encephalopathy. In symptomatic patients without encephalopathy, may discontinue BAL after 2–3 days if symptoms abate.

[c] Ca EDTA for i.m. use should be mixed with 2% procaine HCl in a ratio of 3 parts Ca EDTA to 1 part procaine so that the final concentration of solution is 0.5% procaine.

[d] A less painful alternative for treatment with Ca EDTA alone, often used at Children's Hospital of Philadelphia, has been to dilute the Ca EDTA in 5% dextrose in water to a concentration of less than 500 mg/100 ml, and infuse it intravenously by infusion pump over 1 hr, with monitoring of cardiac rhythm during infusion. When this route is used, the total daily dose (1000 mg/m², or 50 mg/kg in children less than 20 kg) is given in divided doses every 4–6 hr.

ORGANOPHOSPHATES

BACKGROUND

Organophosphates are strongly lipid-soluble insecticides that are commonly applied in sprayed dust or emulsion formulations. These compounds are found in agricultural and home use. Organophosphates are readily degraded in the environment and metabolized in mammals by hydrolic cleavage. Some of these chemicals are "systemic" insecticides, meaning that they are taken up by the roots of the plants and translocated into foliage, flowers and/or fruit.

PATHOPHYSIOLOGY

Compounds of this class can be absorbed by inhalation, ingestion and skin penetration. They irreversibly phosphorylate the enzyme, acetylcholinesterase, in tissues, allowing acetylcholine accumulation at cholinergic junctions in autonomic effector sites (causing muscarinic effects) and in skeletal muscle or autonomic ganglia (causing nicotinic effects).

CLINICAL MANIFESTATIONS

The symptoms of acute poisoning develop during the first 12 hours of contact. These include complaints related to the central nervous system such as: dizziness, weakness, headache, ataxia, blurred vision and miosis initially; the severely intoxicated patient may develop muscle twitching, tremors, mental confusion, or convulsions and coma. Gastrointestinal symptoms include nausea and vomiting, abdominal cramps, and diarrhea. Excessive cholinergic activity may cause patients to sweat profusely and have rhinorrhea, tearing and/or salivation; occasionally, pulmonary edema develops. Severe intoxications cause a toxic psychosis that resembles alcoholism.

A history of exposure to organophosphates and the clinical manifestations discussed above are the best clues to an organophosphate poisoning. A depression of plasma or red blood cell cholinesterase activity provides the most satisfactory and generally available laboratory marker of excessive absorption of organophosphates. A decrease in the cholinesterase activity of the red blood cells is more specific for organophosphate inhibition than is the plasma assay. Although plasma cholinesterase is depressed by liver injury from a variety of causes, and a small percentage of the population has a genetically determined deficiency of plasma cholinesterase activity, a depression of 25% or more is strong evidence of excessive organophosphate absorption. It is important that treatment not be delayed until confirmation of plasma cholinesterase is obtained.

MANAGEMENT

The management of a patient who has ingested organophosphates must always include safeguards against exposure for the individuals treating the patient. If the compound is ingested orally, emesis and/or gastric lavage should be induced; care should be taken that the vomitus not be splashed on the emergency department staff, since the organophosphates are readily absorbed through the skin and mucus membranes. Patients who have been poisoned by the topical application of organophosphates should receive a thorough scrubbing with a soap solution upon admission to prevent further absorption of organophosphates. Additionally, all contaminated clothing must be removed and stored in a plastic bag to protect the institutional personnel. Activated charcoal should be instilled for those individuals who have been poisoned by the oral route, and a cathartic should be administered unless the patient has severe diarrhea.

After decontamination, antidotal therapy begins with the administration of atropine sulfate given in a dose of 0.05 to 0.1 mg/kg to children and 2 to 5 mg for adolescents and young adults. This dosage should be repeated every 10 to 30 min or as needed to obtain and maintain full atropinization, as indicated by clearing of bronchial secretions and pulmonary rales. Therapy is continued until all absorbed organophosphate has been metabolized and may require 2 to 2000 mg of atropine over a course of a few hours to several days. After atropinization has been instituted, severe poisonings should be treated with the addition of pralidoxime. This drug finds particular use in those poisonings characterized by profound weakness and muscle twitching. A dose of 25 to 50 mg/kg should be administered in saline by infusion over approximately 30 min; adults may receive 1 g intravenously. This may be repeated at intervals of 6 to 8 hours if muscle weakness is not relieved. In those individuals with severe poisoning, these dosage recommendations may be doubled.

Organophosphates are usually dissolved in hydrocarbon bases; thus, the clinician should be prepared to treat hydrocarbon pneumonitis if it develops. Also bronchopneumonia complicating the pulmonary edema has been observed in acute poisonings.

Since the organophosphates cause elevated levels of acetylcholine in the plasma, compounds that effect the uptake of acetylcholine and/or its release should be avoided in the management of these patients. Specifically, aminophylline, phenothiazines, and the reserpine alkaloids are contraindicated. In those situations where identification of the ingested insecticides is difficult, consultation may be obtained from the National Pesticide Telecommunication Network (800-845-7633). This network provides an around-the-clock consultation service for advice on pesticides.

PHENOTHIAZINES

BACKGROUND AND PATHOPHYSIOLOGY

The phenothiazines are the most frequently prescribed major tranquilizers. Additionally, phenothiazines are often used inadvisedly to treat nausea and vomiting in young children. The toxic effects of phenothiazines primarily involve the three components of the nervous system: central (CNS), autonomic (ANS), and extrapyramidal (EPS).

The three subgroups of phenothiazines, aliphatic, piperazine, and piperidine, vary in their effects on the different components of the central nervous system. In general, the aliphatic group (e.g., chlorpromazine), cause sedation and hypotension. The piperazine group (e.g., prochlorperazine), have more effects on the EPS. Another general guideline is that as sedation decreases, the effect on the EPS increases.

CLINICAL MANIFESTATIONS

The manifestations of intoxication with these drugs vary from mild to severe. In mild intoxications, CNS signs such as sedation, ataxia, and slurred speech occur commonly. Effects on the EPS include mild salivation and minor extrapyramidal findings, e.g., decreased eye blinking. Dystonic reactions are rare at this level of intoxication. Involvement of the ANS causes constipation, urinary retention, blurred vision and alterations in temperature regulations. Orthostatic hypotension may also be noted with mild intoxication.

In moderate intoxications, the patients may lapse into coma, but usually respond to painful stimuli. EPS effects notable at this level of intoxication include muscle stiffness or "cogwheel" rigidity upon passive movement of the neck, biceps, or quadriceps. Laryngospasm may also occur at this state of intoxication. The ANS manifestations are severe and include acute urinary retention and paralytic ileus; hypotension may be profound.

In the severe overdoses, patients are unarousable to both verbal and painful stimuli. The EPS signs include hyperactive reflexes and flexor Babinski response. Dystonic reactions may occur, involving the head and neck and the cranial nerves (torticollis and opisthotonos). Also, the temperature may rise slightly. The effects of the ANS are life threatening at this state of intoxication. These include dysrhythmias and shock, and may precipitate acute renal shut down.

MANAGEMENT

Treatment hinges on the severity of ingestion. In the mild overdose, hospitalization is not usually necessary. The autonomic signs and symptoms are most often transient and require no treatment. However, the importance of orthostatic hypotension should be stressed with the family. The duration of symptoms depends upon the chemical class of the phenothiazine and its duration of action; in general, they may persist for 24 to 48 hours.

In the moderate overdose or therapeutic misadventure with phenothiazines, the problem of dystonic reactions is particularly distressing. Diphenydramine effectively controls the EPS symptoms in a dose 1 to 2 mg/kg parenterally, repeated within 5 to 10 min if no effect is noted. Subsequently, the same dose may be given either parenterally or orally every 6 hours over the next 24 to 36 hours as needed. The phenothiazines have a long half-life and a delayed elimination from the body; therefore, dystonic reactions may recur after initial treatment. For this reason, oral treatment should be continued for at least 24 hours.

In the case of the severe ingestion, the patient should be managed symptomatically. Pressors such as dopamine (see Chapter 3) may be utilized to correct the hypotension. In those rare instances of hypertension, the use of nitroprusside (see Chapter 4) may be indicated. Attention should be directed to the treatment of temperature instability and other autonomic disturbances.

PLANT TOXICITY IN CHILDREN

Plants are among the more frequently reported accidental ingestions in children. The majority of such ingestions involve common house and garden plants. Fortunately, of the many varieties of such plants, only a small fraction pose a serious toxic hazard.

When a child visits the emergency department following a plant ingestion, a general evaluation should be performed. Unless the plant can be absolutely identified and is known to be nontoxic, the stomach should be emptied, preferably by emesis (if consciousness is unimpaired), since this is more efficacious than lavage in evacuating plant particles. Activated charcoal may also be extremely useful in adsorbing plant toxins. If the plant is subsequently identified and not felt to have serious toxic potential, or if the plant is not available (or recognizable) for identification, the child should be observed for a short period in the emergency department. The child who remains asymptomatic may then be discharged and further observed at home. Children who develop symptoms, or for whom there is strong suspicion or confirmation that the ingested plant poses a potentially serious intoxication, should be admitted for further observation and specific or supportive treatment.

Specific Categories of Plant Toxidromes

Plants with Gastrointestinal Irritation

This group of plants accounts for the majority of plant poisonings in the United States. The range of symptomatology extends from mild oral burning to a severe gastroenteritis syndrome. Representative species include: *Philodendron* and *Dieffenbachia* species (leaves), causing minor mouth and throat burning; pokeweed (roots, stem), *Wisteria* (seeds), spurge laurel (berries), buttercup (leaves) and daffodil (bulbs, accidentally substituted for onions), causing severe vomiting, colicky abdominal pain and diarrhea; and the toxalbumin-containing plants such as rosary pea and castor bean (seeds) which can cause a violent hemorrhagic gastroenteritis leading to profound dehydration and circulatory collapse when the seeds are chewed up. The management of this group of ingestions consists essentially of fluid and electrolyte therapy.

Plants with Digitalis Effects

Several common garden or wildflowers contain digitalis, and have been responsible for fatal ingestions. Chewing on leaves or flowers or swallowing the berries of lily-of-the-valley, foxglove and oleander have all led to such poisonings. Intoxication has even occurred when water from a vase containing these flowers was ingested. Early after ingestion, the child may complain of intestinal symptoms such as mouth irritation, vomiting and diarrhea. As the digitalis is absorbed, typical digitalis effects may ensue, with conduction defects, and at times, serious arrhythmias. Treatment may include atropine for advanced heart block, and diphenylhydantoin for the more serious tachyarrhythmias (see Chapter 43).

Plants with Nicotinic Effects

Several species of plants contain nicotine or closely related alkaloids. Ingestion of wild tobacco (leaves), golden chain tree (seeds) and poison hemlock (leaves, seeds) usually leads to spontaneous vomiting within 1 hour. Salivation, headache, fever mental confusion and muscular weakness may follow, and the child may deteriorate to convulsions, coma, and death due to respiratory failure. Charcoal is especially useful in adsorbing these nicotinic alkaloids. Further treatment consists of intensive supportive care, with anticonvulsants and ventilatory assistance.

Plants with Atropinic Effects

The most common atropine-containing plant in the United States is jimsonweed, which is very widely distributed in this country. Cases have been seen in inner city children who managed to find this weed growing in their neighborhoods, where flora in general is quite scarce!

Symptoms and signs are those of atropinization (see Table 48.5) and include visual blurring, dilated pupils, dryness of the mouth, hot dry skin, fever, delirium or psychosis. Convulsions and coma may follow. Treatment consists of supportive care and, in severe cases, physiologic antagonism with physostigmine (see Table 48.3).

Plants that Cause Convulsions

Convulsions represent the principal toxic effect of some plants. Water hemlock, with its potent cicutoxin, is the main such species in the United States. Within an hour after ingestion, nausea, vomiting and profuse salivation occur. These initial symptoms are followed by tremors, muscle rigidity and multiple major motor seizures. Treatment is with anticonvulsants as for status epilepticus (see Chapter 44).

Mushrooms

Mushrooms cause an estimated 50% of all deaths due to plant poisoning in the United States. The difficulty in accurate identification of mushrooms makes reliance of such identification for appropriate management of ingestions extremely hazardous in the emergency department. Rather, the approach advocated by Lampe will be reviewed here.

Two main groups of mushrooms can be characterized on the basis of the time interval between ingestion and symptom onset. Regardless of the type of mushroom, the initial management for all suspected poisonings includes emesis, charcoal and catharsis.

Onset of symptoms within 6 hours of ingestion usually confers a benign prognosis, although careful attention to fluid and electrolyte management is critical. Most such mushrooms have some early gastrointestinal effects. Some "early onset" mushrooms cause muscarinic effects, usually within 15 min, such as sweating, salivation, colic and pulmonary edema. This syndrome will respond to atropine therapy. Other "early onset" mushrooms will cause drowsiness, followed by mania and hallucinations, usually within 2 to 3 hours of ingestion. Treatment need only be supportive. An additional subgroup of early onset mushrooms produce primarily a severe gastroenteritis syndrome. Management, again, consists of careful monitoring of fluid status.

The second important category of mushrooms, responsible for 90% of mushroom poisoning-related deaths, are those belonging to the *Amanita phalloides* group, in which there is a latent period of 12 hours or so before onset of symptoms. These poisonings have an extremely poor prognosis. Two compounds are known to produce the toxic effects. Phallotoxins act first, causing gastrointestinal symptoms including nausea, vomiting, abdominal pain and diarrhea. Fever, tachycardia and hyperglycemia may also occur during this stage. The gastroenteric phase may be followed by a remission of symptoms for 3 to 5 days. However, during this period, renal and hepatic function deteriorate.

The other toxin, amatoxin, causes renal tubular and hepatic necrosis. In milder cases, only renal damage occurs. With large ingestions, hepatic failure supervenes before the renal pathology has a chance to evolve. Treatment of the gastroenteric phase includes fluid and electrolyte replacement. If renal failure develops, dialysis may be necessary. Hepatic damage may be attenuated by early use (within 36 hours of ingestion) of an investigational drug, thioctic acid (α-lipoic acid), and/or hemoperfusion over charcoal. Precise indications for such treatment modalities must await further clinical trials, although both therapies have recently been recommended.

TRICYCLIC ANTIDEPRESSANTS

BACKGROUND

The ingestion of tricyclic antidepressant compounds is a significant problem in pediatric patients. The availability of these compounds in the household may be the result of therapy for depression for either a parent or a grandparent, or the use of these compounds in the treatment of enuresis in the patient or a sibling.

CLINICAL MANIFESTATIONS

The ingestion of 10 to 20 mg/kg of most tricyclic antidepressants represents a moderate to serious exposure, with coma and cardiovascular symptoms expected. The ingestion of 35 to 50 mg/kg may result in fatality. Children have been reported to be more sensitive than adults to tricyclic antidepressants and often have symptoms at lower doses.

The anticholinergic activity of the tricyclic antidepressants causes many of the clinical manifestations observed in the overdose patient. The cardiovascular effects include supraventricular tachycardia, depressed myocardial conduction, multiple focal premature ventricular contractions, and ventricular tachycardia. It has been shown that a QRS interval of greater than 0.1 sec is associated with a significant morbidity and mortality in these patients; this delay in conduction may progress to complete heart block and cardiac standstill.

Neurologic findings include lethargy, disorientation, ataxia, hallucinations, and, with severe overdoses, coma and seizures. Fever is commonly present initially, but hypothermia may occur later. Additional anticholinergic symptomatology includes decreased gastrointestinal motility, which delays gastric emptying time, and urinary retention from high doses of tricyclic antidepressants. Muscle twitching has been observed and may be associated with decreased deep tendon reflexes. While the pupils may be dilated, they usually respond to light.

MANAGEMENT

The management of children with tricyclic antidepressant overdoses begins with the initiation of emesis or gastric lavage. This dictum holds true even for those patients who present as late as 4 to 12 hours after ingestion. Since tricyclic antidepressants decrease gastrointestinal motility, unabsorbed drug may be left in the stomach for prolonged periods of time. After lavage and/or emesis, the administration of activated charcoal should be performed and a cathartic administered, such as magnesium sulfate 250 mg/kg. Symptomatic patients should be monitored in the hospital for a minimum of 48 hours. A significant addition in the treatment of arrhythmias from tricyclic antidepressants has been the use of sodium bicarbonate to alkalinize the blood to pH 7.4 to 7.5 range. This therapeutic maneuver produces an increase in plasma protein binding of tricyclic antidepressant, resulting in a lower concentration of the free compound which exerts pharmacological effects. If arrhythmias persist, appropriate antiarrhythmic therapy should be instituted, utilizing either propranolol, lidocaine or phenytoin (see Chapter 43). Quinidine or procainamide should be avoided since they may increase heart block in this situation. In the presence of hypotension, many clinicians have advocated the use of norepinephrine infusions. This is based on the observation that the hypotension is the result of norepinephrine depletion secondary to the block of catecholamine uptake caused by tricyclic antidepressants. Other clinicians have reported that dopamine is as effective; however, the occurrence of ventricular arrhythmias has been reported with dopamine.

Perhaps the greatest source of controversy in the management of tricyclic antidepressants concerns the use of physostigmine. Specific indications for physostigmine use are seizures, severe hallucinations, and unresponsive cardiovascular complications, such as hypertension and arrhythmias. The recommended dosage in these situations for small children is 0.5 mg administered slowly intravenously and repeated at 5-min intervals until a maximum dose of 2 mg has been administered. In larger children and adults, a dose of 1 to 2 mg should be infused slowly i.v. and repeated in 20 to 30 min if reversal of symptoms have not occurred. Physostigmine is metabolized within 30 to 60 min and repeated doses are often necessary. At all times, atropine at a dose one-half that of the amount of physostigmine administered should be available to reverse toxic cholinergic effects, which may result from physostigmine administration. The adverse effects of physostigmine include sinus bradycardia, cardiac standstill, heart block, seizures and severe bronchorrhea. During the recovery period, serum electrolytes should also be monitored since the infusion of bicarbonate may cause hypokalemia which may aggravate tricyclic antidepressant induced cardiac arrhythmias.

In many institutions, clinical laboratories can detect the presence of tricyclic antidepressants. While the clinical condition is the primary determinant in survival of the tricyclic antidepressant-poisoned patient, the concomitant use of plasma concentrations may be helpful. Patients who have a tricyclic antidepressant concentration greater than 1000 ng/ml (1 μg/ml) are significantly poisoned and require intensive therapy for 72 to 96 hours. When the plasma concentration falls below 50 to 200 ng/ml, the patient is unlikely to develop severe toxicity. It must be remembered in the treatment of tricyclic antidepressants that these compounds have long half-lives and slow elimination rates; therefore, the therapy for these ingestions is often protracted and intensive.

References

General

American Association of Poison Control Centers, Criteria for Regional Poison Control Programs: *Vet Hum Toxicol* 20: 117, 1978.

Berg MJ, Berlinger WG, Goldberg MS et al.: Acceleration of the body clearance of phenobarbital by oral activated charcoal. *N Engl J Med* 397: 642, 1982.

Bloomer HA, Maddock RK: An assessment of diuresis and dialysis for treating acute barbiturate poisoning. In *Acute Barbiturate Poisoning*, Chap. 15, edited by H. Matthew. Excerpta Medica. Amsterdam, 1971.

Done AK: Clinical pharmacology of systemic antidotes. *Clin Pharmacol Ther* 2: 750, 1961.

Done AK: Pharmacologic principles in the treatment of poisoning. *Pharmacol Phys* 3: 1–10, 1969.

Drug Abuse Warning Network Annual Report: IMS, Ambler, Pa., 1979.

Easom JM, Lovejoy FH: Efficacy and safety of gastrointestinal decontamination in the treatment of oral poisoning. *Pediatr Clin North Am* 26: 827, 1979.

Micik S: Emergency medical services and poison control. *Clin Toxicol* 12; 309, 1978.

Micik S: *Developing Regional Poison Systems*. Health Resources Administration, DHEW, 1981.

Mofenson HC, Greensher J: The unknown poison. *Pediatrics* 54: 336, 1974.

Mofenson HC, Greensher J: Controversies in the prevention and treatment of poisonings. *Pediatr Annu* 6: 60, 1977.

National Clearinghouse for Poison Control Centers: Poison Control Statistics, FDA:DHEW, 1978.

Picchioni AL, Chin L, Verbulst HL, Dieterle B: Activated charcoal vs. "universal antidote" as an anti-

dote for poisons. *Toxicol Appl Pharmacol* 8: 477, 1966.
Project DAWN Annual Report for 1979, DEA-NIDA, 1979.
Rosenbaum JL, Kramer MS, Raja R: Resin hemoperfusion for acute drug intoxication. *Arch Intern Med* 136: 263, 1976.
Temple AR, Veltri JC: Program Guide for Regional Poison Control Programs, Prepared under Contract No. 223-75-3013 for the Public Health Service, FDA:DHEW, 1975.
Temple AR, Veltri JC: One year's experience in a regional poison control center. *Clin Toxicol* 12: 277, 1978.
Winchester JF, Gelfand MC, Knepshield JH, Shreiner GE: Dialysis and hemoperfusion of poisons and drugs—update. *Trans Am Soc Artif Intern Organs* 23: 762, 1977.

Acetaminophen

Piperno E, Mosher AH, Berssenbruegge IA, et al.: Pathophysiology of acetaminophen overdosage toxicity; implications for management. *Pediatrics* 62(Suppl): 880, 1978.
Rumack BH, Peterson RG: Acetaminophen overdose; incidence, diagnosis and management in 416 patients. *Pediatrics* 62(Suppl.): 898, 1978.

Alcohols

McCoy HG, et al.: Severe methanol poisoning—application of a pharmacokinetic model for ethanol therapy and hemodialysis. *Am J Med* 67: 804–807, 1979.
McFadden, et al.: Coma produced by topical application of isopropanol. *Pediatrics* 43: 622, 1969.

Antihistamines

Hestand HE, Teske DW: Diphenhydramine hydrochloride intoxications. *J Pediatr* 90: 1017, 1977.
Schwartz JF, Patterson JH: Toxic encephalopathy related to antihistamine-barbiturate anti-emetic medication. *Am J Dis Child* 132: 37, 1978.

Aspirin

Segar WE: The critically ill child; salicylate intoxication. *Pediatrics* 44: 440, 1969.
Temple AR: Acute and chronic effects of aspirin toxicity and their treatment. *Arch Intern Med* 141: 364, 1981.

Household Cleaning Products and Caustic Agents

Berenson MM, Temple AR: Detergent toxicity, effects on esophageal and gastric mucosa. *Clin Toxicol* 8: 399, 1975.
Krenzelok EP, Clinton JE: Caustic esophageal and gastric erosions without evidence of oral burns following detergent ingestions. *JACEP* 8: 194, 1979.
Landau GD, Saunders WH: Effect of chlorine bleach on the esophagus. *Arch Otolaryng* 80: 174, 1964.
Temple AR, Lovejoy FH Jr: *Cleaning Products and Their Accidental Ingestion*, Soap and Detergent Assoc., New York, 1980.
Temple AR, Veltri JC: Outcome of accidental ingestions of soaps, detergents, and related household products. *Vet Hum Toxicol* 21: 9, 1979.

Hydrocarbons

Anas, et al.: Criteria for hospitalizing children who have ingested products containing hydrocarbons. *JAMA* 246: 840–843, 1981.
Beamon, et al.: Hydrocarbon Ingestion in children; a six year retrospective study. *JACEP* 5: 771, 1976.

Iron

Henretig FM, Karl SR, Weintraub WH: Management of severe iron poisoning with enteral and intravenous deforoxamine. *Ann Emerg Med* (in press).
Jacobs J, Greene H, Gendel BR: Acute iron intoxication. *N Engl J Med* 273: 1124, 1965.
Lacouture PG, et al.: Emergency assessment of severity in iron overdose by clinical and laboratory methods. *J Pediatr* 99: 89, 1981.
Robotham JL, Lietman PS: Acute iron poisoning—a review. *Am J Dis Child* 134: 875, 1980

Lead

Chisolm JJ, Jr: The use of chelating agents in the treatment of acute and chronic lead intoxication in childhood. *J Pediatr* 73: 1, 1968.
Pincus D, Saccar CV: Lead poisoning. *Am Fam Physician* 19: 120, 1979.
Preventing Lead Poisoning in Young Children: A Statement by the Center for Disease Control. USPHS, April 1978.

Organophosphates

Namba T, et al.: Poisoning due to organophosphate insecticides. *Am J Med* 50: 475–492, 1970
Norrel CL: The management of organophosphate intoxication. *South Med J* 68: 335–339, 1975.

Phenothiazines

Gupta J, Lovejoy FH: Acute phenothiazine toxicity in childhood; a five-year study. *Pediatrics* 39: 771, 1967
Lee AS: Drug-induced dystonic reactions. *JACEP* 8: 367, 1977.

Plants

Editorial. *Lancet* 2: 351, 1980.
Lampe KF: Systemic plant poisoning in children. *Pediatrics* 54: 347, 1974.
Lampe KF: Common Poisonous and Injurious Plants. HHS Publication No. (FDA) 81-7006, U.S. Department of Health and Human Services.
Litovitz TL, Fahey BA: Please don't eat the daffodils. *N Engl J Med* 306: 547, 1982.

Tricyclic Antidepressants

Brown TCK: Tricyclic antidepressant overdosage; experimental studies on the management of circulatory complications. *Clin Toxicol* 9: 255–272, 1976.
Callaham M: Tricyclic antidepressant overdosage. *JACEP* 8: 413, 1979.
Petit JM, et al.: Tricyclic antidepressant plasma levels and adverse effects after overdose. *Clin Pharmacol Ther* 21: 47, 1977.

CHAPTER **49**

A. Allergic and Pulmonary Emergencies

GERALD B. KOLSKI, M.D., Ph.D.

B. Cystic Fibrosis

THOMAS F. SCANLIN, M.D.

ASTHMA

BACKGROUND

Asthma is one of the most common problems confronting the emergency department physician. It is estimated that 10 to 15% of the population have had manifestations of asthma. In terms of pediatric patients it is the most common chronic disease and is the leading cause of school absence. Asthma can be associated with a significant morbidity in terms of exercise intolerance and disruption of the family unit.

Asthma is a disease characterized by a hyperreactive airway associated with reversible obstruction of that airway. The degree of reversibility is often taken as a measure of the asthmatic component of the airway obstruction. Methods have been devised to determine the degree of reactivity of the airway.

Inhalation of methacholine and histamine by subjects can be used to quantitate the reactivity of the airway. The dose of histamine or methacholine at which a patient has a significant fall in pulmonary functions is a measure of the reactivity; the lower the dose of histamine and methacholine where there is a drop in pulmonary function, the higher the reactivity of the airway. In addition to histamine and methacholine, exercise challenges have also been utilized. There is a good correlation between reactivity determined by methacholine, histamine, and exercise. The degree of reactivity in the airway may vary with time. Viral infections of the respiratory tract have been associated with increases in reactivity, as have seasonal exposures to pollens in allergic individuals. When reactivity is increased, it appears to be increased for all initiating triggers. The increased response to methacholine and diminished response to β-agonists has led to the postulation of a theory for asthma which involves abnormal autonomic function. In evaluating the initiating causes for asthma, allergy, exercise, infections, irritants, weather changes, and emotions have been the most commonly postulated triggers for individual attacks.

Allergy

The inhalation of a substance to which the patient is allergic initiates bronchospasm by an immune event. The allergic response may be of the immediate type or delayed. The immediate reaction is thought to be secondary to IgE specific to a particular allergen. This IgE is bound to mast cells which on interaction with allergens cause mast cell degranulation (Fig. 49.1). The mediators of anaphylaxis are released, and bronchospasm and an inflammatory response occur. The delayed allergic response to allergens is thought to involve either a delayed response secondary to the initial IgE mediated process or an IgG mediated response. The postulated IgG mediated response involves immune complexes activating the complement system with a subsequent inflammatory response. Patients with a significant delayed reaction characteristically have more hyperreactivity in their airway.

Exercise

Exercise can induce wheezing in patients with asthma. The etiology for the wheezing has been characterized as secondary to a loss of heat from the airway. This loss of heat is exacerbated by hyperventilation and cold, dry air. The exercise itself is not necessary in that hyperventilation without exercise in cold dry air also produces wheezing. Receptors in the airway are thought to sense the heat loss.

Infections

Exacerbation of asthma correlates well with upper respiratory infections, particularly with viral illnesses. Bacterial infections in most studies have not been shown to be associated with significant alterations of reactivity of the airway. Viral infections are thought to precipitate asthma by increasing inflammation, airway reactivity, and mucus production and decreasing the response to β-adrenergic agents.

Chronic infections, especially of the nasopharynx and sinuses, have also been associated with exacerbations of asthma.

Irritants

Sulfur dioxide, cigarette smoke, and ozone are irritants which can cause exacerbation of asthma. These effects appear to be primarily an irritant effect due to the response of receptors in the airway. In addition to the irritant effect, cigarette smoke also decreases mucociliary clearance and increases mucus production.

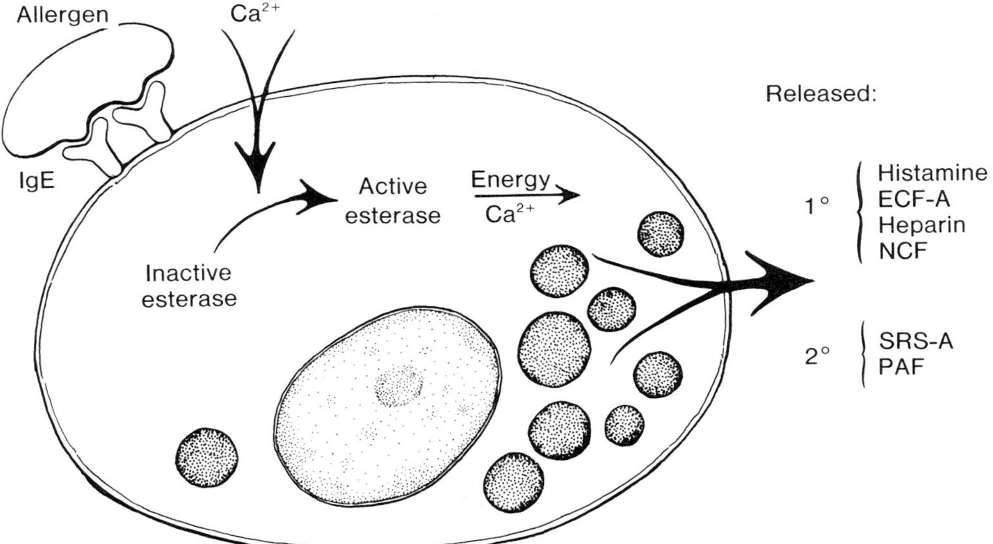

Figure 49.1 Schematic mast cell degranulation on allergen exposure with mediator release. *ECF-A*, eosinophil chemotactic factor of anaphylaxis; *SRS-A*, slow reacting substance of anaphylaxis; *NCF*, neutrophil chemotactic factor; PAF, platelet activating factor.

Weather Change

The etiology for the exacerbation of asthma with weather change is not well understood. Alterations in barometric pressure, air ion concentrations, and mold spore concentrations have all been suggested.

Emotions

Emotions have been often implicated in exacerbations of asthma. Whether this is secondary to central nervous system input into the airway through the vagus nerve or through other mechanisms is not well understood. If the patient is anxious and hyperventilating, then the above mechanism for exercise-induced wheezing might also be the etiology for wheezing with emotions.

Drugs

Drugs, especially aspirin and nonsteroidal anti-inflammatory agents, occasionally exacerbate asthma. Recent information on pathways of arachidonic acid metabolism have shown that in addition to the prostaglandins, arachidonic acid may also be converted to substances called leukotrienes. These leukotrienes are chemicals with slow reacting substance of anaphylaxis-like activity. The implication is that if nonsteroidal inflammatory agents block the production of prostaglandins, more arachidonic acid may be shunted into the production of leukotrienes. In addition to asthma, the nonsteroidal anti-inflammatory agents are associated with nasal polyps and sinus disease.

PATHOPHYSIOLOGY

All of the above mechanisms for triggering an asthmatic attack lead to the final common pathway of exaceration of asthma (Fig. 49.2). The airway in asthma shows smooth muscle hypertrophy, bronchospasm, mucous gland hypertrophy, edema, and mucous plugging. These all contribute to the obstruction seen in asthma. The airway narrowing varies from severe to mild. In treating asthmatics, it is important to remember that there is more to the obstruction than just the bronchospasm. Even in autopsy specimens smooth muscle hypertrophy, increased mucous gland secretion, and mucous plugging are seen in patients without clinical asthma.

It has been proposed that the effect of β-agonists is to increase cAMP (Fig. 49.2) by activation of adenylate cyclase and that this increase in cAMP relaxes the bronchial smooth muscle. Theophylline increases cAMP by inhibiting cAMP metabolism by

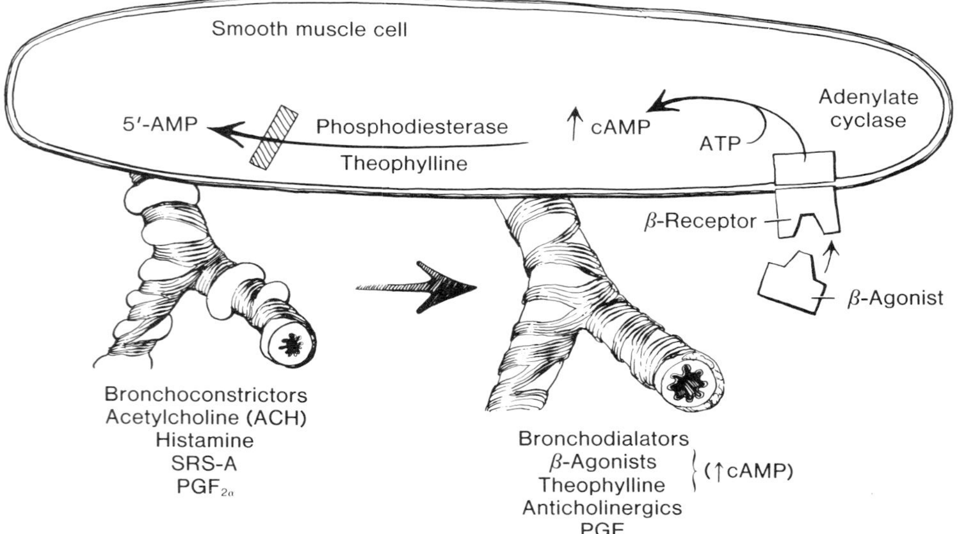

Figure 49.2 Mechanism of bronchoconstriction in asthma. *$PGF_{2\alpha}$*, prostaglandin $F_{2\alpha}$; *PGE*, prostaglandin E. *SRS-A*, slow reacting substance of anaphylaxis

hosphodiesterase. Theophylline and β-ag-nists do not operate through the same mechanism so their effects are synergistic.

:LINICAL MANIFESTATIONS

A patient presenting in the emergency epartment with acute respiratory distress iust have a careful history taken to deter-nine the etiology for the respiratory dis-ess. Asthma should be considered in any atient presenting with recurrent coughing, heezing, shortness of breath or chest ongestion.

The *rapidity* of onset of symptoms, the *equency* of attacks, and the *duration* and *everity* of symptoms should be deter-ined. The *initiating* cause, *associated ymptoms* (e.g., itchy, watery eyes; rhinor-iea; fever), and medications should be de-rmined where possible. The actual brand ame of theophylline medications and haracter of the formulation (e.g. slow-elease capsule, tablet, liquid) should be etermined as well as the time since the ist dose.

The patient's *past history* of severity, ıcluding requirements for steroid therapy, entilatory assistance, or intravenous iso-roterenol, seizures, and cardiorespiratory rrest, should be obtained.

An *environmental history* may be helpful ı determining the initiating cause and the kelihood of continued provocation. The *amily history* is important in a situation here wheezing is observed for the first me. An atopic family history suggests that ı individual is predisposed to asthma.

The manifestations of asthma are those f severe airway obstruction. The obstruc-on can be of both small and large airways. ı order to expire against the obstruction, the first anatomical response is hyperinfla-tion. This hyperinflation allows the airway to remain open on expiration. This is man-ifested by the increased anterioposterior chest diameter characteristically seen in asthmatics. As obstruction increases, expi-ration becomes more prolonged. Initially this may only be evident on force vital capacity maneuvers or on deep inspiration. As the obstruction worsens, increasing res-piratory effort is observed on expiration. This results in the use of accessory muscles of respiration. On auscultation of the chest, rhonchi and wheezes are heard. It is often at a time when the obstruction is not severe enough to cause significant wheezing that coughing may manifest itself. Coughing in fact may be the only manifestation of air-way obstruction. This is probably second-ary to increased mucus production and in-flammation of the airway.

It is very important in clinically following a patient to have some rigorous method of evaluating changes in the respiratory sta-tus. Since there may be many observers, including physician and nursing staff, a well outlined scoring or grading system is useful. The method used at Children's Hospital of Philadelphia involves assessment of cere-bral function, accessory muscle use, inspi-ratory sounds, expiratory sounds, and cy-anosis (Table 49.1). Each of these cate-gories has a score from 0 to 2 with 2 being the most severe. An outline of the scoring system is shown in Table 49.1. This scoring system takes into account the respiratory effort by the patient, the response of the central nervous system to hypoxemia, and the patient's ability to move air on inspi-ration and expiration. With this type of scoring system an organized and observant

able 49.1
linical Asthma Score

	0	1	2
	70–100 in room air	<70 in room air	<70 in 40% O_2
$_{a}O_2$ or cyanosis	None	In air	In 40% O_2
ıspiratory breath sounds	Normal	Unequal	Decreased to absent
ccessory muscle use	None	Moderate	Maximal
xpiratory wheezing	None	Moderate	Marked
erebral function	Normal	Depressed or agitated	Coma

staff should be able to monitor a patient closely. Changes in the scores often herald an approaching complication.

The chest x-ray in uncomplicated asthma shows hyperexpansion of the lungs. The anteroposterior diameter of the chest is increased, and the diaphragms are depressed. Patchy atelectasis may also be seen.

Hypoxemia develops with obstruction, and the patient responds by hyperventilating. This drives the PCO_2 down, and increases respiratory water and heat loss. If there is significant obstruction and the PCO_2 is normal, this is an indication of impending respiratory failure.

If a patient becomes severely obstructed, retention of CO_2 occurs along with profound hypoxemia. As the patient begins to retain CO_2, usually with a score of 5 or greater, the level will rise from low to normal. As ventilation continues to be a problem, more and more CO_2 will be retained. Profound changes in blood gases can occur rapidly and are often heralded by abrupt changes in the asthma score. In addition to arterial blood gases, peak flows, forced expiratory volumes (FEV), and midmaximum expiratory flow rates can be utilized to evaluate the severity of obstruction and the response to treatment (Fig. 49.3). However, pulmonary functions should not be attempted in the severely obstructed child.

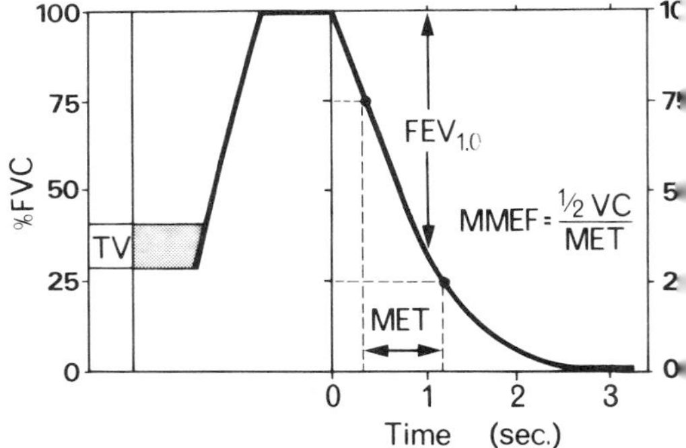

Figure 49.3 Pulmonary function measurements. FEV_1, forced expiratory volume in 1 se[c]; *FVC*, forced vital capacity; *MET*, mid maximu[m] expiratory flow time; *MMEF*, mid maximum ex[piratory] flow rate; *TV*, tidal volume; *VC*, vit[al] capacity.

Table 49.2
Complications of Asthma

I. Central Nervous System
- A. Seizures
- B. Agitation
- C. Somnolence
- D. Syndrome of inappropriate secretion [of] antidiuretic hormone

II. Respiratory
- A. Laryngeal edema or spasm
- B. Pneumothorax
- C. Pneumomediastinum
- D. Pneumonia
- E. Atelectasis

III. Cardiovascular
- A. Dehydration
- B. Hypotension
- C. Hypertension
- D. Arrhythmias
- E. Cardiac arrest

Complications

The complications outlined in Table 49.2 may arise from the disease itself or from the therapy; most frequently they involve the respiratory tract. It is important to distinguish complications from inadequate treatment of asthma as well as from overtreatment. The complications of treatment will be discussed in more detail in the section on Management.

Central Nervous System Disturbances. The most common complication of hypoxemia is a change in sensorium resulting in either a combative child or a very agitated child. A hypoxemic and agitated child does not need sedation, but does need more vigorous treatment of his hypoxemia. Agitation due to anxiety must be distinguished from agitation secondary to hypoxemia. An appropriate scoring and evaluation of the patient's pulmonary status wi[ll] give some idea about the underlying etio[l]ogy.

If the hypoxemia is more severe, seizure[s] may occur. Seizures are a disturbing aspec[t] of asthma therapy, because they furthe[r] hinder an already compromised respirator[y] effort. It is also important in therapy fo[r] asthma to keep in mind that theophyllin[e] is an epileptogenic drug when given in larg[e] enough doses. Seizures are not usually ob[-] served at theophylline levels less than ap[-] proximately 30 mg/ml but, in a patient with an underlying seizure disorder, seizures might occur at lower levels.

Inappropriate Secretion of Antidiuretic Hormone. When there is profound hypoxemia, occasionally there is inappropriate secretion of antidiuretic hormone (see p. 000). This plays a crucial role in managing the fluid status of the patient. Urine osmolality and serum osmolality should be used to evaluate whether the renal response is normal or whether the patient is significantly dehydrated.

Airway Obstruction. Complete obstruction of the upper airway may occur with laryngospasm secondary to an allergen-induced anaphylactic response. In such patients, there is usually evidence for a systemic allergic reaction; thus laryngospasm and laryngoedema respond readily to systemic adrenalin. Because of the hyperreactivity of the airway in asthmatic patients, this may also be a complication of intubation, especially for surgical procedures. Under such situations there is usually no manifestation of a systemic allergic reaction, but the irritation by the endotracheal tube exacerbates the bronchospasm and laryngospasm.

Proceeding down the airway, obstruction of the trachea or main stem bronchi may occur with mucus plugging. This is a frequent complication in children who are significantly dehydrated and have increased mucus production. If the main stem bronchi are affected, one can see atelectasis of an entire segment of the lung. If the mucus plugging occurs further down the airway, atelectasis of smaller segments may occur. Figure 49.4 shows an x-ray of a patient who had atelectasis of a large portion of his left lung. Subsegmental atelactasis is a common complication of status asthmaticus. Infiltrates on chest x-rays are usually secondary to atelectasis rather than lobar pneumonia. Atelectasis can usually be distinguished from pneumonia by the fact that the atelectatic segment shows volume loss, whereas pneumonia is usually a volume expanding lesion.

Pneumothorax and Pneumomediastinum. In addition to atelectasis, the occurrence of a pneumothorax or pneumomediastinum must also be considered in a patient who presents with decreased aeration, either bilaterally or asymmetrically. In the patient with a hyperinflated chest, the chances of a pneumothorax or a pneumomediastinum increase dramatically. Evaluation of the patient must be made rapidly in order to facilitate proper treatment. A pneumomediastinum can progress to a pneumopericardium with cardiac tamponade.

Cardiac Arrhythmias. In the patient who is on numerous agents including inhaled bronchodilators, the problem of cardiac arrythmias may be encountered. The most common reasons for arrythmias are abuse of inhaled β-agonists and the combination of β-agonists, theophylline, and hypoxemia.

MANAGEMENT

The known asthmatic child with an uncomplicated attack needs no laboratory or radiographic evaluations. A chest x-ray should be obtained in a child with a first episode of wheezing to look for other diseases (such as cystic fibrosis or a foreign body aspiration) and in the patient suspected clinically of having pulmonary complications (e.g., pneumonia or pneumothorax). Evidence of severe obstruction, such as markedly decreased inspiratory air flow or an asthma score (Table 49.1) greater than or equal to 5, mandates an arterial blood gas analysis.

The treatment for status asthmaticus revolves around the three causes for obstruction: bronchospasm, mucosal edema, and mucus secretion and plugging. Pharmacotherapy must be utilized to address all of the above. The initial treatment of the asthmatic should include inhaled oxygen. This oxygen should be humidified in order to minimize heat loss from the airway in the hyperventilating patient. In addition to oxygen, therapy should begin with appropriate bronchodilators. The drugs most commonly used for the initial treatment of asthma are subcutaneous epinephrine or terbutaline. The dose of epinephrine is 0.01 ml (1/1000 solution) per kilogram up to a maximum of 0.35 ml. Inhaled β-agonists may be used in lieu of subcutaneous drugs

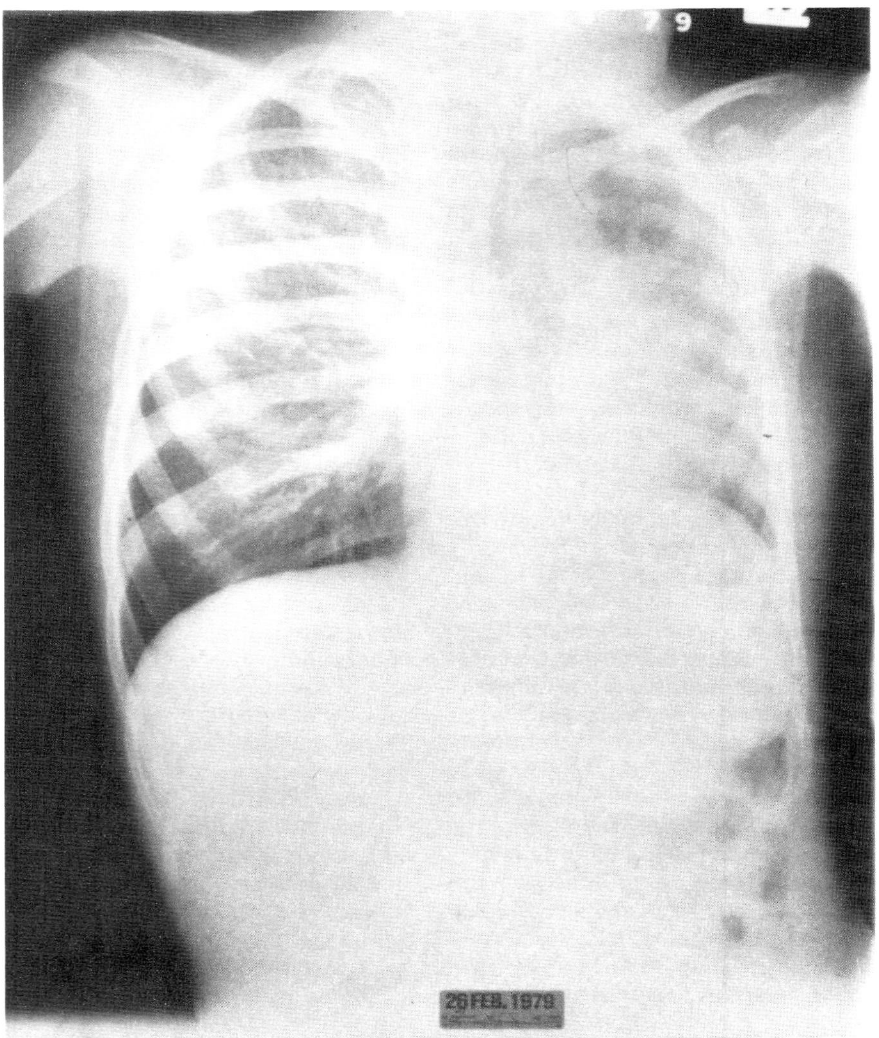

Figure 49.4 Severe atelectases of the left lung in child with asthma.

if adequate ventilation and respiratory effort can be obtained from a cooperative patient. The β-agonists available for inhalation treatment include isoproterenol, isoetharine, metaproterenol, terbutaline, and albuterol. Positive pressure treatments with inhaled bronchodilators should never be used, because of the possibility that the delivery system may cause a pneumothorax or pneumomediastinum. Guidelines for inhalation treatments are given in Table 49.3. Epinephrine and terbutaline subcutaneously or isoproterenol by inhalation, should be given every 20 min for maximum benefi A maximum of three doses is usually ut lized. Studies have shown that inhaled is proterenol and parenteral epinephrine terbutaline have similar bronchodilator c pacities.

Increased bronchodilation is obtained in addition to the aforementioned drug intravenous aminophylline is also given. the patient who is in severe enough distre to potentially require hospitalization d spite catecholamine therapy, an intrav nous dose of aminophylline should be give

Table 49.3
Recommended Protocol for Use of Nebulized Isoproterenol and Metaproterenol

Isoproterenol (inhalation solution 1:200, 5 mg/ml)
1. 0.25 ml in 2.5 ml normal saline for children 2 to 9 yr
2. 0.50 ml in 2.5 ml normal saline for children over 9 yr

Metaproterenol (inhalation solution 5%, 50 mg/ml)
1. 0.20 ml in 2.5 ml normal saline for children 2 to 9 yr
2. 0.30 ml in 2.5 ml normal saline for children over 9 yr

in addition to the other drugs (see Equations 1 and 2). If no aminophylline or theophylline has been taken orally, then a good approximation for how much aminophylline can be given safely is shown in Equation 1, where the bolus dose of aminophylline needed to achieve a serum level of aminophylline is the bolus dose divided by the volume of distribution (Vd). The volume of distribution is approximately 0.5 L/kg. This is a good estimate, varying only in very small children and premature infants. Looking at the equation, it can be seen that a bolus dose of 6 mg/kg of aminophylline will raise the serum level of theophylline by approximately 10 μg/ml. If the desired level is higher than 10 μg/ml, then larger boluses may be utilized. The bolus dose of aminophylline is not dependent on the metabolism of the drug, but only depends on the volume of distribution.

Equations for aminophylline administration are:

$$\Delta\text{Cpo. (change in level)} = (\text{bolus dose/Vd}) \times 0.85 \quad (1)$$

$$\text{Cpss (steady state level)} = (\text{infusion rate} \times 0.85/\text{clearance}) \quad (2)$$

For constant infusion of aminophylline, a calculation based on the patient's daily dose or on a theophylline clearance can help decide what an appropriate infusion should be. Using Equation 2, the theophylline level at steady state is equal to the infusion rate of theophylline divided by the theophylline clearance. If one has a theophylline clearance from previous studies, than one can easily calculate the infusion rate necessary to give a desired serum steady state level. If the patient has had good levels of theophylline on oral doses of medication, one can calculate the infusion rate by dividing the 24-hour theophylline requirement for the individual by 24 in order to estimate the hourly theophylline requirement. This is a reasonable approximation. If the oral medication the patient has been on has not given adequate theophylline levels or if no previous clearances are available, a starting dose of 0.9 mg/kg/hour for adolescents and 1.1 mg/kg/hour for younger children should be utilized. For intermittent bolus aminophylline treatment, the guidelines for therapy should take into account the fact that younger children have a much more rapid clearance of theophylline than do adolescents and adults. The bolus therapy with aminophylline will require similar calculations. A dose of 6 mg/kg every 6 hours or 4 mg/kg every 4 hours gives the same total theophylline dose per day as a 1 mg/kg per hour constant infusion, but will be associated with a higher peak level.

To eliminate errors, a standard method for preparation of the infusion is advisable. The infusion should be made up by multiplying the patient's weight in kg by the desired number of mg/kg/hour (i.e., 0.9 or 1.1 mg) and placing that amount of aminophylline in each 25 ml of diluting solution. The infusion is then run at 25 ml/hour, giving the proper rate of infusion of 0.9 or 1.1 mg/kg/hour.

If theophylline levels are not available, the child should be closely observed for symptoms of theophylline toxicity. These are nausea and vomiting, diuresis, and tachycardia at approximately 20 μg/ml and hypotension and seizures as the levels go above 30 μg/ml. Seizures from theophylline toxicity are extremely difficult to control with anticonvulsant agents. Because of this, the most effective means of controlling theophylline seizures is elimination of the drug. If oral doses of the medication have been taken recently, then lavage, charcoal, and cathartics should be utilized. If the levels are significantly elevated, charcoal hemoprofusion may be necessary in order to eliminate the drug.

It is best to remember that as theophylline levels increase, the enzyme system for metabolism of the drug becomes saturated. With saturation of the liver microsomal enzyme system, the elimination of the drug switches from first order kinetics to zero order kinetics. This means that the amount of drug that can be eliminated per hour is fixed. The fixed elimination will continue until the saturation of the enzyme system is no longer present.

In addition to theophylline, corticosteroids may be necessary, especially for the child who has previously been on such drugs or is obstructed enough to require admission. A dose of 4 mg/kg of hydrocortisone or an equivalent amount of another steroid preparation, should be given.

The child with asthma should receive appropriate fluid management to correct any dehydration that may be present. Patients with status asthmaticus often have vomiting and increased fluid losses from their hyperventilation. It is for this reason that appropriate fluids should be given in order that the patient may maintain the normal turgor of the mucous membranes. It is probably unnecessary for the patient to receive fluids much over maintenance after rehydration. A normovolemic state is to be preferred to a hypervolemic state. With excessive fluid administration, the likelihood of pulmonary edema and hypertension increase.

If the patient does not respond to the initial therapy and shows evidence of increasing respiratory distress and retention of CO_2, then therapy should begin with intravenous isoproterenol. The isoproterenol is begun at a dose of 0.1 μg/kg/min and increased every 15 min by 0.1 μg/kg/min until a response is seen or severe tachycardia occurs. If, despite intravenous isoproterenol at maximal doses, the patient continues to be in respiratory failure, then intubation and ventilation may be necessary. Ventilation in the asthmatic is associated with many complications including pneumomediastinum, pneumopericardium, pneumothorax, atelectasis, pneumonia, and inappropriate antidiuretic hormone secretion. The presence of the endotracheal tube in the trachea may also exacerbate the wheezing.

If the acute episode is reversed with appropriate medication and the patient is ready for discharge from the emergency department, then several goals must be taken into consideration: (1) an effort must be made to remove the trigger, if at all possible; (2) sustained bronchodilation must be maintained with injected long acting epinephrine in the form of susphrine (0.005 ml/kg to 0.15 ml) and oral bronchodilators; and (3) appropate follow-up must be arranged. Theophylline should be given at a starting dose of 5 mg/kg every 6 hours for children older than 1 year and at 4 mg/kg every 6 to 8 hours for adolescents. Additional β-agonists (metaproterenol, 10 to 20 mg every 6 hours) or steroids (prednisone, 1 to 2 mg/kg/day) may be needed.

ANAPHYLAXIS AND ANAPHYLACTOID REACTIONS

BACKGROUND

The systemic manifestation of an allergic reaction is characterized as anaphylaxis, a life-threatening emergency that requires immediate attention. These reactions are usually immediate hypersensitivity reactions that occur soon after antigen exposure. The true anaphylactic response occurs only after a repeated contact with a particular antigen and is the manifestation of sensitization with the particular antigen. It is usually an IgE-mediated reaction where on first exposure to the antigen IgE antibodies are formed. On reexposure to the antigen, symptoms develop.

The development of IgE antibodies is often dependent on both the nature of the antigen and the degree of atopy of the individual. Atopy is a hereditary predisposition to the formation of IgE antibodies. Individuals with atopy may have an increased incidence of anaphylactic reactions. This is not a requirement, however, since patients without atopy have also been known to have sensitivities to pencillin and hymenoptera. The occurrence of anaphylactic reactions to the same antigen in family members is also well recognized. This is one of the reasons why a strong family history of penicillin allergy is often used as an indication for avoiding penicillin therapy.

Every route of exposure from intravenous to oral administration has been associated with anaphylaxis, although parenteral administration tends to cause more severe reactions. The most common etiologies for anaphylactic-like reactions are exposure to hymenoptera, drugs, immunotherapy, foods, radiocontrast media, and blood products.

Penicillin

Penicillin and penicillin derivatives are probably the most common cause of anaphylactic reactions. The reaction may occur following oral or parenteral administration and often occurs in patients that have a negative history for previous reactions. In the patient with a previous history of a reaction, skin testing can often detect those that have IgE antibodies to penicillin. Penicilloyl polylysine (PPL) is used to test the major determinant in penicillin sensitization and detects a majority of the positive patients. Minor determinant sensitization can be detected by using the minor determinants for testing or penicillin G. Penicillin G does not pick up all those patients sensitive to the minor determinants, and testing with it can sensitize a patient.

There is a cross reactivity between penicillin and the cephalosporins, and this must be kept in mind when substituting a cephalosporin for a penicillin derivative in the penicillin sensitive patient.

Insect Stings

Insect sting hypersensitivity is fairly common. The reaction may be local or systemic. The insects usually involved are the hymenoptera (bees, hornets, wasps, yellow jackets) which are common and present throughout the United States. The reactions that occur are predominantly against the venom from the stinging insect. With the use of venoms for hyposensitization, reactions to venom immunotherapy injections have also increased.

Foods

Of the foods incriminated in anaphylactic reactions, the most common are nuts, peanuts, sea food, eggs, milk, and berries. Most fatal anaphylactic reactions from foods occur in the older age group.

Immunotherapy

Injection of extracts of allergens for hyposensitization in highly atopic individuals is still a common cause of anaphylactic reactions. It may occur at extract doses that have previously been tolerated especially during a concomitant seasonal exposure or with changes to a new batch of extract.

Hormones

The use of insulin, ACTH, and other hormones of animal origin has led to the development of sensitization to these agents. The reactions are usually mediated by IgE. The patients are skin test positive to the hormone derived from the particular animal to which they have become sensitive. Desensitization or a switch to another source of the hormone is usually necessary if the hormone is essential like insulin.

Radiocontrast Media

Radiocontrast studies have been associated with a significant number of adverse reactions. The reactions have been associated with urticaria, angioedema, bronchospasm, hypotension, cardiac arrhythmia and arrest. Despite these anaphylactic manifestations, the reactions have not been associated with an IgE-mediated process. They are thought to be secondary to direct effects on basophils causing mediator release or complement activation. Intravenous cholangiograms with meglumine iodipamide (Cholografin) are associated with the highest incidence of anaphylaxis, but almost all iodinated radiocontrast media carry some risk.

Other Drugs

In addition to penicillin and its derivatives, there are a large number of other drugs associated with allergic reactions, some of which are shown in Table 49.4. Some drugs can also cause spontaneous histamine release. The most common of these are morphine, codeine, *d*-tubocurarine, and polymyxin antibiotics.

Other Agents

Inhaled pollens can occasionally be associated with anaphylaxis. Animal danders are also commonly implicated.

PATHOPHYSIOLOGY

Anaphylaxis is the systemic manifestation of an immediate hypersensitivity reaction. This necessitates formation of reagenic antibodies that are of the IgE class predominantly. IgE binds to tissue mast cells and for this reason is called homocytotropic. Bound IgE on cells can then interact with antigen at the cell surface to initiate activation. Antigen must bridge at least two IgE molecules in order to get degranulation of the mast cell. (Fig. 49.5). This bridging of IgE molecules is associated with changes in the phospholipid membrane and with an influx of calcium which activates an esterase and causes degranulation of the mast cell with histamine release. Increases in intracellular cyclic AMP inhibit degranulation; activation of the adenylate cyclase by β-adrenergic agents or inhibition of the degradation of cyclic AMP by phosphodiesterase inhibitors, such as theophylline, leads to a buildup of cyclic AMP.

Table 49.4
Some Drugs Associated with Anaphylaxis and Anaphylactoid Reactions

I. Immune-mediated
- A. Penicillin
- B. Penicillin derivatives
- C. Cephalosporins
- D. Sulfonamides
- E. Local anesthetics
- F. Antiarrhythmic agents
- G. Organic mercurials
- H. Streptomycin
- I. Dyes
- J. Tetracyclines

II. Nonimmune-mediated
- A. Morphine
- B. Codeine
- C. Polymyxin antibiotics
- D. *d*-Tubocurarine
- E. Radiocontrast media

Mediators of Anaphylaxis

The mediators of anaphylaxis can be separated into two groups, preformed and secondary. The performed mediators are histamine, eosinophil chemotactic factor of anaphylaxis, neutrophil chemotactic factor, heparin, neutral protease, and acid hydrolases. Histamine causes contraction of smooth muscle, increased vascular permeability, and an elevation of cyclic AMP. It is inactivated by histaminase and histamine methyltransferase. Eosinophilic chemotactic factor functions as an attractant and deactivator of eosinophils and neutrophils, while neutrophil chemotactic factor has the same role for neutrophils. Heparin is an anticoagulant and also inhibits complement activation.

The secondary mediators of anaphylaxis are slow reacting substance of anaphylaxis (SRS-A) and platelet activating factor. SRS-A, a leukotriene, causes contraction of human bronchial smooth muscle and an increase in vascular permeability. It is deactivated by arylsulfutase A and B. Platelet activating factor (PAF), a phospholipid derivative, is associated in rabbits with the aggregation of platelets. It is deactivated by a phospholipase corroborating its lipid structure. The secondary mediators of anaphylaxis can arise from cells other than the mast cells and may be released by cells activated by the primary mediators of anaphylaxis.

CLINICAL MANIFESTATIONS

The most common manifestations of anaphylaxis are urticaria, angioedema, pruritis, laryngeal edema, hypotension, bronchospasm, hyperperistalasis, and cardiac arrhythmias.

History

Since these reactions are the result of an immediate hypersensitivity reaction, the history should focus on the period of time immediately before the reaction began. The 1- to 2-hour period before the onset of symptoms may offer the key to the etiology of the reaction if it is not obvious. As has

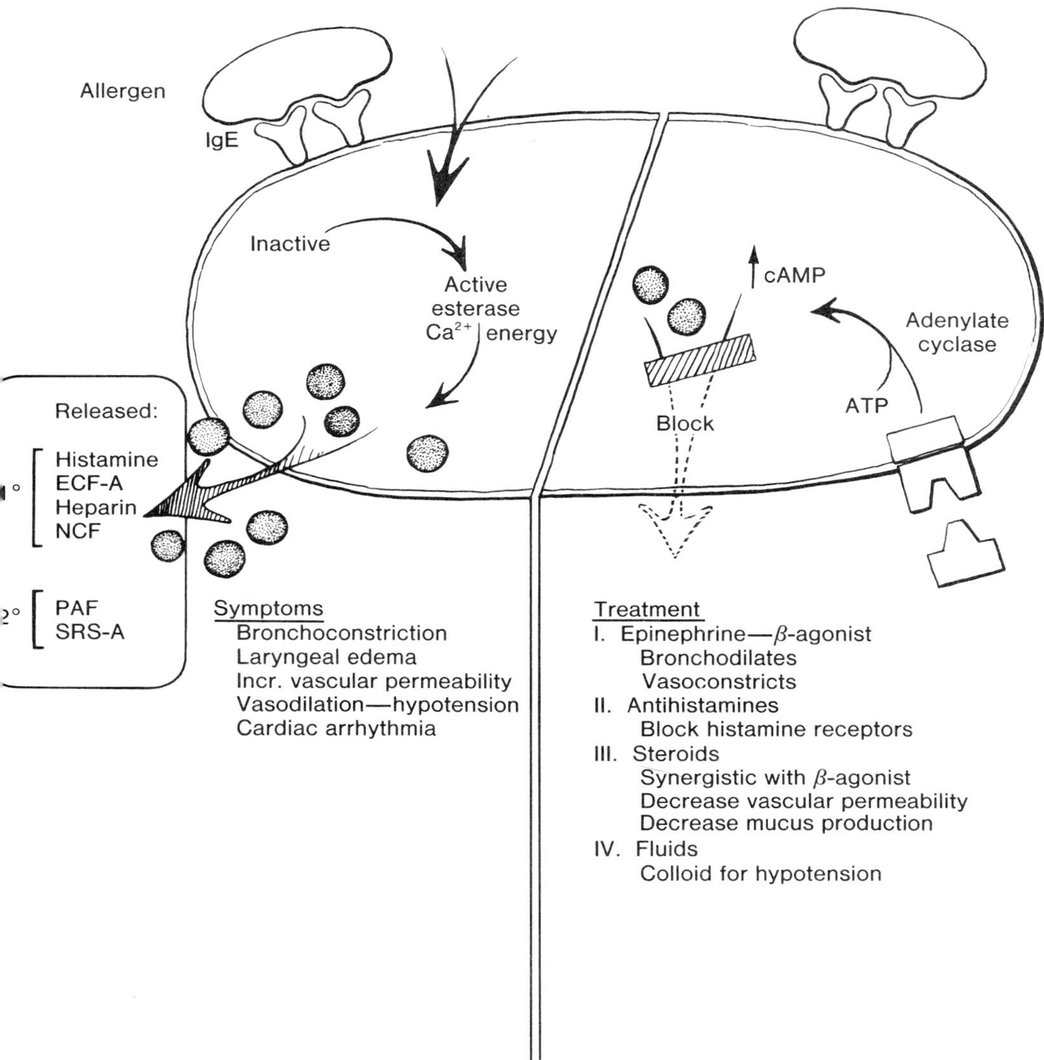

igure 49.5 Mechanism involved in anaphylaxis and the treatment rationale. ECF-A, eosinophil hemotactic factor of anaphylaxis; PAF, platelet activating factor.

een outlined, the common agents that ause anaphylaxis are often evident without nuch questioning. The association of anaphylactic reactions with foods is often less bvious. Although people often pick out a articular food and focus on it as the cause, more detailed dietary history may in fact mplicate something else in the meal that vas not apparent at first. People associate dverse reactions with chocolate when it is ot that common an agent, whereas the nuts in many of these preparations are often the cause of the reactions.

In addition to determining the etiology, the type of reaction and the severity must be ascertained. A history of a change in voice, difficulty swallowing, or dyspnea should give rise to immediate action before seeking any other historical information. Angioedema without pruritus, or a pruritic rash and the finding of a family history of angioedema, point to hereditary angioedema which is secondary to a deficiency of C1 esterase inhibitor.

Physical Examination

The physical examination should focus on (1) vital signs for evidence of hypotension and shock, (2) the cardiac examination for signs of arrhythmia, adequate cardiac impulse, and rate; (3) the airway and lungs for signs of tongue swelling, laryngeal edema, or bronchospasm; and (4) the skin for evidence of altered perfusion, angioedema, and the rash.

Urticaria. Urticaria is a common manifestation of immediate hypersensitivity reactions. In addition to being a sign of immediate hypersensitivity, it is also a manifestation of a number of other disease processes. In the patient with acute urticaria from an IgE-mediated process, the urticaria that develops may be localized to the area of exposure, such as the area around a sting. In addition to the localized urticaria, there may be a systemic reaction. Urticaria is often associated with angioedema which is swelling of the lower dermis and subcutaneous tissues. Angioedema is not usually pruritic, but when associated with urticaria there is pruritus. Angioedema with pruritic urticaria needs to be distinguished from angioedema secondary to processes other than immediate hypersensitivity. The urticarias are usually separated into those that are acute and those that are chronic. Most immediate hypersensitivity reactions are associated with an acute reaction, but chronic recurrent urticaria could be mediated by an unknown antigen that was associated with recurrent exposure. In determining the cause of an urticarial reaction, the classification shown in Table 49.5 is important in deciding what the course of action should be after the control of the episode for which the patient is being treated.

Table 49.5
Urticaria: Classification

- I. *Dermographism*
- II. *Physical Urticaria*
    - A. Cold
    - B. Cholinergic
    - C. Pressure
    - D. Solar
- III. *Familial Urticaria*
    - A. Hereditary angioedema
    - B. Familial cold urticaria
- IV. *Urticaria Secondary to Common Agents*
- V. *Urticaria Secondary to Serum Sickness*

The physical urticarial reactions can be life-threatening, and they should be part of the differential diagnosis of anaphylaxis. *Cold urticaria* is an acute reaction to cold temperatures with hives at the site of cold exposure. Generalized cold exposure such as with immersion in a cold pool can precipitate an anaphylactic reaction with hypotension and shock. The cold urticarias are often acquired and may follow viral infections. There is a familial cold urticaria that is rare and is associated with a delayed onset, leukocytosis and pain that distinguishes it from acquired cold urticaria. *Cholinergic urticaria* is characterized by punctate hives surrounded by an erythematous flare. The reaction can be precipitated by exercise, anxiety, shivers, and temperature change. It has been associated with exercise-induced anaphylaxis and often causes systemic manifestations (i.e., abdominal pain, headaches, etc.). *Solar urticaria* is a reaction to light, often sunlight, with the development of pruritus, erythema, and edema. Solar urticaria can be a manifestation of porphyria. *Pressure urticaria* is associated with hives developing at the site of significant prolonged pressure in areas of the body. It is often associated with tight clothing. Other urticarias such as aquagenic urticaria are rare and are usually not seen in children.

Laryngeal edema is a life threatening swelling of the upper respiratory tract secondary to an immediate hypersensitivity reaction. Any patient who comes in and is unable to speak or has stridor on inspiration, has significant laryngeal edema.

Cardiovascular Signs. The rapid decrease in plasma volume that occurs with anaphylactic reactions may produce hypotension and shock. Rarely, cardiac arrest and arrhythmias occur as complications of anaphylaxis; these are probably secondary ɔ the cardiotoxic effects of histamine and ther mediators.

Smooth Muscle Contraction. Hyper-eristalsis and uterine contractions may oc-ur in anaphylactic reactions. These may resent with abdominal pain or, in the case f pregnancy, premature labor.

MANAGEMENT

Initiation of treatment requires that the irway, heart, vascular system, central ner-ous system (CNS), abdomen, and skin be valuated. These are the focus of treatment s outlined in Figure 49.5. The resuscitative fforts in anaphylaxis require: (1) mainte-ance of an adequate airway, (2) mainte-ance of the circulation with adequate renal nd CNS perfusion, (3) control of any car-iac arrhythmias, and (4) treatment of ur-caria and abdominal symptoms.

Maintenance of the Airway. Laryngeal dema and severe bronchospasm may ob-ruct the airway. The first line of treat-ent is epinephrine, 0.01 ml/kg (1:1000), to maximum dose of 0.4 ml. This acts as utlined in Figure 49.5 in several ways. Its -adrenergic properties cause bronchodila-on and inhibit granule release from mast ells and other inflammatory cells, and its drenergic effects cause vasoconstriction lthough the clinical significance of this roperty is questionable at these doses. pinephrine may be given every 15 to 20 in. If epinephrine does not reverse the ryngeal edema, intubation of the trachea r tracheostomy may be necessary. In pa-ents with hereditary angioedema, epi-ephrine is not effective, and insertion of n artificial airway will probably be neces-ary with life threatening laryngeal swell-g.

Bronchospasm can be treated with in-aled isoproterenol and intravenous ami-ophylline (see under "Asthma") in con-unction with epinephrine, if epinephrine one is not effective. Isoproterenol (0.25 ml oproterenol 1:200/2.0 ml saline at age < 9 ears, 0.5 ml isoproterenol/2.0 ml saline at ge > 9 years) administered by a nebulizer an effective bronchodilator. It works syn-rgistically with epinephrine and aminophylline in dilating the bronchial tree. Aminophylline at 5 to 7.5 mg/kg can be given in an i.v. bolus over 30 min. If bronchospasm does not improve with the above, then intravenous isoproterenol or intubation may be necessary.

Maintenance of the Circulation. In a patient with hypotension, intravenous fluid therapy should begin immediately in addition to epinephrine. Ringer's lactate or normal saline at 20 ml/kg should be given in a bolus and then continuously until adequate perfusion and blood pressure are maintained (Chapter 2). If hypotension remains a problem despite volume expansion, then a central venous pressure (CVP) line should be established; if the CVP is low, more fluid should be administered. If it is high, sympathomimetic agents should be used to increase cardiac output. Since plasma volume may fall by 20 to 40%, large amounts of fluid may be necessary in the resuscitation.

Cardiac Arrhythmias. Decreased cardiac output, arrhythmias, and myocardial ischemia may arise in anaphylaxis. The myocardial ischemia is usually associated with shock. Resuscitation should include the above mentioned treatment for shock, plus efforts at monitoring cardiac function. A CVP line should be placed, and, if the CVP is elevated, pressors such as metaraminol or norepinephrine should be used (Chapter 2).

Urticaria. Diphenhydramine (1 mg/kg i.v., i.m. or, if not severe, p.o.) is the antihistamine which is most commonly used as an histamine antagonist. In the case of cold urticaria, cyproheptadine is the drug of choice (0.25 mg/kg/day), whereas hydroxyzine (1 to 2 mg/kg/day) is preferred for cholinergic urticaria or most of the other chronic urticarias. Corticosteroids in the form of hydrocortisone at 150 to 200 mg intravenously can be given during the acute anaphylactic episode, but will not have significant beneficial effects for 4 to 6 hours.

Determination of the antigen that was responsible for the anaphylaxis is vitally important from the point of view of eliminating it, if it is still present on presentation to the emergency department, and for avoidance in the future. If a slowly absorbed antigen has been injected, the application of a tourniquet and the administration of epinephrine (0.005 ml/kg, 1:1000) at the site will ameliorate the reaction. In a patient who has had a life-threatening episode with an antigen that cannot be totally avoided, an anaphylaxis kit containing preloaded adrenaline should be accessible to the patient at all times.

SERUM SICKNESS

BACKGROUND

The first cases of serum sickness were noted at the beginning of the century. These cases were associated with the injection of horse serum antitoxins to various toxins such as the one causing tetanus. In the years since that time, techniques have developed in order to eliminate use of foreign proteins. Even in recent times, however, some indications still remain for the use of horse serum. Exposure to foreign serum proteins stems from the utilization of reagents like antithymocyte globulin from horses for patients preceding transplanatations or those with abnormal clones of T lymphocytes. In addition to the reactions from foreign proteins, a serum sickness-like illness can occur with various drugs, chemicals, infectious agents, or autologous antigens.

It is often extremely difficult to separate the syndromes that one sees secondary to an immediate hypersensitivity reaction from those due to a serum sickness-like reaction. In both, the clinical manifestations may be fairly similar. In the former IgE is primarily responsible, while the latter is mediated by IgG or IgM immune complexes. In a number of cases, both processes may be involved.

Serum Proteins

Antithymocyte globulins, horse antitetanus toxoid, and human γ-globulin can produce a serum sickness-like picture. In the case of patients with hypogammaglobulinemia receiving γ-globulin, the reaction is thought to be secondary to microaggregates of immunoglobulin. Centrifugation and filtration of the preparation or plasma therapy reduce this complication.

Drugs

If a drug binds to a protein and alters i antigenic determinants, then the new dru protein-complex may act to produce a se rum sickness-like reaction. This can be see with drugs such as penicillin, its vario derivatives and the cross reactive cephal sporins. A significant number of the dru cited as causes of anaphylactic reactio are also implicated in serum sickness-lil reactions. Penicillin, pencillin derivative cephalosporins, sulfonamides, thriourac streptomycin, hydantoins, and *p*-aminosa icylic acid have been incriminated. Becau these drugs are all low molecular weig substances, they cannot act as antigens d rectly but must bind to proteins, usual through their metabolites. For this reas it is often difficult to substantiate sensit zation.

Blood Products

Patients receiving frequent transfusio of cellular elements or blood products su as cryoprecipitate often have reactions the transfusions. The reactions are usual acute and are often associated with ur caria, angioedema, and fever.

Infectious Agents

Infectious mononucleosis, hepatitis B other chronic viral infections can also pr duce a serum sickness-like reaction that often chronic. The reaction occurs wi agents that are not quickly cleared a maintain a significant antigen level. Th may be evidenced by signs of a chron vasculitis.

Autologous Antigens

Occasionally autologous antigens such tumor-associated antigens or autoimmu disease antigens (i.e. double standed DN may lead to clinical manifestations of seru sickness. This is not surprising since th are often associated with immune com plexes in the circulation.

PATHOPHYSIOLOGY

In the classical serum sickness model, a animal is injected with foreign serum pr tein. Seven days later the animal develo the symptoms characteristic of serum sic ness. During the initial period after th injection of the foreign protein, there is a period of antigen excess (see Fig. 49.6). This is a period during which no antibody has been formed. Antibodies develop at approximately 6 to 10 days after the initial antigen was injected, and antibody-antigen complexes may then form. These immune complexes may deposit in the tissues and may also activate complement. Following this period of immune complex formation, there is a period of antibody excess during which there is clearance of antigen from the system. Symptoms develop when there are soluble immune complexes being cleared by the body. The immune complexes can activate complement through their receptors. These receptors fix complement and activate the classical pathway (Fig. 49.7).

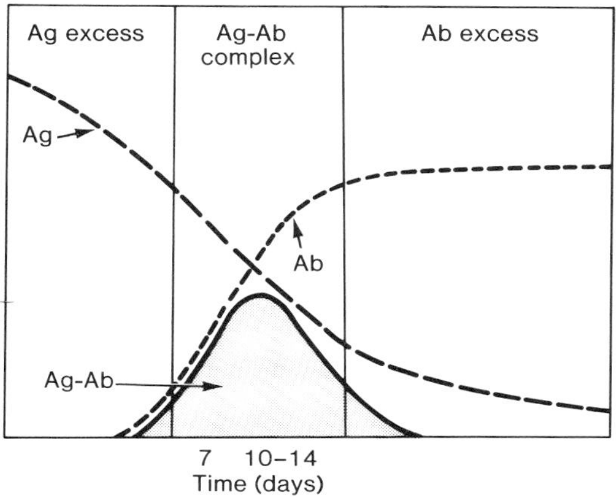

Figure 49.6 Time course of immune complex formation.

The classical pathway of activation begins with the formation of the Clq antibody complex which activates a Cl esterase that cleaves the fourth and second complement components (C4 and C2). The C4 and C2 which have been activated can then cleave C3. It is cleavage of C3 and generation of all of its active components that allows for the activation of the late-acting complement components (C5 to C9). Since the immune complex activation involves the classical components, C4, C2, and C3, their serum concentration decreases. The complement activation generates the anaphylatoxins C3a and C5a which increase vascular permeability, release histamine, and produce bronchospasm. They activate many other cells in the inflammatory process and lead to inflammation around deposits of complexes in various tissues.

Clearance of immune complexes depends on their size and the effectiveness of the reticuloendothelial system. The organ sys-

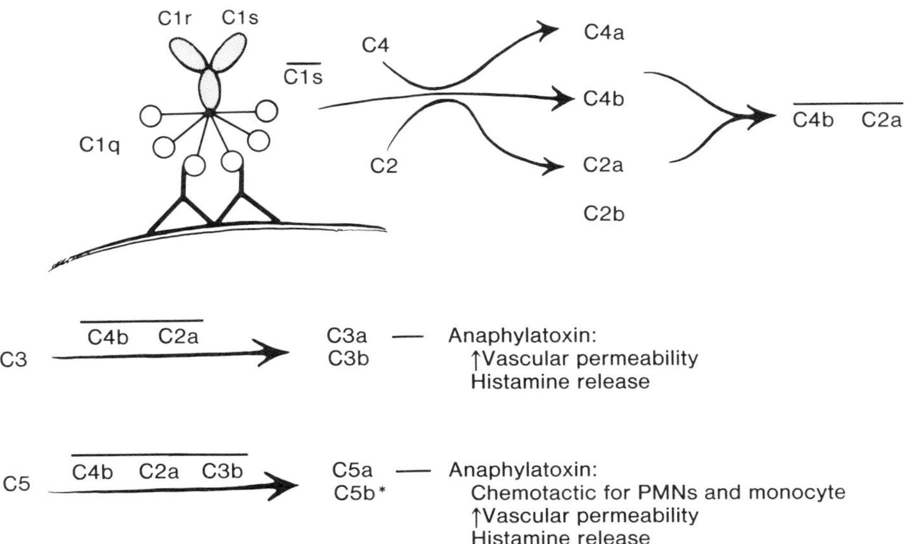

Figure 49.7 Complement activation sequence.

tems that are most vulnerable to damage by circulating immune complexes are those with a filtering membrane. The kidneys are commonly involved, as are the vascular system and choroid plexus.

If serum sickness is due to a primary exposure, the symptoms occur 7 to 14 days after the initial exposure. If there has been a prior exposure, then the second exposure will often result in a more rapid onset of symptoms, usually within 1 to 4 days. It has also been shown in experimental animals that immune complex deposition can be enhanced by concomitant activation of an immediate hypersensitivity reaction because IgE-mediated mast cell degranulation increases permeability, enhancing immune complex deposition. For this reason, these disease processes are not distinct entities, but rather a spectrum from IgE-mediated anaphylaxis at one extreme to IgG- or IgM-mediated immune complex disease at the other. There may be significant overlap with some clinical conditions involving both processes.

CLINICAL MANIFESTATIONS

The clinical manifestations of serum sickness are often indistinguishable from anaphylactic reactions and involve the same agents. The findings include a pruritic rash (maculopopular or urticarial most commonly), angioedema, fever, abdominal pain, lymphodenopathy, arthritis, nephritis, carditis, hypotension, anemia, and rarely neuritis.

History

Since the symptoms are those of an immune complex-mediated process, it is not only important to treat the process, but to determine and eliminate the agent if at all possible. The onset of symptoms occurs 7 to 14 days after a primary exposure; thus, this period of time should be reviewed when trying to ascertain a possible etiology for the process. Since a secondary exposure can produce a more rapid onset of symptoms (1 to 4 days), inquiries about this interval must be made if the source is not obvious; patients are often not aware of primary exposures if they have been relatively asymptomatic. The history should also include information about possible organ system involvement including the CNS, respiratory tract, heart, joints, gastrointestinal tract, urinary tract, and skin. A rash may have changed and evolved with time so it is important to know the nature and course of the rash as well as whether or not it is pruritic. Changes in memory, mood, and school performance may suggest CNS involvement. Abdominal pain, nausea, vomiting, diarrhea, and melena may be signs of gastrointestinal inflammation. Nephritis, arthritis, or carditis should also be considered; the physician should ask about hematuria, flank pain, peripheral edema, joint pain and swelling, and symptoms of congestive heart failure.

Physical Examination

As outlined above, the clinical manifestations of serum sickness encompass almost every organ system. Examination of the skin may show a maculopapular eruption, urticaria, or the palpable purpura of a cutaneous vasculitis, usually seen on the lower extremities. Generalized lymphadenopathy often occurs. Wheezes may be heard on auscultation of the lungs, and a pericardial friction rub may be audible if pericarditis is present. The liver and spleen often enlarge. Characteristically, the extremities are involved; examination of the joints may show erythema, warmth, and an effusion. Rarely, neurologic deficits occur secondary to a vasculitis of the central nervous system.

Laboratory

One should evaluate a patient for manifestation of an immune complex-mediated disease as outlined in Table 49.6. The erythrocyte sedimentation rate may be elevated. A CBC and differential may show a leukopenia or leukocytosis, and the urine may contain cells or casts. The CH_50 may decrease due to complement activation. A C3 and C4 should be determined. Since the complement components are acute phase reactants, they often go up with inflammation. A mild depression of C3 and C4 may be indicative of complement activation and can be followed over time. Any of the tests for circulating immune complexes (e.g., cryoglobulins) may be utilized. A screening

Table 49.6
Possible Laboratory Evaluation of Serum Sickness

Test
Blood Tests
Erythrocyte sedimentation rate
CBC with differential
CH_{50}, C_3, C_4
BUN, creatinine
ANA[a]
Rheumatoid factor (RF)[a]
Hepatic enzymes[a]
Hepatitis B screen[a]
Heterophil antibody[a]
Immune complex assay[a]
Other Laboratory Tests
Urinalysis
ECG
Hematest stool[a]
EEG[a]
CAT scan[a]

[a] Tests to be done at discretion of clinician and depending on likely etiology.

ECG should also be done in any severe cases. Stool evaluation for blood should be performed on patients with abdominal pain or symptoms referrable to the gastrointestinal tract. Headache or focal neurologic deficits can occur, and are indications for an EEG and/or CAT scan.

MANAGEMENT

The treatment of serum sickness requires an understanding of the disease process. Since the usual onset involves only pruritus and rash, treatment is initiated with an antihistamine such as diphenhydramine at mg/kg every 4 to 6 hours orally. If the disease progresses to joint involvement, nonsteroidal anti-inflammatory agents such as aspirin (100 mg/kg/day) are useful. With significant systemic involvement, corticosteroids (prednisone, 1 to 2 mg/kg/day) should be used, continued until improvement occurs, and then tapered as symptoms decrease. If laryngeal edema or life-threatening airway obstruction occurs, epinephrine is indicated as outlined under "Anaphylaxis and Anaphylactoid Reactions."

There must be an effort made throughout the evaluation to determine the antigen responsible, and to remove it if possible. If a slowly absorbed antigen has been injected and symptoms develop at the site, a tourniquet can retard its access to the rest of the circulation, and epinephrine 0.005 ml/kg (1:1000) should be injected locally.

In life-threatening serum sickness with significant circulating immune complexes, plasmaphoresis may play a role, but this procedure has not yet been utilized extensively for treatment of this disease.

CYSTIC FIBROSIS

INTRODUCTION

Cystic fibrosis (CF) is the most common lethal inherited disease among Caucasians in this country. CF is a generalized defect in all of the exocrine gland secretions. Although it is inherited as an autosomal recessive condition, there is no clinical feature or biochemical marker which can reliably identify a heterogygote carrier for CF. Most homozyotes for the disease have the "classical triad" of clinical findings: (1) chronic pulmonary disease, (2) malabsorption secondary to pancreatic insufficiency, and (3) elevated concentration of sweat electrolytes. However, it must be emphasized that there is a great variability in the severity and the course of the disease.

Whether it is mild or severe, the course of CF is generally a chronic progression of the pulmonary disease, and the severity usually correlates with the rate of progression. Many more CF patients are now surviving to adulthood, and they are leading active and productive lives. Several factors contribute to this improving survival including more effective antibiotics, earlier diagnosis and comprehensive care in CF centers. Another important factor in the improving outlook for CF patients is the prompt recognition and aggressive treatment of the serious, acute complications that can occur in this chronic disease.

Since CF affects the exocrine glands which are distributed throughout the body, it is understandable that such a wide variety of symptoms in a number of different organs can be associated with a single disease entity. It will not be possible to discuss all features of the disease here, many of which are chronic rather than acute. However, several of the more common and severe symptoms of CF which are likely to be seen by a physician in an emergency department are listed in Table 49.7. A discussion of the clinical manifestations and treatment of these complications of CF will form the basis of this chapter. If any of these conditions are present in a patient not previously diagnosed as having CF, the patient should be referred for diagnostic evaluation after treatment of the acute episode. The evaluation should include a sweat test performed using the quantitative pilocarpine iontophoresis method.

PATHOPHYSIOLOGY

The exocrine glands are primarily affected in CF. Each of these glands performs a specialized function. Since the basic defect in CF has not been elucidated, it is not yet possible to describe precisely the pathogenesis of this complex disorder. Abnormalities have been found in secreted glycoproteins, calcium metabolism, ion transport, serum factors and the autonomic nervous system. The relationship of these and other abnormalities to the basic defect in CF remains to be defined by further research. Although it involves an enormous oversimplification, it is useful to consider the pathogenesis of symptoms in two large categories. First, viscous secretions result in obstructive phenomena in the respiratory and gastrointestinal tracts. Second, altered reabsorption results in electrolyte losses in the sweat glands.

The abnormally viscous mucous secretions and the chronic colonization of the respiratory tract with bacterial pathogens, predominantly *Staphylococcus aureus* and *Pseudomonas aeruginosa*, appear to be the most important factors in the progressive deterioration of pulmonary function which is characteristic of CF. The interplay of these two factors, mucus plugging and infection, produces a variable amount of hyperinflation, bronchiectasis and atelectasis. Increasing ventilation-perfusion abnormalities and structural changes lead to chronic pulmonary insufficiency. Most CF patients eventually die of respiratory failure complicated by cor pulmonale.

Pancreatic insufficiency occurs with the obstruction and dilatation of pancreatic ducts and the production of viscous, low volume, bicarbonate and enzyme deficient pancreatic secretions. Abnormal intestinal mucins and biliary tract secretions have also been implicated in the intestinal malabsorption and obstruction which are seen in CF.

The high concentrations of sodium and chloride in the sweat of CF patients can lead to acute or chronic electrolyte depletion. The elevated sweat electrolytes are the most important criteria for establishing the diagnosis of CF.

Table 49.7
Common Manifestations of Cystic Fibrosis Requiring Emergency Interventions

- Meconium ileus
- Rectal prolapse
- Intestinal obstruction
- Hypoelectrolytemia with metabolic alkalosis
- Pneumothorax
- Hemoptysis
- Pulmonary exacerbation
  - Cor pulmonale
  - Respiratory failure

CLINICAL MANIFESTATIONS

Presentation

Patients who have CF, but who have not yet been diagnosed as CF, may present with a variety of chronic symptoms. Failure to thrive and a history of chronic respiratory and/or gastrointestinal symptoms is a fairly typical presentation of CF. The respiratory symptoms may vary from a mild, but persistent, cough to recurrent pneumonia and atelectasis. Expiratory rhonchi and low pitched wheezes are sometimes found on auscultation of the chest in CF patients. The atypical asthmatic who has digital clubbing, bronchiectasis or a cough productive of purulent sputum may also have CF.

Frequent passage of pale, bulky, loose, and excessively foul-smelling stools is characteristic of CF. Patients with this presentation are often misdiagnosed as chronic diarrhea or milk allergy. The loose stools often prompt repeated formula changes. Edema and hypoproteinemia may develop in children with CF and especially in those who are receiving a soy protein formula. In addition, a hemorrhagic diathesis resulting from Vitamin K malabsorption has been reported.

In contrast to the more acute manifestations listed in Table 49.7, many of the patients who present with chronic symptoms will not require emergency treatment. However, proper management requires that they be referred for a further evaluation which should include a quantitative pilocorpine iontophoresis sweat test.

Meconium Ileus

CF often presents as intestinal obstruction secondary to meconium ileus in the neonatal period. A typical history is that after the first few feedings the infant develops abdominal distension and begins vomiting. Usually there is a history of passing little or no meconium stool. In addition to the obvious abdominal distension, peristaltic waves may be seen on the abdomen and a mass may be palpable. Three-view radiographic examination of the abdomen should be obtained promptly. The typical findings of uncomplicated meconium ileus include dilated loops of bowel and a bubbly granular density in the lower abdomen. In many cases air-fluid levels will not be seen (Fig. 49.8*A*). If there are associated signs of intestinal perforation, such as calcifications or free air in the abdomen, a laparotomy will be necessary. If there are no signs of perforation a radiographic examination following contrast enema will typically show a microcolon of disuse and impacted meconium in the terminal ileum (Fig. 49.8*B*). Other abnormalities or complications such as volvulus can usually be seen on the barium enema. If complications exist or if there is some doubt, laparotomy should be performed.

In cases of uncomplicated meconium ileus, an enema with diatrizoate methylglucamine (Gastrografin) can be used to clear the obstructing meconium, and surgery may not be necessary.

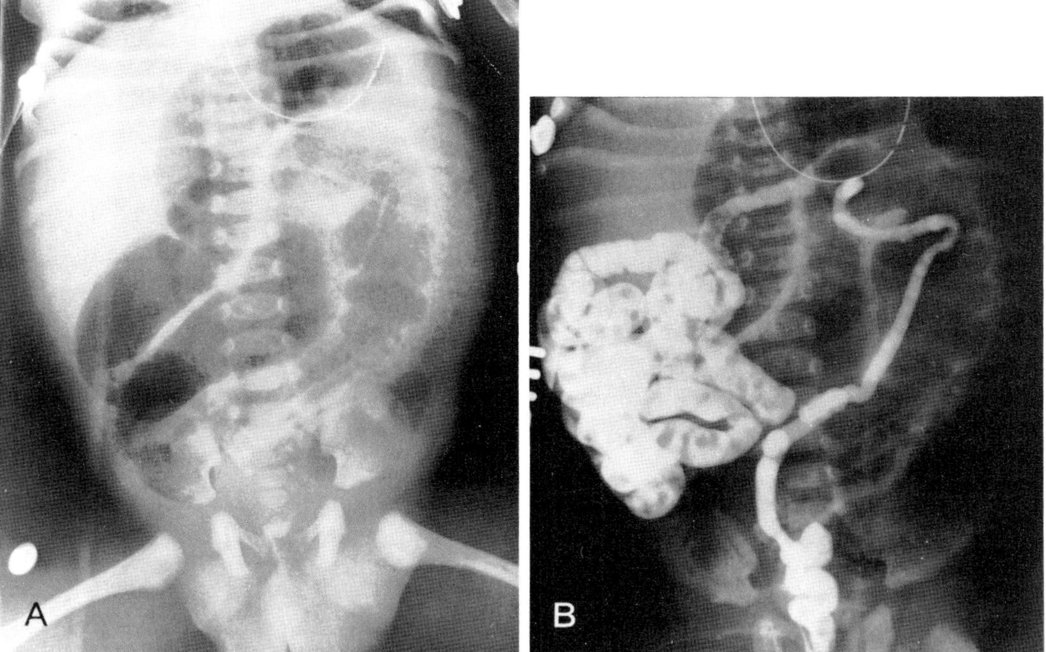

Figure 49.8 (*A*) Roentgenogram of the abdomen showing dilated loops of bowel. Note the absence of air fluid levels. (*B*) Barium enema showing microcolon of disuse and impacted meconium in terminal ileum.

Rectal Prolapse

This condition occurs most commonly in children less than 3 years of age. Although several other conditions may cause a rectal prolapse, the association with CF is frequent and a sweat test is indicated for a child who has had rectal prolapse. In a child who is known to have CF, rectal prolapse usually results when pancreatic enzyme therapy has been inadequate. Although it may be frightening in appearance, the prolapse can usually be easily reduced by placing the infant in a comfortable position and using a lubricated glove for manual reduction. It is only in the unusual situation when an intussusception is responsible for the prolapse that there is a danger of bowel strangulation.

Intestinal Obstruction

Acute or chronic crampy abdominal pain is common in CF patients, and an associated fecal mass in the right lower quadrant is often present. Some patients with this history may present with signs and symptoms of intestinal obstruction, and roentgenograms of the abdomen may show dilated loops of bowel with air fluid levels. Intestinal obstruction occurring beyond the neonatal period in patients with CF is often referred to as meconium ileus equivalent. It has been suggested that the abnormal intestinal mucus in CF patients causes a decreased motility and that this along with a decreased amount of abnormal pancreatic and biliary secretions, results in dry, putty-like stool which cannot pass from the terminal ileum to the cecum. In its mildest form, this situation may be responsible for intermittent abdominal pain. Eventually the fecal mass may cause an obstruction or serve as a leading edge for either an intussusception or a volvulus.

When the roentgenogram of the abdomen shows signs of obstruction, such as dilated loops of bowel and air-fluid levels, a barium or diatrizoate methylglucamine enema must be performed. If a nonreducible volvulus or intussusception is seen, emergency surgery is necessary. If only a fecal mass is present without an associated volvulus or intussusception, medical management using diatrizoate methylglucamine and saline enemas usually results in dissolution of the impacted feces. Because the diatrizoate methylglucamine has a very high osmolarity, the infant must be well hydrated before, during and after the procedure. Fluid balance and serum electrolytes must be monitored closely. A useful technique is to instill a small amount of the diatrizoate methylglucamine as a bolus followed by the diluting water. This often achieves a good result while using a lower total osmotic load. If some progress is made with the first diatrizoate methylglucamine enema, the procedure may be repeated. Pressure (other than hydrostatic) should not be exerted to instill the diatrizoate methylglucamine. External pressure to the infants abdomen is also contraindicated. These procedures should be done in consultation with surgery so that they may be prepared to intervene. In cases of fecal impaction without complete obstruction, enemas and oral administration of either mineral oil or *N*-acetylcysteine (30 ml in 30 ml cola) have been reported to be effective.

Hypoelectrolytemia and Metabolic Alkalosis

Especially during periods of hot weather, the increased loss of sodium and chloride in the sweat of patients with CF may lead to severe and symptomatic electrolyte depletion. Examples of the electrolyte abnormalities which were seen in two infants are shown in Table 49.8. The first patient was

Table 49.8
Hypoelectrolytemia with Metabolic Alkalosis in Cystic Fibrosis Patients

Patient	Age (mo)	Serum Electrolytes (meq/l)				Serum pH
		Na	K	Cl	CO_2	
1	9	123	2.2	49	48	7.60
2	6	125	2.4	55	41	7.63

known to have CF. An intercurrent upper respiratory tract infection occurred during hot weather, and a decrease in oral intake was followed by profound lethargy. Several features of the electrolytes are characteristic of the abnormalities seen in CF. The extremely low chloride and elevated bicarbonate combined with a less severe hyponatremia probably reflect a renal compensation for the increased salt loss in the sweat of CF patients. The second patient presented with a history of an upper respiratory tract infection which progressed to bilateral upper lobe pneumonia and atelectasis during a period of warm weather. Again, an abrupt decrease in oral intake was followed by lethargy. In this second patient who was not previously diagnosed as having CF, the electrolytes provided an important clue for the subsequent diagnosis. In these patients, prompt fluid replacement with isotonic saline is critical; 20 to 30 ml/kg should be given within 15 min if there are signs of shock or within 1 hour in less severely ill patients. Potassium chloride should be administered as soon as urine output is established. However the concentration of potassium should not exceed 40 meq/L. Frequent determinations of serum electrolytes will be necessary to guide further therapy until correction is complete.

Pneumothorax

Sudden onset of chest pain, often referred to the shoulder and sometimes associated with the acute onset of increasing dyspnea and cyanosis, is most likely the result of a pneumothorax in the CF patient. Rupture of a subpleural bleb introduces air into the pleural space. This complication is being reported with increasing frequency in older CF patients, and it is important to realize that recurrences are very common and that tension pneumothorax has been reported in as many as 30% of these cases.

CF patients with a pneumothorax of larger than 10% of the area of the hemithorax should be treated with tube thoracostomy. This procedure should be performed promptly, but care should be taken to prepare the patient and surroundings properly and to consult an experienced surgeon, if one is available. Needle aspiration of the pneumothorax should be avoided unless the patient's condition is rapidly deteriorating as the result of developing a tension pneumothorax (Fig. 49.9).

Hemoptysis

The expectoration of a small amount of blood, usually seen as blood-streaking of the sputum, is a fairly common occurrence in CF patients. Although the first such episode may be very alarming to the patient and parents, there is no need for a major change in the patient's usual home care regimen other than considering an appropriate course of antibiotic therapy to treat any intercurrent pulmonary infection.

Significant hemoptysis has been arbitrarily defined as the expectoration of at least 30 to 60 ml of fresh blood. The mechanism proposed to explain this event is the erosion of an area of local bronchial infection or bronchiectasis into a bronchial vessel. Hospitalization for observation is indicated for significant hemoptysis. If the bleeding persists or increases, vitamin K (5 mg initially), antibiotics and blood transfusions may be necessary. Although it is less common, some patients with CF may have bleeding from esophageal varices secondary to advanced cirrhosis with portal hypertension. It is therefore important to establish whether the source of the bleeding is from the respiratory or gastrointestinal tract.

CF patients occasionally present with an episode of massive hemoptysis with volumes of blood loss ranging from 300 ml to 2500 ml. Massive hemoptysis represents a life-threatening situation and, in addition to instituting the measures described above, the skilled intervention of a team including a bronchoscopist, anesthesiologist, and thoracic surgeon may be necessary to maintain an airway and to locate and ligate the bleeding vessel. Bronchial artery embolization has been described for CF patients, and although there are potentially serious complications, this may be a valuable procedure when conservative measures fail and surgery is not feasible.

Pulmonary Exacerbation

CF patients who experience an increase in respiratory symptoms such as cough and

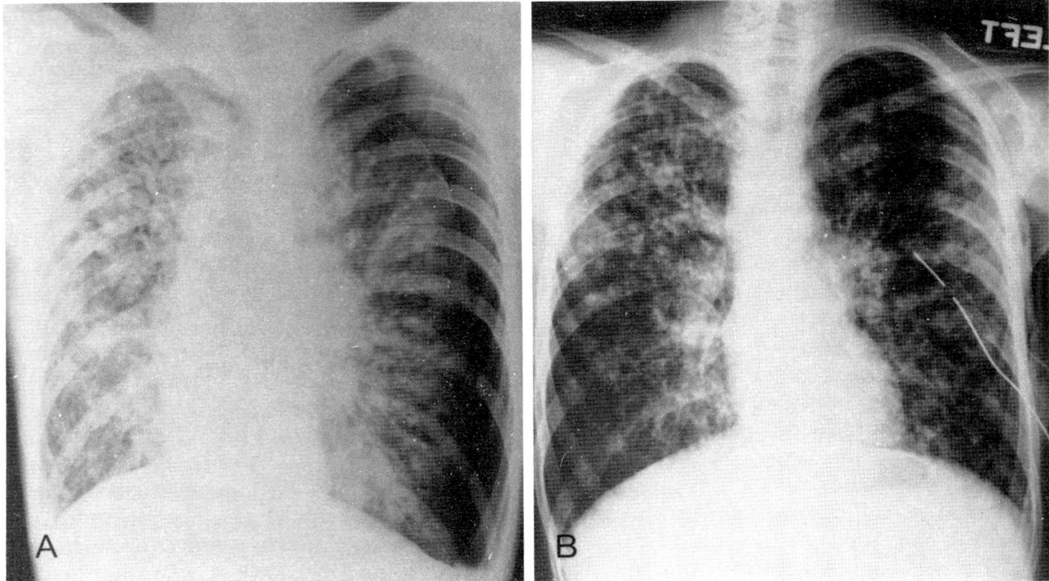

Figure 49.9 (*A*) Chest roentgenogram showing a large left-sided pneumothorax with some shift of mediastinal structures of the right. (*B*) Re-expansion of the left lung after tube thoracostomy and suction.

the rate and effort of breathing require careful evaluation. Often these symptoms will occur after the onset of a mild upper respiratory tract infection. On physical examination the patient will be tachypneic with intercostal retractions and may be cyanotic. Auscultation may reveal areas of coarse rales. A chest roentgenogram should be done to determine if pneumothorax, effusion or local consolidation or atelectasis are present. However, in many cases the roentgenogram will show only diffuse peribronchial thickening with a varying amount of fluffly infiltrates and hyperinflation. It is most helpful in assessing the degree of acute change in the roentgenogram if comparison can be made with previous roentgenograms and if medical personnel who are familiar with patients' previous course can be contacted for advice. The establishment of the network of CF Centers by the CF Foundation for the comprehensive care of CF patients has helped to ensure that such information will be available even on an emergency basis. If such guidance is not available and if either lobar atelectasis, significant respiratory distress, or hypoxia ($PaO_2 \leqq 60$ torr) is present, the patient should be treated in a hospital setting with vigorous chest physiotherapy and antibiotics effective against *S. aureus* and *P. aeruginosa* (until results of sputum culture are available). Oxygen therapy should be guided by arterial blood gas determination.

Diffuse expiratory wheezing and prolonged expiration in a patient with CF suggest the possibility of coexisting asthma. A previous history of respiratory allergy with a good response to bronchodilators provides further support for this diagnosis. If these findings are present, or if the patients show an improvement after a dose of epinephrine (1:1000, 0.01 ml/kg subcutaneously), therapy should be administered as outlined under "Asthma" in addition to treating for CF.

Cor Pulmonale. Patients with CF who have moderately severe pulmonary insufficiency and some degree of hypoxia will eventually develop right ventricular hypertrophy secondary to pulmonary hypertension. However, this is often not detected by a standard electrocardiogram. Increased hypoxia during an exacerbation of pulmonary symptoms in such patients may precipitate an episode of congestive heart failure. In addition to cyanosis, tachypnea and tachycardia, other associated signs are an enlarged, tender liver and in some patients a gallop rhythm, peripheral edema and ascites. Most of these patients will have pronounced digital clubbing which reflects the severity of their pulmonary disease. Rather than the elongated, narrow cardiac silhouette usually seen in the patient with CF, the chest roentgenogram will now show some cardiac enlargement with a prominence of the pulmonary vasculature. Oxygen and diuretics (furosemide 1 mg/kg given intravenously as an initial dose) have been most helpful in addition to starting treatment for the underlying pulmonary disease. Digitalis and pulmonary vasodilators have not been shown to be of proven benefit. However many CF Centers will use digitalis during an acute episode of congestive heart failure and in selected CF patients, e.g., those with recurrent episodes of congestive heart failure and/or significant left ventricular dysfunction in addition to right ventricular dysfunction on echocardiography.

Some consideration must be given to the course of the patient's disease prior to the current episode when anticipating the response to therapy. The patient with a first episode of congestive heart failure precipitated by an acute exacerbation of the pulmonary disease may improve appreciably. However, in a patient in whom the congestive heart failure is superimposed on a course of inexorable deterioration in pulmonary status, there is little hope for a dramatic response.

Respiratory Failure. When a CF patient presents with respiratory failure, i.e. hypercarbia ($PaCO_2 \geqq 55$ torr) in addition to hypoxia, the management decisions become extremely difficult. CF patients in general do not respond as well to mechanical ventilation and have more complications from mechanical ventilation when they are compared to patients with other forms of chronic obstructive pulmonary disease.

If an acute episode such as viral pneumonia or status asthmaticus precipitates respiratory failure in a CF patient who has a history of good pulmonary function prior to the episode, mechanical ventilation should be considered. Factors that play a role in this decision include the patient's level of activity and pulmonary function prior to the episode and also the course of the patient's disease and the expectations of the patient and parents. Adequate, objective guidelines are not currently available, but one large retrospective study found that a history of prior hypercarbia indicated a poor prognosis. It seems reasonable that good pulmonary function prior to the acute episode provides an opportunity for a good result. However, when mechanical ventilation is used for a patient with CF, a skilled intensive care team must be prepared for a potentially difficult course.

When respiratory failure with increasing hypercarbia occurs in a CF patient after a course of progressive pulmonary insufficiency despite adequate medical therapy, mechanical ventilation is not indicated. However, consultation with the physicians providing chronic care for the patient is important before choosing this course.

References

Asthma

Austen KF, Orange RP: Bronchial asthma. *Am Rev Respir Dis* 112: 423, 1975.

Commey J, Levison H: Physical signs in childhood asthma. *Pediatrics* 58: 537, 1976.

Galant SP, Grouncy CE, Duriseti S, Struck L: The effect of metaproterenol in chronic asthmatic children. *J Allergy Clin Immunol* 61: 273, 1978.

Leffert F: Asthma; a modern perspective. *Pediatrics* 62: 1061, 1978.

Leffert F: Management of acute severe asthma. *J Pediatr* 96: 1, 1980.

Leffert F: Management of chronic asthma. *J Pediatr* 97: 875, 1980.

Lulla S, Newcomb RW: Emergency management of asthma in children. *J Pediatr* 97: 346, 1980.

McFadden ER, Kiser R, de Groat WJ: Acute bronchial asthma. *N Engl J Med* 288: 221, 1973.

McFadden ER, Ingram RH: Exercise-induced asthma. *N. Engl J Med* 301: 763, 1979.

Webb-Johnson DC, Andrews JL: Bronchodilator therapy; Parts 1 and 2. *N Engl J Med* 297: 476, 1977.

Wood DW, Downes JJ, Schienkopf H et al.: Intravenous isoproterenol in the management of respiratory failure in status asthmaticus. *J Allergy Clin Immunol* 50: 75, 1972.

Anaphylaxis

Austin KF: Anaphylaxis. In *Immunological Diseases*, p. 885, edited by M. Samter. Little, Brown, Boston, 1978.

Chipps BE, Valentine MD, Kagey-Sobotka A, et al.: Diagnosis and treatment of anaphylactic reactions to hymenoptera stings. *J Pediatr* 97: 177, 1980.

Criep LH, Woehler TR: The heart in human anaphylaxis. *Ann Allergy* 29: 399, 1971.

Franklin EC: The role of cryoglobulins and immune complexes in vasculitis. *J Allergy Clin Immunol* 66: 269, 1980.

Matthews KP: Management of urticaria and angioedema. *J Allergy Clin Immunol* 66: 347, 1980.

Orange RP, Donsky GJ: Anaphylaxis. In *Allergy: Principles and Practice*, p. 563, edited by E. Middleton Jr, E, CE Reed, EF Ellis: C.V. Mosby, St. Louis, 1978.

Serum Sickness

Cochrane CG: Studies on localization of circulating antigen-antibody complexes and other macromolecules in vessels. *J Exp Med* 118:503, 1963.

Cochrane CG, Koffler D: Immune complex disease in experimental animals and man. *Adv Immunol* 16: 186, 1973.

Dixon FJ, Vazquez JJ, Weigle WO, Cochrane CG: Pathogenesis of serum sickness. *Arch Pathol* 65: 18, 1968.

Frick OL: Serum sickness. In *Allergy: Principles and Practice*, p. 574, edited by E Middleton Jr, CE Reed, EF Ellis: C. V. Mosby, St. Louis, 1978.

Kniker WT, Guerra FA, Richards SEM: Prevention of immune complex disease by antagonists of vasoactive amines. *Pediatr Res* 5: 381, 1971.

Trepo CG, Zuckerman AJ, Bird RC, Prince AM: The role of circulating hepatitis B antigen/antibody immune complexes in the pathogenesis of vascular and hepatic manifestations in polyarterities nodosa. *J Clin Pathol* 27: 863, 1974.

Vaughan JH, Barnett EV, Leadley PG: Evidence in man of antigen-antibody complexes and free light chains in the circulation during the acute reaction. *Ann Intern Med* 67: 596, 1967.

Wiggins RC, Cochrane CG: Immune-complex mediated biologic effects. *N Engl J Med* 304: 518, 1981.

Cystic Fibrosis

Davis PB, di Sant'Agnese PA: Assisted ventilation for patients with cystic fibrosis. *JAMA* 239: 1851–1854, 1978.

Fellows K, Khaw KT, Schuster S, Shwachman H: Bronchial artery embolization in cystic fibrosis; technique and long-term results. *J Pediatr* 95: 959–963, 1979.

Rich RH, Warwick WJ, Leonard AS: Open thoracostomy and pleural abrasion in the treatment of spontaneous pneumothorax in cystic fibrosis. *J Pediatr Surg* 13: 237–241, 1978.

Roy CC, Silverman A, Cozzetto FJ (Eds.): Exocrine pancreatic insufficiency. In *Pediatric Clinical Gastroenterology*, Ed. 2, C.V. Mosby, St. Louis, 1975.

Ruddy R, Anolik R, Scanlin TF: Hypoelectrolytemia as a presentation and complication of cystic fibrosis. *Clin Pediatr* 21: 367–369, 1982.

Scanlin TF: Cystic fibrosis; current trends in research. *Clin Chest Med* 1: 423–427, 1980.

Stern RC, Borkat G, Hirschfeld SS, et al.: Heart failure in cystic fibrosis. *Am J Dis Child* 134: 267–272, 1980.

Stern RC, Wood RE, Boat TF, et al.: Treatment and prognosis of massive hemoptysis in cystic fibrosis. *Am Rev Respir Dis* 117: 825–828, 1978.

Taussig LM, Landau LI: Cystic fibrosis. *Semin Respir Med* 1: 167–182, 1979.

Waring WW: Current management of cystic fibrosis. *Adv Pediatr* 23: 401–438, 1976.

Wood RE, Boat TF, Doershuk CF: Cystic fibrosis. *Am Rev Respir Dis* 113: 833–877, 1976.

CHAPTER 50

Gastrointestinal Emergencies

JOHN T. BOYLE, M.D., AND JOHN B. WATKINS, M.D.

MANAGEMENT OF SEVERE UPPER GASTROINTESTINAL BLEEDING

In Chapter 22, we discuss a systematic diagnostic approach to the patient who presents to the emergency department with overt gastrointestinal (GI) bleeding. In this chapter we will discuss the initial resuscitation of the patient with major GI hemmorrhage. Since upper GI bleeding accounts for 90% of major GI bleeding, the medical treatment of the two major categories of upper GI hemorrhage, mucosal lesions and esophageal varicies will be covered in detail. The treatment of severe lower GI bleeding usually involves surgical therapy (see Chapter 59), in addition to the supportive care outlined here.

Resuscitation and Stabilization of the Patient with Severe GI Hemorrhage

Severe GI bleeding is an emergency that requires, from the first contact with the patient, the cooperation of a team including the emergency physician, surgeon, and gastroenterologist.

A patient with overt hemodynamic instability or suspected significant volume loss should be positioned with legs elevated and given nasal oxygen. A patient with hematemesis would have his head elevated 30 to 45° to lessen the chance of pulmonary aspiration of blood. In massive upper intestinal bleeding, protecting the airway with a cuffed endotracheal tube may be lifesaving. The next priority is insertion of *two* large bore i. v. cannulas (14 to 18 gauge in the child; at least 22 gauge in small infants). If there is going to be any difficulty in promptly establishing i.v. access either because of poor veins or poor venous filling, a second physician should be called to do a cut down or subclavian puncture to place a large central venous line.

Immediate blood studies in any patient with severe GI bleeding should include: (1) type and crossmatch, (2) complete blood count (CBC), (3) platelet count, (4) prothrombin time (PT), and (5) partial thromboplastin time (PTT). These studies should be drawn at the time of insertion of the intravenous lines. Arterial blood gases and pH are also important parameters to follow in severe blood loss associated with shock. The hematocrit is an unreliable initial index of acute blood loss since it may be normal or only slightly decreased. Its subsequent fall will depend upon (1) rate and type of fluid replacement and (2) the body's own hemostatic mechanisms, both resulting in renal conservation of fluid and electrolytes and in gradual shifts of fluid from extra- to intravascular compartments. Any patient with or without a previous history of liver disease who presents with GI bleeding associated with an abnormal PT should receive vitamin K, 5 to 10 mg i.m. or i.v., as soon as possible.

Intravenous therapy has two major objectives: (1) restoration of intravascular volume (reflected in blood pressure or pulse) and (2) restoration of oxygen carrying capacity (reflected in hemoglobin and hematocrit values). The former may be accomplished both by nonsanguineous crystalloid or colloid solution or blood products, the latter solely by the infusion of blood. The practical limitations in time required to properly type and crossmatch blood make nonsanguineous solution the mainstay of early resuscitation. In the rare circumstance of massive ongoing hemorrhage where low oxygen-carrying capacity is felt to be an important factor at onset of resuscitation, Rh and type-specific blood can usually be provided in 10 to 15 min. If type-specific blood is not immediately available, O-negative blood may be used. In the vast majority of cases, proper type and crossmatch can be performed while intravascular volume is restored by nonsanguineous solutions. The exact type of solution to be used is controversial. Since studies in both animals and man have shown not only a reduction in intravascular volume but also in extravascular volume in acute blood loss, we prefer to infuse crystalloid solutions such as normal saline or Ringer's lactate at a rate of 20 ml/kg/hour (see Chapter 46) until intravascular volume is minimally restored as indicated by a rise in blood pressure and disappearance of clinical signs of peripheral vasoconstriction. Colloid solutions such as albumin or plasma are used only when blood loss is massive and continuous because in this situation respiratory insufficiency or shock lung may develop with a fall in plasma oncotic pressure. Dextran is to be avoided as it may affect platelet function. Hetastarch is a new artificial colloid available in the United States which is claimed to be as effective and safe as albumin, but at a fraction of the cost. While more experience is needed before its relative effectiveness and long-term safety can be determined, it should be kept in mind for use in the rare Jehovah Witness who presents with acute GI bleeding and refuses transfusion.

Overexpansion of intravascular volume is potentially dangerous, particularly in bleeding varices but also in bleeding gastric or duodenal ulcers. Therefore, following correction of shock and restoration of urine flow, further intravenous volume replacement should be titrated to match continuing blood loss. The decision as to whether or not to begin transfusion depends on the level of hematocrit taken at the time of restoration of blood volume, and on evidence of ongoing bleeding. In a patient who has stopped bleeding, blood transfusion is given to allow some reserve in case of rebleeding. Under most circumstances, slow transfusion to return hematocrit to approximately 30% is recommended to achieve this objective. In this case, packed cells (10 ml/kg, initially) are used to reduce the volume load to the patient. In addition, packed blood cells contain considerably less ammonia than whole blood, an important factor in patients with severe liver disease. In the patient with continuous bleeding, ongoing blood transfusion is the only means of maintaining adequate oxygen carrying capacity. In this case, the rate of bleeding determines the rate of transfusion. A sustained rate of transfusion is recommended and is best achieved with an electrical infusion pump, not by gravity. The risks inherent in massive transfusions are definitely lowered by using packed red blood cells, fresh frozen plasma, proper filters, and blood warmers. Complications of massive transfusions include hypercitraemia, hyperlacticacidemia, hypocalcemia, decreased levels of clotting factors, and thrombocytopenia. To minimize these problems, the patient should be given intravenous calcium and fresh frozen plasma (10 ml/kg) after every 40 to 50 ml/kg of packed cells or whole blood. Similarly, platelets should be monitored after every 40 ml/kg of transfusion and platelet transfusion given as needed.

In any patient requiring intravenous resuscitation for GI hemorrhage, it is highly recommended that a flow sheet similar to that shown in Figure 50.1 be initiated while the patient is in the emergency department. Patients who are in shock at the time of admission should have the urinary bladder catheterized in the emergency department to accurately measure urine output and for early detection of acute tubular necrosis.

Initial Control of Upper GI Bleeding

The initial technique used to control bleeding, irrespective of etiology, is nasogastric lavage. Contrary to common opin-

Patient Name:			Date	
Time	11:00 p.m.	12:00 a.m.	2:00 a.m.	3:00 a.m.
CLINICAL				
Mental Status	Confused	Clear	Clear	Clear
Pulse: Supine	120	100	100	90
Upright	140	105	—	—
Blood pressure:				
Supine	90/60	100/65	110/70	110/70
Upright	70/50	100/60		
CVP		3	5	5
Gastric aspirate	Bloody	Bloody	Clearing	Clear
Stool	—	—		
Urine output	—	10 ml/hr	20 ml/hr	40 ml/hr
LABORATORY				
Hb/Hct	7/20			6/18
Platelets	225,000			
PT/PTT	14/28			11/28
Bun/Creatinine	35/1.4			
Other:	Lytes-WNL pH 7.35 PO_2	Blood culture		PO_2-84
THERAPY				
Blood products		250 FFP	Packed RBL, 500 ml	
Fluids		1500 ml NaCl	1000 ml, 5% dextrose in 0.5 N NaCl	
Pharmacologic Rx		Vitamin K, 10 mg i.v.		
Tamponade				
COMMENTS:		Endoscopy Esophageal varices		Maalox, 45 ml/ p.o. q1h

Figure 50.1 Flow sheet for intravenous resuscitation for gastrointestinal hemorrhage (example).

ion, passage of a nasogastric tube in patients with suspected variceal bleeding does not increase the risk of rebleeding or prolong the original hemorrhage. The importance of lavage in confirming the level of bleeding and estimating the rate of hemorrhage is discussed in Chapter 22.

Whether lavage (either at room temperature or iced) actually controls bleeding is not proven. Although hypothermia has been shown to reduce gastric blood flow in dogs, other studies suggest platelet function is impaired in the cooled canine stomach. At least two recent studies have reported that iced saline lavage is no better than lavage with room temperature saline in decreasing canine gastric ulcer bleeding. Nevertheless, gastric hypothermia is believed by most gastroenterologists to be the safest and simplest way of reducing upper GI bleeding, particularly from the stomach. Gastric lavage with a solution containing norepinephrine (4 ampules in 500 ml lavage fluid) may also induce gastric vasoconstriction and has been reported successful in stopping hemorrhage from a variety of lesions. However, there have been no control studies to establish its efficacy or safety. There is no benefit to be gained by the addition of pitressin or antacids to the lavage solution.

Since only a very small amount of fluid is absorbed from the stomach, it is generally of little importance whether isotonic saline or water is used for lavage. We tend to pour normal saline directly into a container of ice during lavage and keep the patient's head elevated 30°. Most patients can be effectively lavaged with a nasogastric sump tube: 12 F in small children, and 14 to 16 F in older children. Verification of the location of tube in the stomach by injection of 10 cc of air and auscultation over the stomach is essential. Lavage should be continued until the return is either light pink or clear. The recommended volume for each infusion depends on age: 50 ml for infants, 100 to 200 ml for older children. The solution is rapidly infused into the stomach, allowed to stand for 2 to 3 min and then aspirated by gentle suction. Return volumes should approximate input volumes and discrepancies should be recorded. If aspiration meets with significant resistance, either reposition the tube, reposition the patient, or increase the amount of solution introduced. Intensive iced saline lavage of the stomach is a job for two people. One fills and empties the stomach while the other empties and fills the syringes.

There is really no benefit to continuous lavage beyond the first 15 or 20 min if return is not clearing. The tube can be left to gravity or low suction and irrigated every 15 to 30 min to assess the activity of the bleeding. The specific lesion causing the bleedings determines the subsequent management of the patient.

Treatment of Specific Disorders

Mucosal Lesions

Esophagitis, duodenal and gastric peptic ulcer, stress ulcer, gastritis and Mallory-Weiss tears are grouped into one category because, in the acute situation of GI bleeding, all respond to the same treatment.

PATHOPHYSIOLOGY

The most important variable in all these disorders is gastric acidity. A Mallory-Weiss tear is actually a mucosal rent at the gastroesophageal junction caused by forceful vomiting, but gastric acid affects the normal rapid healing of the superficial tear. In the other disorders, gastric acid is the primary mediator of cell damage, erosion, and ulceration.

NATURAL HISTORY

Gastrointestinal bleeding in these disorders, while initially potentially severe, is usually self-limiting, either stopping spontaneously or with iced saline lavage.

EMERGENCY MANAGEMENT

Patients with these disorders theoretically should benefit from diminution of hydrochloric acid and subsequent limitation of pepsin activity. However, there is no evidence that antacids, or the H_2-receptor antagonist, cimetidine, are beneficial during active bleeding. The rationale for antacid use is to prevent potential further damage by gastric acidity to already existing breakdown in the gastric, duodenal, or esophageal mucosal barrier. Antacids have also been shown to prevent stress ulceration in critically ill patients.

If gastric contents clear following initial iced saline lavage, and immediate endoscopy is not planned, gastric irrigation is performed every 15 min for 1 hour, then every hour for 2 to 3 hours. Antacid (15 ml, infants; 30 ml, preschool-age children; 60 ml, school age children) is infused into the tube after every lavage. The dose of antacid is titriated during the hourly monitoring so that gastric pH 1 hour post antacid infusion is greater than 3.5. If the patient is hemodynamically stable and gastric return remains clear for the above period of time, then the tube is electively removed. Persistent nausea or vomiting or the presence of ileus point to the need for continuing drainage.

We do not generally use the H_2-receptor antagonist, cimetidine, to prevent further bleeding in children. Adult studies have shown cimetidine to be ineffective in consistently elevating gastric pH above 3.5. More important, there are no good pharmacokinetic and dose response data in children.

Unremitting mucosal bleeding requires either therapeutic angiography or surgery. Intra-arterial infusion of vasopressin has been shown to be effective in controlling bleeding due to hemorrhagic gastritis. Peripheral intravenous vasopressin is less effective in these conditions than intra-arterial infusion (as opposed to variceal bleeding), but may be tried (see below). For bleeding from a pyloroduodenal ulcer, results with vasopressin are poor, and transcatheter embolization is now considered to be the primary therapeutic modality. The mortality of emergency surgery for ulcer disease is reported to be 15 to 25%.

Other pharmacologic agents are now being evaluated for bleeding control including somatostatin, prostaglandins, and glucagon. At this time, none of these agents has been sufficiently studied clinically to establish efficacy and safety. Endoscopic control of bleeding as discussed in Chapter 22 is also experimental at this time.

Gastroesophageal Varices

Portal hypertension results from relative obstruction of portal venous blood flow. The etiology of portal hypertension may be presinusoidal, sinusoidal, or rarely postsinusoidal (Table 22.3, Chapter 22).

PATHOPHYSIOLOGY

Portal hypertension leads to the development of portal systemic collateral veins, or varices. Portal-systemic collaterals will develop in any area where veins draining the portal venous system are in close approximation to veins draining into the caval system, i.e. submucosa of the esophagus, submucosa of the rectum, and anterior abdominal wall. Esophageal and gastric fundal varices, connecting branches of the coronary veins with branches of the azygous vein, are the most likely to be the site of spontaneous hemorrhage.

NATURAL HISTORY

The majority of gastroesophageal varices bleeding will stop spontaneously. However, there is a high incidence of rebleeding. In series of adults, the mortality from each bleed varies between 25 and 50%.

EMERGENCY MANAGEMENT

If bleeding ceases during the initial nasogastric lavage, the tube should be managed as described above. Even in patients with suspected variceal bleeding, antacids are given in the range of doses used for mucosal lesions.

If bleeding continues despite nasogastric lavage, the two major medical therapies for variceal bleeding include: posterior pituitary extract (vasopressin) and gastroesophageal tamponade. These therapies are reserved for the following two sets of patients: (1) those with endoscopically confirmed variceal bleeding and (2) those with endoscopic evidence of esophageal varices and ongoing bleeding in the absence of mucosal lesion but no confirmation of variceal hemorrhage.

Vasopressin

Vasopressin administration has been well documented to decrease blood flow and pressure through the portal circulation. Indications for vasopressin include continued massive hemorrhage and recurrent bleeding. It is now well accepted that peripheral intravenous infusion is as effective for varices as selective infusion into the superior mesenteric artery during angiography. The dose in children is not well established. We empirically begin infusing 0.1 unit/min and increase the dose by 0.05 unit/min hourly up to a maximum of 0.2 unit/min in children less than 5, 0.3 unit/min in children less than 12, and 0.4 unit/min in adolescents above 12 years of age. Side effects are significant, thus the child must be monitored carefully. Major complications include myocardial ischemia, life-threatening arrhythmias, and limb vasoconstriction or ischemia. Minor complications include water retention with sodium depletion, benign arrhythmias, and acrocyanosis. The vasopressin is usually given in 5% dextrose in water, the exact dilution being based on overall volumes of fluids being infused. It is safest to infuse vasopressin through a large bore, preferably central venous, line. The reported success rate of vasopressin infusion in adults is 50 to 70%. Because of the high rate of rebleeding, once begun the drug is continued at the dose which controls bleeding for a minimum of 12 to 24 hours after all bleeding has stopped. This management plan stems from studies by Johnson et al. showing sustained vasoconstrictive effects of vasopressin on splanchnic vessels in dogs for over 24 hours. However, this is a controversial point as it is also reported that tachyphylaxis develops with prolonged use of vasopressin.

Gastroesophageal Tamponade

Balloon tamponade is a high-risk procedure. It should be considered only in endoscopically proven gastric or esophageal varices. Indications include massive life-threatening hemorrhage, or continued bleeding despite 2 to 6 hours of intravenous vasopressin. Either a Sengstaken-Blakemore (S-B) (Fig. 50.2) or a Linton tube may be used. The S-B tube has both gastric and esophageal balloon tubes, while the Linton tube has a single lavage gastric balloon. Gastroesophageal tamponade is reported to arrest bleeding initially in 50 to 80% of cases. At the same time, the reported incidence of major complications from use of the S-B tube ranges from 9 to 35%. Death directly attributed to the use of the tube has been reported in 5 to 20% of patients on whom the tube was used. Other major complications include rupture or erosion of the esophageal or gastric fundal mucosa, occlusion of the airway by the balloon, or aspiration of secretions resulting from inadequate drainage of the occluded esophagus.

Whenever a tube is used, it should be inserted only by a physician skilled in its use. We prefer the S-B tube (Fig. 50.2). A pediatric tube is used for children less than 11 to 13 years of age; the adult tube is used in adolescents. Passage through the nose is the procedure of choice, but, in small children, passage through the mouth may be necessary. Intranasal cocaine (0.1%) is used for local anesthesia, and vasoconstriction. Each balloon is pretested for air leaks prior to insertion. The tube is heavily lubricated and passed through the nose to its full length; 50 to 100 cc of air is instilled and the balloon pulled up until the resistance of the gastroesophageal junction is encountered. An emergency x-ray is then performed to assure correct balloon position immediately below the diaphram.. Additional air is then instilled into the gastric balloon—up to 150 cc in the pediatric balloon and 250 cc in the adult balloon; the tube is pulled taut and is taped at the nose. In many cases, the gastric balloon alone will stop bleeding by preventing flow of blood from the stomach into the esophagus or by directly occluding a gastric varix. It is absolutely essential to pass a second nasoesophageal tube to aspirate saliva and blood from ongoing esophageal hemorrhage. If esophageal bleeding continues, the esophageal balloon is inflated with air. The volume in the esophageal balloon is determined by the pressure within the balloon which is measured by connecting its inflow tube to a syhygmomanometer. The pressure is maintained at the minimum required to control bleeding with the maximum being no more than 40 mm Hg.

If bleeding is controlled, the balloons are kept inflated for 24 hours. The esophageal balloon is deflated first, then the gastric balloon approximately 1 hour later. The gastric tube is irrigated every 30 min for 1 to 2 hours more and then the tube is pulled.

A patient with an indwelling S-B tube must be transferred to an intensive care unit. A pair of scissors should be kept at bedside; if any respiratory embarassment occurs, the tube should be immediately cut, thereby deflating the balloons.

Ancillary Medical Measures

Once again, it is important to caution about overexpansion of intravascular volume in patients with bleeding varices. These patients should have a central venous line placed and have their central venous pressure (CVP) maintained at 4 to 5 cm H_20. Coagulation abnormalities should be aggressively managed with intravenous vitamin K, fresh frozen plasma, and platelets. We have had the experience of five

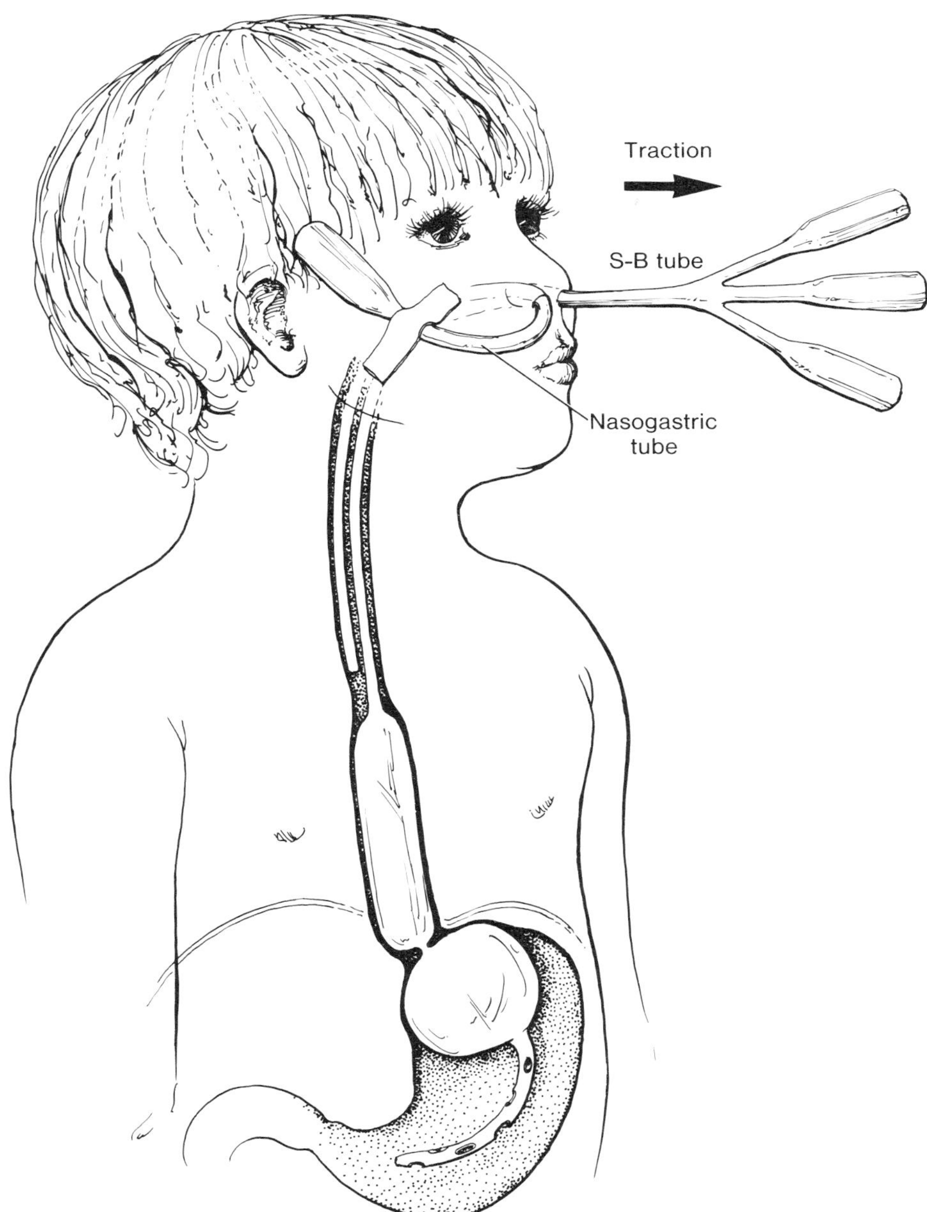

Figure 50.2 Gastroesophageal tamponade.

patients with portal hypertension secondary to both cirrhosis and extrahepatic obstruction present with variceal bleeding associated with sepsis. Therefore, in variceal bleeding, we will draw blood cultures and empirically begin broad-spectrum antibiotics pending culture results.

Management of Bleeding Esophageal Varices Unresponsive to Medical Management

Obliteration of Varices. Percutaneous transhepatic obliteration of gastroesophageal varices with Gelfoam, sclerosing agents, or metal coils is an alternative angiographic procedure for control of variceal bleeding. While this technique may temporarily correct bleeding, several studies have now shown a high incidence of rebleeding within 4 to 6 weeks, and no net overall improved mortality rate, particularly in patients with associated cirrhosis. The procedure may be of use in temporarily arresting bleeding so that the patient may be prepared for elective surgery.

Surgery. The overall mortality following emergency surgery for variceal bleeding is reported to be between 50 and 75%. Therefore, emergency surgery is to be avoided, if possible.

MEDICAL MANAGEMENT OF SPECIFIC DISORDERS PRESENTING WITH LOWER GI BLEEDING

Anorectal Fissures

Anal fissures are the most common proctologic disorder during infancy and childhood. The vast majority occur in infants less than 1 year of age. Anal fissure may result from diarrhea which causes perineal irritation, but more commonly is associated with constipation. The fissure usually starts when passage of a hard stool tears the sensitive squamous lining of the anal canal. Subsequent bowel movements are associated with pain and/or bleeding. Bright red blood is seen coating the stool. The infant begins to withhold stool, leading to increasing constipation and a vicious cycle of hard stools, bleeding, and pain. Anal fissure can be seen by spreading the perineal skin to evert the anal canal. Simply spreading the buttocks to visualize the anal opening is not sufficient. Treatment consists of local skin care combined with stool softeners. Maltsupex (1 to 3 tablespoons/day) or Kondremul (1 to 3 tablespoons/day) can be given to soften the stool. Local care involves sitz baths 4 times a day, a perianal cleasing lotion (Balneol) after bowel movements, and an emollient protective ointment (Balmex) after each bowel movement.

Hemorrhoids

Hemorrhoids are rare in childhood even in patients with known portal hypertension. When they occur, they are almost always "external," involving the external hemorrhoidal plexus, and are most commonly secondary to perianal infection (cryptitis) with spreading to the hemorrhoidal veins. Hemorrhoids are treated with local measures as outlined for anal fissures.

Bacterial Colitis

Bacterial enterocolitis may be associated with rectal bleeding varying in quantity from small to moderate amounts of blood. The diagnosis and treatment of these disorders is discussed in Chapter 45.

Pseudomembranous Enterocolitis

Pseudomembranous colitis is a severe form of inflammatory colitis characterized by the pathologic presence of pseudomembranes consisting of mucin, fibirin, necrotic cells, and polymorphonuclear leukocytes. The entity has been associated with administration of antimicrobial agents of every class particularly clindamycin; however, in childhood the most common are ampicillin and amoxicillin. Pseudomembranous colitis should be suspected in any patient with lower GI bleeding who gives a history of recent antibiotic intake. Recent experimental and clinical studies suggest that the pathogenesis of this condition is related to an enterotoxin-producing *Clostridium difficile* whose overgrowth in the colon might be enhanced by antibiotic therapy. Diagnosis is suggested by recovery of *C. Difficile* from the stool and confirmed by documenting enterotoxin production. The proctosigmoidoscopic finding of yellow plaquelike pseudomembranes in an inflamed colon provides immediate clinical confirmation of the diagnosis. Suspected pseudomembranous enterolitis is an indication of proctosigmoidoscopy in the emergency department.

Cholestyramine (80 mg/kg/24 hours given orally in three divided doses) is now the drug of choice for the treatment of pseudomembranous colitis. Recent studies have shown in vitro that cholestyramine binds the clostridral toxin present in the stool. Oral vancomycin has also been shown to be effective but is extremely expensive and is recommended only in severe cases.

Nonspecific Proctitis

A diagnosis of nonspecific proctitis is made in an otherwise well infant (less than 2), who presents with blood-streaked stools and whose physical examination and stool cultures are negative. Infants with nonspecific proctitis are usually taken off milk products and either observed or, if bleeding is significant, treated with local rectal sterioid (Cortenema, 25 to 100 mg hydrocortisone) or Proctofoam (twice daily for 3 days, then once daily for 1 week). In the majority of patients, bleeding will resolve with the above therapy. Milk products are usually reinstituted 2 to 4 weeks after resolution of bleeding and parents are given Hemoccult cards to send in for monitoring of blood in stool. An unknown but definite number of patients will have recurrence of bleeding not associated with milk products or other food intake. In such patients, further workup with proctosigmoidscopy is necessary. They should be referred to a pediatric gastroenterologist for follow-up.

Juvenile Polyps

Juvenile polyps are benign lesions which begin as sessile growths and become pedunculated. Histologically, they are unique, consisting of proliferated mucous glands and cystic spaces lined by a single layer of epithelium. The surface epithelium is frequently ulcerated with a loss of mucosal surface. They are not inherited. Seventy percent are solitary, 80% are located within 25 cm of the anus, and 30 to 40% are palpable by rectal examination. Patients with palpable polyps should have an air contrast barium enema and upper GI series to search for additional polyps in the GI tract, which may suggest inherited polyposis syndromes. All polyps in reach of the proctosigmoidoscope should be removed for biopsy. Polyps in the proximal colon should be removed by colonoscope for there is a small but definite risk of intussusception. Emergency admission is indicated only if there is significant bleeding.

Henoch-Schönlein Purpura/Hemolytic-Uremic Syndrome

Henoch-Schönlein purpura (HSP) is a systemic vasculitis which may cause edema and hemorrhage in the intestinal wall. GI symptoms may precede the usual cutaneous and urinary tract symptoms and include: abdominal pain (60 to 70%), occult bleeding (50%), gross bleeding (30%), massive hemorrhage (5 to 10%), and intussusception (3%). Children with HSP limited to involvement of the skin and joints can often be managed as outpatients. However, severe abdominal pain or GI hemorrhage are indications for admission.

In the hemolytic-uremic syndrome (HUS), a disorder characterized by the triad of acute microangiopathic hemolytic anemia, thrombocytopenia, and oliguric renal failure, GI manifestations may also occur prior to the onset of any other derangement. Diarrhea, which subsequently becomes bloody, is a prodromal manifestation in 80 to 90% of these patients.

All children with HUS require admission to the hospital. Laboratory studies should be obtained including a CBC, platelet count, PT, PTT, electrolytes, BUN, and creatinine. Intravenous access needs to be secured immediately for the correction of dehydration and the administration of blood products (see Chapter 2).

INFLAMMATORY BOWEL DISEASE

BACKGROUND

The term inflammatory bowel disease (IBD) is used to designate two chronic intestinal disorders of unknown etiology: (1) ulcerative colitis, characterized by inflammation and ulceration confined to the colonic mucosa; and (2) Crohn's disease, manifested by transmural inflammation and frequent granulomas that may affect any segment of the GI tract. Many clinical features are common to both disorders, including diarrhea, GI blood and protein loss, abdominal pain, fever, anemia, weight loss, and growth failure. Extraintestinal manifestations involve the joints, skin, eyes and liver. The onset of both ulcerative colitis and Crohn's disease is usually insidious. The emergency department is not the place to work up a patient for IBD, but the emergency physician should be aware of the acute presentations and complications of IBD.

CLINICAL MANIFESTATIONS/ MANAGEMENT

Acute Presentations of Inflammatory Bowel Disease

Acute Fulminant Colitis. Approximately 10% of children with ulcerative colitis and a lesser percentage with Crohn's disease present with a fulminant onset of fever, abdominal cramps, and severe diarrhea with blood, mucus and pus in the stools. A fulminant episode may also occur in the patient with known disease. There may be associated anemia and dehydration. The presence of abdominal distention, accompanied by diminished or absent bowel sounds, should raise the suspicion of actual or impending perforation, even in the absence of severe pain. Werlin and Grand have classified patients as having severe colitis if they have toxic megacolon or fulfill 4 of the following 5 characteristics: (a) more than 5 grossly bloody stools per day, (b) oral temperature >37.8°C, (c) tachycardia (pulse ≥90), (d) anemia (hematocrit <30%), and (e) serum albumin <3.0 g/dl. The differential of acute fulminant colitis includes acute bacterial enteritis, amebic dysentery, ischemic bowel disease, and radiation colitis.

Emergency Management. All patients with acute fulminant colitis should be admitted to the hospital and have a surgical consultation. Oral intake should be discontinued and an intravenous infusion begun with normal saline until the electrolytes and BUN levels are known. Opiate or anticholinergic drugs are to be avoided as they may precipitate toxic megacolon. The following blood studies should be obtained: CBC, serum electrolytes, BUN, calcium, magnesium, and type and crossmatch. A flat and upright abdominal film are needed to look for radiologic evidence of perforation or toxic megacolon.

Acute Abdominal Pain Strongly Suggesting Acute Appendicitis. Severe abdominal pain often prompts an emergency department visit by the patient with Crohn's disease. There may have been no previous history of abdominal complaints. The pain is colicky with localization in the right lower quadrant or periumbilical area. The abdominal examination may elicit guarding and rebound tenderness. A low grade fever and mild leukocytosis occur frequently.

Emergency Management. When severe abdominal pain occurs in a patient not known to have IBD, surgical consultation is mandatory. An exploratory laporatomy is usually indicated because the diagnosis of appendicitis cannot be excluded. In the emergency department, abdominal x-rays and laboratory studies (CBC, electrolytes, BUN, urinalysis) should be obtained and an intravenous infusion of normal saline started.

Perianal or Enterocutaneous Fistulas. Patients presenting with acute fistulas should be considered to have Crohn's disease until proven otherwise. They should be referred to the proper medical specialist for diagnosis and management.

Complications of Inflammatory Bowel Disease

Toxic Megacolon. The development of massive colonic distention is a rare complication of both ulcerative colitis and Crohn's disease. Toxic megacolon represents a life-threatening emergency with a reported mortality rate as high as 25%. Approximately 40% of the cases occur with the first attack of IBD; another 40% are seen in patients on high dose steroid therapy for fulminant colitis. Toxic megacolon almost always involves the transverse colon. The pathophysiology is felt to be an extension of the inflammatory process through all layers of the bowel wall with resulting microperforation, localized ileus, and loss of colonic tone. The end result is imminent major perforation, peritonitis and overwhelming sepsis. Antecedent barium enema, opiates or anticholinergics may all precipitate toxic megacolon. Clinical features include: (a) a rapidly worsening clinical course usually associated with fever, malaise, and even lethargy; (b) abdominal distention and tenderness usually developing over a period of a few hours or days; (c) temperature ≥38.5°C and a neutrophilic leukocytosis; and (d) an abdominal x-ray showing distention of the transverse colon of more than 5 to 7 cm.

Emergency Management. If toxic megacolon is suspected, arrangements should be made for immediate surgical consultation and admission to an intensive care unit. The patient should discontinue all antidiarrheal and anticholinergic medicines. The first priority in the management of children with toxic megacolon is the treatment of intravascular dehydration and shock. Intensive intravenous therapy with normal saline, albumin, or blood must be sufficient to correct hypotension and assure adequate urine flow. A nasogastric tube, or preferably a Miller-Abbott tube for small bowel decompression, should be placed. The patient should receive intravenous hydrocortisone (10 mg/kg/day) in four divided doses and gentamicin (5 mg/kg/day) and carbenicillin (500 mg/kg/day).

Exsanguinating Hemorrhage. IBD occasionally causes massive lower GI bleeding. Management of the GI bleeding should be performed as described in Chapter 22 and immediate surgical consultation obtained. Severe bleeding from ulcerative colitis is almost always an indication for subtotal or total colectomy, but bleeding from Crohn's disease can often be controlled by a limited intestinal resection.

Intestinal Obstruction. Rarely, Crohn's disease causes complete intestinal obstruction. The patient always gives a history of antecedent abdominal pain, diarrhea, and weight loss. Emergency management includes decompression with nasogastric drainage and intravenous rehydration, initially with normal saline. These patients require admission to the hospital for further treatment and evaluation by a surgeon.

REYE'S SYNDROME

BACKGROUND

Reye's syndrome is a distinct, clinicopathologic entity of unknown etiology which is preceded by a prodromal viral or viral-like illness and is characterized by a rapidly progressive encephalopathy and fatty degeneration of the viscera. Reye's syndrome is now considered by some observers to be among the 10 major causes of death in children aged 2 to 10 years. It is a true pediatric emergency with cerebral complications capable of rapidly reaching an irreversible state; yet it is a syndrome in which all the complex biological events are completely reversible.

Prior to 1977, the mortality rate in Reye's syndrome reached as high as 40 to 50%. Improved physician awareness and prompt treatment have reduced the mortality rate to 12 to 15%. Survival is still directly related to the severity of cerebral edema and increased intracranial pressure. Improved survival in recent years indicates that early recognition and treatment of mild cases may prevent progression of the encephalopathy. Nevertheless, at least 15% of the patients are left with significant neuropsychiatric deficits.

Reye's syndrome affects children of all ages. There is no sex difference. Eighty percent of cases occur between the ages of 1 and 13 years, an age group in which there seems to be a predilection for white suburban children. Fifteen percent of cases occur in infants less than 1 year of age where black, urban children are more likely to be affected. Mortality continues to be high in infancy, reaching 30 to 40%.

Reye's syndrome is a seasonal disease with two peaks: one from late December to early March, and the other from June to early July. There are two epidemiologic patterns: epidemic cases usually associated with influenza outbreaks occurring in older children (median age 11 years), and sporadic cases occurring in younger children (median age 6 years) and associated with numerous other viral agents, the most common of which is varicella.

PATHOPHYSIOLOGY

The pathogenesis of Reye's syndrome is felt to center around a primary mitochondrial injury in all tissues of the body. Abnormally low mitochondrial enzyme activities parallel histopathologic observations of mitochondrial degeneration in virtually every tissue studied by electron microscopy including liver, brain, kidney, skeletal muscle, pancreas and heart. The mitochondrial injury results in decreased activities of enzymes involved in the Krebs cycle, gluconeogenesis, and urea biosynthesis. Most of the clinical features of Reye's syndrome, including lactic acidosis, elevated fatty acids, nitrogen wasting, hyperammonemia, cellular fat accumulation, and cytotoxic cerebral edema may be explained in the context of primary mitochondrial damage.

The etiology of the mitochondrial damage remains unexplained. The disease is consistently associated with a prodromal viral infection, yet the primary pathologic findings do not indicate an acute or chronic inflammatory process. At least four pathogenic mechanisms have been hypothesized, none of which has yet been proven (Table 50.1).

1. Aprille has championed the concept of an intrinsic toxin affecting mitochondrial metabolism following a viral illness. To date, no such toxin has been identified. There was much enthusiasm in the late 1970's when serum from patients with Reye's syndrome was shown to stimulate oxygen utilization in preparations of isolated rat liver mitochondria and to cause mitochondrial swelling. This phenomenon, however, has subsequently been shown to be caused by uric acid, a serum factor known to be increased in Reye's syndrome.

2. A number of investigators have hypothesized an extrinsic toxin such as environmental chemicals (pesticides, organic solvents) or drugs (salicylates, antiemetics) which may alter the host response during the recovery phase of a viral illness.

The similarity of Reye's syndrome to salicylate intoxication has always intrigued investigators. A recent report has documented that salicylates have been consumed more frequently and in larger quantities by patients who developed Reye's syndrome than control subjects and suggested that increasing doses of salicylate relate directly to the severity of Reye's syndrome. Despite the fact that no direct evidence points to salicylates as the specific etiology of the metabolic disturbances found in Reye's syndrome, the American Academy of Pediatrics has recently recommended that aspirin should not be given to children with varicella or those suspected of having influenza.

Table 50.1
Pathogenic Mechanisms Implicated in Production of Reye's Syndrome

Interaction of viral illness with—
1. Intrinsic toxin
2. Extrinsic toxin
   a. Environmental chemicals (pesticides, organic solvents)
   b. Drugs (salicylates, antiemetics)
3. Genetic predisposition
4. Primary metabolic disorder

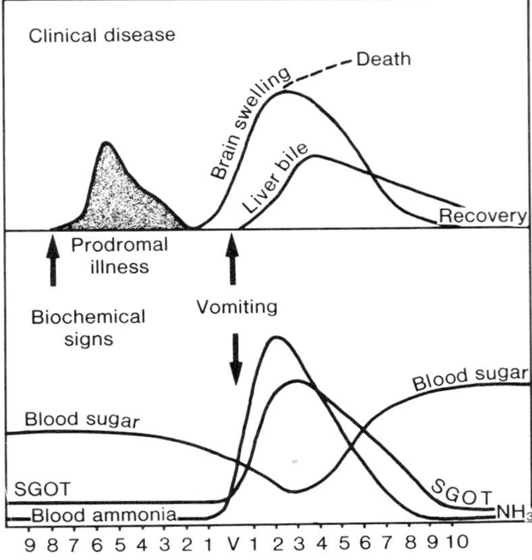

Figure 50.3. Clinical history in Reye's syndrome. (Modified from J. C. Partin: *Gastroenterology, 69:* 511, 1975.)

3. A genetic predisposition has been suggested by rare cases reported in siblings and first cousins, together with a few documented cases of recurrent Reye's syndrome.

4. Finally, there is still the possibility that Reye's syndrome reflects a primary metabolic disorder in lipid and ammonia metabolism which is unmasked following viral exposure.

CLINICAL MANIFESTATIONS

The biphasic clinical history is remarkably constant (Fig. 50.3). There is a history of a recent, usually febrile, illness that is waning or has resolved. Approximately 90% of the children have an antecedent upper respiratory infection and 5 to 7% of cases are associated with antecedent varicella. The abrupt onset of protracted vomiting usually starts within 1 week following the prodromal illness. The vomiting is unresponsive to restriction of oral intake or to antiemetic therapy. It is a somewhat less constant finding in infants less than 1 year of age (86%) as compared to older children (98%).

Coincident with the onset of vomiting (or shortly thereafter), signs of encephalopathy appear. At first, encephalopathy may be manifested by unusual quietness or disinterest. However, there may be rapid sequential progression to irritability, combativeness, confusion, disorientation, delirium, stupor and coma. Seizures are a late sign in older children but may occur during early stages of encephalopathy in infancy (usually secondary to hypoglycemia).

In the emergency department, patients are usually afebrile. Tachycardia and hyperventilation commonly occur. At the initial presentation only 50% of patients have hepatomegaly. The liver usually increases in size during the first 24 to 48 hours after the diagnosis is made. Absence of jaundice and scleral icterus is characteristic and is the major mitigating clinical sign against hepatic encephalopathy secondary to acute fulminant hepatitis. Despite evidence of encephalopathy, there are no focal neurological signs, nor signs of meningeal irritation. The level of coma should be classified as proposed by Lovejoy (Table 50.2).

Table 50.2
Clinical Staging of Reye's Syndrome (Lovejoy)

Stage I.	Vomiting, lethargy and sleepiness
Stage II.	Disorientation, delirium, combativeness; hyperventilation, hyperreflexia, appropriate responses to noxious stimuli
Stage III.	Obtunded, coma, hyperventilation; inappropriate response to noxious stimuli; decorticate posturing; preservation of pupillary, light reflexes and oculovestibular reflexes (doll's eyes)
Stage IV.	Deeper coma, decerebrate rigidity, loss of oculovestibular reflexes, dilated fixed pupils, dysconjugate eye movements in response to caloric stimulation
Stage V.	Seizures, absent deep tendon reflexes, respiratory reflexes, flaccid paralysis

Diagnosis

The diagnosis of Reye's syndrome is suggested by the clinical presentation, supported by characteristic biochemical findings, and confirmed by characteristic histologic findings on liver biopsy. The biochemical evaluation of suspected Reye's syndrome is outlined in Table 50.3. The hallmark of the acute encephalopathy of Reye's syndrome is the associated evidence of liver abnormality. Transaminases (SGOT and SGPT) and blood ammonia are almost always elevated at the time of the onset of protracted vomiting. The range of transaminase elevation is highly variable and has not been shown to correlate well with severity of the disease. Ammonia levels greater than 300 μg/L have been shown to be an indicator of a poor prognosis. The protrombin time is less than 50% of control in at least half the patients, although clinical bleeding is rare and evidence of disseminated intravascular coagulation is absent. The serum bilirubin may be greater than 2.0 mg/100 ml in 10 to 15% of patients; however, the highest reported

Table 50.3
Biochemical Evaluation of Reye's Syndrome

I. Abnormal Studies
- A. Evaluation of SGOT, SGPT (at least 2 times normal)
- B. Elevation of blood ammonia (at least 1.5 times control)
- C. Prolongation of prothrombin time
- D. Hyperammonoacidemia (particularly glutamine, alanine, lysine)
- E. Elevated blood urea nitrogen (BUN)
- F. Ketonuria
- G. Hypoglycemia
- H. Decreased serum bicarbonate
- I. Decreased arterial PCO_2
- J. Bilirubin <3.0 mg/100 ml

II. Normal Studies
- A. Spinal fluid cell count, protein, Gram strain
- B. Platelet count and blood smear
- C. Drug toxic screen
- D. Amylase

value in an accepted case of Reye's syndrome is only 3.5 mg/100 ml. The direct reacting fraction of the total bilirubin usually is greater than 15% of the total. Hypoglycemia is rare, except in children presenting in Stage IV coma and in infants less than 1 year old, in whom the incidence is reported to be as high as 70 to 80%. Azotemia is seen 30 to 40% of the time and ketonuria, 80%. Both are felt to be secondary to starvation and dehydration, from vomiting and poor oral intake. Patients most frequently have a mixed respiratory alkalosis and mild metabolic acidosis. The metabolic acidosis correlates with the level of ammonia elevation and reflects the degree of mitochondrial dysfunction.

Oil red O stain of a frozen section of liver obtained by percutaneous needle biopsy reveals panlobular steatosis, with multiple small droplets of lipid uniformly distributed throughout the hepatocytes. The biopsy is also characterized by insignificant inflammation, rare individual cell necrosis, and minimal bile stasis. These histologic findings are not pathognomonic of Reye's syndrome; however, in conjunction with the classical clinical presentation and biochemical findings discussed above, the liver biopsy proves the diagnosis.

Differential Diagnosis

A number of conditions have now been reported to mimic Reye's syndrome, especially mild or sporadic cases (Table 50.4).

Table 50.4
Mimickers of Reye's Syndrome

I. *Infectious.* Viral encephalitis, varicella hepatitis
II. *Metabolic Disorder.* Urea cycle disorder, carnitine deficiency, β-OH-, β-methylglutaric aciduria, hereditary fructose intolerance, isovaleric acidemia, cystic fibrosis
III. *Drug Intoxication or Idiosyncratic Reactions.* Salicylates, lead, acetominophen, valproic acid, methyl bromide, hydrocarbon, chlordane, disulfiram, ethanol
IV. *Other.* Pancreatic encephalopathy; acute encephalopathy and fatty metamorphosis associated with cold agglutinin autoimmune hemolytic anemia; toxic encephalopathy without liver dysfunction (Gall's syndrome)

These can usually be ruled out in older children by a good history, together with pertinent negative biochemical findings (Table 50.3). The physician should carefully inquire about the child's recent drug ingestion or the possible exposure to environmental toxins. Parents should be asked specifically about the occurrence and frequency of the child's use of aspirin. Inquiries should be made regarding the parents' occupation, hobbies, recent travel, home renovation, and the spraying of pesticides. A past medical history of any head trauma, previous signs of encephalopathy, protein intolerance, muscle weakness, and vomiting associated with fasting should be sought. Family history of neurologic or liver disease is important. All patients with a presumed diagnosis of Reye's syndrome must have a lumbar puncture to rule out meningitis and encephalitis. While a lumbar puncture during acute intracranial pressure spikes (see below) is contraindicated, complications are rare because of the diffuse nature of the cerebral edema. Spinal fluid pressure is usually elevated, and the CSF glucose may be reduced if the patient has been hypoglycemic. A toxicology screen including salicylate levels should be performed on all patients. The absence of jaundice, together with a bilirubin less than 3.0 mg/100 ml essentially rules out the possibility of acute fulminant hepatitis. Absence of a history of abdominal pain, together with a normal serum amylase, rules out pancreatitis. Diffuse intravascular coagulation as a cause for the abnormal prothrombin time is unlikely if there is a normal platelet count and blood smear.

Management

General Overview

Despite the generalized nature of the mitochondrial insult in Reye's syndrome, the brain is the principal organ affected by the syndrome. Increased intracranial pressure (ICP), secondary to cerebral edema, is the major factor contributing to morbidity and mortality in Reye's syndrome. The effectiveness of accurate ICP monitoring via a subarachnoid bolt or intraventricular catheter is now well established. With the ability to monitor ICP, a number of different invasive therapies have been introduced in an attempt to rapidly reduce and control cerebral edema. None of these therapies, including hyperventilation and muscle paralysis using neuromuscular blocking drugs, hyperosomolar agents, high dose barbituates, exchange transfusions, or hypothermia has been clearly established to protect the brain from progressive ischemic insult. Various centers throughout the country advocate differing treatment measures. To date, no controlled studies have been initiated. While ICP monitoring and aggressive treatment were previously reserved for patients reaching Stage III coma, more and more centers are now instituting these measures in Stage II coma, particularly if admission serum ammonia levels are greater than 300 μg/L. The latter, more aggressive, approach demands an accurate diagnosis.

There is considerable controversy surrounding the necessity of doing a liver biopsy in every case to establish the diagnosis. We feel the decision to perform a biopsy must be made based on the physician's judgment of (a) ruling out conditions known to mimic Reye's syndrome and (b) the safety of liver biopsy. We recommend a liver biopsy in order to confirm a diagnosis of Reye's syndrome in the following cases:

1. Sporadic cases outside the usual seasonal occurrence.
2. Infants less than 1 year old.
3. Atypical history or biochemical findings.
4. Any patient sufficiently ill to require ICP monitoring, either by a subarachnoid bolt or by an intraventricular catheter.

If there is a gastroenterologist or surgeon experienced in the performance of liver biopsy, the procedure can be performed safely in even severe cases if the prothrombin time can be reduced to 16 sec or less. The abnormal prothrombin time in Reye's syndrome rarely responds to vitamin K infusion, but usually does improve following fresh frozen plasma. We usually give 5 to 10 mg of vitamin K by slow i.v. push in addition to 10 ml/kg of fresh frozen plasma and then recheck the prothrombin time. If the level improves (to less than 14 sec) then no further therapy is needed. If the value is between 14 and 16 sec, we then have another 10 ml/kg of plasma infusing during the liver biopsy.

The performance of a liver biopsy should never, however, be a prerequisite to the institution of aggressive medical management in the patient with clinical Reye's syndrome who demonstrates rapidly progressing cerebral edema.

Emergency Department Management of Reye's Syndrome

Once the diagnosis is suspected, immediate plans should be set into motion to admit the child to a center with a staff and facilities to monitor intracranial pressure. A hospital without such facilities should not observe a patient in the early stages of Reye's syndrome because too often the progression of the encephalopathy may proceed rapidly, resulting in increased mortality and morbidity. During the first 72 hours, Reye's syndrome should always be managed in an intensive care unit.

The proper initial staging of coma is essential (Table 50.2). The survival of the patient is definitely related to the stage of the disease upon admission. In practice it is difficult to distinguish between Stage II and Stage III coma. However, the reaction of the child to noxious stimuli often serves as a guide. The delirious patient in Stage II will have an appropriate response to noxious stimuli, i.e., if you squeeze behind the ankle of the right foot, the patient will withdraw the right foot. If you squeeze the right foot and the patient moves the left arm, this is usually an indication of Stage III coma.

The management of Reye's syndrome is supportive, since no specific curative therapy is currently available. A treatment plan, based on stage of coma and level of blood ammonia, is outlined below:

1. For Stage I Patients:

a. Draw initial blood studies including a crossmatch for blood (Table 50.3). Measure the serum glucose immediately and then hourly. Hypoglycemia, if present, can usually be corrected early by hypertonic glucose infusion.
b. Perform a lumbar puncture using a small gauge (22) needle.
c. Place a large bore intravenous cath-

eter and give intravenous fluids at a rate of ⅔ maintenance (see Chapter 46). Use a 10% dextrose solution to protect against hypoglycemia. Most Reye's syndrome patients do not present with more than a mild case of dehydration. *It is paramount to avoid early overhydration.*

d. Monitor vital signs every 15 min.
e. Avoid excessive stimulation that may increase the intracranial pressure. Try to keep the patient in a quiet room.

2. *For Stage II Patients with Blood Ammonia <300 μg/L:*
   a. Monitor vital functions with a continuous ECG, indwelling urinary catheter, and arterial line.
   b. Place a nasogastric tube and begin neomycin 50 mg/kg/day (given by nasogastric tube 3 times a day) to reduce blood ammonia.
   c. Begin mannitol (20% solution) 1 g/kg i.v. over 30 min every 6 hours. Mannitol is a hyperosmolar agent which does not cross the blood-brain barrier. Hyperosmolar therapy increases serum osmolarity and actually dehydrates the brain by withdrawing fluid from the tissues. We do not agree with those who feel there is a rebound of cerebral edema following mannitol infusion.
   d. Dexamethasone may be used at a loading dose of 0.2 mg/kg i.v. followed by 0.1 mg/kg every 6 hours. The site of action of steroids on brain edema is still unknown. Although the ICP lowering effect requires 24 hours or more, stabilization of ICP pressure waves and improved intracranial compliance may occur in a considerably less period of time.

3. *For Stage II Coma with Blood Ammonia >300 μg/L, and Stage III, Stage IV, and Stage V Coma*
   a. Elective intubation and manual hyperventilation are required until the patient can be transferred to a unit for mechanical ventilation and intracranial pressure monitoring. All patients should be paralyzed with pancuronium (see Chapter 3).

4. *Acute Spontaneous Intracranial Pressure Spikes:*

   Acute intracranial pressure spikes may occur in the emergency department. Clinical signs include increased hyperventilation, episodic bradycardia, intermittant pupillary dilatation, and decerebration.

   Management of an acute spike in the emergency department should include:
   a. Manual hyperventilation.
   b. Mannitol, 1 g/kg i.v. over 30 min if the patient has not had a dose within 3 hours.
   c. Thiopental (2 to 4 mg/kg i.v.).
   d. Lasix, 1 mg/kg i.v.
   e. Immediate neurosurgical consultation for emergency placement of an intraventricular catheter or decompressive craniotomy if there is no response to medical measures.

ACUTE BILIARY TRACT DISEASE

BACKGROUND

Acute biliary disease occurs only occasionally in childhood and is associated with a wide spectrum of clinical manifestations. Biliary colic and acute cholecystitis are complications of cholelithiasis, which is primarily associated with hemolytic anemias such as sickle cell disease and hereditary spherocytosis. Acalculous cholecystitis, or acute inflammation of the gallbladder in the absense of gallstones, is actually more common than cholelithiasis in children and has been associated with bacterial enteric infections (typhoid, shigellosis, *Escherichia coli*), scarlet fever, pneumonia, mucocutaneous lymph node syndrome, leptospirosis, hepatitis, polyarteritis nodosa, and parasitic infections (ascaris and giardia). Acute cholangitis results from concurrent biliary infection and obstruction and is seen primarily in the pediatric patient who has had surgical correction of congenital biliary tract obstruction (biliary atresia, choledochal cyst).

PATHOPHYSIOLOGY

Biliary colic results from acute transient obstruction of the cystic duct or common bile duct by gallstone(s). Cholecystitis is an aseptic inflammatory process which develops as a reaction to chemical injury triggered by obstruction to the cystic duct by a gallstone. This inflammation is mediated by (a) lysolecithin, which is formed from biliary lecithin by refluxed pancreatic enzyme phospholipase A, (b) refluxed proteolytic pancreatic enzymes, and (c) unconjugated bile salts. The etiology of acalculous cholecystitis is unknown. The condition is commonly associated with gallbladder distention, or so-called acute hydrops of the gallbladder. In infectious syndromes inflammation of the cystic duct and/or enlargement of mesenteric lymph nodes may result in obstruction to bile flow. In vasculitis syndromes such as mucocutaneous lymph node syndrome or polyarteritis nodosa, there may be a reactive serositis or vasculitis with increased mucus secretion by the gallbladder which, when coupled with factors that contribute to bile stasis such as fever, prolonged fasting, ileus, or dehydration, may result in gallbladder distention that in turn may kink the cystic duct. Cholangitis results from secondary bacterial infection by enteric organisms in the face of continued biliary tract obstruction. In cholangitis, the infection may be mild and superficial producing only short-lived symptoms. Alternatively, it may be extensive and progress to suppurative cholangitis with septic shock and formation of hepatic abcesses.

CLINICAL MANIFESTATIONS

The pain of biliary colic is acute in onset, frequently follows a meal, and usually localizes in the epigastrium or right upper quadrant. In children, however, it may be localized to the periumbilical area. Characteristically, the pain rises to a plateau of intensity over 5 to 20 min and persists for a variable duration, usually less than 4 hours (although less than 1 hour in 50% of patients). In contrast to the colicky pain of intestinal or ureteral origin, biliary colic does not worsen in relatively short cyclic paroxysms or bursts, but instead is characterized by its sustained, intense quality. Unlike pancreatitis, the patient tends to move about restlessly and the pain is not improved by changes in position. In addition, referred pain is common, particularly to the dorsal lumbar back near the tip of the right scapula. Nausea and vomiting are commonly associated with biliary colic, but are not severe and protracted as seen with pancreatitis. Mild or low grade jaundice occurs in one quarter of patients, but the serum bilirubin rarely exceeds 4 mg/dl.

Clinically, an attack of acute cholecystitis begins with biliary colic, which increases progressively in severity or duration. Pain lasting longer than 4 hours suggests cholecystitis. As the inflammation worsens, the pain changes character, becoming more generalized in the upper abdomen and increased by deep respiration and jarring motions. The temperature is usually elevated to 37.5 to 39.0°C. Low grade jaundice is present in about one quarter of patients.

Cholangitis should be suspected in the patient who has right upper quadrant abdominal pain, shaking chills, and spiking fever (≥39.0°C) with jaundice (Charcot's triad). The danger of this disorder is that overwhelming sepsis can develop rapidly. Listlessness and shock are characteristic of advanced or very severe cholangitis and usually reflect gram-negative septicemia. It is important to recognize that cholangitis can evolve very rapidly before development of significant jaundice. Clinically apparent jaundice may be absent even in postsurgical biliary atresia patients.

In addition to scleral icterus, nonspecific physical findings which suggest gallbladder disease include: right upper quadrant guarding even to light palpation; Murphy's sign (production of pain by deep inspiration or cough when the physician's fingers are depressing the abdomen below the right costal margin in the midclavicular line and abrupt cessation of inspiration due to pain); and production of pain or tenderness by a light blow applied with the ulnar surface of the hand to the subcostal area. In about one third of patients with cholecystitis, the gallbladder is palpable as a sausage-shaped mass lateral to the midclavicular line. A rigid abdomen or rebound tenderness suggests local perforation or gangrene of the gallbladder.

Laboratory tests are also nonspecific. CBC and blood smear may show evidence of hemolysis. The leukocyte count averages 12,000 to 15,000/cu mm with a neutrophilic leukocytosis. Leukocyte counts above 15,000/cu mm suggest cholangitis. Serum bilirubin rarely exceeds 4 mg/dl and higher values are more compatible with either complete common duct obstruction or cholangitis. Serum transaminases, SGOT and SGPT, and alkaline phosphatase may be mildly elevated. Marked elevation of transaminases may occur with acute complete common duct obstruction. Serum amylase may be mildly elevated without other evidence of pancreatitis. Abdominal flat and upright x-rays may show right upper quadrant calcification of gallstones, particularly in patients with hemolytic anemia or a right upper quadrant mass. Abdominal x-rays are particularly important to rule out perforation.

Conditions to be considered in the differential diagnosis of biliary tract disease include perforated peptic ulcer, pneumonia, intercostal neuritis, pancreatitis, hepatitis, and hepatic and abdominal sickle cell crisis. Therefore, evaluation should also include stool guaiac, chest x-ray, amylase/creatinine ratio, and a peripheral blood smear.

EMERGENCY MANAGEMENT

All patients with suspected acute biliary tract disease should be admitted to the hospital. The exception is biliary colic that has resolved spontaneously, in which case an outpatient evaluation can be pursued. Biliary colic, cholecystitis, and cholangitis are general indications for surgery in patients with gallstones. Conditions associated with acalculous cholecystitis should be evaluated and treated if identified.

General emergency room management includes discontinuation of oral intake, support with intravenous fluids, and surgical consultation. Narcotics should be withheld until a tentative decision regarding early surgery is reached. When given, meperidine 1 to 2 mg/kg is the treatment of choice.

In suspected cholangitis in patients with congenital biliary tract obstruction, blood cultures should be drawn but antibiotics withheld pending liver biopsy for definitive culture. The exception is the clinically septic child in whom antibiotic coverage should be immediately instituted with a cephalosporin, such as cefazolin (100 mg/kg/day), and gentamicin (5–7.5 mg/kg/day).

ACUTE PANCREATITIS

BACKGROUND

Because it is rare in children, the diagnosis of pancreatitis is often overlooked as pathognomonic symptoms are infrequently present. Pancreatitis should be considered in any child with acute or chronic abdominal pain, vomiting and epigastric pain, ascites of obscure origin, and following upper abdominal trauma. Table 50.5 lists the wide spectrum of causes of pancreatitis; in upward of 30% of cases, however, the precipitating factor is unknown. About 50% of cases are associated with either mumps or blunt trauma. Mumps pancreatitis is seldom severe and rarely occurs under the age of 5 years; clinical mumps is present in only 50 to 60% of cases. Most blunt injuries to

Table 50.5
Causes of Acute Pancreatitis in Children

I. *Trauma.* Blunt, penetrating, surgical.
II. *Infectious.* Mumps, coxsackievirus B, hemolytic streptococcus, salmonella, hepatitis A and B
III. *Obstructive.* Cholelithiasis, ascaris, congenital duodenal stenosis, duplications, tumor, choledochal cyst
IV. *Drugs.* Steroids, chlorothiazides, salicylazosulfapyridine, azothiaprine, alcohol, valproic acid, tetracyclines, borates, oral contraceptives
V. *Systemic.* Systemic lupus erythematosus, periarteritis nodosa, malnutrition, peptic ulcer, uremia
VI. *Endocrine.* Hyperparathyroidism
VII. *Metabolic.* Hypercholesterolemia, cystic fibrosis, vitamin A and D deficiency
VIII. *Hereditary*
IX. *Idiopathic*

he pancreas are the result of automobile ccidents or falls from bicycles. Neverthe-ess, since the pancreas is a fixed retroperi-oneal structure, seemingly mild trauma rom small pointed objects, such as sticks r fence posts may transmit a localized hock wave directly to the organ.

ATHOPHYSIOLOGY

Regardless of the initiating event, the athophysiology of acute pancreatitis is robably very similar. Activation of the umerous pancreatic enzymes, including roteolytic enzymes, lipase, amylase, elas-ase, and phospholipase A, produces auto-igestion of the gland. The process may be ocal or diffuse. In mild cases there is nterstitial edema and inflammatory infil-rate without significant cell necrosis. This ype of pancreatitis, called *acute edema-ous pancreatitis*, is by far *the most com-non form seen in children* and is usually elf-limiting and associated with complete ecovery. When the autodigestive process ntensifies with increased inflammation, fat ecrosis, and hemorrhagic changes, the pro-ess is called *necrotic or hemorrhagic pan-reatitis*. This type of pancreatitis is asso-iated with a 20 to 40% mortality and sig-ificant morbidity. It is not clear why the utodigestive process is arrested in some ases and not others, but one factor may be he magnitude of the initial triggering nechanism.

The morbidity and mortality associated vith pancreatitis is related to complications rom the autodigestive process. Fat necrosis f neighboring tissue and saponification of alcium often result from release of pan-reatic lipase. Released proteolytic en-ymes may extend the inflammatory pro-ess into the retroperitoneum as well as eritoneal cavity. Proteolytic enzymes may ctivate kallikrein, a potent vasoactive po-ypepticle which may mediate systemic vas-dilatation and increased vascular perme-bility producing severe hypotension. Sec-ndary infection may lead to abscess for-nation, and walling off of the autodigestive rocess may result in pseudocyst formation.

LINICAL MANIFESTATIONS

Abdominal pain is the most consistent ymptom of pancreatitis and may vary from a tolerable distress to severe incapacitating pain. Onset is typically insidious over sev-eral hours, but may be acute. Pain is usually localized to the epigastrium, although it may radiate to the back (left scapula or either the right or left upper quadrants). The pain is usually described as knifelike and boring in quality and is aggravated when the patient lies on his or her back. Classically, the pain of pancreatitis is *con-stant*, as opposed to colicky pain which waxes and wanes. Nausea and vomiting are the most common associated symptoms. Vomiting may be severe and protracted. Low grade fever (<38.5°C) is present in 50 to 60% of cases. In cases of severe necrotic pancreatitis, the patients may complain of dizziness. Mental aberrations are common in necrotic pancreatitis; patients may act overtly psychotic or present in coma.

Early in the course of the disease, the discrepancy between the severity of the patient's pain and physical findings may be sharp. Patients are usually quiet and prefer sitting or lying on their side with knees flexed. The abdomen may be distended but is not rigid. There may be mild to moderate voluntary guarding in the epigastrium. Re-bound tenderness is rare but a poor prog-nostic sign when present. A palpable epi-gastric mass suggests pseudocyst. Ascites is rare. Bowel sounds may be decreased or absent. Associated physical findings may include: signs of parotitis, mild hepatosple-nomegaly, epigastric mass, pleural effu-sions, and mild icterus. Bluish discoloration around the umbilicus (Cullen's sign) or flanks (Grey Turner's sign) is a poor prog-nostic sign and evidence of hemorrhagic pancreatitis. Signs of overt hemodynamic instability are rarely present at initial pre-sentation. It is particularly important to evaluate patients for clinical signs of hypo-calcemia (Trousseau and Chvostek signs).

Clinical diagnosis is often tentative be-cause the same constellation of symptoms (abdominal pain, vomiting and low grade fever) and signs (abdominal tenderness and guarding) may be mimicked by several other conditions including penetrating pep-tic ulcer, gastritis, biliary colic, acute cho-lecystitis, intestinal obstruction and appen-dicitis.

Currently two easily attainable tests are

used to make a diagnosis of pancreatitis: (1) serum amylase and (2) the amylase-creatinine clearance ratio. Neither of these is specific for pancreatitis, and therefore they must be analyzed in the context of clinical presentation and physical examination. The pillar of laboratory diagnosis is the serum amylase. In acute pancreatitis, the serum amylase increases 2 to 12 hours after the onset of the autodigestive process and returns to normal within 3 to 4 days. Elevations 3-fold greater than normal are always significant, but may not be present when the patient first presents to the emergency department. Likewise, because amylase is rapidly cleared by the kidneys, the level may return to normal within 24 hours of onset even though pain persists. Additionally, elevated serum triglycerides may interfere with the assay and result in falsely normal values. There may also be a number of situations that cause an amylase elevation other than pancreatitis: penetrating or perforated ulcer, intestinal obstruction or infarction, Crohn's disease, pneumonia, hepatitis, liver trauma, acute biliary tract disease, salpingitis, salivary adenitis, renal failure, diabetic ketoacidosis, and benign macroamylasemia. Because of the above problems, a much more useful screening laboratory test is the urinary excretion of amylase, and its relationship to the creatinine clearance. In acute pancreatitis, more amylase is delivered to the urine by way of clearance from the serum than is normally the case. The cause for this increased urinary excretion of amylase is unknown, but the mechanism has been shown to be a reduced tubular reabsorption of amylase. This increase in renal clearance of amylase does not occur in most other situations associated with hyperamylasemia (exceptions being renal failure, burns, and diabetic ketoacidosis). The ratio of renal clearance of amylase to creatinine can be obtained by testing a spot urine and serum sample.

$$C_{amylase}\ (C_{AM})/C_{creatinine}\ (C_{CR})\ (\%) = (\text{urine amylase}/\text{serum amylase}) \times (\text{serum creatinine}/\text{urine creatinine}) \times 100$$

In adults, C_{AM}/C_{CR} over 4 to 5% is diagnostic for pancreatitis. Unfortunately, scant information is available on the sensitivity of the ratio in diagnosing pancreatitis in children. We have observed a number of patients with pancreatitis without an elevated ratio such that in pediatrics a normal ratio cannot rule out a diagnosis of pancreatitis.

Corroborating information for the diagnosis can be obtained by the findings of an elevation of serum lipase and swelling of the pancreas on abdominal ultrasound, but these studies are not usually available to the emergency physician.

EMERGENCY MANAGEMENT

All patients with suspected pancreatitis should be admitted to the hospital. Treatment, however, should begin in the emergency department. The goals of medical treatment include suppression of pancreatic secretion and relief of pain. Morbidity and mortality in pancreatitis are directly related to complications which may already be present at the time of initial presentation. Therefore, agressive early maintenance of intravascular volume and treatment of hypocalcemia, respiratory distress, and suspected infection are mandatory.

The patient's oral intake should be discontinued and i.v. fluids infused at 1.5 times the maintenance rate. Frequent monitoring of vital signs and urine output should be instituted. Continuous nasogastric suction is begun using a sump tube. Aspiration of gastric contents is based on the premise that prevention of delivery of gastric acid into the duodenum will diminish hormonal stimulation of the pancreas. Nasogastric suction also relieves pain and prevents development of ileus. Use of anticholinergics or cimetidine to reduce gastric secretions is controversial and not recommended in the initial management of patients. Pain is treated with meperidine 1 to 2 mg/kg i.m. Morphine or codeine should not be used because they increase spasm at the spincter of Oddi.

Blood studies drawn in the emergency department, in addition to serum and urine amylase and creatinine should include: CBC, electrolytes, BUN, calcium, glucose, SGOT, SGPT, bilirubin, alkaline phosphatase, triglyceride, PT and PTT. Arterial blood gases should be obtained in patients vith tachypnea. A chest x-ray should be btained and evaluated for pleural effusion, nterstitial pneumonic infiltrates, and basiar atelectesis. A flat and upright abdominal -ray is needed to rule out perforation, asites, and pancreatic calcifications.

In the vast majority of cases, maintelance of intravascular volume and relief of ain will result in rapid resolution of sympoms. Prognostic indicators of necrotizing r hemorrhage pancreatitis include: hypoalcemia (<8.0 mg/dl), hyperglycemia >200 mg/dl), clinical shock, elevated henatocrit or BUN, ascites, and $PO_2 < 60$ orr. Such patients should be admitted to n intensive care unit, given sufficient coloid (albumin 0.25 g/kg) to maintain normal ntravascular volume, and have more extenive monitoring with an arterial line and rinary catheter. An arterial PO_2 less than 0 torr is an indication for elective intubaion. Early peritoneal dialysis should be tarted if there is rapid clinical deterioraion.

Antibiotics are not indicated in the initial nanagement of pancreatitis. Pancreatic abess, however, should be considered if temerature is greater than 38.5°C, in which ase broad spectrum antibiotic coverage vith ampicillin (200 mg/kg/day) and genamicin (5 to 7.5 mg/kg/day) are indicated ending the results of blood cultures and liagnostic ultrasound. Emergency surgery s rarely necessary in acute pancreatitis. ndications include control of active intraeritoneal bleeding, suspected abscess, and uspected traumatic transection.

VIRAL HEPATITIS

BACKGROUND

Epidemic jaundice is a disease first decribed by Hippocrates in 337 B.C. Since hen, numerous accounts of epidemics, paricularly during times of war, are well decribed. The current incidence reported in his country in 1973 was 8851 cases anually. This has fallen by approximately 0% within the last 10 years with recogniion of the virus(es) responsible for the isease and the evolution of new techniques or the identification of specific infective gents. Further studies have resulted in the development of a successful animal model for viral hepatitis and in the production of a first generation of effective vaccines. These advances have marked a new era in understanding the pathogenesis of these endemic diseases.

Epidemiological surveillance suggests that type B hepatitis is prevalent in all parts of the world, regardless of the cultural or socioeconomic conditions. However, its prevalence varies with different populations and environments. For example, it is 4 times more prevalent in health care personnel involved in direct patient care; particularly hemodialysis units, institutions for the mentally handicapped and in commercial donors. The magnitude of the type B hepatitis problem is expanded by its ability to produce a chronic carrier state with persistent antigenemia in 5 to 10% of infected subjects. Thus, it may maintain an infectious pool without serial transmission.

It has long been recognized that hepatitis B is transmitted predominately by the parenteral route. Additionally, the presence of virus in saliva, breast milk, urine and genital secretions, plus a demonstrated higher incidence of infection in family contacts, dictates that the infection may spread by other than parenteral inoculation. Today, the majority of post-transfusion hepatitis most likely occurs from a non-A, non-B hepatitis virus yet to be isolated.

Hepatitis A, by contrast, is spread principally by the fecal oral route, although documented parenteral contamination has been demonstrated. There is no chronic carrier state.

CLINICAL MANIFESTATIONS

There are several different distinct clinical presentations of viral hepatitis which vary widely from slight malaise without icterus to a severe fatal disease culminating in hepatic failure. In general, viral type A, type B, and non-A, non-B hepatitis run the same clinical course. However, type B tends to be more severe and may be associated with a serum sickness-like syndrome which develops a week before the onset of jaundice. Fever is the rule; skin lesions are urticarial with a papular acrodermatitis being described in children. The arthropathy is symmetrical, nonmigrating and affects small joints.

In a typical case, a prodromal phase is distinguished in retrospect and is characterized by fatigue, anorexia, and gastrointestinal upset. A mild fever may occur between 3 and 4 days and even up to 2 weeks preceding the onset of jaundice. Hepatitis, at this stage, is usually not suspected unless in the midst of an epidemic. The prodromal phase is followed by fever, chills, headache, arthritis and discomfort, or heaviness in the right upper quadrant with tenderness to percussion. In children, the onset is usually rapid with progression to hepatosplenomegaly over 1 to 3 weeks, most often in less than 9 days. After about 1 week, jaundice becomes evident at the onset, first involving the scleral conjunctivae, and then extending to the face, trunk and extremities. Nearly one third of the children have mucous membrane and nasal pharyngeal symptoms. Pruritus without an associated rash is common.

During the icteric phase, the fever falls by lysis, subjective complaints decrease, and the jaundice becomes more pronounced. Liver enlargement usually increases and is tender. The spleen is nearly always palpable in children and in 25 to 50% of adolescents and young adults. The icteric period lasts from 1 to 4 weeks with nearly all symptoms resolving by 4 to 6 weeks after the onset of jaundice. In 1 to 15% of cases, fatigue and gastrointestinal symptoms may persist. Occasionally, the cholestasis is prolonged for 4 to 6 weeks with increasing pruritus at 2 to 3 weeks. Coexistant drug exposure as a cause of hepatic damage must be ruled out by history; however, the prognosis is usually excellent in viral hepatitis.

Laboratory Findings

Urine and Feces. Bilirubin appears in urine before the clinical appearance of jaundice. Urobilinogenuria is found in the late preicteric phase, but may disappear at the height of jaundice. Reappearance signifies hepatic recovery.

Serum Changes. The serum bilirubin rises, but levels vary widely, and conjugated hyperbilirubinemia occurs even before th total values are significantly elevated. Serum alkaline phosphatase is usually les than 3 times the upper limit of normal fo age. Serum albumin and globulin are usually normal. SGOT and SGPT elevation are useful for early diagnosis in a prodroma phase and for the detection of inapparen cases during epidemics. Peak values occu immediately preceding and after the onse of jaundice. The degree of elevation is no useful in prognosis, and they may remai elevated for up to 3 to 5 months even i patients making an uneventful recovery However, a more prolonged elevation ma necessitate evaluation for chronic liver disease.

Hematological Changes. The icteri stage is marked by leukopenia, lymphopenia, and neutropenia. Anemia and hemolysis may be precipitated in patient with glucose 6-phosphate dehydrogenas (G6PD) deficiency. Aplastic anemia is rar but often fatal.

Serological Changes. Figures 50.4 an 50.5 show the serological changes in hepatitis A and B, the most commonly see types.

Fulminant Hepatitis

This complication, fortunately rare, overwhelms the patient in 7 to 10 days. It ma develop so rapidly that the central nervou system findings of hepatic encephalopath predominate, and the patient presents wit acute behavioral changes and psychosi rather than jaundice. Alternatively, after

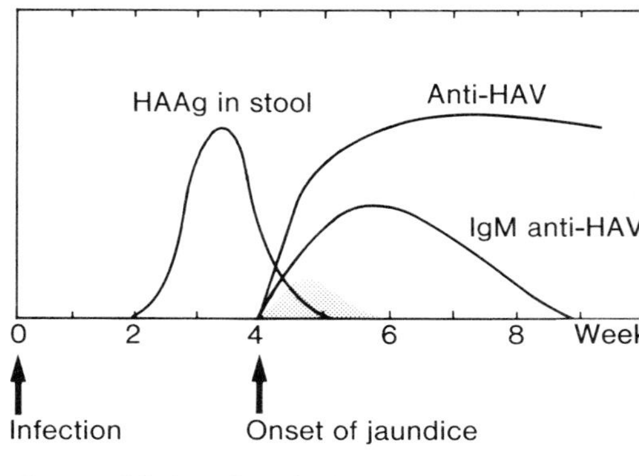

Figure 50.4. Serologic changes in hepatiti A. (HA = hepatitis A; V = virus; Ag = antigen

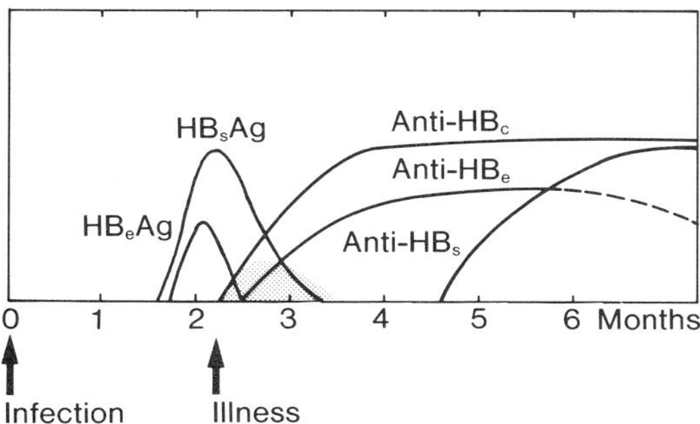

Figure 50.5. Serologic changes in hepatitis B. (HB = hepatitis B; S, C, and E are antigens.)

typical acute onset of viral hepatitis, the patient may become more deeply jaundiced and develop ominous signs including repeated vomiting, fetor hepaticus, mental confusion and drowsiness. A rising fever, hemorrhages, and decreasing liver size are poor prognostic signs. Leukocytosis, in contrast to the usual leukopenia of a viral hepatitis, is often seen. The biochemical changes are those of acute hepatic failure (e.g., hyperbilirubinemia, markedly elevated transaminase values and serum ammonia, and occasionally hypoglycemia). Laboratory indicators of a poor prognosis include a low serum albumin, poor response to parenteral vitamin K without normalization of the prothrombin time, and, possibly, low α-fetoprotein levels. Particular attention should be paid to the possibility of drug toxicity, especially acute acetaminophen overdose, and sepsis. Management requires an experienced staff and meticulous attention to all life-support measures.

MANAGEMENT

There is no specific treatment for viral hepatitis. Management is aimed at the maintenance of adequate nutrition and hydration, avoidance of secondary complications, and recognition of poor prognostic signs. The history should include a search for infectious contacts, drug exposure or venereal exposures. Initial laboratory studies should include determination of serum albumin, bilirubin, SGOT, SGPT, alkaline phosphatase, PT, PTT and acute titers to determine etiology of viral hepatitis (i.e., hepatitis A antibody, HBsAg, HBeAg, and HBsAB) unless the case follows known exposure or it is in the midst of an epidemic. Assessment of the nutritional status and hydration status are all necessary parts of the initial evaluation. Signs of chronic liver disease (ascites, gynecomastia), muscle wasting, vascular spiders or underlying metabolic (Wilson's disease, diabetes) or surgical disease (abdominal pain, cholecystitis, signs of intestinal obstruction) may be indications for hospitalization. Other indications include a severe course of the disease with increasing jaundice 12 to 14 days after the onset of illness, bleeding tendencies characterized by a prolonged prothrombin time uncorrectable by parenteral vitamin K, hypoalbuminemia (3 g/100 ml), dehydration, or a central nervous system disturbance.

IMMUNOGLOBULIN PROPHYLAXIS

Hepatitis A

Immune serum globulin (IsG) is effective in preventing or modifying type A viral hepatitis. When administered within 1 to 2 weeks of exposure in a dose of 0.02 ml/kg intramuscularly, it will prevent illness in 80 to 90% of those patients exposed. It should be given to all close personal contacts, including household members and playmates, who have not already had hepatitis A. School contacts should not be given IsG routinely unless a school-centered epidemic exists. When a common source of infection is identified (for instance, food or water), IsG should be given to all exposed. Previous exposure and demonstration of immunity may be confirmed by the demonstration of anti-HAV antibodies in the serum.

Hepatitis B

The role of hepatitis B immunoglobulin (HBIG) in prophylaxis is still under discussion. Post-exposure prophylaxis reduces the incidence of infection, but may prolong the incubation period and modify the disease. HBIG may be effective for patients with accidental percutaneous (e.g., needle stick) or sexual exposures. The dose is 0.05 to 0.07 ml/kg within 2 days of exposure, followed by a similar dose 25 to 30 days later.

References

GASTROINTESTINAL BLEEDING
General

Katz, LA: Advances in the approach to gastrointestinal bleeding in childhood. In *Digestive Disease in Children*, p. 405, edited by E Lebenthal. Grune & Stratton, New York, 1978.

Law DH, Watts HD: Gastrointestinal bleeding. In *Gastrointestinal Disease: Pathophysiology, Diagnosis, Management* Vol. 2, p. 217, edited by MH Sleisenger, JS Fordtran. W.B. Saunders, Philadelphia, 1978.

Ostrow JD, Mulvancy CA, Hansell JR, Rhodes RS: Sensitivity and reproducibility of clinical tests for fecal occult blood with an emphasis on false-positive reactions. *Am J Dig Dis* 18: 930, 1973.

Roy CC, Morin CL, Weber AM: Gastrointestinal emergency problems in pediatric practice. *Clin Gastroenterol* 10: 225, 1981.

Roy CC, Silverman A, Cozzetto FJ: Symptoms; hematemeses; rectal bleeding. In *Pediatric Clinical Gastroenterology*, Ed. 2, p. 23. C. V. Mosby, St. Louis 1975.

Spencer R: Gastrointestinal hemorrhage in infancy and childhood: 476 cases. *Surgery* 55: 718, 1964.

Upper GI Bleeding

Ament ME: Upper gastrointestinal fiberoptic endoscopy in pediatric patients. In *Digestive Disease in Children*, p. 3, edited by E Lebenthal. Grune & Stratton, New York, 1978.

Bismuth H: Hemobilia. *N Engl J Med* 288: 617, 1973.

Chojkier M, Conn HO: Esophageal tamponade in the treatment of bleeding varices; a decadal progress report. *Dig Dis Sci* 25: 267, 1980.

Eastwood GL: Does early endoscopy benefit the patient with active upper gastrointestinal bleeding? *Gastroenterology* 72: 737, 1977.

Gellis SS: Portal hypertension in early childhood; etiology and diagnostic procedures. In *Liver Disease in Infancy and Childhood*, SR Berenberg. Williams & Wilkins, Baltimore, 1971.

Hastings PR, Skillman JJ, Bushwell LS, Silen W: Antacid titration in the prevention of acute gastrointestinal bleeding. *N Engl J Med* 298: 1041, 1978.

Ivey KJ: Gastritis. *Med Clin North Am* 58: 1289, 1974.

Johnson WC, Widrich WC, Ansell JE, Robbins AH, Nabseth DC: Control of bleeding varices by vasopressin; a prospective randomized study. *Ann Surg* 186: 369, 1977.

Lamiell JM, Weyandt TB: Mallory-Weiss syndrome in two children. *J Pediatr 92:* 583, 1978.

Ponsky JL, Hoffman M, Swayngim DS: Saline irrigation in gastric hemorrhage; effect of temperature. *J Surg Res* 28: 204, 1980.

Priebe HJ, Skillman JJ, Bushnell SL, Long PC, Slien W: Antacid versus cimetidine in preventing acute gastrointestinal bleeding. *N Engl J Med* 302:426, 1980.

Protell RL, Silverstein FE, Gilbert DA, Feld AD: Severe upper gastrointestinal bleeding; I. Causes, pathogenesis and methods of diagnosis. *Clin Gastroenterol* 10: 17, 1981.

Rigberg LA, Ufberg MH, Brooks CM: Continuous low dose peripheral vein Pitressin infusion in the control of variceal bleeding. *Am J Gastroenteol* 68: 481, 1977.

Robb JDA, Thomas PS, Ors Zulok J, Odling-Smee GW: Duodenal ulcer in children. *Arch Dis Child* 47: 688, 1972.

Sernuau J, Nouel O, Belghiti J, Rueff B: Severe upper gastrointestinal bleeding; III. Guidelines for treatment. *Clin Gastroenterol* 10: 38, 1981.

Silen W: The prevention and management of stress ulcers. *Hosp Prac 15:* 93, 1980.

Thoeni RF, Cello JP: A critical look at the accuracy of endoscopy and double-contrast radiography of the upper gastrointestinal (UGI) tract in patients with substantial UGI hemorrhage. *Radiology* 135: 305, 1980.

Lower GI Bleeding

Apt L, Downey WS: Melena neonatorum; the swallowed blood syndrome. *J Pediatr* 47: 6, 1955.

Boley VJ, Brandt LJ, Frank MS: Severe lower intestinal bleeding; diagnosis and treatment. *Clin Gastroenterol* 10:65, 1981.

Bussy HJR, Veale MO, Marson BC: Genetics of gastrointestinal polyposis. *Gastroenterology* 74: 1325, 1978.

DeBartolo H, vanHeerden J: Meckel's diverticulum. *Am Surg* 183: 30, 1976.

George WL, Wolfe RD, Finegold SM: Treatment and prevention of antimicrobial agent-induced colitis and diarrhea. *Gastroenterology* 79: 366, 1980.

Gierup J, Jorulf H, Livaditis A: Management of intussusception in infants and children; a survey based on 288 consecutive cases. *Pediatrics* 50: 535, 1972.

Holgersen LO, Miller RE, Zintel HA: Juvenile polyps of the colon. *Surgery* 69: 288, 1971.

Karmali MA, Fleming PC: Campylobacter enteritis in children. *J Pediatr* 94: 527, 1979.

Katz AJ, Gang DL: A five-year-old girl with skin rash and abdominal pain. N Engl J Med 302: 853, 1980.

Kilpatrick ZM: Gonorrheal proctitis. *N Engl J Med* 287: 967, 1972.

Nugent FW, Veidenheimer MC, Zuberi S, Garabedian M, Parikh NK: Clinical course of ulcerative proctosigmoiditis. *Dig Dis* 15: 321, 1970.

Patterson M, Healy GR, Shabot JM: Serologic testing for amoebiasis. *Gastroenterology* 78: 136, 1980.

Polin R, Pollack PF, Barlow B, Wigger HG, Slovis TL, Santulli TV, Heird WC: Necrotizing enterocolitis in term infants. *J Pediatr* 89: 460, 1976.

Prince AS, Neu HC: Antibiotic-associated pseudomembranous colitis in children. *Pediatr Clin North Am* 26: 261, 1979.

Vantrappen G, Agg HO, Ponette E, et al.: Yersinia enteritis and enterocolitis; gastroenterological aspects. *Gastroenterology* 72: 220, 1977.

Whitington PF, Friedman AL, Chesney RW: Gastrointestinal disease in hemolytic-uremic syndrome. *Gastroenterology* 76: 728, 1979.

INFLAMMATORY BOWEL DISEASE

Binder SL, Patterson JF, Glotzer DJ: Toxic megacolon in ulcerative colitis. *Gastroenterology* 66: 909, 1974.

Farmer RG, Hawk WA, Turnbull RB Jr.: Clinical patterns of Crohn's disease; a statistical study of 615 cases. *Gastroenterology* 68: 627, 1975.

Hartong WA, Aryanitakis C, Scribba RM, et al.: Treatment of toxic megacolon; a comparative review of 29 patients. *Am J Dig Dis* 22: 195, 1977.

Kelts DG, Grand RJ: Inflammatory bowel disease in children and adolescents. *Curr Probl Pediatr* 10:000, 1981.

Soyer MT, Aldrete JS: Surgical treatment of toxic megacolon and proposal for a program of therapy. *Am J Surg* 140: 421, 1980.

Werlin SL, Grand RJ: Severe colitis in children and adolescents; diagnosis, course, and treatment. *Gastroenterology* 73: 828, 1977.

REYE'S SYNDROME

Aprille JR, Austin J, Costello CE, Royal N: Identification of the Reye's syndrome "serum factor." *Biochem Biophys Res Commun* 94: 381, 1980.

Baistreri WF, Buchino JJ: Dehydration, seizures, and hypoglycemia in a four-month-old child *J Pediatr* 97: 689, 1980.

Chapoy PR, Angelini C, Brown WJ, Stiff JE, Shug AL, Cederbum SD: Systemic carnitine deficiency—a treatable inherited lipid storage disease presenting as Reye's syndrome. *N Engl J Med* 303: 1389, 1980.

Corey L, Rubin RJ, Bregman D, Gregg MB: Diagnostic criteria for influenze B-associated Reye's syndrome; clinical vs. pathologic criteria. *Pediatrics* 60: 702, 1977.

Corey L, Rubin RJ, Hattwick MAW: Reye's syndrome; clinical progression and evaluation of therapy. *Pediatrics* 60: 708, 1977.

DeVivo DC: Reye's syndrome; a metabolic response to an acute mitochondrial insult. *Neurology* 28: 105, 1978.

Glasgow AM: Reye's syndrome mimiker. *J Natl Reye's syndrome Found* 1: 104, 1980.

Huttenlocber PR, Trauner DA: Reye's syndrome in infancy. *Pediatrics* 62: 84, 1978.

Lovejoy FH, Smith AL, Bresnan MJ, Wood JN, Victor DI, Adams PC: Clinical staging in Reye's syndrome. *Am J Dis Child* 128: 36, 1974.

Partin JC: Reye's syndrome (encephalopathy and fatty liver); diagnosis and treatment. *Gastroenterology* 69: 511, 1975.

Reye RDK, Morgan G, Baral J: Encephalopathy and fatty degeneration of the viscera; a disease entity in childhood. *Lancet* 2: 749, 1963.

Starko KM, Ray CG, Daminguez LB, Stromberg WL, Woodal DF: Reye's syndrome and salicylate use. *Pediatrics* 66: 859, 1980.

ACUTE BILIARY TRACT DISEASE

Boey JH, Way LW: Acute cholangitis. *Ann Surg* 191: 264, 1980.

Earnest DL: Manifestations and complications of gallstones. *Prac Gastroenterol* 5: 20, 1981.

Holcomb GW Jr, O'Neill JA, Holcomb GW III: Cholecystitis, cholelithiasis, and common duct stenosis in children and adolescents. *Ann Surg* 191: 626, 1980.

Sean HF, Golden GT, Horsley JS III: Cholecystitis in childhood and adolescence. *Arch Surg* 106: 651, 1973.

Way LW, Sleisenger MH: Acute cholecystitis. In *Gastrointestinal Disease: Pathophysiology, Diagnosis, Management*, Vol. 2, p. 1302, edited by MH Sleisenger, JS Fordtran. W. B. Saunders, Philadelphia, 1978.

ACUTE PANCREATITIS

Arvanitakis C, Cooke AR: Diagnostic tests of exocrine pancreatic function and disease. *Gastroenterology* 74: 932, 1978.

Brandborg LL: Acute pancreatitis. In *Gastrointestinal Disease: Pathophysiology, Diagnosis, Management*, Vol. 2, p. 1409, edited by MH Sleisenger, JS Fordtran. W.B. Saunders, Philadelphia, 1978.

Gauthier A, Escoffier JM, Camatte R, Sarles H: Severe acute pancreatitis. *Clin Gastroenterol* 10: 209: 1981.

Jordan S, Ament M: Pancreatitis in children and adults. *J Pediatr* 91: 211, 1977.

Levitt MD: Clinical use of amylase clearance and isoamylase measurements. *Mayo Clin Proc* 54: 428, 1979.

Mallory A, Kern F: Drug-induced pancreatitis; a critical review. *Gastroenterology* 78: 813, 1980.

Pokorny WJ, Raffensperger JB, Horberg FJ: Pancreatic pseudocysts in children. *Surg Gynecol Obstet* 151: 182, 1980.

Warshaw AL: Acute pancreatitis. *Viewpoints Dig Dis* 9: 1, 1977.

Warshaw AL: Surgical aspects of inflammatory pancreatic diseases. *Pract Gastroenterol* 2: 34, 1978.

HEPATITIS

Center for Disease Control: Recommendation of the Public Health Service Advisory Committee on Immunization Practices—Immune Globulins for Protection Against Viral Hepatitis. Hepatitis Surveillance Report No. 42, issued June 1978.

Krugman S, Gocke DJ: Viral hepatitis. In *Major Problems in Internal Medicine*, Vol. XV. W.B. Saunders, Philadelphia, 1978.

Krugman S, Overby LR, Mushahwar IK: Viral hepatitis, type B; studies on natural history and prevention re-examined. *N Engl J Med* 300: 101, 1979.

Sherlock S (ed): Viral hepatitis. In *Clinics in Gastroenterology*. W.B. Saunders, Philadelphia, 1980.

Vyas GN, Cohen SN, Schmid R (eds): *Viral Hepatitis*. Franklin Institute Press, Philadelphia, 1978.

CHAPTER **51**

Environmental Emergencies

ANN E. THOMPSON, M.D.

DROWNING AND NEAR DROWNING

BACKGROUND

Drowning is responsible for approximately 5,000 deaths a year in the United States, affecting all age groups, and affecting males 2 to 3 times more than females. Drowning and near drowning comprise a major component of the problem of childhood trauma, being the second or third most common cause of death in warm, water-oriented parts of the country.

Older infants and toddlers are disproportionately represented in these accidents, and their survival rates are lower. They are singularly vulnerable to immersion in bath tubs, diaper or laundry pails, rain barrels, home swimming pools, and other bodies of water near their homes, indicating the importance of careful surveillance, as well as public safety measures, such as fenced pools. Young teenagers are also at greater risk, probably as a result of decreased supervision by adults and increased bravado. However, coexisting trauma, drug or alcohol use, or intended suicide must be considered in each case.

Submersion accidents may be divided into two groups: drowning, with death occurring within 24 hours; and near drowning, with survival for at least 24 hours. Each of these is further divided according to whether aspiration has occurred.

PATHOPHYSIOLOGY

When a conscious mammal is submerged, either breath holding or laryngospasm occurs. The resulting hypoxemia may lead to loss of consciousness and cardiovascular collapse without aspiration of fluid. Alternatively, frantic struggling may result in gasping while submerged, with subsequent aspiration. If there is pre-existent impairment of consciousness and loss of protective airway reflexes as a result of head trauma, drug ingestion, seizure activity, or cardiac arrhythmia, aspiration is more likely to occur. Thus, it becomes obvious that although most systems may become involved, the major morbidity is in the pulmonary and central nervous systems.

Fresh water aspirated into the lungs is rapidly taken up into the circulation, resulting in a transient rise in circulating blood volume that is quickly redistributed through the body. Even small quantities of water, 1 to 3 ml/kg, cause disruption of surfactant, a rise in surface tension in the lungs, and alveolar instability. Capillary and alveolar membrane damage allows fluid to leak into the alveoli with subsequent pulmonary edema.

Aspiration of salt water (osmolarity > normal saline) does not disrupt surfactant but creates an osmotic gradient for fluid to accumulate in the lung in quantities far greater than that aspirated. In either case pulmonary compliance is markedly decreased, airway resistance increased, pulmonary artery pressure elevated, and pulmonary flow diminished. The result is a drastic fall in PaO_2 secondary to an absolute intrapulmonary shunt; i.e., perfusion of nonventilated alveoli.

In animal studies, aspiration of as little as 2.2 ml/kg of fresh water leads to a fall in PaO_2 to about 60 mm Hg in 3 min, while a similar amount of sea water precipitates an even greater drop to about 40 mm Hg. In human victims even lower levels of PaO_2 are seen. Severe metabolic acidosis is then a consequence of tissue hypoxia. A rise in $PaCO_2$ also occurs but in general can be corrected spontaneously by the victim. Additional trauma to the lungs may occur as a result of aspirated bacteria, gastric contents, and foreign materials.

Hypoxemia, whether secondary to upper airway obstruction (here, laryngospasm), or to impaired gas exchange after aspiration, results in loss of consciousness. If anoxia ensues, irreversible central nervous system damage begins after 4 to 6 min. Some protection is effected by the diving reflex, strongest in infancy and triggered by fear or cold, shunting blood primarily to the brain and heart and affording a few minutes more perfusion. Experience with drowning victims and in cardiovascular surgery indicates that cold water is relatively protective of the CNS, but probably only if immersion hypothermia develops before compromise of oxygenation. The onset of hypothermia is more rapid in young children because of their greater surface-to-volume ratio and is also enhanced by vigorous struggling or swimming and swallowing large amounts of icy fluid. If, however, laryngospasm or aspiration occur prior to a fall in core body temperature and, therefore, cerebral metabolic rate, protection is probably minimal. Anoxia produces acidosis, and restoration of the circulation may result in severe cerebral edema and secondary injury as a consequence of elevated intracranial pressure.

Cardiovascular effects are primarily those expected with myocardial ischemia, severe systemic acidosis, hypothermia, and intravascular volume changes: variable dysrhythmias and myocardial depression. After aspiration of fresh water, there is a transient rise in intravascular volume which is quickly redistributed, later to contribute to problems of cerebral edema and pulmonary function. Aspiration of salt water may cause intravascular depletion as a result of fluid drawn into the lungs along the osmotic gradient.

Electrolyte abnormalities occur after massive aspiration in laboratory animals, but rarely achieve clinical significance in either adult or child victims. Likewise, changes in the hematocrit are not predictable, and those that occur are more closely related to coexisting trauma than the effects of hyper- or hypotonic fluids. Occasionally, however, massive hemolysis may occur.

CLINICAL MANIFESTATIONS

In the first moments after rescue, the appearance of the child who has nearly drowned may range from apparently normal to apparently dead. Body temperature is frequently low, even in temperate, warm-water environments. Respiratory efforts may be absent, irregular or labored, with pallor or cyanosis, retractions, grunting, and cough productive of pink, frothy material. The lungs may be clear, or there may be rales, rhonchi, and wheezing. Infection may develop as a consequence of aspirated mouth flora or organisms in stagnant water, but is not usually important in the first 24 hours.

Respiratory function may improve spontaneously or deteriorate rapidly as pulmonary edema and small airway dysfunction worsen. Alternatively, one may see slow deterioration over 12 to 24 hours.

Neurological asssessment may show an alert, normal child, or any level of CNS compromise. A child may display agitation and combative behavior, blunted responsiveness to the environment, or profound coma with stereotypic posturing or flaccid extremities. Superficial evidence of head trauma may be noted in a few children whose submersion episode was a secondary event.

Initial laboratory evaluation should include CBC, electrolytes, urinalysis, arterial blood gas, and chest x-ray. Results will vary in each, except for predictably profound hypoxemia and acidosis in patients who suffer frank cardiopulmonary arrest or exhibit obvious signs of respiratory distress.

It must be stressed that pulmonary and neurological damage need not occur together. While extensive pulmonary destruction and resultant hypoxemia may cause neurologic damage, all combinations of mild and severe lung and brain damage are possible.

MANAGEMENT

The ultimate outcome of serious immersion accidents depends on the duration of the submersion, the degree of pulmonary damage by aspiration, and effectiveness of initial resuscitative measures. Most victims will appear "dead" on extraction from water: apneic, cyanotic or (deathly) pale, with such intense peripheral vasoconstriction and myocardial depression that the child may be apparently or actually pulseless. Because the majority are salvageable, all children should receive the benefit of excellent cardiopulmonary resuscitation without delay, according to the principles elaborated in Chapter 2. In particular, because of the profound hypoxemia commonly present, they should receive the maximum concentration of supplemental oxygen possible (100%) in transport to an emergency facility. The victim who remains asystolic in the emergency department is almost certain to die or survive only in a vegetative state. Even those rescued with spontaneous ventilation and minimal or no neurologic dysfunction should be given the benefit of supplemental oxygen to minimize the risk of progressive hypoxemia and acidosis with secondary myocardial and cerebral damage. Physical examination is notoriously insensitive to hypoxemia; a seriously hypoxemic child may be alert and talking. Once the child has arrived at an emergency facility (and cardiovascular stability is achieved), further treatment is based on pulmonary and neurologic assessment.

Effective therapy of all aspects of the morbidity of near drowning depends on the reversal of hypoxemia and metabolic acidosis. The pulmonary status is assessed initially with measurement of arterial pH, $PaCO_2$, and PaO_2, and with a chest x-ray (Table 51.1). If oxygenation is normal on breathing room air, then the child can be assumed to have suffered near drowning without aspiration. Observation for 12 to 24 hours with repeat arterial blood gas (ABG) determination excludes the possibility of late deterioration in gas exchange.

Patients with abnormalities of gas exchange and acid-base status but with normal chest radiographs can usually be managed with supplemental oxygen, pulmonary physiotherapy, and bicarbonate therapy. (If base deficit > 10 or $HCO_3^- < 15$, correct with $NaHCO_3$:

$$\text{meq} = (\text{base deficit} \times \text{body weight (kg)} \times 0.6)/2).$$

Additional blood gas analysis should be done to document adequate oxygenation and reversal of metabolic acidosis. Any change in mental status or increase in respiratory distress should also prompt a repeat ABG determination, as either may be the result of arterial hypoxemia. Serial PaO_2 measurements will guide the physician to continue conservative treatment or to intervene with more vigorous ventilatory support as below.

Patients with obvious respiratory distress, hypoxemia ($PaO_2 < 60$ on 60% inspired oxygen), and extensive pulmonary edema or infiltration generally require more vigorous treatment and more extensive monitoring. All should be monitored for heart rate, cardiac rhythm, respiratory rate, and blood pressure. Most will require frequent blood gas analysis and may be more easily monitored through arterial cannulation. Intubation, supplemental oxygen, and continuous positive airways pressure (CPAP, 5 to 15 cm H_2O) should be provided.

If oxygenation is still inadequate, or if ventilatory failure occurs ($PaCO_2 > 50$), intermittent mandatory ventilation (IMV) may be beneficial, while interfering less with cardiovascular stability than controlled ventilation. Once blood pressure is stabilized, fluid restriction (to approximately one-half maintenance rate) and diuretic therapy (e.g. furosemide 0.5 to 1 mg/kg i.v.) may improve gas exchange. In the setting of extensive pulmonary damage, hypoxemia and acidosis, and major intravascular volume changes, pulmonary and cardiovascular components of the disease are intimately entwined and optimum management will require monitoring of blood gases, arterial pressure, and central venous pressure. When lung compliance is severely decreased, oxygenation is tenuous, and posi-

Table 51.1
Pulmonary Assessment after Near Drowning

Presentation	Treatment
Chest x-ray normal ABG[a] normal	Observe ↑ Improvement
Chest x-ray normal ABG: Alveolar-arterial oxygen difference (PaO_2 expected on known concentration of inspired oxygen)	Serial ABG's Supplemental oxygen Diuretics, fluid restriction Monitor heart rate, respiratory rate, blood pressure ↓ Deterioration
Chest x-ray abnormal ABG: Large alveolar-arterial difference	Serial ABG's Supplemental oxygen Diuretics, fluid restriction Monitor heart rate, ECG, respiratory rate, blood pressure Intra-arterial line ↓ PaO_2 60 on 60% oxygen Intubation Continuous positive airway pressure 5 to 15 cm H_2O Consider mechanical ventilation for $PaCO_2 < 50$, persistent hypoxemia Consider antibiotics Monitor heart rate, ECG, respiratory rate, temperature, central venous pressure, consider pulmonary artery catheter

[a] ABG = arterial blood gas.

tive airway pressure compromises cardiac function, pulmonary artery catheterization may provide critical information about cardiac output and oxygen consumption.

The risk of pulmonary infection is always present, but antibiotics should be reserved for proven bacterial infection. Exceptions can be made in the worst cases, where maximal ventilatory support is required, to provide any margin for survival. Steroids have no demonstrated benefit.

Renal function must be maintained. If significant hemoglobinuria exists, forced diuresis is required. Maintenance of an adequate hemoglobin level (>10 g/100 ml) and normal electrolytes is obviously necessary, but, because specific problems will vary from patient to patient in an unpredictable way, an understanding of the principles outlined in Chapters 46 and 47 is essential.

Successful management of pulmonary dysfunction, no matter how dramatic, is only truly satisfying if accompanied by neurologic recovery as well (Table 51.2). Treatment here is substantially more uncertain and controversial.

Patients who are awake, alert, and fully responsive can be presumed to have survived the episode without CNS damage. Only conservative observation for 12 to 24 hours is warranted. Those who are obtunded but rousable and exhibit purposeful responses to pain and a normal respiratory pattern have suffered certain but reversible CNS hypoxia. In these, the goal is to prevent further hypoxic damage by intensive management of the cardiopulmonary disease. Repeated neurologic evaluation is essential. Fluid restriction and diuretic therapy within the limits of cardiovascular stability may decrease the risk of cerebral edema. The use of steroids may be consid-

Table 51.2
Neurologic Assessment after Near Drowning

Group	Description	Treatment
A (alert)	Alert Fully conscious	Observe
B (blunted)	Obtunded but arousable Purposeful response to pain Normal respiratory pattern	Prevent further hypoxic damage Monitor clinical neurologic status Therapy as required for pulmonary and cardiovascular stability Normal temperature
C (comatose)	Comatose, not arousable Abnormal response to pain Abnormal respiratory pattern	Prevent further hypoxic damage
C.1	(Decorticate) Flexion response to pain Cheyne-Stokes respiration	Monitor clinical neurologic status If deterioration occurs: Monitor intracranial pressure Consider cerebral protection.
C.2	(Decerebrate) Extension response to pain Central hyperventilation	Monitor temperature Maintain hypothermia at 30–32°C Control ventilation: $PCO_2 \approx 30$ mm Hg Barbiturate coma Steroids
C.3	(Flaccid) No response to pain Apnea, or cluster breathing	Consider withdrawal of support if no protection from hypothermia

ered, but there is no clear evidence of their benefit in this setting (see Chapter 67). In both of these groups, temperature normalization should be prompt. Assuming effective reversal of coexisting pulmonary damage, neurologic recovery should be complete in these two groups.

Most of the controversy concerns patients in a third group, those who have clearly suffered severe CNS asphyxia. These children are not rousable and can be divided into three subcategories according to neurologic findings: (1) those with decorticate response to pain and Cheyne-Stokes breathing, (2) those with decerebrate response to pain and central hyperventilation, and (3) those who are flaccid with fixed dilated pupils and apneustic breathing or apnea. Again, reversal of hypoxemia and acidosis is critical. If hypothermia exists, it is probably protective and should be maintained at 32°C at least long enough to fully evaluate the child's history and presentation. Beyond this point, the debate centers around the value of initiating measures thought to provide cerebral protection and prevent or treat elevated intracranial pressure.

Avoidance of hypercapnia and resultant cerebral hyperemia is generally accepted, but the value of hyperventilation, neuromuscular paralysis, barbiturate coma, and hypothermia is uncertain. The prognosis for this group is certainly more grim, with a much greater risk of death or severe anoxic encephalopathy, the risk increasing with the depth of coma on presentation. Those in the third subdivision, flaccid with fixed dilated pupils, rarely survive intact regardless of treatment, although coexistent hypothermia has provided some remarkable exceptions. Whether intensive cerebral protection can alter this outcome is vigorously debated. In each case, consideration should be given to the possibility that continued resuscitation will salvage only the cardiovascular system, and that, in these cases, the physician may reasonably discontinue resuscitative efforts.

SMOKE INHALATION

BACKGROUND

Although fire has been the cause of much death and misery throughout human history, the importance of smoke inhalation has only been recognized in the last 40 years. Respiratory complications of smoke inhalation rank with carbon monoxide poisoning as the major causes of early death from fire, accounting for 50 to 60% of the 12,000 fire deaths in the United States each year. While serious pulmonary disease may occur in the absence of cutaneous injury, inhalation injury dramatically increases the morbidity and mortality associated with any given percent body surface area burn.

The severity of carbon monoxide inhalation and respiratory problems is related to the duration of exposure, the occurrence in a closed space (more likely in the very young or elderly victims), the nature of the materials involved, and the products of incomplete combustion. Direct inhalation trauma is further complicated by severe hypovolemic shock, massive tissue destruction, extensive fluid resuscitation, and infection.

PATHOPHYSIOLOGY

Direct thermal injury is usually limited to the upper airway because of the excellent heat exchanging properties of the nasopharynx and the relatively low heat capacity of dry air. Dry air of temperatures >160°C (300°F) has little effect on the lower airway. Greater risk of lower airway damage occurs with steam inhalation because of its greater heat capacity. In addition, continuing combustion of soot particles carried deeply into the lung may extend thermal injury.

Chemical injury can occur at any level of the respiratory tract. Oxides of sulfur and nitrogens combine with lung water to form corrosive acids. Burning wood produces large amounts of carbon monoxide. Combustion of cotton or plastic produces aldehydes which cause denaturation of protein and cellular damage. One, acrolein, is known to cause upper airway irritation at concentratiaons of 5.5 ppm and pulmonary edema within seconds at 10 ppm. Polyvinylchloride releases chlorine and hydrochloric acid, while polyethylene produces hydrocarbons, ketones, and other acids. One of the hydrocarbons, benzene, may anesthetize the upper airway and allow increased passage of toxins and particles. Fire retardants containing phosphorus may actually produce phosgene. Most soot particles are filtered by the upper airway, but those carried into the lung may cause reflex bronchospasm and extend chemical damage by way of substances adsorbed onto the particle surfaces.

Upper airway lesions include actual burns of varying severity as well as severe edema of the nose, mouth, pharynx, and laryngeal structures. Lower airway lesions depend on the toxin involved. Pulmonary disease is complicated by secondary changes related to circulatory, metabolic, and infectious complications, as well as therapeutic interventioins such as endotracheal intubation, oxygen administration, mechanical ventilation, and fluid therapy.

From the infants killed in the Dellwood nursery fire, it was learned that serious respiratory damage may occur in the absence of cutaneous injury. Necrosis of bronchial, bronchiolar, and alveolar epithelium, vascular engorgement and edema, and formation of membranes or casts of the airway produce small and large airway obstruction. If severe surface injury has occurred, then damage to the vascular side of the lungs becomes evident with increased alveolar capillary permeability and hemorrhage, edema, and hyaline membrane formation.

Upper airway edema causes a tremendous increase in the work of breathing as a result of increased inspiratory and expiratory resistance. If airway narrowing is severe or complete, acute respiratory failure with hypercarbia and hypoxemia occurs with subsequent cardiovascular collapse.

Immediate effects of smoke inhalation on the lower airway include loss of ciliary action, mucosal edema, bronchiolitis, alveolar epithelial damage, and impaired gas exchange, particularly oxygenation. In addition, areas of atelectasis or air trapping are produced, leading to worsened ventilation perfusion mismatch and greater hypoxemia. Loss of surfactant activity exaggerates this phenomenon. Hours later, sloughing of tracheobronchial mucosa and mucopurulent membrane formation increase the degree of obstruction and poor gas exchange and the likelihood of infection. Beyond the first 24 hours, all the complications mentioned above result in pulmonary pathology largely indistinguishable from any other cause of the adult respiratory distress syndrome.

CLINICAL MANIFESTATIONS

Concern regarding smoke inhalation is increased by a history of exposure in a closed space. Need for cardiopulmonary resuscitation at the site implies significant carbon monoxide poisoning and/or hypoxia secondary to decreased ambient oxygen concentration or severe airway or parenchymal disease. Determination of the types of materials involved increases the physician's sensitivity to the risk of carbon monoxide poisoning or other toxic effects.

Physical examination showing facial burns, singed nasal hairs, soot in the pharynx, or carbonaceous sputum makes smoke inhalation likely. Any sign of neurological dysfunction, including irritability or depression, should be presumed related to tissue hypoxia until proven otherwise. Signs of respiratory distress may be delayed for 12 to 24 hours, but tachypnea, cough, hoarseness, stridor, decreased breath sounds, wheezing, rhonchi, or rales may be present from the start. Auscultatory findings frequently precede chest x-ray abnormalities by 12 to 24 hours. When radiographic changes do appear, they may be those of diffuse interstitial infiltration or local areas of atelectasis and edema.

As mentioned above, acute respiratory failure may occur at any point, initially related to CNS depression by asphyxia or carbon monoxide, and later to airway obstruction at any level or to parenchymal dysfunction. Arterial blood gas analysis provides the ultimate assessment of effective respiratory function. Xenon lung scanning may give evidence for smoke inhalation but does not add significantly to that obtained by repeated clinical assessment and blood gas determinations in the emergency department. Bronchoscopy can document the extent of inhalation injury and help remove debris, but because the procedure may worsen airway edema and because supportive care is guided by respiratory function rather than the lesions noted during the procedure, most patients can be effectively treated without it.

MANAGEMENT

Initial assessment and resuscitation at the scene of the fire should proceed according to the principles outlined in Chapter 2. Because of the likelihood of carbon monoxide exposure and the difficulty of assessing hypoxemia clinically, all victims should receive the maximum concentration of inspired oxygen possible in transport and in the emergency department until further evaluation is complete (Table 51.3).

Upon arrival in the emergency department, fluid resuscitation and assessment of respiratory function should proceed together. Fluid replacement is most complex when major surface burns have occurred. The details of therapy are elaborated elsewhere but, in general, the goals are stabilization of cardiovascular function without compromise of gas exchange by fluid overload. This is best accomplished by titrating fluid infused against the pulse rate and blood pressure, as well as some measure of central vascular volume such as central venous pressure or, ideally, left atrial pressure (or pulmonary artery occluded pressure) and cardiac output (requiring insertion of a pulmonary artery catheter). Maintenance of central venous prerssure of 6 to 10 cm H_2O or pulmonary artery occluded pressure of 3 to 8 cm H_2O and urine output of at least 0.5 ml/kg/hour should provide adequate tissue perfusion. If pulmonary artery occluded pressure rises and urine output falls, normal or elevated cardiac output calls for the use of diuretics, while a depressed cardiac output indicates the need for inotropic agents. While adequate fluid administration is essential, careful monitor-

Table 51.3
Management of Smoke Inhalation

Initial management
- Remove from contaminated environment
- Cardiopulmonary resuscitation as needed
- Provide 100% supplemental oxygen
- Ensure patent airway

Laboratory determinations
- Arterial blood gas analysis
- Carboxyhemoglobin level
- Chest radiograph

Monitor
- Heart rate, ECG, respiratory rate, blood pressure
- Consider central venous pressure
- Consider pulmonary artery catheterization

Fluids
- 5% dextrose in 0.25 N saline at maintenance rates or less to maintain urine output/ml/kg/hr
- Volume expansion in presence of cutaneous burns: normal saline, lactated Ringer's solution, or 5% albumin to maintain central venous pressure 4–6 cm H_2O

Respiratory management
- Intubation for: (1) upper airway obstruction
  (2) $PaO_2 < 60$ mm Hg on 60% oxygen
  (3) Central nervous system depression with loss of cough and gag reflexes
- Continuous positive airway pressure 5–15 cm H_2O, 60 mm Hg on 60% oxygen
- Intermittent mandatory ventilation for (1) hypoxia unresponsive to continuous positive airway pressure, or (2) $PaCO_2$, 50 mm Hg.
- Humidification of inspired gases
- Meticulous pulmonary toilette
- Consider inhaled or intravenous bronchodilators

ing of the renal and cardiovascular systems allows for the infusion of the minimal amount of fluid needed to maintain the intravascular volume and may decrease the severity of acute pulmonary edema and the risk of delayed pulmonary dysfunction secondary to late fluid mobilization and infection.

Assessment of the airway and respiratory function must proceed simultaneously with cardiovascular stabilization. Thermal injury to the nose, mouth, or face or upper airway compromise (stridor, hoarseness, barking cough, retractions, delayed inspiration, or difficulty handling secretions) indicate the need for direct laryngoscopy. The presence of significant pharyngeal, supraglottic, or glottic edema mandates elective endotracheal intubation. While some may elect to observe closely, worsening edema over 24 hours is likely, and much is lost by waiting until respiratory arrest occurs and emergency intubation through a distorted airway is necessary. Elective tracheostomy may be considered if severe facial burns interfere with securing the endotracheal tube or if airway edema predisposes to additional trauma by the endotracheal tube. However, in the presence of extensive cutaneous burns, tracheostomy dramatically increases the risk of systemic and pulmonary infection.

Serial blood gas determinations should be obtained to guide oxygen supplementation and to assess adequacy of ventilation. The child should be intubated if adequate oxygenation ($PaO_2 \geq 60$ torr) cannot be maintained with an inspired oxygen concentration of 40 to 60%, or if $PaCO_2$ rises above 50 torr. In the presence of small airway edema and disrupted surfactant activity, improved oxygenation may be obtained by providing continuous distending airway pressure. Spontaneous ventilation with continuous positive airway pressure (CPAP) causes less cardiovascular interference, but in the patient with severe CNS depression or very severe pulmonary parenchymal damage, positive end expiratory pressure (PEEP) with intermittent mandatory ventilation (IMV) or controlled ventilation may be necessary. After the first few hours, diuretic therapy (furosemide 0.5 to 1 mg/kg/i.v.) within the limits of cardiovascular stability may also improve oxygenation and pulmonary compliance, leading to more effective ventilation. Reflex bronchoconstriction secondary to chemical and particulate irritation of upper airway reception may contribute to lower airway obstruction. A trial of bronchodilators is reasonable. Nebulized isoetharine (BronKosol 0.5 ml in 1.5 ml normal saline, or isoproterenol 0.25 ml (1:200) in 1.5 ml normal saline) may reduce bronchospasm. If one of these drugs is effective but the duration of action is too short, intravenous aminophyllin is an alternative. An initial dose of 5 to 6 mg/kg followed by an infusion of approximately 1 mg/kg/hour, adjusted according to serum levels, should be effective. In most cases, however, relief of bronchospasm will be most dependent upon removal of secretions and debris from the respiratory tree.

Maximally humidified oxygen should be delivered by mask or artificial airway to prevent occlusion of the airway by inspissated debris. Meticulous pulmonary toilette is essential, with frequent suctioning to remove edema fluid, mucus, and sloughed epithelium which may otherwise quickly occlude the endotracheal tube. The patient with a natural airway should also receive humidified gas mixtures and be encouraged to take deep breaths and cough frequently.

Steroids have not been demonstrated effective in reducing airway edema or decreasing the inflammatory response to smoke inhalation. There is evidence that, when steroids are used, sodium and fluid retention increases, healing is delayed, and bacterial clearance from the lung is decreased. In balance, little argument remains for their routine use.

Similarly, there is no value in the use of prophylactic antibiotics. Institution of antimicrobial therapy should await specific indications, which will rarely occur in the first 24 hours.

CARBON MONOXIDE POISONING

BACKGROUND

As noted previously, carbon monoxide poisoning is one of the most significant causes of early deaths related to fire. However, exposure may occur in a variety of other settings unrelated to accidental fires and some present significant risk to children. Other environments where carbon monoxide poisoning takes place include those with incomplete combustion of wood or coal in improperly vented stoves, exposure to automobile exhaust in closed garages or in cars with faulty exhaust systems, and in station wagons, vans, and trucks with open backs and rear, rather than side-vented, exhaust.

PATHOPHYSIOLOGY

In the normal person, carboxyhemoglobin levels are less than 1%. In smokers, levels of 5 to 10% are common. When carbon monoxide is inhaled, it binds to hemoglobin with an affinity 200 to 300 times greater than that of oxygen. In addition, carbon monoxide shifts the oxyhemoglobin dissociation curve to the left and changes the shape from sigmoid to hyperbolic (Fig. 51.1). As a result, not only is the oxygen content of the blood decreased, but that which is carried is only released at a much lower tissue oxygen level. Thus, the effects of carbon monoxide poisoning are those of tissue hypoxia. When exposure occurs during fires and ambient oxygen is decreased, hypoxemia is even more severe. The effects are intensified by anemia or high altitude. Although oxygen content of the blood is very low, the PaO_2 remains normal. Since carotid body receptors respond to PaO_2, respiration may not be stimulated until very late when metabolic acidosis activates other centers. In patients with tissue hypoxia, cerebral blood flow, cerebrospinal fluid pressure, and cerebral capillary permeability are all increased, predisposing to the development of cerebral edema.

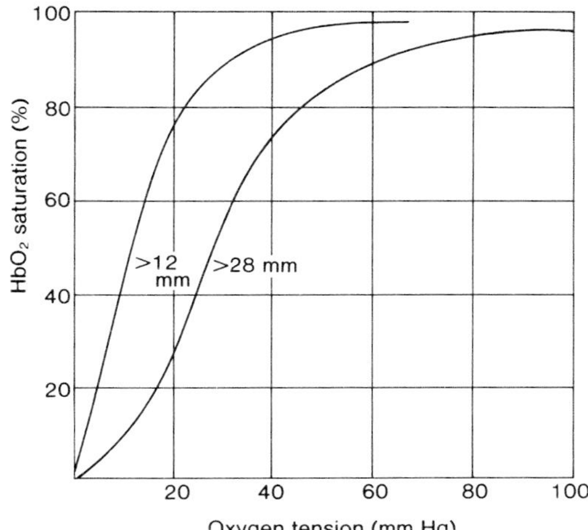

Figure 51.1. Carbon monoxide shifts the oxyhemoglobin dissociation curve to the left and changes its shape. This makes unloading of oxygen in the tissues more difficult and provides an inadequate diffusion gradient.

CLINICAL MANIFESTATIONS

History provides the most valuable clue to the diagnosis. Carbon monoxide poisoning should be suspected in all fire victims and considered in children exposed to other hazards noted earlier. Levels of carboxyhemoglobin as low as 5% in nonsmokers may result in impairment of judgment and fine motor skills. Mild intoxication (20% carboxyhemoglobin) produces headache, mild dyspnea, visual changes, and confusion. Moderate poisoning (20 to 40%) produces drowsiness, faintness, nausea and vomiting, tachycardia, dulled sensation, and decreased awareness of danger. At lower levels, these symptoms are only noted with exertion, but as the fraction approaches 40%, they are present at rest. Between 40 to 60% weakness, incoordination, and loss of recent memory occur, and cardiovascular and neurologic collapse is imminent. Above 60%, coma, convulsions, and death are almost certain.

Classically, physicians are reminded of the "cherry red" or "pink" color of the blood in these patients. However, patients may be red as a result of thermal injury or very pale secondary to vasoconstriction. Both color and respiratory rate may be deceptive and lead the physician away from recognition of severe tissue hypoxia.

Determination of blood levels of carboxyhemoglobin documents the diagnosis and aids in prognosis. Spectrophotometric methods are most widely used clinically. Venous blood may be used because of the high affinity of carbon monoxide for hemoglobin, but an arterial sample provides more precise information about acid-base balance and adequacy of ventilation. The level of hemoglobin should also be determined.

Patients with severe poisoning are peculiarly vulnerable to pressure trauma to skin, subcutaneous tissue and muscle, especially at sites supporting body weight or pinned under fallen objects. The history may suggest which sites are most vulnerable, and pain is an early symptom. Muscle breakdown and myoglobin deposition in renal tubular cells may precipitate acute renal failure.

MANAGEMENT

Most important and obvious is the immediate need to remove the victim from the contaminated environment (Table 51.4). Resuscitation should proceed according to general principles and then, as soon as possible, provide anyone suspected of suffering carbon monoxide poisoning with as close to 100% oxygen as possible. If the patient is breathing spontaneously, this can be accomplished with well-fitting masks supplied with nonrebreathing valves and a reservoir bag. (Simple masks will rarely provide more than 40% oxygen, even if the fresh gas supply is 100%, because of entrainment of room air). The half-life of CO-Hgb is approximately 4 hours, breathing room air at sea level. It can be decreased to less than 1 hour if pure oxygen is inspired. In cases of very severe poisoning, if the facilities for delivering hyperbaric oxygen are available, even more expeditious removal of carbon monoxide is possible. Use of carbon dioxide-containing mixtures (5%) to increase minute ventilation may precipitate respiratory failure if used at the scene

Table 51.4
Management of Carbon Monoxide Positioning

Initial management
- Remove from contaminated environment
- Cardiopulmonary resuscitation as needed
- Provide 100% supplemental oxygen

Laboratory determinations
- Arterial blood gas analysis
- Carboxyhemoglobin level
- CBC, electrolytes
- Urinalysis for myoglobin

Monitor
- Heart rate, ECG, respiratory rate, blood pressure

Treatment
- Correct pH < 7.30 [meq $HCO_2 = (BE \times BW^{a}\ (kg) \times 0.6)/2$]
- Correct anemia Hgb 10
- Continue supplemental oxygen until carboxyhemoglobin 5%
- Decrease oxygen consumption with bedrest, avoid producing anxiety
- Maintain urine output 1 ml/kg/hr

[a] BE = base excess (or deficit); BW = body weight.

where ventilation cannot be well-monitored or assisted. It may be considered under closely controlled situations in the hospital but probably is of little benefit. If metabolic acidosis is present, it should be treated with sodium bicarbonate. Anemia (hemoglobin < 10 g/100 ml) must be corrected to maximize oxygen carrying capacity. If myoglobinemia or myoglobinuria is present, vigorous hydration and forced diuresis with furosemide (1 mg/kg i.v.) and/or mannitol (0.5 to 1 g/kg i.v.) with close attention to urine output may preserve renal function. If hydration and diuresis are ineffective, renal failure should be considered and fluids restricted accordingly (see Chapter 46).

Regression of symptoms should occur in the reverse order of onset. Consciousness may return long before levels of CO-Hgb are in a nonthreatening range. The child should be kept quiet, if possible, to decrease oxygen consumption. He should be observed over a 24-hour period to identify other sequelae of smoke inhalation. There remains concern about long-range neurological problems, although most patients with late sequelae are the ones with a prolonged period of unconsciousness, i.e., those with significant cerebral hypoxia.

ENVIRONMENTAL AND EXERTIONAL HEAT ILLNESS

BACKGROUND

Environmental and exertional heat illness occurs because of excessive heat generation and storage when high ambient temperature prevents heat dissipation by radiation or convection, and sweat evaporation is limited by humidity. The spectrum of illness is broad, including heat cramp, heat exhaustion, and heat stroke, the last an acute medical emergency with significant associated morbidity and mortality.

Heat illness is a serious tropical health hazard, but even in the United States summer heat is implicated in the deaths of more than 4,000 people per year. Epidemic illness is associated with heat waves, as in the Southwest in 1980, but sporadic cases are also common, and the same risk factors apply in both types. The elderly are most vulnerable (more than 80% of cases occur in people older than 50), but heat illness is significant among healthy young people as well. Military recruits, laborers, and athletes working in a hot, humid atmosphere (including hot industrial settings) are notoriously vulnerable. Obesity, physical disability, heart disease, alcohol and drug use increase risk. Pediatricians need to be alert to the special risk to young athletes, children with cystic fibrosis, infants left in automobiles on hot days, and the rare child with congenital absence of sweat glands. Mortality related to acute heat stroke has been estimated to range from 17 to 70%, depending on the severity of heat stress and age of the patient.

PATHOPHYSIOLOGY

Under normal conditions, body core temperature is maintained constant within 0.6°C (1°F) when the environment varies from 9.4°C to 60°C (55 to 140°F) in dry air. This represents a remarkable balance between heat production and heat loss by the body. Heat is produced as (1) a by-product of basal metabolism, (2) a consequence of muscle activity (including shivering), (3) the result of thyroxine effect on cells, (4) sympathetic stimulation of cellular processes, and (5) direct temperature effect on cells. Heat is lost by (1) conduction to objects and air, (2) convection through air or liquid surrounding tissues, (3) radiation of infrared energy, and (4) evaporation.

Conduction to objects represents a small fraction (about 3%) of heat lost. Conduction to air and convection represent another 12% in still air. As air movement increases, the proportion of heat lost by these mechanisms may increase to nearly 60%. Radiant heat losses usually account for 60% of total heat loss. Evaporation normally accounts for 25% of heat lost by the body. However, when ambient temperature is higher than skin temperature, the body gains heat by conduction and radiation and can only lose heat by evaporation. High ambient humidity and the absence of convection currents will decrease the rate of evaporation.

Heat conduction from the body core to the skin is controlled by vasoconstriction of arterioles and subcutaneous arteriovenous anastomoses. These vessels are regulated by sympathetic tone controlled by the heat-sensitive centers of the posterior hypothalamus. Flow through these areas may represent 0 to 30% of the total cardiac output. High flow provides efficient heat transfer from the body core to the skin, which is an effective radiator. Low flow to the skin means that the only route for heat to dissipate from the core is by inefficient diffusion through the insulating skin and subcutaneous tissues.

When body temperature goes up, especially when blood reaching the preoptic area of the anterior hypothalamus is warmer than optimal, impulses from this area increase, traveling via autonomic pathways to the spinal cord and then, through cholinergic fibers, to the sweat glands, resulting in large quantities of sweat production. Circulating epinephrine and norepinephrine, released during exercise and certain emotional states, also increase sweat production.

The sweat gland is composed of two portions. The deep coiled portion actively elaborates a precursor secretion in response to cholinergic stimulation. At low rates of sweating, much of the NaCl contained in the precursor secretion is reabsorbed before the sweat is conducted to the skin surface. At higher rates, flow exceeds the capacity of the duct to reabsorb solute, and substantial total body NaCl depletion may occur.

In the unacclimatized adult, sweating may vary from negligible amounts at rest in a cool, dry environment, to 1.5 liters/hour during vigorous activity in hot weather. Long-term exposure to tropical weather results in a steady increase in sweating rate over approximately 6 weeks, to a maximum of about 4.0 liters/hour. Initially, huge salt losses may occur (15 to 20 g/day). However, aldosterone secretion rises and stimulates active reabsorption of NaCl in the ducts of sweat glands much as it does in the kidney, and salt losses decrease to a normal 3 to 5 g/day.

In the human being, behavioral control over temperature regulation is probably as important as all other mechanisms. When body temperature changes, psychic sensations of being overheated or too cool prompt efforts to correct the situation. One moves out of the cold or into the shade, selects additional or cooler clothing, initiates maneuvers which warm or cool the environment, or alters ones level of activity.

Choice of clothing that traps a layer of air around the body prevents significant heat loss by convection. A reflective inner surface decreases radiant heat loss by more than half. On the other hand, light colored clothing permeable to moisture but impervious to radiant heat from the environment prevents the formation of an insulating layer of air. This allows heat loss by evaporation and prevents radiant heat gain.

CLINICAL MANIFESTATIONS

Three types of heat illness are recognized and represent different physiologic disturbances. *Heat cramp* refers to the sudden onset of brief, intermittent, and excrutiating cramps in muscles after they have been subjected to severe work stress. Cramps tend to occur after the work is done, on relaxing, or on taking a cool shower. Occasionally, abdominal muscle cramps may simulate an acute abdomen. The usual victim is highly conditioned and acclimatized. Typically, these individuals can produce sweat in large quantities and provide themselves with adequate fluid replacement, but inadequate salt replacement. The electrolyte depletion is probably the cause of the cramps.

Most spasms last less than a minute, but some persist for several minutes during which a rock-hard mass may be palpated in the affected muscle. Cramps frequently occur in clusters. Rapid voluntary contraction of a muscle, contact with cold air or water, or passive extension of a flexed limb may reproduce a cramp. Laboratory investigation reveals hyponatremia and hypochloremia and virtually absent urine sodium. The blood urea nitrogen is usually normal but may be mildly elevated.

Heat exhaustion is less clearly demarcated from heat stroke than are heat cramps. In most cases, water depletion predominates because individuals living and working in a hot environment do not voluntarily replace their total water deficit. Progressive lethargy, intense thirst, and inability to work or play are followed by headache, vomiting, CNS dysfunction (including hyperventilation, paresthesias, agitation, incoordination, or actual psychosis), hypotension, and tachycardia. Hemoconcentration, hypernatremia, hyperchloremia, and urinary concentration are typical. Body temperature may rise, but rarely over 39°C. If unattended, heat exhaustion may progress to frank heat stroke.

Heat exhaustion may also occur secondary to predominant salt depletion. As in heat cramp, water losses are replaced but without adequate electrolyte supplementation. Symptoms include profound weakness and fatigue, frontal headache, anorexia, nausea, vomiting, diarrhea, and severe muscle cramps. Tachycardia and orthostatic hypotension may be noted. Unlike heat cramp victims, these patients are typically unacclimatized. Children with cystic fibrosis are included in this group. Because the greater salt losses in their sweat apparently do not respond to acclimatization and aldosterone stimulation of the sweat gland, they are vulnerable to electrolyte depletion, especially while young and unable to meet increased salt requirements on their own. Hyponatremia, hemoconcentration, and markedly diminished urine sodium are consistent findings.

Heat stroke is a life-threatening emergency. It is recognized by hyperpyrexia (≥41°C); hot, dry skin which is pink or ashen, depending on the circulatory state; and severe CNS dysfunction. Frequently, but not invariably, sweating ceases before the onset of heat stroke.

The onset of the CNS disturbance may be quite abrupt with sudden loss of consciousness. Frequently, however, premonitory signs and symptoms exist. These include a sense of impending doom, headache, dizziness, weakness, confusion, euphoria, gait disturbance, or combativeness. Posturing, incontinence, seizures, hemiparesis, and pupillary changes may occur. Any level of coma may be noted. Cerebral spinal fluid findings are usually normal. The extent of damage to the CNS is related to the time and extent of hyperpyrexia and to the adequacy of the circulation. Once the body temperature is lowered, consciousness is usually quickly restored, but occasionally coma persists for 24 hours or more.

Patients able to maintain cardiac output

adequate to meet the enormously elevated circulatory demand are most likely to survive. Initially the pulse is rapid and full with an increased pulse pressure. Total peripheral vascular resistance falls as a result of vasodilatation in the skin and muscle beds. Splanchnic flow diminishes, central venous pressure is low or normal, and cardiac index is elevated at ≥5 liters/min/m^2. If the hyperpyrexia is not corrected, ashen cyanosis and a thin, rapid pulse herald a falling cardiac output. Central venous pressure rises and cardiac index is less than 2 liters/min/m^2. This may be caused by direct thermal damage to the myocardium or may be secondary to marked pulmonary hypertension with secondary right ventricular failure. Even after body temperature is returned to normal, cardiac output remains elevated and peripheral vascular resistance low for several hours, resembling the compensatory hyperemia after ischemia noted in posttrauma, postshock, and postseptic states. Persistently circulating vasoactive substances probably account for this phenomenon.

Severe dehydration is not a necessary component of heat stroke, but may play a role if prolonged sweating has occurred. Electrolyte abnormalities may occur, especially in the unacclimatized victim, if NaCl has not been replaced. In acclimatized individuals, NaCl is conserved but often at the expense of a severe potassium deficit. Polyuria is sometimes noted, often vasopressin-resistant and possibly related to hypokalemia. Acute tubular necrosis may be seen in as many as 35% of cases and probably reflects combined thermal, ischemic and circulating pigment damage. Hypoglycemia may also be noted.

Nontraumatic rhabdomyolysis and acute renal failure have been described as a consequence of a variety of insults including hyperthermia and strenous exercise in unconditioned persons. Clinically, there may or may not be musculoskeletal pain, tenderness, swelling, or weakness. Laboratory evidence includes elevated serum creatine phosphokinase (300 to 120,000) and urinalysis which is Hematest (orthotoludin) positive without RBC's and shows red-gold pigmented granular casts. Typically, serum potassium and creatinine levels rise rapidly relative to BUN. Calcium is initially low, possibly because of deposition into damaged muscle, and then rises to hypercalcemic levels during the diuretic phase a few days to 2 weeks later.

MANAGEMENT

Most cases of *heat cramp* are mild and do not require specific therapy. Rest and increased salt intake via liberally salted foods will be sufficient. In severe cases with prolonged or frequent cramps, intravenous infusion of normal saline is effective. Approximately 5 to 10 ml/kg over 15 to 20 min should be adequate to relieve cramping. Oral intake of fluids and salted foods can then complete restoration of salt and water balance.

Heat exhaustion due to predominant water depletion is treated with rehydration and rest in a cooled or well-ventilated place. If the child is able to eat, he should be encouraged to drink cool liquids and be allowed unrestricted dietary sodium. If weakness or impaired consciousness preclude oral correction, then intravenous fluids are given as in any hypernatremic dehydration.

Exhaustion due to predominant salt depletion also requires rest in a cool environment. Alert, reasonably strong children can be given relatively salty drinks such as consommé or tomato juice and should be encouraged to salt solid foods. Hypotonic fluids (e.g. water or Kool-Aid) should be avoided until salt repletion has begun. Patients with CNS symptoms or gastrointestinal dysfunction may be rehydrated intravenously with isotonic saline or Ringer's lactate. Initial rapid administration of 20 ml/kg over 20 min should improve intravascular volume with return of blood pressure and pulse toward normal. Further correction of salt and water stores should be achieved over 12 to 24 hours. In especially severe cases with intractable seizures or muscle cramps, hypertonic saline solutions may be used.

Treatment of *heat stroke* centers around two priorities: (1) the immediate elimination of hyperpyrexia, and (2) support of the cardiovascular system. Clothing should be removed and the patient should be actively cooled. (Patients should be transported to an emergency facility in open or air-conditioned vehicles.) Placement in an ice bath is the most efficient means of lowering body temperature, but makes other support and monitoring difficult. Massaging with ice, keeping the patient's skin moist, and directing fans onto the patient to increase convection and evaporative heat loss is an effective alternative. Judicious use of phenothiazines, e.g., chlorpromazine 0.05 mg/kg i.v., may help maintain peripheral vasodilatation and prevent shivering thermogenesis. Temperature should be monitored continuously with a rectal probe and active cooling discontinued when rectal temperature falls to approximately 38.5°C.

The type of cardiovascular support to be used depends on the severity of the patient's presentation. If the skin is flushed and blood pressure adequate, lowering body temperature with close attention to heart rate and blood pressure may be sufficient. Although severe dehydration and electrolyte disturbances are uncommon, these should be determined and corrected. Fluids cooled to 4°C hasten temperature correction, but may precipitate arrhythmias upon contact with an already stressed myocardium. Adult patients have rarely required more than 20 ml/kg over the first 4 hours, but precise titration of fluids and electrolytes should be guided by determinations of electrolytes, hematocrit, urine output, and clinical assessment of central vascular volume.

Patients with ashen skin, tachycardia, and hypotension demonstrate cardiac output insufficient to meet the circulatory demand and are in imminent danger of death. Support should be guided by monitoring ECG, CVP, arterial blood pressure (via an indwelling arterial line), and possibly cardiac output determination.

A fluid challenge as described above should be followed by inotropic support (see Chapter 2). Isoproterenol is probably most appropriate: its β-agonist properties increase myocardial contractility and maintain peripheral vasodilatation. Additional fluid resuscitation may be necessary with the initiation of isoproterenol to fill the effective increased vascular space. Normal saline or albumin should be given to maintain the central venous pressure between 6 to 10 and the arterial blood pressure in the normal range. Dopamine or dobutamine may also be effective, infused at rates compatible with inotropic support without vasoconstriction. Agents with α-agonist characteristics (epinephrine, norepinephrine, metaraminal) are not sensible: they cause peripheral vasoconstriction, may further compromise hepatic and renal flow, and interfere with heat dissipation. Digoxin has been recommended by some authors, but is less titratable and may be risky where hypokalemia is possible. Atropine and other anticholinergic drugs which inhibit sweating should be avoided.

Renal function should be carefully monitored, especially in patients who have been hypotensive or in whom heat stroke was precipitated by vigorous exercise. BUN, creatinine, electrolytes, Ca, and urinalysis for protein and myoglobin should be obtained. Once the patient's vascular volume has been restored and arterial pressure normalized, hourly urine output should be followed. If urine output is inadequate (<0.5 ml/kg/hour) in the face of normovolemia and adequate cardiac output, furosemide (1 mg/kg i.v.) and/or mannitol (0.5 to 1 g/kg/i.v.) should be given. If the response is poor, acute renal failure should be suspected, and fluids restricted accordingly. Rapidly rising BUN or K+ should prompt consideration of early dialysis.

Most cases of pediatric heat illness are preventable by means of exercising common sense and by recognition of high risk situations. Hot, humid, still days present the greatest potential for illness. Every pediatrician has encountered infants with fever due to inappropriate bundling. Parents should be educated to avoid overdressing babies.

Infants and young children should never be left unattended in automobiles. Even at moderate ambient temperatures, the temperature in a closed or partially open vehicle rises in a few minutes to well over 37.7°C (100°F). Clothed children on synthetic seat covers not only absorb radiant heat from all automobile surfaces and have little opportunity for convective loss, but are quickly surrounded by moisture from sweating and cannot lose heat by evaporation. Deaths by heat stroke in such young children are reported each year and are entirely preventable.

Young novice athletes are another special case. Coaches and the general public should be aware of the conditions which promote heat loading. Gradual conditioning in hot weather allows acclimatization of the sweat glands and improved metabolic efficiency so that less heat is generated for a given amount of work by muscles. Dehydration should be avoided, recognizing that one does not voluntarily replace fluid losses. Liberal dietary sodium is appropriate, but salt loading risks hypernatremia and severe potassium depletion. Because young athletes are highly motivated, they frequently attempt to exert themselves beyond the level of their conditioning and do not heed premonitory warning symptoms. Any syncopal episode or odd behavior should be viewed as impending heat stroke and should prompt rest, rehydration, and lowering temperature as necessary.

Children with cystic fibrosis and their parents should be educated to replenish salt routinely and especially in hot weather (see Chapter 49). The rare child with congenital ectodermal dysplasia (including absence of sweat glands) must be protected from a warm environment altogether, and may also have to limit physical activity.

Finally, patients who have suffered heat stroke may have permanently impaired heat tolerance. They should be attentive to this possibility to prevent future episodes.

ACCIDENTAL HYPOTHERMIA

BACKGROUND

Most physicians, and perhaps pediatricians in particular, are routinely concerned with elevations of body temperature. However, hypothermia, defined as core temperature less than 35.5°C, is frequently overlooked. Reduced body temperature may be a consequence or cause of many other disorders but is only diagnosed if health care providers maintain a high index of suspicion.

Populations at high risk for hypothermia are similar to those vulnerable to heat illness. Neonates and the elderly are most often affected. Physical disability, especially immobilizing conditions, and drug or alcohol ingestion increase risk at any age. Healthy young people working or playing to exhaustion in a cold environment are also at risk. The rising popularity of cold weather sports is producing more cases of accidental hypothermia. However, environmental conditions need not be extreme, and the diagnosis should be considered even in temperate climates.

Depressed core temperatures may also be the result of primary CNS dysfunction, endocrinopathies, sepsis, protein caloric malnutrition, and a variety of metabolic derangements.

Mortality rates are reported from 30 to 80%, more closely related to the underlying disorder than to the degree of temperature depression.

PATHOPHYSIOLOGY

Body core temperature is normally maintained within one degree of 37°C. As described in the section on heat illness, this represents a fine balance between heat production and loss. When core temperature begins to fall below 37°C, physiologic mechanisms to produce and conserve heat are activated. Hypothalamic stimulation by cooled blood causes increased muscle tone and metabolism and increases heat production by 50%, even before shivering occurs. When muscle tone reaches a critical level, shivering begins, and heat production increases 2 to 4 times basal levels. Nonshivering thermogenesis results when sympathetic stimulation increases the metabolic rate, with increasing oxidative phosphorylation and high energy phosphate production.

Conservation of heat produced is primarily by vasoconstriction of cutaneous and subcutaneous vessels. While body surface temperature, especially of the extremities, may drop nearly to environmental temperature, blood and core structures are protected from ambient air temperature, humidity, and wind velocity. Piloerection also occurs, but in humans is not effective in providing an insulating layer of air surrounding the body. Sweating is abolished, decreasing heat loss by evaporation, unless as a consequence of external moisture.

When any component of the balance between heat production and loss is altered, the risk of hypothermia increases. Neonates, with their large surface to volume ratio and small amount of subcutaneous fat, conserve heat poorly. Also, they are unable to produce heat by shivering. While the capacity for nonshivering thermogenesis, primarily metabolism of brown fat, is intact, oxygen consumption is markedly increased. Hypoxemia may result, as well as metabolic acidosis, hypoglycemia, and hypocalcemia.

While neonates are sensitive to relatively minor deviations from a neutral thermal environment, any child or adult may become hypothermic as a result of more severe environmental stress. Immersion in cold water causes the most rapid fall in body temperature. Struggling or swimming movements increase blood flow to the extremities and hasten hypothermia. In water at 0°C (32°F), death occurs in 15 min, but significant hypothermia occurs even in water at 21°C (70°F).

Exposure to extreme cold is an obvious risk, taxing the body's ability to conserve and produce heat maximally. Voluntary motor activity produces heat, and physically fit, acclimatized persons may be able to increase their activity to balance heat loss even in very cold environments. However, the metabolic cost of physical activity increases in the cold, and less fit individuals quickly exhaust muscle glycogen supplies, are unable to maintain adequate heat production, and are likely to become hypothermic quickly. Wet, windy conditions hasten loss of body heat and may precipitate hypothermia even in temperate environments. Adolescents are psychologically less likely to conserve energy and take preventative or corrective measures, thus increasing their risk of hypothermia.

Once homeostatic mechanisms fail and core temperature falls, predictable physiologic changes take place. If shivering does not occur, basal metabolic rate decreases steadily, reaching 50% of normal at 28°C. As a result, oxygen consumption and carbon dioxide production decline. The oxygen-hemoglobin dissociation curve is shifted to the left, but this is compensated by the decrease in oxygen requirements.

Cardiac output decreases primarily as a consequence of a decreased heart rate. Blood pressure initially rises as a result of vasoconstriction and increased central vascular volume, and then falls, becoming clinically significant below 25°C. A variety of cardiac conduction abnormalities occur, including decreased sinus rate, T-wave inversion, prolongation of ECG intervals, and the appearance of pathognomonic J-waves (Fig. 51.2), which may provide the first clue to the diagnosis. Atrial fibrillation may occur at temperatures under 33°C but is usually not significant. Below 28°C myocardial irritability increases dramatically, and ventricular fibrillation is very likely.

Respiratory depression occurs very late. However, impaired mental status and cold-induced bronchorrhea predispose the patient to airway obstruction and aspiration. Acid-base balance follows no predictable pattern. While respiratory acidosis occurs, metabolic acidosis is also common, as a consequence of tissue hypoxia, increased lactic acid production, and decreased clearance of lactate by the liver.

Intravascular volume diminishes. Cold-induced diuresis occurs secondary to pe-

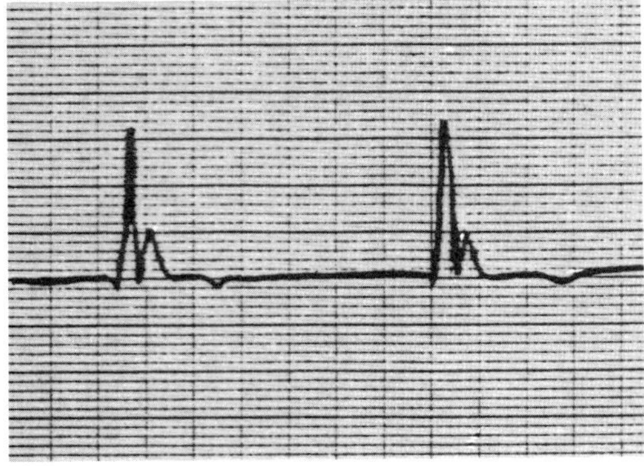

Figure 51.2. J-wave, pathognomonic of hypothermia.

ripheral vasoconstriction and elevated central blood volume and pressure. At lower temperatures, tubular dysfunction allows salt and water loss. As a consequence of acidosis, potassium shifts from the cells and is lost in the urine. Increased capillary permeability results in loss of fluid into the extracellular space. Another consequence of the plasma loss is a rise in hematocrit. White blood cell and platelet counts fall, probably as a result of splenic sequestration. Disseminated intravascular coagulation is sometimes seen.

CNS impairment is progressive. Each fall of 1°C produces a 6 to 7% decline in cerebral blood flow. Increased blood viscosity secondary to plasma loss further contributes to decreased cerebral microcirculation and impaired mentation. Peripheral nerve conduction is slowed and deep tendon reflexes are decreased. Pupils are dilated and sluggishly reactive, if at all, below 30°C. The electroencephalogram progressively deteriorates with falling temperature through high voltage slow waves, to burst suppression patterns, to electrical silence at 20°C.

Gastrointestinal motility decreases below 34°C. The liver's capacity for detoxification or conjugation of drugs and products of metabolism is poor. Insulin release is decreased and serum glucose rises. Frank pancreatic necrosis may also occur, producing clinical evidence of pancreatitis.

CLINICAL MANIFESTATIONS

The diagnosis of hypothermia requires, first of all, that it be kept in mind. A history of sudden immersion in icy water or prolonged exposure to extremely low environmental temperatures is an obvious clue. However, significantly low core temperatures may occur under much less suggestive circumstances. Examples include: victims of trauma found unconscious or immobile on a wet, windy, summer day; infants from inadequately heated homes or others left exposed during prolonged medical evaluation; adolescents with anorexia nervosa; and patients with sepsis, burns, etc. An occasional episode of apparent sudden infant death syndrome may actually be secondary to severe hypothermia, coma, and cardiac arrest. Because the lower limit of most thermometers is only 34.4°C, hypothermia will often go undetected, especially if the thermometer is not shaken down adequately. Low-recording thermometers should be available in the emergency department and intensive care unit. The diagnosis should be borne in mind for any patient with a suggestive history or coma of uncertain etiology.

Physical examination reveals a pale or cyanotic patient. At mild levels of hypothermia, mental status may be normal, but CNS function is progressively impaired with falling temperature until frank coma occurs at approximately 27°C. Blood pressure also falls steadily below 33°C and may be undetectable. Heart rate slows gradually unless atrial or ventricular fibrillation occur. Because of intense peripheral vasoconstriction and bradycardia, the pulse may be inapparent or absent. Below 32°C, shivering ceases, but muscle rigidity may mimic rigor mortis. Pupils may be dilated and sluggishly reactive, if at all. Deep tendon reflexes are depressed or absent. Evidence of head trauma or other injury, drug ingestion, and frostbite should be sought.

Severe hypothermia mimics death. However, life may be sustained for long periods, even after cessation of cardiac function, because of the marked decrease in oxygen consumption. Signs usually associated with certain death, i.e., dilated pupils or rigor mortis, have little prognostic value here. If the patient's history suggests that hypothermia is the primary event, and not a secondary *consequence* of death, resuscitation should be attempted and death redefined as failure to revive with rewarming.

Initial laboratory evaluation should include CBC, and platelet count, clotting studies, electrolytes, BUN and creatinine, glucose, serum amylase, and arterial blood gases corrected for temperature (Table 51.5). Serum and urine should be sent for drug screening.

MANAGEMENT

Therapy for hypothermia can be divided into two parts: general supportive measures and specific rewarming techniques (Table 51.6). The obvious starting place is to document hypothermia and monitor temperature continuously as treatment progresses. The heart rate and rhythm should be monitored continuously and the patient handled very gently, to avoid precipitation of life-threatening dysrhythmias in an exquisitely irritable myocardium. Sinus bradycardia, atrial flutter, and atrial fibrillation are common, but rarely of hemodynamic significance. Spontaneous reversion to sinus rhythm is the rule when temperature is corrected. Ventricular fibrillation may occur spontaneously or as a result of apparently trivial stimulation, especially at temperatures below 28 to 29°C. An attempt at electrical defibrillation is warranted, but frequently ineffective until core temperature rises. Closed chest massage should be initiated and maintained until the temperature is over 30°C, when defibrillation is more likely to be effective. Drug therapy is rarely effective and frought with hazard because of decreased hepatic and renal metabolism.

All patients should be given supplemental oxygen. Patients with respiratory depression or those unable to maintain airway patency as a consequence of profuse secretions or impaired mental status should be provided with an artificial airway and mechanical ventilation if respiratory acidosis is noted. Intubation should be as gentle as possible to minimize the risk of dysrhythmias. Ventilation should be begun at approximately one-half the normal minute ventilation and thereafter guided by arte-

Table 51.5
Effect of Body Temperature on Arterial Blood Gases Measured at 37°C

	For Each Elevation of 1°C	For Each Depression of 1°C
pH	−0.015	+0.015
$PaCO_2$ (mm Hg)	+4.4%	−4.4%
PaO_2 (mm Hg)	+7.2%	−7.2%

Table 51.6
Management of Hypothermia

Initial management
- Provide supplemental oxygen
- Cardiopulmonary resuscitation for asystole, ventricular fibrillation

Laboratory determinations
- Arterial blood gas analysis corrected for temperature
- CBC, platelet count
- Prothrombin time, partial thromboplastin time
- Electrolytes, BUN, creatinine
- Glucose, amylase
- Drug screen

Monitor
- Heart rate, ECG, respiratory rate, blood pressure
- Temperature
- Consider central venous pressure

Treatment
- Correct hypoxemia, hypercarbia
- Correct pH < 7.25, avoid alkalosis
- Correct hypokalemia
- Correct hypoglycemia, 25% dextrose 1 g/kg i.v.
- Observe hyperglycemia
- Temperature ≧ 33°C: passive rewarming or simple external rewarming
  - < 32°C (acute): external or core rewarming
  - < 32°C (chronic): core rewarming
- Fluid replacement:
  - (acute) 5% dextrose in 0.25 N saline at maintenance rates
  - (chronic) Normal saline, 5% albumin, fresh frozen plasma to maintain blood pressure, central venous pressure

rial blood gas analysis. Because of a decreased metabolic rate, carbon dioxide production is low, and usual minute ventilation will produce respiratory alkalosis, increasing the risk of dangerous dysrhythmias. Blood pH and gas tension must be corrected for temperature, or else very misleading results will be obtained. Communication with the laboratory performing the analysis is essential. Table 51.6 shows one set of guidelines for appropriate correction.

Fluid replacement is essential. Relatively little plasma loss occurs in acute hypothermia (as after cold water immersion), but losses may be very great in hypothermia of longer duration. Normal saline or lactated Ringer's solution, warmed to about 43°C in a blood warming coil, is appropriate initially. Further replacement should be guided by electrolyte determinations. If clotting abnormalities occur, fresh frozen plasma (10 ml/kg, see Chapter 47) is a useful choice for volume expansion. As temperature rises and peripheral vasoconstriction decreases, hypovolemia is expected. Fluid volume should be sufficient to provide an adequate arterial blood pressure. If central venous pressure is monitored, care should be taken to avoid placement into the heart where dysrhythmias may be initiated.

Serum glucose should be checked. Hypoglycemia should be treated with glucose (1 g/kg) given intravenously. If, however, hyperglycemia has resulted from impaired insulin release by the hypothermic pancreas, even marked elevations should probably be tolerated to avoid severe hypoglycemia with rewarming. Severe metabolic acidosis should be corrected to maintain the arterial pH at 7.25 or higher, but overzealous correction may worsen hypokalemia and increase the risk of dysrhythmias. If the patient's blood volume is restored and oxygenation maintained, acidosis will be corrected spontaneously as the patient is warmed.

There are numerous methods for rewarming, and no consensus exists as to the best. Passive rewarming implies removal of the patient from a cold environment and maximizing the effect of basal heat production, as with blankets. For patients with mild hypothermia (T > 33°C) this may be adequate.

Active rewarming is divided into external and core rewarming techniques. Electric blankets, hot-water bottles, overhead warmers, and thermal mattresses are simple, easily available sources of external heat. Immersion in warm-water baths is also possible. All of these methods, however, cause early warming of the skin and extremities with peripheral vasodilatation and shunting of cold, acidemic blood to the core. The well-known "after-drop" of core temperature results. Severe hypotension may also occur in chronic cases as vasodilatation increases the effective vascular space. Both the after-drop in temperature and the vasodilatation effect may be minimized if external rewarming techniques are limited to the head and trunk, excluding the extremities. Another risk of immersion in a warm bath is the loss of the ability to monitor heart rate and ECG, or to respond easily if significant dysrhythmias occur. In acute hypothermia, active external rewarming is appropriate, but there is some evidence that in chronic cases (>24 hours) mortality is higher if active external rewarming is used instead of simple passive techniques.

Core rewarming techniques are almost certainly more quickly effective and less likely to be associated with an after-drop in temperature, dangerous dysrhythmias, or significant hypotension. These methods are especially valuable in the setting of severe chronic hypothermia (T < 32°C) where all the fluid shifts previously described are most likely. Peritoneal dialysis with the dialysate warmed to 43°C, and inhalation rewarming with inspired gas temperature maintained at 42 to 46°C are effective and only require equipment available in most hospitals. Hemodialysis, extracorporeal blood rewarming, and mediastinal irrigation require mobilization of sophisticated equipment and personnel. Gastric or colonic irrigation has also been advocated, but placement of the intragastric balloon may precipitate dysrhythmias.

Most patients with hypothermia have a good prognosis. In those with mild temperature depression (>32°C), external rewarming techniques and supportive care based on vital signs, arterial blood gases and pH, and metabolic parameters such as glucose and calcium levels should result in prompt recovery. Patients with temperatures under 32°C, and especially those in whom hypothermia developed over 24 hours or more, require meticulous attention to continuously changing vital signs and metabolic needs. More elaborate core rewarming techniques are appropriate. If the physician remains aware that with each increment in core temperature, a "new" patient emerges, and reassesses management accordingly, many of these children will also do well.

References

Clowes G, O'Donnell T: Heat stroke. *N Engl J Med* 291: 564, 1974.

Conn AW, et al.: Cerebral salvage in near-drowning following neurological classification by triage. *Can Anaesth Soc J* 27: 201, 1980.

Grossman RA, et al.: Nontraumatic rhabdomyolysis and acute renal failure. *N Engl J Med* 291: 807, 1974.

Knochel J: Environmental heat illness, an eclectic review. *Arch Intern Med* 133: 841, 1974.

Modell JH, et al.: Clinical course of 91 consecutive near-drowning victims. *Chest* 70: 231, 1976.

Modell JH, et al.: Near-drowning: Correlation of level of consciousness and survival. *Can Anaesth Soc J* 27: 211, 1980.

Mellins, RB, Park S: Respiratory complications of smoke inhalation in victims of fires. *J Pediatr* 87: 1, 1975.

Reuler JB: Hypothermia: Pathophysiology, clinical settings, and management. *Ann Intern Med* 89: 519, 1978.

Root WS: Carbon Monoxide. In *Handbook of Physiology*, Section 3, Respiration Volume II, p. 1087 edited by Fenn WO and Rahn H. American Physiological Society, Washington, DC, 1965.

Trunkey D: Inhalation injury. *Surg Clin North Am* 58: 1133, 1978.

Ward M: *Mountain Medicine*, pp. 300. Crosby Lockwood Staples, London, 1975.

Wilkerson JA: Hypothermia. In *Medicine for Mountaineering*, p. 152. The Mountaineers, Seattle, 1975

CHAPTER 52

Pediatric and Adolescent Gynecology

JAN E. PARADISE, M.D.

INTRODUCTION

Two general considerations should guide the emergency physician's approach to the young patient with a gynecologic problem. These are: (1) whether the patient has started to menstruate, and (2) whether the postmenarchial patient is sexually active. (Throughout this section, "sexual activity" means coital experience.)

Among premenarchial girls with gynecologic complaints, vaginal infections, urethral prolapse, labial adhesions, and trauma are the most frequently encountered specific problems. A number of other patients have nonspecific genital irritation. In assessing any child with a gynecologic complaint, the physician must be alert to the possibility that sexual abuse is the underlying problem. Girls who have been sexually assaulted by strangers are usually not afraid to report such incidents to their parents, but the girl who has been sexually abused by a relative or family "friend" is much less likely to volunteer the information. She may be brought to the emergency department instead because of unexplained trauma, a vague genital complaint, or a vaginal discharge that proves to be gonorrhea.

Most premenarchial girls should not receive a standard pelvic examination including the use of a speculum and vagino-abdominal palpation, because such an examination is uncomfortable and unnecessary for diagnosis. An exception to this rule is the girl with vaginal bleeding caused by trauma. She must have a thorough examination, since even a serious laceration can produce only mild pain or minimal bleeding at first. Any premenarchial girl with vaginal bleeding and a history of in utero exposure to medicinal estrogen (diethylstilbestrol or another estrogen prescribed for first trimester bleeding) should also have a complete examination, but it is best to refer such patients to a gynecologist familiar with the management of DES-exposed daughters. For the great majority of premenarchial girls, the history, a general physical examination including inspection of the vulva and visualization of the vagina, and culture of a vaginal discharge if one is present, will lead promptly to a diagnosis.

Most young children will cooperate readily for initial inspection of the genitalia if they can be held on a parent's lap. A child over 3 years of age can comfortably lie supine on the examining table and be asked to bend her legs "like a frog does," with flexed hips and knees and with heels touching (Fig. 52.1). For vaginal examination, the child is first asked to "get up on your hands and knees like you are going to crawl." She should then rest her head on her folded arms, facing her parent. The examiner or

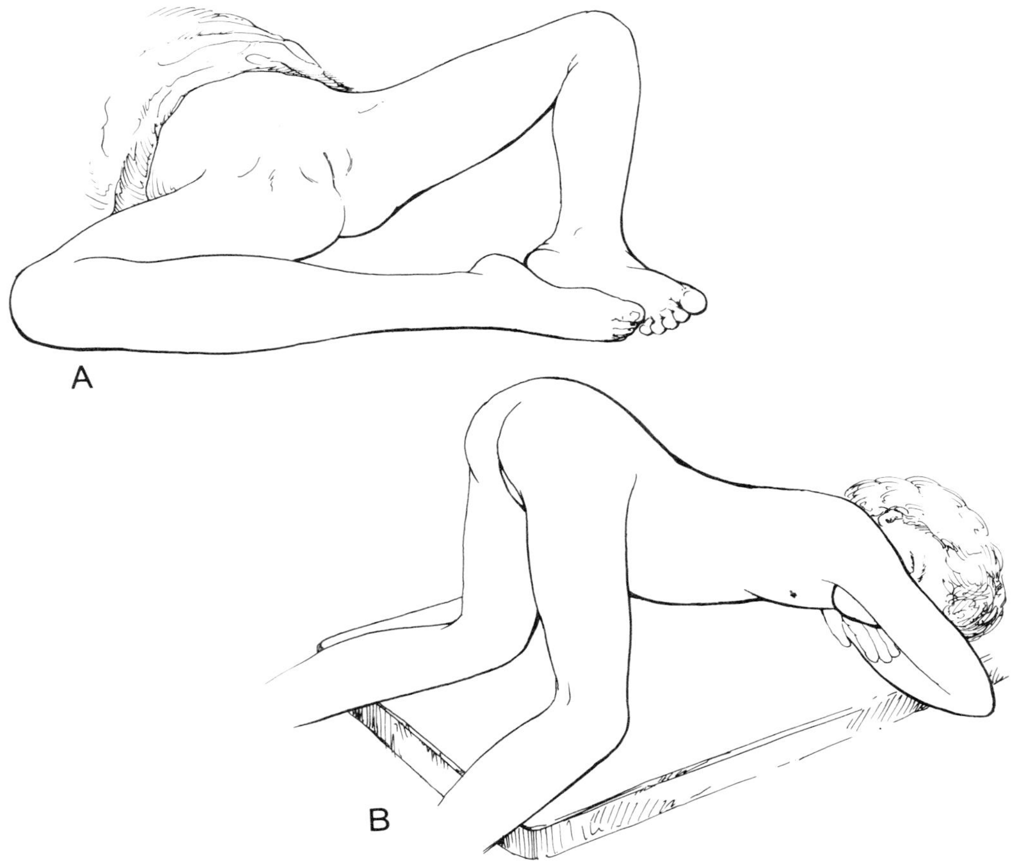

Figure 52.1 (*A*) Girl in the frog-leg position for examination of the external genitalia. (*B*) Girl in the knee-chest position with exaggerated lordosis and relaxed abdominal muscles. The examiner can inspect the interior of her vagina by gently separating her buttocks and labia, using an otoscope without an attached speculum for illumination.

an assistant gently presses the child's buttocks and labia upward and outward. If the child relaxes her abdominal muscles and back at this point, her vagina will usually fall open, permitting inspection with light from an otoscope with no speculum attached (Fig. 52.2). If the child has a vaginal discharge or bleeding, she should then be returned to the supine position so that specimens for culture can be obtained, using either a soft plastic medicine dropper or a cotton-tipped swab moistened with nonbacteriostatic saline solution. Lastly, if the examination of the girl's vagina in the knee-chest position was not satisfactory and a foreign body or a pelvic mass is suspected, recto-abdominal palpation should be performed. A child's cervix is normally felt as a firm, midline button of tissue anterior to the rectum, but the uterus and ovaries should not be palpable.

Obtaining a candid history of previous sexual activity from adolescent girls is not always a simple task, but the emergency department physician can maximize honest reporting by using some basic interviewing principles. First, the teenage girl who asks for a female physician is stating directly what will make her more comfortable. Her request should therefore be honored if it is possible to do so. Secondly, questions to the teenager about sexual activity (as well as

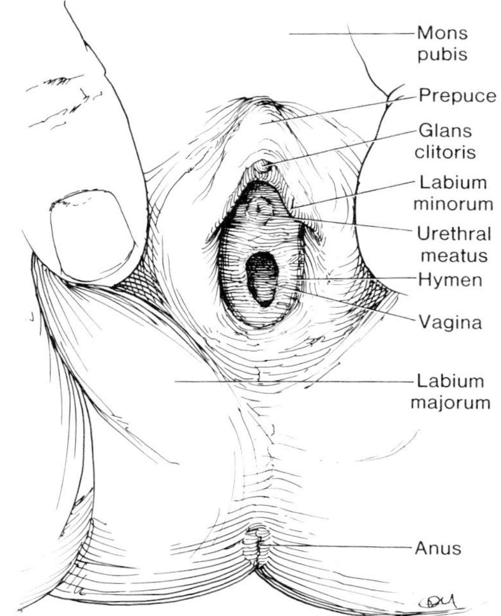

Figure 52.2 Anatomy of the normal female external genitalia.

other potentially sensitive subjects like contraception and substance abuse) should not be asked while a parent is present. This is accomplished more easily by asking the parent to leave the room during the daughter's physical examination. Thirdly, before any questions are asked, it is helpful to assure the teenager that if she wishes, her answers will be kept confidential.[1] Finally, the physician who adopts an empathetic, nonauthoritarian interviewing style is most likely to win the teenager's trust. For general reference, Figure 52.3 indicates the incidence of sexual activity among unmarried adolescent girls surveyed in 1978 and 1979.

Most virginal adolescents with menstrual cramps, mittelschmerz, or vaginal discharge do not require full pelvic examinations, since the likelihood that occult pelvic pathology will be found is very small. Rectoabdominal palpation can be used to evaluate the virginal patient with undiagnosed lower abdominal pain or a mass. However, trauma and vaginal bleeding are indications for pelvic examination, even among virginal patients.

Every sexually active adolescent girl who comes to the emergency department for a gastrointestinal or gynecologic complaint must receive a pelvic examination, since such patients have high rates of pregnancy and sexually transmitted disease. Before the examination, the patient should be given a chance to empty her bladder. If the physician is male, he should always be accompanied by a female chaperone during the examination itself. For female physicians, an assistant is helpful, but a chaperone is not necessary. After the patient is situated comfortably in the lithotomy position and draped, her vulva is inspected, and a small speculum (warmed and lubricated with tap water) is inserted for visualization of her vagina and cervix. A sterile cotton-tipped swab is used to collect endocervical secretions for culture of *Neisseria gonorrhoeae*. After a sample of vaginal discharge for microscopic study has been taken with a second swab, the speculum is removed. If the physician suspects gonococcal infection, urethral and rectal swabs for culture should be taken before bimanual palpation is done, since lubricating jelly can inhibit growth of the organisms. During the bimanual examination, the cervix is assessed for softness, patency of the os, and pain elicited by lateral cervical movement. The size and consistency of the uterus are determined, and the adnexal areas are palpated for masses or tenderness. Lastly, rectovaginal palpation is performed, checking again for masses or local tenderness.

The emergency physician can add an ounce of prevention to the care of the sexually active teenage girl if he or she not

[1] All 50 states have acknowledged the confidential nature of communications between an adult and a physician. This right of confidentiality is extended to minors seeking treatment for certain sex-related problems. Supreme Court decisions in 1976 (*Planned Parenthood of Central Missouri* v. *Danforth*) and 1979 (*Bellotti* v. *Baird*) provided that states can require neither parental consent nor parental notification for minors seeking abortions during the first 12 weeks of pregnancy. This ruling has been extended both by federal agencies that provide contraceptive services and by many states to permit minors to obtain prescription contraceptives without parental consent or notification. No physician has been sued successfully for prescribing a contraceptive for a minor. All states allow minors to obtain treatment for venereal disease without parental consent. However, since local and national policies may change, emergency physicians should become familiar with the relevant current laws of their own states.

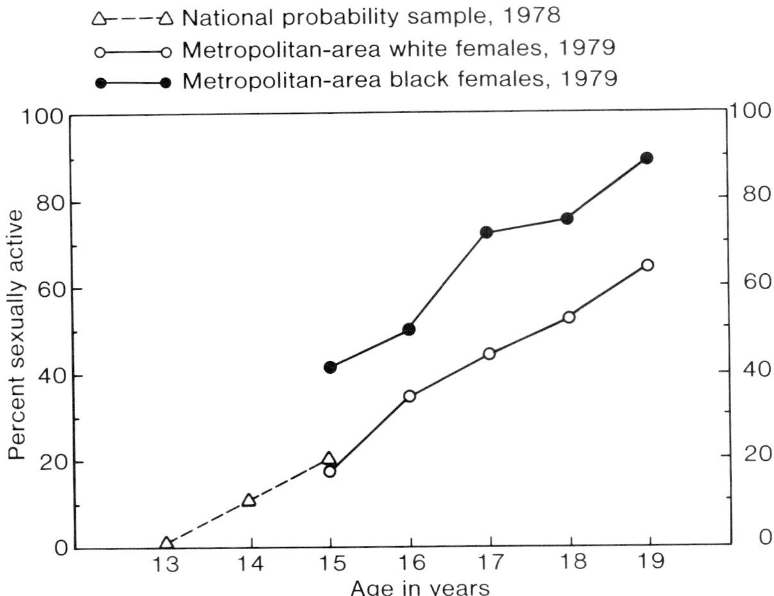

Figure 52.3 Percent of never-married adolescent females aged 13 to 15 years (1978) and 15 to 19 years (1979) who have ever had intercourse. From M. Zelnick and J. F. Kantner: Sexual activity, contraceptive use and pregnancy among metropolitan-area teenagers: 1971–1979, *Fam Plan Perspect* 12: 230, 1980 and from The Alan Guttmacher Institute: *Teenage Pregnancy: The Problem That Hasn't Gone Away*, p. 7. The Alan Guttmacher Institute, New York, 1981.

only provides treatment for the patient's current problem, but also determines whether she has been receiving routine outpatient gynecologic care. For patients without such follow-up, the emergency department can maintain a referral list of appropriate local programs. Most communities have services designed for teenagers that are sponsored by hospitals, health departments, or Planned Parenthood. Similarly, since previously unrecognized pregnancy is a common emergency department diagnosis, it is helpful to establish a procedure so that teenagers who need counselling, prenatal care, and therapeutic abortion can be referred to the appropriate agencies without undue delay or turmoil.

HYDROCOLPOS AND RELATED DISORDERS

BACKGROUND

Definition

In normal females, the vagina provides an outlet for genital secretions and menstrual blood. If the vagina is obstructed, accumulating fluid will eventually distend it, causing symptoms to develop either during infancy or after menarche. During infancy, vaginal distension with mucus secreted as a result of stimulation by maternal hormones is called hydrocolpos or mucocolpos. If the volume of secretions is so large that the uterus is also distended, this condition is called hydrometrocolpos. If an obstructing congenital malformation is not recognized before menarche, menstrual blood will gradually fill the vagina, producing hematocolpos or, less commonly, hematometrocolpos.

Etiology

For hydrocolpos or one of its variations to arise, a female must have vaginal obstruction, a uterus, and a patent cervix. The two most common anomalies with these features are transverse vaginal septum (sometimes called vaginal atresia), and imperforate hymen. Although the embryologic origin of these malformations is not fully understood, they are probably produced between the sixteenth and twentieth weeks of gestation, if the developing vaginal plate fails to perforate at its junction with either the fused paramesonephric (Müllerian) ducts proximally or the urogenital sinus caudally. Most patients with complete agenesis of the vagina (Rokitansky-Küster-Hauser syndrome) have rudimentary uteri or none at all, so that hydrocolpos does not occur.

Epidemiology

Transverse vaginal septum occurs sporadically, with an estimated incidence of between 1 in 2000 and 1 in 84,000 females. However, a few inbred kindreds have been described with transverse vaginal septum, polydactyly, and other recessively inherited anomalies (McKusick-Kaufman syndrome). In one survey, imperforate hymen occurred in 0.1% of full-term female neonates. Epidemiologic studies may be confounded because the two conditions can be confused with each other, and because occasionally, a congenitally imperforate hymen may open spontaneously during infancy.

CLINICAL MANIFESTATIONS

Infancy

Although vaginal obstruction should properly be identified during the initial examination of the newborn female, infants with hydrocolpos often go unrecognized until days or weeks later when they develop the three hallmarks of this condition: a lower abdominal mass, difficulty with urination, and a visible bulging membrane at the introitus. Except in mild cases, the lower abdominal mass consists of the bladder as well as the hydrocolpos itself. The infant strains to micturate or has urinary retention because the urethra is obstructed extrinsically. In more severe cases, infants may also have constipation, hydronephrosis, edema of the lower extremities, and respiratory embarrassment. Inspection of the perineum should immediately indicate the proper diagnosis.

Adolescence

The girl with congenital vaginal obstruction who escapes notice during infancy will not come to attention until late in puberty when she presents with either primary amenorrhea or lower abdominal pain. She will have had satisfactory pubertal developmental until her menarche apparently fails to occur. Accumulating menstrual blood will then eventually produce vague lower abdominal pain that is not necessarily cyclic. As the hematocolpos grows, it will finally interfere with comfortable micturition, producing symptoms of urgency, frequency, or dysuria. The history of amenorrhea and the finding of a lower abdominal mass may lead the physician to suspect a tumor or even pregnancy, but the characteristic appearance of the introitus covered by a bluish bluging membrane is diagnostic of hematocolpos with imperforate hymen (Fig. 52.4). Patients with a high transverse vaginal septum will not be so easily diagnosed since the introitus will appear normal. However, palpation of the vagina will promptly show that it is obstructed, and that the cervix cannot be felt.

Complications

The complication of congenital vaginal obstruction that is most likely to require urgent attention among both infants and adolescents is acute urinary retention. This can of course be managed readily after the primary diagnosis has been recognized. Patients without complete urethral obstruction can instead have variable degrees of hydroureter or hydronephrosis as a result of the chronic extrinsic pressure. Imperforate hymen is usually an isolated anomaly, but other types of obstruction, chiefly transverse vaginal septum, are regularly associated with renal malformations, including hypoplastic or single kidneys, and duplicated or ectopic collecting systems. For these reasons, the patient's laboratory evaluation should include assessment of both renal function and urinary tract anatomy. Endometriosis can be a late complication of severe hematocolpos.

DIFFERENTIAL DIAGNOSIS

The differential diagnosis of hydrocolpos and its variations includes patients with either a lower abdominal or pelvic mass but no vaginal obstruction, and patients with apparent vaginal obstruction. In the former category, the physician simply needs to

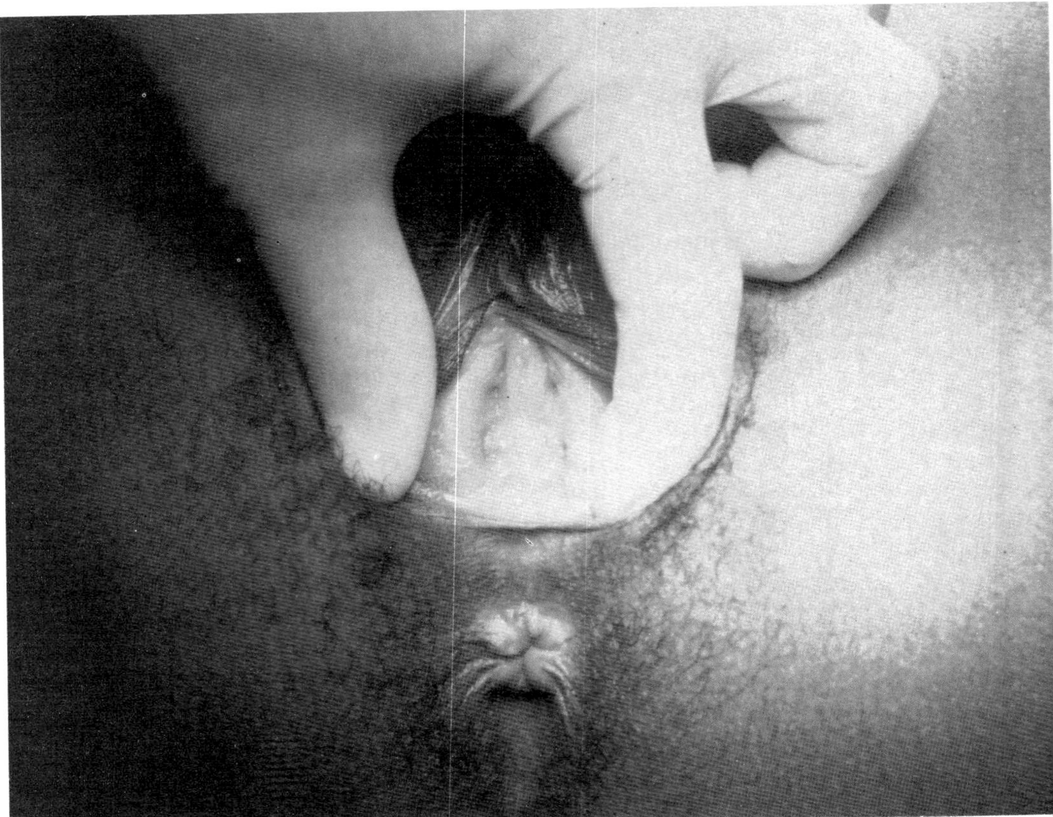

Figure 52.4 Hematocolpos in a 15-year-old patient with an imperforate hymen. The membran bulges at the introitus underneath the labia minora (cf. Fig. 52.5).

demonstrate that the patient has a patent genital tract. The usual measures for diagnosis of the mass can then be undertaken. The latter group includes girls with microperforate hymen, labial adhesions, Gartner's (mesonephric) duct cysts, and rarely, complete agenesis of the vagina and testicular feminization. The microperforate hymen has a tiny orifice just below the urethra, and requires only careful inspection for its diagnosis. Adhesions of the labia minora are superficial to the plane of the hymen, and are characterized by a central vertical line of fusion (see Fig. 52.5). A large vaginal Gartner's duct cyst can resemble an imperforate hymen, but it can be seen to protrude *through* the hymeneal ring, which is itself patent. Patients with complete agenesis of the vagina have only a rugated dimple or shallow indentation at the introitus. A short blind vagina also occurs in testicular feminization, a disorder charac terized by end-organ insensitivity to andro gen. These patients are phenotypic female with an XY karyotype, who undergo breas development at puberty, but lack pubic hai and female reproductive organs.

MANAGEMENT

Patients with congenital vaginal obstruc tion need surgical treatment. Hydrocolpo or hematocolpos complicated by respira tory impairment, compression of the infe rior vena cava, or hydronephrosis must b corrected without delay. The managemen of simple imperforate hymen can be modi fied according to the patient's age. Surger should be scheduled promptly for adoles cents, but can be delayed and performe electively for asymptomatic infants an children.

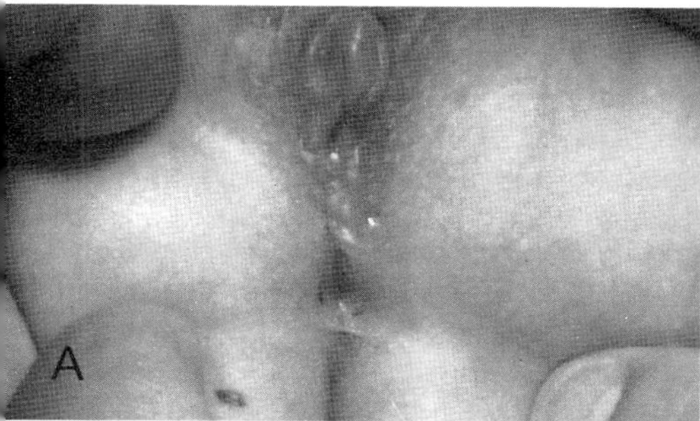

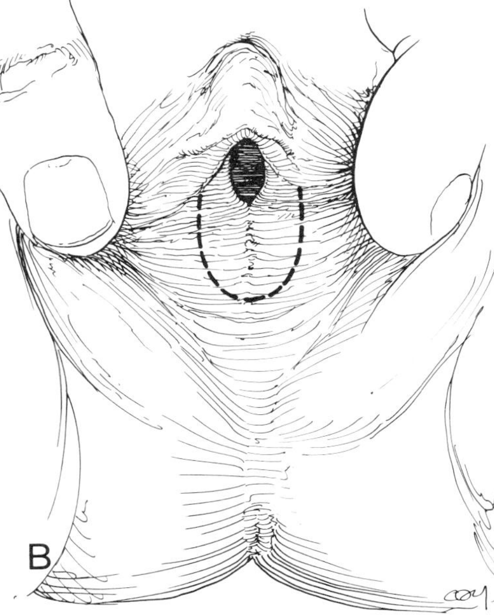

Figure 52.5 (*A*) Labial adhesions in an asymptomatic three-year-old girl. (*B*) A flat surface, a dense central line of fusion, and an opening below the clitoris are characteristic of labial adhesions, which cover the introitus (cf. Fig. 52.4).

LABIAL ADHESIONS

BACKGROUND

Labial adhesions are an acquired attachment of the medial surfaces of the labia minora to each other. The terms labial fusion, synechiae, and agglutination are also frequently used to describe this condition. Although a precise incidence is unknown, clinical experience indicates that labial adhesions are one of the most common gynecological problems among children. Most patients are between the ages of 1 and 6 years, but adhesions have been reported in girls from 6 weeks to 14 years of age. The median age at diagnosis is 2 years.

PATHOPHYSIOLOGY

A cause of labial adhesions has never been established. However, it is generally agreed that they are a concomitant of the child's normally low levels of endogenous estrogen. Without estrogen, the genital epithelium is relatively thin and susceptible to irritation. Possibly following trauma or some other cause of inflammation, the two labial surfaces gradually stick together, with the line of fusion usually advancing anteriorly from the posterior frenulum of the labia minora. Although adhesions are sometimes attributed to previous genital infection, it is uncommon for girls to have either co-existing vaginal infection or a history of one, and vaginal cultures will generally be normal.

CLINICAL MANIFESTATIONS

The parent who notices a daughter's labial adhesions at home usually brings her to the emergency department with a chief complaint that the child's vagina is "closing up." Alternatively, a physician may notice the adhesions first during the child's routine physical examination. The situation is more likely to be difficult if, as occasionally happens, the child is brought to the emergency department for evaluation because another physician has mistakenly informed the parents that their daughter has congenital absence of the vagina or ambiguous gentalia. Imperforate hymen is another notable misdiagnosis. In these cases, the first order of business must be to provide a careful explanation and reassurance for the distressed parents, since the condition itself is essentially minor.

The diagnosis of labial adhesions can be made promptly and confidently by simple inspection of the child's genitalia. When the labia majora are gently retracted laterally, a flat plane of tissue marked by a central vertical line of adhesion obstructs the view of the introitus within (see Fig. 52.5). This thin vertical raphe is pathognomonic of labial adhesions. It is occasionally difficult to detect if the child's adhesions are old and dense. The length of the adhesions is variable, and they can be perforated. They are usually thickest posteriorly, and stop below the clitoris. Even when adhesions appear to have closed the vulva completely, there is generally a pinpoint opening that permits the outflow of urine.

Most girls with labial adhesions are asymptomatic. A few (up to 20%) have associated dysuria, frequency, or refusal to void that may be due either to the obvious mechanical obstruction or to concurrent urinary tract infection. Whether associated urinary tract infections are a cause or an effect of adhesions is uncertain, but they are a recognized complication of the condition. The evaluation of girls with genitourinary symptoms should include a urine culture and the appropriate medical follow-up. Asymptomatic girls need no laboratory evaluation.

MANAGEMENT

Ninety percent of girls with labial adhesions can be treated successfully with a small amount of estrogen cream (Premarin or Dienestrol) dabbed onto the adhesions at bedtime for 2 to 4 weeks. After they have separated, an inert cream (zinc oxide, Vaseline, Desitin) is applied nightly for an additional 2 weeks, to keep the labia apart while healing is completed. It is not necessary to treat asymptomatic girls since the normal increase in estrogen during puberty will produce spontaneous resolution, but many parents prefer that their daughters be treated. Because pharmacies often supply estrogen cream in large tubes, parents should be warned specifically that prolonged use of the hormone can stimulate breast growth in children. Vulvar hyperpigmentation is a common, transient side-effect of treatment.

Labial adhesions should not be separated forcibly unless the child is first sedated or given general anesthesia. The procedure is painful and usually meets with failure since the raw, newly-separated labia promptly adhere again. Topical estrogen cream is a painless, inexpensive, and effective therapeutic alternative.

URETHRAL PROLAPSE

BACKGROUND

Urethral prolapse is the protrusion of the distal urethral mucosa outward through its meatus. Commonly, the prolapsed segment is constricted at the meatus, and venous blood flow is impaired, so that the involved tissue becomes swollen, edematous, and dark red or purplish. If the process is not corrected, the tissue gradually becomes thrombosed and necrotic.

About half of affected females are children before puberty, and most of the remainder are postmenopausal women. Most prolapses during childhood occur in girls between the ages of 2 and 10 years. The observation that black children are particularly predisposed to experience urethral prolapse remains unexplained. Nearly 95% of the 119 affected girls reported in the English-language literature since 1937 have been black. In contrast, race does not appear to be a risk factor for prolapse among postmenopausal women.

Proposed etiologies for urethral prolapse have included sudden or recurrent increases in intra-abdominal pressure (coughing, crying, constipation, lifting heavy objects), local trauma, redundant urethral tissue, neuromuscular dysfunction, and inadequate pelvic support of the bladder neck and urethra, but there has been no convincing evidence to support any of these hypotheses. Cystoscopy has failed to demonstrate anatomic abnormalities in studied patients. Bacterial and viral cultures in a small number of cases have also been negative.

CLINICAL MANIFESTATIONS

Vaginal bleeding or spotting is the chief complaint of 90% of children with significant urethral prolapses. The bleeding is painless, occasionally misinterpreted as menstruation or hematuria, and accompanied by urinary frequency or dysuria in about one-fourth of cases. Only a minority of girls or their parents are aware of the presence of a vulvar mass. On the other hand, it is not rare for the physician simply to note a small prolapse during the routine examination of an asymptomatic child.

On examination of the child's vulva, a red or purplish, soft, doughnut-shaped mass is seen (Fig. 52.6). Most prolapses are not tender, and measure 1 or 2 cm in diameter. By retracting the labia majora posterolaterally, the examiner can often demonstrate that the mass is separate from and anterior to the vaginal introitus, but this may be difficult if the prolapse is relatively large. A small central dimple in the mass indicates the urethral lumen. This dimple can be missed if there is inadequate lighting, active bleeding, or marked swelling of the urethral mucosa. In most cases, the appearance of the prolapse is diagnostic. However, if the diagnosis is in doubt, straight catheterization of the bladder through the mass (using sterile technique) can be performed to demonstrate the anatomic relationships safely and rapidly. No other test is needed for the great majority of patients. If a urinalysis is performed on a spontaneously voided specimen, red blood cells are likely to be found, but urine cultures are routinely sterile. Urethral polyps, prolapsed ureterocele, condylomata acuminata, sarcoma botryoides, and urethral carcinoma may be included in the differential diagnosis, but these entities are far less common in children and lack the characteristically annular appearance of a urethral prolapse.

MANAGEMENT

For the symptomatic patient with a small segment of prolapsed mucosa that looks relatively healthy, warm moist compresses or sitz baths can be recommended initially. The proportion of patients so managed who either will fail to improve or will have a subsequent recurrence is uncertain, but some patients have been reported to improve within 10 to 14 days and remain normal thereafter, thus avoiding surgery. Patients with dark red or necrotic mucosa should be treated within several days by surgical removal of this tissue under general anesthesia. After the diagnosis is confirmed by cystoscopy, the prolapse is excised and the cut edges are sutured together. The procedure is simple and can be carried out in a day surgery unit.

GENITAL WARTS

BACKGROUND

Definition

Genital warts, or condylomata acuminata, are benign fleshy tumors on anogenital skin caused by the DNA-containing human papillomavirus. They are also known

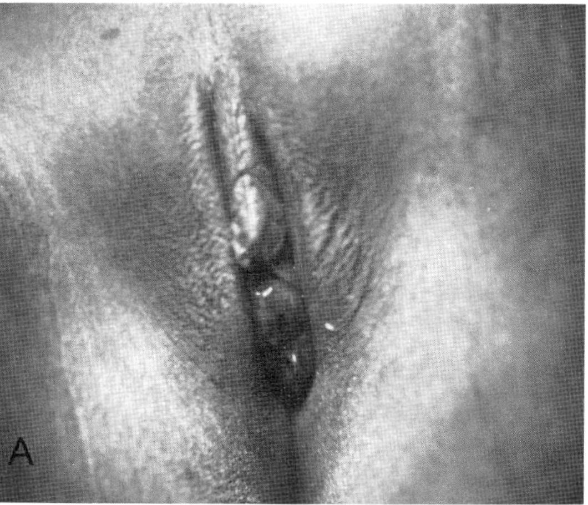

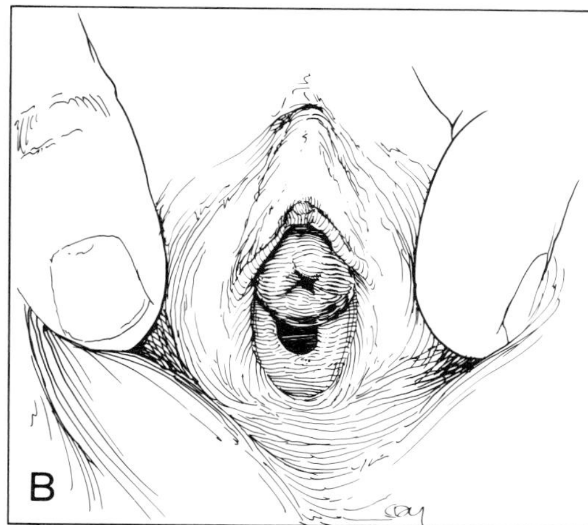

Figure 52.6 (*A*) Urethral prolapse in a 6-year-old girl with "vaginal" bleeding. The vaginal orifice cannot be seen. (*B*) The smooth doughnut shape and central lumen are characteristic features of a urethral prolapse which, if large or swollen, often conceals the vagina below it.

as venereal warts, fig warts, and moist warts. Genital warts must be differentiated from condylomata lata, a contagious manifestation of secondary syphilis.

EPIDEMIOLOGY

Because genital warts are not a reportable disease in the United States, their precise incidence is unknown. In England, however, between 1973 and 1978, the yearly incidence rose from 36.6 to 50.3 new cases per 100,000 population. The age distributions of new patients with genital warts and gonorrhea seen at venereal disease clinics are nearly identical, peaking during the late teens and early twenties when sexual activity with multiple partners is most common. Warts are considered a possible risk factor for the development of vulvar and cervical carcinoma, but substantiating evidence has not yet been reported. Actual malignant transformation of large warts occurs only rarely.

Genital warts are transmitted from person to person by direct skin contact. About two-thirds of the sexual contacts of infected patients will acquire warts themselves. Short-lived warts appear to be more contagious than warts that have been present for 6 months or longer. The incubation period after contact with an infected partner is 2 to 3 months.

Etiology

Although genital warts, common skin warts, plantar warts, and laryngeal papillomas are all caused by the human papillomavirus (HPV), genetic mapping indicates that one HPV subtype with a distinctive DNA pattern may be responsible for causing genital warts. The observation that patients with genital warts are no more likely to have skin warts than matched healthy control subjects also tends to support the notion that genital warts are not just skin warts in an unexpected location.

PATHOPHYSIOLOGY

Grossly, genital warts are hyperplastic lesions that occur at the junction of mucous membranes with squamous epithelium. On microscopic examination, the stratum granulosum contains foci of vacuolated cells. Acanthosis, parakeratosis, and hyperkeratosis are characteristic findings. So-called balloon cells—large multinucleated intermediate cells with perinuclear halos and dense peripheral cytoplasm—can be seen on cytologic examination of cervical and vaginal specimens, and may be pathognomonic for condylomata.

CLINICAL MANIFESTATIONS

Most patients with new warts report that they have noticed bumps in the genital area. Small warts generally do not produce any discomfort, but large perianal ones can interfere with defecation and can be very painful. Intravaginal warts can be friable and cause bleeding. A history of sexual contact may be difficult to obtain since the incubation period for genital warts is relatively long, and since a patient may not have noticed her partner's lesions. If a vaginal discharge accompanies the warts, it indicates the additional presence of vaginitis; warts themselves do not produce discharge.

Warts can occur anywhere on the perineum, but their growth seems to be encouraged by moisture. The most frequent locations in females are the posterior part of the vaginal introitus, adjacent areas of the labia minora and majora, and the lower vagina (Fig. 52.7). On the cervix, obvious warts are less common than dysplastic changes identified by cytologic screening. (In males, warts are usually found on the inner asepct of the prepuce, the glans penis, and the urethral meatus.) Single warts 1 cm or more in diameter, and clusters of seedlings, each a few millimeters across, are both common. They can be velvety and flat, or papillomatous. Large warts often contain distinct cauliflower-like lobulations.

MANAGEMENT

The diagnosis of genital warts is almost always obvious on inspection of the lesions, but evaluation should include a serologic test to exclude syphilis, and, as a matter of course, cultures for gonorrhea. Because warts can be associated with dysplasia of the uterine cervix, a Papanicolaou smear should be obtained in the emergency de-

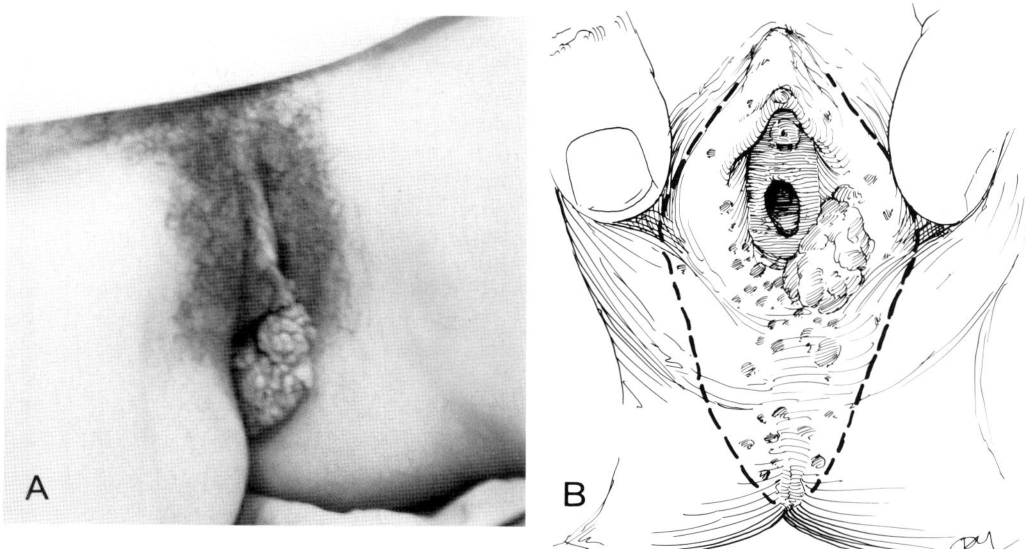

Figure 52.7 (*A*) Large vulvar and perianal genital warts in a 15-year-old patient. (*B*) In females, genital warts are most commonly located along the posterior margin of the introitus, inside the vagina, and on the labia minora.

partment, or the patient should be referred for routine outpatient cytologic screening.

Since genital warts are spread by skin-to-skin contact and since common skin warts have not been shown convincingly to give rise to genital warts, the finding of genital warts in a prepubertal child should prompt an investigation for suspected sexual abuse. Warts in children and those that cause significant discomfort are, respectively, urgent social and medical problems. For the most part, however, patients with genital warts can be managed on a routine basis.

Most genital warts do not regress spontaneously. Podophyllin resin applied topically is the appropriate outpatient therapy for uncomplicated cases. The resin is available commercially in solutions of up to 25% concentration in either alcohol or tincture of benzoin, and is dabbed onto genital warts with a cotton-tipped swab. Except in the case of some perianal warts, topical application is painless. Petroleum jelly can be used as a protective cover for the adjacent normal skin. Patients should be instructed to wash the resin off thoroughly with soap and water within 4 hours after treatment. Applications can be repeated weekly as needed.

Systemic absorption of podophyllin can produce bone marrow suppression, peripheral neuropathy, coma, and death. It is a teratogen, and has been associated with stillbirths when administered late in pregnancy. To avoid these effects, podophyllin must not be used on warts that are large, bleeding, or located on mucosal surfaces. It is absolutely contraindicated during pregnancy. Safe maximum doses of 10% solution are 4 ml for patients weighing more than 40 kg, and 0.1 mg/kg for children. Surgical excision, cauterization, and cryosurgery are alternatives for patients whose warts cannot be treated with podophyllin. Trichloroacetic acid, antineoplastic agents, laser, and autogenous wart vaccine are less widely used remedies.

DYSMENORRHEA

DEFINITION

Dysmenorrhea means painful menstruation. It is considered primary if the pain cannot be attributed to a specific pelvic abnormality such as endometriosis, pelvic inflammatory disease, submucous myomata, or a uterine malformation. Menstrual pain resulting from any underlying disorder is termed secondary dysmenorrhea.

Epidemiology

Among all women, and among adolescents in particular, primary dysmenorrhea is far more common than secondary dysmenorrhea. Estimates of the incidence of primary dysmenorrhea have varied, depending on both the age of the women surveyed and the criterion used for a positive response (any pain, pain that interferes with normal activity, or pain that prompts a visit to a physician). Sixty percent of postmenarchial girls between the ages of 12 and 17 years who participated in the U.S. National Health Examination Survey (1966 to 1970) reported having menstrual pain or discomfort. The prevalence of dysmenorrhea correlated positively with increasing chronologic and gynecologic (postmenarchial) age among the respondents, reflecting the strong association of dysmenorrhea with ovulatory menstrual cycles. At gynecologic age 1, 31% of girls had dysmenorrhea. The proportion by gynecologic age 5 increased to 78%. Data from a number of studies indicate that between 10 and 30% of women are unable to carry out their usual activities during some or all of their cycles because of menstrual pain.

PATHOPHYSIOLOGY

A pathophysiologic basis for dysmenorrheic pain could not be demonstrated until recently. During the 1960's and 70's, numerous investigations indicated that at the end of ovulatory menstrual cycles, prostaglandins $F_{2\alpha}$ and E_2 are synthesized by and released from endometrial tissue. These prostaglandins cause increases in both the uterine resting tone and the amplitude and frequency of myometrial contractions. Uterine contractions that exceed systolic blood pressure produce tissue ischemia and perceptible pain. Intravenous administration of prostaglandins can reproduce the systemic discomforts—vomiting, diarrhea, headache—that often accompany dysmenorrhea. A dose-response relationship has been demonstrated in studies comparing the prostaglandin content of menstrual fluid from women with and without dysmenorrhea, and from individual women during painful and pain-free cycles.

The role of ovarian hormones in endometrial prostaglandin production is not completely understood. Progesterone or its withdrawal appears to enhance prostaglandin synthesis during ovulatory cycles. Conversely, progesterone-impregnated intrauterine devices and the inhibition of ovulation by birth control pills are both associated with decreased prostaglandin production and with relief from dysmenorrhea.

CLINICAL MANIFESTATIONS

Typical primary dysmenorrhea consists of cramping, dull, midline, or generalized lower abdominal pain at the onset of a menstrual period. The pain may coincide with the start of bleeding, or may precede the bleeding by several hours. Many women have associated symptoms that can include backache, thigh pain, diarrhea, nausea or vomiting, and headache. The discomfort usually abates within 48 hours. Because dysmenorrhea is a hallmark of ovulation, adolescents characteristically do not experience dysmenorrhea until after several months of painless, anovulatory cycles. Menstrual pain that begins either at menarche or more than 4 years after regular cycles have been established is less common. The patient with such early or late dysmenorrhea should be assessed carefully for a possible underlying disorder, but she is still more likely to be having simply a particularly early or late onset of fertile cycles. Intrauterine devices often exacerbate primary dysmenorrhea; birth control pills almost uniformly abolish it.

Patients with straightforward dysmenorrhea have normal physical examinations and no associated abnormalities on routine laboratory evaluation. Pelvic inflammatory disease and congenital abnormalities (rudimentary uterine horn, partially obstructed genital duplications) must be included in the differential diagnosis for sexually active adolescents and those with atypical pain or a pelvic mass. Recent investigations indicate that endometriosis and postoperative adhesions are also potential explanations for chronic, cyclic, undiagnosed pelvic pain in teenagers.

MANAGEMENT

The virginal adolescent with a typical history of dysmenorrhea should undergo a routine physical examination including inspection of the external genitalia, but a pelvic examination is not necessary. However, virginal patients with atypical or severe pain should undergo recto-abdominal or one-finger vagino-abdominal palpation. Sexually active adolescents with pelvic pain cannot be adequately evaluated without a complete pelvic examination to screen for pelvic infection and unsuspected pregnancy. No specific laboratory or radiologic evaluation is needed for otherwise healthy virginal adolescents. Pelvic ultrasound or laparoscopy may be helpful in the assessment of patients with uncertain diagnoses or with pain unresponsive to adequate treatment (see below).

The recognition that prostaglandins cause primary dysmenorrhea allows physicians to forego household remedies (rest, exercise, heat, vitamins), minor narcotics, and surgery (cervical dilatation, presacral neurectomy) for its treatment. Because it inhibits prostaglandin synthesis and is well-known and inexpensive, aspirin in the standard adult dose (650 mg q.i.d.) is the mainstay of initial treatment. Other commonly used agents—acetominophen, caffeine, propoxyphene—lack aspirin's specific analgesic action. Aspirin's effectiveness may be enhanced if it can be started 3 days before the expected menstrual period, but adolescents with irregular cycles will have difficulty following this schedule. Contraindications to the use of aspirin include aspirin hypersensitivity, gastrointestinal ulcers, and bleeding disorders.

The nonsteroidal anti-inflammatory drugs listed below are newer and considerably more expensive than aspirin, but they are also several hundred times more potent inhibitors of prostaglandin synthesis. These drugs provide effective treatment for approximately 80% of women whose dysmenorrhea is not relieved by aspirin. For many women, they also reduce menstrual blood loss somewhat. Like aspirin, these drugs can cause gastrointestinal irritation, inhibit platelet aggregation, and prolong the bleeding time. Their use is contraindicated in patients with aspirin hypersensitivity and gastrointestinal ulcers.

Ibuprofen (Motrin): 300 to 400 mg orally every 4 to 6 hours.

Naproxen (Naprosyn): 500 mg once orally, followed by 250 mg every 6 to 8 hours.

Naproxen sodium (Anaprox): 550 mg once orally, followed by 275 mg every 6 to 8 hours.

For the most part, the availability of these drugs makes the prescription of birth control pills and narcotic analgesics for virginal adolescents with dysmenorrhea unnecessary. However, for sexually active adolescents, birth control pills are an obvious and attractive alternative therapy, since they provide both contraception and pain relief.

DYSFUNCTIONAL UTERINE BLEEDING

BACKGROUND

Dysfunctional uterine bleeding (DUB) during adolescence is best characterized as irregular, prolonged or excessive menstrual bleeding associated with anovulation and unrelated to pregnancy. Ovulatory cycles occur in about 20% of adults with DUB, but this phenomenon is uncommon during the teenage years. Terms often used to categorize patterns of DUB are metrorrhagia (irregular or acyclic bleeding) and menorrhagia (excessive duration or quantity of bleeding). Menstrual bleeding that persists beyond 9 days, that recurs at intervals of fewer than 21 days, or that produces anemia is abnormal and warrants attention.

DUB is prevalent at the beginning and end of the reproductive years, paralleling the times when anovulatory cycles are most common. In girls during the first year after menarche, about half of menstrual cycles are anovulatory as judged by the basal body temperature. This proportion decreases gradually, so that only 5% of cycles are anovulatory 10 or more years after menarche. Of course, the majority of adolescents with anovulatory cycles experience self-limited, reasonably cyclic bleeding episodes. Why a small number of girls develop an erratic bleeding pattern is not understood.

PATHOPHYSIOLOGY

From the standpoint of ovarian function, the normal ovulatory menstrual cycle is divided into an initial follicular and a subsequent luteal phase. The parallel phases of endometrial development are called, respectively, proliferative and secretory. At the start of an ovulatory cycle, pituitary follicle-stimulating hormone (FSH) promotes the growth of ovarian follicles. In turn, the rising concentration of estradiol from these follicles stimulates the proliferation of endometrial stroma and glands, has a negative feedback effect on the secretion of FSH, and finally induces a mid-cycle surge of lutenizing hormone (LH) that triggers ovulation. The duration of the preovulatory phase of the menstrual cycle is variable, but it generally lasts about 14 days. After ovulation has occurred, the ruptured ovarian follicle forms a corpus luteum that secretes progesterone as well as estradiol, and levels of both FSH and LH gradually decline. Although progesterone limits the ultimate thickness of the endometrium, it nevertheless promotes further growth of the endometrial secretory glands and spiral blood vessels, so that they become coiled and tortuous. At the end of the corpus luteum's life span (a highly consistent 14 days unless conception occurs) it degenerates, and circulating levels of both estrogen and progesterone fall, eventually stimulating a resurgence of LH and FSH. As hormonal support wanes, blood flow to the secretory endometrium diminishes, and the spiral arterioles constrict and relax rhythmically. The resulting progressive ischemia leads to endometrial necrosis. Menstrual sloughing begins, and the cycle starts over again.

In contrast, during intervals of anovulation, there is no luteal progesterone to limit the endometrium's thickness or to promote its structural integrity. Parts of the endometrial surface undergo growth and sloughing sporadically, without cyclic coordination. The amount of estrogen secreted by ovarian follicles fluctuates unpredictably, and bleeding can occur either because of a fall in estrogen level (withdrawal bleeding) or despite a sustained level of production (breakthrough bleeding). Relatively constant low levels of estrogen tend to produce intermittent spotty bleeding (metrorrhagia). Larger amounts of estrogen cause greater endometrial proliferation and a cyclic pattern of amenorrhea followed by profuse bleeding (menorrhagia) whenever either the endometrial vessels and glands outstrip their stromal support, or hormone levels spontaneously fall. Compared to the 35 to 75 ml of blood lost during a normal menstrual period, dysfunctional bleeding frequently results in the loss of 100 to 200 ml each month. It is no surprise that iron deficiency with depleted marrow stores or outright anemia is a common concurrent problem for patients with DUB.

CLINICAL MANIFESTATIONS

Dysfunctional uterine bleeding has a substantial capacity to disrupt the everyday activities of adolescent patients discomfitted by an unpredictable, urgent need for bathroom facilities and the risk of visible bloodstains. Large amounts of bleeding often provoke considerable fear in patients as well as their parents. These concerns can overshadow the history of the bleeding itself, but the details of the problem's chronology and an estimate of blood loss (in soaked pads per day) will help the physician to assess the severity of the bleeding, follow the patient's clinical course, and gauge her prognosis. The symptoms that characteristically accompany only ovulatory menstrual cycles—mittelschmerz, premenstrual breast tenderness, bloating, mood changes, and dysmenorrhea—should be absent. DUB is classically painless, but an occasional patient with active bleeding may experience crampy pain if a clot or large quantity of blood is passed rapidly. Weakness or fainting should alert the examiner to the possibility of significant blood loss. Pertinent questions should include whether the patient is currently pregnant, whether she uses contraception if she has been sexually active, whether she has an underlying bleeding tendency (thrombocytopenia, von Willebrand's disease, etc.) and whether she was exposed to estrogens prenatally.

The physical examination must start with careful measurement of the patient's vital signs, including a check for orthostatic changes in the pulse and blood pressure. Pertinent signs including pallor, petechiae or bruises that might indicate a bleeding disorder, and hirsutism or obesity consistent with the polycystic ovary syndrome, should be sought and noted. The pelvic examination is likely to be normal except for the presence of bleeding, but it is far better to perform an examination than to rely on history alone, because teenagers are not always candid about their sexual activity, and the apparent DUB may in fact indicate a serious complication of pregnancy. Recto-abdominal palpation can be substituted if necessary for the standard bimanual examination. Ovarian enlargement is an uncommon finding even among adolescent patients with clear-cut polycystic ovary syndrome. The differential diagnosis of DUB is discussed at greater length in Chapter 38.

MANAGEMENT

A determination of the hemoglobin or hematocrit is essential for the emergency evaluation of patients with DUB, since historical estimates of blood loss are notoriously inaccurate. A platelet count should also be obtained since thrombocytopenia is the most common hematological disorder that produces menorrhagia. The history and physical examination should be used to guide the choice of additional laboratory tests. Sexually active adolescents should receive a pregnancy test and a cervical culture for gonorrhea, since the latter may produce otherwise unexplained uterine bleeding. Patients with menorrhagia beginning at menarche, severe hemorrhage, or a history of bleeding problems should undergo further evaluation for possible clotting disorders.

In order of decreasing urgency, management of DUB includes the identification and treatment of the following problems: shock, active hemorrhage or severe anemia, moderate bleeding with mild anemia, and irregular bleeding that produces distress but no anemia. For patients with brisk hemorrhage or hypotension, prompt hospitalization and volume resuscitation as necessary (see Chapter 2) are the first order of business.

Control of the bleeding itself is accomplished with hormonal treatment. Regimens vary according to the severity of bleeding and individual preference, but each is designed first to stop the bleeding, secondly to convert the unstable proliferative uterine endometrium to the secretory state, and finally to allow a self-limited endometrial slough under controlled conditions. (Pregnancy must be excluded in every case before hormonal treatment is begun). Estrogen is used to support the endometrium acutely and stop the bleeding. A progestational agent must be administered simultaneously to produce a secretory endometrium; otherwise the problem will recur predictably whenever the estrogen is stopped. Any of the oral contraceptive pills with 50 μg of either ethinyl estradiol or mestranol and a progestin (Ovcon 50, Ortho Novum 1/50, Norlestrin 1/50, etc) provides a convenient means of administering the two hormones together. Few families will object if the purpose of the medication—hormonal treatment, not contraception—is clearly explained. The dosage for patients with active bleeding and anemia is one estrogen-progestin tablet orally 4 times a day for 5 days. In almost every case, bleeding will decrease substantially within 24 hours and stop within 2 or 3 days. An alternative treatment for hospitalized patients consists of conjugated estrogens, 20 to 25 mg intravenously every 4 hours until the bleeding stops, with a maximum of 6 doses. This must be accompanied by a progestational agent (medroxyprogesterone 10 to 20 mg orally per day for 5 days). If hormonal treatment fails to arrest the bleeding, dilatation and curettage should be performed, but the procedure is not commonly needed.

For patients with only scanty bleeding and a normal hemoglobin who are nevertheless distressed, the oral regimen can successfully be reduced to one estrogen-progestin tablet twice a day for 5 days. It is not medically necessary to treat such patients, however, since the DUB may improve spontaneously. Nausea is a frequent side-effect of estrogen in each of these regimens, and can be treated symptomatically. Vomiting rarely precludes oral therapy. A progestin alone in higher doses (norethindrone acetate 10 to 20 mg/day for 5 days) can be used if estrogen is contraindicated or not tolerated, but the resulting hemostasis is less prompt and less predictable.

In each of these regimens, the hormones are stopped at the end of 5 days. A self-limited, heavy menstrual period will then follow within 2 or 3 days. The family must be forwarned carefully, so that they anticipate this episode and do not misinterpret it as a recurrence of the DUB. This withdrawal bleeding will stop spontaneously within several days. Subsequent therapy must be individualized. A course of medroxyprogesterone (10 mg orally, daily for 5 days) can be used every 6 to 8 weeks to produce a secretory endometrium and a controlled withdrawal flow, if spontaneous menstruation has not intervened. Sexually active adolescents and those with a history of chronic or severe DUB can be cycled on birth control pills, but this regimen has the potential disadvantage of suppressing a hypothalamic-pituitary-ovarian axis that is already poorly synchronized. Iron supplementation is prudent for all patients with DUB; those without frank anemia are likely to have depleted marrow stores of iron. Finally, careful outpatient follow-up is an essential component of management, since treatment may be needed for months or years, and since chronic anovulation is a risk factor for both infertility and the late development of endometrial carcinoma.

VAGINITIS

BACKGROUND

Definition

Vaginitis, or inflammation of the vagina, can be produced by chemical and mechanical irritants, foreign bodies, and a variety of infectious agents including viruses, chlamydiae, bacteria, fungi, protozoa, and helminths. During childhood, vaginitis is characterized by the presence of vaginal discharge, bleeding, or both. After puberty has begun, girls normally have an asymptomatic vaginal discharge; vaginitis is then indicated by the discomfort it produces or by a change in the character of the discharge. The etiology, clinical features, diagnosis, and treatment of common vaginal infections are presented in this chapter. For a more general review of the differential diagnosis of vaginal discharge and bleeding, the reader is referred to Chapters 38 and 39.

Epidemiology

At least half of all premenarchial girls with vaginal discharge visible on physical examination will prove to have specific vaginal infections that warrant antimicrobial treatment. Among prepubertal girls, *N. gonorrhoeae* causes the greatest number of these specific infections. Less frequent offenders include *Shigella* species, *Streptococcus pyogenes*, *Trichomonas vaginalis*, and *Chlamydia trachomatis*. Although staphylococci and *Haemophilus influenzae* are not well-established vaginal pathogens, it is possible that they also produce symptoms and signs in a proportion of colonized patients. *Candida albicans* is the most common pathogen among patients who are pubertal but still premenarchial.

The prevalence of vaginal infections in a population of postmenarchial adolescents depends largely on how many of them are sexually active. Currently, the proportion of never-married teenagers who have ever experienced coitus increases dramatically with age (see Figure 52.3), and is accompanied by a parallel increase in the prevalence of sexually transmitted infections. Precise data are not available since only gonorrhea and syphilis are reportable diseases, but some general observations can be made. Trichomoniasis is transmitted only by sexual contact, and is probably the commonest cause of vaginitis among sexually active teenagers. Overall, it is roughly 3 to 7 times more prevalent than gonococcal cervicitis. For reasons that are unclear, trichomonal infection is significantly more frequent among black than among white patients. Up to one third of patients with trichomoniasis have concurrent gonorrhea, but it is unusual for trichomoniasis and vaginal candidiasis to coexist. Simultaneous infection occurs in fewer than 5% of patients with either of these latter two disorders. Because the etiology of nonspecific vaginitis after puberty remains uncertain, other important characteristics of the disorder, including its prevalence, have been understandably difficult to determine. However, the constellation of symptoms and signs ascribed to nonspecific vaginitis appears to be very common. This diagnostic category accounts for up to one-third of all vaginitis among sexually active young women. The frequency of *Candida* vaginitis depends in part on the prevalence in any patient group of factors that predispose to its occurrence, including the use of broad spectrum antibiotics, corticosteroids, birth control pills, immunodeficiency, diabetes mellitus, and pregnancy. However, candidiasis can also occur in patients who lack these risk factors.

Neisseria gonorrhoeae

CLINICAL MANIFESTATIONS

Prepubertal girls with genital gonorrhea uniformly have an obvious whitish to greenish purulent vaginal discharge that can be pruritic. Asymptomatic vaginal carriage of the gonococcus is rare in children. Because the child's vaginal flora is normally fairly sparse, a Gram-stained smear of the vaginal discharge can provide a rapid presumptive positive diagnosis if, on microscopic examination, at least 8 pairs of typical gonococci can be seen in each of at least 2 polymorphonuclear leukocytes. However, the social and legal implications of the diagnosis of gonorrhea in a child mandate its confirmation by culture as well.

After puberty, higher estrogen levels stimulate the growth of a thick vaginal mucosa that is relatively resistant to infection by gonococci, and lower genital tract infection is localized to the cervix. A vaginal discharge, excessive menstrual bleeding, or symptoms of cystitis may prompt an infected patient's emergency department visit, but the majority of infections will produce no symptoms at all. On pelvic examination, there may be marked central erythema of the cervix, a purulent cervical discharge, or no abnormality. A culture of a single specimen taken from the endocervical canal with a cotton-tipped swab, plated on a selective medium, and incubated properly will identify about 85% of women with uncomplicated gonorrhea. The remaining 15% of patients have urethral, rectal, or pharyngeal infections without cervicitis.

MANAGEMENT

Pharyngeal and rectal swabs for culture of *N. gonorrhoeae* and a serologic test for syphilis should be obtained from every child in whom gonococcal vaginitis is either suspected or confirmed by culture. Girls with confirmed gonococcal vaginitis who weigh less than 45 kg should be treated with oral probenecid (25 mg/kg to a maximum of 1 g) plus a single dose of either amoxicillin (50 mg/kg p.o. to a maximum of 3 g) or aqueous procaine penicillin G (100,000 units/kg i.m. to a maximum of 4.8 million units). Children allergic to penicillin can be treated with spectinomycin (40 mg/kg i.m. to a maximum of 2 g). Tetracycline (40 mg/kg/day p.o. to a maximum of 2 g/day in 4 divided doses for 5 days) is an acceptable alternative for patients allergic to penicillin who are over 8 years of age. *Gonorrhea during childhood mandates a careful evaluation for sexual abuse and a report of suspected child abuse in every case.* All household contacts of the child, both children and adults, should be cultured, since epidemiologic studies indicate that about 25% of them are likely also to have gonorrhea. Hospitalization of the child may facilitate this investigation in some cases.

Adolescents with uncomplicated genital gonorrhea should receive one of the following regimens:

(1) Aqueous procaine penicillin G 4.8 million units i.m., with probenicid 1 g p.o.

(2) Tetracycline 500 mg p.o. 4 times a day for 5 days.

(3) Either ampicillin 3.5 g p.o. or amoxicillin 3 g p.o. in a single dose, with probenicid 1 g p.o.

Patients allergic to penicillin who cannot tolerate tetracycline may be treated with spectinomycin (2 g i.m.).

Every patient with gonorrhea should receive a screening serologic test for syphilis. None of the treatment regimens for gonorrhea will cure established syphilis, but all except spectinomycin are likely to eradicate incubating syphilis. The management of a case of gonorrhea is never complete until the patient's sexual partner(s) has been notified and treated presumptively. A test-of-cure culture should be obtained from every patient within a week after treatment has been completed.

Trichomonas vaginalis

CLINICAL MANIFESTATIONS

A small proportion of vaginally delivered female neonates will acquire trichomonal vaginitis from their infected mothers. Infants harboring only a few trichomonads may never develop the clinical disease, but the remainder will have a thin whitish or yellowish vaginal discharge that appears within 3 to 10 days after birth. Infected babies may be irritable but are otherwise well.

The classic vaginal discharge of trichomonal vaginitis after puberty is pruritic, frothy, and yellowish. However, many infected women do not complain of excessive discharge, and the discharge when it is present may be scant or nondescript. The so-called strawberry cervix with multiple punctate areas of hemorrhage is pathognomonic for trichomoniasis, but is a relatively uncommon finding.

For patients of all ages, the diagnosis can be obtained rapidly if characteristically motile, flagellated trichomonads are seen in a saline suspension of discharge examined microscopically within about 15 minutes after it has been obtained (Fig. 52.8). If a longer delay occurs, the organisms will gradually lose their mobility and normal shape, making them much more difficult to identify. Wet mounts may also be falsely negative in patients who have only a small number of trichomonads present in the vagina. Culture of a specimen of discharge for *T. vaginalis* is the most sensitive diagnostic test. Selective media are commercially available and can be used if the wet mount fails to confirm the examiner's clinical suspicion of infection.

MANAGEMENT

Metronidazole is effective for the treatment of vaginal trichomoniasis. The dosage for infants is 15 mg/kg/day p.o. in 3 divided doses for 7 days. A single oral dose (2 g) is sufficient to treat adolescents. The 7-day regimen is also effective for adolescents (250 mg p.o. 3 times a day), but compliance is less assured. Since trichomoniasis is sexually transmitted, the adolescent patient's partner(s) is also usually treated with either of the 2 dosage regimens. However, this recommendation should be qualified by the realization that most trichomonal infections of the male urethra are asymptomatic and resolve spontaneously within a week or so. A teenage girl's sexual partner therefore need not be treated if coitus is relatively infrequent.

Nausea, vomiting, and an unpleasant taste are common side-effects of metronidazole. Alcohol should be avoided during treatment to prevent the occurrence of more severe abdominal pain, vomiting, flushing, and headache (disulfiram reaction). Because of its possible teratogenicity and mutagenicity, the use of metronidazole should be avoided during pregnancy.

Candida albicans

CLINICAL MANIFESTATIONS

C. albicans is a normal inhabitant of the vagina after the onset of puberty, when estrogen stimulates local increases in both glycogen stores and acidity that appear to enhance its growth. However, if the ecological balance of the vagina is changed by either inhibition of the normal bacterial flora, impaired host immunity, or an increase in the availability of nutrients (broad-spectrum antibiotics, immunodeficiency states, corticosteroids, diabetes mellitus, oral contraceptive pills, pregnancy), the resulting proliferation of *Candida* will produce symptoms in a fraction of affected patients. Because of the importance of estrogen in promoting fungal growth, candidal vaginitis is uncommon among prepubertal girls.

The hallmarks of *Candida* vaginitis are similar in prepubertal and adolescent patients. Intense pruritus and discharge are common complaints. In severe infections, an associated vulvar dermatitis with edema and erythema can occur. "External" dysuria is often produced when urine comes

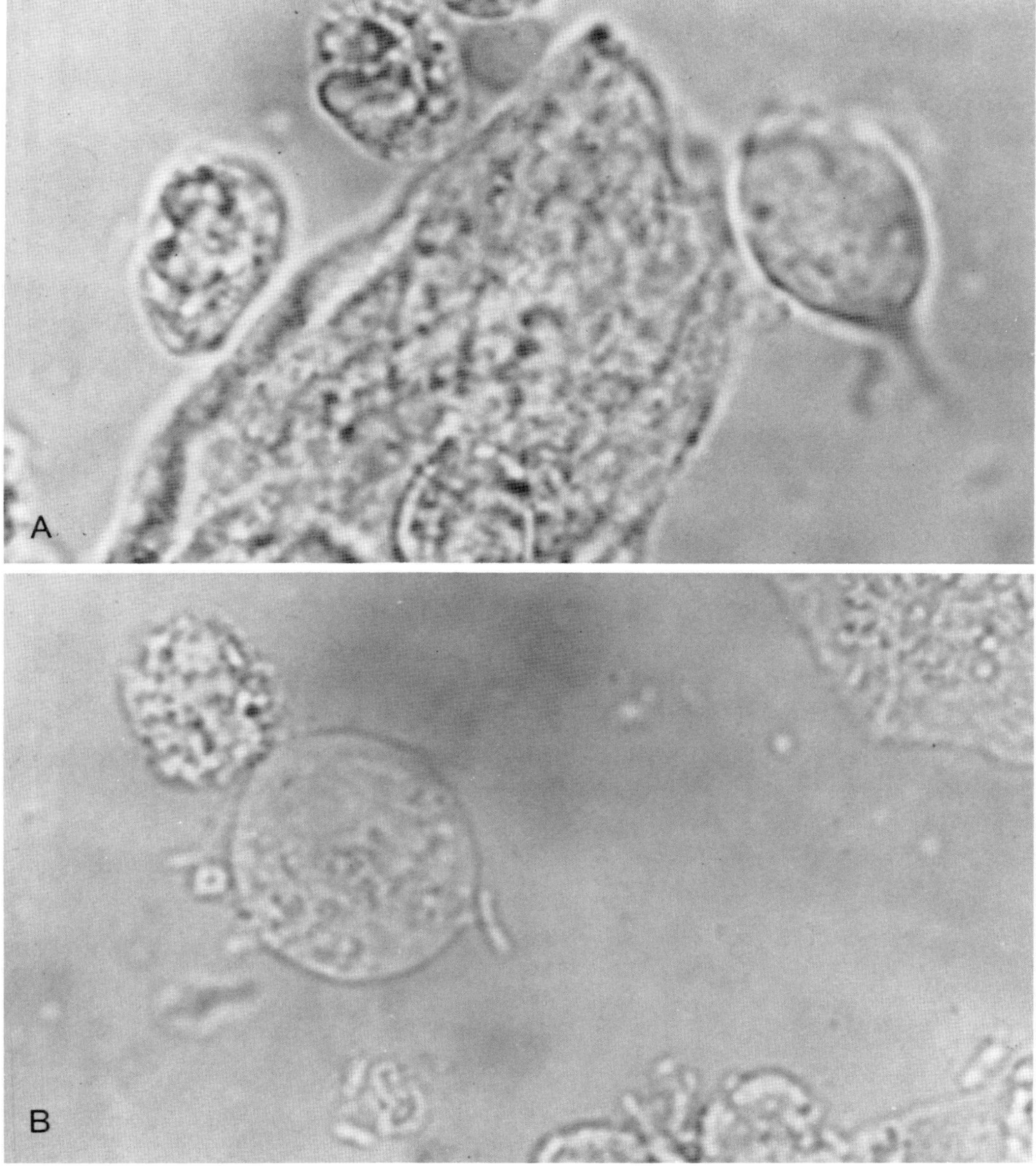

Figure 52.8 (*A*) Trichomonad in the vaginal discharge of a 17-year-old patient with gonococcal pelvic inflammatory disease. The flagellated protozoan is elliptical and somewhat larger than the adjacent polymorphonuclear leukocytes (225× magnification). (*B*) After suspension in saline solution for microscopy, trichomonads gradually become swollen and immobile. This balloon-shaped trichomonad is barely recognizable (225× magnification).

in contact with the inflamed vulva. The vagina itself is red, dry, and has a whitish, curdy discharge that may be so scant as to go unnoticed by the patient.

Microscopic examination of a sample of vaginal discharge suspended in 10% potassium hydroxide to clear the field of cellular debris can provide a rapid diagnosis of candidiasis if hyphae are seen (Fig. 52.9), but such wet mounts have a high rate of false

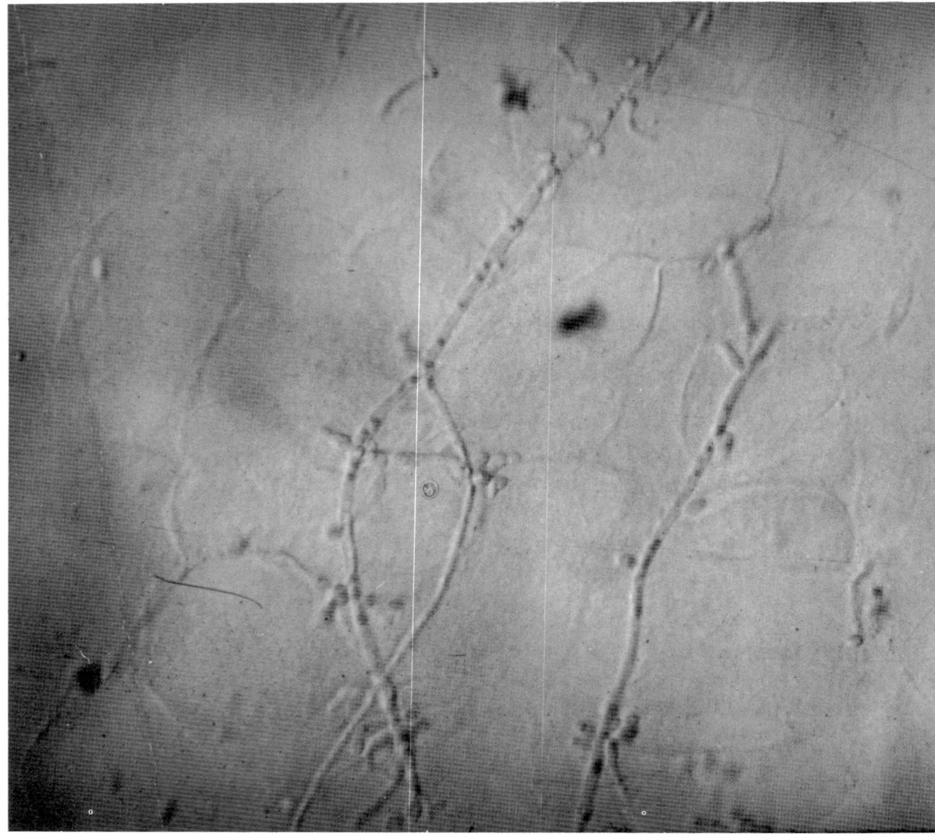

Figure 52.9 Branching hyphae of *Candida albicans* in vaginal discharge suspended in 10% potassium hydroxide. Ghosts of vaginal epithelial cells are also visible (100× magnification).

negative results (approximately 50%). Gram-stained smears of discharge are somewhat more sensitive, since hyphae and yeast cells are gram-positive and more easily visible. Culture can only corroborate or fail to corroborate the clinical impression of candidal vaginitis, since the vaginal flora includes *C. albicans* in about 25% of young women who have no symptoms or signs of infection. Similarly, the culture of patients with classic signs of candidal infection may yield only a light growth of the organism, making heavy growth an inadequate criterion for diagnosis. From these considerations, it is apparent that although the presence of *C. albicans* should be confirmed by laboratory tests, the initial diagnosis and subsequent treatment of this vaginal infection should be guided by the presence or absence of clinical disease.

MANAGEMENT

Topical antifungal agents will cure the majority of patients with candidal infections promptly. The creams are packaged commercially with intravaginal applicators, but some premenarchial and virginal girls can be treated more comfortably by applying cream to the vulva alone. Miconazole cream (one application at bedtime for 7 nights) is effective and allows a short, single course of treatment. Clotrimazole is administered once daily for 7 to 14 days or twice daily for 3 days, and is available in tablets as well as a cream.

Shigella Species

CLINICAL MANIFESTATIONS

Shigella flexneri, *S. sonnei*, and *S. boydii* can produce vaginal infections in infants and children, but do not appear to cause genital disease after puberty. The vaginitis is characterized by a white to yellow discharge that is bloody in half the cases. Associated pruritus and dysuria are not common. One fourth of patients have diarrhea that precedes, accompanies, or follows the vaginal discharge. On inspection, the vulvar mucosa is often inflamed or ulcerated. The diagnosis can be determined by culture of a specimen of vaginal discharge. Rectal cultures are positive in some cases.

MANAGEMENT

Patients with *Shigella* vaginitis should be treated with oral antibiotics chosen on the basis of sensitivity testing. Approximately half of *Shigella* isolates are susceptible to ampicillin (50 mg/kg/day p.o. in 4 doses for 10 days). For patients infected with resistant strains, and patients allergic to penicillin, trimethoprim-sulfamethoxazole (8 mg/kg/day p.o. of trimethoprim in 2 doses for 5 days) should be used.

Streptococcus pyogenes

CLINICAL MANIFESTATIONS

S. pyogenes can be identified in cultures of vaginal specimens taken from about 14% of prepubertal girls with scarlet fever. Most of these vaginal infections produce either no symptoms or minor discomfort, but a few patients develop outright vaginitis with a purulent discharge. Streptococcal vaginitis also occurs uncommonly in girls with neither symptomatic pharyngitis nor scarlet fever. Most of these patients are pharyngeal carriers of streptococci. Streptococcal vaginitis causes genital pain or pruritus, and can mimic candidal or gonococcal vaginitis. A swab of the patient's discharge should be sent for culture to verify the clinical diagnosis, as well as to exclude gonococcal infection.

MANAGEMENT

As for any other infection with Group A β-hemolytic streptococci (*S. pyogenes*), penicillin is the antibiotic of choice. For oral treatment, 25 to 50 mg/kg/day of penicillin V should be prescribed in 4 divided doses for 10 days. If intramuscular administration is preferred, benzathine penicillin is used in a single dose of 50,000 units/kg. Oral erythromycin (40 mg/kg/day in 4 divided doses for 10 days) can be given to children who are allergic to penicillin.

Chlamydia trachomatis

CLINICAL MANIFESTATIONS

Lower genital tract infection with the intracellular parasite *C. trachomatis* is uncommon during childhood, since the organism is acquired by sexual contact. However, approximately 20% of sexually active adult women have been found to have genital chlamydial infections, and a similar prevalence of infection (27%) was observed in a recent study of 31 prepubertal children with anogenital gonorrhea. In women after puberty, genital *C. trachomatis* produces cervicitis that may be either asymptomatic or associated with an increased cervical (not vaginal) discharge. Most of the children with urethral, vaginal, and rectal infections have also been asymptomatic, but there have been reports of prepubertal girls with purulent chlamydial vaginitis. The diagnosis should therefore be suspected in prepubertal girls with vaginal discharge that persists after penicillin or spectinomycin therapy for a prior gonococcal infection, and girls with vaginitis who are known to have had sexual contact. Culture of a sample of vaginal secretions is necessary to confirm the diagnosis; Giemsa-stained smears are not helpful.

MANAGEMENT

Children under 8 years of age with symptomatic chlamydial infections should be treated with either erythromycin (40 mg/kg/day p.o. in 4 divided doses for 10 days) or sulfisoxasole (120 mg/kg/day p.o. in 4 divided doses for 10 days). Tetracycline (40 mg/kg/day p.o. in 4 divided doses for 10 days) is also effective, but should be reserved for children over 8 years of age to avoid possible discoloration of the teeth. Asymptomatic children with genital chlamydial infections are not likely to be identified, but if they are, one of the above treatment regimens should be used, since spontaneous eradication of the organism is not frequent.

Nonspecific Vaginitis

CLINICAL MANIFESTATIONS

The term nonspecific vaginitis, when used to refer to a disorder of prepubertal girls, encompasses a variety of genitourinary symptoms and signs that are sometimes caused by poor perineal hygiene, but that in other cases have no readily identifiable etiology. Genital discomfort, discharge, itchiness, and dysuria are relatively common childhood complaints. When a girl with such symptoms has either a normal vulva and vagina or only mild vulvar inflammation on physical examination, a specific vaginal infection is unlikely, and other possible explanations for the complaint—smegma, pinworms, urinary tract infection, a local chemical irritant, or sexual abuse, for example—should be sought with appropriate questions and laboratory tests. (It should be noted that it is uncommon for commercially available bubblebath to be the culprit.) If, on the other hand, a vaginal discharge *is* present on physical examination, the specific vaginal infections discussed above are diagnostic possibilities, and cultures should therefore be obtained. In reported series of premenarchial girls with vaginitis who have been systematically evaluated, between 25 and 75% are ultimately categorized as having nonspecific vaginitis. The diagnosis should not be made until other entities have been excluded. (A more comprehensive discussion of the differential diagnosis of genital complaints is presented in Chapters 38 and 39.)

Nonspecific vaginitis after menarche is a syndrome that has been attributed to infection with a small microaerophilic, gram-negative coccobacillus currently designated *Gardnerella vaginalis* (previously referred to as either *Haemophilus vaginalis* or *Corynebacterium vaginale*). Evidence for the pathogenicity of *G. vaginalis* in this disorder, first proposed by Gardner and Dukes in 1955, is inconclusive. Some researchers have identified the organism in the vaginal flora of 10 to 30% of virginal young women, sexually active young women with neither symptoms nor signs of vaginitis, and women with nontrichomonal vaginitis. Other investigators have found that cultures of vaginal secretions taken from most women with nonspecific vaginitis have been positive for *G. vaginalis*, whereas those taken from most healthy women selected as controls have been negative. When culture-positive and culture-negative women have been compared, a correlation between the presence of *G. vaginalis* and that of an abnormal vaginal discharge has not always been observed. Whether *G. vaginalis*, like *C. albicans*, is a commensal organism that only produces clinical disease under certain circumstances, or whether it is a pathogen at all, are questions that are not yet entirely satisfactorily answered.

The clinical features of nonspecific vaginitis in postmenarchial women are not distinctive and resemble in part those of trichomonal infection. Patients complain of excessive vaginal discharge or an unpleasant odor, but generally do not have symptoms of mucosal irritation such as burning, itching, or dysuria. The discharge itself is moderate or copious, thin or pasty, and homogeneous. The frothiness of some discharges and a frequent "fishy" or unpleasant odor are characteristics of both trichomonal and nonspecific vaginitis. The vulva, vaginal mucosa, and cervix are not inflamed.

When examined microscopically, a sample of the vaginal discharge suspended in saline may be seen to contain many "clue cells" (epithelial cells with cytoplasm that looks granular because many bacteria are attached to the surface), but only a few polymorphonuclear leukocytes. A gram-stained smear of discharge confirms that the clue cells are studded with gram-negative coccobacilli. Some researchers consider the finding of clue cells pathognomonic of *G. vaginalis* infection; others have observed substantial rates of both falsely positive and falsely negative tests. As in the case of vaginal candidiasis, a positive culture for *G. vaginalis* is not by itself diagnostic, but should rather be used to confirm the presence of the organism in patients with clinical disease. Trichomonal infection is the major diagnostic alternative for patients suspected of having nonspecific vaginitis.

MANAGEMENT

General measures to promote cleanliness and comfort are in order for the premenarchial girl with nonspecific vaginitis. Daily soaking in a bathtub of warm water, either plain or with some baking soda added, gentle perineal cleaning with a soft washcloth, and the use of cotton underwear can be recommended. If she has not been doing so, the girl should be taught to wipe toilet paper anteroposteriorly after having a bowel movement. Using these suggestions, most girls with perineal irritation will be improved within 2 weeks. The remaining patients should be reevaluated to exclude any specific but previously unrecognized disorder. If none is found, these girls may benefit from a brief course of topical estrogen cream (a small amount dabbed onto the vulva nightly for 2 to 4 weeks) to stimulate thickening of the vaginal mucosa so that it is more resistant to local irritation. Parents should be cautioned that estrogen cream is capable of producing breast growth if it is used for a prolonged period of time.

Of the various treatments that have been advocated for nonspecific vaginitis after puberty, only metronidazole (500 mg p.o. twice daily for 7 days) has been consistently effective. Despite initial claims of efficacy for oral tetracycline and intravaginal sulfonamide, neither antibiotic has been successful in subsequent therapeutic trials. *G. vaginalis* is sensitive to erythomycin and ampicillin in vitro, but these drugs fail to produce clinical and bacteriological cures, perhaps because of variable local antibiotic levels or because the vaginal pH is relatively acid. Common side-effects of metronidazole include gastrointestinal upset, headache, and a metallic taste. Metronidazole is contraindicated during pregnancy.

ACUTE SALPINGITIS

BACKGROUND

Definition

Salpingitis is an infection of the fallopian tubes. The discussion below is limited to acute salpingitis caused by sexually transmitted microorganisms ascending from the lower genital tract, and excludes infections that follow childbirth or surgery. The term pelvic inflammatory disease (PID) is often used instead of salpingitis, perhaps to reflect the user's acknowledgment that the clinical diagnosis of salpingitis cannot always be made with certainty. In this section, the terms PID and acute salpingitis will be used interchangeably.

Diagnostic criteria for chronic salpingitis are not standardized, and vary from prolonged or relapsing clinical illness to evidence of long-standing pelvic inflammation (tubal scarring, adhesions) seen at laparoscopy or laparotomy regardless of whether symptoms or signs had been present earlier. For purposes of clinical evaluation, an episode of salpingitis that persists beyond 3 weeks despite antibiotic treatment can properly be considered chronic. If possible, this should be distinguished from repeated episodes of acute infection that are separated by intervals of good health.

Epidemiology

Between 1977 and 1980 there were 400,000 cases of gonorrhea among American women reported annually to the Centers for Disease Control. It is estimated that an additional 300,000 to 500,000 cases each year went unreported. Approximately 10 to 15% of women with cervical gonorrhea will develop salpingitis. The risks of acquiring gonorrhea and salpingitis are not distributed evenly among women, but vary in part according to the hosts' age, race, and contraceptive methods. Age-specific rates of uncomplicated (lower genital tract) gonorrhea are highest for young women between the ages of 20 and 24 years, followed by teenagers between 15 and 19 years. Teenagers between 15 and 19 years are also admitted to the hospital for salpingitis at a rate surpassed only by women 20 to 24 years old. Among nonpregnant adolescents 15 to 19 years old, 3% of all hospital admissions between 1970 and 1975 were for salpingitis or PID.

In every age category, black women have higher rates than do whites of both gonorrhea and hospitalization for salpingitis. Although socioeconomic factors probably account for part of this difference, it also appears that blacks are more likely than whites to be infected with gonococcal strains that are both relatively resistant to antibiotics and more likely to produce salpingitis.

Methods of contraception influence rates of both gonococcal and nongonococcal salpingitis. The risk of PID is 3 to 9 times higher among women who use intrauterine devices (IUD's) than among non-IUD users. This increased risk is concentrated among IUD users who have never been pregnant and those with nongonococcal infections. Compared to no contraceptive method, barrier methods decrease the overall risk of acquiring sexually transmitted genital infections, and oral contraceptives appear to decrease the likelihood that users with cervical gonorrhea will develop ascending infection.

Salpingitis is rarely fatal (0.4% of hospitalized cases), but it does produce significant long-term morbidity. Among previously healthy women, approximately 0.7% of pregnancies are located ectopically; for women with prior salpingitis, this risk is increased nearly sixfold to about 4%. It has been estimated that half of all ectopic pregnancies are the result of tubal damage produced by salpingitis. Similarly, infertility because of tubal occlusion is rare among healthy women, but occurs in 5% and 16% of women who have had, respectively, a single episode of gonococcal or nongonococcal salpingitis. Repeated bouts of PID increase the risk of infertility substantially.

Etiology

Despite meticulous investigations of the microbiology of the cervix, the fallopian tubes, and the pelvic cul-de-sac during health and disease, the etiology of many cases of pelvic inflammatory disease remains uncertain. About one half of patients in the United States with acute salpingitis have coexisting gonococcal cervicitis (Table 52.1). It is customary to attribute the tubal infection in such cases to gonorrhea, but the finding that *N. gonorrhoeae* can be isolated from cultures of fallopian tube or cul-de-sac samples in only about one quarter of these patients has led some investigators to doubt the etiological importance of this organism. On the other hand, the likelihood that fastidious gonococci lose viability in pus may account in part for their low isolation rate from specimens of purulent peritoneal fluid. Studies demonstrating that cul-de-sac aspirates from 50% of patients with acute salpingitis contain enteric bacteria, predominately anaerobes, lend credence to the hypothesis that gonococcal infection of the fallopian tubes is transient, but paves the way for subsequent invasion by endogenous organisms. However, most of these studies are subject to the criticism that specimens obtained during culdocentesis are more likely than those obtained at laparoscopy to be contaminated with bacteria from the vagina or the gastrointestinal tract. Whether anaerobic bacteria play a principal or a supporting role in the pathogenesis of salpingitis is not well established. Considering the information now available, it seems reasonable to conclude that *N. gonorrhoeae* is the primary pathogen in cases of acute salpingitis accompanied by gonococcal infection of the lower genital tract, but that secondary invasion by both aerobic and anaerobic bacteria is likely to complicate long-standing or recurrent episodes.

C. trachomatis has been isolated in pure growth from the fallopian tubes of a minority of patients with acute salpingitis. The development of salpingitis in grivet monkeys whose cervices were inoculated with *C. trachomatis* confirms the pathogenicity of this obligate intracellular parasite. However, a positive cervical culture alone is insufficient evidence for the diagnosis of chlamydial salpingitis, since patients with nongonococcal salpingitis are no more likely than those with gonococcal salpingitis or no salpingitis to have cervical infections with *C. trachomatis*. In addition, concurrent cervical infections with *C. trachomatis* and *N. gonorrhoeae* are not infrequent. Finally, the observation that specimens of peritoneal fluid obtained by culdoscopy are less likely than tubal samples to contain chlamydiae has hampered physicians' ability to diagnose chlamydial salpingitis with certainty except in patients undergoing laparoscopy. As a result, the question of the relative importance of *C. trachomatis* as a cause of acute salpingitis remains unanswered.

Table 52.1
Cervical gonorrhea and peritoneal isolates among women with acute salpingitis, diagnosed and cultured by either laparoscopy (L), or clinical examination and culdocentesis (C).

Study	Method	No. of Patients Studied	Cervical Gonorrhea (%)	Peritoneal Isolates			
				Neisseria gonorrhoeae[a]	Other bacteria[b]	*Chlamydia trachomatis*	Mycoplasmas[c]
Cunningham (1977)	C	76	45 (59)	22	32	–	–
Eschenbach (1975)	C	54	21 (39)	7	27	1	3
Mårdh (1970)	L	50	17 (34)	2	3	–	6
Mårdh (1977)	L	20	2 (10)	1	–	6	–
Sweet (1979)	L,C	26	13 (50)	8	12	0	5

[a] With or without other bacteria. All patients had concomitant cervical gonorrhea.
[b] Excluding patients with intraperitoneal *N. gonorrhoeae*.
[c] With or without bacteria (not *N. gonorrhoeae*).

Because they have been cultured from peritoneal fluid specimens of a few women with PID, *Mycoplasma hominis* and *Ureaplasma urealyticum* (T-mycoplasma) have also been incriminated as genital tract pathogens. In animal models, *M. hominis* appears to produce parametritis and salpingitis, but *U. urealyticum* has not caused disease. Like other sexually transmitted organisms, mycoplasmas colonize the cervices of a large proportion of women attending venereal disease clinics, women with lower genital tract infections, and women with salpingitis. However, their role in the etiology of upper genital tract infection is not yet firmly established.

The relative frequency of salpingitis caused by the various sexually transmitted agents in a given population depends not only on the virulence of the particular organisms and on variations in host susceptibility, but also on the prevalence of lower genital tract infection with each organism. Thus, although *C. trachomatis* and *M. hominis* appear to cause the majority of tubal infections among hospitalized women in Scandinavia where the prevalence of gonorrhea is low, the converse is true of emergency department patients with salpingitis in the United States, where *N. gonorrhoeae* seems to be the primary pathogen in a majority of cases.

PATHOPHYSIOLOGY

Gonococci reach the fallopian tubes by ascending from the cervix along the endometrial surface of the uterus. In the tubal lumen, gonococci release a lipopolysaccharide endotoxin that damages the ciliated epithelial cells, causing them to slough. The bacteria attach themselves to mucosal secretory cells and invade the submucosal connective tissue, stimulating a marked inflammatory reaction. Pus may be spilled out the fimbriated ends of the tubes, producing generalized abdominal symptoms and signs. As the endosalpingitis heals, intraluminal adhesions are formed.

CLINICAL FEATURES

The patient with classic acute salpingitis is an adolescent or young woman with lower abdominal pain and fever that began just after a menstrual period and have persisted for several days. She reports an increased vaginal discharge, and her examination is notable for fever and marked bilateral pelvic tenderness. Her laboratory findings include a modest leukocytosis, an elevated erythrocyte sedimentation rate (ESR), and a positive cervical culture for *N. gonorrhaeae*. However, when the diagnosis of salpingitis is reserved for patients with tubal inflammation that has been confirmed visually at laparoscopy or laparotomy, it is evident that the clinical features of the disease are variable and nonspecific. Among patients with suspected salpingitis who undergo laparoscopy, the diagnosis is verified in only about 65%. Ten percent are found to have other diseases, and 25% have no identifiable pathology. The diseases most often mistaken for salpingitis are acute appendicitis, endometriosis, corpus luteum hemorrhage, and ectopic pregnancy.

Table 52.2 lists the frequency of symptoms, signs, and laboratory findings in patients with visually confirmed salpingitis. Patients with gonococcal salpingitis are more likely than others to have fever, an onset of pain during the first 2 weeks of a menstrual cycle, and a moderate elevation of ESR (16 to 30 mm/hour). Milder, more chronic pain, an ESR above 30 mm/hour, and disproportionately severe tubal inflammation appear to characterize chlamydial salpingitis. Perihepatitis (Fitz-Hugh-Curtis syndrome) consists of right upper quadrant pain and tenderness produced by inflammation of the liver capsule in association with PID. Liver enzyme determinations are usually normal, but an oral cholecystogram may show nonvisualization. Perihepatitis is classically associated with gonococcal infection, but has also been described recently in patients with nongonococcal salpingitis.

No single laboratory test or battery of tests can exclude or pinpoint the diagnosis of acute salpingitis. As indicated in Table 52.2, the majority of patients have a normal white blood cell count and an elevated ESR, but these tests are neither sensitive nor specific. A Gram-stained smear of purulent cervical secretions (obtained after the cervix has been swabbed to remove vaginal secretions) is considered positive for *N. gonorrhoeae* if at least 8 pairs of gram-negative, kidney-bean-shaped diplococci can be seen in each of at least 2 polymorphonuclear leukocytes. Using this criterion, positive cervical smears are specific for the diagnosis of gonorrhea, but the false-negative rate is over 35%.

Table 52.2
Symptoms, signs, and laboratory findings among patients with salpingitis confirmed by visualization.

Finding	Percentage of Patients
Symptoms	
Lower abdominal pain	95
Vaginal discharge	55
Irregular menstrual bleeding	35
Urinary tract symptoms	20
Vomiting	10
Signs	
Fever (>38°C)	33
Marked adnexal tenderness	90
Perihepatitis	10
Laboratory	
WBC ≥12,000	20
ESR 16–30 mm/hr	40
ESR >30 mm/hr	40

The one complication of salpingitis that warrants prompt diagnosis is ruptured tubo-ovarian abscess. About 15% of tubo-ovarian abscesses rupture spontaneously, but abscess formation itself is an uncommon complication of salpingitis, occurring in fewer than 3% of patients. The symptoms and signs of a ruptured abscess may be mild if only a small amount of pus has leaked out, but the usual clinical picture is one of peritonitis and shock. A pelvic mass is palpable in fewer than half the cases. Prompt surgical intervention is lifesaving.

MANAGEMENT

Every patient suspected of having salpingitis should receive a cervical culture for *N. gonorrhoeae* to guide her subsequent therapy and the follow-up of sexual contacts. Additional specimens for culture may be taken from the urethra, the rectum, and the pharynx. About 15% of women with gonorrhea will only have a positive culture from one of these latter sites. Recommendations may change, but at present the high cost and the uncertain significance of a positive result make routine cervical culturing for *C. trachomatis* unfeasible.

The current Centers for Disease Control recommendations (1979) for the treatment of acute salpingitis are listed in Table 52.3. The recognition that chlamydia can cause salpingitis has led to the reclassification of tetracycline from a second-choice antibiotic to one among several equally acceptable options for treatment. However, tetracycline has not been found superior to the penicillin-ampicillin regimen, even for the treatment of nongonococcal infections. Pregnant women should not receive tetracycline. Although an improved response to antibiotic therapy has not been docu-

Table 52.3
Treatment schedules for acute salpingitis (Centers for Disease Control, 1979)

Outpatients	Inpatients
(1) Tetracycline 500 mg p.o. 4 times daily for 10 days	(1) Aqueous penicillin G 20 million units i.v. daily until improvement, followed by either ampicillin or amoxicillin 500 mg p.o. 4 times daily to complete 10 days of treatment
OR	OR
(2) Probenecid 1 g p.o. with a single dose of either (a) Aqueous procaine penicillin 4.8 million units i.m., or (b) Ampicillin 3.5 g p.o., or (c) Amoxicillin 3 g p.o. Followed by either ampicillin or amoxicillin 500 mg p.o. 4 times daily for 10 days	(2) Tetracycline 250 mg i.v. 4 times daily until improvement, followed by 500 mg p.o. 4 times daily to complete 10 days of treatment

mented, it is common practice to remove an IUD if the wearer develops acute salpingitis. An alternative method of contraception should then be provided.

Hospitalization is indicated for any patient with salpingitis whose diagnosis is uncertain, particularly if ectopic pregnancy is a possibility, and for patients with severe clinical illness, including those with fever above 38.5°C, signs of peritonitis, and suspected pelvic abscess. Patients likely to fail a course of oral antibiotics, because of either poor compliance or vomiting, and those whose illnesses have not responded to prior oral antibiotics, are also candidates for inpatient treatment. Finally, hospitalization is recommended for pregnant patients with salpingitis.

The follow-up of outpatients should include a return visit after about 3 days of treatment. The average duration of symptoms among women with gonococcal salpingitis treated with oral antibiotics is 3.4 days; the corresponding interval for nongonococcal salpingitis is 4.6 days. A poor response to therapy should alert the physician to the possibilities of inadequate compliance, abscess formation, or an alternative diagnosis. A reexamination at the end of antibiotic therapy is scheduled to check the patient for residual pelvic tenderness or adnexal masses. If gonococci were isolated initially, a "test of cure" culture is obtained, and the patient is asked whether her sexual partner(s) has been treated. The importance of prompt notification and treatment of sexual contacts of women with gonorrhea deserves particular emphasis. Such men are frequently asymptomatic, and therefore unlikely to seek treatment if contact tracing fails.

References

General

Cowell CA, ed.: Pediatric and adolescent gynecology. *Pediatr Clin North Am* 28: 1981.

Dewhurst J: Practical pediatric and adolescent gynecology. In *Reproductive Medicine* Vol. 1, Marcel Dekker, New York, 1980.

Emans SJA, Goldstein DP: *Pediatric and Adolescent Gynecology*. Little, Brown, Boston, 1977.

Hatcher RA, Stewart GK, Stewart F, et al.: *Contraceptive Technology 1980–81*, Ed 10. Irvington Publishers, New York, 1980.

Huffman JW, Dewhurst CJ, Capraro VJ: *The Gynecology of Childhood and Adolescence*, Ed 2. WB Saunders, Philadelphia, 1981.

Hydrocolpos

Dewhurst J: Malformations of the genital tract. In *Practical Pediatric and Adolescent Gynecology*, p. 51. Marcel Dekker, New York, 1980.

Wenof M, et al.: Transverse vaginal septum. *Obstet Gynecol* 54: 60, 1979.

Reed MH, Griscom NT: Hydrometrocolpos in infancy. *Am J Roentgen, Rad Therapy Nuclear Med* 118: 1, 1973.

Kahn R, et al.: Spontaneous opening of congenital imperforate hymen. *J Pediatr* 87: 768, 1975.

Labial Adhesions

Capraro VJ, Greenberg H: Adhesions of the labia minora: A study of 50 patients. *Obstet Gynecol* 39: 65, 1972.

Aribarg A: Topical oestrogen therapy for labial adhesions in children. *Brit J Obstet Gynecol* 82: 424, 1975.

Urethral Prolapse

Esposito JM: Circular prolapse of the urethra in children: A cause of vaginal bleeding. *Obstet Gynecol* 31: 363, 1968.

Klaus H, Stein RT: Urethral prolapse in young girls. *Pediatrics* 52: 645, 1973.

Owens SB, Morse WH: Prolapse of the female urethra in children. *J Urol* 100: 171, 1968.

Genital Warts

De Jong AR, Weiss JC, Brent RL: Condyloma acuminata in children. *Am J Dis Child* 136: 704, 1982.

Moher LM, Maurer SA: Podophyllum toxicity: Case report and literature review. *J Fam Pract* 9: 237, 1979.

Oriel JD: Natural history of genital warts. *Br J Vener Dis* 47: 1, 1971.

Powell LC: Condyloma acuminatum: Recent advances in development, carcinogenesis, and treatment. *Clin Obstet Gynecol* 21: 1061, 1978.

Dysmenorrhea

Chan WY, Dawood MY, Fuchs F: Prostaglandins in primary dysmenorrhea. *Am J Med* 70: 535, 1981.

Goldstein DP, deCholnoky C, Emans SJ: Laparoscopy in the diagnosis and management of pelvic pain in adolescents. *J Reprod Med* 24: 251, 1980.

Klein JR, Litt IF: Epidemiology of adolescent dysmenorrhea. *Pediatrics* 68: 661, 1981.

Lennane KJ: Social and medical attitudes toward dysmenorrhea. *J Reprod Med* 25(Suppl): 202, 1980.

Ylikorkala O, Dawood MY: New concepts in dysmenorrhea. *Am J Obstet Gynecol* 130: 833, 1978.

Dysfunctional Uterine Bleeding

Aksel S, Jones GS: Etiology and treatment of dysfunctional uterine bleeding. *Obstet Gynecol* 44: 1, 1974.

Altchek A: Dysfunctional uterine bleeding in adolescence. *Clin Obstet Gynecol* 20: 633, 1977.

Speroff L, Glass RH, Kase NG: Dysfunctional uterine bleeding. In *Clinical Gynecologic Endocrinology and Infertility*, ed 2, p 151, Williams & Wilkins, Baltimore, 1978.

VanLook PFA, Hunter WM, Fraser IS, et al.: Impaired estrogen-induced luteinizing hormone release in young women with anovulatory dysfunctional uterine bleeding. *J Clin Endocrinol Metab* 46: 816, 1978.

Vaginitis

Al-Salihi FL, Curran JP, Wang JS: Neonatal *Trichomonas vaginalis*: Report of three cases and review of the literature. *Pediatrics* 53: 196, 1974.

Boisvert PL, Walcher DN: Hemolytic streptococcal vaginitis in children. *Pediatrics* 2: 24, 1948.

Dunkelberg WE, Hefner JD, Patow WE, et al.: *Haemophilus vaginalis* among asymptomatic women. *Obstet Gynecol* 20: 629, 1962.

Farrell MK, Billmire E, Shamroy JA: Prepubertal gonorrhea: A multidisciplinary approach. *Pediatrics* 67: 151, 1981.

Fouts AC, Kraus SJ: *Trichomonas vaginalis:* Reevaluation of its clinical presentation and laboratory diagnosis. *J Infect Dis* 141: 137, 1980.

Center for Disease Control: Gonorrhea: CDC-recommended treatment schedules, 1979. *J Infect Dis* 139: 496, 1979.

Gallagher E: Genital infection in young delinquent girls. *Br J Vener Dis* 46: 129, 1970.

Gardner HL, Dukes CD: *Haemophilus vaginalis* vaginitis: A newly defined specific infection previously classified "nonspecific vaginitis." *Am J Obst Gynecol* 69: 962, 1955.

Heller RH, Joseph JM, Davis HJ: Vulvovaginitis in the premenarcheal child. *J Pediatr* 74: 370, 1969.

Huffman JW: Premenarchial vulvovaginitis. *Clin Obstet Gynecol* 20:581, 1977.

Komaroff AL, Pass TM, Mc Cue JD et al.: Management strategies for urinary and vaginal infections. *Arch Intern Med* 138: 1069, 1978.

McCormack WM, Hayes CH, Rosner B, et al.: Vaginal colonization with *Corynebacterium vaginale (Haemophilus vaginalis)*. *J Infect Dis* 136: 740, 1977.

McCormack WM, Stumacher RJ, Johnson K, et al.: Clinical spectrum of gonococcal infection in women. *Lancet* 1: 1182, 1977.

Milne JD, Warnock DW: Effect of simultaneous oral and vaginal treatment on the rate of cure and relapse in vaginal candidosis. *Br J Vener Dis* 55: 362, 1979.

Murphy TV, Nelson JD: *Shigella* vaginitis: Report of 38 patients and review of the literature. *Pediatrics* 63: 511, 1979.

Oriel JD, Partridge BM, Denny MJ et al.: Genital yeast infections. *Br Med J* 4: 761, 1972.

Paradise JE, Campos JM, Friedman HM et al.: Vulvovaginitis in premenarchial girls: Clinical features and diagnostic evaluation. *Pediatrics* 70: 193, 1982.

Pheifer TA, Forsyth PS, Durfee MA et al.: Nonspecific vaginitis: Role of *Haemophilus vaginalis* and treatment with metronidazole. *N Engl J Med* 298: 1429, 1978.

Rettig PJ, Nelson JD: Genital tract infection with *Chlamydia trachomatis* in prepubertal children. *J Pediatr* 99: 206, 1981.

Rothenberg RB, Simon R, Chipperfield E et al.: Efficacy of selected diagnostic tests for sexually transmitted diseases. *JAMA* 235: 49, 1976.

Sgroi SM: Pediatric gonorrhea beyond infancy. *Pediatr Ann* 8: 326, 1979.

Spiegel CA, Amsel R, Eschenbach D et al.: Anaerobic bacteria in nonspecific vaginitis. *N Engl J Med* 303: 601, 1980.

Acute Salpingitis

Cunningham FG, Hauth JC, Strong JD, et al.: Evaluation of tetracycline or penicillin and ampicillin for treatment of acute pelvic inflammatory disease. *N Engl J Med* 296: 1380, 1977.

Eschenbach DA, Buchanan TM, Pollock HM, et al.: Polymicrobial etiology of acute pelvic inflammatory disease. *N Engl J Med* 293: 166, 1975.

From the Center for Disease Control. Gonorrhea: CDC-recommended treatment schedules, 1979. *J Infect Dis* 139: 496, 1979.

Hein K, Kleinhaus S, Mayers M, et al.: Laparoscopy for presumed nonacute salpingitis: A new look at an old problem. *J Adolesc Health Care* 1: 96, 1980.

Holmes KK, Eschenbach DA, Knapp JS: Salpingitis: Overview of etiology and epidemiology. *Am J Obstet Gynecol* 138: 893, 1980.

Jacobson L, Weström L: Objectivized diagnosis of acute pelvic inflammatory disease. *Am J Obstet Gynecol* 105: 1088, 1969.

Jones OG, Zaidi AA, St. John RK: Frequency and distribution of salpingitis and pelvic inflammatory disease in short-stay hospitals in the United States. *Am J Obstet Gynecol* 138: 905, 1980.

Mårdh P, Weström L: Tubal and cervical cultures in acute salpingitis with special reference to *Mycoplasma hominis* and T-strain mycoplasmas. *Br J Vener Dis* 46: 179, 1970

Mårdh P, Ripa T, Svensson L, et al.: *Chlamydia trachomatis* infection in patients with acute salpingitis. *N Engl J Med* 296: 1377, 1977.

Sweet RL, Mills J, Hadley KW, et al.: Use of laparoscopy to determine the microbiologic etiology of acute salpingitis. *Am J Obstet Gynecol* 134: 68, 1979.

CHAPTER **53**

Endocrine Emergencies

KENNETH R. LYEN, M.R.C.P., DANIEL HALE, M.D., AND LESTER BAKER, M.D.

INTRODUCTION

Endocrine and metabolic emergencies are relatively common in childhood. The diagnosis is often delayed or missed because the symptoms at presentation are usually nonspecific. Consideration of the condition is frequently sufficient to secure the diagnosis. Prompt treatment is critical toward achieving a favorable outcome.

Table 53.1 summarizes the major clinical features, urgent investigations recommended, and treatment of pediatric endocrine emergencies.

DIABETIC KETOACIDOSIS

BACKGROUND

Ketoacidosis is a life-threatening complication of diabetes. The biochemical disturbances include hyperglycemia, elevated blood ketone bodies, ketonuria, and metabolic acidosis. It may be present in up to 30% of newly diagnosed juvenile-onset diabetics and still accounts for about 65% of all admissions of diabetics under 19 years of age. The mortality is small but significant, most reports quoting a mortality rate of under 3% of children presenting with ketoacidosis; ideally, it should be zero.

In established diabetics, diabetic ketoacidosis may be precipitated by acute infection and inadequate insulin. Recurrent episodes are infrequent. In the teenage child emotional factors may play an important etiologic role. Nonketotic hyperosmolar coma rarely occurs in children.

PATHOPHYSIOLOGY (Fig. 53.1)

Insulin deficiency, possibly assisted by elevated counterregulatory hormones such as glucagon, catecholamines, corticosteroids, and growth hormone, leads to both reduced peripheral glucose utilization and increased hepatic gluconeogenesis, which together result in hyperglycemia. This, in turn, leads to osmotic diuresis and dehydration. Insulin deficiency also causes increased release of free fatty acids from adipose tissue, and the free fatty acids are converted into ketoacids in the liver. These are strong acids which readily dissociate in the blood to produce free hydrogen ions. The result is a metabolic acidosis, for which the body tries to compensate by hyperventilation, hence lowering the PCO_2 and plasma bicarbonate ($HCO3^-$).

Intracellular potassium is depleted because of transcellular shifts of this ion brought about by the acidosis and extracellular dehydration. Protein catabolism secondary to anorexia causes negative nitrogen balance and additional efflux of potassium from cells. The potassium is then excreted in the urine during the osmotic diuresis. Volume depletion causes secondary hyperaldosteronism, which further promotes urinary potassium excretion. Thus there is total body depletion of potassium, although

Table 53.1
Summary of Clinical Features, Investigations, and Initial Treatment of Pediatric Endocrine Emergencies

Condition	Major Clinical Features	Urgent Investigations	Initial Treatment
Diabetic ketoacidosis	Polyuria, polydipsia, dehydration, ketotic breath, hyperpnea, nausea, vomiting, abdominal pain, coma	Blood sugar, potassium, pH, urinalysis	0.9% saline 20 ml/kg in first hour i.v., insulin infusion 0.1 unit/kg/hr, later, may need KCl 40–60 meq/L
Hypoglycemia	*Older child:* hunger, sweatiness, dizziness, convulsions, coma. *Neonate:* apnea, hypotonia, hypothermia, irritability, tremor, convulsions	Blood sugar	25% dextrose 1–2 ml/kg i.v. bolus, or 10% dextrose 5–10 ml/kg/min i.v. infusion, glucagon 0.5–1 mg i.m. stat (if hyperinsulinism)
Congenital adrenal hyperplasia	Ambiguous genitalia in females; poor feeding, weight loss, irritability, vomiting, dehydration	Plasma sodium, potassium, sugar, 17-hydroxyprogesterone; consider buccal smear and chromosomal karyotype	0.9% saline 20 ml/kg in first hour i.v., deoxycorticosterone acetate 0.5–1 mg i.m. stat, hydrocortisone 25 mg i.v. stat.
Addisonian crisis	Nausea, vomiting, abdominal pain, weakness, malaise, hypotension, dehydration, hyperpigmentation	Plasma sodium, potassium, sugar, cortisol (for retrospective confirmation of diagnosis)	Hydrocortisone 100 mg i.v. stat, 5% dextrose in 0.9% saline 20 ml/kg in first hour
Hypercalcemia	Headache, irritability, anorexia, constipation, polyuria, polydipsia, dehydration, band keratopathy	Plasma calcium, phosphate	5% dextrose at 2–3 times maintenance rate, furosemide 1 mg/kg stat
Hypocalcemia	Cramps, carpopedal spasms, paresthesias, lethargy, apathy, convulsions	Plasma calcium, phosphate, alkaline phosphatase	10% calcium gluconate 0.5 ml/kg (or 5 mg Ca/kg) i.v. over 15 min
Diabetes insipidus	Polyuria, polydipsia, dehydration, irritability, fever, drowsiness, coma	Paired plasma and urine osmolality and sodium	*Central:* 5% dextrose at 1½ times maintenance rate, 1-desamino-8-D-arginine vasopressin 4 μg/kg nasally *Nephrogenic:* 5% dextrose at 1½ times maintenance
Syndrome of inappropriate antidiuretic hormone secretion	Anorexia, headache, nausea, vomiting, irritability, seizures, coma	Paired plasma and urine osmolality and sodium	*Symptomatic:* 3% saline at 6–12 ml/kg ± furosemide 1 mg/kg i.v. stat *Asymptomatic:* Fluid restriction
Thyroid storm	Goiter, exophthalmos, high fever, tachycardia congestive cardiac failure, delirium, stupor	Serum T_4, TSH	Propranolol 30 μg/kg i.v. over 15 min, Lugol's iodine 15 drops/day orally, propylthiouracil 2–3 mg/kg t.i.d. orally, tepid sponging
Neonatal thyrotoxicosis	Goiter, failure to gain weight, irritability, tachycardia, congestive cardiac failure	Serum T_4, TSH	Propranolol 1 mg/kg t.i.d. orally, potassium iodide 2 drops/day orally, propylthiouracil 2–3 mg/kg t.i.d. orally
Congenital hypothyroidism	Asymptomatic; hypothermia, hypoactivity, poor feeding, constipation, prolonged jaundice, large posterior fontanel	Serum T_4, TSH	L-Thyroxine 37.5 mg/day orally

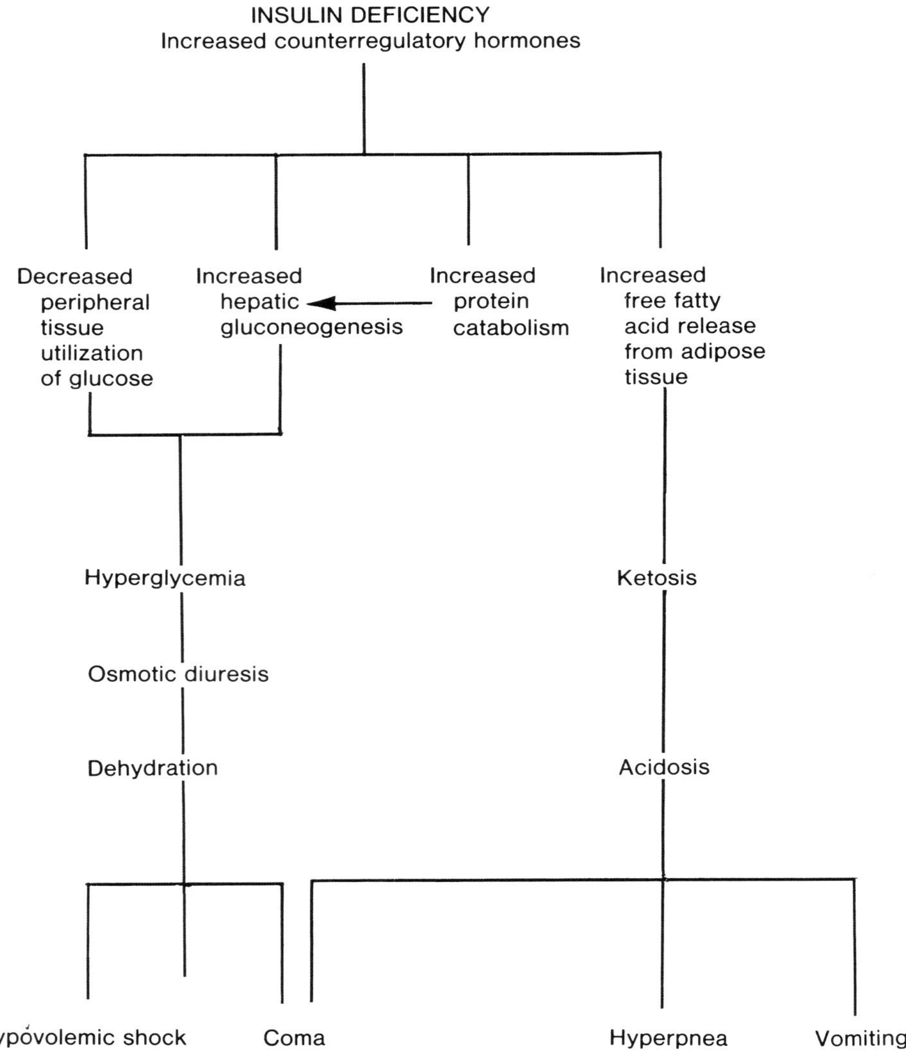

Figure 53.1 Pathophysiology of diabetic ketoacidosis.

the plasma potassium concentration may not reflect this loss at presentation.

CLINICAL MANIFESTATIONS

There is usually a history of polyuria and polydipsia for a few days or weeks prior to the development of overt ketoacidosis in new cases. In established diabetics, the prodrome is usually under 24 hours. Patients may complain of nausea, vomiting, and abdominal pain, and the parents may have noticed some listlessness, tiredness, and anorexia. Fewer than 10% of children are in coma at the time of admission to hospital. The initial diagnosis is usually made on the basis of the history and physical examination alone. However, presenting clinical features can easily be misdiagnosed. Abdominal tenderness may be misinterpreted as appendicitis; hyperpnea may be mistaken as a sign of pneumonia or asthma; and polyuria may be incorrectly diagnosed as a urinary infection. Enuresis, polydipsia or irritability are sometimes wrongly categorized as behavioral problems.

Physical examination should be quick

and efficient, so that urgent treatment can be commenced at the earliest opportunity. The initial focus should be on assessing the degree of dehydration by noting the dryness of the mouth and tongue, and sunken eyes. In severe cases there may be signs of shock, such as a thin thready pulse, cold extremities, and hypotension. More commonly the skin feels warm and dry. The smell of ketones on the breath and the presence of deep sighing (Kussmaul's) respirations reflect the ketoacidosis. The patient's consciousness level should be noted; this may range from full alertness to deep coma. There may be exquisite abdominal tenderness with guarding and rigidity, which may mimic an acute abdomen. Less common findings include an acutely enlarged and tender liver, hypothermia or hyperthermia. The ears, throat, chest and urine should be examined for signs of infection.

Laboratory findings include a serum glucose that is greater than 250 mg/dl and usually 400 to 800 mg/dl, the presence of glucose and ketones in the urine, acidosis (pH $\leq$ 7.3 and $HCO3^-$ $\leq$ 15 meq/L), high or normal plasma potassium, a slightly elevated blood urea nitrogen, and leukocytosis. The latter does not necessarily signify an underlying infection. A useful bedside test to rapidly determine the presence of ketoacidosis is to measure plasma ketones using a crushed Acetest tablet.

MANAGEMENT

The aims of treatment are to address the life-threatening issues. Untreated, diabetic ketoacidosis can kill immediately or within hours of admission, by causing cardiovascular collapse and profound acidosis. Urgent treatment is directed toward expansion of the intravascular volume and correcting the severe acidosis (Table 53.2). Medical intervention carries significant risks of hypokalemia and cerebral edema, which can be prevented.

Rehydration

Fluid replacement should be instituted promptly. In the first hour isotonic (0.9%) saline should be infused intravenously at 20 ml/kg/hour to reexpand vascular volume. Dehydration is always present. In moderate to severe diabetic ketoacidosis it can be assumed that the loss approximates 10% of the body weight at admission. The volume of fluid during the first 24 hours should replace this deficit (deficit = 100 ml/kg) plus the normal daily requirements (see Chapter 46). The type of fluid used should replace the Na lost, which is in the order of 10 meq/kg. The most effective solution that restores circulating volume and improvement of tissue perfusion is isotonic saline for the first 2 to 6 hours, and then 0.5 N saline continued for the remaining 24 hours. After the initial rapid infusion of isotonic saline at about 20 ml/kg/hour, the rate is gradually reduced over the ensuing 24 hours (Table 53.3). The blood sugar usually falls with rehydration alone, even before commencing insulin therapy. No dextrose is included in the initial fluid replacement. However, a 5% dextrose solution should be administered when the blood sugar falls below about 250 mg/dl. Too rapid a replacement of fluids, especially using dilute solutions, can cause cerebral edema. This complication can to a large extent be avoided by careful fluid replacement, and the use of 5% dextrose in 1 N or 0.5 N saline.

Alkali

Whether sodium bicarbonate should be used for correction of acidosis remains controversial. The administration of bicarbonate to correct the systemic acidosis might exacerbate the acidosis in the central nervous system, because the resulting elevated arterial carbon dioxide penetrates the blood brain barrier more readily than $HCO3^-$. This "paradoxical" acidosis of the central nervous system may cause cerebral depression. Therefore opponents to the use of bicarbonate point to this possible hazard and, in addition, draw attention to the other potential complications such as hypokalemia and impaired oxyhemoglobin dissociation with possible aggravation of tissue hypoxia. Most children will spontaneously correct their acidosis during insulin therapy without recourse to alkali therapy. On the other hand, severe acidosis can be fatal. Thus a reasonable approach is to use bicarbonate only when the patient has severe acidosis (pH <7.1) and is unable to compensate adequately by hyperventilation. Such a child would retain CO_2 either be-

Table 53.2
Principles of Management of Diabetic Ketoacidosis

I. Life-threatening complications
- A. *Immediate* (within the first hours after admission)
  1. Cardiovascular collapse
  2. Profound metabolic acidosis
- B. *Short-term* (within 8–24 hr after start of therapy)
  1. Hypokalemia
  2. Cerebral edema

II. Areas of Management Decisions
- A. *Fluids.* Treat hypovolemia with extracellular fluid expander. Use normal saline (154 meq/L) and infuse 20 ml/kg in the first hour. (Avoid hypotonic solutions initially, since they are inefficient volume expanders and may contribute towards cerebral edema.) Continue infusion at this rate until the blood pressure is normal. Total fluid administration in first 24 hr = maintenance + fluid deficit (5–10% body weight). Monitor urine output
- B. *Alkali.* Consider administering $NaHCO_3$ if blood pH 7.10 or lower. Usual dosage, 2 meq/kg $NaHCO_3$ infused over 1–2 hr. Then recheck pH, PCO_2 and HCO_3. (Avoid bolus infusion of HCO_3^-, since this may acutely lower serum potassium)
- C. *Potassium.* Start potassium therapy after the patient urinates (usually 1–2 hr after start of fluid therapy). Potassium replacement should be given as KCl at a concentration of 40 meq/L. If the patient is hypokalemic (≤3.5 meq/L), a higher concentration of potassium, 60 meq/L, may be necessary. Administer high concentrations of potassium only with ECG monitoring
- D. *Insulin.* Low-dose insulin is safe and effective. May be given either as a continuous i.v. infusion (0.1 unit/kg/hr) or an i.m. injection (0.25 unit/kg every 1–2 hr)
- E. *Glucose.* Add 5% glucose to solutions when serum glucose is approximately 250–300 mg/dl. This may be given as 5% dextrose in 0.5 N saline solution

III. Monitoring
- A. *Clinical monitoring.* Blood pressure, pulse, respirations, state of consciousness, fluid intake-output
- B. *Laboratory monitoring.* Obtain initial glucose, electrolytes, blood gases, and BUN. Measure blood glucose every hour initially as guide to insulin dosage. Repeat electrolytes and pH measurementts as necessary

cause of ventilatory exhaustion or because of insensitivity of the respiratory chemoreceptors. In this situation, arterial PCO_2 will be in excess of: $(1.5 \times HCO_3) + 8 \pm 1$. The dose of bicarbonate is 2 meq/kg, and this can be infused over the course of 1 to 2 hours. An alternative method of calculating the amount of bicarbonate needed is to use the formula:

Amount of bicarbonate required (meq) = base deficit (meq/L) × body weight (kg) × 0.3.

Half this amount is given over the course of 2 hours or more intravenously. Boluses of bicarbonate are reserved for the patient in extremis.

Potassium

The initial serum $[K^+]$ is usually normal or slightly high. If the $[K^+]$ is low at the outset, this suggests considerable K^+ depletion, and replacement must be started early. More frequently hypokalemia is seen after the first few hours of treatment with saline and insulin. Thus, potassium is replaced 1 to 4 hours after commencement of fluid replacement, when the plasma potassium level is known. If the serum $[K^+]$ is between 3.5 to 4.5 meq/l, 10 to 20 meq of potassium chloride (KCl) is added to each 500 ml of replacement fluid (20 to 40 meq/L). If the serum $[K^+]$ is less than 3.5 meq/L, 30 meq KCl can be added to each 500 ml (60 meq/L).

Table 53.3
Guide to Treatment of Severe Diabetic Ketoacidosis

Time (hr)	Type of Fluid	Infusion Rate (ml/hr)[a] at Age in Years (weight in kg)				Potassium Replacement (meq/L)	Bicarbonate Replacement	Insulin Infusion rate (unit/kg/hr)
		1 (10)	5 (18)	10 (30)	15 (50)			
0–1	1 N saline	200	360	600	1000	—	If pH <7.1 consider $NaHCO_3$, 2 mEq/kg. Infuse 20–80 mEq over 1–2 hours.	0.1
1–4	1 N saline	180	280	380	500	If K^+ 3.5–4.5 mEq/l: KCl, 40 mEq/l		0.1 (adjust according to blood sugar).
4–12	0.5 N saline or 5% dextrose-0.5 N saline	90	150	220	310	If K^+ <3.5 mEq/l: KCl, 60 mEq/l		
12–24	5% dextrose-0.5 N saline	60	100	145	210			If blood sugar <250 mg/dl, reduce rate to 0.02–0.05

[a] Fluid infusion rate based on the assumption of 10% dehydration + daily requirements: 0–1 hr: 20 ml/kg, 1–4 hr: ⅓ of 24-hr volume, 4–12 hr: ⅓ of 24-hr volume, and 12–24 hr: ⅓ of 24-hr volume.

Insulin

Regular insulin (quick-acting or soluble insulin) is the only insulin appropriate for the treatment of severe ketoacidosis. The current recommendation is either to continuously infuse insulin intravenously or to inject it intramuscularly at hourly intervals. Because of the uncertainties of absorption when the patient is is shock, subcutaneous injections should be avoided in the very ill patient. There is little to choose between continuous intravenous and hourly intramuscular injections. The initial dosage of regular insulin for continuous infusion is 0.1 unit/kg/hour. This can be given by a syringe pump, or diluted in a burette of a pediatric intravenous administration set. There may be some absorption of insulin into the plastic syringe, burette and tubing, but in practice, this does not give rise to difficulties. In any case, the rate of infusion may have to be adjusted according to the rapidity of fall in blood sugar, and improvement in the acidosis. The use of an initial bolus of insulin is advocated by several centers, but there seems to be no practical advantage of giving such a bolus. The dosage for 1 to 2 hourly intramuscular injections is 0.25 unit/kg/dose. Whichever method is employed, the key to success is close monitoring of clinical and biochemical parameters (see below).

Conversion to subcutaneous insulin can be made when the patient is clinically improved, or when the serum glucose falls below about 250 mg/dl. If one is using the continuous infusion of insulin, it may be convenient to continue this for a slightly longer period, until the child is able to start drinking and eating. To avoid inadvertent hypoglycemia with all regimens, the serum glucose should be monitored hourly. When the serum glucose falls below 250 mg/dl, 5% dextrose can be infused, and the rate of insulin infusion reduced appropriately.

Phosphate

Phosphate depletion is almost universal in diabetic ketoacidosis. The clinical significance of this is uncertain. Phosphate is involved in the production of 2,3-diphosphoglyceric acid. Its deficiency can shift the erythrocyte oxygen dissociation curve to the left, and theoretically reduce the delivery of oxygen to the tissues. In a controlled trial, phosphate therapy has been shown to accelerate the regeneration of erythrocyte 2,3-diphosphoglyceric acid, but to have no significant influence on tissue oxygenation or the clinical response in terms of the time taken for glucose, bicarbonate and pH to reach predetermined values. Hence phosphate therapy is probably unnecessary. Moreover excessive phosphate can cause hypocalcemia.

Monitoring

Close monitoring is mandatory. The patient's blood pressure, pulse rate, respiratory rate, and level of consciousness should be observed regularly. The fluid input and output must be recorded accurately. The intravenous fluids should be checked frequently so that pump failure or leakage of fluid into the subcutaneous tissues can be corrected quickly. In the severely ill child, an electrocardiographic monitor is advisable to detect arrhythmias associated with hyper- or hypokalemia.

The serum glucose should be measured at regular intervals until it plateaus at a satisfactory level. The frequency of estimation will vary from individual to individual, but we generally advocate hourly determinations for the first few hours, then 2 to 4 hourly thereafter, depending upon clinical circumstances. Monitoring the serum $[K^+]$ needs to be repeated approximately 2, 6, and 24 hours from the start of therapy, or more frequently if hypokalemia is encountered or bicarbonate therapy is employed. Arterial pH should be obtained before treatment and repeated if bicarbonate therapy is used or contemplated.

When the child is better hydrated and the acidosis resolves, there will be improvement in mental alertness, and symptoms of nausea, vomiting and abdominal pain should remit. Some patients complain of blurring of vision, due to lens distortion caused by fluid shifts with rehydration and correction of hyperglycemia. After a few hours and usually by 12 hours, patients may be able to tolerate oral fluids, at which point rehydration can be continued part orally and part intravenously.

HYPOGLYCEMIA

BACKGROUND

Hypoglycemia is defined as a serum glucose of less than 40 mg/100 ml, whether or not symptoms are present. Hypoglycemia is a chemical finding, and its presence should lead to a diligent search for a cause. A differential diagnosis of hypoglycemia as it may present in the emergency department, is provided in Table 53.4.

The most common cause of hypoglycemia in pediatrics is secondary to insulin therapy for diabetes. Hypoglycemia also frequently accompanies serious systemic disease (e.g., sepsis or Reye's syndrome). Excluding these two categories, virtually all hypoglycemia in children occurs during fasting. Postprandial hypoglycemia is rarely seen in children, except in those who have had prior gastrointestinal surgery.

PATHOPHYSIOLOGY

A constant supply of glucose is necessary to provide energy for cellular metabolism in most human tissues; therefore the maintenance of an adequate blood sugar is critical for normal function. The serum glucose reflects a dynamic balance between glucose input from dietary sources, glycogenolysis and gluconeogenesis, and glucose utilization by muscle, heart, adipose tissue, brain and blood elements.

The liver plays a unique role in the maintenance of a normal serum glucose. When there is adequate glucose intake, it is stored in the liver as glycogen. With fasting, this glycogen is degraded to glucose which is released into the blood stream. In addition, the liver synthesizes new glucose from glycerol, lactate and certain amino acids.

Muscle also contains significant quantities of glycogen as well as protein. Under fasting conditions, the glycogen can be degraded and used endogenously but cannot be released as free glucose into the blood stream. Certain amino acids, particularly alanine and glycine, can be released from the muscle and subsequently used by the liver for gluconeogenesis. During fasting, lipolysis also occurs. The circulating fatty acids thus generated are used to provide a significant proportion of the muscular fuel requirement.

Table 53.4
Causes of Childhood Hypoglycemia

I. Decreased Availability of Glucose
- A. Decreased intake—fasting, malnutrition, illness
- B. Decreased absorption—acute diarrhea
- C. Inadequate glycogen reserves—defects in enzymes of glycogen synthetic pathways
- D. Ineffective glycogenolysis—defects in enzymes of glycogenolytic pathways
- E. Inability to mobilize glycogen—glucagon deficiency
- F. Ineffective gluconeogenesis—defects in enzymes of gluconeogenic pathway

II. Increased Utilization of Glucose
- A. Hyperinsulinism—islet cell adenoma or hyperplasia, nesidioblastosis, ingestion of oral hypoglycemic agents, insulin therapy
- B. Large tumors—Wilms' tumor

III. Diminished Availability of Alternative Fuels
- A. Decreased or absent fat stores
- B. Ineffective mobilization or utilization of fats—carnitine deficiency

IV. Unknown or Complex Mechanisms
- A. Sepsis
- B. Reye's syndrome
- C. Salicylate ingestion
- D. Ethanol ingestion
- E. Adrenal insufficiency
- F. Hypothyroidism
- G. Hypopituitarism

Brain tissue is almost completely dependent on glucose for its energy requirements. Under certain circumstances it can extract a limited proportion of its energy requirement from other substrates (e.g., glycerol, ketones, lactate), although this requires a period of adaptation and does not negate the need for a constant supply of glucose.

Insulin is the primary hormone that regulates the blood glucose level. Insulin stimulates the uptake of glucose and amino acids into skeletal, cardiac and adipose tissue and promotes glycogen and protein synthesis. It inhibits lipolysis and glycogenolysis. The net effect of insulin action is to accelerate the removal of glucose and gluconeogenic substrates from the blood stream. Opposing or modulating the effects of insulin are a number of other hormones including ACTH, cortisol, glucagon, epinephrine and growth hormone. The effects of these hormones include inhibition of glucose uptake by muscle, mobilization of amino acids for gluconeogenesis, activation of lipolysis, inhibition of insulin secretion, and induction of gluconeogenic enzymes. The net effect is to increase the availability of gluconeogenic substrates to the liver, and to increase the accessibility and utilization of nonglucose fuels by other tissues.

CLINICAL MANIFESTATIONS

Prompt recognition of hypoglycemia is important since the risk of irreversible brain damage is great if the hypoglycemia is prolonged or recurs frequently. Any acutely ill child deserves a serum glucose determination because hypoglycemia may accompany almost any illness which interferes with oral intake. Historical evidence may be of help in establishing the cause of hypoglycemia. Since most hypoglycemia in children occurs after a period of fasting, a careful chronology of dietary intake during the preceding 24 hours should be obtained. The possibility of an aberrant ingestion should be considered, since ethanol, propanolol and oral hypoglycemic agents are in common use.

The signs and symptoms of hypoglycemia are nonspecific and are frequently overlooked, especially in the very young child. The clinical findings of hypoglycemia reflect both the decreased availability of glucose to the central nervous system and the adrenergic stimulation caused by a decreasing or low blood sugar. Adrenergic signs and symptoms include palpitations, anxiety, tremulousness, hunger, and sweating. Irritability, headache, fatigue, confusion, seizure, and unconsciousness are neuroglycopenic symptoms. Any combination of these should lead to a careful search for hypoglycemia. Any child presenting with a seizure or unconsciousness should have a serum glucose level obtained.

MANAGEMENT

If hypoglycemia is suspected, blood should be obtained for a serum glucose determination. Rapid screening should be done with one of the glucose-specific chemically coated, plastic strips (e.g., Dextrostix) while awaiting definitive laboratory results. Therapy should be instituted if this screen is suggestive of hypoglycemia. This may lead to some overtreatment since the primary error with the chemically treated strips is underestimation of the serum glucose value. Serum and urine should be obtained and saved for appropriate chemical, toxicologic, and hormonal studies. These values may be of significant use in determining the cause of hypoglycemia. Therapy should not be unduly delayed to obtain these specimens.

The treatment of choice consists of the administration of 0.25 g/kg of body weight of dextrose (2.5 ml of 10% dextrose/kg) rapidly, and the serum glucose should then be maintained by an infusion of dextrose at a rate of 4 to 6 mg/kg/min. Glucagon (1 mg) may be used to treat hypoglycemia known to be caused by hyperinsulinism, but should not be used as part of the routine therapy of hypoglycemia. Cortisol should not be used since it has no acute benefit and may delay the diagnosis of the cause of hypoglycemia.

The adequacy of therapy should be evaluated both chemically and clinically. The serum glucose should be monitored frequently until a stable level is attained. Adrenergic symptoms should resolve quickly. The resolution of central nervous system symptoms may be prolonged, particularly if the child was initially seizing or unconscious. Seizures which do not respond to correction of hypoglycemia should be managed with appropriate anticonvulsants (see Chapter 44). The mild acidosis (pH 7.25 to 7.35) usually seen in hypoglycemia will correct without medical intervention. Marked acidosis (pH <7.10) suggests shock or serious underlying disease, and should be managed appropriately (see Chapter 46).

Any child with documented hypoglycemia should be hospitalized for careful monitoring and diagnostic testing.

ACUTE ADRENAL INSUFFICIENCY

BACKGROUND

Acute adrenal insufficiency occurs when the adrenal cortex fails to produce enough glucocorticoid and mineralocorticoid in response to stress. Patients at risk of this life-threatening event include those who have primary adrenal disease, such as Addison's disease, and those who have adrenal insufficiency secondary to hypothalamic-pituitary lesions (Table 53.5). This emergency has become increasingly common with the widespread use of suppressive doses of corticosteroids in the treatment of such diseases as the nephrotic syndrome, acute lymphoblastic leukemia, status asthmaticus, and others. Acute adrenal crises in infancy are often associated with congenital adrenal hyperplasia, and this is discussed in another section. Infection, trauma or surgery in the susceptible patient precipitates the acute crisis. The diagnosis is largely based on clinical suspicion, and there is usually no time to wait for laboratory con-

Table 53.5
Common Causes of Acute Adrenal Insufficiency in Children

I. *Primary Adrenal Insufficiency*
   - A. Congenital adrenal hyperplasia
   - B. Autoimmunity
   - C. Tuberculosis
   - D. Meningococcal septicemia

II. *Secondary to Hypothalamic-Pituitary Lesions*
   - A. Suppression of ACTH by pharmacological doses of glucocorticoid administration
   - B. Suprasella tumors (craniopharyngioma, dysgerminoma, etc) and their treatment
   - C. Idiopathic hypopituitarism

firmation of the diagnosis prior to commencement of therapy.

PATHOPHYSIOLOGY

The production of adrenal steroids can be impaired by an inborn error of biosynthesis (see section on congenital adrenal hyperplasia). The adrenal gland may be destroyed by an autoimmune process, by an infection such as tuberculosis or meningococcal septicemia, by hemorrhage into the gland, or by surgery. Lack of adrenocorticotropic hormone (ACTH) secretion by the anterior pituitary gland also results in adrenal insufficiency. This may be due to suppression by pharmacological doses of glucocorticoids, to hypothalamic-pituitary tumors such as craniopharyngiomas or dysgerminomas, or to idiopathic panhypopituitarism.

Glucocorticoids are essential for withstanding the stresses of infection, trauma, or anesthesia, but the precise mechanism of this is undetermined. Mineralocorticoids are important for salt and water homeostasis. Aldosterone, the principal mineralocorticoid hormone, promotes salt and water reabsorption in the distal renal tubules and the collecting ducts. It is in turn regulated by the renin-angiotensin system. As the production of aldosterone is not under the direct control of ACTH, adrenal insufficiency secondary to hypothalamic-pituitary causes does not lead to aldosterone deficiency. The production of ACTH is under negative feedback control by glucocorticoids, and therefore primary adrenal insufficiency results in increased ACTH levels which can cause hyperpigmentation.

CLINICAL MANIFESTATIONS

The typical history elicited from a patient with acute adrenal insufficiency is that of nausea, vomiting, abdominal pain, weakness, malaise, and sometimes mental changes or psychosis. In the child with chronic Addison's disease, a history of weight loss, anorexia, easy fatigability, salt-craving, and dizziness or standing, should be sought. Previous neurosurgery to the hypothalamic-pituitary area, steroid therapy, and precipitating factors such as infection, trauma or surgery, should also be ascertained.

Physical examination characteristically shows an ill child with hypotension, dehydration, and, in some cases of primary adrenal insufficiency, hyperpigmentation.

The definitive diagnosis is based on the finding of a low or inappropriately normal serum cortisol level. However, this result is usually not available prior to treatment. Presumptive evidence of adrenal insufficiency is provided by the findings of hyponatremia, hyperkalemia, hypoglycemia, hemoconcentration, mild metabolic acidosis, variable hypercalcemia, and eosinophilia.

MANAGEMENT

Treatment of this life-threatening emergency comprises administration of glucocorticoids and rehydration, in the emergency department. Hydrocortisone 100 mg should be injected intravenously, and then continued at a dose of 25 to 100 mg every 4 to 6 hours. Alternatively, cortisone acetate 100 mg can be given intramuscularly, and then 25 to 100 mg repeated every 6 to 12 hours, or dexamethasone 1 to 4 mg/day may be administered intravenously. Fluid replacement is best given intravenously as 5% dextrose in physiological saline solution at a rate of 20 ml/kg in the first hour and then at 1½ to 2 times the normal maintenance rate until the fluid deficit is corrected.

Mineralocorticoid replacement is not essential in the acute situation, provided fluid replacement is adequate. The patient with continuing salt-wasting will need either deoxycorticosterone acetate, 75 μg/kg in the child under 1 year or 40 μg/kg in the older child, given as a daily intramuscular injection or 9α-fludrocortisone, 5 μg/kg in the child under 1 year or 0.05 to 0.2 mg in the older child orally once daily. Specific correction of the hyperkalemia is usually unnecessary, but if there are associated cardiac arrhythmias, sodium bicarbonate 2 meq/kg can be cautiously infused as 20 to 80 meq over the course of 1 to 2 hours (see Chapter 46). Hypoglycemia is remedied by the use of 5 to 10% dextrose in the rehydra-

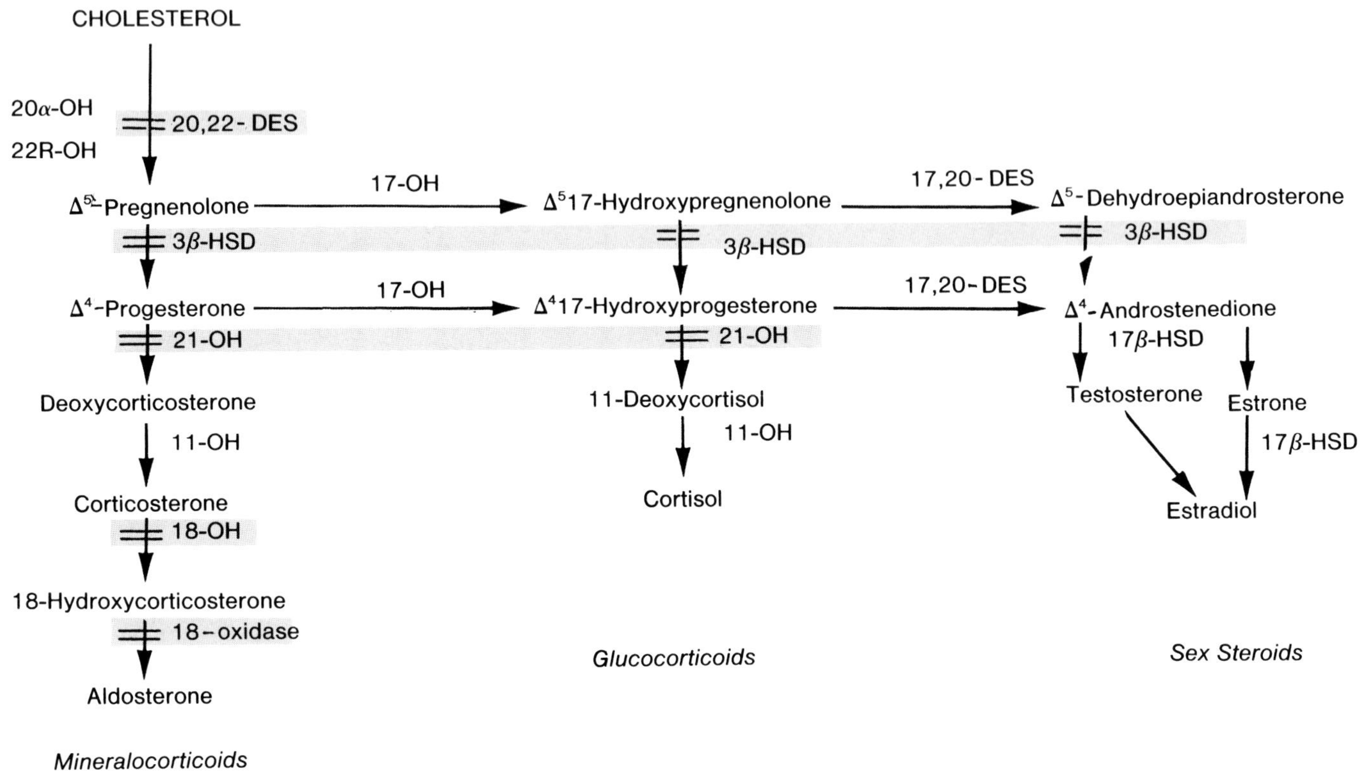

Figure 53.2 Outline of the pathways of adrenal steroid biosynthesis. OH = hydroxylase; DES = desmolase; 3 βHSD = 3 β-hydroxysteroid dehydrogenase; 17βHSD = 17β-hydroxysteroid dehydroxygenase. *Note:* Double bars indicate possible enzyme deficiencies associated with salt-wasting states.

tion fluid, and glucocorticoid therapy also has a hyperglycemic effect. Treatment of precipitating factors such as intercurrent infections is also important.

A clinical response, as judged by improved blood pressure and peripheral circulation and cessation of vomiting, should occur within hours of treatment. The high dose of glucocorticoid hormones may need to be continued for 24 to 48 hours, and then carefully reduced to maintenance values, or stopped completely if there is only transient adrenal insufficiency. Similarly mineralocorticoid therapy, with or without salt supplementation, should be continued at a dosage that maintains normal plasma electrolytes. The patient at risk of adrenal insufficiency should be advised to wear an identification bracelet or necklace.

CONGENITAL ADRENAL HYPERPLASIA

BACKGROUND

Inborn errors of adrenal steroid biosynthesis are grouped under the term congenital adrenal hyperplasia (CAH) (Fig. 53.2). There are two major modes of presentation, both of which might occur in early infancy and require early diagnosis and treatment. The first form of presentation is that of an acute salt-losing crisis, and the second is that of ambiguous genitalia (Table 53.6).

The most common form of CAH is 21-hydroxylase deficiency, which is recessively inherited and accounts for 90% of all cases. Clinically apparent salt-wasting develops in 30 to 70% of patients with this enzyme deficiency. In the United States, the incidence of 21-hydroxylase deficiency is about 1 in 15,000 live births.

PATHOPHYSIOLOGY

The enzymes 21-hydroxylase, 11-hydroxylase, 3β-dehydrogenase, and 20,22-desmolase are involved in the two arms of adrenal steroid biosynthesis (Fig. 53.2). Deficiency of these enzymes can affect both cortisol and aldosterone production. Underproduction of cortisol is sensed by the hypothalamo-pituitary system leading to a compensatory increase of ACTH. The ACTH stimulates adrenal cortical cells to increase production of all of the steroid hormones proximal to the enzyme deficiency. Mineralocorticoid and glucocorticoid insufficiency and the buildup of precursor compounds and their metabolites are responsible for the clinical manifestations of the individual enzyme blocks.

Impairment of the mineralocorticoid synthesis by 21-hydroxylase, 3β-dehydroge-

Table 53.6
Clinical and Laboratory Features of Various Forms of Congenital Adrenal Hyperplasia

Enzyme Deficiency	Clinical Features				
	Newobrn with sexual ambiguity		Salt wasting	Hypertension	Postnatal virilization
	Female	Male			
21-Hydroxylase					
Non-salt-wasting	+	0	0	0	+
Salt-wasting	+	0	+	0	+
11-Hydroxylase	+	0	0	+	+
3β-Hydroxysteroid dehydrogenase	+	+	+	0	0
17α-Hydroxylase	0	+	0	+	0
Cholesterol desmolase	0	+	+	0	0
18-Hydroxylase	0	0	+	0	0
17β-Hydroxysteroid dehydrogenase	?	+	−	−	+

nase, and 20,22-desmolase deficiency can result in salt wasting. Although 11-hydroxylase deficiency also blocks aldosterone production, the immediate precursor to the block, desoxycorticosterone, has potent mineralocorticoid activity. Thus, instead of developing salt loss, patients with this enzyme defect often develop hypertension when older.

There is a buildup of intermediate steroids with androgenic activity in 21-hydroxylase and 11-hydroxylase deficiencies. Females with these defects are virilized in utero and are born with ambiguous genitalia. Males have normal genital development. Deficiency of 3β-dehydrogenase leads to underproduction of both testosterone and estrogens. Boys with this deficiency are undervirilized because of the lack of androgens, whereas girls are mildly virilized probably because of the low estrogen levels. Lack of cortisol renders the patient more susceptible to hypoglycemia and reduces the tolerance to severe stress.

CLINICAL MANIFESTATIONS

Clinical signs of congenital adrenal hyperplasia may be noticed at birth by the discovery of ambiguous genitalia, or betweeen the second and sixth week of life when the baby presents with an acute salt-losing crisis. Salt wasting rarely occurs during the first week of life. The presentation may be slow and insidious, and there may be a history of poor feeding, failure to gain weight, lethargy, irritability, vomiting or loose stools. On the other hand the onset can be fairly sudden where the infant becomes very sick and develops shock within 24 hours. The symptoms are so nonspecific that the initial working diagnosis is often far removed from congenital adrenal hyperplasia. The child may be investigated for pyloric stenosis, meningitis or sepsis.

Examination of the child should include the vital signs and an assessment of the degree of dehydration. In severe cases, there may be signs of shock and metabolic acidosis. The genitalia should be carefully examined. The degree of ambiguity of the genitalia varies considerably. Virilized females may have an enlarged clitoris and fusion of the labial folds. An undervirilized male may have a small phallus and/or hypospadias. It is important to feel the labial-scrotal folds and the inguinal area for the presence of gonads; their presence almost always indicates a male karyotype. Hyperpigmentation of the labial-scrotal folds and the nipples due to excessive secretion of ACTH is occasionally present in the neonatal period. However, it is rarely prominent enough to alert the examiner of its presence until after the diagnosis is established.

In the emergency department, the most urgent investigations are plasma electrolytes and blood sugar. The combination of hyperkalemia and hyponatremia is often the first clue to the diagnosis of congenital adrenal hyperplasia. The plasma potassium is elevated, but in the presence of vomiting and diarrhea the rise may be blunted. Levels between 6 and 12 meq/L are frequently encountered, often without any clinical cardiac dysfunction or electrocardiographic changes. The plasma bicarbonate is usually low, reflecting the metabolic acidosis resulting from the retention of hydrogen ions in exchange for sodium loss. The blood glucose is usually normal; however, hypoglycemia may occur secondary to the lack of cortisol and the reduced caloric intake during the acute illness. Blood should be drawn for 17-hydroxyprogesterone estimation, but treatment must be commenced before the results are available in the child with salt-wasting. The 24-hour urinary 17-ketosteroids and pregnanetriol are elevated in the patient with congenital adrenal hyperplasia beyond the first week of life.

MANAGEMENT

Fluid and Electrolyte Replacement

All children with salt-wasting congenital adrenal hyperplasia should be admitted to the hospital for close monitoring and intravenous therapy. Fluid replacement is a matter of some urgency, as the small infant cannot tolerate severe fluid losses for long. The dehydration in salt-losing congenital adrenal hyperplasia represents urinary losses of isosmotic fluid. Replacement should therefore consist of normal saline

(0.9%). The volume to be replaced should embody the child's daily requirements plus the estimated fluid loss. The initial infusion rate should be more rapid, e.g. 20 ml/kg in the first hour. Fluid input and output should be monitored carefully.

Mineralocorticoid Replacement

Although for a short time, one can keep up with fluid losses with intravenous normal saline, mineralocorticoid replacement will facilitate management. In acute situations, deoxycorticosterone acetate (DOCA) 1 mg should be given i.m. in the emergency department at the time of diagnosis. It does not interfere with subsequent diagnostic tests.

Correction of Hyperkalemia

Babies with congenital adrenal hyperplasia can generally tolerate potassium levels as high as 12 meq/L. Fluid restoration with normal saline is the major and, usually the only, measure needed to lower the potassium. In the presence of arrhythmias, intravenous 10% calcium gluconate can be given for its membrane-stabilizing properties. Therapy with glucose and insulin is contraindicated because of the danger of precipitating hypoglycemia.

Glucocorticoid Replacement

In the sick infant, glucocorticoid replacement is mandatory. Hydrocortisone 25 mg can be given immediately as an intravenous bolus, or cortisone acetate 25 mg i.m. Glucocorticoid hormones can suppress ACTH and the precursor steroids within a few hours of administration, thus rendering diagnosis of 21-hydroxylase deficiency difficult. However, it is better that one keep the child alive by giving the steroid, than unduly delaying treatment for diagnostic purposes.

Correction of Hypoglycemia

Although hypoglycemia is an uncommon complication of congenital adrenal hyperplasia during the acute salt-losing crisis, it should be sought. It is easily correctable by glucose administration intravenously, e.g. by the infusion of 10% dextrose.

Acidosis

Acidosis does not require specific treatment. The low bicarbonate level may take several days to a few weeks to fully correct.

DIABETES INSIPIDUS

BACKGROUND

Diabetes insipidus (DI) is due to an inability of the kidneys to concentrate urine and is characterized clinically by polyuria and polydipsia. Either a deficiency of antidiuretic hormone (ADH) secretion from the hypothalamus and posterior pituitary gland or renal unresponsiveness to ADH can cause this disease (Table 53.7). Most central causes of DI in childhood are acquired and can present at any age. In contrast, the most common etiology of nephrogenic DI in children is the X-linked recessive type and is therefore manifest in males during early infancy. Renal lesions associated with nephrogenic DI can present in later childhood.

Table 53.7
Causes of Diabetes Insipidus in Childhood

I. *Antidiuretic Hormone Deficiency*
   A. Head injury
   B. Meningitis
   C. Idiopathic
   D. Suprasellar tumors and their treatment by surgery and/or radiotherapy:
      1. Craniopharyngioma
      2. Optic nerve glioma
      3. Dysgerminoma
   E. Septo-optic dysplasia
   F. Association with midline cleft palate
   G. Familial (dominant or sex-linked recessive)
   H. Wolfram syndrome (diabetes insipidus, diabetes mellitus, optic atrophy, deafness)
   I. Histiocytosis X (Hand-Schüller-Christian disease)

II. *Nephrogenic Diabetes Insipidus*
   A. Sex-linked recessive
   B. Renal disease
      1. Polycystic kidneys
      2. Hydronephrosis
      3. Chronic pyelonephritis
   C. Hypercalcemia
   D. Hypokalemia
   E. Toxins:
      1. Demeclocycline
      2. Lithium
   F. Sickle cell disease
   G. Idiopathic

PATHOPHYSIOLOGY

ADH is synthesized in the supraoptic and paraventricular nuclei of the hypothalamus. It is transported along nerve axons to the posterior pituitary gland where it is stored. ADH is released in response to increased plasma osmolality, hypernatremia, and decreased right atrial pressure secondary to hypovolemia. The distal convoluted tubules and the collecting ducts of the kidneys respond to ADH by promoting water reabsorption. Lack of ADH (central DI) can be due to a wide variety of hypothalamic pituitary lesions (Table 53.7). Conversely, in nephrogenic DI, ADH levels are normal. The defect resides in the renal collecting tubules which are resistant to the action of ADH. Failure of water reabsorption results in polyuria. A normal thirst mechanism contributes towards fluid balance by promoting adequate fluid intake. However, this balance might not be achieved, and hypertonic dehydration ensues. If such a hyperosmolar state develops abruptly, it may lead to dehydration of neural tissues, which could cause serious neurological sequelae or result in death.

CLINICAL MANIFESTATIONS

Urine excretion is increased both in volume and frequency in the child with DI. In the younger child this may be manifested as enuresis. Provided the thirst mechanism is intact and fluids are accessible, the child can compensate for the water loss by drinking more. One may elicit a history of the child awakening in the middle of the night to drink, and there may be a glass of water kept by the bedside for this purpose. If fluids are not accessible, as in an infant, or if the thirst sensation is impaired by a hypothalamic lesion, hypertonic dehydration develops with drowsiness or irritability, progressing to coma. An unusual mode of presentation is that of unexplained fever.

Physical examination may be normal, or show signs of dehydration, such as dryness of mucous membranes, decreased skin turgor, sunken eyes, and, in an infant, a depressed anterior fontanelle. Hypothalamic-pituitary lesions can give rise to other endocrine abnormalities such as hypothyroidism and growth failure. A craniopharyngioma or optic nerve glioma may affect the visual fields or cause raised intracranial pressure which is indicated by papilledema.

The diagnosis of DI is made by demonstrating the failure of the kidneys to concentrate the urine, which can sometimes be quite difficult in children. Nonetheless an adequate working diagnosis is usually obtained by finding an elevated serum osmolality (normally, <290 mOsm/kg) and a serum Na that is raised or on the high side of the normal range, in the presence of dilute urine (normally, osmolality > 150 mOsm/kg). Blood sugar and serum creatinine are normal.

The definitive diagnosis is made by a formal water deprivation test. However, this test may be both dangerous and unnecessary in the severely dehydrated child; it is performed electively in cases where the diagnosis is uncertain.

MANAGEMENT

Central Diabetes Insipidus

The Severely Dehydrated Child, Serum Na>160 meq/L. Hypernatremic dehydration is associated with a significant mortality, especially in infants. Overly rapid correction of hypernatremia using hypotonic solutions intravenously can cause cerebral edema, seizures and death (see Chapter 46). However, there are no data as to how quickly the serum Na can be safely corrected; hence, treatment remains controversial. Nevertheless most investigators agree that rehydration should be accomplished over a period of 48 hours, and that rapid infusions of hypotonic solutions must be avoided. There are two major schools of thought as to how this emergency should be managed:

1. Rapid intravenous rehydration (over the course of 48 hours) with isotonic (0.9% saline or plasma, at about 20 ml/kg/hour for the first hour, together with 1-desamino-8-D-arginine vasopressin (DDAVP) 0.1 ml, given nasally. After the first 1 to 2 hours, the infusion rate can be tapered to about 1½ times maintenance, and 5% dextrose in 0.25 N saline substituted.

2. Slower rehydration with 5% dextrose or 5% dextrose in 0.25 N saline at about 1½ times maintenance, and DDAVP 0.1 ml given nasally.

The child must be closely observed for changes in the level of consciousness, pulse rate, blood pressure, fluid input and output, urine and serum osmolality, and serum Na. There is a risk of hyperglycemia when 5% dextrose is infused rapidly, which can be avoided by using solutions with lower dextrose concentrations if necessary. DDAVP may need to be repeated if the diuresis persists or reappears. Other antidiuretic agents can also be used, such as aqueous pitressin 0.2 to 1.0 ml (4 to 20 units) intramuscularly or 3 milliunits/kg/min as a constant intravenous infusion. When the child is clinically and biochemically improved, the amount of fluid intake should match the urine output, plus allowance made for insensible losses. This serves to avoid the situation of overhydration inducing further diuresis which might cause the clinician to respond inappropriately by giving yet more fluids and hence perpetuating this vicious cycle.

The Mildly Dehydrated Child, Serum Na<160 meq/L. This is usually a less urgent problem. Rehydration slowly with dilute solutions may be used. Oral or intravenous 5% dextrose given at 1½ times maintenance, is recommended. DDAVP 4 μg/kg (0.05 to 0.2 ml) is given nasally until diuresis recurs, and the dose is then repeated as clinically indicated. The general comments concerning monitoring the child, maintaining fluid balance, and measuring urine and serum osmolality and Na, outlined above, also apply in this situation.

Nephrogenic Diabetes Insipidus

Fluid replacement for a dehydrated child with nephrogenic DI is similar to that for central causes. However, nephrogenic DI does not respond to ADH preparations or analogs. Paradoxically, some benefit may be derived from the use of thiazide diuretics. Chlorothiazide 1.0 g/sq m/day in 3 divided doses, or hydrochlorothiazide 1.0 g/sq m/day in 3 divided doses can be used. The patient's clinical state, fluid balance, urine and plasma electrolytes and Na need to be closely monitored.

SYNDROME OF INAPPROPRIATE ADH SECRETION

BACKGROUND

Excessive secretion of antidiuretic hormone in the face of normal or low plasma osmolality or Na concentration is inappropriate. It further depresses the plasma osmolality and Na concentration. Symptoms, however, are not usually apparent until the plasma Na falls below about 120 meq/L. The overall incidence of the syndrome of inappropriate antidiuretic hormone secretion (SIADH) in childhood is not known, but it is very common in certain disease states. Over 50% of children with bacterial meningitis, about 20% of patients on positive pressure ventilation, and about 70% of children with Rocky Mountain spotted fever develop SIADH.

PATHOPHYSIOLOGY

ADH secretion is stimulated by hypertonicity of the fluid surrounding the hypothalamic osmoreceptors, by volume receptors in the left atrium, and by ill-defined nervous impulses from higher cortical centers. Disorders of the central nervous system (Table 53.8) may cause excessive ADH secretion either by producing some local disturbance of the hypothalamic osmoreceptors or by some undetermined nervous stimuli. Many intrathoracic conditions are also associated with SIADH, probably by stimulating the volume receptors in the left atrium. Physical and emotional stress and severe pain also cause ADH secretion.

Excessive secretion of ADH leads to water retention by the collecting tubules of the kidneys, a mechanism mediated by cyclic AMP. The water retained expands the intravascular compartment, dilutes all plasma constituents, and lowers the plasma osmolality.

CLINICAL MANIFESTATIONS

Most patients with SIADH are asymptomatic. When the plasma Na falls below 120 meq/L, symptoms become more frequent. These range from anorexia, headache, nausea, vomiting, irritability, disorientation and weakness, to seizures and coma, leading ultimately to death. Absence of dehydration is a significant negative finding.

Laboratory investigations for diagnostic purposes must include concomitant serum and urine samples (Table 53.9). There is hyponatremia, hypo-osmolality (serum) and low blood urea nitrogen. In contrast, the urinary osmolality and Na concentration are inappropriately elevated for the hypotonicity of the serum. The plasma uric acid is low, and this has been a useful finding for diagnosis. Radioimmunoassay for ADH is now available and has been helpful in defining this syndrome. However, the length of time usually taken for ADH results to be returned lessens its value for emergency use. The underlying cause of the syndrome should be investigated according to one's clinical judgment. Other causes of hyponatremia, including water intoxication, renal and adrenal salt-wasting states, hypothyroidism, hyperlipidemia, and hyperproteinemia must be excluded. The urine osmolality in water intoxication states is usually low, in comparison to that found in SIADH.

Table 53.8
Some Causes of Syndrome of Inappropriate Antidiuretic Hormone Secretion (SIADH) in Children

I. *Disorders of Central Nervous System*
   A. Infection (meningitis, encephalitis)
   B. Trauma, post neurosurgery
   C. Hypoxic insults, especially in the perinatal period
   D. Brain tumor
   E. Intraventricular hemorrhage
   F. Guillain-Barré syndrome
   G. Psychosis
II. *Intrathoracic Disorders*
   A. Infection (tuberculosis, pneumonia, empyema)
   B. Positive-pressure ventilation
   C. Asthma
   D. Cystic fibrosis
   E. Pneumothorax
   8. Patent ductus arteriosus ligation
III. *Miscellaneous*
   A. Pain (e.g. following abdominal surgery)
   B. Severe hypothyroidism
   C. Congenital deficiency
   D. Tumors (e.g. neuroblastoma)
   E. Idiopathic deficiency
IV. *Drug-induced*
   A. Increased ADH secretion
      1. Vincristine
      2. Cyclophosphamide
      3. Carbamazepine
      4. Adenine arabinoside
      5. Phenothiazines
      6. Morphine
   B. Potentiation of ADH effect
      1. Acetaminophen
      2. Indomethacin

Table 53.9
Criteria for Diagnosis of Syndrome of Inappropriate Antidiuretic Hormone Secretion (SIADH)

1. Hyponatremia, reduced serum osmolality
2. Urine osmolality that is inappropriately elevated (a urine osmolality less than 100 mOsm/kg usually excludes the diagnosis)
3. Urinary Na concentration that is excessive in comparison to the degree of hyponatremia (usually more than 18 meq/L)
4. Normal renal, adrenal, and thyroid function
5. Absence of volume depletion

MANAGEMENT

Symptomatic Children

Patients with seizures attributable to the severe hyponatremia and those who are lethargic or comatose, need urgent treatment. Hypertonic (3%) saline with appropriate amounts of potassium chloride, are infused intravenously at a rate commensurate with urinary losses of sodium and potassium (see Chapter 46). It is probably safer to infuse small amounts of 3% saline, every 10 to 20 min, and to stop as soon as symptoms remit. A single dose of furosemide, 1 mg/kg, can also be administered intravenously. Close monitoring of fluid balance, plasma and urinary sodium, potassium and osmolality is essential. Diphenylhydantoin (Dilantin) in high doses intravenously (5 to 10 mg/kg) inhibits ADH release, and may be of help in the patient with seizures secondary to central nervous system causes of SIADH. The underlying cause of SIADH should be treated where possible, and this is usually accompanied by remission of inappropriate antidiuresis.

Asymptomatic Children

Asymptomatic patients are treated by fluid restriction (50 to 75% of maintenance rate). Once again, frequent measurements of plasma and urine electrolytes and fluid balance are important. When the serum Na rises and urine osmolality falls, the rate of fluid administration can be increased to the regular maintenance rates. The child with chronic or recurrent episodes of SIADH may require treatment with demeclocycline, 10 mg/kg. Again, the underlying cause should be eliminated, if possible.

COMMON THYROID EMERGENCIES

Thyroid Storm

BACKGROUND

Thyroid storm or thyrotoxic crisis is a fulminating intensification of the thyrotoxic state. It is rarely seen in children, and we are aware of only one case report in the literature. In adults, it occurs in about 1% of all thyrotoxic patients. However, the incidence of thyrotoxicosis in children is much less than in adults, and is estimated to be about 1:2000 with a female to male ratio of about 4:1. Therefore almost all information concerning thyroid storm is derived from adult reports. Known precipitating factors include subtotal thyroidectomy in the inadequately prepared patient, trauma, intercurrent infection, and diabetic ketoacidosis. The mortality rate in large series ranges from 20 to 50% of cases.

PATHOPHYSIOLOGY

In thyroid storm, there is a sudden release of thyroid hormone into the circulation. Uncoupling of oxidative phosphorylation and/or increased lipolysis by thyroid hormone contributes to excessive thermogenesis. Insensible fluid loss results from increased metabolism and sweating. Tachycardia is due in part to the hyperthermia, and in part to the direct action of thyroid hormones on the conduction system of the heart.

CLINICAL MANIFESTATIONS

Nearly all reported cases of thyroid storm occur in patients with underlying features of hyperthyroidism. These might include the presence of a goiter and exophthalmos. Fever is nearly always present, and is probably the sine qua non for making the diagnosis; it may rise as high as 41°C. There is marked sinus tachycardia with or without ectopic beats. This cardiac rate may be excessive for efficient cardiac function, resulting in congestive heart failure and hypotension. The latter finding is in contrast to the systolic hypertension frequently found in untreated Graves' disease. The congestive heart failure may lead to hepatic venous congestion and give rise to tender hepatomegaly and jaundice. There is tremulousness and restlessness, mania, delirium, and even frank psychotic behavior. Later, this hyperactive mental state gives way to apathy, stupor and coma.

Laboratory investigations should include serum electrolytes, chest x-ray and an electrocardiogram. The serum T_4 level is raised, as is to be expected, but the level is indistinguishable from that seen with uncomplicated thyrotoxicosis. Therefore one must not await this result before commencing treatment.

MANAGEMENT

The patient should be admitted and urgent treatment should be directed toward the following.

Control of the Tachycardia. A β-adrenergic blocker, such as propranolol, 30 μg/kg, should be given intravenously over 10 to 15 min. Electrocardiographic monitoring for heart rate and arrhythmias is recommended.

Reduction of Body Temperature. Acetaminophen may be used if the hyperthermia is mild. Tepid sponging or use of an ice bath may have to be resorted to when the temperature exceeds 40°C.

Treatment of Hyperthyroidism. Stable iodine is useful in swiftly terminating thyroid hormone release. Lugol's iodine 2 to 3 drops 8-hourly orally, or sodium iodide 125 to 250 mg/day intravenously over 24 hours are doses derived empirically from adult values. Propylthiouracil 6 to 10 mg/kg/day in 3 divided doses, should also be given, although their effect will not be manifest during the emergency. Methimazole 0.6 to 0.7 mg/kg/day in divided doses every 8 hours may be used as an alternative to propylthiouracil.

General Supportive Measures. The child should receive adequate hydration, based on clinical estimates, and replacement of the electrolyte deficits due to gastrointestinal losses from diarrhea.

Administration of Glucocorticoid Hormones. Glucocorticoids are used, and their justification is based on theoretical considerations. Adrenal insufficiency may arise from increased catabolism of glucocorticoids during thyrotoxic states. Moreover dexamethasone has been observed to inhibit the release of hormone from the thyroid, and to increase the conversion of T_4 to reverse T_3 in peripheral tissues, thereby inactivating T_4. Dexamethesone, 0.2 mg/kg, or hydrocortisone, 5 mg/kg, can be administered as a bolus dose parenterally during the acute phase.

Management of Cardiac Failure. If cardiac failure is present, digoxin may be used (see Chapter 43).

Treatment of the Underlying Precipitating Factors.

Peritoneal dialysis, exchange transfusion, and plasmapheresis have all been used in adults, but should perhaps be reserved for those who fail to respond to the more orthodox forms of treatment. Improvement is usually seen within hours of commencing treatment. Full recovery may take a few more days. After the crisis has been resolved, elective thyroid ablation either by surgery or radioiodine must be considered.

Neonatal Thyrotoxicosis

BACKGROUND

This is a rare and potentially life-threatening condition affecting neonates; the diagnosis may, however, escape detection during the newborn's stay in the nursery. The incidence of hyperthyroidism in pregnant women is about 1 in 2000 pregnancies, of which neonatal thyrotoxicosis occurs in about 1 in 70 infants born to these mothers. However, maternal Graves' disease is only present in just over half of affected cases. The sex ratio is about 1 to 1 in contrast to the female predominance in autoimmune thyrotoxicosis.

PATHOPHYSIOLOGY

Neonatal thyrotoxicosis is probably due to transplacental passage of maternal thyroid stimulating immunoglobulins in most instances. The course is self-limiting in the majority of cases, and hyperthyroidism remits within about 6 weeks. Occasionally the disease may run a protracted course, and arise in the absence of maternal thyroid stimulating antibodies. This latter variety may represent a different etiology; its occurrence in families, has led to the postulate that it may have an autosomal dominant mode of inheritance, with a predilection for females.

CLINICAL MANIFESTATIONS

The infant may have a goiter and a staring, lean look. The appetite is increased but there is failure to gain weight. The child may be irritable and tachycardic, and there may be signs of congestive heart failure. Laboratory investigations should include estimations of serum T_4 and TSH. Increased concentration of T_4 in the presence of low or undetectable TSH levels are consistent with the diagnosis. However, in the first few days of life, these thyroid function tests may be unreliable, for values are dependent upon the degree of suppression of the thyroid in utero by maternal antithyroid medication. At the present time, only a few centers are capable of assaying for thyroid-stimulating immunoglobulins. In any case treatment, should not depend upon laboratory findings.

MANAGEMENT

If there is tachycardia and high output cardiac failure, a β-adrenergic blocker such as propranolol 1 to 3 mg/kg/day in 3 divided doses orally, is indicated. Rapid blockade of thyroid hormone release by a saturated solution of potassium iodide, 2 drops/day, can also be given orally. Propylthiouracil, 5 to 10 mg/kg/day, or methimazole, 0.6 to 0.7 mg/kg/day, in 3 divided doses, can also be used. Corticosteroids should be reserved for the severely ill neonate. General supportive measures, such as ensuring adequate hydration and the provision of adequate calories, should be undertaken. The duration of treatment is uncertain and should be based upon serial thyroid function tests. It is anticipated that treatment need only be continued for 6 to 8 weeks in the majority of cases.

Hypothyroidism

BACKGROUND

Children with acquired hypothyroidism do not develop urgent clinical problems and rarely present in the emergency department. However, although strictly speaking not a medical emergency, congenital hypothyroidism has to be recognized early so that prompt treatment might reduce the incidence of mental deficiency associated with this condition. Since the diagnosis is often missed in the immediate newborn period, the emergency physician must be aware of this disorder. Primary screening programs have revealed an incidence in excess of 1 in 5000 live births.

PATHOPHYSIOLOGY

The causes of congenital hypothyroidism are numerous. About one-third of the patients have ectopic glands, and another third have hypoplastic or aplastic thyroid glands. Other causes are uncommon and include dyshormogenesis, maternal ingestion of antithyroid medication, hypothalamic-pituitary disorders, and defects in thyroglobulin metabolism. A significant number of cases have no known cause. Thyroid deficiency results in impaired neurological development, delayed bone growth, myxedema in the subcutaneous tissues and tongue, and a reduced metabolic rate.

CLINICAL MANIFESTATIONS

Clinical signs and symptoms of hypothyroidism are often absent or so subtle as to be overlooked. Severely affected infants may be relatively heavy at birth, have a large posterior fontanelle, manifest hypothermia and hypoactivity, feed poorly, tend to become constipated, and have prolonged jaundice. Thyroid function tests beyond the first 2 days of life are most useful diagnostically. The TSH is elevated in primary hypothyroidism, and the T_4 low or normal for age.

MANAGEMENT

Treatment with L-thyroxine 37.5 mg daily should be instituted as soon as the relevant diagnostic tests are performed. This dose can be adjusted to maintain a T_4 level between 10 and 14 μg/dl, and a TSH value of under 10 microunits/ml after a few weeks of treatment. Both under- and overtreatment must be avoided.

References

Diabetic Ketoacidosis

Burghen GA, Etteldorf JN, Fisher JN, Kitabchi AE: Comparison of high-dose and low-dose insulin by continuous intravenous infusion in the treatment of diabetic ketoacidosis in children. *Diabetes Care* 3: 15–20, 1980.

Johnson DG, Alberti KGMM: Diabetic emergencies; practical aspects of the management of diabetic ketoacidosis and diabetes during surgery. *Clin Endocrinol Metab* 9: 437–461, 1980.

Kogut MD: Diabetic ketoacidosis. *Curr Prob Pediatr* 6: 3–35, 1976.

Moseley J: Diabetic crises in children treated with small doses of intramuscular insulin. *Br Med J* 1: 59–61, 1975.

Acute Adrenal Insufficiency

Himathongkam, T, Newmark SR, Greenfield M, Dluhy RG: Acute adrenal insufficiency. *JAMA* 230: 1317–1318, 1974.

Irvine WJ. Addison's disease. In *The Adrenal Gland*, edited by WJ Irvine. W. B. Saunders, Philadelphia, 1980.

Job JC, Chaussain JL: The adrenals. In *Pediatric Endocrinology*, edited JC Job, M Pierson. John Wiley & Sons, New York, 1981.

Tzagournis M: Acute adrenal insufficiency. *Heart Lung* 7: 603–609, 1978.

Congenital Adrenal Hyperplasia

Brook CGD: Congenital adrenal hyperplasia; pathology, diagnosis and treatment. In *The Adrenal Gland*, edited by VHT James. Raven Press, 1979.

Kaplan SA: Diseases of the adrenal cortex; II. Congenital adrenal hyperplasia. *Pediatr Clin North Am* 26: 77–89, 1979.

Lee PA, Plotnick LP, Kowarski AA, Migeon CJ: *Congenital Adrenal Hyperplasia*. University Park Press, Baltimore, 1977.

Migeon CJ: Diagnosis and management of congenital adrenal hyperplasia. *Hosp Pract* 12: 75–82, 1977.

New MI, Dupont B, Pang S, Pollack M, Levine LS: An update of congenital adrenal hyperplasia. *Recent Prog Hormon Res* 37: 105–181, 1981.

Diabetes Insipidus

Arieff AI, Guisado R: Effects on the central nervous system of hypernatremic and hyponatremic states. *Kidney Int* 10: 104–116, 1976.

Becker DJ, Foley TP Jr: 1-Desamino-8-D-arginine vasopressin in the treatment of central diabetes insipidus in childhood. *J Pediatr* 92: 1011–1018, 1978.

Hendricks SA, Lippe B, Kaplan SA, Lee W-NP: Differential diagnosis of diabetes insipidus; use of DDAVP to terminate the 7-hour water deprivation test. *J Pediatr* 98: 244–246, 1981.

Syndrome of Inappropriate ADH Secretion

Arieff AI, Llach F, Massry SG: Neurologic manifestations and morbidity of hyponatremia: correlation with brain water and electrolytes. *Medicine* 55: 121–9, 1976.

Hantman D, Rossier B, Sohlman R, Schrier R: Rapid correction of hyponatremia in the syndrome of inappropriate secretion of antidiuretic hormone: an alternative treatment to hypertonic saline. *Ann Intern Med* 78: 870–875, 1973.

Kaplan SL, Feigin RD: Syndromes of inappropriate secretion of antidiuretic hormone in children. *Adv Pediatr* 27: 247–274, 1980.

Rivers RPA, Forsling ML, Olver RP: Inappropriate secretion of antidiuretic hormone in infants with respiratory infections. *Arch Dis Child* 56: 358–363, 1981.

Zerbe R, Stropes L, Robertson G: Vasopressin function in the syndrome of inappropriate antidiuresis. *Ann Rev Med* 31: 315–327, 1980.

Thyroid Storm

Galaburda M, Rosma NP, Haddow JE: Thyroid storm in an 11-year-old boy managed by propranolol. *Pediatrics* 53: 920, 1974.

Hoffenberg R: Thyroid emergencies. *Clin Endocrinol Metab* 9: 503–512, 1980.

Machin JF, Canary JJ, Pittman CS: Thyroid storm and its management. *N Engl J Med* 291: 1396–1398, 1974.

Newmark SR, Himathongkam T, Shane JM: Hyperthyroid crisis. *JAMA* 230: 592–593, 1974.

Parks JS: Hyperthyroidism. In *Clinical Pediatric Endocrinology*, edited GCD Brook. Blackwell, Oxford, 1981.

Urbanic RC, Mazzaferri EL: Thyrotoxic crisis and myxedema coma. *Heart Lung* 7: 435–447, 1978.

Neonatal Thyrotoxicosis

Dirmikis SM, Munro DS: Placental transmission of thyroid-stimulating immunoglobulins. *Br Med J* 2: 665–666, 1975.

Hollingsworth DR: Mabry CC: Congenital Graves' disease; four familial cases with long-term follow-up and perspective. *Am J Dis Child* 130: 148–155, 1976.

Lee WNP: Thyroditis, hyperthyroidsm, and tumors. *Pediatr Clin North Am* 26: 53–64, 1979.

Singer J: Neonatal thyrotoxicosis. *J Pediatr* 91: 749–750, 1977.

Hypothyroidism

Barsano CP, DeGroot LJ: Dyshormonogenetic goitre. *Clin Endocrinol Metab* 8: 145–165,1979.

Burrow GN, Dussault JH: *Neonatal Thyroid Screening*. Raven Press, New York, 1980.

Fisher DA, Klein AH: Thyroid development and disorders of thyroid function in the newborn. *N Engl J Med* 304: 702–712, 1981.

LaFranchi SH: Hypothyroidism. *Pediatr Clin North Am* 26: 33–51, 1979.

CHAPTER **54**

Dermatology

PAUL J. HONIG, M.D.

ATOPIC DERMATITIS

BACKGROUND

The definition of atopic dermatitis is a confusing one. Many alternative terms are used to describe the skin inflammation (*dermatitis*) which is chronic and relapsing. Although the eruption may have a variable appearance (erythema, edema, papules, vesicles, serous discharge, and crusting), its constant feature is unrelenting pruritus. The eruption often has a characteristic distribution, depending on age (Fig. 54.1), and frequently occurs in allergic (*atopic*) individuals or those with a family history of allergies (hayfever, asthma, allergic rhinitis). Although many theories relating to etiology exist (genetic, physiologic, pharmacologic, immunologic), the data are conflicting.

Atopic dermatitis affects about 3% of children, beginning at 1 to 2 months of age. Sixty percent of those children who acquire atopic dermatitis will do so by the end of first year of life, 90% by 5 years, 95% by 10 years, and 99% between 10 and 20 years of age. It is difficult to predict the course of an individual case, but only 30% of those who develop the problem during the first year continue to have the disease during childhood. Ninety percent of all children who have atopic dermatitis during childhood will be clear by the time they reach adolescence.

PATHOPHYSIOLOGY

No single theory explains the initiation and progression of atopic dermatitis. There is evidence that a combination of factors is involved in the exaggerated reactivity of the skin, including altered physiologic, pharmacologic, and immunologic mechanisms.

Various studies have found that patients with atopic dermatitis have dry skin. This may be due to increased transepidermal water loss and/or decreased quantities of sebaceous gland derived lipids at the skin surface. There is also an increased sweating response to mecholyl. If this drug is injected into the skin of an individual with atopic dermatitis, it causes blanching rather than the usual erythema. Simple scratching of the skin in an atopic will induce white dermatographism. Finally, the β-adrenergic blockade therapy hypothesizes that reduced function of the β-adrenergic system leads to decreased production of cyclic AMP. This results in increased release of the pharmacologic mediators, such as histamines, producing pruritus and inflammation of the skin.

Abnormalities of immune activity have also been found. Humoral changes include elevated IgE levels and a higher than normal number of type 1 cutaneous reactions to common environmental allergens. Cell mediated abnormalities have been found only during acute flares of the dermatitis. These include: mild to moderate depression

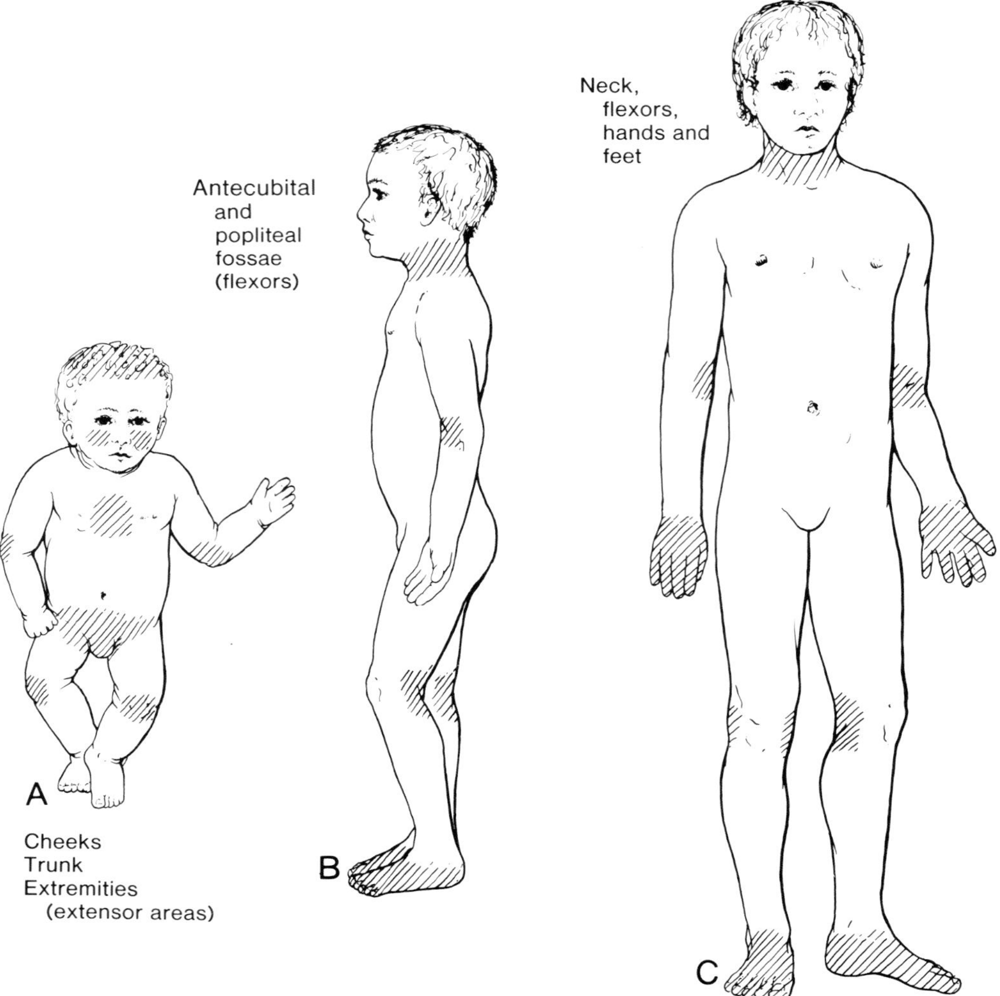

Figure 54.1. Distribution of atopic eczema at varying ages.

of cell mediated immunity, a 30 to 50% decrease in lymphocytes forming E-rosettes, decreased phagocytosis of yeast cells by neutrophils, and chemotactic defects of polymorpho- and mononuclear cells.

CLINICAL MANIFESTATIONS

The age of the patient frequently determines the distribution and appearance of the skin lesions. During infancy the itch-scratch cycle, which usually begins at 2 to 3 months of age, produces the erythematous, exudative lesions that appear on the cheeks and extensor surfaces. At times the process becomes generalized. Near the age of 2 years, the more characteristic flexural involvement occurs. Also indicative of atopic dermatitis are: varying sized patches of hypopigmentation, especially prominent on the cheeks (pityriasis alba) (Fig. 54.2); patchy or diffuse, fine papules (follicular accentuation) (Fig. 54.3), scaling in the scalp with or without hair loss; and hyperlinear palms and soles (Fig. 54.4) which may show desquamation. Involvement of the feet in such a manner often leads to the misdiagnosis of tinea pedis, which rarely occurs in the pediatric population prior to

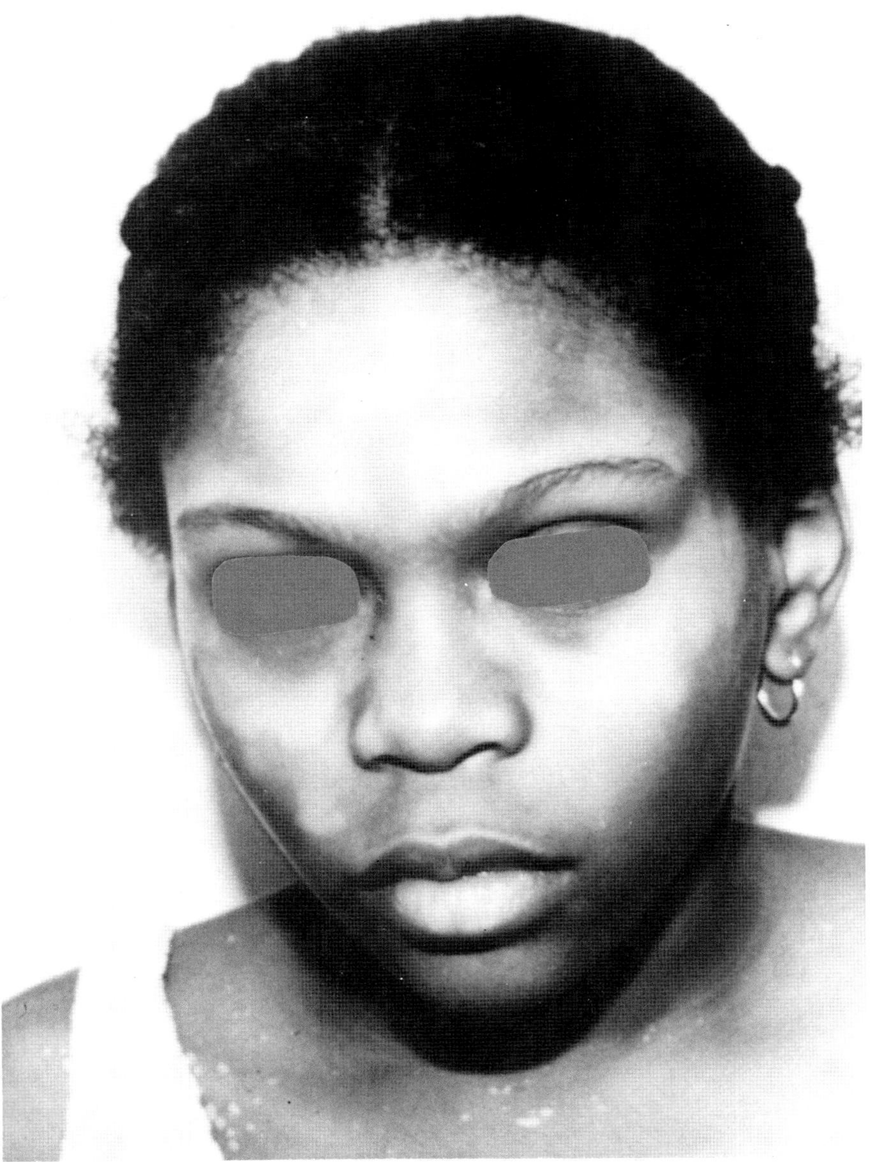

Figure 54.2. Postinflammatory hypopigmentation occurring in child with atopic dermatitis, termed pityriasis alba.

adolescence. During adolescence, the distribution remains the same; however, there is a greater incidence of involvement of the face, neck, posterior auricular areas, and the hands and feet. The major physical findings of chronicity, hyperpigmentation and lichenification, are frequently present (Fig. 54.5).

The diagnosis of atopic dermatitis is based on the presence of pruritus, typical morphology and distribution, and a tendency toward a chronically relapsing der-

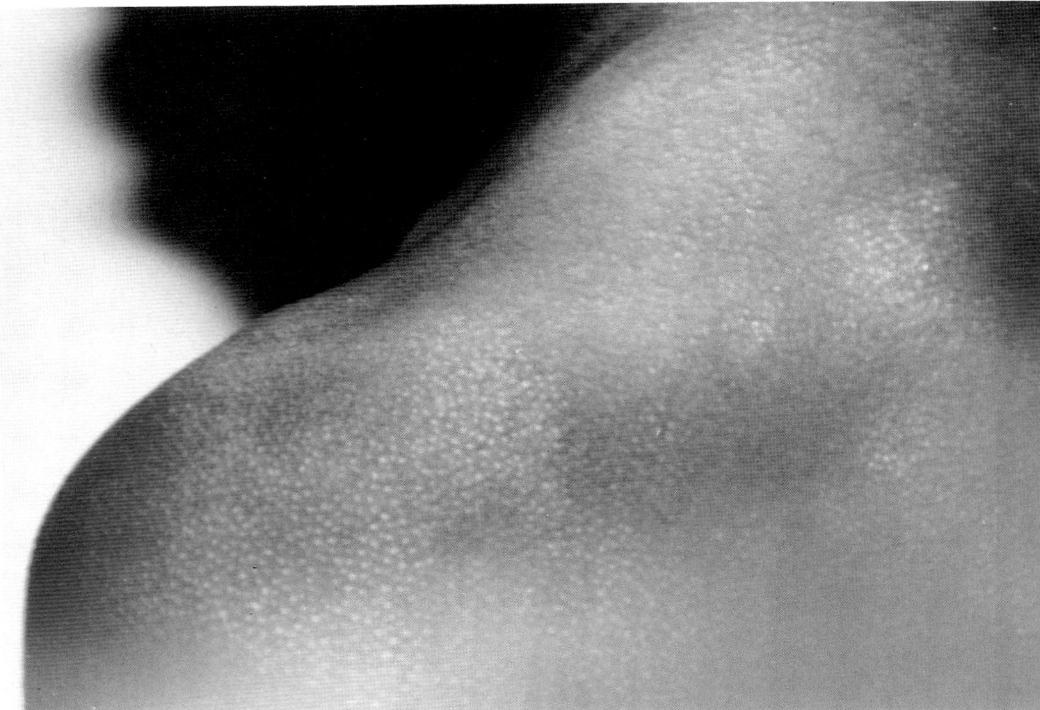

Figure 54.3. Follicular accentuation in a patient with atopic eczema.

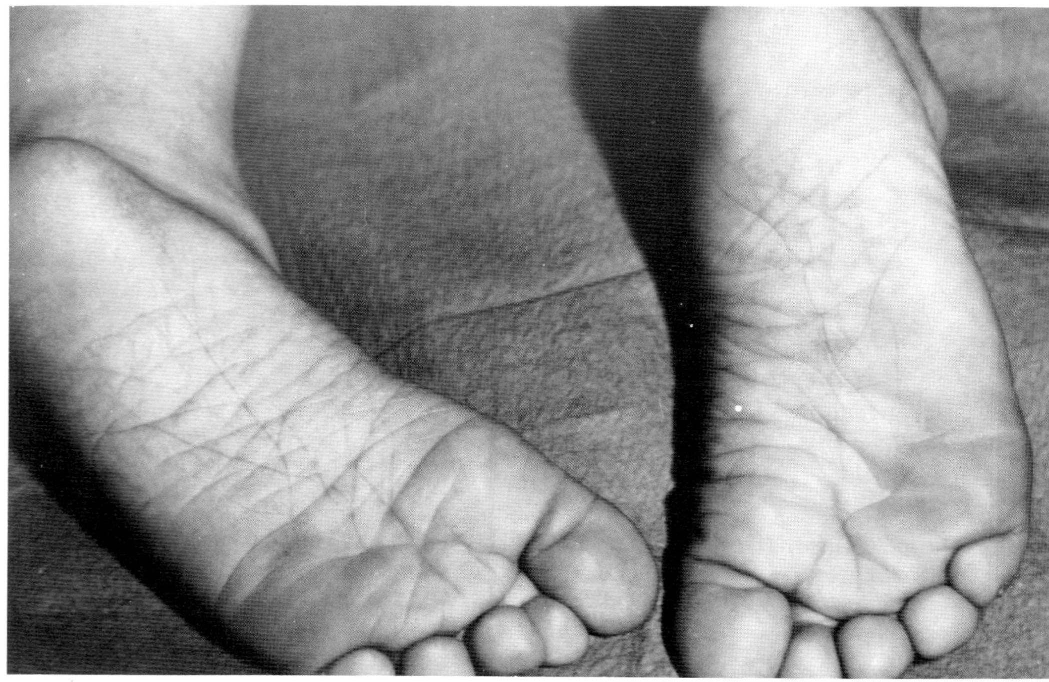

Figure 54.4. A patient with atopic eczema who has hyperlinearity of the soles.

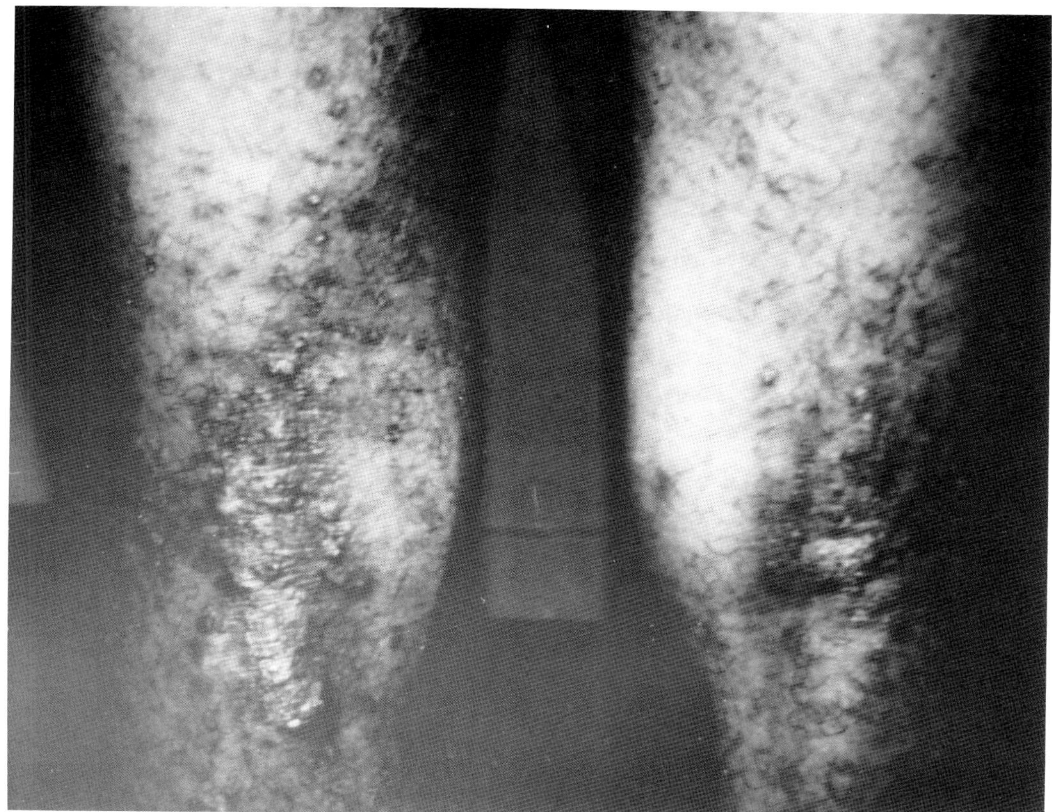

Figure 54.5. Chronic changes of hyperpigmentation and lichenification frequently seen in atopic eczema.

matitis. Other possible features are listed in Table 54.1. Unfortunately, there are no laboratory tests that help in the diagnosis of this disorder. Although eosinophilia and elevated serum IgE levels are present, they are not specific for this condition.

Differential Diagnosis

Atopic and seborrheic dermatitis may be difficult to differentiate when first appearing in a 1- to 2-month-old infant. Both may cause scaling in the scalp or diaper dermatitis. Clues pointing to seborrheic dermatitis include involvement of the flexural and intertriginous areas in the infant, a salmon-colored eruption with greasy, yellow scaling, and the lack of pruritus. Therapeutic clues include a rapid response to antiseborrheic shampoos and steroids in seborrheic scaling of the scalp as opposed to the lack of improvement, slow improvement, or, in fact, worsening of the scaling in the scalp in atopic patients.

Nummular eczema is an eruption that differs from atopic eczema in that the lesions are circular, erythematous, scaling, crusted patches or plaques. The lesions begin as papules and vesicles that spread and coalesce forming the typical coin-shaped patches. Pruritus is variable. Affected individuals usually do not have an atopic background, and IgE levels are generally not elevated. This disorder may be a manifestation of dry skin and, in fact, is aggravated by overwashing, harsh soaps, low temperatures, and low humidity. Decreased bathing, use of mild soaps and topical steroids are generally helpful.

Xerosis, or dry skin, is a condition that is commonly seen in patients who bathe frequently and use harsh soaps. Low temperatures and humidity will exacerbate this disease. Therefore, it is more commonly a problem during wintertime. The rash is pruritic and appears as rough, red, dry, scaling skin. It is similar in appearance to "chapped hands and cheeks" seen in cold weather. Decreased bathing, use of mild soaps, and lubrication of the skin are helpful.

There are also many immune and metabolic disorders associated with a rash that is similar in appearance to atopic dermatitis. These disorders are listed in Table 54.2.

Table 54.1
Diagnostic Features of Atopic Dermatitis

I. *Major*
   A. Typical morphology and distribution
   B. Pruritus
   C. Chronically relapsing course
   D. Personal or family history of atopic disease
II. *Additional Features*
   A. Xerosis
   B. Hyperlinear palms and soles
   C. Follicular accentuation
   D. Pityriasis alba
   E. Scaling of the scalp
   F. Ichthyosis
   G. Tendency toward nonspecific hand and foot dermatitis (pseudo-tinea pedis)
   H. Tendency toward repeated cutaneous infections
   I. White dermographism
   J. Elevated serum IgE
III. *Minor*
   A. Cataracts
   B. Keratoconus
   C. Dennie-Morgan (infraorbital) fold

Complications

Infection of the existing dermatosis is the principle complication in atopic dermatitis. Colonization and infection with *Staphylococcus aureus* is common among atopic children and may account for flares or failure to respond to therapy. Group A β-hemolytic streptococci are also cultured from many individuals with secondarily infected skin.

Viral skin infections also occur more frequently in patients with atopic dermatitis. Whether this is directly correlated to the impaired cellular immunity problem these patients have is not proven. Eczema vaccinatum, once a dreaded and often fatal complication, rarely occurs now since routine smallpox vaccination has been discontinued. The common etiologies for what is termed Kaposi's varicelliform eruption are mainly herpes simplex virus (Fig. 54.6) (eczema herpeticum) or on occasion coxsackievirus infection. Groups of umbilicated vesicles should be cultured for herpes simplex. A diagnostic procedure that may yield a quick answer to the presence of herpes simplex is the Tzanck test (Fig. 54.7). Material from the base of a freshly opened vesicle is scraped for a Giemsa stain. Multinucleated giant cells and balloon cells indicate the presence of herpes simplex. This virus can also cause localized flares of eczema without dissemination. Leyden described culturally proven recurrent local attacks of herpes simplex virus appearing as discrete punched-out ulcerations. The viruses that cause molluscum contagiosum and warts also infect individuals with atopic dermatitis more frequently than the average patient (Fig. 54.8).

Table 54.2
Immune and Metabolic Disorders Causing Rash

Metabolic Disorders	Immunologic Disorders
Phenylketonuria	Ataxia-telangiectasia
Acrodermatitis enteropathica	Letterer-Seiwe disease
Histidinemia	Wiskott-Aldrich syndrome
Gluten-sensitive enteropathy	X-linked agammaglobulinemia
Hartnup's syndrome	Hyper IgE syndrome
Hurler's syndrome	Selective IgA deficiency
	Severe combined immunodeficiency

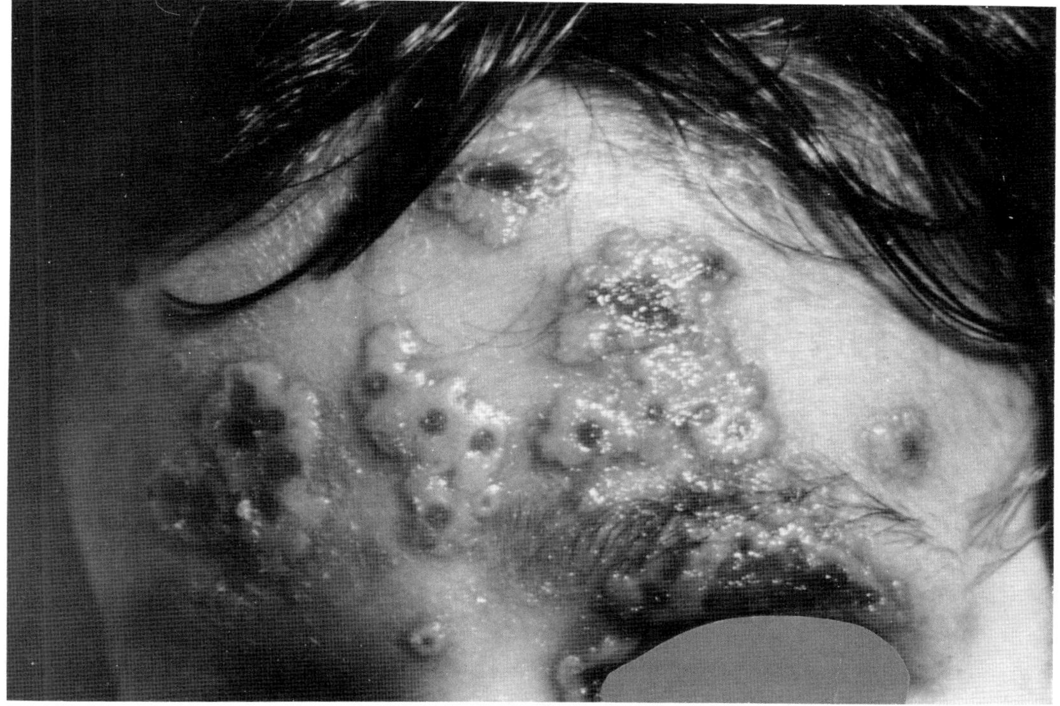

Figure 54.6. Eczema herpeticum.

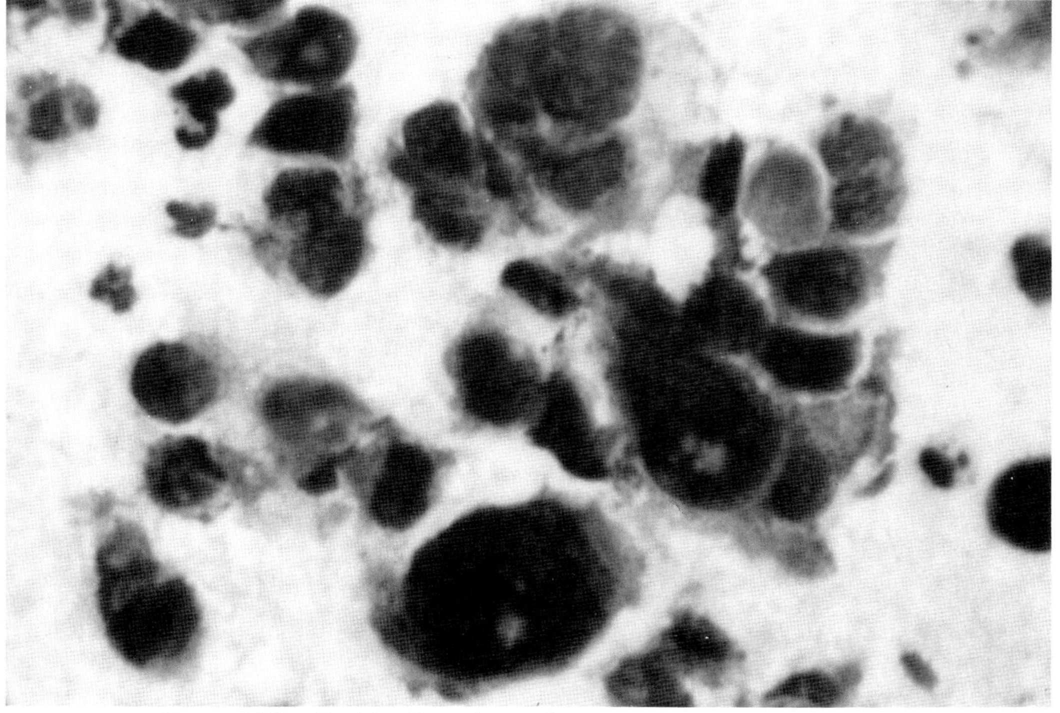

Figure 54.7. Positive Tzanck test demonstrating multinuclear giant cells.

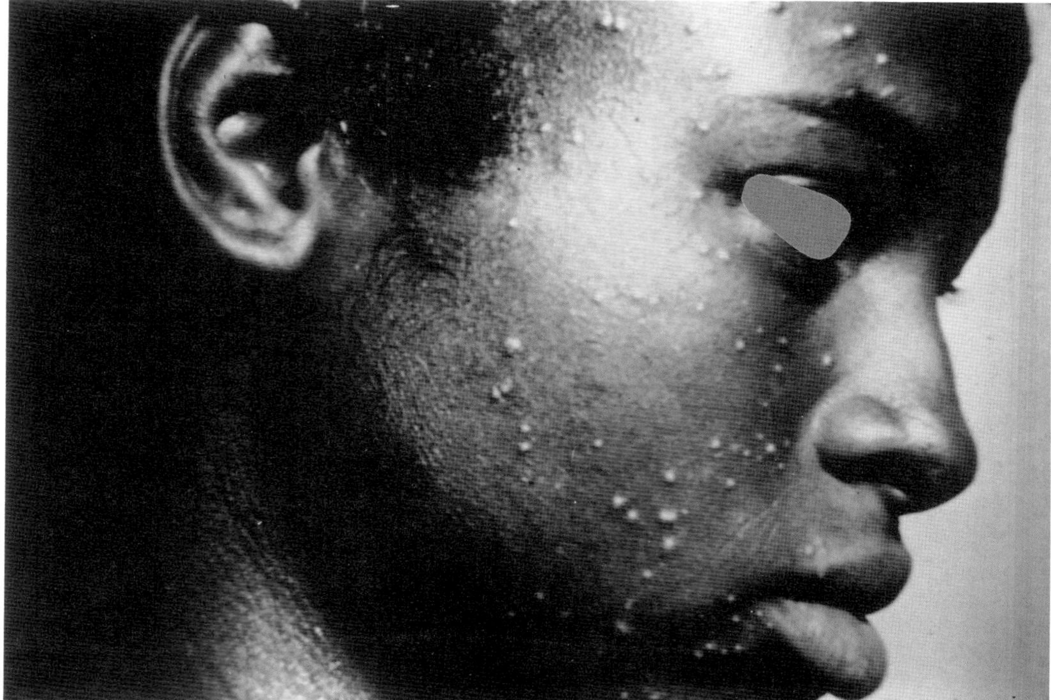

Figure 54.8. An atopic eczema patient whose face is covered with molluscum contagiosum.

MANAGEMENT

Skin tests and hyposensitization are of little value and rarely indicated. Dietary restrictions are controversial and as yet of unproven benefit. There are four main objectives in the treatment of uncomplicated atopic dermatitis: (1) reduction of pruritus, (2) reduction of inflammation, (3) protection of the skin from unknown irritants, and (4) removal of known irritants. Reduction of pruritus can be accomplished in numerous ways. Most important of these is limitation of bathing (at times, to only once per week) and the use of a mild soap (Dove, Tone, Caress). Lubrication of the skin ameliorates dryness which may be a factor in producing pruritus. Finally, antihistamines can be very helpful although, during infancy, soporiphic doses are necessary. Control of inflammation is accomplished with the use of topical steroids (see Table 54.3). During the acute phase, potent steroids should be used to bring the situation under control. Once control is achieved, steroids of mild potency should be used and applied less frequently. Maintenance with the least potent steroid, applied as infrequently as possible, is advisable. However, continued therapy is usually necessary. After control has been maintained for a fairly prolonged period of time, an attempt can be made to

Table 54.3
Potency of Topical Steroids

I. Mild
A. Hydrocortisone 1%
II. Moderate
A. Aristocort ointment 0.1%
B. Cordran ointment 0.05%
C. Synalar cream 0.025%
D. Synalar ointment 0.025%
E. Valisone cream 0.1%
III. Potent
A. Diprosone ointment 0.05%
B. Florone ointment 0.05%
C. Lidex cream or ointment 0.05%
D. Topicort ointment 0.25%

discontinue steroid therapy. Protection of the skin against unknown irritants is best done by covering it. Long sleeve polo shirts and leotards are helpful in preventing dust and pollens from coming into contact with the skin. Removal of known irritants is achieved by environmental control (i.e., no stuffed toys, wool clothing or blankets, or pets); avoidance of harsh soaps; and keeping fingernails short. At times hospitalization for control is advisable and certainly a more desirable alternative then systemic steroids.

Appropriate antibiotics are important in the treatment of secondary bacterial infections. A nontoxic child can frequently be treated orally in the home setting. Since penicillin-resistent staphylococcal organisms are frequently involved, antibiotics such as erythromycin (40 mg/kg/day) or dicloxacillin (50 mg/kg/day) provide suitable coverage. These antibiotics also treat group A β-hemolytic streptococci that may be present. When a child is toxic, intravenous therapy is advisable and, therefore, hospitalization is necessary. Again, penicillinase-resistant antistaphylococcal drugs should be given.

Eczema herpeticum that is localized and has not produced toxicity in a child can be treated symptomatically. It will usually clear in 2 to 3 weeks. With severe infection, especially in young infants, more aggressive therapy may be necessary at a center where adenine arabinoside (Ara-A) is available. A daily dosage of 10 to 15 mg/kg/day by continuous 12-hour intravenous infusion is recommended.

In the event eczema vaccinatum is encountered, vaccinia immune globulin given in a dosage of 0.6 to 1.0 ml/kg intramuscularly is advised. Repeated doses may be necessary.

SEBORRHEIC DERMATITIS

BACKGROUND

Seborrheic dermatitis is the term given to the salmon-colored patches with yellow, greasy scales occurring primarily in the so-called "seborrheic" areas (face, postauricular area, scalp, axilla, groin, presternal area). During childhood seborrheic dermatitis is seen in infants or adolescents. Its onset occurs during the first 3 months of life, and it generally disappears shortly thereafter, only then reappearing in adolescence.

PATHOPHYSIOLOGY

Although sebaceous gland dysfunction is frequently cited as an etiology, the cause of this disorder has not been established. In fact, surface fat levels are normal in seborrheic dermatitis, but their ratio is altered. There is a high correlation between the presence of seborrheic dermatitis and concomitant emotional stress or neurologic disorders.

CLINICAL MANIFESTATIONS

The two common locations of skin involvement during infancy are the scalp ("cradle cap") and diaper area. Most commonly, yellow greasy scales are found over the anterior fontanel. Scaling is concentrated in this location due to the fear some mothers have about rubbing or scrubbing over the fontanel. Many times the scaling is limited to this area; however, not infrequently there is spread to the forehead, eyebrows, nose, ears, and neck. The intertriginous and flexural areas may also become involved. This is especially true of the diaper area (see Fig. 54.14). The child is not irritable, and pruritus does not seem to be present. The prognosis for clearing is excellent, and resolution usually occurs within several weeks to months.

Between the periods of infancy and adolescence, scaling of the scalp usually indicates causes other than seborrheic dermatitis (atopic dermatitis or tinea capitis). In fact, true seborrheic dandruff does not appear until puberty when excessive production of sebum occurs. Most commonly, scaling before puberty and after infancy indicates the presence of atopic dermatitis or tinea capitus (especially *Trichophyton tonsurans*). Differentiation is aided by clinical appearance, cultures, and response to therapy. Atopic dermatitis is frequently made worse with harsh shampoos and responds very slowly to topical steroids. The diagnosis of tinea capitus is best made with cultures (Fig. 54.9). If steroids are used in

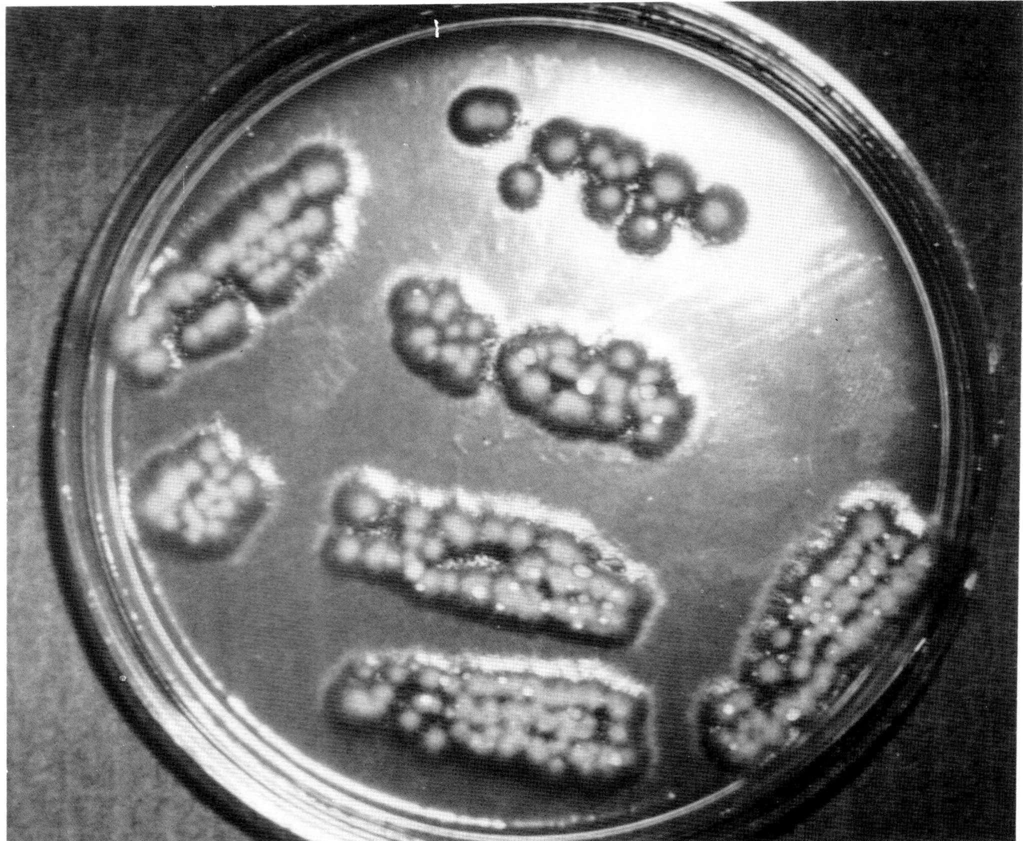

Figure 54.9. Toothbrush implants of scalp brushings that are growing fungus.

the presence of tinea capitus, there will frequently be increased scaling of the scalp secondary to suppressed local immunity of the skin and increased growth of the fungus. Seborrheic dermatitis of the scalp during the adolescent period is very similar in nature to the condition in adults. There is scaling in the scalp and the seborrheic areas are variably involved. Erythema and scaling occur between the eyebrows, on the eyelid margins, and in the nasolabial creases, sideburns, beards, mustache, posterior auricular areas, and aural canals. Rarely, there is secondary infection with monilia or bacteria.

MANAGEMENT

Seborrheic dermatitis of the scalp responds readily to antiseborrheic shampoos (i.e. selenium sulfide) and topical steroids such as fluocinolone acetonide or betamethasone valerate (Table 54.3). In infants, loosening of the scales with a soft toothbrush or fine-toothed comb prior to shampooing frequently hastens clearing of the "cradle cap." Topical steroids are very effective in the treatment of seborrheic dermatitis. Since hairy locations are frequently involved, steroid preparations in the form of lotions or gels are advisable. The strength of the steroid and the frequency of application is determined by the response to therapy. Steroids should not be used for prolonged periods of time on the face because of potential damage to the skin in that area. Secondary infection with bacteria can be treated with appropriate antibiotics. If *Candida albicans* secondarily invades the lesions, topical clotrimizole cream, applied twice a day is useful.

ALLERGIC CONTACT DERMATITIS

BACKGROUND

Allergic contact dermatitis is a cell-mediated reaction to antigenic material in contact with the surface of the skin. The incidence in children is about 1.5%, a considerably lower value than that given for adults. Children below 1 year of age rarely respond to contactants and, until nearly 3 years of age, have a reduced incidence of contact dermatitis.

PATHOGENESIS

An allergen penetrates the stratum corneum (facilitated by trauma at times) and combines with a carrier protein forming the foreign substance that is responsible for the initiation of the sensitization process. This complex is carried via lymphatics to the regional lymph nodes where processing by macrophages occurs. Recognition by T lymphocytes follows; these cells then leave the node, enter the blood stream, and migrate into the skin. When the antigen again comes in contact with the skin, sensitized T lymphocytes combine with the specific foreign material and release inflammatory lymphokines. Six to 18 hours later the characteristic dermatitis occurs.

Table 54.4
Regional Predilection of Varying Substances Causing Contact Dermatitis

I. Head and Neck
- A. Scalp—hair dye, hair spray, shampoo
- B. Ear canal—neomycin
- C. Forehead—hat band
- D. Eyelids—nailpolish, volatile gases, false eyelash cement, mascara, eye shadow cosmetics
- E. Perioral—dentifrices, bubble gum, chewing gum
- F. Ears—earrings, perfume

II. Trunk
- A. Axilla—deodorant, clothing dye
- B. Breasts—metal, elastic in bra

III. Arms. Wrist—cosmetic jewelry (nickel), leather (*p*-phenylenediamine, chrome)

IV. Abdomen. Waistline—rubber dermatitis from elastic in pants, jockstrap (lower)

V. Lower Extremities. Feet—shoe dermatitis

CLINICAL MANIFESTATIONS

The acute onset of linear or geometric areas of erythema, edema, eczematization, and papulovesiculation usually indicates the presence of allergic contact dermatitis. Because skin involvement is limited to areas of contact, the distribution, pattern, and shape of the dermatitis provide important clues for the clinician (Table 54.4). Therefore, a round lesion on the back of the wrist would incriminate a wristwatch; a linear pattern encircling the waist points to the rubber in the waistband of a garment; linear lesions on exposed portions of the body, indicate brushing against the leaves of a poison ivy plant (Fig. 54.10); and extensive involvement of exposed areas of skin suggests an airborne allergen as with ragweed or vaporized oil transmitted in the smoke of burning poison ivy (Fig. 54.11). Generally, the scalp, palms and soles are less permiable to allergens and, therefore, less frequently involved. Involvement of oral mucous membranes is uncommon. As mentioned previously trauma or nonspecific factors such as pressure, heat, and perspiration may predispose the skin to allergic contact dermatitis.

Fisher states that the most common causes of contact dermatitis in order of frequency are: rhus (poison ivy, oak, sumac), *p*-phenylenediamine, nickel, rubber compounds, and the dichromates. Although these conclusions are based on an adult sample, in general, they apply to children except for the substance *p*-phenylenediamine which is found in hair dyes and is probably at the bottom of the list.

Rhus (Poison Ivy, Oak, Sumac)

Rhus dermatitis is the most common allergen involved in the production of contact dermatitis. The poison ivy plant (Fig. 54.12*A*), occurs in all parts of the United States as a shrub or vine, frequently on trees or fences. Poison oak (Fig. 54.12*B*), an upright shrub, appears only on the west coast. Poison sumac (Fig. 54.12*C*), grows as a shrub or tree east of the Mississippi. Seventy percent of the population will become sensitized if exposed to the oleoresin, known as urushiol, contained on the leaf, stem, or root of the plant. The active ingre-

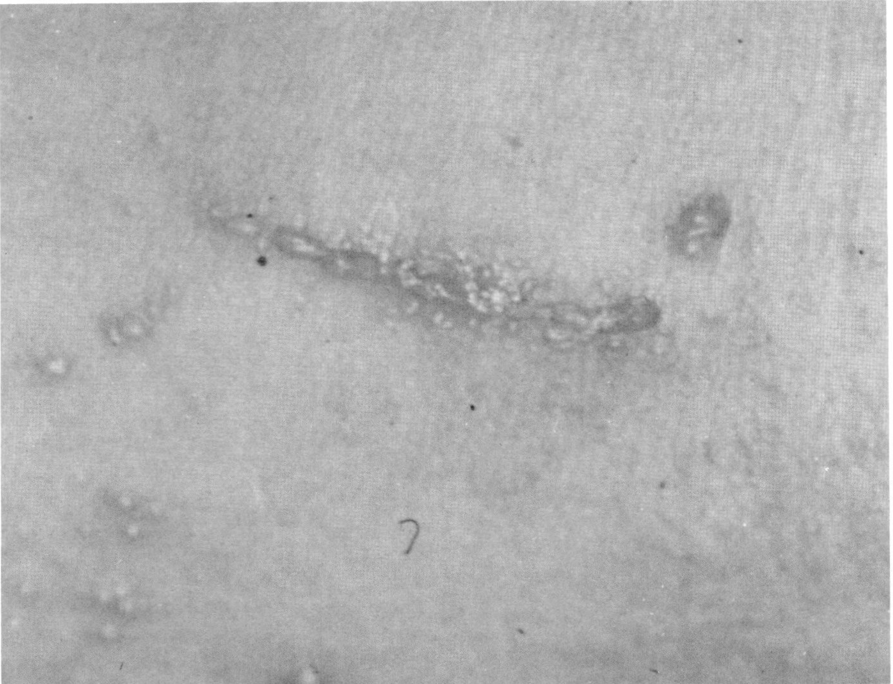

Figure 54.10. Typical linear pattern following exposure to poison ivy plant.

dient in this oil is pentadecylcatechol. The oil can be carried on clothing and pets or by the wind.

Each plant produces an identical redundant eruption. From the time of exposure the average time to the appearance of the rash is 48 hours. At that time, there is onset of pruritus, inflammation, and grouped or linear papulovesicles or bullae. With severe exposure, the face and eyelids become uniformly edematous. The eruption can last from 1 to 3 weeks.

Avoidance of exposure is the best prophylaxis in treatment. However, at times, this is impossible. Once an individual is exposed, contaminated clothing should be removed and laundered, and the body should be bathed with any soap as soon as possible, preferably within 5 to 10 min. Once the oil has been removed, spread does not occur, even from vesicular fluid. Although sequential outbreaks on various parts of the body suggest spread, lesions appearing later in time indicate exposure to a lesser dose of the offending oil initially.

Antipruritic lotions such as calamine are useful. Topical steroids are minimally effective, and topical antihistamines and anesthetics should be avoided because they can be sensitizers. Antihistamines can be helpful. With generalized reactions, oral prednisone 1 to 2 mg/kg once daily in tapering doses over 7 to 10 days is advisable.

Nickel Contact Dermatitis

Nickel dermatitis is frequently seen in the female in response to nickel-containing jewelry. Earlobes are commonly involved because of the popularity of pierced ears. Most articles of jewelry contain nickel, including those made of gold and silver. Any person wearing these items is at risk. Perspiration begins the process by leaching the nickel from the jewelry around the neck, wrist, or the fingers. Treatment consists of removing the offending object, avoiding further contact with nickel-containing jewelry, and application of topical steroids to the affected areas of skin.

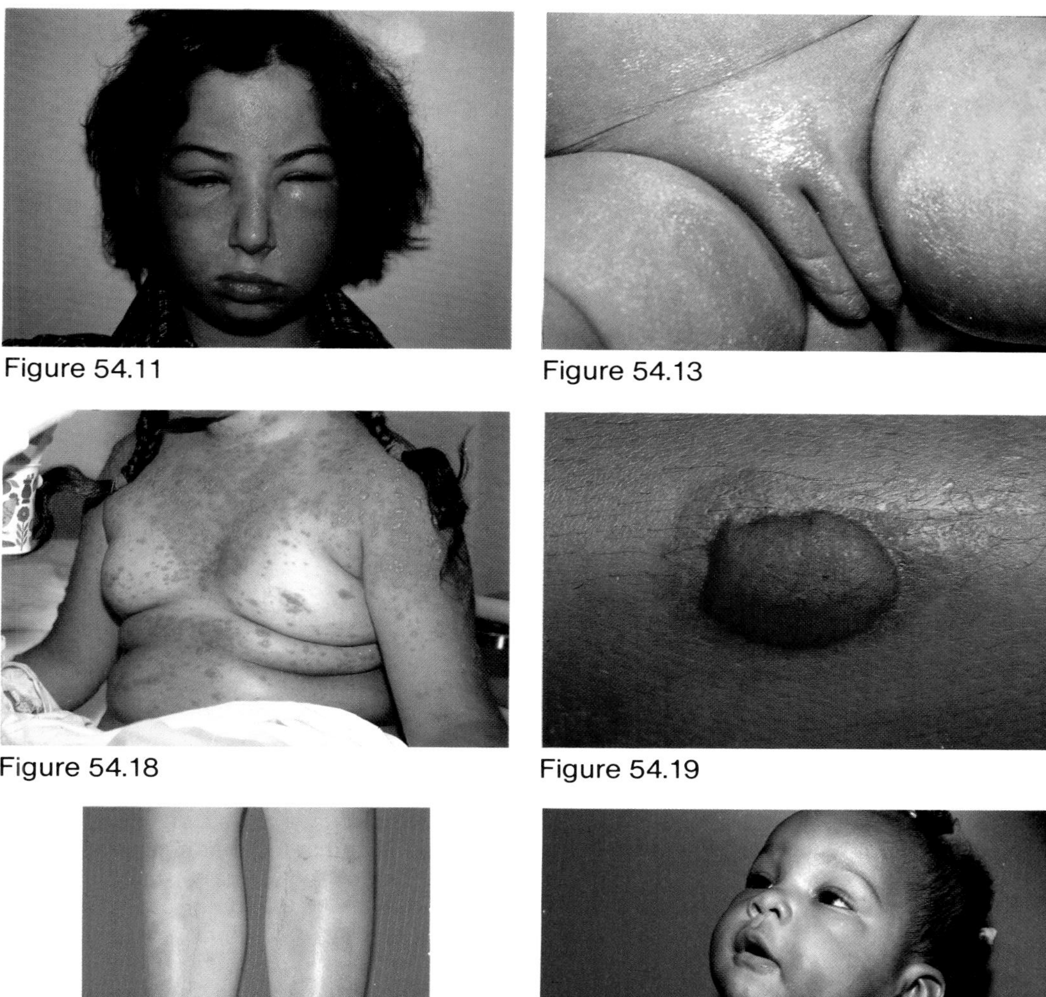

Figure 54.11

Figure 54.13

Figure 54.18

Figure 54.19

Figure 54.20

Figure 54.39

Figure 54.11. Facial edema and inflammation in response to exposure to airborn contact allergen (e.g., vaporized oil in smoke of burned poison ivy plants).

Figure 54.13. Infant with occlusion diaper dermatitis.

Figure 54.18. Same child as seen in Figure 54.17. Note photo distribution of lesions.

Figure 54.19. Hemorrhagic bulla in patient with vasculitis.

Figure 54.20. Extensor surface involved with lesions of erythema nodosum.

Figure 54.39. Infant with popsicle panniculitis of the cheek.

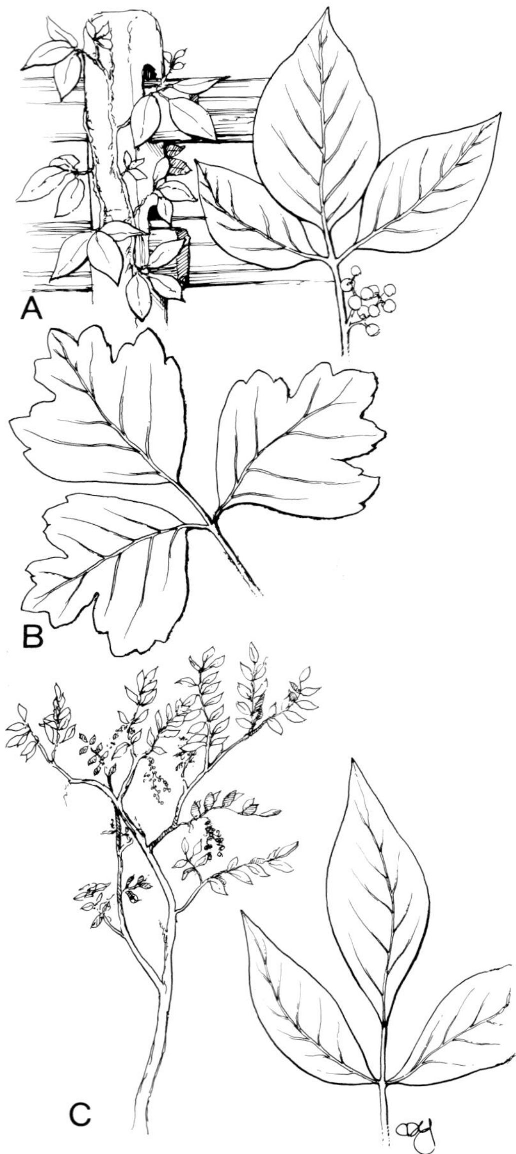

Figure 54.12. (*A*) Poison ivy (*Rhus radicans*), (*B*) poison oak (*Rhus toxicodendron*), and (*C*) poison sumac (*Rhus vernix*).

Shoe Contact Dermatitis

Erythema, blistering, weeping, crusting, or lichenification of the dorsal aspects of the toes and instep of the feet, with sparing of the interdigital webs, suggest the presence of contact shoe dermatitis. The offending agents are usually the rubber, glues, dyes, and tanning agents used in making the shoes. Although not recognized frequently, the problem is common. Those children who sweat freely are more likely to be affected due to the leaching of allergens from the shoes onto the skin. Secondary infection is frequent and an "id" reaction, similar to that seen in tinea pedis, can cause involvement of the hands and other areas of the skin distant from the primary site.

Patch testing kits for shoe components are available to determine specific sensitizing substances. This should be done only after the skin problem is brought under control, and probably by a dermatologist. Control is achieved by avoiding shoes whenever possible, treating secondary infection with appropriate antibiotics, and the use of topical steroids. All antihistamines are helpful for reducing pruritus. An "id" reaction consisting of huge bullae on the hands and feet can occur. The child is frequently unable to walk. Hospitalization and the use of systemic steroids (see section under "Rhus") is necessary.

Cosmetics

Many practicing physicians do not know that nail lacquers (containing sulfonamides and formaldehyde resins) or nail hardeners (containing formaldehyde) are a common cause of allergic reactions on the skin of the eyelids. The skin in this area is thin and permeable. Just rubbing the eyes with the fingers and nails which have the polish on them can induce the problem. *p*-Phenylenediamine, which is contained in hair dyes, will also cause eczematous eruptions of the scalp and face. Finally, ethylenediamine which is found in Mycolog cream (not ointment) may cause allergic contact dermatitis in the diaper area. Therefore, when a diaper rash that is getting better suddenly becomes fiery red, think of sensitization with this substance.

MANAGEMENT

Elimination and avoidance of the causal antigen is the most effective preventive and therapeutic measure. Topical steroids and antihistamines help with the inflammation and pruritus.

With localized involvement, moderate to high potency topical steroids can be helpful in reducing symptoms while the dermatitis clears. With generalized skin involvement, oral steroids are effective in a dose of 1 to 2 mg/kg/day over a 7- to 10-day period. Patch testing should not be done during an acute episode because contact with the allergen may cause worsening of the rash.

DIAPER DERMATITIS

BACKGROUND

Diaper dermatitis is a general term used to describe skin abnormalities beneath the diaper secondary to a variety of causes. The problem is a frequent one in children two years of age or younger who require the use of a diaper. It generally disappears following toilet training.

PATHOPHYSIOLOGY

The pathogenesis of the problem is multifactorial and not clearly defined. The possibilities include the concentration of bacteria or fungi, the action of organisms on the urine, and moisture itself.

There is no firm proof that bacteria play a major role. However, bacterial overgrowth does occur on moist skin with increasing time. In the past, bacteria were implicated in liberating ammonia, a supposedly irritating substance, from urine and raising urine pH. Although this is true, recent studies have shown that the concentration of ammonia and the pH of the urine are the same in patients with or without diaper dermatitis.

Candida albicans is found on the skin in 40% of infants with active diaper dermatitis within 72 hours of the appearance of the rash. Since studies show that this organism is present in less than 10% of infants without diaper dermatitis, *C. albicans* may be playing a significant role. Sources of *C. albicans* include the gastrointestinal tract and secondary implantation from a mother with candidal vaginitis.

Chronic exposure of the skin to moisture, especially under occlusion by the diaper, leads to maceration and alteration of the epidermal barrier with overgrowth of bacteria and *C. albicans*. If there is one major instigating factor, the effect of chronic exposure to moisture is critical to the development of diaper dermatitis.

Another consideration is the predisposition of certain individuals to react more easily and negatively to varying irritants. Generally, those infants with an atopic or seborrheic background are at greater risk for the development and persistence of diaper dermatitis.

CLINICAL MANIFESTATIONS

Differentiation of the various types of diaper dermatitis is difficult. Clues from the history and physical examination are necessary when characterizing the etiology of this problem. The different types of diaper rashes include: (1) occlusion dermatitis, (2) atopic dermatitis, (3) seborrheic dermatitis, (4) moniliasis, and (5) mixed or not diagnoseable rash.

Occlusion Dermatitis (Fig. 54.13). There are two components to this category of diaper dermatitis. The first, friction, occurs mainly on those portions of the diaper area where contact with the diaper is greatest (inner thighs, lower abdomen, and prominent surfaces of the genitalia and buttocks). The rash waxes and wanes and often has a shiny, glazed appearance on the surface of the skin. Occasionally there are associated papules. The second component, trapped moisture, causes the erythema and maceration that occurs in the intertrigenous parts of the diaper area (inguinal, genital, intergluteal, and folds of the thighs). This type of problem is frequently associated with and precipitated by tightly applied diapers, commercial paper diapers (especially those made with plastic edges to prevent leakage around the thighs) and rubber pants put over cloth diapers. Such coverings increase friction and prevent the evaporation of moisture.

Atopic Dermatitis. The appearance of the rash in the diaper area is not different from occlusion dermatitis. It is, however, more chronic and difficult to treat. Exami-

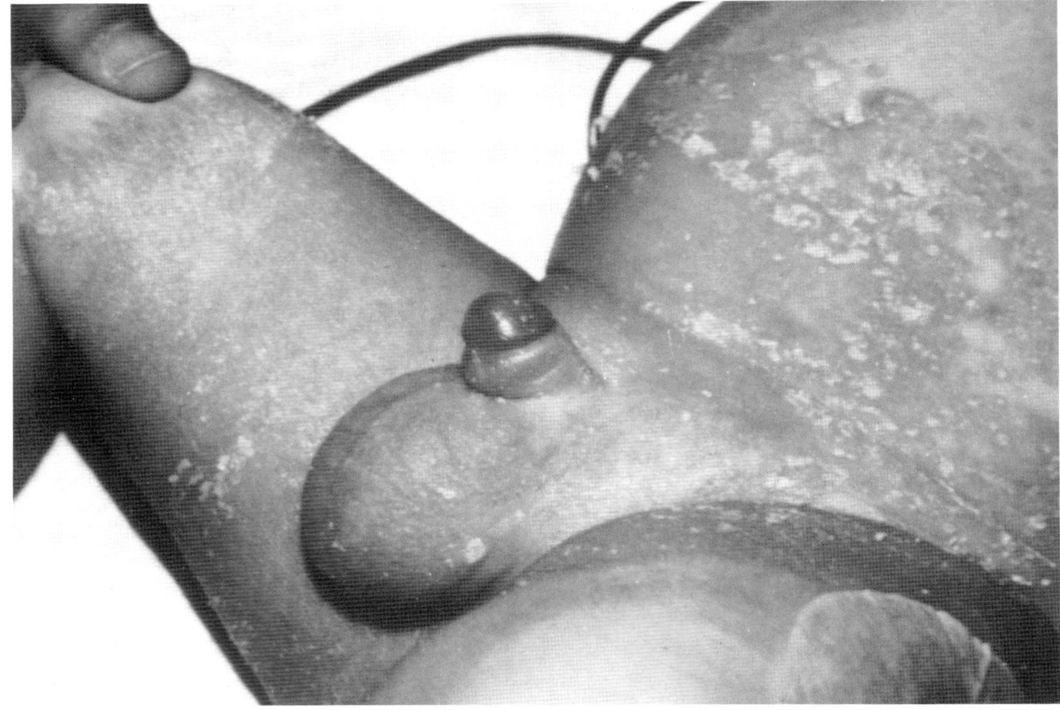

Figure 54.14. Infant with seborrheic diaper dermatitis.

nation may disclose lesions on other body surfaces (cheeks, antecubital and popliteal spaces) typical of atopic involvement, and there is often a family history of atopy.

Seborrheic dermatitis (Fig. 54.14). Generally, the rash has an erythematous base that is salmon-colored and covered with yellow, greasy scaling. Similar involvement of other seborrheic locations such as the scalp, postauricular area, or other flexures helps establish the diagnosis. At times there is a family history of seborrheic dermatitis.

Moniliasis. This is the most characteristic of the diaper rashes. The skin in the diaper area has clusters of erythematous papules and pustules that go on to coalesce into an intensely red confluent rash with sharp borders. Beyond these borders are satellite papules and pustules. At times the infant has concomitant oral thrush. When the problem is chronic and recurrent, seeding from the gastrointestinal tract or from a mother with monilial vaginitis should be considered.

On rare occasions an "id" reaction occurs (Fig. 54.15). Beside the primary monilial diaper rash, there seems to be antigenic dissemination with involvement of the intertriginous areas as well as scattered small patches or plaques of scaling erythema on other parts of the skin surface. Generally, *C. albicans* cannot be cultured from these plaques.

Mixed or Not Diagnosable Rash. Many times there are mixtures of the above categories of diaper dermatitis. Frequently a diagnosis is difficult to make. Secondary invasion with *C. albicans* is common as mentioned. The potential for secondary bacterial infection exists. If blistering occurs, *Staphylococcus aureus* infection should be considered.

MANAGEMENT

Treatment is determined by the etiology of the dermatitis. In general, proper skin care, which includes decreased frequency of washing, the use of mild soaps, and keeping the diaper off as much as possible, will help

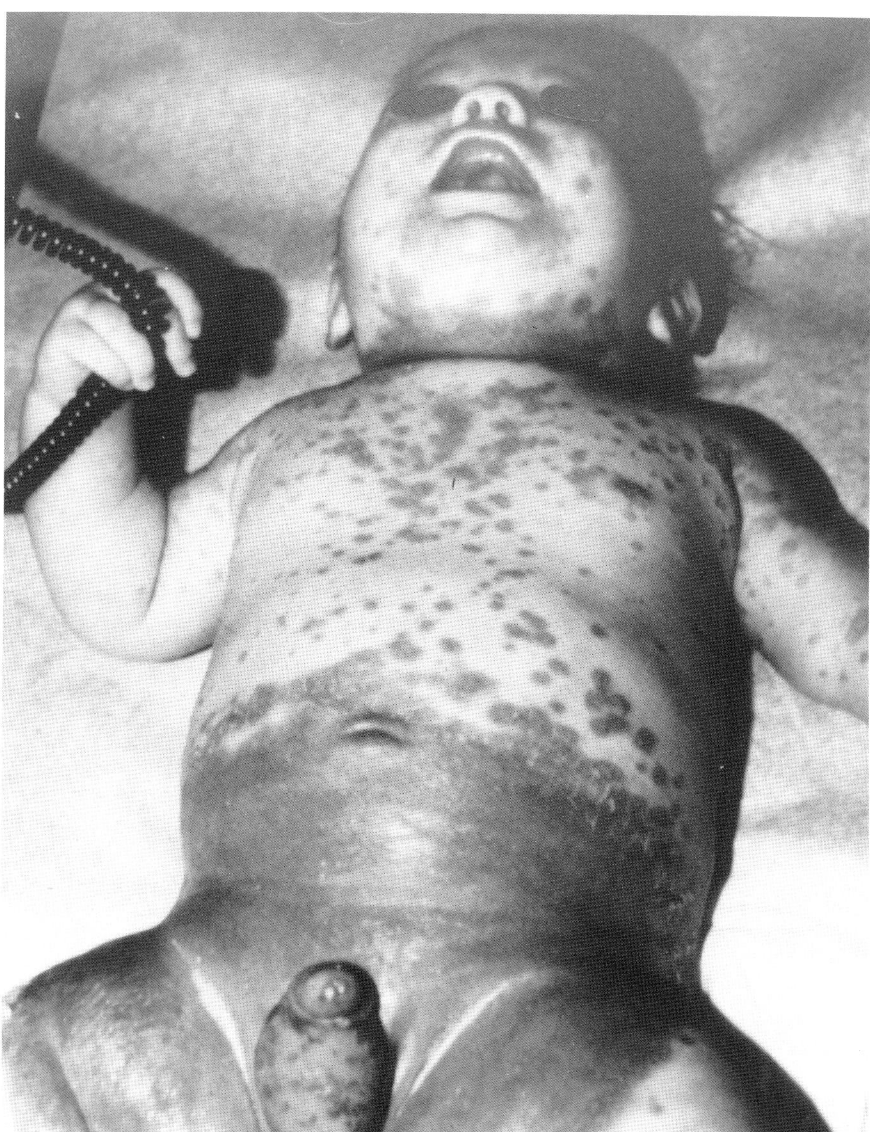

Figure 54.15. Infant with monilial diaper dermatis with "id" reaction.

resolve diaper dermatitis of any etiology. Certainly with occlusive dermatitis avoidance of tightly fitting diapers, plastic covered paper diapers, and rubber pants is important. When atopic dermatitis is present, the use of topical steroids is necessary. It is important to avoid fluorinated or other potent steroids in the diaper area because occlusion by the diaper enhances the steroid effect and is more likely to produce skin atrophy and striae. Therefore, 1% hydrocortisone cream no more than twice daily over a short period of time is recommended. Hydrocortisone (1%) is also very effective for seborrheic diaper dermatitis and can be used intermittently. With monilial diaper dermatitis, the use of preparations such as clortrimazole twice a day is quite effective. If thrush is also present, oral nystatin 200,000 units (2 ml) 4 times a day for 7 days, is advisable. This medication will also be useful if the infant is seeding *C. albicans.* from the gastrointestinal tract onto the skin of the diaper area. Since another potential source of *C. albicans* is from a vaginal infection in the infant's mother, the mother should be questioned for this problem; if a vaginal discharge is present, it should be checked by a gynecologist and treated appropriately. Those patients with "id" reactions, as described before, require oral nystatin, clotrimazole on the diaper and intertriginous areas, and 1% hydrocortisone applied to the plaques. Resolution usually takes 7 to 10 days. Mycolog cream is used for monilial diaper rashes by many physicians. One should be cognizant of the fact that this preparation contains a fluorinated steroid. Also, the cream (not the ointment) contains ethylenediamine which can cause a contact dermatitis as suggested by an acute flare during treatment. Secondarily infected dermatitis, such as bullous impetigo, should be treated with the appropriate systemic antibiotics.

Whether traditionally used diaper creams and ointments are effective is still unproven. Their ability to provide an effective barrier that reduces irritation remains to be established.

DRUG REACTIONS IN THE SKIN

BACKGROUND

When a drug is being taken by a child, any reaction of the skin that is not expected should be considered a drug reaction. Hospitalized patients are more likely (30%) to have a reaction to a drug because of multiple exposures. Approximately 2 to 3% of these inpatients have cutaneous reactions. The rate of adverse effects depend on the particular drug. Arndt and colleagues showed that reactions occur at the rate of 59 per 1000 drug courses for trimethoprim-sulfamethoxazole, while with the use of chloralhydrate, only 0.2 reactions per 1000 courses occurred. When considering all drugs, they found reactions at a rate of 3 per 1000 courses of therapy. Penicillins, sulfonamides, and blood products were responsible for the majority of reactions.

When considering penicillin and its derivatives alone, allergies to these substances affect 1 to 10% of the population. Fatal anaphylaxis occurs in approximately 2 per 100,000 patients taking penicillin. Penicillin reactions appear less frequently in children as is the case with any drug reaction. There is also an increased risk for the development of anaphylactic reactions to penicillin in atopic individuals.

PATHOPHYSIOLOGY

The pathogenesis of such reactions can be on an immune or nonimmune basis. When occurring on an immune basis, any of the four types of immunologic mechanisms (IgE-mediated, immune complex, cytotoxic, cell-mediated) can be involved. However, reactions also occur on the basis of overdosage, specific toxicity, common side effects of a particular drug, or unusual drug interactions. Often pathogenic mechanisms in specific situations cannot be identified.

CLINICAL MANIFESTATIONS

The appearance of drug reactions is nonspecific and may mimic almost any known dermatosis. Therefore, one cannot make a diagnosis of a drug reaction based on the appearance of the rash alone, because the skin can react only in a limited number of ways to many different stimuli. However, certain patterns should make one suspicious of the presence of an adverse reaction.

Laboratory analysis is usually not helpful in the diagnosis of drug eruptions. Peripheral eosinophilia, thought to occur commonly with adverse drug reactions, actually is uncommon. Skin biopsy can be helpful.

Specific Reaction Patterns

Urticaria. Urticaria constitute the most common expression of drug sensitivity. Most commonly, reactions occur within 1 week of drug exposure. When an individual is on multiple agents and has a reaction, one should suspect those agents that were most recently introduced or those medications that are known to be frequently associated with drug reactions (Table 54.5). When questioning for the use of medications, it is important to ask not only about prescription items, but also about over-the-counter preparations. Not infrequently, patients who use aspirin, acetaminophen, laxatives, or ear, nose, or eye drops, do not consider these substances as medications or drugs.

Maculopapular Eruptions Similar to That of a Viral Exanthem. Maculopapular eruptions are the second most common of all drug induced rashes and may be due to many different agents. They are symmetrical and consist of erythematous macules and papules with areas of confluence. There is variable involvement of the palms, soles, and mucous membranes. Purpura may occur. The presence and severity of pruritus is variable. Ampicillin is a medication frequently associated with this type of skin reaction, particularly in patients with infectious mononucleosis.

Table 54.5
Drugs Most Frequently Associated with Allergic Skin Reactions

Trimethoprim-sulfamethoxazole
Ampicillin
Semisynthetic penicillins (carbenicillin, cloxacillin, dicloxacillin, methicillin, nafcillin, oxacillin)
Sulfisoxazole
Penicillin G
Gentamicin
Cephalosporins
Dipyrone
Nitrazepam
Barbiturates
Nitrofurantoin
Glutethimide
Indomethacin

Erythema Multiforme. Erythema multiforme is an acute and frequently recurrent inflammatory syndrome often secondary to drugs (penicillins, sulfonamides, hydantoins, barbiturates) or infections. The skin findings include macules, papules, vesicles, and pathognomonic target or iris lesions (Fig. 54.16). Bullous lesions may also be present. In the more severe cases, constitutional symptoms occur; when mucous membranes are involved, the term Stevens-Johnson syndrome is used (Figs. 54.17 and 54.18). Erythema multiforme consists of two lesion types: (1) macular-urticarial and (2) vesicular-bullous. There is a predilection for the back of the hands, palms, soles, and extensor surfaces of the limbs. The lesions may begin at these sites and then spread diffusely or may begin generalized. In 25% of the patients, the mucous membranes are involved, and in fact, can be the sole site of involvement. The usual sites of mucous membrane involvement are the lips, buccal mucosa, palate, conjunctivae, urethra, and vagina. With severe involvement, the pharyngeal, tracheobronchial and esophageal mucous membranes are also affected. Less common sites are the

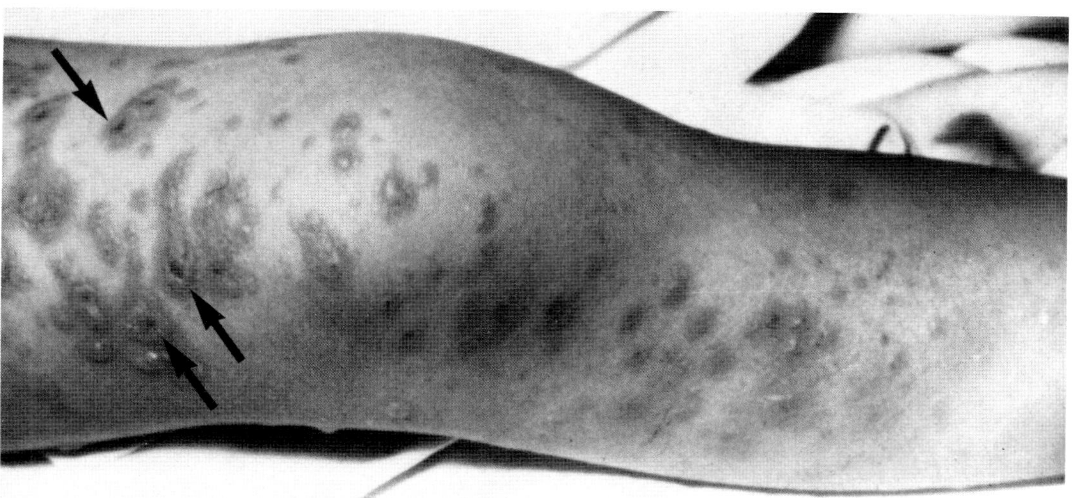

Figure 54.16. Iris or target lesions pathognomonic of erythema multiforme.

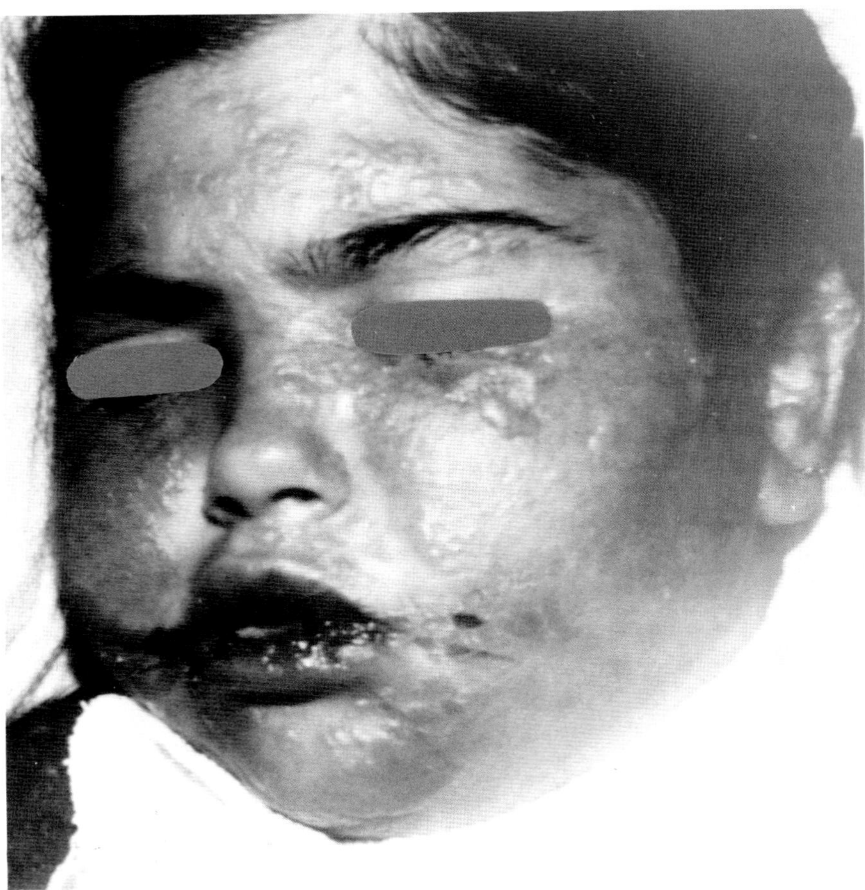

Figure 54.17. Adolescent with Stevens-Johnson syndrome secondary to sulfonamides. Note involvement of mucous membranes of mouth.

anal and nasal mucosa. When the eyes are involved, there may be simple conjunctivitis, severe keratitis, or panophthalmitis, lead to blindness in 3 to 10% of these patients. Therefore, close attention to involvement of the eyes is necessary. Lesions may continue to erupt in crops for as long as 2 to 3 weeks. Death occurs in 3 to 15% of patients.

Vasculitis. The classic lesions of vasculitis are palpable purpura. Although these lesions are characteristic, vasculitis may be manifest by erythematous macules, papules, urticaria, and hemorrhagic vesicles and bullae (Fig. 54.19). The diagnosis is made by skin biopsy which shows leukocytoclasis, endothelial cell necrosis, and destruction of dermal vessels.

Erythema Nodosum. The lesions of erythema nodosum appear as deep, tender, erythematous nodules or plaques of the extensor surfaces of the extremities (Fig. 54.20). They are thought to be hypersensitivity phenomena secondary to infections (streptococcal pharyngitis, tuberculosis, coccidiomycosis, histoplasmosis), inflammatory bowel disease, sarcoidosis, malignancies, and on occasion drugs. The exact immunologic mechanism has not been clarified.

Photosensitive Cutaneous Eruption. When a drug causes an exaggeration of the sunburn response, a phototoxic eruption should be considered. Photoallergic eruptions, however, usually do not occur on first exposure to a medication, because immunologic induction must first occur. Since a hypersensitivity reaction is also involved, the eruption, although concentrated most heavily on sun-exposed areas, can also occur on non-sun-exposed area. Tetracycline and sulfonamides can be involved in this reaction.

Toxic Epidermal Necrolysis (TEN). Drug-induced TEN must be differentiated from an illness caused by a circulating staphylococcal exotoxin (see p. 673). If a child who has TEN has been on drugs chronically or shortly before onset of the rash, is over 6 years of age, or has a mixed rash (i.e. areas with the appearance of erythema multiforme as well as toxic epidermal necrolysis), a biopsy must be done to distinguish between the two disorders. With drug-induced TEN, one sees dermal-epidermal separation on histologic examination. If epidermolytic toxin has been released by staphylococci, epidermal cleavage occurs in the granular layer (see Fig. 54.23). With extensive exfoliation of skin, fluid and electrolyte disturbances may occur and the potential for bacterial sepsis is present.

Fixed Drug Eruption. This term refers to a localized round or oval dermatitis that tends to recur at the same location each time there is exposure to the offending drug. The lesions are generally erythematous and may or may not contain vesicles. They disappear over a period of 7 to 10 days after cessation of the drug, leaving various shades of postinflammatory hyperpigmentation in their place. The discoloration may persist for months or years. Initially, lesions are solitary but then can become multiple; they frequently involve the palms, soles, glans penis, and lips.

MANAGEMENT

Vital to the management of any suspected drug reaction is the identification and removal of the offending drug. Pruritus can be controlled with antihistamines, and open lesions are responsive to compressing. Whenever extensive exfoliation occurs, attention to fluid and electrolyte balance and secondary infection is essential. Although there are no controlled studies to substantiate the efficacy of systemic steroids, most physicians would certainly use them in a seriously ill child. Any patient with mucous membrane involvement should have an ophthalmologic examination to rule out the presence of corneal involvement. Hospitalization should be considered in any patient who has severe involvement of the skin, is toxic, or has extensive exfoliation.

STAPHYLOCOCCAL SCALDED SKIN SYNDROME (SSSS) (TOXIC EPIDERMAL NECROLYSIS)

BACKGROUND

The term toxic epidermal necrolysis (TEN) is often used indiscriminately. In fact, it has very different meanings to the pediatrician and the internist. When used by the pediatrician, it usually indicates a disease process induced by an exfoliative toxin released by *Staphylococcus aureus.* When applied by the internist, a drug reaction is usually suspected. Since the gross dermatologic changes are the same despite different etiologies, this term should be used to indicate only the visible changes. In this way, the physician will approach patients with an open mind and be more likely to consider the alternative possibilities: though rare, a drug-induced TEN in children and bacteria-induced TEN in adults. We will consider staphylococcus-induced TEN or the staphylococcal scalded skin syndrome, in this section. Included under the heading of staphylococcal scalded skin syndrome are bullous impetigo (staphylococcal pustulosis in newborns), scarlatiniform rashes induced by *S. aureus*, and the generalized exfoliative syndrome caused by *S. aureus* seen in newborns (Ritter's disease) or in children (Lyell's syndrome).

PATHOPHYSIOLOGY

The mechanism of these reactions was described by Mellish and Glasgow. They injected coagulase-positive phage group II staphylococci into newborn mice, producing erythema and a positive Nikolsky sign (denudation of skin with gentle rubbing) in 12 to 16 hours, followed by bullae and extensive exfoliation in 16 to 20 hours. Since that time, phage group I and III staphylococci have been implicated also. The disease is felt to occur primarily in children because they lack antibodies against the organism and are unable to metabolize and excrete the toxin as well as adults.

CLINICAL MANIFESTATIONS

The illness begins with malaise, fever, and irritability. The irritability is frequently due to marked tenderness of the skin when touched. Mothers will relate that their infant does not want to be held and cries when handled. A "sunburn" erythema follows which first begins and is most intense around the neck, the intertriginous areas, and periorifically (especially the eyes and mouth). The erythema spreads to varying portions of the skin surface, and the child may be very toxic. With mild involvement of the skin, superficial desquamation (flaking) then follows as after an ordinary sunburn (Fig. 54.21). With severe involvement large sheets of skin sheer away, leaving a denuded, oozing, surface similar to that occurring after a burn (Fig. 54.22). Often the skin can be rubbed off (Nikolsky's sign). Vesicles, pustules, and bullae can also occur during the exfoliative phase. Frequently there is a purulent discharge from the eyes, but no conjunctival injection. Mucous membranes are not involved. Most children do quite well, and clearing of the skin occurs in 12 to 14 days, leaving no residua.

The CBC and urinalysis are not helpful in the evaluation of such children. Although blood cultures should be done, they are usually negative as are cultures of intact vesicles or bullae. At times, *S. aureus* can be grown from exfoliating skin, the umbilicus, circumcision wounds, throat, eyes, ears, nose, or rectum. Histological examination of the skin distinguishes between TEN caused by staphylococci or by a drug reaction. In the staphylococcal scalded skin syndrome, skin clippings or a punch biopsy show separation of the superficial layer of the epidermis subcorneally (Fig. 54.23, *A* and *B*). Patients who have drug-induced TEN will have dermal-epidermal separation (Fig. 54.23, *C* and *D*). Children on medications chronically or shortly before the eruption of the rash, children over 6 years of age, or children with a mixed rash (i.e., areas of TEN and erythema multiforme) should have a skin biopsy done for differentiation.

Etiologies other than *S. aureus* or drugs may produce a similar clinical picture. These conditions include certain fumigants, lymphomas, aspergillosis, irradiation, and graft vs. host reaction. More recently the toxic shock syndrome has been described (see Table 54.6).

MANAGEMENT

Most of the time, TEN is a self-limited disorder. Antibiotics probably ameliorate the course of the disease, but steroids have no beneficial effects. In fact, steroids may exacerbate the dermatitis by increasing the ability of the organisms to proliferate and produce greater amounts of epidermolytic toxin.

Neonates and children less than 1 year of age should be admitted to the hospital and started on intravenous antistaphylococcal antibiotics (cefazolin, oxacillin) after blood cultures are obtained. Additionally, any older child who is toxic or has severe skin involvement with marked denudation should be admitted. Close attention should be paid to state of hydration and electrolyte imbalances when a significant amount of skin is lost. Secondary infection, as in a patient with a major burn, is an important consideration.

Older children with mild involvement limited to dry desquamation, who are not toxic, can be managed on an outpatient basis. These children can be started on oral dicloxacillin or erythromycin and followed closely. Skin care is nonspecific unless extensive denudation occurs; then the use of Silvadene cream is warranted.

BITES AND INFESTATIONS

Children are often bitten by insects (especially mosquitoes and fleas) and at times infested by parasites. The papules, urticaria, blisters, and hemorrhagic lesions pro-

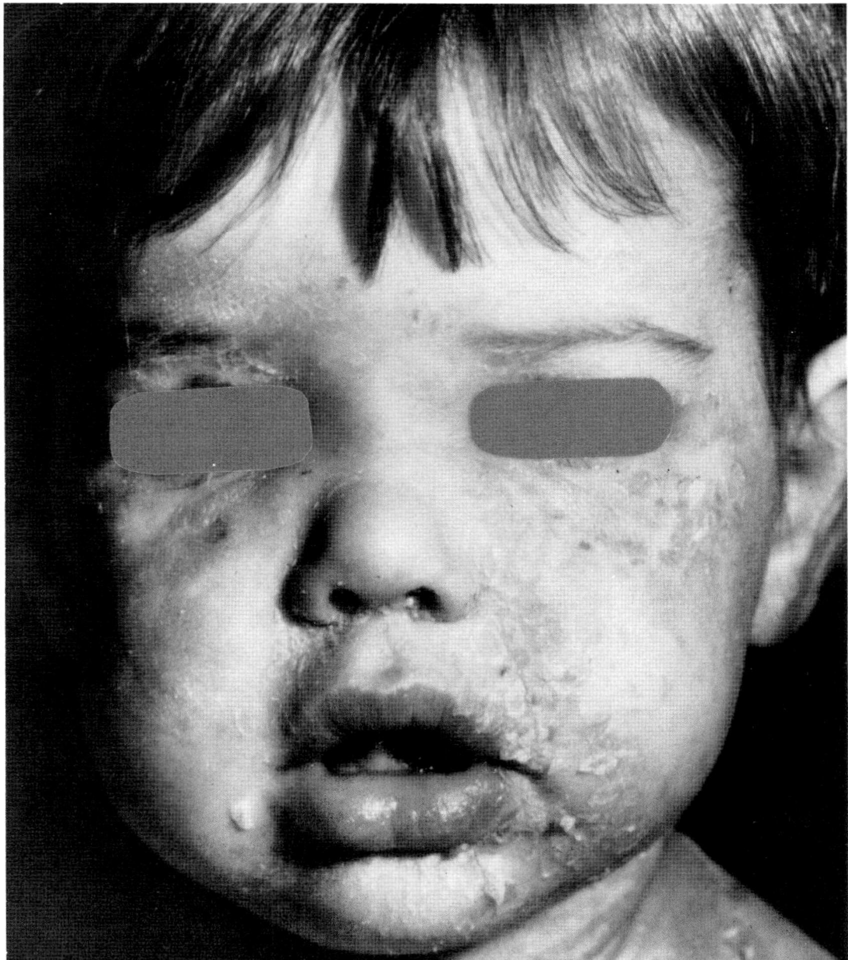

Figure 54.21. Desquamation of skin of face in the staphylococcal scalded skin syndrome (SSSS).

duced are frequently misdiagnosed. The season of the year, area of the country, grouping and appearance (central punctum) of the lesions, and distribution on exposed surfaces provide the clues necessary for diagnosis.

Mosquitoes and Fleas

Mosquitoes are probably the most common cause of insect bites in childhood, followed closely by fleas (Fig. 54.24). Mosquito bites are generally limited to the warm months of the year. On the other hand, flea bites, which predominate from spring to fall, can also occur during the winter months due to cats and dogs living indoors. At times flea bites occur without an animal living in the household. Generally, one should ask for a history of visits to a household that does have pets or whether the patient's family has recently moved into a home in which the prior owners had pets. In the latter situation, fleas can live in carpeting for a long period of time.

The distribution of lesions is a valuable clue in making the diagnosis of mosquito or flea bites. Insect bites generally involve the

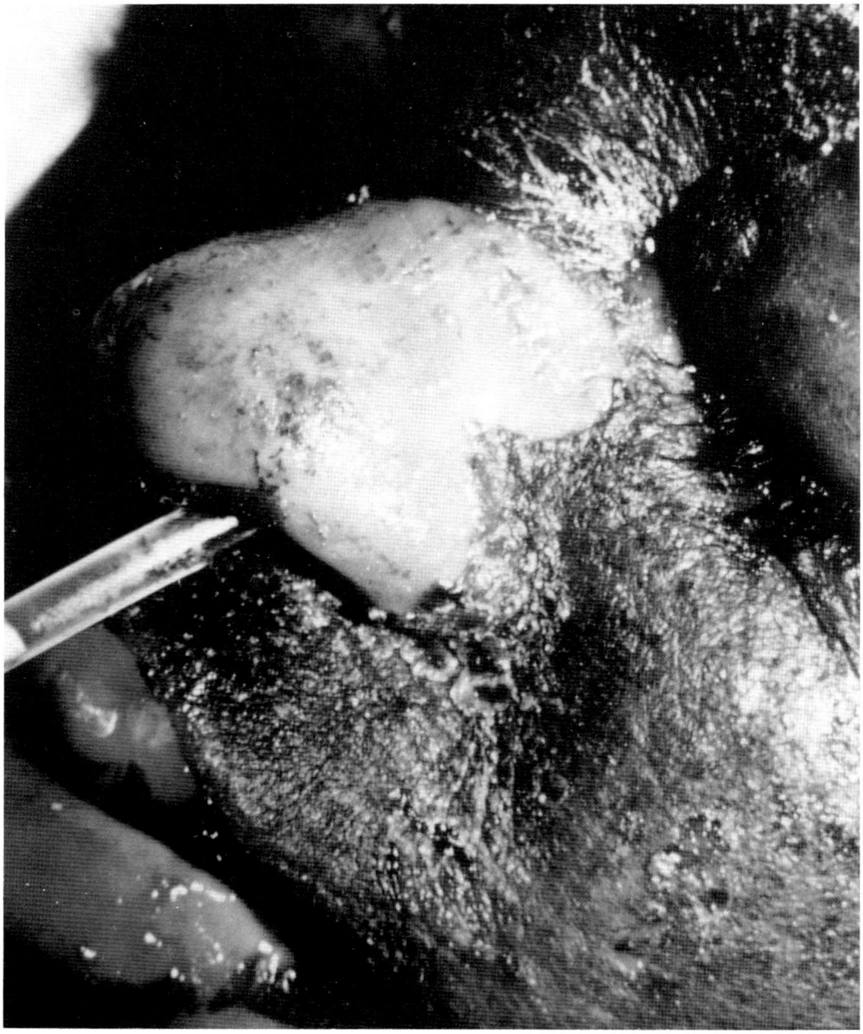

Figure 54.22. Denudation of skin of nose in child with staphylococcal scalded skin syndrome (SSSS).

exposed surfaces of the head, face, and extremities. The lesions are usually urticarial wheals which occur in groups or along a line on which the insect was crawling. On occasion, both mosquito bites and flea bites can cause blistering lesions. These lesions are not due to secondary infection but rather to a violent immune response to the bite. Certainly, excoriation with resulting secondary infection with *S. aureus* or Group A streptococci can complicate a simple bite.

A recurrent papular eruption termed papular urticaria can occur in young children who become sensitized to insect bites. Although the lesions tend to occur on exposed parts of the body, with sensitization, they may appear at sites distant from the primary bite.

Unfortunately, there is no effective treatment for insect bites. Antihistamines, calamine lotion, or topical steroids have a limited or temporary effect. Prevention by the prophylactic use of insect repellents offers

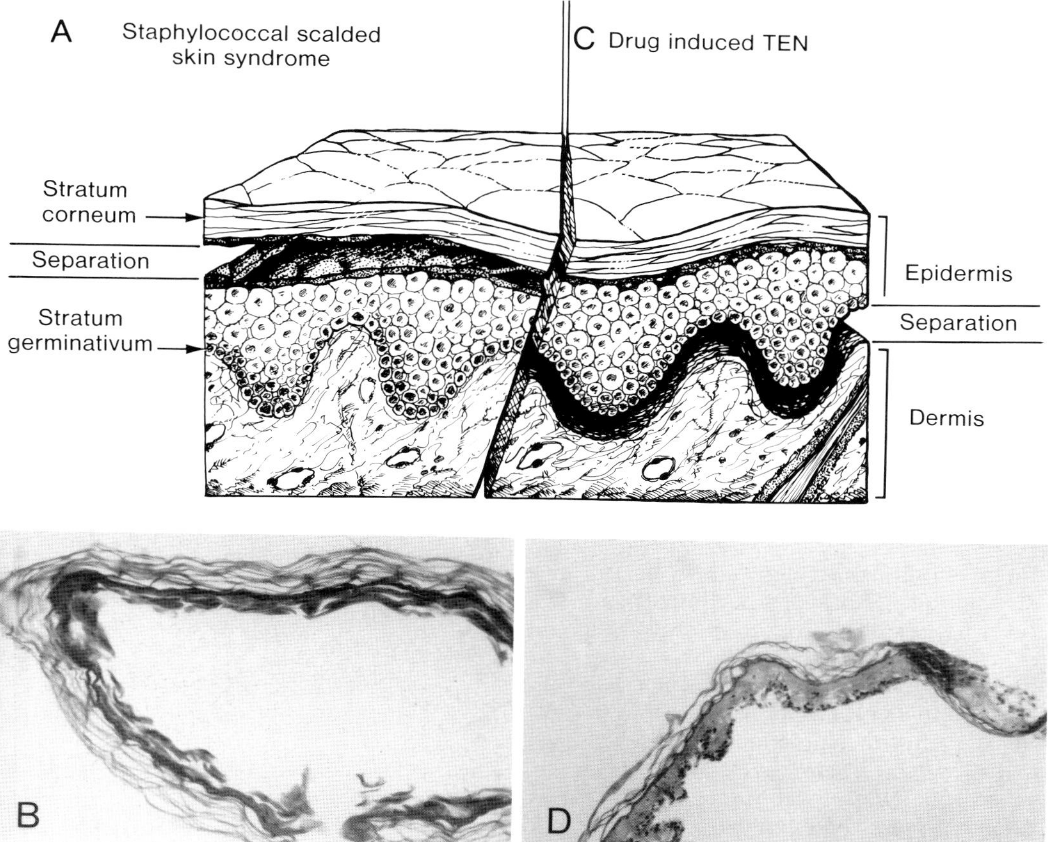

Figure 54.23. (*A* and *B*) Pathology in staphylococcal scalded skin syndrome (SSSS). (*C* and *D*) Pathology in drug-induced TEN.

the best solution. Obviously, elimination of the biting insects by treatment of the homes with insecticides or treatment of the infested animals is important.

Tick bites

Usually, tick bites cause only local reactions. Rarely they are associated with significant systemic illness including Rocky Mountain spotted fever, tick paralysis, and Lyme arthritis.

When ticks are removed it is important not to leave fragments of the mouth parts in the skin. Various methods are recommended for removal of ticks from the skin. These methods include application of a few drops of chloroform to the tick; touching the tick with a hot, previously lighted match; or covering the tick with nail polish, mineral oil, or Vaseline. If mouth parts are left in the skin, they should be removed.

Table 54.6
Toxic Shock Syndrome

Fever
Toxic epidermal necrolysis-like rash
Desquamation (after 10 days)
Hypotension
Vomiting-diarrhea
Hyperemia of the mucous membranes
Sterile pyuria
Elevated bilirubin and enzymes
Low platelets
Disorientation or alteration in consciousness

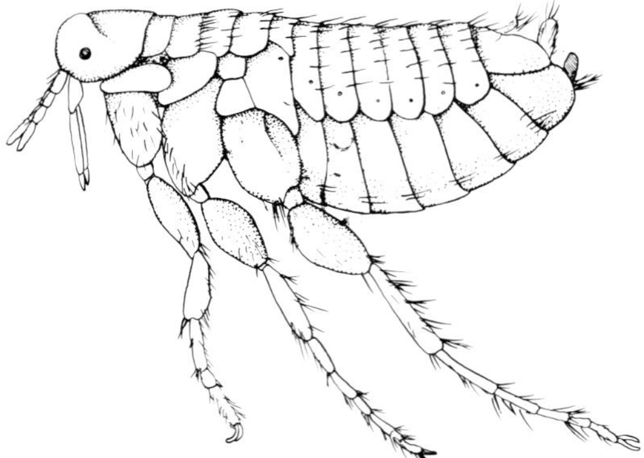

Figure 54.24. Flea (*Pulex irritans*).

Spider Bites

Loxosceles reclusus or the brown recluse (Fig. 54.25), found most commonly in the south central United States, is responsible for most skin reactions caused by the bite of a spider. This spider is quite small, the body being only 8 to 10 mm long, and bears a violin-shaped band over the dorsal cephalothorax. The venom contains necrotizing, hemolytic and spreading factors. The initial symptoms include mild stinging and/or pruritus. A hemorrhagic blister then appears which can develop into a gangrenous eschar. Severe bites can cause a generalized erythematous macular eruption, nausea, vomiting, chills, malaise, muscle aches, and hemolysis. Treatment includes oral steroids within 6 to 12 hours after the bite, antibiotics to prevent secondary infection, and surgical removal of the necrotic area to prevent spread of the toxin.

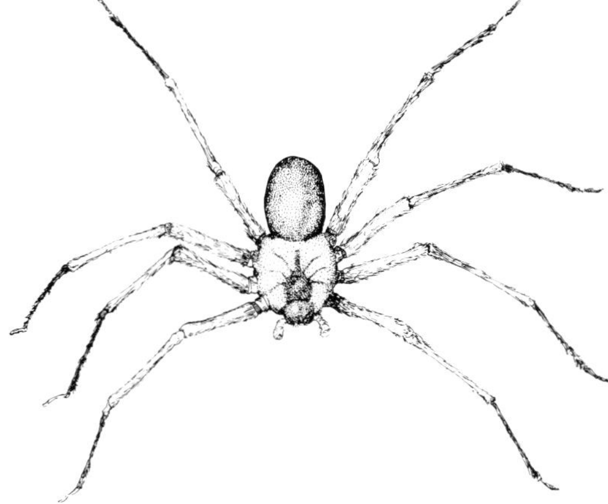

Figure 54.25. Brown recluse spider (*Loxosceles reclusus*).

Scabies Infestation

The cardinal symptom of any infestation with scabies is pruritus. Infants and children excoriate themselves to the point of bleeding. There are two clues to keep in mind when attempting to make this diagnosis: (1) distribution (concentration on the hands, feet, and folds of the body, especially the fingerwebs) and (2) involvement of other family members. It is important not only to ask other family members if they have pruritus but to also examine their skin. In contrast to adults, infants may develop blisters and also exhibit lesions on the head and face.

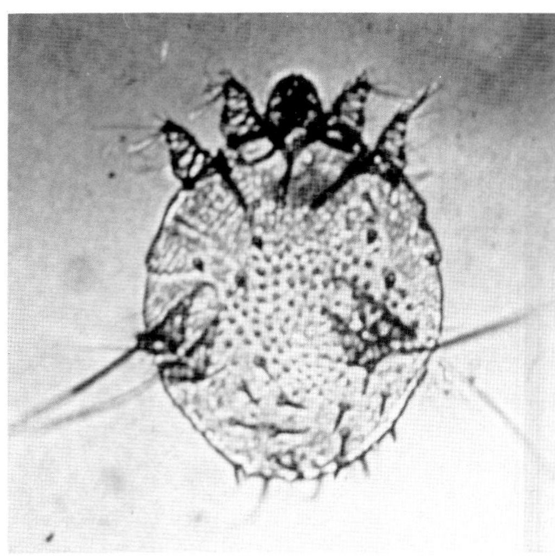

Figure 54.26. Mite which causes scabies (*Sarcoptes scabiei*).

The diagnosis is made by scraping involved skin and looking for mites under the 10× microscope objective (Fig. 54.26). The material necessary to examine the skin for scabies is a glass slide, immersion oil, and a No. 15 scalpel blade. A drop of immersion oil should be placed on the glass slide and the No. 15 blade edge dipped into this oil. The best areas to scrape are the interdigital webs of the hands or tiny linear lesions which represent burrows caused by the mite. A recently described procedure involves the use of fountain pen ink applied to the suspected area of skin. After the surface ink is cleaned away, one can identify the mite burrows by means of the ink which has trickled into them.

Once an infestation occurs, it usually takes 1 month for sensitization and pruritus to develop. Although lindane (Kwell) is an effective treatment, it should not be used in children under 5 years of age, and especially in those under 1 year of age. Because of the relatively large surface area of the young child and the transcutaneous permeability of the insecticide, significant blood levels can occur. The toxin can be concentrated in the central nervous system with the production of seizures. The use of crotamiton (Eurax) is recommended as an alternative therapy in young children and pregnant women. When lindane is used, it should be applied from the neck down, and left on from 4 to 8 hours. It is then showered or washed off. Usually one application is sufficient. If another application is necessary, one should wait for 1 week in young children before reapplying. Crotamiton is applied from the neck down, left on for 24 hours, and followed by an additional application at the end of this period without washing. Finally, after a total of 48 hours, the medication is washed off with soap and water.

Louse Infestation

There are three forms of lice that infest man: the head louse, the body louse, and the pubic or crab louse (Fig. 54.27). The major louse infestation in children involves the scalp and causes pruritis. The female attaches her eggs to the hair shaft. The egg then hatches, leaving behind numerous nits (Fig. 54.28) that resemble dandruff. Secondary infection can occur from vigorous scratching. Body lice generally reside in the seams of clothing and lay their eggs there. They go to the body to feed, particularly the interscapular, shoulder, and waist areas. Red pruritic puncta that become papular and wheel-like then occur. Pubic lice occur in the genital area, lower abdomen, axillae, and eyelashes. Transmission is usually venereal. Blue macules (maculae caeruleae) which are 3 to 15 mm in diameter can be seen on the thighs, abdomen, or thorax of infested persons. These are secondary to bites.

Since the body louse resides in clothing, therapy consists mainly of disinfecting the clothing with steam under pressure. Pediculosis capitus and pediculosis pubis are best treated with lindane. One tablespoon of shampoo is applied to the scalp or pubic area which has been wet with water. Shampooing should be maintained for about 4 minutes and the lather rinsed out. Any nits are removed with a fine-toothed comb.

SUPERFICIAL FUNGAL INFECTIONS OF THE SKIN

Tinea Corporis

Tinea corporis (Fig. 54.29) is characterized by one or more sharply circumscribed scaly patches. The center of the circular patch generally clears as the leading edge spreads out. The leading edge may be composed of papules, vesicles, or pustules. The lesions are most commonly confused with nummular eczema. The diagnosis can be made by scraping the active outer rim of papules and examining the scales with a KOH preparation under the microscope (Fig. 54.30). These lesions do not fluoresce under the Wood's light. The most common offending fungi are *Microsporum canis* and *Trichophyton mentagrophytes*. Treatment with topical antifungal agents such as clotrimazole, miconazole, or tolnaftate produces clearing in 7 to 10 days. Therapy should be maintained for 2 weeks. If improvement does not occur, treatment with griseofulvin, 10 to 12 mg/kg/day in two divided doses, will usually resolve the problem.

Tinea Capitus

Although tinea capitus was commonly caused by the *Microsporum* species in the past, it usually results now from infection by *Trichophyton tonsurans*. The two forms have different clinical appearances. The *Microsporum* species (Table 54.7) generally causes round patches of scaling alopecia (Fig. 54.31). Illumination of a lesion with a Wood's lamp gives a blue-green fluorescence. Kerion formation can occur as a swollen, boggy abscess. The *Trichophyton*

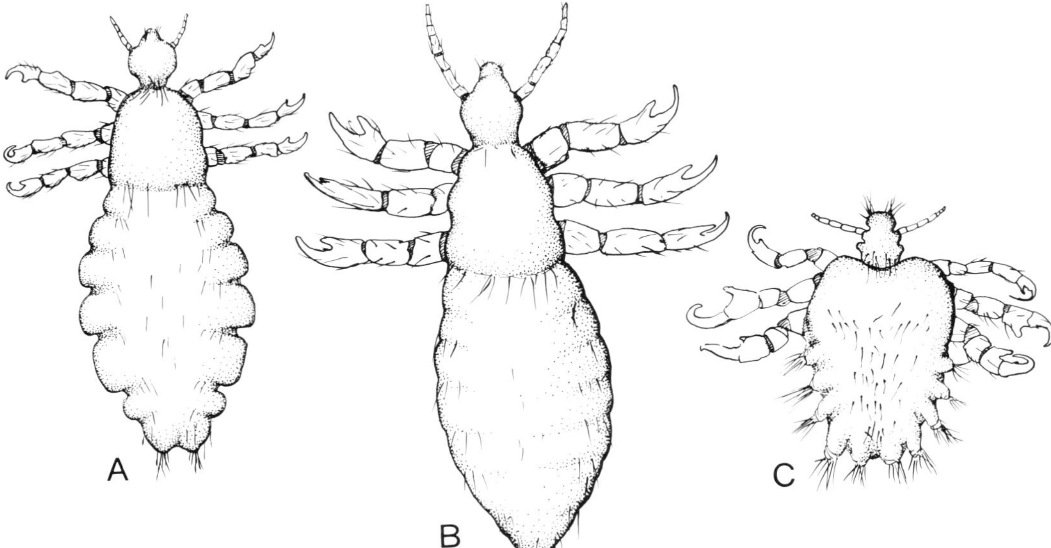

Figure 54.27. (*A*) Head louse (*Pediculus humanus* var. *capitis*), (*B*) body louse (*Pediculus humanus* var. *corporis*), and (*C*) pubic louse (*Phthirus pubis*).

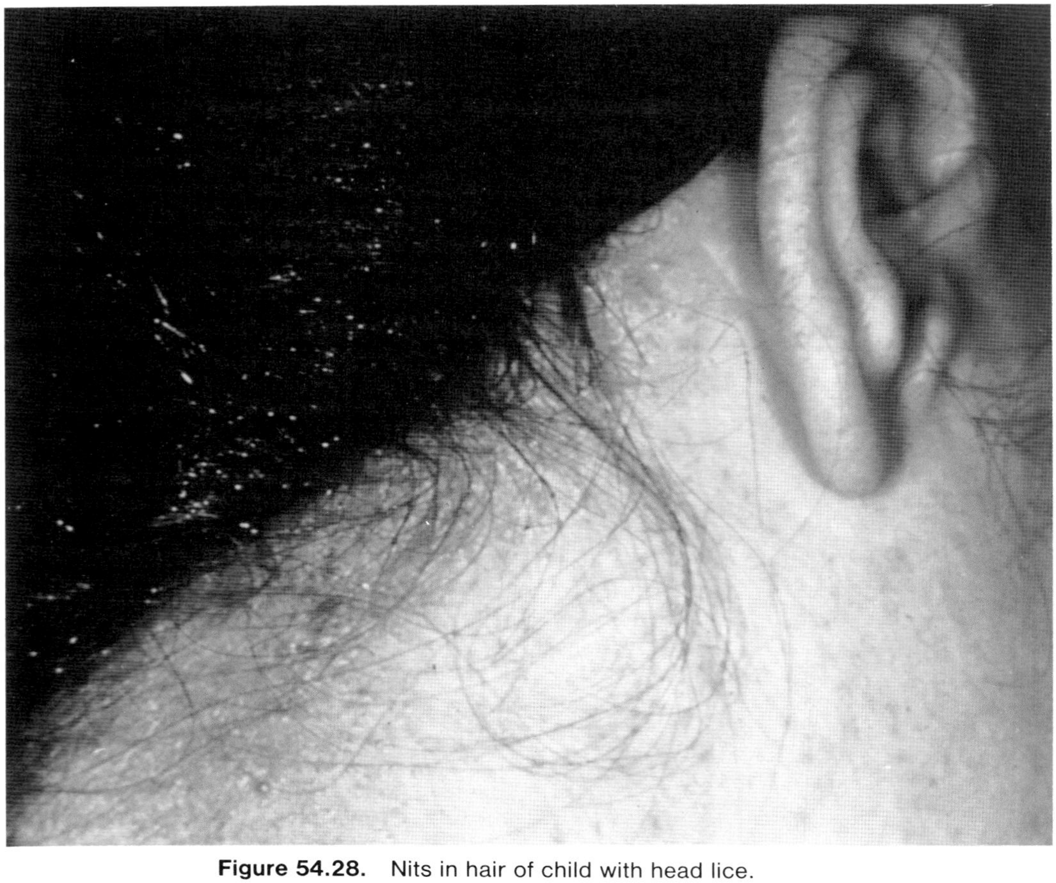

Figure 54.28. Nits in hair of child with head lice.

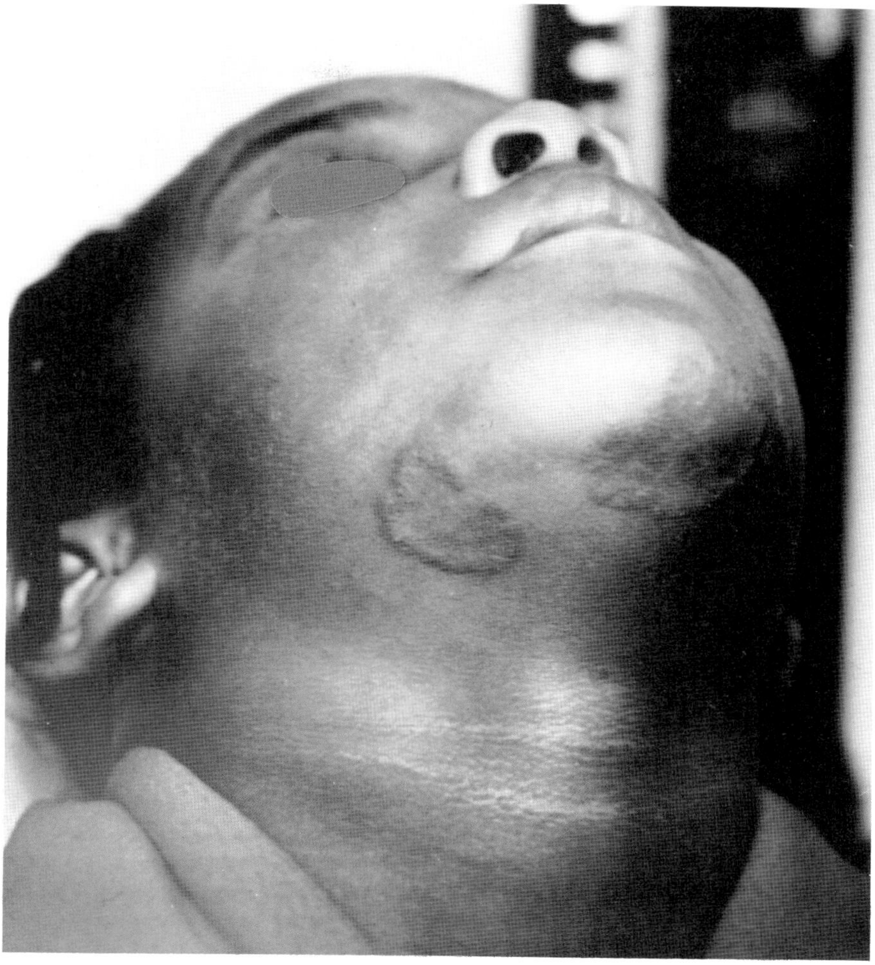

Figure 54.29. Child with tinea corporis.

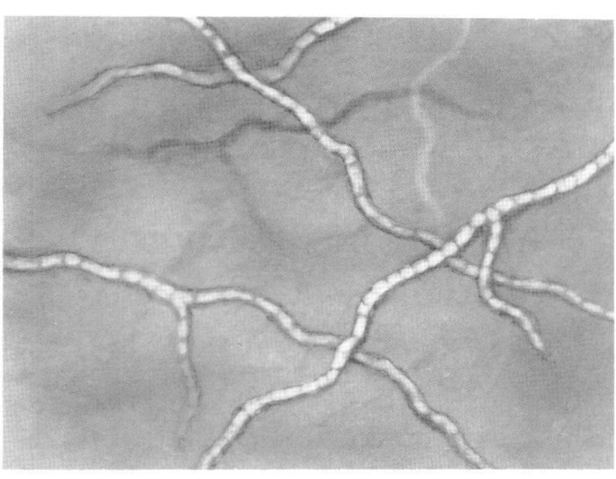

Figure 54.30. Characterization of a positive KOH preparation demonstrating branching hyphae running across the microscope field.

species (Table 54.8) usually causes scattered alopecia, not always oval or rounded; the alopecia is irregular in outline with indistinct margins. Normal hairs grow within the patches of alopecia. At times, the hairs break off at the surface of the scalp, leaving a "black dot" appearance (Fig. 54.32). Diffuse scaling may simulate dandruff, and although minimal hair loss is present it is not perceived. Wood's light examination of the lesion does not produce fluoresence. The organism can cause a folliculitis, suppuration, and kerion formation (Fig. 54.33). Diagnosis is made by culturing the affected scalp area (see Fig. 54.9). One should consider the presence of tinea capitus when a nonresponsive seborrheic or atopic derma-

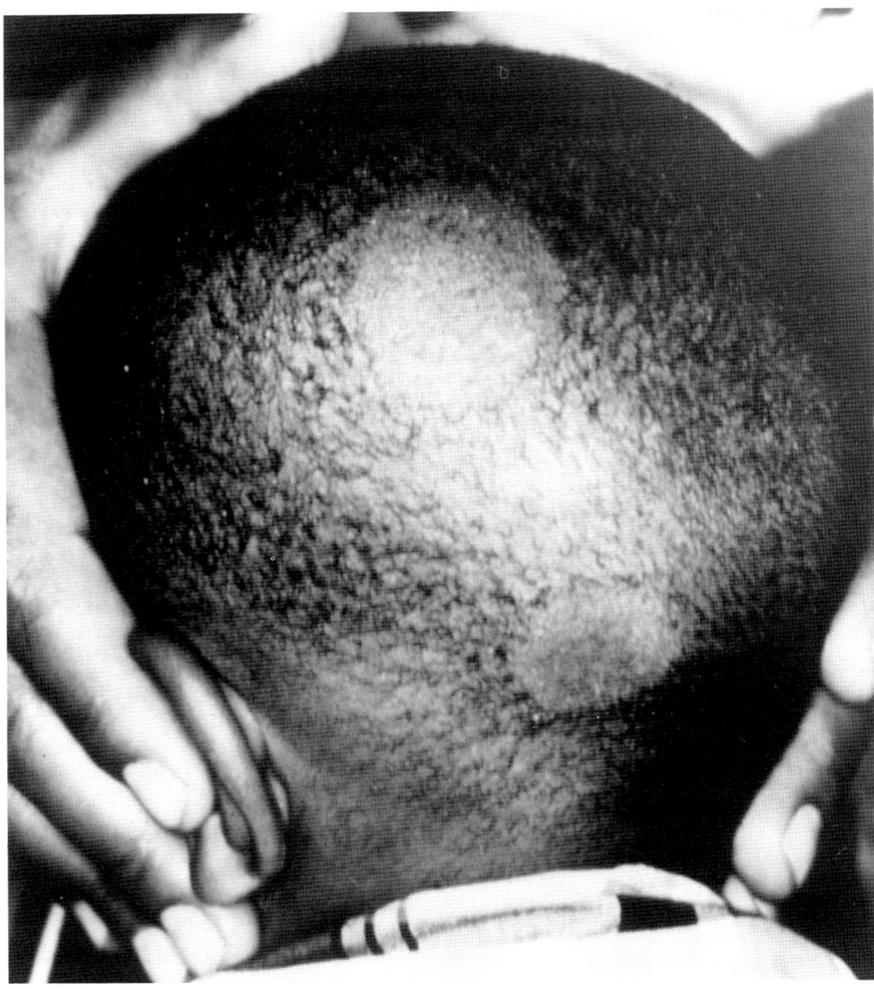

Figure 54.31. Tinea capitus secondary to infection with *Microsporum audouinii.*

titis of the scalp is present, black dots are seen, or increased scaling follows the use of topical steroids. With the use of DTM media a color change occurs in the media (yellow to red) in the presence of a growing dermatophyte. If a kerion is present the swelling (allergic reaction to the fungus) can be controlled by a combination of prednisone and griseofulvin.

In the differential diagnosis of patchy hair loss, as is seen in tinea capitus, one should consider alopecia areata (Fig. 54.34). However, with alopecia areata there is no inflammation or scaling of the scalp. Trichotillomania should also be considered. This is the term given to the habit children develop of rubbing, twirling, or playing with their hair to the point that the hair breaks and is lost in irregular patches. Traction alopecia occurs with certain hair styles. Hair is lost at the margins of the hairline with the ponytail style or frequent use of hair rollers. Tight braiding or corn-rowing can cause hair loss on any area of the scalp. At times, papules or pustules occur where the skin has been disrupted by the traction. Infants who are left on their backs for long periods of time may lose hair at the occiput from the constant friction in that area.

Treatment for tinea capitus consists of

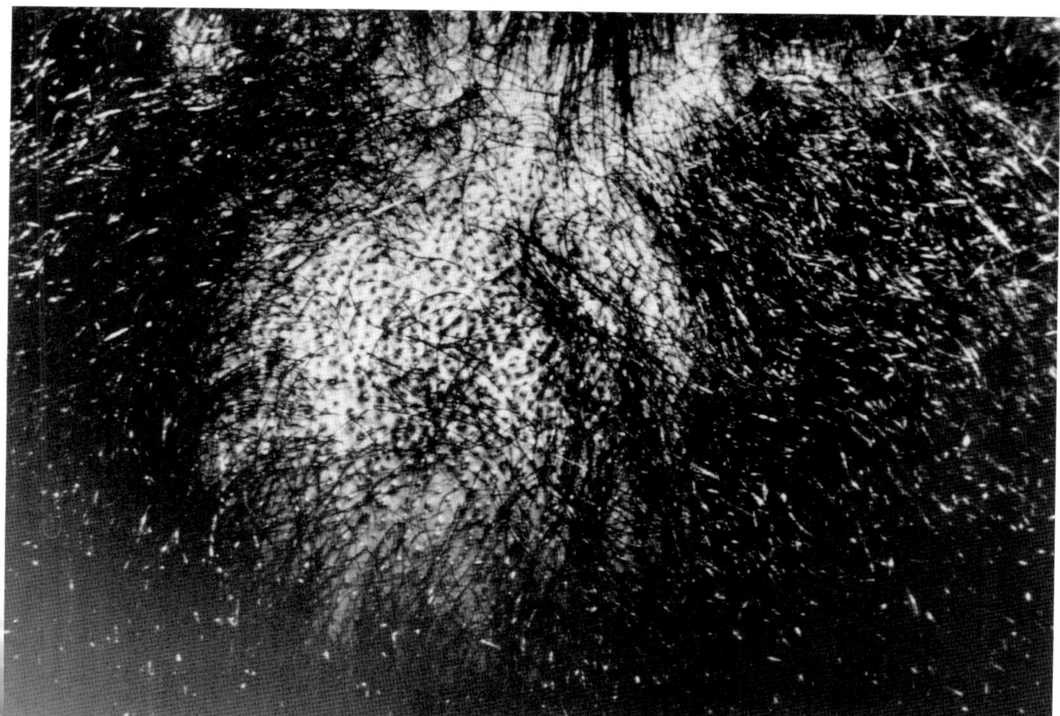

Figure 54.32. "Black-dot" appearance of scalp infection with *Trichophyton tonsurans.*

Table 54.7
Tinea Capitus *Microsporum* Species

Round patches of scaling alopecia
Fluoresce blue-green
Kerion formation

orally administered griseofulvin, 10 to 12 mg/kg/day in two divided doses for 6 weeks. Adjunctive therapy includes the use of selenium sulfide shampoo twice weekly. With the use of this shampoo, shedding of spores is eradicated within 1 to 2 weeks.

Tinea Cruris

Tinea cruris begins as a small red scaling rash in the groin that spreads peripherally and clears centrally. The edges are sharply marginated and scalloped, extending down the thighs. Generally, there is no noticable involvement of the scrotum. This fungal infection is most common in semitropical regions where there is heat and high humidity. Tight-fitting clothes also contribute to the problem by preventing evaporation. Other conditions to consider are seborrheic dermatitis (which usually can be differentiated by involvement of other areas of the body such as the ears, scalp, and eyelids), intertrigo (generally secondary to friction and maceration), contact dermatitis, candidiasis (which usually involves the inner thigh and causes the scrotum to appear bright red) and erythrasma. One should always check the feet to make sure there is not fungal involvement in that area as well. In general, this condition affects only postpubertal children. Diagnosis is made by KOH preparation. Nonspecific measures for treatment include: loose-fitting clothing,

Table 54.8
Tinea Capitus *Trichophyton* Species

Partial scattered alopecia not always oval or rounded
Alopecia irregular in outline with indistinct margins
Normal hairs growing within patch of alopecia
Black dots, diffuse scaling ("dandruff")
Nonfluorescent
Folliculitis, suppuration, kerion formation

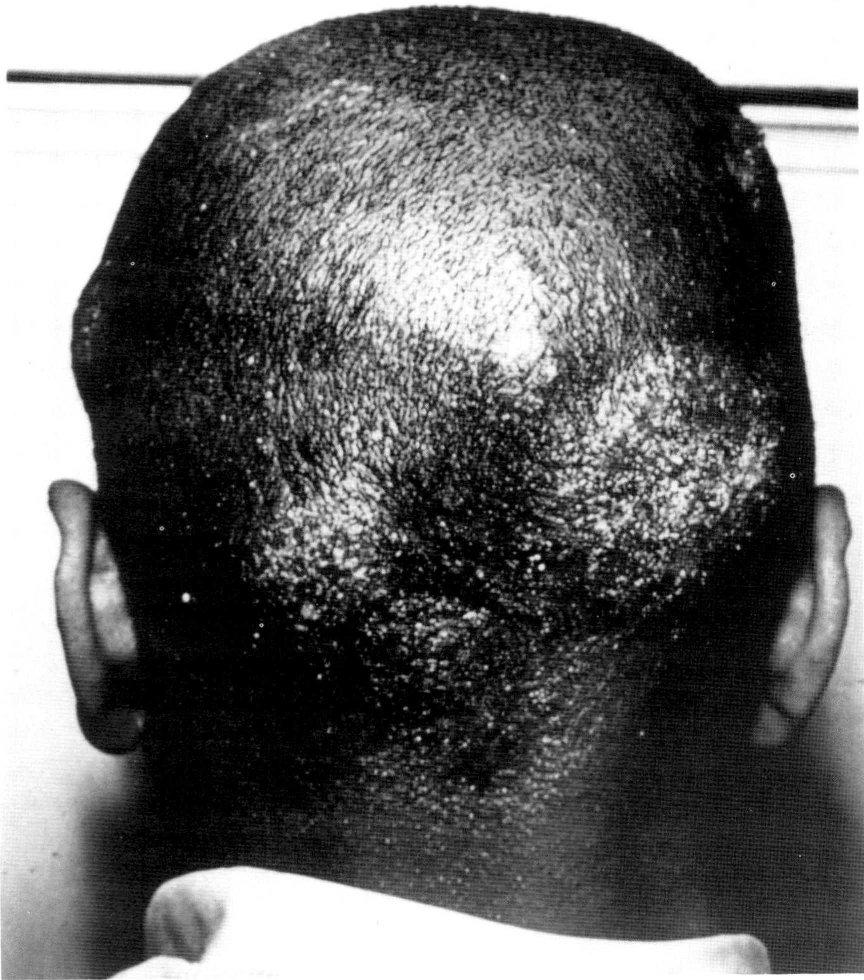

Figure 54.33. Patient with tinea capitus and multiple kerions.

reducing the amount of perspiration by use of dusting powders, and decreasing intake of caffeine-containing foods. Clotrimazole, miconazole, and tolnaftate are useful as topical antifungal agents. Oral griseofulvin may be needed in severe cases.

Tinea Pedis

Tinea pedis is generally due to *Trichophyton rubrum* or *Trichopyton mentagrophytes*. It usually occurs only in postpubertal children. The cracking and peeling of the skin suggestive of tinea pedis in prepubertal children more often indicates the presence of atopic eczema or hyperhidrosis. Tinea pedis is a penalty of civilization, in that it occurs only in those individuals who wear shoes. KOH preparation will demonstrate hyphae, especially when samples are taken from between the fourth and fifth interspaces of the toes. Clinically, the skin has a dry, white hazy appearance and is frequently pruritic. When there is secondary bacterial infection, an odor occurs. At times there is an inflammatory type of lesion (caused by *T. mentagrophytes*) which causes blistering. The presence of an "id" reaction indicates dissemination of antigen

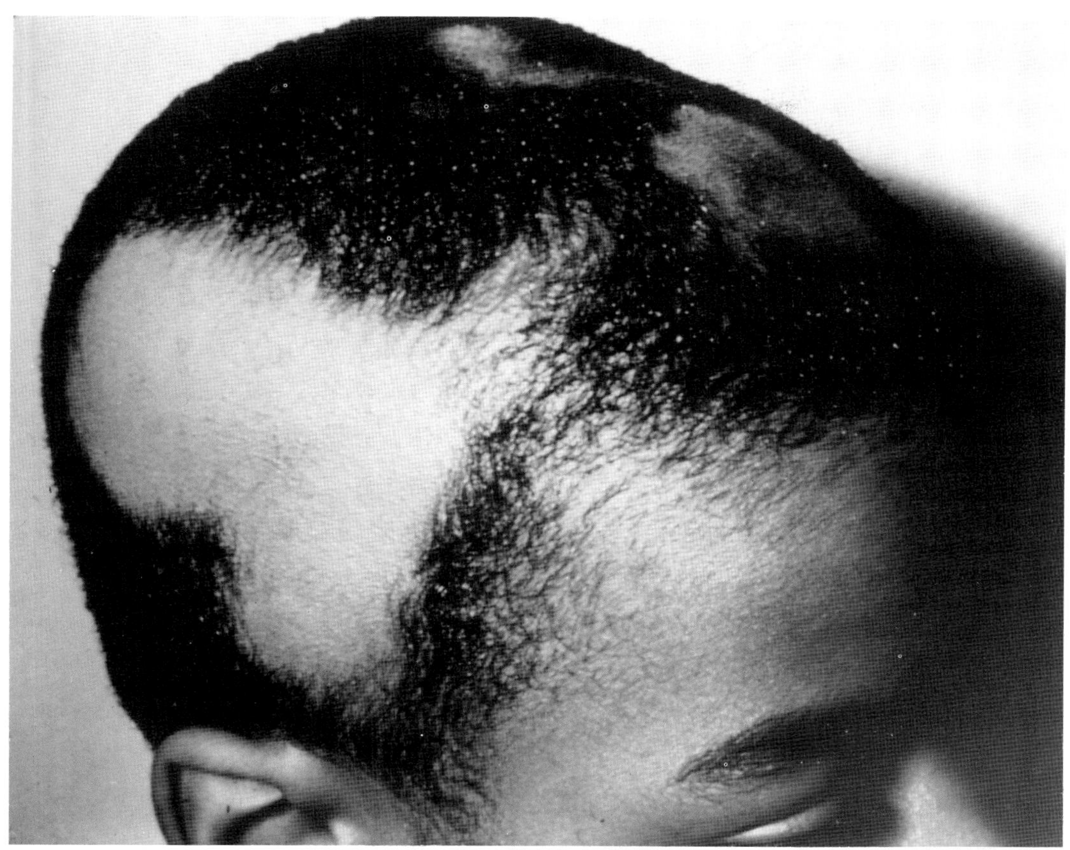

Figure 54.34. Child with alopecia areata.

to other parts of the body, especially the hands.

The differential diagnosis of tinea pedis includes: simple maceration, contact dermatitis, and atopic eczema. Treatment consists of thoroughly drying the feet after washing; the use of dry, clean socks; avoiding caffeine-containing foods to decrease sweating; keeping shoes off as much as possible; and walking barefoot or in sandals. Topical antifungal agents (see under "Tinea Cruris") and/or oral griseofulvin are used to treat this condition.

Tinea Versicolor

Tinea versicolor refers to a superficial infection of the skin caused by *Pityrosporum orbiculare* which produces color changes of the skin; hypopigmentation, hyperpigmentation, and redness (Fig. 54.35). Wood's light examination usually shows yellowish-brown fluoresence. Since moisture promotes growth of the organism, exacerbations occur in warm weather or in athletes who sweat excessively. The infection is difficult to eradicate and frequently recurs. A KOH preparation shows large clusters of spores and short stubby hyphae, frequently referred to as "meatballs and spaghetti."

Treatment consists of lathering the entire body with selenium sulfide shampoo (2½% concentration) after wetting the skin surface in a shower. The lather is left on for 20 min and then showered off. This procedure is carried out multiple times during the first week with decreasing frequency over the ensuing weeks. Maintenance therapy is advisable because of the high incidence of recurrence.

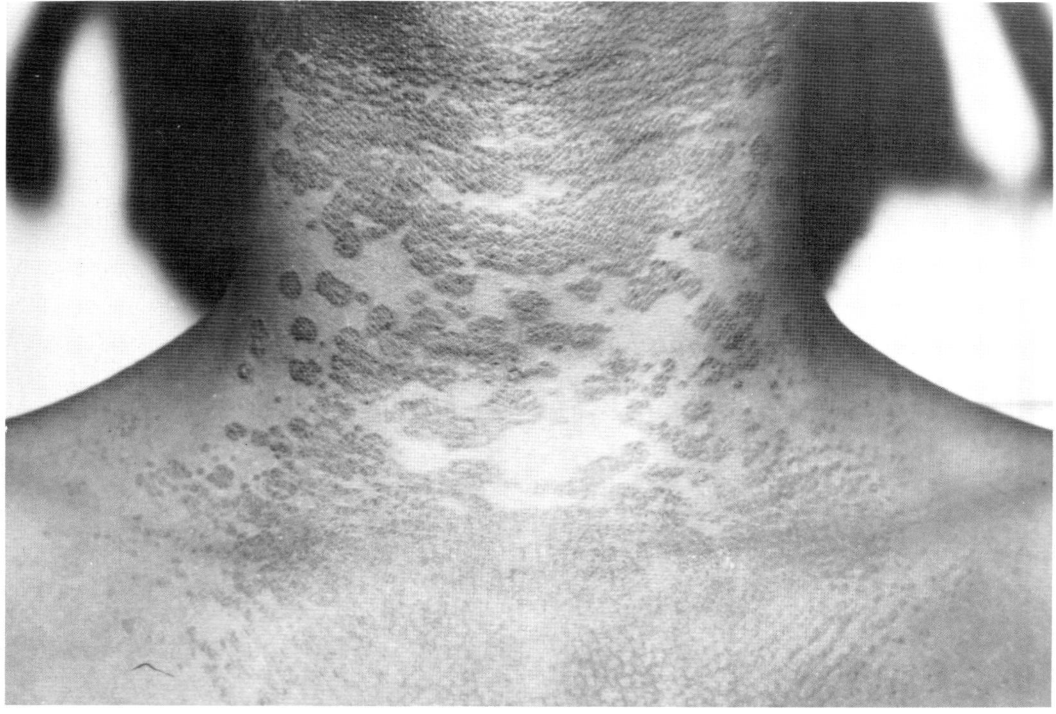

Figure 54.35. Adolescent with tinea versicolor.

PYOGENIC GRANULOMAS

Pyogenic granulomas (Fig. 54.36) are vascular nodules which develop rapidly at the site of an injury such as a cut, scratch, insect bite, or burn. The histologic picture is that of proliferating capillaries in a loose stroma. Although it was thought at first that this lesion was caused by infection of a small wound, the etiology of this lesion has not been established. Pyogenic granulomas occur frequently in children and young adults, usually on the fingers, face, hands, and forearms.

Clinically, the lesions are bright red to reddish-brown or blue-black in color. The vascular nodules are pedunculated, ranging from 0.5 to 2 cm in size. Their surfaces are glistening, or raspberry-like, frequently becoming eroded and crusted. They bleed very easily. Generally, they are asymptomatic. Because spontaneous disappearance is rare, the lesions must be removed by excision, electrosurgery, or cyrosurgery.

URTICARIA

BACKGROUND

Urticaria as a symptom complex is frequently encountered in the pediatric population, occurring in 2 to 3% of all children. In most cases, no etiology is identified. A small number are caused by allergic reactions from the ingestion of drugs or foods (nuts, eggs, shellfish, strawberries). Urticaria also follow viral (Epstein-Barr virus, hepatitis, etc.), bacterial (streptococcal), or parasitic infections. Physical factors can induce urticaria including: dermographism, cholinergic stimulation (induced by heat, exercise, and emotional tension), cold (acquired and familial), and solar exposure. Finally, urticaria may be caused by factors producing a vasculitis and substances causing degranulation of mast cells (radiocontrast material). Episodes of urticaria which last less than 6 weeks are termed transient or acute. The most frequent etiologies are infection, insect bites, drugs, and foods.

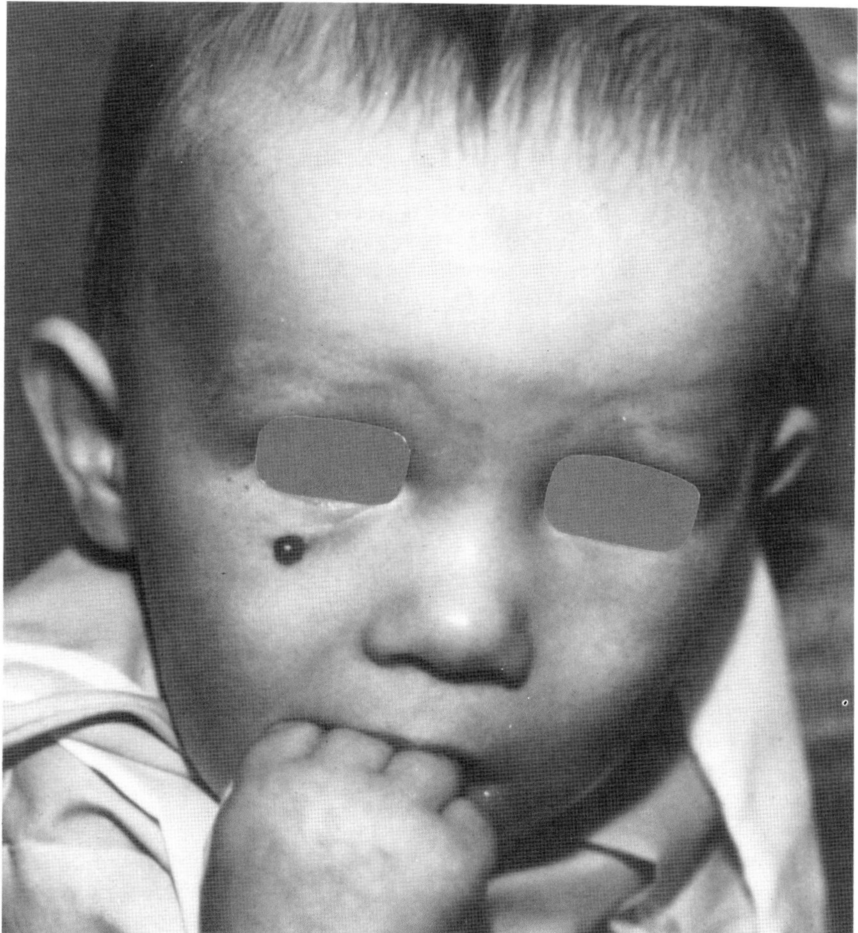

Figure 54.36. Pyogenic granuloma on the cheek of a child.

Chronic urticaria are defined as those that last more than 6 weeks. These include the physical urticarias or urticarial vasculitis.

PATHOPHYSIOLOGY

The lesion itself follows vasodilitation and leakage of fluid and red blood cells from involved vessels. The vascular damage can be caused by such mediators as histamine, complement, and immune complexes. IgE can attach to and cause degranulation of mast cells in sensitized individuals with resulting histamine release. Urticarias are usually acute and transient, but at times, become chronic and recurrent.

CLINICAL MANIFESTATIONS

The typical urticarial lesions are familiar to all physicians. They can be localized or generalized (involving the entire body). At times the lesions are giant with serpentiginous borders. Individual wheals rarely last more than 12 to 24 hours. Most commonly, the lesions appear in one area for 20 min to 3 hours, disappear, and then reappear in another location. The total duration of an episode is usually 24 to 48 hours; however, the course can last 3 to 6 weeks.

MANAGEMENT

Acute relief can be accomplished with subcutaneous epinephrine (1:1,000) 0.01 ml/kg and intramuscular diphenhydramine, 1 mg/kg. Prolonged sympathetic effect can be maintained with Sus-Phrine, 0.005 ml/kg. Oral antihistamines are useful for maintenance therapy for transient urticaria. Hydroxyzine hydrochloride 2 mg/kg/day in 3 to 4 divided doses or diphenhydramine hydrochloride 5 mg/kg/day in 3 to 4 divided doses should be prescribed for at least 10 days.

PITYRIASIS ROSEA

Pityriasis rosea can occur in all age groups but is seen predominately after 10 years of age and only rarely under 5 years of age. The etiology is unknown; however, a viral cause is suspected. Less than 5% of cases occur in multiple family members. In 80% of children, a large, oval solitary lesion known as the herald patch appears on the trunk (Fig. 54.37) prior to the eruption of subsequent lesions. Individual lesions are oval and slightly raised, pink to brown, with peripheral scaling. Because the lesions follow the cleavage lines (Fig. 54.38) of the skin, the backs of patients have a "Christmas tree" appearance. Generally, the face, the scalp, and distal extremities are spared. On occasion, an inverse distribution occurs (lesions on the face and extremities with truncal sparing). The rash is pruritic early in the course but then becomes asymptomatic. It lasts 4 to 8 weeks.

The herald patch can be mistaken for tinea corporis, but a potassium hydroxide preparation eliminates that possibility. When pityriasis rosea appears in adolescence, it must be differentiated from secondary syphilis. Clinical clues are helpful (Table 54.9) but serologic testing is necessary.

Treatment is symptomatic. Antihistamines and topical emollients can help the pruritus.

PANNICULITIS

Erythema Nodosum

Erythema nodosum seems to be a hypersensitivity reaction to infection (streptococci, tuberculosis, coccidioidomycosis, histoplasmosis), inflammatory bowel disease, sarcoidosis, and drugs. The exact immunologic mechanism has not been clarified. The entity occurs predominately in adolescents during the spring and fall. Females are affected more frequently than males.

The lesions of erythema nodosum appear as deep, tender, erythematous nodules or plaques on the extensor surfaces of the extremities (see Fig. 54.20). The sedimentation rate is generally elevated and usually returns to normal with disappearance of the eruption unless an underlying disease is present. The reaction usually lasts 3 to 6 weeks. Treatment should be directed toward the cause when and if established; otherwise, it is symptomatic (aspirin and antihistamines). Hospitalization is not necessary. Corticosteroids should not be used except in severe cases after an underlying infection has been ruled out.

Cold Panniculitis

This entity is secondary to cold injury to fat. During the cold of winter, infants and some older children develop red, indurated nodules and plaques on exposed skin, especially the face. The subcutaneous fat in infants and some children solidifies more readily at a higher temperature than that of an adult because of the relatively greater concentration of saturated fats. Infants who hold ice popsicles in their mouths are also susceptible to this phenomenon (see Fig. 54.39). The lesions gradually soften and return to normal over 1 or more weeks. Treatment is not necessary.

WARTS AND MOLLUSCUM CONTAGIOSUM

Warts

Warts affect 7 to 10% of the population and are one of the most frequent dermatologic problems encountered in pediatrics.

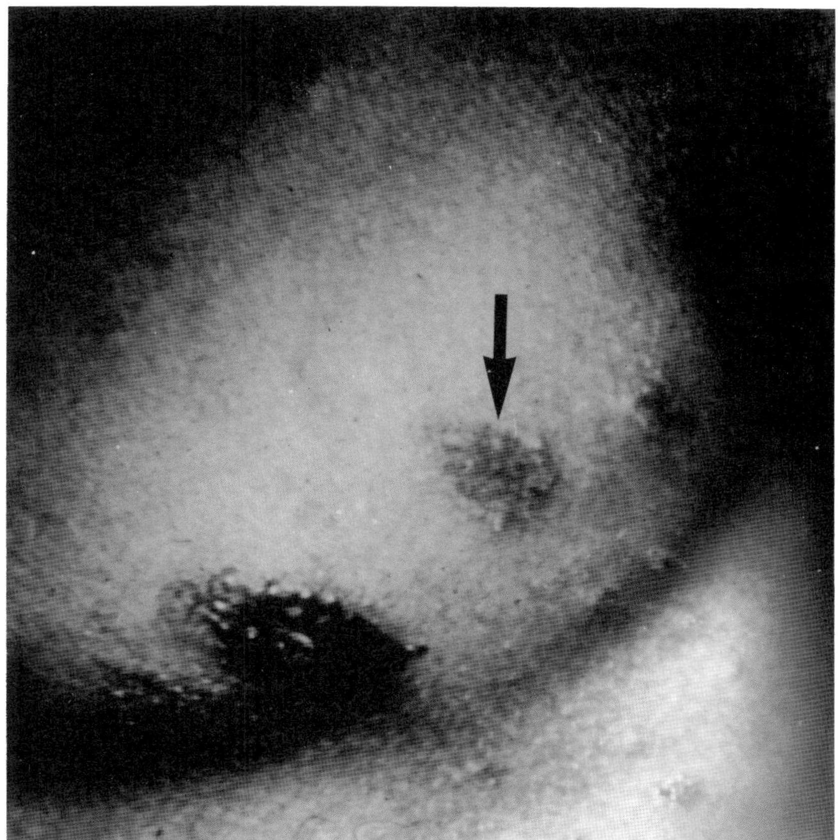

Figure 54.37. Herald patch (*arrow*) in adolescent with pityriasis rosea.

The peak incidence is during adolescence. Sixty-five percent of common warts disappear spontaneously within 2 years, and 40% of plantar warts within 6 months in prepubertal children. However, immunosuppressed patients may have extensive spread of the lesions.

The common wart resembles a tiny cauliflower. The shape of the wart varies with its location on the skin. They may be long and slender (filiform) on the face and neck or flat (verruca plana) on the face, arms, and knees. When located on the soles they are referred to as plantar warts, and when in the anogenital area, condyloma accuminata.

The tendency for recurrence of warts makes the treatment of this condition frustrating. Since most warts disappear spontaneously with time, procedures which are least traumatic for the child should be attempted first (Table 54.10). The simple, nontraumatic method of airtight occlusion with plain adhesive tape for a period of one month has been shown to be successful on many occasions. Topical application of salicylic acid and lactic acid in flexible collodion (Duofilm; Table 54.11) is good for home use, as are some of the over-the-counter preparations (e.g. Compound W). When simple methods are unsuccessful touching the warts with liquid nitrogen for 20 to 30 sec or surgical removal can be attempted. Both procedures are painful.

Plantar warts can be treated with 40% salicylic acid plaster. Circular pieces, slightly larger then the plantar wart, are cut from a sheet of this material. They are

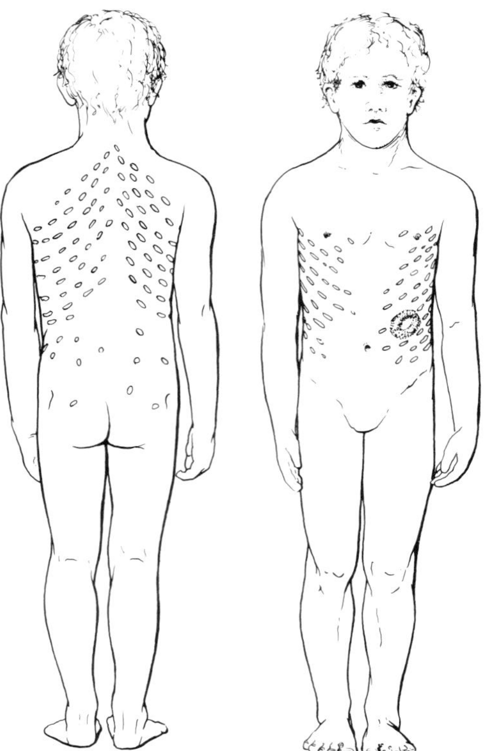

Figure 54.38. Typical distribution of pityriasis rosea.

Table 54.9
Differential Diagnosis

	Pityriasis Rosea	Syphilis
Herald patch	+	−
Ovals follow dermatomes	+	−
Lymphadenopathy	−	+
Mucous-membrane lesion	−	+

placed on the wart and kept in place continuously with adhesive tape for 1 to 2 weeks. At that point the dead tissue is carefully pared away. Treatment is continued until normal skin is seen in place of the wart.

Anogenital warts are treated with 20% podophyllin. This medication is carefully applied to the wart only and washed off in 4 to 6 hours. Severe burning of the skin

Table 54.10
Management of Warts

1. Decrease irritation—cover with tape (1–2 months)
2. Over-the-counter preparations such as Compound W (1 month)
3. Salicylic and lactic acid in collodion (Duofilm) (1 month)
4. Refer to dermatologist

Table 54.11
Use of Duofilm

1. Soak wart for 5 min
2. Dry
3. Surround with Vaseline
4. Apply Duofilm (let dry for few minutes)
5. Cover with tape
6. Repeat twice a day
7. Pare dead skin

occurs if the material is not completely removed.

Molluscum Contagiosum

This lesion, produced by the common pox virus, is a papule with a white center (see Fig. 54.40). It occurs at any age in childhood. It is more frequent in swimmers and wrestlers. Patients with atopic eczema are especially susceptible. Most lesions resolve in 6 to 9 months, but some may persist for more than 3 years. Spread is by autoinoculation.

Lesions can be single or numerous and favor intertriginous areas such as the groin. They are usually 2 to 5 mm in diameter, but several can coalesce and form a lesion 1.5 cm in diameter. They may become inflamed, which sometimes heralds spontaneous disappearance. At times, an eczematous reaction occurs around some lesions, and they can become secondarily infected.

Treatment should be gentle. Removal of the white core will cure the lesion. This can be done by spraying the lesion with ethyl chloride, pricking the skin open over the core with a 26 guage needle, and squeezing the core out with a comedome extractor. Multiple light touches with liquid nitrogen can also be effective. With widespread lesions, nonpainful procedures are preferable.

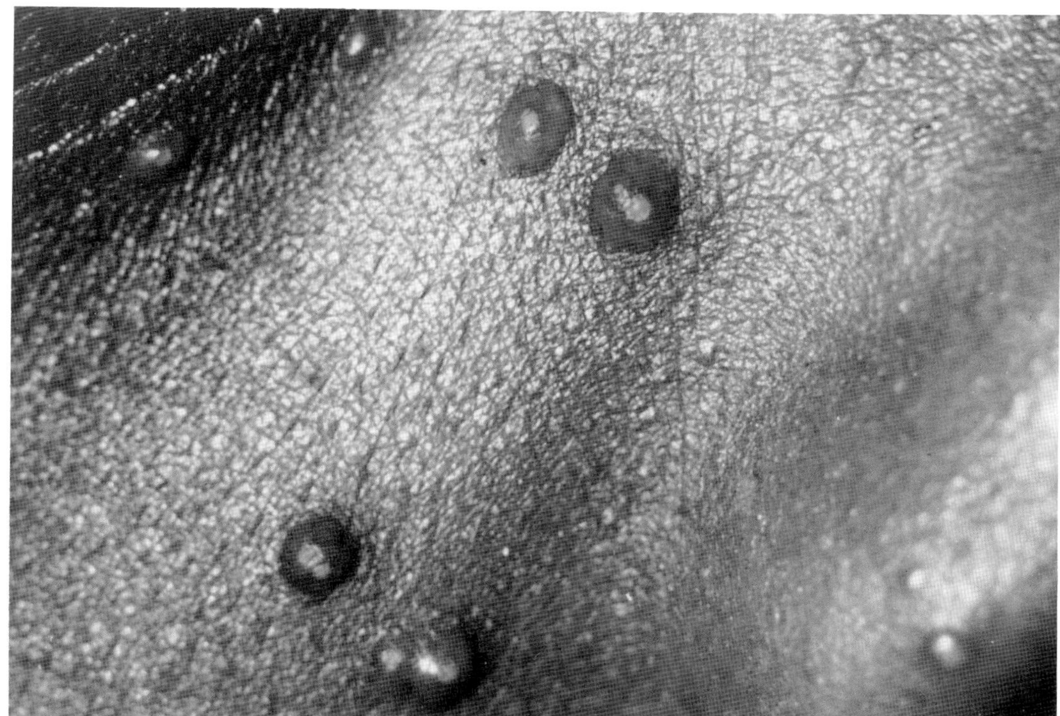

Figure 54.40. Molluscum contagiosum. Papules with white centers that contains the virus.

Application of 0.1% retinoic acid 1 to 2 times daily may induce enough inflammation to cause extrusion of the central core. Multiple painful treatments will cause great fear in the patient and make future visits to a physician difficult for the family.

CONGENITAL HERPES SIMPLEX VIRUS (HSV)

Congenital HSV infection encompasses a broad clinical spectrum ranging from localized cutaneous and mucosal lesions to life-threatening central nervous system and internal organ involvement. Studies have shown that 1% of patients in prenatal clinics have culturally proven HSV type 2 infection of the cervix during the last 20 weeks of pregnancy. This incidence is 3 times that of a nonparous age-matched population. Of this group of infected mothers, only 36% demonstrate clinical lesions consistent with herpes on physical examination. An additional 21% of patients note nonspecific genital urinary symptoms such as dysuria, leukorrhea, hematuria, and pelvic pain. Thus, 44% of pregnant women infected with HSV manifest no clinical signs or symptoms. If maternal herpes infection is culturally proven after the 32nd week of pregnancy, the risk of infection to the infant is 10%. Whereas, most infections are transmitted by direct contact with the infected birth canal during the second stage of labor, there is some evidence to document transplacental infection of the fetus.

The incubation period of congenital HSV infections range from 2 to 30 days following exposure. Lesions present at birth or shortly thereafter have been explained by transplacental passage of the virus. The clinical manifestations of congenital HSV infection are diverse, but over 50% of infected neonates present with external involvement. In vertex deliveries, the scalp is a common site for the vesicles. Conversely, infants delivered by breech often develop lesions of the buttocks and perianal area initially. The lesions are not unlike those seen in older children or adults in that they are grouped tense vesicles arising on an erythematous base. However, the infection may present on the skin as individual vesicles, pustules, bullae, or denuded skin. Unfortunately, when infants have disease limited to the integument, HSV infection is often not considered as a possibility, and instead these children are treated for "impetigo." The correct diagnosis may not be entertained until constitutional symptoms such as fever, hypothermia, poor feeding, irritability, lethargy, and vomiting have appeared. By then, dissemination of the disease has occurred.

Diagnosis of congenital HSV infection should be suspected in any infant less than 1 month of age who presents with a vesicular eruption on an erythematous base. A Tzanck preparation of the base of an unbroken vesicle is an easy and rapid diagnostic tool to aid in the recognition of this potentially lethal disease (see Fig. 54.7). Giemsa, Papinicolaou, or hematoxylin-eosin stains of the smeared preparation of vesicles infected with herpes simplex virus will reveal multinucleated giant cells, intranuclear inclusions, ballooning degeneration, or margination of nuclear chromatin.

The differential diagnosis of vesiculopustular lesions in the newborn includes: bullous impetigo, congenital cutaneous candidiasis, congenital syphilis, neonatal pustulomelanosis, and cytomegalovirus infection. Differentiation of these entities requires the use of Gram stains, KOH scrapings, serologic studies for syphilis, and appropriate cultures. Although many serologic tests are currently available to detect the presence of herpes simplex virus antibodies, none of these studies is valuable in arriving at an early diagnosis of congenital infection. Direct culture of the herpes virus from a lesional vesicle takes 24 to 48 hours for identification.

All infants with suspected congenital herpes simplex should be admitted to the hospital. At present, adenine arabinoside (ara-A, vidarabine) is the most effective antiviral agent available. Given as a steady intravenous infusion over 12 hours for 5 to 15 days at 10 to 20 mg/kg/day it readily crosses the blood-brain barrier and achieves therapeutic levels in the CSF.

DISORDERS OF PIGMENTATION

Hypopigmentation

A dominant form of partial albinism occurs, in which localized areas of skin and hair are devoid of pigment. Ocular albinism is also seen. Two syndromes with albinism are: Waardenberg syndrome (white forelock, heterochromia of the iris, sensorineural hearing loss) and Chediak-Higashi syndrome (immunodeficiency, leukocytes with giant granules.)

Loss of pigmentation can be due to absence of melanocytes as in vitiligo and halo nevi. Vitiligo is a symmetrical, patchy loss of pigmentation. Hair located in areas of vitiligo is often white. Vitiligo can be associated with alopecia areata, pernicious anemia, Addison's disease, hypothyroidism, diabetes mellitus, hypoparathyroidism, and other endocrine disorders. Vitiligo and some of the diseases associated with it may be autoimmune disorders. Antibodies directed against melanocytes have been detected.

Suppression of melanocytic pigment production can cause loss of pigmentation as in postinflammatory hypopigmentation. An example of this is the white patch of hypopigmentation and scaling frequently seen on the face, trunk, or extremities of children with atopic eczema. The ash-leaf macule is a flat hypopigmented (whitish) spot that is present in more than 90% of patients with tuberous sclerosis. In Caucasian patients, they are more easily seen by shining a Wood's lamp on the skin.

Hyperpigmentation

Diffuse hyperpigmentation is associated with Addison's disease, acromegaly, and hemochromatosis.

Pigment deep in the dermis appears gray or blue at the surface of the skin. Mongolian blue spots are an example. The nevus of Ota is dermal pigment in the distribution of the ophthalmic branch of the fifth nerve; this pigmentation can involve the sclera and palate as well.

Certain syndromes are associated with

pigmented skin lesions. Neurofibromatosis is one of these. Patients with this disease have cafe-au-lait spots which are flat, nonpalpable coffee-colored lesions of varying size and shape. When six or more are present, greater than 1.5 cm in size, neurofibromatosis should be considered. The Peutz-Jegher syndrome is a dominately inherited condition which includes freckle-like lesions of the lips, nose, buccal mucosa, fingertips, and subungal areas associated with polyps in the small intestine, stomach, or colon. Melena and intussusception are the chief complications that may develop, usually in the second decade of life. Albright's syndrome should be suspected when one sees unilateral cafe-au-lait spots with irregular borders occurring in the lumbosacral area. Included in this syndrome are boney abnormalities and precocious puberty.

Single or multiple red-brown papules or nodules occurring on the extremities or face of children may have a confusing histology. Although the lesions are benign, they have been frequently misdiagnosed as malignant melanoma. Therefore, the name, benign juvenile melanoma has been assigned to this condition. Other names include Spitz tumors or spindle-cell epitheloid nevi. True malignant melanomas are rare in childhood. They usually arise from congenital pigmented nevi.

References

Fitzpatrick, TB: *Dermatology in General Medicine,* Ed. 2. McGraw-Hill, New York, 1979.

Hurwitz, S. *Clinical Pediatric Dermatology.* W.B. Saunders, Philadelphia, 1981.

Solomon LM, Esterly NB: *Neonatal Dermatology* (in series *Major Problems in Clinical Pediatrics*). W.B. Saunders, Philadelphia, 1973.

Weinberg S, Hoekelman RA: *Pediatric Dermatology for the Primary Care Practitioner.* McGraw-Hill, New York, 1978.

Weston WL: *Practical Pediatric Dermatology.* Little, Brown, Boston, 1979.

Atopic Dermatitis

Hanifin JM, Lobitz WC: New concepts of atopic dermatitis. *Arch Dermatol* 113: 663, 1977.

Leyden JJ, Baker, DA: Localized herpes simplex infections in atopic dermatitis. *Arch Dermatol* 115: 311, 1979.

Pauly, CR, Artis, WM, Jones HE: Atopic dermatitis, impaired cellular immunity, and molluscum Contagiosum. *Arch Dermatol* 114: 391, 1978.

Contact Dermatitis

Fisher, AA: *Contact Dermatitis,* Ed. 2. Lea & Febiger, Philadelphia, 1975.

Gaul LE: Development of allergic nickel dermatitis from earrings. *JAMA* 200: 176, 1967

Drug Reactions

Arndt KA, Jick H: Rates of cutaneous reactions to drugs; a report from the Boston Collaborative Drug Surveillance Program. *JAMA* 235: 918, 1976.

Diaper Dermatitis

Leyden JJ, Katz S, Stewart R, Kligman AM: Urinary ammonia and ammonia-producing microorganisms in infants with and without diaper dermatitis. *Arch Dermatol* 113: 1678, 1977.

Weston WL, Lane AT, Weston JA: Diaper dermatitis; current concepts. *Pediatrics* 66: 532, 1980.

Staphylococcal Scalded Skin Syndrome

Amon RB, Diamond RL: Toxic epidermal necrolysis; rapid differentiation between staphylococcal and drug-induced disease. *Arch Dermatol* 111: 1433, 1975.

Curran JP, Al-Salihi FL: Neonatal staphylococcal scalded skin syndrome; massive outbreak due to an unusual phage type. *Pediatrics* 66: 285, 1980.

Melish ME, Glasgow LA: The staphylococcal scalded-skin syndrome; development of an experimental model. *N Engl J Med* 282: 1114, 1970.

Bites and Infestations

Davis CM, Israel RM: Treatment of creeping eruption with thiabendazole. *Arch Dermatol* 97: 325, 1968.

Ginsburg CM, Lowry W, Reisch JS: Absorption of lindane (γ-benzenehexachloride) in infants and children. *J Pediatr* 91: 998, 1977.

Hershey FB, Aulenbacher CE: Surgical treatment of brown spider bites. *Ann Surg* 170: 300, 1969.

Orkin M, Epstein E, Maibach HI: Treatment of today's scabies and pediculosis. *JAMA* 236: 1136, 1976.

Woodley D, Sawrat JH: The burrow ink test and the scabies mite. *J Am Acad Dermatol* 4: 715, 1981.

Fungal Infections

Esterly NB: Fungal infections in children. *Pediatr Rev* 3: 41, 1981.

Honig PJ, Smith LR: Tinea capitus masquerading as atopic or seborrheic dermatitis. *J Pediatr* 94: 604, 1979.

Rockoff AS: Fungus cultures in a pediatric outpatient clinic. *Pediatrics* 63: 276, 1979.

Urticaria

Mathews KP: A current view of urticaria. *Med Clin North Am* 58: 185, 1974.

Schuller DE, Elvey SM: Acute urticaria associated with streptococcal infection. *Pediatrics* 65: 592, 1980.

Congenital Herpes Simplex

Honig PJ, Holtzwanger J, Leyden JJ: Neonatal herpes simplex infection; report of three cases and literature review. *Arch Dermatol* 115: 1329, 1979.

CHAPTER **55**

Oncologic Emergencies

BEVERLY J. LANGE, M.D., AND STEVEN HALPERN, M.D.

INTRODUCTION

Each year only 1 in 10,000 children develops cancer. And yet, next to accidents, cancer remains the leading cause of death in children over 1 year of age. Fortunately, with carefully planned therapy, at least half the children diagnosed with cancer can now be expected to grow up to be healthy, productive members of society.

Not so much because cancer is potentially fatal, but because it is potentially curable, pediatric oncology concerns all physicians seeing children. It is the pediatrician or the emergency department physician who must first think of cancer and who must decide which child needs a blood count, x-ray, or biopsy. This decision is not always easy because children with cancer complain of the same things that bother most children: fatigue, fever, headache, or pain. After a history, physical examination and appropriate laboratory tests, the emergency department physician may already have sufficient information to make a presumptive diagnosis of cancer. His or her role in the management of the child may consist of sharing this information with the family and then referring the child to a specialist qualified to confirm the diagnosis and undertake the care of pediatric cancer. Occasionally, the emergency department room physician may need to begin supportive therapy that is potentially lifesaving.

Usually, the child with cancer is only mildly to moderately ill at initial presentation. However, some children develop conditions that are threatening to life or function and require immediate intervention. More often, it is the complications of cytotoxic and immunosuppressive therapy that bring children to the emergency department. Life-threatening oncologic problems occur for the following reasons: (1) marrow failure from leukemia, metastatic tumor, or cytotoxic therapy predisposes to infection, hemorrhage, and anemia; (2) lysis of tumor cells causes metabolic derangement; (3) a solid tumor invades or compresses a vital organ; and (4) cancer therapy damages a vital organ.

The chapter is subdivided according to type of malignancy. Acute leukemia is discussed first and in greatest detail because many of the complications of leukemia and its treatment are common to other forms of cancer. The sections on non-Hodgkin's lymphoma and histiocytic diseases follow that on leukemia because these diseases are similar in presentation and pathophysiology. Hodgkin's disease is then compared to non-Hodgkin's lymphoma. Other solid tumors are presented by location: thoracic tumors, abdominal tumors, genitourinary tumors, and tumors of the head, neck, and extremities. Potential oncologic emergencies are emphasized in each section. Antineoplastic therapy is summarized in the last section.

Pain is associated with cancer at diagnosis or cancer that has failed to respond to therapy. The pain of cancer is often severe and can qualify as an emergency.

The management of pain is discussed in Chapter 3 and in the references.

LEUKEMIA

BACKGROUND

Definition

In leukemia excessive numbers of immature malignant white blood cells, "leukemic blasts," replace normal marrow hematopoietic cells. Leukemic blasts leave the marrow, circulate in the peripheral blood and infiltrate lymph nodes, liver, spleen, meninges and soft tissues. Leukemia manifests itself by bone marrow failure and by its infiltration into extramedullary sites. Without treatment leukemia is fatal. Today specific antileukemia therapy and sophisticated supportive care have brought long-term survival to many children with leukemia.

Classification

Leukemia is a group of diseases. The various types of leukemia are classified according to whether the disease is acute or chronic and according to the morphology of the leukemic blasts. Acute leukemia is characterized by a natural history of marrow failure of weeks to months from the time of apparent onset to death. Most childhood leukemia is acute. Chronic leukemia, in contrast, evolves over months to years. Initially there are increased numbers of peripheral blood granulocytes of all stages of maturation, but ultimately blasts predominate ("blast crisis") and marrow failure ensues. Sometimes the distinction between acute and chronic leukemia is not clear. Certain cases of childhood leukemia designated "acute" may in fact be occult chronic leukemia that has progressed to the point where blasts are the dominant cell type.

Morphologic classification of leukemia defines two discrete groups according to the appearance of the blasts: (1) lymphocytic (lymphoid, lymphoblastic, lymphatic) and (2) myelogenous (myeloid, myelocytic, myeloblastic). The distinction is based on the superficial resemblance of the lymphoid blasts to immature or transformed lymphocytes and of the myeloid blasts to normal myeloid or monocytic precursors. Unlike normal myeloid and lymphoid precursors, the leukemic blasts do not have the ability to mature and differentiate in vivo, do not obey the signals that regulate proliferation of normal cells, and make no contribution to the body's immune system.

The distinction between acute myelogenous (AML) and lymphocytic leukemia (ALL) is important: childhood lymphocytic leukemia responds to different therapy and has a substantially better prognosis than myelogenous leukemia. Most childhood leukemia is lymphocytic. Current subclassification of leukemia is presented in Table 55.1.

Epidemiology

Leukemia is the most common malignancy of childhood in the United States. The estimated yearly incidence is about 4 cases/100,000 children aged 0 to 4 years. The peak incidence is between 3 and 6 years. There is a slight male predominance. There does not appear to be any racial predilection. Several "clusters" of leukemia have occurred in the United States, but they appear to be chance phenomena.

Physical agents (e.g. ionizing radiation) and chemical agents (e.g. benzene) can cause leukemia in man, and certain DNA viruses and RNA retroviruses are associated with leukemia in laboratory animals. However, the cause of leukemia in the vast majority of children with AML or ALL is unknown. Extensive epidemiologic investigation has defined certain groups that are at especially high risk of developing leukemia, "the leukemia susceptibles" (Table 55.2).

CLINICAL MANIFESTATIONS AND PATHOPHYSIOLOGY

The symptoms of acute leukemia are the symptoms of marrow failure and tissue infiltration. Marrow failure leads to anemia, thrombocytopenia and leukopenia. Anemia causes pallor, fatigue, and irritability. Thrombocytopenia causes spontaneous bruising, epistaxis, and oozing from gums. Patients with myelogenous leukemia, especially hypergranular promyelocytic leu-

Table 55.1
Classification of Childhood Leukemia

I. Acute Leukemia: > 95%
- A. Lymphoid: 80%
  - 1. French, American and British (FAB) morphologic classification
    - L1. Microlymphoblasts (scant cytoplasm, rare nucleoli)
    - L2. Large lymphoblasts (moderate cytoplasm, 1, 2, 3 or more nucleoli)
    - L3. Large lymphoblast (basophilic cytoplasm, vacuoles, nucleoli, Burkitt's type cells)
  - 2. Immunologic classification
    - Common ALL[a]. Ia surface antigen; common ALL antigen
    - Null cell. No specific surface marker
    - T-cell. T cell antigen, E rosettes
    - B-cell. B cell-monocyte antigen, surface immunoglobulin, F_c receptor, complement receptor
    - Acute undifferentiated leukemia
- B. Myeloid: 15–20%
  - FAB morphologic classification:
    - M1. Myeloblasts with no maturation
    - M2. Myeloblasts with maturation—granules, Auer rods
    - M3. Hypergranular promyelocytic
    - M4. Myelomonocytic
    - M5. Monocytic or histiocytic
    - M6. Erythroleukemia

II. Chronic Leukemia: < 5%
- A. Lymphoid: Rare in pediatrics
- B. Myeloid:
  - 1. Adult form:
    - a. Philadelphia chromosome
    - b. Hemoglobin F, 2–7%
    - c. Marked splenomegaly
  - 2. Juvenile form: Hemoglobin F, 30–70%

[a] ALL = acute lymphocytic leukemia.

Table 55.2
Acute Leukemia: High Risk Groups[a, b]

Group	Risk	Time
Identical twin of leukemic child	1:5	Weeks–months
Polycythemia vera (radiation treated)	1:6	10–15 years
Bloom's syndrome	1:8	<30 years
Hodgkin's disease (radiation and chemotherapy)	~1:10–1:50	Months–10 years
Hiroshima survivors (within 1000 m of hypocenter)	1:60	12 years
Down's syndrome	1:95	<10 years of age
Ankylosing spondylitis	1:270	15 years
Sibs of leukemic children	1:720	10 years
U.S. Caucasian children (<15 years of age)	1:2880	10 years

[a] Other groups include persons exposed to benzene compounds, patients with refractory anemias and chromosomal aberrations, or with ataxia telangiectasia, neurofibromatosis, or chronic myelogenous leukemia (CML).
[b] Most data were adapted from R. W. Miller: *Cancer Research*, *27:* 2420, 1960.

kemia, are prone to central nervous system hemorrhage.

Infiltration of the marrow with leukemic cells can cause bone pain. Joint pain also occurs, but its etiology is obscure. Leukemic infiltration of the reticuloendothelial system can cause adenopathy, hepatosplenomegaly and mediastinal mass (T cell leukemia). In myelogenous leukemia, gingival hypertrophy is seen, and in monocytic leukemia subcutaneous and soft tissue collections of leukemic blasts (chloromas) are not uncommon. Leukemic cells invading the central nervous system can be clinically silent or can produce a meningitic syndrome or spinal cord compression. Extreme leukocytosis can also cause central nervous system symptoms. The presence of high white blood cell count, central nervous system disease, and mediastinal mass are unfavorable clinical presentations.

Table 55.3 shows the clinical and laboratory presentation of 1637 children with ALL. Although the majority of patients do have some hematologic abnormalities, many do not show such profound leukocytosis that a diagnosis of leukemia is certain from the peripheral count. Strikingly abnormal blood counts can also be seen in aplastic anemia, infectious mononucleosis, cytomegalovirus infection, and leukemoid reactions.

Although an experienced hematologist can usually differentiate blasts from atypical mononuclear cells on the peripheral smear, the diagnosis of leukemia is made by marrow aspiration and/or biopsy. The leukemic marrow is hypercellular and contains a monotonous population of blasts. Normal precursors are rare or absent. Generally, it is not advisable to perform the marrow biopsy in an emergency department setting because diagnosis and current management of acute leukemia require karyotyping, surface markers, and special histochemical stains; these studies need to be arranged by the physician who will assume responsibility for the management of the leukemia.

MANAGEMENT

In many instances confirmation of the diagnosis of leukemia is not made in the emergency department. However, when leukemia is the probable diagnosis or the only tenable diagnosis (e.g., white count of

Table 55.3
Acute Lymphocytic Leukemia: Presentation of 1637 Children from 1972 to 1977, Children's Cancer Study Group[a]

Clinical		Laboratory	
Characteristic	Percent	Characteristic	Percent
Age (yr)		Hemoglobin (g/100 ml)	
<2	9	<7	44
2–6	61	7–10	36
7–10	15	>10	20
>10	15	WBC × 10^3/cu mm	
Sex (male)	56	<5	30
Race (white)	85	5–10	24
Adenopathy	61	10–20	15
Hepatomegaly	65	20–50	14
Splenomegaly	57	50–200	12
		>200	5
		Platelets × 10^3/cu mm	
		<50	50
		50–150	32
		>150	18
		Mediastinal mass	5

Adapted from Hammond et al. (1980).

100,000/cu mm with obvious blasts), the emergency department physician or pediatrician should discuss the possibility that a child's disease is leukemia. This is accepted practice provided the physician has laboratory evidence to support the diagnosis, can take time to explain the reasons for concern, and can reassure the family that leukemia is no longer a hopeless disease. After the physician has begun appropriate supportive care, he or she should arrange admission or referral of the child to a hematologist or oncologist. Referral to a specialist or cancer center is important because it has been shown that survival is better when a child is treated at a cancer center or is managed by a specialist according to a current protocol.

Specific treatment of leukemia with chemotherapy should not be undertaken in the emergency department. Immediate antileukemic therapy in a child with a large tumor burden can cause death from hyperkalemia or can precipitate renal failure. Definitive therapy requires medical and emotional support and use of chemotherapeutic protocols designed for specific subsets of leukemia. Typical protocols currently in use for the treatment of lymphocytic and myeloid leukemia are shown in Tables 55.4 and 55.5. These are modified year by year. The goals of therapy are first to achieve a

Table 55.4
Acute Lymphoblastic Leukemia: General Treatment Strategy

Induction	Intensification	Maintenance
Vincristine,	*CNS prophylaxis*	6-Mercaptopurine (6-MP)
prednisone	Intrathecal methotrexate	Methotrexate
±	±	±
L-Asparaginase	CNS irradiation	Vincristine
±	±	Prednisone
Daunomycin	*Marrow consolidation*	±
	Vincristine	Adriamycin
	Prednisone	Cytosine arabinoside
	6-MP	Cyclophosphamide
	Methotrexate	Intrathecal methotrexate
0 1	2	24 60

Time (months)

Table 55.5
Acute Myeloid Leukemia: General Treatment Strategy

Induction	CNS Prophylaxis	Maintenance
Cytosine arabinoside	Intrathecal	Cytosine arabinoside
Adriamycin	methotrexate	6-Thioguanine
or	±	±
Daunomycin	CNS irradiation	Cyclophosphosphamide
±	±	Vincristine
6-Thioguanine	Marrow consolidation	BCNU[a]
±	Cytosine arabinoside	Adriamycin
Prednisone	6-Thioguanine	5-Azacytidine
Vincristine		Steroid
	MARROW TRANSPLANTATION	
0 2–4	2–6	24 44

Time (months)

[a] BCNU = *N*,*N*-Bis(2-chloroethyl)-*N*-nitrosourea.

marrow "remission," i.e. a normal bone marrow, within 1 or 2 months of intensive "induction" therapy and then to maintain the remission. Induction is followed by a period of prevention or treatment of occult central nervous system disease, and then maintenance therapy. Treatment is changed if the disease recurs in the marrow or appears in the central nervous system or testes. Treatment is stopped after several years of continuous remission.

Fortunately, most children diagnosed with acute leukemia do not present with problems that are imminently life-threatening. But, there are some situations at diagnosis and many complications of therapy that demand recognition and immediate intervention. These are discussed in detail below.

Infection and Fever

Infection is the leading cause of death in leukemia. Although fever is a symptom of leukemia itself in 25% of patients, it more often is an indication of infection. In the leukemic patient, significant fever is defined as at least 2 temperature elevations of over 38.4°C in 24 hours or a sustained temperature of ≧39°C for over 4 hours in the absence of an obvious iatrogenic cause. Not only is fever a frequent sign of infection, but the height of the fever correlates with the severity of infection: if it is under 39°C, a positive culture is unlikely; if it is over 39°C a positive blood culture occurs in roughly 25% of patients—often with gram-positive organisms; and if it is over 40°C, gram-negative or polymicrobial septicemia becomes increasingly likely. There are exceptions to the correlation of fever with infection. Some patients in septic shock may have no fever and, in fact, may be hypothermic, and patients who have been receiving corticosteroids for longer than 4 weeks may not manifest fever even with overwhelming infection.

The approach to presumed infection in a child with leukemia is unlike that in otherwise healthy children. It depends on the following variables: the type of leukemia, the status of disease (remission or relapse), the current therapy, the absolute neutrophil count and condition of the patient. Infection is much more common in AML than ALL. For this reason it is common for patients with AML to be hospitalized for the entire 6 to 10 weeks of induction therapy. Infection is more common in relapse than during induction, and is relatively uncommon during remission. Treatment also determines the predisposition to infection and types of infection. Steroids interfere with neutrophil migration and bactericidal function, and they lyse lymphocytes; cytosine arabinoside and Adriamycin or daunomycin cause extensive mucosal ulceration allowing entry of commensual flora into the bloodstream and tissues; central nervous system irradiation causes a transient bactericidal defect.

The Febrile Neutropenic Patient. The most important variable in determining outcome of infection is the degree of neutropenia caused by the disease itself and by many cytotoxic agents. In adults neutropenia is defined as fewer than 1000 neutrophils. In practice, children tolerate neutropenia better than adults, and most can remain free of infection with counts between 500 and 1000 neutrophils. However, below 500 neutrophils, the risk of infection increases; below 200 it becomes more likely; and if the neutrophil count is on its way down from 200 to 0, the risk of infection becomes even greater yet. Duration of neutropenia is also significant. If neutropenia represents a transient dip in the neutrophil count following a high dose of chemotherapy and recovery is likely in a few days, infection is less likely. If infection occurs, the patient's own defenses can usually come to his aid in time. If, on the other hand, the neutropenia is of several weeks duration, overwhelming infection is more of a threat.

Management of fever and presumed infection begins with a careful history. Today most parents of children with leukemia have acquired a remarkable degree of medical sophistication: they can define the precise type of their child's leukemia, name the current therapy, recall recent blood counts, suggest tendencies toward certain recurring illnesses in their child, and often can reliably judge how ill their child is. This historical information is important, because the neutropenia and cytotoxic therapy can mask signs of illness and cause a physician who does not know the child well to underestimate the potential seriousness of the illness.

A thorough physical examination sometimes uncovers the source of fever. In addition to examining the common sites of infection in children, the buccal mucosa, perianal area, and nailbeds, muscles, joints, bones, and former sites of intravenous infusions should be searched. Even an apparently minor swelling or a tear in the mucosal surface or skin can be a source of disseminated infection (Fig. 55.1). Perirectal abscesses, seen frequently in AML, can present with pain and discoloration but no edema. Seemingly insignificant paronychia can be the source of significant bacteremias. Blood and urine cultures should be obtained and a chest x-ray should be taken, but a lumbar puncture is not indicated unless signs of meningitis are present; for unknown reasons, infectious meningitis is rare in leukemic children. If symptoms of meningitis occur, spinal fluid should be obtained for bacterial, fungal and viral cultures and for cytology to rule out central nervous system leukemia.

The accepted practice in treating a febrile neutropenic patient is to begin empiric antibiotic therapy with combinations of intravenous broad-spectrum antibiotics. The choice of antibiotic combination depends on the prevailing patterns of infection and antimicrobial resistance in the area. First line combinations currently in use are listed in Table 55.6. These choices are based on experience: most infections in neutropenic patients arise from the patient's endogenous flora and are caused by invasion of skin (*Staphylococcus aureus*) or intestinal flora (*Escherichia coli, Pseudomonas, Klebsiella, Enterococcus, Serratia*). Antibiotics should be started if the child appears toxic or the neutrophil count is less than 500. Whenever possible, the primary physician should be contacted for advice.

Most patients with leukemia do not pre-

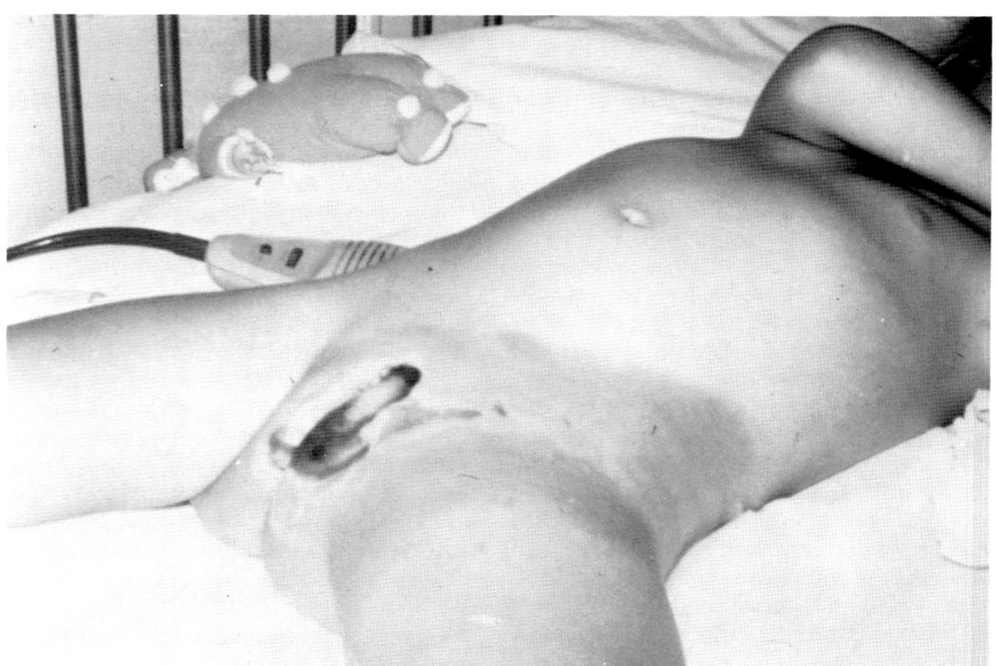

Figure 55.1. Necrotizing perineal cellulitis in 4-year-old girl with acute lymphoblastic leukemia. The patient presented with fever, neutropenia, pain and erythema in the perineum. The lesion and blood culture grew *Escherichia coli.* This lesion resolved with minimal scarring after antibiotic therapy and local debridement.

Table 55.6
Two Antibiotic Combinations Used in Empiric Therapy of Fever and Infection in Neutropenic Pediatric Patient

I. Carbenicillin[a]	500 mg/kg/day i.v. every 4 hr not to exceed 40 g/day
Cephalothin[b]	150 mg/kg/day i.v. every 4 hr not to exceed 10 g/day
Gentamicin[c]	5 mg/kg/day i.v. every 8 hr for those over 10 yr 6 mg/kg/day i.v. every 8 hr for those 5 to 10 yr 7.5 mg/kg/day i.v. every 6 hr for those 1 mo to 5 yr
II. Trimethoprim-sulfamethoxazole[d]	5.0 mg/kg (of trimethoprim) i.v. loading, 1.0 mg/kg i.v./day every 6 hr
Carbenicillin	500 mg/kg/day i.v. every 4 hr

[a] From P. A. Pizzo et al.: *American Journal of Medicine*, 67: 194–200, 1979.
[b] Oxacillin: 150 mg/kg/day i.v. every 6 hours (usually not to exceed 12 mg/day) can be used instead of a cephalosporin where *Staphylococcus aureus* is likely. Cefazolin 100 mg/kg/day i.v. every 8 hours and cefoxitin are under investigation in compromised hosts.
[c] Tobramycin occasionally is more effective than gentamicin against *Pseudomonas aeruginosa* (5–7.5 mg/kg/day every 8 hours). Amikacin, 15 mg/kg/day every 8 hours (maximum 1.5 g/day) should be used for gentamicin-resistant Enterobacteriaceae.
[d] From R. K. Stuart et al.: *American Journal of Medicine*, 68: 876, 1980.

sent to the emergency department with invasive fungal disease unless they are in relapse or have been recently discharged from the hospital after a protracted course of antibiotics or hyperalimentation. Corticosteroids and indwelling catheters also predispose to fungal disease. Fungal overgrowth can present as esophagitis, cellulitis, pneumonitis, meningitis, urinary tract infection, septicemia, or fever of unknown origin. Oral candidiasis (thrush) and esophagitis are the most common infections. Esophagitis presents with retrosternal pain or dysphagia with or without oral lesions (Fig. 55.2). Thrush responds to oral Mycostatin (200,000 to 400,000 units 4 times a day), but esophagitis and other invasive fungal diseases require intravenous amphotericin B.

Bacterial, viral, or fungal infections can cause septic shock in the patient with leukemia. Treatment consists of aggressive measures to maintain intravascular volume and blood pressure (Chapter 2), broad-spectrum antibiotic therapy appropriate for neutropenic patients, and hematologic support with red cells, platelets, and plasma. The use of high dose bolus steroids (30 mg/kg of methylprednisolone) is still controversial.

Interstitial Pneumonitis. Interstitial pneumonitis presents a special problem for the patient with acute lymphocytic leukemia. The most common documented cause of interstitial pneumonitis in ALL patients in remission is *Pneumocystis carinii*, a ubiquitous protozoa. Pneumocystis pneumonia is also the most common cause of death in patients with ALL in remission. It usually presents within the first few months following central nervous system prophylaxis. The onset can be insidious, with a few days or weeks of fever and cough, or it can be fulminant, with rapid development of tachypnea, air hunger, cyanosis and respiratory failure. The lungs are relatively free of adventitious sounds. Classically, the chest x-ray shows an interstitial pattern with pronounced hilar markings (Fig. 55.3).

In the past decade it was considered necessary to document the presence of pneumocystis pneumonia by lung aspirate, tracheal aspirate, or open lung biopsy. The only available antimicrobial for therapy was pentamidine isothionate, a drug with major toxic side effects. However, it has been shown that trimethoprim-sulfamethoxazole, a relatively safe antibiotic, is equally effective in treating pneumocystis (20 mg/kg/day as trimethoprim). The child who is ill or has air hunger, cyanosis, and rapid evolution of his illness, or who lives more than 1 hour away from medical care should be admitted for initiation of therapy, observation and consideration of diagnostic procedures.

Some cases of interstitial pneumonia during the early months of remission do not have a discernible infectious cause. Conceivably they represent toxic pneumonopathies from drugs, such as methotrexate, cytosine arabinoside, or cyclophosphamide, or from infectious agents that are difficult to document.

Common Childhood Infections in the Leukemic Child in Remission. Children with leukemia also acquire common pediatric viral and bacterial illnesses. If the child has been in remission for several months, diseases such as otitis media, urinary tract infection, streptococcal pharyngitis, impetigo, infectious mononucleosis, mumps, influenza, and the ubiquitous upper respiratory infections can be managed as they would be in the otherwise healthy child. However, both varicella and rubeola are dangerous infections in children with leukemia regardless of the status of the leukemia. Pneumonia and encephalitis are major complications. Varicella has a mortality of up to 10% and a major morbidity of 25%. Varicella can be attenuated or prevented by administration of zoster immune plasma (10 ml/kg i.v.) or zoster immune globulin (0.1 ml/kg i.m.) within 72 hours of exposure. These products are available in blood banks or from the Centers for Disease Control in Atlanta, Georgia.

Rubeola can cause a protracted illness that culminates in fatal pneumonia. γ-Globulin (0.1 ml/kg i.m.) provides some protection from rubeola and should be given for exposure, but measles vaccine is contraindicated. Children who have received adequate rubeola vaccination before developing leukemia usually are immune.

Children with leukemia who have varicella or rubeola require close observation, and parents require education about signs of progression. If the child is clinically well, admission is not necessary. If he or she is toxic or shows signs of pneumonitis, encephalitis, liver failure or hemorrhagic exanthem, admission is mandatory.

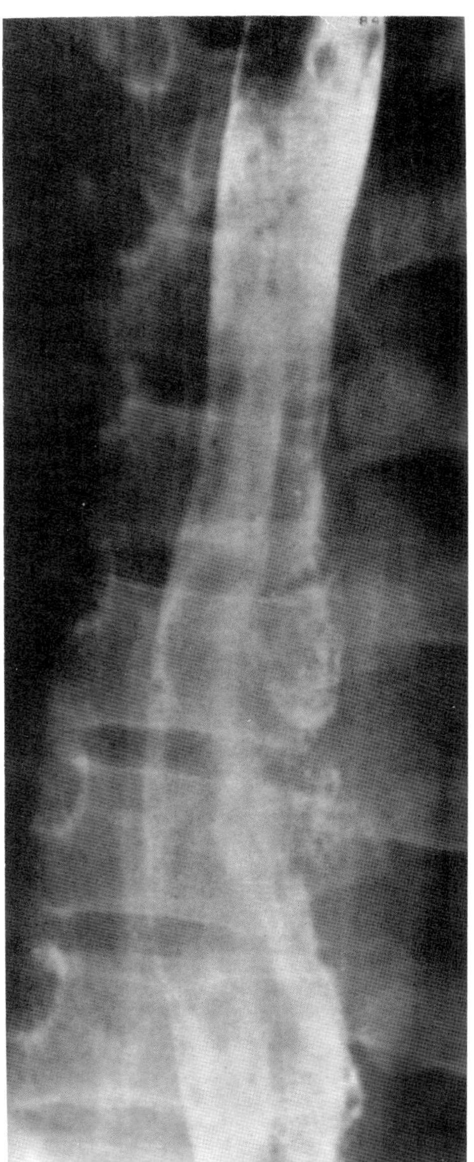

Figure 55.2. Esophageal candidiasis in a 12-year-old boy with acute lymphocytic leukemia (ALL) receiving corticosteroids and broad spectrum antibiotics. Barium swallow shows ulceration and dissection of esophageal mucosa. (Reproduced with permission of Dr. Spencer Borden, Department of Radiology, Children's Hospital of Philadelphia.)

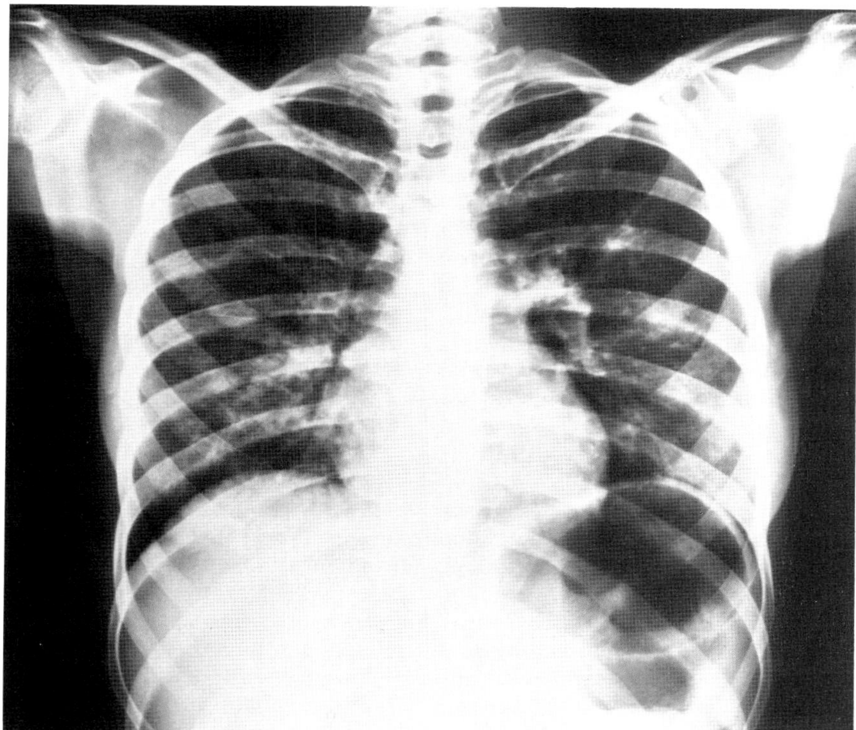

Figure 55.3. *Pneumocystis carinii* pneumonitis in a 13-year-old girl with a 48-hour history of fever and cough. Chest x-ray shows bilateral alveolar infiltrates most prominent at the hila. (Reproduced with permission of Dr. Spencer Borden, Department of Radiology, Children's Hospital of Philadelphia.)

Hemorrhage

Hemorrhage is the second most common cause of death in leukemia. At the time of diagnosis and induction therapy, during relapse, or 5 to 30 days after intensive chemotherapy, thrombocytopenia is common. Spontaneous bleeding can occur at platelet counts below 10,000 to 20,000/cu mm although spontaneous bruising is seen at higher levels in some patients. Other factors contributing to a bleeding tendency include: infection with associated disseminated intravascular coagulation (see Chapter 47), antibiotic therapy which causes hypoprothrombinemia, and aspirin which interferes with platelet function.

In most leukemic children during the early stages of disease, bleeding problems can be controlled with local measures alone (i.e. pressure for epistaxis), or in conjunction with platelet transfusions (0.2 unit/kg of platelets). Epistaxis is sometimes a serious problem that may last for hours, and may fail to respond to pressure. If local measures and platelets fail, packing is a necessary but uncomfortable therapy. Sedation and analgesia may be helpful in controlling the anxiety of a severe bleed.

In some patients with AML at diagnosis, especially those with hypergranular promyelocytic leukemia, a bleeding diathesis may occur at presentation or upon initiation of therapy. Bleeding is generally refractory to platelets. Patients show prolonged prothrombin and partial thromboplastin times, elevated fibrin-split products and drastically shortened fibrinogen half-life. The most common form of bleeding in this situation is in the central nervous system; it is frequently fatal in the first few days of illness. Fresh frozen plasma (10 ml/kg) and cryoprecipitate can help to maintain levels of fibrinogen and clotting factors.

Although there has been no controlled study demonstrating the benefit of prophylactic heparin, heparinization (loading dose, 50 units/kg; then 5 to 10 units/kg/hour to maintain the PTT at twice normal) is usually started before initiation of specific chemotherapy.

Anemia

At the time of diagnosis most children with leukemia are anemic. If the hemoglobin is under 8 g/dl, it is advisable to administer packed blood cells (10 ml/kg over 4 hours) because it is unlikely that that child will have the ability to produce his or her own erythrocytes for several weeks. If, in the absence of hemorrhage, the child presents with profound anemia, i.e. hemoglobin 1 to 4 g/dl, transfusions at the usual rate can precipitate heart failure. Blood should be replaced slowly at 3 to 5 ml/kg over 4 hours, and supplemental oxygen given to enhance oxygen delivery to tissues. Furosemide (1 mg/kg) can help avoid fluid overload or heart failure; however, if the white blood cell count is very high (> 100,000 cu mm), diuretics should be withheld because intravascular dehydration encourages sludging and thrombosis. Exchange transfusion has been advocated by some in these exceptional circumstances. Obviously if hemorrhage is the cause of a very low hemoglobin, fluid and transfusion therapy should be carried out to replace losses quickly (Chapter 47).

Anemia is common in children being treated for cancer and is usually well-tolerated. Most often anemia is a result of chemotherapeutic suppression of normal hematopoiesis. Other causes such as nutritional deficiencies, chronic blood loss, infection, or hemolysis should be ruled out if the anemia is problematic. After induction therapy, routine transfusion for hemoglobin in the range of 7 to 10 g/dl is not advisable unless the anemia is causing symptoms or there is continuing blood loss. If the child is a potential candidate for marrow transplant, blood products from family members should not be used.

Extreme Leukocytosis

Extreme leukocytosis with white blood cell counts over 200,000/cu mm occurs at diagnosis in about 5% of patients with acute leukemia and in chronic myelogenous leukemia. In acute leukemia, extreme leukocytosis predisposes to early bleeding and thrombosis in the central nervous system. It has been suggested that patients with white blood cell counts above 200,000/cu mm should receive prompt cranial irradiation or plasmapheresis, but these are unproven therapies. Patients with chronic myelogenous leukemia (CML) do not have the problem of sludging and thrombosis seen in ALL unless there is a predominance of blasts.

Uric Acid Nephropathy

Some patients with acute leukemia present with an elevated uric acid in the serum caused by spontaneous breakdown of leukemic cells. The excess uric acid precipitates in the renal tubules. Antileukemic therapy accelerates breakdown of leukemic cells; more urates are formed and renal failure can occur. To prevent urate nephropathy, all children with leukemia should receive the xanthine oxidase inhibitor, allopurinol (50 mg p.o. 3 times a day under 6 years; 100 mg p.o. 3 times a day over 6 years) for at least 24 hours before starting therapy. Hydration at the rate of twice maintenance and alkalinization of urine to pH > 6.5 with sodium bicarbonate (40 meq/L) facilitates dissolution of uric acid crystals since uric acid precipitates at pH $\leqq$ 5. Once the serum uric acid is normal and the child is adequately hydrated and producing a dilute urine, specific antileukemic therapy can begin. Bicarbonate is stopped at this time to avoid development of hypoxanthine crystals.

Hypercalcemia

Hypercalcemia occurs in about 2% of patients with acute leukemia. Hypercalcemia is caused by destruction of bone by the malignant cells, by ectopic production of parathormone by the leukemic cells themselves, or by elevated levels of peripheral plasma prostaglandin E_2, vitamin D-like substances, or osteoclast-activating factors. The serum calcium can reach levels high enough to cause anorexia, nausea, vomiting, constipation, lethargy, confusion, coma, tachycardia or bradycardia, and renal failure. The ultimate therapy of leukemic hypercalcemia is treatment of the leukemia. Interim supportive management consists of hydration with normal saline (200 ml/sq m/hour), followed by diuresis with furosemide (1 to 2 mg/kg i.v. every 4 to 6 hours). Monitoring of the cardiovascular status is essential. For indications for corticosteroids, calcitonin, or dialysis in symptomatic hypercalcemia (usually > 15 mg/dl), see Chapter 46. Phosphorus has no role in the emergency situation in the patient with leukemia with acute elevation of calcium and marginal renal function.

Tumor Lysis Syndrome

In patients with large tumor burdens, especially those patients with leukemia or organomegaly and/or with high white blood cell counts, or in patients with non-Hodgkin's lymphoma, institution of therapy can bring about a potentially fatal tumor lysis syndrome consisting of a rapid rise in serum potassium and phosphorus, a precipitous fall in serum calcium and elevations of the serum uric acid, BUN, and creatinine. These abnormalities occur in spite of hydration and allopurinol therapy. Hyperkalemia, the most dangerous abnormality, demands prompt treatment with Kayexalate, insulin and glucose infusion, or dialysis (see Chapter 46).

Syndrome of Inappropriate Antidiuretic Hormone (SIADH)

SIADH is caused by many processes. In children with leukemia SIADH can occur for reasons unrelated to cancer (stress, pulmonary disease, CNS disease, etc.). However, it is most commonly a side effect of vincristine or cyclophosphamide. Treatment is as discussed in Chapter 53.

Spinal Cord Compression

Spinal cord compression occurs in leukemia because of epidural or subarachnoid collections of leukemic cells. Symptoms include radicular pain, back pain, difficulty with urination, paresis or paralysis. Physical examination can be unremarkable or may show tenderness over spinous processes, weakness, hyperactive or later absent deep tendon reflexes, absent superficial reflexes, and inability to walk on the toes or heels. Radiographs may show a collapsed vertebral body, but often they are normal. A myelogram confirms the diagnosis, and therapy consists of immediate corticosteroid therapy (dexamethosone, 0.1 to 0.5 mg/kg every 6 hours) and/or prompt irradiation. Leukemia or lymphoma of the spinal cord do not require laminectomy.

Central Nervous System (CNS) Leukemia

Leukemia can present or relapse in the CNS as diffuse subarachnoid disease. Symptoms include headache, stiff neck, malaise, and rarely fever. Diagnosis is made by finding > 10 leukemic blasts/cu mm in the spinal fluid. Treatment consists of intrathecal methotrexate, reinstitution of chemotherapy similar to that used in induction, and cranial or craniospinal irradiation.

Testicular Leukemia

In males, the first site of relapse can occur in the testes causing a painless hard swelling of one or both testes. Treatment consists of reinduction therapy and irradiation but is not always satisfactory because overt testicular relapse is often a harbinger of marrow relapse.

Encephalopathy

Prevention or treatment of CNS leukemia with irradiation and methotrexate is not without hazard. Approximately 6 weeks after cranial irradiation some children develop profound somnolence. Somnolence lasts 1 to 2 weeks. It may be associated with low grade fever in a child who appears mentally and physically well. In patients treated multiple times for repeated relapse, cerebral white matter degenerates. Mild leukoencephalopathy may present as a learning disability. Advanced disease insidiously causes slurred speech, broad based gait, obtundation, coma, and death. This constellation of symptoms and a CAT scan showing cortical atrophy, degeneration of white matter and extensive intracerebral calcification confirm the diagnosis.

Other causes of encephalopathy include viral encephalitis (especially herpetic encephalitis), or adverse reactions to vincristine, prednisone, L-asparaginase or intrathecal medications. L-Asparaginase encephalopathy causes hemorrhagic or thrombotic cerebrovascular accidents caused by the drug's interference with coagulation. Acute encephalopathy requires evaluation and usually admission.

NON-HODGKIN'S LYMPHOMAS

BACKGROUND

Definition

Non-Hodgkin's lymphomas (NHL) are malignant tumors that originate in lymphatic tissues: lymph nodes, Waldeyer's ring, the appendix, mesentery, Peyer's patches, or rarely the spleen. Sometimes NHL arises in extralymphatic sites such as bone, ovaries or skin. In contrast to NHL in adults, where the disease often remains indolent and localized for years, NHL in children has a tendency to proliferate rapidly and spread outside the primary lymphatic area in weeks or months. Often it metastasizes to marrow and/or the central nervous system. When extensive marrow replacement occurs, the distinction between NHL and acute leukemia may be difficult.

Classification

There is no disease classification that is more controversial than that of NHL. The NHL are classified according to histology, cytology, and immunology. They are also classified according to stage (see under "Clinical Presentation"). The types of lymphoma that are seen in children are almost always poorly differentiated and diffuse (as opposed to nodular), and they efface entirely the architecture of the tissue of origin. In children the malignant cells are often B lymphoblasts, T lymphoblasts, or undifferentiated stem cells.

NHL are also classified according to stage. Stage reflects the tumor burden. A small tumor burden confers an excellent prognosis. The staging system used at St. Jude Children's Research Hospital is well suited to pediatric NHL (Table 55.7). Most pediatric NHL presents as Stage III or IV disease.

Table 55.7
Clinical Staging Classification Suited for Children with Non-Hodgkin's Lymphoma[a, b]

Stage I
- A single nodal or extra nodal tumor with the exclusion of mediastinum or abdomen

Stage II
- A single extranodal tumor with regional-lymph node involvement or two or more nodal areas on the same side of the diaphragm
- A resectable primary gastrointestinal tract tumor (usually ileocecal), with or without involvement of mesenteric nodes

Stage III
- Intrathoracic tumors
- Extensive unresectable intra-abdominal disease
- Paraspinal or epidural tumors
- Two single tumors on opposite sides of the diaphragm

Stage IV
- Any of the above with involvement of central nervous system or bone marrow or both

[a] Marrow involvement is defined as less than 25% replacement by tumor without circulating blast cells. The majority of children have Stage III–IV disease. The most common clinical presentation is intra-abdominal disease.
[b] Adapted from S. B. Murphy: *New England Journal of Medicine, 299:* 1447, 1978.

Epidemiology

NHL usually occurs before puberty or in early adolescence. The incidence falls off in late adolescence and then rises logarithmically with age. The incidence in childhood is 0.5 per 100,000. There is a male predominance of 1.4:1. In adults a small excess of NHL has been reported among anesthesiologists, workers in polyvinyl chloride factories, rubber workers, petroleum refinery workers, arsenic ore refineries, and veterinarians.

Patients with immunodeficiency diseases have an exceptionally high incidence of NHL. The inherited immunodeficiency states associated with NHL include severe combined immunodeficiency, variable immunodeficiency, X-linked hypogammaglobulinemia, IgA deficiency, IgM deficiency, X-linked lymphoproliferative syndrome (Duncan's disease), ataxia telangectasia, Wiscott-Aldrich syndrome and others. In addition, NHL occurs with increased frequency in patients with acquired disorders of immunity including rheumatoid arthritis, systemic lupus erythematosus, sarcoidosis, and celiac disease. NHL develops with increased frequency in renal and cardiac transplant patients, in patients receiving chronic immunosuppressive therapy, and in patients with Hodgkin's disease treated with radiation and chemotherapy.

A special case exists with respect to African Burkitt's lymphoma. This tumor is the most common childhood neoplasm in Uganda, Cameroons, and Congo: that is, in those areas of high rainfall, warm temperature, and holoendemic malaria. African Burkitt's lymphoma is almost always associated with high titers to Epstein-Barr virus (EBV) antigens and with the presence of EBV in the tumor cells. There is a male predominance of 4.7:1.

CLINICAL MANIFESTATIONS AND PATHOPHYSIOLOGY

Localized NHL

About 25% of childhood NHL presents as Stage I or Stage II disease. Presentations include localized swelling in the cervical or inguinal nodes, nasopharyngeal masses, mediastinal masses, bone pain and swelling, and acute abdomen.

B Lymphocyte NHL (American Burkitt's Lymphoma)

Although over half of patients with African Burkitt's lymphoma present with swelling in the jaw, this is an uncommon finding in American patients. Jaw tumors occur in only 20% of American cases and cervical nodal primaries, in about 15%. American Burkitt's lymphoma, usually causes generalized abdominal enlargement, pain, nausea, vomiting, constipation, and, in about half the cases, malignant ascites. In these circumstances the primary tumor is either in the ovaries or retroperitoneal nodes, but kidneys and sometimes bowel are involved.

Burkitt's tumor cells proliferate exceedingly rapidly. Thus tumors grow quickly and tend to extend locally over a number of days to weeks causing ascites, pleural effusion and renal failure. Frequently, they metastasize to the marrow and meninges. Untreated, abdominal American Burkitt's lymphoma is rapidly fatal, usually because of renal failure. When treated, the disease tends to recur within a few months either as abdominal tumor or as leukemia.

Mediastinal NHL

Mediastinal NHL occurs most often in males in late childhood or early adolescence and, untreated, metastasizes to marrow, nervous system and testes. The signs and symptoms of mediastinal NHL may be those of leukemia or may be those of a thoracic tumor (see under "Thoracic Tumors").

MANAGEMENT

Localized NHL

When localized NHL is suspected, the node or mass should be biopsied promptly. Open biopsy is mandatory to evaluate nodal architecture. Prior to biopsy it is advisable to obtain a chest x-ray and blood count to make certain that there is no large mediastinal mass or unsuspected leukemic process. When treated with surgery and chemotherapy with or without irradiation, prognosis in localized NHL is excellent.

Burkitt's Lymphoma with Extensive Abdominal Involvement

When the primary tumor is abdominal, this disease usually constitutes a medical emergency because the cells are proliferating rapidly. The tumor grows day by day, encroaching on vital organs, especially the kidneys. Spontaneous tumor lysis causes metabolic abnormalities, discussed under tumor lysis syndrome (see p. 705). The role of the emergency physician who suspects intra-abdominal Burkitt's lymphoma is to ascertain the hematologic and metabolic status of the child with the following studies: CBC, BUN, creatinine, uric acid, electrolytes, calcium, phosphorus, and liver function tests. Hydration at 3000 ml/sq m/day of 5% dextroxe in water-0.25 N saline solution, alkalinization, and allopurinol (50 mg p.o. 3 times a day for those < 6 years; 100 mg p.o. 3 times a day for those > 6 years) should be started immediately. If renal failure is present, it is necessary to determine whether it is from uric acid nephropathy, tumor infiltration, or obstructive uropathy. An intravenous pyelogram or ultrasound can detect infiltration or compression by tumor. Catheterization should be performed to establish whether the kidneys are forming urine and to rule out bladder obstruction. Treatment of renal failure varies with the cause (see Chapter 46). Immediate antitumor therapy with cyclophosphamide or corticosteroid is contraindicated.

Mediastinal Lymphoma

When the chest x-ray reveals a mediastinal mass and no obvious congenital abnormality or infectious cause is apparent, cancer must be ruled out. Sometimes it is possible to diagnose an NHL by the combination of an abnormal blood count or bone marrow and a mediastinal mass. Other times it is necessary to biopsy a peripheral node or the mass itself. Often open biopsy is a straightforward procedure, but it can be life-threatening. For a discussion of mediastinal masses, see under "Thoracic Tumors," p. 712.

Mediastinal NHL is responsive to combinations of chemotherapy and irradiation and the majority of patients are now long-term survivors.

HISTIOCYTIC DISEASES

BACKGROUND

Histiocytic diseases include a heterogeneous group of benign and malignant disorders in which histiocytes, that is, tissue macrophages, appear to be the dominant abnormal cell type. With some of these diseases, it is difficult to determine whether the histiocytes are benign or malignant because they may appear histologically benign and yet metastasize; conversely, they can appear histologically malignant and behave with relative benignity.

CLINICAL MANIFESTATIONS AND PATHOPHYSIOLOGY

Groopman and Golde have brought order into the classification of histiocytic diseases by grouping them according to their pathophysiology into lipid storage diseases, reactive diseases, and neoplastic diseases. Among the reactive disorders are those diseases formerly called histiocytosis X and familial erythrophagocytic lymphohistiocytosis. Some reactive disorders tend to behave in a malignant fashion. Among the neoplastic group, acute monocytic leukemia and malignant histiocytosis are seen in children and adolescents. Three of the disorders, which behave in a malignant fashion regardless of etiology or pathophysiology, will be discussed: the spectrum of eosinophilic granulomas, familial erythrophagocytic lymphohistiocytosis, and malignant histiocytosis. Monocytic leukemia is considered a form of acute myeloid leukemia (see under "Leukemia").

Eosinophilic Granuloma Syndromes

This group of diseases includes solitary eosinophilic granuloma lesions in bone, multiple eosinophilic granulomas of bone, and disseminated eosinophilic granulomas (Letterer-Siwe). A solitary eosinophilic granuloma presents as a painless or mildly painful swelling in the skull, long bones, ribs, pelvis, or vertebra. X-ray shows a lytic lesion with well-defined borders. Multiple eosinophilic granulomas can arise over weeks, months or years. They can be confined to long bones or may be distributed in the skull in such a way as to cause proptosis, diabetes insipidus, cholestatomas, and loss of teeth (Hand-Schüller-Christian disease). Rare cases of paraplegia caused by vertebral lesions have been described.

Widespread eosinophilic granulomas in bone and soft tissue in an infant comprise Letterer-Siwe disease. Signs and symptoms include failure to thrive, diarrhea, chronic seborrhea, chronic otitis media, purpuric rash, generalized adenopathy and hepatosplenomegaly. The chest x-ray may show interstitial pneumonitis. The blood count may be normal, but marrow involvement or massive splenomegaly can lead to pancytopenia.

Specific therapy depends on the extent of disease. Isolated eosinophilic granulomas can be cured with surgical curettage. If they are in inaccessible but critical areas (e.g. pituitary fossa), low dose irradiation often arrests the process. Diabetes insipidus may require vasopressin (Pitressin) (Chapter 53). Although rare spontaneous regressions have been reported, disseminated histiocytosis requires multiagent chemotherapy: vinblastine, prednisone, cyclophosphamide and methotrexate are active agents. Recently fetal thymic extract has also been shown to induce regression of these lesions.

Familial Erythrophagocytic Lymphohistiocytosis (Familial Histiocytic Reticulosis, Congenital Hemophagocytic Reticulosis)

This is a sex-linked or autosomal recessive systemic disease presenting in early infancy with fever, vomiting, anorexia, irritability and occasionally (25%) with seizures, cranial nerve abnormalities and "bizarre" meningitis. Generalized adenopathy and hepatosplenomegaly are common and a purpuric rash sometimes occurs. Laboratory abnormalities include pancytopenia, hypofibrinoginemia, hyperlipidemia, elevated liver enzymes and hypo- or hypergammaglobulinemia. Biopsy of involved tissues or bone marrow aspiration shows diffuse infiltration by morphologically benign histiocytes and prominent erythrophagocytosis. There is depletion of thymic and lymphoid tissue.

The disease is usually fatal in weeks or months. Transient responses have occurred with vinblastine and prednisone. Plasmapheresis has achieved remission in 2 patients.

Malignant Histiocytosis (Histiocytic Medullary Reticulosis)

This disease presents with fever, adenopathy, hepatosplenomegaly, pancytopenia or leukocytosis. The mean age at presentation is 31 years but the age range is from 1 to 71 years. There is a male predominance and high incidence in certain areas of Africa and Asia. Ten cases have been reported following induction therapy for acute lymphoblastic leukemia. Biopsy of involved tissues reveals infiltration with malignant histiocytes of all stages of maturation. Infiltrates are prominent in the medullary zone of lymph nodes. The distinction between this disease and monocytic leukemia is sometimes impossible. The disease is usually fatal, but remissions have been achieved with cyclophosphamide, Adriamycin, vincristine and prednisone.

MANAGEMENT

The emergency physician's management of the histiocytic disorders consists in suspecting them, recognizing their presentations and handling the complications of the diseases and therapy. Eosinophilic granulomas can usually be diagnosed by an x-ray. The significant problems they can cause are diabetes insipidus (Chapter 53), pathologic fracture or rarely paraplegia. Letterer-Siwe disease can be suspected from the clinical findings. The complications of pancytopenia are the same as in leukemia (p. 697). Massive organomegaly can cause respiratory embarrassment. Irradiation and chemotherapy will usually restore adequate ventilation.

Management of the complications of familial erythrophagocytic histiocytosis and malignant histiocytes is the same as for leukemia. The main problems are marrow failure predisposing to infection and hemorrhage (see under "Leukemia").

HODGKIN'S DISEASE

BACKGROUND

Definition

Like NHL, Hodgkin's disease is a malignancy of the lymph nodes. Usually it begins in a cervical node and spreads in a predictable and orderly sequence from one lymph node region to the next; untreated it progresses to involve organs outside the lymph nodes. In contrast to NHL, spread to the marrow and central nervous system is rare. The malignant cell in Hodgkin's disease is the Reed–Sternberg cell which is thought to originate from either a B lymphocyte or a histiocyte precursor.

Classification

Hodgkin's disease is classified according to the extent of disease at presentation (the stage) and the histology of the involved lymph node. Unlike most other malignancies, Hodgkin's disease is multicellular—i.e. there is clearly more than one cell type present and it appears that it is the interaction of these cells that comprises the malignant process. The accepted histologic classification is a modification of the Rye, N.Y., classification based on the number of lymphocytes, the number of "reactive" cells, the number of Reed–Sternberg cells and the amount of fibrosis. As a general rule, the greater the number of lymphocytes and the fewer the Reed–Sternberg cells, the better the prognosis. The four histologic types are termed lymphocyte predominant, nodular sclerosing, mixed cellularity and lymphocyte depletion. Most pediatric Hodgkin's disease is the nodular sclerosing type.

Epidemiology

The incidence of Hodgkin's disease is similar to that of NHL, 0.6 per 100,000 per year. Although Hodgkin's disease has been reported in infants, it is rare under 5 years of age; there is one peak in adolescence and a later peak in the 6th decade. In the United States Hodgkin's disease tends to occur more frequently in the higher socioeconomic classes. Familial cases of Hodgkin's disease have been reported, and it has been shown the male sibling of a male patient has an increased risk of developing Hodgkin's disease.

There has been much literature about a possible viral etiology of Hodgkin's disease, but these studies have been difficult to confirm. It has been established that Hodgkin's disease patients have higher antibody titers than other children to the viral capsid antigen and early antigen of the EBV and have enhanced excretion of this virus in the oropharynx. However, it appears that these abnormal titers to EBV antigens reflect an altered response to the virus caused by the immunosuppression that is part of Hodg kin's disease and its therapy.

CLINICAL PRESENTATION AND PATHOPHYSIOLOGY

Hodgkin's disease most often manifest as a mass in the neck; about 4% present a masses in the groin. The mass may hav been present for days, months, or year. Some patients initially complain of adenop athy localized to a few lymph node regions others note generalized adenopathy. Ante rior mediastinal masses occur in 50% c patients. Large mediastinal Hodgkin's tu mors can present with the same cardiovas cular or respiratory symptoms as medias tinal NHLs (cf. "Thoracic Tumors"). Mos Hodgkin's disease patients are well ("A symptoms) but 30% present with fever an involuntary weight loss ("B" symptoms At diagnosis the fever may be low or hig grade. The Pel-Epstein fever, a high deb litating fever followed by a drenching swea is usually a sign of very advanced disease

Hodgkin's disease is staged according t the extent of disease and the presence c symptoms: Stage I, one lymph node region Stage II, two nodal regions on the sam side of the diaphragm; Stage III, nodal dis ease (including spleen) on both sides of th diaphragm; Stage IV, nodal disease plu lung, liver, marrow or bone involvemen "A" patients have no symptoms; "B" pa tients have fever and weight loss. The clin ical stage is that which is determined b physical exam and x-ray studies, includin lymphangiogram and/or retroperitonea CAT scan. The pathologic stage refers t the stage as determined by laparotomy wit splenectomy and surgical sampling of ab dominal lymph nodes, liver and bone mar row.

MANAGEMENT

In the past, the majority of patients i the United States underwent staging lapa rotomy and splenectomy. Those with Stag I-IIIA were treated with large fields of i radiation and those with more advance disease were treated with chemotherap combinations (MOPP: nitrogen mustar Oncovin, prednisone and procarbazine, c AVBD: Adriamycin, Velban, bleomyci and 5-(3,3-dimethyltriazeno)-imidazole-4-carboxamide (DTIC)). It has become apparent that with these therapies, most Hodgkin's disease patients can be cured. However, it has been shown that splenectomy carries a high risk of hyperacute pneumococcal infection in children with Hodgkin's disease. Furthermore, irradiation causes major growth disturbances in children under 18. On the other hand, chemotherapy and large field irradiation predispose to the development of leukemia and NHL in about 5% of patients. Awareness of these complications is leading many pediatric oncologists to investigate staging without laparotomy and to the use of different combinations of chemotherapy and lower doses and smaller fields of irradiation.

Special problems that the Hodgkin's disease patient have that represent emergencies are discussed below:

Massive Mediastinal Tumor

The issues regarding biopsy and superior vena cava syndrome tumors in patients with Hodgkin's disease are presented in the next section (see "Thoracic Tumors").

Hyperacute Infection

Today Hodgkin's disease patients should receive pneumococcal vaccine prior to splenectomy. However, most patients do not respond optimally to the vaccine. Furthermore, splenectomized patients are at risk of developing sepsis from strains of pneumococci not in the vaccine and from other encapsulated organisms (*Haemophilus influenzae* and *Neisseria meningiditis*). Many patients are placed on prophylactic penicillin or ampicillin, but this has not been proven to prevent infection.

Hyperacute infection has been reported in as many as 10% children with Hodgkin's disease. Most of these had advanced disease or had had repeated relapses. Children with hyperacute infections develop high fever and cardiovascular collapse, followed by death in at least half the patients. If a patient who has undergone splenectomy or who has had >3600 rad splenic irradiation suddenly develops high fever and appears acutely ill, cultures should be obtained and ampicillin (200 mg/kg/day) and gentamicin (5 to 7.5 mg/kg/day) should be started immediately with careful attention given to maintenance of blood pressure. If the patient is neutropenic as result of therapy, even broader antibiotic coverage is necessary (Table 55.6).

Interstitital Pneumonitis

Interstitial pneumonitis occurs in patients who have had whole lung irradiation or who are immunosuppressed from therapy. The causes are radiation pneumonitis, *Pneumocystis carinii* infection, or toxic reactions to chemotherapeutic agents (cyclophosphamide, bleomycin or procarbazine). If a patient who has had extensive mediastinal irradiation receives steroids as part of chemotherapy and then has the steroid withdrawn abruptly, "rebound" interstitial pneumonia can occur. This entity responds to resumption of steroids, but the use of steroids in radiation and chemical pneumonitis is controversial. Pneumocystis infection is treated with trimethoprim-sulfamethoxazole (p. 701). Symptomatic interstitial pneumonitis in patients with Hodgkin's diseases requires admission to the hospital.

Varicella Zoster

Up to half the children with Hodgkin's disease develop herpes zoster during or after therapy. About 20% develop cutaneous dissemination and 1% develop lethal visceral dissemination. Adenine arabinoside (10 mg/kg/day i.v. infusion) can shorten the course and lessen the risk of dissemination in compromised hosts; thus, these children should be hospitalized to receive therapy. If a child with Hodgkin's disease who has not had chickenpox is exposed to a child with chickenpox, prophylaxis with varicella immune plasma or globulin should be given (p. 702).

Mycobacterial and Fungal Infection

Because of impaired cell-mediated immunity caused by Hodgkin's disease and its therapy, patients are prone to develop fungal or mycobacterial disease in the form of cryptococcal meningitis, invasive mucormycosis, aspergillosis or pulmonary tuberculosis.

Pericarditis

Patients who have received potentially curative radiation to the mediastinum have a small risk of developing postradiation pericarditis, usually occurring 12 to 18 months after therapy but occasionally delayed for 5 to 7 years. If the patient has a pericardial effusion and is asymptomatic, an elective pericardiocentesis is necessary to rule out infection or tumor. Most asymptomatic effusions resolve over about 1 to 1½ years. If the patient with an effusion has symptoms of impending tamponade, pericardiocentesis becomes an urgent procedure (Section VII).

THORACIC TUMORS (Table 55.8)

Anterior Mediastinum

Hodgkin's disease and NHL are the most common malignant tumors in the anterior mediastinum. Other tumors include thymoma, thymic cyst, thymic hyperplasia, teratoma, ectopic thyroid, thyroid carcinoma, lymphangiomas and inflammatory processes such as sarcoid. Half of anterior mediastinal masses are benign. However, most large tumors and masses that cause compromise to the great vessels or cause pleural effusions are malignant.

Large tumors in the anterior mediastinum can cause tracheal narrowing and/or the superior vena cava syndrome. Tracheal compression causes tracheal deviation, stridor, cough, dyspnea, and orthopnea. Compression of the vena cava by tumor may cause headache, neck vein distension, cyanosis of the head and neck, dyspnea, orthopnea, and syncope or cardiovascular collapse. Physical examination may be unremarkable or show a geographic distribution of swelling, persistent fullness of veins in the arm when it is elevated, papilledema, bulging of the chest wall, and pleural effusion. Chest x-ray reveals a mass in the anterior mediastinum (Fig. 55.4). If a tumor

Table 55.8
Thoracic Tumors[a]

Benign	Malignant
Anterior Mediastinum	
Thymic neoplasm	Hodgkin's disease
Teratoma	Non-Hodgkin's lymphomas
Cystic hygroma	Thymoma
Hemangioma	Teratoma
Lipoma	Rhabdomyosarcoma
Middle Mediastinum	
Inflammatory adenopathy	Lymphoma (hilar nodes)
Cardiac neoplasms	Hodgkin's disease (nodes or pericardium)
Pericardial cyst	Neuroblastoma
Posterior Mediastinum	
Ganglioneuroma	Neuroblastoma
Neurofibroma	Ganglioneuroblastoma
Neurenteric cyst	Neurofibrosarcoma
Paraganglioma	
Pheochromocytoma	
Bronchogenic cyst	
Visceral duplication	
Pulmonary Parenchyma	
Fungal or mycobacterial infection	Metastatic tumor
Pseudotumorous infection	

[a] Adapted from P. G. Jones and P. E. Campbell: *Tumors of Infancy and Childhood*, Blackwell Scientific Publishing Co., Oxford, 1976.

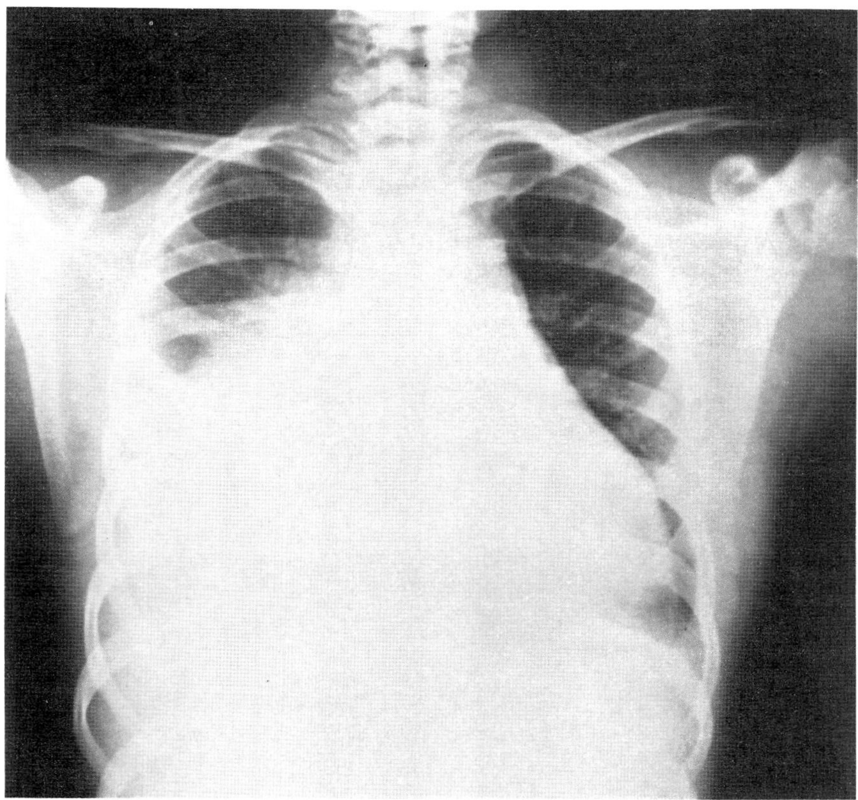

Figure 55.4. Mediastinal lymphoma and superior vena cava syndrome in a 12-year-old girl with a 2-week history of "bulging veins," swelling in the face, and orthopnea. Chest x-ray shows enormous mediastinal tumor, fullness of the vascular structures in the superior mediastinum, bilateral pleural effusion, and subcutaneous edema. (Reproduced with permission of Dr. Spencer Borden, Department of Radiology, Children's Hospital of Philadelphia.)

is causing superior vena cava syndrome in a child or adolescent, it is almost certain to be a malignant lymphoma or Hodgkin's disease.

Superior vena cava syndrome is life-threatening. Often it is ill-advised to try to obtain a histologic diagnosis under general anesthesia because these patients tolerate procedures poorly. Intravenous infusions should be started in the feet if both arms are involved because injections in the arms can cause respiratory distress, thrombosis, or phlebitis (provided venous return is good in the lower extremities). In the unstable patient with superior vena cava syndrome, empiric therapy with radiation (400 rad to midplane for 2 or 3 days) and/or corticosteroids (hydrocortisone, 2 mg/kg every 6 hours) may alleviate symptoms. Either treatment may make later interpretation of histology difficult. Therefore, if the patient can tolerate procedures, effusions should be drained, a marrow aspirate should be done as early as possible (to rule out NHL) and an accessible peripheral node biopsied under local anesthesia.

Middle Mediastinum

Most tumors of the middle mediastinum are benign. Malignant tumors include Hodgkin's disease of hilar nodes or pericardium, less commonly NHL or metastatic tumor such as neuroblastoma, and rarely sarcomas. Many large anterior mediastinal tumors extend into the middle mediastinum. Rarely these large tumors may cause cardiovascular compromise by compression of the vagus nerve, coronary vessels, or pericardial invasion. Spontaneous syncope or syncope with a Valsalva maneuver are clues to vagal involvement. Like the rare patients with superior vena cave syndrome, these patients are poor surgical risks. They require hospitalization and supportive care.

Posterior Mediastinum

Most tumors in the posterior mediastinum are of neurogenic origin: neuroblastoma, neurofibrosarcoma, ganglioneuroblastoma, ganglioneuroma and neurofibroma (Fig. 55.5). Only the first two have malignant potential. The more slowly grow-

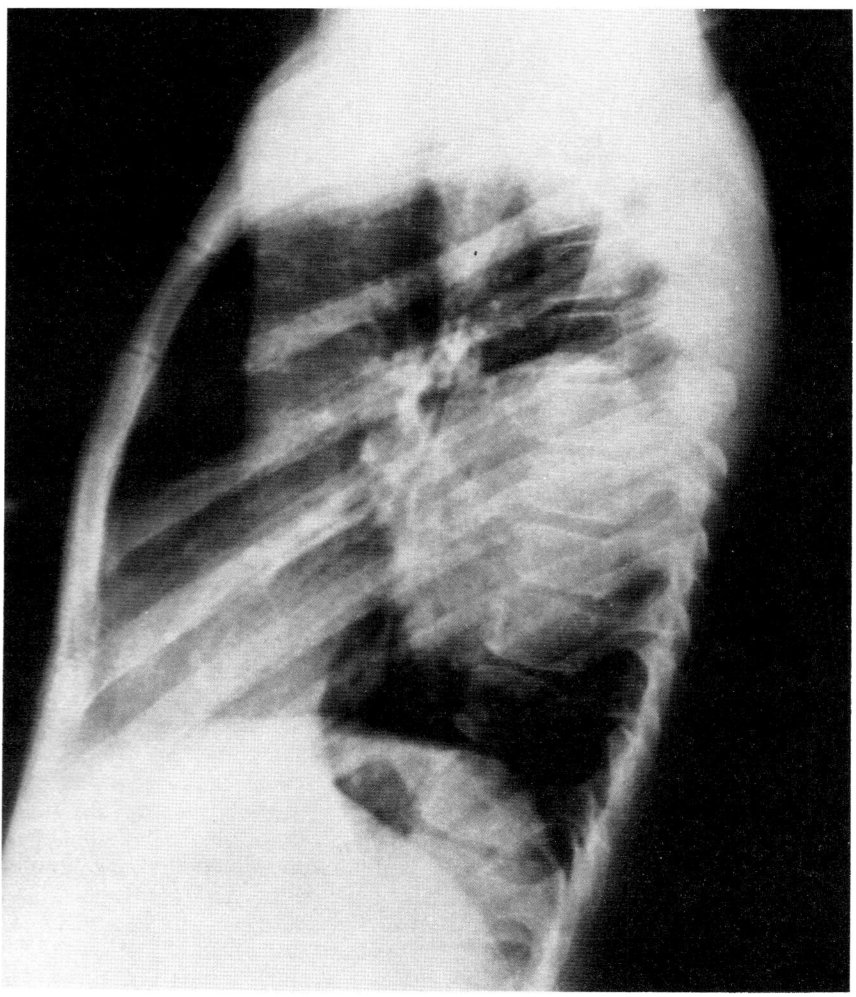

Figure 55.5. Posterior mediastinal ganglioneuroblastoma discovered incidentally on chest x-ray obtained because of chest pain after a fist fight. X-ray shows a large mass apparently originating from region of the spine; widening of spaces between ribs and absence of bone destruction suggest that the lesion has been present for months or years. (Reproduced with permission of Dr. Spencer Borden, Department of Radiology, Children's Hospital of Philadelphia.)

'able 55.9
'umors in Upper Abdomen[a]

Benign		Malignant
	Renal	
Hydronephrosis		Wilms' tumor
Polycystic kidney		Adenocarcinoma
Benign neoplasms		
Renal hypertrophy		
	Adrenal	
Adrenal hyperplasia		Neuroblastoma
Benign neoplasms		Ganglioneuroblastoma
		Adenocarcinoma
		Pheochromocytoma
	Liver	
Hepatosplenomegaly		Hepatoblastoma
Benign neoplasms		Hepatocellular carcinoma
Benign hyperplasia		Metastatic tumor

Adapted from P. G. Jones and P. E. Campbell: *Tumors of Infancy and Childhood*, Blackwell Scientific 'ublishing Co., Oxford, 1976.

ng tumors often may be detected on chest ilms taken for other purposes. Larger, rapdly growing tumors can cause pain and eurologic deficits.

Pulmonary Parenchyma

Nodules ("coin" lesions or "cannonball" esions) in a child with a solid tumor are isually metastatic tumor. In the severely :ompromised host they may be fungus)alls.

ABDOMINAL, GENITOURINARY, AND RETROPERITONEAL TUMORS

Intraabdominal tumors manifest themelves as discrete masses or as generalized bdominal enlargement. The spectrum of ntraabdominal and pelvic tumors is listed n Tables 55.9 and 55.10. Wilms' tumor and ieuroblastoma are the most common inraabdominal malignant tumors in young :hildren. Wilms' tumor presents as a large 'lank mass in a well child and abdominal ieuroblastoma, outside of infancy, as a midine or flank mass in an ill child. Hepatic umors are sometimes associated with sysemic illness. Pelvic sarcomas, teratomas, ieuroblastomas, or lymphomas may first :auses neurologic deficits or abdominal pain. Pelvic sarcomas are discussed under "Soft Tissue Sarcomas."

For most of these tumors, staging usually depends on the amount of tumor that has been removed surgically. Stage I tumors are tumors removed completely. If there is microscopic or gross residual or spread to regional nodes, the tumors are Stage II or III. The most advanced stage (IV) is when distant metastases are present. For each tumor category there is also a classification based on histology. The importance of histology has emerged only recently as survival has improved.

WILMS' TUMOR

BACKGROUND

Definition

Wilms' tumor (nephroblastoma), the most common intrarenal malignancy of childhood, is an embryonal neoplasm of mixed histology. About 5% of Wilms' tumors are bilateral.

Classification

The accepted classification of Wilms' tumor is based on extent of disease after surgery and on tumor histology. The group-

Table 55.10
Tumors of Lower Abdomen and Genitalia[a]

Benign		Malignant
	Retroperitoneum	
Presacral teratoma		Soft tissue sarcoma
Anterior meningomyelocele		Bone sarcoma
Ganglioneuroma		Lymphoma
Lipoma		Neuroblastoma
		Teratoma
	Bladder and Urethra	
Abscess		Rhabdomyosarcoma
Ureterocele		Leiomyosarcoma
Polyp		
Neurogenic bladder		
	Bowel	
Appendicitis		Lymphoma
Feces		Adenocarcinoma
Duplication cyst		Carcinoid
Carcinoid		
	Female Genitalia	
	Vagina	
Cysts		Rhabdomyosarcoma
Hydrocolpos		Clear-cell sarcoma
Hematocolpos		Endodermal sinus tumor
Neurofibroma		
Adenoma		
	Uterus and Fallopian Tubes	
Abscess		Rhabdomyosarcoma
Papilloma		Adenocarcinoma
		Embryonal carcinoma
	Ovary	
Teratoma		Teratoma
Cyst		Dysgerminoma
Granulosa theca cell		Arrhenoblastoma
Fibroma		Adenocarcinoma
Hemangioma		Choriocarcinoma
		Metastatic tumor
	Male Genitalia	
	Prostate	
Abscess		Rhabdomyosarcoma
	Testis	
Hydrocele		Rhabdomyosarcoma
Testicular torsion		Embryonal carcinoma
Orchitis		Seminoma
Teratoma		Leukemia
Leydig or Sertoli cell tumor		
	Spermatic Cord	
Hydrocele		Rhabdomyosarcoma
Hernia		Leukemia
Inflammation		
Adrenal rest		
Benign tumors of connective tissue		

[a] Adapted from P. G. Jones and P. E. Campbell: *Tumors of Infancy and Childhood*, Blackwell Scientific Publishing Co., Oxford 1976.

ng system of The National Wilms' Tumor Study-III (NWTS-3), a multi-institutional cooperative group, is as follows: a Group 1 umor is one that has been resected entirely; Group 2 has microscopic residual; Group 3, gross residual; Group 4, metastatic disease; and Group 5, bilateral tumors. The most favorable histology has a high degree of differentiation of the epithelial elements. Histologically unfavorable tumors are sarcomatous or anaplastic.

An intrarenal tumor similar in presentation to Wilms' tumor clinically but morphologically distinct is congenital mesoblastic nephroma. Mesoblastic nephroma occurs under 1 year of age, is comprised primarily of mesenchymally derived cells, and lacks the malignant elements of Wilms' tumor. It is treated by nephrectomy alone.

Epidemiology

Wilms' tumor occurs in 7.8 per million children under 15 years of age. In children under 5, it is the fourth most common malignancy; 65% of children presenting with Wilms' tumor are under 5 years of age.

There is a significant association between Wilms' tumor and congenital anomalies including aniridia, hemihypertrophy, genitourinary anomalies, hemangiomas, hamartomas, and cardiac anomalies. There are reports of familial cases of Wilms' tumor, as well as reports of families where some of the members had the congenital anomalies listed above while other members had Wilms' tumor.

CLINICAL MANIFESTATIONS AND PATHOPHYSIOLOGY

The majority of patients with Wilms' tumor have an abdominal mass discovered accidently by the parents while bathing or clothing a child or by a physician during a routine physical examination. The mass is deep in the flank and can be either firm or soft. Abdominal pain, fever, anorexia, malaise, vomiting and weight loss are rare presenting complaints. Gross hematuria occurs in less than 25% of patients. Some institutions report hypertension in up to 25% of patients. Hypertension is thought to result from increased renin secretion secondary to compression of the renal artery. By a related mechanism, polycythemia also occurs occasionally in the patient with Wilms' tumor. More often anemia results from bleeding into the tumor. In performing a physical examination, the physician should be particularly attentive to the size of the liver and spleen, the site and size of the mass, blood pressure and the presence of the congenital anomalies listed above. Laboratory evaluation should include complete blood count, BUN, and creatinine. Abdominal x-ray (kidney, ureter, bladder, KUB) may reveal a mass displacing bowel. Intravenous pyelogram (IVP) demonstrates an intrarenal mass distorting the calyces (Fig. 55.6). Ultrasound can detect a mass if the kidney is not seen on IVP.

MANAGEMENT

Children with a presumed Wilms' tumor should be referred to a surgeon experienced in the diagnosis and treatment of this tumor. Definitive therapy for localized disease with favorable histology consists of complete resection and chemotherapy. Surgery, chemotherapy and irradiation are used in patients with advanced disease or unfavorable histology. The chemotherapeutic agents with proven efficacy are vincristine, actinomycin D, and doxorubicin.

Wilms' tumor exemplifies the advances made in pediatric oncology with multimodal therapy: disease-free survival of all patients approaches 90%. Even patients with metastatic disease, bilateral tumors, or unfavorable histology can be treated successfully.

Certain problems that result from therapy may bring the child to an emergency facility. Fever and neutropenia are rare, but, if they occur, the same empiric approach as used in leukemia is appropriate (p. 699). However, in contrast to children with leukemia, children with Wilms' tumor and neutropenia are unlikely to have fatal infection because the neutropenia usually lasts days rather than weeks.

Patients who have received pulmonary irradiation for metastatic disease can develop interstitial pneumonitis several weeks to months after irradiation. The pneumonitis is frequently a combination of radiation pneumonitis and *P. carinii* infection. Admission is necessary and agressive supportive care with antibiotics, including tri-

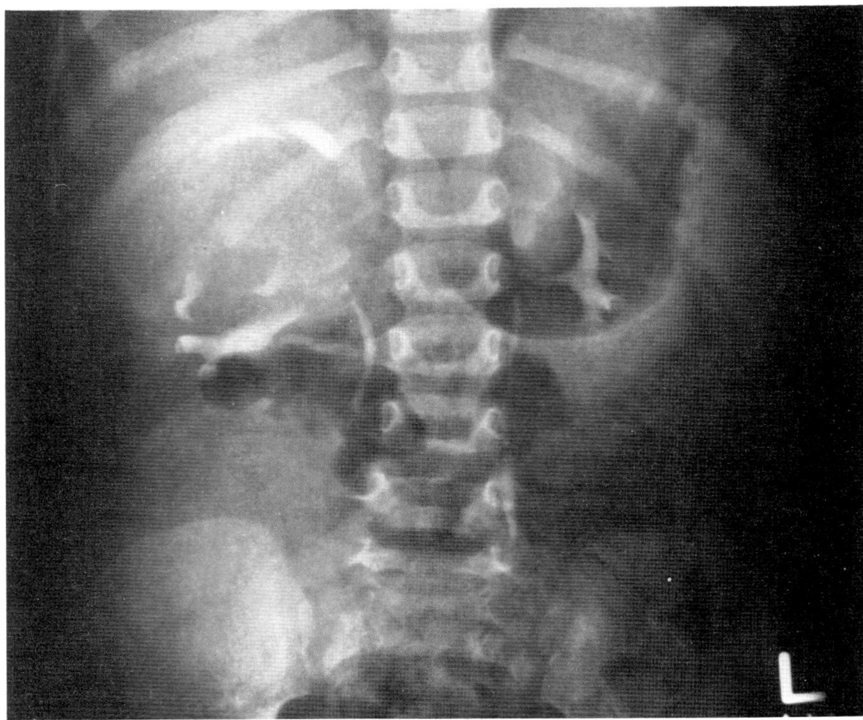

Figure 55.6. Wilms' tumor on the right kidney: intravenous pyelogram shows a large mas splaying the calcyces and displacing the kidney down; bowel gas is scarce in the left uppe quadrant; the left kidney is normal. (Reproduced with permission of Dr. Spencer Borden, Depar ment of Radiology, Children's Hospital of Philadelphia.)

methoprim-sulfamethoxazole, should be instituted.

Delayed complications from the combined use of radiation and chemotherapy can occur months or years after treatment. They include inflammation and then fibrosis of lung, liver, or kidneys. Postradiation hepatitis is often associated with thrombocytopenia. The complications can be either debilitating or fatal; fortunately, they are rare.

NEUROBLASTOMA

BACKGROUND

Definition

Neuroblastoma is a malignant tumor arising from the sympathetic tissue in the adrenal medulla or in the sympathetic chain along the craniospinal axis, in the neck, in the posterior mediastinum (see "Thoracic Tumors"), intraabdominally o in the pelvis. The tumor is composed c small round cells with scant neurofibrilla cytoplasm. The cells may form rosette Neuroblastoma commonly metastasizes t bone, bone marrow, liver, skin, lymp nodes, and uncommonly to lung or to th central nervous system.

Classification

One of several staging and classification based on extent of disease is that of Evan et al. Stage IV-S encompasses a uniqu group of patients with metastatic disease generally well-appearing infants whose pr mary tumor is small with metastases lim ited to liver, skin, and marrow. Most c these patients have spontaneous regressio of tumor, even with a massive tumor bur den. Infants with Stage IV-S appear to hav a tumor that is biologically distinct fro the tumor of older patients with Stage IV disease metastatic to bone and bone marrow.

Epidemiology

After central nervous system tumors, neuroblastoma is the most common solid tumor in childhood. About 50% occur before the age of 2 and about 80% are found in children under 5. Neuroblastoma occurs in approximately 1 per 100,000 children per year under age 16.

CLINICAL MANIFESTATIONS AND PATHOPHYSIOLOGY

About ⅔ of patients present with widespread metastases. Signs and symptoms include irritability, anorexia, weight loss, pallor, and subcutaneous lumps. Adrenal neuroblastoma as well as nonadrenal intraabdominal tumors can cause an abdominal mass palpable on routine physical examination. Involvement of the cervical sympathetic ganglia can cause Horner's syndrome or hoarseness by compressing the recurrent laryngeal nerve. Neuroblastoma arising from the sympathetic ganglia and extending into and out of the intravertebral foramina, a "dumbbell tumor," can cause signs and symptoms of compression of the spinal cord. Skeletal lesions lead to bone pain or pathologic fractures. Periorbital metastases cause proptosis and periorbital ecchymosis, "black eyes." The patients with "black eyes" can be mistaken for battered children (Fig. 55.7). Rarer presentations include opsoclonus-myoclonus or hypertension, tachycardia, skin flush, and

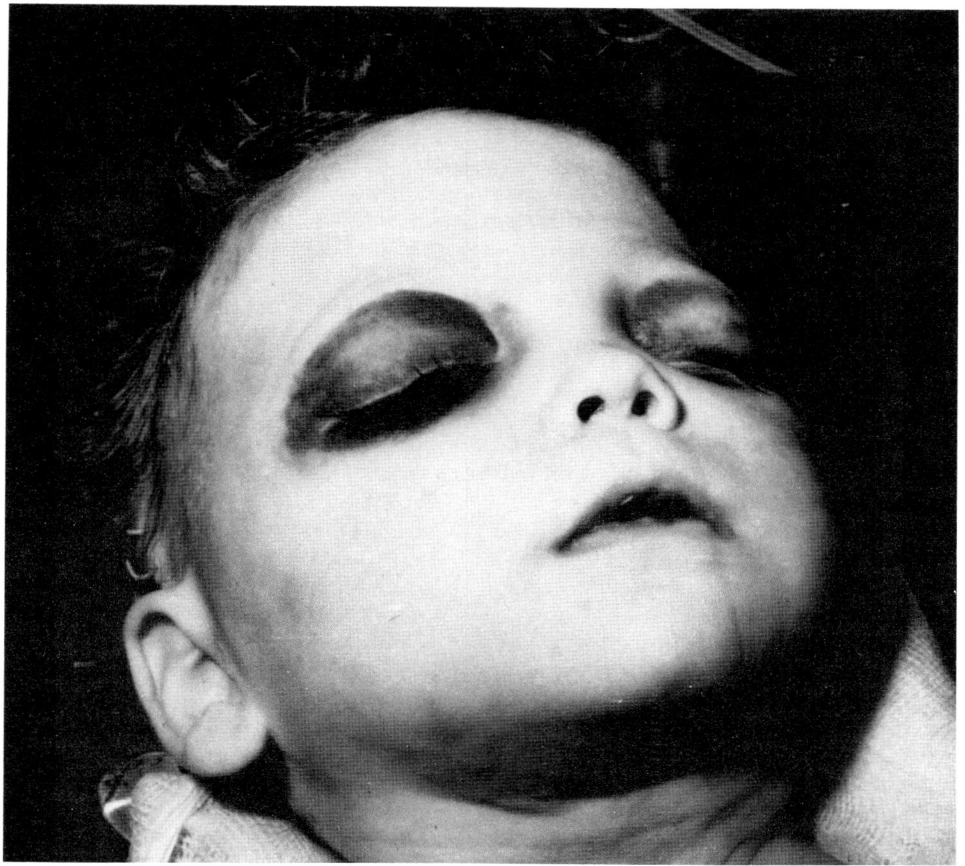

Figure 55.7. Stage IV neuroblastoma causing black eyes in a 20-month-old boy.

chronic diarrhea from excess catecholamine secretion.

An intriguing characteristic of neuroblastoma is its ability to undergo spontaneous regression or to undergo maturation to more benign lesions, ganglioneuroblastoma and ganglioneuroma. Whether all ganglioneuromas were once neuroblastoma is unclear, but it is generally agreed that they have the same cellular origin.

Patients with Stage IV-S present in the first few months of life with gross hepatomegaly or skin nodules. The primary tumor may not be obvious. The emergency department physician who notes massive hepatomegaly in an otherwise healthy looking infant should consider Stage IV-S neuroblastoma in the differential diagnosis.

Radiographs of painful areas in bones may show symmetric lytic lesions of the metaphyses of the long bones. Cortical destruction is seen in flat bones. Skull films may show increased soft tissue over the involved orbit in a child with proptosis. Abdominal radiographs reveal a retroperitoneal mass displacing normal structures. Adrenal primaries commonly have fine calcifications. IVP can show a suprarenal mass that displaces the kidney down and away from its normal axis.

MANAGEMENT

Evaluation of patients with suspected neuroblastoma should include a CBC, IVP, chest radiograph, skeletal survey, bone scan, and marrow aspiration and biopsy. All patients with suspected neuroblastoma should have quantitative evaluation of urinary catecholamines including homovanillic acid (HVA) and vanillylmandelic acid (VMA). Evaluation requires several days and is most efficiently performed in a hospital prepared to treat the tumor.

Treatment of neuroblastoma is directed both toward the tumor itself and complications of the tumor. The treatment of choice of Stage I and II disease is usually surgical removal. In Stage III complete surgical excision is also the treatment of choice, but total resection is usually not feasible in patients with large tumors. Radiation may be used to reduce tumor bulk and for palliation, especially to treat painful bone lesions. Chemotherapeutic agents used to treat advanced neuroblastoma include cyclophosphamide, doxorubicin, DTIC, VM-26, and cis-platinum. Even though the majority of tumors initially respond to therapy, most eventually become refractory to treatment, and the disease is fatal.

Emergency physicians need to recognize special conditions in neuroblastoma.

1. Massive hepatomegaly in a neonate or infant can cause hepatic failure or respiratory embarrassment. These children need to be admitted for supportive care.
2. Dumbbell tumors can cause cord compression. These children need immediate evaluation. Rapidly occurring paraplegia in a child under 5 should be considered neuroblastoma unless another cause has been proven. Treatment consists of laminectomy, surgical removal, and often irradiation.
3. Rarely, airway obstruction can result from large mediastinal tumors.
4. Extensive marrow disease or intensive therapy can cause pancytopenia. In either case, children with neuroblastoma with fever and neutropenia need to be managed similarly to children with leukemia (p. 699).
5. Interstitial pneumonitis caused by *P. carinii* or by viruses such as cytomegalovirus or by therapy (cyclophosphamide pneumonitis) is becoming more common. Admission for evaluation and treatment is advisable in the symptomatic child.
6. Opsoclonus-myoclonus can resemble a toxic drug reaction or neuromuscular disease. This disorder is usually seen in children with limited, surgically resectable disease.

HEPATIC TUMORS

BACKGROUND

Definition

The two major primary liver tumors in children are hepatoblastoma and hepatocellular carcinoma. Hepatoblastomas are of epithelial cell origin and contain osteoid and fibrous tissue. Hepatocellular carcinomas arise from hepatocytes. Liver tumors originate most commonly from the right lobe in the liver. The common sites of metastases are lung and intraabdominal lymph nodes and viscera. Bone and bone marrow spread is unusual.

Classification

Liver tumors are classified according to histology as described above and according to extent of disease as follows: Group 1, complete resection of tumor by wedge, lobectomy, or extended lobectomy as initial treatment; Group 2A, tumors rendered completely resectable by initial irradiation and chemotherapy; Group 2B, residual disease confined to one lobe; Group 3A, disease involving both lobes of the liver; Group 3B, regional lymph node involvment; and Group 4, distant metastases.

Epidemiology

The incidence of primary hepatic tumors in children is 2 per million per year. Hepatoblastoma usually occurs before age 3 years. Hepatocellular carcinoma shows one peak around 4 years of age and a second around 15 years.

There is a strong association between the appearance of cirrhosis and the development of hepatocellular carcinoma, although the association in children is not as strong as it is in adults. Metabolic diseases that cause cirrhosis (von Gierke's disease, Niemann-Pick disease, galactosemia, and chronic hereditary tyrosinuria) can progress to hepatic cancer. Patients who have received anabolic steroid therapy are at risk for developing benign hepatic neoplasms, and a few cases of hepatocellular carcinoma following androgen therapy have been reported.

CLINICAL MANIFESTATIONS AND PATHOPHYSIOLOGY

By far the most common presentation of a hepatic tumor is an enlarging abdomen, an abdominal mass and signs and symptoms resulting from the mass. Anorexia, weight loss, vomiting, pain, fever, diarrhea, and irritability occur. Jaundice is uncommon, but pallor due to chronic disease is seen. Virilization may result from production of chorionic gonadotropin.

MANAGEMENT

The evaluation of patients with suspected liver tumors includes roentgenographic examination of the abdomen, which may show an enlarged liver and occasionally hepatic calcifications; a chest roentgenogram should be taken to look for metastases. Initial laboratory tests should include a CBC and liver function tests (although they are often normal). Further evaluation necessitates admission to the hospital.

TUMORS OF THE FEMALE GENITALIA

BACKGROUND

Definition

Tumors of the female genitalia include primary ovarian tumors and vulvar, vaginal and intrauterine tumors. Most ovarian tumors are cystic and histologically benign. Malignant ovarian tumors are solid, and in children they are usually derived from the germ cells. Malignant tumors of the vulva are usually sarcomas; vaginal tumors are either sarcoma botryoides in younger girls or adenocarcinomas in adolescents.

Classification

The ovarian tumors seen in childhood are dysgerminomas, embryomal carcinomas, endodermal sinus tumors, teratomas, choriocarcinomas, and mixed germ-cell tumors (Table 55.10). The staging system is based on the extent of involvement.

Epidemiology

Ovarian tumors are uncommon, accounting for only about 1% of malignant neoplasms in females under 17 years. Incidence increases with age with approximately 20% occurring between 0 and 4 years, 30% between 5 and 9; 50% between 10 and 14. Menarchial hormonal factors may play a role in development of ovarian tumors.

Female offspring of mothers who received stilbesterol during pregnancy are at risk for developing vaginal adenocarcinoma.

PRESENTATION AND PATHOPHYSIOLOGY

Ovarian tumors are usually large and may be mistaken for pregnancy. They can cause painful ovarian torsion or an acute abdomen, especially if there is hemorrhage or rupture of a cyst; right-sided ovarian tumors may mimic acute appendicitis.

Stromal tumors may produce hormones, causing precocious puberty, vaginal bleeding (granulosa cell tumors), or masculinization (arrhenoblastoma). Ovarian tumors spread by direct extension along the adnexal structures to lymph nodes and the peritoneal surface of the bladder, uretus, sigmoid colon, liver, diaphragm, and small intestine. Rarely these tumors metastasize to lung, liver, and bone. Ascites and pleural effusion are seen with fibroid tumors (Meigs' syndrome); however, fibroids are rare in children and adolescents.

Vaginal sarcomas may present as exophytic masses. Vaginal adenocarcinoma is detected by a routine PAP smear or by the presence of a mass or bleeding.

MANAGEMENT

Girls with suspected genital neoplasms need a thorough physical examination, including careful inspection of genitalia, bimanual pelvic examination, and evaluation of pubertal status. An abdominal x-ray looking for calcification, teeth, and ascites should be obtained, as well as radiographs of the chest and an IVP. Laboratory examinations for ovarian tumors should include measurement of α-fetoprotein, which is produced by embryonal carcinoma and endodermal sinus tumor, and human chorionic gonadotropin, produced by embryonal carcinoma and choriocarcinoma.

TUMORS OF MALE GENITALIA

BACKGROUND

Tumors of the male genitalia include testicular and paratesticular and prostatic tumors. Germ-cell tumors comprise about 75% of the primary testicular tumors. Leukemia can metastasize to the testes. Paratesticular and prostatic tumors are usually rhabdomyosarcomas. Table 55.10 gives the classification of these neoplasms.

There is relatively high incidence of germ-cell testicular tumors in infancy. The incidence falls off after age 4 years and begins to rise again in puberty with a continued increase into early adulthood. A cryptorchid testis has a 30 to 50 times increased risk of developing a neoplasm; 10 to 20% of all testicular cancers arise from a cryptorchid testis. Sarcomas of the male genitalia occur mostly between ages 2 and 10 years.

CLINICAL MANIFESTATIONS

Most testicular tumors present as slowly growing scrotal masses. Occasionally, a patient may have pain. About 25% of the patients have either an associated hydrocele or inguinal hernia. Testicular and paratesticular tumors most commonly metastasize to lung or spread to regional lymph nodes.

MANAGEMENT

Patients with solid testicular or paratesticular masses should be referred to a surgeon with experience in removing pediatric neoplasms. Treatment usually consists of orchiectomy with high ligation of the spermatic cord for germ cell tumors. Sarcomas require chemotherapy and irradiation.

TUMORS OF THE HEAD, NECK AND EXTREMITIES

This diverse group of tumors includes those which present as masses in the brain itself (brain tumors) or near the brain (parameningeal tumors), in the eye (retinoblastoma), or in the neck or extremities. Most malignant tumors on the nasopharynx or middle ear or behind the eye are rhabdomyosarcomas. In the neck, lymphomas are most common (p. 709); sarcomas, neuroblastomas, thyroid carcinomas and metastatic tumors also occur. Soft tissue sarcomas and bone sarcomas are the commonest malignant tumors of the extremities. Tables 55.11 and 55.12 list tumors of the head and neck according to location and malignant potential.

Table 55.11
Swelling and Tumors of the Head[a]

Benign	Malignant
The Orbit	
Inflammation	Rhabdomyosarcoma
Hematoma	Metastatic tumor (Ewing's, leukemia)
Cyst	Neuroblastoma
Pseudotumor	Histiocytosis
Benign connective tissue tumor	Optic nerve glioma
AV fistula	
Thyrotoxicosis	
The Eye	
Coats' disease	Retinoblastoma
Primary hyperplastic vitreous	Dictyoma (medulloepithelioma of ciliary body)
Parasitic infection	Malignant melanoma (iris, ciliary body)
The Ear	
Cholesteatoma	Rhabdomyosarcoma
Polyp	Histiocytosis
Chemodectoma	
The Nasopharynx	
Infection	Rhabdomyosarcoma
Polyp	Lymphoma
Fibrous dysplasia	Esthesioneuroblastoma
Neurofibroma	Craniopharyngioma
Schwannoma	Carcinoma
Angiofibroma	
Rathke's pouch cyst	
Oropharynx	
Benign neoplasms of the tongue, salivary glands, mucous membranes	Soft tissue sarcoma
Inflammation	Parotid carcinoma
	Parotid lymphoma
	Lymphoma

[a] Adapted from P. G. Jones and P. E. Campbell: *Tumors of Infancy and Childhood*, Blackwell Scientific Publishing Co., Oxford, 1976.

CENTRAL NERVOUS SYSTEM TUMORS

BACKGROUND

Definition

Primary central nervous system tumors are those tumors, histologically benign or malignant, which arise primarily in the brain, meninges, or spinal cord. This group of diseases includes many histiologic variants, but only the relatively common primary neoplasms will be discussed. In the past, metastatic brain tumors have been relatively uncommon in children but as chemotherapy changes the natural history of some tumors, cerebral or epidural metastases of rhabdomyosarcoma, Ewing's sarcoma, osteogenic sarcoma and lymphomas are becoming more common.

Table 55.12
Tumors and Swellings of Neck and Extremities

Benign	Malignant
The Neck	
Lymph Nodes	
Adenitis	Hodgkin's disease
Reactive hyperplasia	Non-Hodgkin's lymphoma
Sinus histiocytosis	Metastatic tumor
Salivary Glands	
Calculus	Carcinoma
Angioma	Metatastic tumor
Adenoma	
Midline	
Benign neoplasms	Thyroid carcinoma
Inflammation	Metastatic tumor
Nerve and Connective Tissue	
Cystic hygroma	Rhabdomyosarcoma
Fibromatosis	Neuroblastoma
Ganglioneuroma	Schwannoma
Pheochromocytoma	
Teratoma	
The Extremities	
Benign neoplasms	Soft tissue sarcoma
Trauma	Ewing's sarcoma
Inflammation	Osteosarcoma
	Non-Hodgkin's lymphoma

[a] Adapted from P. G. Jones and P. E. Campbell: *Tumors of Infancy and Childhood*, Blackwell Scientific Publishing Co., Oxford, 1976.

Classification

A number of classification systems have been set up for characterization of brain tumors based on histology, degree of malignancy or location. Histologically, the most common brain tumor is the astrocytoma which comprises about one third of all brain tumors. Astrocytomas are graded according to the degree of malignancy: Grade 1 astrocytoma is histologically benign and Grade 4, glioblastoma multiforme is the most malignant. Seventy percent of astrocytomas are infratentorial, predominantly cerebellar in location.

Medulloblastoma is the second most common histologic types of brain tumor. Medulloblastoma occurs subcortically, arising from germinative cells of the external granular layer of the cerebellum and grows predominantly from the vermis of the cerebellum. Less common brain tumors include gliomas, which occur in the brain stem, and ependymomas, which can occur either in the posterior fossa or in the cerebral hemispheres. In contrast to adult brain tumors, the majority of pediatric brain tumors are infratentorial. For the clinician a more useful classification is one based on the location of the tumors because lesions at specific locations produce corresponding specific neurologic deficits. Table 55.13 lists brain and spinal cord tumors by location. Astrocytomas and ependymomas are the common spinal cord tumors.

Epidemiology

Brain tumors occur in 2 to 4 per 100,000 children yearly. Brain tumors are the most common group of solid tumors. They can occur at any age but their peak incidence is from 5 to 10 years. Gliomas are more common under 5 years, and medulloblastoma is most common around 8 years with a striking male predominance of 4:1. Certain systemic diseases are associated with an increased risk of development of brain tumors: neurofibromatosis with acoutstic neuroma, meningeal fibroma, optic glioma and cerebellopontine angle tumor; tuberous sclerosis with gliomas; von Hippel-Lindau disease with ependymomas; and nevoid basal cell syndrome with medulloblastoma.

Table 55.13
Central Nervous System Tumors[a]

I. *Posterior Fossa*
    A. Astrocytoma
    B. Medulloblastoma
    C. Ependymoma (fourth ventricle)
    D. Brainstem glioma
II. *Third Ventricle*
    A. Craniopharyngioma
    B. Optic nerve glioma
    C. Pineal tumor
III. *Cerebral Hemispheres*
    A. Astrocytoma
    B. Gliomas (Grade 1–4)
    C. Oligodendroglioma
    D. Ependymoma
    E. Choroid plexus papilloma
    F. Meningioma
IV. *Miscellaneous*
    A. Sarcomas
    B. Melanoma
    C. Metastatic tumors
V. *Tumors of the Spinal Cord*
    A. Intramedullary
        1. Astrocytoma
        2. Ependymoma
    B. Extramedullary, paraspinal and epidural tumors
        1. Neurofibroma
        2. Epidermal cysts
        3. Neuroblastoma
        4. Ganglioneuroma
        5. Sarcomas
        6. Leukemia
        7. Lymphoma
VI. *Vertebral Body*
    A. Ewing's sarcoma
    B. Metastatic tumors

[a] Adapted from P. G. Jones and P. E. Campbell: *Tumors of Infancy and Childhood*, Blackwell Scientific Publishing Co., Oxford, 1976.

CLINICAL PRESENTATION AND PATHOPHYSIOLOGY

Ultimately, nearly all brain tumors cause signs and symptoms of increased intracranial pressure (Chapter 67). In fact brain tumors are now a relatively common cause of increased pressure because the incidence of other causes, such as abscesses, is decreasing. The symptoms of increased pressure vary with age. Infants show personality changes, vomiting, lethargy, loss of previously acquired motor skills, seizures, and symptoms of obstructive hydrocephalus. In older children headache is the most common symptom. Early in the course headaches are usually intermittent. A history of headache on arising in the morning should alert the emergency department physician to the possibility of a central nervous system tumor. Vomiting with or without nausea is also a common presenting symptom. Other presenting symptoms include diplopia, dizziness, ataxia, personality changes, motor impairment, speech disturbance, and stiff neck.

Specific tumors cause specific focal neurologic changes. Brainstem gliomas cause cranial nerve deficits usually in the order of VI, V, IX and X. Facial palsies and dysphagia are presenting symptoms; ataxia and hemiparesis follow. Localizing symptoms often occur before increased intracranial pressure in these tumors. Medulloblastoma, because of its midline location, causes truncal ataxia and an unbalanced reeling gait. If medulloblastomas "drop" metastases to the cord, symptoms of cord compression occur. Cerebellar astrocytomas which occupy one hemisphere cause ipsilateral hypotonia and a tendency to fall to the side of lesion. Herniation of a cerebellar tonsil causes headtilt and neck stiffness. Tumors near the third ventricle (craniopharyngiomas, germinomas, optic gliomas, and hypothalamic and pituitary tumors) cause visual impairment, increased intracranial pressure and hydrocephalus. Tumors of the hypothalamus produce the dienciphalic syndrome (failure to thrive, wasting, and inappropriate alertness) in infants and young children. Pineal tumors obstruct the aqueduct of Sylvius, producing increased intracranial pressure and upward gaze paralysis. Cerebral astrocytomas, ependymomas and oligodendrigogliomas cause seizures and hemiparesis.

Spinal cord tumors cause pain at the site of the tumor and neurologic deficits. Depressed motor function, sensory deficit, and hyperreflexia below the lesion may be present. Later, paralysis areflexia and loss of bladder and bowel control may occur (see Chapter 44).

When an intracranial lesion is suspected, a complete neurologic evaluation including eye examination and developmental assessment is mandatory. Diagnostic procedures should be selected not only to help make a diagnosis but to help plan definitive therapy. Computerized axial tomography of the brain is the most practical way to document a mass; injection of water soluble contrast will show enhancement of the mass. In the younger child, plain films of the skull showing split cranial sutures or widening of the sella turcica indicate chronic increased intracranial pressure. Radionuclide scanning may locate supratentorial lesions. Pneumoencephalography and angiography probably are not necessary in diagnosis of brain tumors but may occasionally help the neurosurgeon in planning a surgical approach. Lumbar puncture is rarely useful and may be contraindicated in a space-occupying lesion; lumbar puncture can lead to brainstem herniation. If a lumbar puncture is necessary to rule out meningitis, a small gauge needle should be used and only 1 to 2 ml of fluid should be removed for analysis. The patient should be admitted and observed for neurologic deterioration and prepared for surgery if necessary.

Definitive diagnosis of a brain tumor should be made by biopsy. Attempt at surgical resection is becoming increasingly common because surgery in the hands of experienced pediatric oncologic neurosurgeons appears to be improving the prognosis. Diagnosis of an intramedullary cord tumor is made by myelogram and surgery. CSF cytology or bone scan may suggest extramedullary tumors.

MANAGEMENT

The management of brain tumors requires a team approach that includes a pediatric neurologist, neurosurgeon, oncologist, and radiation therapist. The role of the emergency department physician is one of recognizing central nervous system lesions and stabilizating the patient with life-threatening increases in intracranial pressure. Administration of dexamethasone (0.5 mg/kg/day in 4 divided doses) and diuretics such as mannitol (2 g/kg over 30 to 60 min) may reduce symptoms of increased pressure. Definitive therapy will depend on the size, location, and histology of the tumor. An operative procedure that removes as much of the tumor as possible is obviously the goal except when the tumor is lcoated in deep areas of the dominant hemisphere or the brainstem. Radiation therapy (4500 to 6500 rad) has improved survival in most children with unresectable brain tumors, especially in medulloblastomas, ependymomas, and low grade astrocytomas. Chemotherapy has also been used, but the initial treatment of primary tumors is still considered investigational. Agents that have been used include the nitrosoureas, vincristine, prednisone, VP-16, procarbazine, and nitrogen mustard.

Tumors causing spinal cord compression, whether intrinsic to the cord such as astrocytomas, ependymomas, or chordomas, or extrinsic to the cord, such as lymphomas or sarcomas, demand immediate diagnosis and treatment in the hospital (see cord compression in Chapter 44).

RETINOBLASTOMA

BACKGROUND

Retinoblastoma is the most common primary intraocular malignancy in childhood. Retinoblastoma arises from the nuclear layer of the retina and is of neurological origin. Most cases of retinoblastoma are cured by enucleation. Retinoblastoma occasionally metastasizes hematogenously, to bone marrow, bones, lymph nodes, and liver. It can also spread by direct extension via the optic nerve to the meninges and into the spinal fluid. The staging system for retinoblastoma is based on size, number, and location of lesions in the retina and vitreous.

Retinoblastoma occurs in 1 of 23,000 births. Most patients are diagnosed by 2 years of age. There are two patterns of retinoblastoma: a hereditary form which is inherited as an autosomal dominant with about 60 to 90% penetrance, and a sporadic form. Most bilateral cases carry a high probability of being hereditary. Approximately 35 to 45% of retinoblastomas are hereditary whereas 55 to 65% represent spontaneous mutation.

Some patients with retinoblastoma are at risk for developing osteosarcoma or pineal tumors later in life.

CLINICAL MANIFESTATIONS

Two thirds of the children with retinoblastoma present with a white pupil (leukokoria or cat's eye), often detected by the parents. The white pupil is actually the tumor itself, as it is seen through the vitreous. Other signs and symptoms include strabismus, a unilateral, fixed dilated pupil, decreased visual acuity, a red painful eye due to glaucoma, spontaneous hyphema, proptosis, and heterochromia iridia. In families with known hereditary forms of retinoblastoma, most tumors are detected while asymptomatic because of careful and frequent ophthalmologic examinations.

MANAGEMENT

All children who present with a white pupil or with suspected retinoblastoma need a thorough ocular examination under general anesthesia by an experienced ophthalmologist. The ophthalmologist needs to be able to differentiate other causes of leukokoria (nematode endophthalmitis, persistent hyperplastic primary vitreous, Coat's disease, coloboma, idiopathic retinal detachment, and congenital cataract) from a neoplasm.

THYROID CANCER

BACKGROUND

Thyroid cancers are carcinomas, usually arising in the thyroid gland and less commonly in ectopic thyroid tissue. Thyroid cancer is divided into four histologic subtypes: papillary, follicular, medullary, and anaplastic. Papillary carcinoma accounts for approximately 70% of cancers, and follicular comprises 20%.

Thyroid cancer is very uncommon in children. It is difficult to obtain exact figures regarding the incidence in childhood. It is approximately twice as common in females as in males.

There is a well documented association between previous low dose head and neck irradiation and the development of thyroid cancer. This pattern emerged when it was discovered that many patients with thyroid cancer had received irradiation for such conditions as acne, tonsil enlargement, or thymic enlargement. All persons with previous neck irradiation should have careful neck examinations every 1 or 2 years, and all palpable nodules should be removed surgically.

CLINICAL MANIFESTATION AND PATHOPHYSIOLOGY

Thyroid cancer usually presents as one or more firm, painless nodules in the neck. Occasionally, patients will have symptoms of dysphagia or hoarseness. Thyroid cancer commonly spreads to cervical lymph nodes, and less commonly to lung and bones. Local invasion of the trachea, larynx, or esophagus can also occur. Any patient suspected of having a thyroid nodule should have a radioisotope study of the thyroid with either iodine-123 or technetium-99m pertechnitate. Thyroid scan usually reveals a "cold" nodule, although "hot" nodules can also be malignant. Other evaluations should also include x-rays of the chest and neck, radionuclide bone scans, as well as T_3, T_4, and TSH.

SOFT TISSUE SARCOMAS

BACKGROUND

Definition

Soft tissue sarcomas are derived from mesenchymal tissue: muscle, tendon, nerve, fat, and endothelium. Rhabdomyosarcoma arises from striated muscle and is the most common member of this group in childhood. Less common are fibrosarcoma, neurofibrosarcoma, synovial sarcoma, mesenchymoma, malignant fibrous histiocytoma and leiomyosarcoma.

Classification

Soft tissue sarcomas are classified according to their apparent tissue of origin. Rhabomyosarcoma is further subdivided according to histologic subtype (embryonal, alveolar, or pleiomorphic) and according to the extent of disease after surgery.

Epidemiology

Soft tissue sarcomas can occur at birth. They have a peak incidence at 2 to 6 years of age (median age, 5 years). Sarcoma botryoides of the bladder, prostate or vagina tends to occur in infants; paratesticular sarcomas occur in childhood or adolescence. Soft tissue sarcomas occur at an annual rate of 8.4 per million white children and 3.9 per million black children. They account for approximately 6% of all neoplasms in children.

CLINICAL PRESENTATION AND PATHOPHYSIOLOGY

A sarcoma usually presents as a lump in the soft tissues. The lump may be painless or painful. Specific symptoms depend on the location of the tumor.

Orbital tumors cause rapidly developing unilateral proptosis. Nasopharyngeal tumors can present with recurrent epistaxis, chronic sinusitis, chronic nasal obstruction or dysphagia. Middle ear rhabdomyosarcoma can cause a chronic otitis media, ear pain, cranial nerve palsies, and rarely sarcomatous meningitis. Neck tumors can cause dysphagia, hoarseness, or simply a painless mass in the posterior cervical triangle. Tumors of the bladder or prostate lead to acute urinary tract obstruction or constipation. Sarcoma botryoides of the vagina presents with bleeding or as a polypoid mass protruding from the introitus. Extremity sarcomas usually appear as painless masses.

MANAGEMENT

The role of the emergency department physician is to include cancer in the differential diagnosis of masses in the soft tissues in children and to refer children for prompt biopsy of the mass when a benign lesion has been ruled out. Definitive therapy consists of surgery, chemotherapy, and usually radiotherapy.

BONE TUMORS

BACKGROUND

Definition

A variety of neoplasms occur in bones; many of them are benign. The malignant tumors are sarcomas arising from the cells of the cortical or cancellous bone (osteogenic sarcoma), cartilagenous bone (chondrosarcoma), periosteum (periosteal sarcoma) or reticuloendothelial cells of the marrow (Ewing's tumor).

Classification

Malignant bone tumors are classified according to their cell of origin. The two malignant bone tumors that are of practical importance to the pediatrician are osteosarcoma and Ewing's tumor.

Epidemiology

Osteogenic sarcoma and Ewing's tumor are more common in adolescence than in childhood. However, both tumors have been described in infancy. Sixty percent of osteogenic sarcomas occur just above or below the knee. Both osteogenic sarcomas and Ewing's tumor show a male to female predominance of 1.6:1. The incidence of osteogenic sarcoma in the United States is approximately 0.5 per 100,000 children and that of Ewing's tumor is 0.1 per 100,000. Osteogenic sarcoma shows no racial predilection; Ewing's tumor, in contrast, is exceedingly rare in blacks.

Considerable epidemiologic data have accumulated to show that ionizing radiation causes osteogenic sarcoma. In spite of the extensive epidemiologic data linking radiation and osteogenic sarcoma, most adolescent patients with osteosarcoma have had no excessive exposure to sources of radiation. Likewise, the cause of Ewing's tumor is unknown.

CLINICAL PRESENTATION AND PATHOPHYSIOLOGY

Patients with malignant bone tumors complain of pain or a painful lump. Frequently the pain occurs after a well-remembered episode of trauma. Traumatic hemorrhage into the tumor may fortuitously call attention to a preexisting lesion. Often the pain is more intense at night and may waken the patient from sleep. Patients with osteogenic sarcoma are almost always well. About one third of the patients with Ewing's tumor have a history of systemic symptoms: fever, weight loss, anorexia, and malaise.

When the tumor is in an extremity, physical examination may reveal a hard, tender swelling. Large tumors may feel warm and may have obviously increased vascularity. Disuse atrophy may occur on the affected side.

Trunk lesions, especially those of the pelvis, are difficult to diagnose. Often the mass is buried in gluteal tissue and cannot be appreciated on routine physical examination or on routine x-rays. A meticulous neurologic examination including testing for ability to walk on the heels and toes, to stand on either leg, and to abduct and flex the hips, as well as the symmetry of superficial and deep tendon reflexes may show abnormalities.

Diagnosis of a malignant bone tumor requires an x-ray and a biopsy of the lesion. Radiographs will reveal changes associated with an aggressive destructive process in bone. Early changes include loss of soft tissue fat planes and periosteal elevation (Codman's triangle). Later, one sees an "onionskin" periosteal reaction caused by repetitive episodes of the lesion pushing out the periosteum and the periosteum responding in turn by laying down calcium. Later, normal trabeculation disappears, and areas of lysis are seen. There is no defined sclerotic margin around the area of destruction and it is impossible to know precisely where the tumor begins and ends. Eventually the tumor breaks through the cortex, weakening bone and predisposing to pathologic fracture. The "sunburst" phenomenon of osteosarsarcoma occurs as the tumor blood vessels grow perpendicularly to the shaft of the bone and malignant osteoblasts lay down bone along the vessels (Fig. 55.8). Almost all osteosarcomas are seen on plain x-rays. Some Ewing's tumors may not be obvious: if the history and physical suggest that trauma alone cannot account for the pain, a bone scan is the next radiologic study to order in the search for a cause of pain. Other studies that may be helpful are a CBC, sedimentation rate, and serum LDH in Ewing's tumors, and serum alkaline phosphatase in osteosarcoma. If a presumed malignant tumor is seen, a plain chest x-ray should be taken to determine whether there are obvious metastases.

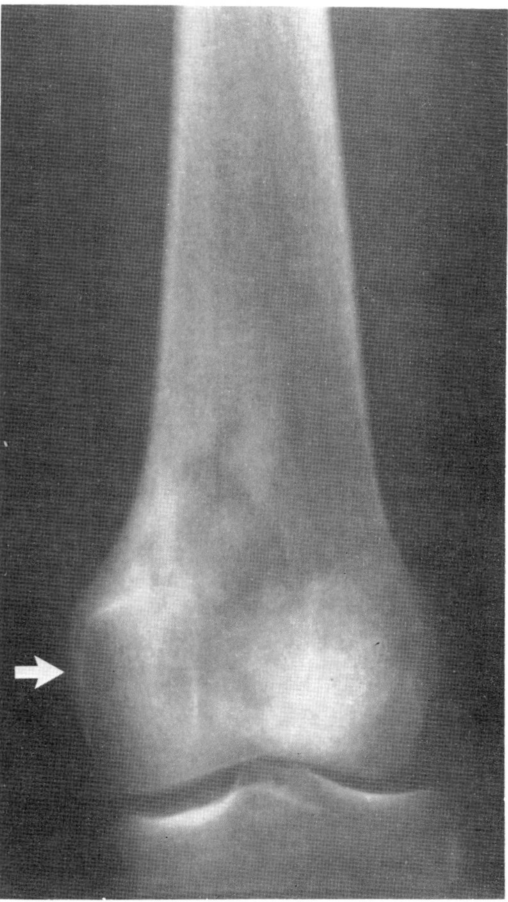

Figure 55.8. Osteosarcoma of the femur in a 17-year-old girl. Plain film of the leg shows lysis of cortical bone and ill-defined zone of transition between destroyed bone and normal bone. There is a slight periosteal elevation (*arrow*).

MANAGEMENT

Whenever the changes of an aggressive bony lesion are seen on x-ray, diagnosing the cause is mandatory. If the clinical find-

Table 55.14
Cancer Chemotherapy

Drug	Class	Clinical Uses	Side Effects	Route of Administration, Schedule/Dose
Actinomycin D (AMD, dactinomycin, Cosmegen)	Antibiotic	Wilms' tumor, Ewing's sarcoma, sarcomas of soft tissue, ovarian tumors	1. Local tissue necrosis with extravasation 2. Nausea and vomiting 3. Myelosuppression 4. GI ulceration 5. Alopecia 6. Radiation "recall"	i.v. push, 0.015 mg/kg day for 5 days, every 3–4 weeks
Adriamycin (doxorubicin)	Anthracycline antibiotic	Acute lymphocytic leukemia (ALL), acute myelogenous leukemia (AML), Ewing's sarcoma, hepatoma, Hodgkin's disease, lymphoma, neuroblastoma, osteosarcoma, ovarian tumors, soft tissue sarcomas, testicular tumors, Wilms' tumor	1. Local tissue necrosis with extravasation 2. Nausea and vomiting 3. Myelosuppression 4. Alopecia 5. Cardiac failure (dose related in range of 450–550 mg/sq m total dose)	i.v. push, 30 mg/sq m/day, 2 × 2–3 days, 75–90 mg/sq m × 1 every 3–4 weeks
Bleomycin (Blenoxane)	Antibiotic	Hodgkin's disease, ovarian tumors, testicular tumors	1. Skin toxicity 2. Fever and chills 3. Nausea and vomiting 4. Alopecia 5. Pulmonary fibrosis (dose related)	i.v. push or drip, i.m., s.q., 10–20 units/sq m/day, every 2–4 weeks
Busulfan (Myeleran)	Alkylating agent	Chronic myelogenous leukemia (CML)	1. Myelosuppression 2. Pulmonary fibrosis 3. Gonadal dysfunction	Oral, 2–12 mg/day, daily
Cis-platinum (*cis*-diammine-dichlorophatinum, CPDD, Platinol)	Heavy metal	Brain tumors, hepatomas, neuroblastoma, osteogenic sarcoma, ovarian tumors, soft tissue sarcoma, testicular tumors	1. Nausea and vomiting 2. Myelosuppression 3. Nephrotoxicity 4. Ototoxicity	i.v., drip, 3–4.5 mg/kg/day or 0.5 mg/kg/day × 5 days, every 3 weeks

Cyclophosphamide (Cytoxan)	Alkylating agent	ALL, AML, Ewing's sarcoma, hepatoma, histiocytosis, Hodgkin's disease, lymphoma, neuroblastoma, osteogenic sarcoma, ovarian tumors, retinoblastoma, soft tissue sarcoma, testicular tumors, Wilms' tumor	1. Nausea and vomiting 2. Myelosuppression 3. Alopecia 4. Hemorrhagic cystitis 5. Inappropriate antidiuretic hormone secretion 6. Gonadal dysfunction 7. Interstitial pneumonitis	Orally, 60–120 mg/sq m daily, i.v., drip, 500–1500 mg/sq m, every 3–4 weeks
Cytosine arabinoside (Ara-C, Cytosar, cytarabine)	Antimetabolite (pyrimidine analog)	ALL, AML, lymphoma	1. Nausea and vomiting 2. Fever 3. Myelosuppression 4. GI ulceration 5. Pulmonary edema	i.v. push or drip, i.m., s.q., i.t., 100–150 mg/sq m/day, 1–7 days, every 2–3 weeks; 30–60 mg/sq m i.t.
Daunomycin (daunorubicin)	Anthracycline antibiotic	AML, lymphoma	See adriamycin	
DTIC (dacarbazine imidazole carboxamide diemthyltriazanol)	Alkylating agent	CML, Hodgkin's disease, neuroblastoma	1. Nausea and vomiting 2. Myelosuppression 3. Fever, chills, myagias 4. Pain with administration	i.v., push or drip, 850 mg/sq m/day × day, 250 mg/sq m/day × 5 days, every 2–4 weeks
5-Fluorouracil (5-FU, Fluorouracil)	Antimetabolite (pyrimidine analog)	Ewing's sarcoma, histiocytosis, osteosarcoma, ovarian tumor, testicular tumors	1. Nausea, vomiting 2. GI ulceration 3. Myelosuppression 4. Alopecia 5. Dermatologic 6. Neurotoxicity (headache, cerebellar ataxia)	i.v. push or drip, 500–600/sq m, weekly
5-Azacytidine	Antimetabolite (pyrimidine analog)	AML	1. Nausea, vomiting, diarrhea 2. Myelosuppression 3. Fever 4. Hepatotoxicity	i.v. 100–400 mg/sq m day, × 5 days, every 3–4 weeks
Hydroxurea (HU)	Antimetabolite	AML, CML, lymphoma	1. Myelosuppression 2. Nausea, vomiting	Oral, 10–20 mg/kg/day, daily

Table 55.14—*Continued*

Drug	Class	Clinical Uses	Side Effects	Route of Administration, Schedule/Dose
L-Asparaginase (Elspar, L-asp)	Enzyme	ALL, lymphoma	1. Allergic reaction 2. Hepatic toxicity 3. Interference with protein synthesis 4. Diabetes mellitus 5. Pancreatitis 6. Cerebrovascular accidents	i.m. or i.v. (must be administered carefully by i.v. route) 6,000–20,000 units/sq m, daily—3 ×/week
Melphalan (Alkeran, L-PAM L-phenylalanine mustard)	Alkylating agent	ALL, CML, Hodgkin's disease, neuroblastoma	1. Nausea, vomiting 2. Myelosuppression 3. Alopecia 4. Stomatitis	Oral: 10 mg/sq m/day, i.v.: in trial
Methotrexate (MTX)	Antimetabolite (folate analog)	ALL, brain tumors, histiocytosis, lymphoma, osteosarcoma, testicular tumors	1. Myelosuppression 2. Nausea, vomiting 3. GI ulceration 4. Hepatotoxicity 5. Dermatologic 6. CNS (leukoencephalopathy) 7. Renal toxicity	i.t.: 6–12 mg, Oral: 10–20 mg/sq m, i.v.: 300 mg–15 g/sq m weekly
Nitrogen mustard (mustargen, HN_2 mechlorethamine hydrochloride)	Alkylating agent	Hodgkin's disease, lymphoma, testicular tumors	1. Tissue necrosis with extravasation 2. Nausea, vomiting 3. Myelosuppression 4. Fever 5. Gonadal dysfunction	i.v.: 6–12 mg/sq m (every 4–6 weeks)
Nitrosoureas (BCNU-Carmustine) (CCNU-Lomustine)	Alkylating agent	Brain tumors, Hodgkin's disease, lymphomas AML (BCNU only)	1. Delayed myelosuppression 2. BCNU—pain on administration 3. Nausea, vomiting 4. Hepatotoxicity 5. Renal toxicity 6. Pulmonary fibrosis	CCNU: oral 100–300 mg/sq m BCNU: i.v. 200 mg/sq m (every 4–6 weeks)

Prednisone (oral) *or* Methylprednisolone (i.v.) Hydrocortisone (oral, i.v.) or Dexamethasome (oral, i.m., i.v.)	Corticosteroid	ALL, AML, histiocytosis, Hodgkin's disease, lymphomas, increased intracranial pressure (dexamethasone only)	1. Cushing's syndrome 2. Increased appetite 3. Diabetes mellitus 4. Acne 5. Aseptic necrosis 6. Hypertension 7. Peptic ulcer 8. Psychiatric symptoms 9. Impaired immunity	40–60 mg/sq m/day—prednisone for leukemia (daily given in 3 divided doses—needs to be tapered when given more than 2 weeks; other corticosteroid doses depends on indication)
Procarbazine (Matulane, ibenzmethyzin)	Alkylating agent	Brain tumors, Hodgkin's disease, lymphomas	1. Myelosuppression 2. Fever, chills, myalgias 3. Dermatologic reactions 4. Nausea and vomiting 5. CNS symptoms, (paresthesia, neuropathy, confusion) 6. Stomatitis 7. Hypersensitivity reactions 8. Teratogenesis	Oral: 50–200 mg/sq m 10–20 days
6-Mercaptopurine (6-MP, Purinethol)	Antimetabolite (purine analog)	ALL, AML, lymphoma	1. Myelosuppression 2. Dermatologic 3. Hepatotoxicity	Orally 75–500 mg/sq m daily at lower doses, every 4–6 weeks at higher doses
6-Thioguanine (6-TG)	Antimetabolite (purine analog)	ALL, AML, lymphoma	1. Myelosuppression 2. Nausea, vomiting 3. Hepatotoxicity	Oral 40–60 mg/sq m (daily)
Vinblastine (Velban)	Vinca alkaloid	Hodgkin's disease, lymphoma, histiocytosis, ovarian tumors, testicular tumors	1. Tissue necrosis with extravasation 2. Myelosuppression 3. Alopecia 4. Neurotoxicity (rarely) 5. Lethargy and depression	i.v. push, 4.0 mg/sq m (every 1–4 weeks)

Table 55.14—*Continued*

Drug	Class	Clinical Uses	Side Effects	Route of Administration, Schedule/Dose
Vincristine (Oncovin, VCR)	Vinca alkaloid	ALL, AML, brain tumors, Ewing's sarcoma, hepatoma, histiocytosis, Hodgkin's disease, neuroblastoma, osteosarcoma, soft tissue sarcoma, testicular tumors, Wilms' tumor	1. Tissue necrosis with extravasation 2. Peripheral neuropathy (pain, loss of deep tendon reflexes, weakness) 3. Constipation and paralytic ileus 4. CNS depression 5. Seizures 6. Inappropriate antidiuretic hormone secretion	i.v. push 1.5–2.0 mg/sq m (maximum dose 2 mg) (weekly—every 4 weeks)
VM-26 (Teniposide)	Epipodophylotoxin	ALL, AML, brain tumors, lymphoma, neuroblastoma, Hodgkin's disease	1. Myelosuppression 2. Hypotension 3. Chemical phlebitis	i.v.: 100 mg/sq m/week, over ½ hr, every 4–6 weeks
VP-16 (Etoposide)	Epipodophylotoxin	Soft tissue sarcoma, AML, lymphomas	1. Myelosuppression 2. Nausea and vomiting	i.v., 50–60 mg/sq m/day, 5 days every 2–4 weeks

[a] s.q., subcutaneously; i.t., inthecally.

ings suggest osteomyelitis, blood culture and culture from the lesions are necessary. If the clinical presentation is more suggestive of tumor, a biopsy is indicated. Ideally, biopsy of Ewing's tumor or osteosarcoma should be performed by an orthopaedic surgeon who has expertise in the total management of neoplastic bone lesions.

Before 1970, patients with osteogenic sarcoma or Ewing's tumor succumbed to pulmonary metastases within months or years. Since the early 1970s adjuvant chemotherapy has been combined with surgery (amputation or en bloc resection for osteogenic sarcoma) or high dose irradiation (Ewing's tumor). Agents used to treat osteogenic sarcoma include vincristine, high dose methotrexate with leucovorin rescue, Adriamycin, and *cis*-platinum. Agents used to treat Ewing's tumor include vincristine, Adriamycin, cyclophosphamide, actinomycin D, and 5-fluorouracil (5-FU). Current projected survival for patients with these tumors is roughly 50%.

The major complications of therapy of osteogenic sarcoma that may bring a patient to the attention of an emergency facility is methotrexate toxicity. Patients treated with high dose methotrexate can develop life-threatening toxicity. Signs and symptoms include diarrhea, vomiting, facial flush, mucosal ulceration. Pancytopenia, hyperuricemia, and renal failure can ensue. Treatment consists of vigorous hydration at twice maintenance fluid rate, alkalinization, allopurinol (if the uric acid is elevated), leucovorin (9 mg every 6 hours), and general support. If the patient has an elevated serum creatinine and cannot maintain oral hydration, admission to the hospital is necessary.

Rarely patients with osteosarcoma develop pneumothoraces. Usually this is an indication that a subpleural metastasis has broken through the pleura. No immediate intervention is warranted unless the pneumothorax is causing respiratory distress.

Patients with Ewing's tumor who have received irradiation and chemotherapy are prone to develop pathologic fractures. These may occur silently or may cause pain and dislocation. Treatment consists of external immobilization. Eventually, many fractures require internal fixation.

Occasionally patients with bone tumors develop fever, neutropenia and sepsis as a result of therapy. The approach to diagnosis is the same as in a child with leukemia (p. 699). Infections in patients with solid tumors are less likely to be fatal than those with leukemia.

CANCER CHEMOTHERAPY

Table 55.14 lists antineoplastic agents, their uses, side effects, doses and route of administration. Most of these agents and irradiation cause some myelosuppression or immunosuppression, and most (except corticosteroids, vinca alkaloids, and bleomycin) cause nausea and vomiting. Attempts to control nausea and vomiting are made at the time of administration by using phenothiazine antiemetics (promethazine or chlorpromazine or 0.25 to 0.50 mg/kg/dose every 4 to 6 hours p.o., i.v., p.r., or rarely i.m.). These antiemetics are not effective in controlling emesis in all patients. Newer agents include droperidol (1 to 2 mg/kg/dose every 4 to 6 hours i.v.) and Metaclopropamide 2 to 3 mg/kg/dose. Tetrahydrocannabinol is also effective in some patients; it is investigational in children. Relaxation therapy or hypnosis help some patients to control their vomiting.

References

Introduction

Altman AJ, Schwartz, AD: Malignant diseases of infancy, childhood and adolescence. In *Major Problems in Clinical Pediatrics*. W. B. Saunders, Philadelphia, 1978.

Catalano RB: The medical approach to management of pain caused by cancer. *Semin Oncol* 2: 379, 1975.

Jones, PG, Campbell PE: *Tumours of Infancy and Childhood*. Blackwell, Oxford, 1976.

Newburger PE, Sallan SE. Chronic pain; principles of management. *Pediatrics* 2: 180, 1981.

Sutow WW, Vietti TJ, Fernbach DJ: *Clinical Pediatric Oncology*. C. V. Mosby, St. Louis, 1977.

Shimm DS, Logue GL, Maltbie AA, Dugan S: Medical management of chronic cancer pain. *JAMA* 241: 2408, 1979.

Leukemia

Aur RJ, Simone JV, Verzosa MS, Hustu HO, Barker LF, Pinkel DP, Rivera G, Dahl GV, Wood A, Stagner S, Mason C: Childhood acute lymphocytic leukemia. *Cancer* 42: 2123, 1978.

Bennett JM, Catovsky D, Danie MT, Flandrin G, Galton AG, Gralnick HR, Sultan C: The morphological classification of acute lymphoblastic leukaemia; concordance among observers and clinical correlations. *Br J Haematol* 47: 553, 1981

Bruckman JE, Bloomer WD: Management of spinal cord compression. *Semin Oncol* 5: 135, 1978.

Chan KW, Steinherz PG, Miller DR: Acute promyelocytic leukemia in children. *Med Pediatr Oncol* 9: 5, 1981.

Cohen LF, Balow JE, Magrath IT, Poplack DG, Ziegler JL: Acute tumor lysis syndrome; a review of 37 patients with Burkitt's lymphoma. *Am J Med* 68: 486, 1980.

Bodey GP, Rodriguez V, Chang HY, Narboni G: Fever and infection in leukemic patients. *Cancer* 41: 1610, 1978.

EORTC, International Antimicrobial Therapy Project Group: Three antibiotic regimens in the treatment of infection in febrile granulocytopenic patients with cancer. *J Infect Dis* 137: 14, 1978.

Garnick MB, Mayer RJ: Acute renal failure associated with neoplastic disease and its treatment. *Semin Oncol* 5: 155, 1978.

Gill FA, Robinson R, Maclowry JD, Levine AS: The relationship of fever, granulocytopenia and antimicrobial therapy to bacteremia in cancer patients. *Cancer* 39: 1704, 1977.

Greaves MF, Janossy G, Peto J, Kay H: Immunologically defined subclasses of acute lymphoblastic leukaemia in children: their relationship to presentation features and prognosis. *Br J Haematol* 48: 179, 1981.

Hammond D, Ather H, Honour RC, Nesbit ME, Miller D, Siegel S, Coccia P: The relative importance of clinical and biologic predictors of outcome in the treatment of acute lymphocytic leukemia. Publication of Children's Cancer Study Group (USC Comprehensive Cancer Center, 1721 Griffen Ave., Los Angeles), 1980.

Hoecker JL, Pickering LK, Groschel D, Kohl S, van Eys J: Current concepts of bacteremia in children with malignancies. *Cancer* 44: 1939, 1979.

Hughes WT: *Pneumocystis carinii* pneumonia. *N Engl J Med* 297: 1381, 1977.

Koeffler HP, Golde DW: Chronic myelogenous leukemia *N Engl J Med* 304: 1201, 1981

Levine AS, Schimpff SC, Graw RG, Young RC: Hematologic malignancies and other marrow failure states; progress in the management of complicating infections. *Semin Hematol* 11: 141, 1974.

Mazzaferri EL, O'Dorisio M, LaBuglio AF: Treatment of hypercalcemia associated with malignancy. *Semin Oncol* 5: 141, 1978.

Myers WPL: Differential diagnosis of hypercalcemia and cancer. *CA* 27: 258, 1977.

Pizzo PA: Infectious complications in the child with cancer; I. Pathophysiology of the compromised host and the initial evaluation and management of the febrile cancer patient. *J Pediatr* 98: 341, 1981.

Pizzo PA: Infectious complications in the child with cancer; II. Management of specific infectious organisms. *J Pediatr* 98: 513, 1981.

Smithson WA, Gilchrist GS, Burgert EO Jr: Child acute lymphocytic leukemia. *CA* 30: 158, 1980.

Stuart RK, Braine HC, Lietman PS, Saral R, Fuller DJ: Carbenicillin-trimethoprim/sulfamethoxazole versus carbenicillin-gentamicin as empiric therapy of infection in granulocytopenic patients. *Am J Med* 68: 876, 1980.

Thomas ED, Buckner CD, Clift RA, Fefer A, Johnson FL, Neiman PE, Sale GE, Sanders JE, Singer JW, Shulman H, Storb R, Weiden PL: Marrow transplantation for acute nonlymphoblastic leukemia in first remission. *N Engl J Med* 301: 597, 1979.

Walzer PD, Perl DP, Krogstad DJ, Rawson PG, Schultz MG: *Pneumocystis carinii* pneumonia in the United States. *Ann Int Med* 80: 83, 1974.

Sallan S, Weinstein H, Nathan D: The childhood leukemias. *J Pediatr* 99: 676, 1981.

Weinstein HJ, Mayer RJ, Rosenthal DS, et al.: Treatment of acute myelogenous leukemia in children and adults. *N Engl J Med* 303: 473, 1980.

Non-Hodgkin's Lymphoma

Berard CW, Greene MH, Jaffe ES, Macgrath I, Ziegler J: A multidisciplinary approach to non-Hodgkin's lymphomas. *Ann Intern Med* 94: 218, 1981.

Murphy SB: Childhood non-Hodgkin's lymphoma. *N Engl J Med* 299: 1446, 1978.

Wollner N, Exelby PR, Lieberman PH: Non-Hodgkin's lymphoma in children. A progress report on the original patients treated with LSA_2-L_2 protocol. *Cancer* 44: 1990, 1979.

Ziegler JL: Burkitt's lymphoma. *N Engl J Med* 305: 735, 1981.

Histocystic Disease

Groopman JE, Golde DW: The histiocytic disorders; a pathophysiologic analysis. *Ann Intern Med* 94: 95, 1981.

Hodgkin's Disease

Aisenberg AC: Current concepts in cancer; the staging and treatment of Hodgkin's disease. *N Engl J Med,* 299: 1228, 1978.

DeVita VT, Simon RM, Hubbard SM, Young RC, Berard CW, Moxley JH, Frei E III, Carbone PP, Canellos GP: Curability of advanced Hodgkin's disease with chemotherapy. *Ann Intern Med* 92: 587, 1980.

Kaplan HS: Hodgkin's disease; biology, treatment, prognosis. *Blood* 57: 813, 1981.

Thoracic Tumors

Lockich JJ, Goodman R: Superior vena cava syndrome; clinical management. *JAMA* 231: 58, 1975.

Perez CA, Presant CA, Van Amburg AL III: Management of superior vena cava syndrome. *Semin Oncol* 5: 123, 1978.

Pokorny WJ, Sherman JO: Mediastinal masses in infants and children. *J Thorac Cardiovasc Surg* 68: 869, 1974.

Theologides A: Neoplastic cardiac tamponade. *Semin Oncol* 5: 181, 1978.

Abdominal, Genitourinary, and Retroperitoneal Tumors

Grossman H: Evaluating common intra-abdominal masses in children—a systematic roentgenographic approach. American Cancer Society Professional Education Publication, 1976.
Sise JG, Crichlow RW: Obstruction due to malignant tumors. *Semin Oncol* 5: 1978.
Belasco J, D'Angio GJ: Wilms' tumor. *CA* 31: 258, 1981.
Breslow NE, Palmer NF, Hill LR, Buring J, D'Angio GJ: Wilms' tumor; prognostic factors for patients without metastases at diagnosis. *Cancer* 41: 1577, 1978.
D'Angio GJ, Evans A, Breslow N, Beckwith B, Bishop H, Farewell V, Goodwin W, Leape L, Palmer N, Sinks L, Sutow W, Tefft M, Wolff J: The treatment of Wilms' tumor; results of the Second National Wilms' Tumor Study. *Cancer* 47: 2302, 1981.

Neuroblastoma

Evans A: Staging and treatment of neuroblastoma. *Cancer* 45: 1799, 1980.
Koop CE, Schnauffer L: The management of abdominal neuroblastoma. *Cancer* 35: 905, 1975.

Hepatic Tumors

Popper H, Schaffner F: *Prog Liver Dis* 5: 636, 1976.

Tumors of Female Genitalia

Anikwue C, et al.: Granulosa theca cell tumors. *Obstet Gynecol* 51: 214, 1978.
Association of Maternal Stilbesterol with Tumor Appearance in Young Women: *N Engl J Med* 280: 352, 1973.
Barber HK: Ovarian cancer in children—guide for a difficult decision. *CA* 25: 234, 1975.

Tumors of Male Genitalia

Exelby PR: Malignant scrotal masses in children. *CA* 163: 24, 1974.
Ise T, Ohtsuki H, Matsumoto C, Sano R: Management of malignant testicular tumors in children. *Cancer* 37: 1539, 1976.
Javadpour N: Germ cell tumor of the testis. *CA* 30: 242, 1980.

Central Nervous System Tumors

Edwards MS, Levin VA, Wilson CB: Chemotherapy of pediatric posterior fossa tumors. *Childs Brain* 7: 252, 1980.
Ertel IJ: Brain tumors in children. *CA* 30: 306, 1980.
Koos ET, Miller MH: *Intracranial Tumors of Infants and Children*. C. V. Mosby, St. Louis, 1971.
Wilson CB: Diagnosis and surgical treatment of childhood brain tumors. *Cancer* 35: 950, 1975.
Catalano JD: Differential diagnosis of white pupil (leukokoria). *Pediatr Ann* 6: 91, 1977.

Thyroid Cancer

Hopwood N, Carroll R, Kenny R, Folety T: Functioning thyroid masses in childhood and adolescence. *J Pediatr* 89: 710, 1976.
Scott M, Crawford J: Solitary thyroid nodules in childhood. Is the incidence of thyroid carcinoma declining? *Pediatrics* 4: 521, 1976.

Soft Tissue Sarcomas

Hajdu SI: Soff tissue sarcomas; classification and natural history. *CA* 31: 271, 1981.
Handler SD, Raney RB Jr: Management of neoplasms of the head and neck in children; I. Benign tumors. *Head Neck Surg* 3: 395, 1981.
Oakhill A, Willshaw H, Mann Jr.: Unilateral proptosis. *Arch Dis Child* 56: 649, 1981.
Raney RB Jr, Handler SD: Management of neoplasms of the head and neck in children; II. Malignant tumors. *Head Neck Surg* 3: 500, 1981.
Raney RB Jr, Chatten J, Littman P, Jarrett P, Schnaufer L, Bishop H, D'Angio GJ: Treatment strategies for infants with malignant sacrococcygeal teratoma. *J Pediatr Surg* 16: 573, 1981.
Suit HD: Sarcoma of soft tissue. *CA* 28: 5, 1978.
Tefft M, Fernandez CH, Moon TE: Rhabdomyosarcoma; response with chemotherapy prior to radiation in patients with gross residual disease. *Cancer* 39: 665, 1977.

Bone Tumors

deSantos L: The radiology of bone tumors. *CA* 30: No. 2, 1980.
Jaffe N: Bone tumors in children. In *Progress in Pediatric Hematology/Oncology*, Vol. II. PSG Publishing, Littleton, Mass., 1978.
Proceedings of the Osteosarcoma Study Group Meeting (Bethesda, Md., January 19, 1977): *Cancer Treat Rep* 62: 187, 1978.
Rosen G, Caparros B, Nirenberg A, Marcove R, Hubos AG, Kosloff C, Lane J, Murphy ML: Ewing's sarcoma; ten-year experience with adjuvant chemotherapy. *Cancer* 47: 2204, 1981.

Cancer Chemotherapy

Dorr RT, Fritz WL: *Cancer Chemotherapy Handbook*. Elsevier, New York, 1979.
Friedman MA, Carter SB: Serious toxicities associated with chemotherapy. *Semin Oncol* 5: 193, 1978.
Krakoff IH: Cancer chemotherapeutic agents. *CA* 31: 130, 1981.
Harris JG: Nausea, vomiting and cancer treatment. *CA* 28: 194, 1978.
Pratt WB, Ruddon RW: *The Anticancer Drugs*. Oxford University Press, New York, 1979.

CHAPTER 56

Rheumatologic Emergencies

BALU H. ATHREYA, M.D., AND CAROLYN L. YANCEY, M.D.

JUVENILE RHEUMATOID ARTHRITIS

BACKGROUND

Juvenile rheumatoid arthritis (JRA) has replaced acute rheumatic fever as the commonest rheumatic disease of children in the Western world. JRA is known to occur throughout the world, though this disease has been reported to be rare in children of Chinese origin. There are approximately 200,000 children with JRA in the United States. Girls are affected more frequently than boys.

This diagnostic category includes a group of syndromes characterized by chronic synovitis. Since there are no laboratory abnormalities which are characteristic of JRA, the diagnosis is made clinically after exclusion of other identifiable diseases associated with chronic synovitis. The American Rheumatism Association has suggested the following criterion for diagnosing JRA: persistent arthritis of one or more joints lasting over 6 weeks in children less than 16 years of age, after other causes of arthritis have been excluded.

JRA has been known to occur following trauma or a systemic infection, but no definite etiological association has been established between those events and the onset of JRA. Extensive investigations to correlate JRA with viral, bacterial or mycoplasmal infections have not been conclusive. The presence of rheumatoid factor (RF) in the serum, a lowered level of complement in the synovial fluid, and lymphocytes in the synovial tissue, suggest that immunologically mediated injury plays a part in the pathogenesis of this disease. There may also be a genetic factor as suggested by the association of JRA with certain types of histocompatibility antigens (HLA).

PATHOPHYSIOLOGY

The pathogenesis of JRA can be divided into an initiating phase and a perpetuating phase. There is minimal information on initiating factors. The mechanism that perpetuates inflammation is better understood and forms the basis for the current modalities of treatment.

Pathologically, vasculitis is prominent in early lesions. In established cases of arthritis, light microscopy of the synovium shows fibrin deposits, hyperplasia and hypertrophy of synovial lining cells and an inflammatory cell response. Increased secretion of fluid results in joint effusions. In uncontrolled and persistent arthritis, synovial villi project into the joint. Thickened synovial membranes may spread from the edges of the joint and grow over the articular cartilage (pannus) and cause destruction of the cartilage.

CLINICAL FEATURES

JRA has been divided into various subtypes based on the pattern of the disease in the first 6 months (Table 56.1). These are polyarticular arthritis (RF positive), polyarticular arthritis (RF negative), pauciarticular arthritis (Type I), pauciarticular ar

Table 56.1
Subgroups of Juvenile Rheumatoid Arthritis[a]

Subgroup	*Sex Ratio*	*Age at Onset*	*Joints Affected*	*Serologic and Genetic Tests*[b]	*Extraarticular Manifestations*	*Prognosis*
Rheumatoid factor positive polyarticular	80% girls	Late childhood	Any joints	ANA 75%, RF 100%	Low-grade fever, anemia, malaise, rheumatoid nodules	>50% severe arthritis
Rheumatoid factor negative polyarticular	90% girls	Any age	Any joints	ANA 5%, RF negative	Low-grade fever, mild anemia, malaise, growth retardation	10–15% severe arthritis
Pauciarticular with chronic iridocyclitis	80% girls	Early childhood	Few large joints (hips and sacroiliac joints spared)	ANA 50%, RF negative	Few constitutional complaints, chronic iridocyclitis in 50%	Severe arthritis uncommon, 10–20% ocular damage from iridocyclitis
Pauciarticular with sacroiliitis	90% boys	Late childhood	Few large joints (hip and sacroiliac involvement common)	ANA negative, RF negative, HLA-B27 75%	Few constitutional complaints, acute iridocyclitis in 5–10% during childhood	Some have ankylosing spondylitis at follow-up
Systemic onset	60% boys	Any age	Any joints	ANA negative, RF negative	High fever, rash, organomegaly, polyserositis, leukocytosis, growth retardation	25% severe arthritis

[a] Modified from J. G. Schaller: In *Clinical Immunology Update*, edited by E. C. Franklin, Elsevier North Holland, New York, 1979.
[b] ANA, antinuclear antibody; RF, rheumatoid factor; HLA-B27, histocompatibility antigen-B27.

thritis (Type II), and systemic type JRA. Pauciarticular arthritis is defined as arthritis involving four or fewer than four joints.

Polyarticular arthritis (both types) occurs more commonly in girls and is characterized by insidious onset, low grade fever, morning stiffness and symmetric polyarthritis of both large and small joints (Fig. 56.1). Fusiform changes of the fingers are seen commonly. Cervical spine involvement occurs in approximately 30 to 50% of patients with this variety of arthritis resulting in neck pain, stiffness and torticollis. Involvement of the temporomandibular joint results in an inability to open the mouth. Involvement of the hip may result in permanent disability. Though both subtypes of polyarticular arthritis have these same features, children with RF positive rheumatoid arthritis tend to be older at the onset of the disease, develop subcutaneous nodules more commonly, have more erosive changes in the joints, develop vasculitic complications more often, and have a poorer prognosis than those with RF negative polyarthritis.

Pauciarticular arthritis (Type I) occurs more often in young girls. Typically it involves one or more large joints (less than 4) with swelling, pain and limitation of range of movement. When the disease involves only one joint, exclusion of infectious arthritis becomes important. Antinuclear antibody (ANA) is demonstrated in the sera of over 50% of these children. They are at high risk for developing iridocyclitis. Since the onset of iridocyclitis is insidious, they may not have symptoms referable to the eye until late in their course, and periodic slit lamp examination of the eye is necessary to detect this complication early.

Pauciarticular arthritis (Type II) occurs more often in preadolescent boys. Though they are classified as JRA, many of them may evolve into one of the spondylarthropathies on long-term follow-up into adulthood. The risk for developing chronic iridocyclitis is negligible, but some of them may develop acute iridocyclitis.

Systemic type JRA occurs most often in the younger age group (less than 5 years), though it is being reported even in adults. Approximately 20% of children with JRA have the systemic type. Clinically these children have high intermittent spiking fevers (39 to 41°C) for several weeks or

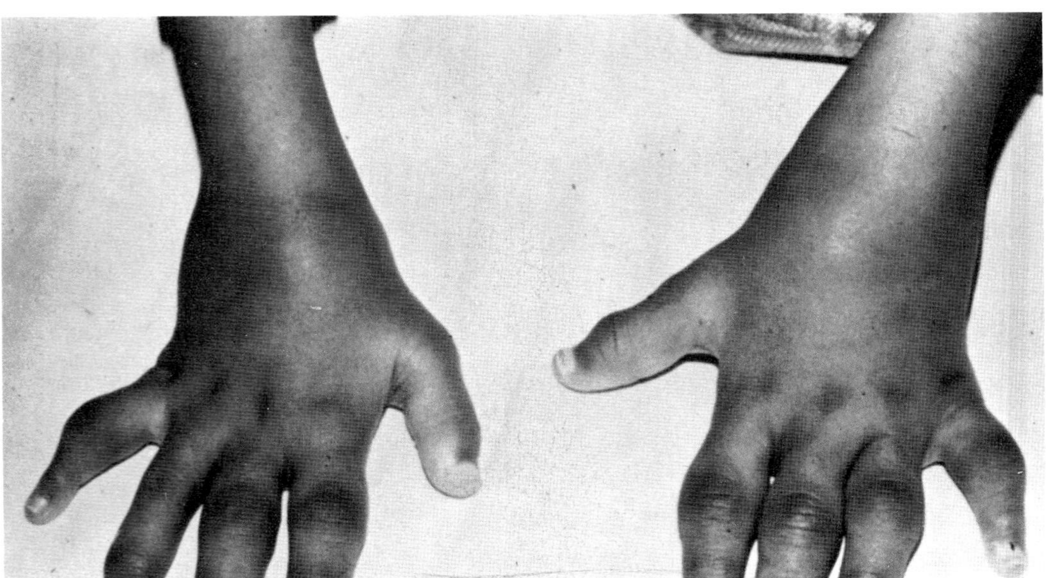

Figure 56.1 Symmetrical involvement of large and small joints of the hands in a child with polyarticular arthritis.

months, an evanescent maculopapular rash (Fig. 56.2), lymphadenopathy, and hepatosplenomegaly. In the early stages, though the child feels stiff and does not move normally, arthritis may not be a prominent feature. Athralgias and myalgias are common. Pericarditis occurs most commonly in this subtype of JRA. On long-term follow-up, systemic features of the disease get less prominent and polyarticular arthritis becomes the major focus of management. The list of differential diagnoses of this group includes various infectious diseases, leukemia and neuroblastoma.

Laboratory and Radiological Features

There is no laboratory test that is diagnostic of JRA. In the polyarticular variety, one subgroup shows RF in the serum. None of the other subgroups of JRA have this marker. Mild to moderate anemia is common in all subtypes, particularly the systemic type. The white count is often elevated. This is particularly true of the systemic type in which counts up to 30,000/cu mm may be seen. Platelet counts are often elevated. Urinalysis is usually normal. There is elevation of levels of acute phase reactants in the serum, and the albumin-globulin ratio is often reversed. The complement level may be normal or elevated. ANA in the serum, particularly in the pauciarticular arthritis, is an important marker for children at risk for iridocyclitis. Radiological features of JRA include soft tissue swelling of affected joints with periosteal

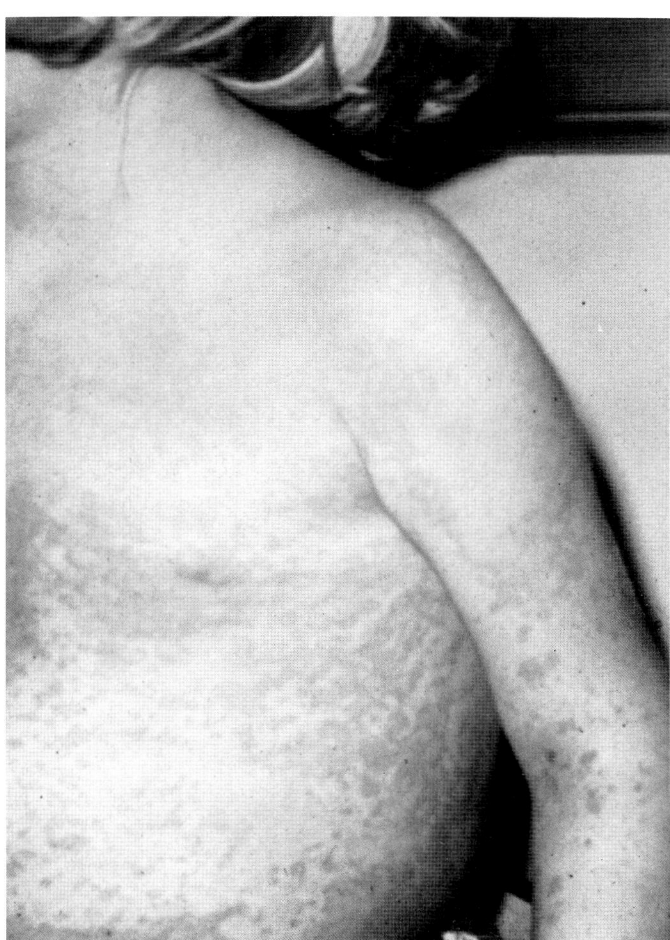

Figure 56.2 Macular rash in a child with systemic type of juvenile rheumatoid arthritis.

new bone formation and osteoporosis of bones close to the affected joints. Later, narrowing of the joint space, erosions, subluxation and ankylosis are seen.

MANAGEMENT

General Management

The comprehensive management of children with JRA requires the skills of several different specialists. The major goal of therapy is to help the child and the family maintain as normal a life as possible. The family and child should know that the majority of children with this disease recover with minimal residual problems. Simple measures such as warm tub baths and the use of sleeping bags at night help control morning stiffness. For children with minimal joint involvement, regular daily activities and modified gym activity are recommended. In the presence of muscle wasting, weakness and developing contractures, an active physical therapy program is indicated. Splinting is indicated to rest actively inflamed, painful joints and to prevent worsening of deformities.

The simplest, safest and most economical agent for the medical management of JRA is aspirin. The usual starting dose is 80 to 90 mg/kg in 3 or 4 divided doses during the waking hours; subsequent drug dosages should be adjusted to achieve serum salicylate levels of 25 to 30 mg/dl. Serum transaminase (SGOT and SGPT) levels should be checked to monitor for aspirin-induced hepatotoxicity, particularly during the first 3 months of therapy. One of the newer nonsteroidal anti-inflammatory drugs (NSAID) may be used in the place of aspirin as the initial agent, in the presence of aspirin toxicity, or in cases of failure of response to aspirin therapy (Table 56.2).

If after an adequate trial with aspirin or one of the NSAID, there is no response, or an inadequate one, a slow acting antirheumatic drug such as a gold compound or D-penicillamine, may have to be added to the basic regimen. Steroids are reserved for children with severe cardiac, pulmonary, or ocular complications and those with fever unresponsive to simple measures. Intra-articular steroids may be used in certain patients with monoarticular arthritis and in children with polyarticular disease who improve with systemic medical therapy except for the persistence of inflammation in one or two joints.

Management of Complications and Emergencies

Fever. Marked elevation of body temperature is characteristic of systemic JRA at the time of the initial presentation. Since the diagnosis of JRA is by exclusion and since fever is a common symptom, all efforts have to be made to exclude infectious diseases and malignancies such as leukemia and neuroblastoma. This requires hospitalization for the first diagnostic evaluation, particularly in infants and young children. Appropriate cultures should be obtained, including cultures of cerebrospinal fluid if

Table 56.2
Nonsteroidal Anti-Inflammatory Drugs (NSAID)

Drug	Dosage Range	Side Effects
Tolmetin sodium (Tolectin)	Start at 15 mg/kg/day; increase to 30 mg/kg/day; maximum daily dose, 1800 mg	Gastric irritation, headache, hematuria
Indomethacin (Indocin)	Start at 0.5 mg/kg/day; increase to 2.5 mg/kg/day; maximum daily dose, 100 mg	Gastric irritation, headache, hematuria
Ibuprofen (Motrin)	Dose not established for children; doses up to 40 mg/kg/day have been used	Gastric irritation, hematuria, transient rash, thrombocytopenia
Naproxen (Naprosyn)	10 mg/kg/day in 2 divided doses; maximum daily dose, 1000 mg	Gastric irritation, headache, rash

indicated. A bone marrow examination for malignancy is needed in most of the patients with systemic type JRA.

In a patient known to have systemic type JRA and on therapy, the appearance of fever is always of concern. The fever may represent recurrence of JRA or an intercurrent infection. If the fever pattern resembles that seen during the earlier course (one or two peaks above 39°C daily), if there are no localizing signs of infection, and if the CBC and urinalysis are normal, treatment may be maintained with the same NSAID or switched to one of the other drugs from the same group (Table 56.2). If the fever is due to a specific infection (such as otitis media or urinary tract infection), appropriate antibiotics should be used. If the patient is currently taking steroids or has received steroids for more than 2 weeks within the previous 6 months, appropriate coverage with steroids (3 times physiologic dosage) is indicated during the period of treatment of the infection (p. 641).

Pericarditis, Myocarditis and Cardiac Tamponade. Pericarditis is an important feature of systemic onset JRA. Marked elevation of temperature is often seen during the course of pericarditis. Common symptoms are chest pain, dyspnea, and inability to lie down flat in bed. Occasionally, there may be no symptoms. On physical examination, a pericardial friction rub may be heard over the left 2nd and 3rd intercostal spaces close to the sternum with the patient supine. If the child has a moderate to large effusion, one may not hear the friction rub but should look for the following evidences of pericardial effusion: edema, tachycardia, weak pulse, distended neck veins, distant heart sounds, palpation of the apical impulse within the border of cardiac dullness, hepatomegaly and congestive heart failure. Occasionally, the effusion can be massive and lead to cardiac tamponade as suggested by pulsus paradoxus of over 12 mm Hg. Myocarditis is rare but can occur. Tachycardia out of proportion to the elevation of temperature, arrythmias, and congestive heart failure are the usual clinical indicators of myocarditis.

If pericarditis or myocarditis is suspected, the child should be admitted and observed closely. Diagnostic studies should include electrocardiogram, echocardiogram and roentgenogram of the chest. The usual changes noted on ECG are: tachycardia, elevated S-T segment and inverted T waves. Roentgenograms of the chest should be obtained to look for straightening of the left border of the heart and cardiac enlargement (Fig. 56.3). Echocardiogram should be performed to document ventricular function, particularly if cardiac tamponade is suspected.

Bed rest and therapy with salicylates or one of the NSAID should be adequate for the treatment of mild to moderate pericarditis. The dose of acetyl salicylic acid is 80 to 90 mg/kg/day in 3 or 4 divided doses; the dose of tolmetin sodium (Tolectin) is 15 to 30 mg/kg/day in 3 divided doses. Steroids (prednisone 2 mg/kg/day) are indicated for the treatment of pericarditis if the effusion is massive leading to tamponade, or if the effusion progresses in spite of adequate therapy with salicylates or other NSAID. Steroids are always indicated for the treatment of myocarditis. In the presence of tamponade or progressive compromise of cardiac function, pericardiocentesis becomes necessary. If the child is acutely ill requiring intravenous fluid support, care should be taken to avoid fluid overload and diuretics should be used early.

Cricoarytenoid Arthritis. In patients with known polyarticular arthritis, cricoarytenoid arthritis may lead to acute airway obstruction. The cricoarytenoid joint is a diarthroidal joint with a synovial membrane and has been reported to be involved in 26% of the adults with rheumatoid arthritis. There is a report of a 3-year-old boy with left cricoarytenoid arthritis who developed airway obstruction and required emergency tracheostomy.

Clinical features of cricoarytenoid arthritis include stridor and hoarseness. The inspiratory stridor may wax and wane and may be present only when the patient is asleep. Hoarseness of the voice may be mild or severe. Some of these patients may also complain of pain in the throat while swallowing and pain in the ears. Since many of

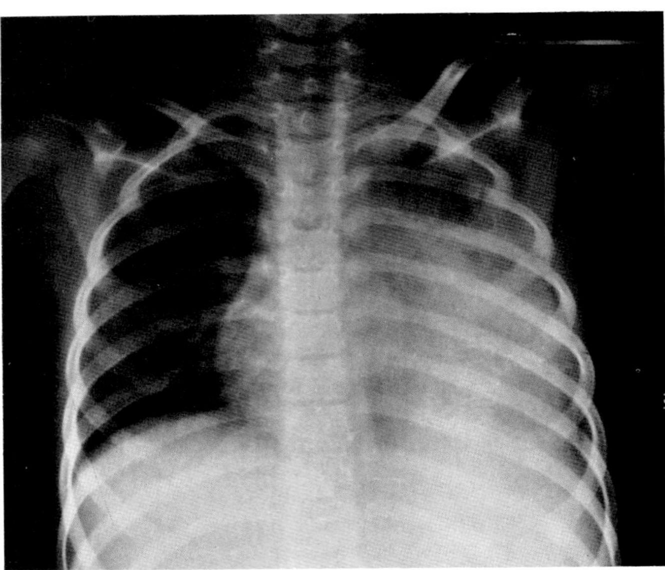

Figure 56.3 Pericardial and pleural effusions in a child with systemic type of juvenile rheumatoid arthritis.

these symptoms and signs are similar to those of severe acute laryngotracheobronchitis, one has to be cautious. Increasing airway obstruction with severe inspiratory retractions demands urgent treatment.

The diagnosis is established on direct laryngoscopy. Redness and swelling of the arytenoid eminences may be observed. Large doses of steroids (prednisone, 2 mg/kg/day) may control acute inflammation of the joints, avoiding emergency tracheostomy. If significant obstruction occurs, intubation should be attempted to establish an airway until swelling decreases; occasionally emergency tracheostomy may be necessary. Even if tracheostomy is done, steroid therapy is indicated so that the tracheostomy can be closed as quickly as possible.

Cervical Spine Involvement. This complication is seen usually in children with established severe polyarticular arthritis. Though cervical spine involvement is known to occur in 30 to 50% of patients with JRA, atlantoaxial subluxation (AA subluxation) and subluxation of the lower cervical spine are less common. In adults, approximately 50% of patients with rheumatoid arthritis have AA subluxation. Clinical evidence of pressure on the spinal cord is seen in 23 to 65% of those with radiological evidence of AA subluxation. Similar figures are not available for children. The incidence of AA subluxation among patients with JRA followed at The Children's Hospital of Philadelphia is 17%.

Neck stiffness is the commonest symptom of cervical spine involvement in JRA. This is often worse in the morning. Severe pain in the neck and referred pain over the occipital and retroorbital areas may also occur. The pain has a dull, aching quality and is often aggravated by neck movement. Torticollis may be the earliest manifestation of JRA in a small number of children. On physical examination, torticollis and/or loss of lordosis of the cervical spine and limitation of range of movement of the neck are the important findings.

Paresthesia of the fingers is the commonest symptom in the presence of spinal cord compression. Weakness of the arms and legs, vertigo, and inability to control the bladder are other complaints which should suggest spinal cord compression. During the initial stages, exaggerated deep tendon reflexes and an extensor plantar reflex are noted. Chronic myelopathy results in muscle atrophy and loss of deep tendon reflexes. A lateral roentgenogram of the neck with the neck in flexion and in extension is required for complete evaluation of the cervical spine. The patient should be asked to actively and slowly flex and extend the neck to tolerance without discomfort; care should be taken not to force these movements. Laminograms and an open-mouth view of the odontoid process may be helpful. On some occasions, computerized tomography may be indicated.

The distance between the anterior surface of the odontoid and the posterior surface of the anterior arch of atlas when measured in a lateral flexion film is usually 4 mm or less. In the presence of AA subluxation, this may be as wide as 10 to 12 mm (Fig. 56.4). Other radiological abnormalities of cervical spine involvement in JRA are: loss of curvature, osteoporosis, erosions and sclerosis of joints, disk space narrowing and altered height to width ratio of the vertebral bodies.

Most children with AA subluxation do not have evidence of spinal cord compression; however, the physician must be aware of this possibility with excessive movement, as for endotracheal intubation. Regular use of a light plastic cervical collar is all that is required to relieve pain and prevent excessive anterior flexion, particularly during automobile rides. In the presence of spinal cord compression with muscle weakness and atrophy, surgical stabilization may be required.

Iridocyclitis. Iridocyclitis (inflammation of the iris and ciliary body) occurs in approximately 10 to 20% of all children with JRA. This can be of acute or chronic onset. The chronic type of iridocyclitis occurs primarily in young girls with the pauciarticular

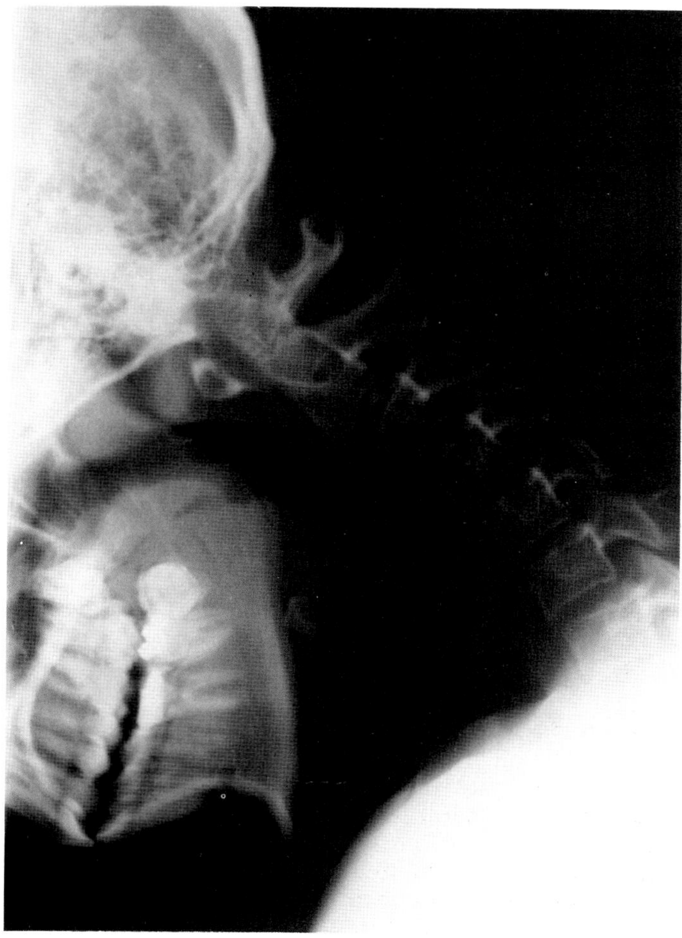

Figure 56.4 Atlantoaxial subluxation in a child with juvenile rheumatoid arthritis. (The distance between the anterior arch of atlas and the odontoid process in the original x-ray was 5 mm.)

type (Type I) of arthritis; the correlation gets even higher with pauciarticular arthritis in girls who have ANA in their serum.

The onset of chronic iridocyclitis is insidious. Symptoms and signs of chronic iridocyclitis are red eye, ocular pain, photophobia, decreased visual acuity, and unequal pupils; however, the majority of these children are asymptomatic. Therefore, all children with JRA, particularly those at high risk for iridocyclitis, should have a routine eye examination as soon as the diagnosis is made and at frequent (3- to 6-month) intervals. In addition, if a child develops one of the symptoms listed above, an immediate slitlamp examination is indicated. The physician in the emergency department may be able to recognize established evidence of iridocyclitis such as band keratopathy, posterior synechiae and cataracts using a +8 or +10 diopter lens in the ophthalmoscope; but slitlamp examination is required to recognize early lesions.

In contrast, the acute onset type iridocyclitis occurs most often in older boys with pauciarticular arthritis and no ANA in their serum. Acute iridocyclitis is characterized by sudden onset of redness, watering, pain and photophobia.

Both these conditions require urgent management, but admission is not necessary. Consultation with an ophthalmologist is essential. The usual treatment includes topical steroids and mydriatics.

Pulmonary Emergencies. In patients with systemic JRA, pleural effusions are known to occur. Other pleuropulmonary manifestations in JRA include pneumonitis, diffuse interstitial disease, lymphoid bronchiolitis and pulmonary arteritis. Occasionally pleural effusion can be massive resulting in respiratory distress. The usual clinical features of pleural effusion are chest pain, cough and dyspnea. On physical examination there is dullness on percussion and diminished breath sounds on auscultation over the area of fluid. A roentgenogram of the chest defines the extent of effusion, and thoracentesis is indicated mainly for diagnosis. Treatment is aimed at the basic disease. Children with this complication require admission for the overall severity of systemic features of the disease rather than for the pleural effusion alone.

Flare of a Single Joint in a Patient with JRA. In a patient known to have JRA and currently receiving anti-inflammatory medication, acute swelling with pain and limitation of range of movement of a single joint raises a major management problem. The differential diagnosis of this situation includes an acute flare of JRA and infectious arthritis.

Physical findings characteristic of infection of the joint are extreme pain, tenderness, erythema and warmth over the joint. The affected joints of JRA appear swollen, warm and stiff; however, they are rarely red. There is usually a pronounced limitation of range of movement of the joint in infectious arthritis. Even a 5° movement may cause severe pain and muscle spasm. In contrast, some range of motion (5 to 10°) is usually possible even with severely inflamed joints of JRA. If the patient is taking one of the steroid preparations, physical findings of inflammation may be masked.

If infection is suspected, aspiration of joint fluid must be performed and the fluid sent for cell count, Gram stain and culture. If there is any doubt about the diagnosis, it is best to obtain blood culture and initiate treatment for septic arthritis. For the acute swelling and pain in a single joint due to JRA, resting for 2 to 3 days using a splint is adequate. Local injection of the joint with steroid (triamcinolone hexacetonide) is sometimes indicated after infection has been excluded.

Ruptured Popiteal Cyst. There are six bursae around the knee joint. Of these, the gastrocnemius semimembranosus bursa is the one that most often communicates with the knee joint. Consequently, in the presence of effusion in the knee joint, fluid may enter the bursa and produce a popiteal cyst (Baker's cyst). Patients with popiteal cysts have a palpable and visible enlargement in the popiteal area best seen with the knee in extension.

Rupture of this popiteal cyst with drainage of fluid into the calf muscles may occasionally present as an emergency. These patients complain of sudden pain in the calf associated with swelling in the leg. On physical examination, they have swelling, erythema, warmth and tenderness of the calf and ankle edema. An effusion in the knee joint and evidence of synovial thickening are present. Homan's sign may be positive; however, there are no palpable venous cords, dilatation of collateral veins or arterial spasm which are signs of thrombophlebitis.

Differentiation of a ruptured popliteal cyst from thrombophlebitis may be very difficult. Consequently, various diagnostic techniques may be needed to establish the diagnosis. Though arthrogram of the knee has been the accepted procedure, ultrasound and intra-articular administration of ^{131}I-labeled albumin followed by scintigraphy have been recently found to be useful noninvasive techniques.

Intra-articular administration of steroids (triamcinolone hexacetonide, 10 to 25 mg) is the recommended initial treatment. If there is no response or if the syndrome is chronic, surgical excision of the cyst is indicated.

Drug Toxicity. It is important to remember that almost all of the drugs used for the treatment of JRA have the potential for serious toxicity. Therefore, if a child with JRA on treatment develops a new symptom, drug toxicity must be considered as one of the causes. Table 56.2 lists the common adverse reactions reported with NSAID. The major side effects from gold compounds are: skin rash, bone marrow suppression with anemia, neutropenia, and thrombocytopenia and nephrotoxicity. D-Penicillamine may cause skin rash, bone marrow suppression, nephrotoxicity, myasthenia gravis, and Goodpasture's syndrome.

SYSTEMIC LUPUS ERYTHEMATOSUS

BACKGROUND

Systemic lupus erythematosus (SLE) is a multisystem disease with great variability in its clinical course. The annual incidence of this disease has been reported to be 7.6 per 100,000 in adults. There is a greater prevalence of SLE among women between the ages of 15 and 64 years (1 in 700), particularly among black women (1 in 245). It is estimated that there are approximately 10,000 to 15,000 children with SLE in the United States.

The much quoted criteria developed by the American Rheumatism Association are listed in Table 56.3. A patient should fulfill 4 of these 14 criteria to be classified as definitely having SLE. However, the clinician is justified in making the diagnosis of SLE in any patient with multisystem disease and circulating ANA after exclusion of disorders resembling SLE.

PATHOPHYSIOLOGY

SLE is a diffuse disease that may involve almost any organ in the body. The histopathology of the skin varies from nonspecific vasculitis in the maculopapular variety of rash, to lesions showing thinning of the epidermis, disruption of dermal-epidermal junction, edema of the dermis, lymphocytic infiltration, and fibrinoid degeneration of the connective tissue in the acute phase of SLE. On immunofluorescent staining, localization of the immunoglobulins and complement in the dermal-epidermal junction of the skin is seen in over 75% of patients; however, this is not specific for SLE. The synovium shows synovitis with fibrinoid de-

Table 56.3
Preliminary Criteria of the American Rheumatism Association for Classification of Systemic Lupus Erythematosus[a]

1. Facial erythema (butterfly rash)
2. Discoid lupus
3. Raynaud's phenomenon
4. Alopecia
5. Photosensitivity
6. Oral or nasopharyngeal ulceration
7. Arthritis without deformity
8. LE cells
9. Chronic false-positive standard serologic test for syphilis (STS)
10. Profuse proteinuria
11. Cellular casts
12. One or both of the following: (a) pleuritis, (b) pericarditis
13. One or both of the following: (a) psychosis, (b) convulsions
14. One or more of the following: (a) hemolytic anemia, (b) leukopenia, (c) thrombocytopenia

[a] From *Bulletin of the Rheumatic Diseases, 21:* 645, 1971.

generation of connective tissue but no pannus formation or cartilage destruction. Major pathological lesions of SLE are noted in the kidney. If light microscopy, immunofluorescence, and electron microscopy are applied to renal tissue in patients with disease, most will reveal some renal pathology. The renal lesions of SLE are classified under the following headings: (1) mesangial neprhitis, (2) focal proliferative nephritis, (3) diffuse proliferative nephritis, (4) membranous nephritis, (5) glomerular sclerosis, (6) vasculitis, and (7) interstitial disease.

Current concepts of the pathogenesis of SLE invoke an interplay of environmental and genetic factors (Fig. 56.5) which lead to polyclonal activation of B cells. Until recently, this particular defect (overactivity of B cells) was considered secondary to low suppressor T cell activity. The current view favors a primary role for polyclonal B cell

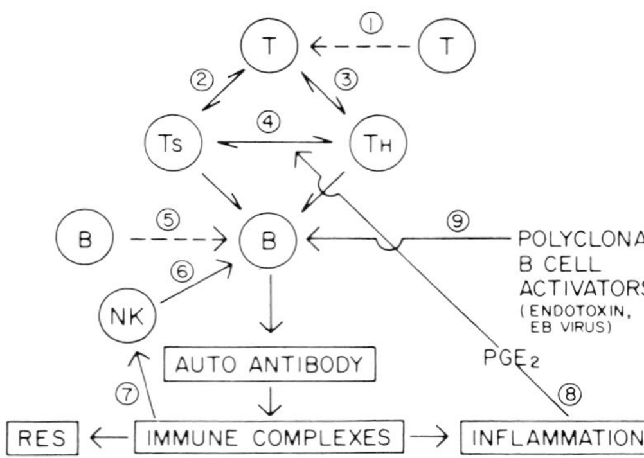

Figure 56.5 Defective immunoregulation in systemic lupus erythematosus. Impaired thymocyte differentiations (*1*); impairment in numbers or function of T suppressor lymphocytes (*2*); or T helper lymphocytes (*3*); defective signals for T help or T suppression (*4*); premature activation of B lymphocytes (*5*); failure to eliminate autoreactive B lymphocyte clones by cytotoxic natural killer cells (*6*); immune complex inactivation of cytotoxic natural killer cells (*7*); interference with regulatory T cells by prostaglandin E_2 (*8*); nonspecific polyclonal activation of preexisting autoreactive B cell clones (*9*). (Reproduced with permission of David Bell, MD, from *Journal of Rheumatology, 8:* 341, 1981.)

activation and consequent production of antibodies to various antigens, including self antigens. These antibodies, in turn, are responsible for circulating immune complexes that deposit in tissues and activate the complement cascade. Release of activation products of complement, such as C5A, which are chemotactic, leads to accumulation of phagocytes. During the process of ingestion of immune complexes by phagocytes, lysosomal enzymes are released which cause local destruction of tissues.

Some of the known environmental factors which precipitate or exacerbate SLE include exposure to sun, exposure to certain drugs (e.g., procainamide) and various types of infections. Clustering of families with discoid lupus and SLE, the occurrence of lupus-like syndromes with certain types of complement deficiencies, the association between SLE and specific HLA subtypes, and the characteristics of SLE-like illness in certain strains of mice support the notion that genetic factors play a part in the pathogenesis.

Current modalities of treatment are directed at controlling inflammation and reducing or modulating the number and function of lymphocytes. Future treatment methods may be capable of modulating and fine tuning specific steps in the immune system.

CLINICAL MANIFESTATIONS

The onset of SLE may be insidious or acute. The initial presentation may include generalized features such as fever, rash, arthritis, myalgia, and weight loss; or features of specific organ involvement such as pericarditis, pleuritis, proteinuria, hemolytic anemia and seizures. Joint involvement is usually symmetrical, involving large and small joints. Cutaneous lesions are present in 85% of patients with SLE. The typical erythematous rash with butterfly distribution over the face occurs in about half the patients at the time of diagnosis. Discoid lesions are less frequent, but when seen are characteristic of SLE (Fig. 56.6). Other types of cutaneous lesions seen in SLE include maculopapular rash, livedo reticu-

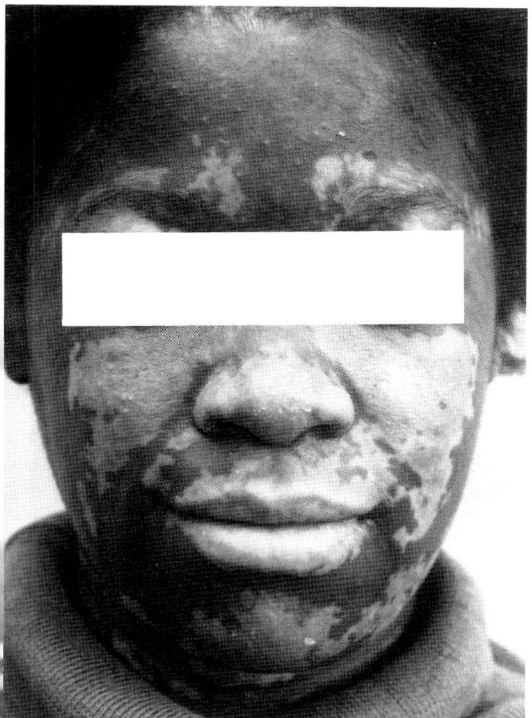

Figure 56.6 Adolescent female with discoid lesions in malar distribution.

laris, Raynaud's phenomena, urticaria, erythema multiforme, and alopecia. Vasculitic skin lesions are reported in about 20% of the patients over the extensor surface of the forearm and on the fingertips. These lesions are tender and may ulcerate. Nodules are less common. Mucosal lesions (macular and ulcerative) may involve the nose or the mouth, particularly the palate (Fig. 56.7).

Evidence of renal disease is present in over 50% of children with SLE at the time of initial diagnosis. If sophisticated investigations were used, probably every patient with lupus would show some abnormalities in the kidneys during the subsequent course. Usually renal disease is asymptomatic, though occasionally edema or hypertension may be clues to involvement of the kidney. Proteinuria, hematuria, and cylindruria are the usual evidences of renal disease.

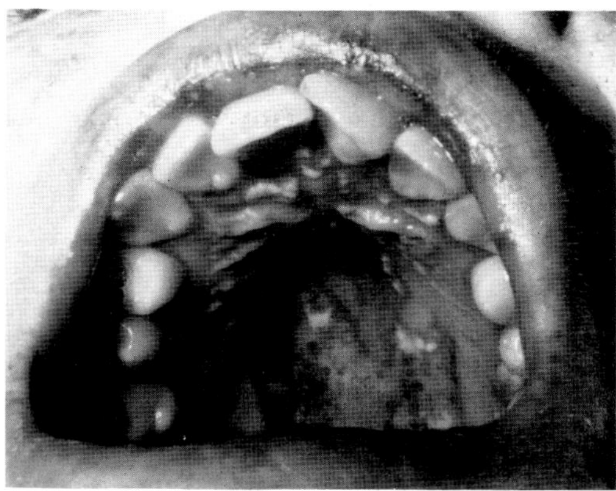

Figure 56.7 Mucosal lesions (macules and ulcers) of the palate in an adolescent girl with active lupus.

Clinical evidence of central nervous system involvement includes headache, seizures, chorea, polyneuropathy, hallucinations, memory alterations, psychosis and behavior disorder. This may occur at the onset or later in the course of the disease.

Pericarditis is the commonest form of cardiac involvement of SLE. Myocarditis is less frequent then pericarditis in SLE, but myocarditis in general is seen more often in SLE than in JRA. Heart murmurs due to valvular lesions are not common in SLE.

Patients with pleuropulmonary manifestations frequently complain of chest pain. Pleural rub is the commonest physical finding. Dullness on percussion of the chest and diminished breath sounds on auscultation indicate the presence of pleural effusion.

Common gastrointestinal (GI) manifestations include nausea, vomiting, and anorexia. Persistent localized abdominal pain should suggest specific organ involvement, such as pancreatitis and gastric ulcer—both of which may occur either due to the disease or secondary to steroid therapy. Malabsorption syndrome may be an occasional manifestation of SLE. Melena should suggest bleeding from the GI tract requiring immediate treatment. Abdominal pain in SLE is not always related to SLE but may be due to other causes such as appendicitis, ruptured ovarian cyst, or pelvic inflammatory disease.

Laboratory Abnormalities

Mild to moderate anemia is common in SLE. Hemolytic anemia associated with a positive Coombs' test is most characteristic. Leukopenia and thrombocytopenia are also commonly seen. The acute phase reactants are elevated in the serum; serum protein electrophoresis demonstrates elevation of α_2-globulin. Proteinuria, hematuria and cylinduria are the usual urinary abnormalities. Renal failure is suggested by elevated levels of BUN and creatinine and reduced creatinine clearance.

The best screening test for the serological diagnosis of SLE is ANA measured by immunofluorescent methods. The demonstration of antibodies to double-stranded DNA, particularly in high titers, is relatively specific for the diagnosis of SLE. Total serum hemolytic complement (CH50) and C3 are often decreased in patients with active disease. An elevated level of anti-DNA antibody with hypocomplementemia correlates particularly with active renal disease.

MANAGEMENT

General Management

There is no specific treatment for SLE. However, the inflammation in various tissues secondary to immune complexes and vasculitis can be controlled with various drugs. Patients with mild disease (fever and arthritis) without nephritis should receive salicylates (80 to 90 mg/kg/day) or one of the NSAID (tolmetin sodium 15 to 30 mg/kg/day). In patients with discoid lupus, hydroxychloroquine (7 mg/kg/day, maximum of 400 mg/day) has been found to be effective when used with caution. Severe systemic features may require treatment with steroids (prednisone 1 to 2 mg/kg/day) to be tapered quickly to the lowest possible dose. Patients with severe disease, particularly those with severe renal or CNS involvement, will require larger doses of steroids (prednisone 2 to 4 mg/kg/day) and one of the immunosuppressive agents (e.g. azathioprine 2 mg/kg/day or cyclophosphamide 2 mg/kg/day). Symptomatic management may be necessary for the treatment of seizures, psychosis, or oral ulcers. Close follow-up is mandatory to look for clinical and serological clues of exacerbations and to monitor drug toxicity. Since the disease often starts in the adolescent age group, total management should include emotional support for the children and their families.

Management of Complications and Emergencies

Fever. When a child known to be on treatment for documented SLE develops fever and an exacerbation of the basic disease, it is hard to decide whether the fever is due to an infection, to a flare of the disease, or to a combination of both. A complete physical examination should be performed, and a CBC and urinalysis obtained, though they may not be helpful. Children with an identifiable localized infection (e.g., otitis media) should have cultures taken from the affected site. Cultures of the blood, cerebrospinal fluid, and all secretions are indicated for children who are acutely ill and in those taking cytotoxic drugs, particularly if no source of fever is apparent.

Infections in SLE. Opportunistic infections account for a large percentage of deaths in SLE and are probably related to the therapy of these patients with steroids and immunosuppressive agents. *Listeria, Candida, Aspergillus, Cryptococcus, Pneumocystis* and the *varicella-zoster virus* are the unusual organisms associated with severe infections in SLE. In addition, septicemia due to gram-negative bacilli is also common.

In patients not on treatment with steroids and cytotoxic drugs, pathogens commonly seen in the immunocompetent host are the frequent offenders. Ordinary infections, such as those of the urinary tract may vary from mild to severe and may produce symptoms suggesting exacerbation of SLE as discussed in the previous section. All patients with SLE and infection need not be admitted. However, acutely ill children and those with pneumonia or meningitis require hospitalization for intravenous antibiotics while awaiting culture reports. Patients with minor infections who are not acutely ill may be treated with appropriate antibiotics given orally. The dose of steroids should be increased to provide at least 3 times the physiological need.

Renal Complications. Since renal disease is a major cause of death in SLE, it is important to establish its presence and severity at the time of diagnosis and periodically thereafter. Symptoms and signs are often minimal. In the presence of nephrotic syndrome, the child may be edematous. Gross hematuria or headache due to hypertension may be the presenting symptom. Laboratory evidence of renal disease includes proteinuria, hematuria, cylindruria, and elevated levels of BUN and creatinine. The presence of these findings in a patient with known SLE requires a more thorough investigation that should include estimation of the protein in a 24-hour urine collection, creatinine clearance, measurement of C3 and anti-DNA antibodies and renal biopsy. In a patient with SLE and documented renal disease, admission is necessary only in the presence of rapidly worsening renal status, acute renal failure, hypertensive crisis, or complications of therapy.

Treatment of renal disease is aimed at improving renal function. Generally, treatment of active disease with the usual doses of steroids (prednisone 1 to 2 mg/kg/day) should be adequate. In the presence of progressive renal failure, the patient should be admitted for aggressive therapy. This should include higher doses of oral steroids (prednisone 3 to 4 mg/kg/day) and an immunosuppressive agent. "Pulse" therapy with methylprednisolone (30 mg/kg in 50 ml of 5% dextrose in water given intravenously over 30 min) and/or plasmapheresis may be indicated in the presence of rapidly progressive renal disease.

Hematologic Complications. Anemia is common in SLE and may be due to many causes. The most common type is normocytic normochromic anemia of chronic disease. Anemia due to GI blood loss may be secondary to the vasculitic process or due to irritation of the GI tract by drugs. These patients often have symptoms of GI irritation and occult blood in the stool; they need further investigation, but the urgency for admission depends on the severity of the bleeding.

Hemolytic anemia in SLE can be related to the disease itself (antierythrocyte antibodies) or related to drugs. Patients with hemolytic anemia often present with pallor, fatigue, jaundice and dark colored urine. Occasionally these patients develop symptoms of cardiorespiratory distress following severe hemolysis and rapid fall in hemoglobin.

Laboratory investigation of anemia of SLE should include CBC, reticulocyte count and examination of the blood smear for red cell size and shape, nucleated red cells and fragmented red cells. Serum levels of iron, iron binding capacity, free erythrocyte protoporphyrin, and bilirubin should be checked. The antibody responsible for autoimmune hemolytic anemia is of the "warm variety," most commonly of the IgG type; IgM type antibody accounts for a small percentage. Since these antibodies, attached to the red cells, may not all be demonstrated by standard Coombs' test, more sensitive assay systems such as the antibody consumption test have to be used to detect antierythrocyte antibodies.

Mild to moderate anemia, whatever the mechanism, can be managed using oral iron preparations and by treatment of the primary disease. Children with a hematocrit of less than 20%, compromised cardiac functions, or complications of SLE need admission to the hospital. Corticosteroids are the most effective agents for the control of autoimmune hemolytic anemia of SLE. Prednisone at 2 mg/kg/day is the initial treatment of choice. Transfusion may be needed for children with a rapidly dropping hemoglobin concentration or congestive heart failure. Management of patients who fail to respond to steroids includes splenectomy and immunosuppressive agents but should not be a major concern for the emergency department physician.

Leukopenia occurs in about 50% of patients with SLE. This may be due to reduction in granulocytes, lymphocytes, or both. A reduction in granulocytes may be secondary to drugs used in the treatment or to peripheral destruction of granulocytes coated with IgG. Children with absolute granulocyte counts of less than 1000/cu mm should be admitted for further studies.

Thrombocytopenia occurs in approximately 25% of patients with SLE. The usual causes of thrombocytopenia are circulating antibodies to platelets and drug-induced bone marrow suppression. Infections should always be remembered as another cause. The presence of purpura and ecchymoses demands immediate investigation. Hemorrhage into one of the internal organs and platelet counts less than 50,000/cu mm are the usual indications for admission to the hospital. Studies should include CBC, examination of blood smear, bone marrow examination, appropriate cultures, and testing of serum for antiplatelet antibodies.

Life-threatening hemorrhage from the nose may be due to the combination of a vasculitic ulcer and thrombocytopenia. These patients may need local packing and HLA matched platelet replacement in addition to high dose steroids. Severe hemorrhage from the lungs may require general measures such as platelet transfusion and steroids, and local measures such as ventilatory assistance and bronchial lavage. Treatment of GI hemorrhage is described on p. 557.

Though very rare, disseminated intravascular coagulation can occur in SLE, with or without associated infection. Therefore, patients with thrombocytopenia and severe bleeding disorder should be investigated for this life-threatening complication.

Central Nervous System (CNS) Complications. Seizures and altered states of consciousness are the most common manifestations of CNS involvement in SLE. Both these symptoms may be due to many causes. Seizures may result from hypertension (due to the disease or complication of steroid therapy), infection (meningitis), or uremia. Coma may be due to meningitis or CNS hemorrhage secondary to thrombocytopenia. Therefore, patients with SLE who develop seizures or altered states of consciousness require admission for evaluation. This should include a thorough examination with special attention to blood pressure and neurologic findings and the following investigations: electrolytes, BUN, creatinine, urinalysis, lumbar puncture including measurement of opening pressure and cultures. Subsequently, both an EEG and a computerized tomography scan should be obtained.

Intravenous diazepam (0.2 to 0.3 mg/kg) is the drug of choice for the initial management of seizures followed by phenobarbital (see Chapter 336). If CNS manifestations are considered to be secondary to active vasculitis, steroid therapy should be initiated (prednisone 2 mg/kg/day). In the presence of deteriorating mental function, methylprednisolone (30 mg/kg in 50 ml of 5% dextrose in water given over 30 min) may be given (pulse therapy.)

Other manifestations of CNS involvement, such as psychosis, may also need inpatient evaluation, but not on an emergency basis. It may be difficult to determine whether the psychosis is secondary to steroid therapy or due to the disease itself. Psychotropic drugs (haloperidol 0.025 to 0.01 mg/kg/day in divided doses) may be used along with large doses of steroids (prednisone 3 to 4 mg/kg) for 1 to 2 weeks. If there is no improvement, steroid dose should be reduced gradually. During this process the patient may need pulse therapy or a cytotoxic drug to keep the disease under control.

Pulmonary Complications. Pleural effusion is the most common of the pulmonary manifestations in SLE. However, pulmonary infections and pulmonary hemorrhage contribute to more serious illness and death in these patients.

Pleural effusion is often bilateral and small. Occasionally it may be massive. The child is often ill with acute manifestations of systemic disease, such as fever, fatigue and poor appetite. Symptoms may be minimal (cough, chest pain) or absent. Chest pain aggravated by deep breathing or coughing is suggestive of pleurisy. On auscultation, pleural rub may be heard. An x-ray is essential to determine the extent of the effusion. If the diagnosis of the cause of pleural effusion is in doubt, pleural fluid should be aspirated. Usually, pleural fluid in SLE is an exudate that shows increased levels of protein and numbers of cells, glucose greater than 80 mg/dl, and low level of lactic dehydrogenase. If the child is known to the physicians and there are no concerns about infections, admission is not necessary. Increasing the dose of steroids, or adding indomethacin (0.5 to 2 mg/kg/day) or tolmetin sodium (15 to 30 mg/kg/day), may be adequate. However, arrangements must be made for close follow-up.

In the presence of moderate to massive effusion, the patient may have dyspnea and tachypnea. Chest pain is not an important complaint. The presence of fluid is easily demonstrated clinically (dullness on percussion and diminished breath sounds), and the roentgenogram of the chest establishes the extent of the effusion. Thoracentesis is often necessary (1) to relieve symptoms, (2) for diagnosis, and (3) to uncover any underlying lesions behind the effusion. Patients with large effusions should be admitted for further observation and management.

Pulmonary hemorrhage is increasingly recognized as a common cause of death in SLE, particularly in the pediatric age group. The cause of hemorrhage can be (1) related to the disease itself—vasculitis or thrombocytopenia; (2) related to the treatment—drug-induced thrombocytpoenia, or (3) related to an infection (e.g., aspergillosis). Differential diagnosis should include pulmonary hemosiderosis and Goodpasture's syndrome. Clinical features of patients with pulmonary hemorrhage include hemoptysis, tachypnea, tachycardia and dyspnea. Rapid deterioration may result in asphyxia and death within 24 to 48 hours. The roentgenogram of the chest shows infiltrates resembling pulmonary edema. There is a dramatic drop in hemoglobin, and the platelet count may often be low. A lung biopsy may be needed in some patients if the hemoptysis is not massive and there is a suspicion of pulmonary infection due to pneumocystitis or aspergillosis. Management should include transfusions and high doses of steroids (2 mg/kg/day) in the hospital. If the bleeding is due to thrombocytopenia, platelet transfusion is indicated. Intubation, tracheal lavage with epinephrine, O_2 therapy and positive end-expiratory pressure (PEEP) may be needed, depending on the severity and progression of the disease.

Occasionally acute lupus pneumonia may be the presenting manifestation of SLE. These patients are often ill with high fever, chest pain, cough, and dyspnea. On examination, rales may be heard throughout the chest. Roentgenograms show a diffuse alveolar exudate. Cultures of the blood and respiratory secretions, bronchial washing, a transtracheal aspirate or a lung biopsy may be necessary to exclude infections.

Supportive therapy should include increased concentrations of oxygen, adequate pulmonary toilet, and antipyretic drugs. High dose steroids (prednisone 2 mg/kg/day) often lead to dramatic improvement.

GI Complications. Peritonitis, an acute abdomen, and GI hemorrhage are the common emergencies associated with SLE. Drug-induced gastric ulcer and pancreatitis also occur. Peritonitis may be either part of the disease itself (serosal inflammation) or due to secondary infection or perforation of the intestines. Patients with SLE and peritonitis should be admitted at once. Symptoms and signs associated with peritonitis are pain in the abdomen, fever, vomiting, diarrhea, abdominal distention, diffuse tenderness, rigidity of the anterior abdominal wall, and hypoactive or absent bowel sounds on auscultation. A rotengenogram of the abdomen may show dilatation of intestinal loops with edema of the wall of the intestines, free air in the peritoneal cavity, or evidence of ileus or obstruction. Aspriation of the peritoneal fluid under strict aseptic conditions is essential. The fluid should be sent for Gram stain and culture. Cell counts over 250 or 300/cu mm should be considered indicative of infection. If peritonitis is of the serous type (a feature of SLE), the patient may be treated with one of the NSAID (e.g., indomethacin 0.5 to 2 mg/kg/day or tolmetin sodium 15 to 30 mg/kg/day). Steroids may be added if there is no response to NSAID or if there is evidence of active systemic disease. Peritonitis secondary to GI perforation should be treated aggressively with surgery and intravenous antibiotics.

An acute abdomen in SLE may be due to bowel ischemia, infarction, or perforation. Occasionally, an intussusception or pancreatitis may also cause this condition. Pancreatitis may be due to the vasculitis of SLE or, more often, complication of steroid therapy. Symptoms of an acute abdomen include sudden onset of abdominal pain, vomiting, and diarrhea which may be bloody. The patient may rapidly go into shock. There is often localized abdominal tenderness, guarding, and rigidity with absent bowel sounds. The patient should be kept hydrated and shock promptly treated in an intensive care setting. A CBC, serum electrolytes, and serum amylase determination should be obtained at once. Stool should be examined for frank or occult blood. A plain rotengenogram of the abdomen may show air-fluid levels or free air under the diaphragm. Paracentesis is essential to rule out infection or hemorrhage secondary to perforation. Gram stain and culture of peritoneal fluid, in addition to blood culture, should be obtained immediately. Infection should be treated aggressively, and the ischemic or perforated area of intestine corrected surgically.

If the serum amylase is normal and pancreatitis (see Chapter 50) is suspected, one should obtain an amylase clearance. An amylase/creatine clearance ratio of over 5 suggests pancreatitis. If pancreatitis is secondary to SLE, steroid therapy is used. If it is secondary to steroids, attempts should be made to withdraw steroids gradually while introducing steroid-sparing drugs, such as one of the NSAID or a cytotoxic drug. During this slow process, the patient may have to be maintained on parenteral hyperalimentation.

GI hemorrhage may be secondary to steroids (stomach), or due to vasculitis of the GI tract (small intestines), or due to thrombocytopenia. The symptoms are abdominal pain, hematemesis and melena if the bleeding is in the upper GI tract, and abdominal pain with melena or blood in the stool if it is from the lower GI tract. The patient may develop massive bleeding leading to shock.

Immediate studies to be obtained in the emergency department include a hematocrit, CBC, serum electrolytes, and type and crossmatch. If bleeding from a gastric ulcer is suspected, endoscopy can confirm the diagnosis. Therapy for a bleeding gastric ulcer includes volume replacement, hourly antacid administration, and cimetidine (20 to 40 mg/kg/day, maximum 1200 mg/day). If active bleeding due to vasculitis is suspected, a technetium scan may help to locate the site of hemorrhage. This is usually followed by celiac axis arteriography to precisely pinpoint the bleeding vessel. The radiologist may be able to inject Pitressin at the time of the angiogram into the bleeding vessel, though systemic Pitressin has also been shown to be effective (see Chapter 50 p. 561).

Often it is difficult to know the nature of an intra-abdominal catastrophe. If plain roentgenograms of the abdomen and peritoneal aspiration suggest infarction or perforation, surgical exploration is required to close the perforation or remove the affected portion of the intestine.

Cardiac Complications. Pericardial effusion and myocarditis are two of the important cardiac complications of SLE that may require emergencv care. The features of pericarditis are similar to those described in JRA and include chest pain, dyspnea, inability to lie flat in bed, and pericardial friction rub. In the presence of massive effusion, cardiac tamponade can occur. The features of cardiac tamponade are weak pulse. distended neck veins, distant heart sounds, and pulsus paradoxus of over 12 mm Hg (see p. 316). Pericarditis with mild to moderate effusion is treated with prednisone, 2 mg/kg/day. Massive effusion leading to tamponade requires pericardiocentesis in addition to treatment with steroids.

Myocarditis is characterized by resting tachycardia out of proportion to elevation of temperature, cardiomegaly without an effusion, congestive heart failure, ST-T wave changes in ECG, and arrhythmias. These patients should be on strict bed rest with monitoring. In addition to treatment of the basic disease (steroids and cytotoxic agents), digoxin and diuretic therapy is often indicated (see Chapter 43).

Raynaud's Phenomenon. Raynaud's phenomenon is characterized by sequential color changes of the extremities on exposure to cold. These color changes start with pallor, followed by cyanosis and then redness. Occasionally, these changes may be troublesome with pain in the extremities and ulceration and loss of tips of the fingers. Patients with gangrene or impending gangrene should be admitted. Minor episodes of Raynaud's phenomenon are treated with avoidance of exposure to cold. The value of vasodilator drugs (e.g., reserpine or tolazoline) is questionable. For severe episodes with impending gangrene, intra-arterial reserpine and sympathetic ganglion block may be tried. These procedures should be done in an intensive care setting.

Hypertension. Hypertension may be part of SLE or secondary to steroid therapy. Mild to moderate hypertension is usually controlled by combinations of diuretics, hydralazine, and propanolol (see p. 447). Diazoxide (5 mg/kg) given intravenously as rapidly as possible as a single bolus is the drug of choice for the treatment of hypertensive encephalopathy.

DERMATOMYOSITIS

DEFINITION AND INCIDENCE

Dermatomyositis (DM) is a relatively rare rheumatic disorder characterized by inflammation of the skin and striated muscle. The disease has a wide spectrum, from mild disease involving mainly the skin to a severe type with a rapid fulminating course. It runs through four different phases in the pediatric age group: (1) a prodromal phase with nonspecific aches and pains, (2) a phase of progressive muscle weakness, (3) a phase of persistent active disease, and (4) a phase of recovery with contractures and calcinosis. The predominance of generalized vasculitis, the occurrence of calcinosis, and the almost negligible correlation with malignancy in childhood DM make this entity different from adult-onset DM. Bohan and Peters's criteria for the diagnosis of DM/polymyositis (PM) are given in Table 56.4.

Table 56.4
Criteria for the Diagnosis of Dermatomyositis (DM)/Polymyositis (PM)[a]

1. Symmetrical weakness of the proximal limb muscles and of anterior neck flexors
2. Evidence of necrosis of Type I and II fibers on muscle biopsy
3. Elevation of serum levels of skeletal muscle enzymes—creatine phosphokinase and aldolase
4. Short, small, polyphasic motor unit potentials with fibrillation, insertional irritability and high frequency repetitive discharges on electromyography
5. Skin rash—characteristic heliotrope rash, scaly erythematous rash over extensor aspects of the joints and periungual erythema

Definite —	4 criteria (PM)
	3 or 4 criteria + rash (DM)
Probable—	3 criteria (PM)
	2 criteria + rash (DM)
Possible —	2 criteria (PM)
	1 criterion + rash (DM)

[a] From A. Bohan and J. B. Peter: *New England Journal of Medicine*, *292:* 344–347, 1975.

PATHOPHYSIOLOGY

Microscopically, the skin in DM shows dermal atrophy, obliteration of appendages, and lymphocytic infiltration. Characteristic lesions in the muscle include a mixture of degenerating and regenerating muscle fibers, variations in muscle fiber size, perivascular lymphocytic infiltration, and perifascicular atrophy of muscle fibers. Angiopathy involving small arteries, venules and capillaries of the skin, muscle, fat and gastrointestinal tract is considered to be characteristic of childood DM.

Viral infections, vasculitis due to immune complex deposition and cell-mediated cytotoxicity against muscle fibers have all been implicated in the pathogenesis of DM, but no primary mechanism has been established.

CLINICAL MANIFESTATIONS

The onset of DM is often insidious with aches and pains in the limbs, low grade fever, general weakness, and edema of the hands, feet, and eyelids. There may be a diffuse and nonspecific rash.

This prodromal stage is followed soon by the acute phase when the characteristic features of DM become evident. The classical triad in the skin includes: heliotrope rash (violaceous) in the periorbital region and occasionally on the forehead; dusky red, scaly lesions (Gottron's lesions) over the extensor aspects of the knees, elbows (Fig. 56.8) and the small joints of the hand; and periungual erythema. The muscular involvement is characterized by pain, tenderness and weakness of proximal muscles in a symmetrical fashion with involvement of the anterior neck flexors and sparing of the facial muscles. The disease may progress to involve the muscles of the palate and pharynx resulting in nasal regurgitation, nasal voice and aspiration. Involvement of the respiratory muscles may lead to a poor cough, pneumonia, and respiratory failure. GI hemorrhage is common at this stage and is associated with abdominal pain, hematemesis and melena.

During the third phase, the disease is often active with exacerbations and remissions, but it is not progressive. This stage may last for 2 to 5 years. The rash over the extremities often becomes dry, scaly, and atrophic (Fig. 56.9). Muscle wasting and weakness persist and contractures are common. Occasionally, children pass from stage 1 to stage 3 insidiously and come to the attention of the physician with contractures and calcinosis. Pronounced muscle wasting, calcinosis, contractures, and pigmentary changes of the skin characterize the recovery phase.

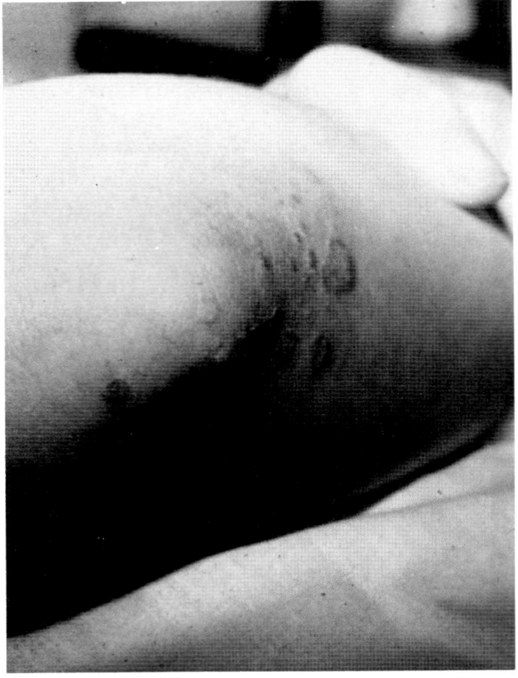

Figure 56.8 Gottron's lesions over the elbow.

MANAGEMENT

General Management:

During the acute phase of DM, it is essential to monitor the function of the palatopharyngeal and respiratory muscles. Frequent suctioning may be necessary to avoid aspiration. If palatal weakness is marked and there is a likelihood of aspiration, nasogastric feeding is indicated.

Treatment with prednisone will bring the myositis under control in most cases. The usual dose is 1 to 2 mg/kg/day in 2 or 3 divided doses. On this therapy, muscle enzymes return to normal levels in 2 to 4 weeks, and clinical improvement usually follows. Once the symptoms are controlled, the steroid dose should be gradually decreased to the lowest possible level. If a patient does not respond to prednisone (1 to 2 mg/kg/day) for over 8 to 12 weeks or if evidence of steroid toxicity develops, it may be necessary to add cytotoxic drugs such as cyclophosphamide (0.5 to 2 mg/kg/day). An alternative approach is to give methylprednisolone, 30 mg/kg over 30 to 45 min (pulse therapy) intravenously. Though plasmapheresis has been reported to be beneficial in some cases, this method of therapy remains experimental at this time. Finally, a comprehensive rehabilitation program is essential.

Management of Complications and Emergencies

The most serious emergencies in DM relate to two systems: pulmonary and GI. In addition, complications occur due to therapy with steroids (e.g., infections and GI hemorrhage).

Pulmonary Complications. Pulmonary emergencies seen in childhood DM include: (1) aspiration secondary to weakness of palatal muscles; (2) progressive weakness of respiratory muscles resulting

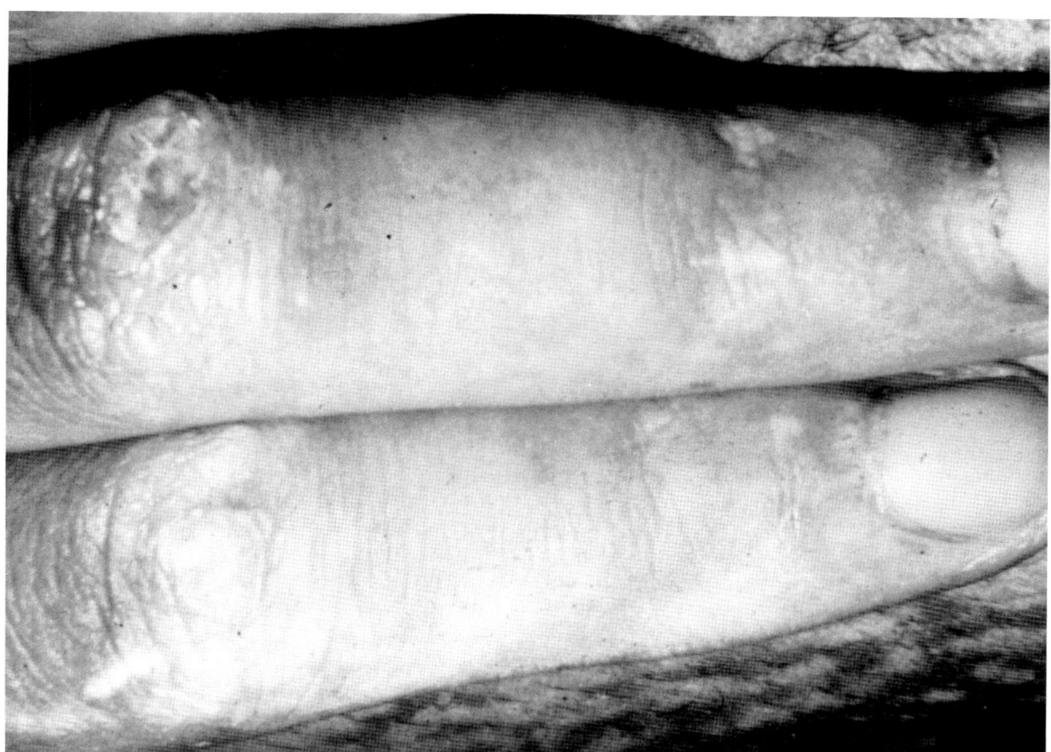

Figure 56.9 Dry, atrophic, depigmented lesions over the extensor aspects of small joints of the fingers.

in difficulty in clearing secretions, atelectasis, and pneumonia; (3) progressive weakness of respiratory muscles resulting in respiratory failure; (4) progressive interstitial disease of the lung; and (5) unusual infections (tuberculosis, *Pneumocystis*) in the immunocompromised host.

The history should provide clues to some of the above listed possibilities. On physical examination, the child with a pulmonary complication is often acutely ill with an elevated temperature. Since fever can also occur with active DM, it is necessary to differentiate fever due to infection from fever due to underlying disease. The patient with respiratory complications is often dyspneic and tachypneic and has a weak cough with no production of sputum. Pooling of secretions in the mouth should suggest the presence of palatal weakness. Each breath is shallow with poor air entry on auscultation. The child cannot complete a sentence in one breath and often pauses between words. On auscultation, rales are heard over various areas of the chest. Cyanosis and clouding of consciousness suggest the onset of respiratory failure.

Children with DM who develop respiratory problems are usually admitted for observation and diagnosis. Those with impending respiratory failure should be cared for in an intensive care unit.

Preliminary investigations should include a complete blood count, urinalysis, serum electrolytes, muscle enzymes and a chest x-ray. Depending on the seriousness of the symptoms and the cooperation from the child, blood gas analysis and pulmonary function studies may be obtained. Pulmonary function studies usually show restrictive disease and a diffusion abnormality. Steroid therapy (prednisone 2 mg/kg/day in 4 divided doses) is the treatment of choice. If the weakness seems to be worsening, an alternative worth considering is the use of methylprednisolone intravenously at 30 mg/kg in a single bolus dose in 50 ml of 5% dextrose in water over 30 to 45 min. During this pulse therapy, blood pressure should be monitored and the infusion stopped if it shows a sudden increase or decrease. Frequent suctioning and nasogastric feeding may be necessary to avoid aspiration pneumonia. If pulmonary problems result from infection, treatment with intravenous antibiotics should be initiated. In addition, sufficient steroids (3 times physiological) are given to protect against adrenal insufficiency. Plasmapheresis is reserved for children who deteriorate even after pulse steroid therapy.

Pneumothorax is another complication known to occur during the course of childhood DM. The usual symptoms are sudden onset of chest pain and tachypnea. Physical examination should indicate the involved side as demonstrated by deviation of the trachea to the opposite side and increased resonance and diminished breath sounds on the affected side of the chest. A roentgenogram of the chest shows air in the pleural cavity. Depending on the extent of the pneumothorax, needle aspiration should be performed or a chest tube inserted.

GI Complications. Vasculitic changes characterized by intimal hyperplasia and occlusion by fibrin thrombi of the arteries and veins of the entire GI tract have been reported to be important pathological features of childhood DM. Resultant ulcerations and perforations can occur anywhere from the esophagus to the large intestine. Symptoms and signs of these complications depend on the site of the major lesion. Bleeding from the esophagus is not common; mediastinitis may be seen occasionally. Massive hemorrhage from the stomach, perforation of the intestine with peritonitis, or slow bleeding from the small intestine are also reported. Occasionally pneumatosis intestinalis and pneumoperitoneum can occur. Steroid therapy may also be a contributory cause of GI bleeding in some cases.

Symptoms of bleeding from ulceration of the upper GI tract are abdominal pain with vomiting and melena. If the bleeding is severe, hematemesis with a sudden drop in the hemoglobin will be the presenting manifestation. Laboratory studies to be obtained include a CBC, electrolytes and BUN. Treatment includes support of circulatory volume, hourly antacids, and cimetidine (20 to 40 mg/kg/day, maximum 1200 mg).

Symptoms of bleeding from the lower portion of the GI tract include abdominal pain, vomiting, a distended abdomen and melena or bright red blood in the stool. In the presence of perforation, abdominal tenderness, guarding of the abdominal wall, and distant or absent bowel sounds are usually found; however, large doses of steroids may mask these signs. The hematocrit can fall precipitously, and roentgenograms of the abdomen may show free air in the peritoneum. If there is active bleeding, a technetium scan to locate the area of hemorrhage is the initial step. This may be followed by an angiogram to localize the actual vessel which is bleeding. The details of the management of hemorrhage from the GI tract are discussed under SLE (p. 747) and in Chapter 50.

Pneumatosis Intestinalis. In a patient with DM, intestinal perforation may go unnoticed and present with pneumatosis intestinalis. This finding may also precede perforation and pneumoperitoneum. Thus, any patient with DM and persistent abdominal pain should be examined radiologically for the presence of pneumatosis intestinalis. Supine and erect abdominal roentgenograms are indicated to demonstrate intramural gas. Patients with this diagnosis require admission and surgical consultation.

Calcinosis. During the period of formation of subcutaneous calcification, children with DM may develop high fever, chills and one or more areas of swelling under the skin. This swelling may resemble an area of cellulitis or abscess formation with warmth, redness and tenderness. After 2 to 7 days, the lesion may break open and extrude calcium at which time the fever subsides. Though this is the natural history of subcutaneous calcification, it is often hard to exclude infectious etiology for the swelling in the early stages before calcium starts to leak out. If doubt exists, needle aspiration of the site may be performed and the fluid examined for calcium crystals and organisms. In the face of uncertainty, it is best to treat for infection with antibiotics until culture reports are available.

Cardiac Emergencies. One of the less common complications of childhood DM is myocarditis. Tachycardia out of proportion to fever may be the earliest evidence of this complication. Involvement of the conduction system by edema and fibrosis leads to electrical abnormalities and arrhythmias. All patients with myocarditis should be admitted for an evaluation that includes an ECG, chest x-ray, and echocardiogram. Supportive management includes judicious and careful use of diuretics and cardiotonic drugs while treatment of the primary disease with steroids is continued.

SCLERODERMA

BACKGROUND

Systemic sclerosis (SS) is a relatively rare disorder occurring in 2 to 12 adults per million per year. It is even less common in children. Morphea and linear scleroderma are more likely to be seen than SS in this age group. Various conditions included under the term "scleroderma" are given in Table 56.5.

PATHOPHYSIOLOGY

The most characteristic microscopic feature of affected areas of the skin is increased thickness and density of collagen in the dermis. In addition, flattening of rete pegs, mononuclear cell infiltrate around small blood vessels and skin appendages, obliteration of skin appendages and hyalinization and fibrosis of arterioles are seen.

The etiology of this disease is unknown, but various theories have been proposed to account for the genetic and environmental factors associated with it. Recently, a unifying theory incriminating a factor toxic to endothelial cells has been proposed. Similarities between this disorder and graft vs. host disease following bone marrow transplantation have opened up many immunological avenues of approach.

Table 56.5
Classifiication of Scleroderma[a]

I. Systemic Sclerosis
- A. Classic disease with bilateral symmetrical diffuse involvement of the skin (scleroderma) affecting face, trunk and proximal as well as distal portions of the extremities; associated with tendency toward relatively early appearance of visceral involvement
- B. With relatively limited involvement of skin, often confined to fingers and face, and tendency to long delayed appearance of visceral involvement (CRST syndrome)
- C. "Overlap" syndromes, including sclerodermatomyositis and mixed connective tissue disease

II. Localized (Focal) Forms of Scleroderma
- A. Morphea (plaque-like, guttate, or generalized; subcutaneous and keloid morphea)
- B. Linear scleroderma
- C. Scleroderma *en coup de sabre*, with or without facial hemiatrophy

III. Chemical-Induced Scleroderma-like Conditions
- A. Vinyl chloride disease
- B. Pentazocine-induced fibrosis
- C. Bleomycin-induced fibrosis

IV. Eosinophilic Fasciitis

V. Pseudoscleroderma
- A. Edematous (scleredema, scleromyxedema)
- B. Indurative (amyloid disease, porphyria cutanea tarda, carcinoid syndrome, phenylketonuria, acromegaly)
- C. Atrophic (progeria, Werner's syndrome, lichen sclerosis et atrophicus)

[a] From *Bulletin of the Rheumatic Diseases, 31:* 1–6, 1981.

CLINICAL FEATURES

Localized scleroderma is more common in children than in adults. The lesions may be one of three types. Morphea is a focal ivory white-patch with a violaceous or erythematous rim; it is often a single lesion on the trunk though generalized morphea also occurs in children. The linear form of scleroderma causes scarring, fibrosis and atrophy (not corresponding to dermatomes) of involved skin with firm binding of the subcutaneous tissues to deeper structures ("hide-bound") and may extend to involve an entire extremity (Fig. 56.10). Linear scleroderma may also affect underlying muscle and bone. This may result in flexion contractures, leg length discrepancies and hemiatrophy of an extremity. A variant of linear scleroderma affecting the forehead is called "en coup de sabre."

SS often presents with cutaneous changes such as tightening of the skin, increased pigmentation, induration, edema and Raynaud's phenomenon. Some of these children may also develop arthritis resembling JRA, muscle weakness resembling DM, and nodules along tendon sheaths. If these features are seen, one should consider the possibility of mixed connective tissue disease (MCTD) in which features of SLE, progressive systemic sclerosis (PSS), DM and JRA overlap.

Serious illness and death can occur in SS. In adults, the major complication is severe uncontrolled hypertension and rapidly progressive renal failure (scleroderma renal crisis). In children this is relatively rare. Other common causes of death in SS are: (1) primary myocardial disease with conduction disturbances, pericarditis and intractable congestive heart failure; (2) pulmonary hypertension secondary to involvement of the pulmonary arteries by the sclerodermatous process; and (3) renal failure with malignant hypertension.

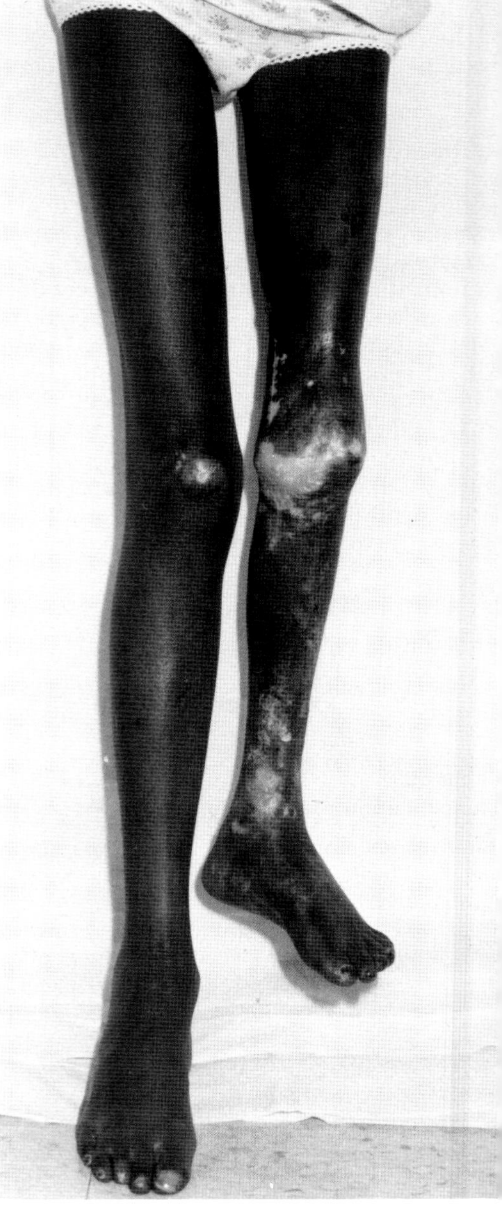

Figure 56.10 Linear scleroderma involving left lower extremity in a 12-year-old girl.

Additional complications of SS are: (1) Raynaud's phenomenon; (2) digital gangrene; (3) nonhealing ulcers most frequently involving the fingers, elbows and malleoli; (4) disordered motility of the distal esophagus with dysphagia and reflux esophagitis; (5) malabsorption syndrome; (6) thrombocytopenia with subsequent cerebral hemorrhage; (7) interstitial lung disease; and (8) cranial nerve involvement with trigeminal sensory neuropathy, facial weakness, and tinnitus.

MANAGEMENT

General Management

Specific therapy for SS is nonexistent at present. However, recent evidence indicates that D-penicillamine may be useful in arresting the progress of the disease if used early in the course. In the presence of prefibrotic stages of interstitial lung disease and pulmonary vascular involvement, steroids (prednisone 2 mg/kg/day) are indicated. If the esophageal sphincter is involved, patients should be advised to sleep with the head comfortably elevated and an antacid may be prescribed. Minor episodes of Raynaud's syndrome are managed with prophylactic measures such as the avoidance of cold exposure and the use of warm clothing. Aggressive physical therapy is indicated to prevent contractures and maintain normal function. Linear scleroderma with involvement of deep structures may lead to contractures of the extremities requiring surgery.

Management of Complications and Emergencies

Cardiac Complications. Tachycardia, arrhythmias, cardiac hypertrophy, congestive heart failure, and angina pectoris are manifestations of myocardial disease; sudden death has also been reported. Even in the absence of symptoms or physical findings, cardiac involvement has been documented in adults with SS using echocardiographic studies. Management of cardiac dysfunction is symptomatic and supportive. There are no specific drugs to arrest the progress of cardiac involvement.

Pulmonary Complications. Pulmonary involvement in SS may be one of three major types: pleurisy, interstitial fibrosis, and primary involvement of the pulmonary vasculature with resulting hypertension. Diffuse interstitial lung disease is often asymptomatic. A dry cough may be the earliest symptom. With progression of the disease, cough and dyspnea become prominent. On examination, rales over both sides of the chest, particularly over the infrascapular area, may be the only finding. With the onset of right-sided heart failure, these patients may have increasing dyspnea, edema of the lower extremities, and evidence of pulmonary hypertension. Early in the course of the disease, even before symptoms appear, these patients show a restrictive pattern on pulmonary function tests and diffusion abnormalities. Roentgenograms of the chest show increased reticulation or "honeycombed" appearance, mainly basal and bilateral. Patients in right-sided heart failure need admission and symptomatic management.

Patients with irreversible pulmonary fibrosis and chronic respiratory failure may also need admission. If patients with well-established pulmonary fibrosis and respiratory failure have upper respiratory infections, they should be treated promptly. Low concentration of oxygen, bronchodilators, and steroids may be helpful. After further investigations, such as roentgenograms, pulmonary function tests, flow scan, diffusion studies and biopsy, these patients should receive steroids (prednisone 2 mg/kg/day) for 6 to 8 weeks, though the value of this therapy is doubtful in established fibrosis. In addition, treatment of right-sided failure is indicated.

Pulmonary hypertension often presents with acute onset of breathlessness. On physical examination these patients are acutely ill with dyspnea. On auscultation, the pulmonic component of the second heart sound is accentuated, and there is a wide or fixed split of the second heart sound. The electrocardiogram shows right ventricular hypertrophy. Echocardiography, right heart catheterization, and lung biopsy are often indicated. Steroid therapy (prednisone 2 mg/kg/day) is the treatment of choice in addition to supportive measures.

Renal Complications. Sclerodermatous involvement of the vessels of the kidney resulting in renal failure is the most common cause of death in SS. Proteinuria and hypertension are early indicators of the patient at risk for renal scleroderma. The development of a microangiopathic hemolytic anemia suggests imminent renal failure. Fortunately, these complications are less common in children then in adults.

Renal failure may set in gradually or acutely in a patient with known renal disease. The syndrome of rapidly developing renal failure with malignant hypertension (scleroderma renal crisis) requires hospitalization and urgent management. Immediate investigation should include urinalysis, measurement of urine volume and urinary electrolytes, serum electrolytes, BUN, creatinine, and plasma renin level. Propanolol is the drug of choice for the treatment of hypertension in this situation, but multiple drug regimens may be necessary (see Chapter 46). Renal dialysis is often life saving for children with hypertension unresponsive to pharmacologic therapy. Maintenance of blood volume is an essential part of management of these patients.

Vascular Complications. Raynaud's phenomenon can be often incapacitating, particularly in cold weather. Symptoms include severe pain in the extremities and loss of sensation in the tips of the fingers. The latter may indicate the onset of gangrene. Patients with gangrene or impending gangrene should be admitted and treated with drugs that block the renin-angiotensin system.

In severe cases, intra-arterial reserpine and sympathetic ganglion block may be tried. Both of these forms of therapy are not of proven value and are associated with complications. Therefore, these procedures should be done only in an intensive care setting. If gangrene has set in, it is best left alone if there is no infection. Spontaneous separation of the tips of the fingers will occur and carries less risk and morbidity than surgical amputation.

GI Complications. Abnormal esophageal mobility with reflux may result in esophagitis. The major symptom of this condition is retrosternal pain which is made worse by certain foods and recumbent position. The pain may be severe and incapacitating. Although children with the complaint of retrosternal pain do not require admission to the hospital, they need an evaluation of their lower esophageal sphincter with esophageal manometry. Those with mild pain and objective evidence of reflux (lower esophageal sphincter pressure of less than 10 mm Hg) are usually treated with simple measures such as antacids 1 hour after meals and 1 hour before bed time and elevation of the head during sleep. If the symptoms are severe, one may need to prescribe cimetidine (20 to 40 mg/kg/day, maximum daily dosage 1200 mg).

POLYARTERITIS NODOSA

BACKGROUND

Polyarteritis is a rare collagen disorder and is often labeled periarteritis nodosa or polyarteritis nodosa (PAN). It primarily involves small and medium sized arteries and falls under the spectrum of necrotizing vasculitis (Table 56.6). It is important to understand that other vasculitities show many clinical and histopathological features of PAN and should be carefully excluded in the differential diagnosis. Major subgroups of PAN in the pediatric age group are infantile polyarteritis, classical polyarteritis nodosa, cutaneous polyarteritis and mucocutaneous lymph node syndrome.

An annual incidence of 0.3 per 100,000 and a prevalence of 0.7 per 100,000 population have been recorded for adults. No such data are available for children. There are two age clusters in the pediatric age group; infants less than 10 months old (in-

Table 56.6
Necrotizing Vasculitis[a]

I. *Small Vessel Vasculitis*
   A. Henoch-Schönlein purpura
   B. Allergic vasculitis
   C. Hypocomplementemic vasculitis
   D. Vasculitis with mixed cryoglobulinemia
II. *Allergic Granulomatous Angiitis*
   A. Churg-Strauss syndrome
   B. Wegener's granulomatosis
III. *Polyarteritis Nodosa*
   A. Classic polyarteritis nodosa
   B. Cutaneous polyarteritis
   C. Infantile polyarteritis nodosa
   D. Mucocutaneous lymph node syndrome
IV. *Giant Cell Arteritis*
   A. Temporal arteritis
   B. Takayasu's arteritis
V. *Vasculitis Associated with Rheumatic Diseases*

[a] From V. Hanson: In *Textbook of Rheumatology*, p. 1342, edited by W. N. Kelly, E. D. Harris, Jr., S. Ruddy, and C. B. Sledge, W. B. Saunders, Philadelphia, 1981.

fantile polyarteritis), and children between 8 and 16 years of age (polyarteritis of childhood). Males predominate in the infantile group. In the childhood variety, males and females are equally affected. In adults, men are more frequently affected than women (3:1).

PATHOPHYSIOLOGY

Characteristically, there are focal and panmural necrotizing inflammatory lesions in small and medium sized muscular arteries, with an increased frequency of involvement at sites of bifurcation. The inflammatory process consists of fibrinoid necrosis and a pleomorphic cellular infiltration with a predominance of polymorphonuclear leukocytes. Thrombosis or aneurysmal dilatation may occur at the primary site.

Hepatitis B antigen, antibody to hepatitis B antigen, and immune complexes containing hepatitis B antigen have been demonstrated in a certain population of patients with PAN. In childhood PAN, a history of antecedent infections with β-hemolytic streptococci has been noted. Such findings suggest that immunological mechanisms are directly or indirectly involved in the pathogenesis of certain types of necrotizing vasculitis.

Soluble antigen-antibody complexes are formed under conditions of antigen excess. These complexes circulate if not cleared by the reticuloendothelial system and deposit on vessel walls. Trapping of immune complexes in the vessel wall activates the complement cascade resulting in release of chemotactic factors. Polymorphonuclear leukocytes attracted by these factors accumulate on vessel walls at the site of immune complex deposition. Lysosomal enzymes released from the polymorphonuclear leukocytes during the process of phagocytosis include collagenase and elastase which damage the vessel walls.

In certain types of vasculidities, cell-mediated immunity seems to play a major part. Sensitized lymphocytes release soluble factors, such as macrophage inhibition factor, which facilitates accumulation of monocytes at sites where antigens are deposited. These cells in turn become macrophages and release lysosomal enzymes causing tissue injury, or transform to epitheliod cells causing granuloma formation.

CLINICAL MANIFESTATIONS

Polyarteritis has a wide spectrum of clinical presentation from mild to rapidly fatal forms. Clinical manifestations in infants (infantile polyarteritis) include prolonged fever following an upper respiratory infection, conjunctivitis, a maculopapular erythematous rash, abdominal discomfort with diarrhea, and aseptic meningitis syndrome. Coronary artery involvement occurs in most infants (80 to 90%). The clinical course is brief, usually approximately 1 month, and the diagnosis is often made on post mortem examination.

Childhood polyarteritis has a more variable clinical course. Common symptoms include fever, generalized weakness, anorexia, arthralgia, arthritis, myalgia, a maculopapular erythematous rash, abdominal pain, vomiting, hematuria, hypertension, and tachycardia. Cutaneous lesions include urticaria, angioneurotic edema, maculopapular eruptions, necrotizing lesions, ischemic changes of the tips of fingers and toes, and ulcerations. Nodules, ulcers, and livedo reticularis are characteristic of the cutaneous form of PAN. With central nervous system involvement, seizures and hemiparesis may occur. Mononeuritis multiplex is a specific form of neuropathy which is often associated with PAN. Proteinuria and an abnormal urinary sediment is seen in 70 to 80% of children with renal disease due to PAN. Impaired renal function and progressive renal insufficiency have been seen with childhood polyarteritis and may be the major cause of morbidity; however, acute renal insufficiency is distinctly unusual. Hypertension, which is a common feature of childhood polyarteritis, may or may not be related to renal involvement. Cardiac disease in childhood polyarteritis is different from that of the infantile variety. Pericarditis, cardiomegaly, and electrocardiographic abnormalities (T-wave changes and left ventricular hypertrophy) are more common than congestive heart failure or myocardial infarction. Pulmonary involvement is rare and usually consists of diffuse pulmonary infiltrates. Occasionally, pulmonary hemorrhage or hemothorax may be the presenting manifestations of PAN due to rupture of aneurysms. Retinal hemorrhages, exudates, and interstitial keratitis are the usual ocular findings in this disease.

Laboratory Studies

Laboratory findings in polyarteritis are nonspecific. Mild to moderate anemia, elevation of the sedimentation rate, leukocytosis up to 40,000/cu mm, elevated α_2-globulin, and diffuse hypergammaglobulinemia are commonly seen. Peripheral eosinophilia has been documented in about 30% of patients. The urinalysis is usually abnormal, proteinuria and hematuria being the most common findings. The complement is usually normal or increased; ANA and RF may be present at low titers.

The diagnosis of PAN is established by demonstrating acute necrotizing inflammation of small and medium sized arteries in the skin or in the muscle. In the absence of available tissue for biopsy, arteriographic demonstration of microaneurysms in the hepatic, renal or the mesenteric arteries is essential to make the diagnosis.

MANAGEMENT

General Management

The initial management of PAN should include steroids (prednisone 2 mg/kg/day in 4 divided doses). A single dose of methylprednisolone, 30 mg/kg in 50 ml of 5% dextrose in water given intravenously over a period of 30 to 45 min (pulse therapy), is a reasonable alternative for the treatment of acute exacerbations, provided the patient does not have elevated blood pressure. In children with moderate to severe generalized activity of the disease, and in those with renal disease, cyclophosphamide (2 to 2.5 mg/kg/day) should be added to the steroid therapy. Supportive therapy includes the use of NSAID (e.g. tolmetin sodium) for fever and arthritis, anticonvulsants, antihypertensives and physical therapy when appropriate.

Management of Complications and Emergencies

The most serious emergencies in childhood polyarteritis are: (1) renal insufficiency with or without acute oliguric renal failure; (2) severe hypertension; (3) cardiac complications such as congestive heart failure, myocardial infarction, and arrhythmias; (4) complications due to involvement of mesenteric vessels of the GI tract (e.g. bleeding, perforation, intussusception, cholecytitis and infarction of the bowel); and (5) central nervous system manifestations.

Renal Emergencies. It is generally agreed that renal disease is the commonest cause of death in patients with PAN. Renal involvement associated with azotemia and hypertension at the time of diagnosis carries a grave prognosis. Arteritis of medium-sized vessels of the kidney and glomerulitis have been described during the course of this disease. Renal arteritis may lead to renal infarction and ischemia or to aneurysm with rupture. Renal infarction with ischemia causes hematuria, hypertension and azotemia. Sudden flank pain associated with gross hematuria should suggest rupture of an aneurysm or a large renal infarction. Severe flank pain followed quickly by gross hematuria, falling blood pressure and hematocrit, and a palpable abdominal mass points to a perirenal or retroperitoneal hemorrhage from a renal artery.

Glomerulitis is accompanied by proteinuria and microscopic hematuria. Azotemia is usually seen late in the course of the disease. Acute renal failure occurs less commonly.

Frequent serial urinalyses, quantitation of total protein in the urine, and measurement of BUN, serum creatinine and creatinine clearance are essential parts of the workup of all patients with PAN. Renal arteriography may help establish the diagnosis in some cases. Renal biopsy may lead to severe complications and is not recommended as a routine procedure.

Management of renal failure is described on p. 450. Rupture of an aneurysm of a renal artery is initially managed with treatment of shock and replacement of volume. Surgical repair of the aneurysm should be undertaken immediately.

Medical treatment for renal disease in PAN includes steroids and immunosuppressive therapy as described earlier in the section on general medical treatment.

Hypertension. A mild to moderate elevation of the blood pressure is a common feature of PAN and is seen in almost all patients. Diuretics, hydralazine, and propranolol are the drugs of choice for the management of hypertension. However, severe hypertension associated with encephalopathy and congestive heart failure will require immediate admission and management (p. 447).

Cardiac Emergencies. Involvement of the coronary vessels by the inflammatory process leads to cardiac manifestations of PAN. Tachycardia, shortness of breath, and weight gain as a reflection of peripheral fluid accumulation may be early signs of cardiac involvement. Chest pain is rare but, when it occurs, should suggest myocardial ischemia. In addition, hypertension which may be primary (due to the disease) or secondary to renal involvement may contribute to strain on the left heart and lead to congestive heart failure. Rarely, one of the coronary aneurysms may rupture resulting in hemopericardium and cardiac tamponade.

Patients with cardiac involvement need not necessarily be admitted. However, those with congestive heart failure, myocardial ischemia, and hemopericardium will require urgent management in the emergency department before transfer to an intensive care setting.

A roentgenogram of the chest, ECG, and M-mode echocardiogram should be obtained immediately. Thallium scan of the heart and coronary angiography may be indicated in certain patients. Supportive medical management includes careful monitoring of cardiorespiratory status, judicious use of intravenous fluids, diuretics, and, when indicated, cardiotonics. Pericardiocentesis may be needed. Treatment of the primary disease with steroids and cytotoxic agents should be continued as described earlier. If hypertension does not respond to diuretic therapy, other antihypertensive agents may have to be added. Serum electrolytes should be monitored since most of these patients will be taking high doses of steroids, diuretics and antihypertensive agents.

GI Complications of Polyarteritis. Abdominal pain is the most common manifestation of GI involvement in PAN. This may be diffuse and nonspecific, or localized and severe. Hematemesis and melena suggest ulceration and hemorrhage. Patients with persistent abdominal pain, hematemesis and melena require immediate admission.

Visceral perforation should be suspected in cases of active systemic disease and unrelenting abdominal pain. Tenderness on palpation of the abdomen, guarding of abdominal wall, and absent bowel sounds are the usual physical findings. Arteritis of specific organs may lead to cholecystitis, appendicitis, and hepatitis. These complications are manifested by localized abdominal pain and tenderness and vomiting. Mesenteric thrombosis with infarction of the bowel may manifest with sudden abdominal pain, vomiting, hematemesis, or hematochezia with shock. Exquisite tenderness of the abdomen and absent bowel sounds are the major physical findings.

Hemorrhage from a ruptured aneurysm (mesenteric, hepatic or renal) with hemoperitoneum is heralded by sudden onset of severe pain, vomiting, tachycardia and shock. The abdomen is tender and tense and bowel sounds are absent.

Initial management includes: (a) volume replacement, (b) decompression of the stomach, and (c) steroid therapy to provide at least 3 times the physiological need, particularly if the patient has been on alternate day steroids or has been recently tapered off steroids. All of these patients will require measurement of intake and output and the following studies: hematocrit, BUN, electrolytes, and plain x-ray of the abdomen. Peritoneal aspiration, abdominal ultrasound, a technetium scan, and angiography of the celiac axis vessels may be indicated in some cases. Surgical consultation should be obtained in the emergency department. In the presence of bleeding aneurysms or infarcted bowel, surgical exploration is manditory.

CNS Complications. Clinical signs of CNS disease are much less frequent than those of peripheral nervous system involvement. Seizures and hemiparesis are the most common manifestations of CNS involvement in PAN and require immediate admission and management. A complete neurological evaluation should be done including measurement of the blood pressure (since hypertensive encephalopathy may be present with seizures) and examination of the fundus to look for evidence of hypertension and intracranial bleeding. Computerized axial tomography and/or carotid angiography may be indicated.

Management of hypertensive encephalopathy (p. 447) and increased intracranial pressure (p. 1012) have been described elsewhere. Surgical correction of a ruptured aneurysm should be undertaken if the bleeding vessel can be localized and is accessible.

KAWASAKI DISEASE
(Mucocutaneous Lymph Node Syndrome

BACKGROUND

Kawasaki disease (mucocutaneous lymph node syndrome or MCLNS) is a recently recognized syndrome resembling infantile PAN. This syndrome, first described in 1967, is characterized by fever, rash, conjunctivitis, mucous membrane lesions and lymphadenopathy. The important aspects of this disease are the following: (a) similarity of clinical features of MCLNS to those of infantile polyarteritis, streptococcosis, rickettsial infections and heavy metal poisoning; (b) similarity of pathological features of MCLNS to those of infantile polyarteritis; (c) 10 to 20% incidence of cardiac disease; and (d) 1 to 2% mortality due to coronary artery disease.

The disease affects children of all races, but there is a preponderance of children of Asian (Japanese) origin (19:1). There is also a possible association between an HLA antigen (HLA BW22 J2) which is common in the Japanese population and MCLNS. Recently an association between HLA-B4 and MCLNS also has been described.

The etiology of this illness is unknown. Most of the clinical features (fever, arthritis, rash, mucocutaneous lesions) and epidemiological characteristics support an infectious etiology. However, no viral or bacterial agent has thus far been isolated. Since the disease has been recognized only recently, and since some of the features (oral lesions, skin lesions, peeling of skin) resemble acrodynia, an environmental toxin has been considered as the possible etiological agent. Indeed, in one study, the urinary mercury level was found to be high in children with MCLNS. The association with certain HLA antigens and the higher incidence of the disease in the Japanese population suggests a genetic factor as partial explanation. Finally, immune complexes have been considered responsible for this disease, but support for this hypothesis is lacking.

PATHOPHYSIOLOGY

The most important pathological changes are found in the heart, particularly in the coronary arteries. The cardiac lesions have been categorized by Fujiwara and Hamashima into four stages depending upon the duration of illness at the time of death (Table 56.7). Most of the deaths occur be-

Table 56.7
Pathology of Kawasaki Syndrome (Adapted from Fujiwara)[a]

State I—Disease duration < 10 days
- Acute perivasculitis of coronary arteries
- Microvascular angiitis of coronary arteries and aorta
- Pancarditis with pericardial, myocardial, endocardial inflammation
- Inflammation of the AV conduction system

Stage II—Disease duration 12–28 days
- Acute panvasculitis of coronary arteries
- Coronary artery aneurysms present
- Coronary obstruction and thrombosis
- Myocardial and endocardial inflammation less intense

Stage III—Disease duration 28–45 days
- Subacute inflammation in coronary arteries
- Coronary artery aneurysms present
- Myocardial, endocardial inflammation much decreased

Stage IV—Disease duration >50 days
- Scar formation, calcification in coronary arteries
- Stenosis and recanalization coronary vessel lumen
- Myocardial fibrosis without acute inflammation

[a] From M. E. Melish: *Pediatrics in Review, 2:* 111 1980.

tween day 11 and day 50, corresponding to the peak of inflammatory changes in the myocardium and coronary arteries. These inflammatory changes lead to myocardial ischemia, arrhythmias, congestive heart failure and death.

In addition, small and medium sized arteries in the kidneys, spleen and testes may show inflammation of the intima and destruction of the media. Aneurysms of the mesenteric, hepatic, subclavian, axillary and brachial arteries and occlusion of middle cerebral arteries have been reported. Skin biopsy specimens taken during the acute phase show dilatation of capillary loops in the papillae, edema of the dermis and perivascular infiltration with lymphocytes, macrophages and mast cells.

CLINICAL MANIFESTATIONS

The principal criteria for the diagnosis of MCLNS are listed in Table 56.8. At least five of the six features should be present to make the diagnosis. However, this syndrome evolves over a 2- to 6-week period and all of the features may not be present at the time the child is seen.

The course of the disease can be divided into three phases. An *acute phase*, characterized by fever, rash, lymphadenopathy, conjunctivitis and oral lesions, lasting from 7 to 14 days. During this phase, swelling of the hands and feet and aseptic meningitis syndrome are also seen. Fever and rash subside at the end of the second week followed by the *subacute phase* which lasts for 4 to 6 weeks (6 to 8 weeks from the onset of illness). During this phase, the important features are irritability, arthritis, thrombocytosis, desquamation, myocarditis, and coronary infarction. Soon these features also subside and the patient enters a *convalescent phase* which may last up to 2 years. During this period the major problems are related to formation of aneurysms of the vessels of the heart and/or other organs.

Fever is the first sign of illness and starts abruptly. All children with MCLNS have fever reaching 40°C (104°F) or more. There may be one or more temperature spikes per day, and this pattern lasts for more than 3 to 5 days, thus differentiating MCLNS from

Table 56.8
Diagnostic Criteria for Kawasaki Disease[a]

I. Fever of 5 or More Days
II. Presence of 4 of the Following 5 Conditions
- A. Bilateral conjunctival injection
- B. Change(s)[b] in the mucus membranes of the upper respiratory tract, such as:
  1. Injected pharynx
  2. Injected lips
  3. Dry, fissured lips
  4. "Strawberry" tongue
- C. Change(s)[b] of the peripheral extremities, such as:
  1. Peripheral edema
  2. Peripheral erythema
  3. Desquamation
  4. Periungual desquamation
- D. Rash, primarily truncal; polymorphous but nonvesicular
- E. Cervical lymphadenopathy

III. Illness Cannot Be Explained by Other Known Disease Process

[a] From *Morbidity and Mortality Weekly Report*, 29: 62, 1980.
[b] One of the items is sufficient for diagnosis.

the usual viral illnesses. Characteristically, the fever persists for more than 1 week (5 to 39 days).

Approximately 96% of children develop bilateral conjunctival injection. This usually starts after the first 2 days and lasts through the febrile period. However, this finding may be transient or mild. There is redness of the bulbar conjunctiva without exudate.

Mucous membrane changes occur in almost all children. These are characterized by redness and fissuring of the lips, redness of the oropharynx and hypertrophy of papillae of the tongue (strawberry tongue). There are no vesicles or ulcers. Fissuring and cracking of the lips with bleeding and crusting may be present for a week or two after the febrile period (Fig. 56.11).

Changes in the extremities are characteristic of this syndrome. Initially, there is brawny edema of the dorsum of the hands and feet with pain and tenderness (Fig. 56.12). The children often refuse to walk or use their hands. The fingers are often swollen and the skin is tight and shiny; the tissue feels firm and resembles the skin in

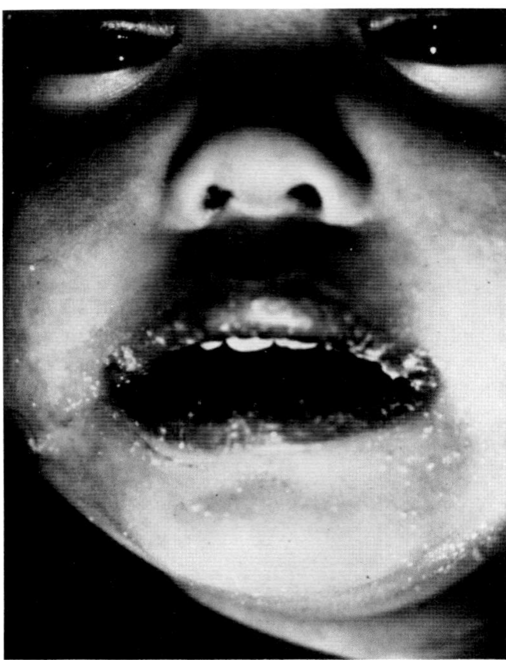

Figure 56.11 Dry, cracked and scaly lips in Kawasaki disease.

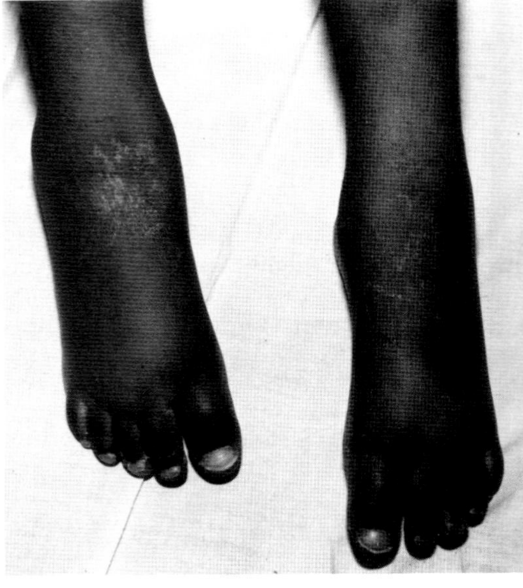

Figure 56.12 Brawny edema of the feet in Kawasaki disease.

scleroderma. The palms and soles are often red. Later in the course of the disease (usually 2 to 3 weeks after the onset of the fever), there is characteristic desquamation of the skin starting around the nails, but involving the entire palm and the sole (Fig. 56.13).

The rash of MCLNS is not diagnostic of the disease but occurs in almost all children during the early acute phase. The rash is usually erythematous and maculopapular or morbilliform, but other types can also

Lymphadenopathy, when it occurs, is often characterized by unilateral enlargement of the cervical node. The nodes are very large and easily visible, but they rapidly decrease in size during the period of defervescence. This finding occurs in less than 75% of children with MCLNS.

Other clinical features include arthritis and arthralgia which occur in approximately 20 to 40% of patients. Both large and small joints are involved. This occurs in the acute or subacute period and lasts for 1 to 2 weeks. The joint fluid has characteristics of an inflammatory effusion. Irritability, crying, sleep disturbances, and lethargy are suggestive of CNS involvement in MCLNS; some children develop coma. The cerebrospinal fluid shows pleocytosis. Diarrhea and abdominal pain are seen in approximately 25% of patients. Features of cardiac involvement will be discussed under "Management of Complications and Emergencies."

LABORATORY FEATURES

Mild transient proteinuria and pyuria are the common urinary findings. The total WBC count is often elevated in the acute phase of the illness; counts up to 77,800/cu mm have been reported. The increase is mainly due to polymorphonuclear leukocytes with both mature and band forms. Elevated platelet counts, as high as 1.8 million/cu mm, are seen in almost all children after the first week of illness with peak levels 2 to 3 weeks after the onset of the illness. The period of thrombocytosis coincides with the period during which coronary artery thrombosis occurs.

The ESR is frequently elevated during the acute phase and reaches normal value 6 to 10 weeks following the onset of fever. Total immunoglobulin levels (IgG, IgA and

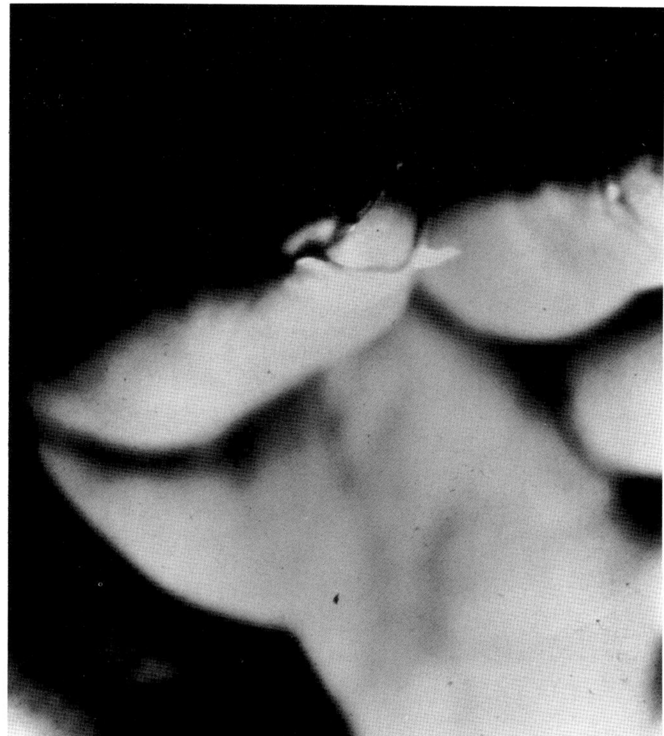

Figure 56.13 Peeling of the skin over the thumbs in Kawasaki disease.

gM) are normal, but IgE levels are often elevated. The sera of these patients do not show antinuclear factor or RF. Levels of total hemolytic complement have been reported to be normal or elevated. When direct bilirubin is markedly elevated together with abdominal distention, hydrops of the gallbladder should be suspected.

MANAGEMENT

General Management

If a child is suspected to have MCLNS, a complete blood count including an absolute platelet count, roentgenogram of the chest, and ECG should be obtained. Children with clinical and laboratory features indicative of high risk for developing coronary artery disease (Table 56.9), and those with clinical, roentgenographic and ECG evidence of heart disease, are usually admitted. Children who are not admitted should be seen biweekly during the first 6 weeks of illness, once a week for 6 more weeks and then every 3 to 6 months for 2 to 4 years. The details of therapy with aspirin and steroids are given below.

Table 56.9
Risk Factors for Coronary Involvement in Kawasaki Disease[a]

Male
Age less than 1 year
Fever over 16 days
Return of fever (2 episodes)
Return of rash (2 episodes)
White cell count over 30,000
Erythrocyte sedimentation rate over 100 mm
Persistent elevation of C-reactive protein
Large heart size
Increased depth of Q wave

[a] From T. Kawasaki: *Japanese Journal of Medical Science and Biology*, *32:* 237, 1979.

Management of Complications and Emergencies

Cardiac Complications. Cardiac involvement of MCLNS is often asymptomatic. Irritability, lethargy and tachycardia are not necessarily indicators of cardiac disease in MCLNS. Tachycardia out of proportion to the fever, distant heart sounds, and arrhythmia should suggest the presence of myocarditis. Myocardial infarction is heralded by the sudden onset of vomiting, pallor and dyspnea. Reduced urine output, edema, dyspnea, enlargement of the liver and rales in the lungs should suggest congestive heart failure which may be due to myocarditis or to myocardial infarction.

Minor ECG abnormalities are observed in over half of the children with MCLNS during the 2nd to 6th week of the disease. These changes include prolongation of the P-R interval, ST-T wave changes, and patterns of left ventricular hypertrophy. Arrhythmias may be an indication of myocarditis or myocardial infarction. In addition, characteristic deep Q waves similar to those seen in adults with myocardial infarction may also be seen (Fig. 56.14).

Echocardiogram may show decreased cardiac contractility, and two-dimensional echocardiography may help visualize aneurysms of the left coronary artery. A coronary angiogram is indicated in patients with evidence of cardiac decompensation and/or those with echocardiographic evidence of aneurysm.

If there is myocardial infarction, the treatment should include pain relief, oxygen therapy, an anticoagulant (heparin), digitalis and diuretics. Aspirin (80 to 90 mg/kg/day in 4 divided doses) is used for control of symptoms particularly in the presence of arthritis, swelling of the hands and feet, and fever. In the presence of pericarditis, aspirin in anti-inflammatory doses is adequate. Steroids (prednisone 2 mg/kg/day) are used in acutely ill children with pericarditis and myocarditis.

Aspirin therapy, once started during the acute phase, is continued for at least 6 to 8 weeks in anti-inflammatory doses. Serum salicylate levels should be monitored. Once the acute period is over, children with no or mild heart disease may be treated with small doses of aspirin (15 to 20 mg/kg/day) for 3 to 6 months. In children who had definite involvement of the heart with heart failure, thrombosis, or valvulitis, aspirin

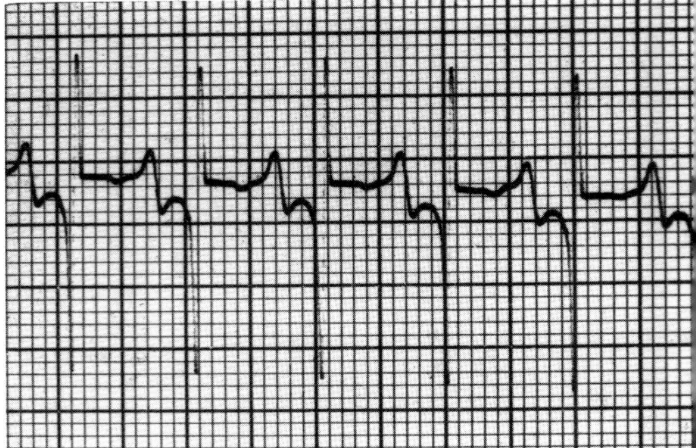

Figure 56.14 Lead III from an ECG on a 15-month-old boy showing deep Q waves in Kawasaki disease.

therapy (15 to 20 mg/kg/day) is usually continued for 1 to 2 years.

Hydrops of the Gallbladder. Another major problem that may prompt an emergency visit during the course of MCLNS is hydrops of the gallbladder. This occurs usually during the early phase of the disease (7 to 14 days). The clinical triad of abdominal pain, vomiting, and right upper quadrant tenderness in a child with MCLNS should suggest the diagnosis. These patients are often icteric, and the serum bilirubin (direct) level is increased. Ultrasonography helps establish the diagnosis. Though there are differences of opinion about the management, it appears that this condition is self-limiting and the chances of perforation are minimal. Therefore, medical management with supportive care and i.v. fluids should be adequate.

Hemolytic-Uremic Syndrome. This complication is rare but can occur during the early phase of the disease (9 to 10 days). Clinical features of hemolytic-uremic syndrome are: petechiae or purpura, easy bruising, melena, pallor, oliguria, proteinuria, hematuria, microangiopathic hemolytic anemia, thrombocytopenia, and an elevated BUN. These patients should be admitted and monitored for their renal, hematological and cardiac status.

Vascular Complications. The pathological process in MCLNS appears to be a generalized vasculitis with intimal inflammation and medial necrosis. Consequently vascular occlusion and aneurysm formation in vessels other than in the coronary system have been reported to occur during the acute illness or during the subsequent 2 to 4 years. Symptoms and signs of these vascular complications vary, depending on the site and the nature of the lesion (occlusion or aneurysm). Occlusion of cerebral vessels may present itself as hemiplegia or seizure. Occlusion of axillary vessels may lead to loss of color, sensation and pulse in the affected extremity. Aneurysms of large vessels may stay asymptomatic until rupture leads to sudden onset of catastrophic symptoms and death. Patients with a history suggestive of MCLNS and symptoms of vascular disease need admission for complete investigation and surgical care.

Acknowledgment. We thank Virgil Hanson, M.D., for his helpful comments.

References

Juvenile Rheumatoid Arthritis

Athreya BH, Doughty RA, Bookspan M, et al.: Pulmonary manifestations of juvenile rheumatoid arthritis. A report of 8 cases and review. *Clin Chest Med* 1: 361, 1980.

Bland JH: Rheumatoid arthritis of the cervical spine. *J Rheumatol* 1: 319, 1974.

Chylack LT, Bienfang DC, Bellows RA, et al.: Ocular manifestations of juvenile rheumatoid arthritis. *Am J Ophthalmol* 79: 1026, 1975.

Jacobs JC, Hui RM: Cricoarytenoid arthritis and airway obstruction in juvenile rheumatoid arthritis. *Pediatrics* 59: 292, 1977.

Leitman PS, Bywaters EGL: Pericarditis in juvenile rheumatoid arthritis. *Pediatrics* 32: 855, 1963.

Miller JJ, French JW: Myocarditis in juvenile rheumatoid arthritis. *Am J Dis Child* 131: 205, 1977.

Schaller JG: The spectrum of juvenile rheumatoid arthritis. In *Clinical Immunology Update*, pp. 71–90, edited by EC Franklin. Elsevier North Holland, New York, 1979.

Schmidt MC, Workman JB, Barth WF: Dissection or rupture of a popliteal cyst. *Arch Intern Med* 134: 694, 1974.

Wedgewood RJ, Schaller JG: The pediatric arthritides. *Hosp Pract* 12: 83, 1977.

Yancey CL, Doughty RA, Cohlan BA, et al.: Pericarditis and cardiac tamponade in juvenile rheumatoid arthritis. *Pediatrics* 68: 369, 1981.

Systemic Lupus Erythematosus

Baldwin DS, Gluck MC, Lowenstein J, et al.: Lupus nephritis; clinical course as related to morphologic forms and their transitions. *Am J Med* 62: 12, 1977.

Budman DR, Steinberg AD: Hematologic aspects of systemic lupus erythematosus. *Ann Intern Med* 86: 220, 1977.

Cathcart ES, Idelson BA, Scheinberg MA, et al.: Beneficial effects of methylprednisolone "pulse" therapy in diffuse proliferative lupus nephritis. *Lancet* 1: 163, 1976.

Decker JL (Moderator): Systemic lupus erythematosus; evolving concepts. *Ann Intern Med* 91: 587, 1979.

Dubois EL: *Lupus Erythematosus*, Ed. 2. University of Southern California Press, Los Angeles, 1974.

Feigin RD, Shearer WT: Opportunistic infection in children; II. In the compromised host. *J Pediatr* 87: 617, 1975.

Hanson V: Systemic lupus erythematosus, dermatomyositis, scleroderma and vasculitidies in childhood. In *Textbook of Rheumatology*, p. 1327, edited by WN Kelley, ED Harris Jr, S Ruddy, CB Sledge. W. B. Saunders, Philadelphia, 1981.

Hunninghake GW, Fauci AJ: Pulmonary involvement in the collagen vascular diseases—state of the art. *Am Rev Respir Dis* 119: 471, 1979.

Rajani KB, Ashbacher LV, Kinney TR: Pulmonary hemorrhage and systemic lupus erythematosus. *J Pediatr* 93: 810, 1978.

Rothfield N: Clinical features of systemic lupus erythematosus. In *Textbook of Rheumatology*, p. 1106, edited by WN Kelley, ED Harris Jr, S Ruddy, CB Sledge. W. B. Saunders, Philadelphia, 1981.

Kaplan D: Treatment of systemic lupus erythematosus. *Arthritis Rheum* 20 (suppl 6): 175, 1977.

Verrier Jones J, Clough JD, Klinenburg JR, et al.: The role of therapeutic plasmapheresis in the rheumatic diseases. *J Lab Clin Med* 97: 589, 1981.

Yancey CL, Doughty RA, Athreya BH: Central nervous system involvement in childhood systemic lupus erythematosus. *Arthritis Rheum* 24: 1389, 1981.

Dermatomyositis

Banker BQ, Victor M: Dermatomyositis (systemic angiopathy) of childhood. *Medicine* 45: 261, 1966.

Bohan A, Peter JB: Polymyositis and dermatomyositis. *N Engl J Med* 292: 344 & 403, 1974.

Cook CD, Rosen FD, Banker BQ: Dermatomyositis and focal scleroderma. *Pediatr Clin North Am* 10: 979, 1963.

Fischer TJ, Cipel L, Steihm ER: Pneumatosis intestinalis associated with fatal childhood dermatomyositis. *Pediatrics* 61: 127, 1978.

Hoare AM, Hawkins CF: Connective tissue disorders affecting the gastrointestinal tract. *Recent Adv Gastroenterol* 3: 96, 1977.

Miller JJ: Late progression of dermatomyositis in children. *J Pediatr* 83: 543, 1973.

Singsen BH, Tedford JC, Platzker ACG, et al.: Spontaneous pneumothorax; a complication of juvenile dermatomyositis. *J Pediatr* 92: 771, 1978.

Sullivan DB, Cassidy JT, Petty RD, Burt A: Prognosis in childhood dermatomyositis. *J Pediatr* 80: 555, 1972.

Sullivan DB, Cassidy JT, Petty RD: Dermatomyositis in the pediatric patient. *Arthritis Rheum* 20 (suppl 2): 327, 1977.

Scleroderma

Bulkley BH, Ridolfi RL, Salyer WR, et al.: Myocardial lesions of progressive systemic sclerosis; a cause of cardiac dysfunction. *Circulation* 53: 483, 1976.

Cassidy JT, Sullivan DB, Dabich L, et al.: Scleroderma in children. *Arthritis Rheum* 20 (suppl 2): 351, 1977.

Cohen S, Snape WJ Jr: The pathophysiology and treatment of gastroesophageal reflux disease; new concepts. *Arch Intern Med* 138: 1398, 1978.

Hoare AM, Hawkins CF: Connective tissue disorders affecting the gastrointestinal tract. *Recent Adv Gastroenterol* 3: 96–123, 1977.

Guttadauria M, Ellman H, Emmanuel G, et al.: Pulmonary function in scleroderma. *Arthritis Rheum* 20: 1071, 1977.

Kornreich HK, King KK, Bernstein BH, et al.: Scleroderma in childhood. *Arthritis Rheum* 20 (suppl 2): 343, 1977.

Mitnick PD, Feig PU: Control of hypertension and reversal of renal failure in scleroderma. *N Engl J Med* 299: 871, 1978.

Porter JM, Snider RL, Bardana EJ, et al.: The diagnosis and treatment of Raynaud's phenomenon. *Surgery* 77: 11, 1975.

Roberts NK, Cabeen WR, Moss J, et al.: The prevalence of conduction defects and cardiac arrhythmias in progressive systemic sclerosis. *Ann Intern Med* 94: 38, 1981.

Teasdall RD, Frayha RA, Shulman LE: Cranial nerve involvement in systemic sclerosis (scleroderma); a report of 10 cases. *Medicine* 59: 149, 1980.

Wasner C, Cooke R, Fries J: Successful medical treatment of scleroderma in renal crisis. *N Engl J Med* 299: 873, 1978.

Young RH, Mark GJ: Pulmonary vascular changes in scleroderma. *Am J Med* 53: 998, 1978.

Polyarteritis Nodosa

Blau EB, Morris RF, Yunis EJ: Polyarteritis nodosa in older children. *Pediatrics* 60: 227, 1977.

Fauci AS, Doppman JL, Wolff SM: Cyclophosphamide-induced remissions in advanced polyarteritis nodosa. *Am J Med* 64: 890, 1978.

Fauci AS, Haynes BF, Katz P: The spectrum of vasculitis; clinical, pathologic, immunologic and therapeutic considerations (NIH Conference). *Ann Intern Med* 89: 660, 1978.

Ford RG, Sickert RG: Central nervous system manifestations of periarteritis nodosa. *Neurology* 15: 114, 1965.

Gillespie DN, Burke EC, Holley KE: Polyarteritis nodosa in infancy; a diagnostic enigma. *Mayo Clin Proc* 48: 773, 1973.

Kielar RA: Exudative retinal detachment and scleritis in polyarteritis. *Am J Ophthalmol* 82: 694, 1976.

Lopez LR, Schocket AL, Stanford RE, et al.: Gastrointestinal involvement in leucocytoclastic vasculitis and polyarteritis nodosa. *J Rheumatol* 7: 677, 1980.

Magilavy DB, Petty RE, Cassidy JT, et al.: A syndrome of childhood polyarteritis. *J Pediatr* 91: 25, 1977.

Reimold EW, Weinberg AG, Fink CW, et al.: Polyarteritis in children. *Am J Dis Child* 130: 534, 1976.

Sack M, Cassidy JT, Bole GG: Prognostic factors in polyarteritis. *J Rheumatol* 2: 411, 1975.

Kawasaki Disease

Ferrino DM, Wolfsdorf JL: Hemolytic uremic syndrome associated with Kawasaki disease. *Pediatrics* 68: 405, 1981.

Fujiwara H, Hamashima Y: Pathology of the heart in Kawasaki disease. *Pediatrics* 61: 100, 1978.

Hiraishi S, Yashiro K, Oguchi K, et al.: Clinical course of cardiovascular involvement in the mucocutaneous lymph node syndrome. Relation between clinical signs of carditis and development of coronary arterial aneurysm. *Am J Cardiol* 47: 323, 1981.

Hosaki J, Abe S, Shoback BR et al.: Mucocutaneous lymph node syndrome with various arterial lesions. *Helv Pediatr Acta* 33: 127, 1978.

Kato H, Koike SK, Yokoyama T: Kawasaki disease; effect of treatment on coronary artery involvement. *Pediatrics* 63: 175, 1979.

Kawasaki T: Clinical signs and symptoms of mucocutaneous lymph node syndrome (Kawasaki disease). *Jpn J Med Sci Biol* 32: 237, 1979.

Landing BH, Larson EJ: Are infantile periarteritis nodosa with coronary artery involvement and fatal mucocutaneous lymph node syndrome the same? Comparison of 20 patients from North America with patients from Hawaii and Japan. *Pediatrics* 59: 651, 1977.

Lipson MH, Ament ME, Fonkastrud EW: Ruptured hepatic artery aneurysm and coronary artery aneurysms with myocardial infarction in a 14-year-old boy; new manifestation of mucocutaneous lymph node syndrome. *J Pediatr* 98: 933, 1981.

Melish ME: Kawasaki syndrome (mucocutaneous lymph node syndrome). *Pediatr Rev* 2: 107, 1980.

Slovis TL, Hight DW, Philippart A, et al.: Sonography in the diagnosis and management of hydrops of the gallbladder in children with mucocutaneous lymph node syndrome. *Pediatrics* 65: 789, 1980.

Yanagihara R, Todd JK: Acute febrile mucocutaneous lymph node syndrome. *Am J Dis Child* 134: 614, 1980.

SECTION IV Surgical Emergencies

CHAPTER 57

Major Trauma

MORITZ M. ZIEGLER, M.D.

INTRODUCTION

Accidents continue to account for close to one half of all deaths in children from the age of 1 to 14 years, exceeding all other causes of childhood mortality and accounting for more than 23,000 deaths in the United States each year. More than one half of these deaths are related to motor vehicle injury. Two out of three childhood accident cases occur in males. The peak accidental age range is between 4 and 12 years, with the highest frequency at age 8. Accidental injury also accounts for approximately 30% of infant deaths.

The mortality rate for children hospitalized following an accident is reported to be low; but this is because one half to two thirds of all trauma deaths occur either at the accident scene or in the hospital emergency department. As many as 18% of hospital trauma deaths are avoidable if a correct diagnosis is made and/or treatment regimen is initially instituted. Combined thoracoabdominal injuries produce an 82% mortality or extremis condition upon arrival at the hospital emergency department. More than one half of these major injuries have associated injuries of the head, chest, and musculoskeletal system. These multisystem injuries require the use of multiple medical disciplines, with varied diagnostic and treatment modalities, to achieve optimal care. These problems clearly place a large burden on the emergency department physician to effect an improvement in outcome from childhood trauma.

A critical factor which influences outcome for the pediatric trauma patient is the recognition that the child's physiologic needs are not the same as those of a small adult. Although the child will usually mount an appropriate physiologic and endocrinologic response to stress, the greater surface area relative to body size results in greater susceptibility to body heat loss and insensible fluid loss. Water, minerals, trace elements, fat and vitamins are all needed in greater maintenance portions in the child. Critically, the growing child has a significantly higher energy-caloric requirement than that of an adult. Equally important to proper tissue repair is the greater total protein and essential amino acid nitrogen requirements which are age dependent.

Whether repair of the malnourished state will influence morbidity and mortality in childhood trauma is speculative, but if adult data examining this question are applicable to the child, then attention to the patient's nutritional status is certainly important. Despite these concerns, children have amazing recuperative powers and are prime candidates for subsequent medical rehabilitation.

BACKGROUND

Etiology of Major Trauma

Automobile-pedestrian accidents account for as many as one half of all childhood accidental deaths, with falls from heights or falls against fixed objects accounting for 25% to 30%, drownings 10% to 15%, burns 5% to 10%, and gunshot wounds, assaults, or ingestions accounting for the remainder. In infancy, however, accidental deaths are more frequently due to poisonings or suffocation rather than automobile accidents. In a 10-year period there will be more than 50,000 accidental deaths reported in children under age 5, while more than 70,000 annual injuries occur as a result of automobile accidents in this younger population. Accident mortality statistics show that the youngest occupant in an automobile will be the most vulnerable in the event of a crash.

Since the United States is a nation in which vehicles are driven on the right side of the road, injuries to the left side of the pedestrian are the most common. The resultant frequency of injured organs include in order: the spleen, genitourinary tract, gastrointestinal tract, liver, pancreas, pelvis, and major vessels. The predominant mechanism of such injuries in children is blunt trauma, but 10% to 20% are penetrating. This is strikingly different than large series of adult trauma patients where as many as 50% will have a penetrating injury. More than one half of the deaths due to such blunt abdominal trauma have an associated major liver injury.

Primary Accident Prevention

With the recognition that accidental injury and death are major public health problems in the United States, educational and legislative programs have been directed toward prevention of this striking morbidity and mortality. Automobile accidents have been reduced by fuel supply-induced lowering of the speed limit to 55 miles per hour. Automobile manufacturers have built vehicles with better safety standards, and the streets are now designed with greater safety for pedestrians. The American Academy of Pediatrics has instituted a program entitled "The First Ride . . . A Safe Ride" in which newborns are placed in infant protective seats within the car upon discharge from the hospital and have such protective devices throughout their growing years. Similarly, some states have initiated legislation to mandate the use of child-automobile restraining devices, thereby preventing the documented increased accident morbidity and mortality induced by permitting a child to ride unrestrained in an automobile.

Educational programs for the public have included intensive training in cardiopulmonary resuscitation and have included variations of the Heimlich maneuver to remove foreign bodies from the upper gastrointestinal-airway systems. Similarly, poison control centers have developed nationwide to assist in the dissemination of information about poisonings and ingestions and to recommend antidotes following an ingestion (see Chapter 48), while the use of child resistant containers has markedly reduced the incidence of accidental ingestions. Fire prevention programs have uniformly both reduced the incidence of fires and improved the methods of evacuation during a fire, and restrictions have been made in the flammability of materials used in making children's clothing. Similarly, water safety and swimming programs have had an impact on the incidence of drowning in the United States, while an awareness of the lead content of paint and the temperature level of hot water have an impact on the incidence of lead poisoning and scald burns, respectively. Public social awareness programs have covered the previously ignored area of child abuse, and the reporting of even suspected child abuse is now a mandatory requirement of all screening physicians (see Chapter 68).

Although these are a telling list of activities designed and proven to reduce the incidence of accidental death, much more specific legislation aimed at child protection is sorely needed.

Secondary Accident Prevention

The establishment of a universal nationwide 911 emergency number has allowed the American citizenry to rapidly report accidents or traumatic events. Police and fire departments throughout the country have established paramedic training and broad based communication networks so that not only can trauma patients be identified, but streetside emergency care can be rapidly and appropriately administered and transportation to the appropriate hospital can be initiated. An additional important development has been the regionalization of trauma care in which patients are not necessarily taken to the nearest hospital, but rather to the most appropriate hospital where the special needs of trauma victims such as children can be readily served.

Organization of the Trauma Service

The regionalization of trauma care in the United States is still in its evolutionary stage. Hospitals have been designated as Level I, II, or III institutions based on both their capability and desirability to care for the multiply injured patient. Level I institutions have a large number of admissions of seriously injured patients and have a high level of skill in the management of such patients, in addition to having ongoing clinical trauma research. Level II facilities are also skilled in trauma care and fill the void in a region lacking a Level I hospital, but such institutions lack the depth of staff specialists and research programs. Level III hospitals also have a commitment to excellence in trauma care but have even fewer specialized personnel and facilities. Under the guidance of the American College of Surgeons Committee on Trauma, the eventual benefit of such a designation plan is to triage appropriate Category I, Category II, or Category III injured patients to these appropriately leveled facilities. Since no one hospital can be expected to have in its immediate geographic area the childhood trauma volume necessary to be an independent and free standing trauma center, regionalization becomes a necessity, utilizing rapid transportation to bring children from afar.

Each institution must develop its own inhouse organizational tree for a trauma service. Such a service needs a well established chain of command with an appropriately designated "captain of the ship," a role which may change hands as additional personnel arrive at the accident scene or in the emergency department. The responsibility of this leadership role in a hospital trauma service is to accept patient care responsibility and organize the multisystem specialists needed to care for the patient's multiple injuries. This organization begins at the scene of an accident, includes the subsequent transport, and includes patient triage following initial evaluation and care once the patient arrives in the hospital emergency department. Subsequently, whether the patient is transferred, admitted to an intensive care unit, or admitted straight to the operating room, a decision will be made by this team leader after consultation with the other varied specialists involved. If at this time it is indeed clear that a single body system is the predominant injury then it is appropriate for this team leader to transfer patient care responsibility to the designated head of a given subspecialty. Figure 57.1 demonstrates a flow diagram of a "response to the traumatized child" at the Children's Hospital of Philadelphia, an example of our organizational schema.

ASSESSMENT AND MANAGEMENT

Prehospital Initial Management (Table 57.1)

Guidelines for the streetside evaluation and treatment of accident victims are well documented by the American College of Surgeons. Obviously, a priority list needs to be established for the logical approach to the trauma victim, priorities which are no different than an approach to the severely and acutely ill emergency department and hospitalized patient. It is also imperative that during injury assessment a simultane-

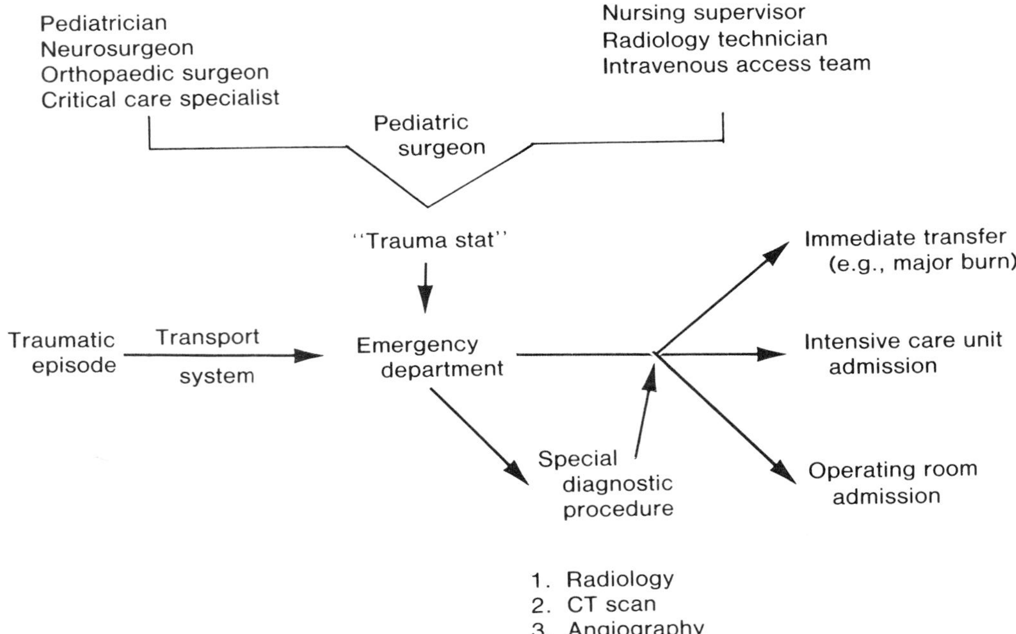

Figure 57.1 Flow diagram depicting an appropriate emergency department response to the traumatized child.

Table 57.1
Pre-Hospital Assessment and Management Guidelines for the Injured Child

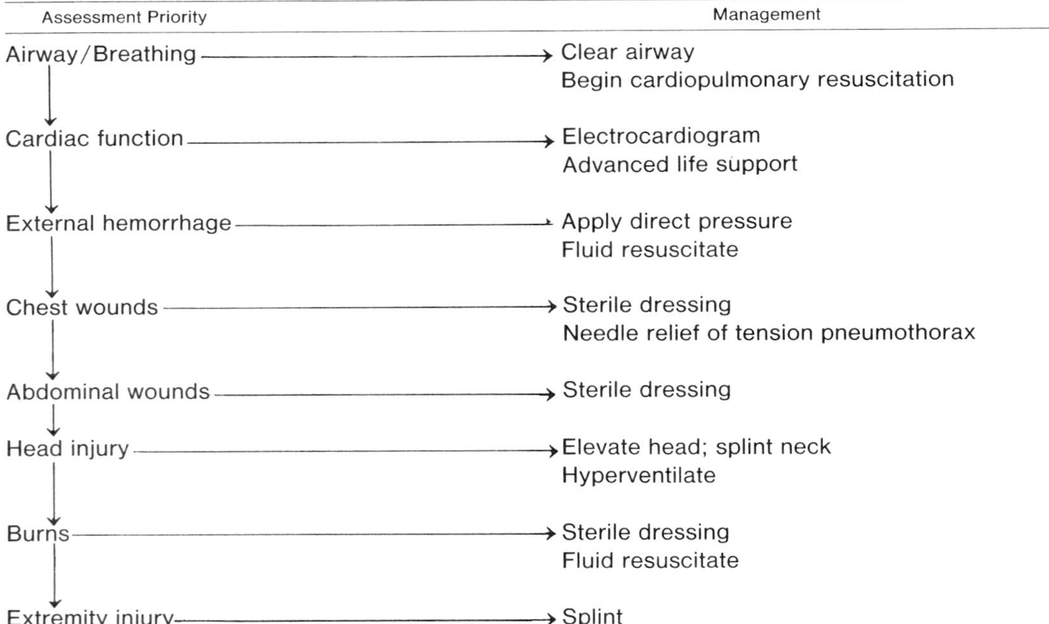

Assessment Priority	Management
Airway/Breathing	Clear airway Begin cardiopulmonary resuscitation
Cardiac function	Electrocardiogram Advanced life support
External hemorrhage	Apply direct pressure Fluid resuscitate
Chest wounds	Sterile dressing Needle relief of tension pneumothorax
Abdominal wounds	Sterile dressing
Head injury	Elevate head; splint neck Hyperventilate
Burns	Sterile dressing Fluid resuscitate
Extremity injury	Splint

Table 57.2
Burn Injury

Classification	Morphology	Appearance	Cause
1st degree	Superficial epidermis devitalized; vasodilatation and vasocongestion	Erythema: blanches on pressure	Ultraviolet exposure; short flash
2nd degree	Epidermal destruction; coagulation necrosis with congestion and fluid collection; skin elements remain viable for regeneration	Painful, erythematous, weeping, blisters, bullae, skin elements white, soft and dry	Short flash or spill scald
3rd degree	All skin elements destroyed; coagulation necrosis of subdermal plexus; capillary thrombosis	Dry, hard, inelastic with visible vein thrombosis	Flame, scald immersion; contact electrical

Table 57.3
Burn Wound Assessment: Body Surface Estimation (Adult versus the Child)

Anatomic Area	Percentage Adult Surface (Greater than Age 10)	Percentage Infant Surface
Head	9	16
Right upper extremity	9	9
Left upper extremity	9	9
Right lower extremity	18	13
Left lower extremity	18	13
Anterior trunk	18	18
Posterior trunk	18	18
Neck	1	4
Total	100	100

ous patient management protocol be initiated in a logical sequence.

The first priorities in managing the traumatized child include resuscitation of cardiopulmonary arrest, control of hemorrhage, treatment of shock, and direction of attention to major thoracic, abdominal, and head injuries. Restoration of the *airway* includes tilting the chin up and forward, pulling the tongue out of the pharynx and cleaning the pharynx of accumulated secretions (see Chapter 1). Artificial ventilation may need to be established by mouth-to-mouth or mouth-to-nose-and-mouth techniques. During resuscitation, the neck should be stabilized if there is any possibility of a cervical spine injury. *Cardiac function* is also an initial priority and must be maintained with external massage if there is no cardiac activity. *External uncontrolled hemorrhage* is best handled by direct pressure, the use of an extremity tourniquet rarely being necessary. A pressurized garment, such as a MAST device, is often beneficial in controlling both external and especially internal venous hemorrhage, and appropriate pediatric sizes are available. Oxygen administration to the patient with major hemorrhage and possible shock is of course beneficial, and an intravenous infusion should be started. If uncontrolled external hemorrhage is associated with a dismembered part, it is imperative to identify and retrieve the amputated part, clean it with sterile saline, wrap it in a sterile bandage and immerse it in ice for transport with the patient to the nearest hospital. If an *impaled object* is protruding from a patient, it is best debrided from surrounding clothing and left in place. *Open chest wounds* raise the possibility of a flail chest, tension pneumothorax, or cardiac tamponade, and such wounds are best covered with sterile dressings. A similar approach is used for *open abdominal wounds*. The use of a modified Trendelenburg position and the use of a MAST suit, if available, provide the best initial therapy of *severe shock*; additionally the patient should receive intravenous fluids and appropriate precautions to maintain body temperature (see Chapter 2). If severe *head injury* is observed at the streetside, early checks and records should be kept of blood pressure, pulse rate, pupils, level of consciousness, the ability to move extremities, a sensory level, and the ability to follow commands. All unconscious patients should be treated as if they have an injury to the spinal cord; they should be supported in static position and during any transfers (see Chapter 67).

Second priority streetside injury management includes both the assessment and treatment of burns and skeletal injury. The *burned child* needs to have an initial appraisal of burn severity including the depth, location, and type of burn (Table 57.2), an appraisal of burned area applying the modified rule of nines for children (Table 57.3), and a determination of whether the injury includes pulmonary, soft tissue or bony damage as well. Burns can be classified in the following categories: *critical*, in which there is a respiratory tract injury, partial thickness burn exceeds 20% of body surface area, full thickness burn exceeds 10% of the surface area, the hands, face, feet or genitalia are included, there is a complicating fracture or soft tissue injury, electrical burns are part of the mechanism, or deep acid burns are present; *moderate*, in which partial thickness is less than 20% and full thickness is less than 2% and does not include the hands, feet or genitalia; and *minor*, in which partial thickness is less than 15% and full thickness is less than 2%. The burn victim should be undressed and sterile covers should be placed over the burn wounds. Intravenous fluid resuscitation is immediately mandatory if the burned area exceeds 20% of the body surface area. In severe burns an NPO status (nothing by mouth) should be promptly instituted, and intravenous fluid resuscitation along with the use of analgesics is mandatory prior to transporting the patient directly to a burn center (see Chapters 2 and 64).

Major *multiple fractures* also rank as a second priority injury. Severe angulations should be straightened, joints should be immobilized, and traction splints should be applied. Compound fracture exposed bone should not be pushed back under the skin. Initial fracture management should also include a check of pulses, pillow splints to elbow and knee joint areas, and the treatment of back injuries with or without cord damage with a back board.

The lowest priority type of injury includes *minor fractures*, *soft tissue injuries*, or *mortal wounds* where death appears certain.

To facilitate data retrieval and clinical research, but most importantly to expedite transportation of the right patient to the right hospital at the right time, the American College of Surgeons, the American Medical Association, and others have developed field categorization scores for such trauma patients. It is important to assess at the scene of the accident and subsequently in the emergency department the extent and severity of a patient's injury. These scores correlate with ultimate morbidity and mortality and serve as useful prognostic indices for patient management. Tables 57.4, 57.5, and 57.6 list three such categorization systems which are applicable to the pediatric patient when appropriate modifications are made regarding the classification of patient age to the infant, preschooler or school-age child. Table 57.7 summarizes age-dependent ranges of vital signs for these categories.

Emergency Department Assessment and Management (see Table 57.8)

Following prehospital evaluation and care of the injured child, the victim is transported to the hospital. A rapid and reproducible schema of immediate, simultaneous, and subsequent evaluation and treatment principles should be applied to every child admitted to the emergency department with major multiple trauma.

General Approach

A "trauma stat" alerting appropriate personnel should be called upon notification of an impending arrival or simultaneous with an unexpected arrival of a multiply injured child in the emergency department, and all participants in the trauma care team should participate in this initial evaluation and initial treatment of the patient (Fig. 57.1).

Table 57.4
Modified Field Categorization of the Trauma Patient

System	Category 1	Category 2	Category 3
Soft tissue	Avulsion type injuries, severe uncontrolled bleeding	Soft tissue injuries with stabilized bleeding	Soft tissue injuries of moderate degree
Fractures	Open fractures, pelvic fractures, severe maxillofacial injuries	Single open or closed fractures	Uncomplicated fractures
Abdomen	Blunt or penetrating abdominal injuries especially when associated with hypotension	Blunt abdominal or penetrating trauma not producing hypotension	No abdominal injuries
Chest	Unstable chest injuries	Multiple rib fractures without flail segments	No respiratory distress
Head and neck, upper respiratory	Severe maxillofacial injuries, open penetrating and blunt trauma to face, neck and cervical spine, multiple facial fractures, injuries affecting vision	Facial trauma with single facial fractures (without airway or major cervical spine involvement)	Simple contusions of the head and neck, nasal fractures
Neurological	Prolonged loss of consciousness, posturing, lateralizing signs open cranial injuries, paralysis	Transient loss of consciousness, oriented to time, place and person	No neurological injuries
Vital signs	Abnormal; skin cool, ashen, pale	Borderline; skin warm to slightly cool	Normal; skin dry, warm

Table 57.5
Modified Field Categorization of the Trauma Patient Based on Assessment of Deranged Physiology

Category	Assessment	Score[a]
Measured capillary return	Normal	2
	Delayed	0
Measured respiratory effort	Normal	3
	Shallow	1
	Retractive	1
	None	0
Eye opening	Spontaneous	3
	To voice	2
	To pain	1
	None	0
Verbal response	Oriented	4
	Confused	3
	Inappropriate words	2
	Incomprehensible words	1
	None	0
Motor response	Obeys command	4
	Withdraws	3
	Flexion	2
	Extension	1
	None	0

[a] Patient with a total score less than 7 should be treated in a Level I facility.

The patient should be admitted to a generous sized area of the emergency department and placed on a multipurpose stretcher where the child should be undressed and examined. It is important that the same examiners serially assess the patient, their first priority being to establish both a logical evaluation and treatment program.

An adequate *airway* must be assured by either elevating the chin and pulling the tongue forward while clearing secretions or by inserting a nasopharyngeal airway or a direct endotracheal tube. Obvious *external hemorrhage* should be treated by direct pressure, the use of tourniquets rarely being indicated. *Intravenous access* is an immediate necessity and, although a large bore cannula is preferred, a small scalp vein needle may prove useful to initial resuscitation. Immediate *laboratory studies* should be done, including a type and cross-match for the blood bank, urinalysis and complete blood count and, where indicated, assessment can also be made of serum electrolytes, blood urea nitrogen, glucose, amylase, and liver function tests. *Hemor-*

Table 57.6
Modified Injury Severity Scale

	Minor—1	Moderate—2	Severe, Not Life-threatening—3	Severe, Life-threatening—4	Critical, Survival Uncertain—5
Neurologic	GCS[a] 15	GCS 13–14	GCS 9–12	GCS 5–8	GCS 4
Face and neck	Abrasion/contusion ocular apparatus; vitreous, conjunctival hemorrhage; fractured teeth	Undisplaced facial bone fracture; laceration of eye, disfiguring laceration; retinal detachment	Loss of eye, avulsion optic nerve, displaced facial fractures, "blowout" fractures of orbit	Boney or soft tissue injury with minor destruction	Injuries with major airway obstruction
Chest	Muscle ache or chest wall stiffness	Simple rib or sternal fracture	Multiple rib fractures; hemothorax or pneumothorax; diaphragmatic rupture; pulmonary contusion	Open chest wounds; pneumomediastinum; myocardial contusion	Laceration of trachea; hemomediastinum; aortic laceration or rupture
Abdomen	Muscle ache, seat belt abrasion	Major abdominal wall contusion	Contusion of abdominal organ; retroperitoneal hematoma; extraperitoneal bladder rupture; thoracic/lumbar spine fractures	Minor laceration of abdominal organs; intraperitoneal bladder rupture; spine fractures with paraplegia	Rupture or laceration of abdominal vessels or organs
Extremities	Minor sprains; simple fractures/dislocations	Compound fracture of digits, displaced long bone or pelvic fracture	Displaced long bone or multiple hand/foot fractures, single open long bone fractures; pelvic fracture with displacement; laceration of major nerves/vessels	Multiple closed long bone fractures; amputation of limbs	Multiple open long bone fractures

[a] GCS: Glascom coma scale.

Table 57.7
Age-related Variations in Normal Vital Signs of the Pediatric Patient Practially Classified as Infant, Preschool and School Age

Vital Signs	0–1 Year (Infants)	1–5 Years (Preschool)	>5 Years (School Age)
Blood pressure	< 80	< 90	< 90
Respiratory rate	25–50	20–30	15–30
Pulse rate	100–140	80–120	60–100

rhagic shock can be promptly treated by utilizing the Trendelenburg position, by the immediate administration of crystalloid solutions, and by the subsequent administration of blood products when they are available. The *cervical spine* should be assumed to be fractured in all unconscious patients or head injured patients, and the cervical spine should be immediately stabilized utilizing sand bags until x-ray study shows that it is uninvolved. The patient should be placed on a *cardiorespiratory monitoring device*, and *vital signs* need to be initially and serially recorded. At this stage it is critical that an adequate and thorough *history* of the nature of the trauma be obtained and that family or witnesses be queried as to the antecedent medical history of the child.

Simultaneously with this initial program, a group of other treatment principles need to be applied. *Long bone fractures* should be promptly splinted. In the face of major trauma, especially in the unconscious child, the *urinary bladder* should be catheterized, a urinalysis should be done to check for the presence of blood, and the urinary output should be monitored. Urethrography is indicated if a *urethral injury* is suspected, this suspicion being especially high if there is gross blood at the urethral meatus, if the patient cannot void, if there is an associated severe pelvic fracture, and if on rectal examination the bladder and prostate gland feel to be separated from the lower urethral structures. The major trauma patient should also have a *nasogastric tube* inserted and the stomach emptied and a prompt and early *chest x-ray* should be obtained. *Tetanus prophylaxis* should be considered if indicated, *tetanus hyperimmune serum* should be given in the face of major soft tissue injury, and *antibiotics* should be administered if specifically indicated. All drugs and other therapy should be recorded on a serial flow sheet by the attending nurse. Similarly, a serial *neurologic evaluation* needs to be obtained, recording the level of consciousness, pupillary reaction, cranial nerve function, extremity motor function, and deep tendon and plantar reflexes.

Specific body systems have specific principles which need consideration in this initial evaluation of the trauma patient in the emergency department. Most importantly, a rising pulse rate and falling systemic blood pressure suggest hypovolemia. Such findings in the unconscious closed head injured child should not be interpreted as being secondary to the head trauma but most likely represent blood loss from an as yet undiagnosed intra-abdominal, retroperitoneal, or thoracic blood losing injury.

Thorax

In the thorax sucking wounds are best treated by application of an air-tight seal with a sterile dressing following preliminary wound exploration. A hemothorax, pneumothorax, or penetrating wound of the chest is most safely treated by insertion of a tube thoracostomy (see procedure in Section VII). In the presence of a tension pneumothorax associated with respiratory distress and mediastinal shift on physical examination, insertion of a needle on the side of the pneumothorax rapidly achieves relief of the tension. A chest tube should then be inserted and placed to water seal drainage with suction applied. If the air leak is large, one should be concerned that a possible bronchial rupture is present.

If multiple rib fractures cause a flail chest, paradoxical respiration might occur, a problem best treated with an endotra-

Table 57.8
Emergency Department Assessment and Management Plan for the Injured Child

Assessment	Diagnosis	Management	Laboratory Study
Airway/Breathing ↓		Clear airway Intubate Ventilate	
Cardiac function ↓		External cardiac massage	Cardiorespiratory monitor
Shock	External hemorrhage →	Direct pressure	CBC
↓	Internal hemorrhage →	Trendelenburg position Establish intravenous access MAST suit	Cross match for one blood volume
Head/Neck injury ↓	Closed head injury Possible cervical spine fracture	Sand bag splint of neck Hyperventilation	Skull film CT scan, head Lateral neck film
Chest injury	Cardiac contusion →	ECG monitor Pericardiocentesis	Chest x-ray ECG Cardiac ultrasound Arterial blood gas
	Hemopneumothorax →	Tube thoracostomy	
	Flail chest →	Intubation/Ventilation	
↓	Sucking wound →	Sterile dressing	
Abdominal injury	Penetrating injury →	Nasogastric tube Serial examination	Plain/Upright x-ray
↓	Blunt injury →	Serial examination Paracentesis with lavage	Tilt table test Amylase Liver function tests Serial CBC
Renal/Urinary injury	Renal contusion/laceration →	Bladder catheterization	Urinalysis Plain abdominal x-ray Intravenous pyelogram
↓	Bladder/Urethral injury →	Delayed catheterization	Voiding cystourethrogram
Musculoskeletal injury	Dismembered part →	Salvage, irrigate and cool	Extremity x-rays Angiography
	Compound fracture →	Sterile dressing; splint	
↓	Boney injury →	Splint, traction	
Soft tissue injury		Irrigate, debride Primary vs. delayed repair	X-ray to exclude foreign body

cheal tube and positive pressure ventilation. If the history relates that there was a severe deceleration injury and chest x-ray demonstrates a widened mediastinum with or without a fractured first rib, a thoracic aortic injury is suggested, and aortography is promptly indicated. If air lucencies suggesting intestine are present on chest x-ray, a ruptured diaphragm is a possibility.

Cardiac tamponade should be suspected if there is a shocklike picture with an elevated central venous pressure or venous engorgement of the head and neck with muffled heart sounds, and prompt treatment utilizing pericardiocentesis is indicated (see procedure in Section VII). If bedside diagnostic ultrasound is available, this study would provide important information to precede such a pericardiocentesis.

Abdomen

The abdomen itself is best evaluated by serial examinations looking for both focal tenderness, involuntary guarding, and for changing girth. In the head injured patient or the patient with altered consciousness, a high suspicion of concomitant intra-abdominal injury needs to be constantly maintained.

In the unconscious child there usually is an absolute indication for abdominal paracentesis with lavage to exclude concomitant intra-abdominal injury. Additional criteria indicating the need for formal diagnostic peritoneal lavage include persistently unstable vital signs following the initial fluid resuscitation, a presentation in or development of a shock state, and the presence of major body system injuries above and below the diaphragm. A lavage should be done under direct visualization of the peritoneum (see procedures in Section VII) and will be considered positive for any of the following reasons: free aspiration of 10 ml or more of gross blood; turbid or bloody lavage fluid which prohibits the reading of newspaper print through the tubing; free egress of lavage fluid through an indwelling urinary catheter or chest tube; presence of more than 500 leukocytes or 100,000 erythrocytes per milliliter on cell count of the fluid; fluid amylase level over 175 units; and either gross stool or food debris in the lavage fluid.

In the presence of either gross or microscopic hematuria, an intravenous pyelogram should be done, and a cystourethrogram is indicated in those children in whom a bladder or a urethral injury is suspected. The intravenous pyelogram (IVP) can be initiated if urgently needed by administering 2 to 4 ml/kg of intravenous 50% diatrizoate sodium (Hypaque—Winthrop) in the emergency department and following the patient with serial abdominal plain films.

Extremities

With extremity injuries the distal pulses should be examined, but the presence of distal extremity pulses does not exclude a concomitant proximal arterial injury. Soft tissue injuries should be thoroughly inspected for both wound foreign bodies and for the presence of devitalized tissue. Generous irrigation and debridement is beneficial in early wound care to minimize contamination before giving consideration to primary or delayed wound closure (see Chapter 58).

MANAGEMENT OF SPECIFIC INJURIES: MAJOR ABDOMINAL INJURY

Penetrating Abdominal Wounds

In adult series of major trauma as many as 50% of abdominal injuries are of the penetrating type, but this ratio is remarkably reversed in the pediatric population. In most series, significantly less than 10% of patients with major abdominal injuries due to trauma are due to penetrating injury. If one extends the age of the pediatric population to the late teenage years, only then does the incidence of penetrating wounds approach the adult 50% figure.

Children with penetrating injuries due to knives or sharp bladed objects may present with a relatively asymptomatic abdominal, lower chest wall, or back wound of entry; or the patient may present in frank hypovolemic shock or even with evisceration through the wound of entrance. These presentations and subsequent evaluation or therapy require a mandatory surgical consultation. The presence of peritoneal signs warrants abdominal exploration, but roentgenographic evaluation may not demonstrate free air even in the presence of hollow visceral injury. Historically, there has been a great deal of enthusiasm for wound exploration under local anesthesia and for sinographic x-rays in which contrast is injected through a catheter secured in the wound of entrance by a purse-string suture. The demonstration of contrast material penetrating the peritoneum suggests a need for formal abdominal exploration; but as more experience is accumulated, it is clear that a great deal of equally objective information may be obtained by serial physical examination alone. The high incidence of false negative local wound explorations and sinograms warrant against their routine use. Selectivity must therefore be practiced in the management of penetrating wounds due to knives, and only those patients having clinical findings of peritoneal irritation or volume loss of an unexplained nature warrant prompt exploration. Such selectivity may be safely practiced with mortality rates less than 2% and morbidity rates less than 10%.

Contrasting with penetrating injuries due to knives, gunshot wounds of the abdomen or wounds of the lower chest potentially entering the abdomen should be treated with greater aggressiveness. All patients should be admitted to the hospital for serial examination. Yet, selectivity can again be practiced, and as many as 5 to 10% of patients can theoretically and practically be observed with conservative management alone. However, the problem with gunshot wounds to the abdomen are that 80% have multiorgan injury, morbidity is high, and the mortality from such injuries is likewise high, at a figure of 12.5%. The presence of peritoneal irritation on physical examination, the demonstration of a hypovolemic state, the presence of free air on radiographic examination, and a positive paracentesis are all absolute indications for operative exploration. The simple presence of a metallic missile within the abdominal cavity does not per se warrant operation. It is clear that in penetrating abdominal injury selectivity should be practiced, but in the presence of gunshot wounds almost all children with such injuries will be explored.

Blunt Abdominal Injury

The appropriate evaluation and treatment of children following blunt abdominal trauma requires serial examinations performed by an experienced, thorough, and suspicious physician. The critical findings on examination are those suggesting the need for operative intervention, namely, a hemodynamically unstable patient with an enlarging abdomen and no other site of intravascular volume loss, peritoneal irritation with involuntary guarding, rigidity, and abdominal wall discoloration, and signs of intravascular volume loss in association with an unconscious patient.

Paracentesis (see procedure in Section VII) is a valuable adjunct for assessing the head injured unconscious patient because in such children the physical examination may be grossly misleading. As a group these patients should not be allowed to sustain major fluid shifts which require high volume rapid replacement because of the potential exacerbation of brain swelling. Paracentesis is also of value in assessing the child with visceral injury of the spleen, liver, or kidney who may be managed nonoperatively if concomitant intestinal disruption can be excluded. The concomitant use of plain roentgenograms, radionuclide scanning, ultrasonography and computerized tomography provide valuable diagnostic adjuncts to the physician evaluating the pediatric trauma patient. Similarly, laboratory data in the form of a complete blood count, serum amylase, serum/urine amylase clearance ratio, urinalysis, renal function and liver function tests are needed in evaluating the blunt trauma patient.

Since the kidneys are more abdominal in location and since left sided blunt injuries are more common, the spleen and kidney become the most frequently injured abdominal organs. A detailed account of each organ system injury follows.

Splenic Injury

The history of the injured spleen and its management dates to almost 600 years ago when the first splenectomy for traumatic injury of the spleen was carried out by Fiorovanti. Subsequently a concept evolved that the injured spleen is the spleen that was best removed, and it had been our standard practice to treat splenic injuries promptly by splenectomy. However, in the last 25 years reports have shown that the spleen may play a critical role, especially in the younger patient, in host protection against bacterial infection. With this as a basis, this entire area has been drastically revised and new options of patient diagnosis and treatment have been devised.

A child with a classic splenic injury has received a blow to his left upper quadrant with or without associated rib fractures, an injury which might occur with a youngster falling forward across the handlebars of his bicycle, as he strikes an immobile object, or as he falls forward off his snow sled. These children may present with pain at the tip of their shoulder, pain in their left upper quadrant, pain in their left chest with breathing, and respiratory distress. Nausea and vomiting are often associated findings which may or may not be due to associated hypovolemia.

The pulse and blood pressure may be normal, but mild tachycardia and hypotension often occur. These findings can be accentuated by placing the patient in an upright posture, such as is done with a classic tilt table test. The pallor, hypotension, and tachycardia are often associated with symptoms of lightheadedness and nausea. On abdominal examination such youngsters may demonstrate abdominal tenderness especially in the left upper quadrant with or without guarding. A Kehr's sign is positive if compression of the left upper quadrant elicits left shoulder pain.

Although laboratory tests and radiographs are often normal in the child with splenic injury, the same tests may demonstrate a falling hemoglobin, an absolute leukocytosis in the 20,000 to 30,000 range, an inferiorly displaced stomach gas bubble or transverse colon, an increased size of the splenic shadow, an effacement of the left psoas shadow, a left pleural effusion, or associated left sided rib fractures. Radionuclide scanning may show a filling defect of the spleen which can be further characterized as a disruption, a tear, or a subcapsular hematoma. This latter highly sensitive technique is noninvasive and is preferred to arteriography which is not a practical tool in the emergency department.

The treatment of a splenic injury classically has been splenectomy. However, in 1957, Smith reported that children with Mediterranean anemia had an increased death rate in the postsplenectomy period. Subsequently it became clear that the spleen had multiple roles including the filtration of particulate antigen, the production of IgM antibody, the production of opsonins, and the regulation of T and B lymphocytes. It was furthermore observed that the younger the splectomized patient, the more susceptible he was to postsplenectomy infection with encapsulated bacteria. The overall mortality in patients losing their spleen secondary to trauma who sustain a postsplenectomy infection is 0.65% which represents a 65-fold increased risk rate compared with the normal population. Because of this risk of serious infection in the splenectomized child, the management of splenic injury has changed dramatically, varying from a complete nonoperative approach, to the repair of the injured spleen, to even the projected autotransplantation of the fragmented spleen.

Surgeons at the Toronto Hospital for Sick Children now strongly advocate the use of nonoperative management of supposed spleen-injured patients. In their series of 49 patients with suspected splenic injury 28 did not require operation. Of the 28 successfully managed by observation alone, 12 had a fall in hemoglobin and required transfusion, 4 had a falling hemoglobin but did not need transfusion, and 12 had no change in their hemoglobin level. As more experience has been gained by this group, they have further revised their "observation only" criteria to the following: patients are admitted to an intensive care unit, they are serially closely observed, and only in the face of suspected injury to other organs or in the face of a greater than 40% blood volume transfusion requirement do they proceed to operative exploration. This form of management, to be successful and

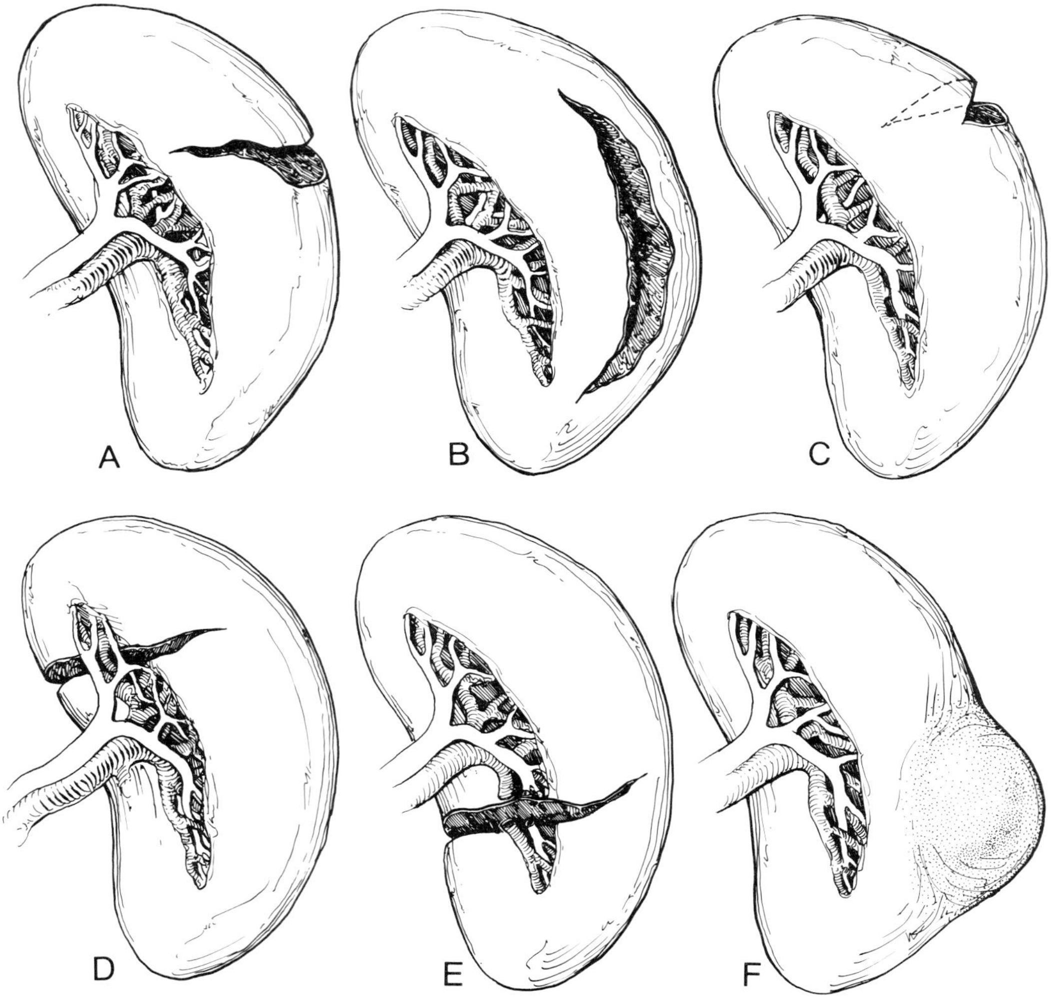

Figure 57.2 Pathophysiology of blunt injury to the spleen. (*A*) Single transverse laceration of free margin, (*B*) vertical laceration of free margin, (*C*) posterior laceration on diaphragmatic splenic surface, (*D*) laceration of splenic hilar surface, (*E*) hilar laceration involving major vascular branches, and (*F*) subcapsular splenic hematoma.

safe, requires exceptionally close scrutiny, serial examination, and the willingness to abandon the conservative plan for prompt operative exploration.

Splenic repair or splenorrhaphy is now a well accepted and technically feasible adjunct in the surgical management of the injured spleen. The anatomic arrangement of the spleen with radial distribution of the vascular system from the splenic hilum permits such splenic repair as does the observation that many splenic tears are not bleeding by the time of exploration. In a series of 17 patients undergoing operation for splenic injury reported from Toronto, 15 underwent spleen repair, 1 underwent splenectomy for a hilar laceration, and 1 underwent splenectomy for associated renal and head injuries. At the time of operation only 7 of these injured spleens were noted to be actively bleeding. Twelve had a single laceration and 5 had multiple lacerations. Fourteen had transverse lacerations, 3 had vertical lacerations, 4 had involvement of the diaphragmatic surface, 8 had the laceration extend toward the hilum, 2 had torn extra splenic vessels, and only 1 patient had fragmentation of the spleen (Fig. 57.2). Useful methods to achieve splenic repair include the application of topical collagen hemostat (Avitene—American Critical Care, McGaw Park, Ill.), various suturing techniques with or without omental wrapping, splenic artery ligation, and splenectomy with a prompt autotransplant to the peritoneal cavity. Patients cared for by surgeons not familiar with such repair techniques are best served by splenectomy.

Because of these management advances, the absolute indications for splenectomy are limited to include a spleen which is completely separated from its blood supply, a patient who has severe associated organ system injuries plus a positive paracentesis and unstable hemodynamics, a patient with a severe head injury who cannot be allowed to tolerate volume shifts and blood loss with volume resuscitation, a patient with increasing blood losses of unknown cause, and a patient who has fecal contamination of his peritoneal cavity. The majority of patients undergoing splenectomy will have a complete uneventful recovery but as many as 70% of patients with splenic trauma have associated injuries of the abdomen, head, chest, or extremities.

These postsplenectomy patients also require a close surveillance with frequent cultures and CBC, prompt, aggressive investigation of a fever, and treatment of any bacterial infections, whether these occur in childhood or in a young adult.

For prophylaxis in the postsplenectomy patient we advocate the use of penicillin 250 mg twice a day for life. Erythromycin may be an appropriate substitute in those children with documented penicillin allergies. Pneumovax vaccine (Merck, Sharp & Dohme) is indicated for prophylaxis even in the patient who has already undergone splenectomy, since antipneumococcal titers will accrue though to a lesser extent and in a slower fashion than in a patient who has an intact spleen.

The postoperative management or post-injury management for patients treated by splenorrhaphy or nonoperatively include bed rest for approximately 10 days. Patients can then be discharged from the hospital on restricted activity returning to full physical activity 6 to 8 weeks following the abdominal injury. After the initial radionuclide scan demonstrating the splenic injury, it is wise to repeat such a scan 6 to 8 weeks later. Scans done prior to that time are unlikely to show significant healing.

Liver Injury

Liver injury is the major cause of mortality from abdominal trauma, accounting for as many as 40% of deaths, particularly in children. In the etiology of accident mortality, the injured liver is second only to head injuries, and the injured liver as a major cause of mortality is often due to an associated injury of the inferior vena cava. Liver injury may be a greater problem in left-sided driving nations where automobiles are likely to strike a pedestrian on his right side.

More than 90% of liver injuries are secondary to blunt trauma and more than 90% of the injuries involve the right lobe. Liver injuries can be classified in increasing severity as subcapsular hematomas, capsular tears, minor lacerations of the parenchyma, deep parenchymal lacerations, and burst liver injuries with or without associated major vascular injury (Fig. 57.3). Anatomically such injuries can be localized to the convex surface of the liver, the anterior, the concave, or the posterior surface of the liver, the latter being the prime site for major associated caval injuries with their attendant mortality.

Patients with liver injury may have right shoulder pain and right upper quadrant tenderness and/or guarding. Hypotension may be present in the face of major blood loss but examination of the stool will rarely reveal traumatic hemobilia with hematochezia. The association of fractured ribs is a common concomitant finding.

Historically, resection of the injured portion of the liver did not become the preferred management choice until the last 30 years. This radical approach awaited definition of the lobar/segmental anatomy of the liver and the use of angiography in the preoperative period. More recently there has been a new enthusiasm for more conservative management of a liver injury with the use of abdominal lavage, serial liver scans, and selection for either observation alone or for operative intervention.

To achieve adequate conservative management, patients must be hospitalized in an intensive care unit and subjected to extremely close scrutiny. In the absence of pelvic or thoracic injuries and signs or symptoms of splenic injury, the source of a patient's hypovolemia must be assumed to be a liver injury. In addition to bedside clinical findings, serial liver scans are needed to demonstrate both injury and subsequent healing; and, until such healing is demonstrated, restricted activity is essential initially as an inpatient and subsequently as an out-patient. The conservative management of liver injury is not dissimilar to that applied to splenic injury.

Operative management of liver injury requires an extremely aggressive operative approach. Preoperative angiography may be especially beneficial in defining the anatomy of the injury and the normal anatomy in terms of the origin and circulation of the right and left hepatic arteries. Such patients require availability of a large volume

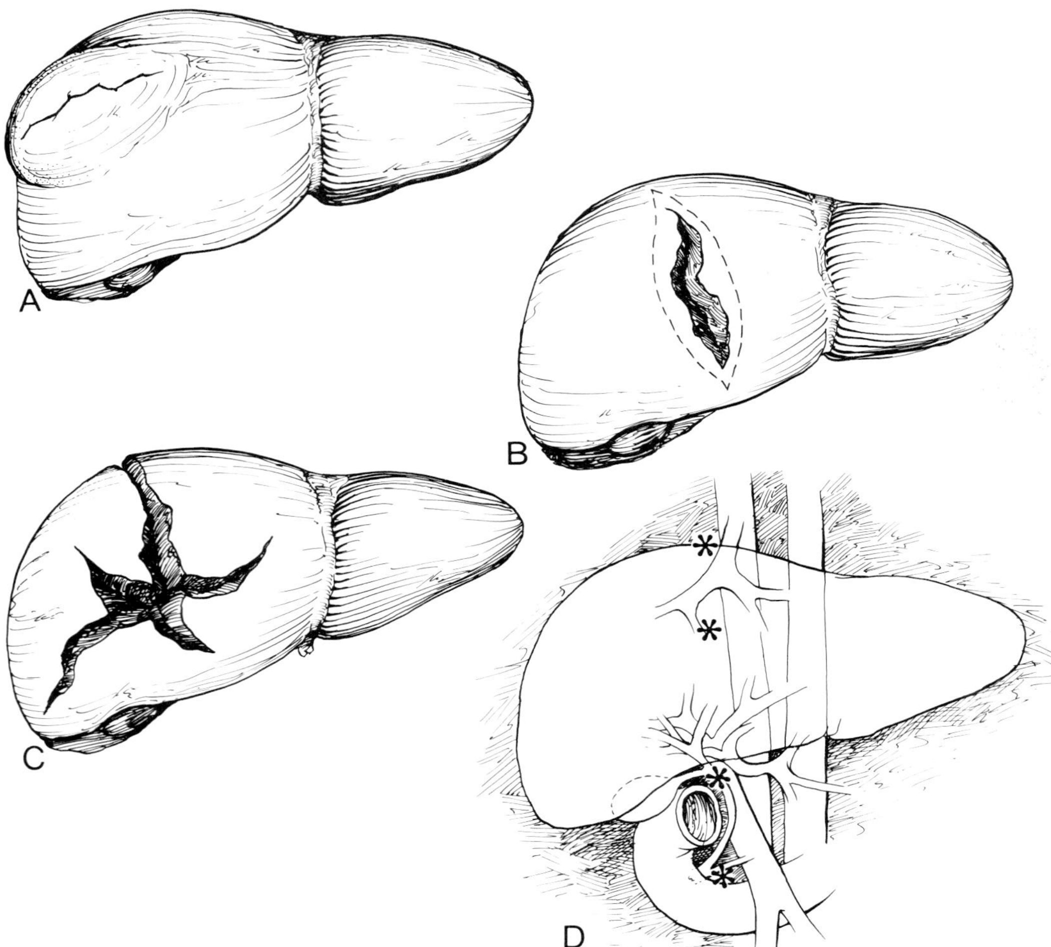

Figure 57.3 Pathophysiology of blunt injury to the liver. (*A*) Subcapsular liver hematoma, (*B*) laceration of liver lobe with adjacent devitalized tissue, (*C*) stellate burst laceration of liver lobe, and (*D*) liver injury may include suprahepatic vena cava, retrohepatic vena cava and portal venous injury (*) and also extrahepatic biliary tree injury (*).

of blood for transfusion (a minimum of one blood volume), and they also require arterial line and central line monitoring in the operating room. Operative treatment may be limited to exploration only, since, if a nonbleeding liver laceration is found, nothing further need be done. Often the injured liver needs debriding and primary suture closure if the laceration is superficial. If the laceration is deep, a debridement and drainage of the site is the preferred treatment. Resection therapy can be done as either a segmental resection, a right or left lobectomy, or as an extended lobectomy or trisegmentectomy as the extent of major lobar injury dictates. Additional treatment modalities include devascularization of the liver in the presence of major liver bleeding with ligation of either the right, the left, or even the common hepatic artery; or treatment may include hepatic arterial embolization with angiographically injected coils or Gelfoam. Extension of the incision into the chest as a sternotomy or anterolateral thoracotomy permits control of both the proximal and distal vena cava which in turn allows placement of an intracaval shunt to facilitate venous return to the right heart in the face of caval injury.

Despite such aggressive therapy for the injured liver, the technical difficulties encountered and problems of associated major vessel injury still produce a high mortality. These patients certainly represent the most severely ill of abdominally injured children.

Biliary Tree Injury

Injury to the extrahepatic biliary system in children, like other aspects of abdominal trauma, is most commonly blunt in origin secondary to right upper quadrant major injury and is most commonly associated with other injuries, particularly to the liver parenchyma. Injury to the biliary tree should be suspected in those children with major right upper quadrant trauma who have blood in their stools. Confirmation of this diagnosis requires the finding of bile in the peritoneal cavity or retroperitoneal space. Such observations may also be due to hepatic parenchymal injury alone. Late presenting biliary tree injury following blunt abdominal trauma include syndromes with anorexia, weight loss, biliary ascites, jaundice and the passage of acholic stools.

The use of operative direct inspection, intravenous cholangiography, or transhepatic cholangiography or direct cholangiography at the operating table are all diagnostic methods to confirm the site of biliary tree injury. It is also possible to do a transduodenal retrograde cholangiographic study by endoscopic technique, a study which allows visualization by contrast injection of the extrahepatic biliary system. The newest diagnostic techniques for biliary tree study involve radionuclide imaging.

Following diagnosis, treatment of biliary tree injuries include direct repair with concommitant ductal decompression through a drainage tube, or a duct anastomosis to a loop of small bowel, usually a Roux-Y choledochojejunostomy. At times cholecystectomy may be combined with such ductal repairs.

Pancreatic Injury

Traumatic pancreatitis is most commonly due to blunt abdominal trauma compressing the pancreas over the body of the vertebral column, resulting in contusion and/or parenchymal disruption with or without ductal disruption (Fig. 57.4). Because of the location of this retroperitoneal structure, associated injuries involving the duodenum, stomach, extrahepatic biliary system and spleen, are all common. Such associated injuries of these structures occur in approximately 50% of patients.

Patients with traumatic pancreatitis most often have diffuse abdominal tenderness, abdominal pain, vomiting, and the findings of the associated injuries. It is not uncommon to palpate a midepigastric mass on abdominal examination secondary to an evolving phlegmon, and it is also not uncommon to find hemodynamic instability which may be due to massive retroperitoneal bleeding or may be due to massive sequestration of third space fluid losses as the pancreatic enzymes are liberated. The presentation with hypovolemic shock secondary to bleeding is uncommon with a pure isolated pancreatic injury, but such a

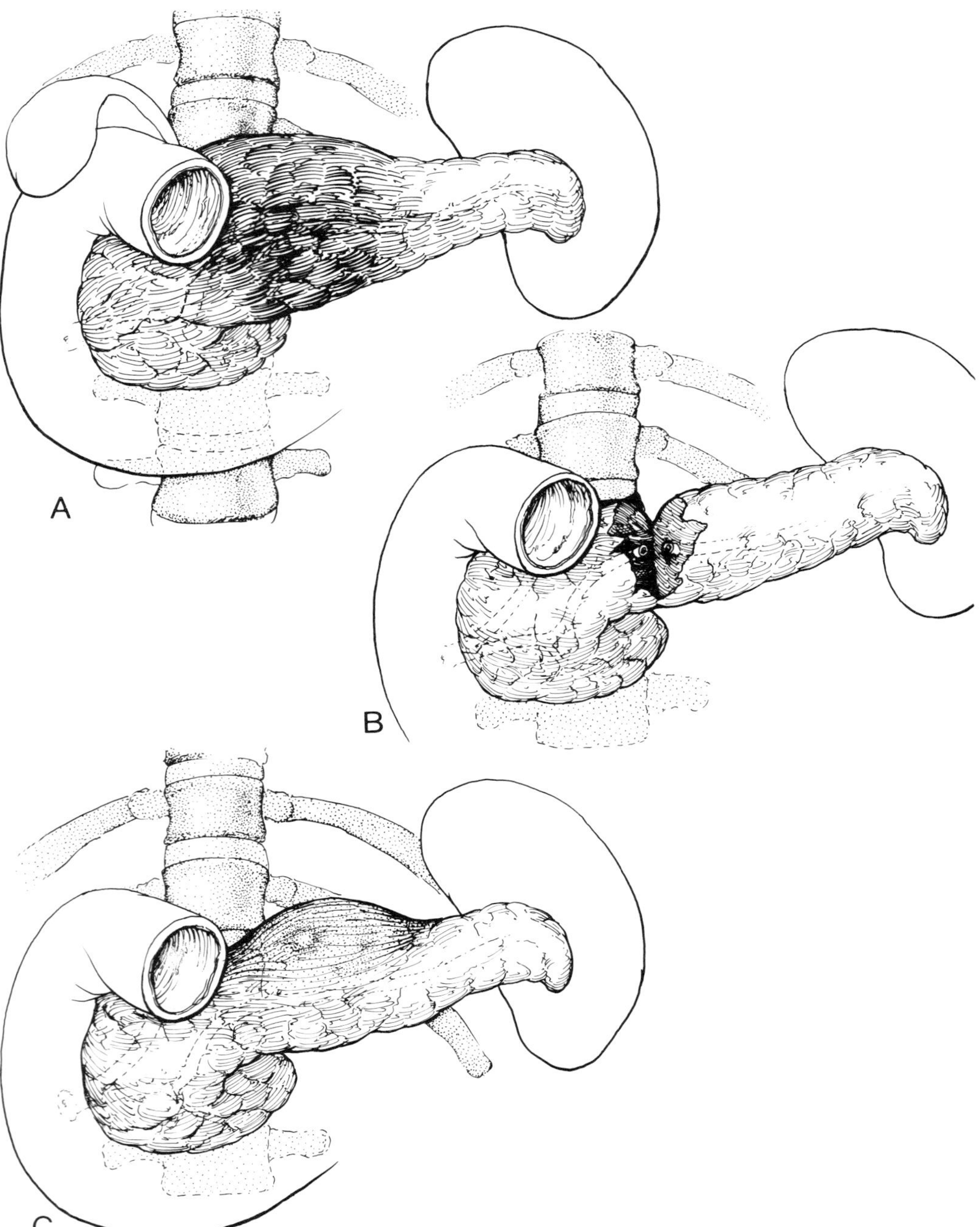

Figure 57.4 Pathophysiology of blunt pancreatic injury. (*A*) Pancreatic contusion and edema, (*B*) pancreatic laceration with ductal disruption, and (*C*) late presenting pancreatic pseudocyst following blunt pancreatic injury with minor ductal disruption.

presentation is more common with associated adjacent major vessel injury.

Laboratory studies to confirm the diagnosis of traumatic pancreatitis commonly rely on the liberation of pancreatic enzymes, usually amylase, since lipase elevation is often delayed until days after the injury. Hyperamalysemia may not occur until 3 to 5 days after pancreatic injury, and the amylase elevation may be missed completely. Because hyperamylasemia itself is a nonspecific finding and may be due to associated renal disease or associated macroamylasemia, a helpful diagnostic adjunct is the measurement of the amylase to creatinine clearance ratio assessing urinary amylase excretion (see Chapter 50). This highly sensitive and specific assay will provide the diagnosis of hyperamylasemia secondary to pancreatic injury. It is also true that an elevated amylase level may be due to a perforated intestine with liberation of pancreatic enzyme directly into the peritoneal cavity. A still more specific confirmation of pancreatic injury is by peritoneal lavage in which the amylase content of the aspirated fluid is elevated, again suggesting the diagnosis of either traumatic pancreatitis or the diagnosis of a perforated viscus.

Roentgenograms may provide confirmation of the diagnosis of traumatic pancreatitis. A barium swallow x-ray shows a widened duodenal C loop, an edematous pancreatic head, and an elevation of the stomach with depression of the transverse colon by a retroperitoneal midabdominal mass. Abdominal sonography is a highly sensitive study for the detection of a traumatically inflamed pancreas, and this study may subsequently be used in a serial fashion to assess alteration of the pancreas due to pseudocyst formation. Specific ductal disruption may also be visualized. The use of endoscopic retrograde choledochopancreatography likewise may show a communicating pancreatic duct and ductal disruption secondary to traumatic injury.

After diagnosis, the preferred treatment of traumatic pancreatitis is medical, if there is no evidence of ductal disruption. The strict use of nasogastric suction to rest the gastrointestinal system is the major treatment modality (see procedures in Section VII). Controversial therapies include the use of anticholinergics, antibiotics, and peritoneal lavage with or without added antibiotics. In addition, a critically important adjunct in the therapeutic protocol is parenteral nutritional support.

Those patients who have findings of traumatic pancreatitis at the time of operative exploration for other intra-abdominal injury can be managed in a variety of ways. The pancreas should be explored after opening the lesser sac and performing a Kocher maneuver of the duodenum to allow thorough palpation of the pancreas from its head to its tail. External drainage with the insertion of sump drains and Penrose drains exited dependently may have great efficacy if there is swelling and edema of the pancreas with evidence of early hemorrhagic change or pancreatic capsule disruption. A distal pancreatectomy with pancreaticojejunostomy of a Roux-Y type or pancreatectomy with ductal ligation is indicated in the face of ductal disruption or a pulverized pancreas lateral to the superior mesenteric vein. It is obvious in children that this should be done with concomitant salvage of the spleen if possible. Partial pancreatectomy may also be done if techncially indicated, removing as much as 85 to 95% of the gland crossing beyond the level of the superior mesenteric vein. It is even possible in children, because of their highly collateralized vascular supply, to do a total pancreatectomy with preservation of the duodenum. This operation is reserved for those severe injuries involving the pancreatic head itself. In very rare circumstances it may be necessary to do an urgent pancreaticoduodenectomy for treatment of traumatic pancreatitis and its associated ductal and/or vascular injuries. The operative finding of a pancreatic head injury with injury to the common bile duct, duodenum, and mesenteric vascular supply poses a tremendous therapeutic challenge. Such major injury requires a great deal of individualization with the aggressive use of primary ductal repairs, stenting, and resection.

Major complications of traumatic pancreatitis in children include the persistence of a pancreatic fistula from the site of ductal disruption which has been purposefully drained or which has spontaneously drained, the development of a pseudocyst which occurs in as many as one third of patients with traumatic pancreatitis accounting for 60% of all pancreatic pseudocysts in children, the development of hemorrhagic pancreatitis which is a severe and often fatal complication, the development of a pancreatic abscess with secondary sepsis, the development of diabetes secondary to pancreatic insufficiency from either injury or resection, and the development of chronic recurring pancreatitis.

Pancreatic pseudocysts present with hyperamylasemia, persistent midepigastric pain, a palpable abdominal mass and vomiting secondary to gastric outlet obstruction. Leukocytosis and fever are often present. The most sensitive technique for the diagnosis of pancreatic pseudocyst is sonography, especially serial sonography. A barium contrast upper GI x-ray can likewise prove helpful to diagnose the presence of a filling defect within the duodenal C-loop compressing the stomach, duodenum and transverse colon. The optimal treatment of a pancreatic pseudocyst includes internal drainage which can be achieved in approximately one half of patients. An interval of 4 to 6 weeks is necessary for the cyst wall to mature, and the cyst can then be decompressed into either the stomach, jejunum, or less preferably, into the duodenum by cystoenteric anastomosis. External drainage utilizing operatively placed single or multiple drainage tubes is necessary in approximately one fourth of patients, and it is even possible to achieve external drainage by placement of a percutaneous sonographically guided catheter. At times, distal pancreatectomy is necessary including the segmental pseudocyst, and at other times a pancreatic pseudocyst will go on to spontaneous but slow resolution. Pseudocysts may be further complicated by abscess formation, by hemorrhage from their wall into the cyst, and by chronicity, developing into chronic pancreatitis.

The mortality of traumatic pancreatitis is directly related to the nature of the injury, the exact anatomic location of the injury, and the associated intra-abdominal problem. The overall mortality of traumatic pancreatitis approaches 1 in 5, but penetrating pancreatic shotgun wounds result in a mortality rate in excess of 50%. Blunt pancreatic trauma has a mortality of 20% while direct stab wound injury has a mortality less than 10%. Mortality is significantly higher in those patients who have pancreatic head injury combined with an injured duodenum and bile duct. Those patients presenting in frank hypovolemic shock likewise have a significantly higher mortality. The major cause of the mortality of traumatic pancreatitis is hemorrhage, pancreatic sepsis, intra-abdominal sepsis, and the associated problems of head injuries, acute pulmonary injury and/or respiratory failure, and acute renal failure in part aggravated by shifts of intravascular volume.

Gastrointestinal Injury

Seemingly trivial blows may disrupt bowel which is filled with postprandial fluid, while more forceful injuries can shear even decompressed bowel at its fixed points at the ligament of Treitz, the ileocecal valve, the ascending and descending colon retroperitoneal reflections, and the peritoneal reflection entered by the bowel at the gastroesophageal hiatus and the distal rectum. Blunt trauma is the most common mechanism accounting for two thirds of such intestinal injuries. The types of injuries include perforation, mesenteric disruption, and traumatic intramural duodenal hematoma.

Perforations of the jejunum, ileum, colon and stomach occur in that order of frequency, and approximately 50% have associated injuries. Diffuse abdominal tenderness with peritoneal signs is most commonly present, and lavage fluid contains bowel content with measured elevated amylase and bilirubin levels; however, x-ray demonstration of pneumoperitoneum occurs in less than 20% of patients.

These injuries require prompt operative intervention for diagnostic confirmation and for repair. The preferred method of repair is an imbrication of damaged but not perforated bowel wall, debridement and closure of small antemesenteric border lacerations, or local resection with primary anastomosis of other intestinal perforations. Colon perforations are best treated by exteriorization because of contamination of the peritoneal cavity, but individual selective management may include primary colonic repair with a proximal protective enterostomy in patients who have minimal peritoneal soiling or especially in patients who have right-sided colonic injuries.

Mesenteric injuries may be minor, involving a laceration in the superficial leaf of the mesentery, to major with disruption of small or even major vascular channels. Mesenteric injury is best treated by reapproximation once hemostasis has been obtained, and assessment must be made of the degree of devascularization of the associated portion of bowel. If major vascular disruption is present involving the superior mesenteric artery or vein then urgent reestablishment of vascular continuity is required. The worst such injury is a superior mesenteric vein disruption which oftentimes is not a retrievable circumstance, the patient succumbing to venous infarction of the entire midgut.

Traumatic intramural duodenal hematomas are secondary to blunt epigastric trauma and result from a disruption of the mucosa and muscularis of the duodenum producing intramural bleeding. Bleeding may be so extensive that rupture of this hematoma may occur into the free peritoneal space; but, more commonly, the hematoma causes compression of the gastric outlet, producing either immediate or delayed obstruction with vomiting. Such patients may also have the associated finding of midepigastric tenderness on palpation. A barium contrast roentgenogram, in addition to showing gastric outlet obstruction with delayed gastric emptying, may show a classic intramural filling defect (Fig. 57.5).

Controversy exists over the optimum management of patients with intramural duodenal hematoma, but it has been our practice to use nasogastric decompression, intravenous nutritional support, and watchful nonoperative management. Such conservative treatment has resulted in success in more than 90% of such patients, the waiting period varying from 1 to 3 weeks. If gastric outlet obstruction persists beyond that time or if there is an associated intra-abdominal injury, then an operative approach to the duodenal hematoma is indicated. Optimum operative therapy is a serosal incision with evacuation of the hematoma and meticulous hemostasis, using fulguration of the small submucosal bleeders. Once this has been achieved, reapproximation of the serosa can be done by suture technique. A less optimal operative management is bypass of the duodenum by a proximal duodenojejunostomy.

Renal Injury

The kidney is the most common solid organ injured when a child sustains blunt abdominal trauma. Of those children sustaining renal injuries secondary to blunt trauma, approximately 40% have other system injury including closed head injuries, spinal cord injuries, fractures, pulmonary injuries, and other intraperitoneal injury. Intraperitoneal injury is especially frequent, involving splenic rupture in approximately 25% of patients who have left-sided kidney injury. The kidney is a highly vulnerable organ to blunt abdominal trauma because in childhood the kidney has a location more anteriorly placed in the peritoneal cavity and since the protecting rib cage and abdominal musculature is less well developed in this age group. In the child with an anatomically normal urinary system, the presence of a lower rib fracture or fracture of a spinal process of the lumbar vertebra should strongly suggest the possibility of a retroperitoneal renal injury. In the face of only minimal abdominal trauma, a major renal injury should suggest the possibility of a coincidental congenital renal anomaly or an intrarenal tumor, such tumors being readily susceptible to minor trauma. It is for these same reasons that children with major renal anomalies should be prohibited from participating in contact sports. As many as 80% of patients with penetrating injury to the kidney will also have other system injury.

The finding of threadlike clots passing via the urethra is almost a sine qua non of major renal injury in childhood. Although some children appear well, they often have flank pain, flank tenderness, and less often peritoneal signs and the presence of a palpable mass. A fluid wave may be elicited on abdominal examination, suggesting urinary ascites, and such patients will likely also have ileus. Shock may be due to either associated sepsis or to a volume deficit secondary to bleeding, and fever may be a part of this presenting picture.

The spectrum of renal injury may be limited to either the kidney proper or to the renal appendages including the renal vascular pedicle or the ureter. Renal parenchymal injuries may be further classified as contusions, small lacerations with an intact capsule, deep lacerations with a disrupted capsule, and deep lacerations penetrating a renal calyx or the renal pelvis (Fig. 57.6). A renal vascular pedicle laceration most commonly presents with shock secondary to

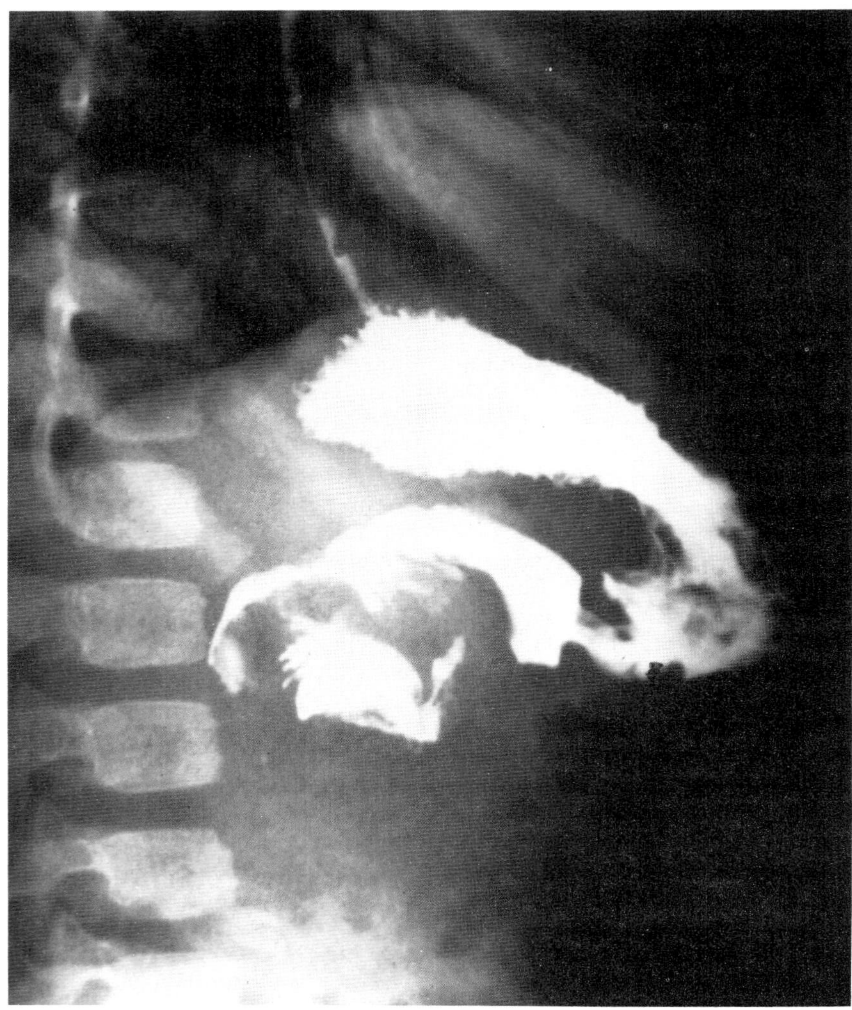

Figure 57.5 Limited upper gastrointestinal barium contrast roentgenogram depicting gastric outlet obstruction secondary to an intraluminal filling defect in the second and third portions of the duodenum. This patient following blunt epigastric trauma was diagnosed as having a duodenal hematoma, and after 3 weeks of nasograstric decompression and intravenous feeding, the patient began to demonstrate normal gastric emptying.

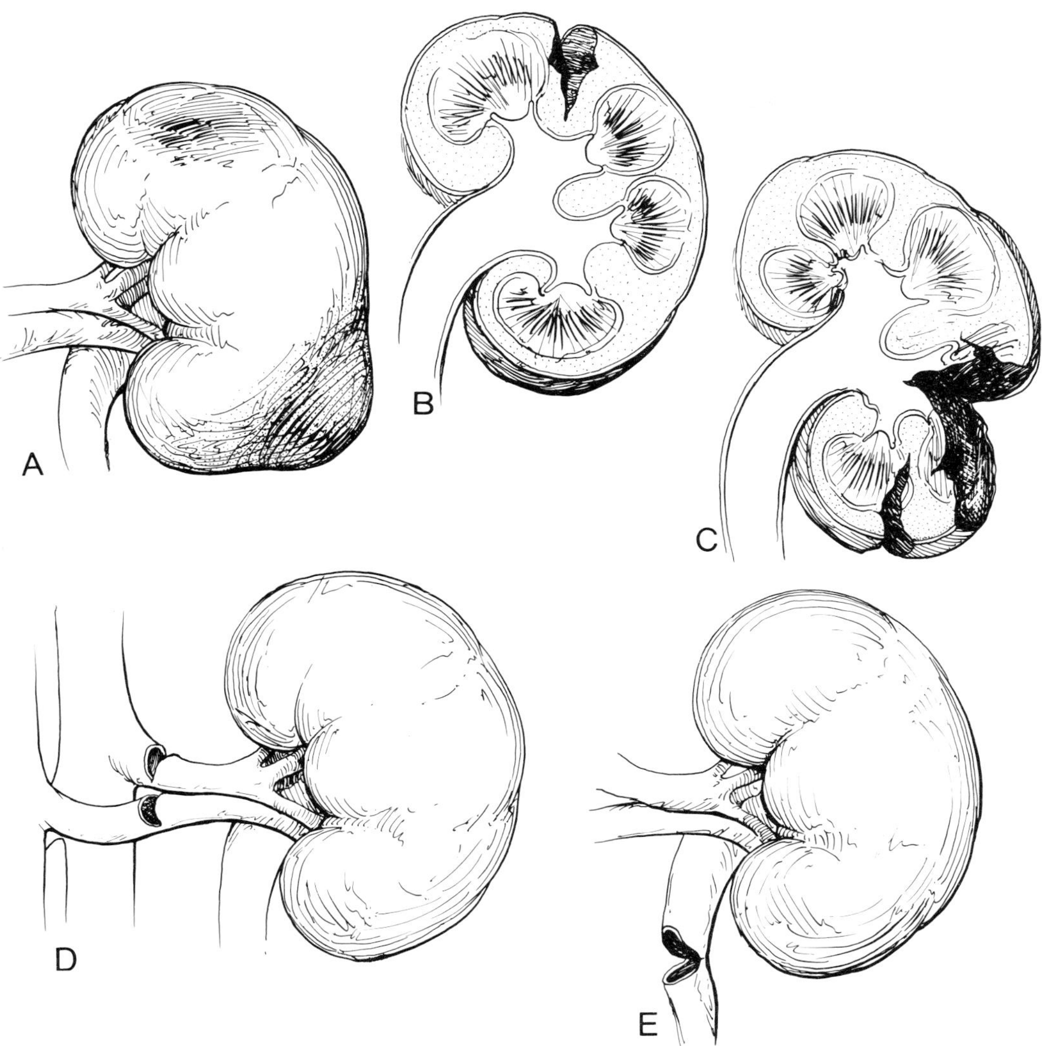

Figure 57.6 Pathophysiology of renal trauma. (*A*) Renal contusion with or without parenchymal hemorrhage, (*B*) parenchymal laceration not involving the collecting system, (*C*) parenchymal laceration extending into the collecting system, (*D*) renal pedicle injury involving the renal artery and vein, and (*E*) ureteric disruption.

both extraperitoneal and intraperitoneal hemorrhage. The ureter itself can be subjected to direct laceration by a penetrating injury, it can sustain a contusion or devascularization by blunt trauma, or it can rupture following a hyperextension injury.

The diagnosis of a renal injury requires classification of both the injured organ plus a confirmation of the integrity of the contralateral kidney. The diagnosis begins with the history and the physical findings as noted and then includes a urinalysis. Urinalysis shows the presence of blood and an increased amount of protein. A urinalysis in which blood is absent does not unequivocally exclude a renal appendage injury secondary to either disruption of the vascular pedicle of the kidney or the ureter itself. In general, the amount of bleeding from a renal parenchymal injury into the urine directly reflects the location of the renal injury, but it is not a direct reflection of injury severity. Plain abdominal x-rays may show obliterated renal and psoas shadows, scoliosis with the concavity toward the injured site, a ground glass appearance of urinary ascites, and a coincident presence of either rib or spinous process fractures of the vertebra. An infusion pyelogram may be diagnostic of renal injury, even in face of hypovolemia. Positive findings include delayed renal function, impaired renal function, extravasation of contrast either within the renal hilum or in the perirenal fat, or pooling of contrast in one area of the kidney also suggesting urinary extravasation. A retrograde ureteropyelogram is helpful especially following an IVP demonstrating nonfunction of the kidneys, in which case a normal retrograde study suggests complete vascular disruption of the renal pedicle. Angiography should be reserved for those patients who have nonvisualization of the kidney or who have a major urinary extravasation in whom flank exploration is indicated. Specifically, angiography will demonstrate extravasation of contrast, displaced or stretched parenchymal or capsular arteries, and vascular narrowing or amputation of occluded or disrupted vessels. Renal scans are useful to assess parenchymal integrity, and sonograms are helpful to show the presence or absence of renal enlargement, perirenal bleeding or urine collections, and the integrity of the urinary drainage system.

It is important to develop a logical evaluation-treatment plan for renal injury. Patients who have blood in their urine require a prompt diagnostic intravenous pyelogram, a study which is best done in the radiology department; however, the IVP can also be done on an unstable patient urgently in the emergency department by administering 2 to 4 ml/kg of 50% diatrizoate sodium intravenously followed by abdominal plain films in 1, 5, and 15 min. Even in the presence of hematuria and flank tenderness, if the IVP is normal, no further intervening therapy is indicated, and conservative bed rest is the treatment of choice until the hematuria has cleared. If a patient has an abnormal IVP with delayed visualization of the kidney or minor extravasation of contrast, again conservative management is indicated. In those patients with either kidney nonvisualization on IVP or with a major urinary extravasation, arteriogram is indicated, and flank exploration is mandatory if vascular interruption is present or if calyceal disruption is severe.

Utilizing these criteria, as many as 80% of renal injured children will be adequately treated by conservative observation and rest alone. Those 20% requiring operation are usually explored for a progressively falling hemoglobin, refractory shock, or clot distention of the urinary bladder following renal injury. The late indications for operative intervention include a perirenal urinoma, recurrent bleeding from the urinary tract, renal infarction with abscess formation, and hypertension secondary to an infarcted and contracted kidney. Only 5 to 7% of all renal injuries result in subsequent nephrectomy, this operation being reserved for those patients with refractory shock and those patients with an irreparable kidney who have had a demonstrated integrity and function of the opposite organ.

Patient problems following renal trauma include those occuring early, such as acute renal failure, secondary hemorrhage, urinary extravasation with or without ascites, shock, and abscess formation. Late sequelae of renal injury include hypertension, stone formation, cyst or hydronephrotic change, caliectasis, arteriovenous fistula, renal atrophy and renal intestinal fistulas.

Bladder-Urethral Injuries

The kidney is located more within the abdomen in children. The distal end of the urinary tract, the bladder, also has a more abdominal location, a factor which renders it more susceptible to blunt and penetrating abdominal injury. In the face of pelvic fracture or sacroiliac joint dislocation, a high suspicion is necessary to show injury to the lower urinary tract. The urogenital diaphragm lying in the juncture of the pubic bones fixes the urethra and makes that structure especially amenable to shearing pelvic forces. With fracture of the anterior pelvis, the anterior and posterior urethra become amenable to such shearing injuries. Similarly, straddle injuries may well injure the urethra as it courses from the bladder in both males and females. Like intestinal injuries which are more prone to occur in the face of a full bowel, a full bladder renders that structure more susceptible to being injured by falls, sharp blows to the abdomen, crush injuries, and penetrating injuries.

On examining the patient with a lower urinary tract injury, the abdominal examination may or may not be positive with peritoneal irritation and a palpable mass. Frank urinary ascites may present with a palpable fluid wave, and peritoneal irritation may exist but not as severely as occurs with fecal contamination of the peritoneal cavity. Close inspection for possible extravasation must be made at the base of the penis, the perineum, and the suprapubic area, noting soft tissue swelling especially

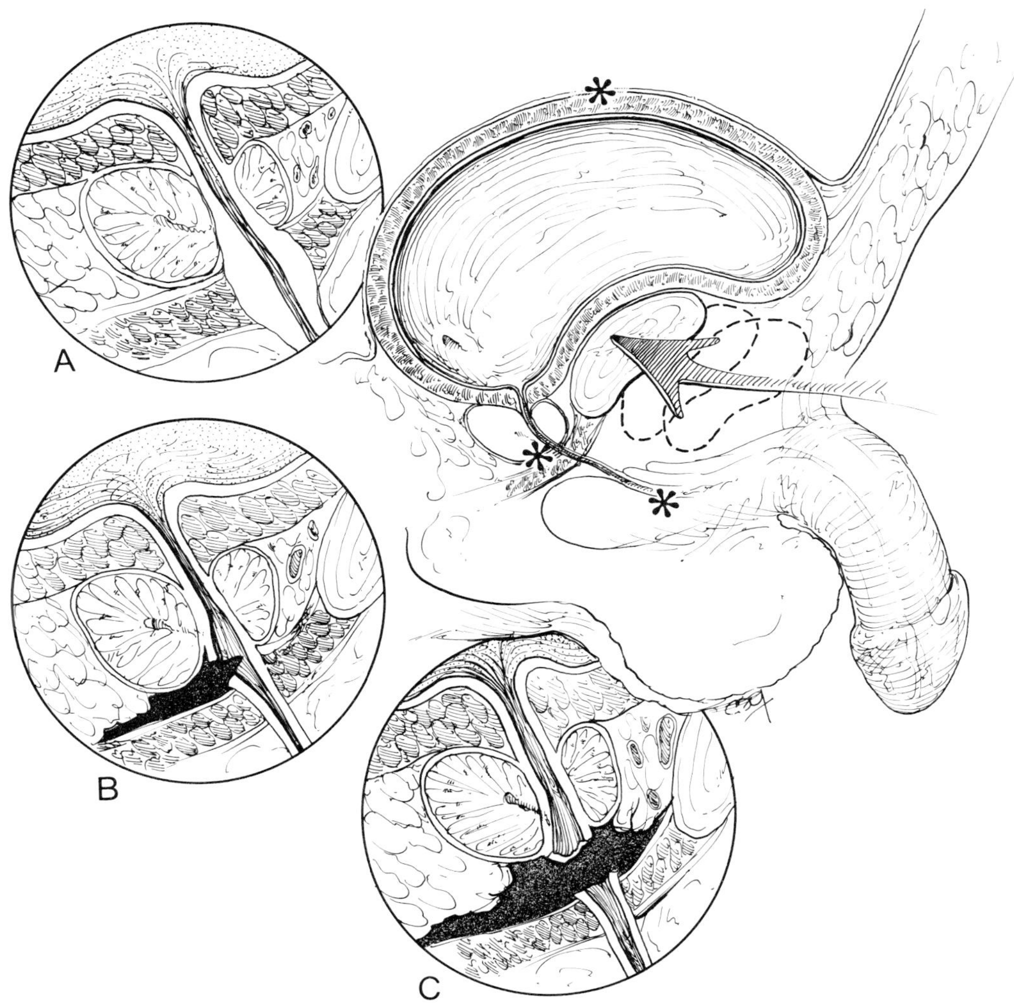

Figure 57.7 Spectrum of urethral trauma following blunt pelvic trauma. (*A*) Urethral contusion should permit catheter placement, (*B*) disruption of the wall of urethra may make catheterization impossible, and (*C*) complete urethral disruption will not permit catheterization and requires diagnostic study with a cystourethrogram.

during voiding. A rectal examination is helpful, especially in males noting an anterior pelvic mass and in detecting disruption and elevation of the bladder and/or prostate gland up and out of the pelvis. This finding is almost diagnostic for urethral disruption.

Evaluation of the patient with a urethral injury is controversial, since the role played by catheterization and by retrograde urethrography varies from one institution to another (Fig. 57.7). Blood at the tip of the urethra suggests a urethral injury, and in such patients a retrograde urethrogram should be done promptly. If there is no blood at the tip of the urethra but the patient has not voided since injury to the pelvis, then gentle catheterization of the urethra is indicated. If the catheter is successfully passed into the bladder, then dye should be instilled and a voiding cystourethrogram done to demonstrate the presence or absence of a disruption of the bladder with or without urinary extravasation. If gentle urethral catheterization is unsuccessful, then a retrograde urethrogram should be done. Throughout these diagnostic and subsequent therapeutic steps in bladder and/or urethral injuries, great detail should be given to the prevention of urinary tract sepsis with the use of sterile technique, urinary suppressant medications, and with the use of prophylactic antibiotics.

The management of a bladder tear may be conservative with transurethral catheterization of the bladder, placing it on drainage for 7 to 10 days. Cystography can then be used to assess timing of catheter removal. Those patients diagnosed as having bladder injury during operation for other injuries or those who have a major extravasation of urine require placement of a suprapubic cystostomy tube.

If the injury is to the urethra itself and catheterization is successful, a 3- to 4-week interval with an indwelling urethral catheter is usually indicated. The decision as to the use of catheter traction is based on the degree of disruption of the urethra and the location of the injury. Whether a urethral injury should be directly repaired using a splint or whether it should be repaired by a delayed urethroplasty is individualized. These patients are especially prone to stricture and its coincident obstructive urinary phenomena with secondary urinary tract infection.

The late sequelae of lower urinary tract injuries can be significant and include urethral strictures with urinary stasis and infection, periurethral fibrotic scarring, urinary incontinence, penile erectile impotence, and infertility.

References

General

American College of Surgeons Committee on Trauma: Multiple trauma; early management in the emergency department. *Bulletin of the American College of Surgeons*, pp. 20–21, February, 1980.

American College of Surgeons Committee on Trauma: Treatment protocol for prehospital management of the trauma patient. *Bulletin of the American College of Surgeons*, pp. 23–27, February 1980.

American College of Surgeons Committee on Trauma: Field categorization of trauma patients and hospital trauma index. *Bulletin of the American College of Surgeons*, pp. 28–33, February 1980.

Champion HR, Sacco WJ, Hannan DS, et al.: Assessment of injury severity; the triage index. *Crit Care Med* 8: 201–208, 1980.

Champion HR, Sacco WJ, Carnazzo AJ, et al.: Trauma score. *Crit Care Med* 9: 672–676, 1981.

Karwacki JJ, Baker SP: Children in motor vehicles; never too young to die. *JAMA* 242: 2848–2851, 1979.

Mayer T, Matlak ME, Johnson DG, et al.: The modified injury severity scale in pediatric multiple trauma patients. *J Pediatr Surg* 15: 719–726, 1980.

Robertson LS: Present status of knowledge in childhood injury prevention. In *Preventing Childhood Injuries*. Report of the Twelfth Ross Roundtable on Critical Approaches to Common Pediatric Problems. Ross Laboratories, Columbus, 1982.

Welch KJ: Abdominal injuries. In *The Injured Child: Surgical Management*, edited by JG Randolph, MM Ravitch, KJ Welch, CD Benson, E. Aberdeen. Year Book, Chicago, 1979.

Blunt Abdominal Trauma

Drew R, Perry JF, Fischer RP: The expediency of peritoneal lavage for blunt trauma in children. *Surg Gynecol Obstet* 145: 885–888, 1977.

Philippart AI: Blunt abdominal trauma in childhood. *Surg Clin North Am* 57: 151–163, 1977.

Penetrating Abdominal Trauma

Freeark RJ: Penetrating wounds of the abdomen. *N Engl J Med* 291: 185–188, 1974.

Wilder JR, Kudchadkar A: Stab wounds of the abdomen; observe or explore? *JAMA* 243: 2503–2505, 1980.

Splenic Trauma

Buntain WL, Lynn HB: Splenorrhaphy; changing concepts for the traumatized spleen. *Surgery* 86: 748–760, 1979.

Ein SH, Shandling B, Simpson JS, et al.: The morbidity and mortality of splenectomy in childhood. *Ann Surg* 185: 307–310, 1977.

Pearson HA: Splenectomy; its risks and its roles. *Hosp Pract* August 85–94, 1980.

Hepatic Trauma

Flint LM, Mays ET, Aaron WS, et al.: Selectivity in the management of hepatic trauma. *Ann Surg* 185: 613–618, 1977.

Frey CF, Trollope M,Harpster W, et al.: A fifteen-year experience with automotive hepatic trauma. *J Trauma* 13: 1039–1049, 1973.

Mays ET: Hepatic trauma. *N Engl J Med* 288: 402–405, 1973.

Pancreatic Trauma

Cooney DR, Grosfeld JL: Operative management of pancreatic pseudocysts in infants and children. *Ann Surg* 182: 590–596, 1975.

Jones RC: Management of pancreatic trauma. *Ann Surg* 187: 555–564, 1978.

Warshaw AL, Fuller AF Jr: Specificity of increased renal clearance of amylase in diagnosis of acute pancreatitis. *N Engl J Med* 292: 325–332, 1974.

Intestinal Trauma

Holgersen LO, Bishop HC: Nonoperative treatment of duodenal hematoma in childhood. *J Pediatr Surg* 12: 11–17, 1977.

Genitourinary Trauma

Uson AC, Lattimer J: Genitourinary tract injuries. In *The Injured Child: Surgical Management,* edited by JG Randolph, MM Ravitch, KJ Welch, CD Benson, E Aberdeen. Year Book, Chicago, 1979.

CHAPTER 58

Minor Trauma and Minor Lesions

JOHN M. TEMPLETON, JR., M.D., AND MORITZ M. ZIEGLER, M.D.

LACERATIONS

BACKGROUND

The presence of a bleeding wound is popularly recognized as a true emergency, so children who have incurred lacerations are generally brought to the emergency department for immediate care.

Approximately 10% of all patients seen in the Emergency Department of Children's Hospital presented for the management of traumatic injuries. Of these 7,440 injured children, 93% were less than 14 years of age and 61% were male. The most common forms of injury were abrasions or contusions (32%) and lacerations (27.6%). Puncture wounds accounted for 3% and foreign bodies for 3.6%. The site of injury was the head and face in 40%, the hand in 12%, and the foot in 5%. The injuries occurred in the following locales: home (63%), street (11%), sports (9%), school (7.5%), and miscellaneous (9.5%).

In treating a child with a laceration, the first priority is controlling blood loss, both before and after arrival in the emergency department. The second priority is protecting the wound. After controlling the bleeding and protecting the wound, the next priority is a thorough assessment of the wound and any associated injuries. The following clinical manifestations serve to guide one's assessment and treatment plans.

CLINICAL MANIFESTATIONS

The emergency physician should consider the following questions in assessing the clinical manifestations of presumed minor trauma:

1. Does the appearance of the wound correlate with the history given? Was the basis of the laceration a blunt or sharp object? Blunt objects suggest the possibility of underlying fractures or crush injury. Sharp objects suggest the possibility of a laceration of deeper structures.
2. Does the history and location of the laceration suggest other possible injuries? Particularly in the neck area, the relatively superficial location and close proximity of multiple organ systems increase the possibility that a serious injury has occurred if the laceration extends through the platysma.
3. Does examination of the wound area suggest deeper injuries, such as the presence of crepitance in the subcutaneous tissue in wounds of the chest and neck?

Tissue Devitalization

All lacerations raise immediate concern regarding the viability of the tissues in and around the wound area. A crush injury-type laceration in particular is more likely to lead to contused devitalized tissue which may require debridement before closure.

Impaired Circulation

In distal body parts such as the fingers, toes, nose, and ears, viability of tissue more distal to the point of injury may be jeopardized as a result of severe proximal vascular compromise. Consideration of circulation is important in two regards: first, to assure hemostasis in the wound; and second, to assure that there will be adequate blood supply at the interface of the wound and to the more distal tissues.

Venous Bleeding

Brisk, continuous flow of dark venous-type blood will indicate that at least a major superficial vein has been injured. Most venous bleeding encountered in lacerations is superficial to the fascia in the area where the laceration occurred. These bleeding veins can generally be safely tamponaded. Subsequently they can be specifically clamped and ligated or sutured.

Arterial Bleeding

More difficult to manage is a wound which demonstrates a major spurting arterial bleed. The amount and rapidity of blood flow often makes it difficult to see precisely the site of the bleeding. It is important to do everything one can to stem potential life-threatening bleeding. In the extremities, in particular, most arterial bleeding can be effectively tamponaded locally; but, if necessary, the bleeding also can be controlled by more proximal occlusion of the involved artery. Such proximal occlusion is generally not well maintained by a tourniquet or even the use of a blood pressure cuff because venous return is also impeded, increasing the amount of bleeding. Also, if the tourniquet or cuff is kept on too long, potential nerve damage may occur. Ideally, one will identify the proximal major arterial component, such as the brachial artery, and tamponade it against the adjacent bone with the use of one's fingers. One should resist the temptation to clamp blindly in the area of a major spurting arterial bleed because these arteries usually travel as part of a neurovascular bundle. Blind clamping of the artery may further damage the artery, and worse, may result in a severe crush injury of an associated nerve. The morbidity of a crushed sensory and/or motor nerve may be much worse than that of the original wound.

Nerve Damage

In the extremities, in particular, potential nerve damage must always be assessed. In the child, complex motor testing of the median and ulnar nerve, for example, may not be possible. Fortunately, in most situations, the possible site at which a nerve injury occurs will involve both motor and sensory function. One can, therefore, usually rely on pin-prick testing to provide an adequate neurological assessment. Only in the severely obtunded or comatose patient will one be unable to show the expected withdrawal reaction in response to pricking the skin with a pin over the distal sensory dermatome distribution in question.

Tendon Injury

Functions such as the ability to extend or flex the fingers also may be difficult to evaluate in the child who is too young to understand or too upset to cooperate. Simple inspection of the natural posture of the hand and fingers, however, will often demonstrate an underlying tendon injury. As seen in Figure 58.1, a flexor tendon injury, particularly involving the superficial tendon, will result in an abnormal posture of the involved finger. Extensor tendon injuries can be demonstrated by showing an inability to withdraw the finger in question from a noxious pin prick on the flexor surface. A wound which is wide enough and deep enough may demonstrate an actual severed tendon. For example, a laceration on the flexor surface of the forearm might reveal the cut end of the tendon when the hand and wrist is placed in full passive flexion.

MANAGEMENT

In general, superficial wounds of the trunk, arms, legs, and scalp can be managed in the emergency department. However, even these superficial injuries require the same rigorous standards for handling damaged tissue as would apply in an operating room. Our goal is to create an ideal environment for early or late primary wound healing. The general principles of wound management are listed in Table 58.1. An optimally treated wound will have less inflammation, more rapid healing, and consequently less scar formation. Discussion of principles of managing facial lacerations can be found in Chapter 64.

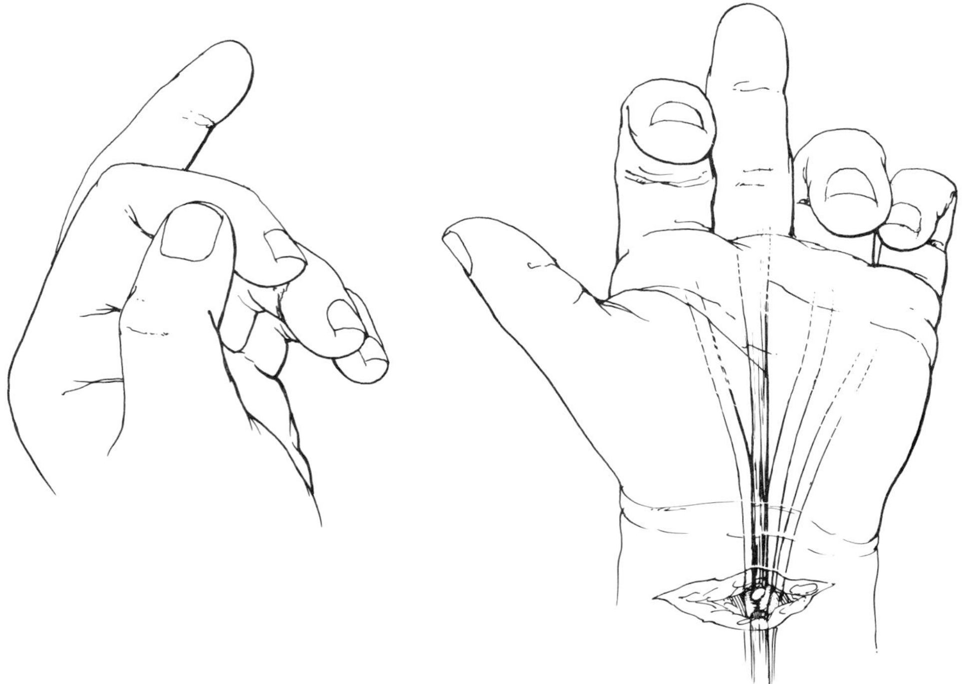

Figure 58.1 A seemingly superficial laceration at the wrist might be treated simply by closure of the subcutaneous tissue and skin unless one appreciates the abnormal posture of the middle finger when the hand is at rest. The loss of normal flexor tone due to a divided superficial tendon results in the involved finger lying in a position of relative extension.

Table 58.1
General Principles of Wound Management

1. *Remove all foreign bodies* (gravel, grass, dirt, clothing, etc.)
2. *Debride devitalized tissue.* Any badly contused or damaged tissue should be debrided back to the point at which normal capillary bleeding is encountered
3. *Avoid leaving a dead space* in the depth of the wound
4. Minimize the final bacterial count in the wound by thorough saline lavage. Use gloves whenever the wound is examined
5. *Maximize the blood supply* to the wound. Do not use anesthetic agents with epinephrine in terminal structures, such as the fingers, nose, or ears. Do not use tourniquets on fingers, and avoid letting the wound dry out from prolonged exposure
6. *Avoid using or placing any noxious material in the wound* which might lead to local tissue damage and increased inflammation. Therefore, when one is soaking a wound such as a cut foot or cut hand, use a mild or dilute antiseptic solution, and rely on mechanical cleansing rather than strong antiseptics

Initial Triage

Calm the Child and Family. One should specifically assure the child and the family that the child will be well taken care of and that pain will be avoided insofar as possible.

Remove Blood. Removal of blood or any bloody items from the area of the wound provides an early visual reassurance that the laceration is indeed being cared for.

Protect Wound from Further Tissue Damage. Until you are actually ready to clean and assess the wound in detail, keep the wound surface covered. Use of a saline moistened gauze pad will prevent the already compromised tissue at the interface of the wound from desiccating and dying.

Apply Pressure. Apply pressure on the gauze pads overlying the wound to tamponade most types of bleeding.

Explore Wound. Explore the wound only when using gloves and mask.

Lavage Wound Thoroughly. Contaminated wounds, in particular, require immediate lavage with copious amounts of sterile saline. Lavage with several hundred milliliters of saline will result in lower bacterial count and potentially less foreign material or devitalized tissue in the wound.

Assess Extent of Injury. Decide as soon as possible whether the wound could be best managed in the emergency department or is extensive and serious enough to warrant repair in the operating room. If there is any doubt, one should not hesitate to arrange for surgical consultation with someone who is more experienced in the management of wounds. The decision to take the child to the operating room will depend on (1) the depth and extensiveness of the wound; (2) the potential for specific injuries to arteries, tendons; and (3) the question of cosmesis particularly when dealing with severe facial injuries.

Preparing the Child

When dealing with children in the setting of an emergency department, one has to keep in mind that one is treating both the wound itself and the child who has incurred the wound. Ideally, the treating physician will have been able to build up sufficient rapport with the child so that the child will not be unduly emotionally traumatized by the experience, and yet, will receive the appropriate optimal care of the wound. In order of importance the factors which make for a quiet, nonstressful repair of a wound in a child are as follows.

A simple open and frank relationship with the child works best. It may help for the child to see enough of his/her wound to understand what one needs to do to "fix it." The child needs to understand that everything will be done to make it as painless as possible. When some pain is anticipated, such as with the installation of anesthetic medication, the child needs to know that the pain is about to occur but that it is limited and will soon disappear. Most children who are 6 years old or older will accept the need for brief mild pain in order to proceed with a painless nonstresful repair of the wound. The two most reassuring features of this rapport are continued verbal and visual interaction. The child who knows and understands each step of the entire wound management process will be the one who will cooperate most readily.

A relaxed helpful parent is always a great reassurance to the child that they will not be harmed. Often a child will more readily accept a parent holding an injured hand or an arm or placing a hand on each side of the face to stabilize a facial wound than he will accept the restraining hand of a stranger. The parent's own verbal reassurance of the child may also help to calm the child. The physician needs to use both intuition and direct questioning of the parent to be sure, however, that the parent feels comfortable enough to assume this role.

A sympathetic but firm nurse or aide can also be a great help. Often, in a few moments, a surprising rapport can be established between the child and the nurse or aide, as "together" they go through the process of getting "fixed up."

Some children, who may only be 3 to 4 years of age, seem to become mesmerized by the whole process of being cared for in the emergency department. With the same approach as suggested for the older child, these children often will be amazingly cooperative. In general, however, for most younger children and for the occasional anxious and uncontrollable older child, some manner of restraint is required. The younger the child, the easier it is to secure most of the noninjured portions of the body in some form of blanket wrap or "papoose" device. Even with such devices, one needs to have sufficient assistance to hold down the injured area to ensure proper sterile draping and precise wound repair.

Preparing the Wound

Once the child has been prepared and the area of the wound has been initially inspected and cleaned, an antiseptic solution can be painted in a wide area around the margins of the wound. It is often difficult to keep the antiseptic solution out of the wound. This is not a problem so long as one remembers to later lavage this material out of the wound. If a final decision has not yet been made, one needs to decide on the basis of a final inspection whether the wound should best be managed by healing by primary intention (restore all tissue layers), healing by secondary intention (by granulation tissue and wound contracture), or healing by delayed primary closure (initial drainage and cleaning followed by subsequent reapposition of the tissue layers). The occasional wounds which one may elect to leave open will be discussed below.

Anesthetic Preparation

As most wounds in an emergency department are repaired by primary closure, one needs to plan for appropriate wound anethesia. Most wounds can be adequately anesthetized by instilling Xylocaine solution (1% in most cases) around the periphery of the wound for a distance of 1 to 1.5 cm by using a fine 25 gauge needle. Since the wound is already open, it is usually less painful to instill the Xylocaine along the interface of the dermis and subcutaneous tissue by slowly injecting the anesthetic as one advances the needle. Using this technique, the anesthetic often advances ahead of the needle resulting in little or no discomfort. Other anesthetic agents and techniques are discussed in Chapter 3. If one is sure of the precise nerve supply to an area in question, one could alternatively perform a regional block by anesthetizing the nerve proximal to the point of the injury.

For finger lacerations it is often helpful, however, to produce a bilateral digital block (see procedure in Section VII), because many areas of injury in a finger will have an overlapping nerve supply from either side of the finger. These finger blocks are best peformed at the level of the web of the fingers. After anesthetizing the skin on each side, one can advance a small 25 or 26 gauge needle through the subcutaneous tissue instilling a small amount of Xylocaine as the needle is advanced. The digital nerves run just superficial to the periosteum of the phalanges. Once the needle hits the periosteum, one should first aspirate and then instill 1 to 2 ml slowly, so as to surround the trunk of the digital nerve with the anesthetic. After approximately 5 to 10 min the anesthetic will have taken effect, and the finger distal to injection site will be well anesthetized.

General Technical Points in Primary Wound Closure

Before proceeding with actual closure of the wound, one should review once again the general principles as enumerated in Table 58.1.

Identify all the layers which have been injured, such as fascia, subcutaneous tissue and skin. Plan to appose each of the lacrated layers as nearly as possible back to its original location.

Select a suture which will have adequate strength but which also will result in as little inflammation of the tissue and skin as possible. In this regard, the use of long lasting absorbable sutures such as Dexon or Vicryl is usually a good choice.

Make sure that, when the sutures are placed, they enter and exit the appropriate layer at the same level so that one margin of the wound will not overlap the opposite margin.

Insofar as possible, minimize the extent to which one uses forceps in repairing the particular tissue layer.

To assure proper alignment, place the first suture in each layer at the midpoint of the wound and then place subsequent sutures lateral to the midpoint.

Skin Closure

A wound which has been well closed in layers does not usually need large or tight skin sutures to complete the closure. The skin in general should be closed with a monofilament nylon. One should aim to appose the skin layers with the minimal amount of tension. One can often use tape strips (e.g. Shur Strips, Steri-Strips, Clearon) in between the sutures to take up much of the tension at the wound margin and thereby minimize the extent to which the sutures may tend to cut into the skin.

Quite acceptable wound repair can be accomplished by using either interrupted or continuous monofilament suturing of the skin. It is important to remember, however, that all wounds after repair go through a stage of inflammation that involves increased edema and swelling. As a result, the suture placed in the emergency department which appeared to be perfectly placed may in fact begin to cut into the tissue over the course of the next few days.

A suture which is particularly effective in apposing the skin edge with a minimum of immediate and delayed tension is a "loop knot" interrupted simple suture. As shown in Figure 58.2, a loop knot involves placement of a surgeon's knot followed by a loop. As a result, when edema develops the sur-

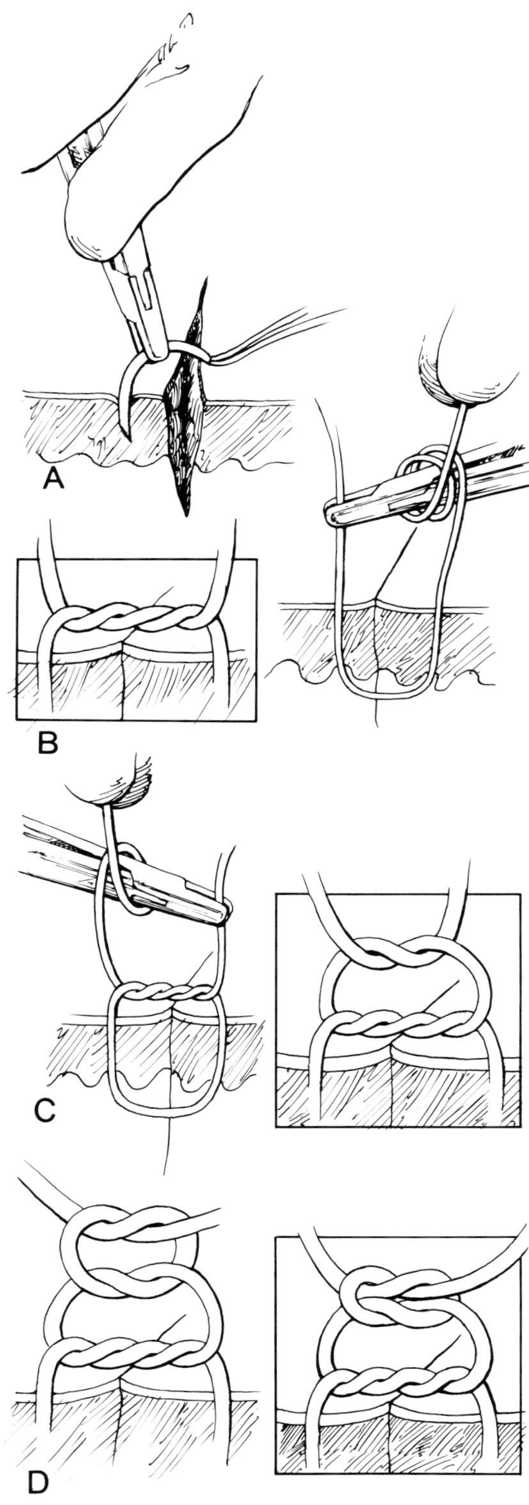

Figure 58.2. Placement of a "loop knot" in conjunction with simple sutures of the skin using an eversion technique. (*A*) The needle enters the skin at a right angle in a way which allows somewhat less skin and more subcutaneous tissue to be caught in the passage of the needle. The needle should incorporate the same amount of skin and subcutaneous tissue on each side. The ideal suture material for placing a "loop knot" is 4-0 nylon. One can also use 5-0 nylon. (*B*) The first knot should be a surgeon's knot drawn down gently so as to barely coapt the skin edges. (*C*) The second tie should be placed so as to produce a square knot but should be drawn down so as to produce an approximate 2-to 3-mm loop. (*D*) The third tie should be placed so as to produce a square knot. This third tie can be secured tightly against the second tie, preserving the loop and allowing for some loosening of the surgeon's knot spontaneously as later edema develops.

geon's knot gives somewhat. This minimizes the garroting effect on the tissue. If one removes sutures, it becomes apparant that there are many wounds in which it is quite difficult to get the sutures out because they have cut so deeply into the skin. A properly placed "loop knot" suture is easily removed, because there is often a free space between the suture and the skin allowing for virtually painless suture removal.

An alternative to the use of full thickness skin sutures is the use of a fine absorbable suture such as Dexon or Vicryl. Such suture materials, however, do elicit an inflammatory response. Furthermore, if these subcuticular sutures are too close to the epithelial layer of the skin, they may extrude before the body has had a chance to absorb the suture material. If one uses subcuticular sutures, it is important to make sure that the suture material is placed on the deeper surface of the dermis and that the epithelial margins are approximated with tape strips.

A third way of managing skin wounds is the use of tape strips (e.g. Shur Strips, Steri-Strips or Clearon) alone. Certainly many simple lacerations that extend barely through the dermis can be managed with local wound cleaning followed by application of an adhesive such as benzoin. The tape strips can be used to obtain wound alignment. One type of soft tissue wound which clearly does best with tape strips is the multiple tangential triangular skin flaps produced when an unrestrained passenger smashes head first into a windshield. Because windshields in the United States are composed of laminated glass and plastic, a smashed windshield becomes a surface with a thousand or more tiny razor blade-like projections. As a result, a patient whose face has smashed into such a windshield may have 50 or more tangential, triangular flap lacerations on the face. After the face is cleaned, one can use a sterile cotton-tipped application to apply small amounts of benzoin, followed by single ⅛-inch tape strips cut to size. Even with the use of tape strips, however, one has to be careful to obtain proper realignment of the dermis and epithelium. If one, for example, pulls too tightly on the triangular flap with a tape strip one may obtain an overlap of the flap on top of the opposite margin of the wound. As a result, the wound will heal with a raised ridge-like area where the overlap occurred.

Special Situations

Because of both function and cosmesis, the face often presents special problems in repairing lacerations in this area. Please refer to Chapters 61 and 64 for further pointers and guidelines in regard to facial lacerations.

Wounds with Flaps. Many wounds are made more difficult by the fact that they are tangential, involving flaps of skin, and subcutaneous tissue of varying depths and varying angles. Particularly difficult are stellate wounds in which two or more corners of the wound have sharp angles at the tip. In apposing such skin margins, it is best to rely on a subcutaneous or subcuticular suture to hold the tips of these stellate flaps together. A single such suture will usually provide good apposition without further damaging or devitalizing the tip of flap. Then along the lateral margins of the wound, other interrupted sutures can be placed to provide further support.

When repairing a wound with a prominent flap, it is important to place the needle in the flap edge first. Then one can move the edges of the flap back and forth until proper alignment with the opposite fixed side is obtained.

Eyebrow Lacerations. Do not shave the eyebrows even when a laceration goes directly through the eyebrow. Repair such wounds as carefully and completely as one would elsewhere. After the sutures are in place, look to make sure that no hairs of the eyebrow are caught inside the wound. If they are, use a needle to simply lift these hairs out of the wound and free of the suture material.

Nose and Ears. One should avoid using epinephrine when anesthetizing these structures. Thorough wound cleansing is essential. The development of a secondary infection and chondritis can be disastrous. Dissolution and loss of all the involved cartilage can occur due to rapidly spreading infections, especially those caused by *Streptococcus.*

Lip and Other Skin Lines. The realignment of skin lines and anatomical margins such as vermilion border of the lip are particularly critical in handling facial lacerations (see Chapter 64).

Scalp. In handling many deep lacerations to the scalp, the amount of bleeding can be prodigious. Often, one cannot tell whether there are specific bleeding vessels which need to be suture ligated before closing the wound. In wounds of the scalp it is quite acceptable to locally instill Xylocaine with epinephrine. As a result, the arteriolar branches in this area will constrict, causing a cessation of arteriolar flow. Larger arteries or veins will not cease bleeding, and therefore, can be more readily identified and secured with sutures. Because the scalp is under significant tension, a certain amount of firmness in tying the skin knots is needed to keep the skin edges together. Because wounds in the hair-bearing area of the scalp are of less cosmetic concern, it is acceptable to tie down the skin suture more tightly than one would do elsewhere. Firm but not strangulating apposition of a wound is also an excellent way to obtain hemostasis.

Dressing

No one would question the need for a strong splint or cast to immobilize a fractured bone; soft tissue wounds benefit just as much from splinting. A wound of the hand will heal more slowly and with greater scar formation, if the hand is allowed to be used actively after the wound has been repaired. All wounds, but particularly those in "active" areas such as the hand, and around the joints, should be carefully dressed after being repaired. This is particularly important for children, as they are likely to quickly resume full activity. A somewhat loose but very bulky splinting type dressing will minimize any motion along the wound interface.

Tetanus Management

The next management consideration is tetanus prophylaxis. Although the amnestic response to a prior tetanus immunization is often quite good 10 years after a complete immunization program, many patients cannot recall exactly when they received their last immunization. If it is clear that the patient has had a prior adequate immunization series, then a booster of tetanus toxoid should be given 5 or more years after a previous dose of tetanus toxoid. In dealing with some children there may be real doubt as to whether the patient has ever had an adequate tetanus immunization. Chapter 45 details tetanus prophylaxis. The use of Hyper-tet is not appropriate for routine outpatient wound management. Occasionally, in wounds associated with massive tissue destruction and contamination, the use of Hyper-tet may be indicated. Patients with such wounds will be admitted to the hospital for further care and management.

Suture Removal

The optimal time to remove skin sutures is when the early fibroblastic proliferation at the wound interface has become strong enough to take the place of the sutures. Sutures left in longer than necessary contribute to unnecessary tissue reaction around the tract of the suture and may therefore contribute to long-term visible cross hatching, so called "railroad ties." The timing of suture removal, therefore, is related to the quality of the blood supply and the tensions at the wound interface. As a general guideline, the more superior portions of the body have better blood supply and seem to heal more quickly. With the exception of the neck, the average time for suture removal increases the lower one gets in the body. Although the neck does not have quite as good blood supply as the face and the scalp, the tensions on neck wounds are not as great as they are in the scalp, which is stretched tightly across the calvarium, or in the face, where so many muscles of expression are involved. Table 58.2 gives general guidelines for removal of sutures from different areas of the body.

In locations of the body where cosmesis is important, one may plan to remove the sutures somewhat sooner than the schedule

Table 58.2
Timing for Suture Removal

Area	Time (days)
Neck	3–4
Face and scalp	5
Eyelids	3
Trunk and upper extremities	7
Lower extremities	8–10

and to reinforce the wound margins with tape strips. One can actually plan ahead for such treatment by placing tape strips in between each interrupted suture at the time the sutures are placed.

Wound Healing by Secondary Intention or by Delayed Primary Closure (DPC)

The decision to leave a wound open for a short period of time or until complete healing has occurred is largely based on concerns about secondary wound infections should one attempt a primary closure. The occurrence of a secondary wound infection results not only in a markedly enhanced inflammatory response but a prolonged period of healing for the wound. In certain areas, such as the face, a secondary wound infection may even become life-threatening if the infection spreads by means of lymphatics and venules into the deeper structures of the head and neck such as the cavernous sinus.

By contrast, if a wound is left open and allowed to heal entirely by secondary intention, the inflammatory response will be prolonged even in the absence of a spreading infection. The resulting scar formation will impair cosmesis and possibly even function. By aiming for an optimal tissue environment for wound healing, one can manage even contaminated wounds in such a manner that will allow for little or no infection risk and rapid healing.

Four examples of wounds where one has to make a decision in regard to infection and primary wound healing are: (1) animal bites, especially human bites; (2) lacerations incurred in a contaminated locale such as a garbage dump or barnyard; (3) lacerations of the feet; and (4) lacerations which occurred many hours before the patient is brought to the emergency department.

When such wounds are large enough that the subcutaneous tissue and even fascial layers are exposed, one would normally prefer after thorough cleansing to close the tissue layers primarily. The subcutaneous tissue, however, has the least good blood supply and the greatest potential for secondary wound infection. If the risk of secondary wound infection seems real, one should leave at least the subcutaneous layer open.

The wound is dressed by placing a moistened fine mesh gauze along the surfaces of the wound and then gently wrapping the area with a bulky dressing. A wound left open in this manner will be able to drain and largely sterilize itself while it is developing early granulation tissue. The use of antiseptic solutions such as Betadine, with the fine mesh gauze will not necessarily improve the ability of the wound to get rid of any potential infection, but such agents are usually somewhat tissue toxic and will, therefore, probably stimulate an enhanced inflammatory response, resulting in an earlier development of healthy granulation tissue.

Open wounds should be checked at least daily or every other day to be sure that no unexpected complications are developing. The fine mesh gauze along the margins of the wound is best removed at about 3 days time. If the development of fresh healthy granulation tissue is not complete at this point, one can apply another layer of fine mesh gauze to the surfaces of the wound with or without an antiseptic solution. Usually by the fifth day, the development of healthy granulation tissue is well advanced. At this point most such wounds can be easily handled by DPC. After meticulously cleansing the wound and sterilely draping it, one can use the same careful techniques as discussed above to obtain closure of the subcutaneous tissue and skin with the combination of sutures and tape strips. In most cases the potential for secondary infection has been eliminated. As a result, these wounds will heal very quickly.

Some potentially contaminated wounds

however, may require primary closure. When cosmesis is involved, such as with an animal bite of the face, it may be appropriate to proceed with a primary repair. In such circumstances, the repair is usually best done in the operating room with preoperative and postoperative intravenous antibiotic coverage. The common procedure of not closing a wound older than 12 hours may be violated for certain low risk wounds. While one might choose, for example, to leave open a 6-hour-old badly contaminated crush wound, an 18-hour-old clean knife wound laceration may be closed safely.

Finally, some wounds are always best left open and allowed to heal entirely by secondary intention. Many puncture wounds of the foot, for example, involve a fairly small laceration. Because of the fibrous structures supporting the skin of the sole of the foot, these wounds already tend to lie in apposition. When the object producing the laceration is unknown or is determined to be contaminated, it may be safer to consider placing a small, sterile wick, e.g., a piece of ¼-inch iodoform gauze, inside the wound in order to keep the skin edges open. After 3 days, one can usually remove the wick, and the subsequent granulation tissue will contribute to rapid healing. If one is particularly concerned about the potential for a secondary infection, one can place a small, sterile rubber drain inside the wound which will facilitate drainage.

The decision to use *antibiotics* for protection against secondary wound infection is based on one's assessment of (1) the amount of tissue destruction, (2) the area of the body injured, and (3) the nature and extent of the contamination involved. Crush injuries are particularly likely to occur when a blunt object hits with force against an underlying bony structure. Areas in which this is particularly likely to occur are the face, skull, and extremities. Beyond the tissue which can be seen in the wound, there may be deeper, hidden areas of tissue destruction. In such cases, the use of antibiotics plus optimal local wound care may help to retard the development of a secondary wound infection.

Certain injuries are of particular concern. These include exposure and contamination of the cartilage of the nose or ears, extensive facial wounds which may involve contamination from adjacent nasal passages or sinus cavities, and wounds in the perineum. Once again, the use of antibiotics may help to retard or avoid a secondary wound infection. Finally, some soft tissue injuries are best viewed as being contaminated beginning at the time of the injury. Such injuries include cases of human bites, or injuries which occur along a roadside or in a trash disposal or barnyard area.

If one is worried enough about a wound to consider using antibiotics, such a patient should probably be admitted to the hospital. The route of the antibiotics in such cases should be intravenous. Although the most common secondary wound infections are due to *Staphylococcus aureus*, it is worth considering a broad enough spectrum antibiotic so that other contaminants may be treated as well. For badly contaminated wounds, one should, therefore, consider the use of high dose intravenous penicillin and tobramycin which will provide a much broader antibacterial coverage than for *S. aureus* alone. As indicated above, the use of antibiotics may be particularly important where one has had to make some compromise in handling the wound for the sake of cosmesis as in the case of a patient with an animal bite to the face.

MINOR LESIONS

Besides lacerations, children are often brought to the emergency department for a variety of minor lesions. Some of these represent true emergencies. Other lesions are not true emergencies but may be considered so by an anxious parent who has just noted an area of discoloration or swelling. The true emergencies are usually associated with pain and/or infection. Conditions such as subungual hematoma, paronychia, subungual splinter, felon, or finger-tip amputation, warrant early definitive care. Other conditions such as lymphadenopathy, branchial cleft sinuses, cystic masses, and lymphangiomas may also present acutely with infection which require urgent care. In general, however, these latter conditions and many others need to be assessed accurately but then may be referred for later definitive evaluation and care.

Subungual Hematoma

A direct focal blow to the tip of the finger or toe frequently causes bleeding at the interface of the nail bed and the nail. The resultant hematoma is usually trapped under the nail. Besides the pain of the trauma itself, the hematoma expands over the course of several hours, heightening the pain. Also, the patient or family is likely to notice a blue-black zone under the nail at the site of the hematoma.

Drainage of the hematoma will provide relief of the pain and clearing of the discoloration. If the hematoma extends almost to the tip of the nail, then a slight separation of the nail from its nail bed will produce drainage. However, more commonly, the hematoma is under the proximal portion of the nail and, such a maneuver will only cause additional pain. Although one can utilize a digital block to lessen the pain, a much more simple and virtually painless maneuver is to produce a hole by cauterization of the insensitive nail directly over the hematoma (see procedure in Section VII). Drainage with relief of pain is almost instantaneous. Because of the potential for secondary infection, one should soak the finger or toe 3 times a day, followed by a light dressing until the underlying space has closed.

Paronychia

The flap of thin epidermis which overrides the base of the nail is called the eponychium (cuticle). In a child, it is particularly thin and therefore vulnerable to generalized trauma during play and specific trauma as with biting or sucking of the fingers. With a break in the epidermal surface, bacterial invasion can occur, leading first to a local cellulitis overlying the base of the nail.

If properly recognized and treated, most infections at this stage can be managed by local hygiene and maneuvers to foster spontaneous drainage. The entire hand should be washed with soap and then soaked for 20 min 3 times a day followed by application of a loose-fitting finger cot which is partially filled with Betadine or Neosporin ointment. The finger cot (or a finger cut from a rubber glove) should be applied so that it does not produce a tourniquet effect at the base of the finger. The continuous contact of the ointment with the inflammed site produces a beneficial maceration of the inflamed skin and spontaneous drainage of the local infection. Usually 2 to 3 days of such treatment is sufficient.

When treatment of an eponychia is delayed or inadequate, or when a foreign body has been imbedded under the cuticle, the patient may develop a true paronychia. This condition involves infection around the base of the nail. In most cases there is an actual collection of pus which is visible under the skin. Local incision and/or debridement of the skin overlying the abscess is usually necessary (see procedure in Section VII).

Some children will present with a far advanced paronychia with extension of pus both deep and superficial to the base of the nail. In such cases the involved portion of the nail will act as a foreign body, thereby perpetuating the infection. One must therefore not only elevate or excise the involved eponychium, but must excise the involved portion of the proximal nail. The attached distal nail may be left in place.

If one fails to achieve adequate excision and drainage, the infection may destroy the nail matrix, the nail bed, and even the underlying phalanx. Drainage of either a superficial or deep paronychia should be followed by frequent warm soaks and antibiotic ointment dressings. Bacteria involved are often mixed, reflecting the diverse causes of this condition. Because staphylococci are commonly involved, dicloxacillin or cephalosporin would be an appropriate first choice for oral antibiotic coverage in more severe cases.

Subungual Splinter

In children the usual subungual foreign body is a wood splinter, although other agents may be involved. Whatever material the foreign body is, the result is penetration of bacteria into a closed space. The presence of the foreign body enhances the local inflammation and acts as an impediment to drainage if infection develops. As with paronychia, the bacteria involved may be mixed and the same serious complications may arise if the problem is inadequately treated.

Many foreign bodies under the nail may not be totally imbedded at the time the injury occurs. Simple picking or probing of the foreign body should be avoided as this usually results in further advancement of the objects. Instead, the nail should be trimmed back as close to the nail bed as possible. Then after thorough washing of the hand, the object often can be caught against the undersurface of the nail with a needle or scalpel tip and gently stroked out from its pocket. When the splinter is deeply imbedded and cannot be gently withdrawn, then direct exposure by scraping a portion of the overlying nail will usually provide adequate access (see procedure in Section VII). After removal of the splinter, the hand should be soaked 3 times a day followed by application of an antibacterial ointment dressing. As with all wounds involving foreign bodies, tetanus coverage should be assured.

Felon

An infection in the pulp of the distal digit is called a felon. Such infections usually arise from small, even unnoticed, puncture wounds of the skin of the distal digit. If the infection stays superficial, an epidermal abscess will result which may be treated by incision and drainage at the center of the visible abscess followed by frequent soaks and antibiotic ointment dressings.

When infection develops deep to the dermis, however, a much more serious sequence of events can develop. Because of the fibrous septa within the pulp of the finger, the infection cannot spread easily. Pressure in the pulp space, therefore, builds up leading to ischemic necrosis of the soft tissue. Since most felons are the result of infection from coagulase positive staphylococci, fat between the septa is often destroyed. The necrotic tissue provides an even more favorable environment for bacterial growth. Long before pointing of the infection and spontaneous drainage occur, invasion of the underlying phalanx with extension along the flexor tendon sheath may occur. The whole finger and even the hand may be jeopardized.

The key to management is early recognition and early drainage. Examination reveals erythema, tenderness, and tenseness of the pulp of the finger. Even without convincing fluctuance, adequate surgical incision and drainage is essential to abort the pathological sequence described above. Incision and drainage should be done in a way which will prevent damage to the digital nerves and avoid troublesome scar formation (see procedure in Section VII). One should therefore not make midline incisions in the volar aspect of the pulp of the finger or transverse incisions along the junction of the distal nail and the tip of the finger. After incision and drainage, the patient should be treated with dicloxacillin. Follow-up within 24 hours is important, to be sure that the infection is appropriately responding. The drain may be removed after 48 hours and the patient begun on frequent warm soaks.

Fingertip Amputations

Because of their inattention, children are prone to crush injuries or amputation injuries of the tip of the finger. Such injuries often involve only the distal ½ of the distal phalanx. They may also involve part or all of the nail bed. In contrast to adults, children have remarkable recuperative abilities with regard to healing an amputated finger tip. Even if bone is exposed or partially amputated, one should at all costs avoid debriding back bone or the nail bed, in order to obtain a skin-to-skin closure. Thorough cleansing and debridement of any necrotic tissue should be followed by application of sterile petrolatum gauze and a bulky dressing to immobilize and protect the finger. More severe or more proximal injuries should be seen as soon as possible by a pediatric hand surgeon. Most lesser amputation injuries, however, will heal spontaneously over several weeks with a remarkable cosmetic and functional result (see Chapter 65).

Cysts of the Face and Scalp

Cysts located about the face and scalp most commonly are inclusion or *dermoid cysts* which may be located either in the midline of the face and head or over the lateral aspects of the eyebrows. Such lesions are subcutaneous in location, varying in size from several millimeters to more than a centimeter in diameter, and are somewhat mobile and nontender. Dermoid cysts should be excised to establish the diagnosis and to prevent erosion of the underlying outer table of the skull. When these lesions are in the midline, preoperative skull x-rays or tomograms are required to rule out the possibility of a dumbbell extension into the cranium. If penetration through the skull is noted, neurosurgical consultation is essential. These benign lesions are not characterized by recurrence, and complications are unlikely.

Sebaceous cysts are related to the hair follicle and glandular oily sebaceous secretions from follicular glands. Sebaceous cysts are prone to infection and for that reason are best treated by surgical excision. Frequently, sebaceous cysts present as a subcutaneous nodule in a hair-bearing area. In this area excision is also required for confirmation of diagnosis and to prevent problems with hair grooming.

Bridge of Nose Lesions

The differential diagnosis of such lesions include a dermoid cyst, an anterior encephalocele, a nasal glioma, or a hemagioendotheloma. *Dermoid cysts* are classic subcutaneous cysts as noted above and can lie in the midline over the bridge of the nose. An anterior encephalocele is associated with a defect in the anterior bony cranium through which protrudes a meningeal-lined cyst arising from within the cranium. These encephaloceles require neurosurgical intervention. A *nasal glioma* is a benign glial tumor characterized by recurrence when resection is inadequate. This lesion should be treated by surgical excision at the time of diagnosis and should not be followed electively. A *hemangioendotheloma* falls into the vascular hamartoma class. It is characterized by spontaneous regression. Therefore, a conservative follow-up approach would be the preferred method of management obviating the need for surgical intervention.

Preauricular Lesions

Preauricular lesions (Fig. 58.3) can be divided into either a simple *pit* with a cutaneous orifice or a *sinus* tract with an associated subcutaneous *cyst* or a deeper tract extending down to the external ear, the auditory canal, or the base of the skull. Some preauricular lesions are simply *cutaneous tags* with or without the presence of a cartilaginous component. Preauricular lesions may be unilateral or bilateral and are quite common in the population at large. In most cases surgical excision is optional. Cutaneous tags themselves can be removed for cosmetic purposes, while sinus tracts and cysts are best treated by operation if there is a previous history of infection or if there is a palpable cystic component in the subcutaneous tissue lying below the pit. If infection does occur incision and drainage is often required to resolve the infection acutely. Then, elective excision can be performed in 1 to 2 months.

Tongue Lesions

Some tongue problems are mild, such as a tongue-tie due to a foreshortening of the frenulum. These may or may not require division of the frenulum. On the other hand, an enlarged tongue, or macroglossia, may be indicative of a lingual thyroid gland located in the posterior one third of the tongue about the foramen cecum. Thyroid in this location represents a failure of descent of the thyroid anlage and may be the sole thyroid in the body. An enlarged tongue may also be due to a lymphangioma involving the tongue. The abnormal lymphatic cysts and channels within are prone to secondary lymphangitis. These acute infections are best managed by antibiotics. Limited surgical excision may eventually be necessary to reduce the tongue size.

Midline Neck Lesions

In the upper midline of the neck the presence of a mass raises several diagnostic possibilities (Fig. 58.3). Under the chin one

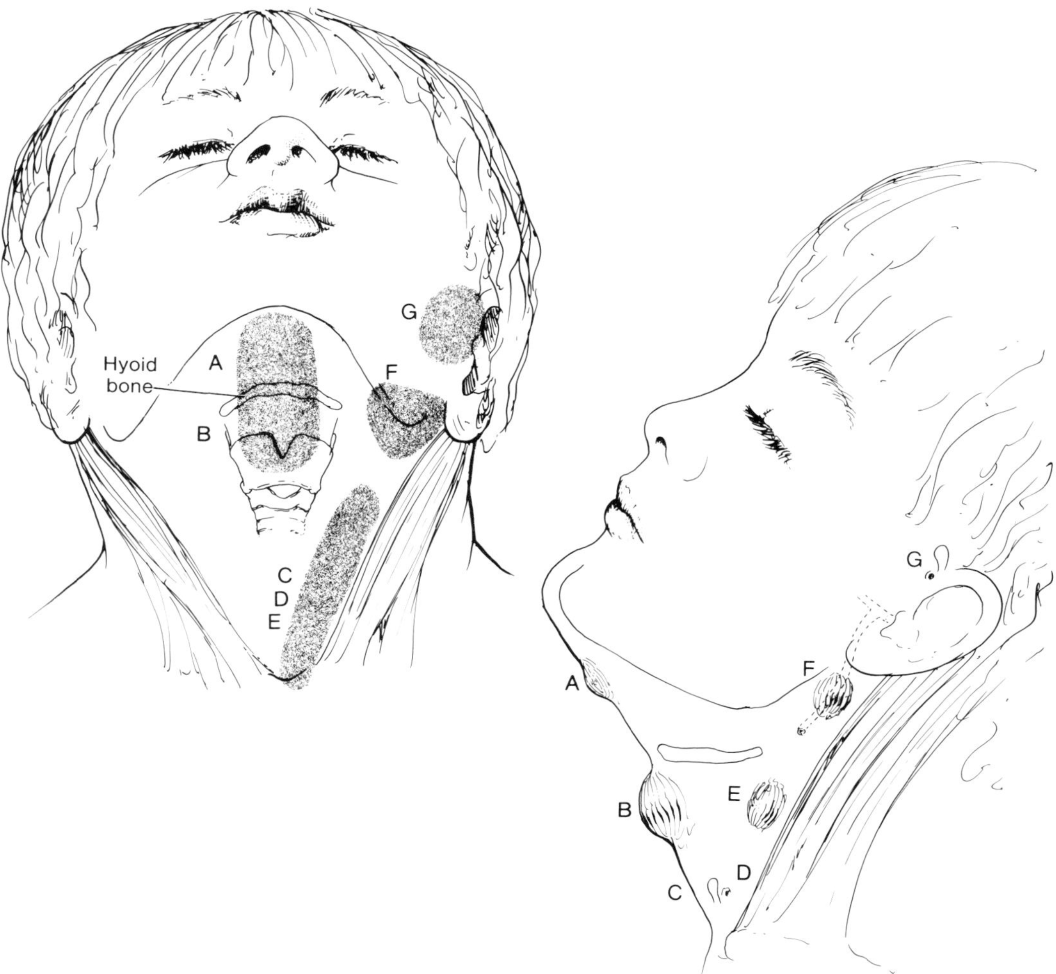

Figure 58.3 Head and neck congenital lesions seen in children in frontal and lateral views. The *shaded areas* denote the distribution in which a given lesion may be found. (*A*) dermoid cyst, (*B*) thyroglossal duct cyst, (*C*) second branchial cleft appendage, (*D*) second branchial cleft sinus, (*E*) second brachial cleft cyst, (*F*) first branchial pouch defect, (*G*) preauricular sinus or appendage.

may palpate one or more enlarged submental lymph nodes which can become secondarily enlarged due to infections in the floor of the mouth or in the perioral area. *Dermoid cysts* may be located anywhere within the midline of the neck, from the mandible all the way to the supraclavicular fossa. These small 0.5- to 1.0-cm lesions occur in the subcutaneous tissue and are mobile and nontender. They commonly are high in the midline of the neck above the area of a classic thyroglossal duct cyst.

A *thyroglossal duct cyst* represents an aberrant cystic remnant occurring during the normal descent of the thyroid gland. It occurs anywhere along the tract from the foramen cecum through the hyoid bone and down to the midline of the neck just above the thyroid cartilage. Such lesions are characterized by a painless midline neck mass. They are prone, however, to infection associated with acute swelling, tenderness, and redness of the overlying skin. These lesions can be confirmed by observing them move when the child swallows or protrudes the tongue. They generally lie in the upper midline of the neck above the level of the thyroid cartilage and below the immediate submental area. On occasion they may present slightly off-center. Thyroglossal duct cysts may contain thyroid tissue which can represent the only thyroid tissue in the neck. Should a solid thyroid mass be identified in the area of the "thyroglossal duct cyst," that mass should not be removed but should be bivalved and returned to a location on either side of the larynx (see Chapter 62).

Indications for operation for a thyroglossal duct cyst include establishing the diagnosis of the soft tissue mass, drainage of an acute pyogenic infection, or excision of a previously infected midline neck cyst. Excision of the cyst should always include the middle one third of the hyoid bone and any sinus tract between the hyoid and the foramen cecum. This method of management avoids recurrence of the lesions.

Thyroid glandular lesions include *goiters* due to hyperthyroidism (toxic goiters), or hypothyroidism (nontoxic goiters). These areas of goiterous involvement may be solitary nodules, or miltinodular. Thyroid neoplasms usually are solitary, nonfunctioning nodules. Thyroiditis may present with multiple nodules, diffuse enlargement, or no change in thyroid size.

Lateral Neck Lesions

The most common neck lesion seen in children is *cervical lymphadenitis* usually due to a suppurative bacterial process. Acute suppurative lymphadenitis is characterized by the onset of swelling and tenderness in the neck with heat and redness overlying the area. It often follows an episode of pharyngitis or otitis. Initially, such lymph nodes can be rubbery hard in texture, but with suppuration they gradually demonstrate central softening as abscess formation occurs. The lymphadenitis is most commonly due to staphylococcal organisms. Treatment, therefore, should include drainage and antistaphylococcal antibiotics. To facilitate the proper selection of antibiotic treatment, drainage can be accomplished by needle aspiration with culture of the aspirate prior to the initiation of antibiotics. Aspiration plus antibiotics and frequent warm soaks is often the only treatment necessary. Sometimes multiple aspirations every 1 to 2 days will be required. If systemic toxicity exists, or if the abscess does not resolve, then formal surgical drainage will be required (see procedure in Section VII).

Mycobacterial lymphadenitis is characterized by a more chronic lymphadenopathy with tenderness and enlargement suggesting an inflammatory process. Any child with a chronic lymphadenopathy of the neck should have a chest x-ray and a tuberculin skin test. Many of these myobacterial infections are due to atypical tubercule bacilli. Even in the presence of fluctuance, drainage will result only in a chronic draining sinus. Total surgical excision of the involved nodes and any sinus tract is the treatment of choice. If culture, histology, and acid-fast stains demonstrate tuberculosis, then long-term chemotherapy will be required (see Chapter 45).

Lymphadenopathy may also be due to neoplastic involvement. In children this usually represents primary lymphoid neoplasms of the *lymphoma* type (see Chapters 27 and 55). Both posterior and lateral cervical nodes may be involved in these processes. Following chest and neck films and skin tests, biopsy of nontender, suspicious nodes is indicated. Metastatic disease to cervical nodes may present as a cervical mass, particularly in children with neuroblastoma. Management of neoplastic involvement of cervical nodes requires a gentle excisional biopsy, microscopic analysis, proper specimen handling for touch preparation and identifying lymphocyte markers, and proper collection for staining and culturing of bacterial, fungal, and acid-fast organisms.

Salivary gland pathology in the lateral neck includes *sialadenitis* of the submandibular or parotid gland with or without secondary abscess formation. These infectious processes are unusual, resulting in systemic symptoms of infection and sepsis, and require prompt antibiotic and even surgical drainage therapy. Salivary glands are more commonly involved by vascular lesions such as hemangioendotheliomas. Rarely these glands may also be involved by neoplasms such as a mixed tumor.

Branchial cysts and *sinus tracts* in the lateral neck occur either in the submandibular triangle and mandibular ramus area (first branchial cleft) or along the anterior border of the sternocleidomastoid muscle (second branchial cleft). Such lesions vary and may consist of a pore in the skin, a subcutaneous cyst associated with that pore, or a proximally ascending sinus tact. Some of these lesions may involve only a subcutaneous cystic component or a solid cartilaginous remnant. If a proximal ascending sinus tract of the second branchial cleft type persists, the tract will pass between the external and internal carotid arteries up to the pharyngeal tonsillar fossa. If, instead, the sinus is from a first branchial cleft type of deformity, the tract may extend into the external auditory canal. Indications for surgical excision include histological diagnosis of the subcutaneous nodule, excision of a cystic mass and/or sinus tract because of the risk of infection, and prevention of the statistically increased likelihood of an in situ carcinoma arising in a branchial cleft remnant.

Torticollis, or wryneck, is commonly associated with breech presentation and a traumatic extraction of the head from the vaginal canal inducing a contusion of the sternocleidomastoid muscle of the infant. Such muscular contusion induces a local hemorrhage followed by an inflammatory healing response which is characterized by fibrosis and thickening of the sternocleidomastoid muscle, limiting its ability to relax and stretch. The result is a palpable nodule within the injured muscle and a twisting of the head and neck. Children with wryneck usually present within the first few weeks of life with an impaired mobility of their head and neck. If uncorrected they may present later in life with hypoplastic development of the neck and face on the same side (see Chapter 28).

A physical examination of the child with torticollis reveals asymmetry of the face and neck, a palpable firm mass in the involved sternocleidomastoid muscle, and tilting of the head toward the injured side with the chin pointing to the contralateral side. The differential diagnosis of wryneck includes neurologic syndromes, Sandifer's syndrome secondary to gastroesophageal reflux, a primary muscle tumor, or even lymphadenitis.

Torticollis is best treated by nonoperative intervention, involving a series of aggressive passive range of motion exercises. Such exercises are done by placing the child in the supine position with the shoulders on a flat surface. While one person holds both shoulders flat, another person rotates the head back and forth through a full 180° range of motion. The 2- to 3-times daily repetition of these exercises for several weeks will slowly begin to loosen the tight muscle and increase the range of motion. Only with failure of such a regimen should operative intervention be necessary. The key to a successful outcome is early treatment before facial asymmetry becomes too severe.

Lymphangiomas of the neck are congenital ectasias of the lymphatic system producing multiple lymphatic cysts ("cluster of grapes"). These ectasias are the result of extensive obstruction of the lymphatic system in the involved area. Lymphangiomas (cystic hygromas) are common in the neck although they can occur throughout the child's body, especially in the chest wall, axilla, and the extremities. These soft tissue tumors vary in size, are spongy, and are filled with a clear yellow fluid. Aspiration of such fluid from the mass will often confirm the diagnosis.

Lymphangiomas are not characterized by spontaneous regression. Rather, they are characterized by a history of recurrent bouts of lymphangitis which result in a gradual coalescence and restriction of their total extent. Nevertheless, even firm lymphangiomas can be diffuse and invade surrounding structures such as adjacent muscle and nerve vascular structures. Discrete lesions lend themselves to conservative excision, either a single or multistage procedure. More extensive disease, as in the case of an entire extremity, is usually best treated nonsurgically.

Vascular malformations of the head and neck are common. These lesions can be located over the nape of the neck as in the classic "stork bites" of the neonate, or they can be located anywhere on the face or neck. *Hemangiomatous lesions* are best classified as *port wine stains* in which there is a purplish discoloration of the skin due to a lesion located beneath the skin's surface. Large port wine stains are best treated by nonoperative means utilizing cosmetic coverage (Covermark). Small areas can be treated with laser therapy with a satisfactory cosmetic result (see Chapter 54).

Capillary hemangiomas are characterized by a raised, reddish lesion which is both visible and palpable. Capillary, or strawberry, hemangiomas usually undergo spontaneous regression after an initial growth phase. The peak of the aggressive growth period is about 2½ to 3 years of age. The apparent progressive growth in size is in reality the opening of more vascular channels. Lesions which might at first be only several millimeters in size can then grow remarkably over the course of several months. In time, however, the central portion of such hemangiomas begins to undergo ischemic changes. The skin develops a whitish sheen and the lesions become less and less palpable. Occasionally some of these infarcting lesions are prone to develop irritation or frank ulceration with bleeding and crust formation. Such problems can usually be controlled by local wound care and hemostatic measures until regression is complete.

Hemangioendotheliomas occasionally have cutaneous involvement with discoloration, but more commonly they are characterized by a soft tissue swelling beneath the surface of the skin. Biopsy often confirms their hemangiomatous nature. Such lesions likewise undergo spontaneous regression of their capillary elements although a stromal element may remain. The preferred treatment, therefore, is conservative observation in anticipation of a spontaneous regression. More active treatment including surgery may be required for those lesions which cause complications such as platelet trapping, cardiac failure, or bleeding. Such complications are characteristic usually of larger lesions. Excision of smaller lesions may be necessary for cosmesis, particularly in those children who are left with a pedunculated stromal mass lesion following spontaneous involution of the hemangiomatous elements.

Cavernous hemangiomas consist of large lakes of vascular channels and are not characterized by spontaneous regression. Physical examination is not as helpful in evaluating these lesions as is a histological biopsy or assessment of larger lesions by means of an arteriogram. Operative intervention for these cavernous hemangiomas is indicated for those lesions which produce symptoms such as heart failure, or which are clearly increasing in size. When these lesions begin to push toward the surface of the skin the child is at risk for exsanguination if a laceration of the involved area occurs.

Venous lakes may occur in the head or neck, especially in the supraclavicular area. When children with venous lakes increase their intrathoracic pressure during Valsalva maneuver, one may see a bulge anterior to the sternocleidomastoid muscle or in the supraclavicular space. Angiography is required to define the underlying pathology. Treatment must be individualized.

Perineal Lesions

Many lesions in the perineum involving the anus, rectum, and genitalia are discussed elsewhere (see Chapters 59 and 63). Several additional conditions and disorders, however, such as rectal prolapse and lesions between the anus and the coccyx may present in the emergency department for care and evaluation.

Rectal prolapse is a condition usually seen in the extremes of life. It involves the extrusion of one or more coats of the rectum. When only mucosa protrudes out the anal opening it is said to be an incomplete prolapse. When all layers of the rectum, including the muscularis and outer surface are involved in the prolapse, it is said to be a complete prolapse. In 90% of children with this condition, prolapse is complete.

The prolapse first presents in children usually between the first and third birthdays. In most cases the cause is idiopathic. However, there are some physiological and anatomical reasons for prolapse to occur in this age group. As toddlers, children enter a period of more and more prolonged standing in an erect position. This occurs at a time when the pelvic and perineal structures may not have obtained full development. The puborectalis sling at this age, for example, is less pronounced than later in childhood. As a result, the rectum lacks the prominent curved passage through the pelvis which is found in the older child or in the adult. Also most toddlers have not yet developed complete competence in the sensory and motor function of their external sphincter mechanism.

Nevertheless there are some conditions which clearly predispose to rectal prolapse. Typically, these conditions are associated with recurring bouts of increased abdominal pressure. Examples of such conditions include marked ascites in an infant, sustained coughing, and excessive straining at stooling as in children with constipation or rectal polyps. Specific disorders which have been associated with rectal prolapse include major neuromuscular disorders of the pelvis as seen in patients with a meningomyelocele or extrophy of the bladder, and malabsorption disorders such as untreated cystic fibrosis or celiac disease.

Initially, rectal prolapse presents as a painless protrusion of the distal rectum during defecation. When the child relaxes, the prolapse usually reduces spontaneously. In time, however, the prolapse may become more pronounced and require manual reduction. When the prolapse becomes severe or prolonged, marked edema and congestion may occur in the exposed rectal bud and hospitalization may be required.

Acute treatment may involve sedation and elevation of the buttocks followed by bimanual reduction with the use of gauze to provide some grip on the rectal bud in order to get it back inside. Once successful reduction has occurred, preventive measures include evaluation for any malabsorption defects and correction of any underlying reason for constipation. Bowel lubricants, such as mineral oil by mouth and the use of an infant-sized toilet seat so that the child can defecate with his feet on the floor, are additonal aids in preventing recurrence. If spontaneous prolapse is a problem between stools, one may tape the buttocks shut in order to apply a sustained pressure to the perianal area.

For particularly severe or unrelenting cases of rectal prolapse, operative maneuvers may be necessary. Under general anesthesia one can instill with a syringe and needle a hypertonic solution such as 30% saline circumferentially in the tissue planes just outside the distal rectum. Then, by keeping the buttocks taped together most of the time, a sterile inflammatory reaction will have time to bind down the distal rectal wall and keep it from prolapsing. Alternatively one can place one or two No. 1 chromic catgut sutures subcutaneously all the way around the perianal area. These sutures can then be tied tightly over an index finger in the rectum until the knot is secure. Finally, in especially difficult cases, it is possible to surgically expose the space between the rectum and the sacrum and pack this area with an absorbable gauze. This technique also relies on a postoperative sterile inflammatory process to bind down the wall of the sacrum.

Pilonidal dimples are common congenital midline indentations of the skin in the area of the coccyx. These dimples may present only as a skin lesion but they may also be associated with a subcutaneous sinus tract leading to a cyst beneath the skin. When the base of the sinus tract is wide and the skin appears intact in the depth of the dimple, prophylactic surgical excision is unnecessary. In the presence of a deeper dimple suggestive of an underlying tract the possibilities for later complications include entrapment of skin secretions and the ingrowth of hair resulting in infection and abscess formation. When a pilonidal defect appears to be associated with a possible tract, therefore, prophylactic excision is warranted. If an acute infection does occur, frequent hot soaks, antibiotics, and possible surgical drainage may be necessary. Once the acute infection is resolved, elective excision of the involved area should take place within 1 or 2 months.

There are two other conditions which may present in the sacrococcygeal area. One is a *tethered spinal cord* which is frequently noted in conjunction with a focal skin abnormality in the midline overlying the sacrum. This skin abnormality might be an otherwise benign appearing skin dimple or a focal hemangiomatous or hairy area. Any such abnormality in this region should be assessed with spine films and a neurosurgical consultation. In children less than 2 to 3 years of age, there may be no signs of symptoms. However, as the child begins to grow in height, tethering of the spinal cord may produce subtle or progressive signs of incontinence, or sensory and motor deficits in the legs. Some of these signs and symptoms are not reversible even after corrective surgery. Early recognition and treatment, therefore, before complications develop is essential.

One other lesion may also present in a seemingly benign fashion in the sacrococcygeal area, namely, a *sacrococcygeal teratoma*. The vast majority of these tumors are benign at the time of birth. Most of them are already so large at the time of birth that they are readily visible and lead to early excision. Some of these lesions, however, may be associated with only subtle changes in the skin and perineum. On external palpation of this area one may perceive only a vague fullness just below the tip of the coccyx. Any child, therefore, with subtle abnormalities in this region should also undergo a rectal examination to assess the possibility of a mass inside the sacrum. The potential for a malignant transformation of these initially benign lesions increases significantly after the third month of life. In some children the tumor will be predominantly within the pelvis. By the time symptoms of constipation and urinary difficuties arise, malignant transformation may have already occurred or the tumor may be so massive as to greatly increase the hazard of surgical resection. Any child with even subtle abnormalities in the sacrococcygeal area, therefore, should have a thorough physical examination, be seen in consultation by a pediatric surgeon, and be considered for possible barium enema, intravenous pyelogram, and ultrasound.

References

Grabb WC, Smith JW (Editors): *Plastic Surgery*, Ed. 3. Little Brown, Boston, 1979.

Koop CE: *Visible and Palpable Lesions in Children*. Grune & Stratton, New York, 1976.

McGregor IA: *Fundamental Techniques of Plastic Surgery*, Ed. 7. Churchill Livingstone, New York, 1980.

Ravitch MM, Welch KJ, et al.: *Pediatric Surgery*, Vol. I and II, Ed. 3. Yearbook, Chicago, 1979.

Sabiston DC Jr (Editor): *Davis-Christopher Textbook of Surgery*, Ed. 11. W. B. Saunders, Philadelphia, 1977.

Schwartz SI (Editor): *Principles of Surgery*, Ed. 3. McGraw-Hill, New York, 1979.

CHAPTER 59

Abdominal Emergencies

HARRY C. BISHOP, M.D., AND LOUISE SCHNAUFER, M.D.

INTRODUCTION

Although some acute intra-abdominal diseases may affect both adults and children, other conditions specifically occur in childhood and are extremely uncommon in the adult population. Appendicitis is similar in both age groups. Disorders such as malrotation and volvulus, Hirschsprung's disease and congenital bowel stenoses affect the younger age group. The emergency department physician must be aware of the unique problems that occur in infancy and childhood and gear his/her thinking to an understanding of the clinical manifestations of these entities. There must also be an awareness and sensitivity to the special techniques for evaluating a child with a potential "surgical abdomen."

The abdominal surgical problems most commonly found in infants and childhood will be discussed under the following categories: (1) diseases producing peritoneal irritation; (2) acute intestinal obstruction; (3) chronic, partial intestinal obstruction; (4) problems producing rectal bleeding; (5) intra-abdominal masses; (6) abdominal wall defects; and (7) foreign bodies of the gastrointestinal tract. Nonsurgical gastrointestinal emergencies are covered in Chapter 50. Chapter 57 deals with major trauma to the abdominal contents. Chapter 5 reviews the diagnostic approach to the child with abdominal pain.

EVALUATION

History

Neither the infant nor the very young child can give a complete history, but it is useful to obtain whatever history from the child is possible. Younger children, for example, are likely to recall recent events. Events somewhat more remote in time may be better remembered by an adult, even though the adult's accuracy may be clouded by his or her emotional state. If a child has been toilet trained for a few years, neither the child nor the parent may be sufficiently attentive to give an accurate history of bowel habits. In general, however, once a child reaches school age, taking a history becomes considerably easier.

In obtaining the history the emergency physican should seek an accurate chronology of events, with direct questions such as: When did the pain start? Where was it felt at first? What happened next? The physician should also obtain a careful history of other symptoms. By asking when the child was last perfectly well, one may get a more accurate assessment of the child's pathophysiology. In this way, one may better evaluate a child with multiple symptoms, such as fever, vomiting, abdominal distension, and any changes in bowel habits, appetite, feeding pattern, or general activity level. One then develops a feeling for the patterns of different diseases in children.

For example, if there is high fever at the onset of the problem, it is more likely infectious in origin (i.e., viral gastroenteritis rather than appendicitis). By contrast, one has to be especially concerned about a possible underlying surgical condition in any child whose *first* presenting symptom is abdominal pain. Visceral pain has a colicky character, and is usually generalized in the upper, middle, or lower abdomen depending on which level of the GI tract is involved. The presence of colic suggests the possibility of obstruction. By contrast, peritoneal pain reflects secondary features of the abdominal disease process, such as fibrinous exudates, inflammation, or bowel perforation. As a result, a child with a surgical abdominal condition may have a clearly perceived shift in the character of the pain from visceral to peritoneal. The development of vomiting following initial symptoms of colicky pain further suggests the possibility of obstruction, particularly if it is voluminous and bilious (see Chapter 4). If the child's illness begins with nonbloody diarrhea it is less likely to be surgical in nature, in contrast to a child with a 3-day history of abdominal pain and fever in whom the onset of diarrhea may be secondary to a pelvic abscess. Diarrhea in the presence of blood may or may not be surgical in nature, but it warrants a very thorough assessment (see Chapters 14 and 22).

Besides detailing the chronology of events and the characteristics of the symptoms, the physician should inquire about any treatments which have been attempted at home, such as cathartics, enemas, or drugs. Frequently these home remedies will have modified the symptoms and their chronology in some way.

It is important not to overlook the past history. For example, a child known to have sickle cell disease may have an acute abdominal crisis as the cause of abdominal pain. The presence of this underlying hematologic abnormality forces the examiner to be more precise in the interpretation of the physical examination. A child with known cystic fibrosis or inflammatory bowel disease may also have frequent abdominal pains that do not require surgery.

Examination

Children vary a great deal in their ability to cooperate during abdominal examination, and very often the physician must make patient, repeated efforts to perform an adequate evaluation. A few minutes spent gaining the child's confidence is important to the child and helpful to the examiner. The best examination is done before the child becomes disturbed by the drawing of blood samples or the performance of a rectal examination. On some occasions, it is very helpful to let the distraught, crying child actually go to sleep; a second examination while the child is sleeping may determine whether or not there is real tenderness. It may also be helpful for the mother to relax the child by holding him on her lap for the examination. On rare occasions, a young child may require sedation with barbiturates in order to improve the reliability of the examination, but one should avoid the use of narcotics which might mask findings of peritonitis. All infants and children should have an examination that is not hindered by the child's clothes. Small incarcerated indirect inguinal hernias can easily escape detection if the entire abdomen is not observed and palpated. Some children need reassurance that being undressed for the examination is important. The child's sense of modesty must be respected whenever possible.

Once the child relaxes, the physical examination should follow an orderly progression: inspection and observation, nontouching maneuvers, abdominal palpation, auscultation, examination of nonabdominal areas, and rectal examination.

The initial step of inspection should focus on the presence of distention, visible bowel loops, and asymmetry. Inspection is very easily done because of the relative prominence of the child's abdomen and thinness of the overlying muscles and subcutaneous tissue. Sometimes observation during a feeding gives important information. The child should be observed in motion; for example, how he behaves when getting on and off the examination table and walking. Nontouching maneuvers include having the child cough or jump up and down while noting any change in symptoms.

Palpation is the most difficult, yet most informative, aspect of physical examination. When possible, the child can initiate his or her own examination by self-palpation. Ask the child to point to the place where the pain is most severe. Avoid the tender area initially but return to palpate it last. There are a number of "tricks" that can be used to facilitate the palpation such as: (1) diverting the child with conversation, (2) palpating with the head of the stethoscope in hand, and (3) palpating while asking the child to take a deep breath. For example, quick withdrawal of a palpating stethoscope may confirm rebound tenderness and the presence of an underlying peritoneal irritation.

Auscultation of the abdomen indicates the state of bowel motility. The presence of normal bowel sounds may not rule out surgical pathology, but a silent abdomen or one with high pitched tinkles and rushes would suggest the possibility of sepsis or obstruction. Auscultation and palpation of nonabdominal areas is quite important. In addition, evaluation of the acute abdomen requires careful examination of the lung fields, testes and scrotum, inguinal regions, femoral triangles, and costovertebral areas. Failure to carefully examine these areas will result in missing important diagnostic clues to nonabdominal problems that may present with abdominal symptoms.

The final step in the evaluation should be a rectal examination. The important technical aspects include: (1) use of generous amounts of lubricant, (2) slow insertion of the examiner's finger as the patient takes slow deep breaths, and (3) palpation of the presumed painful area last. If done carefully and gently, the rectal examination is usually well tolerated by the child. Any stool on the examiner's glove should be tested for the presence of blood.

Laboratory

Laboratory and radiographic studies will vary, depending on the diagnoses that are being considered. Most children accept x-ray studies as "having your picture taken." A urinalysis is an important part of the evaluation of any abdominal symptoms in children. A complete bood count and differential is essential. The need for other tests depends on the child's condition and the diagnostic considerations: BUN, electrolytes, serum amylase, sickle cell prep, etc.

Assessment

Once the history, physical examination and laboratory data are all available, the emergency physician must synthesize them into an overall assessment. If the physical findings are reproducible and consistent in location and character, an accurate diagnosis can often be made and appropriate treatments started. If the findings are both worrisome and equivocal, and do not fit into a comprehensive picture, then the patient should be admitted for observation and reassessment. The sections which follow detail the cardinal signs and symptoms of the common acute surgical problems in children. Initial emergency department management is discussed, but in all cases the definitive treatment requires consultation with a surgeon.

DISEASES PRODUCING PERITONEAL IRRITATION

The physician must perform a careful examination to elicit accurate signs of peritonitis. Tenderness is not necessarily an indication of an intra-abdominal surgical problem in a child. A child with localized peritonitis may have only minimal findings, while a patient with a nonsurgical condition may have severe pain and generalized tenderness. For example, a child with severe colic due to gastroenteritis may, on examination, appear to have genuine peritoneal signs. Such a child may, in fact, only have exaggerated voluntary guarding of the abdominal wall mimicking the true rigidity of peritonitis.

The well-known features of peritonitis, rigidity, spasm, involuntary guarding, and rebound, are as valid for a child as they are for an adult. In a child with abdominal pain, however, one has to be patient and gentle enough in the initial phases of the examination so that signs of peritonitis can be checked repeatedly without breaking rapport with the child. Reproducible anterior peritoneal tenderness in the same location is much more suggestive of peritonitis than deep abdominal tenderness which shifts in location with each reexamination of the child.

Acute Unruptured Appendicitis

Acute appendicitis is one of the most common abdominal surgical conditions seen by the emergency physician or surgeon caring for children. It occurs in all age groups and is particularly difficult to diagnose in its early states and in infants and toddlers. The emergency physician must accurately evaluate the child, and promptly consult a surgeon when the diagnosis is clear or when appendicitis cannot be safely ruled out. Such consultation is especially urgent in younger children in whom perforation can occur within 8 to 24 hours of the onset of symptoms.

CLINICAL MANIFESTATIONS

Usually the child with appendicitis initially complains of poorly defined and poorly localized midabdominal or periumbilical pain. Unfortunately, this symptom is common to many other intra-abdominal, nonsurgical problems. In the young and, to a lesser extent, the older child, vomiting and a low grade fever often occur soon thereafter. Characteristically, the pain then migrates to the right lower quadrant.

Since the position of the appendix may vary in children, the localization of the pain and the tenderness on examination may also vary. An appendix that is located in the lateral gutter may produce flank pain and lateral abdominal tenderness; an inflamed appendix pointing toward the left-sided quadrants may produce hypogastric tenderness; an inflamed low lying, pelvic appendix may not cause pain at McBurney's point but instead cause diarrhea due to direct irritation of the sigmoid colon. Frequently the child with appendicitis will be anorexic, suggesting the presence of nausea even if he or she is unable to verbalize this complaint. Since motion aggravates peritoneal irritation, a child with appendicitis typically prefers to lie still or, when moving, splints towards the painful area.

In the history, one needs to consider other causes of abdominal pain which may appear as appendicitis but, in fact, are nonsurgical. Concurrent GI illness in other family members or friends suggests the possibility of an infectious gastroenteritis. Chronic constipation, urinary tract disease, or an emotional disturbance may also point to an explanation other than appendicitis for the abdominal pain. Cough, fever, and rapid breathing suggest the possibility of a lower lobe pneumonia.

On examination, palpation is usually reliable in demonstrating focal peritoneal signs at the site of the inflamed appendix. If the appendix is in the pelvis or retrocecal area, however, typical anterior peritoneal signs may be absent. The physician can confirm his or her impression of point tenderness by pressing gently in each quadrant and asking the child to indicate which area is most tender. When the inflamed appendix is not close to the anterior abdominal wall, as in the case of retrocecal appendix, tenderness may be more impressive on deep palpation of the abdomen or by palpating in the flank. This impression of focal tenderness can sometimes be confirmed by shaking the child's abdomen or getting him to cough, which often produces a wince of pain at the involved area. Finally, a well done rectal examination may make the difference between deciding to operate or observe the child. One should insert the examining finger as fully as possible without touching the area of presumed tenderness. Then, when the child is relaxed and taking deep breaths, one can gently stroke or indent an area high on the right rectal wall. A sudden involuntary reaction of pain confirms the presence of inflammation. In a child with a history of probable appendicitis for more than 2 or 3 days there may also be a boggy full mass in this location, suggesting an abscess.

A complete blood count in a child with appendicitis usually shows an elevated white count in the range of 11,000 to 15,000 in the first 12 to 24 hours of the illness. As the appendix becomes more gangrenous, the white count rises further, and the differential demonstrates more and more neutrophils and an increasing number of bands. Urinalysis often shows ketosis. If the inflamed appendix lies over the ureter or adjacent to the bladder, there may be a few white cells in the urinary sediment. The presence of numerous white cells and bacteria, on a freshly spun specimen, may indicate an acute urinary tract infection. One must not forget, however, that a child with a chronic urinary tract infection may also develop appendicitis.

If the clinical and laboratory diagnosis of acute appendicitis is quite convincing there is no indication for abdominal x-rays. When the history and/or physical examination is somewhat equivocal, abdominal x-rays may demonstrate two findings if, indeed, appendicitis is present. First, there may be a dilated loop of small bowel in the right lower quadrant suggesting a paralytic ileus. Second, one may find a calcified fecalith in the right lower quadrant. This latter finding would definitely confirm the need for surgery. In fact, there may be some urgency in the need for surgery, since a fecalith may be associated with a more complete obstruction and earlier gangrene with perforation of the appendix. Routine chest x-rays are not indicated unless there is a prior history of pulmonary problems, such as asthma, or unless the signs and symptoms indicate atypical right abdominal pain with splinting respirations. A chest x-ray in such a case may reveal subtle evidence of a right lower lobe pneumonia. With good hydration these subtle findings on x-ray may develop into an early visible infiltrate in a few hours.

Unfortunately laboratory findings do not differentiate mesenteric adenitis, which closely mimics acute appendicitis. A complete approach to the child with abdominal pain is covered in Chapter 5.

MANAGEMENT

The preoperative preparation of a patient with acute appendicitis should include a BUN and electrolytes if the patient has been vomiting or has had poor fluid intake for more than a few hours. If an unexpected anemia is discovered on the CBC, a crossmatch should also be done. Intravenous fluids should be started, with emphasis on replacing the child's deficits as quickly as possible. Protracted GI losses, as with vomiting, may lead to potassium depletion. Therefore, the initial intravenous fluids should contain at least 0.5 N saline with 10 meq of potassium chloride per 500 ml. These fluids can then be altered, if necessary, once the serum chemistries are known. During this period the patient and the family should be psychologically prepared for surgery.

It is very important for the emergency physician to keep in mind the many variations in the way appendicitis can present. As a good rule of thumb, a patient should at least be admitted for observation if there are positive findings in two of the three classical modes of assessment: history, physical examination or laboratory. For example, a child with an excellent history of appendicitis and a high white count should be admitted even if the abdominal examination is normal. Such a child may have perforated his appendix just before the examination with temporary cessation of physical findings. In equivocal situations the key element is follow-up assessment. A child who is admitted can, if necessary, be reexamined every 1 to 2 hours. In a child in whom the possibility of appendicitis seems more remote, one may elect to have the child return for reexamination in the office or in the emergency department. Such follow-up arrangements work best when the parents are reliable and do not live too far from the hospital. Arrangements for follow-up should be quite specific, including time of appointment, the specific doctor to be seen, and a contact phone number in case the child does not return as scheduled.

Perforated Appendicitis

Ideally, once the diagnosis of appendicitis is seriously considered, the patient will have surgery before the appendix has ruptured. Unfortunately some patients, particularly younger children and infants, may arrive for emergency care with an already perforated appendix due to a delay in seeking treatment or in making the diagnosis. Once the appendix has ruptured, there are usually signs of generalized peritonitis, rather than localized peritonitis. In a young child the omentum is flimsy and often incapable of walling off the inflamed appendix. As a result, perforation occurs more quickly, and secondary dissemination of the infection occurs more widely. Although the mortality from appendicitis has decreased, the incidence of perforation in children has remained the same.

CLINICAL MANIFESTATIONS

Within a few hours after perforation has occurred, the child begins to develop increasing signs of toxicity. First the lower abdomen and then the entire abdomen becomes rigid with extreme tenderness. Bowel sounds are sparse to absent. In addition, there are signs of prostration such as pale color, dyspnea, grunting, marked tachycardia and higher fever (39 to 41°C). Rarely the patient may develop septic shock (see Chapter 2) from the overwhelming infection caused by bowel flora.

Initially, the findings may be confused with those of pneumonia, as the extreme abdominal pain may cause rapid shallow respirations and decreased air entry to the lower lung fields. There is impaired excursion of the diaphragm and respiratory failure in some cases. In infants and toddlers, the findings may also be confused with meningitis, as any movement of the child (even flexion of the neck) will produce pain and irritability. The high fever and other signs of prostration may be indications for a lumbar puncture. After the spinal fluid analysis is found to be normal, the suspicion of perforated appendicitis may be heightened.

The laboratory findings in the child with perforated appendicitis often suggest this diagnosis. There is a marked elevation of WBC, usually above 15,000/cu mm and a marked left shift; leukopenia may be seen when perforation has resulted in overwhelming sepsis and septic shock.

MANAGEMENT

Initially, the focus of therapy should be on resuscitation. There must be careful attention to airway, breathing, and circulation (see Chapter 1). The severely septic child may need positive pressure ventilation with high concentrations of oxygen in order to overcome ventilatory insufficiency. Hypovolemia should be immediately corrected with 5% dextrose in either normal saline or Ringer's lactate solution. An alternative volume expander is 5% albumin solution in normal saline. An initial bolus of 20 ml/kg is given over 30 min or until vital signs are restored and the patient produces urine. Metabolic acidosis should be treated with sodium bicarbonate, the dose being determined by the results of the serum electrolytes or more precisely the base deficit from an arterial blood gas (see Chapter 46).

Hypovolemia and acidosis must be treated vigorously until adequate circulation has been reestablished, as measured by the strength of the pulse, blood pressure, skin perfusion, capillary refill in the extremities, and urine output. If it is difficult to reestablish an adequate circulation, a central venous pressure catheter may be helpful in determining the amount of volume needed. Once adequate circulation has been attained, much of the acidosis may correct spontaneously as homeostatic mechanisms are restored.

Additional steps in the management include treatment of infection and further preparation of the patient for surgery. The child should receive broad spectrum antibiotics such as: ampicillin, 200 mg/kg/day and tobramycin, 5 to 7.5 mg/kg/day. Once the emergency physician is certain that the airway can be controlled and the circulation is adequate, relief of pain can be accomplished by using narcotic agents, such as morphine, 0.1 mg/kg. The patient's fever can usually be controlled by the use of a hypothermia mattress, acetaminophen 10 mg/kg/dose per rectum. A nasogastric tube should be placed to evacuate the contents of the stomach and drain ongoing gastric secretions. Several units of blood must be prepared for the operative procedure.

Children with perforated appendicitis can deteriorate quickly. Moreover, the fever, often 40°C or more, may not be controlled until the intra-abdominal infection is drained. Therefore, emergency resuscitation should be quickly followed by operative intervention. At surgery the appendix is removed, the area drained, and other appropriate treatments given. The child will recover more rapidly if this approach is taken than if prolonged medical management is instituted and surgery delayed. On rare occasions one may drain the abscess with the expectation that an appendectomy will be performed at a later time.

Meckel's Diverticulitis With and Without Perforation

Most patients with a Meckel's diverticulum are asymptomatic or, if symptoms do occur, have rectal bleeding from ulceration at the junction of the ectopic gastric mucosa and the normal ileal mucosa, where the diverticulum is attached. A preoperative diagnosis of an inflamed or a perforated Meckel's diverticulum is rarely made but, nevertheless, should be considered in the differential diagnosis of a perforated viscus leading to generalized peritonitis. The diagnosis is usually made in the operating room by the surgeon who finds a normal appendix and then on exploration of the bowel finds a diseased diverticulum within two to three feet of the ileocecal valve (see p. 837 under "Meckel's Diverticulum").

Primary Peritonitis

Primary peritonitis is a bacterial infection of the peritoneal cavity, usually secondary to a blood or lymph borne infection. Although rare, it does occur in children with nephrosis, cirrhosis, or ascites of other etiology, and may mimic appendicitis. Primary peritonitis is usually caused by pneumococcus, Group A *Streptococcus*, and rarely by a gram-negative organism. When due to a gram-negative infection, the portal of entry is usually via the vagina. These occur in girls from 5 to 10 years old in whom the cervix is usually open and the vaginal fluid is not yet acidic enough to retard the ascent of infection.

The clinical manifestations include fever, vomiting, and abdominal pain. The physical examination includes findings of peritoneal irritation. An elevation of the WBC (> 15,000 cu/mm) and left shift are also seen. Often the signs, symptoms and laboratory findings are indistinguishable from perforated appendicitis and thus the diagnosis may be made at laparotomy. If the diagnosis is suspected prior to surgery, the patient should undergo paracentesis. The diagnosis may be confirmed by a Gram stain showing gram-positive cocci, followed by a positive culture. It is important to remember that children with nephrosis or cirrhosis may have appendicitis unrelated to their underlying disease.

Pancreatitis

Although acute pancreatitis is a common condition in adults, it occurs rarely in childhood. The most common cause is abdominal trauma. Pancreatitis produces upper abdominal or periumbilical pain, often radiating to the back. Occasionally, the presentation is that of a patient in shock. Findings which support the diagnosis include: paralytic ileus, distention, and ascites. There is usually an elevated serum or urine amylase. When severe, there is also a decrease in serum calcium. When pancreatitis occurs in a child without a history of trauma one should evaluate the patient for possible congenital abnormalities of the biliary tree or pancreatic ducts, such as abnormal insertion of the main pancreatic duct or the presence of a choledochal cyst. Surgical intervention is rarely indicated in the acute phase. However, active surgical consultation from the beginning is essential in case the patient deteriorates in spite of maximal medical therapy (see Chapter 50). Signs of deterioration or non-response to therapy include persistently low serum calcium, a falling hematocrit, increasing toxicity, and deterioration of the patient's coagulation profile.

ACUTE INTESTINAL OBSTRUCTION

In any child who vomits persistently, particularly if the vomitus becomes bile-stained, the diagnosis of acute intestinal obstruction must be considered. If the obstruction is high in the intestinal tract, the abdomen will not become distended; but, with lower intestinal obstruction, there will be generalized distention and diffuse tenderness, usually without signs of peritoneal irritation. Only if the bowel perforates, or vascular insufficiency occurs, will signs of peritoneal irritation be found. If complete obstruction persists, there may be changes in bowel habits leading to complete obstipation for both flatus and stool. All patients with suspected bowel obstruction should have flat and upright abdominal x-rays (Fig. 59.1). In acute mechanical bowel obstruction, multiple dilated loops are usually seen. Fluid levels produced by the layering of air and intestinal contents are seen in the upright or lateral oblique x-rays.

Intussusception

BACKGROUND

Intussusception occurs when one segment of bowel telescopes into a more distal segment. This is the leading cause of acute intestinal obstruction in infants, and occurs most commonly between 3 and 12 months of age. The most common intussusception is ileocolic but small bowel may intussuscept into itself. Frequently it will be ileoileal at a location close to the cecum. Typically this small bowel intussusception then prolapses through the ileocecal valve (Fig. 59.2). The intussusception continues through the colon a variable distance, occasionally as far as the rectum where it can be palpated on rectal examination. Colocolic intussusceptions are very rare. In infants the lead point for the intussusception may be hypertrophied Peyer's patches. In children older than 2 years of age there is much more likely to be a specific lead point, such as a polyp, a Meckel's diverticulum, a duplication, or a tumor. There may be a

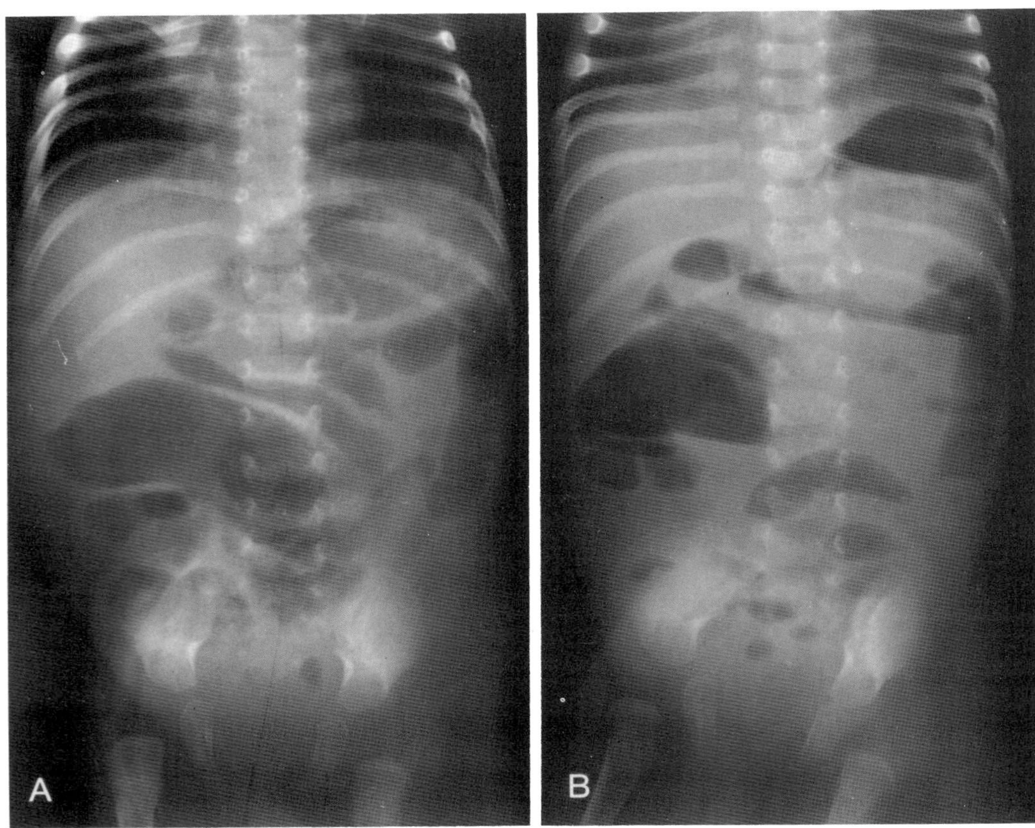

Figure 59.1 (*A*) Flat film of abdomen showing multiple dilated, air-filled loops of bowel. (*B*) Upright film showing air-fluid levels in obstructed loops of bowel.

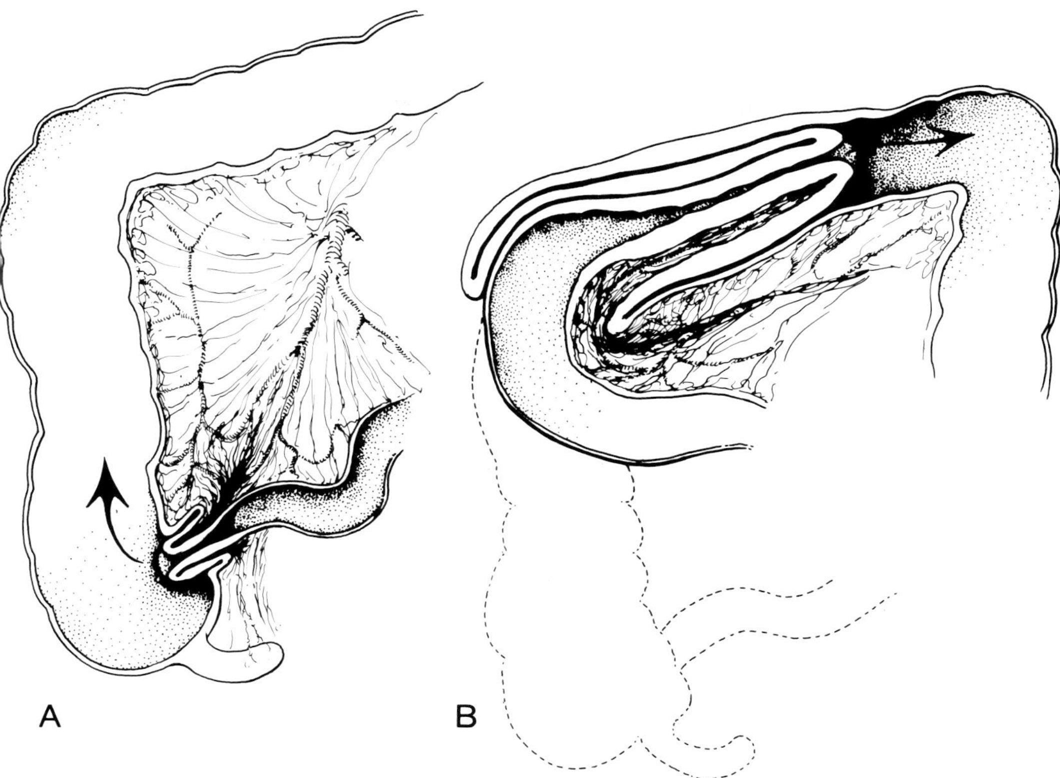

Figure 59.2 Ileocolic intussusception. (*A*) Beginning of an intussusception in which terminal ileum prolapses through ileocecal valve. (*B*) Ileocolic intussusceptum continuing through colon. This can often be palpated as a mass in the right upper quadrant.

diarrheal illness, viral syndrome, or Henoch-Schönlein purpura as a preceding illness several days to a week prior to the onset of abdominal pain and obstruction.

CLINICAL MANIFESTATIONS

The main manifestation of intussusception is crampy abdominal pain. The pain may cause the infant to cry out with episodic spasms of pain or to become still, lethargic and pale. Between periods of pain, the child may return to normal activity. The obstruction leads to vomiting and generalized abdominal distention. Often the intussusception mass can be palpated as an ill-defined sausage-shaped structure if the abdomen is not too distended. The mass is most often palpable in the right upper quadrant.

As the bowel becomes more tightly intussuscepted, the mesenteric veins become compressed, while the mesenteric arterial supply remains intact. This will lead to the production of the characteristic currant jelly stool, which may be passed spontaneously or found on the examining finger. Development of currant jelly stools can occur fairly quickly. Within only a few hours it may be noted on rectal examination. This fact reinforces the need for a rectal examination in any child with unexplained abdominal or GI symptoms. Once the intussusception has become very tight, even the arteries are occluded by the pressure of entrapment. At this point the bleeding lessens, but the bowel can become gangrenous and even perforate, with the development of frank peritonitis.

MANAGEMENT

The patient should be prepared by inserting an intravenous line and a nasogastric tube. Intravenous fluids should be given to correct dehydration. Nasogastric suction minimizes the risk of vomiting and aspiration. Once blood has been sent to the laboratory for CBC, BUN, serum electrolytes, and a crossmatch, the patient should be taken to the radiology department.

In a child with symptoms longer than 6 to 12 hours, flat and upright films frequently show signs of intestinal obstruction, including distended bowel with air-fluid levels. A soft tissue mass in the right abdomen may also be visualized, except when free air is noted, indicating perforation. A barium enema is generally indicated to confirm the diagnosis (Fig. 59.3).

In recent years, hydrostatically controlled barium enema reduction has also been a successful therapy in over half of the cases. Strict guidelines must be adhered to

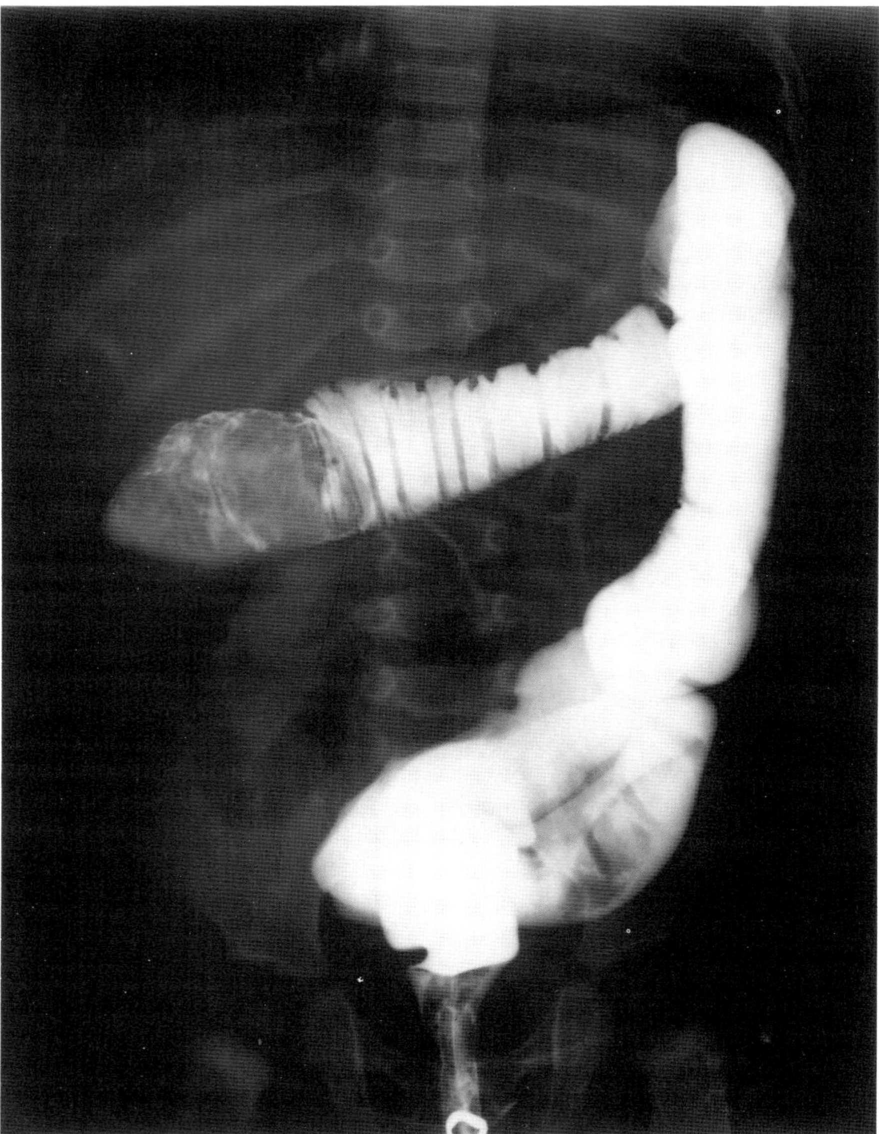

Figure 59.3 Barium enema showing ileocolic intussusceptum in right transverse colon.

in order to avoid perforation when this method is attempted. The barium column should be no higher than 3 feet above the abdomen, and manual palpation of the abdomen during the study is contraindicated. The full reduction of the intussusception is confirmed only where there has been adequate reflux of barium far into the ileum. Otherwise, only the ileocolic component of an ileoileocolic intussusception may be reduced, leaving the ileoileal intussusception unreduced.

Many youngsters with intussusception require emergency surgery, especially if the intussusception has been of long duration or the child shows evidence of gangrenous bowel, including high fever, leukocytosis, marked distention, and general toxicity. If a barium enema seems safe and appropriate, the operating room should be placed on standby and the operating team should be ready to commence immediate surgery if complications develop or the hydrostatic reduction by barium enema is unsuccessful. Preoperative preparation and resuscitation begins in the emergency department and continues during the course of the barium enema. Undue delay may well result in gangrene of the entrapped bowel. The moment surgery is decided upon, the patient should receive broad spectrum intravenous antibiotics.

Incarcerated Inguinal Hernia

Incarcerated inguinal hernia is a frequent cause of intestinal obstruction in the infant and young child. Incarceration occurs more frequently in girls, but usually involves the ovary rather than the bowel. Frequently the patient or his family has no previous knowledge of the presence of a congenital hernia. In children with acute intestinal obstruction, the internal ring area should be carefully palpated for a persistent mass which might be very small. In a youngster, who persistently vomits after a manual reduction of an incarcerated hernia, the possibility of the bowel not being entirely reduced, causing continued obstruction, must be considered. All children with a truly incarcerated lesion should be admitted, even if the hernia has been manually reduced in the emergency department. The purpose of hospitalization is observation and preparation for eventual repair. (See "Inguinal Hernia" on p. 840.)

Incarcerated Umbilical Hernia

Incarceration of an umbilical hernia is a very rare occurrence. If present, there is a persistent and tender bulge in the umbilical hernia sac. If the incarceration is of short duration, a gentle effort might be made to reduce it manually, but frequently it is necessary to prepare the child for urgent surgery. At the time of surgery, the loop of incarcerated bowel should be inspected, rather than letting it drop back into the abdominal cavity, to be certain there has been no vascular impairment. (See "Umbilical Hernias" on p. 841)

Malrotation of the Bowel with Volvulus

BACKGROUND

Malrotation of the bowel is a congenital condition associated with abnormal fixation of the mesentery of the bowel (Fig. 59.4). The bowel, therefore, has a proclivity to volvulize and obstruct at these points of abnormal fixation. Although malrotation with volvulus usually occurs either in utero or during early neonatal life, malrotation can go unrecognized until childhood. This is an extraordinarily dangerous situation, since a complete volvulus of the bowel for more than an hour or two can totally obstruct blood supply to the bowel leading to complete necrosis of the involved segment. When a volvulus involves the midgut, the entire small bowel and ascending colon may be lost, making the patient dependent on intravenous hyperalimentation for survival. The only way to prevent such a catastrophe is to have a high index of suspicion for malrotation in any child with signs of obstruction and to be prepared to get a child with a presumed volvulus to the operating room immediately.

CLINICAL MANIFESTATIONS

Any child with bile-stained vomiting and abdominal pain may have malrotation with volvulus. The pain is usually constant and not crampy. Blood may appear in the stool

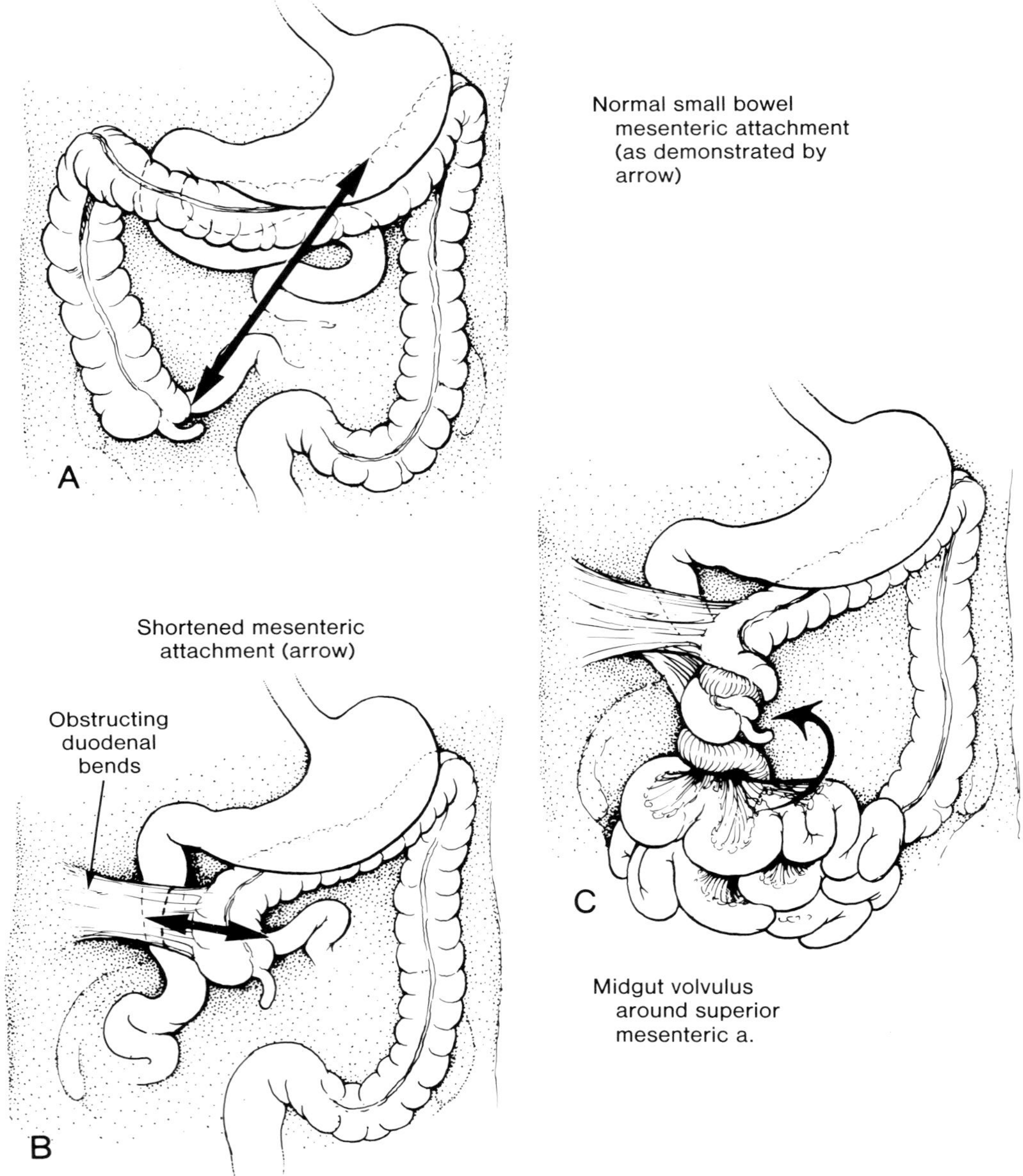

Figure 59.4 Malrotation with volvulus. (*A*) Normal small bowel mesenteric attachment (as demonstrated by *arrow*). This prevents twisting of small bowel because of the broad fixation of the mesentery. (*B*) Malrotation of colon with obstructing duodenal bands. (*C*) Midgut volvulus around superior mesenteric artery due to narrow base of mesentery.

within a few hours and suggests the development of ischemia and possible necrosis of the bowel. Clinically, malrotation can present in several different ways: first, and most dangerous, is the sudden onset of abdominal pain with bilious vomiting with no prior history of GI problems; second, is a similar abrupt onset of obstruction in a child who previously seemed to have "feeding problems" with transient episodes of bilious vomiting; third, is in a child with failure to thrive due to alleged intolerance of feedings. This last example may involve a child who has used a dozen different formulas and in whom the vomiting is chronic and generally unassociated with pain.

On physical examination there may be only mild distention of the abdomen since the obstruction usually occurs so high in the GI tract. On palpation, one may discern one or two prominently dilated loops of bowel. The abdomen may be diffusely tender and yet not have clear signs of peritonitis. On rectal examination the presence of blood on the examining finger is an alarming sign of impending ischemia and gangrene of the bowel.

MANAGEMENT

The key to management is to be suspicious of malrotation and to obtain flat and upright x-rays of the abdomen immediately. The presence of loops of small bowel overriding the liver shadow is very suggestive of an underlying malrotation. When complete volvulus has occurred there may be only a few dilated loops of bowel with air fluid levels. Distal to the volvulus there may be little or no gas in the GI tract. When one is assessing a child for possible malrotation on an elective basis, a barium enema followed by an upper GI series is an acceptable approach. However, in a child with possible acute volvulus of the bowel, a barium enema may take too long to perform and may only show a high cecum which in some infants is a normal variant. By contrast, an upper GI series with 30 to 50 ml of barium will demonstrate within minutes the acute obstruction of the duodenum with the duodenojejunal junction at the midline or to the right of the midline, rather than in its usual position at the ligament of Treitz on the left (Fig. 59.5).

As in the case of a child with presumed intussusception, a child with a possible volvulus should be prepared for immediate surgery. The operating room and operating team should be on standby. Intravenous fluid and electrolyte replacement should begin immediately. A nasogastric tube should be inserted and blood crossmatched. Since this entity can present even in adulthood, every surgeon should understand the pathogenesis and surgical therapy of malrotation. If immediate transfer to a children's hospital cannot be accomplished within an hour, a laparotomy should be performed without delay.

Pyloric Stenosis

Narrowing of the pyloric canal due to hypertrophy of the musculature characteristically occurs in the first born male of a family. It has been shown that there is a familial incidence, particularly if the mother has had hypertrophic pyloric stenosis as an infant. There is a male to female ratio of 5 to 1. The age of onset is usually 2 to 5 weeks. Rarely, the onset may be late in the second month of life. The etiology of this muscle hypertrophy is unknown but its symptomatology, diagnosis and therapy are well defined.

CLINICAL MANIFESTATIONS

Characteristically, the infant does well without vomiting for the first few weeks of life and then starts regurgitating, either at the end of feedings or a few minutes later. The infants are hungry and will eat heartily immediately following such a regurgitation. The vomiting becomes more prominent and eventually becomes more forceful, referred to as "projectile vomiting." The vomitus ordinarily contains just the feeding that has been given and does not contain bile or blood. Occasionally there is some mucus in the vomitus. Infants with pyloric stenosis may also become jaundiced with the onset of the other symptoms. The hyperbilirubinemia usually improves or abates postoperatively for reasons that are not known.

The examination of an infant is best accomplished after the infant's stomach has been emptied. With the child lying on his back, the examiner holds the infant's ankles and flexes his thighs at right angle to the trunk as the mother feeds some warm sugar water with the infant's head turned to the right but not elevated. Once the infant starts to suck, the upper abdominal musculature will relax and the examiner's opposite hand can then gently palpate the upper right abdomen. Palpating under the edge of the liver in an up and down direc-

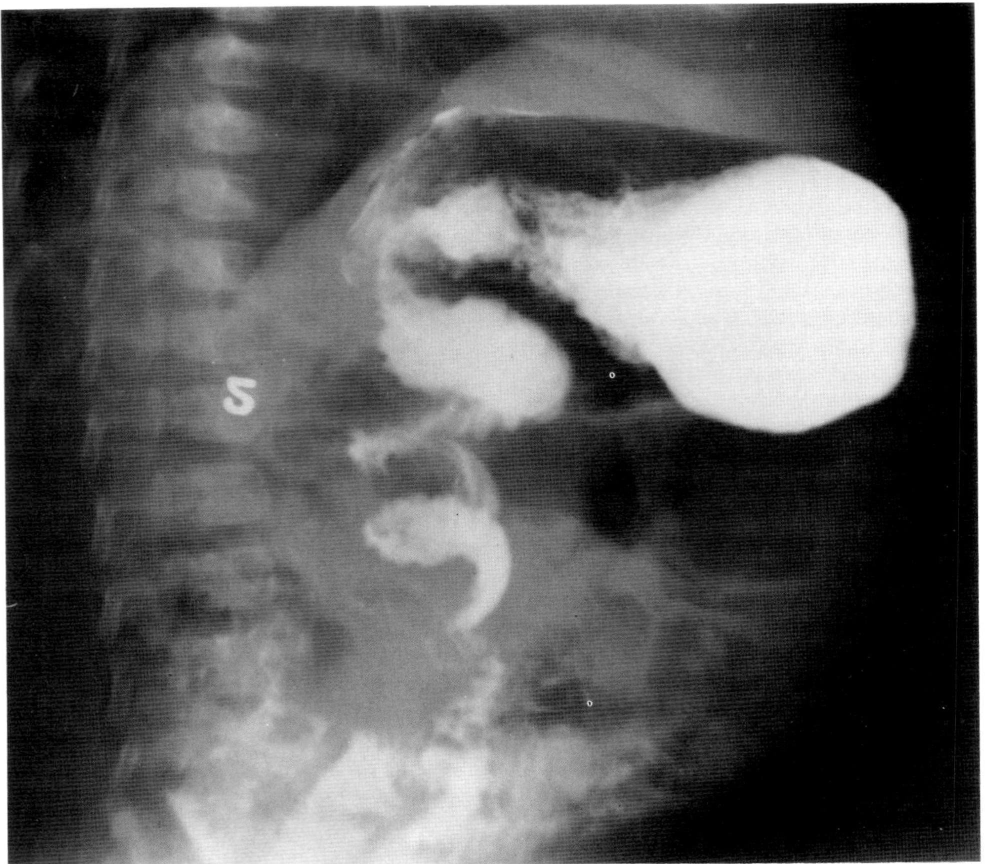

Figure 59.5 Malrotation. Upper GI study showing duodenojejunal junction to the right of the midline, absence of the ligament of Treitz and coiled spring appearance of jejunum.

tion one may discern a firm, fusiform, ballottable mass in the shape of an "olive." If this "olive" is not felt, the stomach can be emptied with a nastogastric tube to allow easier palpation and the examination repeated. Another diagnostic clue is the presence of prominent gastric peristaltic waves that course from left to right across the abdomen.

If there has been vomiting for an extended period of time, the child will show signs of growth failure. There may be an absence of subcutaneous tissue and loose hanging skin. The infant may take on an "old man" appearance with wrinkled skin on the face and body. There will be inadequate weight gain, which may be calculated by knowing that the average child regains his/her birth weight by 10 days of age and therafter 15 to 30 g (½ to 1 ounce) per day.

Serum electrolytes may be abnormal due to gastric losses. The potassium and chloride will be low and serum bicarbonate high. This hypochloremic alkalosis may be profound, with serum chlorides in the 65 to 75 meq/L range. When dehydration becomes severe, the patient may then develop acidosis indicating an advanced and even more dangerous metabolic imbalance (see Chapter 46).

MANAGEMENT

Infants should be hospitalized and rehydrated with appropriate fluid and electrolyte replacement. Initial intravenous fluids should be 5% dextrose in normal saline. Potassium chloride (3 to 5 meq/kg) should be added once urine output has been established. If hypotonic solutions are used, there is significant risk of causing hyponatremia (see Chapter 46). A volume of fluid should be used appropriate to the patient's level of dehydration.

If an "olive mass" is palpable and clear gastric waves are visible, x-ray confirmation of the diagnosis is not needed. If the history of vomiting is not typical and if an "olive" cannot be felt, the patient should undergo a barium upper GI series. The study should be a thorough one in order to eliminate esophageal reflux and malrotation as diagnostic possibilities. In general, pyloric stenosis can be identified by the presence of a "string sign" in the pyloric channel, seen best on oblique projections.

The barium should be evacuated from the stomach after the x-rays have been completed to lessen the risk of vomiting and aspiration. Surgical pyloromyotomy is a most successful form of therapy, and such infants can usually be discharged from the hospital 3 days following surgery. Some infants will have some regurgitation postoperatively due to a temporary relaxation of the gastroesophageal sphincter.

Postoperative Adhesions

Prior abdominal surgery or peritonitis places a child at risk for intestinal obstruction due to adhesions (Fig. 59.6). Such obstruction can occur relatively early in the postoperative course or months or even years later. Suddenly and without warning the child develops abdominal cramps, nausea, vomiting, and abdominal distention. Although most intestinal obstructions due to adhesions do not jeopardize the vascularity of the bowel, occasionally a loop of intestine, caught under a fibrous band, can become gangrenous. Therefore, the diagnosis should be made quickly. All such patients need to be admitted to the hospital and evaluated by a surgeon who should direct the complete management.

CHRONIC, PARTIAL INTESTINAL OBSTRUCTION

Any youngster with intermittent abdominal distention, nausea, anorexia, occasional vomiting, and chronic constipation or obstipation, may have partial intestinal obstruction. There are a number of diagnostic considerations.

Chronic Constipation

This is probably one of the most common causes for abdominal pain, distention and vomiting in childhood. The history, if available from a reliable mother, may attest to chronic constipation; however, occasionally such a child is diagnosed only by palpating a large fecaloma through the intact abdominal wall or a hard fecal mass blocking the anal outlet on rectal examination. Such youngsters may have a history of encopresis and appear malnourished. Chapter 11 covers the diagnostic approach to the child with constipation.

These youngsters should be disimpacted by instilling a generous amount of warm mineral oil per rectum followed by copious saline lavages using a large caliber rectal tube with extra holes. Frequently a gloved finger is necessary to break up a hard fecal mass and allow its evacuation. If the process has reached this stage, it is unlikely that the mother can manage it at home and either emergency department or in-hospital management is necessary to clean out the bowel adequately. Once the bowel has been cleaned, it is important to institute an appropriate regimen to retrain the child and produce better bowel habits.

Aganglionic Megacolon (Hirschsprung's Disease)

In Hirschsprung's disease, there is absence of the parasympathetic ganglion cells of Auerbach's plexus between the circular and longitudinal muscle layers of the colon. The involved segment varies in length, from less than 1 cm to involvement of the entire colon and small bowel. The effect of this absence of ganglion cells produces spasm and abnormal motility of that segment, which results in either complete intestinal obstruction or chronic constipation.

There is a lifelong history of constipation in these children, so it is very important to obtain an accurate account of the child's stool pattern since birth. A child with Hirschsprung's disease typically has never been able to stool properly without assistance (e.g., enemas, suppositories, stimulation with the finger or thermometer, etc.).

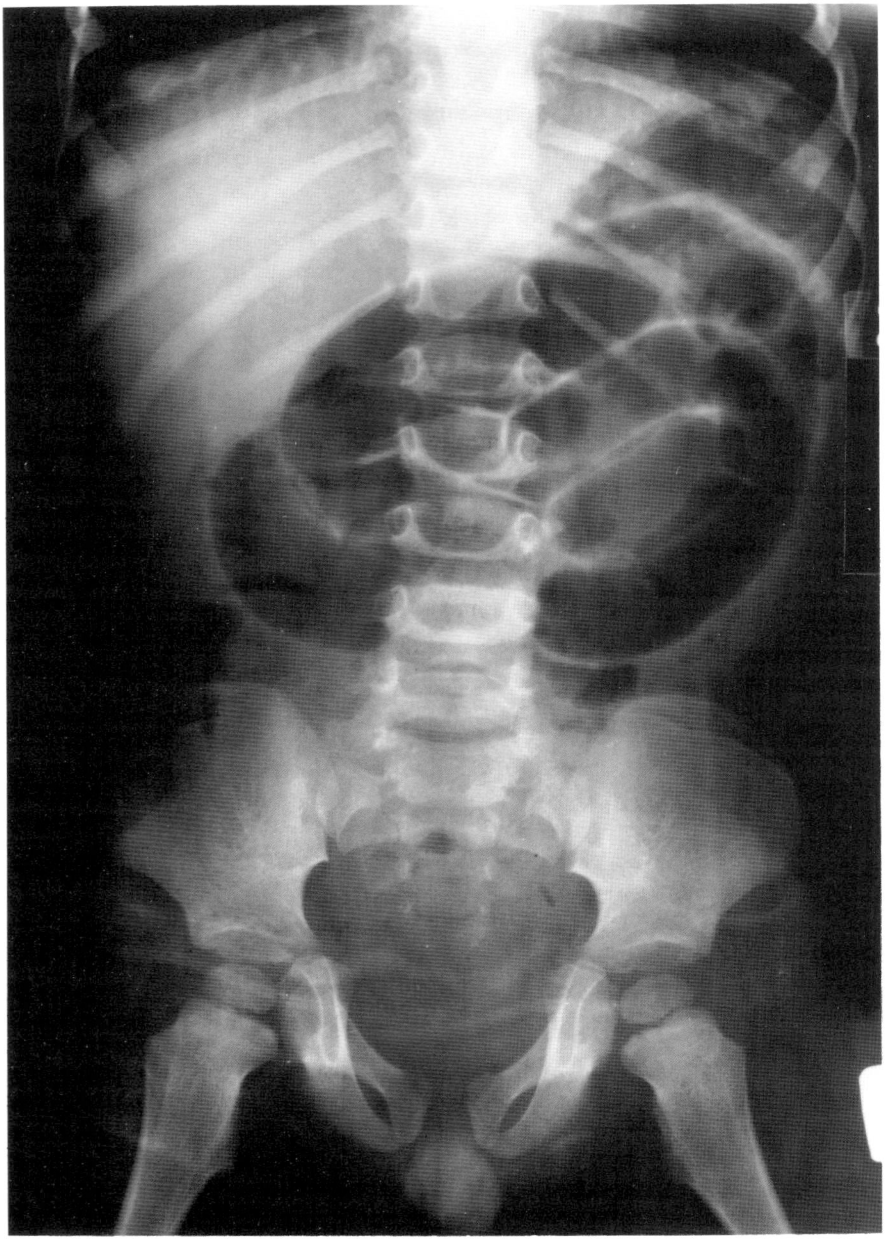

Figure 59.6 Dilated loops of small intestine, absence of air in lower abdomen indicating a high intestinal obstruction due to postoperative adhesions.

Normal stooling is not possible because of the failure of the distal aganglionic bowel to relax. There is usually no history of encopresis as one would find in chronic functional constipation. These youngsters have chronic abdominal distention and are frequently malnourished. Vomiting is uncommon as are other symptoms. Complete intestinal obstruction in Hirschsprung's disease is more likely to occur in early infancy and only rarely in the older age groups.

After flat and upright abdominal x-rays have been obtained, a properly performed barium enema is the best initial diagnostic procedure. There should be no "prep" of the bowel. Ideally there should be no stimulation of the rectum, such as enema or digital examination, for 2 to 3 days before the procedure. The key to diagnosis is seeing a "transition zone" (Fig. 59.7) between the contracted aganglionic bowel and the proximal dilated ganglionated bowel. Stimulation of the rectum shortly before the study may result in decompression of the proximal bowel with loss of definition of the transition zone. When a clear-cut transition zone is seen, it is not necesary to fill the colon with barium more than 12 to 18 inches above the transition point. It is important, however, not to empty the colon of barium at the end of the study. The

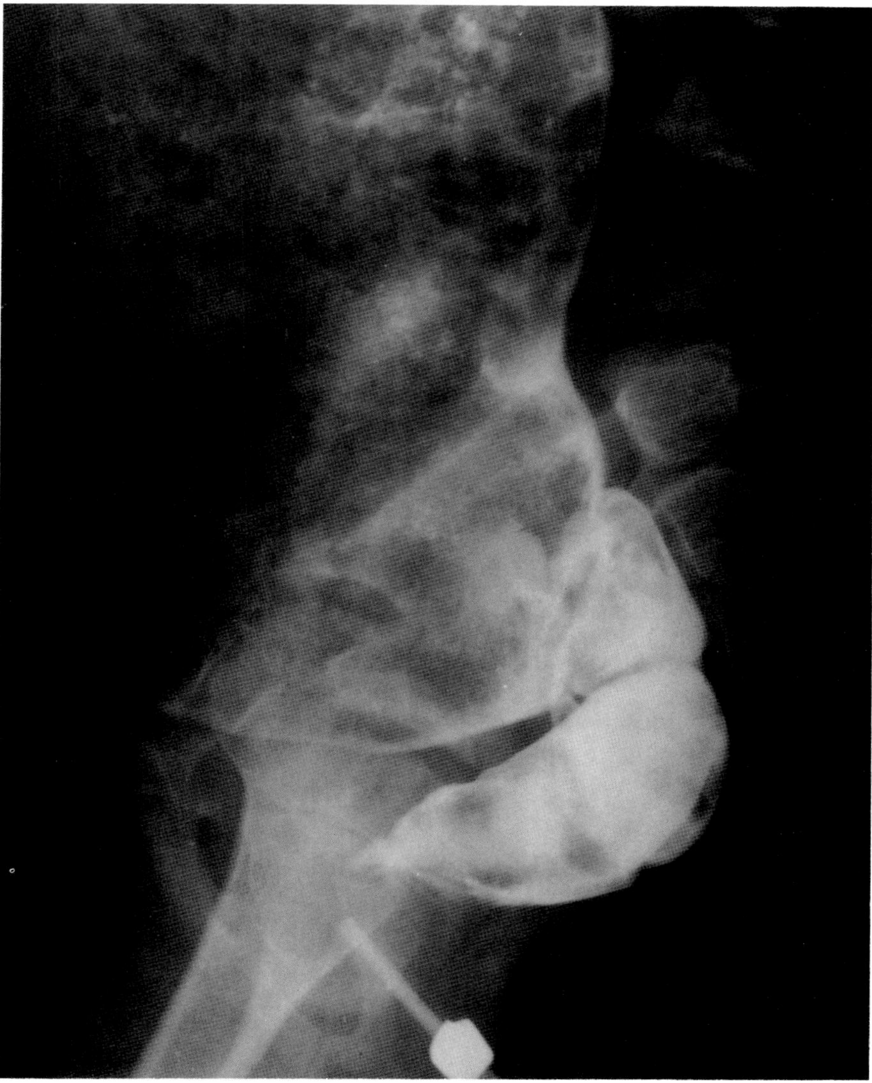

Figure 59.7 Barium enema showing narrow aganglionic segment with proximal megacolon.

presence of retained barium above the transition point 24 hours later will strongly suggest the diagnosis of Hirschsprung's disease.

Anorectal manometrics are helpful in confirming the neurogenic dysfunction of the bowel. In very young infants, however, the manometrics may not be completely reliable. Moreover, in children of all ages an adequately performed suction mucosal biopsy of the rectum 2 cm, or more, above the dentate line can be very reliable in diagnosing Hirschsprung's disease. Because of the complicated evaluation and management of this disease, referral to a pediatric surgeon is recommended.

Duplications

Duplications occur anywhere from the mouth to the anus and produce a variety of symptoms. In the abdomen, there may be a noncommunicating cyst which gradually fills up with secretions and compresses the adjacent normal bowel, producing a palpable abdominal mass or chronic intestinal obstruction. An occasional duplication has a communication, particularly at its distal end, which will produce a large mass that may be confused with the stool mass felt with aganglionic Hirschsprung's disease. Vary rarely a stercorous or a marginal ulcer due to ectopic gastric mucosa may occur, and this produces painless bleeding. After appropriate x-ray diagnosis, surgery is indicated; the surgical procedures vary depending on the locations, size and communications of the anomaly.

Inflammatory Bowel Disease

The older child or adolescent may develop either Crohn's disease or ulcerative colitis and this must be included in the differential diagnosis of chronic intestinal obstruction. Usually there is an antecedent history of changing bowel habits with mucus or blood in the stools, chronic abdominal pain, and weight loss. Chapter 50 covers inflammatory bowel disease in detail.

DISEASE PRODUCING RECTAL BLEEDING

Rectal bleeding is an alarming symptom. It is very important to determine the quantity of bleeding and whether the blood is on the outside of the stool or mingled with it. A "tarry" stool suggests a source of bleeding in the proximal portion of the GI tract and bright red blood a more distal origin. Occasionally the child will have an episode or two of blood with his bowel movements. All patients with rectal bleeding should have a rectal examination. Those with significant hemorrhage require anoscopy, and many should have sigmoidoscopy, or examination through a flexible colonoscope or a contrast barium enema. In some patients, no definite diagnosis may be reached despite extensive studies. In any patient with significant bleeding, however, surgical consultation is indicated. Chapters 22 and 50 discuss further the diagnosis and management of patients with GI bleeding.

Fissures

An anal fissure is probably the most common cause for bleeding, especially in infants. Fissures, however, may occur at any age. There is usually an antecedent history of passing a large, hard stool with anal discomfort. Frequently there is a history of chronic constipation with progressive reluctance of the patient to pass stool, because of the associated discomfort. If bleeding occurs, it usually involves streaking of bright red blood on the outside of the stool or red blood on the toilet tissues. The diagnosis can easily be made by inspection or anoscopic examination, and appropriate measures are taken to relieve the chronic constipation (see Chapter 11). Children may be helped by sitz baths and the application of local anesthetic ointments such as Nupercaine. Rarely does a child require hospitalization or surgery.

Juvenile Polyps

Older infants and children can develop either a single or multiple retention polyps. Usually the polyps occur in the lower portion of the colon and can frequently be palpated on rectal examination. Polyps bleed, although they rarely cause massive hemorrhage. They may intermittently prolapse at the anus or on occasion come free and be passed as a fecal mass associated with bleeding. Colonic polyps may be the lead points for intussusception. Usually, however, polyps are asymptomatic except for the associated bleeding. These are not premalignant lesions, and they tend to be self-limiting.

If a polyp can be felt on rectal examination or viewed through the sigmoidoscope, it may be safely removed, but it is usually not necessary to remove these occurring higher in the colon. This lessens the need for colonoscopy or laparotomy.

Familial Polyposis

Families with multiple adenomatous colonic polyps are rarely encountered. Bleeding is rare. More frequently a colitis type mucous discharge is present. Rectal examination and endoscopy reveal multiple "cobblestone," sessile polyps. These individuals are at risk for neoplasia, since these are premalignant adenomatous polyps. The child should be referred to a pediatric surgeon and gastroenterologist for evaluation and long-term management.

Meckel's Diverticulum

Two percent of the population are born with a Meckel's diverticulum. This is the most common omphalomesenteric duct remnant. The diverticulum is usually located 50 to 75 cm proximal to the terminal ileum. Only 2% of people with a Meckel's diverticulum manifest any clinical problems. The most common complications of a Meckel's diverticulum is a bleeding ulcer. Ectopic gastric mucosa in such patients is usually present in the diverticulum. The acid secretion produces an erosion at the junction of the normal ileal mucosa with the ectopic mucosa. Although bleeding is usually slight, it may become severe and necessitate surgery to remove the offending diverticulum. Small amounts of blood loss over a long period may produce iron deficiency anemia. The bleeding is usually painless. Frequently a patient with massive rectal bleeding and no other abnormal syptoms or signs will require a laparotomy on the assumption that there is a bleeding ulcerated Meckel's diverticulum. Other modes of presentation include diverticulitis, perforation with peritonitis, or intussusception due to the diverticulum serving as a lead point.

Barium studies will usually fail to outline a Meckel's diverticulum. Recently the use of technitium-99m scans with enhancement using pentagastrin stimulation have proved to be especially helped in pinpointing sites of ectopic gastric mucosa in patients with bleeding from a Meckel's diverticulum. These enhanced scans, unfortunately, have only an 80 to 90% accuracy. Therefore, in any child with a major rectal bleed and a negative scan, further workup is required including an arteriogram, if the bleeding continues to be active, or colonoscopy, when the bleeding is not active.

Henoch Schönlein Purpura

Henoch Schönlein purpura is a vasculitic disorder that can produce asymptomatic rectal bleding or abdominal pain and bleeding. Usually there is visible evidence of vasculitis on the skin surface, but initially a patient may have only abdominal pain. Occasionally a child will develop an intussusception due to a submucosal hemorrhage that is acting as a lead point. Other common manifestations are purpuric rash, fever, and joint pains (see Chapter 47).

Other Causes of Rectal Bleeding

Other causes of rectal bleeding include the following: (1) intestinal vascular malformations, (2) intussusception, (3) duplications, (4) inflammatory bowel disease, (5) peptic ulcer with bleding, and (6) portal hypertension with bleeding varices. These topics are covered elsewhere in this chapter and in Chapter 50, "Gastrointestinal Emergencies," or in Chapter 22, "Gastrointestinal Bleeding."

INTRA-ABDOMINAL MASSES

BACKGROUND

Intra-abdominal masses in children can be benign, but, unfortunately, there are also a number of malignant ones. Abdominal masses may be quite silent, even after the tumor has reached a large size. Many intra-abdominal masses are first recognized by the parent or the child's caretaker while the child is being undressed or bathed.

It is very difficult to feel an intra-abdominal mass and outline its limits and its degree of mobility if an infant or child is crying. If the child is fed a bottle with his head turned to one side the infant will relax his abdominal musculature. The physician should then make an effort to carefully palpate the intra-abdominal contents. Since many malignant masses first present as a recent finding due to spontaneous internal hemorrhage, these masses are fragile and prone to rupture. Palpation of the mass, therefore, should be done quite gently and should be strictly limited to as few examiners as possible.

Retroperitoneal masses tend to be fixed, whereas masses attached to mesentery or omentum are mobile and may be shifted to different locations by the examiner. Pelvic masses are frequently fixed and can be often best felt by rectal examination. A presacral mass may narrow the rectum and produce constipation. Abdominal masses present with varying characteristics and may be smooth, nodular, cystic, or rock hard.

Initial evaluation in the emergency department may include flat and upright abdominal films. If, after such an examination, the origin of the mass is unclear or suggests a neoplasm, the patient should be admitted and a workup done without delay. This evaluation often includes intravenous pyelogram, ultrasound, barium contrast studies, and CAT scans. If for some reason it is not feasible to admit the child when he or she first presents with an unexplained mass, careful follow-up arrangements should be made including admission to an appropriate facility within a day or two. There is no place for observation in dealing with unexplained abdominal masses in children.

Nonmalignant Intra-Abdominal Mass

Fecaloma

A lower abdominal mass, particularly one on the left side, is most often related to retained stool, and is more often associated with chronic functional constipation rather than with Hirschsprung's disease. If a mass is found, a careful review of the bowel habits is important. If an abdominal mass is a fecaloma, there will usually be a large bolus of stool that can be felt on rectal examination just inside the anus. The evacuation of the impaction and irrigation of the upper sigmoid colon should cause the mass to disappear. See Chapter 11 for the causes of constipation.

Ovarian Masses

Simple ovarian cysts and solid teratomas are not uncommon and may be asymptomatic even though they have reached a large size. Occasionally the child presents with urinary complaints from the pressure on the bladder or urethra. Granulosa cell tumors of the ovary produce precocious puberty because they are hormonally active tumors and may be malignant. The sudden onset of severe abdominal pain may indicate a torsion of an ovarian mass on a slender pedicle with resultant infarction. They tend to give the impression of rising up from the pelvis and on occasion will lie in the midabdomen or even the upper abdomen. When they are still partially within the pelvis, they usually can be felt by rectal examination. Most ovarian masses are smooth and nontender. X-rays may show calcification in about one half of patients with teratomas. Since an occasional ovarian tumor is malignant in childhood, children with ovarian masses should be promptly evaluated and prepared for surgery (see Chapter 52).

Omental Cysts

Omental cysts are rare, and are usually asymptomatic and can reach gigantic size. It is frequently difficult to differentiate an omental cyst from ascites. There are a number of cases on record where omental cysts have been tapped, on the assumption that they were ascitic fluid. Smaller cysts are more mobile and can be pushed freely into all quadrants of the abdomen. If a cyst volvulizes on its pedicle or has bleeding within it, it may cause abdominal pain or tenderness. Elective surgical excision is indicated.

Mesenteric Cysts

These cysts can occur anywhere in the mesentery but are most frequent in the mesentery of the colon. They tend to be multilocular and are often discovered during a routine examination or after an episode of abdominal trauma with enlargement due to bleeding. They are benign but surgical therapy is indicated, both to confirm the diagnosis and to prevent complications. They can usually be removed with sparing of the bowel, or they can be marsupialized into the general peritoneal cavity where the fluid will be absorbed.

Duplications

GI duplications within the abdomen can occur anywhere along the greater curvature of the stomach, the lesser curvature of the duodenum, or the mesenteric side of either the small or large intestines. They can also be pararectal, rising up out of the pelvis. Duplications that produce abdominal masses are either noncommunicating, and hence gradually enlarge, or communicating in that their secretory lining has a distal communication with the true lumen of the bowel. Except for the rare occurrence of massive rectal bleeding in a child with a communicating duplication, most duplications do not present as emergencies. Instead they present in children either as unexplained abdominal masses or with symptoms of intermittent colic due to partial obstruction of the true lumen of the adjacent bowel. Often the exact diagnosis is not clear until the time of laparotomy.

Malignant Intra-Abdominal Masses

Roughly 50% of the solid malignant tumors seen in childhood occur within the abdominal cavity. They generally occur in the retroperitoneum. The most frequent is neuroblastoma, followed by Wilms' tumor and rhabdomyosarcoma. Other unusual tumors, such as embryonal cell carcinomas (yolk sac tumor) and lymphosarcoma, also occur in young children. Chapter 55 covers oncologic emergencies. As with most malignant tumors, early diagnosis and treatment provide the best prospects for a cure. One must, therefore, have a high index of suspicion for malignancy in any child with a mass or unexplained GI or genitourinary symptoms.

Neuroblastoma

Neuroblastoma most frequently occurs as a tumor in the left or right adrenal gland, but it can develop anywhere along the sympathetic chain or in the pelvis. It has even been found intrarenally. It has the ability to grow extensively, often crossing the midline of the abdomen, and enveloping key vascular and visceral structures. The best cure rates are generally in children who are less than 1 year of age at the time of diagnosis and in whom the tumor is still localized to the point of origin. In such favorable cases the tumor can be totally excised. When widespread dissemination occurs, complete resection is unwarranted because of the risk to other vital structures.

Wilms' Tumor

Wilms' tumor is the most common intrarenal tumor of childhood. Great progress has been made in the last several decades in its management. The tumor can reach a gigantic size before its discovery. Wilms' tumor should be considered in any child who has hematuria even if there is a history of trauma. An intravenous pyelogram is mandatory in a child with hematuria or an unexplained abdominal mass. Further assessment includes ultrasound, an inferior vena cavagram, and chest x-rays to rule out metastases. Surgical removal should not be delayed. Postoperative management with chemotherapeutic agents and selective irradiation is important. These youngsters should be cared for by a team of specialists with thorough knowledge of ancillary forms of therapy.

Rhabdomyosarcoma

Rhabdomyosarcoma can occur anywhere in the abdomen or pelvis where there is striated muscle. Tumors are particularly common in the pelvis, involving the prostate, uterus or vagina and retroperitoneal structures but have been found also in the common bile duct and other unusual sites. These tumors can reach a large size before they become symptomatic and each must be managed individually depending on the site of origin, extent of growth and the degree of spread. Modern selective therapy has greatly improved the survival rate of this highly malignant tumor.

Hepatoma

Hepatomas are fortunately rare. They are usually seen in older infants and young children. Hepatoblastoma is more frequent than hepatoma. They are often discovered accidently when the child is undressed for a bath. The child may feel and act well, yet the tumor is already of a formidable size when first noted. Differential diagnosis should include hemangioendothelioma, hamartoma, and renal and adrenal tumors, especially if they occur on the right side.

Preoperative studies include chest film, intravenous pyelogram, ultrasound and selective arteriography. Survival depends on both complete resection of the primary tumor before metastases have occurred, and intensive prolonged chemotherapy postoperatively. As much as two thirds of the liver may have to be removed.

ABDOMINAL WALL DEFECTS

Inguinal Hernias and Hydroceles

Indirect inguinal hernia is the most common congenital anomaly that is found in children. They are roughly 10 times more frequent in males than in females. There is a strong familial incidence.

CLINICAL MANIFESTATIONS

The child with a hernia may present in different ways. This is determined by the extent of obliteration of the processus vaginalis prior to birth. A child may have a completely open hernia sac, which extends from the internal ring to the scrotum, or a segmental obliteration producing a sac which is narrow at its proximal end, creating a hydrocele either of the tunica vaginalis or spermatic cord. The narrowing of the processus allows the abdominal fluid to seep into the distal portion of the sac. It then becomes entrapped and produces what is clinically recognized as a "hydrocele." It is often difficult for this fluid to egress through the narrow patent process vaginalis back into the abdominal cavity.

At the time of the embryologic closure of the processus vaginalis many fetuses will have some fluid trapped around the testicle in the tunica vaginalis. This is referred to as a physiological hydrocele, which is a normal newborn finding. In such cases the fluid will gradually be absorbed in the first 6 months of life. If, however, an infant or child develops a hydrocele along the cord in the tunica vaginalis sometime after birth, it must be assumed that the processus vaginalis is still patent and in communication with the peritoneal cavity. This patent processus vaginalis represents a hernia sac. Surgical closure of the sac and drainage of the hydrocele is then indicated.

Many infants and children will manifest the classical bulge in the inguinal canal that occurs when straining or crying. This is caused by a loop of intestine distending into the hernia sac. Usually the hernia sac contents reduce into the general abdominal cavity when the straining ceases. If the prolapsing loop of intestine becomes entrapped in the inguinal sac, an incarceration has occurred. This is a true surgical emergency, which could eventually lead to intestinal obstruction and possibly strangulation of the bowel.

Hydroceles of the upper spermatic cord with associated communicating hernias are sometimes difficult to differentiate from an incarcerated hernia. If an empty hernia sac can be felt above the hydrocele, then one can be assured that this is an asymptomatic hernia with an associated hydrocele. However, if the empty hernia sac cannot be felt above the hydrocele and the mass cannot be reduced, the child should be taken to the operating room on the assumption that it probably is an incarcerated hernia that needs to be managed surgically.

MANAGEMENT

Surgeons prefer not to operate on incarcerated hernias in infants and children. Fortunately, strangulation of the entrapped loop of bowel in children occurs relatively late so that, contrary to adult practice, efforts to reduce the incarceration without surgery are usually warranted. When an incarcerated hernia presents in the emergency department the child should be given nothing to eat or drink, mildly sedated, and placed in a Trendelenberg position. Very often this alone will reduce the incarceration. If it does not, bimanual reduction should be attempted. If the child is warm and preferably asleep as a result of the sedation, the reduction is facilitated. The fingers and thumb of one hand should compress the internal ring area while an effort is made with the other hand "to milk" either gas or fluid out of the entrapped bowel back into the intra-abdominal intestines. This relieves the pressure and usually will allow the entire loop of bowel to reduce back into the abdominal cavity. Once the incarcerated hernia is reduced, the child should be admitted. A day or two should be allowed to pass in order to lessen the edema of the area and allow an easier and safer elective herniorrhaphy.

Epiploceles (Epigastric Hernias)

If a discrete mass occurs intermittently about one third of the distance from the umbilicus to the xiphoid, this is usually the result of a weakness of the linea alba through which properitoneal fat protrudes. This defect is known as epiplocele. Such defects are fairly common in infants and usually close spontaneously. In older children the mass may on occasion be tender. If it becomes excruciatingly tender it is a sign that fat has became incarcerated in the hernia. Although there is no great urgency, these small midline defects should be repaired surgically when they become symptomatic.

Umbilical Hernias

Umbilical hernias are very frequent in small infants, particularly those of the black race. Fortunately, most of them tend to close spontaneously and only rarely does incarceration occur. Umbilical hernias can be quite large and unsightly and can have either a small or a large opening through the linea alba. Families need reassurance that watchful waiting is the best course. However if the umbilical hernia fails to close by the age of 4 to 6 years, surgical repair is indicated. Umbilical hernias may be repaired earlier if there is a very large ring which shows no signs of diminishing in size over 1 to 2 years, if there is a thinning of the umbilical skin or if an incarceration has occurred. Hernias that have a supraumbilical component tend not to close spontaneously and may be operated upon at an earlier time of life.

Other Umbilical Defects

Omphalomesenteric duct remnants may persist in either of two forms. When the duct is patent from the ileum to the umbilicus, there is a release of small bowel contents via an opening in the umbilicus. A second form involves a remnant of the omphalomesenteric duct which contains a secreting mucosal patch which is attached to an opening in the center of the umbilicus. Passage of a sterile blunt probe, or instillation of contrast dye under fluoroscopy via the umbilical opening will usually confirm either of these conditions. Once identified, these remnants must be excised surgically. By contrast, some infants present with umbilical granulomas where an excessive amount of granulation tissue has built up following separation of the umbilical cord. In these patients no opening in the granulation tissue can be seen or felt by means of a probe. These granulomas are usually best treated by application of silver nitrate to the granulation tissue. Occasionally two or more treatments are required. After each treatment one should rinse the area thoroughly to prevent burning of adjacent skin. If the granuloma is allowed to persist, it will eventually epithelialize and become an umbilical papilloma (Fig. 59.8).

If the urachus persists following birth it can form a urinary fistula that drains at the umbilicus. This problem is ordinarily noted in the newborn period. Older infants or children may present with drainage at the umbilicus due to persistence of part of the urachus even though connection with the bladder may be obliterated. These urachal remnants also require surgical excision.

FOREIGN BODIES OF THE GI TRACT

When a child ingests a foreign body it causes great family concern. Such ingestions, however, are rarely a problem once the object has reached the stomach. Occasionally a coin or a plastic toy may get impacted at the level of the cricopharyngeus. If these have not moved after a brief period of observation they should be removed with the aid of endoscopy. Foreign bodies that reach the stomach, whether pointed or sharp edged, usually pass completely through the intestinal tract and will be evacuated. Cathartics and other efforts to hurry their transit should not be used.

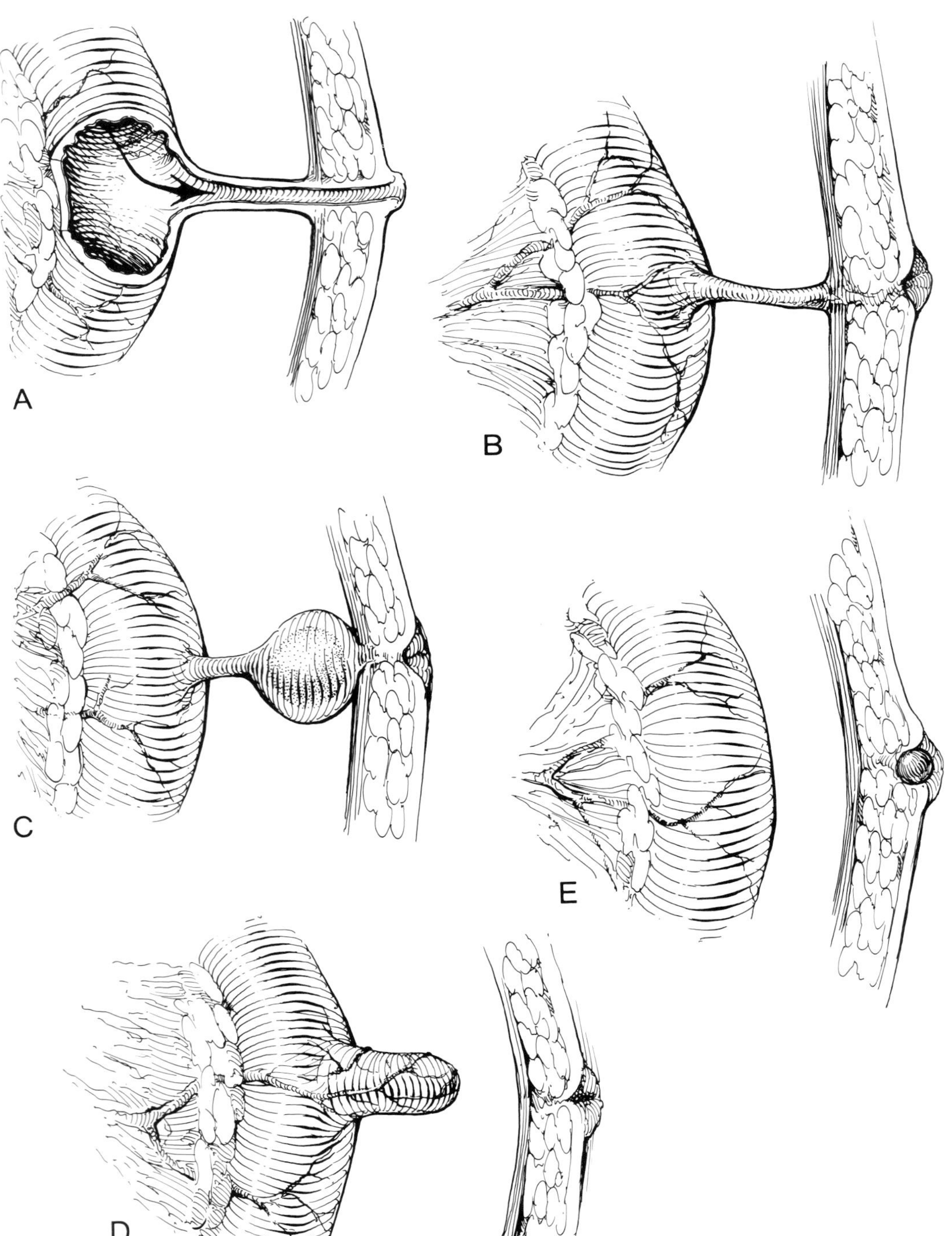

Figure 59.8 Omphalomesenteric remnants. (*A*) Patent omphalomesenteric duct from terminal ileum to umbilicus. (*B*) Closed omphalomesenteric duct with mucosal patch at umbilicus. (*C*) Omphalomesenteric cyst below umbilicus. (*D*) Meckel's diverticulum. (*E*) Umbilical granuloma.

Occasionally, a long, thin foreign body, such as a bobby pin, may not be able to traverse the turn where the duodenum joins the jejunum at the ligament of Treitz. If a foreign body gets entrapped in this area, perforation with local or generalized peritonitis, may occur. When entrapment occurs anywhere beyond the pylorus, surgical removal is indicated either to prevent or to treat local perforation. Occasionally objects, such as straight pins, toothpicks and broom straws, become entrapped in the appendix. When this occurs, the appendix should be removed. Coins may remain in the child's stomach for considerable time and, if they do not become imbeddeed in the gastric mucosa, they will eventually pass, even after a month or more. With the aid of modern flexible endoscopic equipment, foreign bodies in the stomach can usually be removed with ease. Chapter 62 covers pharyngeal foreign bodies.

References

Appendicitis

Bakhda RK, McNair MM: Useful radiological signs in acute appendicitis in children. *Clin Radiol* 28: 193, 1977.

Fine M, Busuttil RW: Acute appendicitis; efficacy of prophylactic preoperative antibiotics in the reduction of septic morbidity. *Am J Surg* 135: 210, 1978.

Golden GT, Shaw A: Primary peritonitis. *Surg Gynecol Obstet* 135: 513, 1972.

Grosfeld JL, Weinberger M, Clatworthy HW: Acute appendicitis in the first two years of life. *J Pediatr Surg* 8: 285, 1973.

Janik JS, Firor HV: Pediatric appendicitis, a 20-year study of 1,640 children at Cook County Hospital. *Arch Surg* 114: 717, 1979.

Intussusception

Gross RE, Ladd WE: Intussusception. In *The Surgery of Infancy and Childhood*, p. 281, edited by RE Gross. W. B. Saunders, Philadelphia, 1953.

Lynn HB: Intussusception. In *Pediatric Surgery*, p. 438, edited by TM Holder, KW Ashcraft. W. B. Saunders, Philadelphia, 1980.

Ravitch MM, McClune RM: Reduction of intussusception by barium enemia; a clinical and experimental study. *Ann Surg* 128: 924, 1948.

Malrotation

Bill HH: Malrotation of the intestine. In *Pediatric Surgery*, p. 912, edited by MM Ravitch et al. Year Book, Chicago, 1979.

Simpson AJ, Leonidas JC, Krasna I: Roentgen diagnosis of midgut malrotation; value of upper gastrointestinal radiographic study. *J Pediatr Surg* 7: 243, 1972.

Stewart DR, Colodny AL, Daggett WC: Malrotation of the bowel in infants and children; a 15-year review. *Surgery* 79: 716, 1976.

Pyloric Stenosis

Benson CD: Infantile hypertrophic pyloric stenosis. In *Pediatric Surgery*, p. 891, edited by MM Ravitch. Year Book, Chicago, 1979.

Ravitch MM: The story of pyloric stenosis. *Surgery* 48: 1117, 1960.

Duplications

Grosfeld JL, O'Neill JA, Clatworthy HW: Enteric duplications in infancy and childhood. *Ann Surg* 172: 83, 1970.

Gross RE: *The Surgery of Infancy and Childhood*, p. 221, W. B. Saunders, Philadelphia, 1953.

Hernias

Bronsther B, Abrams MW, Elboim C: Inguinal hernias in children—a study of 1000 cases and review of the literature. *J Am Med Wom Assoc* 27: 522, 1972.

Lassaletta L, Fonkalsrud EW, Tovar JA, Dudgeon D, Asch M: The management of umbilical hernias in infancy and childhood. *J Pediatr Surg* 10: 405, 1975.

Rowe MI, Copelson LW, Clatworthy HW: The patent processus vaginalis and the inguinal hernia. *J Pediatr Surg* 4: 102, 1969.

Wooley MM: Inguinal hernia. In *Pediatric Surgery*, p. 815, edited by MM Ravitch, Year Book, Chicago, 1979.

Foreign Bodies in the GI Tract

Gans SL, Austin E: Foreign bodies. In *Pediatric Surgery*, p. 116, edited by TM Holder, KW Ashcraft. W. B. Saunders, Philadelphia, 1980.

Loff HS, Allen RD: Management of foreign bodies in the alimentary tract. *J Pediatr* 48: 563, 1956.

Mandell GA, Rosenberg HK, Schnaufer L: Prolonged retention of foreign bodies in the stomach. *Pediatrics* 60: 460, 1977.

CHAPTER 60

Thoracic Emergencies

JOHN M. TEMPLETON, JR., M.D.

INTRODUCTION

Thoracic emergencies in children often result in life-threatening alterations in cardiorespiratory physiology. The etiology of these emergencies are distinct in the pediatric patient. There are a number of congenital defects which are not discovered in the newborn nursery and, thus, may be diagnosed by the emergency physician. Congenital abnormalities which are usually diagnosed at birth are not included in this chapter. There are also many distinctive acquired conditions such as staphylococcal empyema or certain mediastinal tumors which are not usually seen in the adult population.

This chapter will review the pathophysiology and clinical manifestations of thoracic emergencies. The general principles of physical and laboratory assessment are detailed. Subsequent sections cover specific entities within the following categories: (1) airway compromise, (2) violation of the pleural space, (3) circulatory compromise, (4) intrinsic pulmonary lesions, (5) mediastinal tumors, (6) diaphragmatic defects, and (7) chest wall tumors.

PATHOPHYSIOLOGY

Airway Compromise

Airway compromise can occur anywhere in the respiratory tract from the nares and oropharynx to the alveoli. These obstructive emergencies relating to the proximal trachea, larynx, and oropharynx are covered in Chapter 62, "Otorhinolaryngology Emergencies," and in Chapter 1, "Resuscitation."

Compromise of the more distal tracheobronchial tree may be due to either intrinsic or extrinsic obstruction. Examples of intrinsic obstruction include: a tumor within the bronchial lumen (e.g. a hemangioma), a foreign body, or a mucous plug as might occur in a patient with cystic fibrosis. Other forms of intrinsic airway compromise occur due to loss of the integrity of the tracheobronchial tree, as seen in patients with primary tracheomalacia, prior esophageal atresia repair, or lobar emphysema. Patients with extrinsic compromise of the airway usually are symptomatic because of the impingement of a bronchus by some adjacent structure such as a bronchogenic cyst or enlarged lymph nodes.

The physiologic effects of airway obstruction depend on the degree of obstruction. The more severe the obstruction, the greater the impairment of oxygen delivery to the alveoli. When the obstruction is relatively proximal, for example, in the trachea, and is nearly complete, marked impairment of carbon dioxide excretion will also occur. Lobar or segmental obstruction can lead to problems of air trapping, overdistension, and secondary infections. A partial obstruction of a lobe, such as in lobar emphysema, can lead to such massive overdistension of the involved lobe that a tension phenomenon across the mediastinum may occur.

Any impediment to normal opening and closing of the alveoli will predispose the patient to infection. Bacteria, inhaled foreign matter, such as dust, and physiologic bronchial secretions may not be cleared from the lung. Furthermore, there may be impediment to lymphatic drainage. The result is fluid stasis and secondary bacterial overgrowth. Conditions which foster such infections are those with recurrent airway soilage such as tracheoesophageal fistula (H-type), or recurrent vomiting with aspiration. Patients with focal derangements of normal alveolar opening and closing include congenital malformations of the lungs, for example cystic adenomatoid malformation.

Violations of the Pleural Space

Negative Pressure

In a normal thoracic cavity, the pleural space is a potential rather than an actual space. The visceral and parietal pleurae are held in close apposition by a continuous mild negative pressure which creates, in effect, a vacuum. Violations of the pleural space may be caused by the presence of air, fluid, or solid structures (such as tumor). The result is varying degrees of pulmonary collapse producing intrapulmonary shunting and a drop in the PaO_2. When collapse of the lung is complete, the perfusion of the lung is greatly reduced and the degree of shunt may actually be less.

In general, evacuation of air or fluid from pleural cavity with a chest tube reestablishes the physiologic negative pressure between the pleural surfaces. As a result, the lung reexpands and the ventilation perfusion balance is restored. In some chronic situations, which cause the development of a thick peel on the pleural lining, the lung can be fully expanded only by an operative procedure.

Positive Pressure

The development of a positive intrapleural pressure is a more urgent situation than the loss of negative intrathoracic pressure. Positive intrapleural pressure is usually the result of either fluid or air under tension. A tension pneumothorax is one of the more common and serious examples of this positive pressure phenomenon. The condition can become life-threatening when more and more air enters the pleural space and causes not only the complete collapse of the ipsilateral lung, but progressive tension across the mediastinum. When the mediastinum is sufficiently displaced, the venous return from the inferior vena cava is obstructed and circulatory collapse occurs (Fig. 60.1).

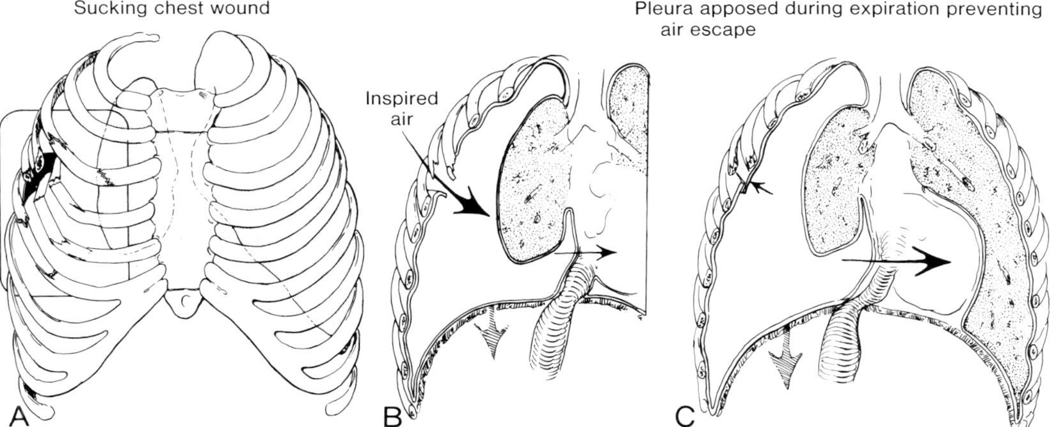

Figure 60.1 The development of a progressive tension pneumothorax as a result of air accumulating in the hemithorax with each inspiration.

Pleural Space Infection

Infection is the third form of violation of the pleural cavity. The pleura is an extensive serosal surface that is able to produce voluminous exudation of fluid in response to inflammation and infection. This exudate is a fertile environment for bacterial growth. Bacteria usually enter the pleural space from an adjacent pneumonia. Because of the extensive size of the pleural space any significant intrapleural bacterial infection (pyothorax) can result in generalized toxemia.

Circulatory Impairment

Thoracic circulatory emergencies in children involve the heart and great vessels. Marked tension phenomenon across the mediastinum or major hemorrhage will impair venous return. If the hemorrhage is within the thoracic cavity, and if the patient requires positive pressure ventilation, the inspiratory intrathoracic pressure may exceed the pressure of venous return. Bleeding from the aorta or one of its major branches, therefore, can produce not only a decrease in the patient's systolic pressure, but also secondary physiological problems caused by increased intrathoracic pressure.

Also, the circulation can be impaired at the cardiac level due to either an intracardiac obstruction or an extracardiac tamponade. Examples of intracardiac obstruction include primary tumors such as rhabdomyosarcoma or metastatic Wilms' tumor. Intracardiac obstruction may also be due to congenital defects that impair the out-flow tract of the ventricles. The more severe intracardiac congenital defects are usually recognized during the neonatal period (see Chapter 43).

CLINICAL MANIFESTATIONS

Dyspnea

Dyspnea in the infant or young child is often observed by the parents although it is not articulated by the patient. The child may communicate dyspnea by becoming agitated and by a look of distress on his face. The rate of respirations is usually increased, but more importantly, the physician will observe retractions and increase use of accessory muscles of breathing. The older child may simply complain of a subjective sensation of being unable to catch his breath.

Tachypnea

Tachypnea is defined as respiratory rate above normal for a patient's age. At rest, a normal newborn infant will breathe 30 to 40 times/min, a rate somewhat faster than an older child. Beyond infancy, however, a rate greater than 30 breaths/min, is abnormal. Emotional states, such as crying or agitation, can greatly affect the child's respiratory rate. Thus, the respiratory rate must be assessed when the patient is at rest. An increased rate of respiration at rest requires further evaluation.

Agitation

This symptom is a generalized phenomenon which can be either functional or organic. Agitation can be a symptom of a serious underlying problem. Patients with ventilatory or circulatory impairment, for example following trauma, may seem to be so agitated that they are unable to be comforted or calmed down. Children who are agitated may thrash about to a sufficient degree to further harm themselves despite the presence of painful unstable fractures. Obviously such patients are responding to a higher sense of alarm than that related to the pain they may feel.

An older responsive child may complain of feeling cold and clammy. In addition, he may express feelings of impending doom. Such symptoms are typical of impending circulatory collapse which is likely to be the underlying basis for his agitation. A patient who complains about both discomfort and distress upon lying down, may also have circulatory impairment. Such symptoms may be expressed by patients with congestive cardiac failure, intracardiac obstructive lesions, or cardiac tamponade due to a pericardial effusion.

Fever, Cough, and Pain

These symptoms are most common to lower airway infections, either viral or bacterial. However, thoracic emergencies may also present with one or more of these symptoms. The child who has a prolonged or severe unexplained fever should have a chest x-ray as a part of his evaluation. There are a number of entities in which secondary bacterial infection draws attention to a primary lesion such as obstructed right middle lobe orifice, cystic adenomatoid malformation of the lung or acute or chronic aspiration.

Determination of the exact nature of the pain or cough may suggest the specific intrathoracic problem. Sudden pain in one hemithorax followed by respiratory distress suggests a spontaneous pneumothorax. Sudden focal chest wall pain followed by local tenderness might indicate a pathological rib fracture. The gradual onset of pain on one side of the chest associated with splinting respirations and fever is typical of a pleural inflammation, while the gradual onset of a gnawing pain over a generalized area without fever might reflect an underlying tumor.

Coughing is a reflection of irritation within the tracheobronchial system. If coughing produces sputum, this should be analyzed for clues to the nature of the problem. A patient who has an unusually foul-smelling breath or produces foul-smelling sputum may have a necrotizing process in the lung. Faintly blood-streaked sputum is common in many pulmonary infections. A patient with significant hemoptysis may have vascular anomalies, sarcoidosis, or cystic fibrosis. A patient who coughs up bilious material may have a bronchobiliary fistula. By contrast, a patient who has acute attacks of coughing, especially during feeding, may have an impingement on the trachea caused by an obstruction in the esophagus or a congenital or acquired fistula between the esophagus and the tracheobronchial tree. The diagnostic approach to cough appears in Chapter 12.

EXAMINATION AND ASSESSMENT

Inspection

A patient with quadriplegia or severe kyphoscoliosis may have an obvious visible explanation for any symptoms of respiratory distress. On the other hand, the findings on inspection may be more subtle. For example, a mild sternal deformity may be associated with an underlying foramen of Morgagni hernia. A child with acute onset of respiratory distress, abdominal pain, and vomiting may be noted to have a scaphoid abdomen. This picture suggests an evisceration of abdominal contents through a diaphragmatic hernia. Splinting due to chest pain may be associated with an acute scoliosis of the thoracic spine. The presence of flaring nostrils, or chest wall retractions, and prominent use of accessory muscles of respiration, all suggest the presence of a ventilatory impairment.

Impairment of oxygenation will be reflected in cyanosis of the fingers, toes, and lips. When there is airway obstruction and an inability to excrete CO_2, cyanosis becomes prominent on both the face and trunk. Engorgement of the neck veins occurs in a patient with cardiac tamponade, while pallor and poor capillary filling in the extremities occurs in a patient in shock. In the traumatized patient, one should examine all aspects of the thorax, neck, and upper abdomen to detect any focal wounds or bruises.

Palpation

Palpation should be gentle and nonthreatening. The area of presumed tenderness should be palpated last during the examination.

In sequence, one should palpate the neck, the precordium, and then the thorax. If the trachea is deviated, there is likely to be a tension phenomenon in the chest on the side opposite to the direction of the deviation (see Fig. 60.1). The presence of a mass in the neck, especially at the thoracic inlet, may reflect a tumor which is impinging on the airway. Subcutaneous emphysema is a finding of significant concern. Subcutaneous air may be palpated in local areas, for example, at the site of a penetrating chest wound. When noted in the neck, however, it usually reflects more serious pathology such as a proximal tear or avulsion of the tracheobronchial tree, or an esophageal perforation.

In palpating the precordium the physician may find that the PMI is significantly deviated away from the side of the thorax in which there is a tension phenomenon. In the presence of pericarditis one may perceive a rub, or in the presence of a pericardial effusion one may not be able to feel a cardiac impulse at all.

When examining the thorax the physician should run his hands gently over the entire thoracic wall looking for any instability. Unilateral tenderness in the upper abdomen may actually reflect a thoracic injury such as fractured ribs in the same sensory dermatome. Last, one can put each hand on either side of the thorax and gently compress the thorax to elicit any tenderness or instability.

Auscultation and Percussion

In an infant or a small child, it is difficult to use auscultation or percussion to distinguish the exact location of the pathology. An infant can have complete collapse of a lung due either to a pneumothorax or a diaphragmatic hernia and yet have seemingly very good breath sounds on that side. Breath sounds on one side can be widely transmitted. Also there is limited thoracic surface area for percussion in an infant. Despite the limitations of these modalities, they remain valuable parts of the examination. One may be able to distinguish a difference in the quality of the breath sounds between the left and right side. One may identify a shift in the heart sounds corresponding to a tracheal shift caused by tension phenomenon in one side of the chest. The presence of diminished heart sounds or unusual heart sounds suggest a pericardial effusion or an intracardiac mass lesion.

In examining the lung fields the physician should assess not only the presence or absence of breath sounds, but the presence of specific sounds such as inspiratory stridor or expiratory wheezes. When such findings are focal they may indicate the site of an impaired bronchus. In an older child a pleural effusion or significant mass can be well delineated by auscultation and percussion.

Laboratory Studies

The sine qua non of evaluating any patient with a thoracic emergency is a good quality chest x-ray. An x-ray of the chest should include posteroanterior (PA) and lateral views done in an upright position unless contraindicated by the patient's condition (e.g. possible injury to the spine). The width of the mediastinum and the degree of mediastinal shift are much better seen in the upright chest x-ray. Moreover, abnormalities in the lung, pleural cavity, and diaphragm are also best appreciated in this view. For example, in the patient with a traumatic rupture of the diaphragm, the true nature of the patient's respiratory distress may not become clear until a proper upright chest x-ray is obtained. Where a pulmonary effusion exists, one can obtain lateral decubitus anteroposterior (AP) views of the chest to determine whether the effusion layers freely or is loculated.

In interpreting the chest x-ray one should distinguish between a diffuse pulmonary problem versus a focal lesion. Hyperaeration of one portion of the lung suggests air trapping in the involved lobe. Hyperaeration of the entire lung field on one side is usually the result of compensatory enlargement of the lung due to atelectasis and loss of lung volume on the opposite side.

Other studies which are indicated in a patient with a thoracic emergency include a CBC and differential WBC, BUN, serum glucose, electrolytes, and an arterial blood gas. Depending on the patient's specific problem, one should also consider obtaining a PT and PTT, a crossmatch, blood cultures, and an assessment of any sputum by Gram stain and bacteriologic culture. Other more involved studies, such as pulmonary function tests, tomograms, barium contrast studies, sonograms, and CAT scans depend on the specific findings.

CONDITIONS ASSOCIATED WITH AIRWAY COMPROMISE

Airway compromise refers to both intrinsic or extrinsic blockage of the major components of the tracheobronchial system to the level of the lobar bronchi. Airway blockage can affect either the expiratory or inspiratory phase of respiration or both phases. Airway compromise also includes those conditions which result in recurrent soilage of the tracheobronchial tree resulting in either a chemical or bacterial insult to the airway and lungs. The conditions discussed below are grouped according to the primary structure occluded.

Tracheal Compromise

BACKGROUND

Aspiration of a foreign body is a relatively common airway problem in children. If the foreign body passes the narrow subglottic area in the larynx, it will pass into one of the main stem bronchi. Depending on the nature of the object aspirated, the patient can develop increasing symptoms over the next few hours or days (see Chapter 62). By contrast, a foreign body which does not pass through the trachea will produce immediate respiratory distress and may result in death even before the child arrives at the hospital (see Chapter 1). Tracheomalacia or extrinsic pressure on the trachea can also cause the signs and symptoms of life-threatening tracheal obstruction.

CLINICAL FINDINGS

Patients with tracheal compromise have symptoms which range from mild to severe. When the symptoms are mild, the underlying etiology for the problem may not be recognized. The patient may have only occasional episodes of respiratory infection thought to be "croup" or bronchitis. In a patient with more moderate symptoms, there may be prominent stridor and wheezing. Such a child may have a past history of hospital admissions one or more times and treatment with mist tent, antibiotics, and physiotherapy.

When the trachea is severely compromised, the child will have a history of stridor at rest. The manifestations include progressive cyanosis and apneic episodes. On physical examination, a child with extrinsic pressure on the trachea may have stridor and wheezing throughout the respiratory cycle, especially over the point of obstruction. By contrast, a patient with an intrinsic weakness of the cartilaginous tracheal rings, as in tracheomalacia, may have more stridor during expiration. Tracheomalacia is a frequent problem in children who have undergone a repair of an esophageal atresia. Even in the absence of symptoms due to tracheomalacia, children with a history of an esophageal atresia repair have a brassy cough throughout their life, indicating some degree of instability involving the membraneous portion of the trachea (see Chapter 35, "Stridor").

MANAGEMENT

If the patient does not require immediate airway management, one should obtain PA and lateral chest and lateral neck x-rays. Spot films taken during fluoroscopy of the trachea during inspiration and expiration may be helpful. On the other hand, if the patient has a life-threatening compromise of the airway, the patient should receive airway management (see Chapter 1). In patients with either tracheomalacia or extrinsic pressure on the trachea, the placement of an endotracheal tube to within 1 cm of the carina is usually sufficient to relieve the symptoms. The patient should then be admitted to the hospital and treated with pulmonary physiotherapy and antibiotics, depending on the x-ray findings. If a mass lesion pressing on the trachea is identified on routine x-rays of the chest and neck, then surgery is required (Fig. 60.2). If no extrinsic lesion is identified, bronchoscopy is indicated to assess the anatomy and integrity of the tracheobronchial tree. If moderate to severe tracheomalacia is noted, the child may require stabilization of the airway with an endotracheal tube. Definitive surgical correction may be achieved when the child is stable.

Bronchial Compromise

BACKGROUND

Bronchial compromise may be caused by an aspirated foreign body (see Chapter 62), congenital lesions, or secondary complications of a preexisting infection. Bronchial

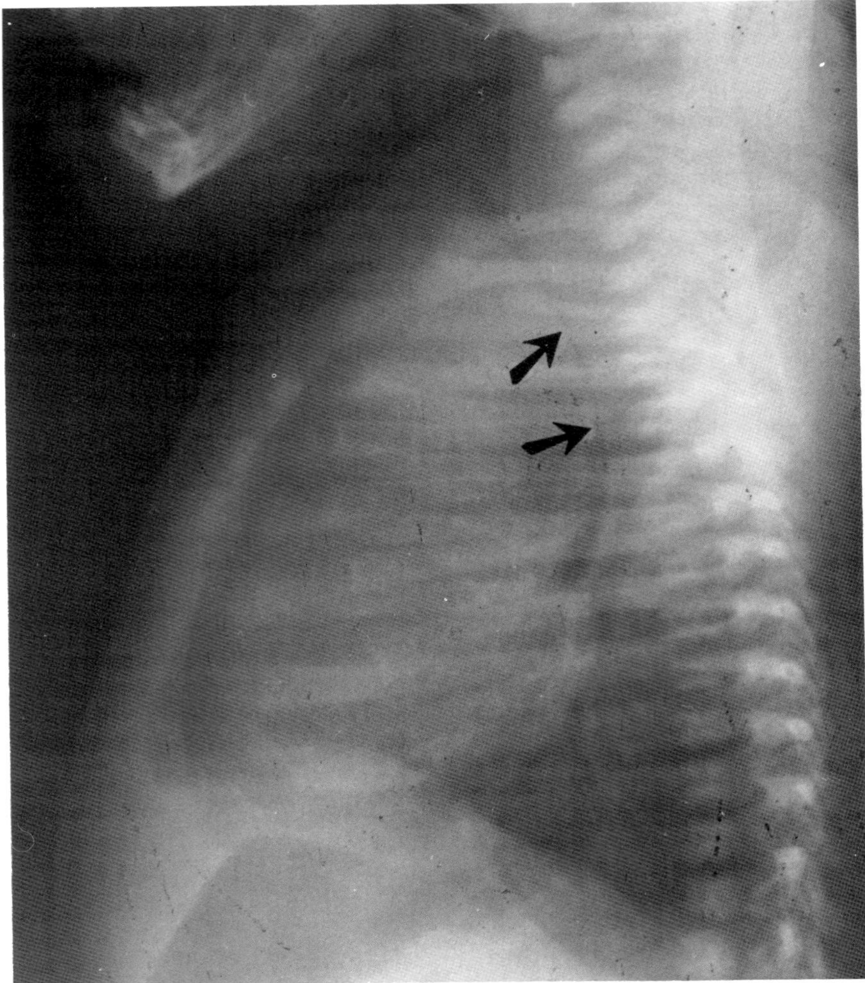

Figure 60.2 An 11-day-old boy was admitted with gasping respirations and cyanosis when crying. A lateral chest film showed severe tracheal obstruction due to a large mediastinal tumor (*arrows*). On bronchoscopy ventilatory impairment was relieved when the bronchoscope reached the level of the carina. A benign teratoma was excised.

compromise is usually associated with one of four mechanisms: (1) complete obstruction of a bronchus as in patients with bronchial atresia, (2) expiratory obstruction of the bronchus as in congenital lobar emphysema, (3) intermittent obstruction of the bronchus as in a bronchogenic cyst or enlarged peribronchial lymph nodes, and (4) recurrent soilage of the tracheobronchial tree. These conditions differ in their pathophysiologic mechanisms, clinical presentations and management.

Bronchial Atresia

CLINICAL FINDINGS

Because there is no communication to the bronchial segments distal to the atresia, patients with this anomaly may not be recognized until they are several years old. Some patients will have a history of episodic upper respiratory infections and wheezing. Those patients with wheezing may have received treatment for presumed asthma. Other patients may be identified during an initial or recurrent episode of apparent pneumonia. Older patients may complain of dyspnea on exertion or unilateral chest pain. On physical examination there may be a complete absence of breath sounds in the involved area.

MANAGEMENT

A chest x-ray (PA and lateral) will usually localize the area of involvement. The findings include localized hyperinflation of the lung in a segmental or lobar distribution. Occasionally one may see a nodular density either in the ipsilateral perihilar region or in the central area of the involved lung field. There is an increased incidence of upper lobe involvement, although, on occasion, the right middle lobe or left lower lobe may be involved. Hyperaeration is presumably a result of communication from the adjacent normal lung through the pores of Kohn and the channels of Lambert.

When an entire lobe appears to be involved, bronchoscopy is the most efficient way to identify the atretic opening to the involved bronchus. In an older child bronchography can be of additional help in outlining the patent and nonpatent bronchial segments.

In addition, other modalities such as ventilation-perfusion scans of the lungs or CAT scans may be useful. The CAT scan, in particular, may demonstrate a solid mass with multiple, well-circumscribed branching channels. This mass represents a mucoid impaction in the atretic bronchus. It is visible on routine chest x-ray because of the surrounding emphysematous lung tissue.

In spite of the hyperaeration, such patients do not develop significant collapse of the adjacent lobes or displacement of the mediastinum. Elective surgery should be performed after any secondary infections have been treated.

Congenital Lobar Emphysema (CLE)

CLINICAL FINDINGS

Although many children with CLE will present within the first few hours or days of life, the majority will not be recognized until beyond the neonatal period. Older children have a somewhat slower onset of symptoms than those who are diagnosed as newborns. Initially, children with CLE may have unexplained tachypnea, increasing wheezing, respiratory distress, or even cyanosis. Some children may present with fever suggesting that infection is the underlying etiology of their problem. On physical examination there may be evidence of decreased breath sounds on the involved side. More impressively, however, there is a deviation of the trachea and the heart away from the side of the involvement. Presumably, much of their distress is due to the tension phenomenon across the mediastinum.

Although the pathogenesis of this entity is not always clear, more than half the patients have either a cartilaginous dysplasia of the involved lobar bronchus or the presence of an approximate 3- to 5-fold increase in the number of alveoli in the involved lobe. This latter condition is known as polyalveolar lobe. Each acinus in this condition is giant in size and has the capacity to trap a considerable amount of air. These two forms of pathology cannot be distinguished either clinically or radiologically.

MANAGEMENT

The key to management is to establish an accurate diagnosis. The chest x-ray, PA and lateral, is essential to the diagnostic process. When CLE is severe, there may be such severe hyperaeration in the involved hemithorax that some examiners are misled to feel that the problem is a tension pneumothorax. However, closer inspection will reveal faint lung markings in the hyperaerated segment and compression and atelectasis of the lower lobe on the involved side (Fig. 60.3). In the vast majority of cases only a single lobe is involved. The single most commonly involved lobe is the left upper lobe. However, patients may also have isolated involvement of the right upper lobe or right middle lobe.

In evaluating and managing a patient with a symptomatic CLE, it is important to avoid positive pressure ventilation by mask or endotracheal tube. Positive pressure will cause further trapping in the affected lobe and result in an even more severe shift of the mediastinum with a possibly fatal out-

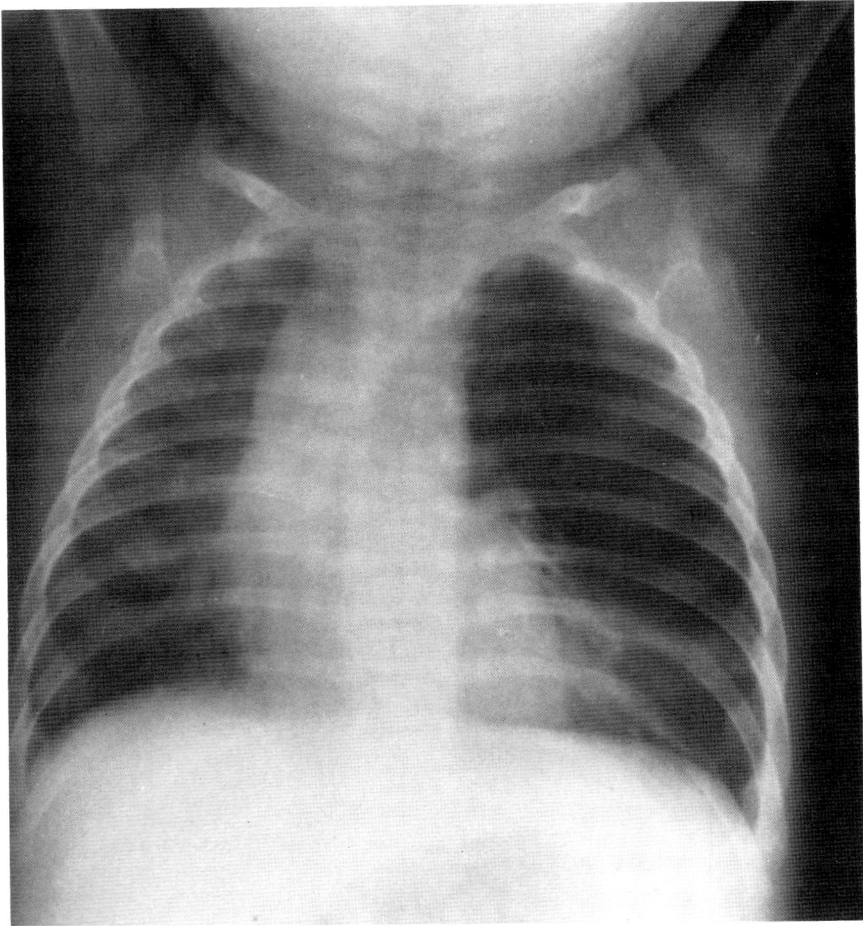

Figure 60.3 Congenital lobar emphysema of the left upper lobe in a 3-month-old girl who presented with decreased breath sounds and rales in this area. Note the secondary compression atelectasis of the left lower lobe.

come. At times, it becomes necessary to take severely afflicted children directly from the emergency department to the operating room for an emergency thoracotomy.

Bronchogenic Cyst

CLINICAL FINDINGS

Bronchogenic cysts can be found in the mediastinum, the lung, or even the neck. Their usual mode of presentation is that of moderate to severe airway obstruction in infants. Their major manifestation in older children is pneumonia. Bronchogenic cysts represent developmental aberrations of the primitive foregut. As such, they can occur anywhere along the tracheobronchial tree.

The central or peripheral location of a cyst will determine its mode of presentation. A mediastinal lesion is likely to produce earlier compression of the trachea or proximal mainstem bronchi. Those children with mediastinal bronchogenic cysts begin to develop recurrent respiratory symptoms such as cough, wheezing, and fever early in life. When carefully examined, such children may have persistent tachypnea and retractions of the chest wall even in the absence of more overt symptoms.

By contrast, only half of the patients with

more peripheral lesions may have respiratory symptoms. The respiratory symptoms are those suggestive of recurrent infections such as fever, cough, and physical findings suggestive of recurrent pneumonia in the same site. These symptoms can occur at any age but commonly the children are older than 2 years before the first respiratory problems develop. Some patients may be poor feeders and have failure to thrive. They may have paroxysms of coughing in conjunction with episodic vomiting leading to the false impression of esophageal reflux. For unexplained reasons, the vast majority of peripheral bronchogenic cysts involve the right lung and right side of the body.

On physical examination the findings reflect either a central or peripheral lesion. Patients with a central lesion and acute respiratory distress have generalized wheezing or stridor heard throughout the lung fields. If the compression occludes one of the main stem bronchi, it is most likely to be on the left side. In an older patient with a more peripheral lesion, the findings are more compatible with a segmental or a lobar pneumonia, including dullness to percussion, splinting respiratory, and focally absent breath sounds.

MANAGEMENT

In both younger and older patients the key to successful diagnosis of this condition is to have a high index of suspicion. Otherwise, a child in whom the symptoms have improved, may be discharged only to experience recurrent and perhaps, worsening symptoms. Routine PA and lateral chest x-rays show a radiopaque mass appearing as a smooth projection from one side of the mediastinum. If a major bronchus is significantly obstructed there may be emphysema of the involved side. Mediastinal cysts are not air filled. By contrast, cysts within the lung parenchyma may contain air and fluid and an air-fluid level within a cystic structure may be seen on x-ray. Presumably this finding is due to a communication which is the result of rupture of the cyst wall into the surrounding lung. The lung on the involved side may also show surrounding pneumonitis.

Once the condition is suspected, the patient should be admitted to the hospital. Further evaluations will document the severity of the patient's condition. If respiratory symptoms are not severe, patients with central lesions should undergo an esophagram and tomograms of the mediastinum. Intubation and emergency bronchoscopy may be indicated in a patient with increasingly severe respiratory distress. One should be prepared, however, to do a definitive surgical resection immediately following bronchoscopy.

A number of other conditions such as cystic hygroma or tumors of the mediastinum may mimic a bronchogenic cyst. If there is intermittent obstruction of a central or a peripheral bronchus, the same management course must be followed. Any tumor involving the bronchus can present with similar clinical and radiological features (Fig. 60.4). There are rare case reports of patients with a chondroma of the bronchus, a carcinoid tumor, a leiomyoma, a mucoepidermal tumor, a rhabdomyosarcoma, and a leiomyosarcoma. The presence of a malignancy will further endanger the child's life. Therefore, any patient presenting with symptoms of a partial, intermittent bronchial obstruction should be evaluated until the underlying basis for the problem is determined.

Right Middle Lobe Syndrome

The right middle lobe has a particular predilection for partial or intermittent bronchial obstruction. As seen in Figure 60.4, one cause for partial obstruction can be a tumor such as a bronchogenic cyst. However, the anatomical location of the right middle lobe and its bronchus make it particularly susceptible to recurrent soilage in patients who aspirate. Moreover, the distribution of lymph nodes in the area of right middle lobe bronchus tend to be circumferential. As a result, when lymphadenopathy develops in response to recurrent bacterial pneumonias, or systemic infections such as tuberculosis, the lymph nodes begin to impinge on the bronchus. As a result, drainage is impaired and bronchiectasis may develop.

Patients with a right middle lobe syndrome have recurrent episodes of atelecta-

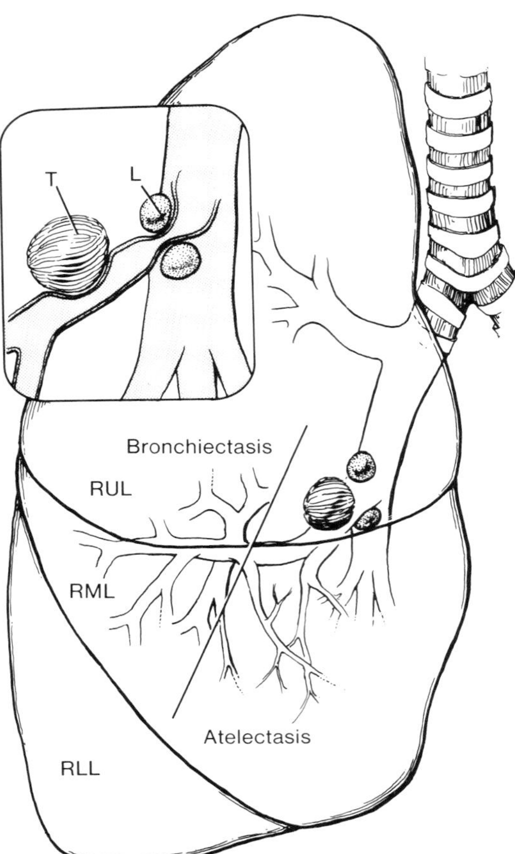

Figure 60.4 Acute and chronic obstruction of a bronchus due to tumor (*T*) or lymph nodes (*L*). When the obstruction is acute, there may only be atelectasis in the distal parenchyma. With chronic obstruction, there may be bronchiectasis due to recurrent pneumonia. The right middle lobe as shown here is particularly prone to bronchial obstruction due to pressure from encircling lymph nodes. *RUL, RML, RLL* = right upper, middle, and lower lobes, respectively.

sis and pneumonia. Generally, these episodes do not respond to physiotherapy and antibiotics if the extrinsic compression on the bronchus is significant. The affected lobe can become a repository of infection which may then seed infection to other portions of the lungs. Any patient with an acute right middle lobe pneumonia should be evaluated thoroughly for evidence of prior illness. Furthermore, such patients should be followed closely as resection of a badly damaged right middle lobe may become necessary.

Tracheobronchial Soilage

BACKGROUND

The tracheobronchial mucosa is an exquisitely sensitive tissue with a surprisingly complex function, including cellular control of infection, production of mucoid secretions, and ciliary motility. While occasional insults to the tracheobronchial tree due to infection or foreign material can be managed without lasting difficulties, continued soilage with chemical irritants can greatly retard the physiological function of the lung. When an infection complicates chemical soilage of the lung, the natural pulmonary defenses break down even further, resulting in serious damage to the lungs and even fatal compromise of the airway.

Esophageal reflux and aspiration are the most common causes of tracheobronchial soilage. Reflux will be considered in the section on esophageal related conditions. The other source of bronchial soilage involves a congenital or acquired fistulous communication of the esophagus with the tracheobronchial tree.

H-type Tracheoesophageal Fistula

CLINICAL FINDINGS

Patients with H-type tracheoesophageal fistulae usually develop symptoms during the first few weeks or months of life after they initially appear to do well. They first present with symptoms of episodic coughing and fever. The x-ray is consistent with a picture of tracheobronchitis or pneumonitis. Patients may be treated with antibiotics and may, in fact, show appropriate resolution of their symptoms. The clue to the underlying condition is continued episodes of the same symptoms and radiological findings. Careful history taking reveals that the episodes of coughing often occur during a feeding. These symptoms may persist in spite of the standard treatment for esophageal reflux: thickened feedings and keeping the patient upright. In time, the child may become cyanotic or develop frank pneumonia and pulmonary collapse. A subtle physical finding is abdominal distention which is due to the presence of a large volume of air in the stomach and bowel. If the stomach is decompressed and the patient fed by gavage feedings, the distention may disappear entirely.

MANAGEMENT

The first step in management is to have a high index of suspicion for the entity. A simple clinical test may be used to support the diagnosis. After passing a nasogastric catheter into the upper thoracic esophagus, place the other end of the catheter under water. If the water bubbles with each respiratory excursion, there is a strong suggestion of a tracheoesophageal fistula. Chest x-rays will not be diagnostic of the anomaly, but are useful in identifying areas of infection or atelectasis. If present, these problems should be treated with physiotherapy and antibiotics.

Selective esophagraphy is a more precise method of diagnosis. The patient is fluoroscoped in a lateral position. The tip of a nasogastric (NG) tube is placed in the lower esophagus. Then, as 1- to 2-ml increments of barium are injected into the esophagus, the NG tube is slowly pulled higher and higher into the upper thoracic esophagus. When the tube reaches the mid or upper thoracic esophagus, a small stream of barium may be seen to ascend through a small fistulous tract between the esophagus and the trachea during deep inspiration. Barium will cause the child to cough and the barium will become alveolized. Fortunately, barium is inert and dense enough that the lungs will be cleared after a few hours of postural drainage. Bronchoscopy with fiberoptic equipment provides an even more precise means of diagnosis.

The treatment of tracheoesophageal fistula is surgical. Most patients are amenable to repair through a cervical approach. Unless there is some contraindication, this approach should always be done through the right, in that the recurrent laryngeal nerve on the right courses towards the tracheoesophageal groove at an angle and does not reach the groove until well above the usual site of the fistula. By contrast, the recurrent laryngeal nerve on the left follows the tracheoesophageal groove from the thorax up into the neck.

While congenital bronchoesophageal fistulas do occur, they usually do not become symptomatic until later in life. These fistulas are smaller and are not as likely to allow esophageal contents to reflux into the tracheobronchial tree. They are often first appreciated in a patient who is intubated for general anesthesia and then develops unexplained massive dilatation of the stomach. In such patients, bronchography and bronchoscopy should enable one to identify the precise anatomy of the lesion.

Bronchobiliary Fistula

CLINICAL FINDINGS

Although patients with this condition may not be identified for 1 month or more after birth, they usually have had the symptom of recurrent coughing. The sputum is often green to yellow. Bile in the tracheobronchial tree in small amounts, is not as irritating as aspirated gastric material. Moreover, bile is usually bacteria-free. As a result, these patients continue to have episodic coughing, and yellow sputum, but may not seem ill. The physical examination of such patients is generally unremarkable.

MANAGEMENT

A small amount of sputum may be analyzed for the presence of bilirubin. An increased sputum bilirubin in a patient with a normal serum bilirubin strongly suggests the diagnosis. Other diagnostic techniques are helpful. A DISIDA (Di-isopropyl imino diacetic acid) scan may demonstrate passage of dye into the thorax. Even if this study is negative, and the diagnosis is strongly suspected, the patient should undergo bronchoscopy. Often the anomalous communication will be seen at the level of the carina or on the proximal surface of one of the mainstem bronchi. One can then catheterize this orifice and obtain a contrast study. The treatment is surgical resection and ligation of the fistula.

Bronchopulmonary Foregut Malformations

CLINICAL FINDINGS

This congenital entity is the result of an anomalous origin of a lobar or a main stem bronchus from the distal esophagus. Most patients are identified shortly after birth because of notable respiratory difficulty. In some patients, however, the communication may be sufficiently narrow or may involve only one lobe, so that it is several weeks before the child develops symptoms. The usual mode of presentation is chronic and persistent cough associated with episodes of pneumonia which do not respond well to antibiotics and physiotherapy.

MANAGEMENT

In most cases, the anomalous communication involves the right main stem bronchus or the left lower lobe bronchus. Therefore, one may suspect this condition when a pneumonia continues to occur in one of these two areas and does not appear to respond to appropriate treatment. The key to diagnosis is an esophagagram which reveals reflux of barium into the involved bronchial system. More than half of the patients have a systemic arterial supply to the involved lung, making it also important to obtain an aortogram. Early diagnosis and surgical correction is important in order to avoid the secondary complications of abscess and empyema development.

Acquired Tracheobronchial Soilage

CLINICAL FINDINGS

Patients with acquired tracheobronchial soilage usually have had an antecedent illness such as infection as the cause of the problem. A patient with recurrent or chronic pulmonary infections may become prone to suppuration within the lung parenchyma or adjacent nodes. These infected areas may subsequently erode into an adjacent bronchus producing purulent soilage of the tracheobronchial tree. Usually patients with such infections are febrile and appear chronically ill. The clinical findings of focal rhonchi and wheezes and consolidation of lung tissue usually point to the site of involvement.

Patients with tuberculosis may develop such severe involvement of mediastinal and bronchial lymph nodes that there is erosion into adjacent structures resulting in a sudden increase in sputum production. Other patients may have paroxysmal coughing whenever they swallow liquid due to a fistulous connection between a bronchus and the esophagus.

Hemoptysis is another form of acquired bronchial soilage. Although patients with bacterial or mycobacterial infections of the lung may have some hemoptysis, major bleeds in children are usually the result of an underlying congenital condition. A patient with significant hemoptysis should be assessed for cystic fibrosis, vascular malformations such as hemangiomata, or pulmonary arterial deficiency. Patients with these disorders develop marked enlargement and tortuosity of the bronchial arteries resulting in prominent vascular ectasias along the mucosal lining of the bronchial tree. When vascular integrity is disrupted, the amount of bleeding which results can be significant enough to require immediate blood transfusion. A more critical complication may occur if the blood is not expectorated rapidly enough and clotting occludes a major air passage.

MANAGEMENT

Chest x-rays (PA and lateral) should be obtained in patients with suspected soilage of the tracheobronchial tree. The presence of focal areas of collapse or consolidation may point to the side of involvement. In addition, a specific abscess with an air fluid level may be identified. Early identification of the site of involvement is important in the event that emergency surgery becomes necessary.

If the patient is stable, cultures of the sputum, obtained by gastric washing, and skin testing should be done. Bronchoscopy is the key to the management; first, to delineate the exact site of involvement, and secondly, to obtain more satisfactory material for culture. If the patient's symptoms suggest a communication with the esophagus, then an esophagagram should also be obtained.

Patients in whom the drainage of bacterial or mycobacterial material into the tracheobronchial tree seems to be resolving with physiotherapy and chemotherapy, can be continued with this medical therapy. However, resection of the involved bronchus and closure of the fistula will be required when there is communication with the esophagus. For those patients with episodes of major hemoptysis the preferred management includes selective arteriographic identification of the enlarged bronchial arteries followed by embolization and thrombosis of these arteries. Resection of an involved lobe or lung may only be temporarily effective if an underlying condition, such as cystic fibrosis exists, as the remaining bronchial tree may soon develop similar vascular ectasias.

Esophageal Related Causes of Airway Compromise

BACKGROUND

In addition to fistulous communication with the tracheobronchial tree, the esophagus can contribute to airway impairment because of its close proximity to the trachea and main stem bronchi and because of the tendency for some children to have reflux aspiration. Any acute or chronic swelling or enlargement of the upper esophagus can result in impingement on the airway. The underlying esophageal disorder may be congenital or acquired. For example, patients who have had esophageal atresia may be prone to tracheomalacia. Furthermore, some scarring may take place at the anastomotic site leading to a thickened bulbous enlargement of the upper esophagus. If food or a foreign body becomes impacted above the anastomosis the result may be pressure on the adjacent airway. In addition, patients with repaired esophageal atresia have high incidence of esophageal motility problems and gastroesophageal reflux. This may be expressed as the late postoperative development of life-threatening cyanotic episodes during, or shortly after, feeding.

A similar phenomenon can occur in children with a significant stenosis or stricture in the upper thoracic esophagus. Occasionally this will occur in an infant born with a relatively thin membranous esophageal stenosis (Fig. 60.5). More commonly, it occurs in children whose prior ingestion of a caustic agent has resulted in scarring and stricture formation.

Certain groups of children have an increased incidence of gastroesophageal reflux such as children with a prior esophageal atresia, and those with psychomotor retardation. In the later group, feeding difficulties, recurrent vomiting, and failure to thrive are often initially mistaken to be a result of the retardation. When subsequent major esophageal and pulmonary complications develop, reflux is often diagnosed.

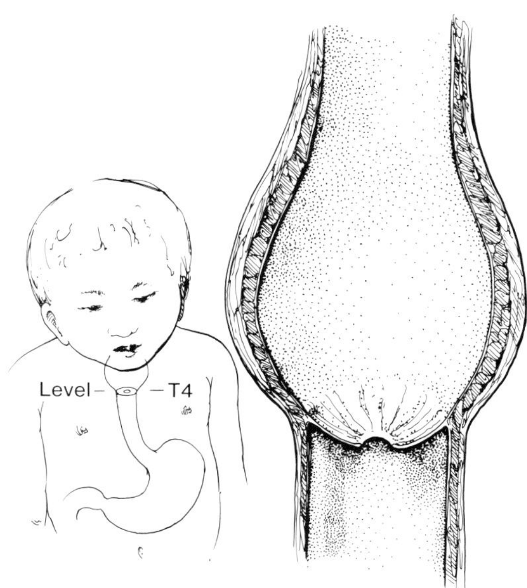

Figure 60.5 A child with chronic partial obstruction of the esophagus due to a congenital web. Similar bulbous enlargement of the proximal esophagus can occur with any type of stricture and result in pressure on the trachea and recurrent regurgitation with aspiration.

Other seemingly normal children may also experience symptoms and signs of gastroesophageal reflux. A patulous connection of the esophagus to the stomach (also termed chalasia) is the anatomical basis for the reflux. The major defect is a loss of the normal cardioesophageal angle (the angle of His) which normally helps to maintain a one-way competence to the gastroesophageal junction. A few children will also have a hiatal hernia. Those with concomitant hiatal hernia are less likely to respond to conservative medical management. Esophageal reflux causes airway compromise when gastric contents reach the hypopharynx and are then aspirated. One of the

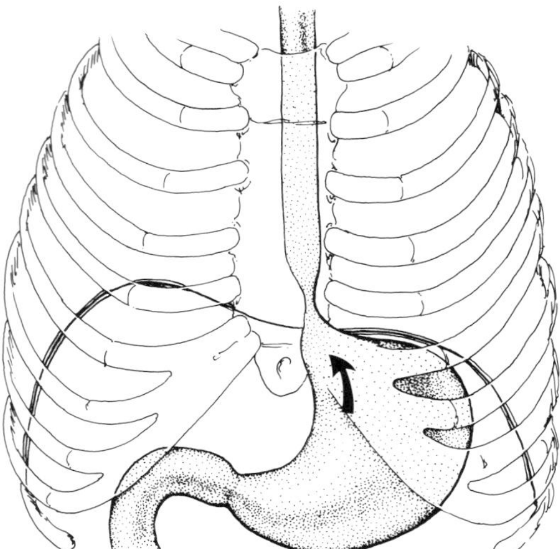

Figure 60.6 Distal esophageal stricture due to prolonged reflux esophagitis. Note the loss of the normal angle between the esophagus and the stomach and propensity for gastric contents to reflux into the esophagus.

advanced complications of chronic reflux is esophageal stenosis, particularly in the distal esophagus. The symptoms of this form of acquired stenosis are severe dysphagia caused by retention of food above the stricture, regurgitation, and worsening aspiration (Fig. 60.6).

CLINICAL FINDINGS

Esophageal disorders may produce any of the following: recurrent vomiting in spite of thickened feedings and upright positioning of the patient, cyanotic episodes during or shortly after feedings, dysphasia, lower thoracic or upper abdominal distress, rumination, recurrent respiratory tract infections, and failure to thrive. In addition, some infants with gastroesophageal reflux will demonstrate recurrent apnea spells. They may come to medical attention during an evaluation for near-miss sudden infant death syndrome. Finally, some children will evidence unexplained iron deficiency anemia, from chronic gastrointestinal blood loss (see Chapter 50).

The many manifestations of esophageal reflux make it an element of the differential diagnosis of many conditions. If esophageal reflux or direct esophageal pressure on the airway is not diagnosed, a number of serious and even life-threatening complications may develop such as nighttime paroxysmal coughing, recurrent episodes of wheezing, prolonged vomiting, failure to thrive, and hematemesis.

MANAGEMENT

Physical examination in most cases is not very revealing. It is helpful sometimes to observe the mother feeding the child so that any symptoms related to feeding may be witnessed by the examiner.

Any child with symptoms related to an esophageal disorder should undergo a barium esophagram and upper GI series. Besides assessing the esophagus and the gastroesophageal junction directly, it is important to identify the possibility of a more distal partial obstruction such as pyloric stenosis, antral web, duodenal stenosis, and malrotation. A hiatal hernia should be readily identifiable by these studies. In addition, a barium esophagram may demonstrate one or more unusual conditions: an esophageal stricture, a diverticulum in the pharyngoesophageal area or thoracic esophageal area, achalasia of the esophagus, or a congenital stenosis and obstruction of the esophagus due to tracheobronchial or pancreatic remnants in the wall of the esophagus.

Even using the most careful radiologic techniques, more than 30% of children with clinically significant gastroesophageal reflux will not demonstrate this reflux on a single upper GI examination. A more in-depth sequence of studies may be necessary including a milk scintiscan, measurement of the patient's lower esophageal sphincter pressures, and monitoring the pH levels of the lower esophagus. Even when reflux is discernible on an upper GI series one should obtain these studies because of their usefulness in planning long-term management of the child.

If studies suggest some other form of esophageal disorder, esophagoscopy is indicated for better anatomical assessment and for biopsy. For example, a patient with a soft, thin congenital diaphragmatic web in the esophagus or an esophageal stricture, following an esophageal atresia repair, will require periodic esophagoscopy and dilatations. In order to avoid strictures in the upper thoracic esophagus caused by or exacerbated by esophageal reflux, it is important to proceed with an anti-reflux operative procedure when significant reflux is present. In children who have esophageal strictures without reflux, a formal resection will be required, if the strictures remain dense and unyielding in spite of repeated dilatations.

Another point in the management of children with esophageal problems is the importance of maximizing overall nutrition prior to surgery. Whether the impaired nutrition is on the basis of partial obstruction or reflux, the child is unlikely to tolerate surgery well until he has developed an anabolic state. While it is possible to provide nutrition by means of NG tube feedings to children with a stricture, such a modality may not work in children with pronounced reflux. One should not hesitate to defer surgery and place the child on central venous hyperalimentation for 3 or more weeks until the child's physical status, serum proteins, and blood counts indicate a good state of nutrition. The time spent on assuring an optimum nutritional state is well spent in view of the significantly lowered morbidity and mortality following surgery in an adequately nourished child.

VIOLATIONS OF THE PLEURAL SPACE

Anything that separates the visceral pleura from the parietal pleura represents a violation of what is normally a potential space. Gas, liquid, or solid substances, or a mixture of these, can be the cause of this separation. The result is a varying degree of "collapse" of the lung. The physiologic effect on the patient will depend upon how severe the collapse and how great the pressure on the adjacent structures of the mediastinum.

Pneumothorax

BACKGROUND

Air can collect in the pleural space acutely or chronically, statically or progressively. Since atmospheric pressure is always greater than intrapleural pressure, any mechanism which allows even momentary communication between the atmosphere outside the chest wall, or the atmosphere within the tracheobronchial tree, can result in a rapid shift of air into the pleural space. Penetrating wounds of the chest are the most common cause for pneumothorax. The penetrating object (a knife, a bullet, or a doctor's needle) may cause injuries of not only the parietal pleura, but often the lung parenchyma. For this reason, many patients with penetrating trauma to the chest will have not only an initial pneumothorax, but an expanding pneumothorax, as more and more air leaks from the surface of the lung.

Nonpenetrating trauma to the thorax can also result in a pneumothorax. For example, a fracture of one or more ribs may result in puncture of the visceral pleura and lung, causing an escape of air from the lung into the pleural space. If the intrapleural pressure increases, air may dissect out through the hole in the parietal pleura and into the chest wall tissues resulting in subcutaneous emphysema. Another form of nonpenetrating trauma is barotrauma which can occur in infants and children who have been ventilated with high inflating pressures via a tight fitting endotracheal tube. A particularly hazardous form of pneumothorax occurs when severe blunt trauma to the chest results in partial or complete tear of a bronchus or the trachea. Usually, patients with more peripheral bronchial tears will immediately develop symptoms of a pneumothorax. If the tear is more central the patient may first develop mediastinal and even cervical emphysema before a secondary rupture occurs into the pleural cavity.

Seemingly spontaneous episodes of pneumothorax may occur in children or adolescents. For example, a patient with one or more emphysematous blebs on the surface of the lung may develop spontaneous rupture resulting in an acute pneumothorax often associated with near complete collapse of the involved lung. In patients with cystic fibrosis, spontaneous pneumothorax is the second most frequent pulmonary complication. It usually occurs in teenage or young adult patients with far advanced diffuse bilateral cystic fibrosis. Another group of children with a high incidence of spontaneous pneumothorax are those with pulmonary metastases, for example, those with osteogenic sarcoma. Many of the metastases occur just below the pleural surface of the lung and, thus, may be the foci for the pneumothorax. Children with staphylococcal pneumonia are especially prone to develop unilateral or bilateral pneumothorax.

If the site through which air enters the pleural cavity seals quickly, and if no fluid or blood collects in the pleural space, a small or moderate pneumothorax will resolve spontaneously. However, some patients may have what appears to be a chronic or static pneumothorax. This usually occurs when there is a slow, persistent leak of air from the surface of the lung. A patient with osteogenic sarcoma metastases to the lung, for example, might continue to have a 5 or 10% pneumothorax.

Two special forms of pneumothorax require emphasis because, if not recognized early and attended to rapidly, these conditions may result in the death of the patient. The first is a tension pneumothorax which results not only in total collapse of the lung but progressive tension across the mediastinum (see Fig. 60.1). Whether the site of entry of the air into the pleural space is through the chest wall, a torn bronchus, or an injured portion of lung, the physiologic result is a one-way valve effect whereby air continues to accumulate in the pleural cavity with inspiration but cannot be extruded on expiration. This phenomenon continues until the intrathoracic pressure on the involved side is so high that no further air can enter the pleural space. This is often the point at which venous return from below the diaphragm is impeded and circulatory failure ensues.

The second life-threatening form of abnormal collection of air in the thorax is massive pneumomediastinum with or without an associated pneumothorax. In extreme cases the tension produced in the mediastinum can be great enough to impair both circulation and ventilation. This much emphysema suggests a major anatomical insult such as a rupture of a major bronchus or the trachea, or a perforation of the esophagus. If the patient survives the immediate physiological insult of air under tension in the mediastinum, the patient will be vulnerable to a disseminating mediastinal infection.

CLINICAL FINDINGS

The symptoms and signs of pneumothorax depend on the size of the pneumothorax and how rapidly it occurred. A patient with spontaneous rupture of an emphysematous bleb may complain of sudden acute pain on the involved side of the chest followed by tachypnea and a sense of shortness of breath. However, he may be found to have only a small (15 to 20%) pneumothorax on x-ray. By contrast, a patient with multiple trauma including blunt or penetrating trauma to the chest, may have so many other injuries that the presence of a pneumothorax is not immediately apparent.

In general, a patient with a pneumothorax will have signs and symptoms of ventilatory impairment—dyspnea, tachypnea, pain, splinting on the involved side, agitation, increase pulse rate, diminished breath sounds and increased resonance on the involved side, and possibly, displacement of the trachea and heart away from the involved side.

MANAGEMENT

The essential components of management involve confirmation that a pneumothorax exists and reexpansion of the lung. Ideally, a patient with a suspected pneumothorax should have an immediate upright PA and lateral chest x-ray. These x-rays are important to determine not only the site and extent of the pneumothorax but any complicating features such as tumor, fluid within the pleural space, or abnormalities of the lungs, diaphragm or mediastinum.

The urgency for treatment of the pneumothorax will depend on the patient's signs and symptoms, clinical circumstances, and the extent of the pneumothorax. For example, a multiple trauma patient who requires an emergency laparotomy should also have a chest tube placed if any degree of pneumothorax is present because, while draped and under anesthesia, there is no assurance that the pneumothorax will not significantly expand, complicating the course of the surgery.

Immediate therapy in a child with a suspected pneumothorax includes: (1) tamponading and obliterating any sucking or open chest wound, (2) inserting a Medicut or Angiocath into the pleural space and evacuating air. If sterile scissors are available, cut one to two side holes near the tip of a 14 to 20 gauge Medicut and then insert the needle with the overriding catheter just into the pleural space. Once inside, the catheter can be advanced and then attached to sterile i.v. tubing and placed to underwater seal. Alternatively one can attach a stopcock to the same setup and attempt to aspirate enough air and/or fluid to improve the patient's pulmonary dynamics. In a patient with a tension pneumothorax, the insertion of the needle and catheter will immediately result in release of the tension on the mediastinum and diaphragm.

Many infants can be effectively managed in this way if the amount of air present in the pleural space is small. However, these temporary catheter devices are small gauge and thus tend easily to develop fibrin plugs. Therefore, in any infant or older child who will require a tube within the pleura for more than a few hours, it is best to proceed with placement of a chest tube through a small incision on the chest (see procedure in Section VII). A size 12 chest tube is best for use in an infant and a size 24 chest tube for a teenager.

Fluid in the Pleural Space

BACKGROUND

Fluid in the pleural space can result from a number of acute or chronic conditions. Acutely, blunt or penetrating trauma to the chest usually produces blood within the pleural cavity. This blood often arises as a result of rib fractures which tear the parietal and visceral pleurae. In such cases, the amount of blood is not great unless an intercostal vessel has been torn. Larger amounts of blood suggest the possibility of direct penetrating injury to the lung, heart, or great vessels. Given the size of the pleural space, it is possible for an older child or adolescent to exsanguinate from blood loss within the pleural cavity.

In most cases of hemothorax, the cause is trauma. Seemingly mild trauma may result in significant hemothorax when there is an underlying congenital malformation, previous pleural disease, or a bleeding disorder. In such cases of unimpressive trauma, the hemothorax is likely to have progressed over several days and will be composed of mainly clotted blood by the time the condition is recognized.

Other fluid collections in the pleural space have nontraumatic etiologies and develop more slowly over a period of a few days. Sterile fluid accumulations in the pleural cavity are mainly a problem because of the degree of pulmonary compromise they produce. Sterile fluids can be a low protein, clear transudate, as in the patient with cardiac failure, or high protein, high fat chylous fluid, as in patients with a leak from the thoracic duct. Chylothorax may be idiopathic or secondary to chronic infection or tumor in the mediastinum. Irritative phenomenon such as viral infections or tumors in the pleural space produce sterile pleural fluid with an elevated protein.

Empyema or pus within the pleural cavity is a particularly serious and, at times, life-threatening situation. The predominant organism is *Staphylococcus aureus*, but rarely may be due to *Streptococcus pneumoniae*, group A *Streptococcus* or *Haemophilus influenzae.* Empyema is usually the result of septicemia, or direct or lymphatic extention from an associated pulmonary infection. When empyema follows accidental trauma or surgery, other bacterial organisms may be involved.

CLINICAL FINDINGS

Small, sterile pleural effusions may be asymptomatic and may only be recognized by x-ray. The more sizeable the effusion, however, the greater the amount of collapsed lung and resultant shunting and hypoxemia. Hypoxemia will cause the patient to develop varying signs and symptoms of respiratory distress including dyspnea, tachypnea, increased use of accessory muscles of respiration, and even cyanosis. As most effusions are not loculated, examination of the chest in an upright position will reveal distant to absent breath sounds and dullness to percussion in the lower lung fields. Using percussion, one can precisely identify the exact level of the effusion.

When there is a chronic condition such as tuberculosis or malignancy, the patient will appear to be chronically ill and may show systemic signs of weight loss. Those patients with a purulent empyema will have high fever and elevated pulse rates, and appear quite toxic.

MANAGEMENT

In any patient with suspected pleural effusion, it is helpful to obtain bilateral decubitus chest x-rays. These views enable one to determine whether the effusion is loculated and to uncover the presence of a tumor or pulmonary lesion otherwise obscured by the fluid. All patients should have a CBC and differential WBC, blood culture, crossmatch, and determination of BUN, sugar, electrolytes, total protein and albumin. However, the most helpful study is an analysis and culture of the pleural fluid. The technique for thoracentesis is given in Section VII.

In most cases, samples of the effusion should be sent for cell count, differential, Gram stain, acid-fast stain, total protein, and a complete set of cultures (aerobic, anaerobic, AFB, fungal). The clinical setting will influence the decision to omit some of these studies or add others. For example, in a patient with an acute hemothorax from trauma, no specific studies of the aspirated blood are indicated. On the other hand, if the patient is suspected of having a malignancy, a generous amount of the fluid should be immediately put into fixative and sent for cytological evaluation. If the fluid appears to be milky, it may be sent for a measurement of its fat content.

After initial studies have been obtained, the physician must decide how to evacuate the remainder of the fluid and keep it evacuated. This will depend on the volume of the remaining effusion and its character. If blood or purulent fluid is present to any significant degree, a chest tube should be inserted to obtain as complete evacuation as possible. Attempts to manage these types of effusions by continued aspirations may lead to clot formation and the development of a thick pleural peel necessitating surgery in the future. Furthermore, full expansion of the lung is the most physiological means of tamponading and obliterating most forms of pleural space compromise, including air leaks, empyema, sterile effusions, hemorrhage, and chylothorax. Smaller effusions which are sterile and free-flowing may be managed with one or two thoracenteses. Much of the success in managing pleural effusions depends on detailed medical management of the underlying process, plus careful attention to adequate nutrition.

Solid Lesions Involving the Pleural Space

BACKGROUND

Solid lesions can be focal and discrete, or they can be diffuse involving much of the pleural space. Although uncommon, these conditions usually warrant urgent attention. Diffuse solid lesions in the pleural cavity are associated with an unyielding collapse of the ipsilateral lung. The basis for these diffuse lesions is traumatic or infectious. Inadequate resolution of blood, serum, or pyogenic fluid within the pleural space will initially result in the formation of loculation of the material and later the formation of a progressively thick fibrous peel. Solid lesions which are more focal and discrete are usually neoplastic. Multiple nodular pleural lesions are usually metastatic. Solitary primary neoplasms involving the pleural space are rare.

CLINICAL MANAGEMENT

The signs and symptoms of a solid lesion involving the pleural space depend on how much lung tissue is compressed and on how much adjacent tissue is involved. A child complaining of shortness of breath, or persistent thoracic pain, should have a chest x-ray. The distinction between diffuse or focal lesion can be made immediately. If the history indicates prior trauma or infection, the patient will most likely require a thoracotomy for removal of the clotted or fibrous peel around the lung. If the patient has one or more focal lesions, a complete assessment for possible tumor sites should be made by using a metastatic bone survey, tomograms, or a CAT scan. Since focal lesions are presumed malignant until proven otherwise, surgery will be required for histological identification and possible excision.

CIRCULATORY COMPROMISE

BACKGROUND

Impairment of the circulation can be caused by one or more of the following mechanisms: (1) impaired venous return, as seen in a patient with massive intra-abdominal hemorrhage, or a severe tension pneumothorax; (2) failure of the heart as a pump as seen in intrinsic lesions of the heart or cardiac tamponade; or (3) failure of systemic perfusion such as a hemorrhage of major pulmonary or systemic vessels within the thorax. Some of these conditions progress so rapidly that in spite of immediate attention the patient may succumb. Penetrating injuries to the root of the lung, or to the heart, are examples of such life-threatening conditions.

Other patients with more slowly progressing circulatory compromise may also have potentially lethal conditions but are more responsive to treatment. Treatment of a patient with a cardiac arrest (Chapter 1), or with multiple trauma (Chapter 57), is described in detail elsewhere. However, there are two clinical situations which require active thoracic intervention. The first is severe progressive cardiac tamponade; the other is the unexplained clinical deterioration of the traumatized patient in spite of appropriate therapy.

CLINICAL FINDINGS

Many of the signs and symptoms of patients with circulatory compromise are discussed above. One should be alert to the following specific findings: (1) evidence of presumed internal or external hemorrhage, especially involving the abdominal cavity; (2) clinical and radiological evidence of a massive hemothorax; (3) penetrating wounds in the region of the heart (even if only the size of an ice pick); and (4) evidence of cardiac tamponade including unremitting shock in a patient with distended neck veins, pulsus paradoxus, and distant to absent heart sounds.

MANAGEMENT

In the emergency department such critically ill patients require the placement of two or more intravenous catheters, providing 100% oxygen, cardiac monitoring, insertion of a Foley catheter and an immediate chest x-ray. If there is evidence of an acute cardiac tamponade, one should immediately perform an emergency pericardiocentesis (see procedure in Section VII). The tamponade may be due to a purulent effusion or a hemorrhage within the pericardium. Regardless of whether blood, pus, or some other fluid is obtained, it is essential to determine if the patient is clinically improved by the pericardiocentesis. If the patient is not improved, it is likely that a large volume of thick clotted material is still present in the pericardium. During the procedure, Ringer's lactate solution (20 to 30 ml/kg) should be rapidly infused in order to produce an elevated venous pressure and thereby enhance cardiac filling in spite of the tamponade.

If shock persists, especially in the presence of increasing bradycardia, one should administer epinephrine (1 μg/kg) to improve cardiac contractility. Such treatment is temporizing and it is likely that the patient will need immediate pericardial drainage. If the clinical presentation and the pericardial fluid suggest an effusion secondary to infection, an immediate incision should be made in the midline below the xiphoid, opening first the linea alba and then the diaphragm, allowing access to the pericardium. The pericardium can then be opened widely and the material within digitally evacuated.

A different surgical approach is indicated for patients with severe thoracic trauma who are continuing to deteriorate in spite of maximal resuscitative efforts. For such patients an immediate thoracotomy in the emergency department may be necessary. This is usually best performed by means of an anterolateral thoracotomy in the 5th or 6th intercostal space. The incision is made on the right side if there is a massive hemothorax on the right side. Otherwise, the left side is preferred because it provides access to the pericardium, the heart, and the distal aorta. The pericardium is opened widely above the phrenic nerve so as not to damage it. Clotted material is evacuated. If a specific cardiac wound is identified, it can be lightly tamponaded until two or three buttress sutures can be placed. If there is massive bleeding from the lung, the root of the lung should be digitally compressed. Finally, a patient with a massive hemorrhage in the thorax or abdomen is helped by temporarily clamping the thoracic aorta as distally as possible. This maneuver often improves systemic circulation above the diaphragm and provides for better coronary filling. Once the patient's vital signs have been stabilized, more definitive surgery can be performed.

INTRINSIC LESIONS OF THE LUNG

The lung may be the site of a number of congenital, as well as acquired, conditions. Many of the congenital conditions, such as absence of a pulmonary artery or agenesis of a lung, are so severe that the child is either stillborn or dies shortly after birth. Other congenital conditions precipitate alarming symptoms in the first few days of life and generally require treatment at that time. A few conditions while present at birth may not produce significant symptoms until several months or several years of life.

Acquired pulmonary conditions in children are usually the result of an acute or a prolonged insult to the bronchial tree. This bronchial insult is often associated with both infection and distal parenchymal destruction of the lung. Such destructive changes can be seen in the following clinical conditions: (1) delayed removal of an aspirated foreign body, (2) chronic aspiration associated with gastroesophageal reflux or inadequate protective mechanisms in the glottis, (3) severe staphylococcal pneumonias, and (4) underlying pulmonary disease such as cystic fibrosis or immunological deficiencies. As a result of any of these conditions, lung abscess or bronchiectasis may develop (see Chapters 45 and 49).

Congenital Cystic Disease of the Lung

BACKGROUND

This disorder, like many congenital disorders in children, has a wide pathological spectrum including: a giant unilocular cyst, a mixed lesion composed of multiple cysts and solid tissue, or a lesion which is composed predominately of solid tissue with only an occasional small cyst. Specific forms of this disease spectrum have been labeled as cystic adenomatoid malformation or lobar sequestration depending on the anatomical, radiological, and clinical features. For the most part, the continuity between these various forms is maintained by histological identification of columnar ciliated bronchial epithelium within the cyst and usually the presence of a communication between the lesion and the bronchial tree.

Congenital cystic disease of the lung is generally unilateral and is not associated with any other congenital disorders. The condition occurs equally on either side and in half the cases arises in a lower lobe. The pathophysiology of this condition may be expressed in two forms. First, air enters the potential cystic spaces through extensive communication with the tracheobronchial tree. If the cystic spaces become quite large and tense, acute respiratory distress and tension across the mediastinum may develop shortly after birth. Second, other patients have lesions which do not trap air very readily and therefore demonstrate limited cyst formation and displacement of adjacent structures. In this latter group symptoms usually develop later in life and the diagnosis may be made in the emergency department during an evaluation for presumed pneumonia.

CLINICAL FINDINGS

The older infant or child with this condition is likely to have recurrent respiratory infections involving the same lobe (Fig. 60.7). Other children may be detected when

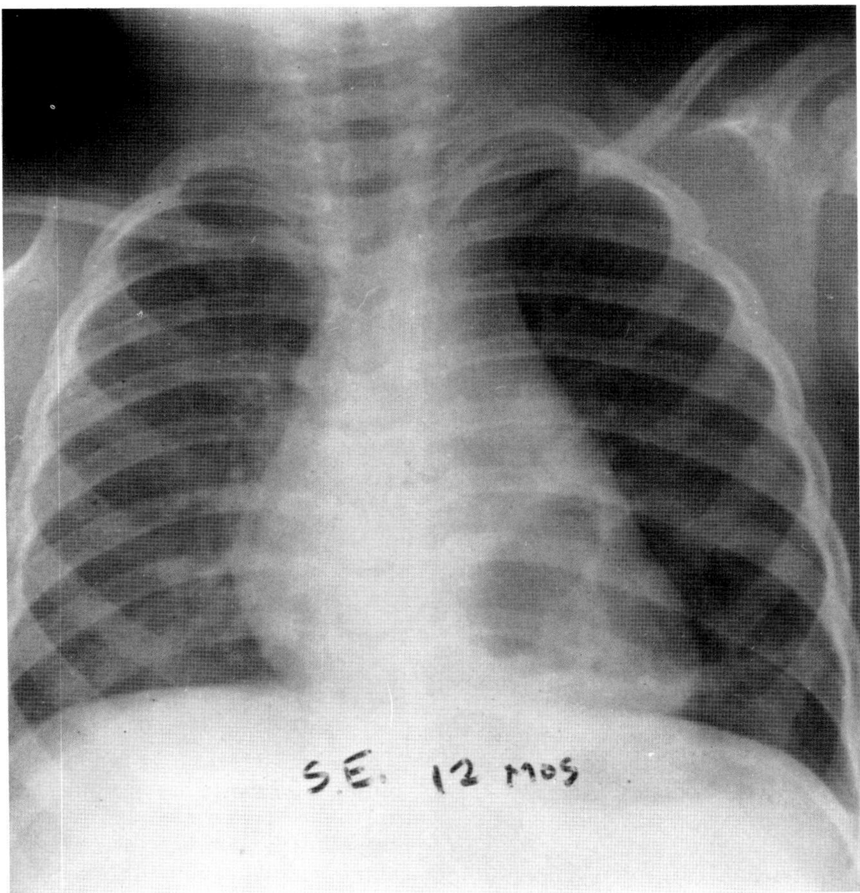

Figure 60.7 Cystic adenomatoid malformation in a 12-month-old girl with recurrent episodes of apparent left lower lobe pneumonia.

an episode of pneumonia does not resolve on appropriate treatment. Their signs and symptoms suggest a focal lobar pneumonia including fever, tachypnea, elevated WBC, dullness to percussion, and production of sputum which has atypical organisms on culture. When the problem has been recurrent, the child may also evidence failure to thrive. Occasionally, a child will appear to have an empyema leading to the inappropriate placement of a chest tube. Despite the chest tube drainage, the child will fail to resolve the empyema until the involved cystic tissue is excised.

MANAGEMENT

In addition to standard chest x-rays, one should obtain bilateral decubitus chest x-rays in order to evaluate any areas with air-fluid levels. Any pathogens identified in the sputum should be treated with appropriate antibiotics. In general, this condition is treated surgically after any acute infectious component has been controlled. Attempted aspiration of the cystic lesions, or placement of a chest tube, is to be condemned as it may lead to spread of infection into the pleural space. In preparing the child for surgery an arterial blood gas determination should be made, and, in an older child, more sophisticated measures of pulmonary function should be made. When the lower lobe seems to be involved, an aortogram should be obtained to identify any possible systemic blood supply. By following this course of evaluation, one is likely to rule out some of the other conditions which may be misdiagnosed, such as a diaphragmatic hernia, post-pneumonic pneumatoceles, or esophageal duplication.

Congenital Pulmonary Arteriovenous Fistula

BACKGROUND

This condition involves a direct communication between a major pulmonary artery and a vein within the lung. The communication is usually in the form of an aneurysmal sac which can vary in size from a few millimeters to several centimeters. Unfortunately, the AV fistulae can be multiple and can involve more than one lobe and more than one lung. When the condition is focal there may be a feeding systemic artery. Pathophysiology depends on the extent of the AV shunting. More severe shunting leads to the earlier recognition of the problem.

CLINICAL FINDINGS

At the time of presentation, the child may have been under treatment for wheezing episodes presumed to be bronchial asthma. As the child develops signs of desaturation, there may be clubbing and cyanosis. Physical examination of the involved area may demonstrate a palpable thrill or atypical flow murmurs. If there are symptoms of hemoptysis and epistaxis, one may find telangiectasias or hemangiomas of the skin and mucous membranes. Evaluation of the family may also reveal the presence of hereditary hemorrhagic telangiectasis (Rendu-Osler-Weber disease) which is present in more than half the patients with congenital pulmonary AV fistula.

MANAGEMENT

Children who are symptomatic from this condition should be evaluated by means of tomography, contrast echocardiography, perfusion scintography, and arteriograms of the pulmonary artery and aorta. Routine chest films show the aneurysmal areas as rounded or lobulated discrete lesions in the midlung field or in the periphery. Usually, these areas are connected to the hilum by one or more linear or tortuous vessels. In the majority of patients, the treatment i resection of the fistula with or without a associated lobectomy. A few patients, un fortunately, have diffuse disease and th extent of any resection is limited.

Miscellaneous Conditions

Other intrinsic lesions of the lung ar quite rare. They often are identified in rou tine chest x-rays which are taken for rela tively mild symptoms. Pulmonary tumor include primary sarcoma, pulmonary blas toma, hamartomas, and teratomas. Funga infections of the lungs are often presume to be neoplasm. Some patients have hyper lucency of one lung, yet on bronchoscop and bronchography have no lesion of th bronchus. A history of hemoptysis in suc patients suggests the need for pulmonar angiography which may reveal absence o pulmonary arterial supply to the involve lung. Hemoptysis in such patients is th result of marked tortuosity and enlarge ment of the bronchial collaterals.

MEDIASTINAL TUMORS

The mediastinum is a common site fo tumors because of its midline location an the highly diverse nature of its content Some entities which affect the medias tinum, such as bronchogenic cysts, are dis cussed above because of their impact o the airway. Malignant neoplasms of th mediastinum are discussed at length in th chapter on oncologic emergencies (Chapte 55).

The most helpful way to classify variou types of mediastinal tumors is by means o routine chest x-rays. Division of the me diastinum into anterior, superior, and pos terior portions is not based on true anatom ical planes but is helpful in categorizin diagnostic possibilities (Fig. 60.8). There i some overlap between the superior and an terior mediastinum in that teratoma or he mangioma may arise in both areas. Fur thermore, a lesion can arise in one are such as the anterior mediastinum and ex tend upward to involve the superior me diastinum.

Approximately 60% of mediastinal tu mors occur in the posterior mediastinum These are mainly composed of enterogen

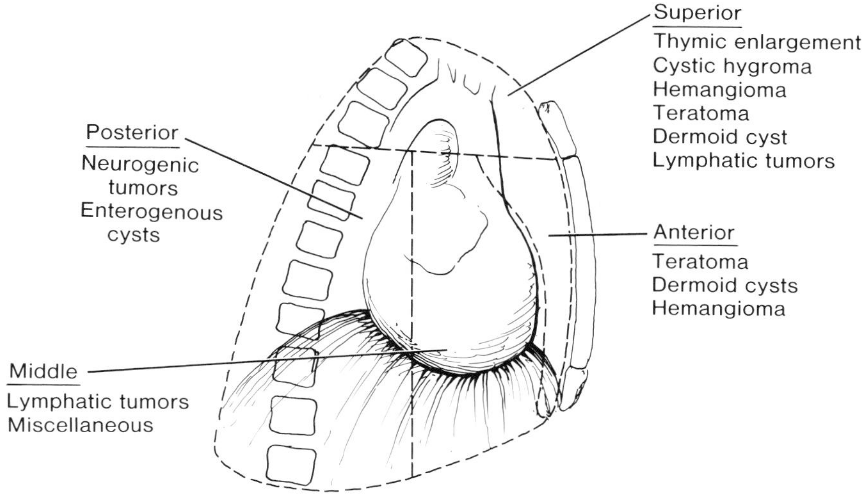

Figure 60.8 Mediastinal tumors in children: differential diagnosis based on anatomical location within the mediastinum.

us cysts or neurogenic tumors, the latter being somewhat more common. Most of these neurogenic tumors are malignant and are composed of neuroblastoma or neuroganglioblastoma. In the anterior and middle mediastinum, and occasionally the superior mediastinum, tumors of lymphatic origin represent the third most common family of mediastinal tumors. Most of these tumors are malignant and are the result of lymphosarcoma, Hodgkin's disease, or leukemia (see Chapter 55).

Enterogenous Cysts

BACKGROUND

These lesions are also referred to as esophageal duplications because of their intimate relationship to the esophagus. Like duplications elsewhere in the GI tract, they are spherical or tubular in shape with the external appearance of bowel. Histologically they are muscle walled and are usually lined by alimentary type epithelium. Enterogenous cysts in the thorax are usually in a posterior mediastinal position. However, they may communicate with the spinal canal, particularly in the presence of vertebral anomalies such as hemivertebrae. Occasionally, these cysts may be attached to a fistulous communication which penetrates through the diaphragm and either ends blindly or communicates directly with the jejunum or the duodenum.

CLINICAL FINDINGS

Lesions in the posterior mediastinum are in a relatively silent area. Therefore, unless symptoms of spinal cord compression develop, enterogenous cysts can become quite large before symptoms arise. Such symptoms include dysphagia, persistent cough, or unexplained pain. Some cysts are lined by gastric mucosa which secretes an acid material that can cause pain and peptic ulceration. Further symptoms may develop should the cyst erode into a bronchus or the esophagus. Dysphasia occurs in those rare enterogenous cysts which are not adjacent to the esophagus but instead occur within the wall of the true esophagus.

MANAGEMENT

The enterogenous cyst is often first noted on routine chest x-rays as a mass in the right posterior mediastinum. An esophagagram will confirm the intimate relationship between the cyst and the esophagus. One should carefully evaluate the spine to eliminate the possibility of a communication with the spinal canal. If peptic ulceration is a feature of the lesion, emergency surgery may be required to control bleeding and prevent a life-threatening mediastinitis.

Teratomas and Dermoid Cysts

BACKGROUND

Dermoid cysts are congenital tumors which are composed entirely of ectodermal derivatives. The lining is composed of squamous epithelium and the sac is often filled with hair and caseous debris. By contrast, teratomas contain all three embryonic germ layers. Teratomas can be solid or cystic and, in spite of their origin in the anterior mediastinum, they can become quite enormous before clinical signs or symptoms develop. As a result, mediastinal teratomas are more frequently identified in adults than in children.

CLINICAL FINDINGS

Symptoms associated with compression of the trachea or heart and great vessels may develop once these tumors have reached a sufficient size (see Fig. 60.2). On occasion, a secondary infection may occur within the cyst which, if untreated, may erode into the pleural cavity or trachea. When this occurs the child may cough up hair as a result of direct extension into the tracheobronchial tree.

MANAGEMENT

In addition to routine chest x-ray, the patient should undergo tomograms and an ultrasound evaluation of the mediastinum. Preoperative diagnosis may be suggested by the presence of teeth or other calcification within the lesion. The therapy is surgical excision which is generally easily performed unless there is malignant conversion or perforation by the tumors.

Thymic Tumors

BACKGROUND

The thymus is located in the anterior and superior mediastinum. Although an enlarged thymus is often identified in an infant's chest x-ray, it is rarely the cause of a thoracic emergency. Most young children with thymic enlargement will show spontaneous diminution in size of the thymus by the time they are 1 or 2 years old. The practice 20 to 30 years ago of treating a physiologically enlarged thymus with radiation therapy resulted in thymic shrinkage, and the subsequent development of thyroid cancer. There are a number of benign and malignant conditions associated with thymic enlargement. If the patient's age clinical presentation, and appearance on x-ray suggests an atypical enlargement of the thymus, a thorough evaluation is essential.

CLINICAL FINDINGS

A patient with a thymic tumor may have no symptoms, or only mild nonspecific symptoms such as persistent cough. On the other hand, some patients will develop progressively severe symptoms of respiratory distress. In such patients, one usually can discern a mass in the neck behind the sternal notch which may be a critical location in regard to tracheal compression.

Other children may have relatively asymptomatic masses which can be palpated in the anterior cervical triangle or under the sternocleidomastoid muscle. Such masses often prove to be thymic cysts that may undergo sudden rapid enlargement as a result of secondary infection or spontaneous hemorrhage.

MANAGEMENT

The indeterminate histological nature of any thymic tumor and its propensity to develop sudden enlargement and respiratory embarrassment necessitates urgent evaluation and treatment of these lesions. In addition to chest x-rays, the patient should undergo fluoroscopy, tomography and a CAT scan to determine both the extent of the tumor and its potential invasiveness. Surgical approach depends on the location of the tumor. Lesions in the anterior mediastinum can be managed by anterior thoracotomy while lesions extending into the cervical area are best approached by median sternotomy. Benign thymomas, common thymic cysts, and thymolipomas are the most common benign lesions. Malignant tumors frequently reflect the lymphatic nature of the thymus and are lymphosarcomas or reticulum cell sarcomas.

Miscellaneous Mediastinal Tumors

Other mediastinal tumors are significantly less common. *Chordoma* may occur in the posterior mediastinum. A *pericar-*

dial cyst may be seen in the middle mediastium as a spherical cystic lesion at the junction of the heart and the diaphragm. This finding in an asymptomatic patient is typical of a benign *pericardial cyst.* Removal of this asymptomatic mass is indicated in order to eliminate the possibility of another tumor. Other rare tumors of the mediastinum can be either benign, such as a *lipoma,* or malignant, such as a *rhabdomyosarcoma.* One particularly difficult tumor to manage is *cystic hygroma* or *lymphangioma* of the mediastinum. Most mediastinal cystic hygromas are found in the superior area but they often directly extend from the cervical area or rarely arise de novo in the anterior mediastinum. Although it is a benign tumor, it may infiltrate widely in the mediastinum and can envelop and separate structures such as the trachea and esophagus. Infection may develop in the lymphangioma leading to acute symptoms of pressure and respiratory compromise. In order to assess the extensive nature of lymphangiomas, the patient's evaluation should include CAT scan and ultrasonography.

DIAPHRAGMATIC DEFECTS

The diaphragm serves two roles: (1) to separate the abdominal from the thoracic viscera and, (2) to contribute to efficient ventilation especially in infants. As a muscular barrier, the diaphragm can fail in either of these two functions.

The vast majority of diaphragmatic hernias are congenital and present within the first 24 hours of life. They occur in the posterior lateral aspect of the diaphragm (foramen of Bochdalek), and on the left, 85% of the time. Diaphragmatic hernias which present later in life include: (1) foramen of Bochdalek types, (2) foramen of Morgagni hernias and, (3) traumatic rupture of the diaphragm. All three of these types produce problems due to pressure on the thoracic viscera, or due to obstruction or strangulation of the herniated structures.

The other form of diaphragmatic dysfunction relates to its role as a primary muscle of ventilation. When there is a large unilateral diaphragmatic hernia, the leaf of the diaphragm cannot contract efficiently during inspiration. Even if the diaphragm is intact, there may be a marked congenital attenuation of the musculature leading to a noncontractile fibrous sheath which extends far into the ipsilateral thorax. Other patients have acquired injury to the phrenic nerve which can result in paralysis of the diaphragm on that side and even a paradoxical ipsilateral elevation of the diaphragm during inspiration (Fig. 60.9).

Late Presentation of a Foramen of Bochdalek Hernia

CLINICAL FINDINGS

Patients may be any age at the time their diaphragmatic hernia is first diagnosed. Often symptoms are the result of an acute change such as a sudden shift of abdominal viscera into the thorax, or an acute bowel obstruction in a portion of thoracic bowel. Congenital diaphragmatic hernias on the right side present later in life, presumably because the liver occludes the hernia. Coughing or a shift in the position of the liver allows the bowel to extend through the hernia defect and to fill some or all of the thoracic cavity. The signs and symptoms in such circumstances are typical of pneumonia including: dyspnea, tachypnea, tachycardia, dullness to percussion, absent breath sounds, and possibly, cough and low-grade fever.

A similar phenomenon may occur on the left side. The spleen, however, is not as effective in blocking the hernia. As a result, the patient may have had loops of bowel in the inferior thoracic cavity for some time without experiencing symptoms. When symptoms do develop they often are those of unexplained bowel obstruction due to a twisting or occlusion of the bowel as it passes through the defect (Fig. 60.10). The patient complains of crampy abdominal pain, anorexia, and vomiting. On physical examination there may be abdominal distention with increased tympany and high pitched rushes. If gangrene or perforation take place, the patient may show signs suggestive of a pneumonia, including focal pleuritic chest pain, splinting respirations, localized dullness to percussion, absent

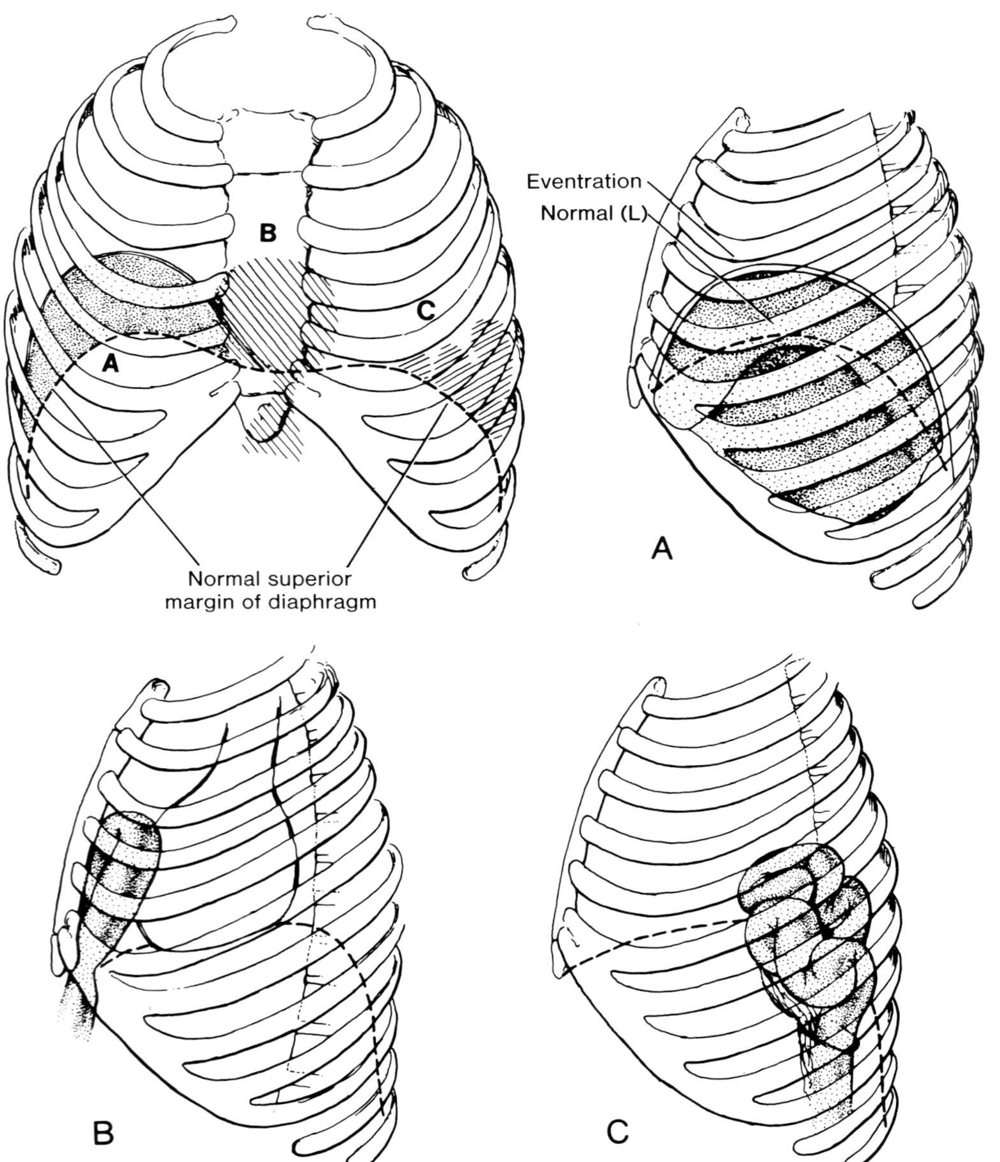

Figure 60.9 Diaphragmatic defects in infants and children. The nature of these defects are often better appreciated on a lateral view of the chest. (*A*) Eventration of the diaphragm, (*B*) foramen of Morgagni hernia, and (*C*) left foramen of Bochdalek hernia.

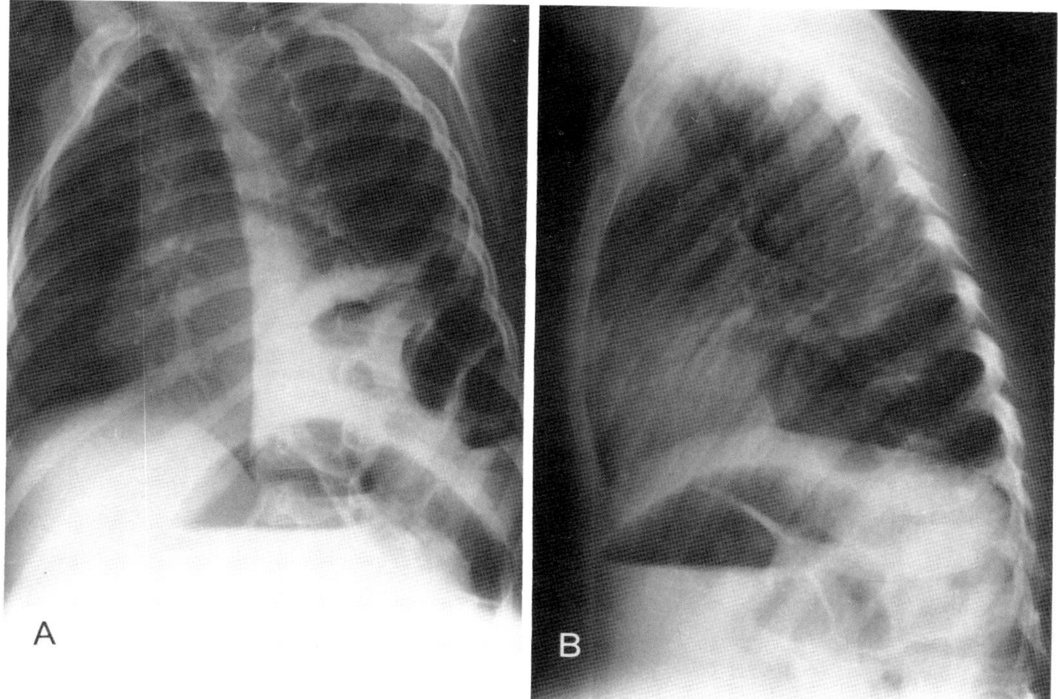

Figure 60.10 A 4-year-old boy admitted with 1-day history of recurrent severe upper abdominal colicky pain with dyspnea and decreased breath sounds in left base. PA (*A*) and lateral (B) chest films demonstrate multiple bowel loops in the lower, posterior left chest, indicative of a foramen of Bochdalek hernia which was subsequently repaired without difficulty.

breath sounds, fever, and an elevated WBC. One remarkable patient who had an asymptomatic herniation of his cecum into the left hemithorax presented with acute gangrenous appendicitis with subsequent perforation.

MANAGEMENT

Patients who express atypical thoracic or GI symptoms should have both chest and abdominal x-rays. Chest x-rays alone may suggest a pneumonic process in a lower lung field and the presence of pneumatoceles, unless one is able to identify continuity between the "pneumatoceles" and loops of bowel below the diaphragm. When a larger amount of bowel extends into the thorax, the anatomic relationships are not so difficult to appreciate. Surgical correction becomes urgent if there are compressive effects on the lung (Fig. 60.11). Also, when obstruction or strangulation of the bowel is the basis for the patient's symptoms, urgent surgery is required to avoid perforation and potentially fatal empyema. If there is any doubt about the diagnosis, the patient should undergo a real-time ultrasound examination of the diaphragm. Other procedures such as barium contrast studies may be helpful but, if the bowel is perforated, may pose an added risk to the patient. Ultrasonography can be done quickly at no added stress to the patient.

Foramen of Morgagni Hernias

CLINICAL FINDINGS

These hernias are in the anterior diaphragm and are located at the attachment of the diaphragm to the under surface of the sternum (see Fig. 60.9). Most foramen of Morgagni hernias are asymptomatic. They are often identified in older children or adults as an incidental finding on a chest

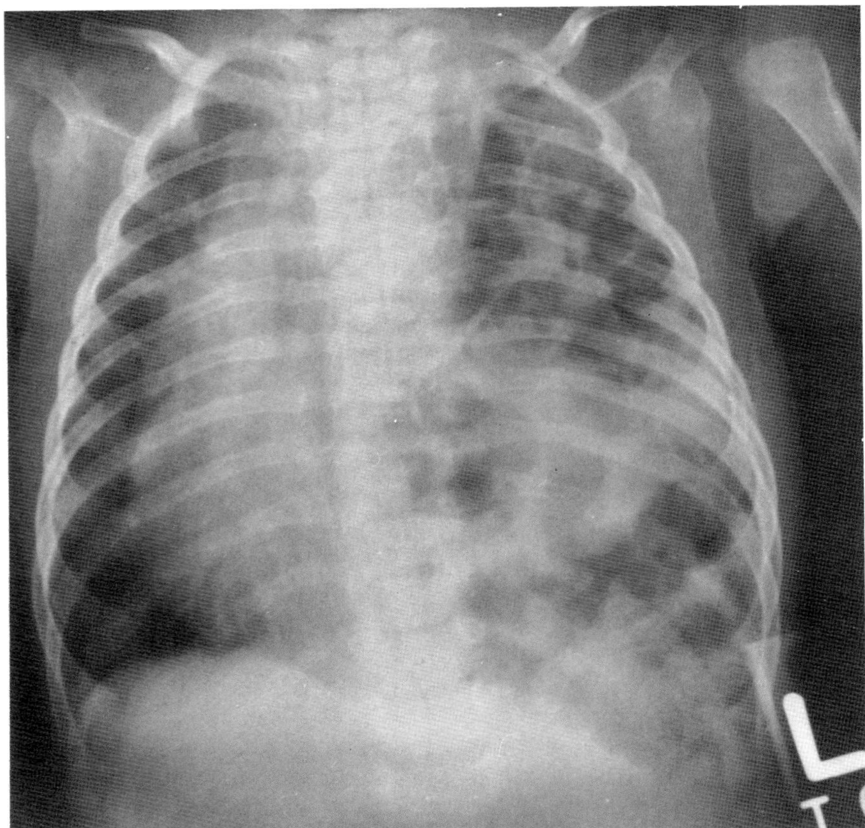

Figure 60.11 A 3½-month-old boy with prior "feeding problems" and sternal retractions. He was admitted with suddenly worse symptoms of vomiting and respiratory distress. A chest film revealed most of the bowel to be in the left chest.

x-ray. The lateral chest film in particular will demonstrate an unusual cystic mass lesion anterior to the heart which may contain an air fluid level. In most cases the loop of bowel which is passed through this hernia is transverse colon. Patients who develop signs and symptoms usually have features of complete or partial bowel obstruction, or a sense of pressure or pain under the sternum.

MANAGEMENT

The main management hazards are: (1) delays in treatment when symptoms are present, and (2) attempts to aspirate a presumed cystic mass without confirming the diagnosis. Real-time ultrasonography is the single best confirmatory test. If the patient is asymptomatic, a barium enema is also a safe diagnostic tool.

Traumatic Herniation of the Diaphragm

CLINICAL FINDINGS

Traumatic rupture of the diaphragm is usually associated with significant blunt trauma to the abdomen and is almost always associated with multiple trauma. Occasional diaphragmatic hernias have occurred as a result of penetrating injuries to the diaphragm from a knife or gunshot wound. The patient's other injuries often necessitate a laparotomy. During the course of laparotomy, diaphragmatic injury is likely to be recognized and repaired. Some patients with lesser degrees of blunt abdominal trauma may appear to be recovering when they develop increasing respiratory symptoms or evidence of GI obstruction.

MANAGEMENT

A supine chest film may suggest a confusing picture interpreted as pulmonary contusion or pleural effusion. This condition, in particular, points to the importance of getting *upright* PA and lateral chest x-rays in the multiple trauma patient. The confusing findings on the supine chest film will often be clarified, as loops of bowel are more clearly identified above the diaphragm. In the past, pneumoperitoneum and contrast studies have been used to confirm this diagnosis; ultrasonography is now the confirmatory diagnostic modality of choice.

Paraesophageal Hernias

BACKGROUND

A paraesophageal hernia involves the protrusion of some or all of the fundus of the stomach through either the esophageal hiatus or through a defect adjacent to the hiatus. Children in whom the hernia is through the hiatus may have had prior nonspecific symptoms of regurgitation or vomiting due to pressure on the distal esophagus. Symptoms of acute distress and esophageal obstruction occur if strangulation or volvulus of the herniated stomach takes place. Patients in whom a discrete hernia defect exists adjacent to the hiatus may have no symptoms until a sudden displacement of stomach through the defect takes place. Esophageal obstruction in these patients is the result of most of the upper stomach being drawn into the thorax as more and more air is trapped within it.

Patients may present with acute symptoms such as tachypnea, tachycardia, splinting toward the left side, and diminished breath sounds in the left lower chest. They may have nonproductive vomiting, and when an NG tube is passed it will clearly not pass beyond the distal stomach (Fig. 60.12).

MANAGEMENT

Chest and abdominal films will show a large air- and fluid-filled protrusion into the left lower thorax. The tip of the NG tube will be seen to have stopped at the distal esophagus. Such a picture is pathognomonic of a herniated and presumably stran-

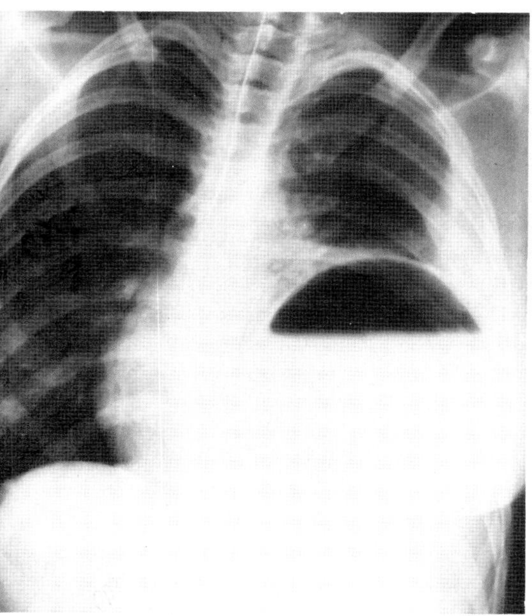

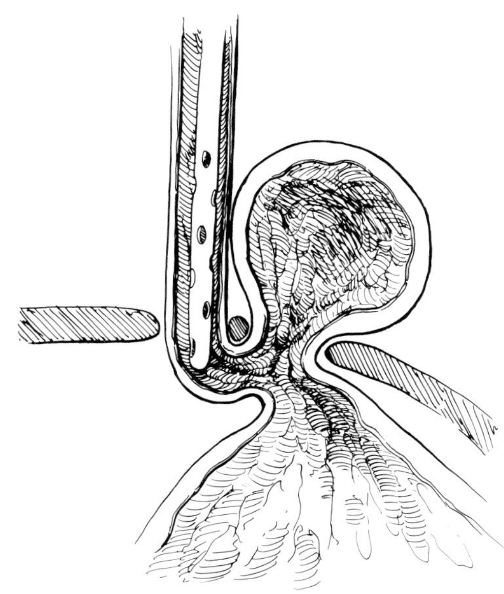

Figure 60.12 A 13-year-old girl developed first right and then left epigastric pain with retching but little or no vomitus. She had grunting respirations. An x-ray revealed a large air and fluid filled mass in the left lower chest. As shown in the diagram, a nasogastric tube would not pass into the stomach.

gulated stomach and is an indication for an emergency laporotomy.

Eventration of the Diaphragm

CLINICAL FINDINGS

The signs and symptoms in this condition depend on the severity of the eventration and whether one or both sides are involved. Left-sided eventrations are more likely to be complete and are, therefore, more likely to be associated with signs and symptoms of respiratory difficulties. The patient may have wheezing, dyspnea, and recurrent respiratory infections. The left lower lung field may be dull to percussion and may have diminished breath sounds, and the mediastinum may be shifted to the opposite side. Major eventrations produce symptoms as a result of progressive attenuation of the diaphragm or acute intestinal distention.

MANAGEMENT

Chest x-rays will usually confirm the presence of a high rounded diaphragm shadow filled with bowel and other viscera involving more than 50% of the thoracic cavity on the involved side. While mild asymptomatic eventrations incidently found do not warrant therapy, major diaphragmatic eventrations should be repaired even if symptoms have not yet developed in order to avoid collapse of the ipsilateral lung (Fig. 60.13).

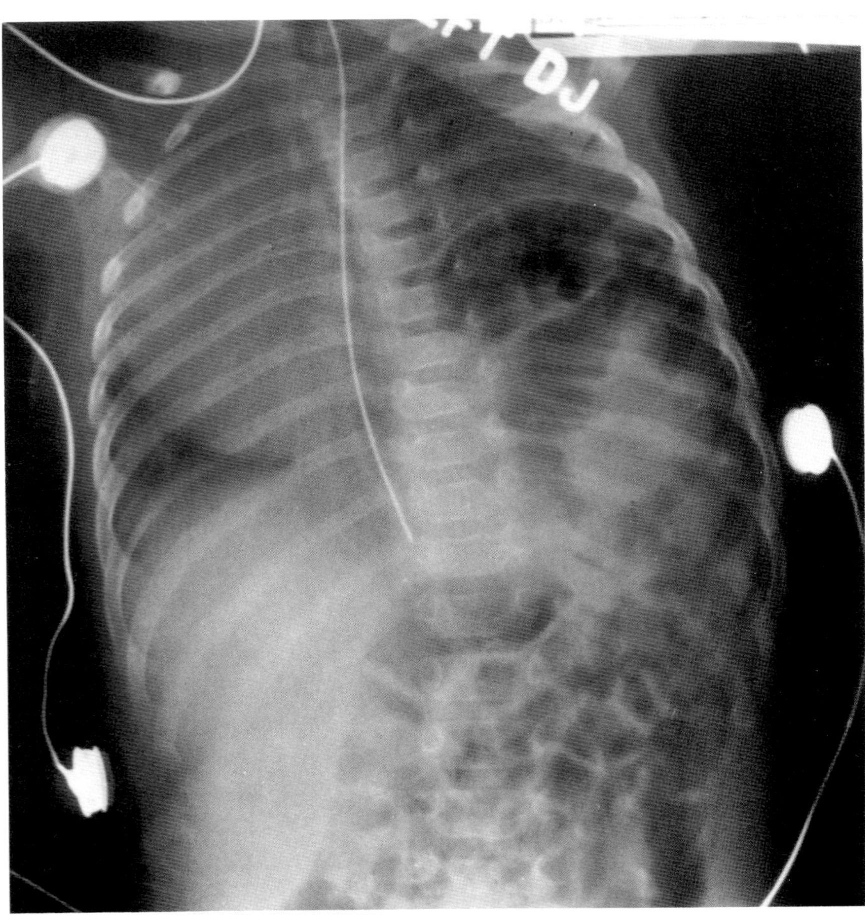

Figure 60.13 This 2-month-old girl was well until 4 days prior to admission. She develope[d] congestion and an apparent URI. She slowly developed increasing dyspnea and was admitted [in] acute respiratory distress. A chest x-ray revealed a high left diaphragmatic eventration with marked mediastinal shift to the right.

Acquired Diaphragmatic Malfunction

CLINICAL FINDINGS

Paralysis of the diaphragm can occur as a result of injury to the phrenic nerve during birth or during a cervical or thoracic operation. In most cases, the paralysis is complete and the symptoms present shortly after the injury occurs. In the newborn a paralyzed diaphragm is particularly debilitating as air exchange is greatly impaired. The mediastinum is so mobile that a pressure differential allows the paralyzed diaphragm to rise paradoxically on inspiration, resulting in a shift of the mediastinum toward the normal side. Infants with only partial paralysis of the diaphragm may be sent home, only to return to the emergency

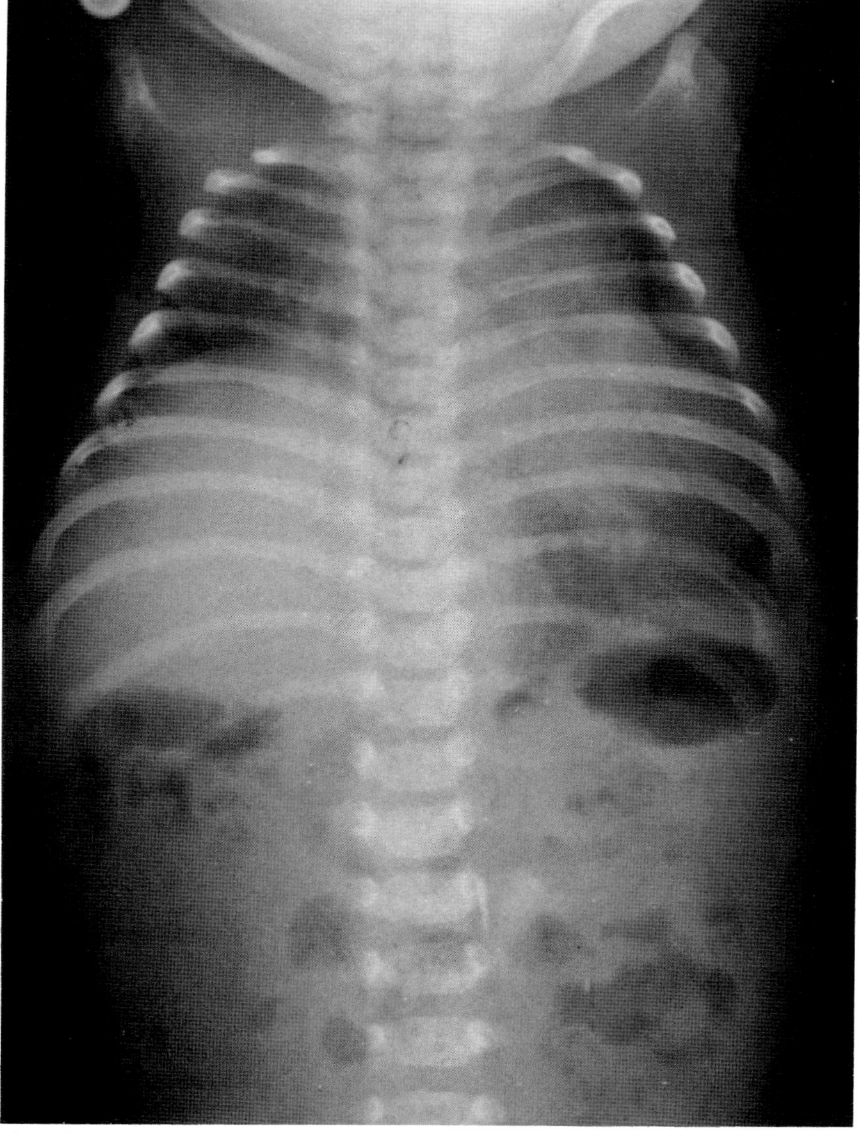

igure 60.14 A 2-month-old girl with a brachial palsy at birth. She initially did surprisingly well ut subsequently developed respiratory distress with cyanosis when out of oxygen. A chest x-ray howed a high attenuated right diaphragm.

department with respiratory distress or pulmonary infection.

MANAGEMENT

As in a child with eventration of the diaphragm, an upright PA and lateral x-ray will indicate the degree of diaphragmatic compromise (Fig. 60.14). Fluoroscopy may demonstrate the paralyzed portion of the diaphragm. If a trial of keeping the child in an infant seat at 60 to 75° elevation does not significantly improve the symptoms, then resection and plication of the attenuated portion of the diaphragm should be performed.

CHEST WALL TUMORS

BACKGROUND

Although chest wall tumors in children are quite uncommon, those tumors which do occur are likely to be malignant. Benign tumors generally arise from the ribs. They include chondromas, osteochondromas, aneurysmal bone cysts, osteoid osteoma, lipoid histocytosis, and giant cell tumors. In some of these tumors the clinical and radiological picture may clearly indicate a benign self-limited process and, thus, observation is appropriate.

If there is question, one should view even a small chest wall mass in a child with great concern. Many of the malignant tumors may be present at birth and some have been identified early in infancy. As a general principle, any chest wall tumor in a child which does not appear to be totally benign should be considered malignant.

CLINICAL FINDINGS

Most benign tumors of the chest wall are generally asymptomatic unless some secondary problem occurs, such as trauma or spontaneous fracture. Many of the malignant tumors, however, are also asymptomatic when they are small. A relatively rapid increase in their size would tend to suggest their malignant nature. If the tumor is associated with pain, local tenderness or signs of inflammation, the lesion is likely to be malignant. This is particularly true for *Ewing's* tumor of the bone which typically involves the lateral aspects of the ribs. Unfortunately, some children with Ewing's sarcoma of the chest wall are treated as if they had an infectious process and, as a result, the tumor mass is far advanced by the time appropriate consultation is obtained.

In addition to Ewing's sarcoma, other

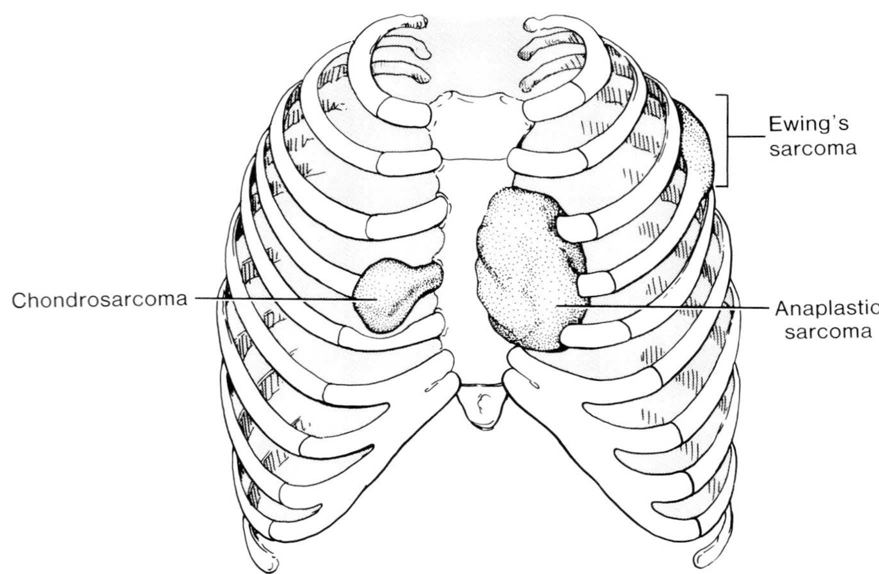

Figure 60.15 Malignant chest wall tumors in children: most common lesions and their usual site of origin.

malignant tumors of the chest wall may tend to have a preferred site of origin (Fig. 60.15). *Chondrosarcoma* typically involves the cartilaginous flat portions of the ribs and, therefore, usually presents in the parasternal areas. *Anaplastic sarcomas* often arise from the sternum. Although these tumors may not have the inflammatory qualities seen in Ewing's sarcoma, most of them will evidence involvement both inside and outside of the chest cavity on chest x-ray. This involvement may include a protruding mass into the pleural space, a pleural effusion, or direct involvement of the underlying lung.

MANAGEMENT

Assessment of these tumors should include tomography, bone scans of the entire body, metastatic bone survey, and a CAT scan of the area involved. Successful treatment of these malignant lesions usually involves three modalities: surgery, chemotherapy, and radiotherapy. If a biopsy is anticipated prior to definitive wide resection, the route of the biopsy should be designed to avoid compromise of the subsequent chest wall reconstruction. Occasional patients with especially extensive tumor involvement have benefited from pretreatment with chemotherapy and radiotherapy before definitive resection was performed. Resection of the tumor and even subsequent recurrences have resulted in disease-free survivals of 15 years or more.

References

Bechamps GJ: Empyema in children; review of Mayo Clinic experience. *Mayo Clin Proc* 54: 43, 1970.

Grosfeld JL, et al.: Primary mediastinal neoplasms in infants and children. *Ann Thorac Surg* 12: 179–190, 1971.

Kendig EL Jr (Ed.): *Disorders of the Respiratory Tract in Children*, Ed. 3. W. B. Saunders, Philadelphia, 1977.

Moser KM, Spragg RC: (Eds.): *Respiratory Emergencies*, Ed. 2. C. V. Mosby, St. Louis, 1982.

Ramenofski ML, et al.: Bronchogenic cyst. *J Pediatr Surg* 14: 219–224, 1979.

Ravitch MM, Welsh KJ, et al. (Eds.): *Pediatric Surgery*, Vol. 1, Ed. 3. Yearbook Chicago, 1979.

Schuster SR, Fellows KE: Management of major hemoptysis in patients with cystic fibrosis. *J Ped Surg* 12: 889–896, 1977.

Schuster SR, et al.: Bronchial atresia; a recognizable entity in the pediatric age group. *J Pediatr Surg* 13: 682–689, 1978.

Schwartz SI, et al. (Eds.): *Principles of Surgery*, Ed. 3. McGraw-Hill, New York, 1979.

Stiles QR, et al.: Pleural empyema in children. *Ann Thorac Surg* 10: 37–44, 1970.

Tapper D, et al.: Poly-alveolar lobe; anatomic and physiologic parameters and their relationship to congenital lobar emphysema. *J Pediatr Surg* 15: 931–937, 1980.

Wolf SA, et al.: Cystic adenomatoid dysplasia of the lung. *J Pediatr Surg* 15: 925–930, 1980.

CHAPTER 61

Ophthalmic Emergencies

GARY R. DIAMOND, M.D.

INTRODUCTION

Ophthalmic emergencies in children are quite common, and most are initially evaluated by nonophthalmologic personnel. Pediatricians and emergency department physicians undoubtedly diagnose more ophthalmic emergencies than do ophthalmologists. Sophisticated improvements have occurred in management of pediatric ophthalmic trauma just as in all aspects of emergency care. This chapter will note these technical advances whenever appropriate, even though they may not be available to the pediatrician or emergency department physician. Familiarity with specialized instrumentation is essential for appropriate management of the emergency ophthalmic patient. Despite easy access to specialized ophthalmic care, a large measure of responsibility for the salvage of a traumatized eye remains with the individual who is first consulted.

The rehabilitation of a child's traumatized eye is potentially a lengthy and complex affair. In order to decrease the potential for amblyopia in children below the age of 7 or 8 years of age, timely clearing of the visual axis and appropriate optical correction is essential in all cases involving perforation of the refracting structures of the eye. Nevertheless, the success of this rehabilitation is to a large degree dependent on the knowledge of the individual who first undertakes care for the ophthalmic trauma.

GENERAL CONSIDERATIONS

Overlooking a vision-threatening ocular injury is a most serious omission of the examining physician (Table 61.1). Occasionally, perforating injuries of the eye are initially undetected because of profound lid swelling or other devastating facial injuries. Treatment will be performed for the latter conditions and only much later is the more serious ocular injury noted. Facial fractures may be repaired without consideration of possible concomitant ocular injury. Careful separation of even the most swollen lids is possible with individual lid speculums but should not ordinarily be attempted by emergency department personnel. This technique permits clear examination of the cornea, and, after appropriate pupillary dilatation, the interior of the globe. Neglect of possible serious ocular injury is understandable in a frightened, struggling child but necessary procedures must be performed nontheless. If necessary, general anesthesia should be undertaken to delineate the extent of the injury and repair be performed at that time. Ophthalmologists are trained to look beyond the lid laceration or periorbital ecchymosis and seek out the occult ophthalmic trauma. Its only surface marker may be injection of the conjunctiva or a small subconjunctival hemorrhage that indicates scleral rupture. If life-threatening injury demands immediate attention, appropriate ophthalmic examination can be performed immediately after these considerations are resolved.

The emergency department setting is quite adequate for a screening eye examination. A list of basic ophthalmic equipment is given in Table 61.2. It is helpful to have this equipment assembled in an ophthalmic kit. Table 61.3 lists useful ophthalmic medications for emergency department use.

Table 61.1
Pitfalls in Management of Ophthalmic Trauma

1. Failure to examine the other eye
2. Failure to check vision in the injured eye
3. Failure to consider globe perforation with external injury
4. Prescribing topical anesthetics
5. Prescribing steroid preparations if diagnosis is uncertain or if herpes simplex infection is possible
6. Use of any ointment when globe perforation is present or fundus examination is indicated
7. Failure to ensure appropriate patient referral or follow-up

Table 61.2
Ophthalmic Equipment for the Emergency Department

Visual acuity charts (Snellen letters, Allen figures, "E" game)
Lid speculums
Saline squeeze bottles for irrigation, sterile
Bottle sterile saline with intravenous tubing for irrigation
Topical anesthetic drops, sterile (see Table 61.3)
Fluorescein strips, sterile
Hand lights, white and cobalt blue
Paper and cloth tape
Eye pads, sterile
Eye patches
Topical ophthalmic antibacterial and antibiotic drops and ointments (see Table 61.3)
Direct ophthalmoscope
Cotton swabs, sterile
pH test strips
Desirable equipment:
- Slitlamp biomicroscope
- Schiötz tonometer with sterilizer

Table 61.3
Useful Ophthalmic Medications for Emergency Department Personnel

- Topical anesthetics
  - Proparacaine 0.5% hydrochloride
    - Ophthaine (Squibb)
    - Ophthetic (Allergan)
- Dilating drops
  - Phenylephrine 2.5%
    - Mydfrin (Alcon)
  - Tropicamide 1%
    - Mydriacyl (Alcon)
- Cycloplegic drops
  - Tropicamide 1%
    - Mydriacyl (Alcon)
  - Homatropine 2% and 5%
  - Atropine ½% and 1%
- Antibacterial drops
  - Sulfacetamide sodium 10%
    - Sulamyd (Schering)
- Antibacterial ointments
  - Sulfacetamide sodium
    - Sulamyd (Schering)
  - Erythromycin
    - Ilotycin (Dista)
  - Polymyxin B-Bacitracin
    - Polysporin (Burroughs-Wellcome)
- Antibiotic drops
  - Gentamycin sulfate
    - Garamycin (Schering)
- Antibiotic ointment
  - Gentamycin sulfate
    - Garamycin (Schering)
- Antihistamine-decongestants
  - Napazoline hydrochloride-pheniramine maleate
    - Naphcon-A (Alcon)
  - Naphazoline hydrochloride-antazoline phosphate
    - Vasocon-A (Cooper Vision)
    - Albalon-A (Allergan)

After a pertinent history is taken, the upper face should be examined with attention paid to possible asymmetry. External trauma should be noted and visual acuity taken with each eye separately, both at distance and near. A choice of visual acuity testing charts should be available for both literate and illiterate children. In the very young infant, fixation pattern with either eye can be tested easily, using an object of interest. The ability of the child to fix and to follow a small toy with either eye is a reasonably accurate measurement of visual acuity. Ideally, emergency department personnel should be trained in the use of the slitlamp biomicroscope but, realistically, examination of the anterior segment of the globe can be undertaken with a small penlight and fluorescein strips. The posterior segment of the eye can be examined with the direct ophthalmoscope familiar to all medical personnel. Ocular motility should be tested, looking for restrictions in movement. Pupillary reaction can also be screened with a penlight. It is appropriate to refer a patient to an ophthalmologist for examination of the posterior segment of the eye if this cannot be performed through undilated pupils and clinical suspicion warrants such examination.

The remainder of the chapter will be divided into traumatic and nontraumatic emergencies, in rough order of urgency. The alert acute-care team will give priority to those children presenting with the more urgent situations, and undertake management as soon as possible.

CHEMICAL BURNS

Chemical burns by acid or alkali are the most urgent ocular emergencies. Alkali penetrates rapidly through the cornea into the anterior chamber, while acids quickly precipitate tissue protein and thus set up physical barriers to their own penetration. Because of this, alkali burns are frequently more disastrous than acid burns. Strong alkali may reach the interior structures of the eye within seconds of contact with the cornea. Alkali combines with cellular membrane lipid and totally disrupts the cells, with softening of ocular tissue.

CLINICAL FINDINGS

Lye (sodium hydroxide or potassium hydroxide), lime (calcium oxide), and ammonia are the alkali burns most frequently seen. The amount of injury is determined by the quantity of alkali, the alkalinity of the material, and the amount of time lapsing before treatment. Initial presentation in severe cases may disclose a pearly white conjunctiva, corneal opacity because of collagen denaturation, and intraocular inflammation. Glaucoma is quite frequent, potentially disastrous and often overlooked.

Acid burns are less common. Most represent battery explosions or accidents in a school chemistry laboratory. The same considerations apply as to alkali burns, with the somewhat less possibility for disastrous result.

MANAGEMENT

Treatment for both acid and alkali burns is simple and urgent. Immediate copious irrigation using whatever liquid available is the mainstay of therapy. Topical anesthetic, such as proparacaine or tetracaine drops, may be placed in the eye and the lids held apart manually or with lid retractors. Irrigation should be performed with normal saline connected to an intravenous tubing set and at least 2 liters of fluid permitted to lavage the tissues. Monitoring of the pH of the fluid in the conjunctival sac can be performed with litmus paper and lavage continued until pH in the conjunctiva is between 7.0 and 8.0. Recheck 5 to 10 min later is essential. Prolonged irrigation can be obtained with constant infusion scleral contact lenses or a catheter anchored in the conjunctival sac. These techniques require an ophthalmologist's assistance. Particulate matter should be removed from the recesses of the conjunctival sac with either blunt forceps or a swab.

Recent suggestions have included immediate anterior chamber irrigation with phosphate buffer to attempt to neutralize the pH in the anterior segment of the eye. The efficacy of this is unknown. Other recent suggestions have included simple anterior paracentesis to remove alkaline material in bulk from the anterior chamber, with uncertain usefulness.

After or during lavage, cycloplegic drops, such as 1% atropine are placed on the eye to dilate the pupil and prevent iris adhesions to either lens or cornea. In addition, these agents may decrease intraocular inflammation. Further management of burns is performed by the ophthalmologist and may include intravenous osmotic agents, oral acetazolamide and steroid therapy.

For severely burned corneas the prognosis is grim. Without adequate moisture and in presence of active collagenase, the cornea will melt and become necrotic. Inflammation can damage the ciliary processes and lead to cessation of aqueous production. All too often, the end result is a disorganized eye, blind and painful. The importance of immediate lavage and thorough painstaking management cannot be overemphasized.

LACERATIONS OF THE GLOBE

CLINICAL FINDINGS

Next in urgency is the perforating corneal and/or scleral injury. The history is most important, as it often provides an indication of the extent of damage. Information should be obtained concerning the description of injury, the weapon used, and whether or not the child was wearing glasses at the time. Often, children are afraid to confess exact details of the events concerned, and thus some detective work may be necessary. It is our impression that children below the age of 6 or 7 years will be somnolent when presenting to the emergency department with a perforation of the eye. After the history has been taken, examination of the lids and other facial structures should be performed. A measure of visual acuity must be attempted, especially in the uninjured eye. If the child is simply uncooperative, a note should be made of this fact on the record. Attention should then be directed to the globe itself. Often the injury site is clearly visible and the eye will appear inflamed, red and tearing. The presence of iris prolapse, manifesting as a fleshy mass on the surface of the eye with a teardrop-shaped pupil should be specifically noted; this is clear indication of a perforating injury (Fig. 61.1). A hand light directed transversely across the anterior chamber will detect a shallow or flat anterior chamber if the iris does not illuminate uniformly by this maneuver (Figs. 61.2 and 61.3). Hyphema is a frequent complicating factor.

MANAGEMENT

As soon as a perforating injury has been diagnosed, or even seriously suspected, a metal or plastic shield should be placed over the eye and the eye not further manipulated. Specifically, no topical anesthetic or antibiotic ointment should be placed in the eye, as the actions of these topical medications inside the eye are potentially damaging. If the history is indicative, x-rays of orbital fractures and intraocular foreign bodies should be obtained. If at all possible, the nontraumatized eye should be briefly examined at this time.

Perforating injury demands specialized ophthalmic care and is a surgical emergency. Surgery should be performed to close the wound as soon as possible. Sensitive ocular tissues quickly become edematous and reapposition is made more difficult. General anesthesia is induced with nondepolarizing agents such as curare so as not to extrude intraocular contents. Depolarizing agents such as succinylcholine are avoided. Surgical repair is performed with microsurgical techniques using very fine sutures and minimally traumatic needles. The eventual outcome from a perforating injury may not be known for a long period thereafter.

In summary, the most important function that the initial treating physician can perform for these injuries is their recognition and thenceforth lack of manipulation of the damaged eye. Rapid progress to the operating room will be rewarded by more precise anatomic closure and better visual and functional results.

HYPHEMA

Hyphema is blood within the anterior segment of the eye and may range from a small clot on the iris, or a few cells floating in the aqueous to a complete filling of the anterior segment of the eye with blood (Figs. 61.4 and 61.5). With rare exceptions, these are secondary to trauma. Children with juvenile xanthogranuloma lesions on the iris, herpes zoster keratouveitis, and intraocular tumors may present with spontaneous hyphema.

CLINICAL FINDINGS

The presence of hyphema should be suspected from the history of trauma and the presentation of a red, inflamed, teary eye. Hand light examination often shows blood

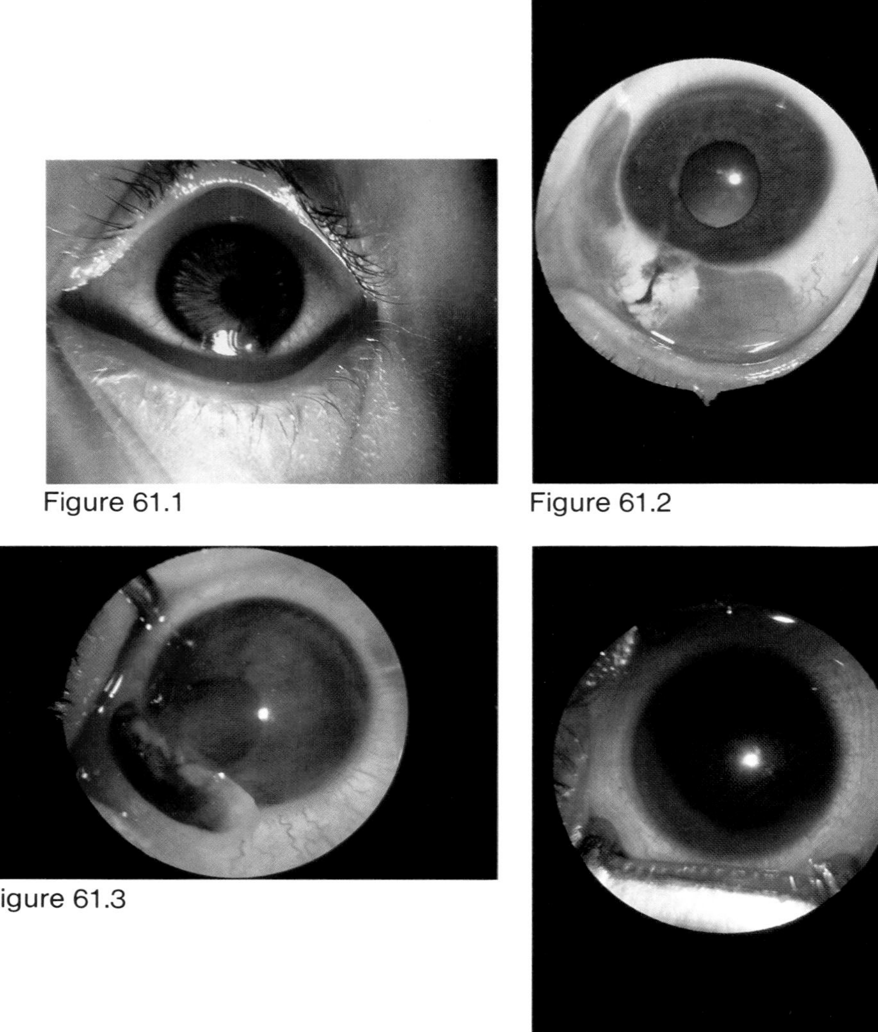

Figure 61.1

Figure 61.2

Figure 61.3

Figure 61.4

Figures 61.1–61.4 **(61.1)** Inferotemporal corneal laceration with iris prolapse. Note similarity to corneal foreign body and subtle iris distortion toward the wound. **(61.2)** Inferonasal perforating corneoscleral laceration with exposure of ciliary body in depth of scleral wound. Note subconjunctival hemorrhage and subtle distortion of pupil toward laceration. **(61.3)** Larger inferonasal perforating limbal laceration with large prolapse of necrotic (strangulated) iris. The anterior chamber is shallow, a small hyphema is present, and the iris is distorted toward the laceration. **(61.4)** Settling hyphema.

in the anterior chamber, but slitlamp examination may be necessary for smaller bleeds. Anatomically, most hyphemas arise in the ciliary body behind the iris and, therefore, the bleeding site is difficult to find. The initial bleed often clears completely, but a more ominous rebleed may occur between 3 and 5 days after the initial

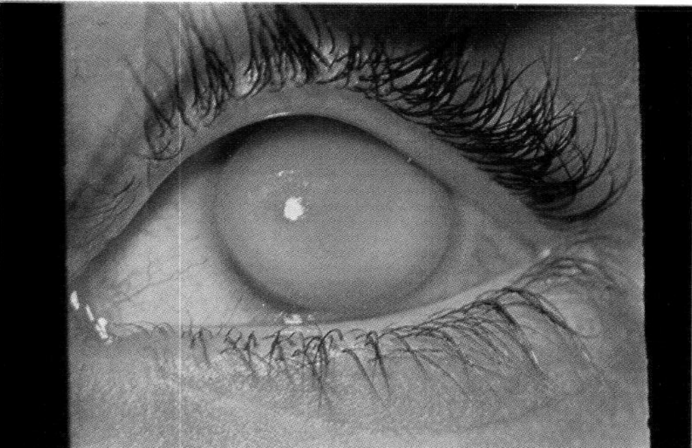
Figure 61.5

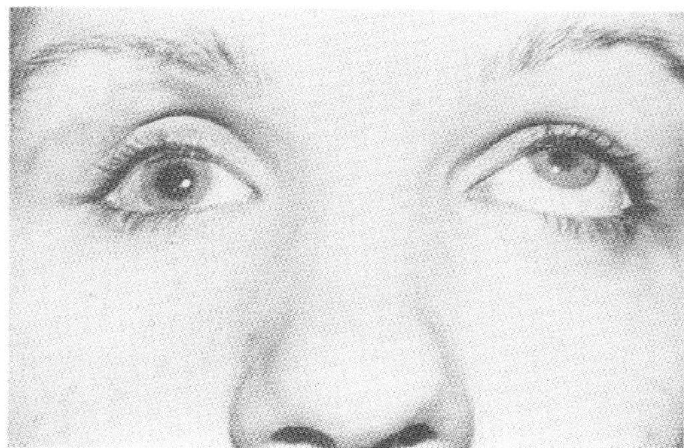
Figure 61.6

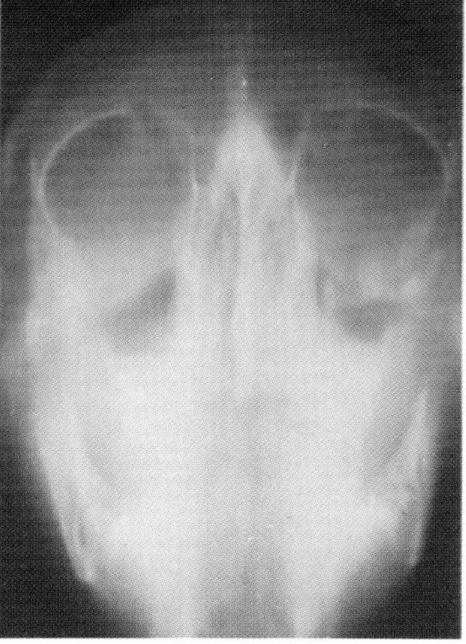
Figure 61.7

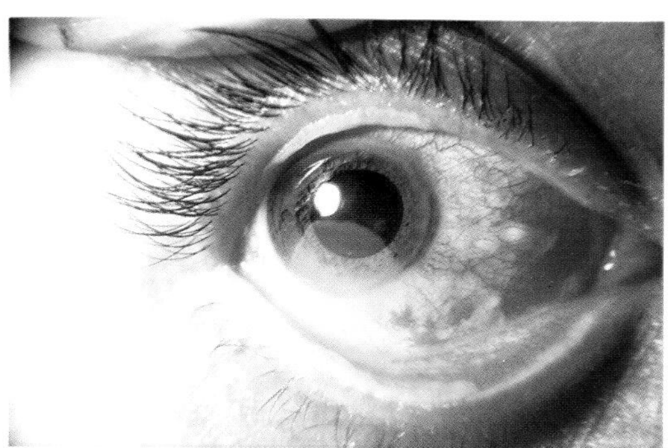
Figure 61.8

Figures 61.5–61.8 **(61.5)** Blood-staining of the cornea after hyphema. **(61.6)** Restriction of upgaze right eye after inferior orbital (blowout) fracture with incarceration of orbital tissue. **(61.7)** Orbital tomogram displaying left orbital floor fracture. **(61.8)** Fluorescein staining of inferior corneal abrasion.

bleed. This may lead to refilling of the anterior chamber with blood, cessation of aqueous flow and glaucoma.

Initial evaluation of the child with hyphema should include a careful history and a high level of suspicion for possible intraocular foreign body. Visual acuity should be tested in both eyes and will often be reduced if there is a hyphema. As complete an examination of the eyes as can be performed should occur, with the exception of any technique that might place force on the eye. Often, an examination of the posterior pole of the damaged eye can be performed at the time of the initial evaluation and, should rebleed occur, this evaluation would then be very useful.

MANAGEMENT

A somewhat empiric management of hyphema has developed which is clinically successful in the vast majority of cases, the components of which may not have clearly proven efficacy. Our approach is to admit the child to the hospital at strict bed rest, except for bathroom privileges and meals.

Sedation is used if necessary to maintain these goals. The head of the bed is kept at 30° in an attempt to have blood settle inferiorly. In the younger child, both eyes may be patched. Atropine 1% drop is utilized 4 times a day for cycloplegia to provide comfort from ciliary spasm and to decrease inflammation. Prednisolone acetate 1% drops or Decadron ointment are used 1 to 4 times a day or even more frequently if inflammation in the eye is severe. The place of systemic steroids is as yet unsettled and contradictory reports have appeared recently in the literature. The child is examined daily at the bedside and in most cases, blood will clear within a few days from admission. Generally, children are permitted to go home on limited activity at the end of 5 days and are given a shield to wear at night for the first week or so. In the event of rebleed, hospitalization is prolonged.

It is vitally important that no child with suspected or proven hyphema be permitted to leave the emergency department without ophthalmologic consultation. Those children who are not treated appropriately run a risk of rebleed and eventual loss of the eye.

ORBITAL INJURIES

CLINICAL FINDINGS

Orbital fractures are not uncommon and are generally signaled by ecchymosis, lid swelling, proptosis of varying degrees and possible ophthalmoplegia from orbital hemorrhage. In addition, subcutaneous emphysema from sinus fracture and localized anesthesia above or below the orbit are frequently seen.

History of trauma should be sought; most orbital injuries are secondary to blunt trauma from a fist, brick, or other large object. Smaller objects generally damage the globe without involving the surrounding orbit.

Visual evaluation of the symmetry of the face can be very revealing, as can palpation of the orbital rim. Presence of subcutaneous emphysema is seen frequently as a result of ethmoid air cell fracture into the orbit. Fractures of the orbital roof may be associated with cerebrospinal fluid rhinorrhea and lateral wall fractures with transection of the optic nerve and profound loss of vision.

Complete ophthalmologic evaluation is performed, including acuity testing in both eyes and examination of the uninjured eye. Pupillary reactions and motility are tested as well as extraocular motility, and evidence is sought for scleral rupture and/or perforating injury of the eye. Classically, orbital floor fracture is associated with inability to elevate the eye, but this latter finding can often be seen simply from swelling within the orbit (Fig. 61.6). Thus it is unusual today for repair of orbital floor fractures to be performed as an emergency. In general, even with radiographic evidence of floor fracture, a period of 2 weeks is permitted to elapse for edema to resolve unless there is obvious enophthalmos or prolapse of orbital contents into the maxillary sinus.

Plain x-rays have a high diagnostic failure rate but, with tomography, floor fracture confirmation can be obtained in more than 90% of cases (Fig. 61.7). It is reasonable to delay the obtaining of tomograms until and if surgical intervention is planned. Thus, it is unlikely that they will be requested by emergency department personnel. Of the available plain film views, the Waters' view of the orbital floor is most useful.

The ophthalmologist will perform a forced duction test if indicated, involving topical anesthesia at the inferior limbus and traction on the eye in an attempt to elevate the eye. If forced ductions are limited, entrapment of orbital contents in a fracture is highly suspicious.

MANAGEMENT

The basic indication for repair of orbital floor fracture is prevention of subjective diplopia and cosmetically significant enophthalmos. If these goals are not relevant to the condition, surgical repair is rarely justified.

Medical management of fractures involves systemic antibiotics if paranasal sinuses are fractured, nasal antihistamine, and decongestant therapy. The major considerations are the ruling out of concomitant injuries to the globe and frontal fossae and caution with regard to repair of floor fractures.

CORNEAL ABRASIONS

Corneal abrasions probably represent the most common pediatric eye trauma. The cause of injury may range from fingernail scratch to thrown foreign body to contact lens overwear to child abuse.

CLINICAL FINDINGS

Soon after injury, irritation may be mild depending on degree of corneal abrasion. Photophobia may be minimal if present. Should a day or so be permitted to elapse, the lids may be profoundly swollen and diagnosis of preseptal orbital cellulitis may be made in error. Occasionally, the abraded area may be noted with tangential flashlight illumination, but fluorescein installation is much more diagnostic. The green color is thought to be secondary to access of the fluorescein to subepithelial corneal tissues which carry a more acidic pH than the tear film (Fig. 61.8). Carefully inspect the upper and lower lids for a retained foreign body which may have caused the abrasion. Caution must always be exercised that a simultaneous perforation injury is not also present.

MANAGEMENT

Once the diagnosis is made, therapy consists of protecting the abraded area from the constant lid up-and-down action so that reepithelialization by sliding and by mitosis of epithelial cells may occur. This may be accomplished by providing antibiotic ointment such as sulfa or bacitracin, or by a semipressure patch. The latter must be placed with strict care to allow for immobilization of the lids but no undo pressure placed on the globe. It is much easier and just as effective in the case of smaller abrasions to instill ointment four times a day and permit healing to occur under protection of the ointment. There is no evidence that ointment inhibits reepitelialization, or that ointment is trapped under healed epithelium with cyst formation.

It is customary for relief of ciliary spasm and photophobia to also instill a cycloplegic. This may well be delegated to the ophthalmologist, or a drop of homatropine 2% or 5% placed in the eye. The duration of cycloplegic effect of homatropine is generally 24 hours and this would not represent an extreme hardship for an older child.

It is important that the eye be examined daily until healing has occurred. Occasionally, damage to the basement membrane which lies just under the epithelium will not permit firm adherence of the epithelial cells to cornea and a recurrent erosion will occur. This requires specialized ophthalmic care and prolonged treatment with ointments, patches, or soft contact lens. Most abrasions heal without sequelae.

CORNEAL FOREIGN BODIES

Foreign bodies in the cornea are also very common in the pediatric age group. These are often small particles of iron or other metallic material but may be vegetable matter, pieces of lead pencil or other objects. Occasionally, these can be irrigated with a gentle stream of saline or brushed off the cornea with a moist cotton swab. Local anesthetic with a drop of topical tetracaine or proparacaine (Ophthaine) is appropriate before attempting removal but this should never be prescribed on a continued basis, as serious corneal injury can occur from prolonged use.

Should simple methods not be successful, then removal by an ophthalmologist using slitlamp magnification is appropriate. Using a spud or small knife, the foreign body is carefully removed. Occasionally, a small child will require general anesthesia or restraint for complete removal. Iron foreign bodies tend to form rust rings which should also be removed to aid corneal epithelial healing.

It is customary after removal of a foreign body to treat with cycloplegic agents such as homatropine 5% four times a day or atropine 1% twice a day and with the same care as a corneal abrasion until healing has occurred. Presence of multiple foreign bodies often requires general anesthesia and detailed compulsive removal, especially if they lie in the visual axis. The possibility of a perforating foreign body should be considered by all initially treating physicians so that these will not be overlooked. X-ray search for a perforating foreign body may be appropriate. Of course, as in all ophthalmic injuries, visual acuity in each eye and a complete examination of the eyes is required.

A disastrous error occurs when a prolapsed iris laying on the surface of the cornea is thought to represent a foreign body (Fig. 61.1). Should the tear-shaped pupil with the point of the tear directed toward the corneal laceration not be appreciated, then manipulation of the prolapsed iris will only cause further deformation of the globe and possible expulsion of intraocular contents. When in doubt, place a shield over the eye and obtain an ophthalmologist's opinion as soon as possible.

TRAUMATIC IRITIS

Traumatic iritis is commonly seen with any of the above examples of ophthalmic trauma. In addition, it may be the only manifestation of trauma.

History is significant for the incident of trauma and following this, photophobia, tearing and redness of the eye are often noted.

CLINICAL FINDINGS

On examination, there may be mild lid swelling and tearing, and the child tends to avoid examination with a light. Because of the spasm of all muscles within the eye and the naturally stronger sphincter of the iris, miosis is often seen. If sphincter rupture has occurred secondary to trauma, however, pupillary dilatation may result. It is difficult to appreciate the inflammation within the eye unless it has settled in the form of hypopyon in the inferior chamber angle. Slitlamp examination is necessary to note the small inflammatory cells and protein manifesting as flare in the slitlamp beam. Careful examination for other ophthalmic trauma such as iridodialysis, subluxation of the lens, and vitreous in the anterior chamber must be noted. In addition, fundus examination should be meticulous, as retinal damage may also be present.

MANAGEMENT

Once perforating injury of the eye and/or intraocular foreign bodies have been ruled out, the mainstays of therapy are cycloplegia and anti-inflammatory agent treatment. In the younger child, atropine drops or ointment, either 0.5% or 1%, 2 to 4 times a day, are useful. In the older child, homatropine or scopolamine may interfere less with daily function. Topical anti-inflammatory agents such as 1% prednisolone acetate drops (Pred Forte) used hourly while awake to twice a day depending on severity of inflammatory response are indicated. An effort is made to decrease frequency of steroids and cycloplegia as soon as inflammation quiets. This is done to minimize side effects of topical steroids, which may include glaucoma and/or cataracts.

Traumatic iritis may always be treated successfully with medical means, but its primary importance as a sign of significant ophthalmic trauma should serve to alert one that more severe underlying damage may be present. All patients with traumatic iritis should be seen by an ophthalmologist as soon as possible for continued management of the iritis as well as its occasional long term complications, such as glaucoma.

SUBCONJUNCTIVAL HEMORRHAGE

Subconjunctival hemorrhages are frequently seen, either spontaneously or in association with blood clotting difficulties (Fig. 61.9). They seem to occur commonly after direct trauma, after prolonged periods of nose-blowing with upper respiratory infection, or after forceful vomiting. They probably represent rupture of the small subconjunctival vessels and appear more ominous than they are.

Unless suspicion exists that the child has a bleeding tendency, no further workup is indicated. After complete ophthalmic examination, reassurance may be given that these always clear within 2 to 3 weeks without sequelae. The larger ones, however, may rarely harbor an occult scleral rupture or avulsion of an extraocular muscle (Fig. 61.10).

True conjunctival hemorrhages are quite rare and present after perforating injuries of the conjunctiva.

LID LACERATIONS

Other than superficial linear injuries involving only the skin of the lid, definitive therapy of the lacerations of the lid requires the skill of an ophthalmologist; however, the emergency department physician should be aware of certain principles of management and diagnosis. Once again, the presence of lid lacerations should alert the emergency department personnel to the possibility of damage to the globe and other adnexal structures.

CLINICAL MANIFESTATION

In most cases, meticulous reapposition of the margins of laceration are sufficient for good cosmetic effect and lid function. There are occasions, however, where large parts of the lid have been avulsed and more definitive plastic surgical procedures are required. Primary attention must be directed to the possibility of damage to the lacrimal drainage tracts, specifically the canaliculi and/or lacrimal sac structures (Fig. 61.11). The physician should be aware that injuries to the medial one third of the lid very often involve these structures, and if both upper and lower systems are involved, the child may require lacrimal drainage surgery, either a dacriocystorhinostomy or a conjunctivodacriocystorhinostomy.

MANAGEMENT

The repair of lid lacerations is emergent but can rationally await the next day's operating schedule if this is more convenient. Some ophthalmologists believe that there is some benefit to a brief delay during which lid swelling decreases, allowing for easier anatomic reapposition.

Upper lid injuries may perforate to the level of the levater aponeurosis, which lies deep to the orbital septum. If orbital fat protrudes on the skin, this possibility is more likely. Ptosis will result if upper lid retractors are not repaired. As always, the possibility of occult globe damage should be forefront in one's mind.

THE BATTERED CHILD

Examination of the eye in the case of suspected child abuse can be very rewarding toward making the appropriate diagnosis. The finding of any of the above evidences of trauma to the eye or adnexal structures strengthens the case. In addition, there are certain findings that are never seen in the eye except after trauma. Many require expert ophthalmological evaluation and the emergency department physician should not hesitate to seek such consultation (see Chapter 68).

Specific traumatic injuries include: choriodal rupture (Fig. 61.12), iridodialysis (Fig. 61.13), and avulsion of the vitreous base. Flame-shaped and blot hemorrhages in the fundus with white centers, so-called Roth spots (Fig. 61.14), are commonly seen in the pediatric population after blunt trauma to the eye. In addition, Purtscher's retinopathy, appearing as profound posterior pole linear retinal hemorrhages with large exudates simulating central retinal vein occlusion, may be seen after crushing thoracic injuries or shaking injuries and may represent sudden increased central venous pressure.

ORBITAL CELLULITIS

The remainder of the chapter will discuss nontraumatic ophthalmic emergencies. The most significant of these is orbital cellulitis, as even in the era of antibiotic treatment orbital cellulitis represents a potentially lethal condition. The prognosis has certainly improved since the development of antibiotics. In the preantibiotic era approximately 20% of the patients with this disease died from meningitis or cavernous sinus thrombosis and another 20% developed blindness.

CLINICAL FINDINGS

The child often looks systemically ill and febrile. Presentation of orbital cellulitis involves all degrees of conjunctival injection, proptosis and lid swelling. A more benign form may be called preseptal cellulitis when involvement includes only the anterior structures of the lids.

Figure 61.9

Figure 61.10

Figure 61.11

Figure 61.12

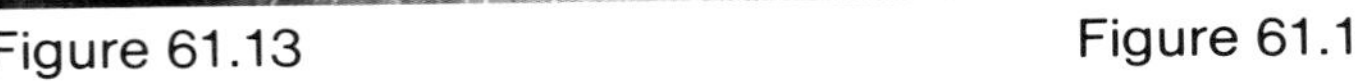

Figure 61.13

Figure 61.14

Figures 61.9–61.14 **(61.9)** Subconjunctival hemorrhage. **(61.10)** Larger subconjunctival hemorrhage, potentially masking scleral rupture or avulsion of extraocular muscle. **(61.11)** Medial upper lid laceration cutting lacrimal canaliculus. Note lacrimal punctum. **(61.12)** Choroidal rupture, circumferential to optic nerve. **(61.13)** Temporal iridodialysis. Note second "pupil" formed by traumatic dehiscence of iris from ciliary body. **(61.14)** Retinal "blot" hemorrhages, in characteristic form with white centers ("Roth" spots) as seen in battered children.

The majority of orbital cellulitis cases are secondary to inflammatory processes in the adjacent sinuses. This is particularly true of the ethmoid air cells, due to the thinness of the bone that separates the medial orbit from ethmoids. In addition, there is free flow of blood between the ethmoidal and ophthalmic veins. The history may include recent upper respiratory tract infection. X-rays will show severe sinusitis or clouding of the sinuses.

MANAGEMENT

The mainstay of treatment is intravenous antibiotic therapy, including agents that are effective against *Staphyloccocus aureus*, the group A *Streptococcus*, and *Haemophilus influenzae*. These are generally continued for 7 to 10 days. The reader is referred to Chapter 45, "Infectious Diseases," for details of management. Frequent examination is necessary to ascertain findings of cavernous sinus thrombosis, which may include pupillary dilatation, paralysis of extraocular muscles and proptosis.

Long-term disability is infrequent but minor abnormalities of extraocular muscle function and/or pupillary reactivity are common.

CONJUNCTIVITIS

The most common cause of red eye and the most common presenting complaint regarding the eye in an emergency department is conjunctivitis. It is helpful to consider conjunctivitis in the pediatric population as divided into ophthalmia neonatorum and conjunctivitis in the older child.

Ophthalmia Neonatorum

In an era in which newborns are discharged from the hospital within a few days of birth, ophthalmia neonatorum has become an outpatient disease. It is unlikely that silver nitrate irritation will present to the pediatrician in the emergency department since it usually occurs in the first 48 hours of life, but this form of chemical conjunctivitis should be considered. The primary concern is to rule out the potentially devastating *Neisseria gonorrhoeae* conjunctivitis.

Neisseria

CLINICAL MANIFESTATION

These children present within the first week of life with profound purulent bilateral discharge and lid swelling. The conjunctivae are red, and the cornea may or may not be clear.

MANAGEMENT

N. gonorrhoeae is one of the few organisms that can penetrate an intact corneal epithelium and lead to perforation of the cornea within a very short period of time. Thus, any purulent conjunctivitis in a child less than 1 month of age should be immediately cultured and smeared for Gram stain to look for the presence of intracellular gram-negative diplococci. A Giemsa stain should also be obtained to help confirm the diagnosis of inclusion conjunctivitis which may also present as a purulent conjunctivitis in this age group.

Should the diagnosis of gonococcal conjunctivitis be strongly entertained or confirmed, the child should be admitted to the hospital and treated with aqueous penicillin, 100,000 units/kg/day, and topical antibiotics as well. Topical antibiotics are much less important than systemic and may consist of fortified aqueous penicillin drops, chloramphenicol drops, or bacitracin ointment. For medicolegal purposes it is unwise to discuss the potential diagnosis with the family unless and until culture and typing of the organism is confirmatory.

Chlamydia

The agent of *inclusion conjunctivitis* is a chlamydial organism which is an obligate intracellular parasite.

CLINICAL MANIFESTATIONS

This conjunctivitis classically presents within 5 to 10 days but may occur as late as 3 months after birth as a purulent conjunctivitis, often bilateral and symmetric. No follicles are noted on the conjunctival surface as newborns do not have the ability to form lymphoid follicles in the conjunctivae.

MANAGEMENT

Diagnosis is made by finding intracytoplasmic inclusions on Giemsa stain or

Wright stain of conjunctival scrapings taken with a blunt spatula. The more epithelial cells that are included in this scraping, the better the possibility of obtaining a positive specimen. The disease is usually self-limited and spontaneous resolution will occur without treatment. There are cases, however, where corneal scarring has resulted leading to decreased vision, and for this reason and because of parental concern children are treated with topical antibiotics for this condition. Sulfonamide, erythromycin or tetracycline ointment are the antibiotics of choice; despite its reputation for causing dental problems in the older child there has never been a reported case of tetracycline ophthalmic ointment causing dental difficulties.

The use of systemic antibiotics for inclusion conjunctivitis is unsettled, despite occasional reports of pneumonitis and other systemic difficulties from this chlamydial organism. Most pediatricians do not presently feel that systemic antibiotics are routinely indicated. If a conjunctivitis fails to improve with topical therapy, oral erythromycin 40 mg/kg/day should be used in addition to topical therapy.

Besides *N. gonorrhoeae* and inclusion conjunctivitis, other bacteria may cause a purulent conjunctivitis in the newborn. Most common of these is *Escherichia coli* although other pathogens are not unusual. It is uncommon for viral conjunctivitis to affect the newborn.

Conjunctivitis in the Older Child

CLINICAL PRESENTATION

In the preschool and early school years viral conjunctivitis is quite common. Often there is an antecedent history of upper respiratory infection, and preauricular and submandibular nodes may be palpated. Usually the initial complaint is that of an itchy, scratch sensation, rapidly progressing to watery discharge. The eyes may be stuck together upon awakening with ensuing swelling of the lids. Photophobia is variable and is dependent upon punctuate epithelial erosions secondary to virus infestation. The process is often bilateral but may be unilateral.

Most ophthalmologists do not believe that routine cultures are necessary for management of viral conjunctivitis if the history and examination is consistent with that diagnosis. It is important, however, to maintain follow-up to be certain that resolution is occurring. The course of viral conjunctivitis involves redness, irritation and photophobia for seven to ten days.

Differential diagnosis includes uveitis, allergic conjunctivitis, and bacterial conjunctivitis. Bacterial conjunctivitis generally presents with a purulent discharge in the older age group, although in the immunocompromised host this may not be evident.

MANAGEMENT

Once the diagnosis has been made, treatment of both bacterial and viral conjunctivitis is supportive. Antibacterial drops or ointment is prescribed for bacterial conjunctivitis based on results of Gram stain and/or culture, and measures are recommended for the patient's comfort. Cold compresses frequently during the day may aid and comfort, and a prescription of an antihistamine-decongestant drop such as Vasocon-A or Naphcon-A is often helpful. Topical steroids and/or anesthetic drops should not be prescribed for conjunctivitis as the risk of damage far outweighs their potential benefits.

GLAUCOMA

Children's glaucoma is rarely seen in an emergency department. When it is, it presents with a red, teary, photophobic eye. The differential diagnosis includes uveitis and conjunctivitis, and the diagnosis is made by the finding of increased intraocular pressure. Therefore, except in rare circumstances, an ophthalmologist's assistance will be necessary.

CLINICAL FINDINGS

The emergency department physician should suspect glaucoma in a child with a history of past trauma, prematurity with retinopathy of prematurity (retrolental fibroplasia, RLF), Marfan's syndrome, or any systemic condition known to be associated with inflammation in the eyes such as juvenile rheumatoid arthritis. The etiologies are varied in these conditions but all represent difficulties in outflow of aqueous from the eye. Examination will disclose a diffusely red, tearing, tender eye. The cornea may be cloudy and microcyst formation may be noted on the corneal surface. Hand light or slitlamp examination may disclose a shallow or nonexistent anterior chamber with iris close to or against the back surface of the cornea. Visual acuity testing should be attempted in each eye and the noninvolved eye examined to the best of one's ability, searching for early evidence of a similar process and therefore a clue to the diagnosis. An enlarged cornea may represent long-standing elevated intraocular pressure in a child under 3 or 4 years of age. Palpation with gentle tactile pressure may disclose a rock-hard eye and solidify the diagnosis of glaucoma.

NONTRAUMATIC UVEITIS

Most children with uveitis presenting to the emergency department will have a traumatic etiology for uveitis, but occasionally a child with sarcoid or known juvenile rheumatoid arthritis will present with this complication. Rarely a child with retinoblastoma will present in this manner. The eye will be red with photophobia and tearing. Closer inspection will disclose a circumlimbal flush. The physician skilled in the use of the slitlamp microscope will see inflammatory cells floating in the anterior chamber and aqueous flare reflecting increased protein content of the aqueous humor. Inflammatory cells may settle on the back surface of the cornea forming keratic precipitates.

Any child with suspected nontraumatic uveitis should be referred immediately to an ophthalmologist for diagnosis and therapy, the mainstays of which are cycloplegia and anti-inflammatory medication as outlined in the section on traumatic iritis.

HORDEOLUM AND CHALAZION

These two conditions are seen frequently by the emergency department physician and represent localized lid inflammations.

CLINICAL MANIFESTATION

The chalazion is a primarily noninfectious inflammation of the meibomian glands in either the upper or lower tarsal plate of the lid. The lipid secretion from the glands creates in some individuals an inflammatory reaction which may then become superinfected with bacteria. These present as nodules ranging in size from very small to quite large in upper and lower lid. Hordeolum represents an infection of either the Meibomian or other lid glands with, most commonly, *S. aureus* or a nonhemolytic *Streptococcus*. These lesions tend to be more inflamed than the chalazion and more diffuse.

MANAGEMENT

Treatment is conservative with warm compresses for 15 min 4 times a day and topical antibiotic, either sulfonamide drops or ointment. Most will resolve in 7 to 10 days, but some may need to be surgically excised if resolution does not occur. Individuals with a tendency toward chalazion formation will have recurrent episodes. Should either hordeolum or chalazion persist beyond 7 to 10 days, consultation of an ophthalmologist is indicated.

References

Birch-Hirshfeld, cited by Duke-Elder S: The ocular adnexa. In *Textbook of Ophthalmology*, Vol 5, pp. 5420–5423. C.V. Mosby, St. Louis, 1950.

Blanton FM: Anterior chamber angle recession and secondary glaucoma; a study of the after-effects of traumatic hyphema. *Arch Ophthalmol* 72: 39–43, 1964.

Brown SI, Tragakis MP, Pearce DB: Treatment of the alkali-burned cornea. *Am J Ophthalmol* 74: 316–320, 1972.

Brown SI, Weller CA: The pathogenesis and treatment of collagenase-induced diseases of the cornea. *Trans Am Acad Ophthalmol Otolaryngol* 74: 375–383, 1970.

Emery JM, von Noorden GK, Schlernitzauer DA: Orbital floor fractures: long-term follow-up of cases with and without surgical repair. *Trans Am Acad Ophthalmol Otolaryngol* 75: 802–812, 1972.

Escapini H: Trauma to the cornea. In *The Cornea: World Congress*, pp. 300–315, edited by JH Krug Jr, JW McTigue. Butterworth, London, 1965.

Fedukowicz, HB: *External Infections of the Eye*, pp. 38–44. Appleton-Century-Crofts, New York, 1963.

Forster RC: Ophthalmia neonatorum. In *Clinical Ophthalmology*, Vol 4, Ch. 6, pp. 1–9, edited by T Duane. Harper & Row, Hagerstown, Md., 1975.

Fueger GM, Milauskas AT, Britten W: The roentgenologic evaluation of orbital blow-out fractures. *AJR* 97: 614–617, 1966.

Harley RD: Ocular manifestations of child abuse. *J Pediatr Ophthalmol Strabismus* 17: 5–13, 1980.

Jarett WH, Gutman FA: Ocular complications of infections of the paranasal sinuses. *Arch Ophthalmol* 81: 683–686, 1969.

Khodadoust AA, Silverstein AM, Kenyon KR, Dowling JE: Adhesion of regenerating corneal epithelium; the tole of basement membrane. *Am J Ophthalmol* 65: 339–348, 1968.

Lemp MA: Annual review—corneal and sclera. *Arch Ophthalmol* 35: 1077–1088, 1962.

Lippas J: Continuous irrigation in the treatment of external ocular diseases. *Am J Ophthalmol* 57: 298–305, 1964.

Locatcher-Khorazo D, Seegal BC: *Microbiology of the Eye*, pp. 241–252. C. V. Mosby, St. Louis, 1972.

Paterson CA, Pfister RR, Levinson RA: Aqueous humor pH changes after experimental alkali burns. *Am J Ophthalmol* 79: 414–419, 1975.

Paton D, Goldberg MF: Management of ocular injuries. W. B. Saunders, Philadelphia, 1976.

Rakusin W: Traumatic hypehma. *Am J Ophthalmol* 74: 284–292, 1972.

Read J, Goldberg MF: Comparison of medical treatment of traumatic hyphema. *Trans Am Acad Ophthalmol Otolaryngol* 78: OP799–OP815, 1974.

Read J, Goldberg MF: Blunt ocular trauma and hyphema. *Int Ophthalmol Clin* 14: 57–95, 1974.

Tenzel RR: Trauma and burns. *Int Ophthalmol Clin* 10: 55–69, 1970.

Wilson LA: Bacterial conjunctivitis. In *Clinical Ophthalmology*, Vol. 4, Ch. 5, pp. 1-9, edited by T Duane. Harper & Row, Hagerstown, Md., 1975.

Yasuna E: Management of traumatic hyphemas. *Arch Ophthalmol* 91: 190–191, 1974.

CHAPTER **62**

Otorhinolaryngology Emergencies

WILLIAM P. POTSIC, M.D., AND STEVEN D. HANDLER, M.D.

INTRODUCTION

The ear, nose, and throat are common sites for infection and trauma and the sources of acute pain. This makes the head and neck region one with which the emergency medicine specialists must be familiar as they will be called upon to evaluate it frequently. Although the presenting complaints may seem extremely distressing to the patient and cause considerable anxiety for his parents, the diseases prompting the visit are rarely life threatening. This chapter will include disorders of ear, nose, nasal sinuses, oral cavity, pharynx, esophagus, larynx, trachea, and neck.

EAR

Methods of Examination

Every emergency department should have an otoscope with good illumination, wax loops, illuminated head light and otologic forceps.

Examination of the ear begins by inspection of the auricle and surrounding areas. The external meatus should be visualized directly with a bright light after it is fully opened by pulling the pinna posteriorly and superiorly. The tragus may be displaced forward by traction on the skin in front of the ear with the examiner's other hand. The ear canal can then be examined with a pneumatic otoscope using the largest speculum that will fit in the meatus painlessly. Wax or debris occluding the ear canal should be removed with a curette or by repeated irrigation with body temperature water (see procedure in Section VII). Irrigation of the canal should not be done if a perforation of the tympanic membrane (TM) is suspected.

The TM should be evaluated for its appearance but the examination should not stop there. Part of the middle ear contents can often be seen through a translucent eardrum. Mobility should be assessed with the pneumatic otoscope. Pneumatic otoscopy is performed by applying positive and negative pressure to the TM with the pneumatic otoscope fitted tightly into the ear canal. The ear pressure can be varied by squeezing a rubber bulb or blowing through a tubing connected to the otoscope head (see procedure in Section VII).

Crude hearing acuity can be tested with a ticking watch or a 512 Hz tuning fork. The sound should be heard equally in each ear. However, this does not rule out a bilateral equal hearing deficit. If the tuning fork is applied to the forehead, it should be heard equally in both ears. If it is then heard only in one ear, it signifies either a conductive loss in the ear that hears the tone or a sensorineural loss in the opposite ear. Audiometry is required for accurate definition of hearing.

Infection

Acute Purulent Otitis Media

Acute purulent otitis media (APOM) is one of the most common head and neck infection in children. It may occur as an isolated infection or as a complication of an upper respiratory infection. Secretory otitis media (SOM) (noninfected fluid in the middle ear) and immune deficiency states predispose children to recurrent acute otitis media.

The most common organisms causing acute otitis at all ages are *Streptococcus pneumoniae*, *Haemophilus influenzae* and less frequently, Group A β-hemolytic *Streptococcus*. Gram-negative organisms may occur in patients who are under 8 weeks of age or immune suppressed.

CLINICAL MANIFESTATIONS

APOM should be suspected in any child who is irritable or lethargic. The pain develops rapidly and is severe. Spontaneous perforation of the TM with serosanguineous drainage may occur in less than hour after the onset of pain. APOM is easily diagnosed by pneumatic otoscopy. The TM is hyperemic and there is decreased mobility. As the drum becomes more edematous, the landmarks may become unrecognizable. Infection with *Mycoplasma pneumoniae and other bacteria cause* blebs on the lateral surface of the drum. The vesicles of bullous myringitis are filled with clear fluid and are very painful. The appearance of the TM in APOM does not differ significantly from viral acute otitis media.

Complications of Acute Otitis Media

The complications of APOM may also be encountered in the emergency department. The purulent exudate that fills the middle ear space causes a conductive hearing loss. The congealed exudate may organize and stimulate hyalinization and calcification leading to tympanosclerosis (white patches in the TM).

Spontaneous perforation of the TM usually produces a small hole that heals rapidly; however, large perforations may occur that do not heal after the infection has cleared. Ossicular necrosis may also occur, causing a persistent conductive loss. As the TM heals following a perforation, skin from its lateral surface may be trapped in the middle ear forming a cyst (cholesteatoma) that expands and destroys the structures of the middle ear and surrounding bone.

Facial nerve paralysis may occur suddenly during APOM. The nerve paralysis may be partial or complete when the child is first examined. The facial nerve usually recovers complete function if appropriate intravenous antibiotic therapy is administered and a wide myringotomy for drainage is carried out immediately.

APOM may cause inflammation in the inner ear (serous labyrinthitis). This causes mild to moderate vertigo without a sensorineural hearing loss. Bacterial invasion of the inner ear (suppurative labyrinthitis) causes severe vertigo and sensorineural hearing loss.

Pus always fills the mastoid during APOM causing radiographic opacification, but acute suppurative mastoiditis (acute coalescent mastoid osteomyelitis) may develop, causing destruction of the mastoid air cell system. As the infection spreads to the postauricular tissues, the swelling that occurs displaces the auricle laterally and downward from its normal position. The pus may extend through air cells to the medial portion of the temporal bone causing third cranial nerve paralysis, deep retroorbital pain and otorrhea (Gradenigo's syndrome). Pus may also break through the mastoid tip and extend into the neck (Bezold abscess).

The most common intracranial complication of otitis media is meningitis, which may be associated with severe sensorineural deafness and irreversible vestibular damage. Less commonly associated complications are cerebritis, epidural abscess, brain abscess, lateral sinus thrombosis, and otitic hydrocephalus. Overt or impending intracranial complications should immediately be evaluated by a neurologist and a computed tomogram (CT) should be obtained.

MANAGEMENT

The treatment of uncomplicated APOM is oral antibiotic therapy with amoxicillin 25 to 50 mg/kg per 24 hours in 3 divided doses for 10 days. Systemic or local antihistamine-decongestant preparations are of no proven value. Patients with complicated APOM should also be treated with a wide inferior myringotomy for drainage. The incision should extend from the anterior inferior quadrant to the posterior inferior quadrant (see procedures in Section VII) Tympanocentesis (see procedures in Section VII) should be performed for Gram stain and culture in neonates, immune suppressed patients, and in cases where antibiotic therapy is not affecting resolution of the infection. Patients treated on an emergency basis for APOM should be referred for follow-up examination 2 weeks after therapy is started.

Patients with suspected or identified complications of APOM should be referred to an otolaryngologist.

External Otitis

External otitis usually follows swimming and is often referred to as "swimmers ear." Ear canal trauma or foreign bodies may also contribute to the development of external otitis.

Otitis externa may be localized or diffuse. Localized external otitis is caused by an abscessed hair follicle in the outer ⅔ of the ear canal. These abscesses are caused by *Staphylococcus aureus*.

Diffuse external otitis is caused by *Pseudomonas aeruginosa*, *Staphylococcus*, fungi or a mixture of gram-negative and gram-positive organisms. Viral external otitis is usually caused by herpes simplex or herpes zoster.

CLINICAL MANIFESTATIONS

The diagnosis of external otitis is usually easily made by external inspection and otoscopy. Otoscopy may be painful and visualization of the eardrum may be impossible because of edema of the canal walls. External otitis usually begins with itching and fullness that progresses to a severe pain. The pain is worsened by chewing or touching the ear. The external canal is red, edematous, and narrowed. A foul smelling, purulent discharge is usually present. There may also be surrounding cellulitis and regional cervical adenitis may be present. Rarely, necrosis of surrounding tissue occurs (malignant external otitis). Malignant external otitis occurs in debilitated patients who have diabetes or are immune suppressed. It may cause extensive tissue necrosis and can be rapidly fatal if not treated immediately with antibiotics and surgical debridement.

MANAGEMENT

If the abscess in localized external otitis is about to drain spontaneously, it should be opened at the tip with an 18 gauge needle, or an 11 scalpel blade. Drainage results in immediate relief of pain. Antibiotic therapy with erythromycin, dicloxacillin, or cephalosporin should be administered for 10 days. The treatment of diffuse external otitis is to use antibiotic ear drops containing neomycin, polymyxin, and hydrocortisone, 4 drops 3 times daily, in the affected ear for 10 days. Before the drops are started, the pus and debris should be cleaned from the ear canal with gentle suction, a curette, or cotton-tipped applicators. If the meatus is nearly swollen closed, a wick of gauze soaked in antibiotic ear drops should be gently advanced into the ear canal with a forceps (Fig. 62.1). It should be left in place for 24 to 48 hours while the infection is being treated with antibiotic ear drops that also contain a topical steroid to decrease edema and inflammation. Systemic broad spectrum antibiotics should be used if cellulitis or regional cervical adenitis is present. No water should be permitted to enter the ear canal during the 10 days of therapy.

Chronic Otitis Media

Chronic otitis media is persistent perforation of the tympanic membrane acquired or iatrogenic (by tympanostomy tube) with or without active infection. When infection is present the organism is usually *P. aeruginosa* or *S. aureus*, and it causes a profuse foul smelling discharge. Any acquired perforation may be associated with a cholesteatoma (white skin-lined cyst) that destroys the structures of the ear as it expands.

CLINICAL MANIFESTATIONS

Chronic otitis media is easily diagnosed by otoscopy. A perforation of the eardrum is easily seen and the white pearly, flaky

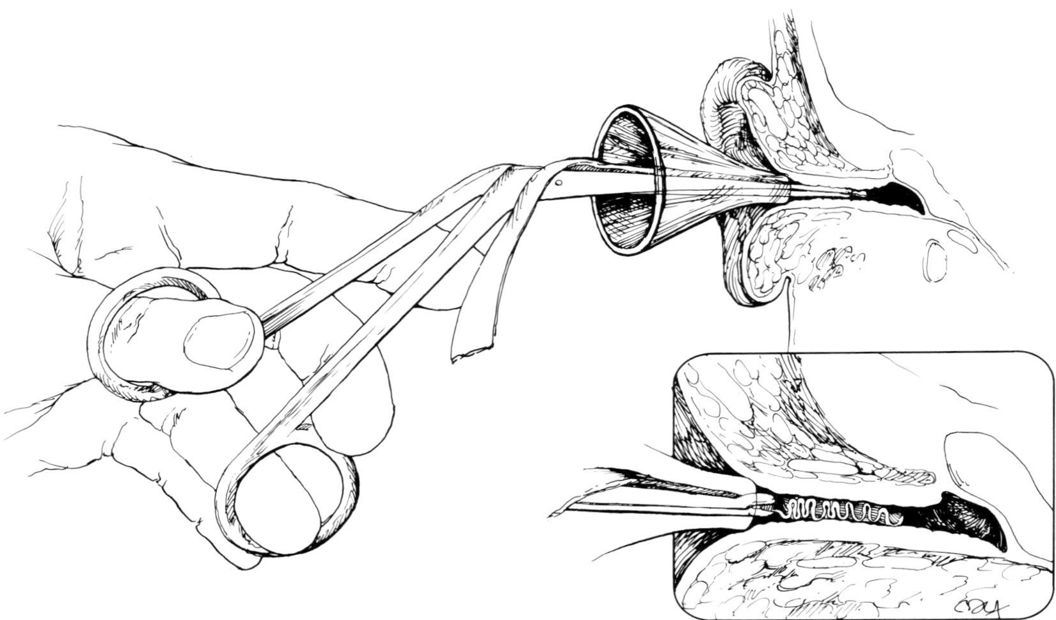

Figure 62.1 Gauze wick (¼'' × 1½'') being placed in ear canal to facilitate topical treatment of otitis externa.

debris from a cholesteatoma may also be present.

MANAGEMENT

Systemic antibiotics are of limited value unless there is regional cellulitis or cervical adenitis. When used, amoxicillin 25 to 50 mg/kg per 24 hours in 3 divided doses, should be administered for 10 days.

The perforation and cholesteatoma will require surgical correction.

The complications of chronic otitis media with infection are the same as those that occur in acute otitis media including intracranial spread of the infectious process. In addition, with repeated infection a progressive sensorineural hearing loss is likely to develop.

Infection of the Pinna

The pinna may become infected in a fashion similar to skin surfaces anywhere else on the body (refer to "Infectious Disease," Chapter 45). Preauricular sinuses may occasionally be infected with *S. aureus* and should be treated with antistaphylococcal penicillin or cepholasporin for 10 days. If an abscess forms, it should be drained surgically.

Foreign Bodies

Foreign bodies in the ear canal are common in children. Solid objects such as stones, beads or paper are the most frequently encountered, but live insects may also enter the ear canal. Foreign bodies should be removed as soon as possible and as safely as possible. Most objects can be gently rolled out of the external meatus with an ear curette or grasped and removed with an otologic forceps (see procedure in Section VII). However round or occluding objects may be removed by irrigation of the canal with room temperature water. The stream is directed along the side of the foreign body bringing it to the external meatus (see procedure in Section VII). Insects should be killed with alcohol or drowned in mineral oil before they are removed from the ear canal by the techniques already described. Objects resting against the TM are best removed by irrigation to avoid injury by manipulation.

Care must be taken to remove the foreign material without causing pain, because if the removal is unsuccessful, a general anesthetic will almost certainly be necessary for removal by the otolaryngologist.

Trauma

External Trauma

External ear trauma is common in children. External blunt trauma is caused by an athletic injury, from a fall, or from a direct blow to the ear. Blunt trauma to the ear may result in simple ecchymosis or may disrupt perichrondrial blood vessels with subsequent hematoma or seroma formation. These collections form a smooth bluish colored mass on the lateral surface of the ear that obscures the normal contour. Hematomas and seromas must be evacuated immediately to prevent cartilage necrosis (see procedure in Section VII). Lacerations of the pinna should be closed using the same surgical principles applied to repairing lacerations in other areas of the body. Earrings in pierced ears may be torn from the lobule. These lacerations should be closed like all skin lacerations, reestablishing the normal anatomy.

Thermal injury of the external ear occurs frequently because the ear protrudes from the head and is exposed to burns and cold. Burns of the ear should be treated in the same fashion as burns in other parts of the body. Frostbite is suspected when the ear is pale and painful on warming. The frostbitten ear should be rewarmed rapidly by applying warm soaked cotton pledgets at 38 to 40°C; the ear should be completely thawed and never recooled.

Middle Ear Trauma

A slap to the head may result in perforation of the TM but traumatic perforation of the drum is usually caused by poking an object in the ear canal. The structures of the middle ear may also be damaged by the penetrating object. The ossicles may be fractured and a perilymph fistula may develop in the footplate of the stapes. This causes immediate vertigo and a sensorineural hearing loss. The facial nerve may be injured and cause facial paralysis. Traumatic perforations of the tympanic membrane must be examined microscopically to be certain that the edges of the perforation do not fold into the middle ear. If they do, skin may grow into the middle ear and a cholesteatoma will develop. Clean perforations with margins that do not fold into the middle ear usually heal spontaneously in 2 to 3 weeks. Systemic antibiotics are not necessary, unless the ear was contaminated by the injury. Traumatic perforations associated with vertigo, sensorineural hearing loss or facial nerve paralysis require urgent exploration of the middle ear by an otolaryngologist.

Sudden Hearing Loss

Sudden hearing loss is not a common complaint in the emergency department, but it requires prompt attention if it is determined to be a sensorineural loss. Sudden conductive losses almost never occur without a known antecedent event such as head trauma, infection or wax occlusion of the ear canal. History and otoscopy can usually establish the cause of the conductive hearing loss. However the etiology of sudden hearing loss is more deceptive when the history is unrevealing and otoscopy is normal. Tuning fork testing will help to confirm the presence of a sensorineural hearing loss.

Sudden hearing loss that occurs following an airplane trip, scuba diving, straining or head trauma is highly suggestive of a perilymph fistula. These fistulas leak perilymph from around the oval window or round window. They cause a fluctuating sensorineural loss and require surgical exploration of the middle ear for repair.

Sudden sensorineural deafness may occur without a history suggestive of a fistula and without otoscopic abnormalities. This is often caused by viral infection of the cochlear labyrinth. Measles and mumps are notorious although now infrequent causes of sudden sensorineural deafness. Other viruses may injure the cochlea as well. There may be no systemic symptoms or signs of viral infection. These patients may have partial or complete recovery of hearing over a several week period. Initial therapy includes bed rest and aspirin to decrease platelet aggregation and to maintain patency of the cochlear blood vessels. Many other treatments have been proposed but are of uncertain efficacy.

Vertigo

Sudden vertigo is very disturbing and a child may be brought immediately to the emergency department because his parents think he is having a seizure. Vertigo may follow dysfunction of any part of the vestibular system from the labyrinth to the vestibular cortex.

Pressure and infection in the middle ear may cause vestibular dysfunction and inner ear inflammation (serous labyrinthitis) which produces either vague unsteadiness or vertigo. The child may present with serous otitis media, acute suppurative otitis media, or chronic otitis media. The conductive hearing loss and the dizziness resolve when the middle ear pressure is normalized or the inflammation subsides. If bacteria invade the inner ear (suppurative labyrinthitis), severe vertigo and a profound sensorineural hearing loss result. Measles and mumps may also infect the inner ear causing vertigo.

Chronic otitis media (perforation of the TM) may be associated with a cholesteatoma that has invaded the bony wall of the labyrinth. Pneumatic otoscopy will produce vertigo by transmitting the pressure directly to the inner ear.

Perilymph fistulas occur most often following barotrauma, blunt head trauma, or straining produce vertigo that fluctuates in severity. However, head trauma may also cause labyrinthine concussion or hemorrhage (hemorrhagic labyrinthitis) resulting in vertigo. Cerebral injuries involving the temporal lobe also can cause vertigo.

A common cause of sudden vertigo is vestibular neuronitis. The etiology is uncertain and the vertigo resolves spontaneously over several weeks. There are no accompanying signs or symptoms. The etiology of Ménière's disease (endolymphatic hydrops) is also unknown and is fortunately very rare in childhood. The symptoms are intermittent vertigo, tinnitus, and fluctuating hearing.

Other causes of sudden vertigo in children are benign paroxysmal vertigo of childhood and retrolabyrinthine lesions such as tumors, demyelinating diseases and temporal lobe seizures.

Vertigo is *only* a symptom of an underlying disease. Emergency treatment should consist of searching for the underlying disease as well as providing symptomatic relief. Vertigo is rarely associated with a life-threatening illness. Since sensorineural hearing loss usually accompanies serious causes of vertigo, its absence can provide some level of confidence that no life-threatening disease is present. See Chapter 16 for further discussion.

Neoplasms

Neoplasms of the external ear are as varied as the tissue types of the auricle and are not difficult to diagnose because they are so visible. Neoplasms of the middle and inner ear are rare but bear mentioning because they are so frequently missed until they are beyond treatment. External canal and middle ear tumors are most often brought to the physician's attention because of painful secondary infection that responds poorly to conventional treatment. The examiner may overlook a tumor, assuming that it is granulation tissue caused by an infection. If an ear infection does not respond appropriately to treatment or is associated with any abnormal tissue, a tumor should be suspected, and any abnormal tissue biopsied. Inner ear tumors are usually neurofibromas of the eighth nerve that cause progressive sensorineural hearing loss, increasing vertigo, and increasing fifth nerve anesthesia. These signs or symptoms should prompt suspicion that an acoustic neuroma is present.

Inner ear tumors are very deceptive in their early stages and are rarely detected until they cause either hearing loss, vertigo or focal neurologic signs.

NOSE AND PARANASAL SINUSES

Methods of Examination

The external nose and anterior portion of the nasal cavities can be examined by direct visual inspection. A nasal speculum and directed light source are necessary to permit good visualization of the anterior septum and inferior and middle turbinates. In younger children, the examiner's thumb can elevate the mobile nasal tip to allow adequate inspection of the anterior nasal structures. Vasoconstrictors such as 0.25% phenylephrine (2 or 3 drops) can be applied to the nose to shrink the mucosa and allow a more complete examination. The posterior nasal structures and nasopharynx can be seen with the aid of a nasopharyngeal mirror or a fiberoptic telescope placed in the nose or the posterior oropharynx (Fig. 62.5). Patency of the nasal cavities in the neonate can be assessed by the passage of small rubber catheters through the nose and into the pharynx. Palpation is also important in the evaluation of nasal and facial trauma. Tenderness to palpation over the sinuses is a common sign of acute sinusitis.

A careful examination of adjacent areas is important when evaluating sinus disease. Dental pathology must be detected in the search for a possible cause of a bacterial maxillary sinusitis. An examination of the orbit with assessment of visual acuity and ocular mobility should be performed to detect possible orbital complications of sinus disease.

Transillumination of the maxillary sinus can be performed by placing a small penlight in the patient's mouth and having him close his lips around it. In a dark room, the light should be transmitted equally through the maxillary sinuses to both anterior cheeks. Inequality of the transmitted light indicates a difference in aeration of the sinus but this could be caused by fluid, a mass lesion or hypoplasia of one maxillary sinus. Because of the lack of specificity of this technique, radiographic techniques have largely replaced transillumination in the evaluation of sinus disease.

Radiographs are indispensible in evaluating diseases of the nose and sinuses. Plain films (sinus or facial series) are used to evaluate nasal and sinus trauma, or to detect the presence of a mass or fluid in a sinus. Polytomograms and CT scans are indicated for more precise and detailed evaluation of tumors or fractures of this area.

Infection

Infections of the nose and paranasal sinuses are most often a component of the common upper respiratory infection (URI). The symptom complex of fever, nasal congestion/rhinorrhea, and headache is most often caused by a viral agent. Physical examination will reveal swollen, often erythematous nasal turbinates. The rhinorrhea can be clear or white in color. Facial tenderness is usually absent. Viral rhinitis requires little more than supportive care with hydration, rest, antipyretics and oral antihistamines and/or decongestants. Topical decongestants are to be avoided because of their tendency to cause rebound congestion as their vasoconstricting effect on the nasal mucosa wears off.

Bacterial infection of the nose and paranasal sinuses is a more serious condition and requires a careful examination and prompt treatment. Bacterial sinusitis should be suspected when the nasal discharge is thick yellow to yellow-green. Tenderness over the face may indicate clinical involvement of one or more of the paranasal sinuses. While transillumination can be useful in detecting the presence of sinusitis, the diagnosis is usually confirmed radiographically. Gram stain of the material will reveal many polymorphonuclear leukocytes (PMN) and the causative organism. Since the most common organisms responsible for bacterial rhinosinusitis are *H. influenzae* and Group A *Streptococcus*, amoxicillin 25 to 50 mg/kg/day for 10 days is the treatment of choice.

Complications of acute sinusitis, such as orbital cellulitis, facial cellulitis/abscess or meningitis, require admission to the hospital for appropriate intravenous antimicrobial therapy and possible operative intervention. Otolaryngologic consultation should be obtained in the evaluation of these patients with complicated acute sinusitis; a surgical drainage is often needed.

One complication of chronic sinusitis, the sinus mucocele, can cause a child to present to the emergency department with acute symptoms. Mucoceles are expansile cystic lesions that occur secondary to a long-standing blockage of a sinus ostia. The lesion evolves over several months or even years, but the child will present with the sudden onset of signs and symptoms usually related to an acute infection of the mucocele. These include pain and swelling secondary to osteomyelitis of the frontal bone, inferior and lateral displacement of the globe with proptosis, limitation of ocular mobility, and chronic nasal/postnasal discharge. Radiographs (plain films and tomograms) are often needed to determine the presence and extent of a mucocele. The patient should be referred to the otolaryngology service for appropriate intravenous antimicrobial therapy and surgical drainage.

Any child presenting to the emergency department with a history of persistent (after what would appear to have been an adequate course of appropriate treatment) rhinosinusitis should have a careful search for predisposing causes. Foreign bodies, choanal atresia, neoplasms, septal deviation, dental disease, adenoid hypertrophy, allergic polyps or immune-deficiency states may all present with recurrent or persistent rhinosinusitis.

Trauma

Facial trauma occurs frequently in children as a result of play activities, contact sports and automobile accidents. The abundance of facial soft tissue and the soft nature of their bony facial skeleton make most of these injuries minor. Any child with facial trauma should be assessed for associated, possibly more serious, injuries to the cervical spine, central nervous system and chest (see Chapter 57, "Major Trauma").

Nasal Trauma

The nose, because of its prominent position on the face, is subject to frequent trauma and accounts for the majority of facial injuries in children. Trauma to the nose most often causes ecchymosis and edema of the overlying skin. However, a direct blow to the nose can fracture the nasal skeleton with resultant deviation and/or depression of the nasal bones and septum. The deformity should be readily apparent by clinical examination, but the postinjury edema may prevent its recognition for several days until the swelling has subsided (Fig. 62.2). A step-off or bony irregularity may often be detected in these patients. Radiographs of the nose may demonstrate these fractures but are of little help in the management of the child. Epistaxis commonly accompanies nasal trauma but has usually stopped by the time the child reaches the emergency room. Persistent or severe bleeding may require local pressure, topical vasoconstrictors or nasal packing (see under "Epistaxis"). The presence of any associated ocular injury such as hyphema or retinal detachment must be detected and ophthalmologic consultation obtained.

In assessing the nasal injury, the emergency department physician must determine the nature and extent of trauma to the overlying skin, the nasal skeleton, and the nasal septum. Otolaryngologic consultation should be obtained in all but the most straightforward (i.e. no deviation,

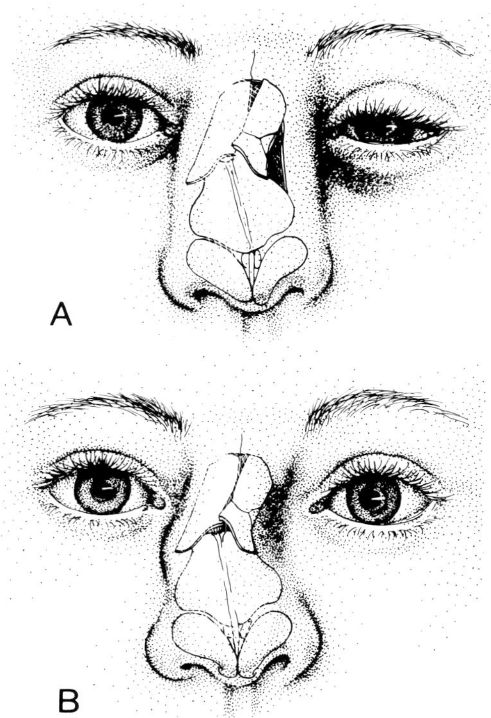

Figure 62.2. (*A*) Postinjury edema may mask underlying nasal bone deformity. (*B*) Nasal deformity becomes manifest as edema subsides.

minimal swelling, no septal hematoma) cases. The amount of nasal deviation and/or depression should be noted. Since this can be masked by the postinjury edema, it may be necessary to see the child again in 3 to 4 days when the swelling has subsided to allow an accurate determination of nasal deviation and/or depression.

The presence of a septal hematoma must be recognized as soon as possible after the injury. A septal hematoma will appear as a bulging of the nasal septum into the nasal cavity. Accumulation of blood between the septal cartilage and its overlying mucoperichondrium will deprive the cartilage of its blood supply. Otolaryngologic consultation should be obtained if a septal hematoma is suspected. The hematoma is drained as soon as possible and the mucoperichondrium packed back against the septal cartilage to restore its blood supply (see procedure in Section VII). If the hematoma is left for any length of time, septal abscess and cartilage destruction will occur. A saddle nose deformity is the result of an improperly treated septal hematoma.

If there is no septal hematoma or associated ocular or intracranial injuries, the deviated nose and septum can be reduced by the otolaryngologist when the swelling has subsided enough to permit an accurate evaluation of the nasal deformity. If more than 7 days elapse between the time of injury and the attempt at reduction, the fracture fragments will begin to form a strong fibrous union in their deviated positions making reduction difficult. Antimicrobials (usually amoxicillin 25 to 50 mg/kg/day for 7 days) are generally administered to these patients to prevent complications from occurring in what is almost always a compound fracture (i.e. open into the nasal cavity).

A clear, watery rhinorrhea occurring after nasal trauma may be cerebrospinal fluid (CSF) which would indicate a skull fracture, usually through the cribriform plate. If the patient leans forward allowing the nasal drainage to drip onto a piece of paper, a characteristic target pattern will often appear with a blood stain in the center of the drop and a clear halo of CSF around it. CSF is high in glucose and this can be detected with the use of a glucoseoxidase test paper (used in urinalysis). Care must be taken in interpreting these tests, however, because normal nasal mucus can look like CSF and the oxidizing substances present in nasal and lacrimal secretions may give a false positive reaction. If CSF rhinorrhea is suspected by history or clinical examination, the child should be admitted and placed at bed rest with his head elevated in an attempt to decrease the leak. Further diagnostic studies such as tomograms, CT scans and isotope scans can be performed to confirm the diagnosis of CSF leak. Antimicrobials are generally administered to prevent the occurrence of meningitis.

Sinus Trauma

Fractures of the paranasal sinuses may occur as isolated injuries or in association with trauma to the nose and orbital structures. Fractures of the ethmoid sinus or anterior wall of the maxillary sinus usually occur as a result of blunt trauma to the nose or cheek, respectively. The otolaryngologist should assist the emergency department physician in evaluating these injuries. Subcutaneous crepitation may be felt in the cheek or around the eye. Radiographs may demonstrate air in the cheek or orbit, or air-fluid levels. After determining the absence of associated ocular injury, the patient is usually placed on oral antimicrobials (usually amoxicillin 25 to 50 mg/kg/day for 7 days) and observed as an outpatient until the crepitation resolves.

Facial Trauma

Blunt trauma to the orbit may result in the force being transmitted through the globe to break the orbital floor (roof of maxillary sinus) or the medial orbital wall (lamina papyracea of the ethmoid sinus). These "*blowout*" fractures are discussed in detail in Chapter 61, "Ophthalmic Emergencies."

Fractures of the malar bone can occur, affecting the orbital floor and the maxillary sinus. A complete *malar* (incorrectly called "trimalar" or "tripod") *fracture* is present when the malar bone fractures at the infraorbital rim, zygomatic arch and frontozygomatic suture (Fig. 62.3). Isolated malar fractures can also occur at the zygomatic arch or the lateral wall of the maxillary sinus. Significant swelling and ecchymosis usually occur over the involved cheek and eye. Hypesthesia of the cheek is often present secondary to trauma to the infraorbital nerve at the orbital floor or rim. While facial asymmetry occurs as a result of inward displacement of the malar eminence, this may be masked by edema over the fracture area. A step-off may be palpated at the orbital rim and, occasionally, at the frontozygomatic suture area. Diplopia can be present as a result of entrapment of orbital contents if the fracture extends into the orbital floor. Radiographs are useful in detecting the fracture sites and the amount of displacement of the malar bone. Otolaryngologic consultation should be obtained to assist in the evaluation of these injuries.

More severe fractures of the midface can occur as a result of high velocity injuries, usually related to vehicular (automobile, bicycle) accidents. *LeFort fractures* comprise a group of midface fractures that present with a depressed midface, malocclusion, and can extend into the orbits and intracranial cavity. Mobility of the maxilla with stabilization of the forehead is pathognomonic of a LeFort fracture (see Fig. 64.9 in Chapter 64). Severe hemorrhage can accompany these fractures and may require nasal and/or pharyngeal packing. CSF rhinorrhea may occur as a result of fracture that extends through the cribriform plate. The patient with a LeFort fracture should be admitted to the hospital for care and observation. Multidisciplinary cooperation between otolaryngology, ophthalmology, plastic surgery, oral surgery, and neurosurgery is often mandatory for proper treatment of these patients. (See Chapter 64, "Plastic Surgical Emergencies," for more detail.) Tracheotomy may be indicated if the hemorrhage or edema of the facial structures compromises the airway and prolonged intubation is anticipated. Tracheotomy in children should be performed over an indwelling endotracheal tube and in the operating room.

Barotrauma

There is normally a direct open communication between the paranasal sinuses and the nasal cavities that permits prompt

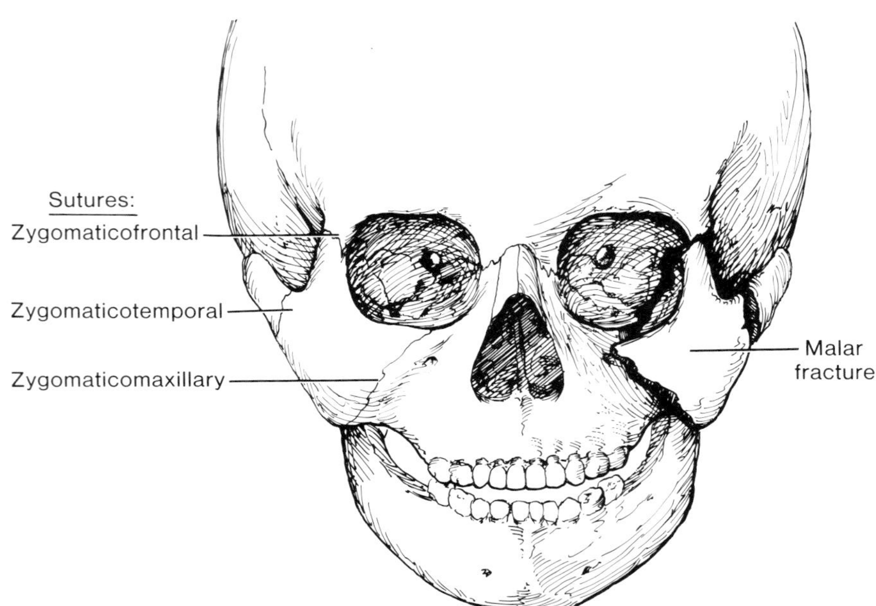

Figure 62.3 Malar fracture (note three fracture sites).

equalization of changes in ambient pressure. If a sinus ostia is obstructed, changes in ambient pressure may not be transmitted to the affected sinus cavity (most frequently the maxillary sinus though the frontal sinus may be affected in older children and adolescents), and barotrauma can result. As the child descends in an airplane (or during an underwater dive), the increased ambient pressure is transmitted to the cardiovascular system and thus to the vessels of the mucosal lining of the sinus. The mucosa becomes edematous and vessels engorged. If the sinus is obstructed and has not equalized the air pressure, a large differential pressure occurs between the sinus mucosa and its air-filled cavity. This results in a rupture of the blood vessels within the mucosa and bleeding into the sinus. The child will usually complain of cheek pain and may demonstrate epistaxis (of sinus origin). The treatment for this condition involves amoxicillin 25 to 50 mg/kg/day for 7 days (to prevent infection of the blood-filled sinus), antihistamine-decongestant therapy to restore the normal physiologic communication between the sinus and the nasal cavities, and the avoidance of further barotrauma. The rare case that does not respond to this regimen should be referred to an otolaryngologist for further evaluation and treatment.

Foreign Bodies

Nasal foreign bodies are common in children. While these children are usually brought to the emergency department with the history of putting an object into the nose, the presence of a foreign body may often be unsuspected and may be discovered only during evaluation of a child with persistent, unilateral, foul-smelling, purulent rhinorrhea. This is such a common mode of presentation for these problems that any child with a foul-smelling unilateral nasal discharge (even without a history of placing an object in his nose) should be considered to have a nasal foreign body until proven otherwise. The foreign body is usually visible on anterior rhinoscopy. However, purulent secretions may have to be suctioned from the nose before the object is seen. Radiographs are of limited value because most of the foreign bodies are radiolucent (paper, cloth, sponge, food, etc.).

If the object is located in the nasal vestibule, the emergency department physician may attempt to remove it (see procedure in Section VII). The child should be adequately restrained and the necessary equipment including a nasal speculum, directed light, suction, small hooks and forceps available. An otolaryngologist should be consulted if the foreign body cannot be removed easily. Hygroscopic foreign bodies, such as beans, may swell with nasal secretions and become very difficult to remove. The foreign body should never be pushed or irrigated into the nasopharynx, where it could be aspirated by the struggling child. Antimicrobials (usually amoxicillin 25 to 50 mg/kg/day for 7 days) are administered to prevent (or treat) an infection in this already traumatized area.

Chronic Nasal Obstruction

Obstruction to the normal passage of respiratory gases can occur with a variety of conditions, and will give the sensation of a blocked or "stuffy" nose. Temporary partial obstruction of one nasal cavity at a time occurs normally in the nasal respiratory cycle. Prolonged blockage, however, is not physiological, and one should search for an etiology.

While most instances of nasal obstruction cause only mild feelings of discomfort, some children may present with a history of obstructive apnea ("Pickwickian syndrome") and even cor pulmonale. A history of trauma or foreign body can lead one to the reason for the obstruction. A careful examination of the nasal cavities and pharynx is often necessary to determine the cause of the obstruction. Septal deviation, nasal tumor, and turbinate hypertrophy related to allergy and/or infection are frequent causes. Adenoid hypertrophy, nasopharyngeal tumor (lymphoma, rhabdomyosarcoma) and choanal atresia (unilateral or bilateral) can all present with nasal obstruction. Examination and radiographs of the nasopharynx may be useful in the evaluation of the blocked nose. If the etiology of the obstruction is not apparent after the above maneuvers, referral should be made to an otolaryngologist to perform a complete examination of the nose and nasopharynx.

Epistaxis

Epistaxis is a relatively common occurrence in childhood, and may cause significant anxiety in both the child and his parent. Although bleeding occasionally occurs secondary to the mucosal maceration caused by upper respiratory infections, nose-picking accounts for the great majority of recurrent epistaxis. (A more complete discussion on the differential diagnosis is presented in Chapter 20, "Epistaxis".) The usual site of bleeding is the anterior nasal septum (Kiesselbach's or Little's area) (Fig. 62.4).

A complete history is an important step in the proper management of epistaxis. Site of bleeding (one or both sides of the nose), frequency, bleeding from other places, history of trauma, and family history of bleeding are all important factors to know in this evaluation. A careful examination of the nose should be performed to identify the site and cause of the bleeding. Good lighting, suction and material for cauterization and packing should be readily available (see procedure in Section VII). Topical vasoconstrictors such as phenylephrine (0.25%), epinephrine (1:1000), or cocaine (1 to 5%) can be used to shrink the nasal mucosa to allow better visualization of the nasal cavity and may slow or even stop the bleeding. Simple pressure by squeezing the nostrils together is usually sufficient to stop most epistaxis. Occasionally, a roll of cotton placed under the upper lip will stop bleeding by compression of the labial artery. If pressure is not successful, cauterization with silver nitrate sticks or packing of the nose is performed (see procedure in Section

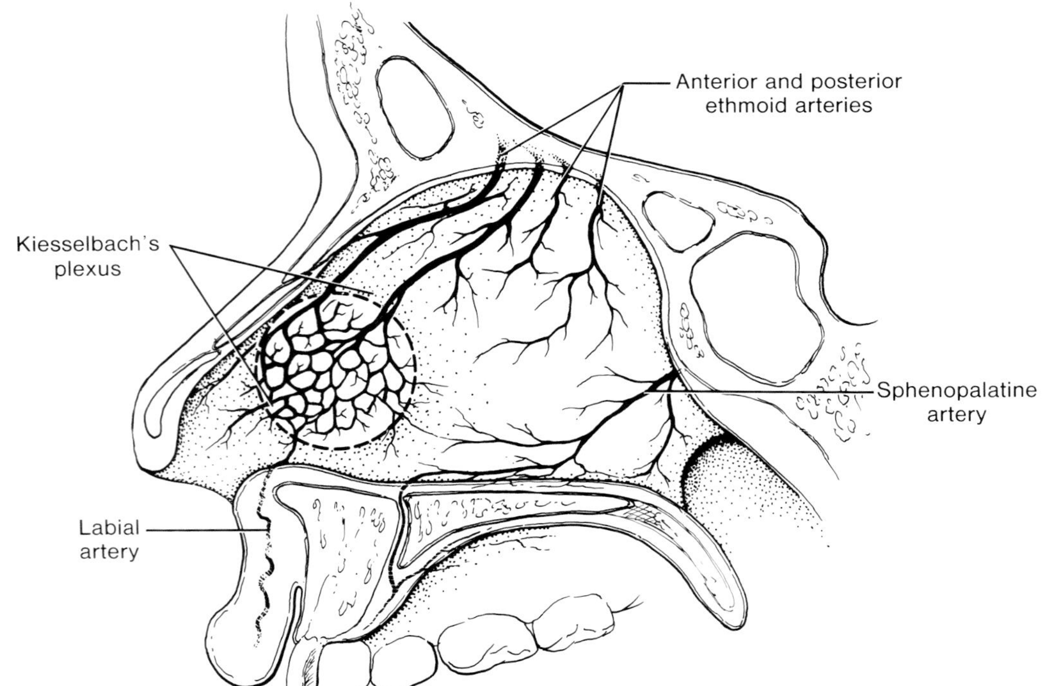

Figure 62.4 Vascular supply of nasal septum. Note prominence of vessels that form Kiesselbach's plexus.

VII). Absorbable packing such as oxycellulose (Surgicel) is usually adequate for most epistaxis and has the advantage of not requiring removal.

Further treatment should also be directed toward preventing the child from continuing to traumatize his nose, resulting in further bleeding. Using a vaporizer to increase the humidity in the child's room and applying Vaseline to the anterior septal areas twice daily can aid in healing the irritated nasal mucosa and preventing recurrent epistaxis. Fingernails should be cut short.

Severe or recurrent episodes of epistaxis require the assistance of an otolaryngologist in their diagnosis and management. Epistaxis that does not stop with simple pressure or oxycellulose packing may require a more substantial anterior nasal pack of Vaseline-impregnated gauze. A posterior nasal pack (using gauze or a Foley catheter) may be necessary in managing severe epistaxis that originates in the posterior nasal cavity or nasopharynx. (See procedure for nasal packing techniques in Section VII.)

If the epistaxis recurs despite the above treatment, an otolaryngologist should be consulted to look for other causes for the epistaxis. Nasal septal deviation or perforation, sinusitis, tumor (nasal, nasopharyngeal or sinus) Rendu-Osler-Weber disease (hereditary hemorrhagic telangiectasia), and nasal foreign body can all present with epistaxis. Blood dyscrasias such as hemophilia, idiopathic thyrombocytopenia purpura, von Willebrand's disease, and those hematologic conditions associated with leukemia or the administration of chemotherapeutic agents may lead to severe epistaxis. Treatment consists of correcting the underlying hematologic problem in addition to the previously described local measures. Recurrent or severe bleeding may require more extensive cauterization or even ligation of dilated vessels on the septum.

Neoplasms

Neoplasms of the nose and sinuses are uncommon in children. They may present as mass lesions or as chronic/recurrent rhinosinusitis. When a neoplasm is suspected, the child should be referred to an otolaryngologist for a complete evaluation of the nose and sinuses that is a prerequisite to the proper treatment of these lesions.

Hemangiomas are the most common benign neoplasms of the head and neck in children and frequently occur on the skin near or on the nose. Since hemangiomas often go through a period of rapid growth for the first 12 to 18 months of life before they begin to involute, a period of observation is recommended prior to considering surgical excision for cosmetic reasons. Recurrent bleeding, thrombocytopenia, skin breakdown and cardiac failure are some indications for early intervention. *Papillomas* are viral-induced verrucous growths that are the most common neoplasms of the aerodigestive tract. When they appear in the nose, they are most often found on the nasal septum. Simple excision or fulguration is the preferred treatment for these lesions. *Fibro-osseous disorders* include *osteomas*, *giant cell granuloma*, *fibrous dysplasia*, *fibroma* and the *"brown tumor" of hyperparathyroidism.* After blood tests to rule out hyperparathyroidism, treatment consists of simple excision or sculpturing for cosmetic purposes and for relief of nasal or sinus obstruction.

Malignant tumors of the nose and sinuses in children include *rhabdomyosarcoma*, *lymphoma*, *esthesioneuroblastoma* (*olfactory neuroblastoma*) and, rarely, *metastatic lesions* from primary tumors below the clavicle. These lesions can present with a mass in the nose or orbit, nasal congestion, epistaxis or clinically apparent cervical adenopathy. If a malignancy is suspected, the child should be admitted to the hospital for a complete evaluation and possible biopsy.

ORAL CAVITY, PHARYNX AND ESOPHAGUS

Methods of Examination

The oral cavity and oropharynx are directly visible with the aid of a tongue blade. A head light or brightly lighted flashlight is required for this examination. The tongue should be displaced down and forward with

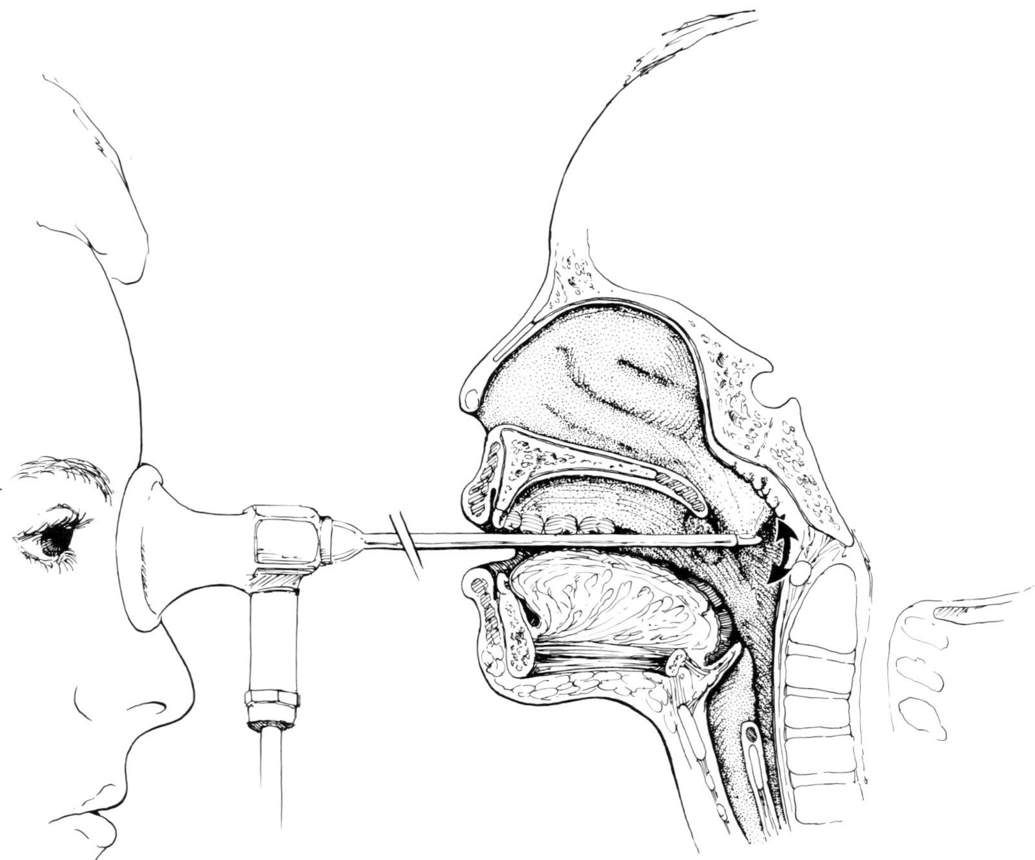

Figure 62.5 Fiberoptic telescope in place to view nasopharynx or hypopharynx, and larynx.

the tongue blade placed on the anterior two thirds of the tongue to avoid gagging. The examination of the nasopharynx, hypopharynx and esophagus requires special instrumentation. The nasopharynx and hypopharynx can be examined indirectly with a mirror of pharyngoscope (Fig. 62.5). This latter procedure requires special skills and is best left to the otorhinolaryngology consultant. Examination of the esophagus requires direct visualization with an esophagoscope under general anesthesia. Palpation of the hypopharynx and nasopharynx should not be performed as it is uncomfortable to the child and potentially dangerous.

Radiography contributes minimally to the examination of the oral cavity and oropharynx because these areas are visible by direct examination. The nasopharynx and hypopharynx are very well outlined by air contrast and the esophagus can be coated with barium contrast. The lateral neck radiograph is very useful to visualize the nasopharynx and hypopharynx.

Infection

Stomatitis

The most common infectious lesion of the oral cavity is the aphthous ulcer. The ulcers are often recurrent, may appear singly or confluent, and can cause severe stomatitis. The exact etiology of aphthous ulcerations is unknown but is believed to be infectious.

Herpes simplex can cause severe gingivostomatitis while the pharynx is relatively spared. On the other hand *coxsackie virus* infection (herpangina) causes severe ulcerative lesions of the pharynx but not the anterior mouth. These viral infections cause severe oral pain and inability to eat. They are self-limited and require only symptomatic relief. (Refer to Chapter 45, "Infectious Diseases.")

Candida albicans oral infection (thrush) usually appears as white patches with surrounding inflammation on the oral mucosa. It frequently occurs in newborns, immune suppressed patients and patients on antibiotic therapy. Nystatin is an effective treatment. The dose is 200,000 units (2 ml) 4 times a day for 14 days.

Acute necrotizing, ulcerative gingivitis ("trench mouth") causes painful, bleeding gums. Vigorous brushing of the teeth and gums with a soft brush will promote rapid healing. Antibiotics are of limited value.

Pharyngitis

Viral pharyngitis is by inspection indistinguishable from bacterial pharyngitis. Only a throat culture can differentiate these infections. The degree of erythema and exudate may vary on the pharynx and tonsils. Pharyngeal infections may spread to the peritonsillar area causing cellulitis. The affected tonsil bulges forward and medially to touch the uvula. If pus localizes in the peritonsillar space, a peritonsillar abscess is formed. The peritonsillar abscess will also cause trismus. Suspected abscess formation requires immediate consultation with an otorhinolaryngology specialist.

Retropharyngeal and Parapharyngeal Infection

Retropharyngeal and parapharyngeal lymph nodes may also be involved during pharyngitis and progress to abscess formation. Retropharyngeal abscess is usually easily seen on the lateral neck x-ray (Fig. 62.6). Peritonsillar, retropharyngeal and parapharyngeal abscess must be treated by intravenous penicillin and surgical drainage.

One must always keep in mind that unusual infections like actinomycosis, mucormycosis, and syphilis may present in the oral cavity. Actinomycosis causes oral-cervical fistulas, and mucor causes necrosis of the palate. Syphilis can present in many ways (ulceration, raised lesion etc.), and has no characteristic appearance.

Lymphoid hyperplasia (enlarged tonsils and adenoids) can cause severe airway obstruction with intermittent sleep apnea. If right heart strain or somnolence are present, a tonsillectomy and adenoidectomy may be required urgently.

Trauma

Oral cavity trauma is usually caused by biting the inside of the cheek or tongue. This is very painful and can cause a laceration or hematoma formation. Treatment of self-inflicted bites is rarely needed but a laceration may require suturing if it bleeds excessively or is severe enough to alter intraoral anatomy or physiology (i.e., breathing, deglutition or speech).

Children also may have oropharyngeal lacerations or puncture wounds when they fall with an object, such as a stick, in their mouths. Penetrating wounds of the pharynx may cause injury to the deep structures of the neck. The carotid artery, jugular vein and cranial nerves may be injured. If major vessel or cranial nerve injury is suspected, urgent surgical exploration of the neck must be considered.

Caustic substances (lye or acid) may be ingested causing burns anywhere from the lips to the stomach. Burns of the oral mucosa appear as patches of erythema, blebs, or ulcerated areas. Although caustic burns are usually visible in the oral cavity and pharynx, large skip areas may exist. The absence of oral or pharyngeal burns does not rule out esophageal injury. If there is a history of caustic ingestion, an esophagoscopy should be performed 6 to 12 hours later to establish the presence of esophageal burns, regardless of the condition of the oral cavity and pharynx. Since burns occur very rapidly, the child should not be given any oral antidote in the emergency room department.

Caustic substances may burn the larynx when ingested and can cause rapidly progressive edema and respiratory distress. Orotracheal intubation for acute airway management should be done if necessary in the emergency room. A tracheotomy should be performed as soon as possible after the

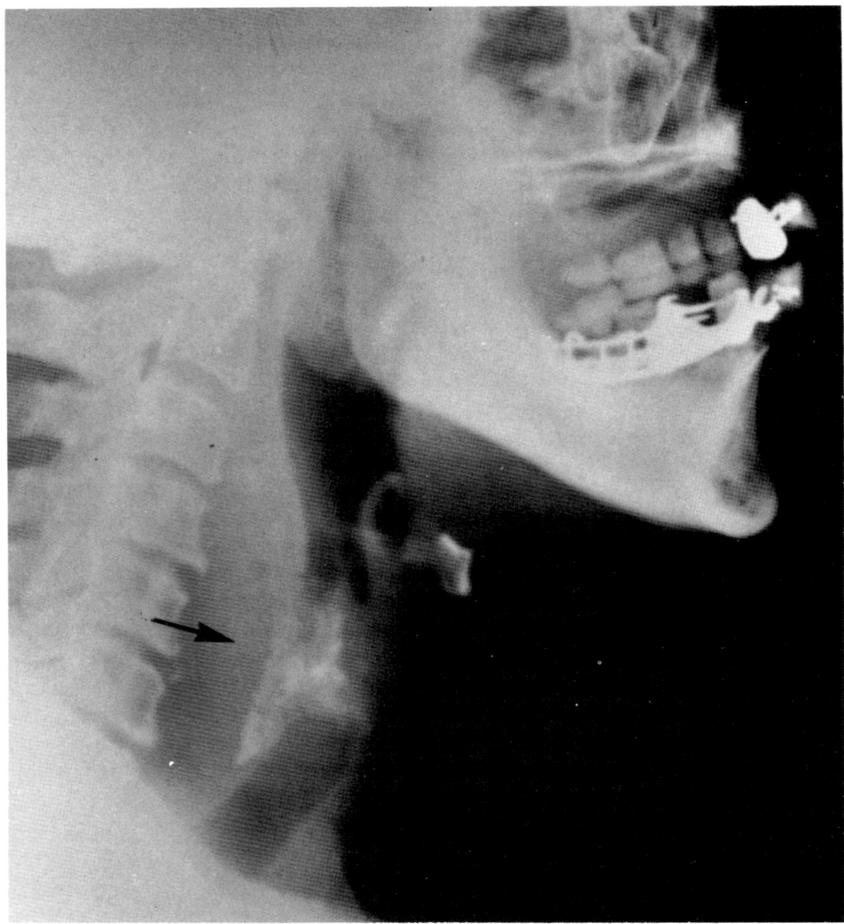

Figure 62.6 Lateral neck radiograph demonstrating retropharyngeal abscess (*arrow*).

intubation to minimize laryngotracheal stenosis.

Foreign Bodies

Foreign bodies in the oral cavity and pharynx are not common because of the child's protective reflexes. The tongue is very sensitive and can detect sharp foreign objects that are then spat out. The gag reflex frequently expels foreign material from the pharynx, but sharp objects like fish bones, pins and pieces of plastic may get stuck in the oral mucosa, tonsils or pharynx (Fig. 62.7). If visible, and if the patient is cooperative, a foreign body they may be removed with a clamp or forceps.

Objects of all types may lodge in the hypopharynx or esophagus. Esophageal foreign bodies generally lodge at the areas of natural narrowing of the esophagus. The most common sites are the cricopharyngeal area, thoracic inlet, arch of the aorta and gastroesophageal junction. If the child can breathe and talk, no attempt should be made to remove the object in the emergency department. The safest method of removal is endoscopically, utilizing a general anesthetic. If the child is gagging and unable to breathe, the Heimlich maneuver should be used (refer to Chapter 1, "Resuscitation"). If this is not effective, emergency intubation or tracheotomy may be required to bypass the obstructing object.

Lateral neck and chest radiographs will demonstrate radiopaque hypopharyngeal and esophageal foreign bodies. Plastic and other nonradiopaque objects cause the same foreign body sensation (something stuck in the throat) but are not visible on x-ray. Young children often have dysphagia and drooling because of painful swallowing.

Although ingestion of a foreign body usually causes gagging and choking that lasts for several seconds and subsequently subsides, the initial episode may take place unobserved by an adult. Thus, unexplained dysphagia or drooling should initiate a search for a possible foreign body.

Neoplasms

Benign and malignant neoplasms occur in the oral cavity, pharynx, hypopharynx, and esophagus. Benign neoplasms in the oral cavity may rise from the mucosa or underlying tissues. Minor salivary gland tumors, hemangiomas, lymphangiomas, pyogenic granulomas and neurofibromas are

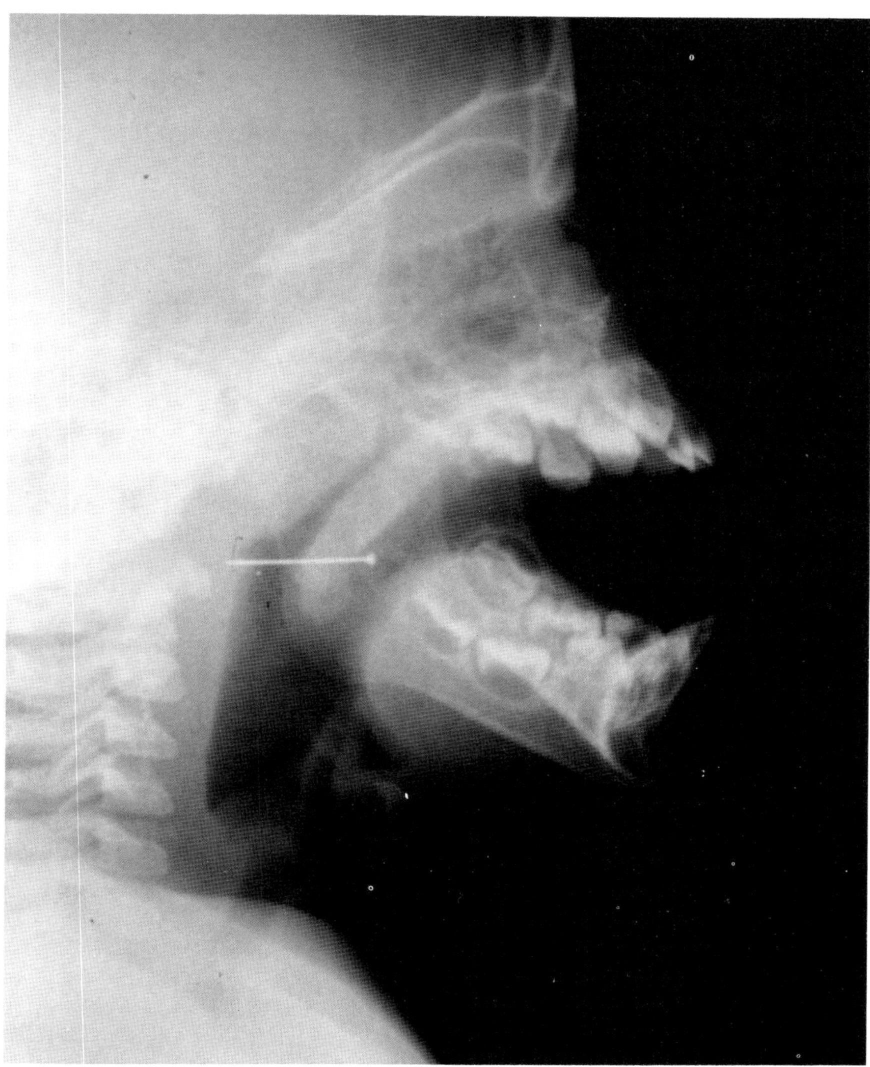

Figure 62.7 Lateral neck radiograph of a straight pin lodged in pharyngeal wall.

found in the oral cavity but rarely present as an emergency.

Nasopharyngeal angiofibromas occur in prepubescent males and cause nasal obstruction. They may present in the emergency department as massive epistaxis. Posterior packing is required to control the hemorrhage that may be life-threatening. (See procedure in Section VII.)

Malignant neoplasms are rare but can occur throughout the oral cavity, pharynx and esophagus. *Rhabdomyosarcoma, lymphoma* and *squamous cell carcinoma* (lymphoepithelioma) are the most common lesions and rarely present as emergencies unless there is extensive hemorrhage or a compromised airway.

Biopsy of oral, pharyngeal and esophageal tumors is best done in the operating room where adequate exposure and control of hemorrhage is most effectively obtained.

LARYNX AND TRACHEA

Methods of Examination

Examination of the larynx is often difficult in the young child. Frequently, however, the tip of the epiglottis may be visualized when the tongue is protruded during the examination of the oropharynx. Indirect examination of the larynx can be performed using a laryngeal mirror or telescopic endoscope. Vocal cord mobility, the structure of the larynx, and the presence of laryngeal masses can usually be assessed in this manner in a cooperative child 3 years of age or older. The otolaryngologist should be consulted to perform this examination on the child presenting to the emergency department with symptoms related to the larynx.

Lateral and anteroposterior plain radiographs of the neck can provide significant information about the larynx and upper trachea. While xeroradiographs offer more precise detail of the airway by virtue of their property of edge enhancement, the extra radiation exposure involved may make this a less desirable study. Tomograms and CT scans are very useful in examining the fine detail of laryngeal and tracheal structures, but the general anesthetic required to keep the child still for these examinations restricts their use to very specific instances. Fluoroscopic examination of the larynx is one method of evaluating the movements of the vocal cords during phonation and respiration. Vocal cord paralysis and laryngomalacia can often be identified in this manner. Contrast studies can also be used in the evaluation of laryngeal function. A barium swallow is useful in detecting aspiration related to vocal cord paralysis, posterior laryngeal cleft, or tracheoesophageal fistula.

Infection

Viral laryngitis is often a component of the common URI described previously in this chapter. Laryngeal involvement is indicated by a hoarse, raspy voice. This is related to edema of the vocal cords secondary to the inflammation. Airway obstruction is rare in viral laryngitis. Symptomatic treatment with humidification, antipyretics, analgesics, throat gargles and voice rest is recommended while the disease runs its natural course. When the viral infection involves the subglottic space, a more serious clinical problem appears. *Laryngotracheobronchitis (croup)* is a common, and potentially life-threatening, infection occurring in early childhood. The diagnosis and management of croup is discussed in other chapters of this book ("Stridor," Chapter 35; "Infectious Diseases," Chapter 45).

Bacterial laryngitis does occur but is not nearly as common as its viral counterpart. It is also very difficult to distinguish bacterial laryngitis on clinical grounds from a similar infection of viral etiology. Etiologic agents responsible for bacterial laryngitis include *Staphylococcus* and *H. influenzae.* Treatment consists of the same measures recommended for viral laryngitis with the addition of the appropriate antimicrobial agents. The otolaryngologist is rarely required to perform a direct laryngoscopy to to confirm the diagnosis or to aspirate secretions for therapeutic and diagnostic purposes.

Diphtheria may involve the larynx, in addition to other areas of the upper aerodigestive tract. The diagnosis is suspected by the presence of a membrane covering the pharynx and larynx that leaves a raw, bleeding surface when it is removed. The diphtheria membrane can compromise the laryngeal airway to cause obstruction requiring endoscopic removal of the membrane and/or tracheostomy, in addition to antimicrobial therapy.

Bacterial infection of the supraglottic larynx can cause a symptom complex with potentially life-threatening airway obstruction. *Epiglottitis* (more appropriately termed *supraglottitis*) is an infection of the supraglottic larynx that is caused most often by *H. influenzae*, type B. The diagnosis and management of epiglottitis is discussed in other chapters in this book ("Stridor," Chapter 35; "Infectious Disease," Chapter 45).

Neoplasms

Neoplasms of the larynx and trachea are uncommon in children. The otolaryngologist should be consulted to assist the emergency department physician in the management of these patients.

The most common neoplasm of the larynx in children is the *laryngeal papilloma*. This is felt to be a viral-induced neoplasm that has a predilection for the upper aerodigestive tract and the larynx in particular. The disease usually appears in the child between 2 and 5 years of age with persistent or worsening hoarseness and, occasionally, airway obstruction. If papillomas are suspected as the source of hoarseness in a child, the otolaryngologist should be consulted to perform the indirect or direct laryngoscopy required to confirm the diagnosis. A lateral neck radiograph may demonstrate a soft tissue mass in the area of the larynx. (Fig. 62.8). The course of the disease is characterized by multiple cycles of growth and regression until a spontaneous remission occurs, usually around puberty. The otolaryngologist's goal in managing these patients is to maintain a good voice and unobstructed airway by repeated excision of the papillomas.

Hemangiomas may occur in the larynx, primarily in the subglottic area. As with most juvenile hemangiomas, these lesions present in the second to sixth month of life and can enlarge over several months to cause significant airway obstruction. Episodes of stridor may be precipitated by a URI. The presence of cutaneous hemangiomas in an infant with stridor should suggest to the emergency department physician the possibility of a subglottic hemangioma. Hemangiomas appear as posterior subglottic masses on lateral neck radiographs but the diagnosis must usually be confirmed by laryngoscopy performed by an otolaryngologist. Since most hemangiomas of infancy tend to involute after an initial period of rapid growth during the first 1 to 2 years of life, close observation has been advocated as the only treatment of those lesions which are causing minimal symptoms. If there is severe, persistent or recurrent respiratory distress, intervention is indicated. Tracheostomy, systemic corticosteroids and CO_2 laser excision are some of the modes of treatment presently being advocated.

Malignant neoplasms of the larynx are uncommon. They include *rhabdomyosarcoma*, *chondrosarcoma* and *lymphoma*. These tumors present with varying degrees of hoarseness and respiratory obstruction. If a laryngeal malignancy is suspected, the otolaryngologist should be asked to perform indirect and direct laryngoscopy to confirm the laryngeal problem and to obtain tissue for histologic identification of the tumor.

Trauma

Laryngeal trauma can occur in a variety of ways. Blunt or penetrating injuries of the larynx can result in mucosal lacerations, laryngeal hematomas, vocal cord paralysis, or fractures of the thyroid and cricoid cartilages. Proper treatment requires prompt recognition of the presence and nature of a laryngeal injury and protection of the airway. Patients with laryngeal trauma present with varying degrees of neck pain, hoarseness, hemoptysis and airway obstruction. Physical examination of a child with blunt trauma can reveal anterior neck tenderness, crepitation and absence of the normal prominence of the thyroid cartilage or "Adam's apple" (Fig. 62.9). The otolaryngologist should be called upon to perform an indirect examination of the larynx on the child with a suspected laryngeal injury. A direct laryngoscopy may be required in

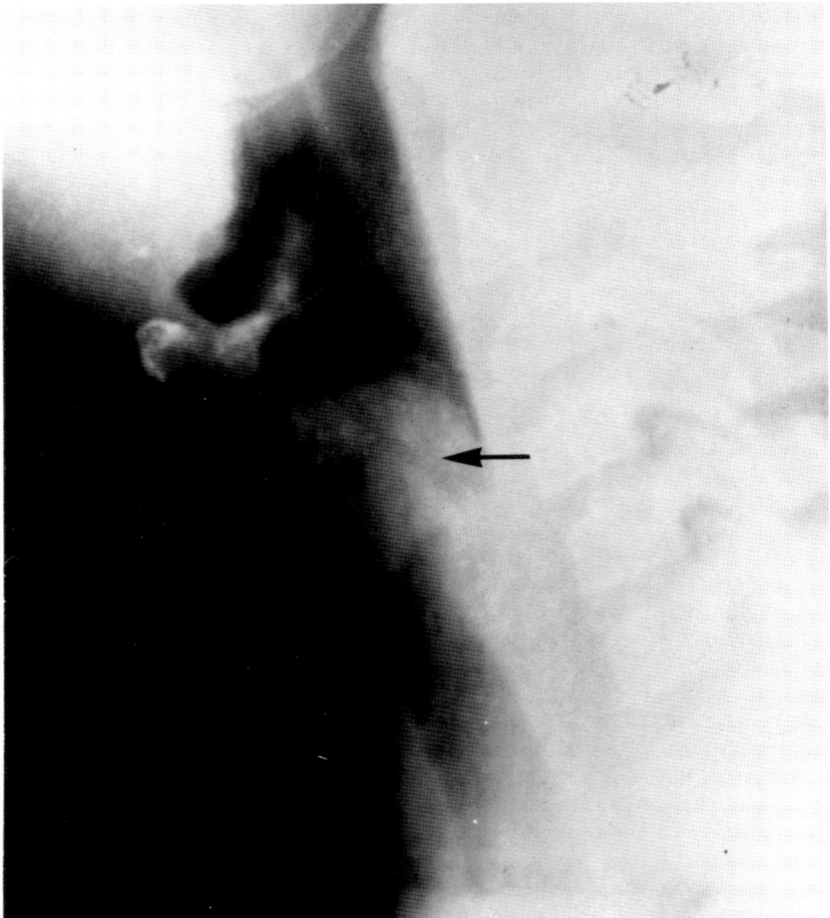

Figure 62.8 Lateral neck radiograph demonstrating soft tissue density (*arrow*) at level of larynx. Direct laryngoscopy revealed this to be papilloma.

those instances where a foreign body is suspected, or there is a significant laryngeal injury with respiratory distress. The otolaryngologist should be prepared to intervene with intubation, tracheostomy and/or surgical exploration of these laryngeal injuries.

Ingestion of *caustic substances* can cause severe burns of the larynx and pharynx; airway obstruction may occur secondary to the edema related to this injury. Laryngeal burns should be suspected in the child with hoarseness or stridor after caustic ingestion. The child should be hospitalized and otolaryngologic consultation obtained. If signs of respiratory distress (tachypnea, stridor) occur, the child should be taken to the operating room where endoscopy is performed and an artificial airway, usually a tracheostomy, placed.

Foreign Bodies

Foreign bodies may become trapped in the laryngeal inlet causing acute upper airway obstruction. The child will usually present with severe coughing, hoarseness and significant respiratory distress. If the child is able to phonate, air is moving through his larynx, indicating only partial obstruction. "Back blows" or the Heimlich maneuver should *not* be performed in these children, since this may cause the foreign body to lodge more firmly in the larynx and convert a partial obstruction into a complete one. The child should be taken immediately to the operating room where the otolaryngologist can perform the direct laryngoscopy necessary to remove the foreign body. If the child is not able to speak, he may be totally obstructed by the foreign body. In this case, a true emergency exists and "back blows" or the Heimlich maneuver may be lifesaving. Care must be taken in performing the Heimlich maneuver in young children because of the potential hazard of liver laceration. Emergency laryngoscopy, intubation, or tracheostomy are rarely required, and only if the above maneuvers are unsuccessful.

Foreign bodies that pass the larynx to lodge in the trachea or proximal bronchi can present problems in diagnosis and management. Usually a history of coughing or choking on food (for example, a peanut or raw carrot, etc.) or toy is obtained. The child is often in no acute distress but may demonstrate a mild cough and/or wheezes. Inspiratory and expiratory stridor are characteristic of tracheal foreign bodies. Unilateral wheezes and decreased, or even absent, breath sounds are often seen with unilateral bronchial obstruction. Since most of the foreign bodies are radiolucent, they are not identifiable on radiographs. However, a difference in aeration of the lungs will often help to detect the presence and identify the site of a bronchial obstruction. Volume de-

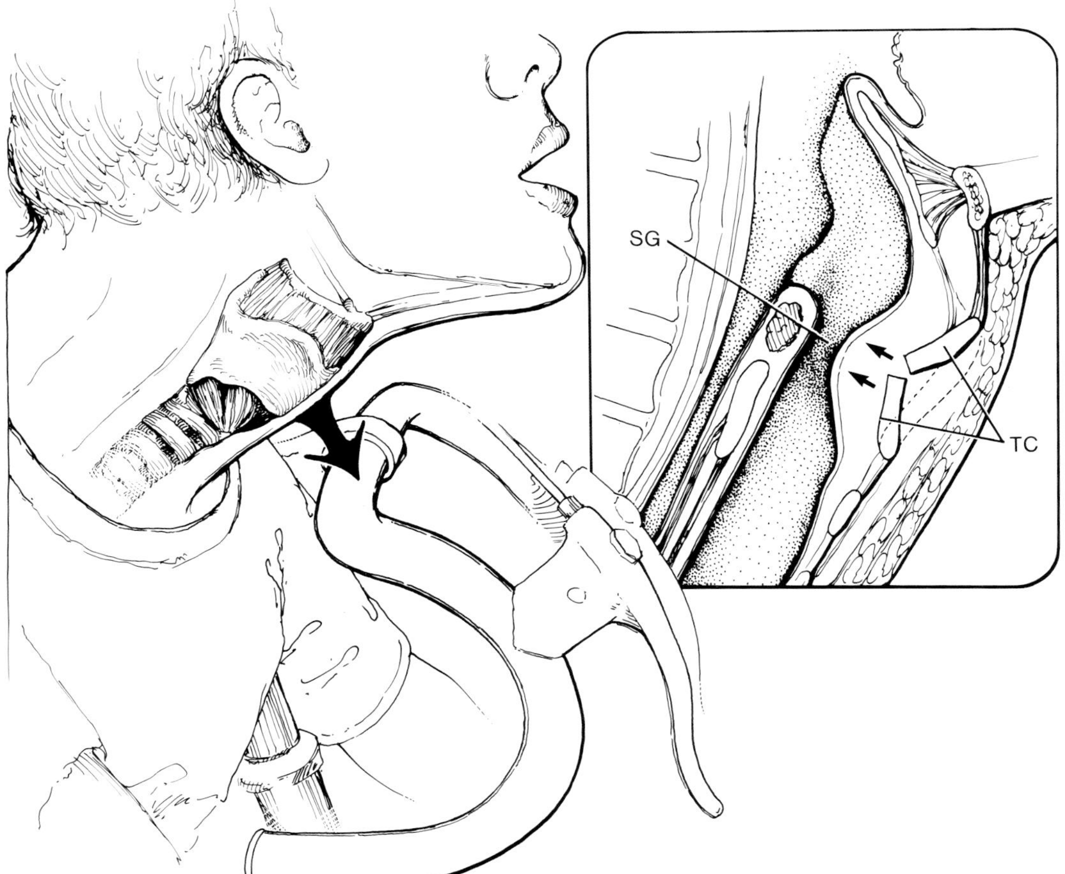

Figure 62.9 Loss of thyroid cartilage prominence and associated acute airway obstruction secondary to laryngeal fracture. *SG*, narrowed subglottic space; *TC*, fracture of thyroid cartilage.

crease, atelectasis and infiltrate are often seen on plain chest films. Hyperaeration (air trapping) secondary to a ball-valve effect of the foreign body is best seen by comparing inspiration and expiration films (Fig. 62.10). If the child will not cooperate to obtain these views, right and left lateral decubitus films can often demonstrate the same phenomena. A normal chest radiograph, however, does not rule out the possibility of a foreign body. If a foreign body is suspected (by history, clinical or radiographic examination), the child should be admitted and otolaryngologic consultation obtained to perform the endoscopy necessary for its prompt and safe removal.

Stridor

The differential diagnosis and emergency management of a child presenting with stridor is discussed in detail in Chapter 35, "Stridor."

NECK AND ASSOCIATED STRUCTURES

Methods of Examination

Visual inspection and palpation provide the basis for examination of the neck and its enclosed structures. The head should be erect during the examination with the normal prominence of the sternocleidomastoid muscle on each side. Anterior projection of the thyroid cartilage or "Adam's apple" is seen in postpubescent males. Palpation of the neck is performed to assess the normal structures in the neck and to detect the presence and nature of any cervical masses. Examination of the two sides is done simultaneously so they can be compared to one another. The examiner should be able to grasp the thyroid cartilage and move it gently from side to side without any discomfort to the patient. Immobility or significant pain may indicate the presence of laryngeal pathology. Crepitation of the neck indicates free air in the tissue planes of the neck from perforation of a hollow viscus. Passive and active range of motion of the neck should be complete in all directions. Restriction in movement may be caused by tender cervical adenopathy, cervical spine disease, spasm or fibrosis of the sternocleidomastoid muscle or meningeal irritation (Kernig's sign). Arterial pulses of equal strength should be palpable in the carotid artery on each side of the neck. The carotids can also be auscultated for evidence of bruits.

Radiographs are often invaluable in the examination of the neck. Plain anteroposterior and lateral views provide significant information in the evaluation of cervical problems. The presence of masses projecting into and compromising the airway can be detected. Air between the muscle planes of the neck indicates a perforation of a hollow viscus such as the pharynx, esophagus, larynx, trachea or pulmonary alveolus. Sinus films, by identifying a neoplasm or sinusitis, are often helpful in determining the etiology of a neck mass.

Infection

Cervical adenitis is the most common cause of a neck mass in a child. The lymphatic system of the neck drains the internal cavities of the head and neck (ear, nose, mouth, pharynx, sinuses, and larynx) as well as the skin and associated adnexal structures of the face and scalp. Regional cervical lymph nodes respond when there is a primary infection in any area of the head and neck. Since certain groups of nodes drain specific sites in the head and neck, the location of the swollen and infected lymph node can often help the practioner to identify the area of the primary infection. Ear infections most often drain to the infra-auricular nodes; pharyngeal infections (e.g. tonsillitis) usually present with jugulodigastric node involvement; and posterior cervical nodes often accompany nasopharyngeal infections (e.g. adenoiditis).

Cervical adenitis is uncommon secondary to brief, uncomplicated viral URI. Tender and enlarged nodes occur more frequently as a result of bacterial infection of the head and neck with the ears and throat responsible for a large portion of these. Since *Streptococcus* species are the etiologic agents in the majority of bacterial infections in the head and neck, the infected

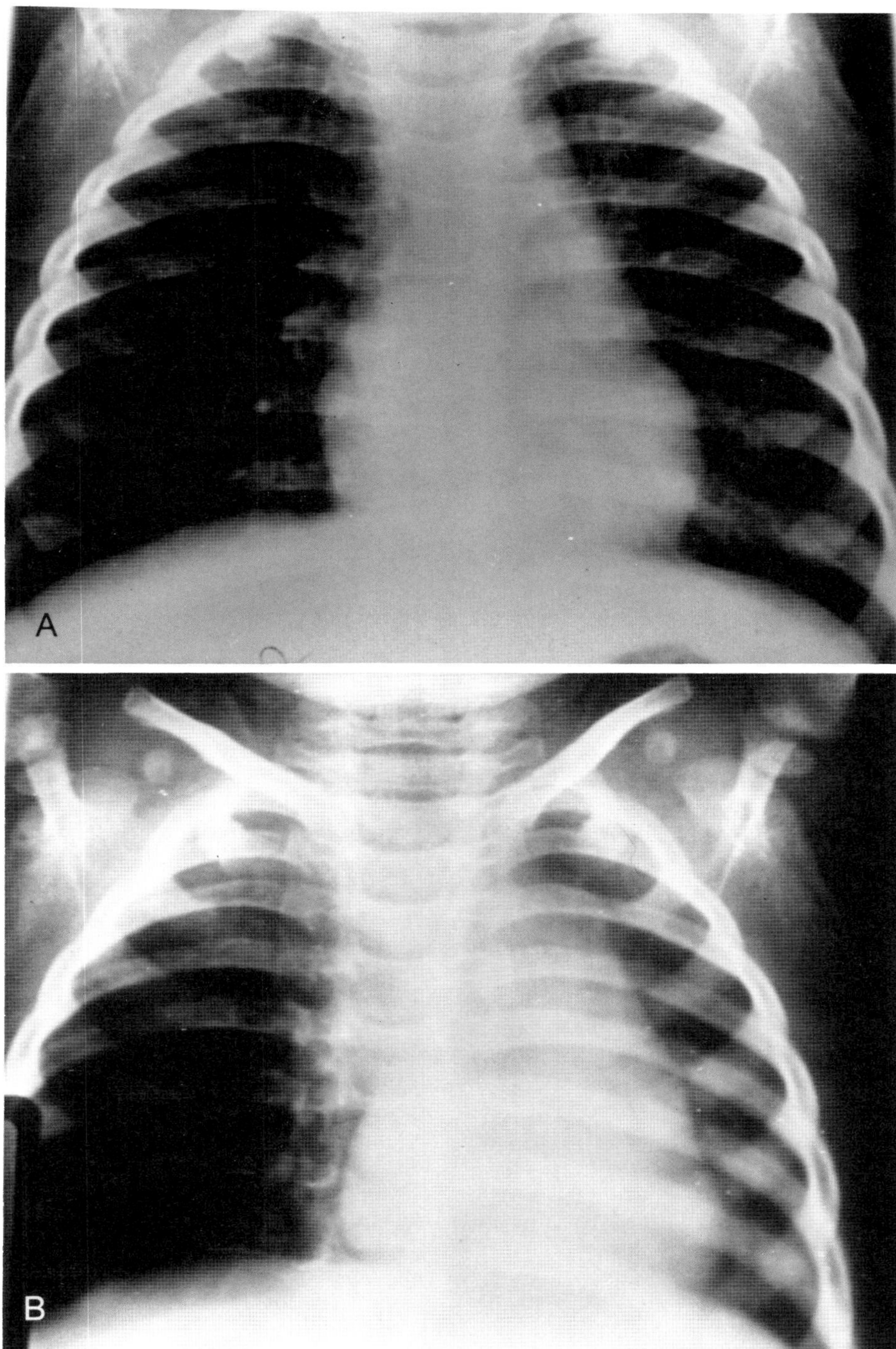

Figure 62.10 Chest radiograph of child with bronchial foreign body. (*A*) Inspiratory film demonstrates normal aeration bilaterally. (*B*) Expiratory film shows hyperaeration on the right secondary to air trapping by the foreign body in the right mainstem bronchus.

lymph nodes will usually contain the same organisms. Treatment with oral penicillin (or amoxicillin) will usually clear the primary infection and cause regression of the enlarged lymph nodes. Culture of the nasopharynx, throat or aspirate of the cervical node can assist the physician in the choice of antimicrobial agents.

While most children will respond to the above therapy, there is a small group of children whose nodes progress to suppurative cervical adenitis. Studies of children hospitalized with cervical adenitis have shown a predominence of *S. aureus* as the causative agent. This high incidence of staphylococci is probably the result of selecting out patients who have not responded to a course of oral antimicrobials effective against the more commonly occurring *Streptococcus* species. Therefore, if cervical adenitis has not responded to the primary antimicrobial treatment, agents should be added which are effective against *S. aureus* (erythromycin, dicloxacillin, or cephalosporins).

A child who has demonstrated rapid enlargement of cervical nodes, poor response to oral antimicrobials, cellulitis of the overlying skin, abscess formation, or signs of toxicity (high fever, malaise, dehydration), should be admitted to the hospital for treatment with intravenous fluids and antimicrobials. Surgical consultation should be obtained in the management of these complicated cases in which needle aspiration, incisional drainage, or biopsy (for possible neoplasm) may be required.

Retropharyngeal or *parapharyngeal nodes* are commonly involved with inflammatory processes that originate in the pharynx. Sore throat, dysphagia and stiff neck are some of the symptoms that can accompany markedly enlarged pharyngeal nodes. Retropharyngeal nodes can be noted overlying the cervical spine during examination of the oropharynx. They also appear as widening of the retropharyngeal soft tissues on lateral neck radiographs. Parapharyngeal nodes are seldom detected clinically unless they enlarge sufficiently to deviate the tonsil and pharyngeal wall medially. Treatment of enlarged pharyngeal nodes consists of intravenous antimicrobials (usually penicillin), observation of the child's airway, and possible biopsy if resolution does not occur with treatment or if a malignancy is suspected.

A collection of purulent material within the tissues of the neck, a neck abscess, requires prompt and specific treatment. The most common cause of a neck abscess is breakdown or necrosis of an infected lymph node. Purulent material may be located within a single node or may accumulate between several adjacent nodes. Once the process of cervical adenitis has progressed to the point of abscess formation, treatment is evacuation of the infected material and the prevention of further spread of the infection. The child is hospitalized, and intravenous antimicrobials are administered which are effective against *S. aureus* (antistaphylococcal penicillin). Otolaryngologic consultation is obtained to perform a needle aspiration or incision and drainage to evacuate and culture the infected material.

Deep neck abscesses are uncommon in children but can be extremely dangerous when they occur. *Parapharyngeal abscess* occurs when purulent material collects in the parapharyngeal space lateral to the pharyngeal constrictors and medial to the vascular compartment of the neck. Necrosis of parapharyngeal lymph nodes or lateral extension of a peritonsillar abscess are the two main sources of this infection. The child with a parapharyngeal abscess presents with a stiff neck, high fever, malaise, dehydration, and other signs of toxicity. He usually has dysphagia and may not be able to swallow his own saliva. Physical examination reveals diffuse swelling and tenderness of one side of the neck but fluctuance is seldom appreciated. Intraoral examination may demonstrate medial displacement of the lateral pharyngeal wall and tonsil. Lateral neck radiographs are usually not helpful in evaluating this disease process. If left to progress, the parapharyngeal abscess can involve the adjacent vascular structures in the neck, descend into the mediastinum, or spontaneously rupture into the pharynx causing aspiration of purulent material.

Otolaryngologic consultation should be obtained to assist the emergency room physician in the evaluation of a patient with a parapharyngeal abscess. Appropriate treatment consists of hospitalization, intravenous fluids, antimicrobials effective against *S. aureus* (antistaphylococcal penicillins) and drainage of the abscess.

Retropharyngeal abscess occurs as a result of the necrosis of retropharyngeal lymph nodes or secondary to perforation of the pharynx or esophagus. Purulent material collects between the retropharyngeal and prevertebral layers of the cervical fascia, also known as the *danger space.* This potential space extends from the base of the skull to the mediastinum, thus allowing for extensive spread of the infection. Presenting symptoms are similar to those associated with parapharyngeal abscess. Lateral neck radiographs will demonstrate widening and bulging of the retropharyngeal space (Fig. 62.6). Treatment consists of hospitalization, intravenous fluids, antimicrobials effective against *S. aureus*, and drainage of the abscess.

Salivary gland infections should be considered in the differential diagnosis of a cervical mass suspected to be infectious in origin. Both viral and bacterial agents can be responsible for the infection, with the former being much more frequent. Mumps (endemic parotitis) is the most common salivary infection in children. While the parotid gland is involved in over 85% of the cases, the submandibular gland may also be involved with the viral infection. The infection presents with acute painful swelling of the involved gland or glands. There is erythema around the intraoral orifice of the salivary duct and the saliva expressed is generally clear. Treatment is symptomatic with clear fluids, antipyretics and analgesics as necessary.

Bacterial infections of the salivary glands will present with signs and symptoms similar to those associated with cervical lymphadenitis. Neonatal parotitis and, less commonly, submandibular sialadenitis usually occur in a 3- to 4-week-old child after a systemic illness has caused dehydration. The affected gland is very swollen and abscess formation may occur. Purulent material may be expressed from either Stensen's or Wharton's duct by massage of the affected salivary gland. Otolaryngologic consultation should be obtained. The child is hospitalized for treatment with intravenous antimicrobials effective against *S. aureus* (antistaphylococcal penicillin) and evacuation of any collection of purulent material. Recurrent or chronic infections of the salivary glands are usually related to some predisposing factor. Management should include the detection and correction of these conditions.

Neoplasms

Neoplasms of the neck, both primary and metastatic, occur in children. If a cervical neoplasm is suspected, a head and neck surgeon should be consulted to perform a complete examination of the head and neck (including nasopharyngoscopy, laryngoscopy and hypopharyngoscopy) that is a prerequisite to proper management.

The *hemangioma* is the most common neoplasm of the head and neck in children. While they are more common on the skin of the face and scalp, lesions can occur on the skin of the neck and involve deeper structures such as the parotid gland. The diagnosis of cutaneous hemangiomas of the cervical skin is usually obvious on physical inspection; the lesions are red to reddish-purple, flat or raised, blanch with pressure and increase in size with crying or straining. Deep-seated lesions without cutaneous manifestations may require special diagnostic aids such as angiography, thermography and biopsy to confirm the diagnosis.

These juvenile hemangiomas demonstrate a cycle of rapid growth for the first 12 to 18 months of life. Slow regression and even total disappearance occurs over the next year or two. Because of this natural history, once the diagnosis of hemangioma is made, the preferred treatment is close observation. Lesions that grow rapidly to produce complications such as airway obstruction, skin necrosis, hemorrhage, high-output cardiac failure or thrombocytopenia require more active intervention. The child should be admitted and surgical consultation obtained. Treatment modalities presently advocated include systemic corticosteroids, cryotherapy, CO_2 laser excision, sclerosing agents, surgical excision and rarely radiation therapy.

Lymphangiomas are uncommon benign lesions of the neck. Cystic hygroma is the most common type of lymphangioma found in the neck. These lesions consist of multiple cystic spaces filled with lymph and, occasionally, blood. They present most commonly as large lateral neck masses in neonates. The diagnosis is often obvious on physical examination of a large cystic lesion that transilluminates. The natural history of these lesions is usually one of progressive growth and enlargement. Lymphangiomas can fluctuate in size secondary to a concurrent infection of the head and neck or hemorrhage into a cyst. Small, stable, asymptomatic lesions can be managed by close observation. Surgical excision is the treatment of choice for all large symptomatic lesions, with several staged procedures often being required. Aspiration of a large cyst (or cysts) can temporarily decompress a lesion, but is not a substitute for definitive surgical excision. Large cystic hygromas may cause feeding difficulties or respiratory distress in the newborn and may necessitate early surgical intervention which can include tracheostomy and gastrostomy.

Less common benign neoplasms of the neck in children include *teratomas, paragangliomas (carotid body tumors, glomus tumors), neural sheath tumors (neurofibromas, neurilemomas),* and *thyroid* and *salivary gland neoplasms.*

The most common malignant neoplasm of the neck in children is *lymphoma,* being almost equally divided into *Hodgkin's* and *non-Hodgkin's* types. The disease may be localized in the neck or be a part of a more generalized disorder. Physical examination will often reveal multiple firm, rubbery, unilateral or bilateral nodes. If the diagnosis of lymphoma is suspected, otolaryngologic consultation should be obtained for a careful examination of the oral cavity, pharynx and paranasal sinuses to look for a primary or associated lesion. This not only aids in the evaluation of the extent of the lymphoma but may also locate a site from which a biopsy can be obtained without the morbidity of a neck exploration.

Cervical lymph nodes may present with neoplasm metastic from a nonlymphogenous primary tumor. *Thyroid carcinoma, squamous carcinoma of the nasopharynx* and *malignant melanoma* may all present first with enlarged cervical lymph nodes. These nodes tend to be hard, singular and may be fixed to underlying structures. Surgical consultation should be obtained to perform a complete examination of the head and neck to search for a primary lesion. Biopsy of the node is usually required for diagnosis.

Rhabdomyosarcoma is the most common soft-tissue sarcoma of the head and neck in children, and its frequency of occurrence in the neck is second only to that in the orbit. The child will usually present with a history of rapid enlargement of a painless neck mass. The mass itself is hard, often diffuse and poorly mobile. While diagnosis of the rhabdomyosarcoma is often suspected from the history and physical examination, biopsy is usually required for confirmation.

Many other malignant neoplasms can also occur in the neck. These include *soft-tissue sarcomas* other than rhabdomyosarcoma, *malignant fibrous histiocytoma,* and *neuroblastoma.*

Neck Mass

The differential diagnosis and emergency room management of the child with a neck mass is presented in detail in Chapter 27, "Neck Mass."

Torticollis (Wry Neck)

The differential diagnosis and emergency room management of the child with torticollis or stiff neck is presented in detail in Chapter 28, "Neck Stiffness."

Trauma

Neck trauma can be an isolated injury or only one part of a multisystem insult. In evaluating trauma of the neck, the emergency department physician should search for evidence of associated injuries to the vertebral column, head, chest, and abdomen. Management of these potentially more serious injuries may take precedence over the treatment of the cervical trauma.

Neck injuries are usually divided into

blunt and penetrating types. *Blunt trauma* is by far the most common type of injury of the neck, with vehicular (automobile, motorcycle, bicycle) accidents and sports-related activities accounting for the majority of these occurrences. A *bruise* or *hematoma* of the soft tissues of the neck is the most common lesion resulting from blunt injury to the neck. A tear of a small blood vessel allows blood to extravasate and infiltrate adjacent soft tissues. The child will complain of pain and swelling in the affected area. A bluish discoloration of the overlying skin often is not present at the time of the acute injury but will appear 1 or 2 days later. These injuries are most often self-limited and will resolve spontaneously within several days. Heat and rest may aid in this recovery process.

Severe blunt trauma can result in injuries requiring more involved care. A progressively enlarging neck mass following cervical trauma may indicate persistent hemorrhage from a large blood vessel. Surgical consultation should be obtained. An angiogram followed by surgical exploration and ligation of the bleeding vessel may be required in these cases. The airway may become compromised in these patients requiring endotracheal intubation or tracheostomy.

Cranial nerve deficits indicate a serious injury of the deep tissues of the neck or base of skull and require careful neurologic evaluation with possible neck exploration.

A potential late sequela of vascular injury is an *arteriovenous fistula*. Its diagnosis is suggested by a pulsatile mass appearing several weeks after an injury. Surgical exploration and resection of the fistula is the treatment of choice.

Penetrating injuries of the neck pose many difficult problems both in evaluation and management. Once again, severe associated injuries may require treatment first. The nature of the injury must be determined during the initial evaluation: Length of knife, caliber of bullet, number of entrance and exit wounds, apparent course of the missile, etc. The status of the airway should be ascertained; the presence of respiratory distress, stridor, hemoptysis, subcutaneous emphysema or hoarseness can all indicate possible airway injury. A complete neurological examination must be performed to detect injuries to the spinal cord, cranial and other peripheral nerves.

Excessive hemorrhage, absent pulses and an expanding neck mass are all signs of significant vascular injury. Pressure on the bleeding site, angiogram, and surgical exploration may be necessary parts of the management of these injuries. While some authors feel that any neck laceration or penetrating injury that is deep to the platysma muscle requires surgical intervention, most feel that surgical exploration should be performed selectively in those patients who demonstrate signs or symptoms of significant vascular or airway injury.

Blunt trauma to the anterior neck can also result in laryngeal injury, which has been discussed earlier in this chapter. An otolaryngologist should be consulted if there is any suspicion of laryngeal or tracheal injury. He is able to perform the indirect and direct laryngoscopy required to determine the extent of the damage and is prepared to intervene with laryngoscopy, bronchoscopy, endotracheal intubation and tracheostomy as they become necessary for airway management and protection.

The *sternocleidomastoid tumor of infancy* is the most common cause of torticollis in the newborn. Not really a neoplasm, this condition is thought to be related to perinatal trauma. The histopathology of this condition appears to start with a traumatic hematoma within the sternocleidomastoid muscle. The hematoma begins to organize leading to fibrosis of the surrounding damaged muscle during the third or fourth week of life. At this time, a mass is noted within the substance of the sternocleidomastoid muscle. Conservative management, with heat and passive range of motion exercises, is recommended to hasten resolution of the process and to prevent fibrotic shortening of the sternocleidomastoid muscle and resultant torticollis. If the lesion does not begin to recede after 1 to 2 months of this conservative management, surgical exploration and resection of the fibrous mass and lengthening of the sternocleidomastoid muscle may be required.

References

Austin DF: Trauma as it affects the temporal bone. *Laryngoscope* 78: 938–943, 1968.

Banks W, Potsic WP: Elusive unsuspected foreign bodies in the tracheobronchial tree. *Clin Pediatr* 16: 31–35, 1977.

Banks W, Potsic WP: Unsuspected foreign bodies of the aerodigestive tract. *Ann Otol Rhinol Laryngol* 87: 515, 1978.

Batsakis JG: *Tumors of the Head and Neck; Clinical and Pathological Considerations*, Ed. 2. Williams & Wilkins, Baltimore, 1979.

Burket LW, Lynch MA: *Burket's Oral Medicine*, Vol. 7. J.B. Lippincott, Philadelphia, 1977.

Busis SN: Vertigo in children. *Ear Nose Throat J* 57: 20–26, 1978.

Garfinkle TS, Handler SD: Hemangiomas of the head and neck in children; guide to management. *J Otolaryngol* 9: 439–450, 1980.

Handler SD: Maxillo-facial injuries. In *Athletic Injuries to the Head, Neck and Face*, edited by J Torg. Lea & Febiger, Philadelphia, 1982.

Handler SD, Raney RB: Management of neoplasms of the head and neck in children; I. Benign tumors. *Head Neck Surg* 3: 395–405, 1981.

Healey GB: Acute sinusitis in childhood. *Int J Pediatr Otorhinolaryngol* 2: 11–20, 1980.

Jones JH: *Oral Manifestations of Systemic Disease.* W. B. Saunders, Philadelphia, 1980.

Krugman ME, Canalis RF, Konrad HR: The sternomastoid "tumor" of infancy. *J Otolaryngol* 5: 523–529, 1976.

Lane RJ, Keane WM, Potsic WP: Pediatric infectious cervical lymphadenitis. *Otolaryngol Head Neck Surg* 88: 332–335, 1980.

Levitt GW: Cervical fascia and deep neck infections. *Otolaryngol Clin North Am* 9: 703–716, 1976.

May M: Civilian neck injuries; a review. *Ear Nose Throat J* 59: 5–18, 1980.

Montgomery WW: Surgery of the trachea. In *Surgery of the Upper Respiratory System*, Vol 2, pp. 315–372. W. B. Saunders, Philadelphia, 1973.

Northern JL: *Hearing in Children.* Williams & Wilkins, Baltimore, 1974.

Olsen KD, Carpenter RJ, Kern EB: Nasal septal trauma in children. *Pediatrics* 64: 32–35, 1979.

Potsic WP: Management of trauma of the external ear. In *Otolaryngology*, edited by G English. Harper & Row, New York, 1980.

Potsic WP: Middle ear effusions; the thin and thick of it. *Bull NY Acad Med* 53: 806–808, 1977.

Raney RB, Handler SD: Management of neoplasms of head and neck in children; II. Malignant tumors. *Head Neck Surg* 3: 500–507, 1981.

Rankow R: *Diseases of the Salivary Glands.* W. B. Saunders, Philadelphia, 1976.

Senturia BD, et al.: Recent advances in otitis media with effusion. *Ann Otol Rhinol Laryngol* 89 (Suppl 68): May–June 1980.

Senturia BD, et al.: *Diseases of the External Ear.* Grune & Straton, New York, 1980.

Senturia BD, et al.: Recent advances in antimicrobial therapy for infection of the ear, nose and throat—head and neck. *Ann Otol Rhinol Laryngol* 90 (Suppl 84): May–June 1981.

Sessions RB: Nasal hemorrhage. *Otolaryngol Clin North Am* 6: 727–744, 1973.

CHAPTER 63

Urologic Emergencies

HOWARD McC. SNYDER III, M.D.

INTRODUCTION

The act of voiding and the appearance of their genitals are aspects of their lives with which children rapidly grow familiar. Disturbances of either are a great source of concern to them and their parents. This may result in a trip to the emergency department in a high state of anxiety, requiring the emergency physician to be familiar with the problems to be discussed in this section. Reference should be made to Chapter 34, "Scrotal Pain/Swelling." In this chapter, we include (1) penile problems, (2) testicular problems and (3) urinary tract infections. Renal trauma is covered in Chapter 57, "Major Trauma."

PENILE PROBLEMS

Penile Care in the Uncircumcised Male

As it is being increasingly realized in America that there are only rare medical indications for circumcision, there are increasing numbers of uncircumcised children who may be seen in the emergency department. It is surprising how few physicians know how to care for uncircumcised boys. It is important to realize that, in male infants, adhesions between the glans and the foreskin are normal. The foreskin is not normally retractable in this age group. No effort should be made to strip the foreskin back in infants as this not only produces undue pain for the child, but may also result in a raw surface with consequent inflammation and scarring. Between age 2 and 4, there is spontaneous lysis of the adhesions in 90% of children. It is extremely rare for the young male to have any adverse hygenic consequence from leaving the foreskin in place until spontaneous lysis of the adhesions takes place. The small, whitish lumps which may be seen and felt beneath the foreskin represent only desquamated epithelium and need not be removed. When a boy is able to retract his foreskin, usually between 4 and 6 years of age, but sometimes later, he may be taught to withdraw the foreskin and carry out normal hygiene as part of bathing.

Phimosis and Paraphimosis

Phimosis exists when tightness of the distal foreskin precludes its being withdrawn to expose the glans. While inflammation of the foreskin from severe chronic ammoniacal rash or infection may lead to scarring and a true phimosis, this is not common in children. More often, normal penile adhesions are confused with phimosis.

In the uncircumcised male, if the foreskin is retracted behind the glans and left in this position, venous congestion and edema of the foreskin will result, which will make it very difficult to reduce the foreskin to a normal posion. This condition of a swollen, retracted foreskin is termed *paraphimosis.* The application of ice and steady local manual compression will usually reduce the edema and permit manual reduction of the paraphimosis. If this fails, then a surgical division of the foreskin to permit reduction is indicated. This usually may be accomplished with sedation and local anesthetic. If surgical reduction of the foreskin is required, it should be followed a few weeks later by a circumcision. Education in the care of the uncircumcised male will reduce the incidence of this condition.

Balanophosthitis

This term is used to describe an infection of the foreskin which may extend onto the glans. This is a cellulitis and has its origin from a break in the penile skin. This may be the result of local trauma or may, in the older boy, be associated with poor penile hygiene. Scarring following the inflammatory reaction may lead to true phimosis. The acute infection is dealt with adequately by warm soaks and the administration of an appropriate antibiotic, usually ampicillin (50 to 100 mg/kg/24 hours in 4 doses). It is unusual for a child to be unable to void secondary to this condition, although he may be more comfortable voiding while in a tub of warm water. After resolution of the acute infection, the youngster should be examined again, and, if true phimosis is present, a circumcision is advisable. One episode of balanophosthitis with a normal retractable foreskin does not indicate a need for a circumcision. However, if a child has recurrent infections, then a circumcision would be in order.

Penile Swelling

While most penile swelling will be painful and be the result of either infection as described above or trauma to be described later, occasionally a child will be seen who has isolated penile edema which is either non- or minimally tender. This may result from an insect bite, with local edema secondary to histamine release. A history of a bite or the finding of a small punctate lesion may give the clue to diagnosis. Painless penile edema may be seen with a generalized allergic reaction or as part of the manifestation of a general edematous state secondary to renal, cardiac, or hepatic problems. Here the diagnosis is suggested by evidence of this dysfunction in these organ systems on general examination.

Priapism

Prolonged painful penile erection unaccompanied by sexual stimulation is termed priapism. While in the pediatric age group this entity may be caused by trauma or leukemic infiltration, it is most commonly seen in black males with sickle cell disease. A sickling crisis that thus involves the corporal bodies does not necessarily need to be related to symptomatic sickling elsewhere in the body. Sickling of the erythrocytes produces sludging and stasis in the erectile tissue of the corporal bodies. This stasis leads to further hypoxia, acidosis and more sickling. The thick dark sludge which is formed prevents detumescence of the erectile tissue and thus causes priapism. It is speculated that an inflammatory reaction to this material may lead to fibrosis of the erectile tissue. Impotence may result.

While previous recommendations to treat priapism have ranged from ice or hot packs, estrogens, and spinal anesthesia to radiation therapy, the best treatment for priapism associated with sickle cell disease now appears to be hydration and hyper- or exchange transfusion in order to reduce the percentage of hemoglobin S to 30 to 35%. This should be accomplished rapidly and is usually possible within 24 hours. Because of reduced sickling and better venous flow in the erectile tissue, there is usually rapid relief of pain and subsequent gradual detumescence over the next few days. If significant pain persists in spite of reduction of the hemoglobin S, then a surgical procedure to produce detumescence is appropriate. This is rarely needed. While priapism has been documented to lead to impotence in some cases, this is rare in priapism related to sickle cell disease unless the patient has been subjected to a surgical procedure. It may be that the more difficult cases are the ones most likely to come to surgical treatment and thus impotence may reflect the basic disease rather than the type of treatment.

Meatal Stenosis

Meatal stenosis is a problem almost exclusively of circumcised males and follows an inflammatory reaction around the meatus, usually caused by an ammoniacal irritation such as produced by a typical diaper rash. Meatal stenosis is rare in the boy who has a circumcision after becoming continent. Many times appearances are deceiving. The meatus may appear to be stenotic, but may be functioning very adequately. Significant meatal stenosis causes spraying of the urinary stream or dorsal deflection of the stream. Only if these symptoms are present is surgical treatment of the meatus warranted. Meatal stenosis is not a cause of frequency, enuresis or urinary tract infection. When indicated, we carry out a meatotomy in our office after the infiltration of a small amount of Xylocaine with epinephrine into the ventral edge of the meatus. A general anesthetic is generally not necessary or indicated.

Penile Trauma

Direct injury. The most common source of direct injury to the penis comes from the toilet seat falling on the penis of a little boy who is learning to stand at the toilet to void. Although the resulting penile edema may be quite notable, it is rare for a significant injury to the corporal bodies or urethra to take place. Parents may be concerned that the child will be unable to void. This generally is not a problem, although the child may be more comfortable voiding in a tub of warm water. The only treatment required is warm soaks and expectant observation. It should be recalled that a child who has any form of a genital injury may be a victim of sexual abuse (see Chapter 68).

Zipper injury. Boys often seem to be in a hurry and sometimes fail to get their penis or foreskin completely back in their pants before they pull up the zipper. This results in the entrapment of penile skin or foreskin in the teeth of the zipper. The teeth may be so engaged that it is not possible to simply unzip the zipper. Often the problem may be dealt with very simply as shown in Figure 63.1. The median bar of the zipper may be cut with a pair of wire cutters which will permit the two halves of the zipper then to fall apart, releasing the entrapped skin. Local infiltration of Xylocaine will make this much less traumatic to the child. Only rarely will a general anesthetic be required. After the zipper is removed, the penis may become quite edematous, but generally nothing more than warm soaks is required for further treatment.

Strangulation. The penis may be encircled by a constricting ring formed by hair, just as takes place with digits. Many times the cause of the problem is not immediately evident because local edema may hide the ring of hair. The edema is produced by venous engorgement which will take place early, following the development of this type of a constriction around the penis. Once the source of the problem has been identified, therapy requires the division of the hair and the release of the constriction. This may require a general anesthetic. Pediatric urologic consultation is advisable. A urethrocutaneous fistula or even the loss of the penis has been reported, but this is quite rare. How the hair comes to encircle is generally unknown, but it should be remembered that this has been occasionally reported as a form of sexual abuse.

TESTICULAR PROBLEMS

BACKGROUND

Primordial germ cells take their origin from the entoderm of the yolk sac. By the fifth week of intrauterine life, they have reached the ventromedial portion of the urogenital ridge, the portion destined to form the testis. A mesodermal cord, the gubernaculum, comes to be attached to the bottom of the testis at the epididymis and runs to the bottom of the scrotum. With rapid growth of the trunk, the testis comes to lie adjacent to the internal ring by the third month of gestation. The testis remains at this location until the seventh month when, preceded by a fold of peritoneum (the processus), the testis moves down the inguinal canal and reaches its final scrotal position shortly before birth.

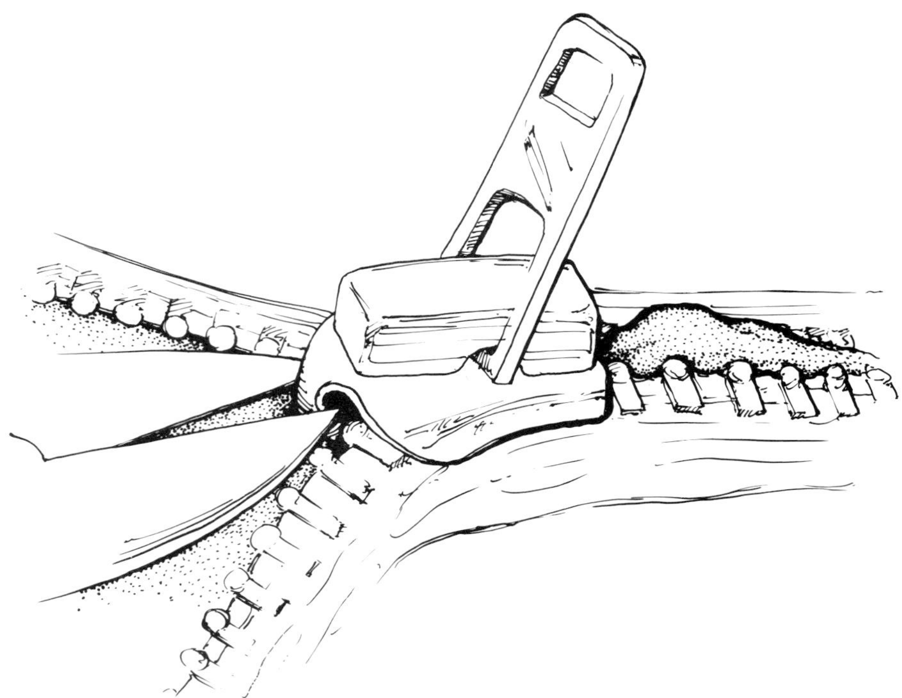

Figure 63.1 Penile zipper injury: a wire cutter may be used to cut the median bar of the zipper, releasing the two sides of the zipper and freeing the penis.

This fact accounts for the higher incidence of undescended testis in premature boys. The gubernaculum appears to have an important role in testicular descent, although the exact nature of its role remains incompletely understood.

Refer to discussion of the acute scrotum in Chapter 34 for acute conditions involving the testis.

Retractile Testis

In the physical examination of the child in the emergency department, an empty scrotum on one or both sides is a frequent finding. While the testis may be found to be truly undescended, more often it is merely a retractile testis. In the boy with a retractile testis, the active cremaster muscle attached to the small prepubertal gonad is able to draw the testis up into a position near the pubic tubercle. When the testis enlarges at puberty, it will assume a scrotal position permanently, as the cremaster is no longer able to draw it out of its more normal position. The diagnosis of a retractile testis is made by being able to milk without difficulty the testis down into a position in a dependent portion of the scrotum. It is not adequate merely to be able to pull the testis into the upper corner of the scrotum. In obese youngsters, it may be difficult to get a grasp on the testis in order to be able to pull it down. It is worthwhile putting a youngster in a "catcher's position" where the testis is pushed down to where it may be able to be grasped and drawn into the scrotum. If a scrotal position cannot be achieved, the youngster should be referred to a pediatric urologist or general surgeon.

Undescended Testis

True undescended testes are seen in 4% of newborn males. This instance decreases to 0.8% by 1 year of age, indicating that some undescended testes do descend after birth. Spontaneous descent rarely occurs after 1 year. While it may be appropriate to continue to observe an infant who has an undescended testis for a few months, the child over 1 year of age should have pediatric urologic or pediatric surgical consultation.

Testicular malignancy and infertility are increased in the male with an uncorrected undescended testis. By electron microscopy, it is possible to demonstrate degenerative changes in the undescended testis by 1 year of age. Early referral to a pediatric urologist or pediatric surgeon for orchidopexy (before age 2 and preferably near 1) appears advisable, as data are now accumulating that indicates early surgery may decrease the incidence of both testicular malignancy and infertility.

Usually an undescended testis is asymptomatic. However, in a position against the abdominal wall, it may be more subject to trauma than when freely mobile in the scrotum. The undescended testis also is malfixed and may undergo torsion more easily than a normally descended one. The boy who presents with an acutely tender groin mass with an ipsilateral empty scrotum may have a torsion of his undescended testis. The physician must consider the differential diagnosis of an incarcerated inguinal hernia or acute hydrocele of the cord. Prompt surgical treatment is required in order to prevent infarction of the testis with torsion.

Varicocele

Varicoceles are an abnormal dilatation of the cremasteric and pampiniform venous plexuses surrounding the spermatic cord. They generally present as an asymptomatic scrotal swelling about the time of puberty and are rare in the prepubertal boy. Almost all are of congenital origin and affect the left testis. The anatomic problem is a defect in the valves of the spermatic vein which, on the left, drains directly into the left renal vein. Why varicoceles are often not noted until a boy approaches puberty is unclear. Usually no evaluation or therapy is indicated. If the varicocele does not disappear when the child lies down, this suggests a varicocele secondary to obstruction of the left renal vein and an intravenous pyelogram is appropriate. If the boy complains of pain, urologic referral for ligation of the varicocele is appropriate. This is not frequently necessary.

In adult males, varicocele has been occasionally shown to be associated with infertility, presumably secondary to defective spermatogenesis caused by the increased temperature produced by the nest of veins surrounding the testis. The testis on the affected side may be smaller or softer under these conditions. As up to 19% of adolescent males have small, asymptomatic varicoceles, it does not appear logical to suggest that all varicoceles which are seen in young boys need ligation. Controversy exists on this point, however, and no good prospective studies have been reported to help identify the boys who should have their varicoceles surgically treated.

URINARY TRACT INFECTIONS

BACKGROUND

Urinary tract infections (UTI) rank as the second most common form of bacterial infection in children behind upper respiratory problems. Between 1 and 2% of infants and children have bacteriuria at any given time, and 5% of all girls will have UTI during their school years. Except in the newborn, in whom UTI may be caused by hematogenous spread of bacteria to the kidneys, most UTI result from fecal bacteria on the perineal skin ascending the urethra. The short female urethra, with resultant ease of bacterial contamination of the bladder, accounts for the higher incidence of UTI in girls.

A UTI may be defined as the multiplication of bacteria in the urinary tract. Normally, urine from the bladder and upper urinary tract should be sterile. The concept of "significant bacteriuria" ($>10^5$ organisms/ml of one colony type) in a clean voided midstream specimen is based on the statistical likelihood that this colony count is associated with the actual presence of bacteria in the bladder. A colony count of $>10^5$ organisms/ml of a single type suggests infected urine with an 80% confidence level. Reliability can be increased to 95% if a second culture confirms the presence of the same bacteria type with identical antibiotic sensitivity; 10^4 to 10^5 bacteria/ml is an equivocal result and requires repeat culture. Less than 10^4 organisms/ml, or the presence of several different organisms, suggests no infection, or contamination of the specimen.

CLINICAL MANIFESTATIONS

Particularly in the infant, UTI may produce very nonspecific findings. The urine may be cloudy or have a foul odor. There may be a history of unexplained fevers, general irritability or failure to thrive and gain weight normally. Gastrointestinal symptoms are frequent, and many times the youngster with a urinary tract infection is felt to have gastroenteritis or a food allergy. A high index of suspicion is required. If a urine culture is not obtained, the source of the child's problem will be missed.

In the older child, symptoms may point more directly at the urinary tract. Frequency, urgency and dysuria are produced by inflammation of the bladder and urethra. A previously toilet-trained child may begin to have "accidents." Particularly in girls, hematuria may be seen. Although symptoms do not provide a completely reliable way of differentiating cystitis from pyelonephritis, the presence of systemic findings, such a as high fever and malaise or abdominal/flank pain, suggests renal involvement. A UTI, especially when chronic, may also have few, if any, symptoms.

It is important to emphasize that in children anything which irritates the urethral meatus may produce dysuria and occasional urgency and frequency (see Chapters 17 and 37). The source of the irritation may be a tight or moist bathing suit or underwear or an ammoniacial-type rash. Bubble bath or other soap in contact with the urethral meatus may not only produce these symptoms, but, by producing inflammation, contribute to the ascent of bacteria up the urethra and the development of true infection. In order to avoid being confused by noninfectious etiology of symptoms, it is important that an actual UTI be demonstrated by urine culture and not diagnosed by history and urinalysis alone.

Escherichia coli is the most frequently isolated organism responsible for UTI in children, constituting 80 to 90% of the total. This is due to the prevalence of this organism in gastrointestinal tract flora, as well as its short mean generation time which enables it to multiply rapidly once it has entered the bladder. The other organisms commonly found can be seen in Table 63.1.

MANAGEMENT

The first step in management is to *make an accurate diagnosis.* The presence of pyuria does not provide an accurate criteria for the diagnosis of a UTI. At least 20% of children with pyuria do not demonstrate significant bacteriuria. In any febrile illness, mobilization of the peripheral leukocyte pool may be adequate to produce the presence of white cells in the urine. Conversely, a child with bacteriuria occasionally does not demonstrate pyuria. Bacteria demonstrated by Gram stain of an unspun urine specimen are more reliably indicative of a UTI. However, it is difficult to determine if one bacteria or several different contaminants are present. Thus, culture of the urine must continue to be the benchmark for the diagnosis of a UTI in children.

The *obtaining of an adequate urine specimen* for bacterial culture is the most critical step in diagnosing a UTI. A clean voided specimen obtained as a midstream catch after the washing of the periurethral area is the preferred technique in the toilet-trained child. Simple soap and water washing of the periurethral area is preferred as antimicrobial soaps or solutions may become mixed with a voided specimen and lead to a false negative result.

Table 63.1
Bacteria Commonly Causing Urinary Tract Infections

Escherichia coli
Klebsiella pneumoniae
Streptococcus faecalis (enterococcus)
Proteus species
Pseudomonas aeruginosa
Staphylococcus epidermidis

In the infant, obtaining an adequate urine specimen is more difficult. Specimens collected in a plastic bag (U-bag) attached to the perineum are rapidly contaminated by perineal bacterial skin flora. If a culture from a bag is sterile, it is acceptable. However, the demonstration of bacterial growth must be confirmed by some other means before a bona fide UTI can be presumed to be present. The most reliable way to obtain a confirming specimen of urine is by means of suprapubic aspiration of urine from the bladder. This is not a dangerous procedure and has a reliability approaching 100%. The procedure for performing suprapubic aspiration is covered in Section VII. In the female, a specimen obtained by urethral catheterization is an acceptable alternative. If it is essential that the first specimen be the definitive one for diagnosis of UTI, as in the infant undergoing septic workup, then the primary use of these techniques is justified.

When symptoms strongly suggest the possibility of a UTI, we recommend beginning *antibiotic therapy* as soon as an adequate urine specimen for culture has been obtained. The matter of just a day or two before the institution of antibiotics may make a difference in the degree of pyelonephritic scarring which takes place. If the urine culture turns out to be negative, then the antibiotics may be stopped. Table 63.2 lists the most commonly used outpatient antibiotics for urinary tract infections.

Trimethoprim-sulfamethoxazole in a dose of 1 ml/kg/day in 2 divided doses is also an excellent drug; however, we reserve it for more difficult cases. Methenamine mandelate is not useful unless there is urinary statis and acid urine, and accordingly has little role in most childhood UTI. Tetracycline is not recommended in the child under 8 years of age because of its potential for discoloration of the teeth. When the organism causing UTI is sensitive to the antibiotic selected, the urine is usually rapidly sterilized. It is advisable to repeat a culture 48 hours after starting an antibiotic. The continued presence of infection suggests inaccuracy of the sensitivity, noncompliance or obstruction.

Table 63.2
Antibiotic Agents for Urinary Tract Infections

Drugs	Oral Dose (mg/kg/day)	No. of Doses
Sulfisoxazole	120	4
Nitrofurantoin	5–7	4
Amoxicillin	50–100	3
Cephalexin	25–50	4

If a child is sufficiently toxic to warrant *hospitalization*, the intravenous administration of antibiotics is appropriate. The drugs of choice while cultures are pending are a cephalosporin or aminoglycoside, singly or in combination.

The duration of therapy has been subject to recent debate, with some evidence emerging that 1 to 3 days of therapy may be as efficacious, especially in the treatment of infection confined to the bladder, as the conventional 10-day course of antibiotics which most continue to recommend. Follow-up cultures should be routinely carried out.

Other factors in the treatment of UTI involve high fluid intake with regular and frequent voidings to promote bladder washout of bacteria. Avoiding constipation helps to ensure better bladder emptying. Good perineal hygiene, including wiping from front to back after a bowel movement, is important. Eliminating pinworms prevents a source for inflammation, excoriation and secondary increase in perineal skin flora. Bubble bath by producing inflammation at the meatus may promote the ascent of bacteria and should be avoided. Acidification of the urine with oral vitamin C or juices high in citric acid content may be useful by producing an acid urine in which bacteria multiply less rapidly.

Follow-Up of UTI and Radiographic Investigation

A suppressive dose of antibiotics should be begun following the acute phase of full dose treatment. It is customary to use ⅓ to ½ the dose of antibiotic used for actue treatment, usually administered in a once-a-day evening dose. Suppressive antibiotics will reduce the likelihood of recurrent infection pending urologic consultation and radiographic investigation.

The routine radiographic evaluation of a urinary tract infection is by means of a voiding cystourethrogram (VCUG) followed by an intravenous pyelogram (IVP). Usually these studies are carried out about 2 to 4 weeks after the acute treatment of a UTI; however, failure of a child to respond promptly to appropriate antibiotic therapy should lead to the urgent performance of an IVP to rule out urinary obstruction. The cystogram must include a voiding phase, or significant pathology may be missed, particularly vesicoureteral reflux which may be evident only on voiding films. In the usual child with a UTI, cystoscopy contributes little to the initial investigation, so we do not routinely carry this out.

All boys should be investigated after their first urinary tract infection. In little girls, previous recommendations were to wait until a second infection had taken place before recommending urographic investigation. Kunin's data demonstrate that after one UTI, there is an 80% likelihood of a second episode of bacteriuria and that half of these children will be asymptomatic. It thus appears justified to carry out radiographic studies after a first documented infection in girls as well as boys.

In approximately 50% of infants and 30% of older children, an anatomical abnormality will be found in association with a UTI. The most common finding is vesicoureteral reflux. Reflux permits infected urine to ascend to the kidney where pyelonephritic damage may occur. With linear growth of the child, many milder cases of reflux may spontaneously cease, leaving surgical management primarily for the more severe cases. These decisions are best made in consultation with a pediatric urologist.

In the child who has no abnormality demonstrated by IVP and VCUG, the parents can be reassured that while the child may have a symptomatic problem from cystitis, there is little likelihood of renal damage. Occasionally, if a child has frequent episodes of symptomatic cystitis, suppressive antibiotics are justified in order to reduce the morbidity of these infections. Although the reason these children develop frequent UTI remains to be fully clarified, in many the problem fortunately appears to lessen with time.

Acute Urinary Retention

A patient with acute urinary retention is unable to empty the bladder even though it is full. In children, as adults, this may be due to a urethral obstruction. Congenital lesions, such as urethral valves, or acquired lesions, such as post-traumatic strictures may lead to urinary retention. In these cases, a careful history will often elicit symptoms of a weak stream or difficulty initiating the stream. Children who have any form of urethral irritation and dysuria may voluntarily retain urine. This is a different situation and needs to be differentiated carefully from organic obstruction causing retention. For the child with voluntary retention, usually gentle massage of the lower abdomen combined with a soak in a warm tub will lead to spontaneous evacuation of the bladder. It should be remembered that a child is able to voluntarily hold urine for longer periods than would be suspected. Up to 12 hours is not unusual. Unless the child has a history suggestive of an organic obstruction or has a palpably enlarged bladder which has not been able to be emptied by massage and warm tub soaks, we would not consider instrumenting the child's urethra. Pediatric urologic consultation would be advisable before undertaking such maneuvers.

Penile Problems

Baron M, Leiter E: The management of priapism in sickle cell anemia. *J Urol* 119: 610–11, 1978.

Kinney TR, Harris MB, Russell MO, Duckett JW, Schwartz E: Priapism in association with sickle hemoglobinopathies in children. *J Pediatr* 86: 241–2, 1975.

Oosterlinck W: Unbloody management of penile zipper injury. *Eur Urol* 7: 365, 1981.

Osborn LM, Metcalf TJ, Mariani EM: Hygenic care in uncircumcised infants. *Pediatrics* 67: 365–367, 1981.

Rifkind S, Waisman J, Thompson R, Goldfinger D: RBC exchange phoresis for priapism in sickle cell disease. *JAMA* 242: 2317–2318, 1979.

Seeler RA: Intensive transfusion therapy for priapism in boys with sickle cell anemia. *J Urol* 110: 360–361, 1973.

Wallerstein E: *Circumcision: An American Health Fallacy*. Springer, New York, 1980.

Testicular Problems

Bierich JR, Giarola A (Eds.): *Cryptorchidism.* Academic Press, London, 1979.

Dubin L, Amelar RD: Varicocelectomy as therapy in male infertility: a study of 504 cases. *J Urol* 111: 640, 1975.

Fonkalsrud EW, Mengel W: *The Undescended Testis.* Yearbook, Chiago, 1981.

Oster, J: Varicocele in children and adolescents: an investigation of the incidence among Danish school children. *Scand J Urol Nephrol* 5: 27, 1971.

Scorer CG, Farrington GH: Congenital deformities of the testis and epididymis. Butterworths, London, 1971.

Urinary Tract Infections

Kaye D (Ed.): *Urinary Tract Infection and Its Management.* C. V. Mosby, St. Louis, 1972.

Kunin CM: *Detection, Prevention and Management of Urinary Tract Infections.* Lea & Febiger, Philadelphia, 1979.

Stamey TA: *Pathogenesis and Treatment of Urinary Tract Infections.* Williams & Wilkins, Baltimore, 1980.

CHAPTER **64**

Plastic Surgical Emergencies: Facial Injuries and Burns

LINTON A. WHITAKER, M.D.

INTRODUCTION

The emergency department physician sees numerous injuries to the face, many minor burns to all areas of the body, and some major burns. Thus, a basic knowledge of plastic surgery principles can be beneficial. This chapter will cover the evaluation and management of the common injuries to the face and treatment of burns. It will also give guidelines as to which injuries are appropriate for management in the emergency department and which are not.

Several points will first be made, and not repeated later in this chapter. Patients who have suffered significant facial trauma, resulting from any etiology, always have the potential for occult injuries elsewhere. In particular, the cranium, cervical spine, larynx, thorax and abdomen are always at risk. Even in the presence of grotesque facial injuries, attention must be directed elsewhere once airway stability is assured.

The airway should be cleared and examined and a determination made of the risk to it from subsequent swelling or bleeding. Because of the tremendous local blood supply, lacerations of the face or mouth can fill the pharynx with blood. Also, teeth or foreign bodies can be pushed into the pharynx from the blow. Suctioning, and a search for foreign bodies in the pharynx, is therefore important. Loss of support, because of fracture to the mandibular arch, can allow the tongue to fall posteriorly and occlude the airway in a comatose patient. If urgent, a towel clip may be placed through the tip of the tongue allowing it to be pulled outward and thereby relieve the obstruction.

If a patient who is initially alert and cooperative becomes drowsy or agitated the airway may be closing off. This patient may attempt to sit up, thereby clearing or improving the airway. If other injuries do not preclude this, the patient should be allowed to sit.

It is the extremely rare situation that requires tracheostomy on an emergency basis. Most airway problems can be handled with oral or nasal airway tubes, endotracheal intubation, or, as previously mentioned, traction on the tongue. As a rule tracheostomy should be reserved for the operating room.

Although edema of the tongue, pharynx larynx or neck may be insignificant at first it can be progressive and substantial. Therefore, such patients with potential airway occlusion should be frequently checked, both in the emergency department and following admission.

The cervical spine is of concern, not because of its immediate threat to life, but because of the potential consequences if an injury there is ignored. The head and neck should be treated delicately until an injury to the cervical spine is ruled out. If there is any question, the head should be stabilized by sandbags or with the use of an attendant's hands, until a lateral film of the complete cervical spine can be obtained to rule out a spine injury. See Chapter 67 for a more complete discussion.

The final point relates to tetanus immune status. Although not of immediate concern, the date of the patient's most recent immunization should be determined and a tetanus toxoid booster given if needed. This includes patients with lacerations, burns, or abrasions. Guidelines for reimmunization are given in Chapter 45, "Infectious Diseases."

FACIAL INJURIES

BACKGROUND

The etiology of facial injuries is varied. Three broad categories include accidents in or about the home, vehicular accidents, and assault. In the pediatric age group, injuries are relatively more frequent in the home. Falls against various objects account for a large number of injuries in children. Depending upon the fall, the injury can vary from a small abrasion to a substantial laceration, or even a fracture. As children grow, begin riding bicycles, and playing sports, the severity of the injury tends to increase.

CLINICAL MANIFESTATIONS

Fractures of the mandible can occur in any of a number of areas (Fig. 64.1) (symphysis, body, etc.). When one fracture is found, another should be looked for, particularly in the area of the neck of the condyle. Anesthesia of the teeth and lower lip is a sign of fracture with entrapment of the inferior alveolar nerve. Once fractures occur, segments of the mandible can be pulled out of their normal position by the local musculature. This will result in a change in occlusion, which the patient will notice. A frequent facial fracture in younger children is the mandibular subcondylar fracture (Fig. 64.1). This can be secondary to a fall, with the child striking his chin. Growth disturbances are possible with this fracture. It should be carefully looked for clinically and on x-ray. Pain and/or difficulty opening the mouth are important signs.

The so-called blowout fracture of the orbit is a response to a compression of the

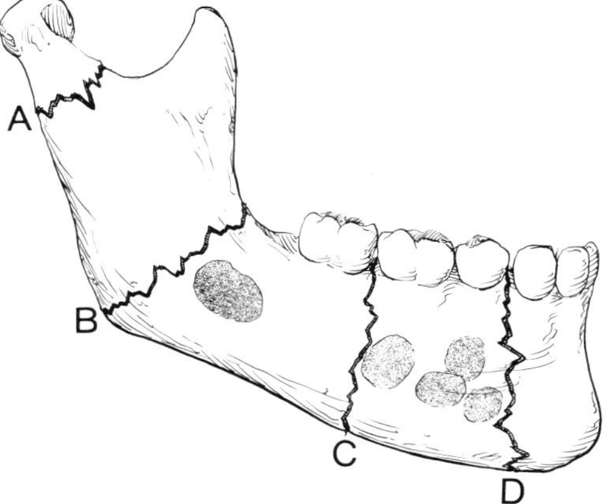

Figure 64.1. Examples of various types of possible mandibular fractures. A child's mandible with unerupted dentition is shown. (*A*) Subcondylar fracture, (*B*) fracture at the angle, (*C*) body fracture, and (*D*) symphyseal fracture.

orbital contents (Fig. 64.2). The orbital floor is broken through when force is applied to the eye itself. On x-ray, a Waters' view, or a posteroanterior view shows opacification of the maxillary sinus (Fig. 64.3) It should be noted that the maxillary sinus is frequently not seen well until about 4 years of age. With the increased orbital volume, the eye tends to drop in the orbit, producing enophthalmos and a lowering of the eye.

Because of their prominent position on the face, the nasal bones are the most frequently fractured when all age groups are considered. The fracture can be difficult to detect clinically because of the edema that is often present. X-rays will sometimes be helpful. A concomitant injury is the septal hematoma. Bleeding can occur beneath the septal mucosa. If left unrecognized it can cause necrosis of the septal cartilage with resultant loss of support.

Zygomatic fractures occur in response to a blow to the malar area. A malar ("tripod") fracture (Fig. 64.4) involves fractures across the zygomaticofrontal suture, infraorbital rim and zygomaticotemporal junction. This can produce a shift of the malar eminence. It may be difficult for the patient to open his mouth. If the infraorbital or superior alveolar nerves have been traumatized, there may be anesthesia of the nasolabial area or maxillary teeth.

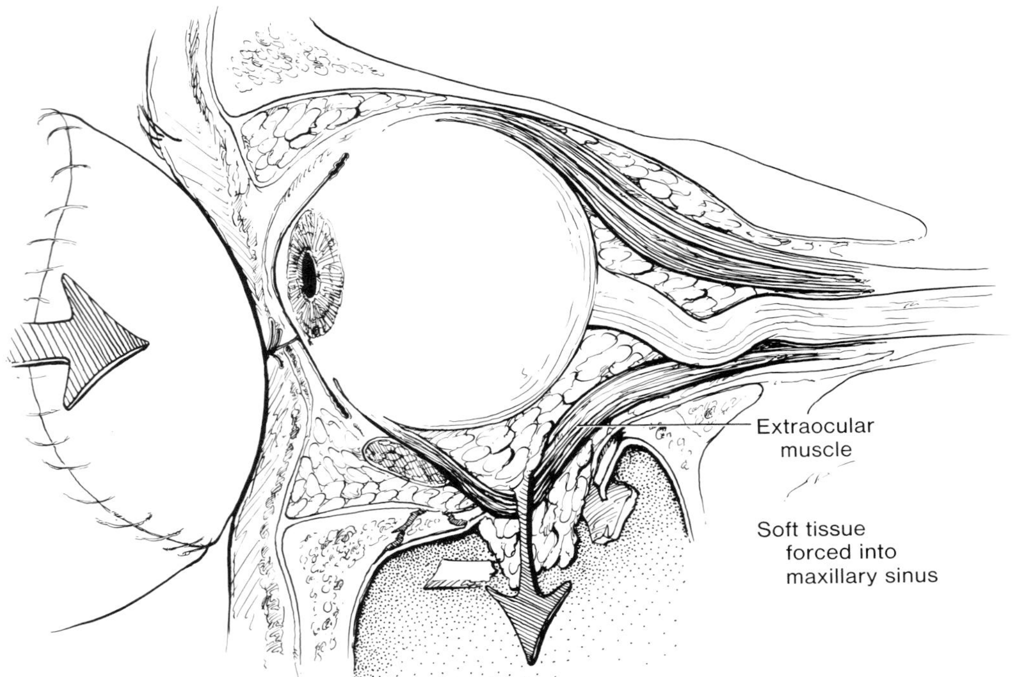

Figure 64.2 Mechanism of blowout fracture. In a sagittal view, a ball is shown striking the eye deforming it and causing increased pressure of the intraorbital contents. The periorbital fat is forced through the floor of the orbit. There can be retropositioning of the eye (enophthalmos), lowering of the eye, and extraocular muscle entrapment as a result.

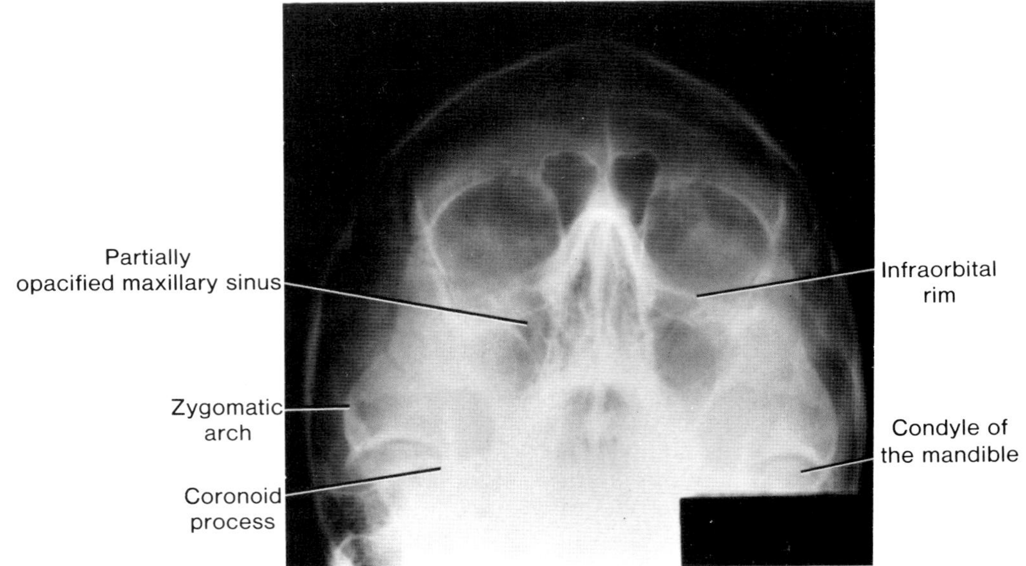

Figure 64.3 Waters' view of the skull demonstrating a number of important facial bone structures. Note the clouded right maxillary sinus in conjunction with a malar fracture on patient's right side.

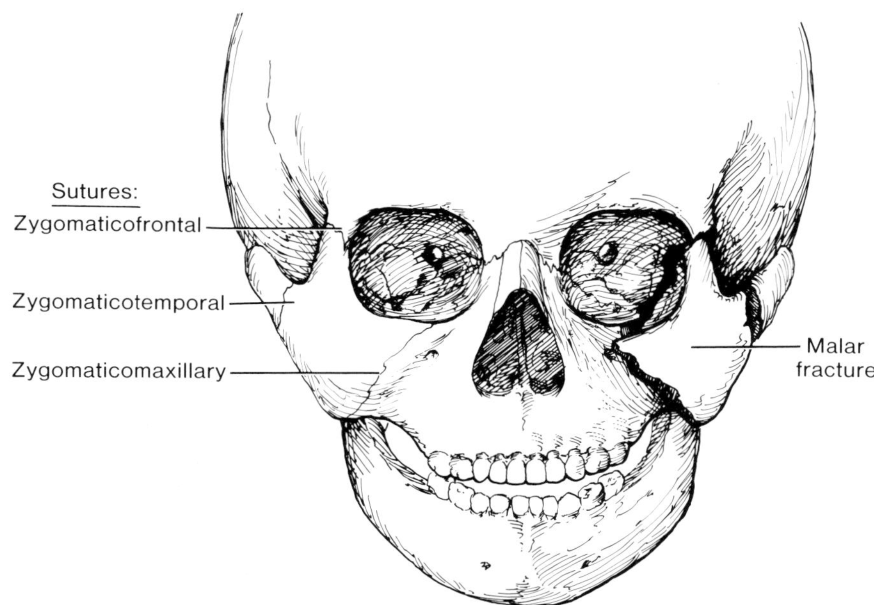

Figure 64.4 Zygomatic sutures and a malar fracture are shown. Fractures do not necessarily occur at these points. The zygomaticofrontal suture separation occurs most frequently.

Lacerations are usually more straightforward in their presentation. They can, however, involve local structures aside from the skin. A deep laceration can transect various branches of the facial nerve or the parotid duct (Fig. 64.5). This will result in an inability to move a given area of the face, or in saliva entering the wound rather than the mouth.

As flaps of tissue are separated from their natural bed, their viability is compromised. Blood supply is dependent upon the base of the flap. It follows that the distal-most portion of the flap (tip) is most at risk. If the flap has a very narrow base and is raised at a superficial level, there is less circulation in comparison to a broad, thick, flap.

The edges of a simple, linear type of laceration may also be at risk, if the injury was of a crushing type. The tissue at the margins may have been totally or partially destroyed by the crushing force, negating the presence of a healthy, broad, vascular bed.

MANAGEMENT

The keys to successful management include: (1) making a complete assessment of the injury including history, physical examination, and radiographic studies; (2) determine the guidelines for plastic surgical consultation; and (3) following specific guidelines.

Assessment

Since many facial injuries will eventually result in the victim filing a law suit against an automobile owner, pet owner, etc., it is important for the emergency department physician to obtain a complete, detailed history. If the patient is not able to give an adequate history, an observer of the accident should be sought and questioned. Pictures of the injury should be taken and made part of the chart.

For purposes of treatment, the mechanism and instrument of injury and the likelihood of contamination should be determined. For example, did a sharp blade cause a clean wound with healthy margins, or did the head of the patient strike a blunt object in an automobile that crushed the skin and ripped it open? Is there likely to be glass or debris from the road within the wound? How was the wound treated prior to arrival at the hospital, and how long ago

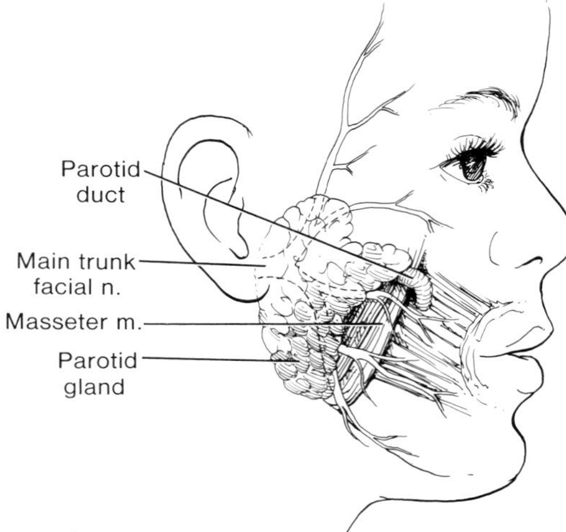

Figure 64.5. Deep lacerations to to the cheek can injure the facial nerve, parotid gland, or parotid duct. The facial nerve becomes more superficial as it branches and proceeds distally. Distal nerve injuries can thus occur with more superficial wounds.

did the injury occur? These are important questions to be answered, if possible, during the history.

Examination

Soft Tissue Injuries

Abrasions of the face should be evaluated for size, area, likely depth of the wound, presence of foreign bodies, and exposure of underlying structures. These are all important points that the primary physician and consultant will need to know in formulating a treatment plan. It is sometimes difficult to determine how deep is a particular wound. For example, the wound may have to be thoroughly cleansed of debris before an adequate evaluation can be made. Local anesthesia will frequently need to be given before this can be done.

Probably the most frequently seen laceration of the face is the simple, linear laceration. When this has been done with a sharp object and is relatively superficial, it is a fairly simple problem. However, when the injuring object was blunt (or sharp, but at an angle), different problems exist. The configuration of the laceration may be a U- or V-shaped flap, or it may be stellate (i.e., several lacerations emanating from a central point). (Fig. 64.6)

The major concern here is the viability of the flap. The wound margins should, therefore, be examined for discoloration and capillary refill. Depending on the mechanism of the injury and depth of the laceration, the entire flap could be lost. These flaps must, therefore, be handled gently during cleaning and evaluation.

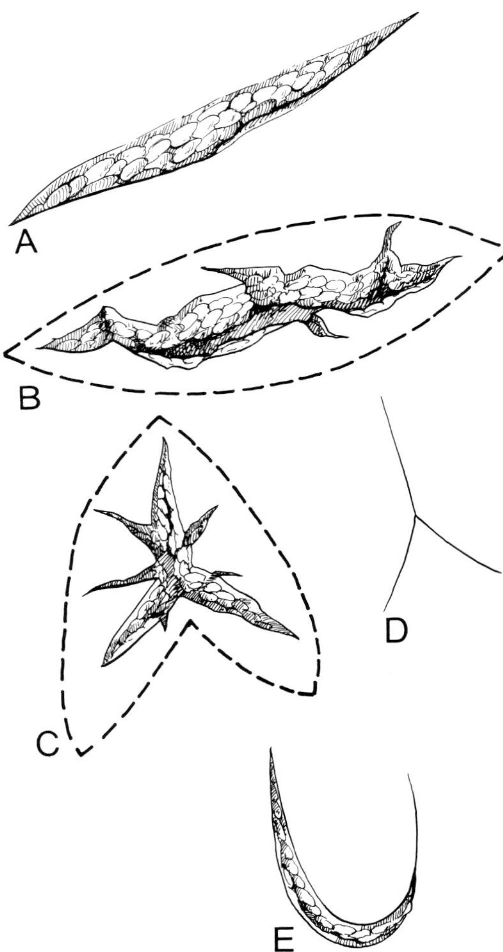

Figure 64.6. Variation in laceration injuries and suggestions for management: (*A*) simple laceration, (*B*) ellipical excision of damaged wound margins, (*C*) and (*D*) excision and closure of stellate laceration, and (*E*) flap-type laceration.

Prior to exploration of any wound it is usually advisable to administer some type of local anesthesia. The most frequently used is 1% Xylocaine with 1:100,000 or 1:200,000 epinephrine solution. The epinephrine should not be used if there is any question of tissue viability or the injury involves an end organ, such as the tip of nose or the margin of the ear. Maximum doses of Xylocaine are 4.5 mg/kg for plain solution (maximum dose 300 mg) and 7 mg/kg with solution with epinephrine (maximum dose 500 mg). This can be injected through the wound itself, if feasible, in order to lessen the discomfort to the patient. A fine (27 gauge) needle should be used and the solution injected slowly as the needle is passed distally. Consideration can also be given to p.o. or i.v. sedation, such as diazepam. This frequently lessens the patient's apprehensions, and it makes both evaluation and treatment much easier for the patient and the doctor. If an airway or CNS problem exists, sedatives or narcotics are inadvisable.

An attempt should be made during the initial evaluation to determine if foreign bodies are present within the wound. Some are obvious, but others are not. Profuse irrigation and careful probing are necessary. Glass in small pieces is difficult to find. Some glass will not show up on routine x-rays. In cases where there is a reasonable suspicion for more glass being present, a xeroradiogram may be helpful; but there is concern about the amount of radiation to which the patient is subjected with this study. It may, therefore, be inadvisable in children.

With deep lacerations of the face, the likelihood of injury to underlying structures is increased. The facial nerve and parotid duct are the structures most subject to injury. The facial nerve lies buried deeply at its exit from the stylomastoid foramen and injuries here at the main trunk are rare. As it courses through the parotid gland to reach the facial muscles, it becomes more superficial. If the patient is conscious, it is easy to determine if any branches have been injured by having the patient move the various facial muscles (wrinkle forehead, close eyes tightly, whistle, smile). Similarly, if a laceration has come across the midcheek and Stensen's (parotid) duct has potentially been injured, a check of the papilla intraorally on the buccal mucosa of the cheek at the second maxillary molar will reveal the presence or absence of saliva. If there is none, a search of the wound must be made.

Puncture wounds secondary to a bite or a sharp object can be evaluated relatively simply, since they are limited in size. However, this must be done with some diligence, since a foreign body can be implanted relatively deeply and can be hidden by a small flap of tissue. Therefore, an effort should be made to probe the wound, after anesthetizing if needed, and determining if flaps of skin have been invaginated into the wound. If they have been, they should be gently elevated. Larger complex lacerations will usually not be handled by the emergency department physician, but a detailed description of the injury will be helpful to the consultant, when called.

The mouth should be thoroughly examined for lacerations of the mucosa or the tongue, injury to the palate and loose or missing teeth. Persistent bleeding points may cause problems in the comatose patient who cannot protect his airway or in an awake child who simply continues to swallow the blood until vomiting occurs. Chapter 66, "Dental Emergencies", details specific oral injuries.

Two areas of potential "quiet" soft tissue injuries involve the ear and nose. The subperichondral hematoma of the ear is most frequently seen in boxers and wrestlers, and characterized by a swelling of the conchal (concave) area of the pina. With any blunt trauma to the nose, a nasal speculum should be used to examine the septum for a septal hematoma. Gentle palpation of the septum with an instrument will differentiate hematoma from fracture displacement. The importance of looking for these injuries is that they can be treated easily. If the injuries are missed they can cause permanent deformities.

Bony Injuries

If enough force has been absorbed to fracture a facial bone, except for isolated nasal bone fractures, other areas of the head and neck must be thoroughly examined. The cranium, cervical spine, and peripheral neurologic status are all important. Cervical spine x-rays are mandatory. Leakage of clear fluid through the nose or the ear may be suggestive of cerebrospinal fluid leak. Weakness of an *entire* facial nerve when no lacerations are present is suggestive of a temporal bone fracture, which may not be obvious on x-ray.

Examination begins with observation (Fig. 64.7). The patient should be observed full face and also from the top of the head. Particular attention should be directed at any asymmetries. This will reflect either edema on one side or a depressed fracture on the other. Any differences will be assessed in the second or palpation stage of evaluation. In particular the malar prominence and zygomatic arch are well seen from above. Deviation or flattening of the nose should be obvious. Periorbital ecchymosis and rounding of the medial canthi, with depression of the nasal bones, indicate a severe injury to the area of the nasal bones (Fig. 64.8).

During observation, careful examination of the eyes is extremely important. Even if there is considerable edema present, the lids should be opened and the eye examined for injuries. Gross visual acuity should be checked and charted. The patient's extraocular motions should be checked and any evidence of orbital entrapment noted, including the direction of the immobility. Also, if possible, a determination should be made as to whether there is any enophthalmos, and any difference in eye level (see Chapter 61).

Inspection of the mouth is important in the evaluation of possible jaw fractures. The patient should be asked to bite down and then asked if his bite feels normal. Observation should be made as to what type of occlusion the patient has (i.e., is there a crossbite deformity, anterior open bite deformity, etc.). Altered occlusion is usually indicative of a maxillary or mandibular fracture. The floor of the mouth often becomes ecchymotic if there has been a fracture of the mandible. If the patient experiences pain upon opening the mouth, suspicion is also raised for a mandibular fracture. If the patient complains of preauricular pain on opening, and the jaw deviates to that side, a subcondylar fracture is likely.

Gentle palpation is the next step in evaluation. To be orderly, this may begin cephalad and progress caudad. The forehead and supraorbital rims are first palpated for any depressions. Here, and around the orbits themselves, note should be taken if there is any subcutaneous emphysema, indicating that a fracture has occurred through one of the sinuses. Careful comparison should be made during palpation side to side. If there are asymmetries, it must be decided if this is because of a depression on one side or an elevation on the other side. Nearly always, it will be because of a depression on the injured side.

The zygomatic arches should next be followed from the zygomatic process of the temporal bone anteriorly across the arch to the malar area and then across the inferior orbital rims. The arch of the zygoma is one area that can become raised beyond its normal level because of buckling outwardly from a blow to the malar eminence. The arches, when palpated simultaneously, can be compared side to side even when considerable edema is present. Step offs of the infraorbital rim should be noted. The nasal dorsum, if fractured, can be mobile but may be in numerous small fragments and difficult to palpate.

Maxillary fractures are checked for by grasping the anterior maxilla in the area of the incisors and attempting to move it. Alveolar fractures should be looked for in the same fashion. Fractures of the mandibular body can sometimes be digitally palpated along the lingual aspect of the mandible intraorally. Gross fractures and step offs are usually easily palpable. The body of the mandible can be grasped on either side, with the right hand of the examiner on the left body and the left hand on the right body of the mandible. The index and long fingers can be placed within the mouth and the thumbs in the submental area. An attempt is then made to produce an abnormal motion in the mandible by torquing the bodies in opposite directions. Light pres-

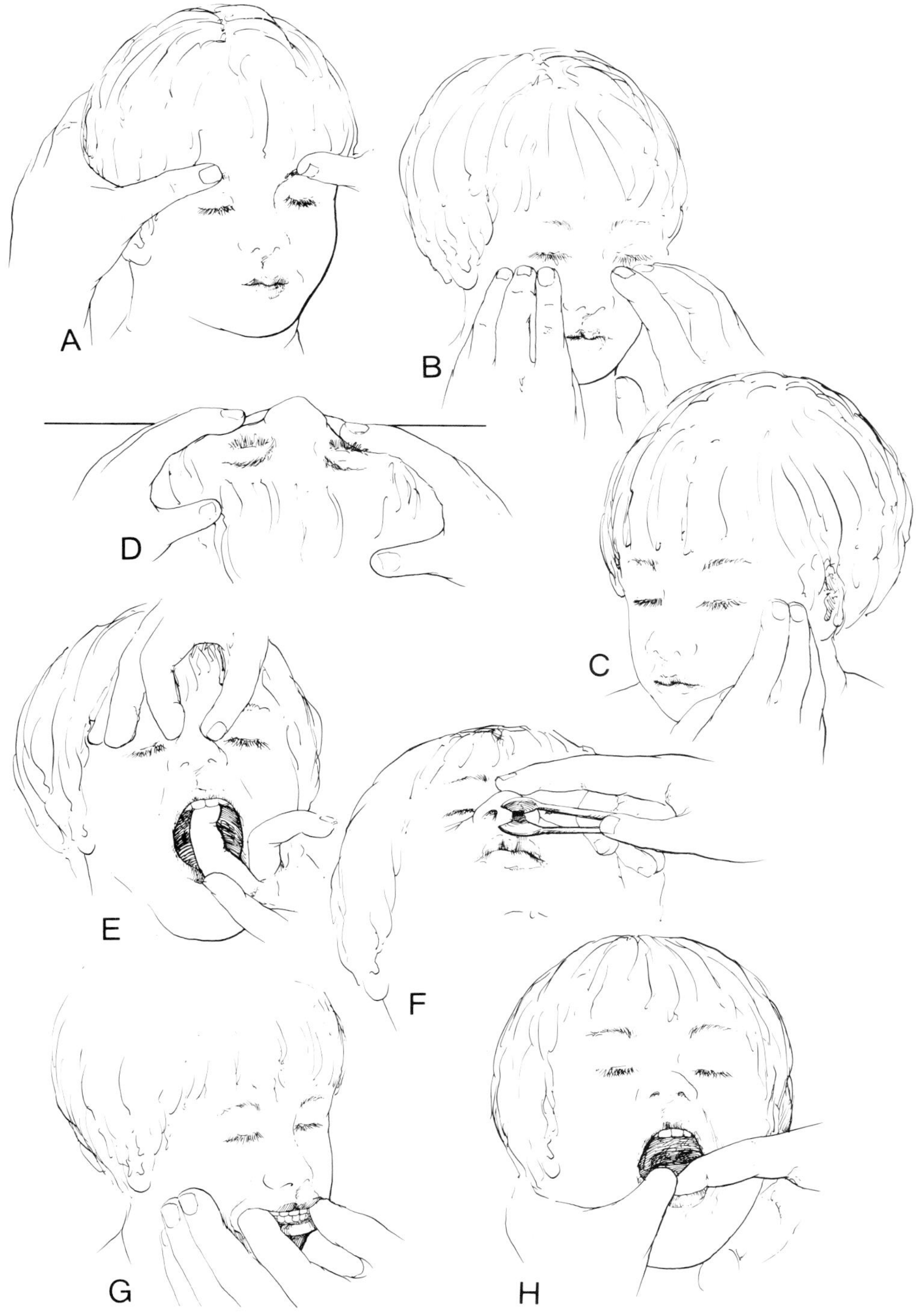

Figure 64.7 Sequential steps in examination for facial fractures. (*A*) The supraorbital ridges are palpated while steadying the patient's head. (*B*) The infraorbital ridges are lightly palpated using the index, middle, and ring fingers to determine symmetry or fractures. (*C*) The zygomatic arch is palpated on each side to determine continuity and the possible presence of displaced fractures. (*D*) The infraorbital rims, zygomatic bodies, and maxilla are palpated and examined from the top of the head to determine depressions and fracture displacements. (*E*) The nasal bone and maxilla are examined for stability and possible fracture displacement. (*F*) The nose is examined intranasally to determine placement of the nasal septum and possible displacement of nasal bones or disruption of nasal mucosa. (*G*) The occlusion is observed to determine any disturbances of normal teeth relations. (*H*) The mandible is palpated, then distracted to determine sites of discomfort and possible mandibular fractures.

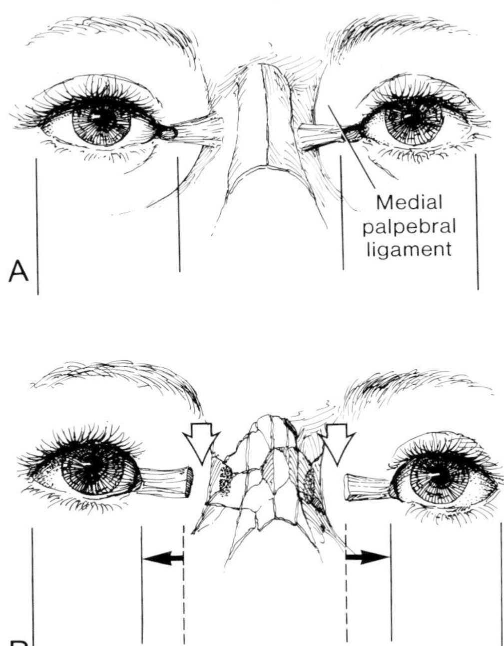

Figure 64.8. Mechanism of telecanthus. (*A*) Normal attachment of medial palpebral ligament to medial aspect of orbital wall. (*B*) Trauma producing comminution of the nasal and orbital bones allows the ligaments to drift laterally, resulting in rounding of the medial canthus.

sure in the preauricular area may help delineate a subcondylar fracture. The patterns of facial fractures as described by LeFort emphasize common points of weakness in the facial skeleton (Fig. 64.9).

The patient should be checked for anesthesia of the cheek (involvement of the infraorbital nerve from orbital rim fracture) and the lower teeth and lip (inferior alveolar nerve can be injured from a mandibular body fracture). After thorough observation and palpation, the examiner usually has a good idea as to the specific area of injury and frequently will be able to predict what the x-rays will show.

Radiographic Studies

The Waters' view (occipitomental) is the most useful x-ray (Fig. 64.3). It provides a good view of the orbital rims (particularly the inferior orbital rim) and the maxillary sinuses. The posteroanterior view of the face and of the mandible is also useful (Fig. 64.10). It, along with a lateral view of the face, provides a good view of the mandible on that side as well as a view of the sinuses and nasal bones (Fig. 64.11). With blowout fractures, the floor of the orbit is fractured, and periorbital contents are pushed into the maxillary sinus. Using these three views, the vast majority of facial bone fractures can be detected. Supplemental views of the mandible can be done if fractures of the mandible are suspected but not seen on routine views. For example, oblique views of the mandible remove overlapping of one body of the mandible over the other and allow a clear view of each body and ramus. The Panorex view, if available, shows the mandible in its entirety and is also very good for both a view of the condylar regions bilaterally and the temporomandibular joints. X-rays specifically for the nasal bones can also be ordered if the injury is limited to this area. Submental views can be helpful in viewing the zygomatic arches. (Fig. 64.12).

GUIDELINES FOR CONSULTATION

There are many cases in which management of a specific injury is not best handled in the emergency department. A phone call to a consultant can clarify the issue. The following can be used as very general guidelines as to what degrees of injuries should be handled by the primary physician in the emergency department and which should be left to the specialist. Clean, simple lacerations of the face without significant injury to the wound margins or underlying structures can usually be handled by the primary physician. Of course, there are other factors that come into play, namely the expertise of the primary physician and the amount of time that is available to spend on the particular patient. Also, the family or patient will sometimes ask that a specialist do the repair. This request can usually be handled adequately with an explanation that the specialist has no different techniques that will be used to close the wound. A call might nonetheless be placed to the specialist to advise of the situation and ask follow-up instructions. There are, of course, those individuals who will demand a specialist in spite of all explanations

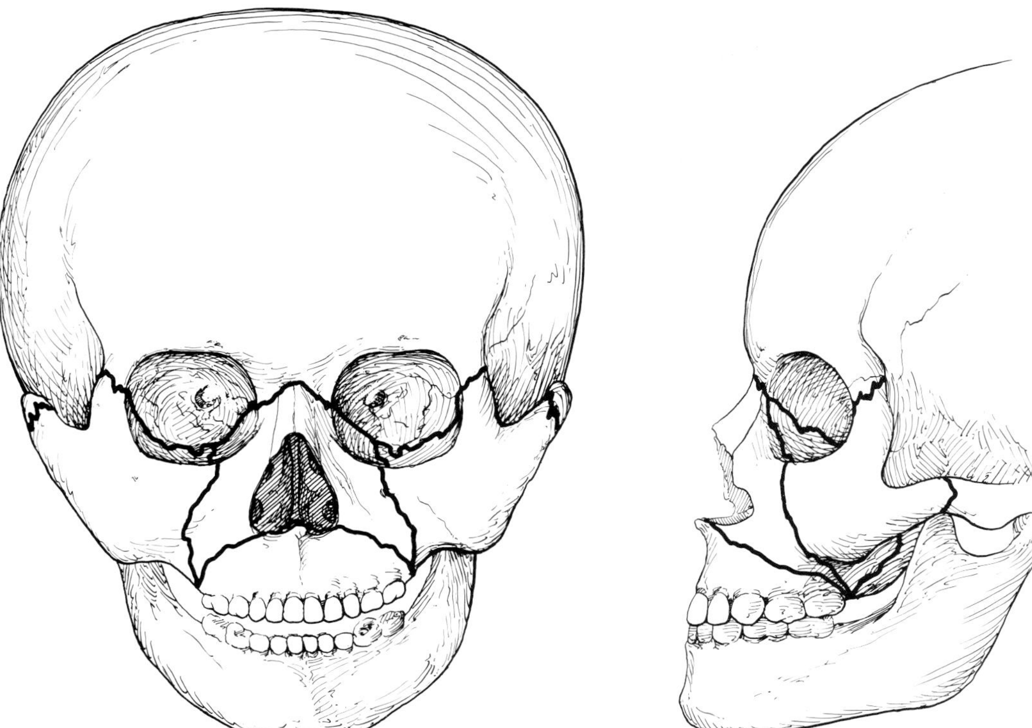

Figure 64.9 LeFort classification of fractures. With Type 1, the maxilla is separated from its attachments. Type 2 (pyramidal) produces a mobile maxilla and nose. With Type 3 (craniofacial dysjunction), all attachments of the midface to the skull have been separated. Traction on the anterior maxilla will produce motion up to the inferior orbital rims and zygoma. These fractures are not mutually exclusive. For example, a LeFort 1 can be present with a Type 2 or Type 3. LaFort 2 may exist on one side with a Type 3 on the other side.

and also those specialists who will insist on doing the repair themselves.

When there is evidence of a deep structure having been injured (namely a major motor nerve branch or a glandular duct), this injury should be left to the specialist for repair. Underlying facial bone fractures are not a contraindication to repair of a skin wound. Frequently, the repair of the facial bone fracture will not be done at that time, or if it is nondisplaced the possibility exists that nothing will be done. Therefore, after discussion with the specialist, repair of the skin wound may sometimes be done primarily.

Other injuries that should probably not be handled primarily are those in which there is a substantial amount of devitalized tissue, or in which a significant amount of tissue has been avulsed. These wounds will quite frequently require flaps or shifting of tissue that are best done in the operating room. In wounds that have a substantial amount of bleeding that cannot be easily controlled by carefully clamping an obvious bleeder, the wound should simply be covered (after cleaning) with moistened gauze and, if possible, pressure placed on the wound until a specialist can see the patient. Attempting to blindly clamp an area within a wound that is actively bleeding is inadvisable, since there is an attendant risk of injury to sensory nerves, facial nerve branches and underlying structures.

SPECIFIC MANAGEMENT PROBLEMS

Lack of cooperation on the part of the patient, even when adequate sedation has

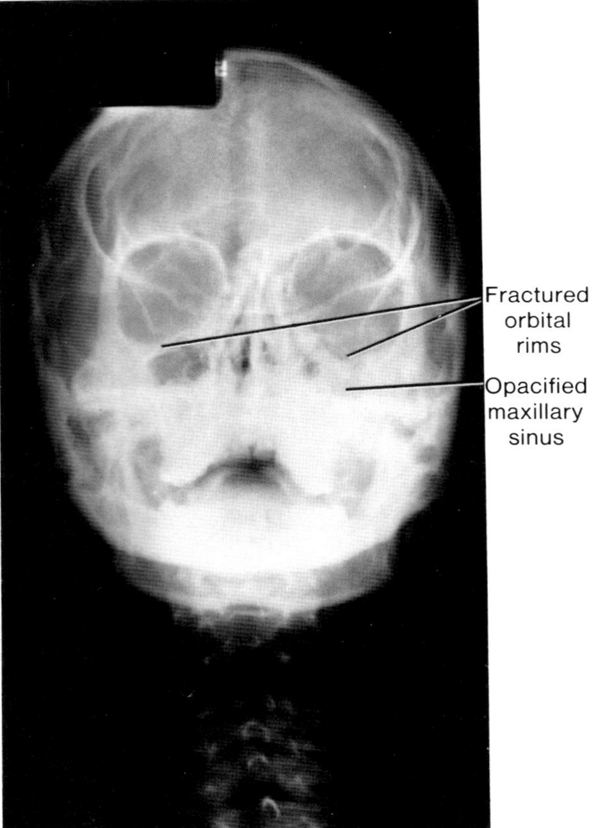

Figure 64.10 Postero-anterior view of the face and mandible demonstrating fractures of the right and left inferior orbital rims and an opacified left maxillary sinus.

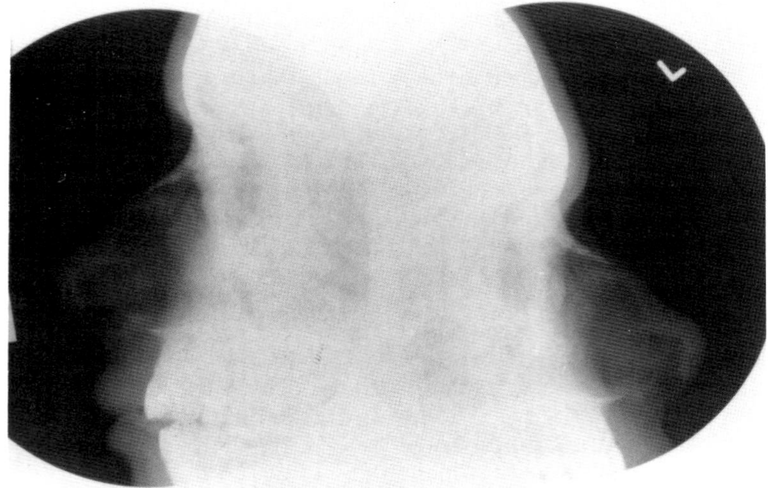

Figure 64.11 Lateral view of the face demonstrating a fracture of the nasal bone with minimal displacement.

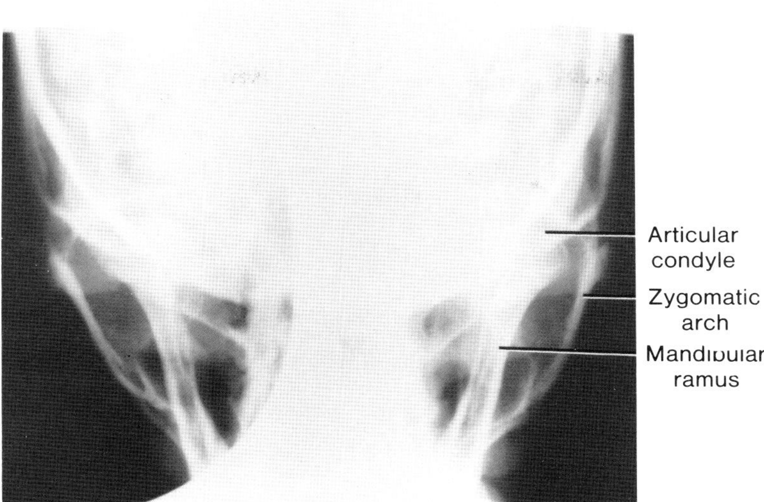

Figure 64.12 A modified submentovertical x-ray that clearly shows both zygomatic arches as well as the ramus of the mandible. This view is especially useful to determine fractures of the arch and mandibular rami. In the illustration shown, the arches and rami are normal, and the articular condyles can be seen.

been given, may be a contraindication to emergency department management. Facial wounds in small children can usually be handled by restraining the child, either wrapping them in a sheet or using a "papoose." Sedation, of course, can also be given to children when airway problems or internal injuries are not a concern.

A clean, sharp laceration can be closed up to 24 hours after the injury. A different situation exists when the wound was created by a contaminated object, or by a human or animal bite. These wounds should be cleaned thoroughly. The patient may be started on prophylactic antibiotics and should be advised to see their private physician or specialist on a daily basis. The wounds can still be closed at 4 to 5 days after the injury. Fresh animal or human bites or contaminated puncture wounds can be primarily closed in the emergency department if managed properly.

Treatment will be covered, beginning with the most simple injuries and going on to the complex types. Minor abrasions can be handled in the emergency department. The area involved should be cleaned by washing with a mild soap solution and covering with an antibiotic ointment or cream, either Polysporin or Silvadene. The patient should be advised to keep the area clean by washing 1 to 2 times a day and then recovering with the antibiotic ointment or cream. An alternative is to dress the wound with a petrolatum gauze type dressing and advise the patient to leave the wound closed.

Deeper abrasions are of more concern. If there is any possibility of a full or nearly full-thickness skin loss, even of a small area, a consultant should be contacted. He might advise simple cleaning and coverage, but should see the patient within 24 hours and evaluate for possible skin graft. Another concern with deeper abrasions is foreign body implantation. Injuries on road and gravel can implant particulate matter which will cause permanent tattooing if not removed initially. After the area is anesthetized, it can be gently scrubbed. If particles are deeper, a No. 11 scalpel blade can be used to remove them. When abrasions of the nose or ear are deep and cartilage is exposed, a specialist will be needed.

There are no "secrets" to achieving good closure of a facial or any other wound. If the basic elements of wound closure are known to the physician, the only other important points are that adequate time be taken with the closure and that adequate attention be given to detail. As with all wounds, those on the face should be closed in layers with a deep layer of absorbable suture, usually 4-0 or 5-0 size, and a fine suture in the skin, usually a monofilament nylon of 5-0 or 6-0 in size. Sterile skin tapes should be used in place of sutures only in superficial wounds. They can also be used to cover a closed wound. Factors that will contribute to a poor appearance following wound closure are: (1) infection, (2) leaving devitalized tissue within the wound, (3) failure to close the deeper aspects of a wound adequately, (4) excess tension on the skin margins, (5) leaving sutures in too long, (6) mishandling of the tissue during closure, and (7) failure to evert the wound margins.

How then to effect a good closure? (1) Make certain that the wound has been adequately cleaned and all foreign material removed. All cleaning agents are toxic to exposed wounds, therefore, they should be rinsed *well* with saline after cleansing. (2) Devitalized tissue (subcutaneous or skin) should be excised prior to closure. Leaving deep devitalized tissue can lead to drainage and infection with resultant wound separation. (3) All but the most superficial wounds should be closed in layers. If deep layers of the face are inadequately closed, a depression will be left which brings attention to the wound when it is healed. There are areas where a depression is hard to avoid (e.g., a wound extending across the margin of the mandible), but usually it should be possible to leave the wound actually slightly higher than the surrounding skin. (4) The skin should be essentially closed *before* skin stitches are applied. If the wound is extensive, it may require three layers in closure. A vertical simple suture that catches the lower dermis will approximate the wound edges together (Fig. 64.13). If the skin stitch is either tight or pulled down tightly because of carelessness, cross-hatch marks will be left. This should be avoided. Leaving sutures in too long will also produce cross-hatching. Patients should, therefore, be advised upon discharge from the emergency room as to when sutures should be removed. Almost no facial stitches should stay in longer than

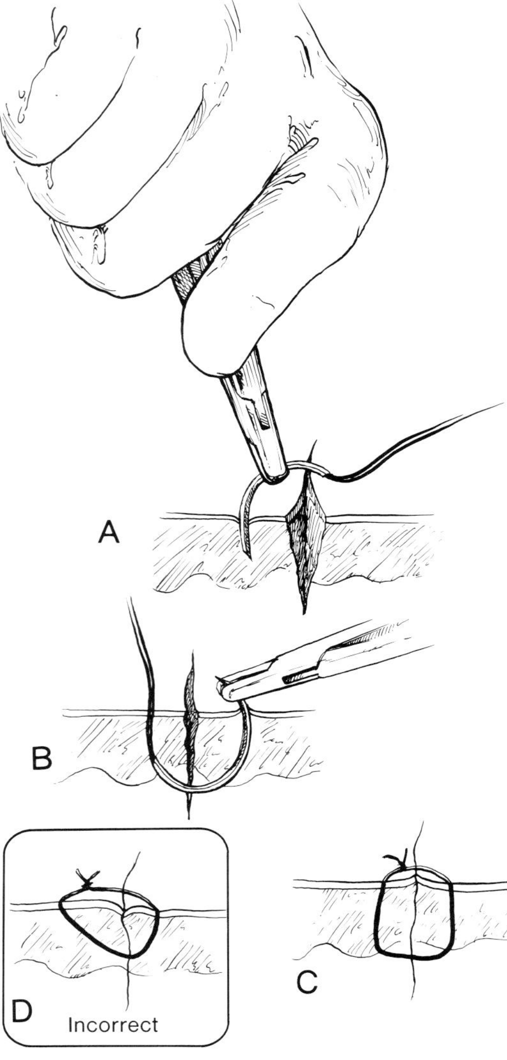

Figure 64.13. Correct suture technique. (*A*) The needle holder is held with the hand well pronated, and the needle entering the skin at a right angle and near the wound margin. (*b*) The needle crosses the wound at the same level on each side, and exits at the same angle and distance from the wound margin as the other side. (*C*) The suture is tied with minimal tension to one side of the wound. (*D*) Incorrect placement of a suture. It is inserted at a shallow angle, too far from the wound margin. The wound, therefore, is inverted.

5 days. Eyelid sutures should come out in 3 days. Mucosal stitches should be done using absorbable suture material and simply left in place. (5) Excising devitalized tissue is fruitless if more tissue damage is produced in the closure of the wound. That is, forceps should be used delicately, so that the skin is not crushed during closure. If possible, skin hooks should be used when handling the skin, or a fine forceps. (6) Every attempt should be made to evert the skin margins. This can only be done if a conscious effort is made to put the needle into the skin at a right angle or greater, and coming out of the skin at the same angle. There is a tendency, particularly when the physician is in a rush, to do the opposite and have the needle enter and exit at a shallow angle. An everted wound, as it heals, will flatten out to the same level as the surrounding skin. However, a noneverted wound will tend to become depressed as it heals. Usually, interrupted sutures are used in the closure of facial lacerations.

Treatment of complex wounds is simply an extension of the precepts given for simple wounds. It may be difficult to determine with stellate or other types of complex lacerations which tissue came from where. However, with close observation and by trial and error shifting, the tissue can be returned to its normal position. The question in these types of lacerations is whether tips or flaps or narrow strips of tissue will be viable. This determination becomes easier with experience; however, if there is any question, tissue should usually be left in place. Simple bites and puncture wounds should be left to heal secondarily or excised or closed. If it is decided to excise the wound because of contamination, an elliptical excision should be done paralleling the relaxed skin tension lines as diagrammed (Fig. 64.14).

Facial fractures in the emergency department are a diagnostic rather than a treatment problem. Treatment is rarely done in the emergency department. Once confirmatory x-rays have been done, the specialist should be contacted. With fractures of the nose, the specialist may in fact advise simply that the patient be sent home to follow up with them after a short interval. Antibiotics are not necessary for closed facial fractures.

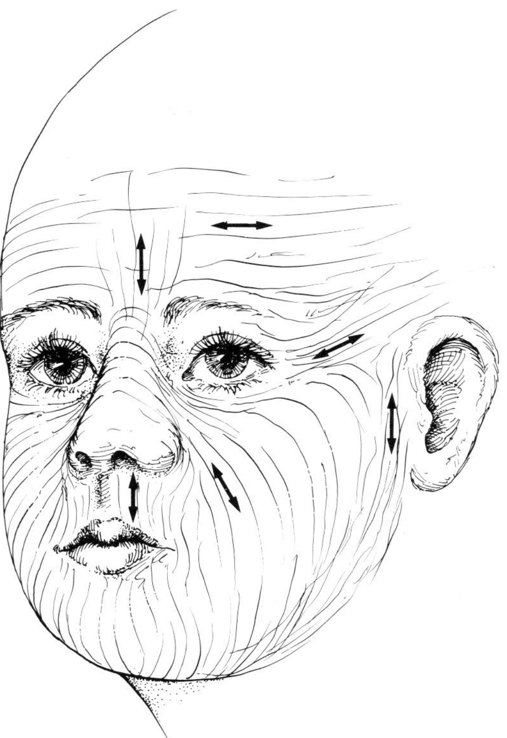

Figure 64.14. The illustration shows the natural pattern of skin creases that occurs with aging. If a circular type of wound needs to be converted to an elliptical shape for closure, an attempt should be made to have the wound parallel these lines.

By area, specific important points will be reviewed.

Forehead. If a laceration extends across the anterior hairline or across the eyebrow, shaving of the hair should *not* be done because this will make it difficult to carefully match up the skin margins.

Eyelids. Injuries to the eyelids are described in Chapter 61, "Ophthalmic Emergencies."

Nose. Full thickness defects caused by laceration through the skin of the nose and extending through the ala into the nose should probably be handled by a specialist. Those that do not extend completely through can be handled adequately in the emergency department. The cartilages, if lacerated, should be returned to their normal position by suturing with fine chromic suture and the soft tissue and skin closed over these. Notching of the ala should be avoided.

Lips. If a laceration extends across the mucocutaneous junction, careful attention must be given to matching up the white line which is the segment between the skin and the mucosa. This is sometimes difficult when the wound margins are irregular. If this is the case, closure must be left for the specialist.

Cheeks. Lacerations across the posterior cheek can potentially injure the parotid gland, facial nerve, or parotid duct. If the substance of the parotid gland has been exposed, nothing need be done to repair it. A specialist should be contacted, however. It may be advisable to insert a small drain, followed by a pressure dressing after the wound is closed.

Mouth. With the tremendous blood supply to the mouth, substantial bleeding may occur with mucosal lacerations. These are usually controlled by suturing of the laceration. With lacerations to the tongue, however, especially if they are deep, edema can occur in the tongue and pharynx at a later time and potentially obstruct the airway. Consideration must, therefore, be given to admission and observation of the patient.

Ears. Simple lacerations of the ears can be sutured as with simple lacerations elsewhere. When the cartilage is exposed, it should be covered by soft tissue in the repair. If the cartilage itself has been split, an attempt should be made to repair it using an absorbable stitch such as chromic. If the full thickness of the ear has been lacerated it should be repaired in layers, using nonabsorbable suture in the skin and absorbable suture in the cartilage and other soft tissues.

In conclusion, the physiology of normal wound healing should be enhanced, not impeded, by the way in which the tissue is handled and in which the repair is performed.

BURNS

BACKGROUND

About 3.6 million visits to physicians are made each year for the assessment and treatment of burns. Children make up a high percentage of these visits. More than 2,500 deaths in children occur annually as a result of burns, more than die from cancer each year. Three times this number suffer severe and prolonged disability due to burns. Most children with burns are initially seen in an emergency department. Before departing for the hospital, family or paramedics may telephone for advice on management and transportation of the burned child.

The vast majority of burns (about 80%) occur from accidents in the home, particularly when children are the victims. In children under 3 years of age, scalding is the most common type burn. This occurs from the spilling of hot food or liquid, or from immersion in a hot bath. Some burns are inflicted. Chapter 68 covers the management of the abused child and his/her family. Scald burns usually result in partial thickness injuries except in infants or toddlers in whom the skin is quite thin. Children over 3 years of age are more frequently burned by ignited clothing. These flame burns usually result in large areas of full-thickness injury.

CLINICAL MANIFESTATIONS AND PATHOPHYSIOLOGY

Surface burns to the skin result in destruction of the epidermis and varying thicknesses of the dermis. First degree burns involve only the epidermis, second degree burns extend into the dermis, and third degree burns involve the entire epidermis and dermis to the level of the subcutaneous tissue. So-called fourth degree burns involve muscle, tendons, and bone (Fig. 64.15). Third degree burns are also called full-thickness, while first and second are referred to as partial thickness. (The epidermal appendages are not destroyed in the partial thickness injury, but they are in full-thickness burns.)

Capillary permeability is markedly in-

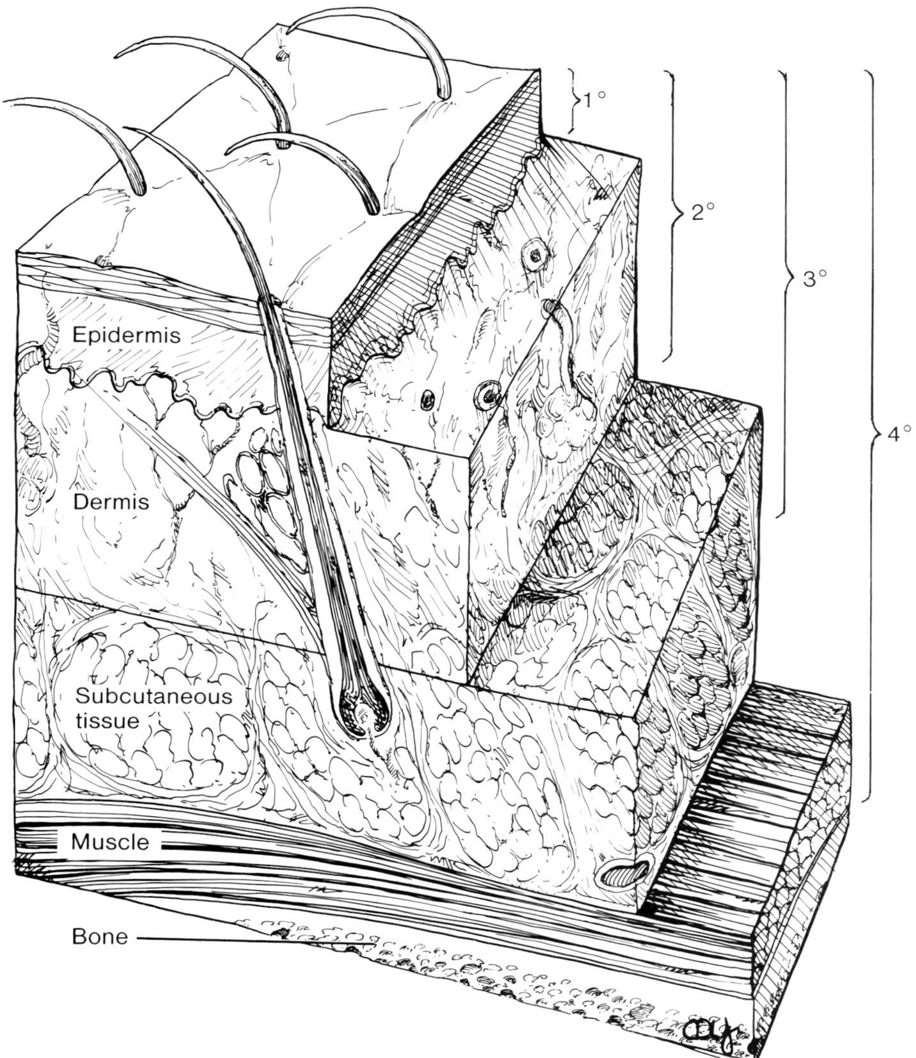

Figure 64.15 Degree of burn wound depth. First degree involves only epidermis; second degree extends into the dermis; third degree into subcutaneous tissue; and fourth degree to muscle, tendons, or bone.

creased in the burn patient, especially so in deep second or third degree burns. Capillary permeability is limited to the involved areas and burns less than 30% total body surface area, but is generalized in burns greater than 30%. This permeability results in a large loss of fluid from the intravascular compartment into the extravascular space. The resultant edema, plus loss of fluids through the wound itself, necessitate large amounts of fluid to be administered in the resuscitation of a burn victim.

Multiple physiological derangements often occur as a result of burns. With dehydration and hypoperfusion, peripheral tissues produce an excess of lactic acid. The result is systemic metabolic acidosis. This effect is magnified by the effects of hypothermia. The kidneys are particularly at risk, not only from hypovolemia and possible acute tubular necrosis, but also from toxic damage if the burn injury produces hemoglobinemia. The potential for pulmonary injury occurs in all fires, especially those in closed spaces. Frequently, death occurs with relatively little surface evidence of burn injury due to carbon monoxide poisoning, toxic products of burning plastics, and direct chemical tracheobronchitis. Finally, reflux ileus, in any child with a major burn, can result in abdominal distension, vomiting, and aspiration.

CLINICAL ASSESSMENT

History

All sources of information should be questioned thoroughly—the child, family, paramedics, etc. One should determine the patient's age, preexisting medical conditions, the possibility of airway damage or other significant injuries, and the mechanism and extent of the burn injury itself. Evasive answers or history that does not support the injuries noted might suggest child abuse. Also, one should document the time the injury occurred and any therapy provided prior to arrival at the hospital.

Physical Examination

The emergency physician begins with evaluation of the patient's sensorium, ventilation, and circulation. An inhalation injury is suggested by the presence of carbonaceous sputum, pharyngeal edema, bronchorrhea, hoarseness, and facial burns including singeing of the eyebrows, eyelashes, and nasal hairs. Rhonchi and stridor are later signs of airway injury. The disoriented or obtunded child may have inhaled toxic products or may have severe carbon monoxide poisoning. Symptoms of headache, dizziness, and nausea in the presence of tachycardia, tachypnea, and red skin and mucous membranes also suggest probable carbon monoxide poisoning.

Impairment of circulation can be systemic in a child with inadequate fluid resuscitation. It can also be regional in a child with circumferential burns of an extremity. Peripheral pulses and capillary filling must be documented both on admission and at frequent intervals as occlusion of arterial flow may produce irreversible ischemic changes.

Once all of the body systems have been assessed for the injury, one should next weigh the patient and then focus on the burn injuries. Estimation of burn depth and the percentage of total skin involved are important in both triage and prognosis of the burn victim. First degree burns produce only erythema of the skin. Second degree burns can be shallow or deep. When shallow, the burn is characterized by blebs beneath which the skin is weeping, pink or red, and sensitive. When deep, the exposed dermis is whitish in color, soft, and sensitive to pressure. Full-thickness or third degree burns are tan to dark in color, firm, dry, and anesthetic; thrombosed vessels can be seen beneath the surface. Charting of the distribution and percentage of second and third degree burns should be done carefully. The "rule of nine" is cumbersome in a child because children have relatively large heads and smaller lower extremities than do adults. Figure 64.16 shows a modification by O'Neill of the Brooke Army Burn Center diagram as applied to children. It is easy to follow and readily provides an accurate summation of the total areas of second and third degree burns.

Finally, specific attention should be paid both to the pattern of the burns and the specific areas of the body involved. Symmetrical scald burns to the lower body suggest an intentional immersion of the child in hot water. Injuries unrelated to the burns, such as ecchymosis or cigarette burns, also suggest child abuse.

The eyes should be examined for evidence of any direct burn injury or for the presence of foreign bodies, contact lens, extraocular motor function, and visual acuity. Fluorescein can be used if a corneal injury is suspected. The ears should be examined for possible exposure of cartilage. A secondary infection of the cartilage can lead to its complete destruction. Major burns of the perineum are infection prone and they increase the hazard of long-term indwelling urinary catheters.

MANAGEMENT

The first management decision is often made at the scene of the injury, namely, which institution will best serve the child and how should he be managed until the

Area	Birth 1 yr	1–4 yr	5–9 yr	10–14 yr	15 yr	Adult	2	3	Total
Head	19	17	13	11	9	7			
Neck	2	2	2	2	2	2			
Ant trunk	13	13	13	13	13	13			
Post trunk	13	13	13	13	13	13			
R buttock	2½	2½	2½	2½	2½	2½			
L buttock	2½	2½	2½	2½	2½	2½			
Genitalia	1	1	1	1	1	1			
R U arm	4	4	4	4	4	4			
L U arm	4	4	4	4	4	4			
R L arm	3	3	3	3	3	3			
L L arm	3	3	3	3	3	3			
R hand	2½	2½	2½	2½	2½	2½			
L hand	2½	2½	2½	2½	2½	2½			
R thigh	5½	6½	8	8½	9	9½			
L thigh	5½	6½	8	8½	9	9½			
R leg	5	5	5½	6	6½	7			
L leg	5	5	5½	6	6½	7			
R foot	3½	3½	3½	3½	3½	3½			
L foot	3½	3½	3½	3½	3½	3½			
						TOTAL			

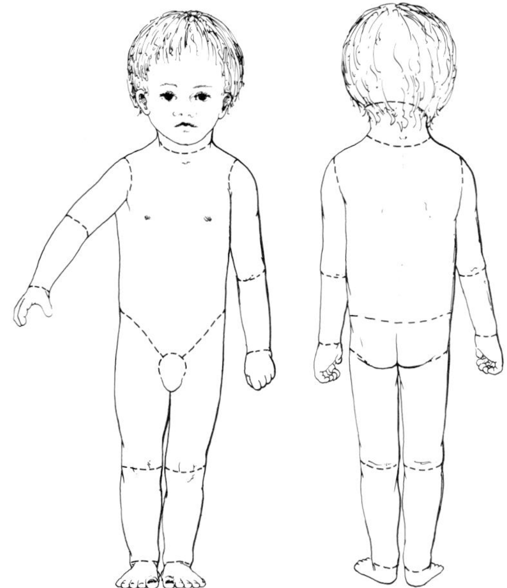

Figure 64.16 Estimation of surface area burned based on age. This modification by O'Neill of the Brooke Army Burn Center diagram shows the change in surface of the head from 19% in an infant to 7% in an adult. Proper use of this chart provides an accurate basis for subsequent management of the burned child.

arrival at the hospital. Any smoldering, wet, or chemically contaminated clothes should be removed. Dressings should not be applied. Instead, the child should be wrapped first in a sterile (or clean) sheet and then in blankets to conserve body heat.

Depending on time and distance, the hospital of choice should be one which is best equipped to handle the child's most severe injuries. For example, a severe pulmonary injury may be more critical than a 20% burn of the trunk. In general, critically injured children should be stabilized and then referred to a regional children's hospital or a designated burn center.

The decision to admit a child with a burn will depend not only on the nature and extent of the burn, but also on the feasibility of caring for the child at home. Even relatively severe first degree burns should not require hospitalization in most cases. However, if the child shows signs of toxicity, hospitalization may be required for intravenous fluids, sedation, and analgesia. Admission is indicated for any child with second degree burns of greater than 10% of the body surface area, or in the case of severe burns of the face, perineum, or an entire hand or foot. Except for small burns (2 to 3 cm or less, in noncritical areas), any child with a third degree burn should be admitted. Children under 2 years of age should be admitted with lesser burns, because they may react to the injury with ileus or refusal to feed.

Admission to a community hospital is appropriate for children with burns in noncritical areas of the body; when second degree burns are limited to 10 to 20% of the body; and when third degree burns involve 10% or less of the body. Transfer to a children's hospital or specialized burn center is recommended for the following situations: (1) a young child with partial thickness burns of 20% body surface area or greater, (2) an older child or adolescent with 25% body burned surface area or greater, (3) most electrical burns, (4) major concomitant injuries, or (5) significant respiratory tract involvement. In these circumstances, aside from functional morbidity or cosmetic considerations, appropriate emergency care and optimal in-hospital management is imperative to avoid mortality.

Outpatient Care

First degree burns, even when severe, can usually be well managed at home. Analgesics, and the application of cool, moist towels or cool baths, usually provide symptomatic relief. Caution should be exercised with the very young child or infant, as hypothermia may result from overzealous cooling. The young child is prone to hypothermia because there is a large body surface area in relation to body weight.

Once a child with a minor second or third degree burn has been evaluated in the emergency department, the following treatment steps may be followed. The wound should be cleansed with a mild soap, and rinsed with sterile saline. Any intact bullous lesions should be left alone. For those bullae that have ruptured, or are likely to, the excess devitalized tissue should be trimmed away. Even in the presence of intact bullae, the protective barriers of the skin are at least partially diminished.

Inadequate treatment of seemingly minor burns can result in infection and bacterial invasion and proliferation in the deeper layers of the remaining dermis. Secondary infection can result not only in delayed healing, but possible destruction of the underlying dermis. A partial thickness burn wound may then become a full-thickness wound that will require eventual skin grafting. Therefore, the goal in treating all burn wounds is rapid healing without infection. In order to suppress bacterial invasion, a topical antibacterial agent is required. After cleansing the wound, Silvadene cream is applied lightly over the burn area. Subsequently the burn should be washed gently with warm water, and fresh Silvadene applied twice daily. For pain, codeine or meperidine may be given orally in small doses. A 3- to 4-day follow-up appointment should be arranged with a physician experienced in burn care.

Most minor burns, especially those on the face and neck, can be treated using an open technique, that is, with no dressings. One may elect to use an occlusive dressing for awkward areas such as the hands or feet, or for an active child who may rub off the Silvadene. In these situations, one may apply a nonadherent petrolatum guaze over the Silvadene and then cover with bulky gauze dressings and roller gauze. Elevation of burned extremities will minimize any edema formation. If the parents are reluctant to change the dressings, this may be done every other day by a physician. Removal of the dressings is least painful when they are soaked off with warm water.

Prophylactic antibiotics are not indicated unless the child has a coincident bacterial infection. If the margins of the burn wound become red or tender, there may be a secondary staphylococcal or streptococcal infection. Infection is more likely to occur in burns treated by a closed technique. The burn should be cultured and local care changed to frequent cleansing and open treatment with Silvadene. Antibiotics should be given to treat both staphylococci and streptococci until culture results are evaluated. Even after early epithelialization of the burn has occurred, continued follow-up care will be required to assure optimal healing.

Inpatient Care

The treatment of major burns may begin at the scene of the accident. On arrival to the emergency department, all clothing should be removed immediately, especially in cases of flame or chemical burns. While an emergency department staff thoroughly washes all the wounds with warm sterile saline, the physician should rapidly complete a general physical examination to detect any life-threatening injuries or secondary problems. Examples of such problems include acute airway compromise or carbon monoxide toxicity in cases of flame burns, or cervical spine injuries or a pneumothorax in cases of multiple trauma. Attention to these problems takes precedence over definitive care of the burn wound.

Next, fluid resuscitation should be initiated. An intravenous catheter should be inserted percutaneously in an unburned area if possible. In a small child, a well placed 20 or 22 gauge plastic catheter provides adequate vascular access. The optimal intravenous fluid is Ringer's lactate given at a rate of 4 ml × percent burn × weight in kg over the first 24 hours. Half of this volume should be given in the first 6 to 8 hours. Subsequently, fluid rates will depend on the patient's response as determined by vital signs and urine output. A urinary catheter should be inserted in the child's bladder when the burns are in excess of 20% of body surface area. With a urinary catheter one can adjust fluid administration so as to maintain an average urine output of 1 ml/kg/hour. Because of the burn patient's marked increase in capillary permeability, colloid should not be administered in the first 24 hours.

Admission laboratory studies should be obtained including a CBC, BUN, creatinine, electrolytes, calcium, amylase, and liver function tests. These studies are important as a baseline for subsequent evaluation of fluid shifts, renal status, and liver function. An initial chest x-ray should be followed by daily chest x-rays to assess any early or delayed pulmonary changes. Frequent urinalyses should be performed to determine the specific gravity and to check for pigment such as free hemoglobin or myoglobin. The presence of hemoglobinuria suggests a potential life-threatening insult to the kidneys which must be promptly recognized and treated (see Chapter 46, "Renal and Electrolyte Emergencies"). In children with flame burns, one should send blood samples for type and crossmatch, arterial blood gas measurements and carboxyhemoglobin levels.

Airway management in the child with a known or potential inhalation injury should include giving humidified oxygen by mask at high flow rates until the arterial blood gas results or carboxyhemoglobin levels are known. Treatment with oxygen can then be adjusted accordingly. If the physical examination suggests an insult to the tracheobronchial tree, the child should be admitted to the intensive care unit even if the area of surface burns is small. If the child develops progressive airway distress, an endotracheal tube should be inserted immediately before edema of the head and neck structures becomes too severe. Tracheostomy in children can be difficult and should virtually never be done in the emergency department. Moreover, tracheostomy poses added pulmonary risks in any patient with a burn. (See Chapter 51 for detailed management of smoke inhalation and carbon monoxide poisoning).

When the airway is assured and the cervical spine is not in jeopardy, one should then insert a No. 10 to 16 gauge nasogastric tube in order to empty the stomach contents. If little material is obtained and if the burn area is small (e.g. 10 to 20%), the nasogastric tube may be removed. The child should be kept NPO (nothing by mouth) for at least 24 hours, however, until any ileus has resolved.

The next management step is the definitive care of the burns. Besides cleansing with sterile saline, one should debride any loose tissue. If vital signs are satisfactory and pain is a problem, one may administer intravenous narcotics, such as meperidine, 1 mg/kg. One should not use intramuscular medications because of their unpredictable absorption, except for tetanus toxoid for the child who has not had a booster shot in the last 5 years.

After accurate charting of the depth and extent of the burn wounds, all second and third degree burn areas should be covered with Silvadene cream. The use of occlusive dressings, as described above, has the advantage of keeping the Silvadene in place and lessening fluid and heat losses due to evaporation. If the child on the inpatient service has to be transported to another hospital, occlusive dressings may be necessary. Dressings are cumbersome to change. As long as the child's environment can be kept warm, and his fluid status in balance, the use of open treatment allows for frequent (once a shift) cleansing of the wound and reapplication of fresh Silvadene. Covering the child with sterile sheets and blankets over a cradle is essential when using open treatment.

Antibiotics are not given in the emergency department unless required for treatment of some other problem (e.g. bacterial pharyngitis or otitis media). If the child is to be transported to another facility, a physician and/or an intensive care nurse should accompany the patient. Proper supplies and medication should be included to ensure safe transport.

ELECTRICAL INJURY

Electrical burns differ from flame, scald, or chemical burns in their potential for unrecognized, even life-threatening internal injuries. Although the entrance and exit wounds may be relatively small, there is usually deep tissue destruction. Because of the tendency of the current to pass along blood vessels, direct injury to adjacent muscle, nerves, and bone can occur. Moreover, thrombosis of numerous blood vessels can result in extensive infarction and necrosis of these structures. Except for the entry or exit site on a hand or foot, the skin over the extremity may appear to be spared in spite of extensive underlying necrosis of muscle. Viability of the entire extremity may be at risk if pulses, skin color, and capillary refill are poor. Hence, most patients with electrical burns should be admitted to the hospital.

Fluid resuscitation is not based on the amount of injury to the skin. Much larger amounts of Ringer's lactate may be required than predicted by the surface burn formula because of large areas of hidden injury. One should infuse fluid at a rate which will preserve a vigorous diuresis. A dark red urine will indicate probably acute myoglobinuria due to massive muscle injury. Management of myoglobinuria is covered in Chapter 46, "Renal and Electrolyte Emergencies."

One special type of electrical burn is almost unique to children, namely, burns of the corner of the mouth This results from chewing on an electrical cord or extension socket. Saliva causes a short circuit, which results in an electrical arc at extremely high temperatures. The burn of the oral commissure can be of varying degrees.

Depending on the age of the child and the extent of the burn, they can be treated as inpatients or outpatients. Acute debridement of the wound is generally not recommended. The wound should be allowed to demarcate (approximately 2 weeks after the injury) and treatment done at that point, or when the necrotic tissue sloughs (by 4 weeks). Initial management involves local gentle washing 2 or 3 times a day followed by the application of Neosporin ointment. The wound should be left open. If the child is sent home, early follow-up by a plastic surgeon or burn specialists is important. The parents should be advised that bleeding from the labial artery may occur when the necrotic tissue begins to separate 5 to

9 days after the injury. They should be instructed to pinch the lip near the bleeding point and to bring the child to the emergency department if this occurs.

CHEMICAL INJURIES

Chemical burns in children are more likely to result from an accident with household cleaners rather than industrial-type chemicals. It is important to determine the agent with which the child was burned and also the likelihood of ingestion.

As with flame burns, all clothing potentially involved should be removed. Then, the wound should be copiously irrigated with water or physiological saline. If it appears the process is ongoing, a continuous irrigating bath might be set up.

The depth of the burn may be difficult to determine, and, in fact, may get deeper with time. Thus, it is again difficult to use a formula for fluid resuscitation. Fluid replacement should be generous, assuming no prior cardiovascular or renal disease. Burn surface should be treated with Silvadene to minimize secondary invasion (see Chapters 48 and 62).

COLD INJURIES

Frostbite results from exposure of a body area (usually a hand or foot) to below freezing temperature. Actual freeing of tissue results in breakdown of cell membrane integrity, protein denaturation, and changes in enzyme function. The tissue surrounding a frozen area can show ischemic changes secondary to thrombosis and microvascular stasis.

There can be varying degrees of injury to the skin, subcutaneous tissue, and connective tissue. A wound that is first pale and doughy, but then develops rubor, mild edema, and a return in sensation with warming, is a superficial injury. Vesicle formation indicates a deeper injury. An injured part with deep frostbite is cyanotic, hard, and without any sensation. Warming will not produce hyperemia, but instead a mottled cyanotic appearance. Extreme swelling and pain develop over a period of hours in most frostbite injuries. Severe frostbite can also involve muscle and bone.

Treatment of acute cold injury involves rapid rewarming of the involved areas. If possible, the injured area should be immersed in a warm bath at 40 to 43°C for 20 min. If an extremity is involved, it should be elevated to reduce edema after being warmed. Once rewarming is completed, it should not be repeated even if the injured area becomes cool. In cases of severe cold injury, acute treatment with regional intra-arterial infusion of reserpine has been very effective. With both rapid rewarming and intra-arterial infusion, early treatment is imperative in order to maximize salvage of the injured tissues.

Most superficial cold injuries can be treated on an outpatient basis. No special care is necessary. Deeper injuries necessitate hospitalization of the patient for treatment of pain and local wound care (see Chapter 51).

References

Artz C, Moncrief J: *Burns*. W. B. Saunders, Philadelphia, 1979.

Grabb W, Smith J: *Plastic Surgery*. Little Brown, Boston, 1979.

Harris JH: *Radiology of Emergency Medicine*. Williams & Wilkins, Baltimore, 1981.

O'Neill JA: Evaluation and treatment of the burned child. *Pediatr Clin North Am* 22: 407–414, 1975.

Schultz RC: *Facial Injuries*. Year Book, Chicago, 1977.

Schwartz GR: *Principles and Practice of Emergency Medicine*. W. B. Saunders, Philadelphia, 1978.

Zook E, et al: *The Primary Care of Facial Injuries*. Publishing Sciences Group, Littleton, Mass., 1980.

CHAPTER 65

Musculoskeletal Injuries

HENRY H. SHERK, M.D.

INTRODUCTION

Anatomic and physiologic differences between the skeletal structures of children and adults make fracture treatment in children almost a separate discipline from treatment of similar injuries in adults. The skeletal structures of a child include epiphyses, perichondral rings, thick periosteal sleeves, porous bone and other adaptations which allow for growth and which, in turn, cause bony injuries to respond differently. Treatment in an adult aims toward union of the fracture without deformity or loss of motion in the involved joints; but, in children successful treatment has the additional end point of allowing normal growth. Success in achieving these goals requires prompt recognition and correct treatment at the time the child presents for emergency care. The purpose of this chapter is (1) to provide a brief description of the relevant differences between the skeletal systems of children and adults and (2) to present guidelines of diagnosis and treatment for specific injuries.

GENERAL PRINCIPLES

Structure and Physiological Differences between Musculoskeletal Systems of Children and Adults

In utero, bones form from mesenchymal anlage which first chondrify and then ossify. At birth most long bones have developed an ossified diaphysis, and at or soon after birth the ends of the bones, the epiphyses, also ossify (Fig. 65.1). With growth, the ossification centers rapidly increase in relative size, diminishing the extent of the remaining cartilaginous portion of the bone. The cartilaginous plate or physis contains the germinal chondrocytes which, by reproducing themselves, cause the bone to increase in length. At the end of growth the ossification center of the epiphysis and the ossified tissue of the metaphysis fuse, crowding out the last germinal chondrocytes (Fig. 65.2). While enchondral ossification with germinal layer cellular proliferation of the physis causes the bone to lengthen, membranous ossification in the periosteum enlarges the bone circumferentially causing an increase in diameter. The periosteum in children, therefore, contains many more cells and is much thicker than in adults. The rapid production of ossified tissue in the bones of children causes a greater cross sectional area of the bone to consist of Haversian canals, an anatomic fact which in turn makes children's bones more porous and more bendable.

The structure of a given bone, of course, changes with age, and the bone naturally approaches the adult configuration as the child grows older. Infants and young children, therefore, have less ossified tissue, wider epiphyseal plates, and thicker periosteum than older children and adolescents. Change in anatomy dictates different responses to similar types of trauma in different age groups. In young children, for ex-

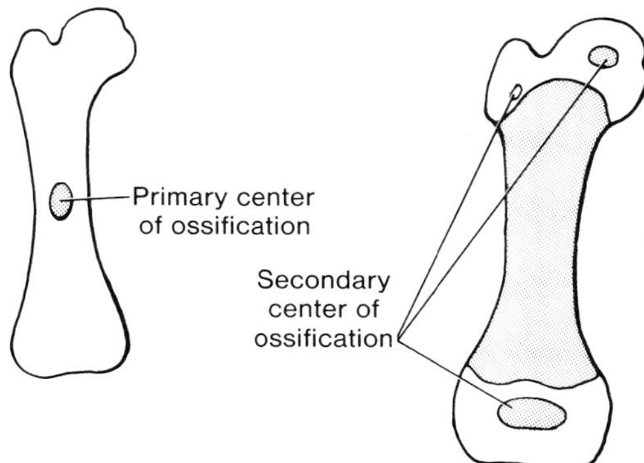

Figure 65.1 On the *left*, the bone has just begun to ossify the cartilaginous model, in utero. On the *right*, at or shortly after birth, ossification has filled in the diaphysis and begun in the epiphysis.

ample, bending stresses on diaphyseal bone produce injuries which reflect the porous, bendable nature of the bone. Minor stresses produce bending deformities or buckle fractures while greater stresses cause greenstick fractures or complete fractures without the comminution noted in the denser, less elastic, bone of adults. Moreover, the thick periosteum about the diaphysis of children's bone acts as a tube attached to both proximal and distal fragments linking them together and tending to limit displacement. The periosteum and elastic recoil of the bone itself can cause diaphyseal fractures to snap back into nearly normal alignment, making it difficult to appreciate the degree of displacement that existed at the moment of fracture or indeed in some cases if a fracture occurred at all. The anatomy of the diaphysis and the physical properties of the bone in the diaphysis dictate the patterns of fracture in response to given stresses and also require certain steps during treatment which absolutely control the outcome and prognosis. Once a buckle or greenstick fracture has returned to nearly normal alignment, muscle pull can cause it to redisplace; so greenstick fractures especially must be broken through and then briefly overcorrected to prevent recurrent and progressive deformity.

The actively osteogenic periosteum about the diaphysis in children forms callus

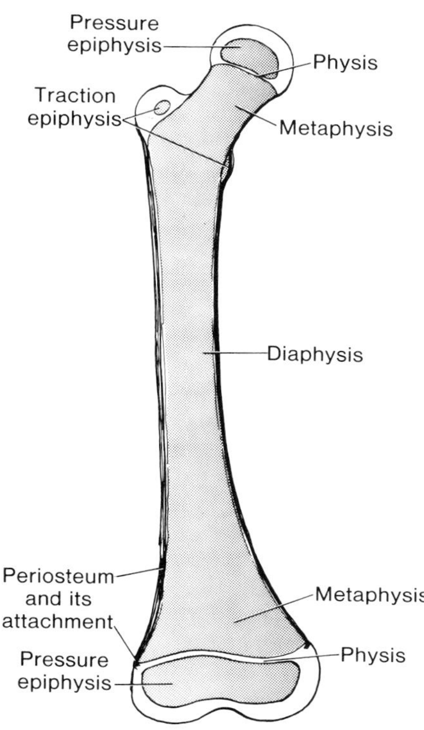

Figure 65.2 Diagrammatic representation of the progression of ossification of the femur later in childhood.

very soon after injury and, within a few days, most such fractures have enough stability to preclude manipulation or change in position. Consolidation and remodeling go forward very quickly and, in young children especially, one cannot detect residuals of even severe displacement after a few months. This potential, of course, diminishes with age, and some fractures in adolescents require the same type of treatment as an adult. Thus the functional adaptation of a shaft fracture varies inversely with the age of the patient, but in young children nonunion of the shaft fracture rarely if ever occurs.

At the ends of the bones, the periosteum forms a thick cuff around the physis. This thickened cuff, called the perichondral ring, provides for the stability of the epiphysis on the diaphysis, binding the former to the latter. The epiphysis projects irregularly into the metaphysis in a number of so-called mammilary processes, and this irregular contour of the ossification front between the epiphysis and epiphyseal plate also increases the stability of the epiphysis on the metaphysis. The perichondral ring and mammilary processes, however, depend on intact periosteum to maintain the normal anatomic configuration of the epiphysis, metaphysis and diaphysis. Fractures of the ends of the bone associated with tears of the periosteum release the perichondral ring from its attachments, and the epiphysis under these circumstances can shift in position relative to the metaphysis and the shaft of the bone.

The ligaments of the joints attaching one bone to another, however, have greater mechanical strength in children than the perichondral rings and epiphyseal plates. The powerful ligaments and strong attachment of these ligaments to the ends of adjacent bones thus make the joints of children the most stable element of the bone-joint-bone biomechanical construct, so trauma of the musculoskeletal system in children, as a result, rarely causes dislocations. Stresses across the knee in young adults, however, do cause ligamentous injury or dislocations. Children respond to similar stresses with epiphyseal displacement, and older adults, with osteoporotic bone, develop fractures. Injuries of the epiphyseal plate in children have such fundamental importance, however, that they must be considered separately.

Physeal Injuries

When stress applied to the ends of a child's bone overwhelms its mechanical integrity the bone structure fails in one of several ways. Certain applied stresses twist, shear, or avulse the epiphysis, and these usually produce a complete separation of the epiphysis from the metaphysis. This is the Type I epiphyseal injury of Salter and Harris. Translational stresses directed laterally push the epiphysis off the metaphysis and usually a triangular piece of metaphysis stays with the epiphysis (Salter and Harris Type II). Both of these mechanisms produce a plane of cleavage through the zone of provisional calcification of the epiphyseal plate. This sparing of the germinal layer of the plate in these two types of epiphyseal injuries allows the germinal layer of the physis to resume normal cellular reproduction and growth, once the effects of the injury have resolved. Patients with these two types of epiphyseal plate injuries have good prognoses for the resumption of normal growth without deformity (Fig. 65.3).

In Salter and Harris Type III injuries, the separation of the zone of provisional calcification extends only part way through the epiphyseal plate. The fracture line then passes directly through the epiphysis into the joint. In Type IV fractures the plane of separation extends through the epiphysis, epiphyseal plate, and metaphysis. The Salter and Harris classification also includes Type V fractures which occur as a result of axially loaded compressive stresses. This mechanism crushes and obliterates the germinal layer of the epiphyseal plate, so the Type V injuries have a poor prognosis for the resumption of normal growth. The surgeon has little control of the almost inevitable growth arrest caused by Type V fractures, but recognition and proper treatment can prevent growth problems caused by bony bridging across the epiphyseal plate in Type III and Type IV injuries.

Principles of Diagnosis and Treatment

A history of injury and clinical deformity makes diagnosis easy. X-rays merely confirm the diagnosis. The emergency physician, however, must follow pre-established guidelines to avoid errors. The initial examination should document the neurovascular status of the limb. The fractured limb should be splinted for comfort and protection prior to transfer. X-rays should always include the joint above and below the fracture to avoid missing an associated dislocation. Both clinical and radiographic evaluation of the rest of the limb may also be required to avoid overlooking an associated injury. X-rays taken in two projections will keep the diagnostician from missing a fracture with deformity in only one plane (Fig. 65.4).

Frequently fractures do not present so clear-cut a picture, and diagnosis of a fracture may require additional effort. Epiphyseal separation with minimal displacement

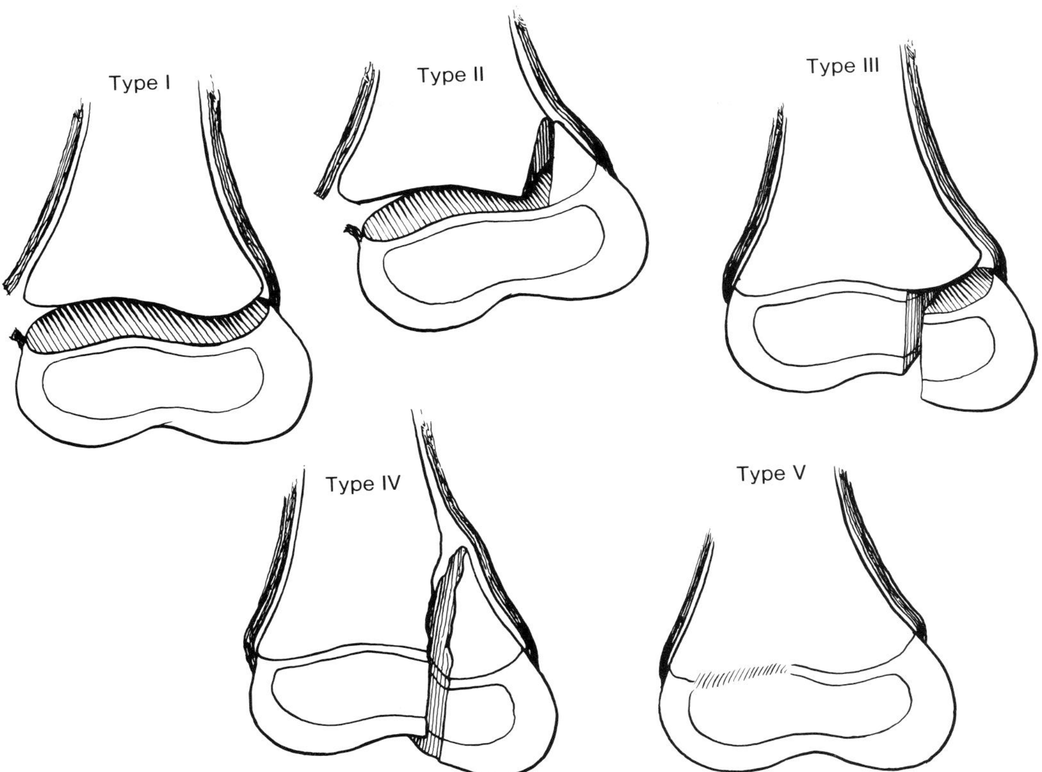

Figure 65.3 Diagrammatic representation of the Salter classification of epiphyseal plate injuries. The prognosis for growth disturbance worsens from Type I through Type V (see text).

and fractures involving unossified epiphyses, for example, may cause the unwary to miss a severe injury. X-rays of both limbs for comparison of the injured with the normal extremity will help avoid this mistake.

Finally, the clinical picture is all important. Pain and swelling should arouse suspicion and cause one to splint the limb and re-evaluate it subsequently with additional films.

Several basic principles must guide the course of treatment. First, the person treating fractures in this age group has the advantage that the child's healing and remodeling powers can compensate for imperfect alignment to a much greater degree than in an adult. Armed with the knowledge that the fracture will almost certainly heal and that growth and development will obliterate many deformities, the physician can use several other criteria in deciding whether to continue the quest for a more perfect alignment. The age of the patient is one of the most important considerations, since infants and young children obviously have more time and greater potential for correcting malalignments than an adolescent whose epiphyseal plates have almost closed. Another factor is the type of deformity. Rotational malalignment and lateral angulation do not self-correct, while bayonet apposition and anteroposterior angulation in the plane of joint motion do tend to correct to a large degree (Figs. 65.5 and 65.6). Another consideration is the closeness of the fracture to the epiphyseal plate. Metaphyseal injuries close to the plate correct malalignment much more satisfactorily than fractures in the midshaft. The distance of the fracture from the growth plate thus also influences the decision to repeat an effort to get better alignment.

Fractures in children rarely require open reduction and can be immoblized without

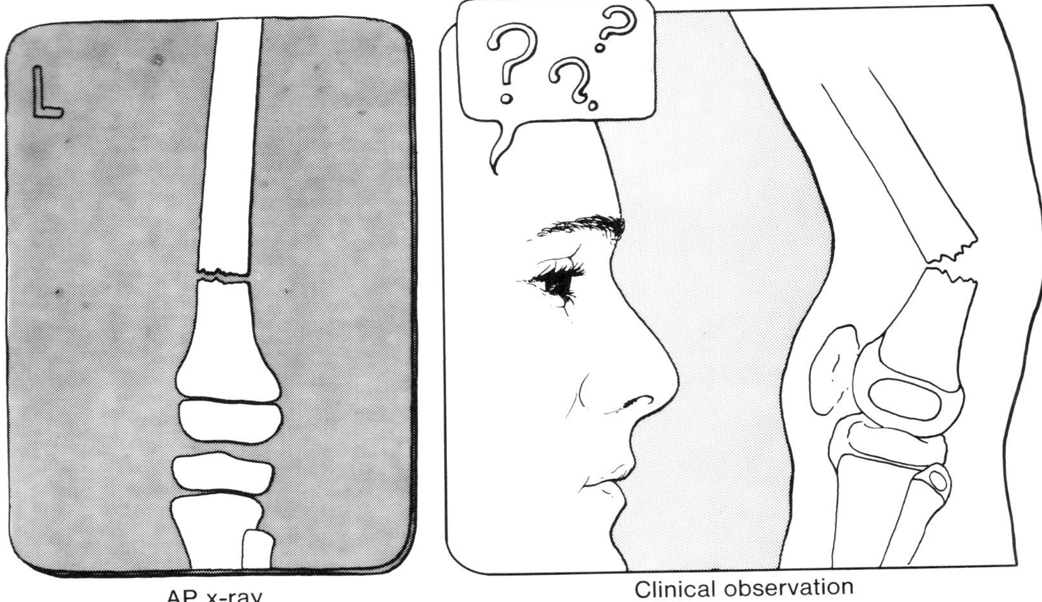

Figure 65.4 Diagnosis of a fracture depends on clinical assessment with careful evaluation of roentogenograms taken in two planes.

fear of stiffness after removal of the cast. Physical therapy in postfracture pediatric patients has less of a role than in adults.

Open fractures in children require observance of the basic principles that apply to adult compound fractures. These injuries present the emergency department team with a true emergency, and the patient must receive immediate treatment. The fracture itself must be splinted and covered with sterile dressings while the patient is evaluated for airway problems and shock. Only after these factors have been stabilized, can the orthopaedist proceed with treatment of the fracture. The techniques of debridement and irrigation of the wound, reduction and fixation of the fracture, whether to close the wound, and appropriate antibiotic treatment do not usually concern the emergency physician. Vehicular accidents or other major violence often cause multiple system injuries, and an open fracture under these circumstances must take its proper place in the line-up of priorities (see Chapter 57). The emergency department physician, therefore, must recognize the open fracture, splint it, dress it and otherwise protect it while he treats the whole patient.

INJURIES OF THE UPPER LIMB

Fractures of the Clavicle

A child with a "broken collar bone" has a good prognosis for trouble-free healing. A posterior figure-of-eight splint or harness keeps the shoulders back and makes patients with this injury comfortable. Parents can change the splint themselves from time to time during the 2 to 3 weeks that it takes the fracture to heal. This injury never needs an open reduction.

Sternoclavicular and acromioclavicular injuries present somewhat different problems. Swelling and pain over the sternoclavicular joint in the pediatric patient usually represents an epiphyseal separation of the medial epiphysis of the clavicle. Strapping with the same type of device used for treatment of a clavicular fracture supports the shoulder girdle and allows the separation to heal. Occasionally in older children and adolescents the clavicle might dislocate on the acromion. If separation is complete, the patient might need a surgical repair but

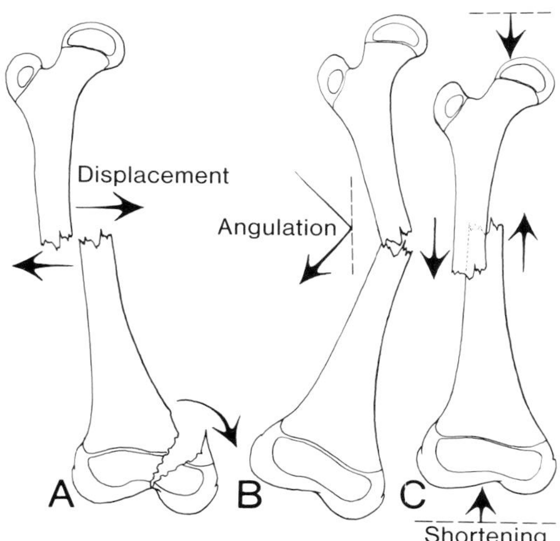

Figure 65.5 Diagrammatic representation of the deformity caused by a fracture; (*A*) displacement vs. (*B*) angulation; and overriding with shortening (*C*).

often, with minor sprains, strapping suffices.

Fractures of the Proximal Humeral Epiphysis

Children and adolescents with shoulder injuries usually have Salter II epiphyseal separations of the proximal humerus.

Actual dislocations of the shoulder joint tend to occur in a slightly older age group. The injury usually occurs when the child falls backward with the arm extended. The periosteum anterolaterally at the junction of the epiphysis and metaphysis is thinner than posteriorly and the epiphyseal plate is cone-shaped, pointing upward, backward and medially. This anatomic structure makes the proximal humerus susceptible to fracture, with anterior angulation at the level of the plate. Since most of these injuries are minimally displaced such patients when seen in the emergency department usually have only pain, swelling, and ecchymotic discoloration. With severe displacement, however, the distal fragment can cut anteriorly through the deltoid muscle. The spike of bone on the distal fragment is very sharp and one can easily palpate it anteriorly in such cases. These fractures can even compound from within, cutting out

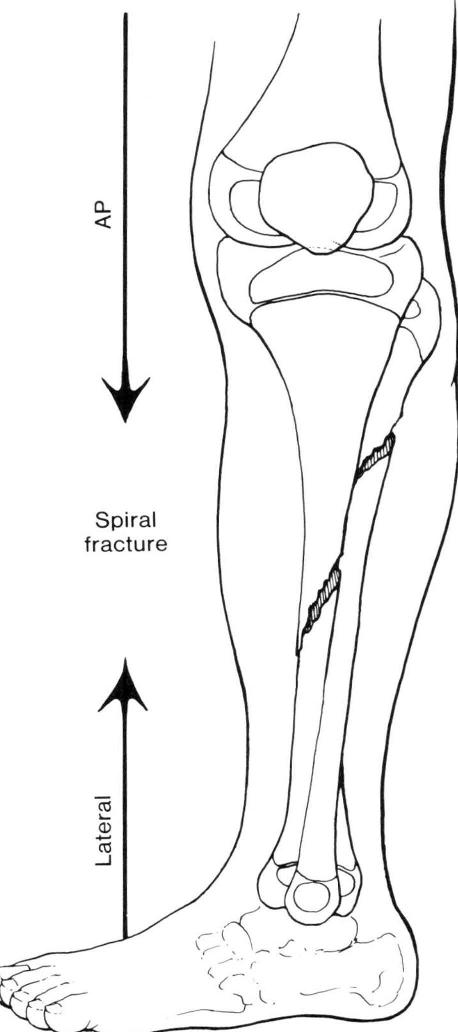

Figure 65.6 Diagrammatic representation of rotational deformity in a spiral fracture. Slight overriding and displacement are acceptable but angulation or rotational malaligment are not. Reduction must correct the latter two or the patient will have permanent deformity.

through the skin anteriorly (Fig. 65.7). An anteroposterior (AP) x-ray of the shoulder establishes the diagnosis. Sometimes the metaphyseal wedge of bone which remains with the epiphysis in the Salter II injury is quite prominent, and the injury looks like a proximal shaft fracture instead of an epiphyseal separation. AP x-ray alone may

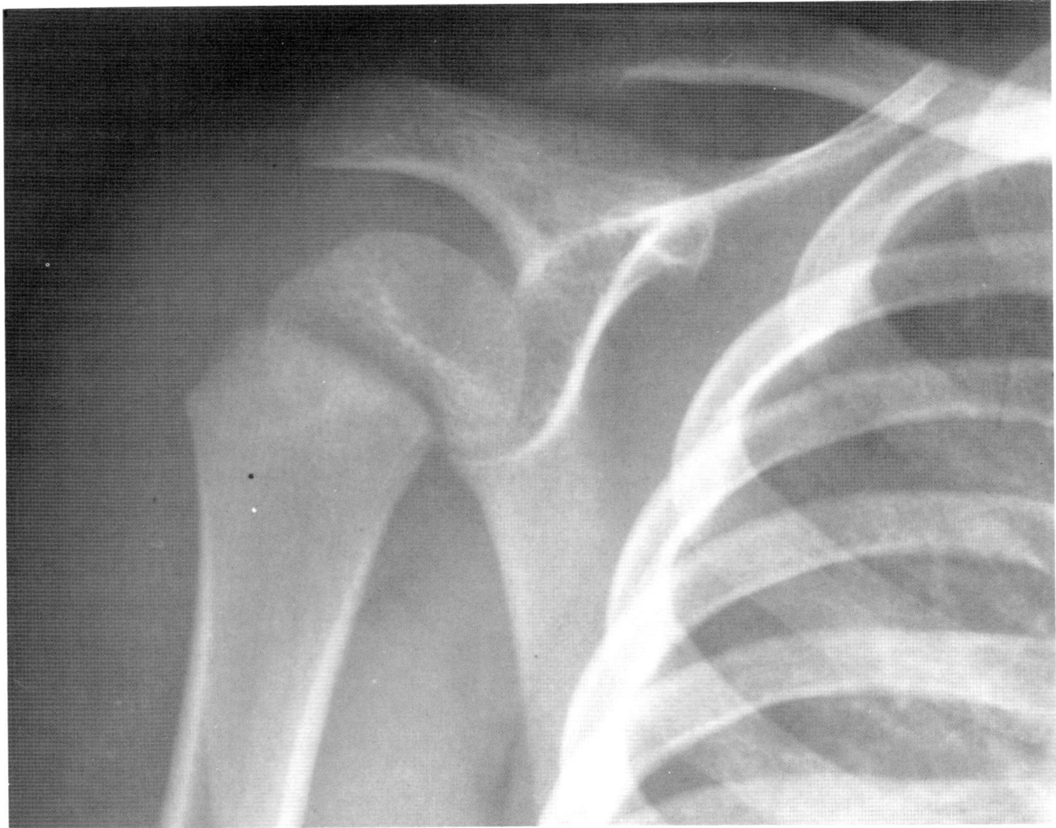

Figure 65.7 Fracture of proximal humeral epiphysis. The roentgenogram showing a typical Salter II fracture of the proximal humeral epiphyseal plate. There is anterior angulation of the fracture site and often one can palpate the sharp distal fragment anteriorly. (Courtesy of J. Gregg, M.D.)

belie the severity of the injury since the fracture angulates in the sagittal plane, and only a lateral view of the proximal humerus obtained with a transscapular or transthoracic projection will reveal the severity of the deformity.

Recognition of the fracture is important, since untreated anterior angulation promptly heals in the position of deformity. Such patients can have permanent limitation of shoulder flexion. Others with untreated damage to the epiphyseal plate can end up with marked shortening of the humerus.

Most fractures of the proximal humeral epiphysis are minimally displaced, and treatment can consist of a collar or cuff or sling until union occurs. More severely displaced fractures, however, require that the distal fragment be brought up into flexion to align the distal fragment with the flexed proximal fragment. The patient's arm can be held in this "salute position" in a shoulder spica cast until union occurs, usually 4 to 5 weeks. In the very occasional case when the biceps tendon is caught and interposed between the two fragments, open reduction and pin fixation may be required.

Fractures of the Humeral Shaft

Spiral fractures of the humerus in newborns can occur as a result of difficult delivery. These are not rare injuries. In older babies the presence of this type of injury suggests parental abuse (see Chapter 68).

In children and adolescents the injury results from direct trauma to the arm. A primary concern is the possibility of damage to the radial nerve where it spirals around the humeral shaft posteriorly. Loss of sensation on the dorsum of the web space between the thumb and forefinger and paralysis of finger and wrist extension establishes the presence of the radial nerve deficit. Usually, however, function in the nerve returns after union of the fracture occurs and a 12- to 14-week wait before exploration of the nerve is justifiable. In children especially a conservative course of treatment is preferred, and exploration of the radial nerve on an emergency basis is only justifiable if the deficit occurs during the course of treatment.

The periosteal sleeve about the humerus, especially in younger patients, is very thick and, even with bayonet opposition or some angulation, union of these fractures is prompt. External support with plaster splints for several weeks in children usually holds the upper arm stably enough to permit union to occur. In infants and babies a soft dressing, wrapping the arm to the torso for 2 weeks, is usually sufficient. Nonunions of humeral shaft fractures in infants and children are virtually unheard of (Figs. 65.8 and 65.9).

Supracondylar Fractures of the Humerus

A child with a supracondylar fracture of the humerus has an acute and serious problem which requires immediate and effective emergency care. The more severe the displacement the more serious the problem (Fig. 65.10).

Most such fractures are so-called extension injuries, in which the distal fragment moves posteriorly on the proximal fragment. The direction of displacement causes the brachial artery and vein to stretch over the sharp edge of the proximal fragment, and subsequent bleeding, hematoma and swelling further narrow the diameter of the vessels. The combination of direct injury to the vessels and swelling in the fascial compartments of the forearm can produce a severe compartment syndrome. Untreated, the muscles of the forearm can develop ischemic myositis and, subsequently, ischemic necrosis. After the death of the muscles the necrotic and degenerated remnants form fibrotic scar tissue. This tissue in turn gradually engulfs the nerves and what viable muscle is left. The subsequent contracture of the forearm scar tissue produces a clawlike deformity which is the familiar Volkmann's contracture.

Clinically the most significant sign of ischemic myositis is pain. In patients with supracondylar fractures the pain is usually in the forearm, and passive extension of the fingers increases the degree of pain considerably. Usually the patient holds the fingers in a flexed position and resists efforts to manipulate the fingers into extension because this maneuver is so uncomfortable. The presence or absence of the radial pulses is of itself not confirmatory. Poor perfusion of the extremity distal to the injury produces pallor, sometimes cyanosis, and loss of sensation. These findings have greater significance than the strength of the radial pulse itself.

Treatment of a flexion injury or a minimally displaced extension injury can usually be conservative with splinting or some other form of external support. Patients with minimal or no displacement, however, require careful observation, and there is a good argument for admitting them for 24 hours to ensure the maintenance of perfusion of the forearm and hand and muscle viability.

Displaced supracondylar fractures of the humerus require emergency treatment. In the past, treatment was usually closed, with manipulation of the fragments under general anesthesia. More recently, however, open reduction and internal fixation with Kirschner wires has been found to provide prompt stability and maintenance of good position (Fig. 65.11). Patients who have this done do require a second minor procedure for removal of the Kirschner wires, but the prompt stable reduction outweighs this inconvenience as well as the theoretical risk of infection, the complications of anesthesia, and the hazards of emergency surgery.

Cubitus varus, or gun-stock deformity, has in the past also been a complication of supracondylar fractures. Often in treating patients with severely displaced fractures, surgeons were forced to concern themselves more with the vascular status of the arm. As a result less than optimal position of the

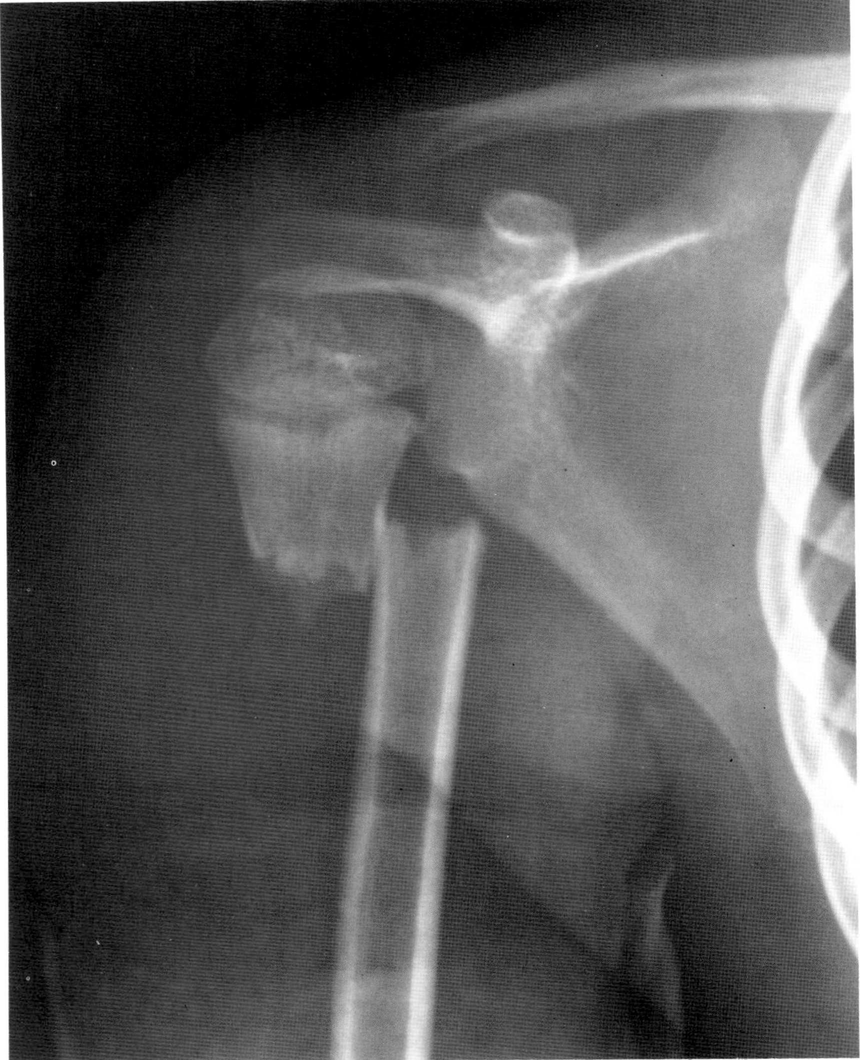

Figure 65.8 Fracture of the proximal humerus. This degree of bayonet apposition healed perfectly in a special cast in 2 months.

fracture was frequently accepted because of the problems with an impending Volkmann's contracture. With open reduction and internal fixation, however, a subsequent cubitus varus deformity is unlikely and treatment of the vascular problems can proceed without the concern that the patient could develop deformity as part of a tradeoff in treatment (Fig. 65.12). With the stable anatomic reduction and internal fixation, the vessels are protected from impingement on sharp fragments and swelling resolves more quickly. The net effect is that a patient is less likely to have a Volkmann's contracture after the operative reduction and fixation.

When findings of impending Volkmann's contracture persist despite the stable reduction, however, the patient may require emergency fasciotomy and arterial exploration. For this reason, these patients require continued observation for several

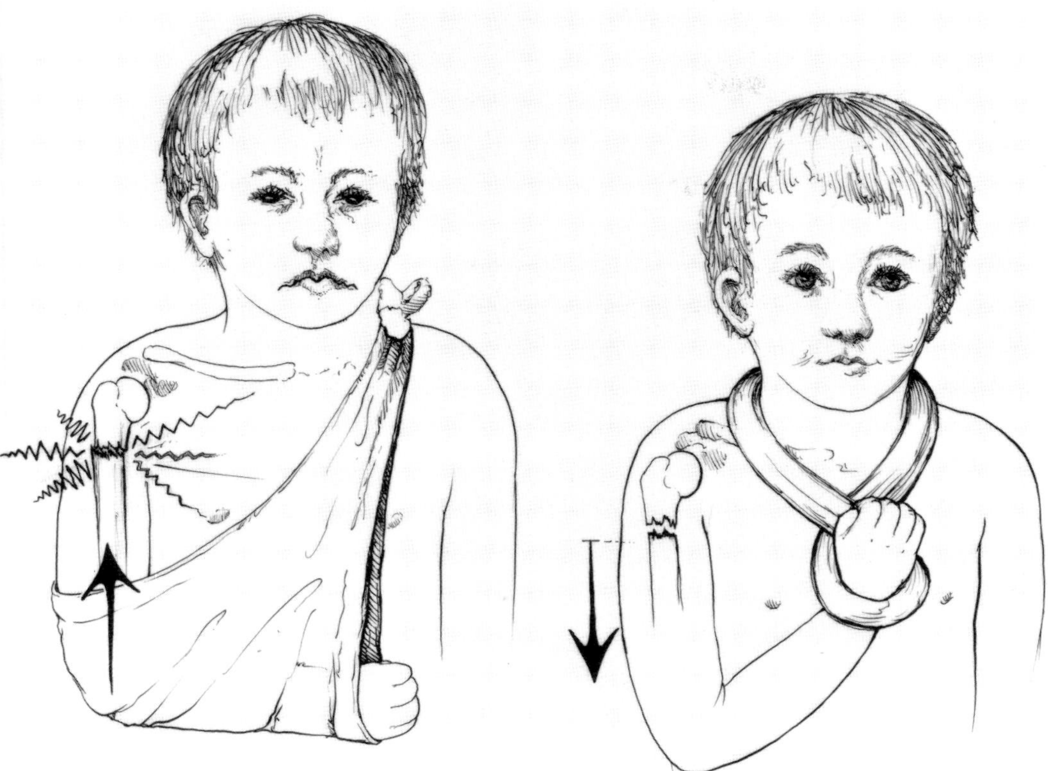

Figure 65.9 Undisplaced fractures of the humerus can be treated with a sling and swathe.

days in the hospital after any type of treatment.

Elbow Injuries in Children

Fractures involving the elbow joint in children very often require open surgery. They require prompt and accurate diagnosis on the part of the emergency physician to avoid releasing such patients from the emergency department. These injuries in general do not have as much potential for severe irreversible ischemic muscle necrosis as noted in the section on supracondylar fractures of the humerus, but they do present the complications of growth disturbance, deformity, late neurologic impairment and joint stiffness.

Recognition of the injury and awareness of its potential should prompt the emergency physician to make arrangements for admission and proper treatment. Injuries under consideration are: (a) fracture of the capitellum, (b) epiphyseal separation of the medial humeral epicondyle, (c) fracture of the medial humeral condyle, (d) fracture of the olecranon, and (e) fracture of the neck of the radius (Figs. 65.13 and 65.14).

Patients who have sustained *fractures of the capitellum* have Salter IV epiphyseal injuries. The fracture line extends from the elbow joint proximally across the epiphysis of the distal humerus and thence proximally into the metaphysis. This fracture has major adverse consequences when it escapes detection, since malunion may result from even minimal displacement. Unless the fracture is opened, accurately reduced, and stably fixed, patients develop severe cubitus valgus, joint stiffness and, probably most disabling of all, a traction palsy of the ulnar nerve. As the elbow drifts gradually into worsening valgus, the ulnar

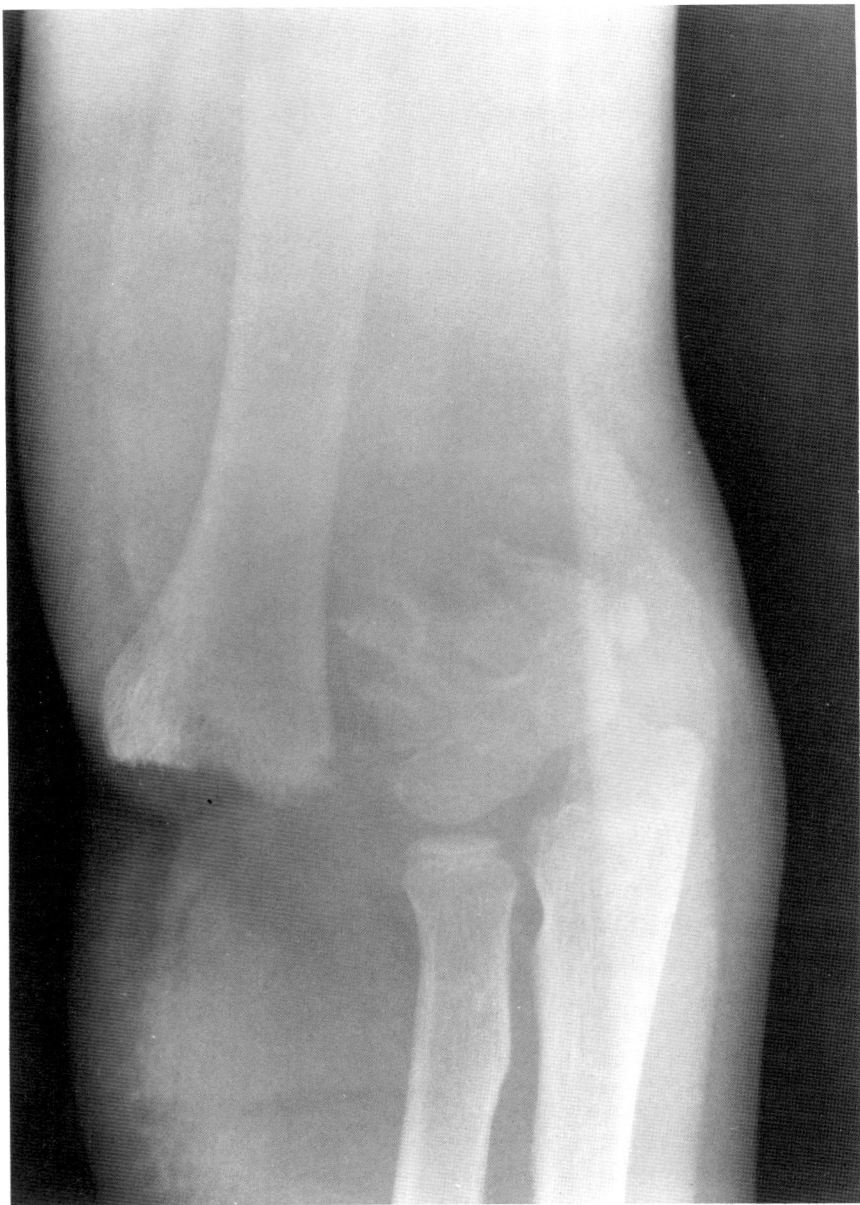

Figure 65.10 A roentgenogram of a badly displaced supercondylar fracture of the humerus. A child with this degree of displacement can develop severe ischemic necrosis of the forearm muscles. This patient requires immediate reduction and close postoperative follow-up to avoid that complication.

nerve is stretched behind the medial epicondyle, and the patient develops paresthesias and loss of sensation in the fourth and fifth fingers and paralysis of the intrinsic muscles of the hand (Fig. 65.15).

Prompt recognition of the fracture depends on accurate assessment of the x-ray of the injured elbow in a patient who has fallen and who complains of pain, swelling, and tenderness over the lateral side of the

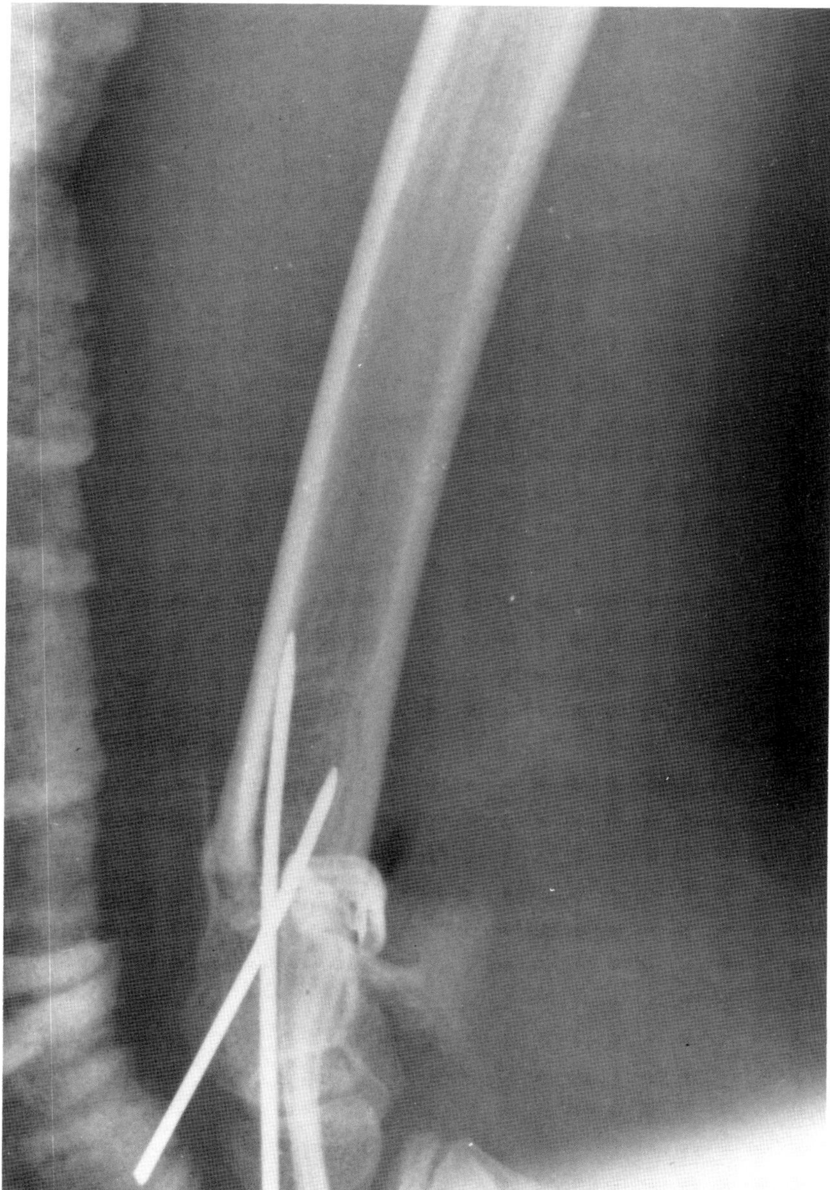

Figure 65.11 A lateral roentgenogram showing good alignment after open reduction and internal fixation with Kirschner wires. The patient recovered without neuromuscular sequella or deformity.

distal humerus. Awareness of the possibility of the injury is usually all that is required, since the fracture is readily evident on an AP x-ray. Nevertheless, comparison views of the normal and injured sides will facilitate diagnosis. Certainly patients with major displacement require admission but probably even those with minor displacement should be admitted for reduction and internal fixation to avoid the late complications described. Patients who have undisplaced fractures of the capitellum require splinting of the elbow and careful follow-up to ensure that the capitellar fragment does

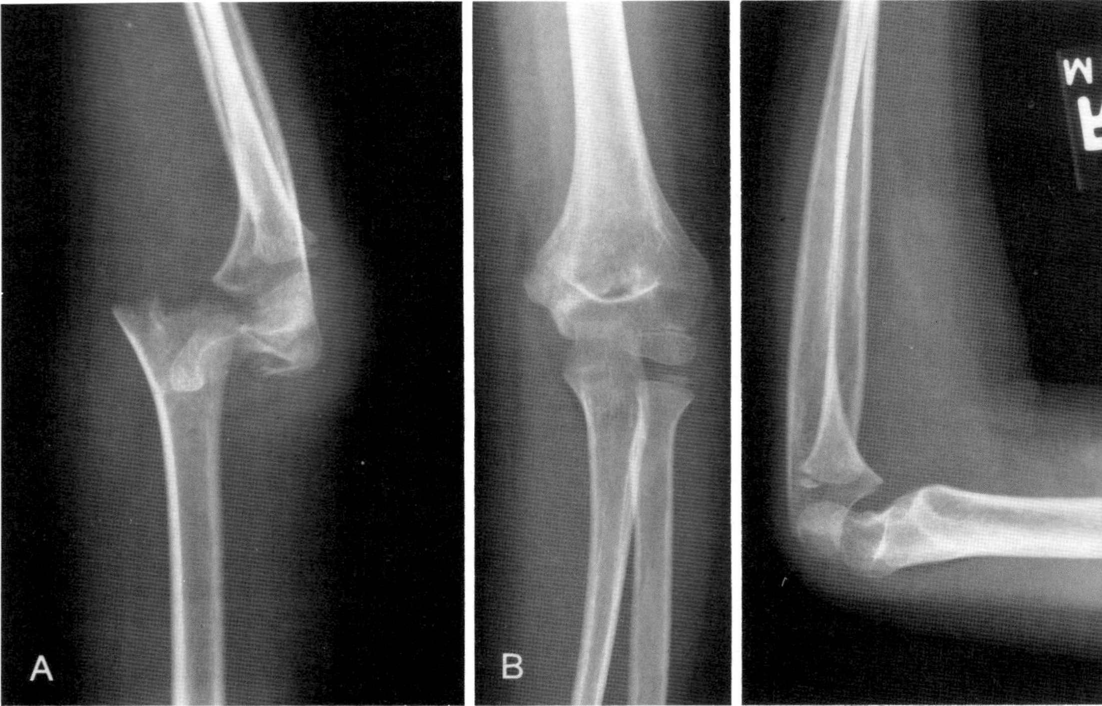

Figure 65.12 (*A*) Roentgenogram of a displaced supercondylar fracture of the humerus. (*B*) Lateral roentgenogram showing slight rotational malalignment. The fracture healed, the patient avoided a Volkmann's contracture but had a decrease in the normal carrying angle.

not lose its satisfactory alignment. If its position shifts even a little, the fracture should be stabilized (Fig. 65.16).

Fractures of the medial humeral condyle are very rare in children, but they have the same potential for producing deformity noted in fractures of the capitellum. The difference, of course, is that the inevitable nonunion on the medial side of the distal humerus causes the elbow to go into a cubitus varus position later on in the months after the injury has occurred.

The primary consideration in the diagnosis and treatment of *medial epicondylar injuries* is the relationship of that structure to the ulnar nerve which passes just behind it on the medial side of the elbow (Fig. 65.17). Fractures of the medial humeral epicondyle in general require open reduction and internal fixation only when they compress the nerve, causing ulnar nerve symptoms and signs. Usually minimal displacement (less than 1 cm) does not result in ulnar nerve involvement, and treatment with splinting for several weeks will permit the swelling and pain to subside and union of the epicondylar epiphysis to occur. Displacement of more than 1 cm, however, reflects more serious injury and may require open reduction. The surgeon must remove the epicondyle from a position which compresses the nerve and stabilize it with pins to maintain position until the fracture heals.

Some patients with medial humeral epicondylar injuries have absorbed enough violence to cause lateral dislocation of the elbow, and a spontaneous reduction results in trapping of the epicondyle within the joint.

X-rays of a child with this injury will reveal an extra density in the joint space and an absence of the medial humeral condyle from its accustomed position. These children have had major injuries. Removal of the epicondyle from the joint space with

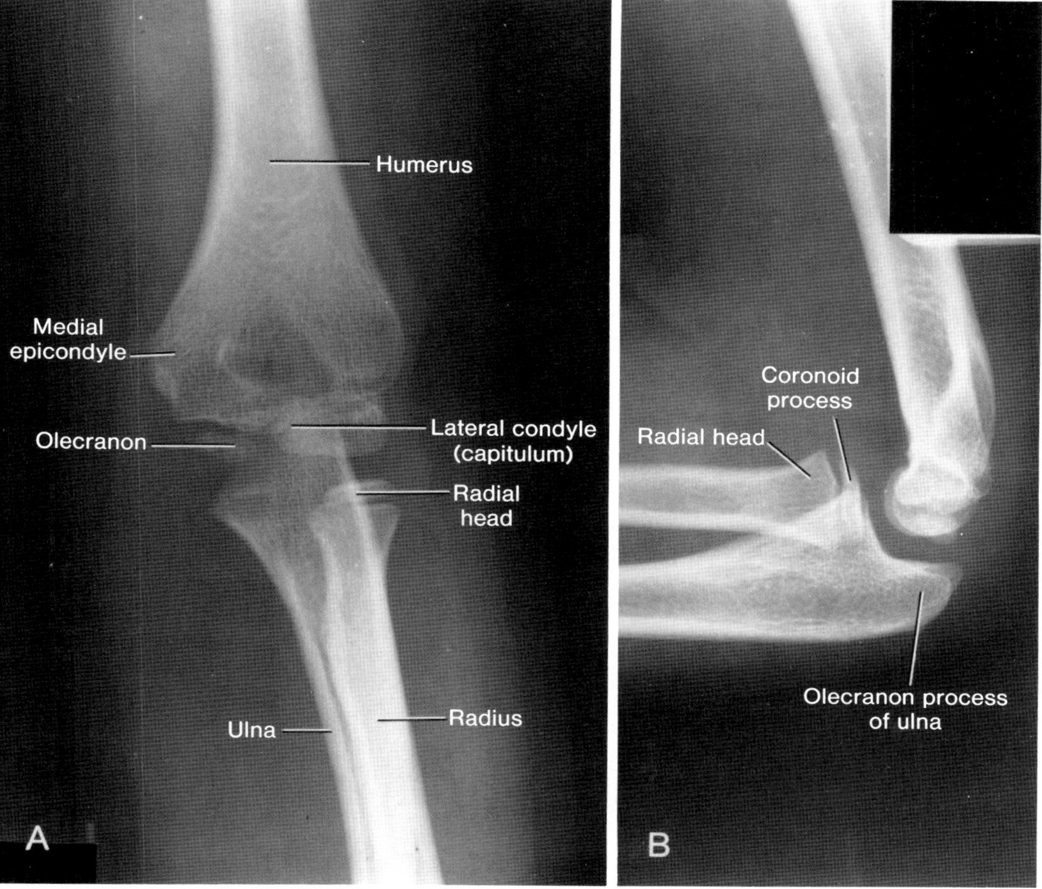

igure 65.13 (*A*) Anteroposterior roentgenogram of normal elbow in a child. (*B*) Lateral roentenogram of normal elbow.

nternal pin fixation is required to prevent evere late disability.

Proper treatment of the injury, of course, lepends on correct diagnosis of the injury n the emergency department. Careful reiew of comparison views will help in making the right diagnosis. One final point rearding medial epicondylar fractures resulting from elbow dislocation is that the child as marked swelling with bleeding into the oft tissues of the elbow and forearm. A hild with this injury, therefore, has the otential for developing a compartment yndrome and Volkmann's contracture. Splinting with a noncompression dressing, dmission to the hospital, and careful obervation of the limb, as described for impending Volkmann's contracture will permit one to institute proper treatment without delay if necessary.

Fractures of the olecranon in children are more often the result of direct violence than in adults, in whom sudden excessively vigorous triceps contracture avulses the olecranon from the distal ulna. In older children or adolescents, in whom the pattern of injury more closely approximates that of adult patients, open reduction and tension band wiring may be required to reestablish the continuity of the extension mechanism of the elbow. Olecranon process fractures are rather rare in pediatric emergencies and, while recognition usually poses no problems after review of the x-rays, dif-

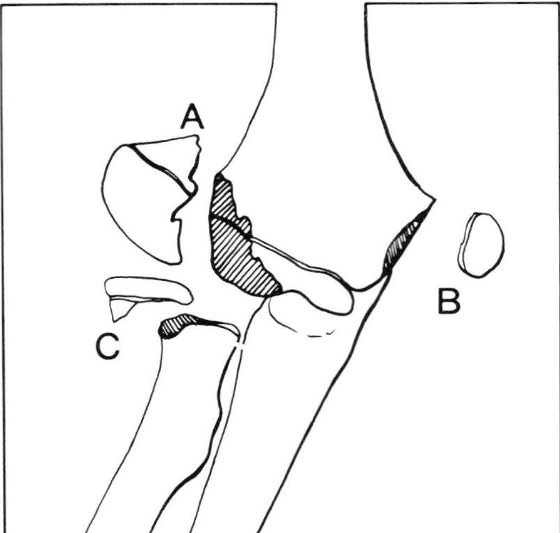

Figure 65.14 Drawing showing the common types of elbow injuries in children. (*A*) Fracture of the capitellum, (*B*) separation of the medial humeral epicondyle, and (*C*) fracture of the head of the radius.

ferences of opinion regarding the best treatment may arise (Fig. 65.18).

Radial neck fractures require open reduction if they have angulated more than 30°. Left untreated, a badly angulated radial neck fracture may not remodel enough to prevent limitation of pronation and supination of the elbow. Usually, in these cases, the force of injury causes the proximal radial epiphysis to displace on the epiphyseal line, taking a small metaphyseal wedge with it. Thus, the injury is really a Salter II epiphyseal separation, and growth disturbances are unusual regardless of treatment. Adult patients with displaced radial neck fractures or comminuted radial head fractures require arthrotomy and removal of the fracture fragments. Removal of the radial head in pediatric patients, however, produces growth arrest proximally and severe radial shortening and forearm bowing. Radial head excision should not be done in pediatric patients.

One other common elbow injury often seen on an emergency basis is a radial head subluxation or nursemaid's elbow. This injury results from a tear of the periosteal attachment of the annular ligament, the structure which maintains the radial head in its relationship with the proximal ulna and capitellum. Typically a parent or babysitter has pulled a young child (usually less than 5 years old) by the arm when the arm was extended and pronated. The child immediately complained tearfully of pain in the elbow sometimes radiating to the wrist and refuses to move the arm out of pronation and slight flexion. One can reduce the subluxation by supinating the forearm and extending the elbow (see procedure in Section VII). Immobilization is required only if the subluxation recurs repeatedly.

Fractures of the Forearm and Wrist

These injuries are among the most common fractures in children and comprise up to 20% of all of the fractures noted in this age group. A busy emergency department, therefore, will probably treat large numbers of such cases, so it is well to have a systematic approach to diagnosis and treatment. Clinically the diagnosis is usually easy, with the child presenting with a history of injury, swelling, pain and unmistakable clinical deformity. Probably the most important diagnostic consideration is the need to obtain films that include the elbow and wrist joint in at least two projections. Occasionally the force that produces a fracture of an ulnar diaphysis also dislocates the radial head. The resultant injury (Monteggia fracture) leaves the patient with severe disability even after satisfactory fracture healing, if the physician misses the diagnosis of radial head dislocation (Fig. 65.19).

One can avoid this mistake by routinely obtaining AP and lateral x-rays that show clearly the status of the elbow and wrist joints. In the emergency department, recognition of the Monteggia fracture is the most important factor in its management, since this complex injury usually requires admission and careful follow-up. In general, patients with this injury should not be simply casted and discharged.

Many fractures of the wrist and forearm, however, can be treated in the emergency department, depending, of course, on the degree of force which caused the injury,

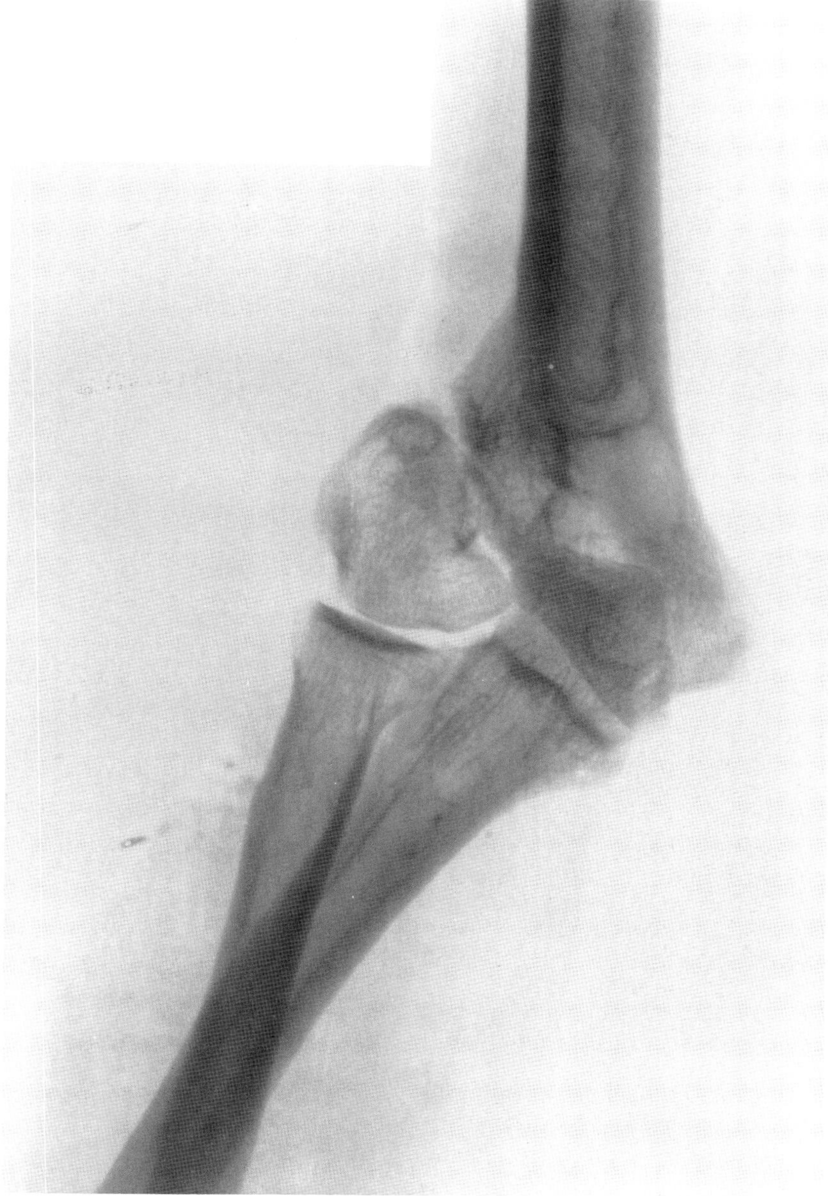

Figure 65.15 Fracture of the capitellum untreated has a bad prognosis. This AP roentgenogram shows the nonunion in an adult, mistreated as a child. The nonunion of the capitellum caused a valgus deformity of the elbow with contraction neuritis on the ulnar nerve.

amount of soft tissue swelling and amount of displacement of the fragments.

An *undisplaced torus fracture*, for example, justifies support in a well-molded short arm cast and discharge home. Even this minor injury, however, can present difficulties in treatment, such as cast problems (swelling with potential neurovascular impairment) and rarely displacement in the cast after swelling has resolved. Careful fol-

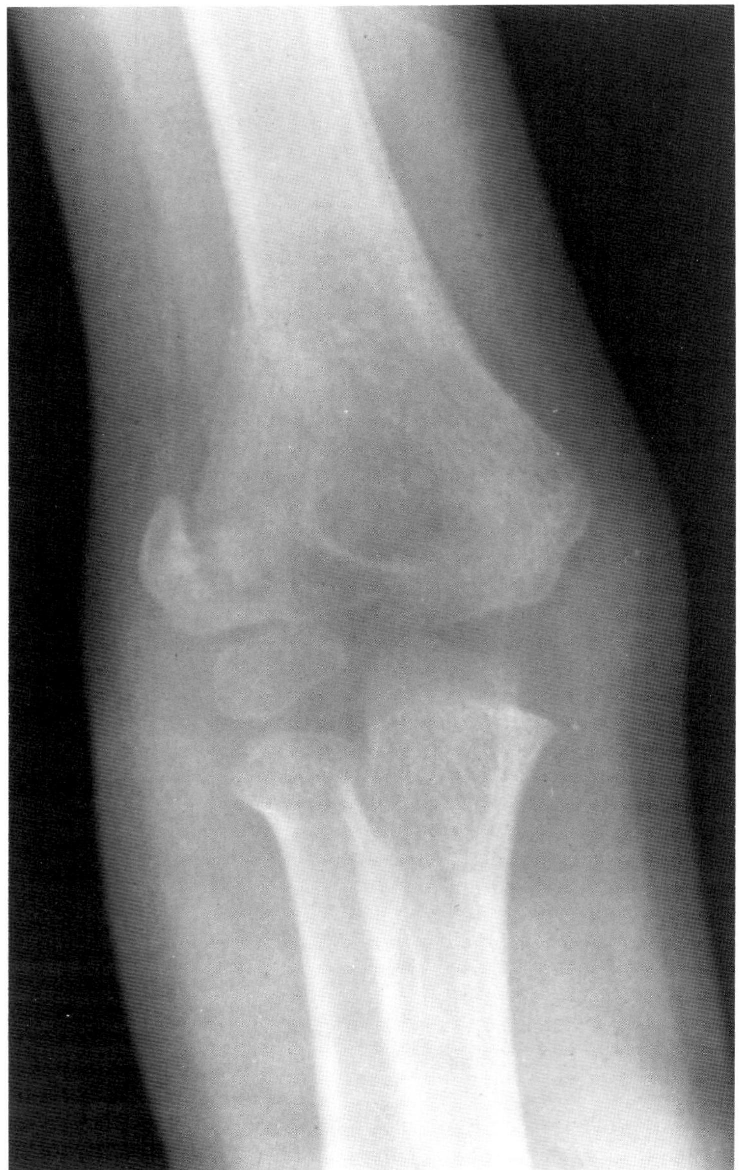

Figure 65.16 AP roentgenogram in a child showing a minimally displaced fracture of the capitellum. This injury usually requires internal fixation to avoid a nonunion.

low-up can prevent these complications, and the parents of a child who has been casted should always be given adequate instructions to ensure subsequent care.

Minor buckle fractures of the distal radius may be difficult to demonstrate in routine AP and lateral views. A child with pain and swelling over the distal radius after a fall, with negative AP and lateral x-rays, should probably be sent back to the x-ray department for oblique views. These are more likely to reveal an undisplaced buckle fracture, than the routine x-rays. It is embarrassing to discharge a child without having established the diagnosis of a "broken arm."

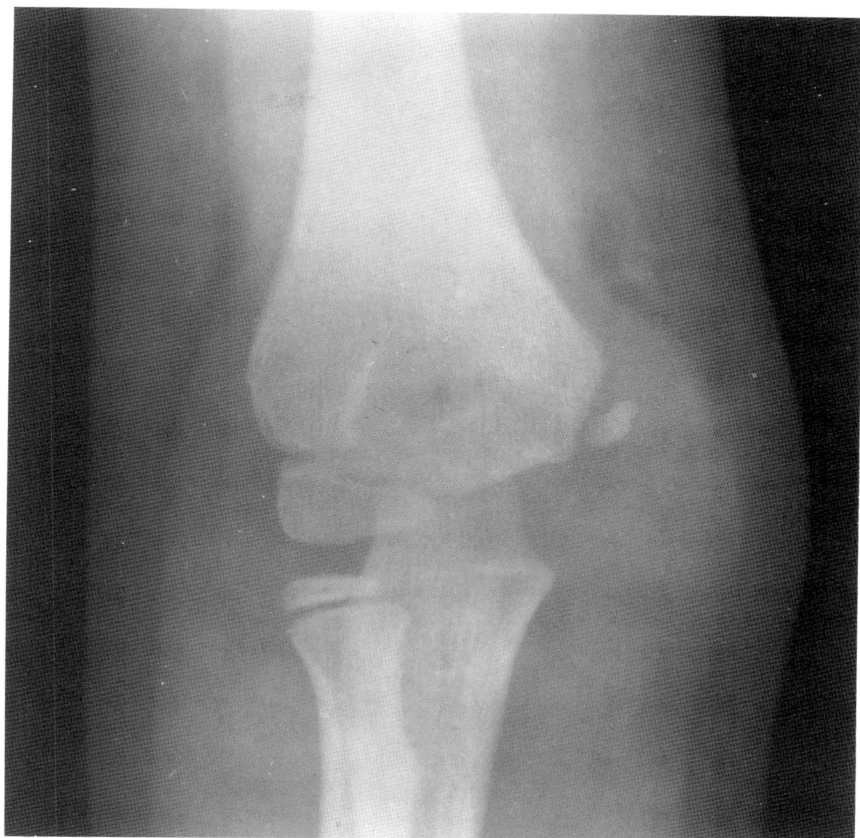

Figure 65.17 AP roentgenogram showing slight displacement of the medial humeral epicondyle. Occasionally patients with these injuries develop ulnar nerve signs and require reduction and fixation of the fracture. Occasionally the fragment remains in the elbow joint after a dislocation and must be removed.

Displaced fractures of the forearm usually require reduction. In the past a 30° angulation has been thought to remodel in young children under 7 years, but the promised restoration of normal alignment by growth and development always comes slowly and occasionally not at all. Most orthopaedic surgeon, therefore, prefer to reduce fractures which have even a mild degree of malalignment. Local anesthesia usually suffices, and admission to the hospital is usually not necessary. Satisfactory follow-up arrangements and suitable instructions for cast care are, of course, mandatory.

More *severely displaced forearm and wrist fractures* usually need more aggressive treatment. Greenstick fractures maintain an intact cortex on the concave side, and unless the treating physician breaks through this intact cortex, the bone will gradually bend further and further into the deformed position (Fig. 65.20).

Displaced fractures of both bones require a formal manipulation and are occasionally quite difficult to align. In general, such patients have a good deal of pain and swelling, and local anesthesia makes both worse. While circumstances vary, many orthopaedists prefer to admit a child with an undisplaced forearm fracture and carry out the reduction under general anesthesia, instead of injecting the hematoma with a local anesthetic.

Fractures of the distal radial physis with dorsal displacement of the epiphysis are

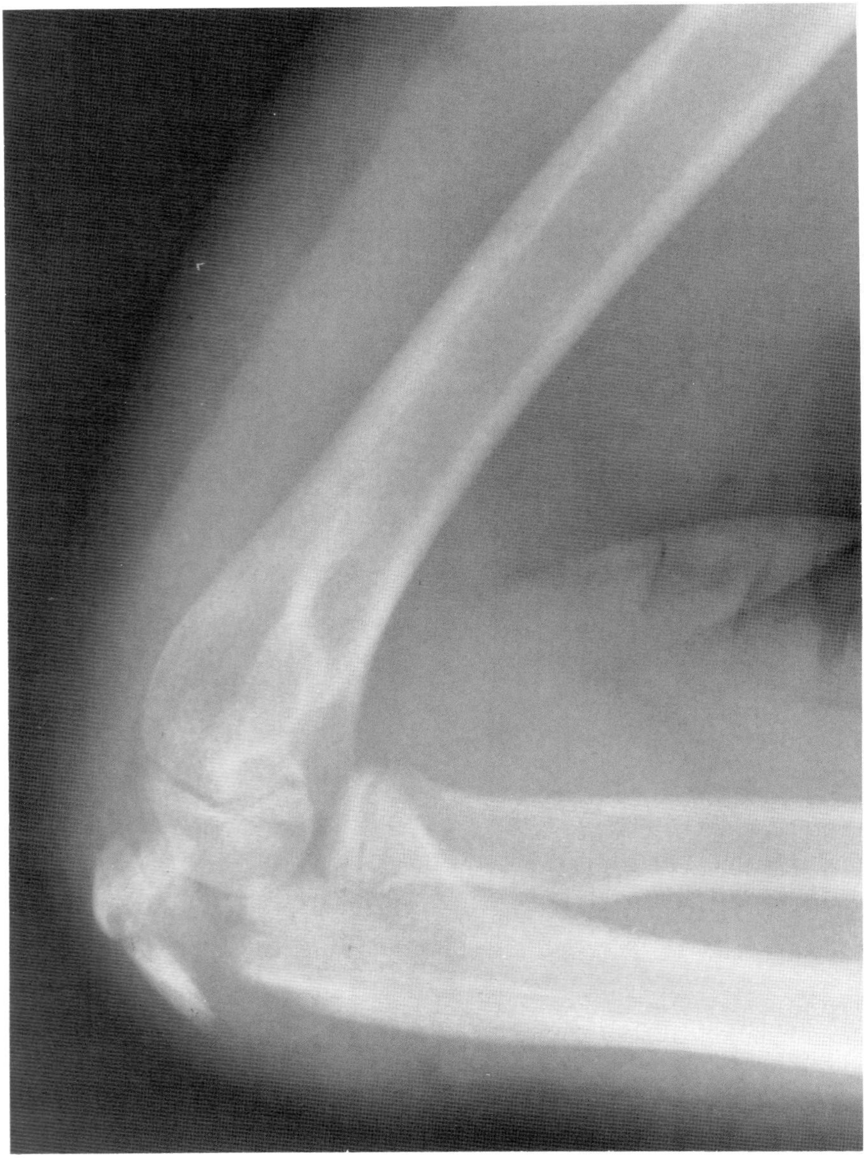

Figure 65.18 Fractures of the olecranon as shown in the lateral roentgenogram may need open reduction and tension band wiring.

very common injuries and usually occur in adolescents and older children. These are usually Salter II injuries, and, since the germinal layer of chondrocytes of the epiphysis is not damaged, a growth disturbance rarely occurs. The clinical and radiographic picture usually easily makes the diagnosis. The fragments early on after the injury have a very unstable interface and one can usually easily reduce the displacement.

A discussion of emergency care of fractures does not need to include much information on the technical details of their management. Nevertheless circumstances may require the physician who sees the

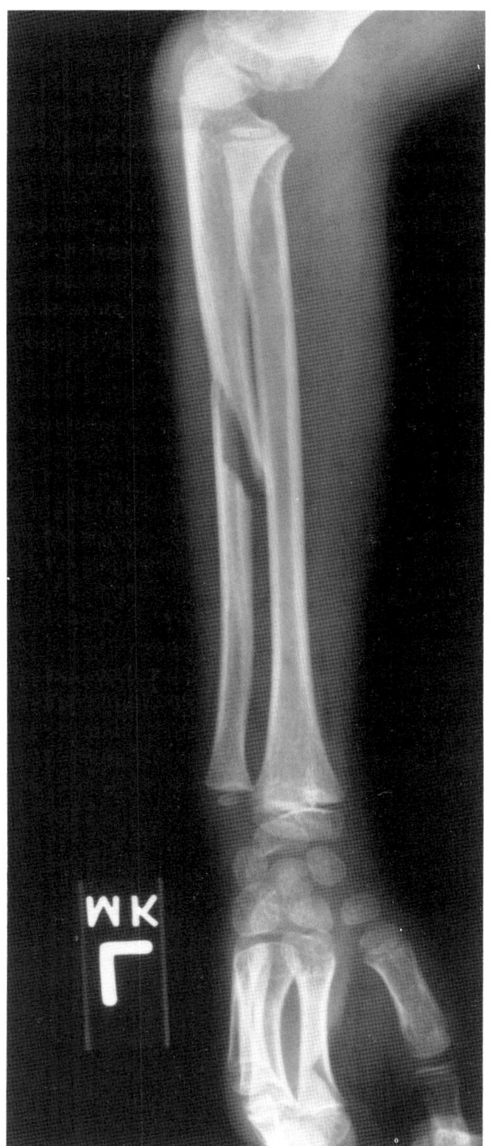

Figure 65.19 Roentgenogram showing a fracture of the ulna and radial head dislocation (Monteggia fracture). Always x-ray the wrist and elbow in children to avoid missing a dislocation associated with the fracture.

patient on an emergency basis to provide definitive treatment. That individual should, of course, familiarize himself with basic cast technique in advance, before working on a restless, agitated child with a painful fractured forearm. Briefly, one must pad the cast well. He must mold the cast as he applies it and not wrap it on circumferentially as a perfect circle in cross section. The round cast does not immobilize well. The child should keep the arm at the desired position while the cast is being applied to keep the cast from wrinkling and cutting into the child's swollen arm. The physician must emphasize follow-up to the parents and see that subsequent x-rays document good alignment of the fragments. Finally he should warn the parents in advance that the fracture may need a second reduction if it loses position. Forearm and wrist fractures heal rapidly and the physician has the opportunity to correct re-displacement after the initial reduction for only about 10 days. It is useful to keep this in mind when ordering follow-up films, because the fracture will quickly become too well-healed to permit re-manipulation.

Hand Injuries

Fractures of the Hand and Fingers

The emergency care of *hand fractures* in children begins with accurate diagnosis. The emergency physician should ask about the history, of course, to make a determination regarding the degree of violence to the hand, the mechanism, and the time the injury occurred. As with other pediatric injuries, however, the parents and the children may mislead the doctor, either intentionally or unintentionally. Diagnosis, therefore, depends on the physical examination and x-ray evaluation. Swelling and tenderness localize the area to which the physician should direct his attention in evaluating the films. In making the diagnosis of finger fractures before taking an x-ray of the injured hand, the emergency physician should check the patient for malrotation of the finger (Fig. 65.21). In the extended position the malrotation is not obvious, but when the fingers flex one will overlap the other if malrotation is present.

The physician must remember that children have epiphyses of the proximal end of each phalanx and epiphyses at the distal end of each metacarpal, except the thumb metacarpal (Fig. 65.22). The thumb meta-

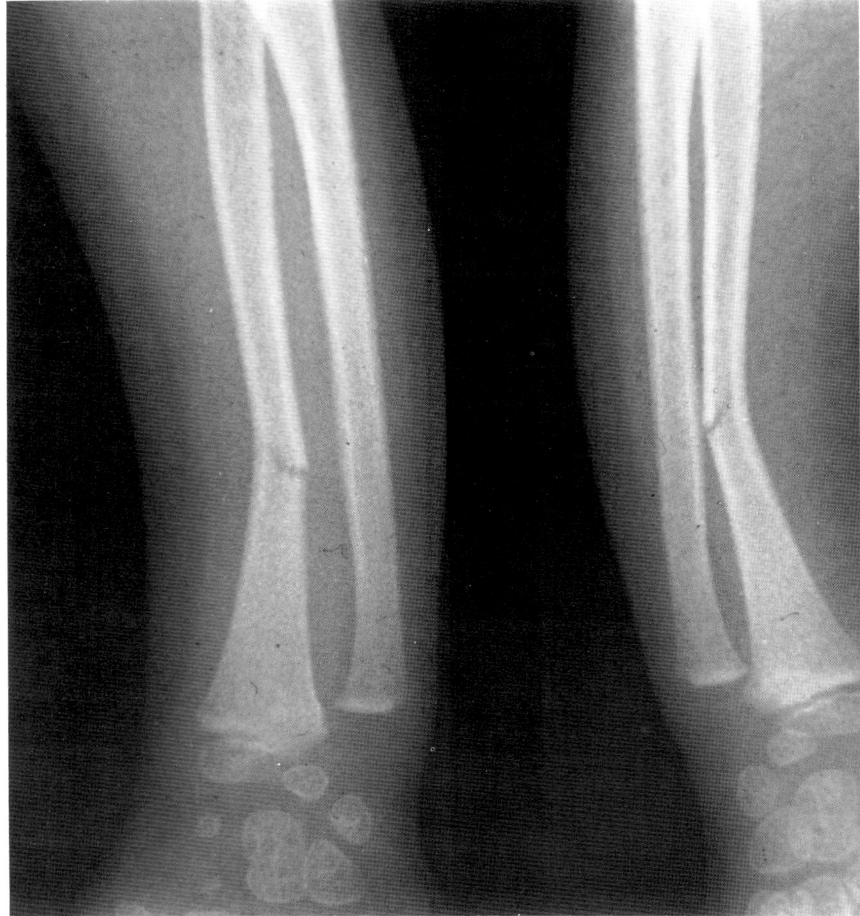

Figure 65.20 Greenstick fracture of the forearm. This injury requires a manipulation to break through both cortices to prevent reangulation. (Courtesy of J. Gregg, M.D.)

carpal has its epiphysis at the proximal end of the bone, since developmentally the thumb metacarpal is a phalanx and the greater multangular is its metacarpal. Rarely, however, metacarpals can have epiphyses at both ends. The emergency physician should also remember that the carpal bones ossify at varying times during childhood and not let himself be confused by the varying appearances of the carpus.

Because carpal bones have a large cartilaginous component, they rarely fracture in the childhood years. Only older boys who sustain navicular fractures provoke concern in this regard, and such patients may need careful review of oblique wrist films to make this diagnosis. If pain and tenderness over the navicular in such a patient does not have the accompanying positive x-ray, the doctor should probably immobilize the wrist and thumb anyway, to protect the navicular, and re-x-ray the wrist in 10 days. If the x-ray is negative then, the patient can discontinue the use of the cast; but, as often as not, the second film will reveal a fracture and the patient will need another 6 weeks of immobilization to avoid the consequences of nonunion and avascular necrosis of the navicular fracture.

Finger fractures in children are very common. Despite the seemingly minor nature of such injuries they can cause persist-

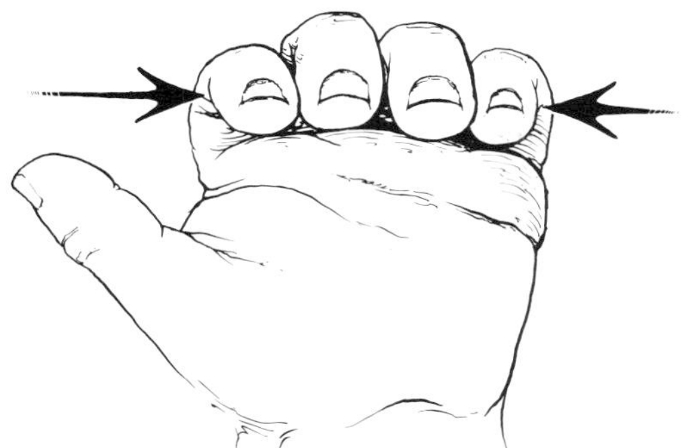

Figure 65.21 Checking for malrotation of the fingers will occasionally establish the diagnosis of a rotated phalangeal or metacarpal fracture. In this position, the fingers all point in the same direction normally but study them to determine if one overlaps another abnormally.

ent disability unless properly treated. Several basic principles deserve mention in this regard. Splinting a child's hand can try the resourcefulness of the physician. When closed reduction and splinting fail, reduction and pin fixation of fracture fragments may better secure the fragments. The position in which the hand is splinted also influences the success of closed techniques. At 90° of flexion the metacarpal phalangeal joint holds the collateral ligament at its maximum length and tension. If the finger on the metacarpal drifts back toward extension in the splint the collateral ligaments shorten, and this may cause metacarpal phalangeal joint extension contractures. The interphalangeal joints, however, require splinting in only 15% of flexion since that position maximally stretches their col-

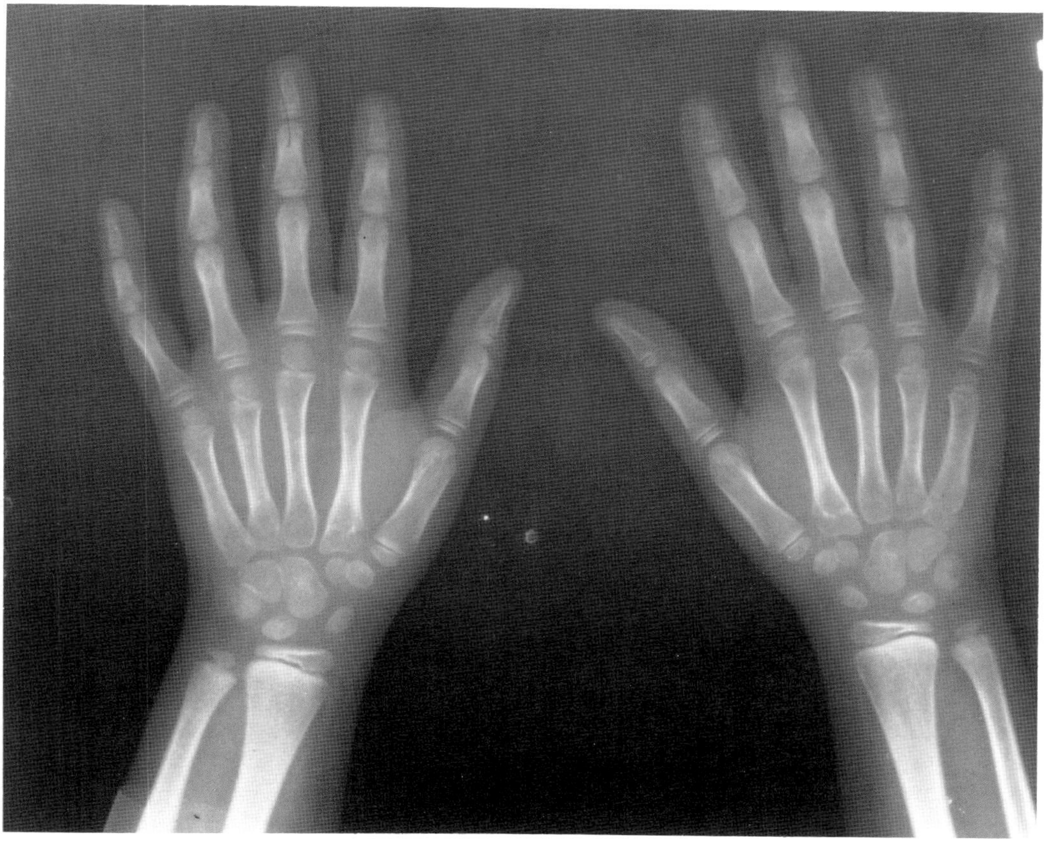

Figure 65.22 AP roentgenogram showing the normal epiphyseal plates in the proximal ends of the phalanges of the fingers and distal ends of their metacarpals. The thumb metacarpal, however, has the growth plate proximally.

lateral ligaments, preventing flexion contractures of the interphalangeal joints when splinting is discontinued. The grasp position formerly suggested as the "position of function" promotes extension contractures at the metacarpal phalangeal joints and flexion contractures of the interphalangeal joints. This position, therefore, should not be used. (Figs. 65.23–65.25).

Thoughtlessly slamming a door and unsupervised playing with machines such as kitchen blenders produce lacerations and *crush injuries of the distal phalanx.* Most of these injuries self-heal and need only washing, irrigation, occasionally an absorbable suture, and sterile dressings. Injuries of the nail bed, however, may need careful surgical repair to prevent permanent deformity of the finger nail. Some finger tip amputations, especially in older children and adolescents, may need skin grafting. It is surprising, however, how well younger children heal badly fractured and lacerated finger tips. Such injuries in young patients justify very conservative treatment.

Mallet finger deformities often result from epiphyseal separation in young children. These injuries can be treated merely by splinting in hyperextension for a few weeks with a small malleable splint. In adolescents, however, the extensor tendons tend to avulse a fragment of epiphysis in the proximal part of the distal phalanx, and these injuries occasionally require open reduction and Kirschner wire fixation.

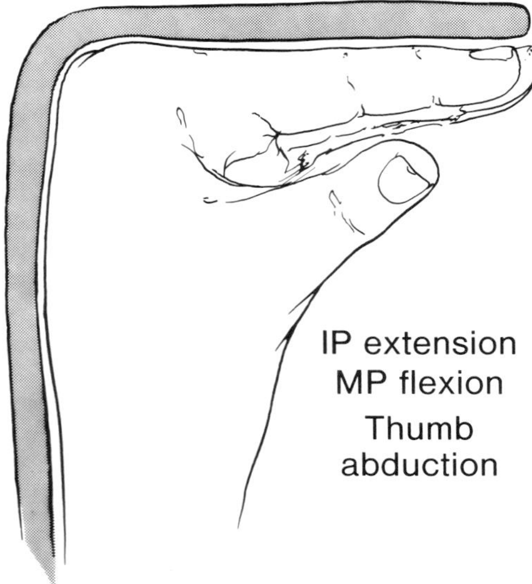

Figure 65.23 The hand should be splinted in this position to prevent extension contractures of the metacarpal phalangeal (*MP*) joints and flexion contractures of the interphalangeal (*IP*) joints.

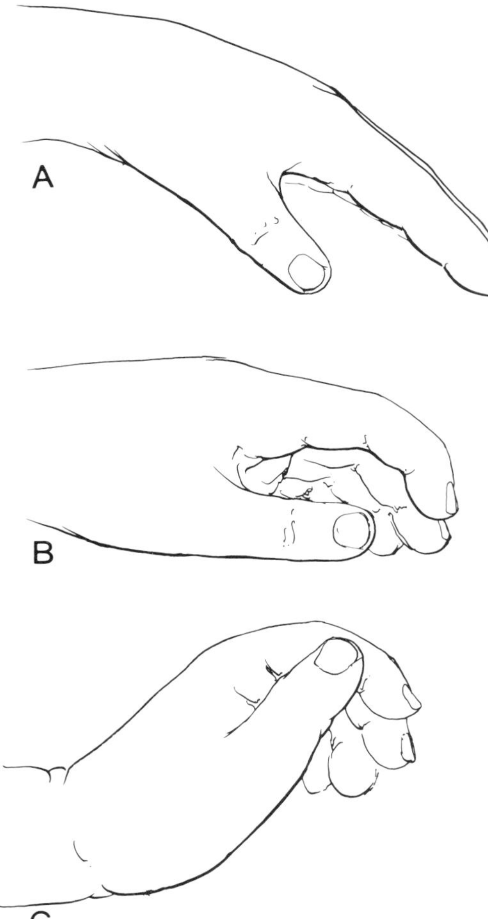

Figure 65.24 Splinting the hand in these three positions (*A*,*B*,*C*) tends to promote recurrence of deformity and joint contractures.

Fractures of the shaft of the phalanx in children angulate dorsally or volarly depending on their location relative to the insertion of the flexor digitorum profundus tendon. A fracture distal to the insertion of the tendon flexes the proximal fragment, so that in splinting the fracture after reduction

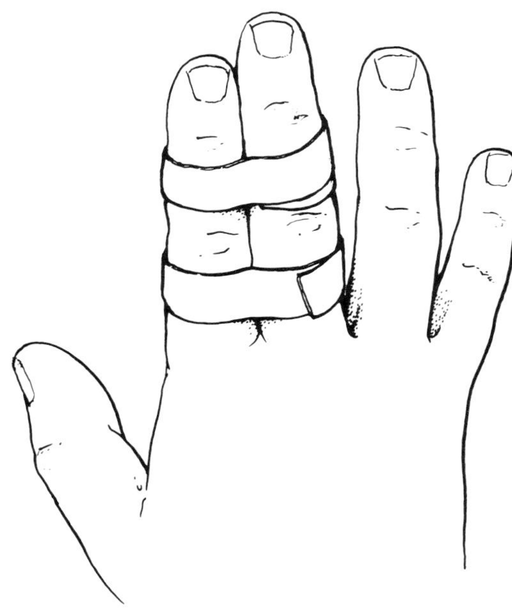

Figure 65.25 "Buddy taping" is a convenient way to splint undisplaced fractures of the fingers but more severe injuries require more aggressive treatment (see text).

one must hold the distal fragment in flexion. When the fracture occurs proximal to the insertion of the flexor digitorum sublimus, the proximal fragment goes into extension because of the pull of the central slip of the extensor tendon. These injuries require splinting in extension.

Fractures of the head of the distal end of the middle phalanx may angulate laterally or medially. This malalignment can be permanent. If closed methods do not maintain correction, the patient may escape permanent malignment only at the cost of open reduction and Kirschner wire fixation.

Fractures of the proximal phalanx of the fingers most often respond satisfactorily to closed reduction and splinting, with the proximal interphalangeal joints in extension and the metacarpal phalangeal joints in flexion. The proximal phalanx may require a more aggressive approach with open surgery and Kirschner wire fixation only if the head of the phalanx is irreversibly displaced or if a spiral fracture of the shaft proves too unstable to remain reduced after satisfactory splinting. Fractures at the base of the proximal phalanx with lateral angulation, particularly of the little fingers are common injuries in patients who have been grasped by the little finger and pulled to the ground in rough play or in sports like football. One can reduce this fracture by placing a pencil between the fourth and fifth digit (for example) and pushing the distal fragment toward the radius. The pencil acts as a fulcrum over which one levers the displaced fracture.

Metacarpal fractures in adults are very common injuries, and result from fist fights, punching a wall and other direct blows. These injuries do not occur as frequently in children, except possibly in older boys. They heal rapidly in both children and adults with conservative treatment. Aggressive open reduction and internal Kirschner wire fixation produces a good deal of discomfort and often considerable joint stiffness.

Thumb fractures in children most often involve the base of the metacarpal and occasionally include a dislocation of one of the fragments. This injury is the familiar Bennett's fracture. Children and adults need adequate fixation to prevent permanent changes at the carpometacarpal joint which in turn would cause subsequent joint stiffness and arthritis. Closed reduction and percutaneous Kirschner pin fixation is an easy way to control this problem.

Patients with thumb injuries should also be evaluated for avulsion of the collateral ligament of the metacarpal phalangeal joint. The ligament in children tends to pull away the base of the proximal phalanx of the thumb, causing a Salter III injury of the epiphysis of the proximal phalanx. Without reduction and pin fixation of the fragment, such patients will develop an angular deformity with growth and will also experience disabling instability of the metacarpal phalangeal joint of the thumb.

Soft Tissue Injuries

Older boys engaged in vigorous athletics often sustain a puzzling irreducible *dislocation of the metacarpal phalangeal joint* of the finger or thumb. The dislocation can even compound through the skin, and the patient can present with a markedly hyperextended digit fixed in the dislocated position, a small volar laceration, and the shiny metacarpal head visible through the skin defect. A sudden gentle snap would appear to reduce the dislocation but will not, because the metacarpal head is caught beneath the thick volar plate. This reduction needs the surgical extraction of the plate fro between the metacarpal head and the base of the proximal phalanx, and usually this can only be done in the operating room. If, therefore, the initial attempt at closed reduction in the emergency department is unsuccessful, the emergency physician should make arrangements for the patient's admission to the hospital for definitive care.

Tendon and nerve injuries in children follow the same general guidelines used for handling these injuries in adults. Since childrens' tendons and nerves are so much smaller, however, the surgeon usually needs better magnification and finer technique. Obviously such injuries do not lend themselves to emergency department repair and, in general, all children with tendon and/or nerve lacerations should be admitted (Fig. 65.26).

As in adults, extensor tendon injuries heal well after primary repair. Extensor tendon lacerations over the dorsum of the proximal phalangeal joint of a finger, however, may require reattachment to the base of the middle finger to prevent a boutonniére deformity. Flexor profundus tendon injuries in children can usually be repaired primarily if the injury was caused by a sharp knife or razor blade, although tenolysis may be subsequently required. Crushing tendon lacerations caused by such devices as power saws or escalators produce crushing injuries of the digits with open fractures and severe tendon disruption. This type of trauma, of course, does not lend itself to primary tendon repair. Such patients need emergency debridement, fracture stabilization, antibiotics, wound care and splinting. When the tissues have healed and the severe swelling has subsided, a surgeon can perform a late secondary procedure including possibly a tendon graft.

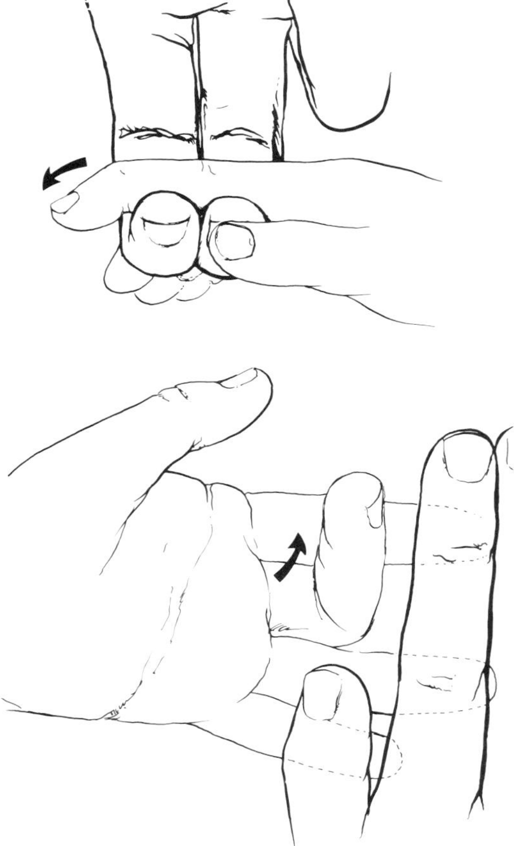

Figure 65.26 Diagnosis of flexor tendon injuries. Flexion of the distal finger joint with the proximal joint extended tests for profundis injury. Flexion of the proximal joint with the adjacent fingers extended tests for sublimis injury.

Mutilating Multiple Injuries

Mutilating *multiple injuries* of the hand, with or without amputations of the digits and metacarpals, present a special problem in reconstruction and rehabilitation. In the emergency situation the physician should do everything possible to maintain viability of as much tissue as possible. Replantation techniques with microsurgery now make replantation of amputated digits possible. The emergency department physician, therefore, should determine where this service is available and make arrangements for prompt transfer. Replantation requires that the amputated digits be kept cool during transfer. Do not pack them in ice until the replantation procedure can begin since freezing destroys their viability. The injured hand itself requires the usual sequence of cleansing, debriding the gross contamination, sterile dressing, splinting, and elevation. The patient should also be started on intravenous antibiotics after culture of the wound has been obtained.

Hand Infections

Other authors have discussed felons and paronychias and this section will briefly present the following: (1) collar button abscess, (2) deep space infection, and (3) tendon sheath infection.

Collar Button Abscess

A collar button abscess presents in the web space between two fingers. It usually begins on the palmar surface but because the palmar skin is more dense and the fascia less yielding, the swelling and abscess formation presents dorsally. This type of abscess can delude the physician who only incises and drains the hand on the dorsum. The dangerous part of the abscess remains undrained on the palmar aspect of the hand. Without adequate decompression, it will spread proximally through the lumbrical canal into the midpalmar space. Collar button abscesses require two short longitudinal incisions, one dorsal and one volar for adequate drainage.

Deep Space Infections

These infections occur in the space between the flexor tendons and the fascia covering the metacarpals and the osseous muscles. A fibrous septum extending from the fascia beneath the flexor tendons to the third metacarpal divides the deep space into the thenar and midpalmar space.

Midpalmar space infections produce massive swelling of the hand, severe pain, and an intense systemic response. Tissue motion of the third and fourth fingers is exquisitely painful. A curved volar incision extending over the space from the distal flexion crease at the third metacarpal phalangeal joint will satisfactorily evacuate this space.

Thenar space infections cause massive swelling on the thumb side of the palm of the hand and restrict motion of the thumb and index finger. A curved incision roughly parallel to the first dorsal interosseous muscle on the palm provides access to the space for drainage, but the proximity of the motor median nerve should make one cautious in using this approach.

Deep space infections do not occur very often. Increased awareness of the adverse consequences of hand infections and the common use of antibiotics early on in such cases has made them less common.

Tendon Sheath Infections

Extension of infection from pulp infections or contaminated puncture wounds of the fingers can cause the development of an abscess in a tendon sheath. Patients develop massive swelling of the involved finger or thumb and have severe pain with attempted passive motion. Left untreated the infection can cause sloughing of the tendon. It also will extend proximally into the palmar spaces or in the case of the fifth finger and thumb into the ulnar or radial bursa of the wrist. The physician can incise the abscess through a midlateral approach on the finger supplemented by a short transverse incision on the volar surface of the metacarpal phalangeal joint. These two incisions provide access to the tendon sheath and permit one to pass a small catheter down the tendon sheath for irrigation and drainage.

If the infection has extended proximally into the radial and ulnar bursae of the wrist the surgeon can pass a catheter proximally and distally to irrigate and drain the infection in the sheath.

Surgery on the infected hand should not usually be done in the emergency room. These cases require general anesthesia, and the controlled environment of the operating room. Children with deep hand infections are usually quite sick and should certainly be treated with intravenous antibiotics selected on the basis of culture and antibiotic sensitivity. Postoperative care, splinting in the functional position, and proper rehabilitation of the hand are additional factors which affect the outcome of these cases. The recognition of the type of infection, its location, necessary treatment, and prognosis will enable the emergency physician to start the patient in the right direction.

SPINE AND PELVIS

The anatomy of the vertebrae in children dictates the nature of the fractures and dislocation which patients in this age group sustain. The vertebra change from cartilage to bone by ossifying from the primary ossific nuclei, one in the center of the vertebral body and one in each neural arch. These ossific nuclei spread throughout the vertebra and fuse at the neurocentral joint. During early adolescence the secondary ossific nuclei appear, one at the tip of the spinous process, one at the tip of each transverse process, and one in the vertebral end plate on the cranial and caudal surface of the ossific nucleus of the centrum. The attachments of the nucleus pulposus to the vertebral end plate have much greater mechanical strength than the attachment of the vertebral end plate to the ossific nucleus of the centrum. Stresses applied (usually flexion or extension) to the spinal column, therefore, cause the distortion to occur at the weakest place, namely the ossification front between the vertebral centrum and the vertebral end plate. Thus fractures and dislocations of the spine, particularly in young children, are primarily soft tissue injuries with major tearing of the posterior longitudinal and interspinous ligaments associated with separation of the end plates from the primary ossific nucleus of the vertebral body. Indeed quadriplegia and paraplegia may occur without gross changes being noted on x-ray in younger patients. The emergency physician must look for slight malalignment, fanning of the spinous process and possibly minor fractures of the neural arch to make the diagnosis of vertebral injury.

Cervical Spine

In younger patients below 6 or 7 years, the odontoid process has not fused to the second cervical vertebral body. In children in this age group the ossification front between the dens and axis vertebra appears weaker even than the interface between the lower vertebral bodies and their end plates. Possibly for this reason, the common injury of the cervical spine in young children is a separation of the dens from the body of the axis. This injury has a good prognosis when it is promptly recognized and treated. Union occurs after the reduction of the fracture by manipulation of the head into extension and maintainance of position for 8 to 10 weeks in a Minerva jacket (Fig. 65.27).

Rotary atlantoaxial subluxation is another cause of acute neck pain in children. Often, these patients have a history of recent upper respiratory infection. After a minor injury, the child may develop a fixed torticollis and complain of severe upper neck discomfort. X-rays may show an increase in the atlantoodontoid interval, but occasionally diagnosis may require a CT scan (Fig. 65.28).

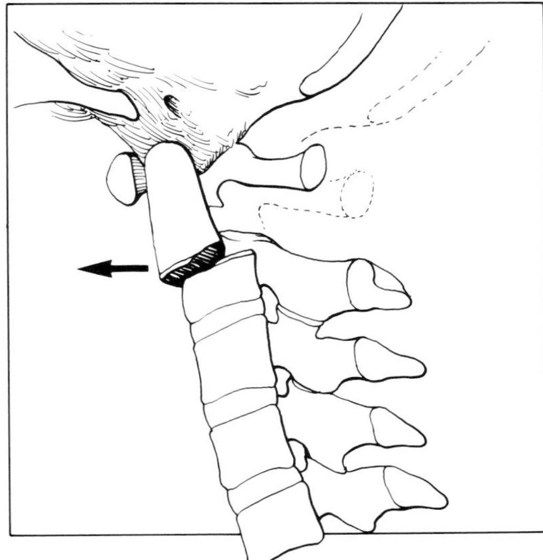

Figure 65.27 Diagrammatic representation of odontoid fracture in children with forward displacement of the dens epiphysis on the vertebral body of the axis.

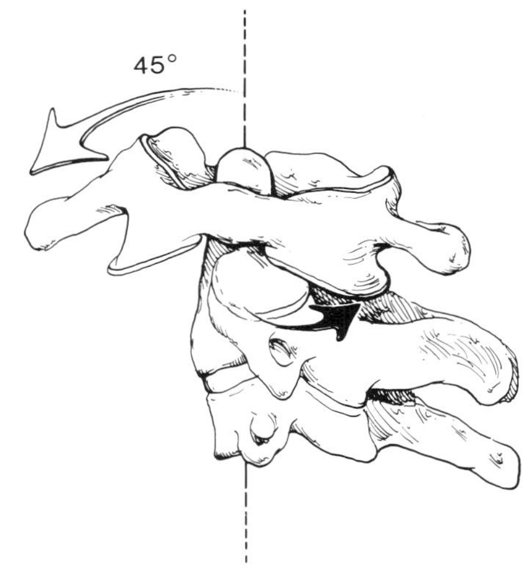

Figure 65.28 Rotary atlantoaxial subluxation often follows upper respiratory infection and a minor injury. These children have fixed painful torticollis. Usually external support relieves symptoms but occasionally they need reduction first and occasionally even a surgical fusion.

Older children participating in gymnastics and football usually develop cervical subluxation in the lower cervical spine at the C5-C6 or C6-C7 levels. Fracture of the facet joints do not occur often in this age group, but such injuries usually do cause disruption of the secondary ring ossification center of the vertebra on which the dislocation has occurred. The change in the shape of the subjacent vertebral body, the elasticity of the remaining ligaments, and the apparently slow healing of the torn interspinous and longitudinal ligaments combine to make these injuries very unstable. They may require fusion after reduction.

One of the most tragic injuries in pediatric practice is the bursting fracture of a vertebra noted in high school football players. The use of the hard shell plastic helmet and face guard has made players unafraid to use their heads as weapons in spearing, blocking and tackling. The sudden forces generated by these activities can place such severe axial load on the cervical vertebrae that they can explosively disrupt a vertebral body, causing a bursting fracture. The retropulsion of bone and disk material into the spinal canal causes an anterior cord syndrome or complete quadriplegia. Sadly these injuries offer little hope for recovery. Emergency care of these patients consists of prompt, accurate appraisal of cord injury and the level of quadriplegia if present.

The physician must place sand bags about the head and neck to prevent motion while the patient is being transferred. One should not struggle with a football helmet. It is better to have heavy metal shears on hand to remove the face guard and slip the helmet off to prevent motion of the neck. When the initial evaluation has been completed, the emergency physician could provide for more complete protection of the neck by applying Gardiner tongs and placing the patient in skeletal traction. The technique is easy to learn and quite useful. Definitive care of the neck injury should procede along established lines after the patient has left the emergency department.

Thoracolumbar Spine

Injuries of the thoracolumbar spine which cause fractures of the vertebra also produce stretching and tearing of the soft tissues surrounding and supporting the vertebrae. Classification, treatment, and prognosis of these injuries depend on whether or not the bones and soft tissues have been disrupted enough to permit the vertebrae to displace one on another when subjected to physiologic stresses.

Most of these injuries occur in older pediatric patients after the appearance of the secondary vertebral epiphysis. Most result from compression forces placed on the vertebral body without extensive soft tissue disruption. X-rays in these patients reveal mild wedging of the vertebrae with some distortion of the vertebral end plates. When the x-ray changes result from a severe injury and the patient comes for emergency care with a documented history of trauma, the physician can make the diagnosis of a compression fracture. The x-ray may resemble Scheuermann's disease (Fig. 65.29), but the latter does not usually follow trauma and produces chronic back pain with gradual onset, as opposed to the sud-

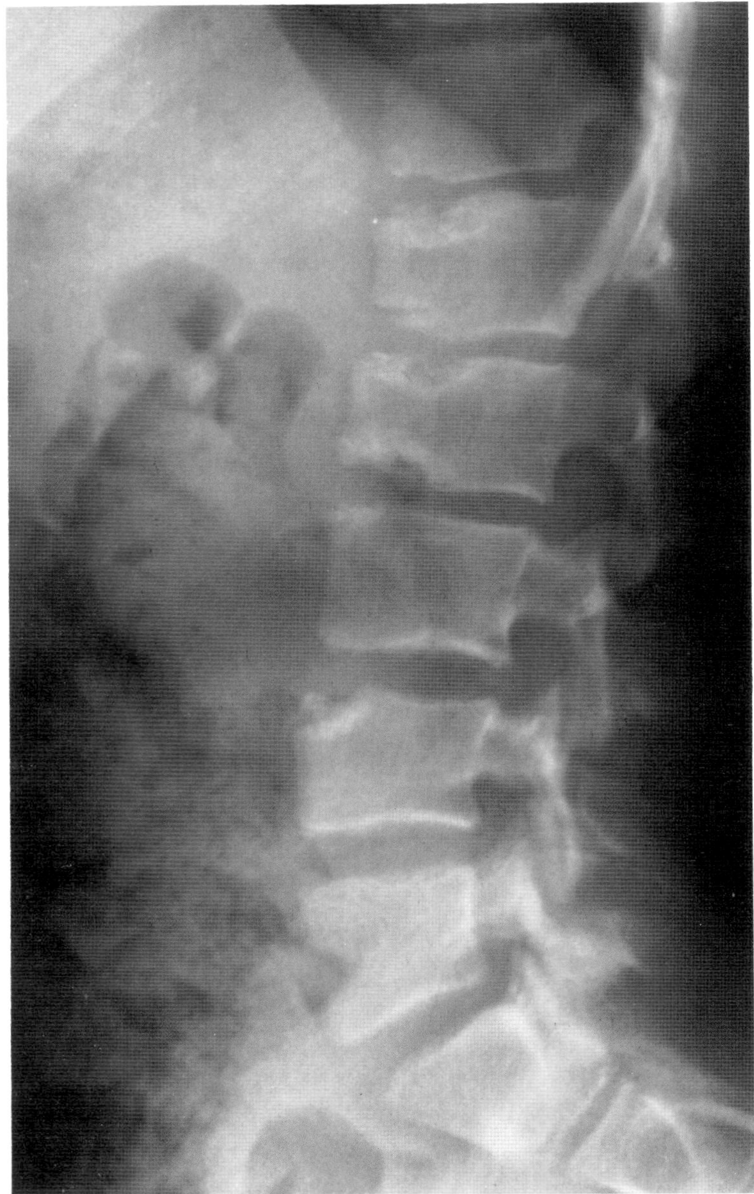

Figure 65.29 Lateral roentgenogram showing changes of Ş̧cheuermann's disease. One might confuse these changes with infection or tumor.

den severe pain of a real fracture associated with acute injury. Trauma patients usually have fallen from a height or had a sports injury. They usually do not have neurologic changes, and they respond well to bed rest and analgesics. Occasionally a patient with this type of fracture may develop an ileus for a few days, and the emergency evaluation of the spinal injury patient should include examination for bowel sounds, abdominal distention and tenderness. Reviews of large series of such patients however, has shown that the vertebrae usually reconstitute themselves satisfactorily and that aggressive reduction and postural exercises do not contribute to the usually good end result.

Another cause of back pain in emergency pediatric practice is "diskitis." This condition is actually an osteomyelitis of the vertebral end plate and usually easier to differentiate because of its sudden onset without injury, febrile course, elevated white count, and sedimentation rate.

High speed vehicular trauma usually causes more severe injury to the thoracolumbar spine. This type of trauma occurs most often in older adolescents who present with fracture dislocations involving the facet joints, lamina, and the vertebral end plate. The injury also disrupts the anterior and posterior longitudinal and interspinous ligaments so that the fragments on either side of the fracture line easily shift back and forth on each other. Severe neurologic damage can accompany this unstable relationship between the elements of the fracture and prompt reduction and stabilization offers the only chance to minimize neural damage and prevent worsening of the paraplegia. These major injuries often accompany multiple system trauma, and the emergency room physician must treat the whole patient under these circumstances (see Chapter 57).

Pelvic Fractures

Fractures of the pelvis fall into two categories: stable and unstable. The stable fractures in children most often follow over exertion in athletics. Patients come to the emergency department with swelling, pain, and ecchymosis at the site of a traction epiphysis, the anterior-superior iliac spine most often, but frequently also at the anterior-inferior iliac spine and sacral tuberosity. The vigorous stretching required by the sports program causes the muscle involved to avulse its bone attachment, the sartorius in the case of the anterior-superior spine; the straight head of the rectus femoris; the anterior-inferior spine; and the hamstrings for the ischial tuberosity. These are benign injuries. They almost invariably heal without sequelae and do not require surgical reattachment or excision of the bony fragment. Patients do not need admission to the hospital and respond well to rest, ice, and analgesics until the symptoms subside (Fig. 65.30).

Isolated fractures of the pelvic ring do not disrupt the stability of that structure and are classified as stable fractures. In children, these injuries are much less common than in elderly adults. Normal development of the pelvic ring moreover can confuse the differential diagnosis. For example, the junction between the ossification centers of the inferior pubic ramus and inferior ischial ramus frequently looks like a stress fracture, but in younger patients this linear lucency is a normal finding. In addition the apophyses of the ischial tuberosity, anterior-superior and anterior-inferior spines may present abnormal appearances suggesting acute injury or infection. The physician evaluating these x-rays on an emergency basis must exercise caution not to overdiagnose.

Forces which break apart the pelvic ring produce unstable fractures. Major trauma usually produces these injuries, and this degree of violence often causes damage to the structures contained within the pelvis as well. Thus the emergency evaluation of a child with an unstable fracture of the pelvis must include examination for injuries of the bladder, urethra, lower genital tract, and lower gastrointestinal tract. The emergency physician must remember that patients with this type of injury have been badly hurt. They often lose massive amounts of blood in the retroperitoneal tissues and need adequate replacement of volume for treatment of shock. They face the whole spectrum of life-threatening conditions such as disseminated intravascular coagulation, shock lung, and thromboembolic problems.

Following the initial assessment and treatment of the injured child, the emergency physician should attempt to classify the pelvic fracture and provide emergency care which will not worsen the soft tissue injury or further damage the patient. In general, forces directed from front to back cause separation of the symphysis pubis and disruption of either the sacroiliac joint or wing of the ileum adjacent to the sacroiliac joint. These fractures cause the pelvis

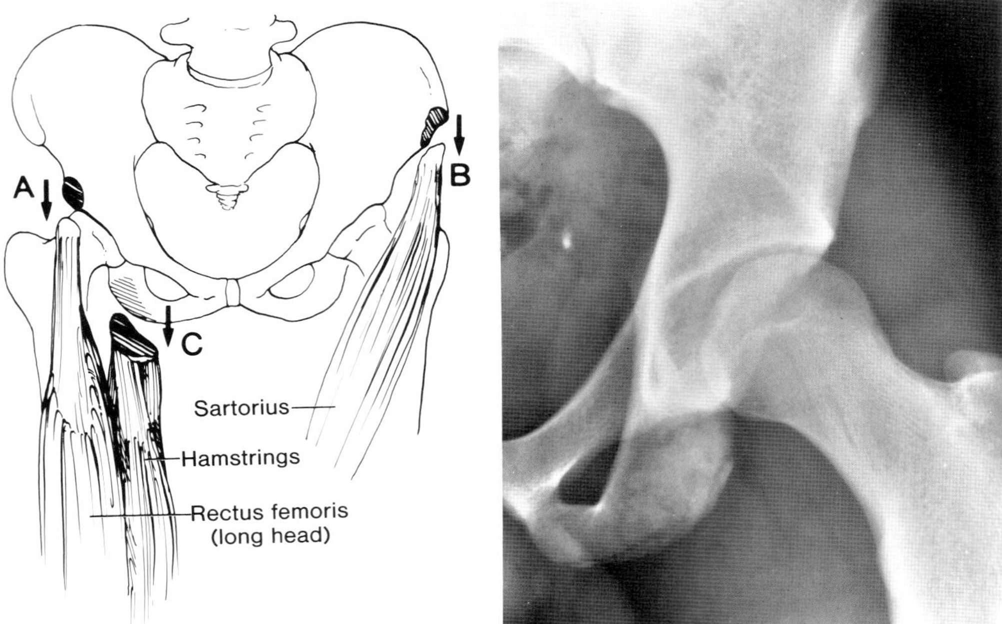

Figure 65.30 (*Left*) Diagram showing the common avulsion injuries of the pelvis. These are common in adolescent athletes: (*A*) anterior inferior iliac spine, (*B*) anterior superior iliac spine, and (*C*) ischial tuberosity. X-rays show the ossific density of the traction apophysis away from its normal location. These patients almost invariably recover with conservative treatment. (*Right*) AP roentgenogram showing developmental changes in the ischial tuberosity.

to open up, with possibly wide diastasis of the symphysis. Such patients can benefit from a pelvic sling or closed reduction by side-lying. The sling or side-lying position tends to close the pelvic separation (Fig. 65.31*A*).

With lateral compression injuries, however, the pelvic ring collapses, so a sling or side-lying would tend to worsen the displacement, further injuring the soft tissues contained within the pelvis. In addition, some patients struck from the front by a violent force sustain fractures of the superior and inferior pubic rami on each side of the symphysis. The whole anterior arch of the pelvis can comprise the free-floating fragment, and lateral compression in these patients would also tend to collapse the pelvic ring. Patients with lateral compression fractures require leg traction on the side of the fracture for emergency care (Fig. 65.31*B*). Patients with anterior arch fractures with a free-floating fragment should be placed supine with the hips slightly flexed to relax the abdominal muscles, in an effort to prevent superior or posterior displacement of the fragment by the rectus abdominis muscle.

Some difficult pelvic fractures in children might lend themselves to stabilization with a Hoffman apparatus or some other type of external fixation. To date there has been little experience reported in this regard, but since these techniques have proved so useful in adults there seems little reason why they should not be utilized in children.

INJURIES OF THE LOWER LIMB

Hip Injuries

Traumatic dislocations of the hip in children are rare injuries. Major violence usually produces them, although a few of the several hundred reported cases have followed a trivial fall. Physical examination after injury reveals shortening and fixed rotation of the lower limb, internally for the more common posterior dislocations and

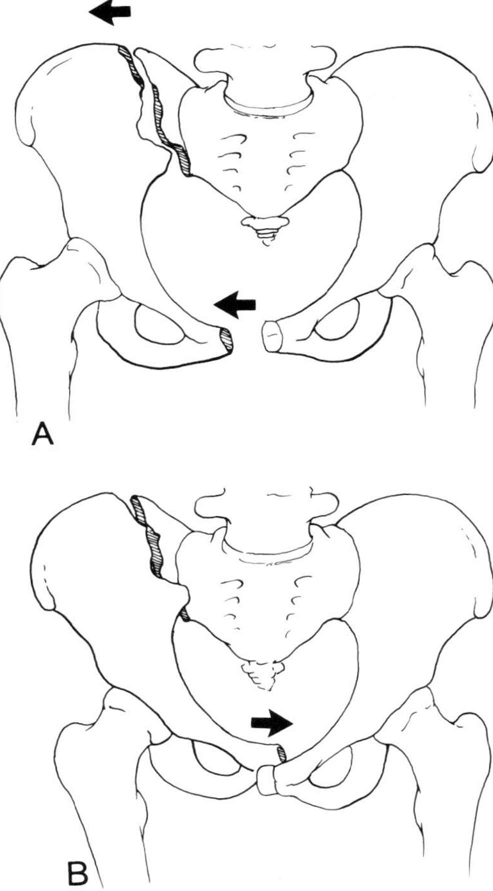

Figure 65.31 Diagrammatic representation of unstable pelvic fractures. In (*A*), the pelvis has been forced open and lateral compression in a sling or side lying might close the pelvic ring. Such treatment would worsen the displacement shown in (*B*) which requires traction or an external fixation.

externally for the rare anterior dislocations. Central dislocations through the floor of the acetabulum into the pelvis may not have a rotational deformity.

An AP x-ray confirms the diagnosis. When the hip dislocates as a result of trauma, the femoral head often fractures the wall of the acetabulum as it leaves its normal relationship with that structure. In adults, detection of the size and location of the acetabular fragment poses special problems. Patients must roll up into an oblique position to permit visualization of fragments from the acetabulum, and they usually complain of a good deal of discomfort when they try to do this. The pediatric patient presents the physician with even more trouble in this regard. First of all, the acetabulum has not completely ossified in younger patients and, secondly, children find it more difficult to cooperate with painful x-ray studies after injury. If there is a question that acetabular fragmentation complicates the hip dislocation, the physician should probably request a CT scan of the pelvis to make the diagnosis.

Without prompt and correct diagnosis and treatment, patients with traumatic hip dislocations develop avascular necrosis of the femoral head and late degenerative arthritis. Even with the best possible treatment, however, there is about a 10% incidence of this complication. Delay in reduction past 12 hours causes this incidence to rise sharply. One can reduce most posterior hip dislocations with traction, flexion, and rotation and most anterior dislocations with abduction and extension. If the acetabulum is intact, the hip will remain stable, and the patient will not require traction or immobilization. With acetabular wall injury severe enough to cause postreduction instability, the patient must have open reduction, internal fixation of the fragments, and skeletal traction for 6 weeks to prevent redislocation. Fragments of bone left in the hip joint produce degenerative arthritis very quickly. Patients with this result from their injury will need referral for open surgery and debridement of the hip joint. The emergency treatment of these patients, of course, does not include the open reduction; but the first doctor handling such a patient must have an awareness of the injury, recognize the complications of acetabular injury, and be prepared to do a prompt closed reduction if specialized help is not very soon available. The prompt reduction of a dislocated hip has two other objectives besides the prevention of late avascular necrosis. Patients with traumatic hip dislocations have intense pain and the prompt relocation relieves this and thus eliminates one of the causes for shock. In addition, the dislocated femoral head can damage the sciatic nerve, and these patients will less likely develop this complication if the physician reduces the dislocation without much delay.

Fractures of the hip in children fall into two broad groups, transepiphyseal and cervicotrochanteric. The former injury is very rare and most patients with displacement of the hip at the subcapital location have a pre-existing *slipped capital femoral epiphysis*. The history in these patients almost always reveals previous hip pain with activity. An injury superimposed on the slipped capital femoral epiphysis can cause the neck to separate completely from the head, leaving the patient with severe displacement. These injuries almost always occur in adolescent patients and if neglected leave the patient with marked physical impairment (Fig. 65.32). An emergency physician must carefully evaluate the adolescent who limps into the department complaining of hip pain. If the patient has slight shortening and an external rotational contracture at the hip, he or she almost certainly has a slipping of the capital femoral epiphysis. X-rays will show varus and posterior displacement of the femoral head on the neck. These patients require admission to the hospital and stabilization of the hip with pins to prevent further displacement or the sudden severe displacement caused by an associated injury. If and when the latter occurs, the child will not likely walk into the emergency department but will be carried on a stretcher. Treatment in the cases with complete epiphyseal separation is more difficult and less likely to succeed.

Cervicotrochanteric fractures of the hip

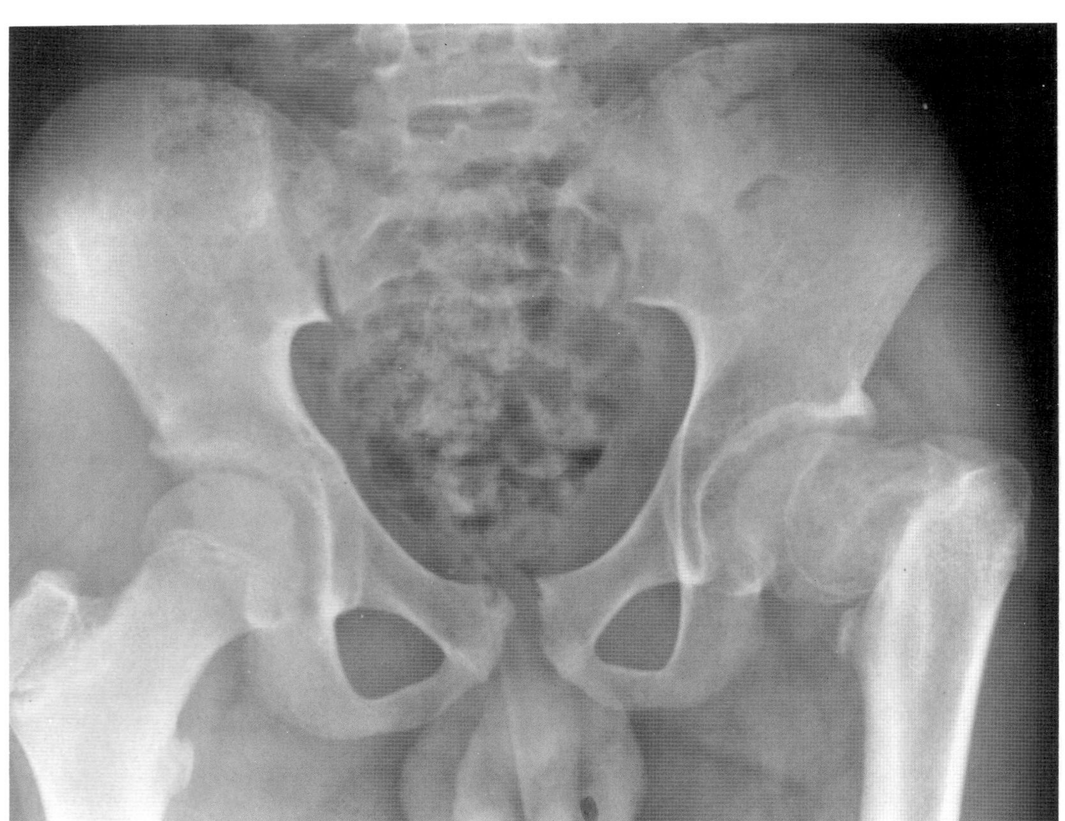

Figure 65.32 Roentgenogram showing the deformity caused by a neglected chronic slipped capital femoral epiphysis on which was superimposed an acute traumatic slip. The patient will have permanant severe deformity.

usually result from major trauma, almost always vehicular, since young children walking into the street are just tall enough to be struck by an automobile bumper at this level. If the fracture has not displaced at all, the physician can treat this injury closed by immobilizing the child in a spica cast. Even a little displacement, however, precludes this type of treatment because the hip goes gradually into varus, regardless of traction or cast support. The pull of muscles on the fragments causes the deformity to almost inevitably worsen (Fig. 65.33). Open reduction and internal fixation with pins prevents deformity and patients with cervicotrochanteric fractures must have this type of treatment (Fig. 65.34). Reconstructive osteotomies after the patient has developed a malunion do not work well and should be made unnecessary by correct treatment in the first place. Until the surgery can be scheduled, the patient can be made comfortable by extension traction. A child who has been struck by a car, and who has been injured badly enough to sustain a major long bone fracture, may also have airway problems, abdominal, intracranial, and other injuries. The whole child requires treatment.

Fractures of the Shaft of the Femur

The history of a child with a fracture of the femoral diaphysis will give the emergency physician an idea of the degree of trauma and the nature and possibility of associated injury. A young child who has fallen on a rug at home has much less of a chance of a ruptured spleen, for example,

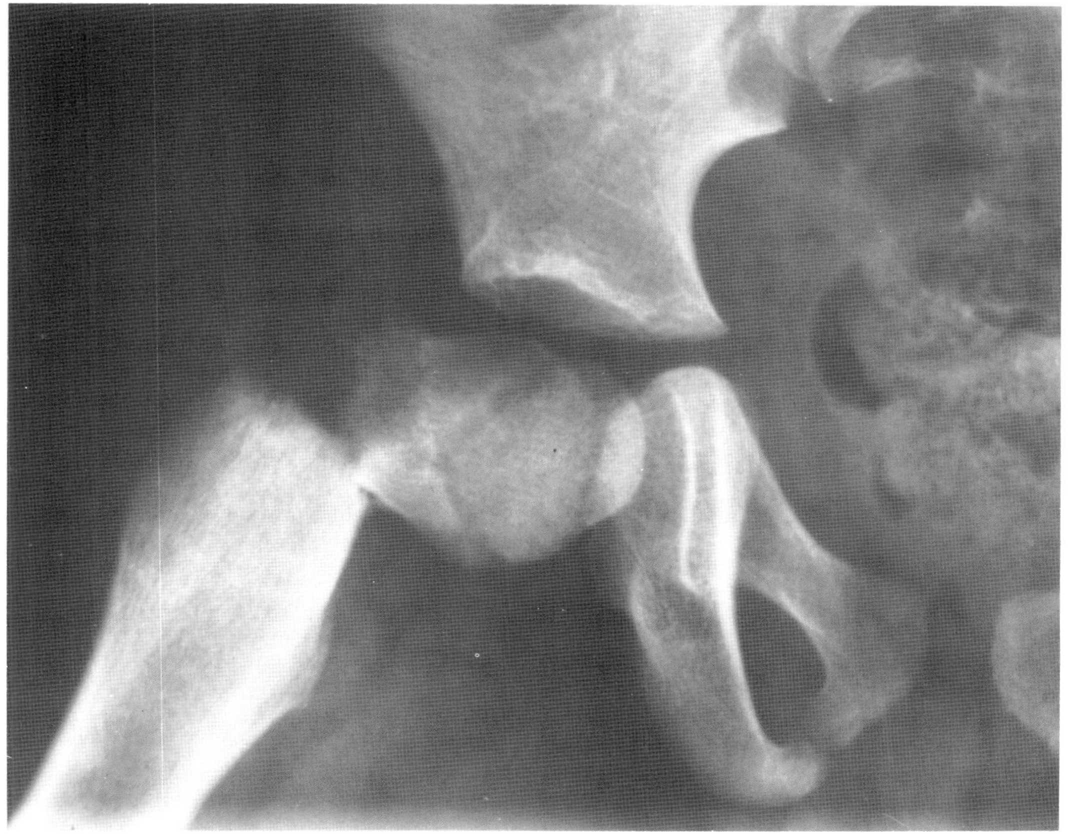

Figure 65.33 Roentgenogram of a badly displaced cervicotrochanteric hip fracture. These injuries do not do well with conservative treatment.

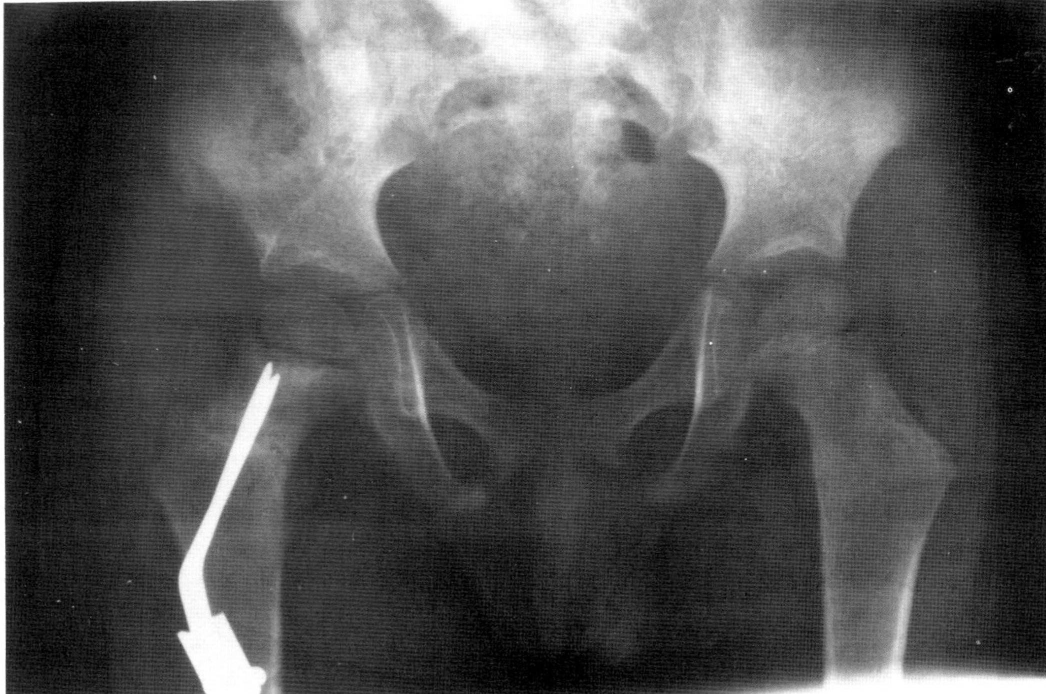

Figure 65.34 Roentgenogram showing the preferred technique for reduction and stabilization of the fracture shown in Figure 65.32. Without internal fixation these fractures produce severe varus deformities.

than a 16-year-old who has just wrecked his car. The emergency evaluation and treatment should proceed coincidently with a check for airway and shock. The physician on the scene of the accident should splint the fracture with Thomas splints, if available, or boards and pillows if that is all he has on hand. In the hospital, treatment depends on the age of the child and the degree of displacement of the fracture (Fig. 65.35).

At any age in infancy and childhood undisplaced fractures of the femoral diaphysis heal well with initial treatment of spica cast immobilization. If the emergency physician must carry out definitive care to this degree because of the unavailability of a fracture surgeon he should remember to immobilize proximal third fractures in 45° of flexion and 20° of abduction. Muscle forces acting on the proximal fragment of proximal femoral fractures pull the proximal fragment into that position, and one must align the distal fragment accordingly. Forty-five degrees of knee flexion will relax the hamstring and put the hip or knee on the same plane to balance the spica when the child lies flat in bed. Fractures of the mid and distal shaft do not require the same degree of flexion in the spica.

The orthopaedic literature reflects some disagreement regarding the best treatment for displaced fractures of the femoral shaft in babies under 2½ years of age. Bryant's traction gained wide acceptance in the past but its use carries the risk of damage to both the normal and fractured extremity. The traction straps (Fig. 65.35) and circumferential wrapping which hold them in place can gradually tighten and produce ischemic changes in both lower legs. Amputation and Volkmann's contractures of both lower legs have resulted from Bryant's traction, and for this reason many orthopaedists treat infants and very young children with immediate closed reduction and spica cast fixation. Fractures of the femoral shaft in this age group heal so rapidly and remodel

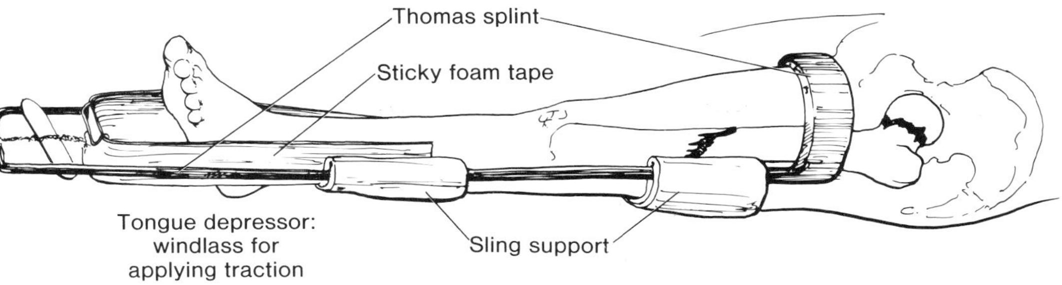

Figure 65.35 Diagrammatic representation of a method for emergency splinting of a fractured femur.

so well that the risk of major and irreversible iatrogenic injury to the normal as well as the injured limb does not justify the use of Bryant's traction in young children.

In older children displaced femoral shaft fractures do require traction to prevent rotational and angular deformity. Skeletal traction with a pin in the distal femur, with the lower leg supported in a short leg cast, holds the thigh and leg in 90° of flexion at the hip and 90° of flexion at the knee. This traction method pulls the fragments into good alignment promptly and makes children comfortable very quickly. It does cause occasional complications, however. Infection about the Kirschner wire in the short-term can force discontinuation of skeletal traction and may rarely make curettage and antibiotics necessary. One can prevent this problem by careful attention to asceptic technique in the emergency department when the pin is inserted. If the traction pin violates the epiphyseal plate, it can cause premature closure and growth arrest. Careful placement of the traction pins can minimize the chances of these complications.

Russell's traction offers an alternative to skeletal traction, but it has the disadvantage of placing traction on the skin of the leg. The circumferential wrappings cover the thigh and lower limb and make it difficult to inspect the injured area. This type of traction also seems to need frequent readjustments and is harder to maintain.

Either traction method should pull the fragments into alignment with not much more than 1 cm of overriding. This degree of shortening will self-correct with growth. However, children have little ability to correct angular and rotational deformity, therefore, the orthopaedist must make occasional adjustment of the traction to prevent angular and rotational deformities.

Children over 10 and adolescents have less growth and remodeling potential than babies and younger children. Unless the initial treatment achieves end to end apposition and suitable alignment, the patient will have permanent shortening and deformity. In late adolescence one can occasionally achieve this goal only by treating the fractures with plates or intramedullar rods. The emergency physician obviously does not get involved with this, but the initial treatment makes these measures possible and facilitates the orthopaedic surgery.

Injuries of the Knee

Knee pain in children severe enough to cause a pediatric emergency arises from numerous causes. The emergency physician must remember, for example, that hip disease can cause knee pain. The sciatic, obturator and femoral nerves supply both joints. Legg-Perthes disease, slipped capital femoral epiphysis and other conditions which cause synovitis and effusions in the hip joint can cause pain which extends from the hip down the thigh and into the knee. The child cannot localize the pain well and tells his parents and doctor that his knee hurts. History taking, therefore, must include questions about hip pain when the child complains of symptoms referrable to the knee. Examination of such a patient also must evaluate the range of motion of both joints and tenderness over the hip as well as the knee. One should also measure the circumferences of the thighs to check the patient for quadriceps atrophy. More than half an inch of atrophy of the thigh suggests some chronicity of the condition with which the child presents.

Most children who present for emergency treatment of knee pain have a history of injury. If the child has not been hurt, however, the physician must consider such entities as septic arthritis (see Chapter 45), rheumatoid disease (see Chapter 56) with a painful effusion, or the less acute conditions such as osteochondritis dissecans and Osgood-Schlatter's disease.

The course of the illness, x-ray examination, and, if necessary, arthrocentesis of the knee with appropriate evaluation of the aspirate makes diagnosis easy most of the time. Comparison x-ray films of the uninvolved knee may be helpful in distinguishing between an injury and normal variation in the appearance of the epiphysis.

X-rays also show changes in soft tissues. If the patient had a penetrating injury the emergency doctor should look for foreign bodies in the joint, such as needles or pieces of glass, and should also determine if there is air in the suprapatellar pouch. If the films are negative and one suspects a major injury, slight varus or valgus stress on the knee might establish an epiphyseal separation of the distal femoral epiphysis.

One should look for the following injuries when the child complains of knee pain after injury: (1) supracondylar fracture of the femur, (2) separation of the distal femoral epiphysis, (3) fracture of the tibial spine, (4) injury of the patella—either fracture or dislocation, (5) avulsion of the tibial tubercle, and (6) proximal growth plate injury of the tibia (Fig. 65.36).

Supracondylar fractures of the femur when undisplaced heal quickly with immobilization in a cast. Displaced fractures at this location, however, present major problems in treatment. Displacement of the fracture can compromise the popliteal artery and vein. If vascular damage is suspected the emergency physician should get help from the appropriate specialist quickly. These fractures also pose problems with reduction and maintainance of reduction, and they challenge the resourcefulness of the physician charged with their definitive care.

Epiphyseal separations and fractures of the distal femoral epiphysis have served as the model for this type of injury from the standpoint of classification and prognosis. Surprisingly, relatively few patients seem to have this type of fracture. Salter Type I and II epiphyseal injuries can be reduced relatively easily and held in plaster until healing occurs. The other types of epiphyseal injuries, Types III, IV and V, have a much poorer prognosis for growth arrest and angular deformity. Accurate reduction lessens the chance of a bad result, and one might achieve this only with open surgery.

For the emergency room doctor or for the pediatrician looking at the x-rays of an older child with a painful swollen knee, recognition of a *fracture of a tibial spine* should present no difficulty. The x-ray shows the tibial spine to be raised up and off from the tibial plateau, sometimes up into the intercondylar notch of the femur. In younger children the diagnosis may be more difficult if the spine has not yet ossified. The knowledge that the lesion exists prepares one for making the diagnosis. The anterior cruciate ligament attaches to the anterior tibial spine, and the child with the injury has anterior-posterior instability. Because of the painful hemarthrosis the young patient may find it hard to cooperate with a physician trying to test for a drawer sign, however, and one may have to rely on the x-ray to make the diagnosis. The technical details of open reconstruction and differences of opinion regarding the need for the same do not involve the emergency department doctor. The team there has fulfilled its obligation to the patient by recognizing the fracture and splinting the knee. Occasionally also one can make a patient with a hemarthrosis more comfortable by aspirating the knee. If definitive treatment cannot take place for several days, one should consider doing this.

A child or adolescent who comes to the doctor for emergency treatment of a *dislocated patella* may recount a history of numerous previous dislocations. Usually these have reduced spontaneously or the patient

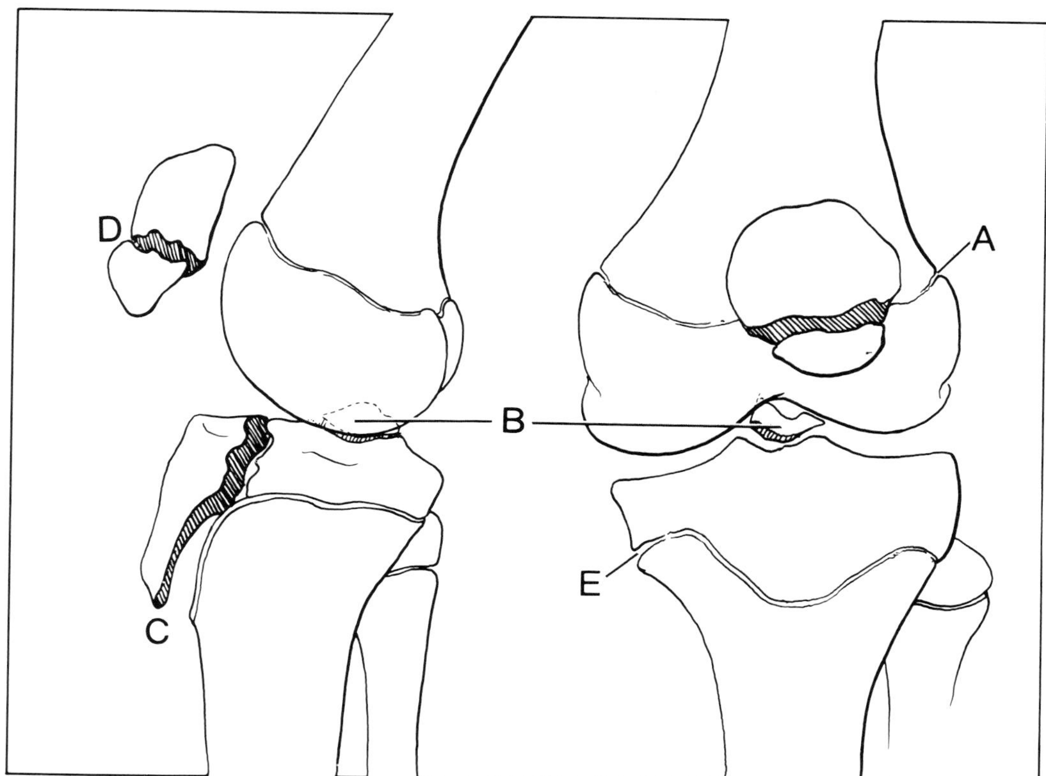

Figure 65.36 Injuries about the knee in children occur at the: (*A*) distal femoral epiphyseal plate, (*B*) tibial spine, (*C*) tibial tubercle, (*D*) patella, and (*E*) proximal tibial growth plate.

has learned how to reduce the patella himself. If the patient cannot get the patella back in position, the physician may have to apply lateral pressure on the patella while extending the knee. A patient who has dislocated the patella for the first time may have much more swelling and pain, and hardly let the doctor touch the bone.

Treatment of recurrent dislocations of the patella is a subject on which authorities differ. Usually support of the knee in a knee immobilizer splint suffices for emergencies although the patient whose patella has dislocated for the first time may feel more comfortable in a cylinder cast. In reviewing the films of these patients, the doctor should also look for an ossific density medial to the patella, beneath it, or possibly in the suprapatellar pouch. A broken osteochondral fragment of the medial patellar facet causes this. Its presence implies the need for an arthrotomy, removal of the loose fragment, trimming of the medial patellar facet, and realignment of the extensor mechanism.

Fractures of the main body of the patella do not occur very often in pediatric practice. One should show caution in overdiagnosing a bipartite patella as a fracture. Undisplaced patellar fractures, however, usually heal with support, while transverse or comminuted fractures with separation need open reduction. An avulsion fracture of all or part of either the superior or inferior pole of the patella may pose a special problem. Occasionally, these injuries do not manifest themselves on initial x-ray. In time they may separate slightly and cause an extension lag. Follow-up x-ray on patients with this type of injury 4 to 6 weeks later make the diagnosis (Fig. 65.37).

Older children and adolescents can *avulse the tibial tubercle* with forceful quadriceps contraction against an external

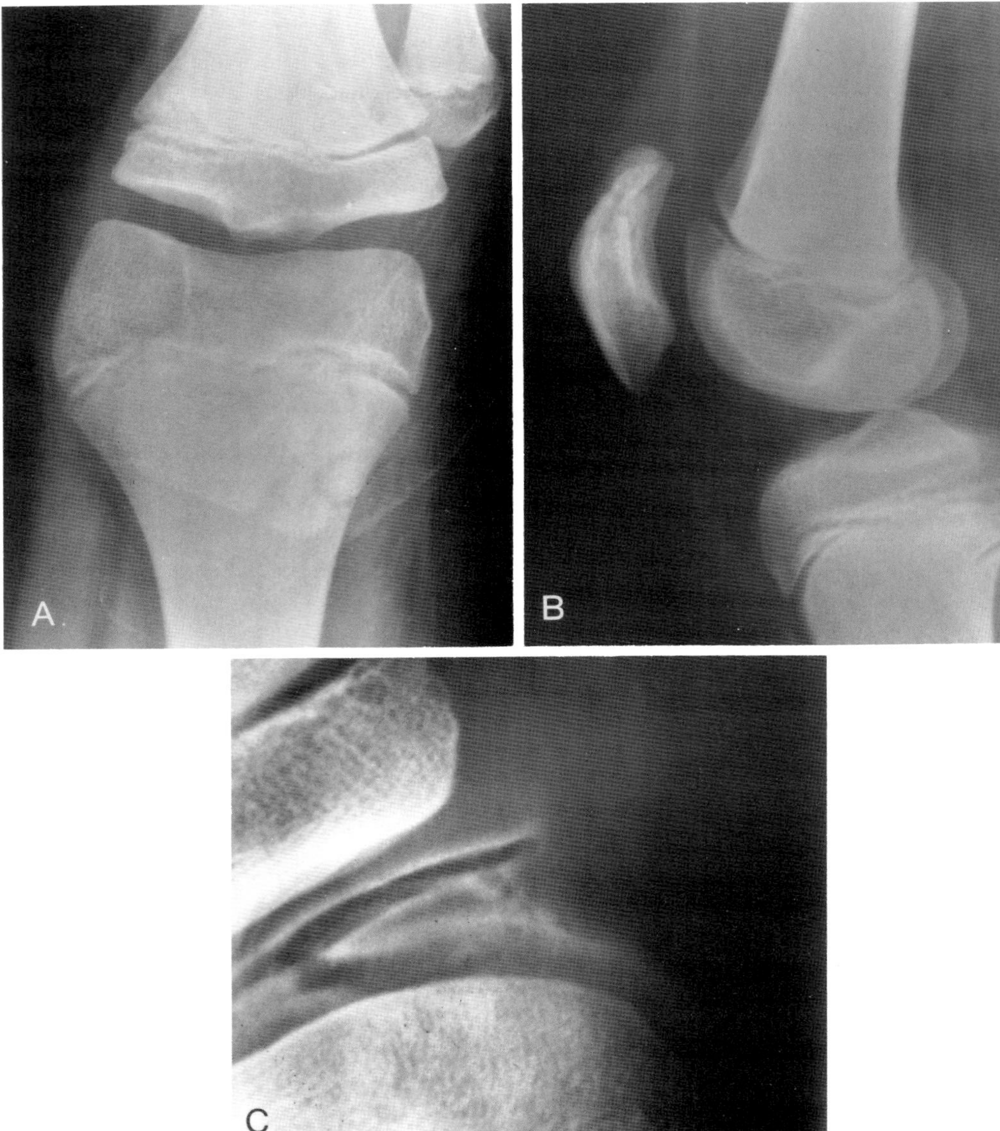

Figure 65.37 Roentgenogram showing end result in a fracture of the patella in a child. The initial film was negative and the proximal pole fracture escaped detection. The arthrogram also shows a tear in the medial meniscus. This is a rarity since internal derangements of the knee do not commonly occur in this age group.

force which is flexing the knee. Athletics usually produces this type of trauma and often patients have a previous history of Osgood-Schlatter's disease. One suspects the diagnosis in a patient who is unable to extend the knee after the type of injury described and in whom one finds swelling, ecchymosis, and pain at the site of the insertion of the infrapatellar tendon. The diagnosis is made by x-ray.

Displacement of the proximal tibial epiphysis is an unusual injury. When it does occur, however, one must realize that a compartment syndrome might accompany it. The patient may need an emergency fasciotomy and vascular repair if the initial examination reveals pain with passive dorsiflexion of the toes. These injuries also involve the epiphyseal plate, and patients may have an angular deformity growth at the knee or develop a leg length inequality because of the injury. The inequality might be overgrowth of the tibia instead of shortening.

Fractures of the Tibia

Fractures of the tibial diaphysis usually do not present such a problem in diagnosis. The child has usually had a major injury; examination shows swelling and tenderness, usually deformity, and occasional crepitus. X-rays, of course, confirm the diagnosis. Initial evaluation should also document the status of the nerve and blood supply. Usually the definitive cure of these injuries requires admission to the hospital, although one can immobilize an uncomplicated undisplaced fracture in a cast and discharge the patient to outpatient follow-up. When the violence of the injury has produced extensive comminution, soft tissue damage, or an open fracture, many surgeons will advise the use of external fixation.

Evaluation of a fracture of the proximal tibial metaphysis might have major long-term consequences (Fig. 65.38). This injury produces a linear radiolucency in the medial side of the proximal tibial metaphysis, and the fibula remains intact. Early on, swelling in the fascial compartments can cause ischemic myositis, and the patient with this problem may require a fasciotomy for decompression. Valgus deformity and overgrowth can occur in the long-term despite adequate care, and the treating physician should alert the patients that this complication might develop. The late deformity that results from this fracture may, in fact, be so bad that an osteotomy of the tibia and fibula might be the only alternative. Parents find it easier to accept such complications if the physician who treats the child warns them in advance that this might happen.

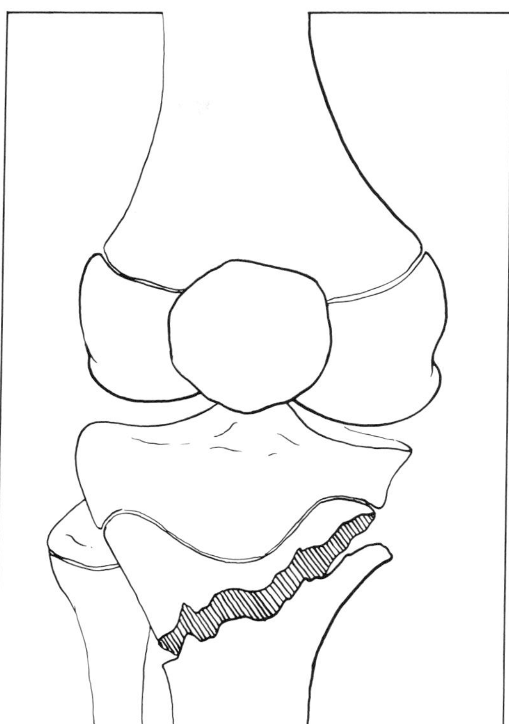

Figure 65.38 Proximal tibial metaphyseal fractures in growing children can cause severe valgus deformity of the knee due to asymmetric epiphyseal plate development after the injury.

Stress reaction of bone (so-called stress fractures) in older children and adolescents can also present problems in diagnosis to the physician who sees a child with this problem on emergency basis. Such children often do not recall a specific injury and cannot explain why they should have swelling, discomfort, and tenderness over the proximal tibial shaft. X-rays reveal a radiolucent line and periosteal reaction, and the specter of osteogenic sarcoma or osteomyelitis frequently arises. On close questioning one can often learn that the child has recently begun to engage in vigorous exercises or some other unaccustomed activity. Differentiation of a benign healing stress fracture from the far more serious problems noted requires a laboratory evaluation including: CBC, sedimentation rate, alkaline phosphatase, serum calcium and phosphorus levels and tomography. The bone scan does not help in this differentiation because all of the conditions noted produce increased uptake of technetium or gallium. A CT scan, however, might reveal a soft tissue extension of a sarcoma, sequestrum, involucrum, or some other clue which would rule out a stress fracture as the cause of the symptoms and findings. If by exclusion the child does have a stress fracture, treatment in a long leg walking cast for 6 weeks allows full healing.

Injuries of the Ankle and Foot

Young children do not often sprain their ankles. Swelling and tenderness more often reflect distal fibular or tibial epiphyseal separation. X-rays may not establish the diagnosis unless one stresses the ankle joint but usually one need not go this far. A short leg cast for a few weeks will permit symptoms to subside.

The adolescent athlete on the other hand may tear the ligaments of the ankle when the growth plates have nearly fused. With major disruption of the ankle ligaments patients run the risk of multiple painful recurrences unless the ankle is placed in a cast until the ligaments heal.

Displacement of the components of the ankle results from the same stresses and mechanisms as ankle fractures in adults. The clinical examination in such patients obviously suggests the diagnosis when the child is brought into the emergency department or office with a deformity after an injury. One should review the x-rays of such a patient carefully for evidence of epiphyseal injury (Figs. 65.39 and 65.40), which might cause subsequent growth arrest and progressive deformity. In patients with Salter Type III or IV epiphyseal injuries, open reduction and internal fixation mgiht offer the best opportunity to avoid the late complications. The emergency physician should

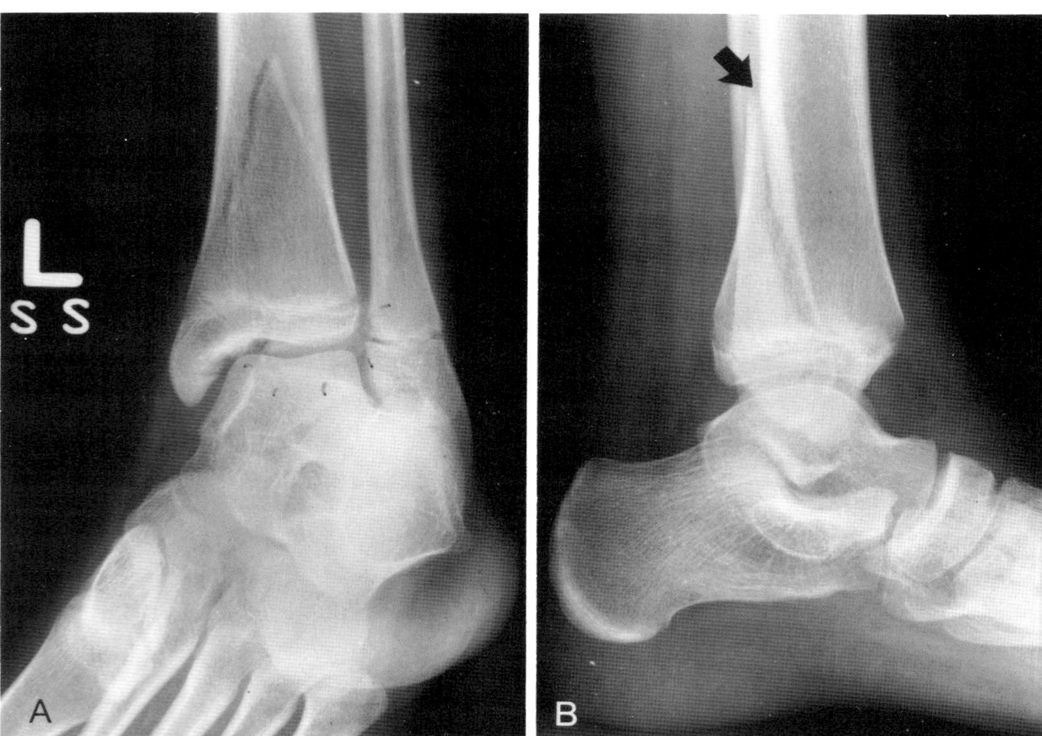

Figure 65.39 Fracture of the distal tibial epiphyseal plate usually occur in three planes and since they are Salter Type IV injuries, they can have a poor prognosis for growth arrest with shortening or deformity. (Courtesy of J. Gregg, M.D.)

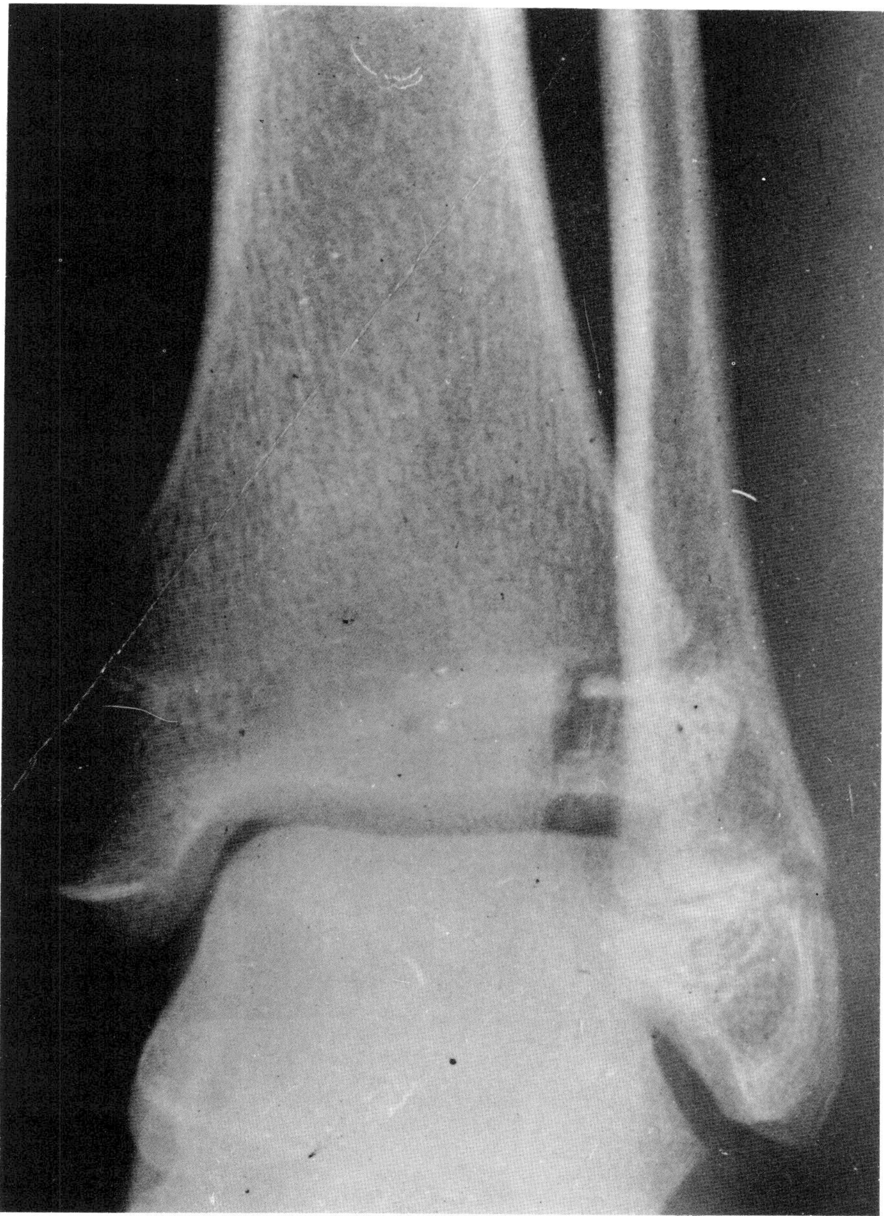

Figure 65.40 Roentgenogram showing the Tilleaux fracture of the distal tibial epiphysis. (Courtesy of J. Gregg, M.D.)

recognize epiphyseal injuries and relate their prognostic significance to the child's parents.

Emergency care consists of reduction of gross deformity to protect the neurovascular supply of the foot. Usually children only need sedation to permit this, and they feel much more comfortable when it has been accomplished. A well-molded and well-padded posterior splint and elevation maintain position and minimize swelling until definitive treatment is available electively.

Hindfoot fractures in children do not occur very often. Probably the cartilaginous covering of the ossific nucleus of the tarsal bones protects the tarsals from injury, unless major violence has caused extensive disruption of the foot and leg. With lesser degrees of injury, the ankle and tibia seem to absorb the stress and more often fractures occur in these locations.

The emergency care of fractures of metatarsals and phalanges in children usually consists simply of splinting until the fracture has healed. In the case of metatarsal injuries this might require a short leg walking cast for 3 or 4 weeks. Phalangeal fractures in children usually need only splinting of the toe by taping it to an adjacent digit.

Penetrating injuries of the foot in children sustained, for example, by stepping on a nail alarm parents who all seem to have heard about "lock jaw." If there is any concern at all about a retained foreign body, one should order an x-ray but usually external care of the penetrating wound suffices after removal of the object. Tetanus prophylaxis has virtually eliminated the possibility of tetanus, but the emergency physician must check the child's records to ensure that this prophylaxis has been received. The child should report back for subsequent follow-up and, if local infection develops, one can treat it accordingly. Routine antibiotic prophylaxis and surgical exploration, however, is not usually required, unless the penetrating wound has caused obvious local tissue injury and contamination.

References

General Principles

Blount WP: *Fractures in Children.* Williams & Wilkins, Baltimore, 1955.

Pollen AG: *Fractures and Dislocations in Children.* Churchill Livingstone, Edinburgh, 1973.

Rang M: *Childrens Fractures.* J. B. Lippincott, Philadelphia, 1974.

Sharrar W: *Pediatric Orthopaedics & Fractures.* J. B. Lippincott, Philadelphia, 1971.

Tachdjian MO: *Pediatric Orthopedics.* W. B. Saunders, Philadelphia, 1972.

Fractures of the Proximal Humeral Epiphysis

Dameron TB, Reibel DB: Fractures involving the proximal humeral epiphysis. *J Bone Joint Surg* 51A: 289, 1969.

Neer CS, Horowitz BS: Fractures of the proximal humeral epiphyseal plate. *Clin Orthop* 41: 24, 1965.

Sherk HH, Probst C: Fractures of the proximal humeral epiphysis. *Orthop Clin North Am* 6: 401, 1975.

Supracondylar Fractures of the Humerus

Childress HM: Transarticular pin fixation in supracondylar fractures of the elbow in children. *J Bone Joint Surg* 54A: 1548–1552, 1973.

D'Ambrosia RD: Supracondylar fractures of the humerus—prevention of cubitus varus. *J Bone Joint Surg* 54A: 60–66, 1972.

Flynn JC, Matthews JG, Benoit RL: Blind pinning of displaced supracondylar fractures of the humerus in children. *J Bone Joint Surg* 56A: 263, 1974.

Griffin PP: Supracondylar fractures of the humerus. Treatment and complications. *Pediatr Clin North Am* 22: 477, 1975.

Shifrin PG, Gehring HW, Ingleias LJ: Open reduction and internal fixation of displaced supracondylar fractures of the humerus in children. *Orthop Clin North Am* 7: 573, 1976.

Fractures and Other Injuries About the Elbow

Buxton St JD: Fractures of the head of the radius and capitellum including fractures in childhood, *J Bone Joint Surg* 20: 709, 1938.

Conner AN, Smith MGH: Displaced fractures of the lateral humeral condyle in children. *J Bone Joint Surg* 52B: 460, 1970.

Dunlop J: Traumatic separation of the medial epicondyle of the humerus in adolescence. *J Bone Joint Surg* 17: 577, 1935.

Jeffrey CC: Fractures of the head of the radius in children. *J Bone Joint Surg* 32B: 314, 1950.

Spellman O: Subluxation of the head of the radius in children. *Acta Orthop Scand* 28: 311, 1959.

Stelling FF: Traumatic dislocation of the head of the radius in children. *J Bone Joint Surg* 37A: 1116, 1955.

Fractures of the Forearm and Wrist

Borden S: Traumatic bowing of the forearm in children. *J Bone Joint Surg* 56A: 611, 1974.

Peiro A, Andres F, Fernanadey-Esteve F: Acute Monteggia lesions in children. *J Bone Joint Surg* 59A: 92, 1977.

Tomkins DG: The Monteggia fracture. *J Bone Joint Surg* 50A: 1109, 1971.

Wilson JC: Fractures and dislocations in childhood. *Pediatr Clin North Am* 15: 659, 1967.

Hand Injuries

Bennett JE: Skin and soft tissue injuries of the hand in children. *Pediatr Clin North Am* 22: 443, 1975.

Eaton RG: Hand problems in children; a time table for management. *Pediatr Clin North Am* 14: 643, 1967.

Leonhard MH, Dubrovcik P: Management of fractured fingers in the child. *Clin Orthop* 73: 160, 1970.

Strickland JW: Bone, nerve, and tendon injuries of the hand in children. *Pediatr Clin North Am* 22: 451, 1975.

Wakefield AP: Hand injuries in the child. *J Bone Joint Surg* 46A: 1226, 1964.

Spinal Injuries and Fractures of the Pelvis

Aufdermaur M: Spinal injuries in juveniles. Necropsy findings in twelve cases. *J Bone Joint Surg* 56B: 513, 1974.
Fielding JW, Hawkins RJ: Atlantoaxial rotatory fixation. *J Bone Joint Surg* 59A: 37, 1977.
Holdsworth F: Review article. Fractures, dislocations and fracture dislocations of the spine. *J Bone Joint Surg* 52A: 1534, 1970.
Hubbard DD: Injuries of the spine in children and adolescents. *Clin Orthop* 100: 56, 1974.
Quimby WC: Fractures of the pelvis and associated injuries in children. *J Pediatr Surg* 1: 353, 1966.
Sherk HH, Schut L, Lane JM: Fractures and dislocations of the cervical spine in children. *Orthop Clin North Am* 7: 593, 1976.
Watts HG: Fractures of the pelvis in children. *Orthop Clin North Am* 7: 615, 1976.

Fractures of the Hip and Femur in Children

Aadalen RJ, Weiner DS, Hoyt W, Herndon CH: Acute slipped capital femoral epiplysis. *J Bone Joint Surg* 56A: 1473, 1974.
Canale ST, Bourland WL: Fracture of the neck and intertrochanteric region of the femur in children. *J Bone Joint Surg* 59A: 431, 1977.
Edvarken D, Syversen SM: Overgrowth of the femur after the fracture in children. *J Bone Joint Surg* 58B: 339, 1976.
Griffin PP: Fractures of the femoral diaphysis in children. *Orthop Clin North Am* 7: 633, 1976.
Irani RN, Nicholson JD, Chung SMK: Long term results in the treatment of femoral-shaft fractures in young children by immediate spica immobilization. *J Bone Joint Surg* 58A: 945, 1976.
Miller WE: Fractures of the hip in children from birth to adolescence. *Clin Orthop* 92: 155, 1973.
Pennsylvania Orthopedic Society: Traumatic dislocations of the hip in children. *J Bone Joint Surg* 50A: 79, 1968.

Injuries In and About the Knee

Aitken AD, Magill HK: Fractures involving the distal femoral epiphyseal cartilage. *J Bone Joint Surg* 34A: 96, 1952.
Crawford AH: Fractures about the knee in children. *Orthop Clin North Am* 73: 639, 1976.
Crosley EB, Insall J: Recurrent dislocational of the patella. *J Bone Joint Surg* 38A: 9, 1976.
Deliyannis SN: Avulsion of the tibial tuberosity; report of two cases. *Injury* 4: 341, 1973.
Larsen RL: Epiplyseal injuries in the adolescent athletic. *Orthop Clin North Am* 4: 839, 1973.
Macnab I: Recurrent dislocation of the patella. *J Bone Joint Surg* 34A: 957, 1932.
Meyers MH, McKeever FM: Fracture of the intercondylar eminence of the tibia. *J Bone Joint Surg* 41A: 214, 1959.
Salter RB, Harris WR: Injuries involving the epiplyseal plate. *J Bone Joint Surg* 45A: 587, 1963.

Fractures of the Tibia, Ankle and Foot Injuries

Cooperman DR, Spiegel DG, Tharos GS: Tibial fractures involving the ankle in children. *J Bone Joint Surg 60A: 1040, 1978.*
Demas MB: Stress fractures in children. J Bone Joint Surg 45B: 528, 1963.
Papas AM: Fractures of the leg and ankle. *Orthop Clin North Am* 7: 657, 1976.
Salter RB: Injuries of the ankle in children. *Orthop Clin North Am* 5: 147, 1974.
Spiegel PG, Cooperman DR, Laros GS: Epiplyseal fractures of the distal ends of the tibia and fibula. *J Bone Joint Surg* 60A: 1046, 1978.
Trott AW: Fractures of the foot in children. *Orthop Clin North Am* 7: 677, 1976.

CHAPTER 66

Dental Emergencies

LINDA P. NELSON, D.M.D., M.Sc.D., AND JACK H. NEFF, D.D.S.

ASSESSMENT OF DENTAL EMERGENCIES

It is important to remember that the oral cavity is an integral part of the child. Thus it follows that the emergency physician must apply the same basic medical tenets that apply to all emergencies. Care of the pediatric maxillofacial/dental emergency should follow the same sequence as any other emergency procedure. An initial general assessment must include airway patency, breathing adequacy, and cardiovascular status. Control of bleeding, assessment of the degree of shock, neurologic status and notation of other injuries must all be done sequentially.

Life Support

The most common cause of airway obstruction in the child with facial injuries is the accumulation of blood in the oral cavity and pharynx. Unconscious children may not be able to cough or swallow, thereby easily obstructing their airway. A fractured mandible may cause the tongue to fall posteriorly and create obstruction. A tooth aspirated by a child can also cause airway obstruction. The mouth should be gently suctioned clean, and, if the mandible is displaced, it should be pulled gently forward by bilateral digital pressure at the angles. If the tongue of an unconscious child is still a problem in obstruction, an oropharyngeal or nasopharyngeal airway can be attempted. Chapter 1 details the procedures for establishing a patent airway. If endotracheal intubation fails, a tracheostomy must be performed.

The soft tissues and bones of the lower and midface are well vascularized and bleed profusely when injured. Controlling hemorrhage is best accomplished by ligating any vessels that are easily visualized. Many of the vessels of the face will retract when severed. If the vessel cannot be visualized, it is better not to dissect and increase the size of the injury, but rather to apply moderate amounts of direct pressure. Another initial treatment consideration is the management of any signs of shock. If shock persists, one must remember that more than one body system may be injured (see Chapter 2).

History

A complete history should be taken as soon as possible. Facial emergencies are often very dramatic and result in the patient being unable to give the history. Informants other than the patient may have to be questioned. Nevertheless, a good history and physical examination are paramount to any treatment considerations. One key question of dental significance is the history of immunizations. Many facial traumatic injuries occur with concomitant soft tissue injuries, and the need for tetanus prophylaxis is based upon the history of immunization. Antibiotic prophylaxis may be indicated in the child with congenital heart defects or prior cardiac surgery in order to prevent subacute bacterial endocarditis (Chapter 43, "Cardiac Emergencies," presents the AHA guidelines in Table 43.12). In addition, based on past medical history, antibiotic prophylaxis may be indicated in children who have certain hematologic, oncologic or endocrine disorders (i.e., sickle cell disease, leukemia, diabetes). The history should also give the physician an indication of the pre- and post-injury neurologic status. A thorough neurologic assessment must be made as early as clinically possible. The risk of neurologic injury is high in all head and neck trauma.

Physicial Examination

Children with facial injuries are usually frightened and acutely apprehensive. Hence, the initial contact with the child should be authoritative and reassuring. The examination should be organized to include inspection, palpation, percussion and auscultation of both extra- and intraoral aspects.

Extraoral Examination

Inspection. The extraoral examination should start with inspection. Note the symmetry of the face in the anterior view, as well as in profile. A sharp loss of symmetry is often associated with a jaw fracture or dental infection. Inspect for any nasal or orbital misalignments. Carefully note the location and nature of any swollen or depressed structure. Inspect for any fistulous tracts which may present as a large focal "pimple." Look for any hematomas, ecchymoses, foreign bodies or ulcerations. Note the color and quality of the skin. Ask the child to open and close his mouth while facing you. Look for any deviations of the mandible during function or speech. If the child is unable to open or close his mouth due to pain, do not use force to gain access as this could increase the extent of injury. Inspect for any increase in the vertical dimension of the face. Ask the child to look up at the ceiling while the observer looks up from a vantage point below the child's chin. Note any asymmetry of the face. Inspect for lip competency, the ability of the lips to cover the teeth. Loss of competency may indicate displacement of the teeth due to trauma or distortion of soft tissues due to cellulitis of a maxillary anterior tooth.

Palpation. Gentle preauricular digital palpation bilaterally should be the next point of the examination. Feel the temperomandibular joints (TMJ) as the child opens and closes. There should be equal movement on both sides without major deviations. On each side, feel the body of the ramus; then move anteriorly, to the orbital rim, checking to be sure it is continuous and intact. Move bilaterally medially to the inner canthus of the eye, palpating to ensure continuity. Come across the zygoma to the nose and palpate for any mobility or discontinuity. Move back to the preauricular region and then along the posterior border of the mandible. Palpate for any discontinuity, soft edematous swellings or point tenderness. Move to the angles of the mandible, then to the symphyseal region and finally palpate the major lymph nodes of the neck. Any notation of paresthesia or hypoesthesia (numbness) of the lips may indicate a fracture. Figure 66.1 shows the main nerve supply to facial structures. However, in the absence of a history of trauma, unilateral paresthesia is highly suggestive of malignancy. Note the temper-

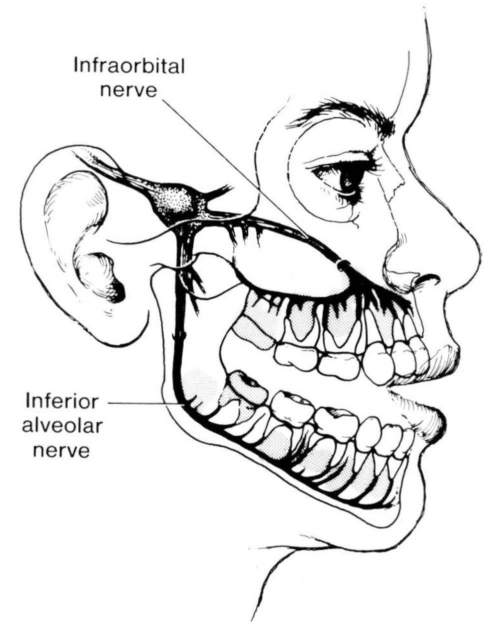

Figure 66.1. Infraorbital and inferior alveolar main nerve supplies to teeth.

ature of the skin; warmth often indicates infection.

Percussion. Usually percussion is not recommended for maxillofacial injuries. However, when there is a chief complaint of pain in the maxilla, percussion of the maxillary sinuses may be necessary in the absence of an odontogenic origin to further rule out sinus pathology.

Auscultation. Listen for crepitus as the child opens and closes his mouth, at the same time palpating the TMJ. This may indicate TMJ pathology.

Intraoral Examination

Inspection. A good light is essential for the intraoral examination. Inspect the color and quality of the lips, gingivae (gums), mucosa, floor of the mouth, tongue and palate. The gingiva should be pink, firm and stippled (like a grapefruit skin). The mucosa should be pink, moist and glassy in appearance. The floor of the mouth should be flat and well vascularized, although gray-blue in color. Hematomas or mucosal ecchymoses in the floor of the mouth or vestibular area are highly suggestive of fractures. Inspect the mouth for any swellings of soft tissue which may be bluish in color due to vascularization and/or hematoma. Note any inflamed, ulcerated, or hemorrhagic areas. Note any foreign bodies or denuded areas of bone. Denudation of alveolar bone often indicates a chronic osteomyelitis. Watch as the child opens and closes his mouth and note any obvious movement of traumatically malposed teeth. Traumatically displaced teeth often produce the complaint that the child's teeth do not feel quite right when he closes. The same complaint may be expressed by a child when a primary tooth is mobile and about to normally exfoliate. Figure 66.2 shows key eruption times for primary and secondary teeth. Exfoliation of primary teeth is often confused with traumatic injuries. Inspect for any chipped or missing teeth. If a tooth is chipped or missing, check for any fragments of teeth or foreign bodies in adjacent soft tissue lacerations. If the child's teeth are missing, yet no bloody socket is present, check the eruption/shedding timetable (Table 66.1). Also look for any grossly decayed teeth since these may be intimately associated with either an intra or extraoral fistulous tract or intra or extraoral cellulitis.

Palpation. Using your thumb and index finger, palpate the base of the alveolar ridge for any soft tissue swellings, discontinuity, or mobility. This should be done circumferentially in all four quadrants. Palpate the palate for any swellings or point tenderness. The masseter muscle should be palpated intra- and extraorally by placing the index finger extraorally and the thumb intraorally and rolling the muscle sequentially. Using a gauze pad, the tongue should be held and lifted gently to better visualize and examine its dorsal, ventral, and lateral aspects. The lips should be palpated for any swellings or nodules. The quality of the swellings should be noted, i.e. fluctuance versus induration. The teeth should be palpated for mobility, point tenderness or fragmentation. Abscessed teeth are often more mobile than surrounding teeth. Look for any purulent exudate during palpation. Palpate for any erupting teeth.

Percussion. The teeth should be individually percussed with the end of a mouth mirror handle or tongue depressor. Mobile, abscessed, or vertically fractured teeth may be hypersensitive and often sound dull upon percussion. In addition, grossly decayed teeth, with or without abscess formation may be hypersensitive to percussion.

Radiographs. Radiographs are a valuable supplement to the clinical examination. It may be difficult, however, to obtain diagnostically perfect radiographic surveys in a child with acute maxillofacial/dental injuries. Table 66.2 indicates the radiographic view which would be the preferred diagnostic aid for dental trauma and/or pathology.

DENTAL TRAUMA

Dental trauma and infection occur in a variety of forms which can be confusing to the primary care provider. The emergency physician needs to know which injuries can be managed without dental consultation, which will need follow-up care and which need emergency dental care. Table 66.3

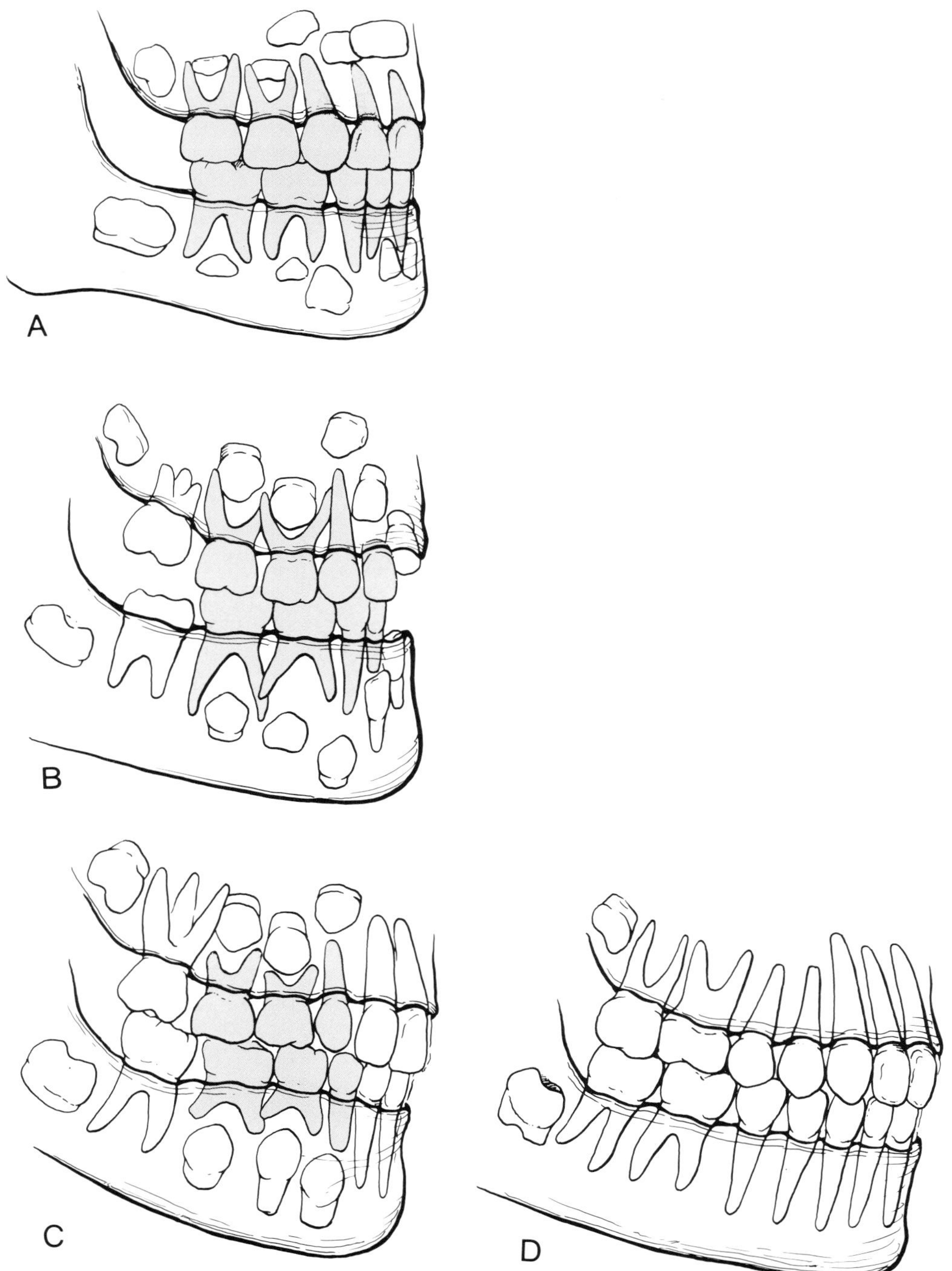

Figure 66.2 (*A*) At *age 3*, 20 primary teeth should be erupted. The permanent teeth are in various stages of calcification underneath and behind the primary teeth. (*B*) At *age 6*, 16 primary teeth should be present. The permanent 6-year molars should be erupting distal to the last primary molar. The permanent anterior central incisors should be erupting. (*C*) At *age 9*, 8 to 12 primary teeth should still be present. The permanent 6-year molars should be totally erupted and in occlusion. The permanent anterior central and lateral incisors are totally erupted and are most prone to fracture at this time. (*D*) At *age 12*, 28 permanent teeth should be present. Only teeth not present should be third molars (wisdom teeth).

Table 66.1
Eruption Schedule for Specific Teeth[a]

A. Primary Teeth				
	Eruption at Age (months)		Shedding at Age (years)	
	Lower	Upper	Lower	Upper
Central incisor	6	7½	6	7½
Lateral incisor	7	9	7	8
Cuspid	16	18	9½	11½
First molar	12	14	10	10½
Second molar	20	24	11	10½
Incisors	Range ±2 months		Range ±6 months	
Molars	Range ±4 months			

B. Permanent Teeth[b]		
	Age (years)	
	Lower	Upper
Central incisors	6–7	7–8
Lateral incisors	7–8	8–9
Cuspids	9–10	11–12
First bicuspids	10–12	10–11
Second bicuspids	11–12	10–12
First molars	6–7	6–7
Second molars	11–13	12–13
Third molars	17–21	17–21

[a] Adapted from M. Massler and I. Schour: *Atlas of the Mouth and Adjacent Parts in Health and Disease*, The Bureau of Public Relations Council on Dental Health, American Dental Association, 1946.
[b] The lower teeth erupt before the corresponding upper teeth. The teeth usually erupt earlier in girls than in boys.

Table 66.2
Radiographic Diagnostic Aids

Radiographic View	Diagnostic Aid for:
Right and left lateral oblique	Fractured body and ramus of mandible
Anteroposterior view of mandible	Fracture of mandibular condyles and symphysis
Towne's	Fractured condyles
Waters'	Maxillary fractures
Intraoral x-rays	
Panoramic	Maxillary and mandibular fractures and related pathology
Occlusal	
Periapical/bite wing	Tooth fractures and pathology; alveolar fractures and pathology

shows the types of injuries referred for dental consultation by the Children's Hospital of Philadelphia Emergency Department during the period 1978 to 1981. This section will detail the management of those dental injuries which are most commonly seen in the pediatric emergency patient.

Soft Tissue Lacerations

Lacerations were found to be the most commonly referred traumatic injury by the

Table 66.3
Dental Emergencies at Children's Hospital of Philadelphia 1978 to 1981

Injury	Total	Percent of Total	Specifics
Soft tissue laceration	319	30	167 lip, 47 tongue 108 mucosa/palate/frenum
Fractures (tooth)	208	20	63 primary dentition 145 permanent dentition
Abscess/cellulitis/ toothache	186	17	107 primary dentition 79 permanent dentition
Displacements	156	15	97 primary dentition 89 permanent dentition
Avulsions	132	13	88 primary dentition 44 permanent dentition
Orthodontic/appliance	35	3	20 space maintainer
Jaw fracture	15	1	8 mandibular 7 condylar, maxillary zygomatic
Alveolar fracture	13	1	
Total	1064	100	

Children's Hospital of Philadelphia Emergency Department physicians to the dental service. Management of injuries to the soft tissues of the oral cavity follow the same emergency care principles used for other soft tissue injuries in the body. Lip injuries swell alarmingly even after minor trauma, but the edema usually resolves without treatment. Lacerations of the tongue bleed profusely due to the richness of the tongue's vascularity. However, as with lip injuries, it is not usually necessary to ligate specific vessels since the bleeding will usually stop with direct pressure and careful deep suturing. The injured area should be thoroughly examined for foreign bodies. To identify a possible foreign body in a deep laceration of the tongue or lip, an intraoral x-ray should be ordered prior to suturing. If chipped teeth are present x-ray examination becomes even more important. The decision to primarily repair a laceration of the oral cavity of the face that is more than a few hours old will depend on the relative risk of secondary infection (see Chapter 58). Special attention should be given to the lip injury which is to be sutured. Suturing of the lip must be done carefully to achieve a precise approximation of the edges of the vermillion border so as to avoid a disfiguring scar. If necessary the lip must be debrided like any other laceration and the skin closed with 5-0 or 6-0 proline. Even with superficial lip lacerations, care must be taken to ensure an even border. Deep lip lacerations are sutured with 4-0 chromic and then with 5-0 or 6-0 proline for the vermillion border. If the lip laceration is through and through, debridement may be necessary. The depth of the wound can be approximated with chromic, but only the external wound should be closed primarily. In children under the age of 5 we prefer to use 3-0 chromic on the deeper mucosal aspects of the lip and 4-0 chromic on the superficial aspects. In children over 5 years of age, 3-0 chromic is used on the deeper mucosal aspect of the lip and 4-0 silk on the superficial edges. Most tongue lacerations heal without suturing. When necessary tongue lacerations are usually sutured with 2-0 chromic if superficial and 3-0 chromic in deeper wounds. With tongue lacerations, it is important to consider the excessive muscular movements which will pull at the sutures; therefore, tongue sutures should be made deeper into the musculature than sutures placed elsewhere in the body. Most superficial mucosal injures are sutured with 3-0 or 4-0 silk. If the mucosal laceration is deep 3-0 chromic can be utilized.

Injuries to the Teeth

These account for 20% of dental emergencies at Children's Hospital of Philadelphia. Traumatic dental injuries occur at these peak ages: (a) as the toddler becomes ambulatory (ages 1 to 3), (b) as the child enters school (ages 7 to 10), and (3) in the adolescent (ages 16 to 18) engaged in athletic activities.

Berkowitz, Ludwig and Johnson categorized traumatic dental injuries into two groups: (1) injuries to the teeth—hard dental tissues and pulp and (2) injuries to the periodontal structures—periodontal ligaments and alveolar bones. Figure 66.3 indicates the relative positions of these structures. Andreason further categorized traumatic fractures of the teeth into complicated and uncomplicated fractures.

Injuries to Hard Dental Tissues and Pulp

Uncomplicated tooth fractures are confined to the hard dental tissue (enamel, dentin, cementum). Clinically there may be a jagged edge of tooth. The fracture line may appear very deep but there is *no sign of bleeding* from the central core of the tooth. The child may complain of sensitivity, especially to cold air and fluids. Emergency treatment is aimed at protecting the pulp even though no frank pulp exposure is noted. The dentist should be called as soon as possible to place a dressing of calcium hydroxide over the exposed dentin for thermal and chemical insulation and for prevention of pulp necrosis. Later, an aesthetic plastic acid-etched restoration can be placed. The prognosis for uncomplicated tooth fractures is usually quite good.

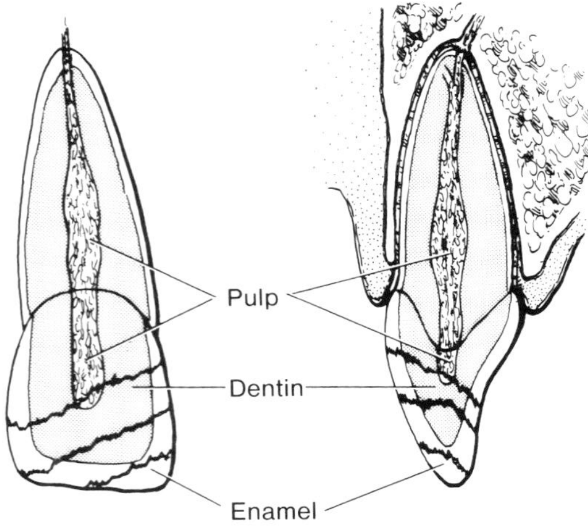

Figure 66.3. The anatomy of a tooth which should be considered during a traumatic injury. Enamel fracture, no emergency treatment; dentin fracture, emergency treatment as soon as convenient; and pulpal fracture, emergency treatment as soon as possible.

A *complicated tooth fracture* involves the pulp of the tooth. By definition, hemorrhaging is noted from the central core of the tooth. In order to best preserve the viability of that tooth, dental pulpal treatment must be initiated within 45 min of the traumatic exposure. Prognosis depends upon the size of the exposure (less than 1 mm pulp exposures carry the best prognosis) and the time interval between the trauma and therapy. Thus it is important to call the dental consultant as soon as possible to institute pulp therapy.

In any injury resulting in fragmentation of teeth, the emergency department physician should attempt to account for all of the fragments. Soft tissue lacerations, especially of the lower lip should be evaluated clinically, and if necessary radiographically, to rule out embedded tooth fragments. Infection and poor wound healing are the sequella of such an oversight.

Crown root fractures are generally seen after the tooth has reached root-end completion. These fractures usually involve maxillary anterior teeth. The child may clinically have a displaced crown in which the tooth seems to be mobile and extruding from the socket. Definitive diagnosis depends upon intraoral dental radiographs; therefore, immediate dental consultation is needed.

Injuries to the Periodontal Structures

The tooth is held in the socket by slender elastic and collagen fibers collectively known as the peridontal ligament. These fine, slender threads are easily broken with trauma to the teeth. Proclined or prominent maxillary anterior teeth are usually more susceptible to this type of traumatic injury. Clinically the physician will note increased mobility or displacement of the affected teeth. If asked, the child will be able to point to an affected tooth, because of the tooth's heightened sensitivity. Periodontal injuries may be further subdi-

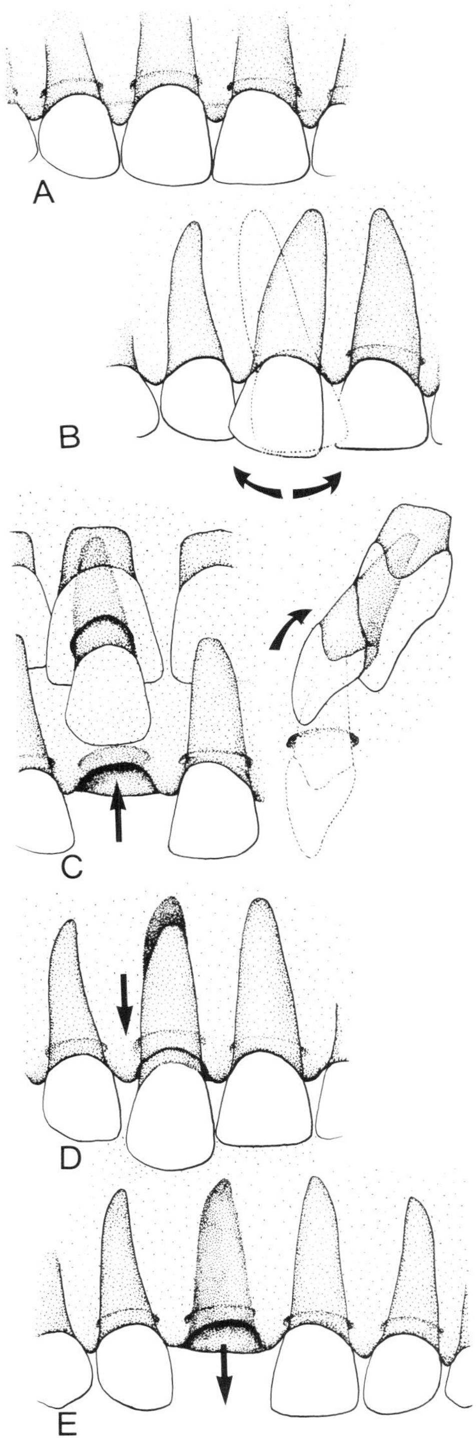

vided into five clinical types: concussion, subluxation, intrusion, extrusion and avulsion, as noted in Figure 66.4.

Concussion is usually of minor damage to the periodontal ligaments. Teeth sustaining concussive injuries exhibit no displacement or excessive mobility. They are very percussion sensitive when tapped with the blunt end of a metal instrument such as an intraoral mirror. No emergency treatment is indicated for such injuries. If there is any question of a more serious dental injury an immediate dental consultation should be arranged.

Subluxation is usually more damaging to the periodontal ligaments. There is excessive mobility in the horizontal and/or vertical direction, but no displacement within the dental arch. The tooth is usually quite percussion sensitive. The child will often complain that his teeth feel unusual when he bites down. Since subluxated teeth, especially in the permanent dentition, should be immobilized with an acrylic splint, this type of injury should be referred to the dental service as soon as possible.

Intrusion, although usually seen in the primary dentition, has been seen frequently in the permament arch. Intruded teeth are teeth pushed up into the socket. Intruded teeth may give the false appearance of being avulsed. In order to confirm intrusion and to rule out avulsion an intraoral dental x-ray is indicated. The intruded primary tooth must be evaluated for its proximity to the developing permanent tooth. Again immediate dental consultation and treatment are necessary. In addition, compression fractures of the alveolar socket and anterior nasal spine may be seen radiographically. The prognosis for teeth sustaining intrusive injuries is quite poor due to pulpal strangulation which occurs upon impact.

Extrusion is manifested clinically as a vertical displacement out from the alveolar socket. Usually the anterior maxillary tooth

Figure 66.4. The various types of trauma to the peridontal structures. (*A*) Concussion, (*B*) subluxation, (*C*) intrusion (if a primary tooth is intruded note location of developing permanent tooth bud), (*D*) extrusion, and (*E*) avulsion. Refer emergencies (*B*) through (*E*) to the dental staff as soon as possible.

is extruded and displaced lingually causing a fracture of the labial wall of the alveolar socket. These permanent teeth must be realigned and immobilized as soon as possible by a member of the dental staff. Extrusive injuries in the primary dentition usually necessitate extraction in order to avoid potential injury to the permanent tooth bud during realignment. The prognosis for extruded teeth is usually good if treatment is rendered promptly.

Avulsion is the term used to describe a tooth which has been completely knocked out. Be sure to account for all avulsed teeth. Radiographs may show the teeth to be actually intruded, ingested, or aspirated. The best prognosis exists if therapy is instituted in less than ½ hour postavulsion. The emergency department physician or the parent should (as seen in Fig. 66.5): (1) find the tooth; (2) determine if this is a primary tooth by checking the age of the child and the table of tooth eruption. If it is a primary tooth, do not reimplant; (3) gently rinse the tooth, do not scrub the crown or root; (4) insert the tooth into the socket, its normal position. Do not be concerned if it extrudes slightly. If the parent, or if the physician cannot reimplant the tooth, have the child hold the tooth under his/her own tongue. If the child is too young, have the parent place the tooth under his/her own tongue. Milk or saliva is the best medium to maintain the peridontal ligament vitality; (5) go directly to the dentist for immobilization (acrylic splint). Dental follow-up is mandatory to prevent ankylosis and resorption of the root. Avulsed primary teeth are generally not indicated for reimplantation due to the close proximity of the permanent tooth to the socket.

Orthodontic Trauma

This often results from loose wires or ligatures which are attached to orthodontic brackets or bands. These emergencies should be seen by the dental service as soon as possible in order to alleviate any discomfort and lessen the risk of aspiration. If no discomfort is noted and there are no loose foreign bodies, the definitive treatment can often be delayed until a more convenient time.

Mandibular Fractures/Dislocations

Although the incidence of facial fractures (other than nasal) in children is rather low, the most common facial bone fractured in children is the mandible. Mandibular jaw and alveolar fractures account for only 2% of the total dental emergencies in the Children's Hospital of Philadelphia survey. The initial head and neck physical examination and radiographs should confirm the diagnosis of mandibular fractures. Initial attention must be focused upon airway patency, control of hemorrhage, shock, and neurologic assessment.

The emergency physician must be knowledgable in the diagnosis of mandibular fractures. Kruger has compared the mandible to an archery bow, which is strongest at its center and weakest at its ends. Thus most fractures will occur at the neck of the condyles. Vulnerability of the jaw itself predisposes certain areas to fracture, i.e., deep impacted teeth or unerupted 6-year molars make the angle of the mandible vulnerable. Remember to examine the teeth for any changes in occlusion, or raised or depressed fragments. Areas of bleeding, tears, or sublingual ecchymosis are clues to mandibular fractures. Pain upon opening, especially if the child is unable to open his mouth fully, often indicates mandibular fracture. The unilateral condylar fracture should be suspected in the presence of a deviation of jaw toward the affected side upon opening.

Radiographic views detailed in Table 66.3 should be ordered. In the pediatric patient a mandibular fracture generally necessitates hospital admission. The appropriate consulting service should be called upon to stabilize the fracture using either open or closed reduction. Figure 66.6 shows a patient in intermaxillary fixation.

Dislocation of the TMJ occurs when the capsule and temporomandibular ligament are sufficiently relaxed to allow the condyle to move to a point anterior to the articular eminence during opening. Dislocation can be unilateral or bilateral and often accompanies a history of extreme opening of the

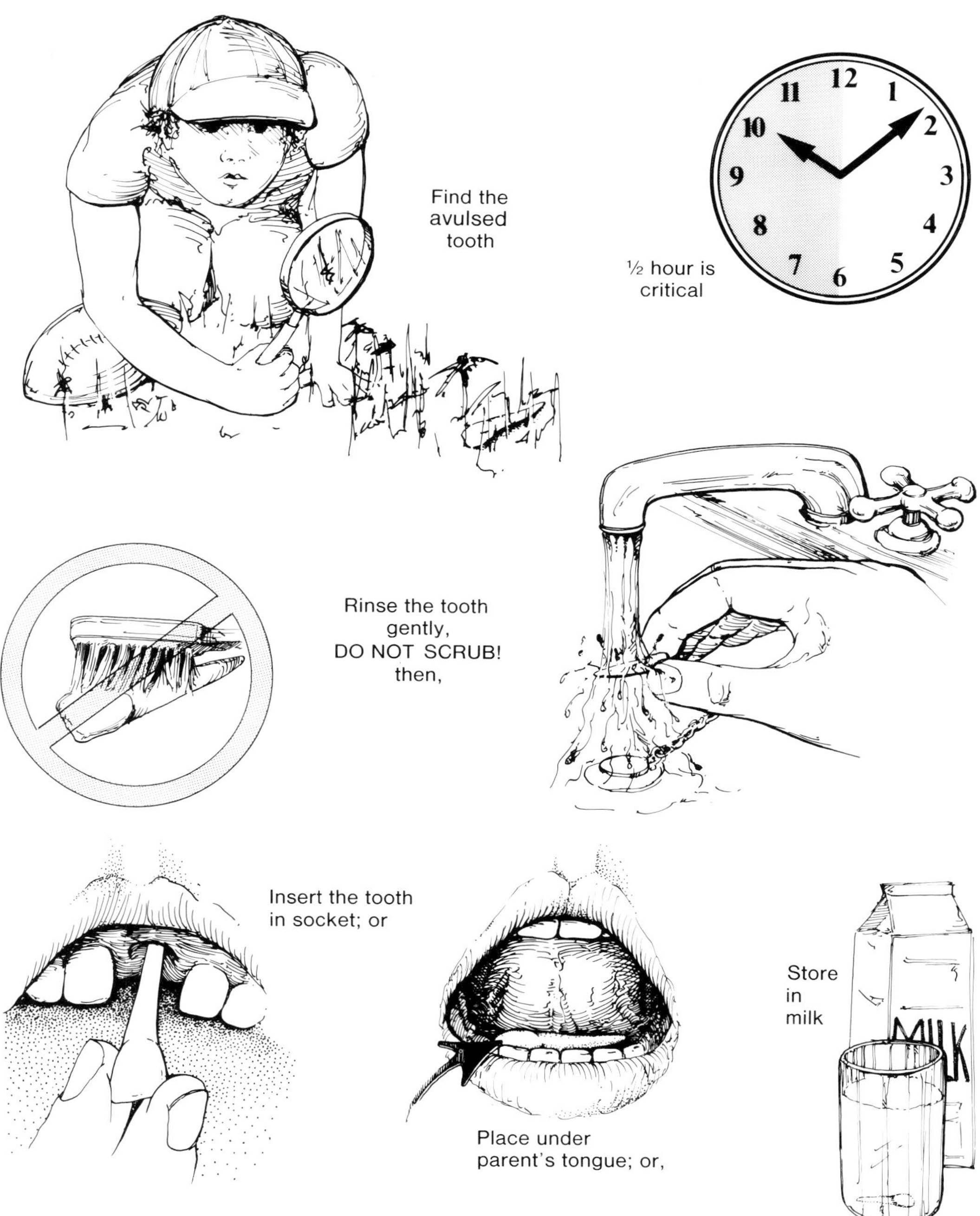

Figure 66.5 If a child looses or avulses a tooth. (*A*) Find the tooth. (*B*) Determine if it is a primary of permanent tooth by checking Table 65.2. If it is a primary tooth—DO NOT RE-IMPLANT. (*C*) Gently wash but do not scrub the tooth. (*D*) Insert the tooth back into the socket or place in milk and take immediately to the dentist. Remember you only have 30 min to preserve the vitality of the tooth.

mouth, i.e., deep yawn or following a long dental treatment session. Reduction is accomplished by standing in front of the patient and pushing downward and forward on the occlusal surfaces of the posterior teeth. This will cause a net posterior positioning of the mandible which will jump the condyles back into the glenoid fossa. The dentist or emergency physician should wrap his thumbs with gauze before placing them on the occlusal surfaces of the teeth in case the child suddenly occludes when the condyles resume their normal position.

Premaxillary or anterior maxillary alveolar bone fractures are a common finding associated with maxillary anterior tooth displacements or avulsions. By gentle digital manipulation the labial plate of bone can often be guided back into position under local anesthesia. (Infiltration with 2% lidocaine with epinephrine is usually used.) Splinting the loose teeth and suturing the gingival tissue will hold the bone fragments in place. After infiltration of local anesthesia and digital manipulation, the bone fragment can be held in place by aluminum foil (3 thicknesses) molded over the teeth and alveolar ridge. This emergency splint will be held in place by having the child bite down. A dental consultant should be contacted as soon as possible for fabrication of a more permanent dental splint. Figure 66.7 shows an acid-etch composite splint in place. Mandibular and other facial fractures are covered also in Chapter 64, "Plastic Surgical Emergencies."

Electrical Burns

Electrical burns of the mouth occur when children bite on electrical cords. The saliva in the child's mouth acts as a conductor to complete the circuit. When seen in the emergency department the first consideration is the patient's respiratory status. Next, the patient should be assessed for the presence of shock or other injuries possibly masked by the burn. Although the commissure of the mouth is most likely affected, the tongue, alveolar ridge, and floor of the mouth are occasionally involved. The majority of these children can be initially managed on an outpatient basis. A bland soft,

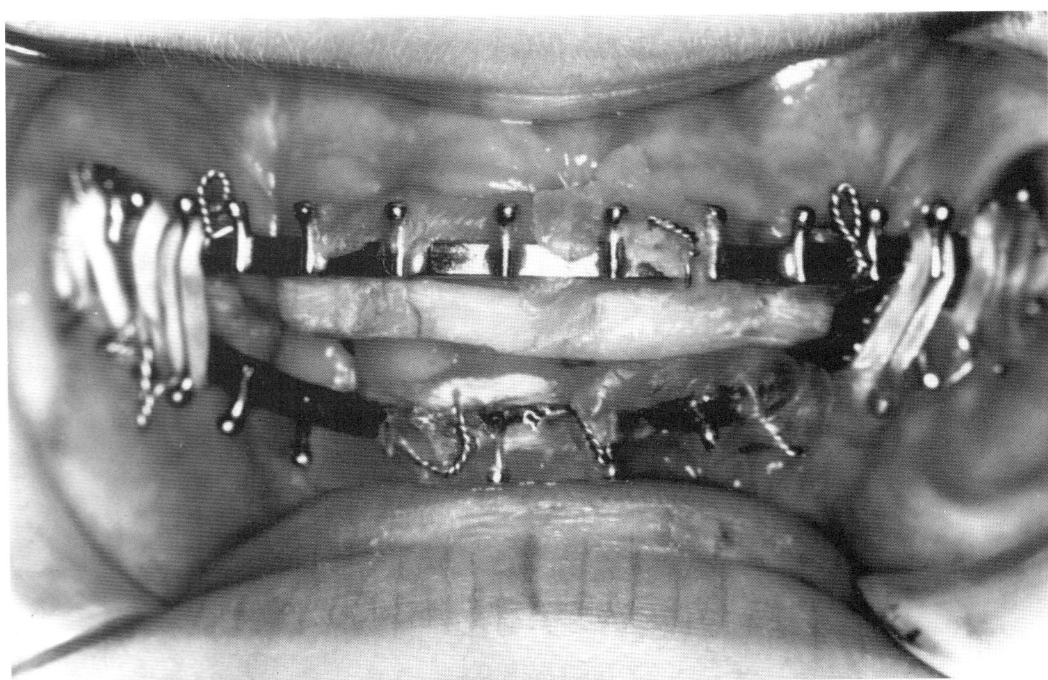

Figure 66.6 An example of a child in intermaxillary fixation for treatment of a mandibular condylar fracture.

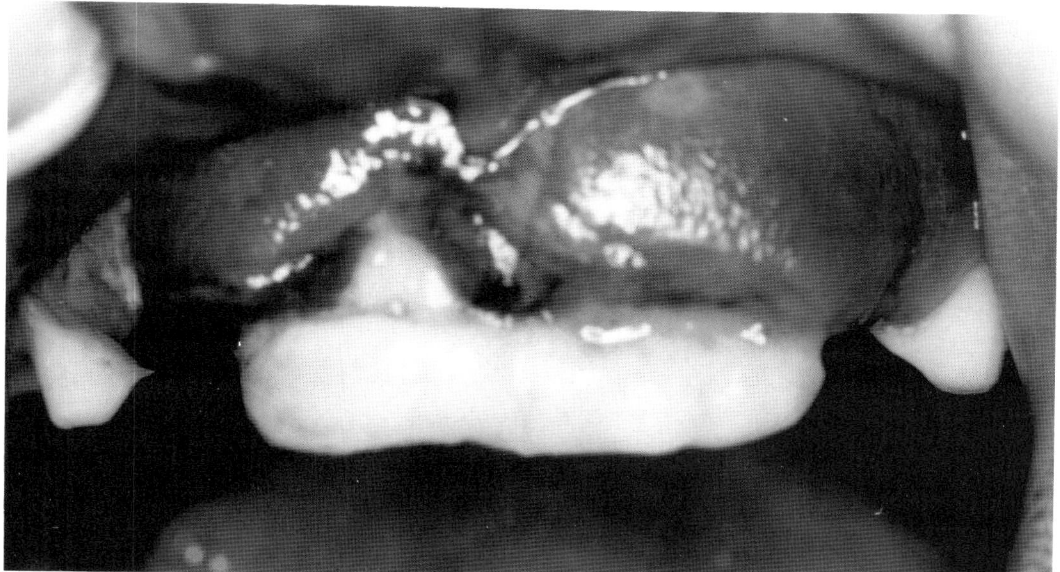

Figure 66.7 An example of an acid etch composite splint in place.

cold diet is initially recommended. If refusal of food and dehydration are a problem, the child will require admission to the hospital. Meticulous oral hygiene using a toothbrush with or without toothpaste must be used 3 to 4 times a day as well as hydrogen peroxide and water (1:1) rinses. With severe burns of the lips and mouth, it is likely that severe arterial bleeding will occur 5 to 8 days after the burn occurs. One should instruct the parent on the method for digitally compressing the labial artery or consider elective admission to the hospital for wound management.

POSTEXTRACTION COMPLICATIONS

Hemorrhage

It is expected that any extraction site may ooze for 8 to 12 hours after the extractions. However, it is important to check for a history of any prior bleeding episodes to rule out a systemic hematologic abnormality.

Emergency treatment includes the following steps.

1. Gauze sponges should be folded and placed over the socket with biting pressure for 30 min. If unsuccessful:
2. Dip a teabag in hot water and allow to cool, then place over the socket. The tannic acid in the teabag may control a bleeding socket. Repeat Step 1. If unsuccessful:
3. Administer local anesthesia (2% Xylocaine infiltration) and suture the socket edges with 3-0 silk and repeat Step 1. If unsuccessful:
4. Remove sutures and pack the socket with ¼-inch gauze. Resuture the socket and repeat Step 1.
5. Check the CBC and coagulation profile

Infection

Postextraction infection is rare in children but if present is seen as erythematous, edematous socket edges. A purulent exudate may be evident. Emergency treatment includes warm, oral saline rinses and antibiotic therapy. Penicillin is the treatment of choice (see section on dentoalveolar abscess for dose and duration).

Alveolar Osteitis

Alveolar osteitis or dry socket is a painful postoperative condition produced by disintegration of the clot in a tooth socket. This condition is usually seen in adults. It usually follows (72 hours) mandibular extractions and is very painful. Emergency dental treatment is variable but the immediate goal is relief of pain. At the Children's Hospital of Philadelphia, the socket is packed with ¼-inch iodoform gauze or Bipp's paste (bismuth, iodoform, benzocaine, and petrolatum). Oral analgesic medication is prescribed.

ORAL INFECTIONS

In our study of dental emergencies at the Children's Hospital of Philadelphia, oral infections and toothaches accounted for 17% of all emergency department referrals to the dental service. It is important to remember that the infant, or small child who is in pain, very often cannot localize the pain. A complete history from the parents and a thorough oral examination are mandatory. Figure 66.3 is a diagram of the normal tooth.

Odontalgia—Simple Toothache

The child will often complain of diffuse mouth pain and may not be able to point to a specific tooth. The emergency physician may note a grossly carious tooth. Swelling or inflammation in the surrounding soft tissue may be present. The tooth will be percussion sensitive but will not exhibit excessive mobility. Analgesics such as acetaminophen or codeine may be prescribed and a dental referral made for the next day.

Dentoalveolar Abscess

Dental abscessess are frequent in children due to the high incidence of dental caries in the population and the morphological characteristics of the primary tooth and immature permanent tooth. In the dentoalveolar abscess the etiologic factors are gross decay, trauma, or an inadequately restored tooth. Suppuration is usually confined to the bone around the apex of the tooth. If the infection is long standing, it can perforate the bony plate adjacent to the root of the involved tooth and spread into the subperiosteal area and then to the surrounding soft tissues. Infection in a child's jaw can spread rapidly due to the bone's wide marrow spaces.

The clinical manifestations of a dentoalveolar abscess in a child are:

1. *Pain*—The tooth is very painful to percussion and may exhibit spontaneous painful episodes.
2. *Mobility*—The tooth may have a greater than normal degree of movement in the socket when palpated with digital pressure bucco-lingually.
3. *Swelling*—The soft tissues surrounding the tooth may or may not be edematous and may or may not be erythematous.
4. *Temperature*—The child may have temperature elevation and general malaise, although this manifestation is quite variable.
5. *Fistulous tracts*—These appear clinically as a pimple-like lesion on the gingiva or face when the abscess has been present for a long time. The lesion should be gently milked, in order to express any purulence.
6. *Lymphadenopathy*—Major lymph node enlargement can occur at any time during the infective process.
7. *Extrusion*—The tooth may become extruded due to abscess expansion.

The first step in treatment is to identify the abscessed tooth. This can be accomplished by using the clinical examination and appropriate radiographs. Note the location, extent, and quality of any swellings. Note any fistulous tracts both intra- or extraorally. In cases of facial swelling or lymphadenopathy due to acute dentoalveolar abscess the antibiotic of choice is penicillin (or erythromycin, if there is a known allergy to penicillin). The initial dose is 1 g p.o., followed by 500 mg every 6 hours until the patient can be seen by a dentist. (For children under 60 lb (27 kg), the penicillin dose is initially 500 mg, followed by 250 mg every 6 hours.)

Penicillin-sensitive streptococci and anaerobic organisms predominate as the cause of acute dentoalveolar abscesses. If there is a facial cellulitis over the maxilla extending toward the inferior border of orbital rim or if there is a mandibular cellulitis, which might be a potential cause of airway compromise, the child should be admitted to the hospital. Treatment for facial cellulitis is covered in Chapter 45, "Infectious Diseases." Other factors to consider in determining the need for hospital admission include the child's ability to take fluids and the parent's level of cooperation for follow-up dental care. In addition to antibiotics, warm oral saline rinses should be used. Heat should *not* be applied extraorally. Extraoral heat will cause the abscess to point extraorally and thus produce an exterior fistula. Mild analgesic therapy such as acetaminophen is usually sufficient. This can be augmented with codeine for extreme pain. Immediate dental consultation should be obtained in order to make an opening into the offending tooth to establish drainage, to incise a fluctuant mass, or to remove the tooth. As with infection elsewhere in the body, the basic surgical principles of treatment must be utilized: (1) remove the cause and (2) establish drainage. An abscessed primary tooth must be vigorously treated, as such infections can effect changes in the unerupted permanent tooth bud, causing an enamel defect. When the affected tooth erupts the enamel may be discolored or pitted. In complicated cases a cellulitis or abscess can cause severe systemic consequences, including cavernous sinus thrombosis, airway obstruction, brain abscess, and septicemia.

In some cases, there may be a need for additional consultation with infectious disease experts especially in a situation in which systemic disorders render the child more susceptible to infection.

Pericoronitis

This is an infection surrounding an erupting tooth. It is usually associated with erupting molars in the adolescent patient (see Table 66.1). Symptoms usually include pain distal to the last erupted tooth in the dental arch. Erythema is usually present and localized to the gingiva in the retromolar area. Lymphadenopathy, trismus, and dysphagia are also noted. There may or may not be an elevation in body temperature. It is not unusual to see or palpate the cusps of the unerupted tooth breaking through the gingiva. The patient may complain of an inability to completely close his mouth due to the edematous gingiva. Otalgia is often a related complaint.

Emergency treatment includes antibiotics. Penicillin is usually the drug of choice (for dose, see dentoalveolar abscess) when there is a fever or lymphadenopathy. Warm oral saline rinses are also helpful. Antibiotics should be continued until definitive treatment is achieved which may include extraction of the impacted tooth. This treatment can be accomplished during a scheduled dental visit.

Primary Herpetic Gingivostomatitis or Herpes Simplex Virus (HSV) Type I

This communicable childhood disease is not a true dental emergency but is a common cause of emergency department visits. The child is usually a preschooler who complains of intense pain or simply stops eating, drinking, or talking. History is characteristic in that the child usually runs a very high fever 3 to 5 days prior to any clinical oral findings. At the Children's Hospital of Philadelphia, we have noted a higher incidence of primary herpes during periods of emotional stress (i.e., hospital admission) or during seasonal changes (October, July). The child may complain of headaches, malaise, nausea, regional lymphadenopathy and/or bleeding gums. The physicial examination includes gingival inflammation and areas of spontaneous hemorrhage. One or two days later, yellowish, fluid filled vesicles develop. The vesicles rupture spontaneously leaving extremely painful ulcers, covered by a gray membrane surrounded by an erythematous halo which may become crusted, as seen in Figure 66.8.

If necessary, a definitive diagnosis can be made upon isolation of HSV in tissue culture (although this is rarely indicated). Emergency treatment includes reassuring the patient. The disease, like recurrent herpes labialis, is self-limiting with a duration of 7 to 14 days. Dehydration and weight loss are concerns; therefore, milk shakes, ice cream, and liberal quantities of clear fluids should be encouraged. The young child with extensive lesions may require hospitalization for intravenous hydra-

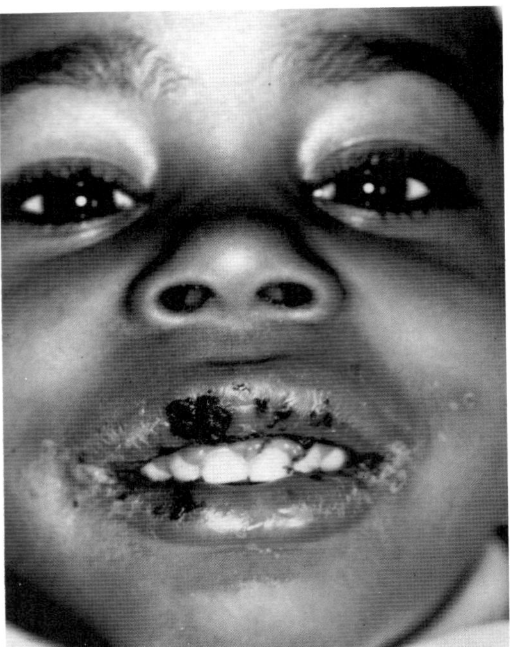

Figure 66.8. A child with typical crusted extraoral lesions of late primary gingivostomatitis.

tion. The use of viscous Xylocaine intraorally may help if administered prior to meals. The unpleasant taste sometimes negates the topical anesthetic quality of medicament. Secondary infection, although rare, is of concern for those children who may be immunosuppressed.

Acute Necrotizing Ulcerative Gingivitis (ANUG), Vincent's Disease, Trench Mouth

This disease is characterized by increases in the fusiform bacillus and *Borrelia vincenti*, a spirochete, coexisting in a symbiotic relationship. The patient (usually 15 years of age and up) complains of soreness and point-tenderness at the gingiva and often tells the physician that they feel as if they cannot remove a piece of food which is painfully stuck between their teeth. Children will also complain of a metallic taste in their mouth and of bleeding gums. Upon examination, there is an immediately obvious fetid odor to the breath. The gingivae are very hyperemic and the usually trian-

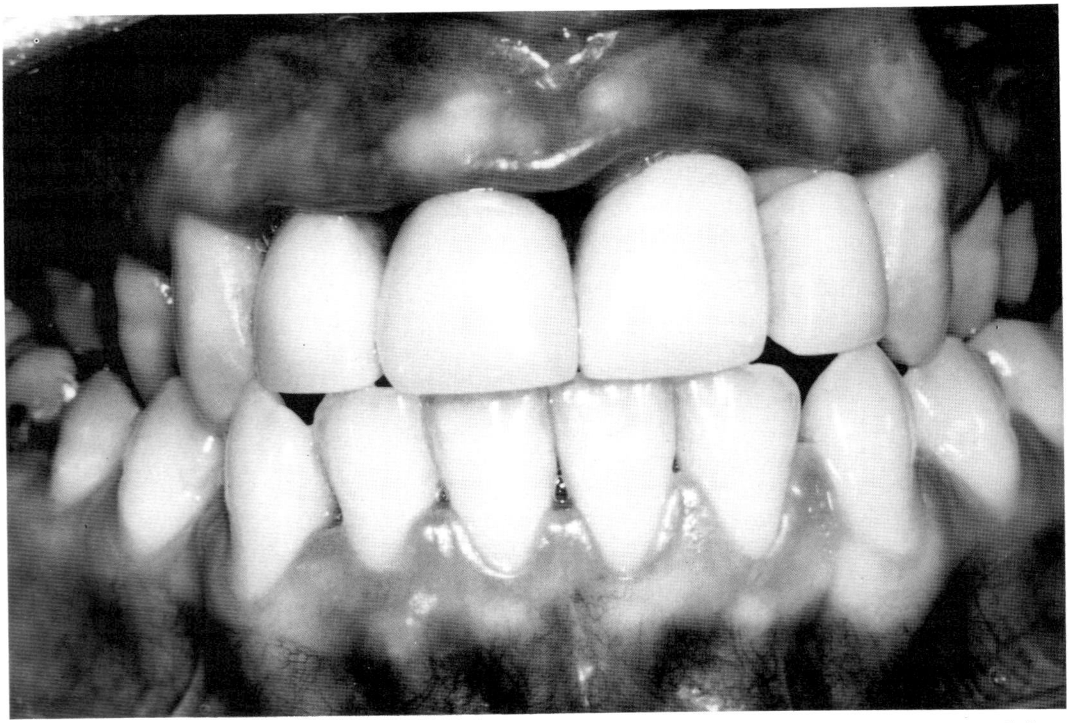

Figure 66.9 A child with typical "punched out" gingiva—pathognomonic for acute necrotizing ulcerative gingivitis. (Courtesy of Dr. Mark Snyder.)

gular gingiva between the teeth is "punched out" (see Fig. 66.9). There is intense pain upon probing and a gray, necrotic pseudomembrane may cover some areas of gingiva. It is extremely rare to find ANUG in a young child, but a mistaken diagnosis is often made by physicians, confusing this disease with primary herpes gingivostomatitis. Primary herpes is usually seen in children at ages 3 to 5 and ANUG is characteristically seen in young and adults (age 15 to 35). Emotional stress is linked to the onset of both disease processes. The adolescent should be advised to brush the teeth as often as possible and use frequent hydrogen peroxide mouth rinses. Diluted 1:1 with warm water, the hydrogen peroxide is vigorously swished and forced between the teeth as frequently as possible throughout the acute phase. Due to the rapidity of tissue destruction and sensitivity of the organisms, penicillin should be prescribed for the first week. When the acute phase is over, the patient should be sent to the dentist for a thorough debridement of the area.

References

Andreason JO: *Traumatic Injuries of the Teeth.* C. V. Mosby, St. Louis, 1972.

Berkowitz R, Ludwig S, Johnson R: Dental trauma in children and adolescents. *Clin Pediatr* 19: 3, 1980.

Croll T, et al.: Rapid neurologic assessment and initial management for the patient with traumatic dental injuries. *J. Am Dent Assoc* 100: 530–534, 1980.

Guralnick W, Donoff R: *MGM Textbook of Emergency Medicine*, edited by EW Wilkens. Williams & Wilkins, Baltimore, 1978.

Kruger G: *Textbook of Oral Surgery*, Ed. 4. C. V. Mosby, St. Louis, 1974.

McCarthy F: *Emergencies in Dental Practice Prevention and Treatment.* W. B. Saunders, Philadelphia, 1979.

Sanders B: *Pediatric Oral and Maxillofacial Surgery.* C. V. Mosby, St. Louis, 1979.

Schultz RC: *Facial Injuries*, Ed. 2. Yearbook, Chicago, 1977.

Shafer W, Hine M, Levy B: *A Textbook of Oral Pathology.* W. B. Saunders, Philadelphia, 1974.

Zook EG: *The Primary Care of Facial Injuries.* PSG Publishing, Littleton, Mass.

CHAPTER 67

Neurosurgical Emergencies

DEREK A. BRUCE, M.B., CH.B., LUIS SCHUT, M.D., AND LESLIE M. SUTTON, M.D.

There are many problems of neurological origin which present to the emergency department physician. The difficulty, especially in children, is that the signs and symptoms of neurological disease may be very similar to those of more common pediatric diseases. Fortunately, the majority of the neurological presentations are not truly emergencies, and patients can be safely referred to the necessary specialty clinics for further investigations. There are, however, acute diseases affecting the brain, spinal cord and peripheral nervous system which require immediate recognition and therapy. It is these diseases of particular pertinence to the neurological surgeon that will be discussed here. While it is most appropriate to consider the presentations under the usual categories of disease (congenital, traumatic, neoplastic and infectious), the acute problem produced by many of these different processes, however, has the same pathophysiology, that of acute intracranial hypertension.

RECOGNITION OF ACUTE INTRACRANIAL HYPERTENSION

A clear understanding of the events leading to elevated intracranial pressure (ICP) and the potentially lethal outcome thereof is vital to supplying the correct emergency care. Acute intracranial hypertension, with or without displacement of cerebral tissue (herniation) can result from: trauma; acute intracranial hemorrhage from aneurysm, arteriovenous malformation or tumor; acute hydrocephalus, either primary or secondary; infection; or tumor. The diagnosis and treatment of the elevated ICP is the most frequent and urgent of all the neurosurgical emergencies.

The intracranial space contains three components: blood, brain and cerebrospinal fluid (CSF). Since the volume inside the cranium is essentially fixed to acute changes in volume, even in the child with open sutures, an expansion of one component within the cranium must be offset by a reduction of the others. In simple terms,

$$V \text{ blood} + V \text{ brain} + V \text{ CSF} + V \text{ other} = \text{constant}$$

where *V other* represents any additional intracranial mass (e.g., tumor or hemorrhage).

The initial compensation for an increase in intracranial volume of one compartment is displacement of CSF out of the head into the distensible spinal dural sac. If the CSF pathways remain patent, a further increase in intracranial volume is associated with displacement of ventricular and subarachnoid CSF out of the cranium into the venous drainage, especially the sagittal sinus.

The response of the cerebral blood volume (CBV) is a little more complex. The greatest blood volume is in the pial veins and this volume can be displaced, providing there is no obstruction to venous outflow. As further increase in intracranial volume occurs and the ICP rises, the cerebral perfusion pressure (CPP) decreases [CPP=SAP (systemic arterial pressure) minus ICP] and cerebral vascular pressure autoregulation produces arteriolar dilatation in an effort to maintain normal cerebral blood flow (CBF). CBF equals CPP divided by CVR (where CVR represents cerebrovascular resistance). The arteriolar dilatation results in an increase in intracerebral blood volume. Thus, there is a biphasic response of the CBV to changes in ICP, with initially a decrease in volume followed by an increase.

The brain itself is viscoelastic in its properties and can be displaced and compressed to some degree. Displacement can occur from one compartment of the cranium to the other, if there is a differential pressure between the two compartments. This differential pressure may be brief, as in the rapid expansion of an epidural hematoma, or prolonged, as in the case of a growing tumor.

HERNIATION OF THE BRAIN

There are three major loci of brain tissue herniation. One is under the falx cerebri from one side of the supratentorial space to the other. This typically affects the cingulate gyrus and clinically is associated with loss of leg function, as a result of compression of one or both anterior cerebral arteries. Symptoms, however, may be lacking at the time of presentation, especially in patients in coma.

The second area for cerebral herniation, and the most frequently identified, is at the tentorial edge from the supratentorial to the infratentorial compartment. The portion of brain herniating is usually the perihippocampal gyrus of the temporal lobe including the uncus. The herniation is associated with compression of cranial nerve III, usually unilaterally, compression and distortion of the upper brainstem and cerebral peduncles, and stretching and distortion of the feeding vessels arising from the basilar artery. The involvement of these structures is responsible for the typical signs and symptoms of transtentorial herniation. Clinically, the complaints are of headache, the result of distortion of the dura and the basal cerebral vessels, followed by deterioration of consciousness. This later event is the result of compression or ischemia of the reticular formation located in the upper brainstem. The clinical signs are decreasing consciousness, followed by dilatation of one pupil, usually that on the side of the herniating brain (80%). The pupillary dilatation is the result of nerve III compression; and, if the herniation is not reversed, motor nerve III paresis will occur, best seen as loss of medial deviation of the ipsilateral eye and ptosis. The next sign of rostral/caudal herniation is the development of decerebrate posturing or hemiparesis of the contralateral extremities. This is due to ischemia of the cerebral peduncle, as a result of compression and distortion by the herniating temporal lobe. The side of motor involvement is more variable than that of pupillary involvement and is contralateral to the mass lesion in only 50% of cases. If the herniation is permitted to continue, then dilatation of the opposite pupil will occur, followed by motor involvement of the opposite side, alteration of respiration, and, only as a terminal event, bradycardia, systemic hypertension and respiratory arrest. This chain of events is common to all lesions, producing a transtentorial herniation if left untreated. As noted, the earliest symptom is headache; the earliest signs, deteriorating level of consciousness and pupillary change.

In young children below the ages of 4 years, bradycardia is a frequent early sign of impending herniation and elevated ICP and should always be taken seriously in any patient suspected of sustaining an acute neurological insult. *It is imperative that every emergency room physician suspect and diagnose transtentorial herniation as the signs become apparent, because failure to diagnose and reverse the herniation at an early stage may lead to a fatal outcome.* When the compression has been sufficiently severe for a long enough period, evacuation of any mass lesion or relief of the intracranial hypertension may be followed by hyperemia of the brainstem and secondary hemorrhages into the brainstem from which recovery is impossible. This irreversible stage may be reached in minutes, and recovery seems to be dependent on the degree of neurological function present at the time of relief of herniation (i.e., the patient with fixed pupils and bilateral decerebrate posturing is much more likely to die despite relief of the herniation than a child with diminished consciousness and only a dilated pupil). Children tolerate brainstem compression produced by the herniation syndrome better than do adults and an attempt should always be made to relieve the herniation even at a late stage. The herniation discussed above is usually from the supratentorial to the infratentorial space and occurs as a result of a focal mass lesion, diffuse brain swelling or edema, or acute hydrocephalus. However, a very similar clinical syndrome is seen when the tentorial herniation is upward from the infra- to the supratentorial space. The most frequent setting for upward herniation is a child with a posterior fossa mass lesion, usually tumor, and significant hydrocephalus. If the supratentorial pressure is relieved too rapidly by ventricular CSF drainage, then a differential pressure develops, with decompression of the posterior fossa contents up through the tentorial notch resulting in the signs and symptoms of transtentorial herniation. While this is uncommon, it has to be recognized and the posterior fossa mass decompressed. Frequently, the diagnosis is not correctly made and the signs of herniation are treated by further removal of supratentorial CSF with clinical worsening each time this is done.

The third area for cerebral herniation is at the foramen magnum. The herniated brain is the cerebellar tonsils. These produce compression of the medulla oblongata and upper cervical spinal cord with associated signs and symptoms. The symptoms in an awake patient are neck pain, with relief provided either by extension of the neck if bilateral herniation or head tilt if there is unilateral herniation. Vomiting is frequently present. There may be no clinical signs referrable to the foramen magnum area or there may be episodes of bradycardia, systemic hypertension, downbeat nystagmus, and pupillary dilatation which occur with flexion of the neck. Herniation at the foramen magnum is difficult to diagnose on clinical examination and the diagnosis is suspected from the history: morning headache, vomiting, stiff neck or head tilt. The danger of missing such herniation is of sudden respiratory and/or cardiac arrest, resulting from acute compression of the medulla and its vital respiratory and cardiovascular centers. This type of herniation usually occurs following chronic or subacute complaints and is most often due to posterior fossa tumor or diffuse brain swelling (e.g., Reye's syndrome).

Acute elevation of ICP can also lead to sudden cardiorespiratory arrest as a result of ICP becoming equal to SAP, resulting in no cerebral perfusion. The danger of an acute wave of ICP is always present, even in a patient with a subacute or chronic history suggestive of elevated ICP. As noted above, the initial response of the intracranial contents to an increase in one of the components is a reduction in volume in the others and, as a result, no increase in pressure, but the response of the ICP to increasing intracranial volume is an exponential one (Fig. 67.1). It is important for the emergency room physician to understand the implications of the volume/pressure curve shown. By the time patients become symptomatic from ICP, they are already on the steep portion of the curve. Thus, they are at risk for sudden, severe elevations of ICP.

Further, in patients with a disturbance of their ICP to volume compensatory mechanism the state is dynamic, not static; and a

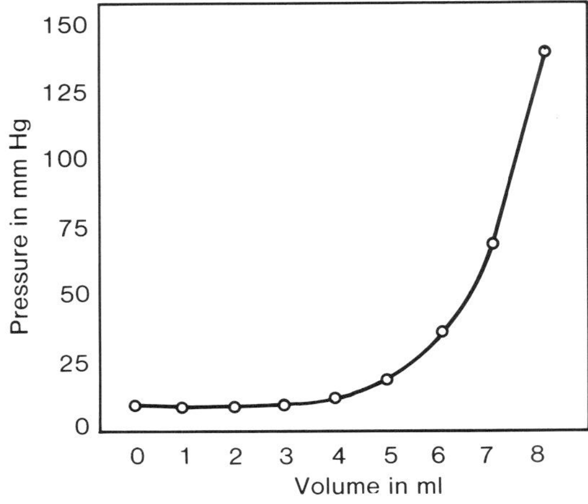

Figure 67.1. Relationship between intercranial volume and intercranial pressure.

sudden increase in volume produced by a rise in the CO_2 (as in sleep or by sedation) or a rise in cerebral blood volume following a seizure may exhaust the residual compensatory mechanisms and result in a fatal rise in pressure. This point is stressed because, even though the patient may tolerate one seizure or one episode of increased $PaCO_2$, there is no guarantee that another similar incident will be equally well-tolerated. When signs of increased ICP are present or increased ICP is suspected from the history, a lumbar puncture (LP) can be dangerous, because the withdrawal of CSF may permit further brain displacement to occur. In general, when acute intracranial hypertension is suspected, a CT scan should be obtained prior to LP.

CLINICAL MANIFESTATIONS

It is clinically impossible to guess the level of ICP, because the symptoms are intermittent and, as noted above, the pressure elevations are intermittent. Certain symptoms, however, must be taken seriously. A history of morning headache and vomiting or the same complaints occurring during sleep, intermittent headaches of such severity as to produce screaming or crying, complaints of transient visual loss associated with headache, or episodic decreases in level of consciousness associated with headache, all suggest ICP waves. Episodes of headache lasting 15 to 20 min, associated with pallor and obtundation is typical of an ICP wave. The clinical examination can be helpful but frequently is not, and the absence of definite signs cannot be used to discard the significance of the clinical history. Further study is indicated even in the absence of physical findings.

The best confirmatory sign of intracranial hypertension is papilledema. However, papilledema may never occur, depending on the anatomy of the veins and the subarachnoid spaces around the optic nerve. Thus, the absence of papilledema does not negate the presence of increased pressure. In children below age 8 to 10 years, chronically elevated ICP or acutely elevated ICP can produce separation of the cranial sutures. This leads to a change in the usual nonresonant note produced by percussing the head to a hyper-resonant, cracked-pot sound (i.e., positive Macewen's sign).

Unilateral or bilateral cranial nerve palsies can occur as a result of either focal herniation or diffusely elevated ICP. In the former, the ipsilateral nerve III is the most frequently involved, whereas when diffusely elevated ICP is present (e.g., hydrocephalus), nerve VI is most frequently affected. Cranial nerve II may be involved as noted above, showing papilledema, retinal hemorrhages or optic atrophy from long-standing pressure. It is rare for other nerves to be involved by intracranial hypertension, but neck pain may be associated with cerebellar tonsillar herniation as may vertical nystagmus.

MANAGEMENT

In the awake patient, diagnosis of intracranial hypertension can be difficult with the history being the most reliable indicator. In the unconscious patient, however, the ability to diagnose elevated ICP from the clinical examination is nearly impossible, in the absence of either papilledema or bulging, tense fontanel. When the history suggests intracranial hypertension, the first step is to obtain a definite diagnosis. Fortunately, the introduction and availability of the CT scanner has markedly improved the capabilities of obtaining an early, safe, and definitive diagnosis of lesions of the brain and, most recently, spinal cord. Nonetheless, there is still value in obtaining a plain skull x-ray. In children, evidence of erosion of the laminae dura of the sella turcica, increased sulcal markings, splitting of the cranial sutures and abnormal calcification may all confirm the diagnosis of elevated ICP or an intracranial mass. Routine brain scan is not nearly so specific a test as the CT scan and will not diagnose hydrocephalus or posterior fossa tumors. Emergency arteriography or pneumoencephalography are rarely required in the modern age.

The treatment of acute deterioration due to intracranial hypertension will depend upon the clinical picture and the suspected diagnosis. The initial approach in all patients, however, is preservation of an open airway, hyperventilation with 100% O_2, and elevation of the head 25 to 30°. A normal PaO_2 and decreased $PaCO_2$ will both reduce cerebral vasodilation, decrease CBV and acutely lower the ICP. When hydrocephalus is present, acute drainage of CSF from the ventricular system may be necessary. When a mass lesion is present, the use of dehydrating agents, such as mannitol and furosemide, may also be required. These treatments will be discussed under the various specific conditions outlined below.

TRAUMA

Acute head trauma can affect either the brain or its coverings. Injury to the scalp will be discussed elsewhere in this book. It is important, however, prior to suturing the scalp wound to manually palpate the underlying bone to rule out fracture and ascertain the cause of the laceration. When a sharp object has produced the wound, careful visualization of the skull is required for evidence of penetration.

Skull Fracture

Linear Fractures

Linear skull fractures are rarely neurosurgical emergencies. The importance of a linear fracture on skull x-ray is mainly a reflection of the degree and type of traumatic impact trauma. Simple linear fractures require no therapy. If the fracture crosses the grooves of the middle meningeal artery or the venous sinus, hospitalization and observation may be necessary because of the risk of delayed hemorrhage. If there is real concern about this, a CT scan will clarify the matter. The majority of children who are awake with linear skull fracture do not require CT scan, however. If the fracture is in a noncritical area, and if the child is conscious, hospitalization is usually not required.

When evidence of CSF leakage is present either from the nose or ear, skull films may be helpful in showing linear fracture passing into the cranial base. With CSF leakage, we do not routinely use antibiotic coverage. The CSF leakage is rarely a neurosurgical emergency, and these leaks will almost invariably stop within 3 to 7 days.

The commonest complication of linear skull fracture is subgaleal hematoma, which may become very large and fluctuant from postinjury a few days to as long as 2 weeks postinjury. This fluid, when in combination with skull x-ray showing a linear fracture, is often thought to be CSF. It is not CSF, and the collection should never be tapped or aspirated unless there is frank evidence of infection. The liquefied blood is an excellent media for bacterial growth, and the risks of aspiration are significant. The blood, if left in situ, will be reabsorbed and no significant loss of iron will occur.

Depressed Skull Fracture

Closed, depressed skull fractures are rarely neurosurgical emergencies. Only if there is evidence of focal seizures or focal neurological deficit under the fracture site will it be necessary to consider immediate surgery. In the others, good skull x-rays will delineate the extent of the fracture and, if the depression appears greater than the width of the tables of the skull, CT scan will reveal the degree of depression intracranially and the extent of underlying brain involvement. These fractures are corrected once full consciousness has been regained. An exception to this is the child in deep coma in whom intracranial hypertension is suspected. If there is a large depressed fracture with the possibility of extensive laceration of the underlying dura, then correction of the depression may be necessary to avoid progressive herniation of brain out through the torn dura with resulting secondary infarction.

Compound Depressed Skull Fractures

These lesions are treated like other compound fractures. The skin is cleaned and the wound gently irrigated with saline. In these lesions, CT scan is a better study than plain x-rays since it shows the bony fragments, the underlying cerebral injury, and other injuries sustained in the cranium. The emergency treatment of a compound depressed fracture is to secure hemostasis from the wound edges, which is most easily done with Raney clips, and gentle irrigation with saline followed by Betadine. For antibiotic coverage we usually use initially only oxacillin in doses of 150 mg/kg/day. It is also necessary to check the tetanus immunization status of the patient. If significant bleeding is occurring from the herniated brain or deep to the bone and cannot easily be controlled, then the child must go directly to the operating room. In the child who is conscious without evidence of other cerebral lesions, plain skull x-rays may be adequate before going to the operating room. If the child is unconscious, it is safer to obtain a CT scan first to evaluate the rest of the intracranial contents and rule out other intracranial lesions prior to opening the cranium. We generally replace the bone by performing craniotomy rather than craniectomy and always close the underlying dura mater.

Traumatic Unconsciousness

The immediate response to the child rendered unconscious from trauma is to follow the ABC's of resuscitation: *A*irway, *B*reathing, *C*irculation. The airway is manually cleared with finger and gauze, then suctioned gently to prevent gagging or vomiting. If an oral airway is used, it must also not produce gagging or vomiting. Once the airway has been opened, adequate ventilation will usually occur spontaneously. Manual hyperventilation by mask with 100% O_2, using bag and mask, is usually adequate to ensure moderate hypocapnia and normoxia. Gentle pressure on the cricoid cartilage will prevent inflation of the stomach and guard against regurgitation and aspiration of gastric contents during manual ventilation. Because of the risk of associated spinal trauma, IT IS NOT NECESSARY, and may be dangerous, to hyperextend the child's neck. If there is severe oro-pharyngeal trauma, and if there is also an apparent spine injury, then an emergency tracheostomy may be indicated.

A rapid neurological examination includes: all the elements of the Glasgow coma score (most valuable in children over 3 years of age) (Table 67.1); pupillary responses, direct and consensual; pupil size; cold-water calorics, after examining the ears to rule out hematoma of the external meatus, perforation, or bleeding; and the patient's spontaneous ventilatory status. A child who remains unconscious requires a portable lateral neck x-ray and, if this is normal, will then be intubated using the same techniques as would be used in the

Table 67.1
Glasgow Coma Scale

Eyes open	
Spontaneously	4
To speech	3
To pain	2
None	1
Best verbal response	
Oriented	5
Confused	4
Inappropriate	3
Incomprehensible	2
None	1
Best motor response	
Obey commands	6
Localize pain	5
Withdrawal	4
Flexion to pain	3
Extension to pain	2
None	1

Teasdale, G. & Jennett, B.: Assessment of coma and impaired consciousness. A practical scale. *Lancet*, 2: 81–84, 1974.

operating room in patients suspected of having intracranial hypertension. This includes hyperventilation with 100% O_2 and intravenous administration of thiopental, 3 to 5 mg/kg, if systemic arterial pressure is normal and hypovolemia has been corrected. This is followed by pancuronium, 0.2 mg/kg i.v. Gentle pressure over the cricoid cartilage will prevent gastric regurgitation, and laryngoscopy and endotracheal intubation can be performed under these controlled conditions. A nasogastric tube is then placed and the stomach contents aspirated. Hyperventilation to $PaCO_2$ around 25 torr is performed. If the vital signs are stable and there is no evidence of multiple trauma or abdominal injury, the child is transported for CT scan. In children with Glasgow coma score (GCS) of 5 or less, we also insert a radial artery catheter to monitor arterial pressure and a frontal subarachnoid pressure monitor in the emergency department prior to transporting the patient. Early elevated ICP is the commonest cause of primary death resulting from major head trauma in children. The sooner the ICP can be monitored and accurately controlled, the better the outlook for the child.

The child who shows evidence of herniation syndrome or rapidly deteriorating consciousness following head trauma requires:

1. Immediate intubation as described above and hyperventilation to $PaCO_2$ 20 to 25 torr
2. Head-up tilt 30°
3. If the history is suggestive of a mass lesion (e.g., focal trauma, minor disturbance of consciousness at the time of injury, swollen boggy temporal area) and the signs of focal neurological change (e.g., large pupil or hemiparesis), then mannitol in a dose in of 0.5 mg/kg is given i.v. over 3 to 5 min. The mannitol is given after hyperventilation has been established
4. An ICP monitor is inserted if there is no improvement in the clinical state
5. CT scan obtained as soon as the child is stable.

Shaking Injury

In children under 1 year of age admitted in coma with bulging fontanel, fixed pupils and either extensor posturing or flaccidity associated with retinal hemorrhages, the diagnosis of shaking is almost always the correct one. After intubation and hyperventilation, bilateral fontanel taps are performed. These must be lateral by at least 2 cm from the midline to avoid the large draining veins. Often, 5 to 20 ml of bloody, nonclotting subarachnoid fluid is obtained. The removal of this fluid is frequently associated with return of the pupil size to normal, decrease in motor tone, and softening of the fontanel. These children then require immediate CT scan. The CT scan findings are rarely impressive and usually show a small posterior interhemispheric subdural hematoma. Further surgery is rarely necessary in this group of children, and the treatment consists of careful control of the ICP in the intensive care unit (ICU) setting. In children who are unconscious but without decerebrate posturing or bulging of the fontanel, fontanel tap is not necessary, but the child should be taken directly to the CT scan once an airway is established.

In children who rapidly recover consciousness following head trauma without focal neurological deficit, the degree of pre- and post-traumatic amnesia, the return or not of full intellectual ability, and the history and type of trauma are all used to decide whether admission and observation are necessary. Whenever a suspicion of a mass lesion is present, CT scan should be performed.

Shock and Head Trauma

In general, shock should never be ascribed to head trauma and other causes of bleeding should be sought (e.g., abdomen, chest, long-bone fractures, etc.). There are, however, some rare exceptions to this rule in childhood. Children under 1 year of age who develop an epidural hematoma associated with a large fracture can decompress the hematoma into the scalp sufficiently to produce anemia and shock (Fig. 67.2). Young children with large CSF spaces (e.g., hydrocephalus or porencephaly) can lose sufficient blood into the cranial cavity to develop acute anemia and occasionally shock. Occasionally, the infant can develop a sufficiently large subgaleal hematoma to develop anemia but, as the bleeding is slow, shock does not occur. These are rare exceptions but the general rule stands true that shock is not due to head trauma.

Acute Brain Swelling

The response of the childhood brain to trauma appears to be quite different from that of the adult. Acute subdural hematomas and cerebral contusions are much less common, and the phenomenon of acute diffuse brain swelling much more common. In children with GCS of 8 or less following head trauma, 50% will show a CT scan pattern of acute diffuse brain swelling. This shows up on CT scan as small ventricles and narrowing or absence of the perimesencephalic and basal cisterns. Studies have suggested that this pattern is not due to cerebral edema but to acute cerebral congestion with an increase in blood flow and blood volume. The clinical history of patients showing diffuse swelling varies from acute and continuous unconsciousness from the time of trauma to those who are unconscious, show some evidence of improvement, and then deteriorate rapidly. Focal neurological signs can occur as well as the pattern of herniation at the tentorial notch.

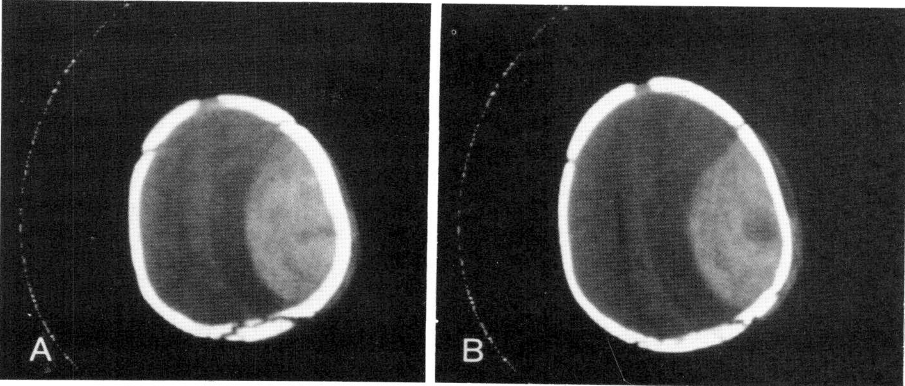

Figure 67.2 Large epidural hematoma in 5-month-old child showing decreased density in the underlying brain suggesting infarction.

Because of the frequency with which diffuse swelling is seen and the infrequency with which mass lesions or cerebral contusions are seen, our prime emergency therapy in children following head trauma is hyperventilation. The decrease in $PaCO_2$ produces a decrease in cerebrovascular diameter, decreased cerebral blood flow and cerebral blood volume. This is the most rapid and efficient way of lowering the ICP in this group of children. We do not routinely use mannitol as part of the resuscitation, since mannitol transiently increases cerebral blood flow and, therefore, may potentially worsen the situation. Mannitol is given, however, when there is suspicion of an expanding mass lesion, particularly where an epidural hematoma is suspected. Even in this circumstance, we hyperventilate the patient first prior to giving the mannitol. While the acute brain swelling may be self-limiting, it will occasionally be progressive and cause death within hours following trauma. Because of this, an aggressive management approach is always indicated.

Spinal Cord Injury

Acute spinal cord trauma fortunately is uncommon in children but becomes increasingly frequent in the later years of teenage when motorcycle accidents play a major role. When examining a patient for evidence of spinal cord injury, the history is extremely important as an alerting sign for the physician about the risk of spinal cord trauma. This is especially true in the patient who is admitted unconscious. Head trauma, when sustained through a fall of significant height or an automobile accident, should be considered one component of craniospinal trauma and all resuscitative efforts and movement of the child should be done while taking all precautions to keep the spine in alignment and the head in the neutral position. When the child is being moved, one attendant's responsibility should be to control the head while the others move the rest of the spine as a log.

Physical examination of the patient with spinal cord injury will vary depending on the completeness of the lesion and level of the lesion. When the patient is awake, there may be complaints of numbness or inability to move the arms or legs. When the injury is high, C5 or above, respiration will be involved because of paralysis of both the intercostal muscles and involvement of the phrenic nerves. Under normal circumstances, an injury above C4 is incompatible with survival unless artificial ventilation is begun soon after the injury. The vital signs may show evidence of low blood pressure and tachycardia which may be the result of the sympathetic impairment as a result of spinal cord injury or may be the result of other blood loss. Examination of the abdomen is difficult in patients sustaining spinal cord injury above the midthoracic level, since this inteferes with sensation coming from the superficial structures of the abdomen, although vagal sensation remains intact. Difficulties in examining the abdomen are also encountered because of the frequent acute ileus that occurs following cord injury giving a distended, nontender abdomen which may simply be due to air and ileus or may be due to hemorrhage. Frequently, abdominal lavage will be necessary to clarify the issue. When respiratory function is impaired, manual hyperventilation with a bag, mask and oral airway is usually possible long enough to obtain spine x-rays. If adequate ventilation cannot be sustained and the stability of the cervical spine is unknown, then emergency nasotracheal intubation without extension of the neck or emergency tracheostomy, again avoiding hyperextension of the neck, will be necessary. Blood pressure control is usually easily achieved by elevation of the feet and legs or a compression (MAST) suit. Portable x-rays of the cervical spine or thoracic and lumbar spine are then obtained. Medications usually play little role, but large doses of steroids are generally given in a dose of 1.5 mg/kg of dexamethasone or 5 to 10 mg/kg of Solu-Medrol. A nasogastric tube is inserted to relieve the gastric distention and a Foley catheter will be required to drain the bladder.

In the conscious patient, the physical examination may be directed by the patient's complaints and cooperation. In a patient who is unconscious or one who has a high cervical injury, position of the upper extremities is most helpful in suggesting the level of damage. Flexion at the elbows suggests that the C5 root supplying biceps is intact and functional and the C6 route supplying mostly triceps is malfunctioning, thus permitting flexion with inability to extend the elbow and no function below C5. Extension at the elbows with the ability both to flex and extend the elbow joint suggests a lesion at the C6-C7 level and is usually associated with preserved extension of the wrist and fingers. Preservation of finger flexion and wrist flexion suggests intactness of the C8 route and level around T1. Preservation of motor function in the upper extremities with loss of function in the lower extremities suggests a thoracic or lumbar level. With central cord injury, the function of the lower extremities may be preserved in the face of absent upper extremity function. This type of injury is usually due to hyperextension with central cavitation and loss of gray matter but with preservation of the long white matter tracts.

Examination of reflex function in the child with spinal cord injury is likely to show preservation of reflexes above the level of injury and usually complete absence of reflexes in the early stages post injury. When partial cord damage is sustained without cord shock, then reflexes may be hyperactive and positive Babinski seen. Spinal cord shock is the state of flaccidity of muscle tone with absence of reflexes in that portion of cord below the level of injury. Because of the tendency of the motor examination to sometimes reflect greater neurological damage than is actual, sensory examination in these patients is extremely important. Careful examination both of proprioception, deep pain, light touch, pin prick, hot and cold are all necessary since sensation is frequently preserved in the face of spinal cord shock. The importance of a careful examination is to reflect whether the injury is a complete lesion (i.e., no sensory or motor function below a level) or incomplete. Even in children, the presence of a complete lesion with absolutely no sensory or motor function below the level of injury carries with it an extremely poor prognosis, although we have seen children who have indeed recovered some significant function from this state. Because of the poor prognosis, a diligent effort must be made to be sure on sensory examination that there is no deep pain or proprioception left. An incomplete lesion (i.e., preservation of some function) may be associated with complete recovery.

The role of therapy, which involves immediate stabilization of the spine and efforts to treat acute swelling, is to prevent progression of hemorrhage and swelling and to prevent the conversion of an incomplete lesion to a complete one. In the cervical region, the best way to acutely stabilize the spine is the insertion of skeletal traction with tongs in the head. In children 3 years and older, we use Gardiner tongs which are put in under local anesthesia and then secured in the skull. In younger children, pin fixation may be impossible because of the thinness of the cranium. In this case, sandbags on either side of the head during transport, followed by the application of some kind of cervical collar, may be the best stabilization that can be obtained acutely. In the infant, the definition of spinal cord injury when associated with severe head trauma may be impossible. A high suspicion of spinal cord trauma is necessary. In the child who is thrown about inside an automobile, the incidence of major high cervical trauma is high and any child admitted following such an injury with flaccid paralysis must be suspected of having high cervical spine injury. As noted above, lateral x-rays and AP of the spine are mandatory. In the cervical region this must include the C7-T1 junction. Frequently, in the small child the only evidence of abnormality is separation either of C1 from C2 or C2 from C3.

Once the level of the lesion has been defined, further studies may be valuable. CT scan of the spine will show evidence of narrowing of the canal and bony impingement on the spinal cord. This would be an indication for surgical decompression. Emergency myelography is valuable when spine x-rays are normal but there is evidence of worsening neurological deficit, or when a fixed deficit is present with normal spine films suggesting the possibility of acute disc protrusion. Both of these may be indications for surgical decompression. The final major indication for early surgery is in penetrating injuries of the spinal cord. These require surgical exploration.

In summary, the emergency care of the child with spinal cord trauma is immediate resuscitation of the airway, stabilization of the spine, identification of the level of injury and administration of large doses of corticosteroids. The most significant single factor in preservation of the incomplete lesion appears to be early stabilization of the spinal canal.

Peripheral Nerve Injuries

The two common situations in which major peripheral injuries occur in children are in association with laceration and with fracture dislocations. While peripheral nerve injuries are rarely treated acutely from the neurosurgical standpoint, a recognition of injury to the nerve, its careful documentation and appropriate early care are paramount to the later outcome from the injury.

Part of the examination of any child with a laceration in the region of a major peripheral nerve is a careful motor and sensory examination of the extremity distal to the injury. In small children, this can be difficult because of fear and pain producing lack of cooperation. Because of the inability to perform an adequate examination, such lacerations must be closed under good light with adequate cooperation from the patient to allow exploration of the area and visualization of any surrounding neural structures. When the child is uncooperative or restless, then general anesthesia may be required. Unless the laceration is produced by a sharp, clean instrument, primary nerve suture is rarely performed. The free nerve ends should be tagged and approximated to facilitate later repair.

The acute exploration of nerve palsies is performed when open reduction of the fracture is required but only rarely in simple fractures and dislocations.

The most important aspect of peripheral nerve injuries is careful documentation of the area of sensory and motor dysfunction so that careful follow up can accurately ascertain whether improvement is occurring spontaneously.

CONGENITAL ANOMALIES PRESENTING AS NEUROSURGICAL EMERGENCIES

Hydrocephalus

It is uncommon for infants with undiagnosed hydrocephalus to present primarily to the emergency department physician. In older children, however, both acute and chronic hydrocephalus may present with severe headache, vomiting, or disturbed consciousness. The pathophysiology of elevated ICP has been discussed earlier. Clinical examination may show: papilledema; nerve VI palsy, from the globally elevated ICP; difficulty with upward gaze due to compression of the collicular plate region by a distended third ventricle; increased tone in the lower extremities with hyperactive reflexes and positive Babinski. The reason for the increased tone abnormality is stretching of the fibers running to the legs around the dilated ventricles. The head circumference is often increased and a cracked-pot percussion (positive Macewen's sign) may be elicited. Plain skull x-rays may be helpful and may show separation of the cranial sutures, erosion of the bone in the floor of the sella turcica, or increased sulcal markings. The sulcal appearance is often seen up to age 14 years and can be difficult to interpret, while the other findings all signify increased ICP. The next step is to obtain a CT scan. If the patient is admitted in coma or if there is an acute episode of severe bradycardia, pupillary dilatation, apnea or bradypnea with alteration of consciousness, it may be necessary to relieve the ICP directly by tapping the ventricles before full resuscitation can be performed.

The initial management is mask hyperventilation. If there is no improvement, in patients with split sutures it is often possible to pass an 18- or 20-gauge spinal needle through the cranial suture and tap the ventricular system directly. This will immediately relieve the elevated ICP and may lead to rapid restoration of normal consciousness. These episodes are produced by pressure waves in which the ICP rises close to the blood pressure. They are a harbinger of potentially lethal deterioration and are an indication for immediate diagnosis and treatment.

Probably the most frequent presentation of hydrocephalus in the emergency room is the child with previously shunted hydrocephalus in whom either a shunt infection or shunt obstruction is suspected. The history may be of repeated headaches, particularly in the morning; stiff neck; screaming spells associated with headache; episodes of obtundation; nerve VI palsy; trouble with upward gaze. The signs will be similar to those discussed above. In the child under 1 year of age with an open fontanel, the diagnosis of shunt obstruction is relatively easy: full, bulging fontanel with a shunt that pumps poorly. There may be no abnormal signs elicited in the older children. The value of a shunt with a pumping system is that the functional status of both the proximal and distal end of the shunt can be easily checked. It takes time and familiarity with the workings of the various shunt systems to be able to ascertain function accurately.

The next step in examination of possible shunt obstruction is to obtain an x-ray evaluation of the entire length of the system, so that the position and intactness of the various components can be checked and evidence of elevated ICP looked for on the skull x-ray. If the diagnosis remains in doubt, CT scan will delineate ventricular size and indicate the adequacy of shunt function. If the child is admitted in coma or suddenly deteriorates in the emergency room or complains of severe head pain, the shunt must be tapped. This must be done under complete sterile conditions by someone experienced in the working and anatomy of the particular shunt system involved (see procedure in Section VII). Three pieces of information must be obtained. The first is the pressure of the fluid in the shunt system. This is easily measured by using a 23-gauge butterfly needle and simply holding the tube vertically to observe the height to which the CSF column rises. If the pressure is elevated, CSF is withdrawn until a normal pressure is reached. The second piece of information is to ascertain that fluid is easily obtained from the ventricular end of the system, thereby establishing patency of the proximal portion. When there is choroid plexus in the ventricular tubing, small amounts of CSF may flow spontaneously and when aspiration is attempted little or no fluid is obtained. This is an indication of upper end obstruction or very small ventricles. The third is to be certain of the drainage pressure of the distal portion of the shunt. This is done by occluding the ventricular end, permitting the withdrawn CSF to flow out the distal end of the shunt, and observing the height of the CSF column in the scalp vein tubing at which the flow stops. The visual appearance of the withdrawn fluid is important and sampling has to be done with measurement of cell count, Gram stain, sugar, protein and culture.

If the proximal end of the shunt is obstructed such that CSF cannot be withdrawn, then therapy will depend upon the patient's clinical status. If the patient is awake with intermittent or constant headache but no history of bradycardia, apnea, or opistotonic posturing, dexamethasone in a single dose of 0.5 to 1 mg/kg and 30 mg/kg of Diamox are given. CT scan is obtained and the child taken to the operating room for repair of the shunt. If the child is in coma or if episodes suggesting intracranial pressure waves are occurring, it may be necessary to tap the lateral ventricle directly either through the fontanel if patent or by passing a spinal needle through a burr hole and down the ventricular cannula. Once the pressure is relieved, correction of the shunt malfunction needs to be undertaken immediately. Whenever there is any suspicion of shunt malfunction, the neurosurgeon should be notified.

In summary, the suspicion of a blocked shunt represents a neurosurgical emergency. The exact site of malfunction needs to be rapidly ascertained, medication to relieve intracranial hypertension given, CT scan obtained and the shunt malfunction corrected at the earliest possible time.

Shunt Infection

While the majority of shunt infections occur within the first month after surgery, delayed infections do occur and may present to the physician in the emergency department. When a child with a shunt presents with fever or irritability, a full examination to evaluate the possible role of infection elsewhere is always necessary. It is uncommon for shunt infection to produce a very sick child, and the florid signs of stiff neck, high fever, thin pulse all suggest true meningitis with bacteremia rather than low-grade shunt infection. The physical examination is rarely helpful unless there is evidence of erythema or frank pus around the shunt system. The common use of ventriculoperitoneal shunts means that abdominal pain and tender ileus or rebound tenderness may be the only signs of a shunt infection. Generally, the presence of a shunt infection does not interfere with shunt function and, therefore, the shunt pumps normally. In children with an open fontanel, bulging of the fontanel may occur due to the increased temperature, increased outflow resistance to CSF, ventricular irritation with increased CSF production, and abdominal irritation with increased intraabdominal pressure and decreased CSF reabsorption. Another cause for distal sluggish shunt function in the face of infection is an increase in protein around the distal valve with sluggish opening. The definitive diagnosis is made by tapping the shunt under full sterile conditions. This should only be done after other causes of fever have been eliminated and is most certainly not indicated in every child with a shunt who presents with a fever.

In children with communicating hydrocephalus, an LP is advised before the shunt is tapped since the diagnosis may be confirmed by the former study and avoid the necessity of tapping the shunt. In children with noncommunicating hydrocephalus in whom central nervous infection is suspected, if the shunt tap shows no evidence of infection, an LP should also be performed since true meningitis can occur without ventriculitis. The emergency department treatment of shunt infection is to begin the appropriate antibiotic and hospitalization of the child.

Arteriovenous Malformations and Aneurysms

The other major congenital anomaly that presents as a neurosurgical emergency is rupture of an arteriovenous malformation (AVM) with acute interparenchymal cerebral hemorrhage and/or subarachnoid hemorrhage. The major symptom of acute intracranial hemorrhage is sudden onset of excruciating headache. Complaints of sudden onset of "the worst headache I have ever had" must be taken seriously, since this may be the only early symptom of early subarachnoid hemorrhage. Interparenchymal hemorrhage is often associated with the sudden onset of focal neurological deficit or acute unconsciousness. However, both signs may be delayed for hours to days after the hemorrhage, depending on the size, location and rate of formation of the hematoma. Also, focal neurological deficit may occur initially with no disturbance of consciousness. There is then a gradual deterioration of level of consciousness which, not infrequently, is assumed to be psychogenic in origin.

If the acute bleeding occurs near the cerebral cortex, then seizures may be part of the early presentation. There is rarely any significant past history. The sudden onset of headache followed by deteriorating level of consciousness, with or without seizures or focal neurological deficit, suggests intracranial hemorrhage until proven otherwise.

In the noncomatose patient, an i.v. line needs to be inserted and CT scan obtained. In the comatose patient or the patient who is showing rapidly progressive neurological deficit or alternating level of consciousness, the ICP must be lowered to prevent progressive cerebral herniation. If the patient is awake, mannitol in a dose of 0.5 to 1 g/kg is given over 5 min plus 1 mg/kg of dexamethasone or 5 to 10 mg/kg of methylprednisolone. If the patient is in coma with no eye opening or speech, then endotracheal intubation using sodium pentothal, pancuronium, hyperventilation and 100% O_2 is necessary before this patient can be safely transported to CT scan. LP should not be performed before the CT scan whenever an intracranial mass lesion is suspected.

Acute subarachnoid hemorrhage in childhood may occur as a result of interparenchymal hemorrhage with rupture into the subarachnoid space or into the ventricular system or may occur *per primum* as a result of rupture of an AVM or aneurysm. In adults, aneurysmal rupture is frequently associated with transient loss of consciousness, followed by stiff neck and headache. In children, particularly those under 5 years, onset of unconsciousness is uncommon with leakage into the subarachnoid space; and, more frequently, seizure, focal neurological deficit or general increased irritability will occur. A high suspicion of intracerebral or subarachnoid hemorrhage is based on an adequate history, since the focal or general neurological findings may be minimal.

NEOPLASM

Brain tumors in children usually present with a chronic history but may present to the emergency department with the sudden onset of acute symptoms. There are three types of symptoms: acute onset of disturbed consciousness, acute onset of cranial nerve palsy, or severe, recurrent headache. Taking the last presentation first, the headache is usually a reflection of elevated ICP. However, dural irritation from tumor may also produce headache. As mentioned previously, complaints of headache on waking suggest intracranial hypertension. The other types of headaches and complaints that are likely to be associated with intracranial hypertension have been discussed previously. Certain tumors, especially those in the sellar and parasellar region are more likely to produce nonspecific headache. The repeat appearance in the emergency department of a child with complaints of headache requires investigation. As a minimum, skull x-rays and frequently CT scan will be necessary.

Physical examination of the child suspected of harboring an intracranial mass must always include good fundoscopy to seek evidence of papilledema. Frequently, this is the only definitive positive finding. Other symptoms will be dependent on the site of the tumor and may vary from focal neurological deficits, visual field cuts, to disturbed consciousness. While these children may appear quite stable, those with headache and papilledema are at significant risk for rapid deterioration, and we suggest immediate skull x-rays followed by CT scan. LP should be delayed until after CT scan and is often not indicated until treatment of the intracranial pressure is well underway.

Acute cranial nerve palsies may occur as a result of intracranial tumors and be responsible for the presentation of the child to the emergency room with complaints of diplopia. The two reasons for cranial nerve involvement are either direct tumor compression or invasion or diffusely elevated intracranial pressure. The commonest nerve involvement by direct tumor invasion is cranial nerve VII followed by nerve VI. The tumor most frequently responsible is a glioma within the brainstem. There is usually no history suggestive of elevated ICP, but, not infrequently, the parents have noted a personality change preceding the onset of the cranial nerve palsy. Physical examination, in addition to the cranial nerve involvement, may reveal weakness, sensory loss or ataxia due to involvement of other tracts within the brainstem. In these patients there is no need for emergency therapy unless there is interference with swallowing or respiration. Differential diagnosis will include Guillain-Barré syndrome, post-viral encephalitis and intoxicants of various types. The child clearly needs to be hospitalized and worked up with neuroradiological investigations and lumbar puncture for diagnosis.

The final presentation is the acute onset of altered consciousness and may be the result of a seizure, acute elevated ICP, hydrocephalus or acute hemorrhage into the tumor. We have found that 10% of brain tumors in childhood present with acute hemorrhage. Repeated episodes of altered consciousness with irritability must arouse the suspicion of brain tumor. If LP consistently shows red cells without any positive culture, recurrent tumor hemorrhage must be suspected. The presentation and treatment of acute intracranial hypertension and acute hydrocephalus have been discussed above.

Spinal Cord Compression

Children with spinal cord compression rarely present in the emergency department, but patients complaining of spinal or radicular pain, acute weakness of the extremities, or difficulties with bladder or bowel control are likely to have acute spinal pathology, and one of the etiologies is tumor. When a child is seen with the complaints of either stopping walking, weakness of the lower extremities, bladder or bowel incontinence a very careful neurological examination is indicated. Frequently, the apparent indifference of the patient to the observed paralysis is taken to indicate hysteria. Hysterical paralysis is extremely uncommon in children and the clinical finding must not be dismissed on this basis. The physical examination should include palpation and percussion of the spine to seek areas of tenderness (suggestive of epidural abscess). The patient's neurological state at the time of therapy is the most important single factor in the prognosis for recovery. The better the neurological examination, the better the chances of recovery. Because of this, we encourage an early investigation of spinal cord dysfunction. In patients with known malignant disease, complaints of back and leg pain and weakness are indications for immediate myelography. Similarly, in any patient in whom there is a chance of compression of the spinal cord being responsible for the neurological picture, plain spine films, CBC and myelography should be performed as soon as possible and any compressive lesion treated by the most appropriate method. The rapidity of investigation will depend upon the patient's history and neurological status. A history of chronic back pain or radicular pain with the rapid progression of neurological deficit is an indication for immediate myelography. Compressive lesions of the spinal canal may rapidly become irreversible as neurological function disappears. Thus, a high index of suspicion of treatable pathology is required and, as noted above, when the history and physical exam suggest rapid progression, studies should be performed acutely.

In summary, the most frequent neurosurgical emergency is that of elevated ICP. This can occur with a variety of pathological lesions of the central nervous system. The ability to recognize and treat intracranial hypertension and cerebral herniation syndrome is crucial to the practicing emergency room physician. The majority of other acute neurosurgical conditions must be recognized and further decision on care made after consultation with the attending neurosurgeon.

References

Bruce DA: The pathophysiology of increased intracranial pressure. In *Current Concepts Scope Publications.* Upjohn Co., Kalamazoo, Mich., 1978.

Bruce, DA: Special considerations of the pediatric age group. In *Management of Head Injuries*, edited by PR Cooper. Williams & Wilkins, Baltimore (in press).

Bruce, DA: Current management of pediatric brain tumors. Current Concepts in Oncology (in press).

Bruce, DA, Berman WA, Schut L: Cerebrospinal fluid pressure monitoring in children; physiology, pathology and clinical usefulness. *Adv Pediatr* 24: 233–290, 1977.

Bruce DA, Gennarelli TA, Langfitt TW: Resuscitation from coma due to head injury. *Crit Care Med* 6: 254–269, 1978.

Bruce DA, Alavi A, Bilaniuk LT, Dolinskas C, Obrist WA, Zimmerman RA, Uzzell B: Diffuse cerebral swelling following head injuries in children; the syndrome of "malignant brain edema." *J Neurosurg* 54: 170–178, 1981.

Bruce DA, Sutton LN, Schut L: Acute brain swelling and cerebral edema in children. In *Brain Edema*, pp. 125–245, edited by M de Vlieger, SA de Lange, JWF Beks. John Wiley & Sons, New York, 1981.

Laurent JP, Bruce DA, Schut L: Hemorrhagic brain tumors in pediatric patients. *Childs Brain* 8: 263–270, 1981.

Raphaely R, Swedlow D, Downes J, Bruce DA: Management of severe pediatric head trauma. *Pediatr Clin North Am* 27: 715–727, 1980.

Schut L, Bruce DA: Recent advancements in the treatment of head injuries. *Pediatr Ann* 5: 80–104, 1976.

SECTION V Psychosocial Emergencies

CHAPTER 68

Child Abuse

STEPHEN LUDWIG, M.D.

Child abuse is a complex phenomenon resulting from a combination of individual, familial, and societal factors. The common denominator in all these factors is parental behavior destructive to the process of normal growth, development, and well being of the child. Abuse may be subdivided into four categories: (1) physical abuse, (2) sexual abuse, (3) neglect, and (4) emotional abuse. Each form of abuse has individual characteristics of family dynamics, clinical manifestations, and management.

The task of the emergency department physician is a difficult one. The physician must first maintain an open mind to the possibility that abuse occurs on a frequent basis. Thus, abuse should be included in the differential diagnosis of any injury or any unusual physical or psychological complaint. Second, the physician must identify signs of suspected abuse. Next, there must be skillful management of the family in a way that will protect the child while maintaining the parents' motivation for help. Finally, there needs to be a thorough understanding of the legal requirements for reporting abuse to the proper social service or police authority.

The demands of managing a case of child abuse may be lessened by sharing the responsibility with other health care professionals. The skills of nursing and social work staff are invaluable. The child abuse field has been a model for multidisciplinary collaboration. Such collaboration is most productive if begun in the emergency department. It is also helpful to establish an institutional or departmental protocol for the management of abuse cases. This relieves the emergency department physician from having to reconstruct a complete management plan for each new case. Having a standard protocol to follow allows the physician more time to concentrate on the individual needs of the patient and parents.

To the unfamiliar observer the easy solution to all abuse cases is to "take away the child and put the parents in jail." This commonly held treatment philosophy would be practiced more if it were truly a panacea. However, the alternative forms of child care (i.e., institutional care, foster care, adoption) are each fraught with their own hazard. With the use of well organized community services, abusive behavior can be controlled while the child and family receive therapy.

There may be support for the notion that parents bring their abused child to the emergency department motivated to seek help for their child and for themselves. It is a rare parent who feels no remorse about his or her abusive behavior. The severity of injuries inflicted is often overestimated as a result of this guilt. The emergency department physician must neither overlook or mismanage the opportunity. Sharp focus should be maintained on the twin goals of case management—protect the child and preserve family life.

PHYSICAL ABUSE

BACKGROUND

Physical abuse is the most often reported form of child abuse. Definitions of physical abuse vary from state to state. Operationally the definitions vary from institution to institution, and indeed from person to person. It is important to note that even the definition of physical abuse is a definition in transition. Over the past century there have been many advances in the "rights of the children." Enactment of child labor and compulsory education laws have been important steps forward. As the history of abuse is traced through the centuries, the forms and the definitions of abuse have changed. Definitions currently used are likely to continue to change with time. The present widespread medical interest on abuse was stimulated by C. Henry Kempe with the introduction of the term "battered child syndrome" in 1962. It was only as recently as 1968 that the last of the 50 states enacted child abuse legislation.

Standard to most definitions of physical abuse is the concept of injury that has occurred through nonaccidental means. The Pennsylvania law is typical of many and defines physical abuse as "injury primarily caused by an act or omission which: (1) significantly jeopardizes the child's safety, (2) significantly impairs the child's physical functioning temporarily or permanently, or (3) is accomplished by physical evidence in a continuous pattern of unexplained injuries." The National Center on Child Abuse has defined physical abuse as: "Child abuse which results in physical injury, including fractures, burns, bruises, welts, cuts and/or internal injuries. Physical abuse often occurs in the name of discipline or punishment, and ranges from a slap of the hand to use of objects...."

The true incidence of abuse is unknown. Many cases go unrecognized and unreported. Estimates for all forms of abuse vary from 500,000 to 4,000,000 cases per year in the United States. Physical abuse accounts for 60 to 65% of reported abuse. Several studies have estimated that 10% of children under 5 brought to the emergency department with traumatic injury are victims of child abuse. There may be as many as 2000 abuse-related deaths per year in the United States.

Although there is question as to the true incidence of abuse, there is no doubt about the escalating number of reports. Table 68.1 shows the number of reports during two 5-year periods in Pennsylvania, as well as the number of deaths for the same periods. Pennsylvania established a statewide reporting registry in 1975. Most authorities feel the increase in reports is due to an increase in awareness and ease of reporting, as well as to a rise in the true incidence of abuse.

DYNAMICS

Many factors contribute to the reasons a parent abuses a child. Helfer's formulation of the necessary elements are shown in Figure 68.1. The factors include a parent

Table 68.1
Physical Abuse and Deaths: Substantiated Cases in Pennsylvania

Year	No. of Cases	Deaths
1969	540	27
1970	695	33
1971	890	36
1972	1,007	28
1973	1,503	28
Total:	**4,635**	**152**
1976	2,664	20
1977	3,920	21
1978	3,652	38
1979	3,699	33
1980	3,187	30
Total:	**17,122**	**142**

who is capable of abuse, a child who actively or passively becomes the target, and a crisis which triggers the angry response. Green has added to this triad the concept that the process must exist in a society which condones or even encourages violence, and in particular violence against children.

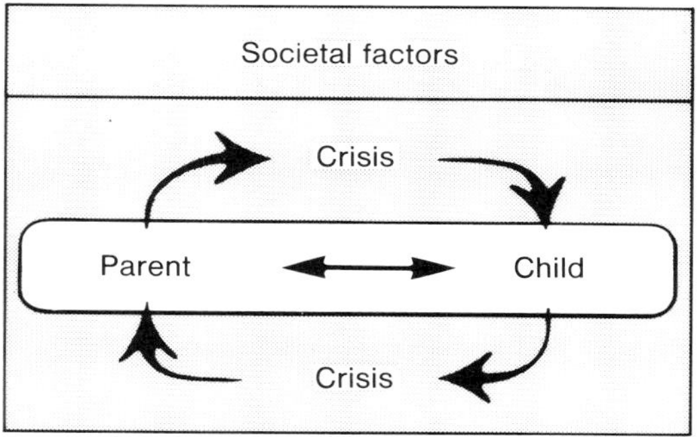

Figure 68.1. Essential elements of child abuse. (Adapted from R. E. Helfer: *Child Today, 4:* 28 1975.)

Some of the factors which contribute to the parents' abusive potential are listed in Figure 68.2. Stress and lack of specific child rearing information and experience play dominant roles. The combination of these factors causes many parents to misread normal childhood behavior as defiant or provocative and to react with a violent, destructive response. The typical example is the parent who is angered by the 1-year-old's refusal to become toilet trained. The child's contribution to abuse may be real, as in the case of negative behavior or disparate temperament, or imagined by the parent (e.g. "he's just like his father"). Children with prolonged neonatal hospitalization, handicapping conditions, or developmental delays are at increased risk. The

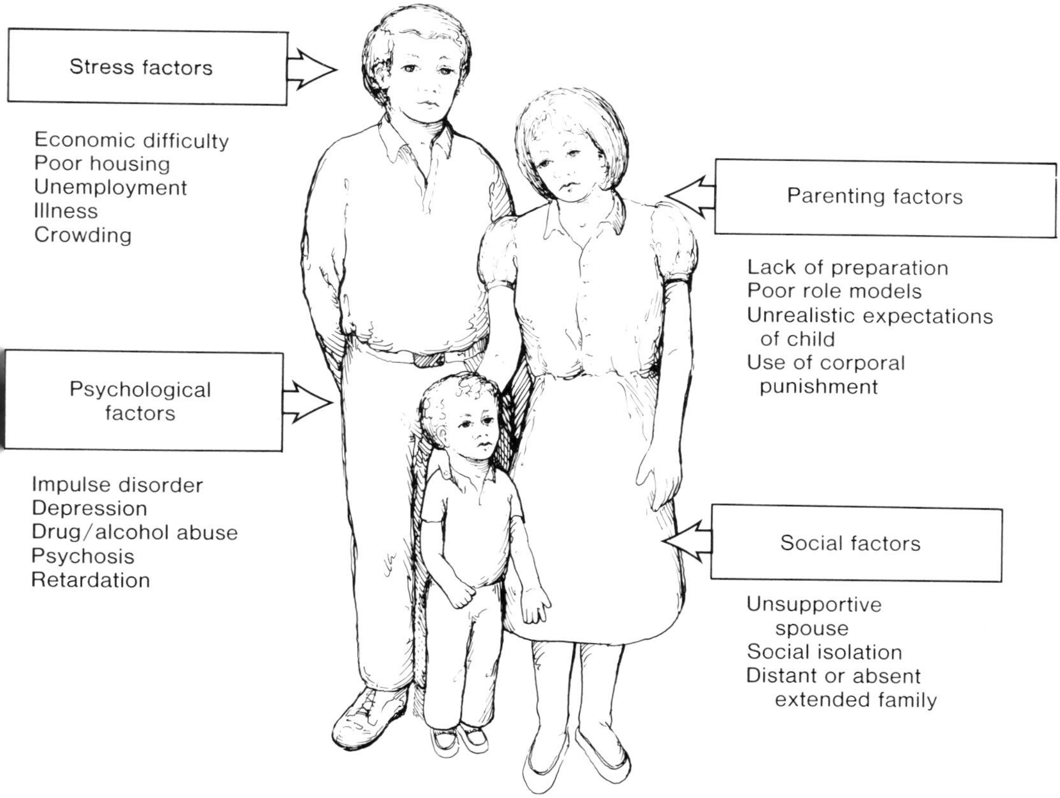

Figure 68.2 Risk factors which contribute to abuse and neglect.

crisis which initiates abuse varies tremendously. It may be unrelated to the child, such as the stress of a family member's death or economic disappointment. However, often it is because the child's behavior does not meet parental expectations. The crisis is identifiable as the spark that ignites the existing potential for abuse.

MANIFESTATIONS

The manifestations of physical abuse may affect any body system. Thus the emergency physician must be prepared to recognize a variety of signs and symptoms. Abuse may also be seen by any subspecialist physician. Injuries seen in abused children at the Children's Hospital of Philadelphia between 1976 and 1979 are shown in Figure 68.3.

Integument

The skin is the most commonly injured body organ. Cutaneous injuries may be divided into nonspecific and specific traumatic lesions, burns, and hair loss. Of the nonspecific traumatic injuries, the *bruise* or *contusion* is the most frequently seen. Although bruises are also frequent in nonabused children, they usually have a different distribution and appearance. Accidental injuries occur most commonly on the extremities and forehead. As bruising moves centrally and becomes extensive, the likelihood of abuse rises. Contusions undergo recognizable stages of healing. This process of resolution is shown in Figure 68.4. It is important to date the bruise and compare it to the history provided. A prothrombin time (PT), partial thromboplastin time (PTT), and platelet count should be obtained if the issue of "easy bruisability" has been offered as a possible explanation. Other nonspecific cutaneous injuries include lacerations, punctures, and abrasions. Important for the evaluation of any nonspecific injury is (1) the history of injury, (2) the age and developmental level of the child, (3) the presence of other old or new injuries, (4) the interaction between the parents and child, and (5) the interaction between the parents and the emergency department staff.

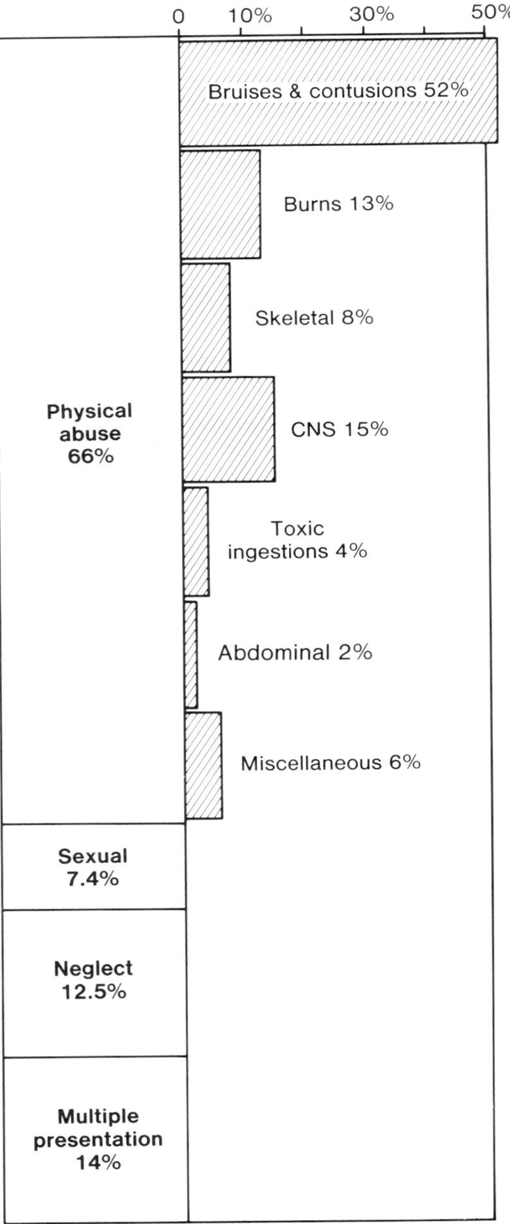

Figure 68.3. Types of child abuse injuries seen at Children's Hospital of Philadelphia 1976–1979. (Courtesy of Dr. M. Zeigler.)

Specific skin injuries are those that clearly reflect the method or object used to inflict the trauma. Loop-shaped marks are readily visualized following a beating with an electric cord or wire. Linear marks may be seen from a belt or paddle injury. Rope

Color	Age
Red Reddish-blue	Not more than 24 hr
Dark purple Dark blue	1–4 days
Greenish Yellow-Green	5–7 days
Yellowish Brown	7–10 days
Normal tint Disappearance	1–3 weeks

Figure 68.4. Estimation of the age of a cutaneous bruise. (Adapted from E. F. Wilson: *Pediatrics, 60:* 103, 1977.)

burns result in circumferential marks on the wrists, ankles, or around the neck when a child has been bound. Another common specific integument lesion is a hand print on the side of the face or on the upper arms. Human bites appear as circular lesions 1½ to 2 inches in diameter. Forensic dentistry is able to match the skin lesion with the dentition of the alleged perpetrator. Some specific skin lesions are shown in Figure 68.5.

Burns of the skin may be caused by abuse or neglect. Burns account for 5% of the cases of physical abuse. In particular, tap water scald burns which occur in an immersion pattern (Fig. 68.6) often have nonaccidental trauma as their etiology. Immersion burns are likely to be inflicted by an abusive parent when they occur on a child who is being toilet trained. Other indications of abuse are: (a) a delay in seeking treatment, (2) a history of the child being unsupervised, and (3) the child being brought to the hospital by the parent who was not present at the time the burn occurred. In attempting to match the physical findings of the burn with the available history, several factors must be appreciated. The extent of the burn depends on the temperature of the water, duration of exposure, thickness of the skin involved, and presence or absence of clothing. Water temperature 130°F (54°C) or greater will cause a full thickness burn with only a 30-sec exposure. Because palms and soles are thick they will frequently be spared. Clothing tends to keep the hot water in contact with the skin and causes more severe burns. Burns presumably caused by falling or thrown fluids should produce droplet or splash pattern. When the child evidences several small bullous lesions, the main differential diagnosis is a second degree burn versus bullous impetigo. This differentiation is easily made by Gram stain and culture of a bulla.

Other burns may occur through contact with a hot solid rather than a hot fluid. Cigarette burns are the most common of this type. If the history given is of a child brushing against a cigarette or of hot ashes falling on the child, the resulting injury should be a nonspecific first or second degree burn. When a cigarette is extinguished on the child's skin, the injury is a burn which is 8 to 10 mm in diameter and indurated at its margin. A healed cigarette burn is indistinguishable from any other circular skin lesion such as impetigo, ichthyma, or vesicles. Burns from radiators, hot plates, curling irons, or standard irons will imprint the shape of the hot object.

The final category of integumental injury is *injury to the hair.* Traction alopecia is seen when a parent pulls the child by the hair. Usually the scalp is clear, differentiating this lesion from tinea capitis, seborrhea, and scalp eczema. Alopecia areata produces a lesion in which the hair is uniformily absent. In the cases of traction or traumatic alopecia, patches of broken hair remain.

Skeletal

The skeletal system is also commonly traumatized when children are physically abused. As previously mentioned, it is important to match the history of injury with the physical findings. It is also important to consider the mobility and strength of the child in order to identify suspicious injuries.

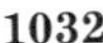

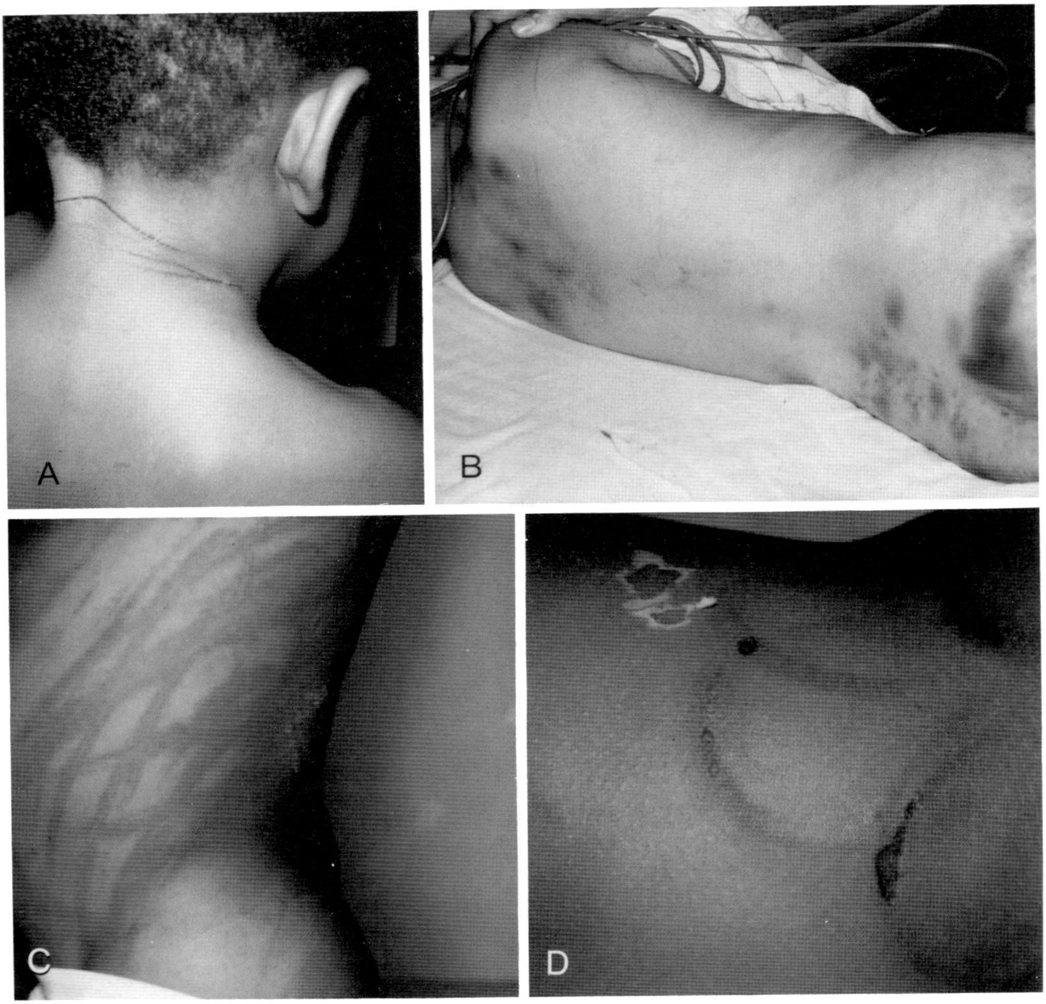

Figure 68.5 Cutaneous manifestations of child abuse. (*A*) Strangulation mark, (*B*) bruises at various stages of healing, (*C*) linear loop-shaped marks, and (*D*) multiple loop-shaped marks.

The radiologist needs to review the patient's past x-rays in order to identify the child with multiple visits to the hospital for fractures. When suspicion of abuse is high, a radiographic skeletal survey should be obtained to ascertain condition of the entire skeletal system. Some of the indications for a radiographic skeletal survey are listed in the management section of this chapter. We have often performed a skeletal survey on a young child with an obvious fracture only to find multiple old fractures. The skeletal survey provides information on the type, location, and age of fractures as well as presence or absence of some bone diseases.

Bone injuries may be of several types including: simple transverse fractures, impacted fractures, spiral fractures, metaphyseal fractures, or subperiosteal hematoma. Radiographs of some of these injuries are shown in Figure 68.7. To explain a transverse fracture, the history should be that of a direct force applied to the bone. It is often difficult to differentiate the true etiology of this type of fracture. The impacted fracture

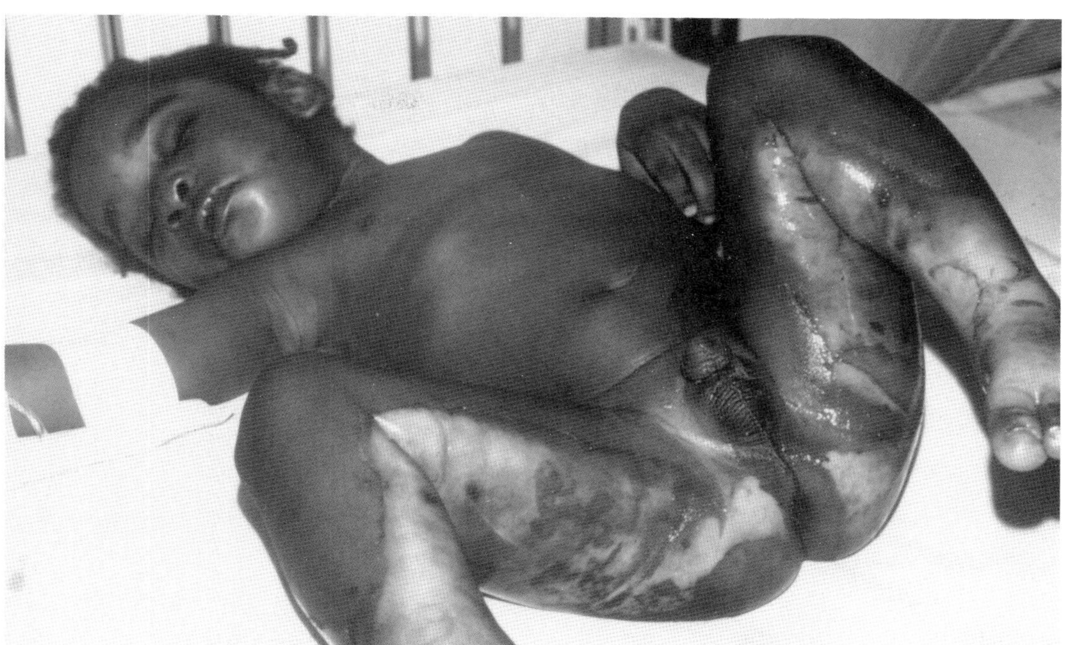

Figure 68.6 Hot water burn in an immersion pattern.

should have an accompanying history of force along the long axis of the bone, such as the child falling on his/her outstretched hand. In the case of a spiral fracture, there should be a history of twisting or torque during the traumatic event. Metaphyseal chip fractures occur when the extremity is pulled or yanked; because the periosteum, which is most tightly adherent at the metaphysis, causes small bone fragments to avulse. Metaphyseal chip fractures are almost exclusively caused by abuse.

Subperiosteal hematomas produce a characteristic radiograph. The elevation of the periosteum is visualized as a linear opacification running parallel to the bone surface. Subperiosteal hematomas are produced by direct trauma to the bone. A caution is that in up to 10% of small and premature infants, there may be symmetrical periosteal elevation along the tibia or humerus which is not caused by abuse. The reason for this finding is unknown, but it should not be confused with abuse.

The location of the fracture is important in the identification of abuse. The fracture of a clavicle or the dislocation of a radial head are common accidental injuries. However, when the femur of a young child is fractured, or when ribs are fractured, the suspicion of abuse increases. Ribs which are fractured along the axillary line are broken by an anterior-posterior force. Ribs which are fractured anteriorly or posteriorly are injured by a side-to-side compression of the thorax. The history of injury must be matched to the physical finding. Other uncommon and, therefore, suspicious fractures are located in the vertebrae, sternum, pelvis, or scapulae. Uncommon fractures need to be carefully evaluated unless there is a clear history of significant trauma, such as an automobile accident.

The age of a fracture may be estimated from the amount of callous formation and bone remodeling seen on the radiograph. Dating of fractures is not an exact science, as there are many confounding variables such as the child's age, location of the fracture, and nutritional status. Nonetheless, the child who presents with an acute fracture, and has a second fracture with a callus, stands out as one who has sustained more than one episode of trauma. The usual

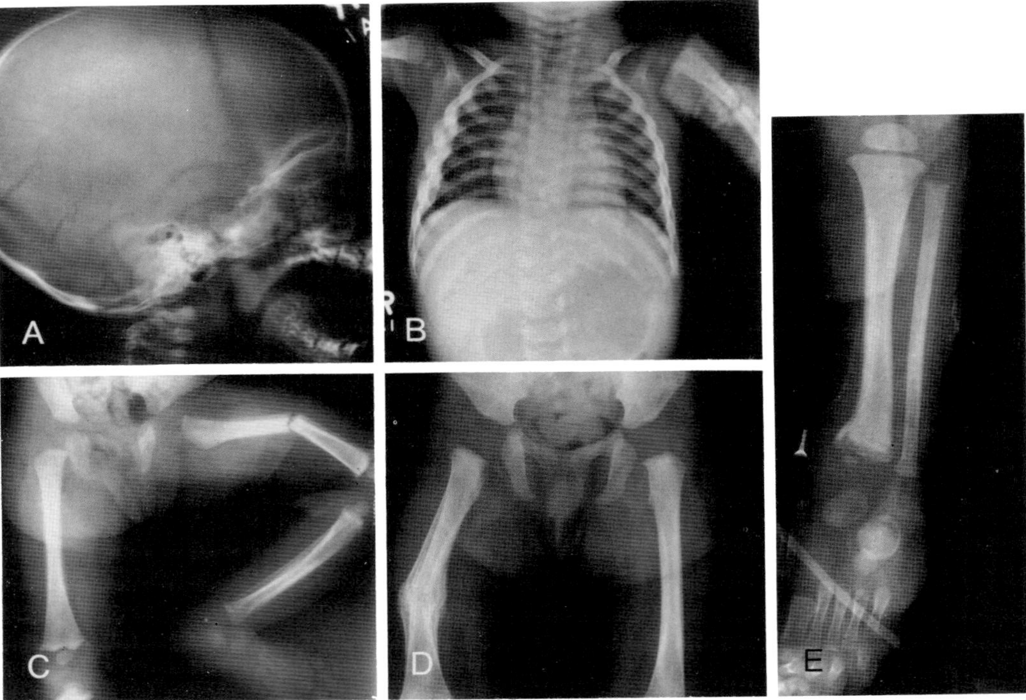

Figure 68.7 Radiographic findings of child abuse. (*A*) Multiple skull fractures in an infant; (*B*) left humerus fracture and multiple old healing rib fractures; (*C*) left femur fracture and metaphyseal chip avulsion fractures of the right distal femur; (*D*) healing fracture of the right femur with callus formation, and periosteal new bone formation; and (*E*) "bucket-handle" deformity of healing distal tibial epiphyseal fracture.

long bone fracture may take 7 to 10 days to form callus and several months for complete healing. In the acute stages of injury, soft tissue swelling should be seen for 2 to 3 days. It is impossible to date skull fractures in the same way.

Whenever a young child sustains multiple fractures, the differential diagnosis must be widened beyond accidental trauma and abuse to include osteogenesis imperfecta, infantile cortical hyperostosis, scurvy, syphilis, osteoid osteoma, neoplasms, rickets, hypophosphatasia, and osteomyelitis. All of these conditions are much less common than abuse and can be ruled out by the appearance of the bone on the radiograph, and by the levels of calcium, phosphorus, and alkaline phosphatase in the serum.

Central Nervous System

Injuries to the central nervous system are the main cause of child abuse deaths. These injuries may be subdivided into two categories: (1) direct trauma and (2) shaking injuries.

Direct trauma is inflicted by striking the child with an object or by dropping or throwing the child against a wall or onto the floor. The extent of the resulting trauma depends on the amount of force used, the surface contacted, and the age of the child. The child may be brought to the emergency department with a small subgaleal hematoma or in coma. Injuries may vary from scalp contusions to intracerebral hematomas.

One will frequently obtain a history of a young infant falling off a bed or dressing table. The precise extent of injury from this type of fall is unknown, but several reports suggest that even uncomplicated skull fracture are as uncommon as 1 to 2% of cases. If the injury is more severe and the only history is of a fall from bed, suspect abuse.

Another scenario is that of a child who

sustained trauma 1 week prior to the emergency department visit. The visit is prompted by the parent noticing a soft spot on the child's cranium. This sequence may occur when the initial scalp hematoma so rapidly expanded that it had a bony consistency. It is only with degradation and softening that the parent now perceives the hematoma. Although a delay in seeking treatment is a well recognized red flag for child abuse injuries, this case provides a plausible explanation.

In all children younger than 1 year of age, who have a history of head trauma, skull x-rays are recommended. Infants are most vulnerable to serious sequelae. If a fracture does exist and there is reason to suspect abuse, a skeletal survey should be obtained also. For the diagnostic methods to be used for more serious head injuries, the reader is referred to Chapter 67, "Neurosurgical Emergencies."

Shaking injuries characteristically cause serious central nervous system damage without evidence of external trauma. The infant's relatively large head size and weak neck muscles are predisposing factors for whiplash injury. The shearing and contusive forces that result from shaking the infant produce this type of injury. Specific lesions that occur include hematomas, subarachnoid hemorrhages, or brain contusions, particularly in the occipital lobe. The child may present with lethargy and a "septic" appearance, with seizures, or in a coma. The physical examination is otherwise unremarkable except for retinal hemorrhages (Fig. 68.8*A*). Occasionally bruises on the upper arms or shoulders point to the sites where the child has been grasped. Lumbar puncture produces grossly bloody or xanthochromic spinal fluid. If computerized axial tomography is available, it will show the characteristic findings of occipital contusion and intrahemispheric blood (Fig. 68.8*B*). This form of abusive behavior by the parent is usually triggered by the infant's persistent crying. Occasionally, excessively rough forms of play may result in shaking injuries.

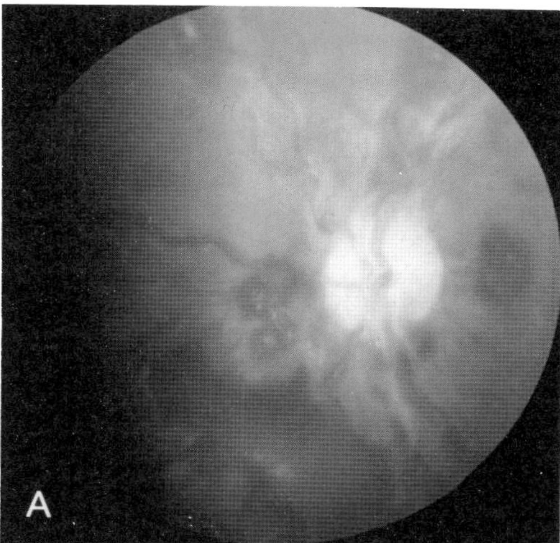

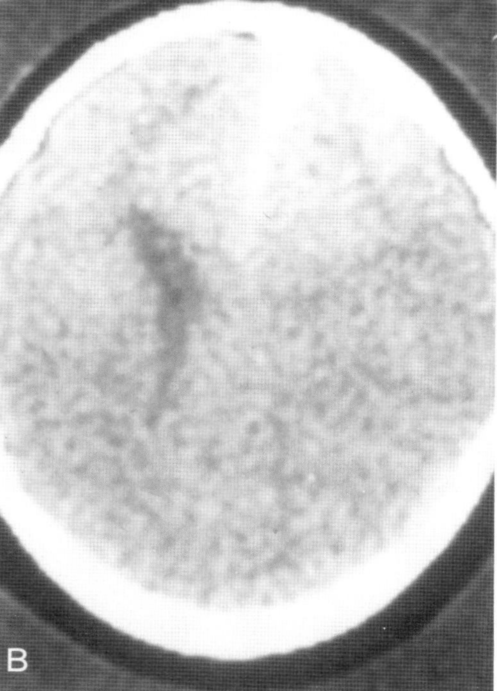

Figure 68.8. Manifestations of the whiplash shaking injury. (*A*) Retinal hemorrhages as seen on fundoscopic examination and (*B*) computed tomogram showing intrahemispheric subdural bleeding and right cortical brain swelling.

Gastrointestinal System

Gastrointestinal injuries are relatively uncommon abuse manifestations. Of all the gastrointestinal injuries, mouth trauma is perhaps the most common. Small infants may sustain a tear of the frenulum resulting from "bottle jamming." In the older child, dental trauma may be a sign of abuse.

Other gastrointestinal system manifestations are more medically serious and generally result from blunt trauma to the abdominal contents. This form of abuse ranks second to head trauma in accounting for abuse related deaths. Rupture of the spleen and laceration of the liver cause the child to present with an acute abdomen or in shock, with no external source of bleeding. The identification and management of these emergencies is covered in the surgical section. A less dramatic presentation is the afebrile child with persistent bilious vomiting from a duodenal hematoma with small bowel obstruction. The etiology is blunt abdominal trauma. Documenting an elevated serum amylase is important in providing tangible evidence of abdominal trauma in cases that lack any radiographic finding or abdominal wall bruising. Elevation of the serum amylase may also identify those cases which should be followed for possible development of a pancreatic pseudocyst.

Cardiopulmonary System

Abuse may be manifested in cardiac or pulmonary trauma. There are no injuries which are characteristically abuse induced. Pulmonary contusion, pneumothorax, hemothorax, cardiac tamponade, and myocardial contusion may all occur occasionally. Specifics of identification and management of these problems are covered in Chapter 60, "Thoracic Emergencies."

Genitourinary Systems

Common genitourinary complaints such as hematuria, dysuria, urgency, frequency, and enuresis may be the presenting sign of abuse. These problems may result from direct trauma, sexually transmitted infections, or emotional abuse. Some aspects of genitourinary manifestation are covered subsequently under "Sexual Abuse." As for direct trauma, any part of the genitourinary system may be involved, from the renal parenchyma to the urethral meatus. Penile trauma which does not have an adequate explanation may be an alerting sign of abuse. Traumatic hematuria is managed as described in Chapter 57, "Major Trauma."

A life-threatening renal manifestation may be the occurrence of rhabdomyolysis and myoglobinuria. With extensive deep soft tissue and muscle trauma, myoglobin may be liberated in quantities sufficient to cause acute renal failure. Such children present with dark or tea-colored urine that tests positive for blood with urine dipstick but has no visible red blood cells on microscopic examination. Serum myoglobin levels confirm the diagnosis, and the serum CPK reaches extremely high values. Prior to using hypertonic intravenous contrast materials in the child with Hematest positive urine, myoglobinuria should be considered and ruled out. The patient with possible myoglobinuria and acute renal failure must not be given potassium-containing intravenous solutions.

Sensory

All of the sensory organs are vulnerable to physical abuse. Included are ocular, nasal and otic injuries. The eye may sustain a number of different forms of injury including periorbital ecchymosis, corneal abrasion, subconjunctival hemorrhage, hyphema, dislocated lens, retinal hemorrhages, or detached retina. Each of these lesions is discussed in Chapter 61, "Ophthalmic Emergencies." A careful history of injury is important when treating any of these conditions.

Injury to the nose may result in simple hemorrhage or fracture and disfigurement of the nasal structures. The external ear may show evidence of contusion. In particular, ecchymosis on the internal surface of the pinna may result from "boxing" the ear and crushing it against the skull. A direct blow to the ear may also cause hemotympanum and perforation of the tympanic membrane. In such cases it is important to also consider hemotympanum on the basis of basilar skull fracture. The presence of discoloration behind the ear (Battle's sign) may be a further indication of a basilar skull fracture. Again the reader is referred to Chapter 67 specifically dealing with these aspects of emergency care.

Unusual Manifestation

Rarely the emergency physician will be confronted by one of the unusual abuse manifestations. Cases of toxic and nontoxic ingestions, electrolytic disorders such as hyponatremia and hypernatremia, foreign bodies, and multiple serious infections may be the result of abuse. In all these situations, the parent actively abuses the child by feeding, instilling, or injecting harmful substances or objects to the child's body. We have cared for children with a toxic ingestion who have revealed that their parent forced them to ingest the substance. The most common toxic ingestants of this type are alcoholic beverages that are given or forced upon the child in order to either quiet the child or to demonstrate "manly" qualities.

Other drugs may be used to poison the child. There have been several case reports of parents who have placed their children on high salt or water-only diets as a form of punishment. Such children may present with signs of hypernatremia or hyponatremia, possibly with seizures. Foreign bodies have been found in every orifice, as well as under the skin and in fingernail beds.

There have been several cases of Munchausen syndrome in which a parent has inflicted illness upon their child rather than feigning or inducing illness themselves. Cases of ficticious fever, hematuria, and even sepsis have resulted from this form of abuse. Although rare, the unusual manifestations of abuse should be considered when more common causes of these problems cannot be identified.

MANAGEMENT

The management of a child abuse case is difficult unless the emergency physician has a previously prepared, well structured protocol. If reports of abuse are not a daily occurrence, it is important to have an institutional policy that serves as a guide to the mechanics of management. Consultants from different disciplines such as nursing and social work provide invaluable assistance. Multidisciplinary approach simplifies the initial decision making and subsequent case management. The steps in the protocol are shown in Figure 68.9.

Suspect Abuse

The first step is to decide if there is a reasonable likelihood of abuse. There are many shades of suspicion, thus making the term imprecise. Although every traumatic injury should be suspected as abuse, the physician has the onerous task of deciding how much suspicion is necessary in order to take some action (i.e. report). In order to establish the level of suspicion, data are gathered by obtaining a complete history, performing a thorough physical examination, comparing the history and physical examination, observing interactions, and obtaining laboratory studies and/or radiographs. Then, the physician can formulate a differential diagnosis and assign a rank to abuse. Indications of abuse in the history and physical examination and observational data must be used like building blocks that are added until they achieve a certain threshold of suspicion. When the threshold is reached, a report of suspected abuse must follow.

A detailed *history* is always important. As in many other medical situations, this is initiated by asking some general open-ended questions as to "what happened?" If the child has sufficient verbal skills, the first questions are directed at him/her. General inquiries must then be followed with specific requests for information; however, a harsh interrogation will only alienate the family. Some specific historical indications are listed in Table 68.2.

As with the history, the *physical examination* must be thorough. The signs of physical abuse have been detailed in the section on clinical manifestations. A thorough examination serves as a means to uncover these findings. Although there is a great temptation to merely glance at a small contusion on a child's face, such a cursory examination will fail to reveal possible linear and loop-shaped marks on the upper thighs and buttocks. Table 68.3 lists some of the important physical examination features that are indicators of abuse.

After completion of the history and physical examination, the next step is to *compare* the two. Does the stated history match the physical findings? Does the history make sense? Does the history correlate with the developmental level of the child? Answers to these important questions may add further elements of suspicion. This step of comparing history and physical examination is done in a subconscious way by

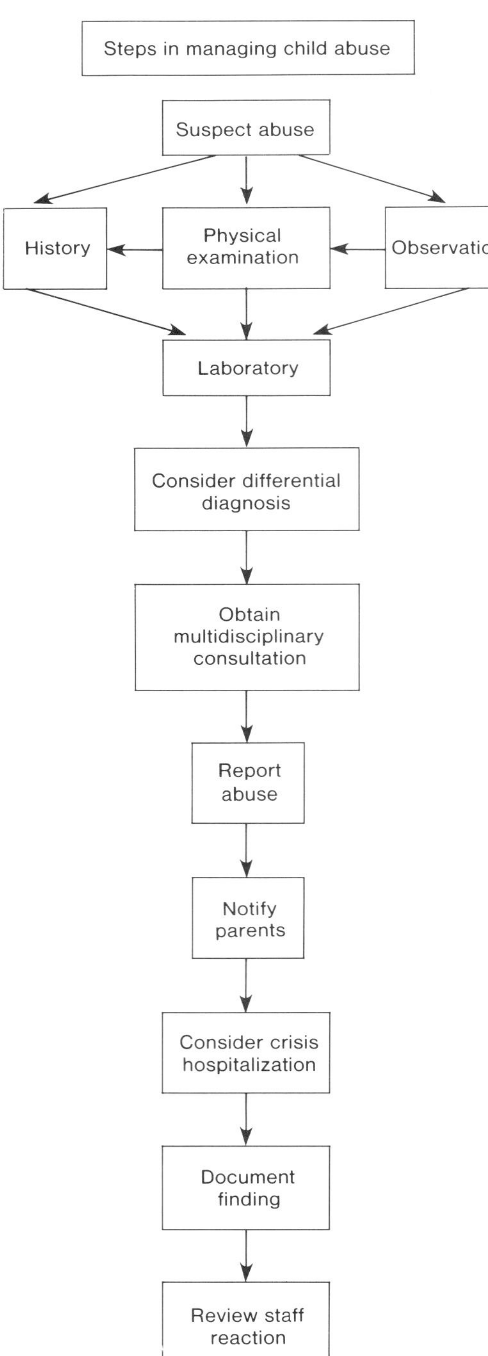

Figure 68.9. Procedure for emergency department management of suspected physical abuse.

Table 68.2
Historical Indicators of Abuse

1. Is the history one of inflicted injury?
2. Is there an absence of history, a "magical" injury?
3. Could the injury have been avoided by better care and supervision?
4. Are there inconsistencies or changes in the history?
5. Is there a history of repeated injury or hospitalization?
6. Was there a delay in seeking medical care?
7. Does the history overestimate or underestimate the injury?
8. Is there a past medical history of prematurity, failure to thrive, failure to receive adequate medical care such as immunization?

Table 68.3
Physical Indicators of Abuse

1. Does injury match the history of injury?
2. Are there pathognomonic injuries such as looped wire marks, cigarette burns, etc.?
3. Are there multiple injuries?
4. Are the injuries at various stages of healing?
5. Are there different injury forms, for example, burns and fractures?
6. Is there evidence of overall poor care?
7. Has poisoning been documented in a young child?
8. Is there evidence of failure to thrive without a history of symptoms or physical findings?
9. Are there any visual or unexplained physical findings?

most practitioners. Physicians often attempt to match the patients' degree of symptoms with the presence or absence of physical findings, particularly in patients with psychosomatic complaints. In child abuse cases, it should be a conscious, well defined step, as it is vital to establishing suspicion. In some cases, a lack of consistency is obvious, such as the parent who claims that burns on her child's buttocks occurred when he inserted his finger in an electric socket. Other situations may be less clear such as the injury being attributed to hot plastic seat covers on an automobile. Although the latter explanation has in fact been reported as a case of accidental injury, it rarely explains burns on the buttocks.

Laboratory data and radiographs are another source of indicators of abuse. The laboratory studies employed are few and, for the most part, document the obvious or rule out other disease states. Biochemical, hematologic, and urinary studies that are used appear in Table 68.4 along with their indications. Radiographs document a specific bony or soft tissue injury. They may provide a comprehensive and longitudinal record of osseous injury at any site in the skeletal system. Although there are no precise indications for ordering a skeletal survey, some relative indications are: (1) any child less than 1 year old presenting with a fracture, (2) any child with severe or extensive fractures, (3) any child who has a history of more than one fracture, and (4) a history in the child or the family of "soft" or easily broken bones.

During the period of time occupied by the history, physical examination, and performance of laboratory studies, the physicians should be cognizant of the *interactions* among family members and between the parents, the child, and the emergency department staff. Such an awareness often uncovers subtle indicators of abuse. The observation of parents arguing vehemently on the way to the radiology department may be a clue. The parent who appears to be distant from both the child and the physician is also suspect. While the parent who is intoxicated or incoherent never fails

Table 68.4
Laboratory and Radiographic Indicators of Abuse

Studies	Indication
Hematologic	
Prothrombin time (PT)	Bleeding disorders
Partial thromboplastin time (PTT)	Bleeding disorders
Platelet count	Bleeding disorders
Complete blood count (CBC) including red cell indicies	Blood loss, nutritional anemia
Biochemical	
Blood urea nitrogen (BUN)	Dehydration
Creatine phosphokinase (CPK)	Muscle injury
Amylase	Abdominal trauma
Electrolytes, osmolality: calcium/phosphorus/alkaline phosphatase	Dehydration, water intoxication
Toxicology screen	Poisoning
Urine	
Specific gravity	Dehydration
Blood	Renal or genital trauma
Ferric chloride	Poisoning
Radiographic	
Skeletal survey for trauma	Periosteal elevation
Bone Scan	Subperiosteal hemorrhage
	Metaphyseal chip fractures
	Epiphyseal separation
	Spiral fractures in nonambulatory patients
	Fractures in various stages of healing
	Rib fractures
	Unusual fractures
Upper gastrointestinal series	Duodenal hematoma
Computerized tomography scan	Head trauma, shaking injury

to gain staff attention, such individuals are in the minority of abusive parents. Observation of the child is important as well. All abused children are not withdrawn, passive, and depressed. On the contrary some will be quite competent, outgoing, or "pseudomature." The observed state of the child will depend on several factors: the length, frequency, and severity of abuse; the developmental level and age of the child; and the amount of positive interaction the child's parents and extended family have had between abusive episodes. Frequently, physicians are surprised that the child does not immediately vocalize the nature and extent of the abuse and ask for asylum. Such statements by children are actually rare and occur mainly in the adolescent patients. Children are loyal to their parents. Abusive parents may be only episodically abusive and at other times nurturant and loving. Young children may have no framework for comparison and may accept the abuse as the norm. Somewhat older children may understand and dislike the abuse but may fear the consequence of reporting it even more. In the child's mind, it may be better to live with the pain of abuse than to face the unknown of institutional or foster placement.

The final step in establishing a threshhold level of suspicion is to review the differential diagnosis. At this point in the management scheme, the physician must add up the indicators and arrive at a judgment. If the process does not lead to a clear determination, most state laws imply that it is more prudent to report than not to. Remember that physicians are asked to report *suspected*, not proven, abuse. The major differentiation is between accidental and nonaccidental trauma. The other elements of the differential diagnosis are all uncommon diseases including: (1) bone diseases such as osteogenesis imperfecta, osteoid osteoma; (2) hematologic disorders such as idiopathic thrombocytopenic purpura and hemophilia; (3) neoplasms; (4) metabolic disorders such as rickets or scurvy; (5) infections such as syphilis or osteomyelitis; and (6) syndromes in which there is an absence of pain sensation such as spina bifida or congenital indifference to pain. All occur with much less frequency than abuse but deserve consideration; simple laboratory and radiographic studies will confirm or deny these diagnoses.

A special note should be made of the child less than 6 months old who is brought to the hospital dead. In this situation the central differential diagnosis exists between sudden infant death syndrome (SIDS) and child abuse. Victims of SIDS may appear to have bruising as a postmortem change. Clearly, their parents have no adequate explanation for the death. In this situation the presumption should always be SIDS. Most localities will require an autopsy to be performed. If not required, the physician should insist on a postmortem examination and wait for the autopsy to ultimately make the differentiation. Interrogating parents in cases of SIDS about the possibility of abuse can produce untoward psychological harm. With the death of a child, supportive emergency department treatment becomes paramount and suspicions of abuse can be pursued by the medical examiner and law enforcement personnel.

Multidisciplinary Consultation

If consultation with a nurse, social worker, or physician with more extensive experience in the management of child abuse is available, it should be obtained. The advantages of consultations are many. They allow for (1) information sharing, (2) joint decision making, (3) planning, and (4) mutual support. Planning an approach to the family and subsequent case management is very useful. This brief consultation will enable the physician to feel more secure in making decisions about matters which are generally unfamiliar and often value laden. Joint interviewing is not only time efficient but gives the family a uniform approach from the professional staff.

Reporting

Once the suspicion of abuse has been established and consultations obtained, the next step is reporting. Although laws vary from state to state, most have common elements. The emergency physician should become familiar with his/her current state law. The definition of abuse is central to each of the reporting laws. A stated age will define a child. The laws will also specify who *must* report (mandated reporters),m and who *may* report (nonmandated reporters). For most mandated reports there is both a penalty (beyond malpractice) for failure to report and protection from liability if the report of suspected abuse turns out to be unfounded once investigated. Finally, the law will dictate to whom and how the report should be made. Generally, reports are made to Child Protective Services Agencies, to police departments, or to some combination of law enforcement and social work personnel. Many states now have statewide central registries for receiving reports.

Notifying the Parents

An important, but often avoided, step in case management is notification of the parents. It is often forgotten, because it is a difficult interpersonal task. Nonetheless, it must be done. Nothing will make parents more resistant to change than completing a "routine" emergency department visit, only to later receive notification that the physician has filed a suspected child abuse report. There are some specific guidelines that will be helpful in avoiding this breech of trust. The overall approach to the parents must be based on *concern for the child.* Stress concern for the child, not accusation. Do not confront the parent or attempt to seek an admission of guilt. Many times the parent in the emergency department may not be the abusive parent and may know as little about the episode as the hospital staff. Explain your requirement as a mandated reporter to report all *suspected* cases. However, stating the requirement should not be used as a replacement for your desire to report. In many states, the reporter is required to report all injuries that are not fully explained. This requirement may also be stated to the parent. It is important to use the words "child abuse report." this is not a time to "soft pedal." However, child abuse does represent a range of behaviors, from the parent who overvigorously disciplines to the parent who sadistically tortures. Often parents have not seen themselves as abusers, and an explanation of the range of abuse is helpful in demonstrating how your report applies to them. Parents are fearful of what a child abuse report means and of what will happen. Therefore, it is worthwhile explaining what will be the consequences of your report (e.g. "a social worker will call and come to visit you in 1 or 2 days").

The physician's natural fear is that the parent will have a dramatic and hostile reaction. The emergency physician can expect a wide variety of reactions from hostility to virtual thanks. In order to minimize the angry reactions, the physician should stress the focus as being concern for the child. This is a perspective which will put the physician on common ground with the parent. An angry reaction will be more likely if guilt or fear is increased. This may be visualized as a feedback relationship. Stoking the fire by increasing the parents' guilt or fear will result in a flare of angry emotion directed at the staff, the child, or the other spouse. Figure 68.10 shows this relationship.

Although there does not need to be any formal notification of the child, often the child may be aware of what is happening and may even ask some pointed questions. The physician may wish to discuss the report with the child. The physician should stress the outcomes of protection and help for the child and family. The emergency department staff should never be accusatory or belittling of the parent.

Crisis Hospitalization

In some cases of abuse, the family crisis will be at such an acute level that hospitalization is necessary. The physician must ask, "Is the home safe?" If there is any question that the child's environment poses

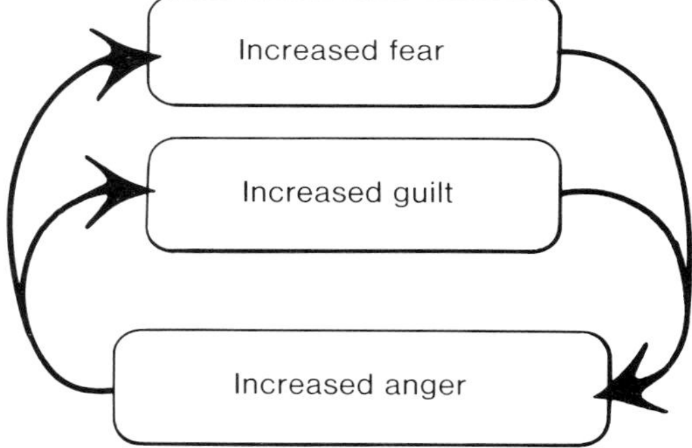

Figure 68.10. The cycle of fear, guilt and anger.

a danger, then the child should be admitted no matter what the extent of his/her injury. Some state laws have included protective custody sections that allow physicians virtual police powers in detaining a child for protection. In other states the physician may need to obtain parental consent for admission. This is yet another difficult task. As with reporting, the approach to the parents must be honest and nonaccusatory. The reasons for admission are to observe the child and allow for time to evaluate the possibility of such an injury happening again. The focus must be the physician's concern for the child's health. In hospitalizing the child, the physician also makes a statement about the seriousness of the situation and the depth of his/her concern. Most hospitals will not have the resources to hospitalize every abused child, nor is it necessary or advisable to do so in every case. Factors which favor sending the child home are (1) a concerned relative or neighbor available to support the family, (2) a solution to the inciting crisis, (3) parental acceptance of responsibility, (4) prompt (less than 24 hours) CPS or police response, (5) a first episode or minor degree of abuse, and (6) an alternative environment (e.g. grandmother's house). If the physician is unable to hospitalize the child and there are lingering doubts, a specific agreed upon return appointment for the next day may be a solution. If the family is unable to organize sufficiently to keep the appointment, then there is grave concern, and emergency CPS or police involvement should be requested.

Documentation

Throughout each step of case management, documentation is important. The record of this visit is both a medical and a legal document. A precise description of the injuries enhances its value, and small sketches are also helpful. Photographs are invaluable in documenting extensive injuries. While some states require parental permission for photographs, other jurisdictions allow photographs to be taken without parental consent. Photographs may be used in court to illustrate, for a judge or jury, injuries which would be difficult for most witnesses to describe. Even if the photographs are not admissable in court, they serve to refresh the memory of the physician for testimony. Often court proceedings may not take place for several months after the emergency department visit.

Written descriptions of an injury are adequate for less extensive trauma. Include as much detail as possible. The record of the history should be as factual as possible. Conclusions or impressions should not be listed. For example, rather than recording "the child looked fearful," it is better to describe the physicial components or behaviors that prompted that judgment under standard court room procedure. Include direct quotes from the child or parents. Quotes from another person are generally considered hearsay and are disallowed. When such quotes are included in the text of a business (medical) record they become more acceptable. General legibility and, in particular, a clearly written signature are always important record requirements. At the time of the emergency department visit, detailed record keeping seems to be a burden and waste of time. When a case record requires review prior to court testimony, good documentation is a necessity.

Staff Reactions

Child abuse triggers many emotions in the physician and in all the emergency department staff. There is obviously sadness and pity for the child and, frequently, anger for the parent. There may be a general feeling of disbelief, "How can this happen?" The case management plan described above requires that each emergency department staff be professional in their control of these emotions. The offhand comment of a clerk or the whispering between nurses can undermine the work being done with the family. If a staff member is too upset by abuse, he/she should be relieved of the responsibility of working in such situations. There is no place for the physician or nurse who openly attacks the family or who is blatantly accusatory. Only after having experience with large numbers of cases is there the appreciation of abuse as a very negative, but a very understandable, human response. With such perspective, the physician can become less angry and more zealous in attempting to provide constructive case management.

If problems of staff reaction exist, as they often will, there are several corrective actions to be taken. At times, a brief meeting of the involved staff can be called after the family has been discharged from the department. This allows the staff an immediate opportunity to ventilate their feelings. In-service education serves the same purpose, providing forum for staff to discuss their personal feelings about abuse as well as their past case experiences. Emergency department staff are always involved in the negative aspects of identifying and reporting abuse and never see the long-term treatment and rehabilitation phase. If a therapist, or better yet, a family, can present this side of abuse to the staff, it engenders more positive attitudes. Staff will frequently displace this anger to the "incompetence" of Child Protective Services Agency or "leniency" of a family court judge. It is important to put such scapegoating into the proper perspective. Again, in-service education and case reviews are useful. The integrity of the entire treatment team, both in hospital and the community, must be maintained in order to accomplish the difficult goals of protecting the child and preserving family life.

SEXUAL ABUSE

The sexually abused child is another difficult psychosocial emergency for the emergency physician. The state-of-the-art in identifying and managing cases of sexual abuse is far less developed than that for physical abuse. Most child abuse centers are reporting increasing numbers of sexually abused children. Perhaps from this increase in reported cases will be produced new information and understanding. Of all our societal taboos, those which prohibit incest are the strongest. This leads to denial and makes even basic recognition of the problem more difficult. As with the physically abused, the sexually abused child engenders a great deal of emotion from the health care professionals in the emergency department. Treatment issues for both the child and the perpetrator are more complex. Working in a multidisciplinary fashion with nursing and social work staff is important. It is clear that the effects of this form of abuse may be profound but may not be expressed as symptoms for many years. Prompt diagnosis, humane emergency management, and referral to long-term treatment resources are the goals of the emergency physician.

BACKGROUND

The term "sexual abuse" congers up images of a violent, forced, sexual attack of children. Although public media present the problem as the psychopathic criminal luring children on their way home from school by offering them candy, such stereotypes are the exception. This has prompted Sgroi and others to suggest the term "sexual abuse" be changed to "sexual misuse." This new term presents a more realistic image of what occurs in most sexual abuse cases. Commonly, there is an existing relationship between the perpetrator and victim. The misuse of that relationship is central to the sexual abuse of the child. The relationship may be a familial one such as father-daughter, a household relationship such as mother's live-in paramour and child, or a more casual relationship, such as that with a neighbor. Most often, there is no overt violence, although there may be threats of violence as a consequence of the child revealing the act to another person. The term sexual misuse is also more encompassing as it includes the misuse of children for prostitution and pornography. Although the suggested terminology change is based on several sound points, most state laws use the term, "sexual abuse"; thus, this chapter will conform to that tradition.

The National Center for Child Abuse and Neglect defines sexual abuse as: ". . . contacts or interactions between a child and an adult when the child is being used for the sexual stimulation of the perpetrator or another person. Sexual abuse may also be committed by a person under the age of 18 when that person is either significantly older than the victim or when the perpetrator is in a position of power or control over another child." Sexual abuse has traditionally been more the domain of police and other law enforcement personnel. A number of specific legal definitions should be understood and used precisely. Each state defines these terms independently as well as legislates the age of consent. Emergency physicians must be aware of their local laws. In Pennsylvania for example, the age of consent is 18 years. Sexual abuse terms are defined as follows.

Rape. A person commits a felony when he engages in sexual intercourse with another person not his spouse:

1. By forcible compulsion
2. By threat of forcible compulsion that would prevent resistance by a person of reasonable resolution
3. Who is unconscious or
4. Who is so mentally deranged or deficient that such person is incapable of consent.

Statutory Rape. A person who is 18 years of age or older commits a felony when he engages in sexual intercourse with another person not his spouse who is less than 14 years of age.

Involuntary Deviate Sexual Intercourse. A person commits a felony when he engages in deviate sexual intercourse per anus, or per os, or any form of sexual intercourse with another person:

1. By forcible compulsion
2. By threat of forcible compulsion
3. Who is unconscious
4. Who is mentally deranged or deficient
5. Who is less than 16 years of age.

Indecent Assault. A person who has indecent contact (any touching of the sexual or other intimate parts of the person for the purpose of arousing or gratifying sexual desire in either person) with another not his spouse, or causes such other to have indecent contact with him is guilty of indecent assault.

Incest. A person is guilty of incest, if he knowingly marries or cohabits or has sexual intercourse with an ancestor or descendant, a brother or sister of the whole or half blood or an uncle, aunt, nephew or niece of the whole blood. These relationships include blood relationships without regard to legitimacy and relationship of parent and child by adoption.

Promoting Prostitution. A person who knowingly induces or encourages a child to engage in prostitution.

The true incidence of sexual abuse is unknown. The statistics for substantiated cases in Pennsylvania from 1976 through 1980, are shown in Table 68.5 as an example of the recently documented upward trend in number of reports. The National Center on Child Abuse/Neglect estimates that the current annual incidence of sexual abuse is between 60,000 and 100,000 cases per year. Most estimates do not include those children who are victims of pornographic exploitation and child prostitution.

DYNAMICS

Sexual abuse encompasses a number of different sexual acts committed by different perpetrators for different reasons. Thus, no single theory can explain the dynamics. In an effort to simplify the interactions and make them understandable in light of behaviors seen in the emergency department, the physician should consider intrafamilial versus extrafamilial sexual abuse. The intrafamilial category includes incest in all its forms as well as sexual abuse by significant, though perhaps not legal, members of the family. Sexual abuse between a girl and her

Table 68.5
Forms of Abuse—Percent Pennsylvania Substantiated Reports, 1976–1980

Year	No. of Cases	Physical (%)	Sexual (%)	Mental (%)	Neglect (%)
1976	3872	64.3	9.1	3.8	22.6
1977	6183	64.6	10.4	4.0	21.0
1978	5961	61.0	11.0	3.0	25.0
1979	5621	66.0	15.0	2.0	17.0
1980	5827	65.0	21.1	1.9	11.5

mother's paramour would be included in this category. Extrafamilial abuse occurs between adults and children or adolescents and children who have no familial relationship.

There is great controversy about the dynamics of intrafamilial abuse. Professionals are themselves divided into two theoretical camps. One group theorizes that sexual abuse is the sole responsibility of the perpetrator, usually a male adult. Advocates of this position contend that the abuse results from an inability of the individual to control his sexual impulses or to establish age appropriate adult relationships. A second group sees the problem more as a family responsibility. In this model, it is the disturbed relationship between the adults that expresses itself in the male parent (or parent equivalent) crossing generational lines for sexual gratification. Theorists in this camp often point to the mother's passive sanction of the abuse, even to the point of being informed about the incest and still allowing it to continue over long periods of time. Obviously the two theories point to very different treatment strategies. According to the first, the solution is to simply remove the male perpetrator to jail or a mental hospital. The second group would prescribe therapy for the entire family to reorder the relationships such that the adults are able to meet their own needs and the children are protected. These professionals would contend that, where the male adult is removed, the mother will soon find a replacement.

The dynamics of extrafamilial abuse are less well understood. The rape of a child by a stranger, like the rape of an adult, is a crime of violence. Such attacks are triggered by extreme anger, and a child may be selected as more easy prey. In other cases of extrafamilial abuse, some of the dynamics are still based on the misuse of a relationship although in this case the relationships are more casual. Perhaps the most common is the sexual abuse that occurs between neighbors or between a babysitter and the child being watched. These episodes frequently involve adolescent perpetrators. The abuse dynamic may be an abuse of a power relationship, an uncontrolled sexual curiosity, or a combination of these factors. As the age difference between the child and the perpetrator widens, the more pathologic the dynamic becomes. As the perpetrator increases in age, there is expectation that socialization will instill more self-control. Certainly, the sexual exploration that occurs between children of the same age is not sexual abuse, although on occasions an uninformed parent may consider it as such.

CLINICAL MANIFESTATION

The manifestations of sexual abuse may occur at a time shortly after the abuse has occurred or at a time more distant from the event. The manifestations may be influenced by there being a single episode or a pattern of repeated encounters. Finally, the manifestations may be dependent on the age and maturity of the child.

The manifestations may be divided into four categories as shown in Table 68.6. These are specific physical findings, specific behavioral manifestations, nonspecific physical complaints and nonspecific behavioral complaints.

Specific Physical Complaints

Bruising on the upper thigh, lower abdomen, or genitalia is a rare finding in childhood sexual abuse. The child is not usually injured as she/he is often used for stimulation, masturbation, or genital contact that involves no force. Nonetheless a physical injury to the genitalia should elicit a suspicion of sexual abuse. For children with even small vaginal lacerations, a detailed history of injury should be obtained. Straddle injuries do produce genital trauma and are the most common form of accidental genital injury to little girls. In males, accidental penile trauma may occur from zipper accidents or from a toilet seat that falls. Beyond these common accidental situations, the emergency physician should scrutinize the history given. The premenstrual child who presents with vaginal hemorrhage may be bleeding due to a vaginal laceration that is not visible on external examination. Prompt surgical or gynecological consultation should be obtained to identify and repair this injury.

Table 68.6
Identification of Sexual Abuse

Physical Complaints	Behavioral Complaints
Specific	*Specific*
Genital injury	Inappropriate knowledge of adult sexual behavior (explicit descriptions on sexual play)
Bruises	Compulsive masturbation
Lacerations	Excessive sexual curiosity
Rectal laceration	
Vaginal/urethral discharge	
Vaginal/rectal pain	
Pregnancy	
Nonspecific	*Nonspecific*
Anorexia	Excessive fear
Abdominal pain	Nightmares
Bedwetting	Phobias
Dysuria	Refusal to sleep alone
Encopresis	Runaways
Evidence of physical abuse	Aggression
	Suicide
	Any abrupt change in behavior

The presence of venereal disease in a prepubertal child is a specific finding of sexual abuse until proven otherwise. Studies by Branch and Paxton and others have shown that when instances of prepubertal gonorrhea were carefully investigated for etiology, the source of the infection was through sexual contact, most often in the child's home or in a relative's home. Gonorrhea may occur in the genitourinary tract, rectum or oropharynx, and cultures should be obtained from all three sites. When gonorrhea is culture proven, it should be pursued as sexual abuse. At times when there is only a history of sexual contact, or when nonspecific symptoms are present, laboratory confirmation of a gonorrheal infection can further substantiate the case. Parents may bring their child to the emergency department for the complaint of vaginal discharge. Gonorrhea may also present as a number of less well defined symptoms such as vaginal pain, itching, urinary frequency, or enuresis. Venereal diseases other than gonorrhea are far less common but may be transmitted to children through sexual abuse.

The pregnant adolescent may be a victim of incest. It is important to try to obtain a specific history of conception. Frequently the focus of case management centers on how the adolescent plans to notify her parents or whether she considers abortion or adoption as options. If the issue of paternity is not pursued, instances of sexual abuse will escape detection.

Specific Behavioral Complaints

The most common clinical manifestation is a positive history of sexual abuse. The child who gives a clear detailed story of sexual encounter with an adult evidences a specific behavioral manifestation. Reports of suspected abuse may be based on history alone since children do not make such allegations lightly. Most nonabused children are not knowledgeable in the details of sexual encounters. The detail of the history will vary with the age and language development of the child, but even children of 3 or 4 years are able to make simple statements about someone touching their genitals.

Some children will manifest behaviors in their play or in their conversation that will indicate that they have been exposed to sexual experiences, and perhaps abused. These signs are less specific than a clearly stated history, but are significant enough to require further explanation. For example, the young child who discusses orogenital contact may be demonstrating a specific behavioral manifestation. There should also be concern about children who wish to fondle their parent's genitals as an expression of affection. These behaviors are usually learned. All children will manifest sexual curiosity and may engage in some form of masturbation. When either of these behaviors appear in excess, they deserve investigation. Sexual abuse may be the cause.

Nonspecific Physical Complaints

The physician should keep sexual abuse in the differetial diagnosis for many complaints. Sexual abuse may present as pain in the abdomen, thighs or genitals, dysuria, pain on defecation, hematuria, or hematochezia. Abuse may manifest as a change in habits such as urinary frequency, enuresis, constipation or encopresis. Other complaints may be vaginal discharge, or chronic sore throat. The etiology of each of these complaints may be any number of things. For example, looking at a group of children with enuresis, sexual abuse is an uncommon cause of the complaint. Nonetheless sexually abused children are regularly brought to emergency departments with nonspecific complaints. If sexual abuse is not considered, it will go unnoticed.

Nonspecific Behavioral Complaints

The final group of clinical manifestations include unexplained changes in the child's behavior. In this group are included relatively minor behavioral changes, such as the recent acquisition of nightmares or phobias, or major changes, such as school truancy and adolescent runaways. Children who bear no physical evidence of their abuse and in whom no physical symptoms develop may express themselves behaviorally. Many will demonstrate changes in one or more of the important spheres of their life: at home, in school or with peers. This is exemplified by a 5-year-old girl who begins avoiding contact with her father and other male relatives following an abusive episode with a friend of the family. The sudden change in school performance unexplained by the teacher, social withdrawal and isolation may also be nonbehavioral manifestations. Like the nonspecific physical complaints, these behavioral complaints may be caused by a number of other things as well. Sexual abuse is likely to produce a behavioral change in children old enough to comprehend the wrongness and shame of the situation.

MANAGEMENT

The primary goals in case management of the sexually abused child are to identify and report the abuse and to avoid the secondary abuse phenomenon. Secondary abuse phenomenon refers to the physical examination that is so overzealous that it assumes a rapelike quality in the mind of the child. Also to be avoided are parental or staff reactions that make the child feel responsible or blamed for the abuse. The following paragraphs offer techniques in management in order to identify suspected sexual abuse, and gather enough documentation for legal purpose in a manner that is humane for the child and supportive for the family.

Interviewing the Parent

Parents may present the problem of sexual abuse either directly or indirectly. For the parent who is direct (i.e. "my child's been raped") it is important to provide a controlled, quiet environment because he or she will be upset and angry. It may be necessary to limit what is said in front of the child. With such parents the interviewer's tasks are calming, limiting, and clarifying. The indirect parent brings the child for complaints such as those detailed in the section on nonspecific physical or behavioral manifestations. With this parent, the task of the interviewer is to bring the possibility of sexual abuse into the open. It is surprising that once the topic is nominally broached it becomes apparent that the parent has often already given it consideration. With both types of parents it is important to explore both their concerns and their information in detail.

Interviewing the Child

Beyond standard history taking from the parents, the emergency physician must always obtain history from the child. This is difficult for several reasons: (1) the level of

Table 68.7
Developmental Issues in Managing the Sexually Abused Child

Age	Developmental Issues		Fears	Techniques
0 to approximately 3 yr	*General:* Dependent on protection of adult Little or no ability to label time or sequence events Language only partially intelligible May not be able to identify body parts Toilet training in process	*Sexual:* Normal self-exploration of genital area is pleasurable Confused if this behavior is labeled "wrong" or "dirty" If sexual abuse is not painful, it may be accepted By age 3 curious about genitals of others	Terrified of painful assault Terrified of losing protection of adult	Keep parent present during interview Use dolls to: Point to body parts Do actions
Preschool, 3–6 yr	Language skills better Able to sequence events Gender differentiation established Cannot tell time but can have established time concepts "before or after"	Sexually curious Younger children exhibit bodies Modesty develops Vocabulary of sex parts and body functions After abuse there may be masturbation, sexual play	Confused over incident Frightened by parents' anxiety and anger Feel they are "bad" for causing parents to be upset Behavior changes and phobias may develop, e.g., fear of dark, fear of strangers	Ask children to draw pictures Use doll or puppet play to note response
School age	*General and Sexual:* Sexual interest increases but usually more curious than erotic Discomfort discussing their bodies, especially outside family Extremely modest with strangers and often with parents Abusive incident may have been pleasurable and nontraumatic		Abuse is perceived as sexual, may feel "sex is wrong" Often have been threatened by adult perpetrator Guilt about what they did vs. guilt over getting adult and family into trouble Fear about their bodies feel "dirty" or "different" after incident	Use same sex interviewer Do not assume correct knowledge of body, a physically mature 10-year-old is not necessarily emotionally mature, or well informed Give reassurance of their nonresponsibility for the abuse Give praise for having reported incident Encourage child to talk about parents' reaction Mobilize family to support victim

Adolescent	Strong urge to conform and be "normal" Knows what is and is not socially acceptable Developing body image and self-esteem is very fragile Conflict between the need to assert independence, and the need for adult protection and approval	Forcible nature of sex is terrifying even to a sexually active adolescent Grief over loss of virginity Feeling that he/she is dirty or abnormal Fear of unavoidable further encounters with perpetrator Fear that a homosexual encounter may have lifelong consequences	Stress the normality of the victim—not branded for life Use charts or models Victims need to know that you have seen others with similar experiences who have recovered well Mobilize active family support Be available—give victim your phone number at work, or social worker's number Victim advocate groups very helpful

(Adapted from J. Michaelson, J. Paradise & S. Ludwig)

language development of the child, (2) the level of psychosexual development of the child, (3) the desire not to contaminate what may be important evidence, (4) the apprehension of the child and parent, and (5) the awkwardness and apprehension felt by the interviewer in discussing sexual matters with a child. The first steps are to obtain a quiet, private place and to decide if you wish the parent to be present. Based on previous history taking from the parent, one can gauge the parent's level of emotional composure. This is a useful criterion to decide whether or not they should be present. If the parents are excluded, it is prudent to have another third party, e.g. a nurse or social worker, present. An initial discussion of topics, other than the alleged abuse, comforts the child. Information about school, peers, and family adjustment is important in looking for nonspecific behavioral manifestations, and this preliminary conversation will also help to evaluate the child's developmental level. Table 68.7 briefly outlines normal sexual developmental stages and appropriate interviewing techniques for each level.

In focusing the conversation on the abuse, one technique may be to ask the child why her parents brought her to the hospital. Another approach that is more appropriate for younger children is to establish common vocabulary, by asking the child the term used for her genitalia. Children will offer a rich variety of terms and may have no understanding of "vagina" or "penis." One 4-year-old girl told us "he tried to put his pencil in my pocketbook." In eliciting and using a common language, the physician gets to the point of the interview more easily.

If the parental history and surrounding circumstances are credible, it is best to phrase inquiries to obtain the details of the abuse rather than to ask the child to make the initial allegation. For example, the physician may want to directly ask "How did Uncle Tommy touch your pee pee (vagina)?" rather than "Did Uncle Tommy touch you?" If questions are phased in a yes or no format, a one-word response will be given. Obtaining detail is important in order to add credibility to the history. It is also important in guiding the physician to significant aspects of physical examination, evidence collection, and treatment.

With a preverbal child it is helpful to use anatomically correct dolls (Table 68.7). These will allow the child to play out the episode. Similarly, some children may choose to draw a picture which will tell the story or which may be used by the interviewer to initiate the interview.

Emotional Support

Throughout the interview and in all contacts with the child, it is important to stress the rightness of her decision to discuss the abuse. A child will feel conflict about revealing a secret, especially one that has been long standing. The patient may also feel conflict in sensing that her actions may be provoking a great deal of emotional turmoil. Often the child will have a relationship with the perpetrator and will realize that this may alter or end the relationship. At times, she is aware or is made aware that she is getting the perpetrator "in trouble." Reaffirm the importance of what the child has revealed and focus the wrongdoing on the perpetrator. It is likely that the child has been threatened not to tell. Thus, it is important to bring the nature of the threats into the open and to offer protection to the child. Finally many children will have fears about the abuse. Common fears are shown in Table 68.7. The physician may anticipate and address these fears based on the child's development.

Physical Examination

The physical examination may be a point of significant trauma for the child. The examination should be conducted in a standard fashion with all parts of the body examined. The position of the child will depend on their age and comfort. Many young children will want to be examined while sitting in their parent's lap. In examining the genitalia of young girls either of two positions is recommended. One is a frog leg posture while sitting on an adult lap. Alternatively, the child can lie prone with knees tucked under the thorax.

In the prepubertal girl only the external genitalia need to be examined. If there appears to be even minimal vaginal bleeding from a more internal source, exploration and repair of this is a procedure that is best done under general anesthesia in the operating room. Examination in the emergency department should be deferred. In the pubertal child, a full genital examination should be performed. This may be modified if it is the girl's first speculum examination and it proves too difficult. Chapter 52, "Gynecologic Emergencies," details physical examination techniques.

Examination of rectum and oropharynx needs to be carefully performed, particularly if the history suggests that these were sites of sexual contact. Other physical findings to note carefully are any contusions, abrasions, or lacerations in nongenital areas. Common sites for these signs of trauma are upper thigh, buttocks, and upper arms.

If the physical examination proves too traumatic for the child, the physician is faced with a significant dilemma. The choices are to further traumatize the child or to do an incomplete examination and inadequate evidence collection. As with all dilemmas, there is no obvious best choice. We would caution against physically or psychologically traumatizing the child. Often there will be no physical evidence and the history, if detailed enough, may be sufficient. The guiding principle should be primum non nocere.

Evidence Collection

The type of evidence to be collected, the collection methods used and the procedures for processing the results will vary from locale to locale. The specimen collecting procedures at the Children's Hospital of Philadelphia have been reviewed by the Philadelphia Police Department and District Attorney. The protocol is listed in Table 68.8.

Whatever the specifics of a particular jurisdiction, some general principles should be followed. It is important to establish a standard protocol so that each new case does not force the emergency physician to reformulate the entire process. The department should have on hand either standard

Table 68.8
Evidence Collection for Sexually Abused Children

Test	Indications
1. Gonococcal cultures Pharynx Vagina or cervix Rectum	History of contact *OR* Loss of consciousness *OR* Poor History
2. Urine pregnancy test	Postmenarchal patient
3. Pap smear	If speculum examination is done
4. 2 swabs: 1 in 0.5 ml saline 1 smear on glass slide	Each body area with seminal secretions by history or examination
5. Saliva sample: spit; or swabs in 0.5 ml saline	As control for Test (4) *OR* Oral-genital contact
6. Venipuncture	
Rapid plasma reagin test	Same as for (1)
3–5 ml of serum for blood group antigens	As control for (4) and/or (5)
7. Foreign pubic hairs and controls	If present (must be *plucked*)

"rape kits" or some modification thereof. The kits should contain all the necessary tubes, slides, swabs, etc. Evidence collection should be performed with another health care professional present, either a nurse or social worker. A standard for marking the specimens should be established including the patient's name and medical record number. Finally, the protocol should include a procedure for a specified person to take the specimens to the laboratory and to officially have them received or logged in by the laboratory. This detail becomes important in the court proceedings against the perpetrator. For example, nothing is more unsatisfying than seeing an alleged perpetrator go unconvicted because the hospital cannot be legally sure that a positive gonorrhea culture belongs to the victim in question.

Documentation

Careful record keeping cannot be stressed too strongly. As with the collection and processing of evidence, emergency department records can make or break a case. At the Children's Hospital of Philadelphia, we have developed a separate form that guides the examining physician to include all the pertinent information (see Chapter 75, pp. 1180–1182). All the aspects of record keeping mentioned in the section on physical abuse apply. In particular there should be careful recording of what the child said in his or her own words. Such questions may be the mainstay of any legal actions to be taken. Good records not only help the police and lawyers involved but will also help the physician review the case prior to a hearing which may not take place for 6 months.

Reporting

In most jurisdictions sexual abuse is a criminal offense. Thus, all cases are reported to the police. In some jurisdictions when the abuse has occurred in the home, or during a time when parental supervision was lax, a civil report to the Child Protective Services Agency may also be required. This is another detail that needs to be specified according to local guidelines and included in an emergency department procedure. In the event of a criminal (police) report, a civil (child abuse) report, or both, the parent needs to be informed that such reports are being made. The physician or social worker must spell out for the parent what will be the practical consequences of the reports.

Preparing the Parent

Beyond notifying the parent about reporting the sexual abuse, there is a great deal of additional preparation that must be given. Many workers believe that, for the young child, the parental reaction to sexual abuse may have as important a role as the abuse itself in producing subsequent manifestations. Parents need to be aware of this. All parents will be upset. All parents will be angry. Some parents may express disbelief or the feeling that "this could not be happening to me." Parental reactions will vary if this is an intrafamilial or extrafamilial abuse. Social worker consultation and collaboration for this aspect of case management is essential.

The first step is to focus the parent's attention on the child. Especially in situations of father-daughter incest or surrogate father-daughter incest, the maternal reaction may be more self-centered initially. In directing the parents' attention to the child, the physician returns the parent to a more comfortable traditional role and opens many important issues to which the parent must attend. Review with the parent that manifestations of sexual abuse may be physical and/or psychological. The physical manifestation may seem minor to the physician, but parents must be specifically told that whatever the injury it can be repaired with no impairment of the victim's sexual functions as an adult. Stress that soft tissues can be repaired, and gonorrhea, if present, can be treated. Parents must be told that the psychological outcome in part will relate to their reactions to the situation. Their role must be to provide comfort, support and reassurance to the child.

Methods of supporting the child have been raised previously in this section. These techniques must be used by the parents. Unfortunately, parental anger and blame may sometimes be displaced onto the child. It is the child who has set off an emotional time bomb by revealing the abuse. For example, parents may openly say "I told you not to play with those children down the street" in a case of extrafamilial abuse. In cases of intrafamilial abuse, there may be an even more damaging undercurrent that the child lured the adult into the abuse. Statements such as "I knew she would end up no good" or "I told her never to walk around the house in her underwear" are not uncommon. All attempts to place responsibility or blame on the victim need to be eliminated. The ultimate responsibility was that of the perpetrator no matter what the behavior of the child.

Some parents may focus their anger clearly on the perpetrator but wish to "take the law into their own hands." Parents should be cautioned about leaving the emergency department in order to find and confront the perpetrator. This is a police responsibility. The parental role is to provide safety for the child. Parental ire can be cooled by pointing out that their own arrest for assault of the perpetrator will not benefit their child.

Yet another common parental reaction is to want to institute a number of life-style changes. Parents may want to change their place of residence, change the child's school, or quit their jobs to be able to guard the child 24 hours a day. The emergency department staff should stress that what is best for the child is to return to as normal a life-style as possible. Change is always difficult for children and the stress of entering a new school or meeting a new set of friends is a burden the sexual abuse victim does not need. Parents should be cautioned about limiting the amount of open conversation with friends and relatives that the child may overhear. The victim's desire to discuss the abuse should regulate how much abuse-related conversation should take place between family members. Some children may want repeated reassurances about their parents' approval and about their future safety. Other children may wish to let the episode be forgotten and return to school and play. If the sexual abuse triggers disruption and chaos in the parents' life and disapproval of the child, it will surely have psychological ramifications. The best prognosis will result if the parent can show their concern in a way which will assure the child of approval, protection, and a resumption of a normal life-style.

Hospitalization

There are two indications for hospitalizing the sexually abused child: (1) severe injury requiring treatment and (2) an unsafe home. However, outpatient management of sexual abuse victims is always preferable, if at all possible. The rationale is to avoid victimizing the child twice. If an adult male has been the intrafamilial perpetrator, he should be removed from the home, so that the child may return. Children who are hospitalized because the home is unsafe feel that they are being sent away for their wrongdoing. Another message hospitalization transmits is that the parent is incapable of providing protection. Both of these messages are harmful to the child's psychological adjustment.

If indeed a parent is incapable of providing protection, then the provisions of most child abuse statutes will allow the physician to assume protective custody and hospitalize the child independent of the wishes of the parent.

Treatment

Whether the child will be hospitalized or discharged from the emergency department, there are two treatment issues to consider: (1) gonococcal prophylaxis and (2) diethylstilbestrol (DES) treatment for pregnancy prophylaxis. If the abuse has occurred less than 48 hours prior to the hospital visit, then gonococcal prophylaxis is recommended. Within this time period, cultures for *Neisseria gonorrhoea* may prove negative, even if a true infection is incubating. In abuse that has occurred greater than 48 hours prior to the visit, the choices are either to treat all children prophylactically or to culture the genitalia, anus, and throat and await culture results. This choice will in part depend on the reliability of the microbiology laboratory in recovering *N. gonorrhoeae* (which is a fastidious organism) and the ability to provide follow-up treatment for positive cultures. Treatment regimens recommended are shown in Table 68.9. The advantage of using oral amoxicillin over intramuscular penicillin is that it avoids another source of trauma to the child, and experience has shown it to be as efficacious.

The question of DES treatment is more controversial. Most children can be eliminated from consideration if they have not yet reached menarche. Another group may

Table 68.9
Treatment for Suspected Gonorrhea Infections In Prepubertal Children: Indication—for All Cases with History of Sexual Contact[a]

1. Amoxicillin dose:
    - If <40 kg, give 50 mg/kg p.o. in one dose
    - If >40 kg, 3.0 g p.o. in one dose
    - With probenecid:
        - If <40 kg, 25 mg/kg p.o. (maximum 1 g)
        - If >40 kg, 1 g p.o.
2. In case of penicillin allergy:
    - If child 8 yr: Spectinomycin 40 mg/kg i.m.
    - If child 8 yr: Tetracycline:
        - If <40 kg, 40 mg/kg/day p.o., in 4 divided doses × 5 days
        - If >40 kg, 500 mg p.o. q.i.d. × 5 days

[a] *Note:* Amoxicillin and tetracycline will probably treat incubating syphilis. Spectinomycin will not.

be eliminated based on the nature of the abuse. If the abuse took the form of fondling, and there was no ejaculate produced by the perpetrator, DES does not need to be used. In the pubertal child in whom there was active penetration at a mid-menstrual cycle time, DES or another effective "morning-after" pill should be employed to avoid pregnancy. The dose of DES is 25 mg twice a day for 5 days. Many centers will obtain informed consent for the use of this drug because of the possibility of inducing congenital anomalies in a fetus were the patient to become pregnant before their next menstrual period. It is always important to document that there is not an existing pregnancy prior to using DES. Also important is to warn the adolescent about the common side effect of gastrointestinal upset, change in menstrual cycle, vaginal discharge, and breast tenderness.

Referral and Follow-Up

All sexually abused children will need some form of referral and will need careful follow-up care. Referral may initially be to the hospital social worker for monitoring of the child's symptoms and the family's ability to cope with this stress. In some locales volunteer self-help groups organized for women who have been raped may provide support to the child victim and parent. Referral for more in-depth mental health counseling will depend on the (1) symptoms manifested by the child, (2) state of family organization, (3) length of time the abuse has occurred, and (4) age of the child. In general, the older the child and the longer the abuse has occurred, the more likely this represents a serious mental health problem. Follow-up health care visits should be arranged, hopefully, with an informed and sympathetic practitioner who can continue the humane and supportive care initiated in the emergency department.

NEGLECT

Child neglect is the most prevalent form of child abuse. When neglect is blatant it is easily recognized and reported. More often, neglect is not obvious and goes undetected for long periods of time. Although the manifestations of neglect are less dramatic than those of physical abuse, the long-term effects may be more destructive to the child. The indolent nature of child neglect makes it a serious public health problem. For the emergency department staff, neglect cases are difficult as they require that certain value judgments be made. The balance between supporting the independent rights of the child and maintaining the privacy and sanctity of family rights is a delicate one. With neglected children the questions are: How much should the family be doing? How much are they capable of doing? How much support from the community or society do they require?

As with the other forms of child abuse, the management of child neglect cases is made easier by working with a multidisciplinary team. In the emergency department the team would generally consist of the physician, nurse and social worker. Particularly in situations where the line between adequate child care and neglect needs to be drawn, the diversity of personal and professional opinions adds credibility to decision making and lessens the burden on the single practitioner.

BACKGROUND

The definition of child neglect is difficult, as there are no societal standards for child care. This creates a situation in which parents and professionals are left to define their own standards. The vagueness of definition produces many problems. Defining "abandonment" (the ultimate neglect) is an excellent example of the difficulties encountered in setting standards. There is no societal norm for either the age of the child left alone or the duration of time. Thus, if a parent leaves a 3-year-old unattended in an apartment several hours, most neighbors and professionals would consider that neglect. But what if the child were 10 years old, and the parent was gone for 20 min? Then the situation becomes less clear. Many states have tried to partially define the condition by making it dependent on a physical manifestation in the child. Thus, the child left alone who stays out of trouble is not neglected. The one who burns himself and cries to the point that the neighbors become aware is neglected.

The National Center for Child Abuse and Neglect uses the following definition: "Child neglect refers to acts of omission; specifically, the failure of a parent or other person legally responsible for a child's welfare to provide for the child's basic needs and proper level of care with respect to food, clothing, shelter, hygiene, medical attention, or supervision."

There are other apparent societal conflicts in defining neglect. One conflict centers on the relationship between neglect and poverty. This relates to the questions asked previously and the issue of what should the family be doing versus what are they economically capable of doing. Certainly, poverty may be coincident with neglect, but they are distinct issues. There is the example of the majority of poor families who do find a way to provide the material essentials and more importantly the emotional essentials. There is the contrasting example of families who are middle or upper class who are neglectful. Another conflict is based on the failure to recognize the evils of excess. The child who is underfed and wasted is promptly labeled "failure to thrive." The child who is overfed to the point of obesity may face as many serious consequences. The child who is developmentally delayed from understimulation may be labeled neglected. The child who has psychosomatic illness from being stressed to overachieve also deserves recognition. The term neglect generally refers to underprovision on the part of the parent. Overprovision may be as deleterious, and this presents a serious conflict to the definition of neglect.

The true incidence of neglect is not ascertainable. Vincent DeFrances of the American Humane Association suggests that the incidence is 10 times that of physical abuse. Table 68.5 shows the incidence of neglect in Pennsylvania. The actual decrease in percentage of substantiated neglect cases may reflect the difficulty in confirming the diagnosis. The age distribution is weighted toward the younger child who is obviously more dependent on the parents for care. The incidence of neglect of older children is probably as great, yet it goes unrecognized and unreported.

DYNAMICS

The dynamics of child neglect have been explained by several different theorists. Some theories are based on pure individual dynamics. These point to the immature, overwhelmed, overstressed parent who responds by withdrawal. Polansky has well documented and labeled this the "apathy futility syndrome." Theories which have a more social orientation point to the societal pressures and to the existence of poverty. David Gil considers all children existing on a welfare stipend as neglected and recommends a change in the distribution of societal resources as a solution.

Most theories would support the notion that the neglectful parent does not see him/herself as such. Most parents are caught up in a neglectful life-style that is self-perpetuating. Most neglect is not purposeful. It just happens. Studies have clearly shown that women who fail to seek prenatal care are also likely to not obtain health care for their children. In the parents view, it is a pattern of living that seems to be the norm. This facet of the dynamics of neglect is important to the emergency department management.

MANIFESTATIONS

The manifestations of neglect are countless. The manifestation may be tangible, such as the weight loss of a child whose diet has been inadequate, or intangible, such as the psychological effects of unsatisfactory relationships. A categorization of neglect can be made by looking at the standard functions of the family and then considering the failure to fulfill these functions. A family must (1) provide and distribute material goods—food, clothing, and shelter; (2) ensure health; (3) promote safety; (4) socialize and educate; and (5) provide emotional support, security and love. The manifestations of neglect may occur in one or more of these functional areas. The most commonly reported manifestations are (1) nonorganic failure to thrive—a lack of food and feeding skills, (2) medical neglect—a failure to provide needed health care, (3) abandonment—total neglect generally viewed as a lack of supervision and as a safety hazard, and (4) truancy and school avoidance.

Failure to Thrive

The term failure to thrive has been used as a diagnostic wastebasket to group a number of diseases and disorders that result in growth failure. Growth failure is generally measured in weight, length, and head circumference as compared to standard growth curves for these parameters. Growth failure may be defined as measurements that fall below two standard deviations for age or patterns that cross percentile lines and do not follow the normal lines of growth. Patients diagnosed as failure to thrive may be subcategorized into three categories: (1) organic, (2) nonorganic, and (3) overlap group. Organic refers to those children whose failure to thrive is based on a physical cause such as congenital heart disease, renal disease, or a genetic abnormality. Nonorganic refers to the group whose growth failure is environmentally related. When these children are hospitalized and fed standard diets, they grow rapidly and thrive. Within the group of nonorganic failure to thrive patients, there are a substantial number of neglected children who may be brought to the emergency department for care. The overlap group refers to patients where there is a combination of physical and environmental factors. An example might be a physical condition which so overstresses a family that they cannot function and thus neglect the child in some aspect of the feeding process.

In recognizing the nonorganic failure to thrive patients the following factors are suggestive. *History*: (1) an idealized feeding history, (2) a chief complaint and history that do not identify the child's growth pattern as a problem, (3) no description of losses such as vomiting or diarrhea, and (4) failure to give a history of a schedule or scheduled pattern of feeding, e.g. baby eats about every 4 hours. *Physical examination*: (1) measurements in which weight is more depressed than length which is more depressed than head circumference; (2) other signs of neglect such as poor hygiene, diaper rash, flat and balding occiput etc.; (3) dull, apathetic facies; (4) body posture of an understimulated child; (5) excessive oral self-stimulation; and (6) developmental delay particularly in the social adaptive and language areas. *Parental observation*: the parent who (1) has a disinterested attitude; (2) does not respond to child's needs, e.g. react to crying; (3) lacks concern about health issues; and (4) appears to be a drug or alcohol abuser. These are shown in Figure 68.11.

Medical Neglect

The differentiation between medical neglect and noncompliance is often difficult. The key to differentiating them is to ask "Has identifiable harm come to the child?" If a parent fails to complete a course of therapy prescribed by a physician, noncompliance exists. However if the failure to give medication results in further illness in the child, then medical neglect exists. The manifestations of medical neglect can be documented and reported as such. Noncompliance merely results in a worsening doctor-patient relationship. It may be difficult to prove that the failure to give medication, attend follow-up appointments or obtain a procedure directly resulted in damage to the child's health. Often there are intervening variables such as the complexity of the disease (e.g. the exacerbations of an asthma attack) or the proven efficacy of the treatment. The emergency department is often the central place for identifying the manifestations of medical neglect. Good documentation of prescribed treatments and good communication with the source of the child's ongoing health care are important.

Abandonment

Local jurisdictions may dictate the length of time a child must be without supervision before he or she is legally abandoned. Often these cases will come to the emergency department as the result of a neighbor's call or the initiative of a relative who is aware of the neglect. At times the situation may become apparent as the emergency department attempts to obtain permission to treat a child and has difficulty locating a parent or responsible adult. Manifestations of abandonment include (1) physical findings such as excessively dirty diapers, poor hygiene or hoarse cry; (2) excessive hunger documented by unusual intake; and (3) dehydration as documented by urine specific gravity or blood urea nitrogen. Other manifestations may relate to lack of supervision and protection and may include burns, ingestions, or repeated accidents. Children with all of these manifestations may be brought to the emergency department for treatment. Good case management will result in their identification.

Truancy

This manifestation of neglect may be less commonly recognized in the emergency department. The section on school avoidance ("Psychiatric Emergencies," Chapter 70) details many of the aspects of this complex psychosocial emergency. The emergency physician may recognize truancy as a neglect problem in the situation where the truant child presents with multiple somatic complaints. As the complaints are explored and no organic basis found, the parent may be instructed to return the child to school. A failure to comply with this aspect of treatment constitutes medical neglect. For the child who makes frequent emergency department visits, neglect needs to be considered.

MANAGEMENT

The management of cases of child neglect follows the principles detailed in the phys-

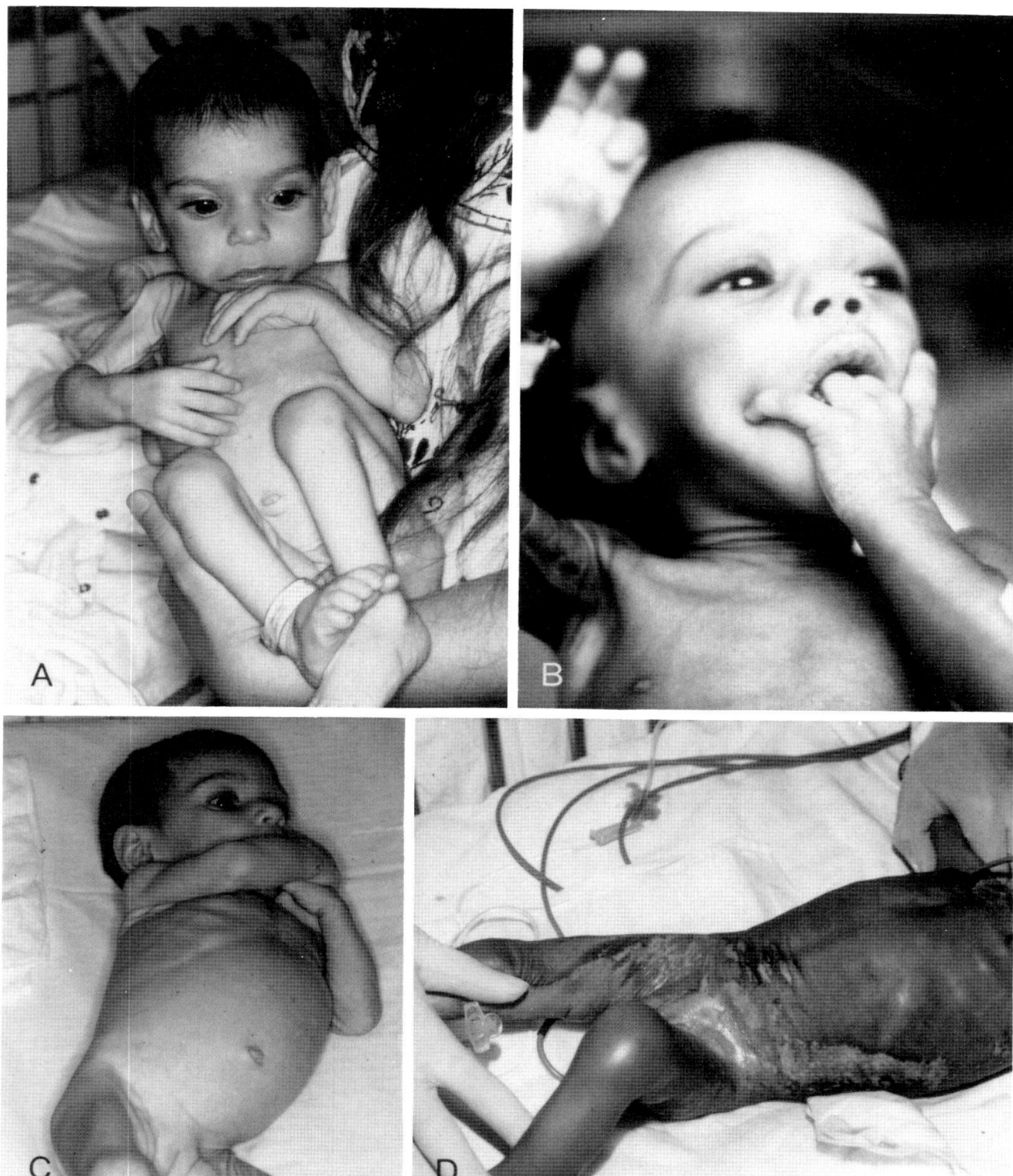

Figure 68.11 Physical signs of failure to thrive. (*A*) Dull, apathetic eyes which avoid eye contact; (*B*) oral self-stimulatory behavior; (*C*) wasted extremities and protuberant abdomen, (*D*) severe diaper rash as a sign of overall neglect.

ical abuse section. The steps are (1) suspect and recognize neglect manifestations, (2) obtain multidisciplinary consultation, (3) report the neglect, (4) inform the parents, (5) determine need for hospitalization, and (6) arrange follow-up. These steps will be reviewed so as to underscore those aspects unique to neglect.

Suspect Neglect

As with other forms of abuse, it is the open mind of the physician which allows neglect to be recognized. Because the manifestations are more subtle than with physical abuse, recognition is more difficult. The physician can overcome this difficulty only by obtaining a more detailed history and observing the parent-child interaction. In-depth social work evaluation can often uncover previous reports of neglect or involvement with child welfare agencies. Piling the building blocks of suspicion to the height of a threshold point may be more difficult as the size of each block may be smaller and less dramatic than in physical abuse.

Multidisciplinary Consultation

Because much of defining neglect is value laden, it is vital to use multidisciplinary consultation. Such consultation can broaden perspectives on "normal" lifestyles and child rearing practices. The difficulty any single professional feels in making a value judgment can be shared by a group. The multidisciplinary consultation may be made with someone outside the emergency department. Speaking with a school teacher, nurse or counselor may be very informative. A public health nurse or visiting nurse may have worked in the family's home and have excellent insights. Any multidisciplinary consultations will be of value.

Reporting

Most states provide that reports of child neglect go to the Child Protective Services (CPS) Agency. Some states will have joint police and social work (CPS) reporting. Criminal charges under the rubric of "endangering the welfare of another" may be brought against some neglectful parents. However, the greatest number of neglect cases come under the supervision of CPS. Police involvement becomes almost essential in cases of abandonment, and police have special skills in locating a missing parent.

Informing Parents

Informing the parents is more difficult in cases of neglect. Responses may either be active or passive. The term "neglect" often triggers an active and angry response. This occurs because neglectful parents feel they are trying to parent as best as they can. Their perceptions of the neglect is different from those of the emergency department staff. This invariably creates conflict and evokes guilt and anger. When informing the parent, the focus should be on the child. The physician may need to verbally recognize the positive efforts of the parent. Nonetheless if the result in the child is inadequate, action needs to be taken to help the child. Taking this approach will often direct the parents' energy toward the child and sufficiently quiet emotional reactions.

The passive response may be equally disquieting to the physician. It may be seen in parents who are overwhelmed, inadequate personalities, depressed, intoxicated, or retarded. It may be difficult to separate these parental problems from one another. The physician may incorrectly assume that the parent does not care what happens to the child because of the lack of any response. With extremely passive parents, it may be difficult to even engage them in conversations. It is helpful to approach the withdrawn parent with simple questions that do not directly relate to the neglect. Often by initiating a neutral conversation the physician can learn about the parental problem. Asking the parent to perform a task that requires reading or writing may also be instructive. When informing the parent of the neglect report does not trigger active resistance, the physician may be left with an uneasy feeling that the communication was not clearly understood. However, repeat explanations may not stimulate more parental response.

Hospitalization

The need for hospitalization is dependent on several factors. Certainly if the child's physical condition warrants treatment, hospitalization is indicated. For example, a child failing to thrive in the first 6 months of life should be hospitalized. Another indication relates to the degree of parental dysfunction. If the parents are assessed as being so overwhelmed, withdrawn, depressed or inadequate that they are unable to assume parental responsibility, the child should be protected regardless of his/her current physical status. A third indication stems from the chronicity of neglect. Because of the indolent nature of neglect it may be necessary for the physician to make a point of hospitalizing a child in order to dramatize a chronic or recurrent situation. The final factor in determining the need for hospitalization is the time required for community agency response. If the report of neglect triggers an immediate investigation and institution of therapeutic services then the need for hospitalization will be diminished. The response to neglect reports will vary from community to community.

Follow-Up

It is very important in cases of neglect to arrange follow-up care to a physician or clinic. Often the step of informing the receiving physician is overlooked. Hopefully, the staff providing the long-term care will be one with the capacity to closely monitor patients and to become aggressive about failure to keep appointments. The treatment of neglected children is often a long and frustrating process. Thus, special referral resources should be sought. Attempts to provide treatment in standard health care facilities may be doomed as the passive and indolent character of neglect affects the child.

EMOTIONAL ABUSE

Emotional abuse is the form of child abuse that most seriously and most often affects children. With every episode of physical or sexual abuse, there is a negative psychological message being inflicted. The child is told "You are bad!" and often comes to believe this. When the bruises, burns and broken bones are healed, psychological injury may remain untreated. The neglected child also feels devalued and unloved. Emotional abuse always accompanies other forms of abuse and at times is inflicted independently.

Yet, this form of abuse is the least well understood. Furthermore it is unusual that a report of suspected abuse is based solely on emotional abuse. It is difficult to gather enough objective data to prove that emotional abuse has occurred. Courts and legal authorities remain unconvinced that a given parental behavior or set of behaviors can be shown to be responsible for effects in the child. Emotional abuse rarely results in a psychosocial emergency. More often, like neglect, it is a chronic impediment to normal growth and development.

BACKGROUND

Emotional abuse has been defined in many different ways. The National Center for Child Abuse and Neglect defines it simply: "Child abuse which results in impaired psychological growth and development. Frequently occurs as verbal abuse or excessive demands on a child's performance and results in a negative self-image on the part of the child and disturbed child behavior." The Pennsylvania Child Abuse Law provides for reporting serious mental injury which is defined as ". . . a psychological condition determined by a psychologist, psychiatrist or pediatrician, and caused by the acts or omissions of a parent or person responsible for the child's welfare which: (1) renders the child chronically and severely anxious, agitated, depressed, socially withdrawn or in reasonable fear of his/her life; (2) makes it extremely likely that the child will be chronically and severely anxious, agitated, depressed, socially withdrawn, or be in reasonable fear that his/her life is threatened; or (3) seriously interferes with the child's ability to accomplish age appropriate developmental milestones or school or community tasks or peer relations."

The Pennsylvania Law identifies some of the potential manifestations of emotional abuse but leaves the difficult issue of a child's behavior as "caused by" an act or omission on the part of the parent. The issue of causality hampers the reporting of emotional abuse. In Pennsylvania there has been a decline in the number of emotional abuse reports as shown in Table 68.5.

The incidence of emotional abuse is unknown. There are not even reasonable estimates of its frequency. It must be the most frequent form of abuse, as it occurs with all other forms of abuse and neglect as well as independently.

DYNAMICS

Emotional abuse occurs when a parent attacks, belittles, humiliates, or devalues a child. Such behavior is not the infrequent reaction of a normal angry parent. It is an often repeated message to the child. An emotionally abusive parent appears to be determined to verbally destroy their child. The reasons for this behavior are many. All of the dynamics responsible for physical abuse may be operative for emotional abuse. Frequently there is a strong component of poor parental self-image. The child either threatens the parent or reflects unwanted parental characteristics. In either case, the parent is unable to withstand the stress and attacks the child. When there are many children in a family, a parent may scapegoat the one child with whom they most identify. At times the child may be identified with another family member such as an estranged father or a grandparent.

Helfer has capsulized the intergenerational nature of emotional and physical abuse in his "World of Abnormal Rearing" formulation. (Fig. 68.12). The child who is told repeatedly that he/she is "bad" and "worthless" will eventually accept it. Once the belief that "I'm no damn good" exists, the child's behavior will match the expectation. Ultimately the poor self-image will be reflected in the inability to choose friends, a mate, and to accept help. The cycle is completed with poor parenting and emotional abuse of the next generation of children. The intergenerational potential for emotional abuse makes it a serious public health problem.

MANIFESTATIONS

Emotional abuse manifests in many forms including children who are excessively withdrawn and passive and those who are aggressive and acting out. The manifestations are so varied that it is difficult to identify any constant characteristics of the emotionally abused child. In order to identify emotional abuse, the physician must witness family interactions on repeated occasions. It is not often that the emergency department physician has the opportunity for such comprehensive evaluation.

Infrequently, more direct presentations of emotional abuse may be seen in the emergency department. Some children may seek hospital asylum because of excessive fear of their parents. Adolescent "runaways" may include a subset of children who are emotionally abused. Developmental delay may be recognized in the emergency department but rarely can the cause of the delay be identified. Finally, children with drug or alcohol abuse may be a high risk group for prior emotional abuse. The effects of emotional abuse closely parallel the findings in children with substance abuse, e.g. poor self-image, difficulty in establishing relationships.

Another group of emotionally abused children frequently seen in the emergency department are youngsters caught in the conflict between estranged parents. These victims have been called "Yo-Yo" children because they are pulled between arguing parents. At times the children are virtually kidnapped by one parent. These presentations to the emergency department will be based on one parent's attempt to document the poor parenting or neglect of the other. The misuse of the child as a pawn in the marital dispute constitutes emotional abuse. Despite the credibility and motivation of the parent in the emergency department, emotional abuse should be reported to remove the child from the middle.

MANAGEMENT

The management principles for emotional abuse are the same as those for other forms of abuse. In order to substantiate emotional abuse, documentations of behavior must be precise. The physician, nurse, and social worker must record observed interactions in behavioral terms while using a minimum of subjective assessments and personal conclusions. Recording significant statements from the parties is good documentation. It may be necessary to cite a pattern of abuse or repeated episodes of abuse in order to strengthen a report.

It is often difficult and painful for parents to see themselves as emotionally abusive.

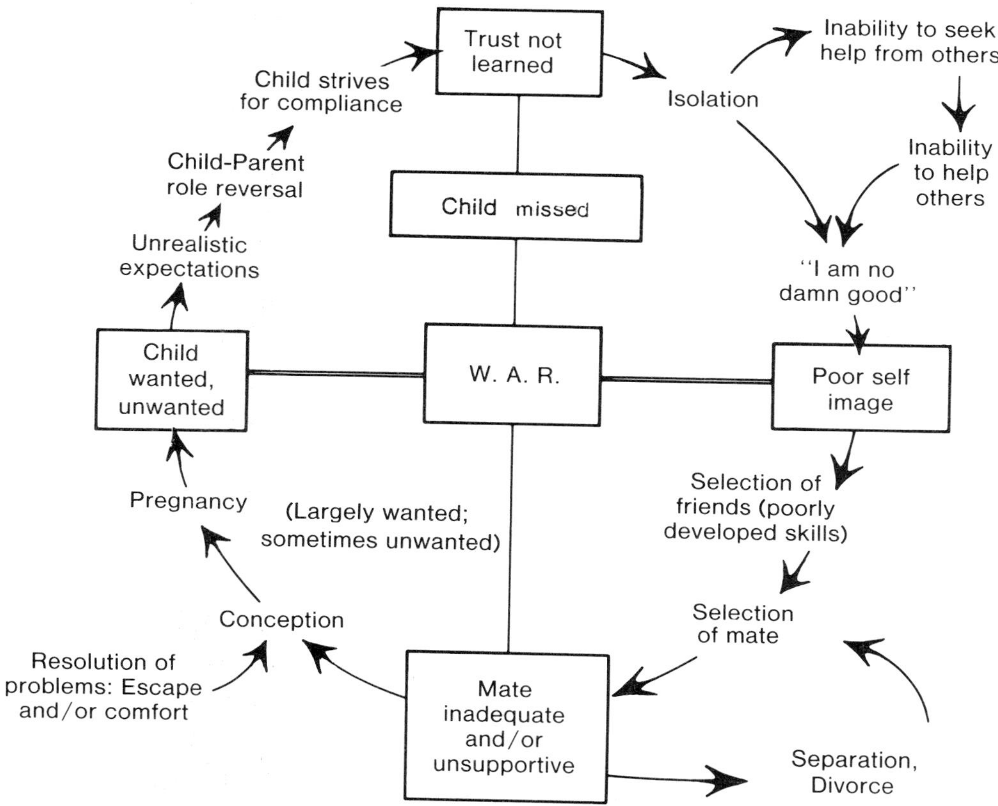

Figure 68.12 World of Abnormal Rearing (W.A.R.) (Adapted from R. E. Helfer.)

Thus, informing the parent in a constructive and sensitive way is very difficult. The informant must keep the discussion child-focused and nonaccusatory. Child welfare agencies and the family court system also have difficulty in identifying and treating emotional abuse. As the rights of children become more well established and standards for child care more widely accepted, management of cases of emotional abuse will become less difficult.

References

General

Gil DG: *Violence Against Children: Physical Abuse in the U.S.* Harvard University Press, Cambridge, Mass., 1970.

Goldstein J, Freud A, Solnit AJ: *Beyond the Best Interests of the Child.* The Free Press, New York, 1973.

Green FC: Child abuse and neglect; a priority problem for the private physician. *Pediatr Clin North Am* 22: 329, 1975.

Helfer RE: Why most physicians don't get involved in child abuse cases and what to do about it. *Child Today* 4: 28, 1975.

Helfer RE, Kempe CH: *The Battered Child,* Ed. 2. University of Chicago Press, Chicago, 1974.

Kempe CH, Helfer RE: *Helping the Battered Child and His Family.* J. B. Lippincott. Philadelphia, 1972.

Kempe, CH, Helfer RE: *Child Abuse and Neglect. The Family and the Community.* Ballinger, Cambridge, Mass., 1976.

Kempe CH, Silverman FH, Steele BF, Droegmuller W, Silver HK: The battered child syndrome. *JAMA* 181: 17, 1962.

Ludwig S: A multidisciplinary approach to child abuse. *Nurs Clinic North Am* 16: 161, 1981.

Newberger EH, Reed RB, Daniel JH, et al.: Pediatric social illness; toward an etiologic classification. *J Pediatr* 60: 178, 1977.

Schmitt BD (ed.): *The Child Protection Team Handbook.* Garland Publishing, New York, 1977.

Wilkerson, AE (ed.): *Rights of Children.* Temple University Press, Philadelphia, 1974.

Physical Abuse

Caffey J: On the theory and practice of shaking infants. *Am J Dis Child* 124: 161, 1972.

Eisenbrey AB: Retinal hemorrhage in the battered child. *Childs Brain* 5: 40, 1979.

Ellerstein NS: The cutaneous manifestations of child abuse and neglect. *Am J Dis Child* 133: 906, 1979.

Ellerstein NS (ed.): *Child Abuse and Neglect: A Medical Reference.* John Wiley & Sons, New York, 1981.

Feldman KW, Schaller RT, Feldman JA, et al.: Tap water scald burns in children. *Pediatrics* 62: 1, 1978.

Helfer, RE, Slovis TL, Black M: Injuries resulting when small children fall out of bed. *Pediatrics* 60: 533, 1977.

Kogertt MS, Swischuk LE, Fagan CJ: Patterns of injury and significance of uncommon fractures in the battered child syndrome. *AJR* 121: 143, 1974.

O'Neill JA, Mescham WF, Griffin PP, et al.: Patterns of injury in the battered child syndrome. *J Trauma* 13: 332, 1973.

Rogers D, Tripp J, Bentovima et al.: Non-accidental poisoning; an extended syndrome of child abuse. *Br Med J* 1: 793, 1976.

Schwartz S, Woolridge SD, Stege D: Oral manifestations and legal aspects of child abuse. *J Am Dent Assoc* 95: 586, 1977.

Slosberg E, Ludwig S, Duckett J, Mauro AE: Penile trauma as a sign of child abuse. *Am J Dis Child* 132: 719, 1978.

Sopher IM: The dentist and the battered child syndrome. *Dent Clin North Am* 21: 113, 1977.

Thomas PS: Rib fractures in infancy. *Ann Radiol* 20: 115, 1977.

Touloukian RJ: Abdominal visceral injuries in battered children. *Pediatrics* 42: 642, 1968.

Zimmerman RA, Bilaniuk LT, Bruce D, et al.: Computed tomography of craniocerebral injury in the abused child. *Radiology* 130: 687, 1979.

Sexual Abuse

Branch G, Paxton R: A study of gonococcal infections among infants and children. *Public Health Rep* 80: 4, 1965.

Burgess AW, et al.: *Sexual Assault of Children and Adolescents.* Lexington Books, Lexington, Mass., 1978.

Kempe CH: Sexual abuse, another hidden pediatric problem. *Pediatrics* 62: 382, 1978.

Peters JJ: Children who are victims of sexual assault and the psychology of offenders. *Am J Psychother* 30: 398, 1978.

Searles RM: Incest. *Pediatr Clin North Am* 22: 633, 1975.

Sgroi SM: Sexual molestation of children. *Child Today* May–June 18, 1975.

Emotional

Elmer E: *Fragile Families, Troubled Children. The Aftermath of Infant Trauma.* University of Pittsburgh Press, Pittsburgh, 1978.

Elmer E, Gregg GS: Developmental characteristics of abused children. *Pediatrics* 40: 596, 1967.

Galdston R: Observations on children who have been physically abused and their parents. *Am J Psychiatry* 122: 440, 1965.

Green AH: Psychopathology of abused children. *J Am Acad Child Psychiatry* 17: 92, 1978.

Martin HP: *The Abused Child. A Multidisciplinary Approach to Developmental Issues and Treatment.* Ballinger, Cambridge, Mass., 1976.

Neglect

Burgess RL, Conger RD: Family interaction in abusive, neglectful and normal families. *Child Dev* 49: 1163, 1978.

Giovannoni JM, Billingsley A: Child neglect among the poor; a study of parental adequacy in families of three ethnic groups. *Child Welfare* 49: 196, 1976.

Homer C, Ludwig S: Categorization of etiology of failure to thrive. *Am J Dis Child* 135: 848, 1981.

Hufton IW, Oates RK: Non-organic failure to thrive; a long-term follow up. *Pediatrics* 59: 73, 1977.

Polansky NA, Borgman RD, DeSaix C: *Route of Futility.* Jossey-Bass, San Francisco, 1972.

Polansky NA, Chalmers MA, Buttenwieser E, Williams DP: *Damaged Parents: An Anatomy of Child Neglect.* University of Chicago Press, Chicago, 1981.

Sills RH: Failure to thrive; the role of clinical and laboratory evaluation. *Am J Dis Child* 132: 967, 1978.

CHAPTER **69**

Sudden Death or Catastrophic Illness: Family Considerations

JOEL E. FRADER, M.D., AND JOHN SARGENT, M.D.

INTRODUCTION

People in our society react in a distinctive fashion to the catastrophic illness and/or death of a child: they are overwhelmed. We are no longer primed to accept the high infant or childhood mortality of the era before antibiotics and modern emergency medical care. We no longer learn cathartic rituals or socially patterned behavior for coping with major childhood medical problems. Yet, tens of thousands of children die each year from sudden infant death syndrome (SIDS), or as accident victims, or increasingly, as victims of homicide or suicide. These, and the many more with serious acute illnesses or injury, are brought to emergency departments for care, resuscitative efforts, or pronouncement of death. Emergency medical personnel must be prepared to help the families, as well as the sick children.

A medical crisis in a child evokes special feelings and behavior in us. Sudnow, a sociologist who has studied large municipal hospital emergency departments, has written that emergency department staff members routinely adjust the degree of their resuscitative attempts on the basis of the patient's age: ". . . the time which will elapse between that point at which breathing noticeably ceases and the heart audibly stops beating and when the pronouncement of death is made, will differ according to [the patient's] age." As adults, we are expected to provide proper care and supervision for children. Thus, we experience the loss, or threat of such loss, of a child's life as the breaking of a special trust. This special relationship between children and adults, especially within the family, requires us to pay systematic attention to the needs of grown-ups, particularly parents, who are close to sick or dying children.

Kubler-Ross and others have delineated the grief of the dying. Much of that work can be applied to situations faced in emergencies when a child has died or is gravely ill. Families and others close to the patient experience a range of emotional reactions. They may *deny* the illness or death, be *angry* at what has happened, attempt to *bargain* to revive or preserve the child's life, become overtly withdrawn or *depressed*, and eventually *accept* the grim reality.

Some concrete manifestations of these responses and suggestions for their management can be found below. The current understanding of the grief work of parents was developed by careful observations of the families of children with chronic fatal diseases. The many reports or studies about parents of children who have died of SIDS have taught us about the evolution of emotional reactions over days, weeks, or months. However, our knowledge is more limited with regard to helping families cope with the immediate stresses of medical catastrophe or death.

Relatively little has been done to elucidate the immediate stress or turmoil that families experience while in emergency facilities. Thus, there is much that is controversial or even contradictory in the literature. The following paragraphs offer a reasoned approach based on knowledge of the field and clinical experience. We urge emergency medical personnel to develop an organized, practical method for helping families of acutely ill, dying, or deceased children. This will be more easily accomplished and the advice offered here will be more useful if employed by a regular team that self-consciously and critically reviews its activities periodically.

MAKING CONTACT

Of primary importance is the rapid establishment of clear communication with the family. The parents and others should not be left totally unattended outside closed emergency department doors, while a team of doctors and nurses attends to the patient. Experienced personnel should engage the family immediately, ask if anyone else should be notified of the illness or accident, and provide, as much as possible, a private setting for further discussion. The importance of family liaison by an experienced individual, be it nurse, physician, or social worker, cannot be overemphasized. Families in crisis may tax the skills of even those who are most resourceful at providing support to others.

As quickly as practical, a physician who has appraised the medical situation should report available facts directly to the family. The doctor can then answer and ask questions. Keep in mind that a medical history from the family may provide crucial information in the management of the patient. Ideally, the physician informing the family should maintain contact throughout the family's stay in the emergency department. Continuity and consistency minimize confusion and permit the family to develop a much needed relationship.

To whatever extent reasonable, the family should be spoken with as a group. If this cannot occur, the emergency department's staff should communicate directly with each parent. In the midst of the medical turmoil and uncertainty that inevitably accompanies critical injury, illness, or death, family members cannot be expected to absorb, accurately recall, and then transmit information to spouses or other key figures.

Emergency facilities are often chaotic. For parents worried that a child is dead or dying, it is especially important to ground conversations with them in the "here and now." Concreteness can be very helpful. Emergency department staff members should introduce themselves with names, position (e.g., staff physician, head nurse, etc.), and professional relationship to the patient and/or family. Thus, a social worker or nurse should state that he or she is there to attend to the family's needs. An attending physician, at some point, should let the family know that she or he is responsible for the child's medical care. This provides a substantive statement that the patient has personal care and establishes the need for the doctor to return to the child.

Families deserve clear and concise statements of fact. If the child has been pronounced dead, this information should be provided directly. No amount of "soft-pedaling" will attenuate the parents' reaction to the truth. Straightforwardness should not be confused with brutality, however. Cold, disinterested statements, followed by the physician's flight from contact unnecessarily add to the parents' pain. Social and psychological studies of patient and family satisfaction and malpractice suit patterns suggest that physicians whose attitudes may be interpreted as uncaring are much more likely to be sued than more compassionate appearing colleagues, regardless of their medical-technical competence.

When immediate announcements of death are not in order, emergency department personnel who are with the family should make every effort to provide periodic short, lucid summaries of the child's condition, as it is perceived, and actions being taken to help the patient. The number of emergency department personnel who provide information to the family should be minimized. This will help avoid inconsistencies and discrepancies in what is told to the parents. It is useful to request that the parents state their assessment of the situation. Having them give their view provides an opportunity to evaluate their understanding and correct any misconceptions they articulate.

As mentioned before, a careful medical history can be very valuable. Eliciting information about a bleeding tendency could be very helpful with an injured child. For a child with cardiovascular collapse a history of recent contact with military personnel could be a clue to fulminant meningococcal disease. Determining possible exposure to chemicals or access to drugs might lead to life-saving treatment of a toxicologic emergency. Aside from providing information which may aid diagnosis or treatment, giving a history can be a therapeutic experience for the family. In telling the medical team about their child, parents participate in the treatment. The family should be told the value of their contribution. Recognition of their own role may decrease the feeling of separation from the child and the helplessness they feel while emergency medical measures are being instituted.

PROVIDING SUPPORT

Having heard the history, therapeutic listening has only begun. Families may experience a gamut of emotions and behaviors when a child's life is threatened. Grief reactions can be quite physical and frightening for parents. They may feel weak or short of breath and have unusual sensations, including hallucinations or a physical sense of being removed from others around them. The emergency department staff needs to anticipate the possibility of parents reporting such experiences. Family members should be reassured as necessary that these sensations are to be expected and will pass with time. It may be helpful to interpret the symptoms as signs of attachment to the injured, sick, or dead child and the experience as an indication of how the parents feel the child as a part of themselves. In addition, they may be told it is all right to openly express or demonstrate their grief while in the emergency department. Parents may also find themselves visualizing images of the child from time to time. These mental pictures may be of the child when they last saw him or her well, in a hospital bed, or in some favorite place or activity. These "visions" are not indications of impending craziness or "losing one's mind." Wishes by parents that they, rather than the child, were sick or dead are also normal. Such thoughts are not truly suicidal; they do deserve a reassuring response.

Those who work with parents of dying/dead children find it helpful to encourage parents to review the place that their child has had in their lives. Often parents will recall special moments that they have shared with their son or daughter, their hopes and plans for the child, perhaps times when the boy or girl has misbehaved or angered the parents. Though telling these stories may be intensely sad for everyone, it focuses the family's thoughts on the child, helping to make the current situation more real.

During the time that parents and others are talking, the staff should observe family interaction. If the parents make frequent eye or body contact, complete sentences for one another, and indicate balance and reciprocity in their behavior, the family will likely do well. Professional intervention, in the form of encouragement to the parents to attend to each other's needs, may be advisable if family members stand or sit apart, seem not to heed the words of others, persistently interrupt others, or pursue widely divergent thoughts with the staff.

ALLAYING GUILT

Inevitably the parents' thoughts turn to guilt. Family members find ways to feel responsible for the accident, illness, or incident that led to the injury, suffering, or death. Moreover, parents often assume that others—spouse, grandparents, or medical personnel—also blame them. If the family does not express guilt freely, one should not assume that it is not there. The doctor, nurse, social worker, or other emergency department professional must raise this issue with the family. It is important to do this in a way that does not suggest accusation. It may be reasonable to say something like, "Parents in your situation may blame themselves for their child's death (illness). Do you have any thoughts of that sort?"

Parental guilt involves a sense of having failed the child. Even when there was no way to predict or prevent the event leading to the child's difficulty—as in SIDS—parents feel they ought to have known something was wrong and acted to change the outcome. The parents' fantasies may even lead them to believe that they were directly responsible for an injury or death. Stories such as those related by Bergman and Beckwith in their writings on SIDS are not uncommon. One parent wrote the Seattle, Washington, SIDS Center: "I told everyone that I had smothered her sometime during the night." Thus, whenever possible, parents should be disabused of the many myths about causes of death or disease that are pertinent to the situation. For example, families should be told that SIDS is not caused by suffocation, choking, or similar mechanisms.

Because misinformation is extremely widespread, it is useful to ask families their ideas about the etiology of the child's problem. It should not be assumed that the family's thinking parallels common medical ideology. An open mind and an attentive ear concerning parental fantasies or concerns about what has happened to their child must be maintained.

It is helpful to let parents know that their guilt is expected and understandable and that it is not an aberration. One might add that accidents or sudden illness are features of life. Parents might be reassured that they could not possibly have anticipated or eliminated all the risks of normal existence without excessive protection of their child and the consequent throttling of a child's growth and independence. The parents might also be warned that their extended family, neighbors, or other acquaintances may not be so understanding. In the event that they encounter such hostility, parents should be told to avoid arguments and to urge the offender to contact the medical team for enlightenment.

Emergency department personnel should not expect that their comforting words will have an immediate palliative effect. Such a belief will inevitably lead to staff frustration and disappointment. Parents may not even "hear" the reassurance at the time. Explanations or instructions may need to be repeated many times. However, families frequently relate that words said to them in the midst of crisis are recalled later with good effect. Parents will remember that the emergency department staff did not accuse or threaten them. Assuming the family respects the medical professionals that they encountered, this may be instrumental in easing their pain.

It may not always be possible to truthfully absolve the guilt. Parents or others may, in fact, be responsible for the child's difficulty. They may have been negligent in preventing an accident, delayed in seeking needed medical care, or actually inflicted harm. Should this be the case, it is not appropriate to be glibly reassuring. Nor, however, is the emergency department the place for confrontation. A high level of self-consciousness should be maintained in such situations. Monitoring one's thoughts and deeds should allow the doctor, nurse, social worker, or other professional to excuse himself or herself when personal feelings overtake the interaction with the family.

A therapeutic approach to justifiable guilt and anger is not fostered by disingenuous comforting. A better outcome is likely with acknowledgment of responsibility where it exists and an effort made to have the family recognize that part of their grief work will be accepting the facts of the case. It may be helpful to consider the reason the parent acted as he or she did. In situations where one parent has been caring for a child when an accident occurs, it is often the case that the absent parent harbors angry feelings toward the "negligent" parent. In one recent case in our institution, a father told us of his desire to put his wife's hand into the house's main electrical supply as punishment for her "allowing" their son to be accidentally electrocuted in the bathtub. Only after open discussion of his feelings with his wife and the physician was he able to accept her remorse and give up his desire to punish her. It made a difference to the father that his wife had meant no harm to the child. Again, it may be wise to encourage expression of this anger when it does not arise spontaneously. One need only reflect to the family that such feelings are normal and common and deserve to be aired to allow for many parents to feel comfortable in speaking up.

Another kind of anger may also be important. Anguished families may lash out, sometime uncontrollably, at the medical staff. Health professionals may find themselves accused of incompetence, of being uncaring, or of lying to the family. If there is no rational basis for such hostility, the providers must resist taking the comments personally and search for any specific meaning that the accusations might have. For instance, if the family feels that the doctors are not adequately assessing the medical situation, one might ask them if they have had previous disappointing experiences with the medical profession. Simply asking why the parents feel the way they do may bring forth an expression of sadness. If no exploration of the anger bears fruit, it is often helpful to simply reiterate the feelings, saying: "It must be very hard for you to have your child so sick (or dead)."

If empathic expressions do not seem helpful, it is important to remember that listening to or simply sitting with the family may be all that is necessary. Silence may be a very valuable therapy. The verbal orientation of middle or upper class health professionals may be quite alien to some families. The family may simply need time to assimilate all that is happening to them. The doctor, nurse, or social worker who finds him or herself talking animatedly with little reaction from the family should take notice. Self-examination may lead to the realization that one's own anxiety or discomfort are interfering with the parents' ability to experience the tragedy in their own way. Finally, defensive or punishing withdrawal from the suffering family is not justifiable and there is virtually no reason to respond to the family's anger in kind.

CULTURAL AND SOCIAL INFLUENCES

Medical care professionals may have considerable difficulty with the many different ways people respond to stress. This is especially true now that people from virtually all backgrounds use the scientific medical care system. That is, many ethnic and social groups who previously shunned hospitals now turn to medicine as a last resort. People may no longer be completely content with traditional, cultural, or religious rituals or behavior patterns in the face of what the dominant culture defines as a medical crisis. Thus, it is important to be open and sensitive to the background and preferences of distraught or bereaved families. One family may wail and moan while another sits stony faced and silent. Each reaction may be culturally conditioned and psychologically healthy. Medical professionals should also take care to avoid imposing preconceived notions of behavior based on the family's socioeconomic group or ethnic heritage. Individual and family responses to sudden and grave illness or death of a child are very idiosyncratic. Much disservice has been done by well meaning health professionals who have misinterpreted Kubler-Ross's stages of grieving and gotten upset with dying patients or bereaved loved ones who do not "complete" all stages of the death and dying "protocol." Emergency department personnel should not commit similar errors because of ethnic stereotypes.

The unpredictable nature of people's responses has two very practical implications. First, individuals should be given the opportunity to define their own needs. Thus, a parent may desire a very detailed and technical explanation of the resuscitative efforts being undertaken or the cause of a death. Another relative may want only broad and simple descriptions. Second, and related, needs within a family may vary tremendously. It is ill advised to assume that because one parent wishes to cry openly with you that the other will want to also. One may wish to talk in relatively intellectualized terms about the child or their own feelings. Parental differences, however, may correspond to sex-role stereotypes. Fathers characteristically have greater difficulty expressing grief and requesting emotional support. They may need explicit permission to do more than "carry" others through the stressful time by maintaining worldly routines. These differences between parents are a potential source of discord and should be addressed directly. The emergency department staff member responsible for family counseling should ask how the family has dealt with crisis in the past. He or she should then ask how that experience can help family members to understand and support one another. If obvious conflict emerges in response to this question it should be discussed openly.

In this age of frequent separation and divorce, the staff should be aware of parent's hostility to one another and each parent's legal relationship to the child. In the event of conflict, the legal guardian, of course, must be respected. However, whenever possible any necessary consent should be sought from both parents.

If only one parent of a divorced or separated couple is present, an offer to contact the other family member should be made. If this is declined, the staff member should determine how and when the parent in attendance plans to notify the absent mother or father. The answer may help emergency department personnel evaluate the couple's relationship and thus provide clues to the emotional reactions of the parent before them.

The stress of a serious illness or death may arouse feelings of loss associated with the failed marriage. Parents who previously cooperated well in joint child-rearing following divorce may suddenly express great anger at one another. In such a situation, the staff should attempt to focus parental attention on the child's immediate needs and each parent's part in meeting those needs. The parents might also be individually encouraged to seek their own help and support during the crisis.

There is a difference between assessing family members' behavior patterns in response to crisis and inappropriate intervention which may break down defenses. An assessment is necessary for matching the staff's efforts with the parents' needs and desires. There is rarely a right or wrong way to react to the threatened or actual loss of one's child. Unless the particular defensive style of the family members interferes with what individuals must actually do to help their child (e.g., refusal to give consent for emergency treatment) or themselves (such as accepting safe transportation home), parents and other relatives are entitled to their own methods of coping. There is no ideal grief.

ORGANIZING SOCIAL SUPPORT

Despite numerous warnings in the literature, well intentioned emergency department personnel commonly react to help family stress in reflexive ways. These actions include calling clergy from institutions of the family's religious organization, assuming that the presence of other family members is desirable and helpful, and thinking that the child's primary physician should be, or wants to be involved and that such involvement would be welcomed. It is essential to inquire about the family's actual wishes in these matters.

Catastrophic illness or death may lead some parents to feel very angry with God and to reject any involvement with a minister, priest, or rabbi. For other families, prayer or contact with the clergy may be welcomed. One need only ask.

Relatives are not always supportive. In a recent incident in our institution, a sister-in-law approached the mother of a nearly drowned boy and asked how the mother could have allowed this to happen to her nephew. Some family members may themselves require so much reassurance or care that their presence or participation is a burden. Not all families "come together" in times of need. Responsible medical professionals will not only ask the child's parents if they want help from others, but also monitor family interaction once a family gathers.

The role of the primary physician (or other primary care practitioner) can be quite complex. Almost every pediatrician has encountered tales of parents who bring SIDS victims to an emergency department crying that the baby had just been seen by the doctor and/or had an immunization. These parents are apt to be very angry. They may not want, at that time, to have anything to do with the "offending" physician. There is no reason to force them to do so. But three actions are essential here. First, the doctor, physician's assistant, or nurse practitioner should be informed of what has happened and the family's feelings. Second, careful explanation of the unpredictable and capricious nature of SIDS (or meningococcemia or epiglottitis, whatever the issue) must be given. Third, the family should be told that, because their doctor was involved with the child, he or she may be an important source of help in the days ahead.

There is another important aspect of primary physician involvement. It is not uncommon for doctors to experience considerable guilt and conflict when a patient suffers from a sudden catastrophe; even experienced pediatricians are not exempt from feeling that they may have prevented a SIDS death. When a child later dies abruptly or following heroic treatment in a tertiary care center, the primary physician may feel that he or she should have seen the patient sooner. Such guilt may inhibit the doctor from being an effective source of support for the family, even if the child's relatives bear no hostility. Thus, an apparently disinterested or unhelpful response from the primary care professional upon being notified of a patient's major medical problem should not occasion a judgmental reaction from the emergency facility staff.

SEEING THE PATIENT

Families may be helped in other ways. Of prime importance is the opportunity for parents to be and/or have physical contact with their child, whether undergoing treatment or dead. It is best to offer this choice without assuming that the family will actually want to see or touch the boy or girl. With a child who is critically ill, it is necessary to explain, in so far as possible, what to expect. Tell the family what equipment is in use, what tubes or catheters invade the child's body, and what the various personnel are doing. If a child's appearance is distorted because of accident or medical intervention, warn the parents ahead of time. After this verbal introduction, some family members may decide not to see the child. If so, let them know that the reality may not be as bad as they imagine, but it is not wise to force the issue. Those who elect to see the child will likely need to have the medical and technical information reviewed once they are in the treatment area. Encourage the family to touch the child. Parents may need permission to hug a dead baby, comb the hair of their comatose toddler, or otherwise behave as loving parents in the alien medical environment. It is essential that parents understand they have the opportunity to hold, speak to, or otherwise have contact with their child. It is often observed that this increases the parent's sense that the child is still real, not merely the object of the staff's activity. Remember that the parents will be feeling especially helpless at this point; their caring and protecting functions have been taken over by the medical professionals. Whatever the parents can do to retain their special relationship with the child will be helpful. Be certain to tell the family of any plan to move the child, such as to the operating room, intensive care unit, or an area where diagnostic tests will be done.

Much of the same advice applies to the situation when a child has died. The family should be told how the child will appear and feel when they touch their son or daughter. Many people are very frightened of dead bodies and have specific superstitions or beliefs about the deceased. It may be helpful to inquire about these and to ask if the family has any questions prior to seeing the body. Again, it is not wise to insist that parents actually see the child. While many believe that seeing and touching or more prolonged contact with the body helps families to accept the death, there is no established evidence that forcing such an encounter in any way aids the grieving process. As in other situations, the staff members' preconceptions have no place in dictating family behavior.

BEYOND THE DEATH

After a child has died, parents are often at a loss about what to do. The gamut of services that should be offered by the emergency department staff is quite broad. Initially, regardless of religious belief, many parents welcome or feel the need for some sort of cleansing ritual. This may be a few moments of silence together, the saying of a prayer, or simply a formal goodbye to the child. Opportunity for these should be provided.

Beyond this, many things need attention. Arrangements for funerals and/or burials must be made. It may be necessary to consult with law enforcement agencies (in the case of accident or suspected homicide), health department officials, or private legal counsel. Parents who have come to the hospital in ambulances need transportation home or to other shelter. Relatives and friends must be contacted. It is extremely helpful if a quiet and private place can be available for any of these activities.

AUTOPSY

The emergency department personnel should be familiar with state and local laws concerning the need to report a death to the medical examiner or coroner. In some areas, all sudden deaths must be referred to the authorities. In other places, the medical examiner need only be contacted when there is suspicion of death by other than "natural causes." In any case, whenever doubt exists, the responsible emergency department staff member should check with the proper authority prior to discussing autopsy with the family. This could avoid confrontation should the family refuse a postmortem examination, but the medical examiner later claim jurisdiction and decide to order the autopsy.

Assuming that there are no legal restrictions concerning autopsy the emergency department physician should be clear about why he or she is requesting the examination. Berger has lucidly summarized the personal and social values of autopsy. The parents may be told that in the case of sudden, unexplained death an autopsy may provide information that will affect other living or future family members through the discovery of hidden (inherited) congenital anomalies. (Congenital anomalies are among the five leading causes of death in children up to the age of 14 in Philadelphia.) For infants, Beckwith has said that 10 to 15% of all autopsies following sudden death will reveal a cause that does not fit the *classic* findings of SIDS. Some of these findings may have genetic implications; others, such as meningococcemia, may raise a public health concern. The information may well help the parents accept (when it is true) that they could not have altered the tragic course of events.

Some families may respond to the suggestion that autopsies may provide valuable information that may help parents and children in the future. This can be the case if the child has died following diagnosis of and treatment for illnesses where the disease process and/or the therapy are poorly understood. It is also true where accidents are the presumed cause of death. Autopsy information may lead to suggestions or legislation for improved safety devices or development of new treatments for the immediate postinjury period.

When autopsy is elective, permission for autopsy is best obtained in person in a straightforward manner. As in other situations, it is helpful if consent is sought by the emergency department physician who has established the closest relationship to the family. The views of both parents should be solicited, if possible. If there is disagreement, the family's questions should be answered and they should be offered an opportunity to discuss the matter privately. The family should be informed that they may be able to specify restrictions on the examination. If permission for an optional autopsy is declined, the reasons for refusal should be requested. Only if the refusal is based on misunderstanding of what is being asked should vigorous attempts be made to dissuade the family.

FOLLOW-UP

Before the parents of a child who has died leave the emergency department, it is imperative arrangements be made for follow-up with the families. Suggestions in the literature for when to see the family vary tremendously. One can find recommendations for a first phone call or visit in as few as 2 or 3 days, to as long as 6 months. If there is to be an autopsy, the next contact with the family could be to discuss preliminary findings. This is especially important in the case of unexplained sudden death. Most workers in this field agree that a session with the family should take place within a month. At that meeting, there should be a review of the circumstances of the death, the parents' and doctors' actions and emotions in response to the death, and any new information that is available. Pathology departments should be informed of the planned meeting and encouraged to have materials available by the appointed time.

In the event of sudden infant death, if there is a SIDS team in the area, the family should be told to expect a call and/or visit from the nurse or family worker. It may also be helpful to suggest phone contact between an emergency department staff member and the family shortly after the funeral. That time tends to be especially hard as the gathered extended family and friends return to normal activities. Parents and immediate family may be left, for the first time, to face their grief, now compounded by loneliness. Thus, a supportive conversation with a hospital staff member may be welcomed.

Whether additional meetings of the emergency department personnel with the family, beyond the first follow-up visit, would be helpful must be assessed on a case by case basis. Many variables will affect the decision, including: the family's relationship to the emergency department staff and other health care professionals; the distance the family lives from the emergency facility; the family's coping at the time; and whether other supports are available. In any case, three suggestions may be helpful. First, the family should be provided with the names and telephone numbers of key figures involved with them and the child at the time of death. The family needs to know that they may call when they have questions or wish to talk. Second, arrangements should be made for an appropriate professional to evaluate the family's function between 6 and 12 months following the death. Only at that time can one begin to differentiate between natural continued sadness from the loss and potentially dangerous depression. By that time, family members should be moving toward reintegration with normal life patterns and improved effectiveness in work and daily activities. Their sleeping and eating patterns should be more regular, they should be less irritable, etc. Third, the family may be told about community resources, such as the Society of Compassionate Friends, that may be helpful to the bereaved.

CONCERNING OTHER CHILDREN

A word should be said about counseling families about the effects of childhood death on siblings. It is currently fashionable to recommend that the approach to other children should be matched to the child's developmental level. Unfortunately, many parents lack the energy or creativity for this effort in the midst of intense grief. Some parents will, in fact, ask medical professionals for assistance. A few general rules may be safely offered. Children, like their parents, may imagine the circumstances of a dead or dying child to be worse than the reality. If siblings are available to see their brother or sister in the emergency department, they too should be offered the chance to do so. As with their parents, they should not be forced to see or touch the body. The same open opportunity should apply to funerals and burial services. Children of this multimedia age are exposed to images of death very frequently. Even quite young boys and girls often have ideas about death that are astonishingly sophisticated. In any event, attempts to "protect" siblings from the sadness and misery are usually in vain. Their parents' behavior and the absence of the dead child will surely inform them that all is not well. Efforts to exclude children from important family rituals or to hide the grieving may only lead to fantasies that the surviving sibling is somehow responsible for the tragedy. There may also be resentment for being excluded from obviously important family activities. This fear of the hidden is exaggerated by natural childhood fantasies that involve harm or death to family members.

Parents should be reminded that childrens' questions should be met with candor. When siblings ask about death, they should be given simple, direct answers. Children should not be told that a brother or sister has "gone to sleep," "been taken by God because he or she was so good," or given similar euphemisms. These deceptions may lead to fears of going to sleep, as slumber is then equated with death, to conflicts about good behavior or pleasing God, and other confusions of immature minds. The importance of answering questions does not imply the need to give extensive lectures, nor a need to imply that the adults fully understand death. Detailed diatribes may be overwhelming and frightening to the children. As recently stated by Lorenzen and Smith, ". . . answers are not what the children need as much as to talk with someone and to be reassured that they are not alone."

ORGANIZATIONAL ISSUES

Encountering death or major devastating illness is only somewhat easier on medical professionals than on families. This is especially true for emergency facilities where dying or critically ill or injured children are seen frequently. Though one can "become expert" or develop professional defenses with the experience of working with the families of many suddenly dead or catastrophically ill children, sadness and a sense of failure can be expected with each new tragic event. Given the likelihood that confrontations with mortality will have a major emotional impact on the staff, it is wise to develop, in advance, clear-cut plans for the treatment of the children and their families. Such plans will reduce the chaos of the moment and may help ease staff tension by providing a concrete set of activities. A check list of actions and procedures in the event of a death and/or a flow sheet for various contingencies may be useful (see Chapter 75, p. 1183).

Because of the need for sensitivity and the ability to function under significant pressure, it is best that responsibilities be clarified for each member of the emergency department team. Each person, whether permanent staff or trainee, should know what to do when. It may be best to spell this out in some detail. It might be specified that initial contact with and support of the family should be the responsibility of a staff nurse or social worker, or that an attending physician is expected to report to the family within 5 minutes of the patient's arrival. The point here is that deaths and resuscitations disrupt routines and may well produce confusion. In the worst of circumstances, everyone stands around the child's stretcher gaping with little organization or leadership, while the family is cut off outside, without knowledge or support. Clear protocols may improve this all too frequent circumstance.

A related point is that staff members must be aware of their own limitations and should not be assigned nor accept responsibility in areas where they are not confident and effective. This requires a high level of self-consciousness and a reliable amount of observation and feed-back among the staff. Competence in working with these families depends, in part, on the achievement of some degree of acceptance of death. The effective medical professional cannot maintain an inflexible notion of the "correct" behavior of families faced with tragedy. Substantial efforts should be made to monitor one's own performance and those of colleagues in these situations. In this regard, it may be wise to allow "recovery time" for staff members involved in an unsuccessful resuscitation. A period of 15 to 30 minutes might be set aside for those who wish an opportunity to reflect on the experience or escape from the emergency department.

Constructive self-criticism can be useful. Regular sessions for review and teaching ("in-service" education) should be instituted. The handling of deaths and resuscitations should be discussed at regular intervals. These sessions should have a specific method and time set aside for talking about psychosocial issues. Team members should evaluate their performance in working with the family, just as they scrutinize how well intravenous access was obtained or medication given. If this is not done, it is quite likely that the discussions will be exclusively biotechnical in nature. Defensive avoidance of the difficult emotional issues should not be permitted. In this regard, the presence of someone with skills in group dynamics and family counseling may be extremely helpful.

A crucial part of this educational effort is

explicit attention to the feelings and beliefs of the staff. Because the death or near death of children is so troubling, staff members suffer from the same self-doubt, hostility to others (whether a child's family or medical team colleague), and depressing helplessness as do the parents. These feeling can and should be worked through. Without opportunity to do so, it is difficult to sustain a sense of effective group action; resentment and covert undermining of others may emerge. Staff members should be alert to signs of "burnout." Loss of job effectiveness and satisfaction, irritability, persistent lateness or frequent sick leave, the appearance of drug or alcohol problems and the like, may signal the need to change an individual's responsibilities. Such behavioral manifestations of discontent may be unrecognized by the unhappy worker; an empathic, rather than a confrontative, approach will likely be successful. Skillfully led group sessions can help clarify mutual interdependencies and foster a sense of shared purpose and achievement. Ultimately, of course, such team building will improve patient and family care.

References

Berger L: Requesting the autopsy; a pediatric perspective. *Clin Pediatr* 17: 445, 1978.

Bergman AB: Psychological aspects of sudden unexpected death in infants and children; review and commentary. *Pediatr Clin North Am* 21: 115, 1974.

Bergman AB, Pomeroy MA, Beckwith JB: The psychiatric toll of the sudden infant death syndrome. *GP* 11: 99, 1969.

Binger CM, Ablin AR, et al.: Childhood leukemia; emotional impact on patient and family. *N Engl J Med* 280: 414, 1969.

Friedman SB: Psychological aspects of sudden unexpected death in infants and children. *Pediatr Clin North Am* 21: 103, 1974.

Friedman SB, Chodoff P, Mason JW, Hamburg DA: Behavioral observations on parents anticipating the death of a child. *Pediatrics* 32: 610, 1963.

Kennell JH, Slyter H, Klaus MH: The mourning response of parents to the death of a newborn infant. *N Engl J Med* 283: 344, 1970.

Kubler-Ross E: *On Death and Dying.* Macmillan, New York, 1969.

Lindemann E: Symptomatology and management of acute grief. *Am J Psychiatry* 101: 141, 1944.

Lorenzen M, Smith L: The role of the physician in the grief process. *Clin Pediatr* 20: 466, 1981.

Mandell F, McAnulty E, Reece RM: Observations of paternal response to sudden unanticipated infant death. *Pediatrics* 65: 221, 1980.

Sahler OJF (Ed.): *The Child and Death.* C. V. Mosby, St. Louis, 1978.

Smialek Z: Observations on immediate reactions of families to sudden infant death. *Pediatrics* 62: 160, 1978.

Sudnow D: *Passing On: The Social Organization of Dying.* Prentice-Hall, Englewood Cliffs, N.J., 1967.

Weinstein, SE (Ed.): Mental Health Issues in Grief Counseling—Summary of Proceedings: Mental Health Issues Related to Sudden Infant Death Syndrome. DHEW Publication No (HSA) 80-5264, Rockville, Md., 1979.

CHAPTER **70**

Psychiatric Emergencies

GORDON R. HODAS, M.D., AND JOHN SARGENT, M.D.

INTRODUCTION

In contemporary American society, the emergency department of the hospital has become a major community resource. It is open 24 hours each day, professionally staffed, and utilized by the community for assistance in dealing with a multitude of physical, social, and emotional problems. The emergency department is the setting for the initial evaluation of a variety of difficulties of children and their families, including acute and chronic illnesses with their emotional sequelae, psychophysiological conditions, family crises, and the entire spectrum of emotional and behavioral disorders. Emergency department visits of children with social and emotional difficulties have been estimated to have more than doubled in the past 10 years. Although there may be significant disagreement between the medical staff and the community concerning appropriate uses of the emergency department, the emergency department staff must, nevertheless, respond to the problems which are brought to it. Therefore, physicians working in emergency departments must master the skills of psychiatric diagnosis, crisis intervention, and disposition planning.

Crisis and Crisis Intervention

Psychiatric emergencies are best understood as crisis situations. Crisis involves the acute development of circumstances or events that render the usual coping and adaptive patterns of an individual or social unit inadequate. Most crisis situations during childhood are handled effectively by the child's family. However, in some instances the child's behavior or the overall situation becomes unmanageable. It is at such a point that professional help is sought, and the child may be brought to the emergency department. Typically, the family members feel overwhelmed and helpless. There may be severe anxiety, disagreements among various caretakers, and disruption of previously stable family relationships.

Psychiatric emergencies in childhood may be defined as crises in which the adults around the child no longer are able to help him to master his anxiety and no longer provide support and control of his emotional reactions and behavior. Any psychiatric emergency in childhood implies a failure of effective interaction of the child and his caretakers. For example, the suicidal child is seen by his family as being uncontrollably self-destructive and needing professional help. However, his suicidal state also reflects the family's inability to assist him in developing alternatives other than suicide. Comprehensive assessment and treatment of psychiatric emergencies in childhood should involve the participation of the child's family. In this way the family, with professional support, can resume its role in guiding the child's emotional and behavioral development.

Psychiatric crises are not just times of intolerable stress for the family; they are also unique opportunities to bring about change. When a family brings a child to the emergency department with an emotional problem, the crisis created by the problem has overcome the usual tendency to deny difficulties and maintain the status quo. Because family coping patterns are failing and denial is lessened, intervention at this time can be used to modify rigid patterns and to create alternative solutions. Thus, family crises are nodal points where the possibility for family change is maximized and where interventions can extend beyond the amelioration of the presenting concern and have lasting impact.

It follows that the goal of the emergency department physician is not to merely alleviate the crisis per se but to use the crisis to create meaningful change. The physician will need to maintain within the family a sense of urgency which will enable them to respond positively. The emergency department physician therefore needs to be able to assess the immediate crisis and to appreciate through observation and history taking how the family has become ineffective. Crisis intervention techniques in the emergency department address not only the presenting complaint but also the underlying problems which have given rise to it.

Requirements of the Emergency Department

The ability to respond effectively to psychiatric emergencies of children and families requires special capacities of the emergency department. The emergency department should have a pre-existing relationship with a mental health team that is committed to providing child psychiatric consultation around the clock. The emergency staff must be capable of collaborating effectively with this mental health team. Requests for psychiatric consultation should provide a clear statement of the *problem* and the *goal* of the consultation. To enable adequate response, the degree of *urgency* of each request should be clearly stated. When the consultant arrives, the emergency department staff should describe in detail their findings and any interventions made thus far. The emergency physician and the consultant should discuss how to proceed throughout the remainder of the emergency department visit. Such clarification will not only be useful in the current situation, but will also foster mutual respect in the future.

Adequate physical space is another requirement of the emergency room. There should be a designated place where psychiatric emergencies can be assessed, where interruptions will be infrequent. This room should have seats for each family member and the emergency physician. The availability of a separate room for psychiatric emergencies enables a mood of concern and deliberation to be achieved. The emergency department should also have a holding or observation room where certain children, such as those recovering from overdoses or those being stablized on psychotropic medication, can be observed and evaluated regularly. Such a room should be adequately staffed by nurses as well as security personnel when indicated, and the capacity for using restraints should also be present.

The emergency department should also have relationships with various psychiatric inpatient units so that hospitalization, when needed, can be arranged efficiently. Of particular value are brief, crisis-oriented inpatient units which involve the child and the family in problem focused treatment. The staff should be thoroughly familiar with the procedures for psychiatric hospitalization, including the specific legal requirements for involuntary commitment. In certain situations, such as children recovering from medically serious suicide attempts, medical hospitalization may be necessary. The hospital should have specific guidelines for the management of psychiatric patients on medical floors.

Finally, the emergency department should have relationships with other social agencies and an awareness of relevant laws. The police should be aware of which children to bring to the emergency department for psychiatric assessment and should be prepared to remain in the emergency department until adequate security has been arranged. Relationships should be developed with temporary shelters and other crisis intervention centers, insuring effective referrals when necessary. Staff should be aware of child protective laws and the procedures for emergency intervention in situations of abuse and neglect.

Physician Responsibilities and Skills

The responsibilities of the emergency physician with psychiatric emergencies are:

1. To rapidly identify a crisis situation
2. To assess the nature and degree of stress for child and family
3. To develop specific approaches to the stressful situation, which may include:
   a. Utilizing a psychiatric consultant as the clinical situation requires, or
   b. Arranging appropriate disposition independently.

In order to effectively fulfill these responsibilities, the physician must possess a variety of clinical skills and the ability to block out other concerns when responding to psychiatric emergencies. The physician must be able to display empathy for the child's and family's distress. Once the family senses the physician's concern, they will be more responsive. The physician will need to handle the family's anxiety and uncertainty by approaching the family crisis calmly and systematically. In so doing, he establishes the leadership and authority which will enable the family to discuss their problems freely and to consider and act on his recommendations. Throughout the emergency department visit, the physician will need to foster the belief among family members that improvement in their situation will be achieved through appropriate changes in family members' behavior and relationships.

Another important skill of the emergency department physician involves the ability to obtain and assess relevant information about the child, family, and their community supports. This is covered subsequently under "Evaluation of Psychiatric Emergencies."

Family Responsibilities

A childhood psychiatric emergency implies a failure of effective interaction of the child and his caretakers. In our society, the child's caretaker has the major responsibility for promoting his growth and development. In many instances the child's caretakers are his parents; but, in some situations, grandparents, extended kin, foster families, and state agencies have legal custody of the child. It is essential for the emergency physician to establish who the child's actual caretakers are and to try to involve as many of them as possible in the emergency room. When evaluating the child, the caretakers, and their relationships with each other, the emergency physician should assess the degree to which the parents (or other caretakers) are meeting their responsibilities.

The first of these parental responsibilities involves providing support and nurturance, especially to younger children, such that an emotional bond is established between child and parent. When such an attachment is present, the child will desire parental approval and will usually respond to parental authority. Second, the parents need to provide enough socialization to set limits on the child's behavior. The physician will assess whether the limits chosen are appropriate, too rigid, or too weak. Third, the parents should promote their child's efforts in age-appropriate tasks. These include consistent school attendance and performance, learning to relate to peers, and assuming greater autonomy within the family as the child grows older. Fourth, the parents should try to instill a sense of competence and mastery in the child at each developmental level. This will allow the child to successfully integrate new knowledge and new experiences. Finally, parents should assist their child in coping with unexpected failures and losses. These may include academic disappointment, family disruption, and disability due to physical illness. By keeping these family responsibilities in mind, the emergency physician can assess families in crisis, determining which functions are being met and which are absent.

Working with Strengths

The emergency physician working with a family in crisis must look not only for problem areas but also for areas of competence in both the child and family. It is these areas of strength that form the basis for a successful treatment plan which enables the family to master the crisis. Typically, families in a crisis underutilize existing abilities as they pursue a narrow range of responses to the problem at hand. Through history-taking, observation of family interaction, and assessment of the way that the family relates to the physician, it is possible to identify the family's assets. Once recognized, these skills will enable the parents to be more confident and competent in dealing with their child. A family that has successfully raised its children up until now should also be able to respond effectively to new challenges that the children present. A family that has successfully dealt with aggressive behavior in a child in the past can utilize some of that previous experience in responding to the current crisis. A family with a disruptive or destructive child that successfully has brought the child to the emergency room, where he sits quietly, has more parenting skills than they may realize. It is the role of the emergency physician to help the family recognize their capabilities at a time when confidence is at its lowest level.

EVALUATION OF PSYCHIATRIC EMERGENCIES

The evaluation of acute psychosocial emergencies can be divided into four sections (Table 70.1). *Orienting data and relevant history* will indicate the general living situation and previous psychosocial adaptation of the child or adolescent patient. It will also provide a complete description of the presenting crisis, including apparent precipitants. *Medical history and physical evaluation* will determine the child's current physical status. The *mental status examination* of the child will provide information about the patient's current psychological well-being. A *family evaluation*, utilizing both history and observation of the family's behavior during the emergency department visit, will enable the physician to determine the family's ability to respond to the child's distress. By integrating these sources of information, the emergency physician will be well equipped to understand the crisis and to pursue appropriate treatment alternatives.

Table 70.1
Types of Necessary Information

1. Orienting data and relevant history
2. Medical history and physical examination
3. Mental status of the child
4. Family evaluation

Table 70.2
Orienting Data

Age of child, sex, race
Grade in school, name of school
Family address, type of neighborhood, parental occupations
Family composition:
- One or two parent family; approximate ages of parents
- Siblings of patient and their ages
- Other family members, if any, living in the home
- Other significant relatives and caretakers

Table 70.3
Relevant History

History of presenting crisis and apparent precipitants
Past episodes or other major psychosocial problems
Psychiatric treatment, past or current, for child or family
School performance of child
Child's relationships with siblings and peers

Orienting Data and Relevant History

Psychosocial orienting data, as shown in Table 70.2, provides information that enables the physician to appreciate the basic living situation of the child and family. This information can be quickly obtained and includes the age, sex, and race of the child, the child's grade in school, and the address and type of neighborhood where the family lives. Family composition includes who lives at home, what are their relationships to each other and to the identified patient, and who are the primary and secondary caretakers.

Relevant history, as shown in Table 70.3, builds upon the identifying information to provide a more complete description of the presenting problem. Historical information should include a thorough understanding of the current crisis and its apparent precipitants, as well as similar problems in the past and previous psychiatric involvement for either child or family. The recent school performance of the child and the adequacy of his relationships with peers and with family members should also be determined.

The history of the current crisis should be obtained directly by asking family members in turn to give their account. Usually, it is best to begin with the parents and other adults in the room. The physician must also obtain the child's version of the current difficulties. If the family does not provide a coherent history, it is the responsibility of the physician to guide the interview by interrupting respectfully and asking relevant questions. The physician can ensure his understanding of the problem by periodically summarizing what family members have said and then checking its accuracy. When accounts and opinions differ among family members, this should be made explicit. When important issues like suicidal thinking and severe depression are not brought up, the physician should inquire about them directly. This will reassure the family that their distress is understood and will enable the emergency physician to have all the relevant information needed for his assessment. As the physician gains control of the interview and obtains the necessary information, his own sense of confidence in dealing with the crisis will increase.

Medical Status of the Child

The physical status of the child must be determined during the emergency assessment. There are many diseases, as well as acute intoxications, that can mimic psychiatric disorders. In addition, psychiatrically impaired children may also have concomitant medical problems. Therefore, it is extremely important that the emergency physician obtain a thorough medical history of the child including current medication and possible medicines available to the child, followed by a complete physical examination including assessment of neurologic functioning. This information will be used in conjunction with the psychological aspects of the assessment to provide a complete picture of the child.

Mental Status of the Child

Evaluation of the child's mental status takes place throughout the entire emergency room visit. The mental status examination provides a psychological profile of the child at the same time that it assists in determination of psychiatric diagnosis. Generally, it is not necessary for the physician to perform a formal mental status examination of the child, since the relevant data emerges from history taking, the physical examination, and the interactions that the child has with family members and with the physician during the emergency assessment. It is important, however, that the emergency physician have a systematic and thorough understanding of the mental status examination. Table 70.4 lists the major categories of the mental status examination. These will be described as they apply to emergency psychiatric assessment.

Orientation. The level of consciousness and orientation of the child is the first area of assessment. The child not under the influence of drugs or with severe organic illness should be oriented in all spheres: person, place, time, and situation.

Appearance. The physical appearance of the child reveals important information about both the way the child feels about and cares for himself and the supervising

Table 70.4
Child Mental Status Examination

Orientation
Appearance
Memory
Cognition
Behavior
Relating ability
Speech
Affect
Thought content and process
Strengths
Synthesis of evaluation

care by the family. The examiner carefully observes such factors as physical size, personal hygiene, choice of clothes, neatness, grooming, posture, and gait.

Memory. The child's memory can be evaluated while listening to the history and through direct questioning. Impairment of memory in a child is strong indication that his emotional and behavioral disturbance may have an organic cause.

Cognition. Intelligence, fund of knowledge, and the ability to think and reason are evaluated while talking with the child. Intelligence and fund of knowledge need only be categorized as adequate or inadequate for the child's age.

Behavior. The child's behavior can be observed throughout the visit. Activity level may be at appropriate age level and goal directed, too rapid and random (hyperactive), or too slow and diffuse (psychomotor retarded). Behavioral tendencies are revealed in the child's talking with the examiner and in interactions with various family members. Psychotic youngsters may respond to people as objects and use objects in non-goal directed and bizzarre ways. Nonpsychotic children may behave in angry, aggressive ways which can usually be distinguished from psychotic children by the negative or resistant nature of the behavior. The child's ability to control his behavior in response to the examiner's or family's request should be carefully noted.

Relating Ability. The capacity of the child to relate to the examiner is a key element in the mental status evaluation. The examiner is, in a sense, a window to the outside world, and the degree to which a positive relationship can develop during the assessment suggests the child's current capacity for forming relationships in general. The examiner should be concerned with what occurs at any moment during the evaluation and, even more importantly, how the interaction evolves during the course of the visit. To what degree does the child offer eye contact and speak spontaneously? How trusting does the child appear to be, and to what degree does the child appear to desire the examiner's approval? On the other hand, is the child too friendly and open, suggesting extreme neediness? The child's cooperativeness and tendency to alter his mood in response to the examiner's support are important components of his capacity to relate.

Speech. Speech includes such elements as spontaneity, coherence, articulation, and vocabulary. As such, the category of speech overlaps with the capacity to relate, the quality of thought processes, and the level of intelligence. Poor vocabulary and articulation may suggest mental retardation, psychosocial deprivation, specific language disabilities, or combinations of the above.

Affect. The child's affect, or predominant feeling state, is assessed informally during the course of the interview. Fluctuations of affect according to changes in content and interactions should be carefully observed, with more serious concern raised by children whose affect does not change as different subjects are discussed. Depressed children may show both sad and angry affect, which suggests the way in which the child sees both himself and the external world. Some children become so well defended that their affect appears flat and constricted. Frankly psychotic children, in addition to blunted affect, show an inappropriate response to internal and external events, such as smiling while serious topics are discussed.

Thoughts. Thoughts include both thought processes and thought content. The evaluation of the preceding categories necessarily yield much information on thinking. Thought process involves the coherence and goal directedness of verbal communication. Evasiveness and guardedness must be distinguished from the looseness of associations of the psychotic child or adolescent. Loose associations have no logical coherence or connection with previous statements. Thought content involves the major themes that emerge as the child talks spontaneously and responsively to the examiner. If themes of violence and insecurity are present, are other more hopeful and positive themes also present? Such information can often be obtained by eliciting fantasy material, such as three wishes, personal goals, and views of the future. Self-concept, when low, may become apparent as persistent themes and fantasies are pursued. Thorough screening also involves determining the possible presence of psychotic phenomena (hallucinations, delusions, and ideas of reference) and present or past suicidality or homicidality.

Strengths. The purpose of any child's mental status examination is not only to screen for possible deficits but also to search for strengths and areas of competence in the child. Thus, it is crucial that the examiner determine areas of interest, competence, and motivation of the child. These strengths will go undiscovered unless specifically looked for. Thus, the role of the evaluation extends beyond assessment; it also involves, through the identification of strengths, the beginnings of positive interventions.

Synthesis. After the component parts of the mental status examination have been determined, the physician should integrate them into a comprehensive picture of the child. For example, a 14-year-old child presents to the emergency room fully alert and oriented but disheveled and malnourished. His cognitive abilities appear to be intact, but his actions are slow and labored. The child's thinking shows no evidence of incoherence, but themes of disappointment emerge from the conversation. The boy relates to the physician in a withdrawn manner, and appears to be preoccupied. The data from this mental status examination suggest that the adolescent described is depressed. This impression should then be integrated with historical, medical, and family information as the examiner plans appropriate treatment.

Family Evaluation

Physicians, while performing emergency assessments, explaining results of evaluations, and developing treatment plans, always deal with both the ill child and his family. Recommendations will depend in part on the physician's impression of the family and of how effectively the family will carry out the required treatment. In order to assess families, the physician needs to have an organized framework to guide the evaluation process (Table 70.5). The goal of a family evaluation for childhood psychiatric emergencies is to determine the methods that the family uses to help its members when distressed, the adequacy of these efforts, and the possibilities for new alternatives that will help the family to cope successfully with the current crisis. In obtaining the history from the family and proceeding with the assessment, the emergency physician should keep in mind these specific aspects of family functioning so that he can evaluate the family systematically during the emergency department visit.

Table 70.5
Family Evaluation

Family mental status
Family hierarchy and leadership
Protectiveness vs. encouragement of autonomy
Capacity for conflict resolution
Family problem-solving capabilities
Relationship with the physician
Ability to utilize community supports

The Family Mental Status

Just as it is important to know the child's mental status, the emergency department physician must also determine the mental status of the rest of the family. This can be done as the physician observes the family members and listens to their presentation of the history. The history should be coherent and logical, and should follow a temporal sequence. Families which do not present an organized history may have serious difficulties resolving crises. Family members under the influence of drugs or alcohol may not be fully alert and oriented. Their history may not be at all clear. A depressed parent will appear withdrawn and downcast. He may be so preoccupied with his depression that he does not focus effectively on the child's problem, or he may describe the problem in extremely hopeless terms.

While anxiety, distress, and even anger may be appropriate responses to a psychiatric emergency, parents should be able to utilize the physician's support to control these responses so that the crisis can be approached systematically. When this does not occur, the emergency physician should consider psychiatric consultation. Other indications for psychiatric consultation include the presence of psychosis or other severe psychiatric disturbance in a parent or caretaker. When the family presents a disorganized history, the physician can indicate that he is confused and ask for clarification. He can also suggest that only one person talk at a time, and can repeat back the history given and ask the family to confirm it. When these attempts to provide structure to the family fail, psychiatric consultation will be needed.

Hierarchy and Leadership in the Family

The family is a social system that requires acknowledged leadership which is consistent and whose direction is followed. Generally in American nuclear families, the parents are the acknowledged leaders with the responsibility to set rules that are respected and followed by the children. In many families, grandparents live nearby and help with the children, but they are expected to defer to the parents' plans and approaches. In other families, however, especially single-parent families, a grandparent may function as caretaker while the parent is away at work and the parenting responsibility is shared. In order for effective collaboration to occur, the specific roles for each caretaker must be explicit and agreed upon.

In two-parent families, specific parental roles and expectations must also be made explicit. In this way, undermining of one parent by the other is avoided and family rules are enforced consistently. Children are allowed to voice complaints, with the understanding that the parents are the final arbiters. In providing leadership, the parents utilize both closeness and distance in relation to the child at different times. The relationship between any parent and child involves closeness—the ability to be loving, nurturing, and supportive, and also involves distance—the ability to set and enforce limits and the willingness to allow the child some independence.

The emergency physician should be concerned when either excessive closeness or excessive distance characterizes the relationship between parent and child. An overly close relationship between parent and child may interfere with the parent's ability to establish and enforce rules. The parent may hold back either because he is unable to get angry at his child or because he fears upsetting the child by taking a firm stand. Overly close relationships are common in single-parent families, but may occur in two-parent families as well. Such relationships may be revealed in the emergency department when child and overinvolved parent are sitting close to each other (and apart from other family members, if present), when the parent answers for the child or describes how the child feels rather than encouraging the child to speak for himself, and when the parent uses the pronoun "we" while describing difficulties pertaining to the child individually.

The emergency physician can assess an overly close parent/child relationship in several ways. He can suggest that child and parent not sit so close to each other or can have the child switch seats with another family member. He can ask parental permission to speak with the child in the presence of the family, with only the child speaking for himself. He can point out the nature of the overly close relationship to the other parent and ask whether this is of concern to the less involved parent. When these interventions fail, psychiatric consultation is in order.

Excessively distant relationships occur in some disorganized families when parents are so involved with their own problems that the needs of the child are neglected. In such families the child is given more autonomy than is age appropriate, and rules are either nonexistent or enforced inconsistently. Such families may be unable to focus on the child's problem. The parents may be primarily concerned about the effect of the child's problem on their lives, and less concerned about the child's distress. The child may be scapegoated by the parents as the source of all the problems. Statements by such parents include "Why are you doing this to me?" "I have better things to do than to be in the emergency room with you," and "If it weren't for you, things would be going smoothly." Disengaged or underinvolved parents may also appear apathetic and unresponsive to the child's disturbed behavior.

In responding to an underinvolved family, the emergency physician should create an intensely serious mood and emphasize the gravity and danger of the situation. In some cases this will create a crisis that enables family members to actively respond to the child's distress. In other situations, however, the caretakers will remain unresponsive. When this happens, psychiatric consultation is required and hospitalization may be necessary.

Protectiveness vs. Autonomy

All relationships can be placed on a continuum of involvement, with intimacy at one pole and disengagement at the other. Effective parenting requires avoidance of the extremes and the capacity to shift from one position to another at different times and in different situations. As described above, some families have an overly close relationship between the child and one parent. This may occur in any family where there is significant conflict between the parents or between parent and other caretakers, e.g., grandmother. In addition, overinvolvement with a child may occur in families with a special child, such as one with a physical handicap or chronic physical illness. Parents in such families may be overprotective of the child, assuming functions for the child and speaking for the child. Overprotectiveness toward the child may involve primarily one parent or may involve the entire family. In such families conflict is often avoided, in order that the child not get upset. The child also may avoid disagreement out of concern for his parents. A consequence of parental overprotectiveness is diminished autonomy on the part of the child, who tends to be more involved with adults than with peers. In such situations, the child's development of independence is often significantly delayed.

Underinvolved families, on the other hand, provide insufficient protection and support for the child. The child learns not to expect parental support, and may present as unsocialized with a conduct disorder, or as depressed and possibly suicidal.

With overprotective families, the emergency department physician can assess the family's flexibility by suggesting that the child speak for himself and that the parents increase their expectations. When the overprotectiveness is rigid and severe, the physician may request psychiatric consultation as a way of initiating ongoing therapy for the family. With disengaged families that fail to respond to the physician's statement of urgency, psychiatric intervention should be pursued.

Conflict Resolution vs. Conflict Advoidance

All families have disagreements among their members. In some families disagreements are acknowledged and confronted directly, while in others potential conflict is consistently avoided. Some families disagree openly but are unable to reach a constructive resolution. The capacity of the family for conflict resolution is an important area for the emergency physician to assess, because unresolved disagreements typically lead to chronic hostility, undermining, and ineffective parenting. Families that tolerate and resolve disagreement are usually more open in their discussion of family problems, whereas conflict-avoiding families utilize a great deal of denial. In some families the presence of conflict becomes apparent as the history is given. Family members provide differing accounts of the history and may interrupt and contradict each other. The tension in the room increases and the physician may start to feel anxious. In such circumstances the emergency physician can indicate the need to hear from each family member one at a time and suggest that everyone take a turn. He can also summarize the family's account as he goes along, confirming information at the same time that tension in the room is controlled.

Families that are unable to resolve conflict usually have significant marital problems. The parents, unable to deal effectively with each other, instead become overinvolved with one of the children. The child may have a chronic illness, may be either the oldest or the youngest, or may be chosen for another reason. The child gets caught in the marital struggle of the parents, in part through their efforts and in part through his own desire to remain close to the parents and keep them together. This child frequently develops physical and psychiatric symptoms and may present to the emergency department with the family.

The emergency physician may observe several possible patterns of conflict avoidance. The parents may agree that the only problem in the family is the child, and that, were it not for him, everything would be fine. However, the physician notes that the parents do not look at each other or talk to each other. Their one common ground of agreement is the scapegoated child and his symptoms. In a related pattern, the parents suppress all conflict by focusing excessive concern on the symptomatic child, who is seen as vulnerable and weak. This frequently occurs in families with a child with psychosomatic symptoms, where the child is overprotected and his symptoms are exacerbated by family conflict. The third pattern involves parental utilization of the child and his symptoms as the battleground for all parental and spouse disagreements. The parents deny the existence of any disagreements except those related to the identified patient, about whom they disagree openly and angrily.

The emergency physician will request psychiatric consultation when inability to resolve conflict has seriously impaired the functioning of the family and the child. Psychiatric involvement should also be sought when patterns of conflict avoidance occur in conjunction with other aspects of family dysfunction described in this section.

Capacity for Problem Solving

Families in crisis usually try to solve their problems by attempting the same solutions over and over again. They perceive other remedies as currently inaccessible or impossible. As a result, the family's repertoire of behaviors becomes extremely limited and their responses to problems are stereotyped and rigid. As the physician pursues historical information and observes the family, he looks for signs of flexibility and strength. The physician asks about the family's previous attempts to solve the presenting problem and seeks their ideas on how to approach the difficulty now. While offering his observations, the physician notes whether his ideas are accepted or rejected. When asking family members to behave differently now, he observes how hard they try to change and evaluates the probability that these changes will enable the family to manage their crisis.

In order to change, disagreeing parents must find a way to put aside their differences in the interest of the child and the family. These parents must develop a mutually acceptable plan for responding to their child's unsatisfactory behavior. Thus, the parents must soften their rigid and polarized positions. For example, a father who harshly states that the child needs strong punishment and a mother who is adamant about not upsetting the child must both change their positions. The emergency physician will try to help the parents to find an acceptable middle ground so they can resume control of their family. When these attempts fail, psychiatric consultation should be sought.

Relating to the Physician

The emergency physician should place considerable confidence upon his overall impression of the family and how they relate to him. Do family members maintain eye contact with the physician, or do they avoid looking at him and display guardedness or a sense of hostility? Families that accept the physician's expression of interest and concern are more likely to benefit from the emergency department visit. Families that are suspicious of the physician's motives and unresponsive to his input will probably gain less from emergency interventions. The emergency physician needs to recognize that those families that antagonize him the most may also be the families that most need his (and the psychiatrist's) interventions. When feeling anger toward the family, the physician must decide if these feelings should be expressed. For example, the physician may feel offended by a family that repeatedly criticizes a child whom he likes. He may feel like rebuking the family for being unfair and want to defend the victimized child. However, such feelings, if acted upon, would only compound the problem, since the family would single out the scapegoated child even more when the physician is no longer present. On the other hand, in other circumstances, expressing one's feelings may be extremely helpful. For example, the physician may tell denying parents that his ideas are being rejected too readily. Such a statement may lead the family to reconsider the validity of the physician's statements.

Utilizing Social Support

Some families come to the emergency department feeling isolated, overwhelmed, and exhausted. Frequently such families have not utilized all of the family and community resources available to them. Effective crisis intervention for psychiatric emergencies involves not only emergency room treatment but also effective disposition planning for the family. The emergency room staff should determine what untapped community resources are available to the family. The parents should be asked about relatives or neighbors who might be able to help them. Families that have previously mobilized community supports should be commended by the emergency physician for their competence and resourcefulness. Very often this support by the physician stimulates the family to recognize their capacity to address the crisis.

Integration

In following the above guidelines for family evaluation, the emergency physician completes the necessary data for understanding the family in crisis. By integrating the history, the physical examination, the child's mental status, and the family assessment, the emergency physician will be able to intervene effectively to the benefit of both child and family.

DEPRESSION

BACKGROUND

The appreciation of depression in childhood and adolescence as a highly significant problem has increased greatly in recent years. Depression can refer to the symptom of feeling sad or can describe a symptom complex or syndrome which includes cognitive and physiological components in addition to affective ones. Depression implies more than momentary sadness, and involves a pervasive inflexibility of sad mood, accompanied frequently by self-deprecation and suicidal ideation. Depression also implies a change in functioning from an earlier state of relatively good adjustment, rather than a temperamental or personality type.

Since there is no generally agreed upon definition of depression, incidence figures vary according to the definition used, as well as the nature of the population studied. In one study of high school students aged 11 to 15 years in suburban Boston, 33% of these early adolescents were felt to have moderate to severe symptoms of depression. Other estimates put the incidence of depression in children and adolescents in the 20% range. The incidence of depression is higher in children with school problems, including learning disabilities and attention deficit disorder, and in children with significant medical problems. Since most children with depression come to the emergency department with another chief complaint (somatic symptoms, school problems, or behavior problems), the physician must keep in mind the possibility of depression in all children seen with recurrent or vague somatic complaints.

There is considerable evidence to suggest that a genetic predisposition exists for depression, particularly severe depression. Depressive episodes may be triggered by environmental events of significance to the child.

The depressed child typically experiences a profound sense of helplessness, feeling unable to improve an unsatisfactory situation. The child may be experiencing frustration and failure at home, at school, and with peers. Negative outcomes reinforce the child's negative self-image, which contribute in circular fashion to more negative outcomes.

CLINICAL MANIFESTATIONS

Depression presents differently at different stages of development. In infancy, depression is usually due to loss of mother and/or lack of nurturance, and presents as a global interference of normal growth and physiological functioning. Thus, some of the manifestations of depression in infancy would include apathy and listlessness, staring, hypoactivity, poor feeding and weight loss, and increased susceptibility to infection.

During latency, depression can present as part of a syndrome, or may be masked by other presenting symptoms. Petti describes the two key features in childhood depression as dysphoric mood and self-deprecatory ideation. Dysphoric mood is manifested by looking or feeling sad and forlorn, being moody and irritable, and crying easily. Self-deprecatory thoughts are reflected by low self-esteem, feelings of worthlessness, and suicidal ideation. Depression in this age can also present as other common symptoms, including multiple somatic complaints, school avoidance or underachievement (including learning disabled children or children with attention deficit disorder), angry outbursts, runaway behavior, phobias, and firesetting.

Depression in adolescence presents more like adult onset depression. The major symptom is a sad, unhappy mood and/or a pervasive loss of interest and pleasure. Other symptoms may include a change in appetite, change in sleep behavior, and psychomotor retardation or agitation. Also present in many depressed teenagers are loss of energy, feelings of worthlessness or excessive guilt, decreased ability to concentrate, indecisiveness, and recurrent thoughts of death or suicide. Depression in adolescence can also present with somatic complaints, academic problems, promiscuity, drug or alcohol use, aggressive behavior, and stealing. Many teenagers with behaviors like these are unaware of their depression, since it is not on the surface. Others simply deny the painful depressive affect. By talking with these patients about their lives at home, at school and with peers, the underlying depression usually becomes apparent.

MANAGEMENT

Once any presenting medical concerns have been dealt with, the three major goals in the management of depression involves (1) determining suicidal potential, (2) uncovering acute precipitants, and (3) making an appropriate disposition.

The emergency treatment of depression can usefully be thought of as the prevention of suicide attempts. The task of the physician is to carefully determine whether or not any suicide attempts have been made and whether suicidal ideation is present. The physician should not be hesitant about asking the child about suicidal deeds, thoughts, or wishes. Such questions represent a positive confrontation of the problem of depression and are unlikely to catalyze a subsequent suicide attempt. In fact, questions about suicide may actually provide a sense of relief for the depressed child.

The physician should attempt to determine possible acute precipitants of the current depression, since this will guide subsequent recommendations. The duration of the depression should be determined, as well as the family response. It is important to assess overall adjustment at home, in school, and with peers, and to look for the strengths of child and family for use in the treatment plan.

When suicidal ideation is present, the emergency department physician should request psychiatric consultation. A decision can then be jointly made regarding outpatient or inpatient treatment. Whether or not suicide is an imminent danger, the task of the physician is to create a sense of hope that things will improve. In order to do this, the physician must form a solid doctor-patient relationship with child and family. Outpatient management can be utilized when adequate social support is present. It is important that the parents first acknowledge the existence of depression in the child and then come to understand that the solution will involve a strong commitment on their part, including at times their participation in family therapy. The physician can begin the process by helping the family to draw up a list of areas in the family that will need to be addressed. Another area frequently needing attention with a depressed child is the school. School consultation as therapy begins may provide valuable information about the child and can help the child to obtain academic remediation when needed. The emergency physician can assure child and family that school difficulties will be addressed in outpatient therapy.

Psychotropic drugs, in particular the tricyclic antidepressants, have been used in adolescent depression. They are not approved for use in children, and there is controversy over whether to use such medication in children under 12. In general, it is not advisable for emergency physicians to prescribe antidepressant medication, since they have a high potential for serious damage through overdose and their desired mood elevating effect generally requires several weeks to take effect. In addition, the act of prescribing medication in the emergency department may decrease the likelihood of family members pursuing ongoing outpatient mental health treatment.

With adolescents, the antidepressants may be used adjunctively as part of the treatment. With drugs such as Tofranil (imipramine) and Elavil (amitriptyline), the usual starting dose is 25 to 50 mg. This may be gradually increased to as much as 100 mg/day in children. In some adolescents, doses in the adult range of 150 to 200 mg/day are needed. The emergency physician should be aware of the major side effect of antidepressant medications. Of concern with tricyclics is the possibility of arrhythmias, especially when doses exceeding 10 mg/kg of body weight are used. Cardiac arrhythmias are reportedly less common with Sinequan (doxepin), and the newer agents, Ascendin (amoxapine) and Ludiomil (maprotiline), a tetracyclic drug. The most common side effects of antidepressant drugs are drowsiness and those due to the anticholinergic effects of these drugs which include dry mouth, constipation, and blurred vision. These side effects sometimes improve as the drug is continued; in other cases, reduction in dosage may be necessary. Chapter 48, "Toxicologic Emergencies," covers the management of specific toxic ingestions.

SUICIDE ATTEMPTS

BACKGROUND

Suicidal behavior involves thoughts or actions which may lead to self-inflicted death or serious injury. A distinction is made between suicidal ideation and suicidal attempts in which a deliberate attempt to take one's life occurred.

There is reason for alarm about the increasing trend toward suicidal behavior by children and adolescents. Suicide attempts by ingestions occur 5 times more often than all forms of meningitis in children between the ages of 5 to 14 years. Suicide attempts have been estimated to account for 44% of all psychiatric emergencies in children and almost 50% of all adolescent psychiatric emergencies.

Incidence figures of suicide tend to be low, because many suicide attempts are either not reported or are called "accidents." In addition, it is impossible to determine how many accidental deaths, particularly car accidents, are in fact suicides. The problem is compounded with latency aged children, since National Vital Statistics do not classify suicide as a cause of death in children under 10 years. Despite these limitations in data gathering, suicide is now known to be the third leading cause of death, after accidents and homicide, in persons between 15 and 24 years. During the period 1965 to 1975, the rate of attempted suicide in this age group doubled. For children between 10 and 14 years, the rate of completed suicide reportedly tripled in the years from 1955 to 1975. Suicide attempts have been reported in children as young as 5 years old. In a study by Pfeffer of latency aged children between 6 and 12 years sequentially admitted to a child psychiatry inpatient service, 72% of the children were found to have suicidal ideas, threats, or attempts. In another study of children ages 7 to 17 years seen in an outpatient psychiatry facility, over 80% of depressed children had suicidal ideation at one time during their depression.

It has been estimated that girls attempt suicide at least 3 times more often than boys but that boys succeed twice as often. Overall, 80% of suicide attempts are by ingestion, but a recent study of latency aged children showed a strong preference for jumping in contemplated and actual suicide attempts.

Suicide can be seen as the final common pathway for a variety of situations in which the child experiences a pervasive sense of helplessness, with a perceived absence of alternative solutions. To the distressed child, suicide appears to be the only solution to his problems and also to the family's problems. Most suicide attempts occur in depressed children. Others occur with children experiencing major losses, such as serious illness or death in the family. A small but significant percentage of suicide attempts occur in psychotic children and adolescents. These may be deliberate (due to hopelessness) or accidental (due to impaired judgment and reality testing).

A factor that complicates the discussion of suicide in children is their differing conceptions of death at various ages. Up to age 5, death is seen as a reversible process in which the activities of life still occur. From 5 to 9 years, the irreversibility of death is beginning to be understood but death is personified, rather than seen as an independent event. It is not until about age 9 that death is seen as irreversible in the adult sense of being both final and inevitable. Even then, however, the child may imagine his own death as being reversible. Under such circumstances, a suicide attempt may have a different meaning than with an adult, where suicide corresponds to a definite end of one's life.

CLINICAL MANIFESTATIONS

In latency aged children, certain risk factors have been identified that distinguish children with suicidal behavior from other children with emotional problems. Suicidal children are likely to be depressed and hopeless. Self-esteem is low, and they see themselves as worthless. The wish to die is present, as are preoccupations with death. The family history may include past episodes of parental depression and suicidal behavior. Suicidal children tend to view death as temporary and pleasant rather than irreversible.

Teicher has pointed out that suicide in teenagers is usually not an impulsive act. Prior to the suicide attempt there have been problems in the family for at least 5 years. These include a parent or close relative attempting suicide, many residential and environmental changes, and unexpected separations from meaningful relationships (divorce, separation, or death). With the onset of adolescence, an escalation phase occurs in which frustration results from the teenager's desire for autonomy and his belief that his parents do not understand. The teenager withdraws or rebels, becoming alienated from his parents at a time when he really still needs them. The scene is then set for the final stage, in which some precipitating event leads to the suicide attempt. The precipitating event may be a peer rejection, the breakup of a romance, an unwanted pregnancy, and problems in school (it was found that 36% of children attempting suicide were not enrolled in school at the time of their suicide attempt).

Table 70.6 indicates the high risk situations for suicidal behavior in which direct questioning about suicide should occur. The first two situations immediately alert the physician to the danger of suicidal behavior. The other situations involve a different chief complaint masking possible suicidal ideation or behavior. All accidental ingestions should be screened for the possibility of a suicide attempt. Overtly depressed children are at risk for suicide, as are depressed children who present with somatic complaints. Children who have acted violently are also at risk, since violence can be turned inward. Psychotic children present a special problem and may present with inadvertent suicide attempts, the result of impaired judgment, hallucinations, and delusions of persecution. The isolated withdrawn child may harbor suicidal thoughts, which will only be uncovered by direct questioning.

MANAGEMENT

Assessment

The emergency room physician should specifically ask about suicidal thinking in all high risk children. When an actual attempt has taken place, the physician should attend to any medical needs such as suturing, lavage, and managing physical repercussions of overdoses. Then he should conduct his own assessment as well as requesting psychiatric consultation.

We disapprove of the dichotomy sometimes drawn between suicide "attempts" and suicide "gestures." We regard all sui-

Table 70.6
High Risk Situations for Suicide

Suicide attempt just made
Suicidal threat made
"Accidental" ingestion
Child complains of depression
Medical concerns but child appears depressed
Aggressive violent behavior
Psychotic child
Significant withdrawal by child

cidal behavior as suicide attempts, which are best evaluated by appreciating the medical *lethality* of the act and the suicidal *intent* of the child. The lethality of a suicide attempt by itself may be misleading, since suicidal children may miscalculate, causing at times greater harm than was intended and at other times less harm than was intended. As an example, the child who takes 10 tablets of his mother's tricyclic antidepressant medication, Tofranil 100 mg, could make a fatal miscalculation, since 1,000 mg of Tofranil can cause fatal arrhythmias in children. On the other hand, a child who takes 10 aspirins may be far more suicidal than the lethality of his ingestion would suggest. In general, more violent methods of attempted suicide (hanging, shooting, jumping) usually reflect greater suicidal intent. But the physician cannot conclude that attempts with low lethality are not serious attempts until he has specifically asked about the child's suicidal intent—e.g. just how seriously the child wanted to end his life.

In addition to asking directly about suicidal intent ("When you took those pills, what were you hoping would happen?"), the physician should gather as much information as possible about the attempt itself in order to help him infer the degree of suicidal intent on the part of the child. Did the child take all the pills that were available, did he expect to wake up, did he tell anyone after taking the pills, did he leave a suicide note? Now that he is awake, is the child pleased or displeased to be alive? Does he intend to try again?

Children who threaten suicide without making an actual attempt should also be questioned carefully about suicidal intent. How long has the child considered suicide, what methods are planned, when will this take place? Has the child ever made previous attempts? How about other family members? There should be particular concern with psychotic and depressed children, especially when the parents appear unable to supervise the child.

The physician should ask the child and family about possible precipitating events, in order to determine what changes in the environment may be needed. The strengths of the family should be assessed, to determine if sufficient social support exists to allow for outpatient management.

Evaluation for Hospitalization

There are no universally agreed upon criteria for when to hospitalize a child with suicidal behavior and when to manage on an outpatient basis. Garfinkel and Golombek have identified seven areas to assess in order to determine whether or not hospitalization is indicated (Table 70.7).

Social set involves the degree of privacy that the child had at the time of the attempt. Did he tell anyone before or after the attempt, or did he take pains to set up a situation in which detection was unlikely? *Intent* may be reflected in a suicide note left by the child, by the degree of detail of the suicide plans, and by direct questioning of the child regarding his suicidal intent at the time of the attempt and at the time of examination. The choice of *method* also helps in the assessment of the suicide attempter. Was a method with high lethality used or desired? Did the child understand the likely outcome of the method used? With an ingestion, were all available pills consumed? The *history* will reveal both the presence of past suicide attempts by the

Table 70.7
Areas to Assess Following a Suicide Attempt

Social set
Intent
Method
History
Stress
Mental status
Support

child and past attempts by other family members. The evaluation of the *stressful precipitating events* is important in planning disposition, as is the *mental status* of the child in the present and in comparison to the past. Finally, the degree of *support* expected from within the family and outside the family (peers and teachers) must be assessed. The decision to hospitalize the child is made when the child's safety is still in doubt after these questions have been answered.

In general, we believe that any suicide attempt deserves a thorough assessment by the emergency physician and a complete psychiatric consultation. Hospitalization should be utilized under the following circumstances: (1) the physician has had difficulty in gaining the cooperation of the child and family, (2) the child had made a serious suicide attempt and continues to have strong suicidal intent, (3) the child is psychotic, (4) the family appears unable to provide necessary supervision and support to the child, and (5) there is rapid denial by child and family of the significance of a serious suicide attempt.

Initiating Treatment

The basic goal in dealing with suicidal behavior in a child is to increase the commitment on the part of child and family to finding alternative solutions to the problems that have arisen and to increase communication between parents and child.

The parents should be encouraged to let the child know that they disapprove of suicide and want to see their child survive. The family should be told that, whether or not hospitalization is employed, they still have the primary responsibility for their child. The child should be told that he has a responsibility to himself and his family to keep himself alive.

If inpatient treatment is required, the child and family should be informed about how the hospital works and what to expect. The goals of the hospitalization should be discussed, and the role of the family in the treatment emphasized. In many states voluntary consent forms need to be signed. In instances where the parents or the child do not agree to hospitalization, involuntary commitment may need to be utilized. Whenever possible, the child and family should be accompanied to the psychiatric hospital by the consultant psychiatrist so that the transition to the psychiatric facility is made smoother.

Outpatient management of suicidal behavior becomes feasible when: (1) the child and family are cooperative and engageable, (2) the attempt was not too serious, (3) the child is not actively suicidal or psychotic at the time of the evaluation, and (4) the family can take responsibility for the child until formal psychiatric treatment is begun the next work day. Before sending a family home, the psychiatrist or emergency department physician should have the family formulate a concrete plan concerning how they will manage the child. The expectations and responsibilities of each family member, including the suicidal child, should be spelled out.

Outpatient psychotherapy can begin immediately with emergencies that occur during the work day. When outpatient treatment cannot begin until the following day, the physician should give the family a therapist's name or the name of the "intake person" at the mental health agency. This personalizes the agency and increases the chances that the family will follow through. The family should be instructed to use the physician's name as the source of referral and should be reassured that the physician will contact the agency prior to the family's call. This will also enable the agency or the psychiatrist to contact the family if the family fails to follow through in making an appointment to be seen.

PSYCHOSIS

BACKGROUND

Psychosis is the term used to describe severe disturbances in a patient's mental functioning. It is manifested by marked aberrations in cognition, perception, mood, impulses, and reality testing. Thoughts and feelings are not well integrated and acted upon, perceptions may become distorted so that the world is seen as threatening, and mood may become ecstatic or despondent. Behavior may also become extremely agitated and potentially violent, or excessively withdrawn to the point where the patient does not recognize and attend to his physical needs. It is important to remember that psychotic patients are actively attempting to regain control over their mental capacities and are trying to understand and deal with highly unusual thoughts, perceptions and impulses. Their subjective experience very often is one of helplessness and extreme anxiety.

Psychosis in childhood and adolescence can be divided into two groups based on etiology—organic psychosis and psychiatrically based psychosis. Psychiatrically based psychosis in children and adolescents has four major causes. These are: (1) infantile autism with onset prior to 30 months of age, (2) pervasive developmental disorders with onset between 30 months of age and 12 years of age, (3) adult type schizophrenia with onset in adolescence, and (4) manic depressive illness with onset in late childhood or adolescence. Emergency management of organic psychosis and the four major types of psychiatrically based psychosis will be described below.

Table 70.8
Medical Conditions Which May Lead to Psychosis

Central nervous system lesions
- Tumor
- Brain abscess
- Cerebral hemorrhage
- Meningitis or encephalitis
- Temporal lobe epilepsy

Cerebral hypoxia
- Pulmonary insufficiency
- Severe anemia
- Cardiac failure
- Carbon monoxide poisoning

Metabolic and endocrine disorders
- Electrolyte imbalance
- Hypoglycemia
- Hypocalcemia
- Thyroid disease (hyper and hypo)
- Adrenal disease (hyper and hypo)
- Uremia
- Hepatic failure
- Diabetes mellitus
- Porphyria

Rheumatic diseases
- Systemic lupus erythematosus
- Polyarteritis nodosa

Infections
- Malaria
- Typhoid fever
- Subacute bacterial endocarditis

Miscellaneous conditions
- Wilson's disease
- Reye's syndrome

Table 70.9
Exogenous Substances Causing Psychosis Following Ingestion of Significant Quantity

- Alcohol
- Barbiturates
- Antipsychotics (e.g., phenothiazines)
- Amphetamines
- Hallucinogens—LSD, peyote, mescaline
- Marijuana
- Phencyclidine (PCP)
- Quaalude
- Anticholinergic compounds
- Heavy metals
- Cocaine
- Corticosteroids
- Reserpine
- Opiates (e.g., heroin, methadone)

Organic Psychosis

Differentiation of organic psychosis as a separate class does not imply that other (psychiatrically based) psychosis is completely independent of brain processes. On the contrary, it is assumed that all psychosis is associated with aberrant brain function. The term organic psychosis merely implies that the cause of the aberrations in mental functioning is known and resolution of the psychosis is dependent upon improvement in the underlying organic derangements. Psychiatrically based psychoses, on the other hand, are those in which specific organic causes have not yet been determined. The causes of organic psychoses can be acute or chronic illnesses, trauma, or intoxications with an exogenous substance (see Table 70.8 and 70.9).

CLINICAL MANIFESTATIONS (see Table 70.10)

The child or adolescent with an organic psychosis will present to the emergency department in an agitated and confused state. The child's orientation to time and place will very often be disturbed, and he may be highly distractible with significant disturbance of recent memory. There will be evidence of bizarre and distorted thoughts, and disconnected ideas may be juxtaposed. The child may also have significant difficulty controlling his behavior, and may persist in activities without regard for personal safety. The child may get up to leave the room without saying where he is going or why he needs to leave. Intellectual functioning may also be impaired, and the child may be unable to concentrate on simple reading or arithmetic tasks.

The child with an organic psychosis may experience visual hallucinations, which may be quite frightening in nature. Auditory hallucinations, more common in schizophrenia and manic-depressive illness, are rare in organic psychoses. As a result of their impaired reality testing, organically psychotic children and adolescents are often extremely difficult to control and may strike out at family or staff when attempts are made to control their behavior.

An accurate and thorough history is essential in the evaluation of any child or adolescent for psychosis and is also helpful in appreciating its underlying cause. A complete medical history will help determine if the organic psychosis is a concomitant feature of an already existing chronic illness (e.g., lupus cerebritis), a result of medication prescribed to treat an ongoing disease, (e.g., steroids for lupus erythematosus), or a result of a drug ingestion (e.g., amphetamine psychosis). Typically, an acute intoxication or drug ingestion causes the acute onset of psychosis and represents an abrupt change from the child's previous psychological functioning. The possibility of alcohol use must also be considered in the etiology of organic psychosis, and the history should explore the possibility of trauma. In general there are no specific features of the mental status examination which differentiate the various causes of organic psychosis.

The physical examination is often extremely helpful in both differentiating organic from psychiatrically based psychosis and in determining the underlying etiology of an acute organic psychosis. Fever is likely to be present in infections, while tachycardia is often associated with chronic illness or intoxication. The general physical examination will give indications of pulmonary, cardiac, liver, or autoimmune disease, and the neurologic examination will assist in the diagnosis of central nervous system disease. Abnormalities of reflexes or of motor, sensory, or coordination systems always require complete neurologic evaluation. Signs of increased intracranial pressure may be indicative of a cerebral vascular accident, central nervous system tumor, or cerebral edema. Signs of autonomic dysfunction such as pupillary abnormalities are often indicative of acute intoxication.

In instances of suspected organic psychosis, laboratory evaluation should include a complete blood count, urinalysis, serum electrolytes, calcium, blood urea ni-

Table 70.10
Differentiating Features of Organic and Psychiatrically Induced Psychosis[a]

Evaluation Feature	Organic Psychosis	Psychiatric Psychosis
Onset	Acute	Insidious
Pathologic autonomic signs	May be present	Absent
Vital signs	May be abnormal	Normal
Orientation	Impaired	Intact
Recent memory	Impaired	Intact
Intellectual ability	May be impaired	Intact
Hallucinations	Visual	Auditory

[a] Children with psychosis regardless of cause will have impaired reality testing, inappropriate affect, thought disorder, poor behavior control and disturbed relating ability.

trogen and blood glucose. Serum, urine, and gastric aspirate should be obtained for toxicology screening. Other laboratory and radiologic studies will depend upon abnormalities noted in the history and physical examination. If central nervous disease is suspected, skull x-rays, computerized tomography, and a lumbar puncture may be necessary. Liver function studies, thyroid studies, and other specialized and specific laboratory tests may be obtained as required.

MANAGEMENT

The management of the child or adolescent with organic psychosis involves first and foremost diagnosing the underlying cause. Medical treatment is then pursued as indicated for the specific organic condition. We believe that any child with a suspected organic psychosis should be admitted to a medical inpatient unit for diagnostic evaluation and treatment. This is especially important, since organic psychosis may be a transitory condition in a child or adolescent whose illness or intoxication is progressive and life threatening.

Other important components of the management of a psychotic child involve controlling the child's behavior, preventing injury to himself or others, and alleviating the child's fear and anxiety. This should be attempted first through supportive statements indicating the physician's appreciation of the child's condition and his distress. Specific instructions to the child (i.e. "Try to relax and look at your mother") may also be effective. Frequently, such interventions succeed in calming and protecting the child, but since the child is distractible and anxious, instructions may need to be repeated frequently.

Antipsychotic and sedative medications affect the child's neurologic status and therefore should be used only when the medical diagnosis is known with certainty and when it is clear that the medication will not worsen the underlying disease process or potentiate the intoxication (see below for specific medications and dosages for psychosis). In most instances when direct behavior control is essential, the child should be placed in arm and leg restraints. While in restraints, the patient should be attended by staff or family members and provided frequent orienting statements and explanations of the need for restraint.

Infantile Autism and Pervasive Developmental Disorder of Childhood

These disorders are extremely rare, occurring at a rate of approximately 2 cases per 10,000 children. Both are approximately 3 times more common in boys than in girls. Due to the infrequency of these disorders and the chronicity of their course, it is unusual for children with either infantile autism or pervasive developmental disorders to present in an emergency department undiagnosed. However, children with these disorders may present in the emergency department for the treatment of intercurrent illnesses or an acute exacerbation of the child's behavior.

Infantile Autism

The major differentiating feature between infantile autism and pervasive developmental disorder of childhood is the age of onset. Autism always has an onset prior to 30 months of age. Children with autism have a generalized lack of responsiveness to other people and a failure to develop normal attachment behavior. They do not develop relationships but play alone, often showing stereotyped behavior and using objects in bizarre, inappropriate ways. The austistic child becomes extremely upset if objects in his environment are disturbed or changed. Language development is impaired or absent. Only 30% of autistic children have an I.Q. greater than 70 and some have underlying illnesses such as maternal rubella syndrome or previous encephalitis or meningitis. Many autistic children also have coexisting seizure disorders. The course of infantile autism is generally chronic, with two thirds of all autistic children remaining severely handicapped throughout life.

A comprehensive psychiatric and educational program is essential for autistic children. If an autistic child seen in the emergency department is not participating in such a program, outpatient psychiatric referral is indicated. The use of antipsychotic medication in the treatment of autistic children is controversial and should only be used in conjunction with ongoing psychiatric treatment. Acute psychiatric hospitalization is rarely necessary. In instances of extremely disturbing behavior or acute agitation, sedation with either chloral hydrate (30 mg/kg) or diphenhydramine (1 mg/kg) may be helpful. If the parents are disturbed by their child's immediate behavior and the child is in psychiatric treatment, phone contact with the psychiatrist may be helpful to both the emergency room physician and the family.

Pervasive Developmental Disorders

Pervasive developmental disorder of childhood is the new term for such entities as childhood schizophrenia, symbiotic psychosis, and atypical psychosis. It has onset after 30 months of age and prior to 12 years of age. Children with this disorder often have extreme anxiety and severe emotional reactions to minor difficulties, with inappropriate affect and extreme mood lability. Abnormalities of speech, hypersensitivity to sensory stimuli, peculiar posturing, and self-mutilation may also occur. Children with a pervasive developmental disorder also have severe, sustained impairment of attachment and social relationships.

These children, like autistic children, require comprehensive psychiatric and educational treatment. However, since many respond better to antipsychotic medication than autistic children, medications such as thioridazine or haloperidol are frequently used. With the acute exacerbation of a pervasive developmental disorder, psychiatric hospitalization may be necessary, both to provide assistance to the parents and to develop or modify a comprehensive treatment program. Families with acute concerns about their child's behavior should receive psychiatric consultation.

Schizophrenia

Schizophrenia frequently has its onset in adolescence and occurs in approximately 0.5% of the population. It is equally common in males and females, and is more prevalent among family members of known individuals with the disease. It is hypothesized that one feature of schizophrenia is an excess of dopamine activity in the brain.

CLINICAL MANIFESTATIONS

Symptoms of schizophrenia involve impairment of basic psychological processes, including perception, thinking, affect, capacity to relate, and behavior. Impaired thought content includes delusions (strongly held beliefs involving the self with no basis in reality), such as delusions of persecution and external control. For example, an adolescent with schizophrenia may feel that others can read his mind and can insert thoughts into his mind. Markedly illogical thinking occurs. Speech is frequently characterized by loose associations, where ideas shift from one subject to another entirely unrelated subject without the speaker recognizing that the topics are not connected. Auditory hallucinations are common, and may include direct commands for suicide or for violence to others. Affect may be blunted and flat, or inappropriate and bizarre. Sudden and unpredictable changes in mood may occur. These teenagers may appear extremely agitated or may be quite withdrawn, speaking only in monosyllables and describing only concrete objects. Schizophrenic patients typically have marked distortions of their identity and their abilities, and demonstrate behavior that is not goal-directed.

Families with schizophrenic adolescents have been noted to have disturbances in communication among family members. There may also be marital difficulties between the parents. Parents may have noted progressive emotional difficulties in the adolescent without seeking assistance and may be frightened about the teenager's bizarre behavior. Often the family is disorganized, and relationships between parents and the affected teenager are superficial, distant, and confused. The family will require clear explanations of the child's condition, proposed treatment, and the essential need for their active participation.

The history often reveals a prodromal phase in which there is social withdrawal, peculiar behavior, failure to look after one's appearance, and marked reduction in performance in school or work. This is followed by an acute phase in which the symptoms described above develop, sometimes but not always a result of an acutely stressful event. The overall course of schizophrenia is often chronic and associated with remissions and exacerbations. Exacerbations often occur when treatment is suspended. Some individuals, however, who experience a schizophrenic-like acute psychosis recover completely with appropriate treatment and experience no further deterioration.

MANAGEMENT

The management of an acute schizophrenic episode should always take place in collaboration with psychiatric consultation. Patients with suicidal or homicidal ideation should receive psychiatric hospitalization. Psychotic patients from chaotic or disorganized home environments should also be hospitalized for initial treatment. In the absence of suicidal or homicidal ideation, when parents or caretakers are responsible, can appreciate the child's condition, and feel capable of managing the child at home, antipsychotic medication can be begun in the emergency department and outpatient psychiatric treatment initiated. At times, an examining psychiatrist in the emergency department may choose to defer initiation of antipsychotic medication for a manageable schizophrenic adolescent until emergency evaluation at the appropriate mental health center takes place. In situations where the adolescent is acutely agitated and potentially violent, antipsychotic medication and/or physical restraint should be utilized in the emergency department.

Commonly used antipsychotic medications, their trade names, relative potency, and usual dosage ranges are listed in Table 70.11. We suggest that the physician become familiar with the use of these drugs in emergency situations. High potency antipsychotic medications, such as haloperidol or trifluoperazine, rapidly reach therapeutic blood levels and produce less sedation than low potency drugs, such as chlorpromazine and thioridazine. However, high potency antipsychotics have a greater incidence of extrapyramidal effects which can be reversed by administration of the appropriate medication (see below). When the emergency physician and the consulting psychiatrist agree to use antipsychotic medication in the emergency room, we recommend that haloperidol be used. Dosages of 5 to 10 mg haloperidol (p.o. or i.m.) for adult-size adolescents (approximately 70 kg), or 2 to 5 mg haloperidol (p.o. or i.m.) for smaller children, should be administered every 30 to 60 min up to a maximum dose of 40 mg, until the patient's state of agitation lessens, or until he becomes sedated. The patient's vital signs, general condition, and possible side effects should be monitored frequently. If the patient does not respond to this medication regimen, inpatient psychiatric hospitalization will be necessary. If significant improvement occurs and side effects are not present, the patient can be discharged to outpatient psychiatric treatment. He should then be maintained on a daily oral dose of medication equivalent to the amount used in the emergency department. Careful outpatient follow-up of such patients is essential.

Table 70.11
Antipsychotic Drugs

Generic Name	Brand Name	Estimated Equivalent Dosage (mg)	Total Daily Dosage (mg)
Phenothiazines			
Chlorpromazine	Thorazine	100	50–1000
Thioridazine	Mellaril	100	50–800
Trifluoperazine	Stelazine	5	5–30
Fluphenazine	Prolixin	2	1–20
Butyrophenone			
Haloperidol	Haldol	2	2–40

The major side effects of antipsychotic medication are extrapyramidal symptoms including acute dystonic reactions (abnormal muscle tone or posturing), akathisia (motor restlessness), and parkinsonian effects (rigidity, tremor, slowed movement, and loss of balance). Acute dystonic reactions are best treated by the intravenous or intramuscular administration of diphenhydramine (25 to 50 mg), followed by a daily maintenance dose of benztropine (1 to 2 mg/day p.o.). We recommend that adolescents begun on high potency antipsychotic medication on an outpatient basis be treated prophylactically with benztropine (1 to 2 mg/day p.o.) to prevent side effects. Patients placed on antipsychotic medication should be clearly informed of possible side effects and instructed to return to the emergency room or to the responsible mental health professional should such symptoms develop. Attempts should be made later in treatment to lower the dosage of antipsychotic medication and discontinue the use of the antiparkinsonian agent.

Manic-Depressive Illness

Manic-depressive illness occurs in approximately 0.5% of the population. Onset is usually prior to 30 years of age, and occurs infrequently during late childhood or adolescence. Since depression is discussed in detail elsewhere in this chapter, this section deals only with manic psychosis.

CLINICAL MANIFESTATIONS

The patient with mania has a distinct period of predominantly elevated, expansive, and irritable mood. There is a marked decrease in need for sleep, high distractibility, hyperactivity and pressured speech, and emotional lability. These patients also exhibit what is called flight of ideas—a nearly continuous flow of accelerated speech with abrupt changes from topic to topic usually based on understandable associations, distractions, or plays on words. Unlike the loose associations of the schizophrenic, the flight of ideas of a manic patient retains logical connection from one idea to the next but moves quickly from one topic to another. The manic patient may at times have a remarkably inflated self-esteem, with uncritical self-confidence and marked grandiosity. This grandiosity may also include delusional ideas. The individual may be aggressive, and may be combative. He may go on buying sprees or pursue other reckless behaviors. Manic patients usually have a history of previous depressive episodes, but an acute manic episode in adolescence may be the initial presentation of the disorder. There is usually a family history of psychiatric disturbance in patients with manic-depressive disorder. Typically, manic patients report feeling extremely good, and they are brought to the emergency department against their will. However, underneath this superficial presentation, the patient has extremely low self-esteem and self-confidence.

The differentiation of mania and schizophrenia in an initial episode of psychosis in adolescence may at times be quite difficult. Hyperactivity, distractibility, and expansive and euphoric mood are often helpful in identifying manic individuals. Both groups may have auditory hallucinations and delusions, but someone listening to the speech of the manic adolescent should recognize the flight of ideas and their connection with each other.

MANAGEMENT

When an adolescent is suspected of having manic-depressive illness or an acute manic episode, psychiatric consultation should be obtained and psychiatric hospitalization initiated. Involuntary commitment may be necessary. Since the treatment of mania includes the long-term use of lithium carbonate, which takes time to take effect and which requires careful blood monitoring to assure therapeutic levels, psychiatric hospitalization is necessary. Initial emergency treatment of the agitated manic patient may require the use of restraints and the acute administration of antipsychotic agents such as haloperidol, in doses equivalent to those used for schizophrenic adolescents. The physician should also be aware that some patients on lithium may present with signs of lithium overdose including nausea, vomiting, muscle weakness, ataxia, tremor, slurred speech, blurred vision, and confusion or somnolence.

SCHOOL REFUSAL

BACKGROUND

School refusal, also called school avoidance and school phobia, entails a child's not attending school, but expressing somatic complaints which keep him at home. Usually, some somatic complaint is used as the justification for school absence, with the child just "too sick" to be in school. School refusal involves the knowledge and complicity of the family. A parent, usually the mother, is aware of the child's school absence and has endorsed his being home, in part because the parent may consider the child to be physically ill.

School refusal is an important condition with which the emergency department physician should be familiar. Usually it is not the presenting complaint. Typically, one or more physical complaints bring the child to the emergency department and information about school attendance is not offered. The physician must maintain an "index of suspicion" in a child with recurring complaints for which no organic etiology is apparent.

On rare occasions, school refusal may be the presenting concern of a parent. The mother may bring her child, stating that for a specified time she has been unable to get her child to school. Attempts to force the child have been ineffective, either because the child refused to go, got sick in school and was sent home, or caused such family upheaval that eventually the parents gave in. In such a circumstance, school refusal represents a true emergency and should be responded to as such.

There are no specific prevalence figures for school refusal, but the condition is not uncommon. It probably occurs more often than diagnosed and may be easily missed. The problem is not confined to a specific population or socioeconomic group and can occur across ethnic, religious, and class lines.

Chronically ill children have been considered high risk for school refusal, though many physically ill children are determined to attend school regularly despite their disability. The child with vague undiagnosable somatic complaints is more likely to fit the school refusal pattern. So-called vulnerable children and special children may also be school refusers. The former were ill at an earlier point in their lives, but parental overconcern remains. The latter are children who were very much wanted by their parents, such as a child born to an older couple who had problems conceiving. The love and attention given to the child can easily yield to overprotectiveness, setting the stage for the development of school refusal. It has been noted that school refusal tends to occur in families with an orientation toward illness and disability; so it is not uncommon for one or more parents to have past or present illnesses, physical complaints, or hospitalizations. The presence of marital problems may also contribute to the development of school refusal.

CLINICAL MANIFESTATIONS

Certain school attendance patterns are suggestive of but not necessary for the diagnosis of school refusal. More absences occur in the fall, when school begins, than in the spring. There is often a reluctance to return to school after weekends and holidays. There may be a lessening of somatic complaints on weekends and over the summer. Similar sporadic attendance patterns may often be elicited at some other time in the child's past. In other instances, however, school refusal may develop in a child who has previously given no cause for concern. Only specific questions asked routinely of every child and parent about school attendance will yield the necessary information. Such questions should be quite specific, addressing not just recent school attendance but the pattern over the entire year. In this way, the diagnosis will be made on the child who missed several days of school per week with good grades, as well as the more easily diagnosed child who has missed several consecutive weeks or months of school.

Schmitt has formulated a diagnostic triad of the clinical manifestations of school refusal: (1) vague physical symptoms, (2) normal physical and laboratory findings, and (3) poor school attendance. The child may have one or more complaints. Schmitt has also pointed out how many of the symptoms are reflective of depression and anxiety. This is consistent with the fact that many children with school refusal also are depressed. The symptoms which may be present include fatigue, insomnia, transient pallor, a smothering feeling (hyperventilation), palpitations, tension headaches, dizziness, syncope, and a variety of gastrointestinal complaints. Most common is nonspecific abdominal pain. Anorexia in the absence of weight loss may occur, as may diarrhea. Nausea may occur with or without associated vomiting. A clue to the psychogenic nature of the vomiting is that it sometimes follows stressful events. The serious complaint of vomiting should not mislead the physician into an overly extensive workup that iatrogenically reinforces disability. Similar considerations apply to the skeletal complaints that may occur—bone pain, joint pain, and back pain. Such tentative diagnosis as "possible rheumatoid arthritis" should be avoided. Other possible symptoms that may mask the school refusal syndrome include chest pain, dysmenorrhea, muscle weakness, coughing, tics, and recurrent sore throats.

Certain characteristics of the family with school refusal have been identified. Berger described four important elements. (1) An overprotective infantilizing attitude toward the patient exists. The child is excused from family responsibilities, and his wishes are quickly granted. (2) There is a belief in the physical or emotional vulnerability of the mother. This belief is fostered by the mother herself, who may voice fear of an emotional breakdown and complain of various physical symptoms. (3) The fathers in such families tend to be isolated and devalued. They are seen as disinterested and unreliable, perhaps even as violent. There may be underlying marital tension. (4) It has also been found that, in many families with school refusal, a major change in family composition, frequently the departure from home of an older sibling, has occurred. This focuses new attention on the identified patient.

Other characteristics of families with school refusal have also been noted. An illness orientation is revealed by physical complaints in other family members as well as frequent somatic references in verbal communication. The closeness between the mother and child may be manifested by the mother's frequent use of "we" when talking about the child. Active undermining by the parents may at times be observed.

MANAGEMENT

The major responsibility of the emergency department physician is the detection of school refusal. The diagnosis will be made by having a higher index of suspicion for children with vague somatic complaints and by routinely inquiring about school attendance patterns.

While the emergency department physician cannot guide the entire treatment of school refusal, he can get the process going. The physical examination should be done in the presence of the parents in a thorough manner, with the physician emphasizing the absence of physical findings. Appropriate, but not excessive, laboratory work should be performed, and medication should not be prescribed. After acknowledging the genuineness of the child's symptom so that there is no misunderstanding that the child is "faking it," the physician should provide a firm and unequivocal statement to the family that the child has no serious illness. He should then make sure that the family understands what he has said and accepts it. In this way, misunderstandings or disagreements can be confronted directly, thereby decreasing the likelihood of subsequent doctor-shopping by the family. The emphasis is then placed on the child learning to function in spite of his symptoms.

Once school refusal is recognized and the possibility of organic disease ruled out, the principal goals in the treatment of school refusal are: (1) getting the child back to school rapidly and (2) addressing underlying family problems that contributed to the development of the problem.

We recommend that the *parents* rather than the physician tell the child that he needs to return. In this way the family takes responsibility for the resolution of the problem from the beginning of the intervention. The parents should be encouraged to work closely together to achieve their desired goal. In this way, underlying marital tensions are addressed without making them explicit. Both parents need to be addressed as responsible and crucial family members.

The emergency department physician will vary his recommendations concerning the child's return to school according to the severity of the problem. Uncomplicated cases of preadolescent school refusal can be managed by the emergency physician himself, the primary care physician, or referred to a pediatric colleague. With severely depressed or psychotic teenagers, it is appropriate to obtain psychiatric consultation. It is important for the emergency physician to clarify with the family who is the responsible physician who will supervise the child's return to school. Ideally, the less disturbed child should return to school within several days' time. A follow-up appointment should be scheduled for the day that the child returns to school. The emergency physician should resist any possible request of child and family to condone or underwrite the child's continued absence from school.

CONDUCT DISORDERS

BACKGROUND

A child with a disorder of conduct engages in repetitive, socially unacceptable behavior, without evidence of medical or other psychiatric disorder. The diagnosis of conduct disorder implies a continuing pattern of disruptive or deviant behavior, rather than isolated antisocial acts. The behavior may involve violence and aggression (e.g., vandalism, mugging, assault, and rape), or may involve behavior that is socially unacceptable but nonaggressive (e.g., truancy, running away, lying, stealing, substance abuse). A disorder of conduct, therefore, involves more serious behavior than ordinary mischief and pranks of children and adolescents. Since violent and other unacceptable behaviors may be performed by children with medical illnesses and intoxications, these must be ruled out before the diagnosis of conduct disorder can be made. Similarly, since children with psychosis and depression can also behave in socially unacceptable ways, these serious psychiatric disorders must also be considered and eliminated prior to diagnosing a conduct disorder (see Chapter 72).

The incidence of violence in youth has been steadily increasing, to the point where there are now estimated to be 500,000 youngsters in detention in the United States yearly. In addition, it has been estimated that 1 in every 9 children will appear in Juvenile Court before his 18th birthday, and that more than 1 million youths are currently runaways from home. Delinquent behavior is 5 times more common in boys than in girls, and boys are more likely to demonstrate violent behavior directed against others.

There is disagreement within society about whether to regard children and adolescents with conduct disorders as psychiatrically impaired and needing treatment, or as delinquent and needing detention or incarceration. Probably only a small percentage of violent and aggressive children are brought to emergency departments for psychiatric evaluation. Many are taken by police to detention centers, while others commit their unacceptable behavior without receiving legal or medical attention. There is also no consistent agreement as to the appropriate criteria for taking such children to an emergency department as opposed to juvenile center. In actual practice, certain factors probably influence the choice of disposition, such as age (younger children are more likely to receive medical evaluation), class (middle and upper class children are more likely to be taken to an emergency department), race (white children are more likely to be taken to an emergency department than black children), and nature of the infraction (children with aggressive acts directed outside the family are more likely to be taken to detention). Aggressive children should always undergo an emergency medical and psychiatric evaluation any time there is reason to suspect an intoxication, underlying medical condition, or other psychiatric disorder.

CLINICAL MANIFESTATIONS

Children with conduct disorders typically have poor adjustment at home and in the community. Peer relationships are absent or superficial, based more on what the child can get from the other person rather than a sense of empathy. The child thinks primarily about himself, trying to manipulate situations to personal advantage without significant concern for the feelings and needs of others. He is unlikely to extend himself for others when there is no immediate advantage for him. When the child with a conduct disorder is apprehended, there is little sense of remorse or guilt, but rather a sense of anger at being detected. Such children rarely accept responsibility for their own actions, but instead tend to blame others for their mistakes.

School attendance of children with conduct disorders is often sporadic, and academic performance is often poor. This may be due to a variety of factors, including lack of interest and discipline, but may also be due to specific learning disabilities and an attention deficit disorder, which are remediable and require attention.

The child or adolescent with a conduct disorder shows low frustration tolerance, irritability, and temper outbursts. He may be reckless in behavior and project an image of "toughness." Smoking, drinking, drug use, and precocious sexual activity may all occur. In addition to possible legal difficulties, the child may have other problems, including school suspensions, drug dependence, venereal disease, pregnancy, and physical injury from accidents and fights.

The presence of a conduct disorder implies a failure of the child's environment to enforce familial and societal rules consistently. As a result, the child comes to believe that he can act as he chooses, and does not develop control of impulses. The specific pattern of inadequate limit-setting varies in these families, but the families share in common an inconsistency in enforcing rules and do not hold the child accountable for his behavior. In some families discipline may fluctuate from being half-hearted at times, to being harsh and even physically abusive at other times. Parental role models may show poor impulse control themselves and disregard societal norms. In some families one parent is the enforcer while the other tends to protect and excuse the child, while in other families the parents may shift roles in protecting the child. In these situations, parental undermining enables the child to persist in avoiding responsibility for his behavior. As a result, the child or adolescent comes to expect that, somehow, he will survive or be excused from any repercussions of his behavior.

In addition to inconsistent limit-setting, the families of children with conduct disorders often have other difficulties. They tend to be poorly organized, with the roles and expectations of various family members often unclear. There may be parental separations and divorce, mental illness, and alcohol or drug abuse. Parental criminality and incarceration occur in some families. Families with aggressive and impulsive children frequently do not know how to effectively utilize social service resources, and may consider themselves helpless in controlling their child and in dealing with the world at large.

When taken to the emergency department, almost invariably by some outside agent (police, parent, or other caretaker) against his will, the child with a conduct disorder may be angry, hostile, uncooperative, and may even be violent. The child or adolescent may refuse to answer questions directed to him but quickly interrupts to defend himself while others are speaking. At other times, the child may present with a superficially smooth and pleasant facade, hoping to persuade the physician and authorities of his innocence. Often, once the child realizes that he will not be permitted to act out or manipulate in the emergency department, he may settle down and cooperate.

MANAGEMENT

The goals for managing aggressive and disruptive children in the emergency room are (1) to ensure the safety of the child, family, and staff; (2) to rule out possible medical conditions and severe psychiatric disorders before making the diagnosis of conduct disorder; and (3) to gather sufficient information to make an appropriate disposition.

The safety of the child and staff and the control of the child's unacceptable behavior must be achieved in the emergency department. In many instances the disruptive behavior occurred and ended prior to the child's coming to the emergency department and there is no problem in gaining the child's cooperation. In other instances, however, the child may remain combative and aggressive in the emergency department. Dealing with such a problem requires the presence of adequate security staff and a quiet space where attempts to control the patient will not disrupt the remainder of the emergency department. The patient should be told firmly that he is in the hospital for medical and psychiatric evaluation and that he will not be permitted to harm himself or others. He should be informed that he is expected to cooperate with the staff and to control his behavior. The child's parents, if present, should be asked to assist in controlling the child. The child can be reassured that he will get a chance to tell his side of the story completely. These interventions usually are sufficient to gain the child's cooperation.

When the child remains aggressive and threatening in the emergency department, an adequate number of security staff should be summoned. If the child still cannot be calmed, physical restraints should be used. This is accomplished by several security personnel laying the child down on a cart and applying leather arm and leg restraints with soft cuffs. Often, the external control established by the use of restraints helps the child or adolescent to feel safe and regain personal control. It is uncommon for nonpsychotic aggressive patients to require psychotropic medication, and none should be given until possible medical conditions and intoxications have been ruled out. When needed for children 12 years and older, chlorpromazine (25 mg i.m.) or haloperidol (5 mg i.m.) can be used, and psychiatric consultation should be sought.

The history and physical examination will assist in ruling out medical conditions and intoxications. The presence of ongoing medical conditions should be specifically asked about, as should any recent alcohol use or drug ingestion. Where indicated, specimens for toxicologic screening should be obtained. Epilepsy can be ruled out as the cause of the abnormal behavior in the presence of a normal neurological examination and the absence of an aura, abnormal neurologic signs, or postictal phenomena.

The history and mental status examination will enable the diagnosis of psychosis or depression, when present, to be made. A history of withdrawal and social deterioration suggests emotional antecedents of the current disturbed behavior. Hallucinations, delusions, and loose associations suggest psychosis, while sad affect, crying, and possible suicidal ideation indicate the presence of severe depression.

With this information available, the emergency physician can now consider appropriate treatment and disposition of the patient. Children with medical conditions and acute intoxications are best managed through medical hospitalization. The presence of psychosis or depression requires psychiatric consultation and possible hospitalization. Psychiatric consultation and hospitalization should also be considered in cases of severe, chronic conduct disorders. For intervention to be effective with such children, the family must support the idea of hospitalization, indicating their willingness to participate and to pursue the difficult process of altering persistent patterns of disturbed behavior. The child should agree to follow the rules of the institution and agree to attempt to control violent impulses. The hospitalization can be explained as an opportunity for the child to learn to behave in more socially acceptable ways while the family learns to enforce rules and control their child's behavior more effectively. In less severe cases, outpatient psychiatric treatment can be recommended and initiated to achieve these same objectives.

Involuntary hospitalization should be used when the child's condition continues to pose a threat to himself or others, or when overt homicidal or suicidal ideation is present. When the child is not suicidal or homicidal and refuses to make a commitment to work in psychotherapy, and when the family refuses to support the proposed psychiatric hospitalization, referral to the juvenile justice system may be appropriate.

ATTENTION DEFICIT DISORDER

BACKGROUND

Attention deficit disorder refers to a syndrome found in toddlers and latency aged children, characterized by a pervasive difficulty in maintaining attention and goal-directed behavior. The condition, previously called hyperkinetic syndrome and minimal brain dysfunction, has been relabeled, "attention deficit disorder," because the primary source of difficulty is believed to be inattention. Attention deficit disorder (ADD) has an incidence of between 5 and 10% of school-aged children, occurring 10 times more often in boys than girls. ADD is presumed to have an underlying neurologic etiology. Some cases of ADD may be inherited while others may be a consequence of prenatal or perinatal difficulties. It has been estimated that ADD occurs in up to 50% of latency-aged children receiving psychiatric treatment, making it the most common cause of chronic behavioral problems for this age group. The peak age range for referral of ADD children is between the ages of 8 and 10.

It is important for the emergency department physician to be familiar with ADD, since many of the children so affected become depressed and may make suicide attempts. In adolescence, antisocial behavior may mask ADD, which the physician should consider in evaluating children with conduct disorders. Since identification and treatment can produce significant improvements in the clinical picture, it is important that the diagnosis not be missed.

CLINICAL MANIFESTATIONS

ADD can occur in the presence or absence of hyperactivity, although more commonly it occurs with associated hyperactivity. Wender has described the various possible components of the ADD picture. The *attentional difficulties* occur both at home and in school, and are often more severe in school. The child has difficulty fixating attention. This manifests itself as an inability to persist for long periods in any activity and, in extreme form, may involve a frenetic movement from activity to activity. Rather than persisting in school work and other tasks, the child often appears not to be listening to the teacher, and discipline may be a problem.

Impulsivity is another essential characteristic of ADD. The child has difficulty with self-control, exhibiting behaviors that get him in trouble with parents, siblings, teachers, and peers. At home the child typically has outbursts and temper tantrums, and enforcement of discipline may be quite difficult. Lack of self-control may also be manifested through stealing, lying, playing with matches and other forms of acting-out.

Hyperactivity is usually part of the ADD picture. As with attentional difficulties and impulsivity, hyperactivity tends to be worse in a group situation than at home or in a one-to-one interaction. This characteristic creates a difficulty in the diagnosis of ADD, since the telltale signs are least likely to occur during an individual assessment by the physician. In one study, 75% of children referred for hyperactivity did not exhibit this behavior in the doctor's office. Therefore, the most important diagnostic clue is the history as related by parents and school teacher. However, it is not the absolute amount of activity that distinguishes the ADD child from a normally active child, but the aimless, non-goal-directed quality of the activity.

The child with ADD may have associated *neurological deficits* or "soft signs," but these are not necessary for the diagnosis. It has been estimated that up to two thirds of ADD children have motor incoordination as manifested by deficits in gross and fine motor skills. Impairment of fine motor skills may be manifested in inability to tie shoe laces and poor handwriting. Poor eye-hand coordination may be reflected in difficulties with sports, while difficulty riding a bicycle suggests an impaired sense of balance. Various *perceptual problems*, including right-left discrimination problems, problems with spatial orientation, problems of sensory integration, and problems of processing various types of information, all may be present and may contribute to learning problems. Specialized psychological and educational tests are used to detect these deficits.

The *personality* of the ADD child is frequently labile, with fluctuations in mood and a tendency toward overreaction and temper tantrums. It is important to appreciate the low self-esteem and possible depression that may be present in these children, a result of academic failure, conflicts at home, and peer and sibling rejection. In acute situations, the depression may find expression as suicide attempts or violent behavior. ADD children are a high risk group for self-destructive behavior. The sense of sadness will frequently be apparent to the physician as he looks beyond the cocky bravado of the ADD child who tries to hide his sense of frustration and inadequacy.

Family problems are typically present in the families of ADD children. The child may provoke the parents and is difficult to discipline. Conflicts with siblings may occur. If the parents become overly concerned with the problem child, marital strain and blaming may result.

MANAGEMENT

The principal responsibility of the emergency physician is to appreciate the possibility of an ADD in children who present with other problems and make the diagnosis. The physician is then in a position to clarify the meaning of this disorder with the family and to restore hope for improved behavior and adaptation of the child by making a psychiatric referral when indicated. The history is the most reliable diagnostic indicator. Once the presumptive diagnosis is made, appropriate referral and treatment can follow.

The treatment approach to ADD should be comprehensive and multimodal. It is best managed by a physician who has a long-term relationship with the child and family. Stimulant medication may be helpful in alleviating the symptoms of ADD. The physician should also be aware that academic achievement and emotional well-being require attention to the child's individual style of learning and a supportive interpersonal environment.

Although stimulant medication should not be prescribed in the emergency department, it is important to have a familiarity with the commonly used drugs. The three principal stimulants are methylphenidate (Ritalin), *d*-amphetamine (Dexedrine), and pemoline (Cylert). Tricyclic antidepressants have also been successfully used in the treatment of ADD but constitute a second line of medication and are not approved by the FDA for this purpose. In general, response rates to the stimulant medications are over 75%. Methylphenidate is given in typical median effective doses of 40 mg/day, but doses as low as 0.3 mg/kg/day (10 to 15 mg/day) have been shown effective. A typical dose of *d*-amphetamine is 20 mg/day, while the usual effective dose range for pemoline is 56.25 to 75 mg/day. The principal short-term side effects of the stimulants are appetite suppression and insomnia. The principal concerns of long-term use of stimulants are suppression of weight gain and linear growth. However, it appears that rebound growth occurs when the medication is discontinued. Since the best indication of adequacy of dosage of medication is the classroom and not the home, it is essential that close communication be maintained between physician and teacher.

In addition to medication, other areas of deficit for the ADD child and his family should be addressed. Learning may improve with the use of medication, but, if the child is far behind academically, tutoring or other remediation should be utilized. With a specific learning disability as revealed by diagnostic evaluation, a special classroom or special school may be indicated. Family therapy sessions may be of benefit in some cases, to help the parents to deal more effectively with the child and to confront other family issues unrelated to the condition. Family therapy can also help the parents improve the child's self-esteem as overall family functioning improves.

DISORDERS OF INFANCY

Excessive Crying

Excessive crying in an infant is a frequent presenting complaint in the emergency department. Usually parents learn to discriminate between the various cries of their baby and to respond with appropriate relief and comfort. By the age of 3 months, crying is generally of short duration and a baby is readily comforted. However, in a few infants, crying without underlying physiologic difficulty continues to be severe and intractable. Parents dealing with this symptom often will be noted to be exhausted and frustrated, and may also describe difficulties in feeding their infants and marked disruptions in their child's sleep patterns.

An appropriate emergency evaluation includes complete medical history and physical examination to rule out underlying physical causes of distress for the infant as described in Chapter 13. While examining the baby, the physician may note that the child is easily excitable and difficult to comfort.

In young infants, excessive crying has been called colic and it can be expected to decrease with time, ceasing by 3 to 4 months of age. In some infants, however, the crying may persist and there will be serious disruptions in parent-infant relationships. Parents in these families may be insecure, and their inability to effectively feed or calm their infants may lead to further insecurity, discouragement, and tension. Parents may be further troubled by impulses to physically harm their babies in response to their frustration. Prematurity and prolonged separation between mother and infant may have been underlying factors in the development of the symptom. Families presenting in the emergency department may feel isolated and have limited support. Other underlying parental difficulties may include disturbed marital relationships, parental depression, and unsupported single parenthood. The disorder itself is recognized by the child's excitability and the parents' anxiety and tension during the emergency room evaluation.

MANAGEMENT

Appropriate treatment involves first and foremost an appreciation of the situation and the level of difficulty felt by the parents. Supportive acknowledgement by the emergency physician of the stress confronting the parents and of their genuine desire to be effective with their child is usually greatly appreciated. Statements about the specific temperamental qualities of the child and about how common excessive crying is in infancy are also quite reassuring.

When the parents are not too exhausted and overwhelmed, or when alternative sources of support and caretaking are available to them, often the problem can be managed on an outpatient basis. Parents should be informed not to overstimulate their baby and can be shown effective ways of handling and feeding the child. Follow-up well child care should be arranged so that the family receives intensive support from the primary care physician and allied professionals such as nurse practitioners, visiting nurses, and social workers. With this support, the family can become more effective in interrupting the vicious cycle of infant crying, parents becoming tense, and infant crying again.

In other cases, where a high degree of parental tension and exhaustion from the crying is present, a brief hospitalization of the infant may be necessary. Hospitalization should be proposed in a positive way rather than as a sign of parental defeat. The mother should be asked if she wishes to stay with her infant. If she feels an immediate need for rest at home, that is acceptable as long as the mother agrees to participate actively during the remainder of the child's hospitalization. In general, formula changes and the use of medication are not recommended in the emergency treatment of excessive crying.

Sleep Disorders

Infants and young children have varying patterns of sleeping. Some are noted to wake easily and others to need only small amounts of sleep while the majority of children during infancy and early childhood sleep through the night. It has been estimated that up to 20% of 1-year-olds wake regularly during the night. The exact causes of sleep disruption in young children remain undetermined but it is felt that low sensory threshold, high activity level, increased irritability and adverse emotional factors in the home may lead to the development of disturbed sleep patterns. A concern about an infant's sleep pattern may be an underlying reason for emergency department visits with minor physical complaints. The emergency department physician should be alert to the possibility of sleep disorders when evaluating young children in the emergency department. Since this is a problem which causes significant anxiety and exhaustion in the parents and can lead to disruptions of maternal-infant attachment, it is important that sleep disorders be appreciated and appropriate treatment initiated.

Infants with sleep disorders often have difficulties going to bed or getting to sleep and may frequently be found to sleep in the parents' bed. These children also are noted to be highly active, extremely intense, irregular in their behavior patterns, and difficult to comfort. The physical examination and medical history will be noncontributory with an isolated sleep disturbance; however, when evaluating children with sleep problems, it is extremely important that any associated physical difficulties or underlying medical illness are ruled out. In some cases, a history of perinatal difficulties or prolonged hospitalization following birth may be obtained. Parental depression and insecurity may also be noted during the emergency department evaluation.

MANAGEMENT

As in the case of persistent crying, the most important part of the emergency evaluation is identifying the problem and conveying to the parents that, with time and appropriate treatment, the child's sleeping behavior will become more regular and less disruptive to family living. Usually, the identification of the problem and the commitment to develop an effective treatment plan are extremely helpful to parents in the emergency department. It is rare that children with isolated sleep disorders require hospitalization, and the initial approach to therapy should again be referral to ongoing primary care with effective social support. Underlying family difficulties or parental depression may require mental health treatment.

Most children with sleep disorders awaken during the night and return to sleep after comforting. Parents should be advised to avoid overstimulation of the child during the night, and sedative medication is rarely necessary. If extreme parental exhaustion is a problem, the possibility of utilizing alternative caretakers should be investigated, and methods of the parents' sharing the care might be suggested. If sedation is viewed as an absolute necessity by the physician, chloral hydrate (30 mg/kg) or diphenhydramine (1 mg/kg) may be administered to the child. Sustained use of sedative medication should only be utilized as part of an ongoing treatment program for the infant and his family. Chapter 72, "Behavior Problems," discusses other sleep disorders.

Attachment Disorders

Occasionally, infants will be seen in the emergency department who are noted to be withdrawn and apathetic. These infants demonstrate severe disturbances of attachment with their primary caretakers, often have feeding disturbances, and may fail to thrive. The most significant disability of these children is a dramatic failure of social development. They do not track with their eyes and they smile infrequently. They do not interact with caretakers in age-appropriate fashion, and facial responsiveness may be entirely absent. The child may be noted to be weak, have poor muscle tone, and a feeble cry. The child will demonstrate little spontaneous activity, sleep excessively, and have a generalized lack of interest in the environment.

The cause of attachment disorders in infants is a continuing lack of adequate caretaking. Features which interfere with maternal-infant bonding are frequently noted in the history. These may include marked maternal depression and isolation, maternal indifference toward the infant, and history of prolonged separation between mother and infant following birth due to perinatal difficulties. Infants who are temperamentally placcid, who make their needs known quietly, often have more difficulties in the presence of maternal depression or maternal preoccupation than more active and responsive infants.

Underlying chronic illness may also lead to the development of social withdrawal and apathy. Also, children with physical problems in infancy may be more difficult to care for and parental reactions to the child's illness may interfere with attachment. Children with mental retardation, although they develop slowly, do not generally demonstrate the profound apathy of the child with an attachment disorder. Furthermore, children with retardation receive generally adequate caretaking and do not fail to thrive.

MANAGEMENT

Children with attachment disorders require complete medical evaluation together with careful investigation of their environment. Such children are frequently seen in the emergency department for minor physical complaints and may not be receiving regular pediatric care. Thus, it is extremely important for the emergency department physician to recognize attachment disorders and to make effective referrals for ongoing health care for child and family. In instances where parental apathy accompanies severe failure to thrive, hospitalization may be necessary to initiate needed changes and to plan continuing treatment. It is important for the physician to recognize that attachment disorders and the associated failure to thrive are often reversible once adequate caretaking is instituted and maintained. If the physician suspects that the child's problems are a result of actual abuse or neglect, he must report the situation to the appropriate agencies (child neglect is discussed in detail in Chapter 68).

FIRE SETTING

Virtually all of the children in our society develop a fascination with fire and may experiment with it at a relatively early age. For most children this is transient and consists mainly of playing with matches or lighting small fires. However, some children may persist with fire setting behavior and may actually plan to set larger fires which are destructive to both people and property. At this point, the child is demonstrating evidence of a significant psychiatric disorder and requires intensive treatment. The exact incidence of firesetting is unknown but serious repetitive fire setting is felt to be uncommon in childhood and adolescence. In general, fire setting is a symptom of serious underlying emotional difficulty and is frequently associated with other disturbances of behavior and impulse control. It is also associated with significant anger and aggressiveness on the part of the child. The family background of fire setting children is likely to be highly chaotic. These children may have had multiple contacts with social agencies in the past, and some may have been placed outside the home in foster homes or institutions. Although the exact percentage of fire setters with underlying attention deficit disorder is unknown, many of these children are described as having been hyperactive with significant learning problems and with long-standing truancy from school.

MANAGEMENT

The clinical manifestations of fire setters in the emergency department are similar to those of other children with conduct disorders as previously described. Effective emergency department evaluation should always consider psychiatric hospitalization. It is extremely important that, as psychiatric hospitalization is arranged, the facility is informed about the child's previous fire setting behavior so that appropriate behavior monitoring and safety measures can be employed and an effective admission achieved.

References

General

American Psychiatric Association: *Diagnostic and Statistical Manual of Mental Disorders,* Ed. 3, 1980.

Anderson, WH: Psychiatric emergencies. In *Massachusetts General Hospital Textbook of Emergency Medicine.* Williams & Wilkins, Baltimore, 1978.

Bristol JH, Giller E, Dougherty JP: Trends in emergency psychiatry in the last two decades. *Am J Psychiatry* 138: 623, 1981.

Gerson S, Bassuk E: Psychiatric emergencies; an overview. *Am J Psychiatry* 137: 1, 1980.

Glick, RA, Myerson AT, Robbins E, Talbot JA (eds.): *Psychiatric Emergencies.* Grune & Stratton, New York, 1976.

Golan N: Short-term crisis intervention; an approach to serving children and their families. *Child Welfare* 50: 101, 1972.

Goodman JD, Sours JA: *The Child Mental Status Examination.* Basic Books, New York, 1967.

Greenspan SI: *The Clinical Interview of the Child.* McGraw-Hill, New York, 1981.
Khan, AU: *Psychiatric Emergencies in Pediatrics.* Year Book, Chicago, 1979.
Langsley DG: Crisis Intervention. *Am J Psychiatry* 129: 725, 1972.
Langsley DG, Kaplan DM: *Treatment of Families in Crisis.* Grune & Stratton, New York, 1968.
McIntire J, et al.: Suicide and self-poisoning in pediatrics. *Adv Pediatr* 24: 291–309, 1977.
Minuchin S: *Families and Family Therapy.* Harvard University Press, Cambridge, Mass., 1974.
Morrison GC (ed.): *Emergencies in Child Psychiatry.* Charles C Thomas, Springfield, Ill., 1975.
Rappaport J: *Community Psychology: Values, Research, and Action.* Holt, Rinehart & Winston, New York, 1977.
Rosenbaum CP, Beeke JE: *Psychiatric Treatment: Crisis, Clinic, Consultation.* McGraw-Hill, New York, 1975.
Rotenberg MB: Psychiatric emergencies in pediatrics. *Pediatr Digest* 21: 33, 1979.
Shader R (ed.): *Manual of Psychiatric Therapeutics.* Little, Brown, Boston, 1975.
Simons J: *Psychiatric Examination of Children,* Ed. 2. Lea & Febiger, Philadelphia, 1974.

Depression

Carlson G, Cantwell D: Unmasking masked depression in children and adolescents. *Am J Psychiatry* 137: 445–449, 1980.
Cytryn L, McNew D: Proposed classification of childhood depression. *Am J Psychiatry* 129: 149–155, 1972.
Cytryn L, et al.: Diagnosis of depression in children; a reassessment. *Am J Psychiatry* 137: 22–25, 1980.
Kashani J, et al.: Current perspectives of childhood depression; an overview. *Am J Psychiatry* 138: 143–153, 1981.
Petti T: Depression in children; a significant disorder. *Psychosomatics* 22: 444–447, 1981.
Renshaw D: Suicide and depression in children. *J School Health* 44: 487–489, 1974.

Suicide

Duncan J: The immediate management of suicide attempts in children and adolescents; psychological aspects. *J Fam Pract* 4: 77–80, 1977.
Garfinkel BD, Golombek H: Suicide and depression in childhood and adolescence. *Can Med Assoc* 110: 1278–1281, 1974.
Hofman A: Adolescents in distress; suicide and out of control behavior. *Med Clin North Am* 59: 1429–1437, 1975.
Mattsson A, et al.: Suicidal behavior as child psychiatric emergency. *Arch Gen Psychiatry* 20: 100–109, 1969.
McAnarney E: Suicidal behavior of children and youth. *Pediatr Clin North Am* 22: 595–604, 1975.
McIntire M, et al.: Suicide and self-poisoning in pediatrics. *Adv Pediatr* 24: 291–309, 1977.
Pfeffer C: Suicidal behavior of children; a review with implications for research and practice. *Am J Psychiatry* 138: 154–159, 1981.
Pfeffer C, et al.: Suicidal behavior in latency-age children. *J Child Psychol Psychiatry* 18: 679–692, 1981.
Teicher J: A solution to the chronic problem of living; adolescent attempted suicide. In *Current Issues in Adolescent Psychiatry,* pp. 129–147, J Schoolar (ed.). Brunner Mazel, New York, 1973.
Wells C, Stuart I (eds.): *Self Destructive Behavior in Children.* Van Nostrand Reinhold, New York, 1981.

Psychosis

Kessler K, Waletsky JP: Clinical use of the antipsychotics. *Am J Psychiatry* 138: 202, 1981.
Werry JS (ed.): *Pediatric Psychopharmacology: The Use of Behavior Modifying Drugs in Children.* Brunner-Mazel, New York, 1978.
Wiener JM: *Psychopharmacology in Childhood and Adolescence.* Basic Books, New York, 1977.

Attention Deficity Disorders

Saccar C: Drug therapy in the treatment of minimal brain dysfunction. *Am J Hosp Pharm* 35: 544–552, 1978.
Safer D, Allen R: *Hyperactive Children: Diagnosis and Management.* University Park Press, Baltimore, 1976.
Wender P: Minimal brain dysfunction in children; diagnosis and management. *Pediatr Clin North Am* 20: 187–202, 1973.

Conduct Disorder

Kashani JH, et al.: Patterns of delinquency in girls and boys. *J Am Acad Child Psychiatry* 19: 300, 1980.
Lewis DO, et al.: Violent juvenile delinquents; psychiatric, neurological, psychosocial and abuse factors. *J Am Acad Child Psychiatry* 17: 307, 1980.
Rada RT: The violent patient; rapid assessment and management. *Psychosomatics* 22: 101, 1981.

School Avoidance

Berger H: Somatic pain and school avoidance. *Clin Pediatr* 13: 819–826, 1974.
Schmitt B: School phobia—the great imitator; a pediatrician's viewpoint. *Pediatrics* 48: 433–442, 1971.
Nader PR, et al.: School phobia. *Pediatr Clin North Am* 22: 605–716, 1975.

Other

Gruber AR, Heck EG, Mintzer E: Children who set fires; some background and behavioral characteristics. *Am J Orthopsychiatry* 51: 484, 1981.
Pruett KS, Leonard WF: The screaming baby; treatment of a psycholophysiological disorder of infancy. *J Am Acad Child Psychiatry* 17: 289, 1978.
Richman N: A community survey of characteristics of one-to-two year olds with sleep disruptions. *J Am Acad Child Psychiatry* 20: 281, 1981.

CHAPTER 71

Adolescent Emergencies

MARJEANNE COLLINS, M.D.

INTRODUCTION

Adolescence is a period of change, a bridge from childhood to adulthood. Each age carries its own developmental tasks and, with the orderly achievement of those tasks, new rights and responsibilities. The goals of adolescence are individuation from previous dependency, a move toward peer group identity, development of sexual identity, the ability to think abstractly, to fulfill such long-term goals as occupational choice, and move from peer group relationships to intimate ongoing relationships with the opposite sex. This period of emotional growth precipitates many maturational crises. The teenager who has successfully negotiated infancy, preschool and latency years is in the best position for a successful resolution of the turmoil produced by the developmental process of adolescence. A supportive family who can provide the right mix of freedom and restriction provides a necessary lifeline. The teenager who has not successfully negotiated prior developmental tasks will be at a greater risk for a difficult adolescence.

Even normal adolescence is not an equally smooth process for all teenagers. Daniel Offer's prospective study of white, middle class, midwestern adolescent males in the 1960s gives us one of our best descriptions of normal adolescence. From his study, it is known that normal adolescents can be categorized into one of three modes of development. He defined the three modes as *continuous growth, surgent growth* and *tumultuous growth.* About one fifth of the students he studied fell into the continuous growth group, one fifth into the tumultuous growth group and one third the surgent growth group. The remainder had overlapping developmental patterns. Students in the continuous growth group developed from adolescents to young men with a smoothness of purpose and self-assurance in their progression toward a meaningful and fulfilling adult life. They had a realistic appraisal of their own abilities and were able to postpone gratification and work in a sustained manner for a future goal. The students in the surgent growth group also functioned adaptively but differed in the amount of emotional conflicts. More energy was consumed in the process of mastering developmental tasks than was evident for the continuous growth group. At times they functioned well, at other times they were immobilized. Therefore a cycle of progression and regression occurred. The tumultuous growth group is typical of the characterization of adolescence by the public. These are the students who go through adolescence with internal turmoil which manifests itself in overt behavioral problems in school and at home. In males this is often school truancy, difficulties with authority figures, drug abuse, and risk taking behavior. All the same behavior can occur in adolescent females in

Table 71.1
Pubertal Development Scale[a]

A. FEMALES

Stage	Pubic Hair	Age in Years −2 S.D. +2 S.D. Mean	Breasts	Age in Years −2 S.D. +2 S.D. Mean	Comments
1	None; prepubertal		Prepubertal; elevation papilla only		
2	Long, lightly pigmented, downy; along labia	9.27 14.11 11.69	Breast bud stage; elevation breast and papilla as small mound and enlargement of areolar diameter	8.95 13.25 11.15	Onset of breast and pubic hair development more or less simultaneous; initiation of height spurt will soon follow
3	Increased in amount and pigmentation; curly; still limited to labia	10.16 14.56 11.69	Breast and areola show further enlargement with no separation of contours	9.97 14.33 12.15	Menarche usually occurs about this time or 1½ years after onset of breast development; axillary hair first appears here or in stage 5
4	Adult in type; covers mons and extends about halfway out to inguinal regions	10.83 15.07 12.95	Areola and papilla project to form a secondary mound above the level of the breast itself (variable; not always present)	10.81 15.31 13.11	Height spurt begins to decelerate
5	Adult in type, quantity, and lateral distribution; extending out to thighs	12.17 16.65 14.41	Mature with projection of papilla only due to recession of general contour of entire breast	11.85 18.81 15.33	Growth almost complete and most epiphyses closed; may grow 1–2 cm more

Table 71.1—*Continued*

B. MALES

Stage	Pubic Hair	Age in Years −2 S.D.	Mean	+2 S.D.	Penis and Testes	Age in Years −2 S.D.	Mean	+2 S.D.	Comments
1	None; prepubertal				Prepubertal; testes approx. 2–2.5 cm in length				
2	Long, lightly pigmented, downy; at base of penis	11.36	13.44	15.62	Testes definitely enlarged; pigmentation and thinning of scrotum; penis beginning to enlarge	9.50	11.64	13.76	Testicular enlargement is earliest sign of puberty and antecedes pubic hair appearance by about 1½ years
3	Increased in amount and pigmentation; curly; still limited to base of penis	11.86	13.90	15.98	Further enlargement of testes and penis, particularly in length	10.77	12.85	14.93	Height spurt initiates at about this time; 50% may have downy facial hair at corners, upper lip, and on cheeks in front of ears
4	Adult in type; extends about halfway out to inguinal regions	12.20	14.36	16.52	Further enlargement of testes and penis, particularly in circumference	11.73	13.77	15.81	Axillary hair appears here or in stage 3; facial hair only slightly increased but extends across lip; beginning deepening voice; deceleration height spurt
5	Adult in type, quantity, and lateral distribution, extending out to thighs	13.04	15.18	17.32	Adult size, may appear disproportionately in boys who have not yet attained full skeletal growth	12.72	14.92	17.12	Upper lip hair conspicuous; may have sparse chin hair; body hair continues developing well into twenties; growth in height may continue significantly past stage 5 in some

[a] Adapted from A. Hoffman et al.: *The Hospitalized Adolescent; A Guide to Manageing the Ill and Injured Youth.* Macmillan, New York, 1976. From J. M. Tanner: *Growth at Adolescence*, Ed. 2. Blackwell, Oxford, 1962; and A. W. Root: Endocrinology of puberty, *Journal of Pediatrics*, *83:* 1–19, 1973.

turmoil but more commonly sexual acting out is the most common risk taking behavior.

All these behaviors have physical as well as psychosocial sequelae. Teens may get involved with the law or sustain significant physical injury as a result of irresponsible social behavior. Pregnancy and venereal disease are common and potentially devastating outcomes of irresponsible sexual behavior.

Table 71.2
Prevalence (Percent Ever Used) And Recency of Use of Seven Types of Drugs[a]

	1969 (High School 9–12)		1977 (Seniors Only)	
	Ever used	Weekly	Ever used	Monthly
Marijuana	21	6	56	35
Hallucinogens	7	1	14	4
Amphetamines	10	2	23	4
Heroin	2	1	18	0.3
Sedatives	6	1	17	5
Alcohol	81	23	93	71
Cigarettes	66	36	75	38

[a] From NIDA Study Drug Use Among American High School Students 1975–77, Publication No. (ADM) 78-619, DHEW, Washington, D.C., 1977.

Teenagers with chronic diseases are at even higher risk for maladaptive patterns of adolescent development due to the interference of their disease state with the accomplishment of developmental tasks. In addition, teenagers with chronic disease often experience delayed puberty, which results in an inappropriate Tanner stage for age, relative to their peer group (see Tanner stage, Table 71.1). Offer's study also pointed out how important is the role of well adjusted parents as facilitators of adolescent development. Adolescents also have more difficulty making the transition to adulthood when society is in turmoil, as during the war in Vietnam.

This chapter will cover the major psychosocial problems of adolescence which are likely to be encountered in the emergency department, including (1) drug abuse, (2) anorexia nervosa, (3) runaways, and (4) chronic organic complaints.

DRUG ABUSE

BACKGROUND

Adolescents who fall into Offer's surgent or tumultuous growth patterns will be more

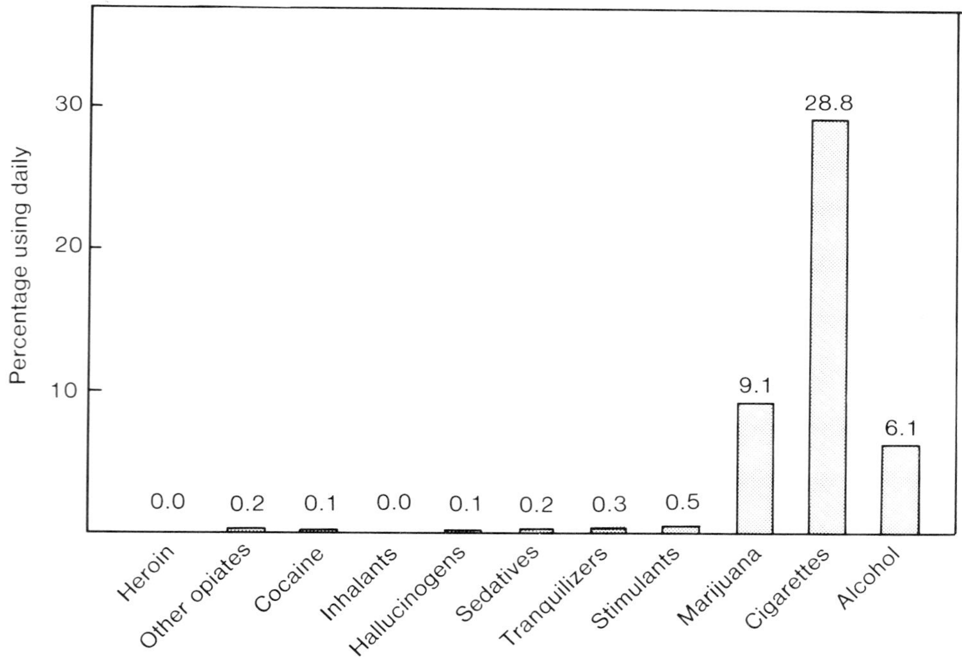

Figure 71.1 Daily use over 30 days of drugs commonly abused by adolescents.

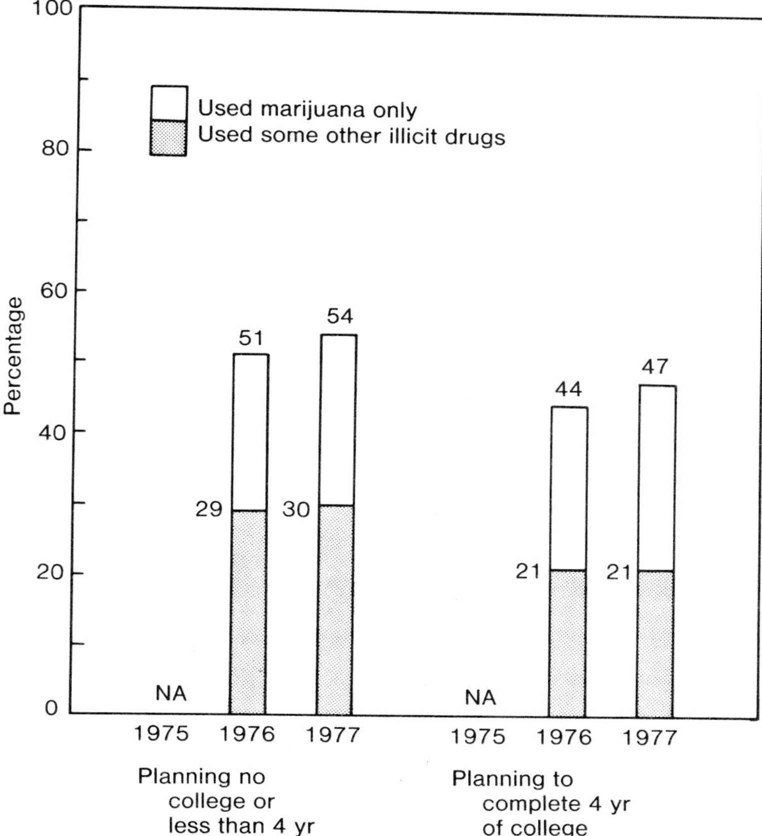

Figure 71.2 Comparison of 2-year trend of illicit drug use in college-bound and non-college-bound adolescents.

at risk for drug experimentation and possible abuse. Similarly, family and community factors (peer group pressures, school environment, religious commitment of family and adolescent) become additional risk or support factors.

In a study by the National Institute of Drug Abuse a comparison was made between drug use by high school students in 1969 and 1977. This study showed a percentage increase in the weekly use of marijuana, hallucinogens, amphetamines, sedatives, and alcohol (Table 71.2). The data clearly demonstrate that the largest substance problems stem first from the licit drugs, alcohol and tobacco, and then the illicit drugs, in order of decreasing frequency of use, marijuana, amphetamines, tranquilizers, sedatives, hallucinogens, inhalants, cocaine, opiates, and heroin (Fig. 71.1).

With respect to adolescent attitudes about drug use, 75% felt that marijuana use should not be treated as a criminal offense. In addition, 65% felt that it should be legal to sell marijuana. There was also a decline in the proportion of seniors who favored legal prohibition of use in public or private of any of the illicit drugs.

The annual prevalence of illicit drug use by adolescents with plans for college for 1977 is shown in Figure 71.1. Among high school seniors not planning to enter college, 30% used some illicit drug other than marijuana and 54% used marijuana only (Fig. 71.2). Of students planning to go to college 21% used some illicit drugs other than marijuana and 47% used marijuana only.

DYNAMICS

Jessor et al. abstracted the personality, social and behavioral data from the sample of junior and senior high school youth surveyed in the National Drug Study in 1974 and tested its correlation with their problem behavior theory. Their theory develops the hypothesis that proneness to drug use can be determined by an analysis of a set of psychosocial attributes that include personality, environmental and behavioral factors. In this framework, drug use is considered as an instance of a larger class of problem behavior (behaviors that elicit negative sanctions from the larger society). Within each of these three systems (personality, environment, behavior), the theory predicts the likelihood of occurrence of problem behavior for a given adolescent according to the presence of certain specified variables. The correlations of these attributes with problem behavior replicated across sex, age and ethnic groups. Donovan and Jessor had previously found that alcohol abuse could be predicted by this theory. Adolescents who use marijuana (but are not problem drinkers) and adolescents who are problem drinkers (but have not used illicit drugs) were similar in their mean score on the majority of personality, environment and behavioral variables. This establishment of psychosocial risk factors for adolescent problem behavior means that engaging in any problem behavior may be associated with engaging in others as well. In addition, although there is general proneness to problem behavior, what determines the specific behavior engaged in may be the specific exposure to it, the specific support for it in the environment, or the specific models for it.

There is no way of predicting whether teenage problem drinking and drug abuse will "mature out" as does a lot of other adolescent problem behavior. It is clear, however, that, for most adolescent abusers of drugs and alcohol, treatment modalities such as family therapy have more to offer than drug rehabilitation programs or straight detoxification and return to the environment without follow-up. Role models among parents and friends need to be assessed as well as the problem teenager.

CLINICAL MANIFESTATIONS

The drug-abusing teenager comes to the attention of the emergency department via an accidental overdose, a suicidal gesture, suicide attempt, or for evaluation of bizarre behavior. The patient's physical status can cover the spectrum from fully awake and responsive to comatose or even convulsing. Table 71.3 provides a quick reference summary of the common drugs of abuse, their symptoms, toxic levels and duration of action.

Initial history from patient, family or friends must specify drugs taken and estimate quantities. Table 71.4 gives the common terminology for street drugs. A determination must be made as to whether the patient is suffering from a drug effect or a withdrawal syndrome. The first responsibility of the emergency department physician is to provide vital life support for impending or actual shock and respiratory or cardiac arrest. This is covered in Chapter 1. Convulsions can occur as a drug side effect or as part of a withdrawal syndrome. Standard anticonvulsant management should be used, except in the case of barbiturate withdrawal in which case barbiturates should be increased and then more gradually tapered.

MANAGEMENT

General Treatment of Drug Overdose

The comatose or near comatose state associated with drug overdose, often compounded by absence of history, is a potentially life-threatening situation. Rappolt et al. have formulated a specific drug arousal therapy consisting of 0.4 mg/ml naloxone (0.8 to 1.6 mg i.v.), activated charcoal slurry 100 to 120 g via large bore orogastric tube instillation, glucagon 1 to 2 mg i.v. and, in selected cases, doxapram 1 to 2 mg/kg i.v. It can be used early in treatment while establishing life support. If early awakening of these patients occurs there are several important advantages. Need for prolonged intubation can be eliminated, a history can be obtained and the overall stay can be shortened.

Activated Charcoal

Activated charcoal is a first line treatment of any confirmed or suspected drug overdose. If the patient has an intact gag reflex and is responsive to voice, a slurry of

Table 71.3
Drug Abuse: Toxicity and Therapy[a]

Drug of Abuse	Symptoms and Signs of Drug Abuse	Diagnosis	Therapeutic Dose	Toxic Dose	Toxic Serum Level	Half-Life
Cannabis Group (marijuana; hashish; Δ9-THC; hash oil)	Pupils unchanged; conjunctiva injected; blood pressure (BP) decreased on standing; heart rate increased; increased appetite, euphoria, anxiety; sensorium often clear; dreamy, fantasy state; timespace distortions; hallucinations rare. Significant airway obstruction with heavy smoking, decreased force expiratory volume (FEV) and decreased vital capacity. Major psychiatric toxic effects: 1. Panic reaction most frequent 2. Psychotic reactions (especially in patients with underlying psychopathology) 3. Toxic delirium (disorientation, confusion, memory impairment) in heavy users 4. Amotivational syndrome (probably due to depression)	Blood urine levels		20 mg Δ9-THC or 1 g cigarette of 2% Δ9-THC produces effects on mood, memory, motor coordination, cognitive ability sensorium, time sense		*1st phase*, minutes, → distribution in lipid-rich tissues; *2nd phase*, (1½–2 days, until mobilized from lipid-rich tissue
Hallucinogens	Pupils dilated (normal or small with PCP); BP elevated, heart rate increased, hyperactive tendon reflexes, increased temp, flushed face, euphoria, anxiety or panic, paranoid thought disorder, inappropriate affect, time and visual distortions, visual hallucinations, depersonalization.					
LSD	Psychosis with hyperalertness; changes in body image; sense of profound significance, delusions; hallucinations (also with amphetamines), visual perceptual distortions due to peripheral effects of LSD on visual system.	Blood, urine levels		20–25 μg produce CNS effects; 0.5–2 μg/kg produce somatic symptoms; between 1 and 16 μg/kg intensity of pathophysiologic effects proportional to dose	Variable	3 hr
PCP	Cyclic coma, extreme hyperactivity, violent outbursts, bizarre behavior, amnesia, analgesia, nystagmus, gait ataxia, muscle	Blood, gastric contents, urine (but level does		1 cigarette (PCP) = 1–100 mg. Psychosis may last several	Individual variability (~0.1 μg/ml)	3 days

Table 71.3—*Continued*

Drug of Abuse	Symptoms and Signs of Drug Abuse	Diagnosis	Therapeutic Dose	Toxic Dose	Toxic Serum Level	Half-Life
	rigidity. Dystonic reactions, grand mal seizures, tardive dyskinesia, athetosis, bronchospasm, urinary retention, diaphoresis, hypoglycemia. Increased uric acid, increased CPK, increased creatinine, increased SGOT/SGPT—heralds onset of rhabdomyolysis (can go to renal failure). Hyperuricemia disapproprotionate to CPK	not correlate with toxicity)		weeks after 1 dose. Fatal dose = 1 mg/kg; <5 mg = hyperactivity; 5–10 mg = stupor, coma; >10 mg = respiratory depression, convulsions		
CNS Stimulants						
Amphetamines	Pupils dilated and reactive. Increased BP, pulse, temperature, cardiac arrhythmias; dry mouth; sweating; tremors; sensorium hyperacute or confused; paranoid ideation; impulsivity; hyperactivity; stereotypy; convulsions, exhaustion	Blood level, urine test	5 mg t.i.d.	**1. Variable 2. Rare under 15 mg 3. Severe reactions have occurred at 30 mg 4. 400–500 mg not uniformly fatal 5. Tolerance is striking, chronic user may take 1700 mg/day without ill effects**	Variable	3 hr
Cocaine	1. Excitement, restlessness, euphoria, garrulousness 2. Increased motor activity, physical endurance due to decreased sense of fatigue 3. Increased tremors, convulsive movements 4. Increased respiration, pulse, blood pressure, temperature, chilld 5. Dilated pupils, intense vasoconstriction	Urine, serum	Anaesthesia—1 ml of 5% solution for surface anaesthesia (=50 mg or less)	Fatal dose may be as low as 30 mg. Ingested cocaine less toxic than by other routes		1 hr (after p.o. or nasal route)
CNS Sedatives (barbiturates, chlordiazepoxide, diazepam, flurazepam, glutethimide, meprobamate, methaqualone)	Pupils normal or small (dilated with glutethimide). Blood pressure decreased, respirations depressed. Drowsy, coma, lateral nystagmus, confusion, ataxia, slurred speech, delirium. Convulsions or hyperirritability with methaqualone overdosage. Serious poisoning rare with benzodiazepines alone	Serum level				

Barbiturates (Secobarbital) (Seconal)	As above	Serum level	30–50 mg, 3–4 ×/day	100 mg per dose	30 μg/ml	19–34 hr
Chlordiazepoxide (Librium)	As above	Serum level	5–20 mg, 3–4 ×/day	25 mg	8 μg/ml	8–25 hr
Diazepam (Valium)	As above	Serum urine	2–10 mg, 4 ×/day	15 mg or greater		20–90 hr
Flurazepam (Dalmane)	As above	Serum urine	15–30 mg		0.12 μg/ml (fatal)	47–100 hr
Glutethimide (Doriden)	As above	Serum level	125–250 mg, 1–3 ×/day	>500 mg (acute intoxication, 3 g)	2 mg/100 ml (but even below, full ICU support may be required)	5–22 hr
Meprobamate	As above	Serum level	400 mg, 4 ×/day	>800 mg	150 μg/ml	6–17 hr
Methaqualone (Parest, Somnafae)	As above	Serum level	100 mg, 4 ×/day	200–400 mg	10 μg/ml	20–60 hr
Narcotics	Pupils constricted (may be dilated with meperidine or extreme hypoxia); respiration depressed to absent with cyanosis; BP decreased, sometimes shock; temperature reduced; reflexes diminished to absent; stupor or coma; pulmonary edema; constipation; convulsions with propoxyphene or meperidine					
Heroin	As above	Serum	3 mg[b]	—	—	1½ hr[d]
Morphine	As above	Serum	10 mg[b]	60 mg = toxic[c] 200 mg = fatal dose[c]	—	3 hr[d]
Codeine	As above	Serum	120 mg[b]	800 mg = fatal dose[c]	1.1 μg/ml	2 hr[d]
Methadone	As above	Serum	7.5–10 mg[b]	100 mg = fatal dose[c]	1.6 μg/ml (fatal)	18–97 hr[d]
Propoxyphene	As above	Serum	65 mg every 4 hr[b]	500 mg = fatal dose[c]	2 μg/ml (fatal)	3–12 hr[d]
Anticholinergics (atropine, belladonna, henbane, scopolamine, trihexphenidyl tricyclic antidepressants, benzotropine mesylate)	Pupils dilated and fixed, heart rate increased, temperature increased, blood pressure decreased. Drowsy coma, flushed, dry skin and mucous membranes, erythematous skin, amnesia, disoriented, visual hallucinations, body image alterations	Urine test				

Table 71.3—*Continued*

Drug of Abuse	Symptoms and Signs of Drug Abuse	Diagnosis	Therapeutic Dose	Toxic Dose	Toxic Serum Level	Half-Life
Atropine	As above		0.5–1 mg	5 mg		24 hr
Belladonna	As above		0.6–1 mg	5 mg		24 hr
Scopolamine	As above		0.6 mg	5 mg		24 hr
Imipramine (Tofranil)	As above		100–200 mg/day	>500 mg		8–16 hr
Amitriptyline (Elavil)	As above		75–200 mg	>500 mg	5 μg/ml	32–40 hr
Desipramine	As above			1 g	10 μg/ml	12–54 hr

[a] From R. H. Dreisbach: *Handbook of Poisoning*, Lange Medical Publications, Los Altos, Calif., 1980.
[b] Dose is amount given subcutaneously that produces same analgesic effect as morphine 10 mg subcutaneously.
[c] Doses given higher for addicts.
[c] Duration is for subcutaneous dose. Intravenous dose peak is more pronounced and overall effects have shorter duration.

100 to 120 g of activated charcoal in 9 oz of water is given. In a more obtunded patient, an orogastric tube (30 to 36 French Ewald in the adult, proportionately smaller for the child) is passed with the chin anteflexed on the sternum. The stomach should be lavaged with 300 ml normal saline, a 100 to 120 g slurry of activated charcoal instilled and the tube clamped. Although the activated charcoal does not adsorb all substances equally, it is completely nontoxic. Nonpolar, large molecules are most rapidly adsorbed. Table 71.5 lists the substances that are well adsorbed by charcoal and those that are not adsorbed. Systemic adsorption of any agent is dependent upon its own dissociation constant and the existing pH of the gastrointestinal tract so that charcoal present in the gut can have a beneficial effect for several hours postingestion. In addition, agents such as tricyclics, phencyclidine and glutethimide undergo enterohepatic and/or enterogastric recirculation and may be trapped in their transit through the small intestine. Therefore, a repeat dose of activated charcoal 100 to 120 g in a 9 oz of water every 4 hours in the presence of continued symptoms is appropriate.

Glucagon

Glucagon stimulates the adenylcyclase system which activates liver phosphorylase thus producing rapid glycogenolysis. It also stimulates gluconeogenesis and converts ATP to cyclic AMP with the release of energy. Glucagon apparently produces a distinct inotropic effect in the heart as glucagon decreases end diastolic filling pressure and improves myocardial performance in the normal heart. Its use in the comatose or nearly comatose patient is for its probable inotropic effect on the heart, to treat the 0 to 2% of overdose victims who will be diabetic (comparable incidence to nondrug using population). Empirically Rappolt et al. have discovered that glucagon i.m. or i.v. often results in lightening of clinical coma within less than one minute.

Doxapram

Doxapram is a respiratory stimulant which exerts it action through the peripheral carotid chemoreceptors. It has been

Table 71.4
Drug Use Terminology[a]

Term/Meaning(s)

Abbotts—Nembutal (pentobarbital) capsules, each marked with the manufacturer's name: "Abbott"
Acapulco gold—Very potent marijuana
Almes [or Aymes, cf Amys]—Amyl nitrite
All-Star—Multiple-drug user
Angle mist—PCP (phenylcyclidine)
Animal—LDS (lysergic acid diethylamide)

Baby—Marijuana. A small, irregular drug habit, as in: A 'baby' habit
Bad seed—Peyote buttons
Bam—Amphetamine pill/capsule. Amphetamine prepared for injection
Barbs—Barbiturates, no specific brand name, jagged edges of old hypodermic needles
Beans—Benzedrine (amphetamine)
Belly habit—Opiate addiction
Benny jag—To be high on amphetamines
Big C—Cocaine
Big Harry—Heroin
Black cadillacs—Biphetamine (dextroamphetamine and amphetamine) 20 mg capsules
Black Dex—Biphetamine (dextroamphetamine and amphetamine) 20 mg capsules
Black Russian—Dark, very potent, hashish, possibly mixed with opium
Blanco—Heroin
Blue Berkley—LSD, similar to "Blotter," in which LSD drops are put on one-inch squares of blue paper and left to dry. This allows for easy transport of drug, and ingestion when paper is taken by mouth
Blue microdot—LSD applied in liquid form to vitamin C tablets and left to dry, forming a blue dot in the middle of the tablet
Bombita/Bombito—Amphetamine or cocaine prepared for injection
Brown—Mexican heroin
Brown mescaline—Brown powder, reported to contain mescaline
Brow stuff—Opium
Busy bee—PCB

Candy—Cocaine, sometimes known as a "nose candy;" any drug
Cartwheels—White, double-scored, amphetamine tablets, usually from illicit manufacturers
Chalk—Amphetamine tablets, usually from illicit manufacturers. These tablets have a white, gritty appearance, like chalk
Channel—Vein used for injection
Chicago green—Marijuana mixed with opium
Chiva—Heroin
Co-pilots—Amphetamine tablets/capsules
Cotton habit—Irregular heroin nabit
Courage pills—Barbiturates
Crank—Amphetamine, usually from an illicit manufacturer
Cross—Amphetamine, usually from an illicit manufacturer, which is white, in tablet form, and double scored
Crossroads—See "Cross" (above)
Crosstops—See "Cross" (above)
Crystal—Amphetamine in powder form; PCP in solid form

Deuce—A $2.00 packet of heroin
Dice—Methamphetamine, possibly Desoxyn
Dirt—Heroin
DOA—PCP
Dollies—Methadone
Downers—Amytal (amobarbital) capsules; Doriden (glutethimide)
Downs—Dalmane (flurazepam hydrochloride)
Drivers—Amphetamine, short from "truckdrivers;" a term used to identify amphetamine
Dust—Cocaine, heroin, PCP, or morphine
Dusting—Mixing heroin and/or PCP with marijuana for smoking

Electric kool aid—LSD mixed with punch
Elephant—PCP
Endurets—Preludin (phenmetrazine hydrochloride), prolonged-action tablets

F-40s—Secondal (secobarbital), 100 mg capsules, which are mixed with the ID code "F-40"
F-66—Tuinal (amobarbital sodium and secobarbital sodium), 200 mg capsule, which is marked with the ID code "F-66"
'Fit—Equipment for injecting drugs
Fives—Amphetamine tablets, 5 mg each
Flea powder—Highly diluted heroin
Footballs—Amphetamine tablets in oval form. (Dilaudid (hydromorphone) tablet
Fours—Tylenol (acetaminophen) with codeine—4 (60 mg of codeine per tablet)
Fuel—Marijuana sprayed or mixed with insecticides then smoked

Gin—Alcoholic beverage; cocaine
Gold—Very potent marijuana, short for "Acapulco gold"
Gold dust—Cocaine
Golf balls—Barbiturates
Goon—PCP
Gorilla pills—Tuinal (amobarbital sodium and secobarbital sodium)
Green—Dexamyl (dextroamphetamine sulfate and amobarbital) tablets/capsules. Low-grade marijuana from Mexico
Green hearts—Dexamyl (dextroamphetamine sulfate and amobarbital) tablets, 5 mg each

Table 71.4—*Continued*

Term/Meaning(s)
Greenies—Dexamyl (dextroamphetamine sulfate and amobarbital) tablets/capsules
Gun—Hypodermic needle used to inject drugs
Gutter—Vein used to inject drugs
Hard candy—Heroin; by extension, any "hard" drug
Harry—Heroin
Hearts—Three-sided, heart-shaped amphetamine tablets
Heaven dust—Cocaine
Hog—PCP, chloral hydrate
Hootch—Marijuana
Hooter—Marijuana
Horn—To sniff a drug
Horse—Heroin
Horse hearts—Benzedrine (amphetamine sulfate) tablets
Horse tranquilizer—PCP
Ice cream habit—Irregular drug habit
Incentive—Cocaine
J—Marijuana
Jellies—Chloral hydrate
Killer weed—PCP mixed with marijuana and smoked
Kool aid—LSD mixed with punch
Krystal—PCP in solid form, amphetamine in solid form
Lady snow—Cocaine
Leaper—Amphetamine, no specific brand
Lightning—Amphetamine, no specific brand
Lilly—Seconal (secobarbital)
'Line—Short for "Mainline;" a vein used to inject drugs
'Luding out—Using methaqualone, either Quaalude or Sopor; using methaqualone, either
Magic mist—PCP
Merck—General term for high-grade drugs
Mexican brown—Heroin of average strength
Mexican reds—Red capsules, imported from Mexico, reported to contain secobarbital
Mexican yellows—Pentobarbital, possibly Nembutal, possibly imported from Mexico
Miss Emma—Morphine
Move-star drug—Cocaine
Nail—Hypodermic needle used to inject drugs
Nose candy—Cocaine
Orange hearts—Dexedrine (dextroamphetamine sulfate) tablets
Paris 400—Parest (methaqualone hydrochloride) capsules, usually 400 mg each
Peace kill—PCP
Pimp—Cocaine
Pinks—Seconal (secobarbital) capsules; Darvon (propoxyphene hydrochloride) capsules
Pink ladies—Seconal (secobarbital) capsules
Poppers—Amyl nitrite
Purple haze—LSD in tablet form, PCP in purple tablet form
Quaas—Quaalude (methaqualone)
Red & Greys—Darvon (propoxyphene hydrochloride) capsules
Rippers—General term for amphetamines
Rock—Cocaine in solid form
Rockets—Marijuana
Rocket fuel—PCP
Roses—Benzedrine (amphetamine sulfate) tablets
Sherman's—PCP cigarette
Short flight—Combination of Coridicin (aspirin, chlorpheniramine maleate, and caffeine) and
Snort—Inhale cocaine or heroin
Society high—Cocaine
Speedball—Combination of amphetamine and cocaine or heroin for injection
Stardust—Cocaine
Strawberry mescaline—Reddish-brown powder, reported to contain mescaline
Superjoint—Marijuana mixed with PCP
Super Quaalude, Sopor, Quaas, 'ludes—Parest (methaqualone hydrochloride)
Tecata—Heroin
Texas reefer—Long, fat, marijuana cigarette, also called a "Bomber"
THC—Tetrahydrocannabinal, possible PCP
Thrusters—Amphetamine, no specific brand name
Thai stick—Asian marijuana mixed with opium and tied to a reed
Tie stick—Marijuana mixed with opium and tied to a popsicle stick
Truck drivers—Amphetamine
Water—Methamphetamine mixed with water for injection
Weekend habit—Irregular drug use
Weekend warrior—Irregular drug user
White cross—Amphetamine tablets, from illicit manufacturers, which are white, and double scored
White dexies—Amphetamine tablets from illicit manufacturers
White horizon—PCP
White horse—Cocaine
White stuff—Heroin, cocaine, morphine
Wobble—PCP
Yellow bam—Methamphetamine; possibly Desoxyn
Yellow jackets—Barbiturates
Zeeters—Amphetamine

Table 71.5
Therapeutic Use of Activated Charcoal

Substances Well Adsorbed
Acetaminophen
Amphetamines
Antimony
Antipyrene
Arsenic
Aspirin
Atropine
Barbiturates
Benzodiapines
Cantharides
Cocaine
DDT (chlorinated hydrocarbons)
Digitalis
Dilantin
Glutethimide
Iodine
Ipecac
Malathion
Meprobamate
Mercuric chloride
Morphine
Muscarine
Nicotine
Opium
Oxalates
Parathion (organic phosphates)
Penicillin
Methylene blue
Phenol
Phenolphthalein
Phenothiazines
Phosphorus
Potassium permanganate
Propoxyphene
Quinine
Selenium
Silver
Stramonium
Strychnine
Sulfonamides
Tricyclic antidepressants
Substances Poorly (or Not) Adsorbed
Common electrolytes
Iron
Mineral acids or bases
Alcohols
Cyanide
Most solvents
Most water-insoluble compounds

rejected in medical circles along with older analeptics. Rappolt et al. have been using doxapram in their treatment of over 1200 street drug abusers since the late 1960s. No serious side effects such as hyperthermia or convulsions have been noted. Patients with prolonged respiratory depression and presumed acidotic changes were excluded. Doxapram was found to be safe and to improve respiratory effort in overdose patients with respiratory depression. Patients were also noted to be moved to a lighter level of obtundation with oropharyngeal reflexes, consciousness and cerebral function often restored within seconds. After initial response some relapse was common but not to the original depth of coma or depressed state. Their dosage is as follows:

1. 1.0 to 2 mg/kg i.v. push
2. 0.5 to 1 mg/kg repeated in 5 min
3. 0.5 to 1 mg/kg at 15-min intervals if indicated × 2 doses
4. If patient continues to respond, then relapses, a drip infusion of 2 mg/kg/hr in 5% dextrose in water can be started.

The therapeutic ratio (convulsive dose/ventilatory stimulant dose) is about 70:1 as compared to 2 or 4:1 for the other analeptics.

Naloxone

Naloxone, a pure narcotic antagonist is the broadest acting, safest and most effective of any true antidote drug now available to emergency medical personnel. It is effective against all opiates and opiate derivatives. It effectively reverses opiate-like depression of Darvon, Talwin, Percodan, Diluadid, Nalline, Lomotil and the antidiarrheal, Imodium. Naloxone is a synthetic cogener of oxymorphone and is devoid of morphine agonist or depressant effects. It has no significant side effects except narcotic withdrawal symptoms in the addicted individual. These symptoms include gastrointestinal upset, tachycardia, hyperpnea, mydriasis, rhinorrhea, diaphoresis, sialorrhea, increased blood pressure, anxiety, restlessness, discomfort, hyperalgesia. These symptoms are not life threatening to teenagers and adults but can be fatal to an infant born to an addicted mother. Withdrawal symptoms, if observed during acute overdose treatment, should be treated with short-acting i.v. narcotics. The serum half-life of naloxone is 1 hour, its duration of action 1 to 4 hours. Initial reversal of narcosis may then revert to coma requiring ongoing reassessment and readministration of naloxone.

The mechanism of action of naloxone is by competitive displacement of narcotic analgesics at central narcotic receptor sites. It can be used as a challenge test with a poor history. Pediatric dose is 0.02 mg/kg/dose up to 0.5 mg/dose. If no veins are available, naloxone can be given to adults as 4 ml i.m. (1.6 mg), 2 ml in each deltoid muscle or 2 to 4 ml sublingually deep into the floor of the subglossal fossa. A repeat dose of 2 ml should be given in 5 min. If a lightening response occurs, it is then appropriate to give an additional 2 ml i.v. every 2 hours for 2 doses. CNS depression secondary to pentazocine (Talwin) and propoxyphene (Darvon) requires high doses of naloxone to get a therapeutic effect. Rappolt has also observed that, in the higher dose naloxone regimen, patients in coma from ethyl alcohol may lighten their coma. He interprets this to mean that naloxone in higher doses is a direct CNS arousal agent.

Disposition

After the patient's initial assessment and medical stabilization, an assessment must be made of the severity of the drug use problem. Six questions should be asked in order to assess this severity.

1. Is the patient a drug abuser? Establish what drugs have been used, what frequency and for what duration.
2. Any withdrawal symptoms experienced? (sedative hynotics or opiates)
3. What is the pattern of use? Is drug used when available socially or does teenager actively seek sources of the drug?
4. What is the developmental stage of the adolescent? Any suggestion of conflict, overcompensation, incongruencies?
5. What role is drug use playing? Are drugs used as part of a social situation, to ease social interaction or as a maladaptive method of integrating adolescent development?
6. Any difficulties in life function areas or medical problems resulting from drug use?

Once the severity of the drug problem has been established, it is essential to arrange a treatment program. Primary care physicians are often comfortable managing intermittent drug users with no life area problems. Compulsive users or anyone who has experienced withdrawal must be referred to a residential program. Steady users who have had major life area problems require referral to an outpatient therapist or an outpatient treatment program. It is important to remember that, if family problems emerge as a significant reason for the drug abuse, family therapy is more appropriate than individual psychotherapy.

Specific Drugs

The major categories of drugs of abuse that require the physicians familiarity with the whole spectrum of their physiologic effects are (1) hallucinogens (phencyclidine, LSD, marijuana); (2) stimulants (amphetamines, cocaine); (3) central anticholinergics; (4) sedatives (barbiturates, benzodiazepines, glutethimide); (5) opioids (morphine, codeine, heroin, methadone); and (6) alcohol. In addition, it is useful to be aware of what street drugs are popular in a given area at a particular time, since these are constantly changing.

Hallucinogens (Psychedelics)

There is no definite line that divides psychedelics from other classes of centrally active drugs such as anticholinergics, cocaine and amphetamines. These drugs can also produce illusions, hallucinations, delusions, paranoid ideation and altered mood and thinking. The feature that distinguishes the psychedelic agents is their capacity to induce states of altered perception, thought and feeling that cannot otherwise be experienced except in dreams or states of religious exultation. The psychedelic state is described as including vivid and unusual sensory experiences with a diminished control over what is experienced. Sensations take on profound meaning and there is a decreased ability to differentiate oneself from the environment. Most of the drugs in this category of psychedelics are related to the indolealkylamines (such as LSD, psilocybin, dimethyltryptamine and diethyltryptamine), to the phenylethylamines (mescaline), or phenyllisopropyl amines (amphetamines).

Phencyclidine (Angel Dust, Busy Bee, Elephant)

PATHOPHYSIOLOGY

Phencyclidine (PCP) was developed in the 1950s as an animal anaesthetic and for a short time as a general anaesthetic in man. It rapidly fell into disuse because of the delirium that patients felt when they emerged from anaesthesia. Sporadic abuse occurred in the 1960s but in the 1970s it became popular for smoking or snorting. Easily synthesized, it has recently been one of the most prevalent street drugs. It is often misrepresented as LSD, mescaline or marijuana (≜9-tetrahydrocannabinol). Chemically PCP is an arylcyclohexylamine. This group of drugs have CNS stimulant, CNS depressant, hallucinogenic and analgesic actions.

PHARMACODYNAMICS

There is great individual variability in the metabolism of the drug. In general 0.1 mg/ml is a toxic serum level. One cigarette may contain 1 to 100 mg depending on the source. A fatal dose is in the range of 1 mg/kg; 5 to 10 mg may produce stupor and coma; greater than 10 mg respiratory depression and convulsions. The half-life lasts 3 days during which time patients show cyclic symptoms as the drug is mobilized from fat stores to the serum. PCP is well absorbed following all routes of administration. Only a small amount of the drug is excreted unchanged.

The concept that PCP interferes with the association pathways linking the cerebral cortex with deeper structures in the brain thus diminishing the ability to integrate sensory input into meaningful behavior is generally accepted. Bizarre behavior and loss of pain sensation are consistent with this action.

A 1977 survey indicated that 14% of all 18 to 25-year-olds had used PCP at least once. About one half of current users claim to use it once a week. Some drug abusers use the drug for 2 to 3 days straight without sleeping or eating. The drug may be sprinkled on tobacco, marijuana or parsley and is smoked after making it into a cigarette. Chronic users may ingest up to 1 g in 24 hours.

CLINICAL SYMPTOMS

Small doses of PCP produce a subjective sense of intoxication with staggering gait, slurred speech, nystagmus and numbness of the extremities. Users may exhibit sweating, catatonic muscular rigidity and a blank stare. They may also experience changes in body image, disorganized thought, drowsiness and apathy. Heart rate and blood pressure may be elevated. There is hypersalivation, sweating, fever, repetitive movements and muscle rigidity on stimulation. At higher doses prolonged coma, muscle rigidity and convulsions may occur. Psychotic states can occur that can be long lasting. In one study 25% of those with a schizophrenic-like reaction were seen again for a similar syndrome in the absence of PCP. Users apparently use it for the increased sensitivity to external stimuli, stimulation, mood elevation and a sense of intoxication. The typical high from a single dose lasts 4 to 6 hours and is followed by an extended coming down period.

Tolerance develops to the behavioral and toxic effects. Some chronic users complain about craving after stopping the drug. Chronic users also report persistent difficulties with recent memory, speech, and thinking that lasts from 6 months to 1 year after stopping. Personality changes such as withdrawal, isolation, anxiety, nervousness, and depression have been reported.

MANAGEMENT

Unfortunately the serum test for PCP does not correlate with toxicity. Treatment must be initiated on the basis of clinical observation and history. Initial treatment for ingestions includes emptying the stomach by gastric lavage or emesis and attaching the patient to continuous gastric suction to lessen gastroenteric recirculation. A quiet room is essential and vital signs must be monitored and supportive measures administered as indicated. Restraints should be avoided if possible because they may predispose to rhabdomyolysis in a thrashing patient. The skeletal muscle injury that causes the rhabdomyolysis is felt to be a result of excessive involuntary isometric motor activity rather than a direct effect of PCP on skeletal muscle. Severe rhabdomyolysis can lead to acute myoglobinuric renal failure. Acidification of the urine (pH below 5.0) and diuretics are known to enhance urinary excretion of the drug but will exacerbate the course of developing rhabdomyolysis. Therefore, it is important not to acidify the urine until creatine phospokinase, creatinine, SGOT, SGPT and uric acid results are known to be normal. If these tests show increases and the urine has a positive test for hemoglobin without red blood cells, the patient should be assumed to have rhabdomyolysis and treated (see Chapter 46, "Renal and Electrolyte Emergencies").

In a review of 27 confirmed cases of PCP poisoning, 3 patients developed rhabdomyolysis and 2 progressed to acute renal failure. Both patients had received ammonium chloride acidification measures before diagnosis. Diazepam 5 mg every 6 hours should be used for hyperactivity and hydralazine 25 to 50 mg b.i.d. for hypertension. If psychotic behavior persists, haloperidol 2.5 mg b.i.d. plus 1.2 mg Cogentin daily should be used.

LSD (Animal, Blue Berkley)

PATHOPHYSIOLOGY

LSD and related psychedelic drugs such as psilocin, mescaline, dimethyltryptamine (DMT) have actions at multiple sites in the CNS from the cortex to the spinal cord. In addition, scientists have produced dozens of cogeners of indoleamine and phenethylamine that cause subjective symptoms similar to LSD. Some of the best described effects involve agonistic actions at presynaptic receptors for serotonin (5-hydroxytryptamine) in the midbrain.

PHARMACODYNAMICS

In man the somatic symptoms of dizziness, weakness, drowsiness, nausea and paraesthesias are observed after one oral dose of 0.5 to 2 mg/kg. Between the dose range of 1 and 16 mg/kg the intensity of the psychophysiological effects of LSD is proportional to the dose. A high degree of tolerance to the behavioral effects develops after 3 to 4 daily doses. Sensitivity returns after a drug-free interval. Withdrawal phenomena are not seen after abrupt discontinuation. Deaths attributable to *direct* effects of LSD are unknown, although fatal accidents and suicides occur during states of intoxication.

CLINICAL SYMPTOMS

In general, the somatic effects are sympathomimetic such as pupillary dilatation, increased blood pressure, tachycardia, hyperreflexia, and increased body temperature. Doses as low as 20 to 25 mg can produce CNS effects such as euphoria, visual perceptual distortions, alteration of subjective time so that time passes slowly, lability of mood, or even an acute panic episode. Hallucinations and psychosis with hyperalertness is commonly seen. The entire syndrome begins to clear in 12 hours. The psychedelic state includes a heightened awareness of sensory input, often accompanied by an enhanced sense of clarity but a diminished control over what is experienced. Often there is a feeling that one part of the self is a passive observer while another part receives vivid sensory input. There is a diminished ability to separate one object from another, or to separate self from the environment. There is an enhanced sense of oneness with mankind or the cosmos.

In general, LSD does not lead to repetitive use over time. It is used mainly by the more affluent, artistic, or college students.

MANAGEMENT

Clinical management involves placing the patient in a quiet room. Someone who knows the patient may quietly talk down and reassure the patient during the time of the vivid perceptual distortion or panic attack. The patient's loss of boundaries and fear of fragmentation or self-disintegration creates a need for a structuring or a supporting environment.

Marijuana (Gold, Hootch, Grass, Pot, Reefer, Hash)

PATHOPHYSIOLOGY

The flowering tops of the female marijuana plant contains the highest concentration of the active constituent, Δ9-tetrahydrocannabinol (THC). Within minutes after smoking this material perceptual, behavioral and emotional states become altered. All of the absorbed THC is excreted in metabolized form. Metabolites have been identified in blood, urine, feces and saliva. The clinical effects are mainly due to Δ9-THC and 11-hydroxy-THC. The mechanism of action is unknown.

PHARMACODYNAMICS

It is estimated that no more than 50% of THC in a marijuana cigarette is actually absorbed. Pharmacologic effects begin immediately. However, the onset of effects occurs at 0.5 to 1 hour after oral administration and peak effects may not occur until the 2nd or 3rd hour and correlate well with plasma concentrations. THC is 3 times more potent when smoked than when taken by mouth. Tolerance develops to drug-induced changes of mood, tachycardia, decrease in skin temperature, increase in body temperature, decrease in intraocular pressure, and impairment of performance on psychomotor tests. Tolerance to cardiac effects develops rapidly and decays rapidly.

Abrupt discontinuation of cannabinoids after chronic use of high dosage is followed by irritability, restlessness, nervousness, decreased appetite, weight loss, insomnia.

CLINICAL SYMPTOMS

The most prominent effects in man are on the central nervous system and cardiovascular system. Descriptions of effects can be misleading because of differences due to dose, route of administration, subjective experience, and expectations. Oral doses of 20 mg of Δ9-THC produces effects on mood, memory, motor coordination, cognitive ability, sensorium, time sense, and self-perception. There is an increased sense of well-being or euphoria accompanied by feelings of relaxation or sleepiness when subjects are alone. With oral doses of Δ9-THC equal to several cigarettes, short-term memory is impaired, and there is a deterioration in capacity to carry out tasks requiring multiple mental steps to reach a specific goal. This effect on memory dependent goal-directed behavior has been called temporal disintegration and is correlated with a tendency to confuse past, present and future and with depersonalization, a sense of strangeness and unreality about one's self. Performance of simple motor tasks and simple reaction times are unimpaired until higher doses are reached. More complex processes including perception, attention, information processing are impaired by doses equivalent to one or two cigarettes. Marijuana smokers frequently report increased hunger, dry mouth and throat, more vivid visual imagery and a keener sense of hearing. Touch, taste and smell seem to be enhanced. Altered time perception is a consistent effect of cannabinoids so that minutes seem like hours. Higher doses of Δ9-THC can produce frank hallucinations, delusions and paranoid feelings. Thinking becomes confused and disorganized. Anxiety reaching panic proportions may replace euphoria, often as a feeling that the drug-induced state will never end. With high enough doses the clinical picture of a toxic psychosis with hallucinations, depersonalization and loss of insight can occur. Because of the rapid onset of effects when marijuana is smoked and low Δ9-THC content of marijuana grown in the United States, most users can regulate their intake to avoid the excessive dosage that produces these unpleasant effects. Marijuana may cause an acute exacerbation of symptoms in stabilized schizophrenics. Cardiovascular effects include an increase in heart rate, an increase in systolic blood pressure and a marked reddening of the conjunctivae. Chronic smoking of marijuana and hashish is associated with bronchitis and asthma, even though the acute response to Δ9-THC is one of bronchodilatation.

The amotivational syndrome described in chronic marijuana users describes people who become complacent and withdrawn and demonstrate a decrease in work output and lessening of interest in their surroundings, career or school life.

MANAGEMENT

In general the only treatment required is discontinuation of the drug. In the patient with a psychotic reaction or acute toxic delirium, a sedative such as diazepam 5 mg by mouth or intramuscularly may need to be used. These acute symptoms should improve with drug abstinence over 4 to 6 hours.

Stimulants (Amphetamines, Cocaine, Dextroamphetamine, Methamphetamine)

Amphetamines

PATHOPHYSIOLOGY

Amphetamine or racemic β-phenylisopropylamine has powerful CNS stimulant actions, in addition to the peripheral α and β actions common to indirectly acting sympathomimetic drugs. Unlike epinephrine it is effective after oral administration and its effects last for several hours. Amphetamines have been used medically to treat narcolepsy, obesity, fatigue, parkinsonism, and poisoning by CNS depressants. The pharmacologic effects include an increase in systolic and diastolic blood pressure, often a reflex slowing of heart rate, contraction of bladder sphincter and dramatic CNS stimulation. Its mechanism of action in the CNS is by releasing biogenic amines from their storage sites in the nerve terminals.

PHARMACODYNAMICS

The therapeutic dose is in the range of 5 mg t.i.d. The toxic dose is variable but is rarely less than 15 mg. Severe reactions have been reported at 30 mg, yet doses up to 400 to 500 mg are not uniformly fatal. Tolerance is striking and the chronic user may take 1700 mg a day without ill effects. The half-life is about 3 hours.

CLINICAL SYMPTOMS

The psychic effect of amphetamines depends on the dose, mental state and personality of the individual. In general 10 to 30 mg causes wakefulness, alertness, decreased sense of fatigue, elevation of mood, with increased initiative, self-confidence, ability to concentrate, elation, euphoria and increase in motor and speech activity. Physical performance in athletes may be improved. Prolonged use of large doses is followed by depression and fatigue. In general, amphetamine accelerates and desynchronizes the EEG. It has an appetite suppressant effect through its action on the lateral hypothalamic feeding center. However, tolerance to this dose develops quickly; therefore, the effect is insufficient to reduce weight over a period of time.

The acute toxic effects of amphetamine are usually extensions of its therapeutic actions and as a result of overdosage. The central effects induce restlessness, dizziness, tremor, hyperactive reflexes, talkativeness, tenseness, irritability, weakness, insomnia, fever and euphoria. In addition, confusion, assaultiveness, anxiety, delirium, paranoid hallucinations, panic states and suicidal or homicidal tendencies can occur, especially in patients with an underlying mental illness. However, these psychotic effects can be elicited in anyone if amphetamine is ingested for a prolonged period. Cardiac toxicity includes flushing, palpitation, anginal pain and circulatory collapse. Gastrointestinal effects include dry mouth, anorexia, nausea, vomiting, diarrhea and abdominal cramps. Severe overdoses terminate in convulsions, coma and cerebral hemorrhages. Psychological dependence occurrs with chronic use. Tolerance develops rapidly to the anorexigenic effect and to the mood effect. All the sympathomimetics have similar CNS effects but not identical mechanisms of action. The subjective effects of the CNS sympathomimetics are dependent on the user, the environment, the dose of the drug and the route of administration. Although tolerance to the CNS effects occurs, a toxic psychosis may occur after weeks to months of continued use of amphetamine drugs.

Chronic intoxication with amphetamine causes symptoms similar to those of acute overdosage. The most common serious effect is a psychotic reaction with vivid hallucinations and paranoid delusions often mistaken for schizophrenia. Recovery is usually rapid after withdrawal of the drug but occasionally the condition becomes chronic. In such persons it is possible that the amphetamine has hastened the onset of incipient schizophrenia.

MANAGEMENT

Treatment of poisoning from this general group should consist of removing the ingested drug by gastric lavage or emesis followed by preventing absorption with activated charcoal and saline catharsis. Specific treatment consists of administration of chlorpromazine 1 to 2 mg/kg. This may be repeated as necessary to control the marked CNS excitation and the concomitant hypertension. If this is not adequate to control hypertension α-adrenergic blocking agents such as phenoxybenzamine (1 mg/kg i.v.) and nitroglycerin (0.4 mg sublinqual) or sodium nitrate 60 mg i.v. can be given. Since up to 45% of ingested drugs will appear in the kidneys unchanged, ample fluids are essential. Peritoneal dialysis can be used in severe amphetamine poisoning. If convulsions are imminent a short-acting barbituate should be given i.v. Treatment of chronic poisoning requires sedation, usually with barbituates, drug withdrawal and a program of psychotherapy.

Cocaine

PATHOPHYSIOLOGY

Cocaine occurs in the leaves of *Erythroxylon coca* and other species of erythroxylon trees indigenous to Peru and Bolivia where the leaves have been used for centuries by the natives to increase indurance and promote a sense of well being. Chemically cocaine is benzoylmethylecgonine. Ecgonine is an amino alcohol base closely related to tropine, the amino alcohol in atropine.

PHARMACODYNAMICS

The relief from fatigue that occurs with cocaine use results from central stimulation which masks the sensation of fatigue. Cocaine is also pyrogenic. The onset of "cocaine fever" is often preceded by a chill. It potentiates the excitatory and inhibitory responses of sympathetically innervated organs to norepinephrine and epinephrine by blocking the uptake of catecholamines at adrenergic nerve endings. This explains why cocaine, unlike other local anaesthetics, produces vasoconstriction and mydriasis. The most important pharmacologic action is its ability to block the initiation or conduction of the nerve impulse following local application. It is still used as a local anaesthetic in the upper respiratory tract. For surface anaesthesia 1 ml of 50% solution (50 mg or less) is used. A fatal dose may be as low as 30 mg. Ingested cocaine is less toxic than by other routes. Its half-life is 1 hour after an oral or nasal dose. Some cocaine is excreted unchanged in the urine and can be diagnosed on paper chromatography.

Cocaine is absorbed from all sites of application including gastrointestinal mucosa and other mucous membranes. Smuggling of illicit drugs via the oral-fecal route may lead to severe toxicity such as seizures and cardiorespiratory collapse if the container ruptures. If smuggling is suspected, a flat plate may show opaque densities within the bowel highlighted by a gas halo. Dry cocaine powder is sometimes mixed with epinephrine to make "cocaine mud" for application on the nasal mucosa. This provides a dangerous potentiation effect.

CLINICAL SYMPTOMS

Cocaine's most dramatic clinical effect is stimulation of the CNS. In man this is manifested by a feeling of well-being and euphoria often accompained by garrulousness, restlessness, excitement, and a sense of clarity. After small amounts of cocaine, motor activity is well coordinated. However, as the dose is increased, tremors and even tonic-clonic convulsions may result from stimulation of lower motor centers and enhancement of cord reflexes. If vasomotor and vomiting centers are stimulated, emesis may occur. Central stimulation is followed by depression. If the vital medullary centers are depressed, death results from respiratory failure.

Initially small doses slow the heart rate through central vagal stimulation. After moderate doses the heart rate is increased, probably from a combination of central and peripheral CNS effects. Although blood pressure may finally fall, there is at first a rise in blood pressure due to sympathetically mediated tachycardia and vasoconstriction. A large intravenous dose of cocaine can cause immediate death from cardiac failure due to direct toxic action on heart muscle.

MANAGEMENT

Symptoms improve upon discontinuation of the drug. In the absence of a positive history of abuse it is important to look for erosions or burns of the nasal mucosa. There are no preparations of cocaine for internal use or for injection.

In the event of a massive intoxication secondary to ingestion, intensive care unit monitoring is essential with appropriate treatment for such complications as respiratory depression, seizures and cardiovascular collapse.

Central Anticholinergic Syndrome

(See Table 71.6 for specific agents.)

PATHOPHYSIOLOGY

Increasingly physicians are called upon to manage toxic states resulting from the use of drugs or ingestion of plants with anticholinergic properties. Compounds such as antidepressants, antihistamines, ophthalmologic preparations, antispasmodics and belladonna alkaloids are in widespread use for a variety of medical reasons. In addition, several over-the-counter drugs can produce anticholinergic toxicity. These compounds exert their anticholinergic effects by antagonizing acetycholine competitively at the neuroreceptor site. The main peripheral effects are on the myocardium, smooth muscle, and exocrine glands. These effects include tachycardia, mydriasis, facial flushing, hyperpyrexia, cardiac arrhythmias, urinary retention, dry mucous membranes, decreased sweating, and decreased or absent bowel sounds. The central effects, which are less well known, include delirium, anxiety, hyperactivity, seizures, visual hallucinations, illusions, disorientation and recent memory impairment.

Table 71.6
Drugs and Chemicals That May Produce the Central Anticholinergic Syndrome

1. *Antidepressants*: amitriptyline (Elavil), imipramine (Tofranil), doxepin (Sinequan, Adopin)
2. *Antihistamines*: chlorpheniramine (Ornade, Teldrin), diphenhydramine (Benadryl)
3. *Ophthalmologic Preparations*: cyclopentolate (Cyclogel), tropicamide (Mydriacyl)
4. *Antiparkinson Agents*: propantheline (Probanthine), clidinium bromide (Librax)
5. *Antiparkinson Agents*: trihexyphenidyl (Artane), benztropine (Cogentin), procyclidine (Kemadrin)
6. *Proprietary Drugs*: Sleep-Eze (scopalamine, methapyrilene), Sominex (scopalamine, methapyrilene), Asthma-Dor (belladonna alkaloids), Excedrin-PM (methapyrilene)
7. *Belladonna Alkaloids*: Atropine, homatropine, hyoscine, hyoscyamus, scopolamine
8. *Toxic Plants*: Mushroom (*Amanita muscaria*), bittersweet (*Solanum dulcamara*), Jimson weed (*Datura stramonium*), potato leaves and sprouts (*Solanum tuberosum*), deadly nightshade (*atropa belladonna*)

PHARMACODYNAMICS

The pharmacodynamics vary according to the specific drug ingested. The antidepressants are particularly difficult to treat because they get deposited in fat tissue and are then mobilized into the serum over a 72-hour period. It is essential to watch patients for 72 hours even if the serum level is low.

MANAGEMENT

The management of a patient with a known central anticholinergic syndrome is a challenge. It is not possible to predict the toxicity of the anticholinergic drug from either the blood level or the ingested dose. The patient requires close monitoring in an intensive care unit that is prepared to provide ventilatory support for coma, anticonvulsants for seizures, and antiarrhythmic drugs for cardiac arrhythmias. Although physostigmine is known to be a specific antidote, its use is controversial. Physostigmine can produce bronchospasm, increased respiratory secretions, muscle weakness, bradycardia, hypotension, and seizures. It is recommended that physostigmine be reserved for coma with respiratory depression, uncontrollable seizures or severe hypertension. The adult dose is 1 to 2 mg i.v. at a rate of 1 mg/min. The trial dose can be repeated in 10 to 15 min up to a maximum of 4 mg. The pediatric dose is 0.5 mg i.v.

slowly, and repeat every 10 min up to a maximum of 2 mg. The lowest effective dose may be repeated every 30 to 60 min if symptoms recur (as is often the case) over 60 to 80 hours. If physostigmine toxicity occurs, treat with atropine i.m. or i.v. at one half of the physostigmine dose given.

CNS Sedatives: (Barbiturates, Benzodiazepines, Meprobamate, Glutethimide, Methaqualone)

PATHOPHYSIOLOGY

The barbiturates and other sedatives reversibly depress the activity of all excitable tissues. The CNS is exquisitely sensitive so, when given in sedative or hypnotic doses, barbiturates have little effect on skeletal, cardiac or smooth muscle. If depression is extended, serious deficits in cardiovascular and other peripheral functions occur. The incidence and prevalence of the abuse of benzodiazepines, meprobamate, glutethimide and methaqualone greatly exceeds opioid abuse. In general, the antianxiety effects of barbiturates and benzodiazepines are similar to, but not identical with, alcohol.

PHARMACODYNAMICS

The barbiturates may have euphoriant effects that are similar to morphine. With this group of drugs it is difficult to draw the line between appropriate use, abuse, habituation and addiction. The pharmacologic characteristics of each drug are largely determined by the chemical nature of the side chains on the barbituric acid. In general, agents with long side chains possess a short duration of action and high potency and are mainly excreted by hepatic degradation. Agents with shorter side chains exhibit longer duration, less potency and are mainly excreted by the kidneys. (See Table 71.7 for pharmacologic characteristics of barbiturates.) The duration of action of any barbiturate is determined by a complex interrelationship between dose, rate of absorption, rate of metabolic degradation or excretion of active drug, drug tolerance and a rate of removal of nonmetabolized and active drug from the central nervous system. Table 71.8 gives serum barbiturate levels at which a conscious state is expected to return. However, the depth of anaesthesia depends on the concentration of the drug in the brain, not in the blood, and serum levels are not absolute guides to therapy.

All barbiturates are bound by plasma proteins affecting their removal by the kidney, hemodialysis, or peritoneal dialysis. Patterns of nonmedical use vary and range from infrequent sprees of intoxication to compulsive daily use. Introduction to this form of drug use may be through street use or drug trade, but commonly it is initiated through a physician's prescription for insomnia or anxiety. Dependence can go unrecognized for months by both the patient and physician. Signs of drug dependency are missed as it is assumed that the return of symptoms such as anxiety, tremulousness and insomnia signals a return of the original anxiety. Barbiturates are often

Table 71.7
Physicochemical Properties of Common Barbiturates[a]

Generic Name	Proprietary Name	pK	Lipid Partition Coefficient[b]	Plasma Protein Binding (%)	Fatal dose (g)	Fatal Plasma Concentration (mg/100 ml)
Long-acting (>6 hr)						
Barbital	Veronal	7.74	1	5	10	15
Phenobarbital	Luminal	7.24	3	20	5	8
Intermediate-acting (3–6 hr)						
Amobarbital	Amytal	7.75				
Butabarbital	Butison	7.74				
Short-acting (<3 hr)						
Pentobarbital	Nembutal	7.96	39	35	3	3.5
Secobarbital	Seconal	7.90	52	44	3	3.5

[a] From J. M. Arena: *Poisoning*, Ed. 4, p. 379. Charles C Thomas, Springfield, Illinois, 1976.
[b] Between methyl chloride and an aqueous buffer. Higher coefficients reflect greater solubility in lipid.

Table 71.8
Barbiturate Blood Levels at Conscious Return[a]

Barbiturate	Level (mg/100 ml)
Long-acting (lethal 10–12 mg/100 ml or greater)	5–9
Barbital (Veronal)	
Phenobarbital (Luminal)	
Mephobarbital (Mebaral)	
Diallylbarbituric Acid (Dial)	
Intermediate-acting (lethal 4 mg/100 ml or greater)	2–4
Amobarbital (Amytal)	
Aprobarbital (Alurate)	
Butabarbityal (Butisol)	
Butethal (Neonal)	
Hexethal (Ortal)	
Vinbarbital (Delvinal)	
Short-acting (lethal 2 mg/100 ml or greater)	1–2
Cyclobarbital (Phanodorn)	
Pentobarbital (Nembutal)	
Secobarbital (Seconal)	
Hexobarbital, sodium (Evipal)	
Thiamylal, sodium (Surital)	
Thiopental, sodium (Pentothal)	

[a] *Note*: These figures are approximate and from limited studies. Wide variations are possible and the clinical class of the barbiturate must be known if the quantitative assay is to be of value. Variable factors are the age of the patient, previously established drug tolerance, and coexisting unrelated illnesses. Relatively low levels may be associated with a fatal outcome in elderly or debilitated patients and much higher levels can be tolerated by individuals who are chronic users of these compounds. In the final analysis the depth of anesthesia depends on concentration of the drug in the brain, not in the blood, and serum levels therefore are unreliable as *absolute* guides to therapy. (From J. M. Arena: *Poisoning*, Ed. 4, p. 383. Charles C Thomas, Springfield, Illinois, 1976.)

used in combination with amphetamines because together they produce more elevation of mood than with either drug alone. In 1977 18% of young adults reported nonmedical use of sedatives and 2.5% reported some use in the month prior to the survey. Short-acting barbiturates such as pentobarbital (yellow jackets) or secobarbital (red devils) are preferred to long-acting agents such as phenobarbital. Diazepam is also a widely abused drug. Chlordiazepoxide is rarely abused because of its minimal euphoriant action and slow onset. The amount of hypnotic taken daily varies considerably but a range of 1.5 to 2.5 g of short-acting barbituate daily is common. Because tolerance develops to most of the actions of this group of drugs there may be no apparent signs of chronic use. However, some patients attempt to maintain a state of intoxication that resembles alcohol intoxication.

CLINICAL SYMPTOMS

The patient exhibits a general sluggishness, difficulty in thinking, slowness and slurring of speech, poor memory, faulty judgment, emotional lability, and short attention span. Irritability, quarrelsomeness, and moroseness are common. Untidiness in personal habits, hostile and paranoid ideas, and suicidal tendencies may be observed. Clinical descriptions of chronic high doses of meprobamate, glutethimide, methaqualone, diazepam and chlordiazepoxide are similar. Barbiturate doses in the range of 400 mg daily for 3 months produce withdrawal symptoms upon discontinuation. Over the first 12 to 16 hours, as concentration in blood declines, the patient seems to improve but becomes increasingly restless, anxious, tremulous and weak. Abdominal cramps, nausea and vomiting may occur, orthostatic hypotension develops and neurologic signs such as hyperactive deep tendon reflexes, and tremors of the hands develop. Convulsions, when they occur, are seen after 48 to 72 hours of abstinence for short-acting barbiturates and after 7 to 8 days of abstinence for longer acting barbiturates. More than one half of patients who have a seizure go on to develop delirium. Anxiety mounts, visual hallucinations of a persecutory nature develop, and disorientation for time and place occurs. During the delirium between the 4th and 7th day post abstinence, agitation and hyperthermia can lead to exhaustion, cardiovascular collapse and death. The withdrawal symptoms from meprobamate, glutethimide, methaqualone, benzodiazepines are similar. In its mildest form the withdrawal syndrome from depressants may consist only of paroxysmal EEG abnormalities, rebound increases of rapid eye movement sleep, insomnia or anxiety. In addition, greater physical dependence will lead to tremulousness and weakness, and severe depressant withdrawal will cause grand mal seizures and delirium.

MANAGEMENT

Because of the drug's availability, barbiturate poisoning is a major clinical problem with death occurring in 0.5 to 12% of cases. Although tolerance to the CNS effects develops in chronic users, the lethal dose is not different from that of nonusers. Thus accidental overdoses can easily occur in chronic users, especially in combination with opioids or alcohol. The barbiturates with short half-lives and high lipid solubility (such as pentobarbital and secobarbital) are more potent and toxic than the long acting compounds such as phenobarbital and barbital. For practical purposes poisoning with intermediate agents like amobarbital and butabarbital is comparable to long-acting agents. Optional treatment of sedative overdose includes continuous monitoring in an intensive care unit with intubation and ventilator support as indicated. If less than 24 hours have passed post ingestion, gastric lavage with saline should be performed after intubation and charcoal placed in the stomach. Dialysis or hemoperfusion may be indicated.

Opioids (Morphine, Codeine, Heroin, Methadone, Propoxyphene)

PATHOPHYSIOLOGY

In the late 1960s heroin use increased dramatically in the United States and Great Britian. Reasons for this included increased availability, increased social acceptance, and increase in the adolescent population due to the post war baby boom.

In the United States there are three patterns of opioid use and dependence. The first begins as medical treatment and constitutes a small number of the addicted group. The second group starts with experimental or recreational drug use and progresses to more intensive use. Adolescents and young adults (males outnumbering females) are introduced to the drug by other users. The third pattern involves individuals who are on methadone treatment programs. When group values support opioid use and pure drugs are easily available, a high percentage of users become physically dependent. This was observed among the military in Vietnam. Physicians, nurses and related health professions have an addiction rate many times higher than in other groups with comparable education. Morphine and related opioids produce their major effects by combining with receptors in the brain and other tissues. Its effects include analgesia, drowsiness, change in mood, respiratory depression, decreased gastrointestinal motility, nausea, and vomiting. The opiate receptors appear to be the normal sites of action of several endogenous opioid like substances including endorphins.

PHARMACODYNAMICS

Generally the toxic dose for a nonaddicted person who is not in pain is around 60 mg. Serious symptoms are experienced after doses of 100 mg and doses above 200 mg carry a serious prognosis. Death may occur as a result of marked respiratory depression and consequent anoxia. Ninety percent of ingested or injected morphine is excreted in the urine and the remainder in the feces. The half-life of morphine is about 3 hours.

CLINICAL SYMPTOMS

Morphine causes constriction of the pupils. Extremely high doses of morphine can produce convulsions although the mechanism is not clear. Respiration is depressed, even in therapeutic doses, by a decrease in responsiveness of brainstem respiratory centers to increases in carbon dioxide tension. Therapeutic doses of morphine have no effect on blood pressure or cardiac rate or rhythm. When blood pressure falls, it falls as a result of hypoxia. Opioids dilate capacitance blood vessels and thereby decrease the ability of the cardiovascular system to respond to gravitational shifts. Thus, sitting or standing can produce orthostatic hypotension.

Morphine and related drugs have extensive effects on the gastrointestinal tract. They decrease secretion of hydrochloric acid, decrease tone and motility in the stomach and duodenum, decrease pancreatic and biliary secretions, decrease peristaltic waves in the colon and increase colonic tone to the point of spasm. In addition, the tone of the anal sphincter is augmented. Therapeutic doses of morphine and codeine can also cause an increase in pressure in the biliary tract. In turn these can produce epigastric distress and biliary colic. Therapeutic doses of morphine increase tone and amplitude of contractions of the ureter as well. Large doses of morphine can produce constriction of the bronchi and can exacerbate asthma.

The opiates are readily absorbed from the gastrointestinal tract, nasal mucosa, and the lung. The usual route of administration is by subcutaneous or intramuscular injection. The effect of a given dose is less after oral administration as the drug is initially metabolized in the liver. The duration of action is usually longer with oral administration. True allergic reactions such as urticaria, contact dermatitis, or anaphylaxis are rare. The presence of coma, pinpoint pupils (except with anoxia when they are dilated) and depressed respiration suggest opioid poisoning. Deliberate or accidental overdose is common among addicts. The finding of needle marks on the body further suggests this diagnosis. Mixed poisonings are also common, especially with alcohol or barbituates. In order to confirm the diagnosis, chemical analysis of urine and gastric contents should be done. Atypical symptoms such as mania, delirium, or convulsions are infrequently noted.

MANAGEMENT

The first management step is to ensure adequate ventilation of the patient. If necessary gastric lavage should be done immediately and followed with a 1-g slurry of activated charcoal. The narcotic antagonist naloxone (0.4 mg for adolescents, 0.01 mg/kg for young children) should be given intravenously. This dose can be repeated after 2 to 3 min up to 3 doses. If pulmonary edema occurs, it may be countered by positive pressure ventilation. Naloxone can precipitate a withdrawal syndrome that cannot be suppressed in patients who have developed physical dependence. Comatose patients can also develop respiratory obstruction due to soft tissue relaxation in the upper airway. Management of the airway is described in Chapter 1. In severe toxicity the cardiovascular system is depressed and requires supportive measures. Hypotension with tachycardia requires vasopressors. Additional measures consist of maintenance of proper fluid and electrolyte balance, maintenance of normal temperature and frequent change in position to obviate secondary pulmonary complications. Gastrointestinal effects such as nausea and vomiting can be severe. If persistent, they can be relieved by an antiemetic, such as Dramamine or Thorazine 50 mg i.m. every 4 to 6 hours.

Even with gradual reduction in dosage most addicted patients will have symptoms of withdrawal. Methadone substitution is now the standard technique for withdrawing a patient from opioids. With the patient under observation, 15 to 20 mg of methadone are given (by mouth if not vomiting, otherwise intramuscularly) at the first appearance of withdrawal symptoms such as sleeplessness, jitteriness, irritability, malaise, pain and fatigue. If symptoms are not suppressed, additional methadone can be given each time withdrawal symptoms reappear. It is rare to require more than 80 mg over the first 24 hours. Usually 1 mg of methadone substitutes for 4 mg morphine, 2 mg heroin, or 200 mg meperidine. A reduction of 20% of total daily dose per day is well tolerated and causes little discomfort. Mild abstinence symptoms may persist for some days after the last dose of methadone.

Alcohol

The widespread use of alcohol by teenagers is accompanied by widespread abuse. In a 1974 national survey, 30% of high school students said that they had been drunk in the preceding month and 7% drunk 4 or more times. Another indicator of alcohol abuse by teenagers is provided by the Department of Justice Uniform Crime Report of 1973 which shows arrests for persons under 18 for alcohol-related offenses (drunken driving; liquor law violations, drunkenness) increased 135% during the period 1960 to 1973. Arrests for driving while intoxicated increased in this age group more than 400%. In 1975 the National Institute of Alcohol Abuse and Alcoholism conducted a national survey to determine alcohol use among junior and senior high school students in the United States. Alcohol use was defined by five categories from the students self-reported behavior.

1. *Abstainers*—do not drink or less than once a year = 27%.
2. *Infrequent to light drinkers*—those who drink once a month = 33%.
3. *Moderate drinkers*—those who drink once a week with small amounts per occasion or those who drink 3 to 4 times a month with medium amounts (2 to 4 drinks) on each occasion = 15%.
4. *Moderate to heavy drinkers*—those who drink at least once a week with medium amounts (2 to 4 drinks) each occasion or 3 to 4 times a month with large amounts (5 to 12 drinks) each occasion = 11%.
5. *Heavy drinkers*—those who drink once a week with 5 to 12 drinks per occasion = 11%.

According to this survey, at least 40% of U.S. junior and senior high school students can be classified as moderate or heavy drinkers. As many as 28% may be problem drinkers (drunk 4 or more times in the last year) and have experienced negative consequences in two life areas such as school, family, work, peer group as a result of drinking. Although more adolescent boys than girls are drinkers, the number of girls who drink is increasing, as in the number of drinkers age 13 and under. Approximately 24% of adolescents age 13 are classified as moderate drinkers.

The pathophysiology, pharmacodynamics, clinical symptoms and management of alcohol intoxication are covered in Chapter 48, "Toxicologic Emergencies."

ANOREXIA NERVOSA

BACKGROUND

The basic definition of anorexia nervosa is a greater than 25% weight loss due to refusal to eat. Usually an associated amenorrhea precedes, occurs coincidentally with, or follows the weight loss. There is an associated disturbance of body image of delusional proportions, a disturbance in the accuracy of perception of cognitive interpretation of stimuli arising within the body with failure to recognize nutritional needs, and a paralyzing sense of ineffectiveness that pervades all activities. The patient experiences herself as responding only in response to other people's demands and not as doing anything for herself.

Cases have been reported from childhood to senility but the majority cluster in the teens and the twenties. The incidence in females is 10 to 20 times that of males. Crisp has estimated that 1 in 100 English boarding school girls ages 16 to 18 suffer from anorexia nervosa. It has been reported in all ethnic groups but does not occur in underdeveloped countries where there is real starvation. It is also extremely rare in poor families.

Anorexia nervosa is not a new disease, although the real incidence is certainly increasing. The grave of Hungary's Saint Margaret who died at 27 years of age of severe inanition secondary to a refusal to eat stands as a historical tribute to the disease. The first detailed medical descriptions were those of Hobbes in 1668. Gull ushered in the modern day interest in the disease when he published a series of cases in England in 1874. The etiology of this disease was initially felt to be a psychogenic malnutrition. However, later, with the description of panhypopituitarism by the German pathologist Simmonds, physicians began to attribute the disease to a primary endocrinopathy. This controversy remains unresolved, although the endocrine manifestations of the disease have been thoroughly described and are felt to be secondary to starvation. The cerebral cortex is felt to inhibit hypothalamic function, possibly mediated by increased dopamine. To date there is no proof of any neurotransmitter abnormalities in anorexia nervosa.

DYNAMICS AND PATHOPHYSIOLOGY

Typically these girls are persistent, perfectionistic, the best child in the family. Although they are good students, highly motivated, they are often shy and lacking in self-confidence. They often start a diet with a group of friends (about 30% are initially overweight), but become obsessed with losing weight and fearful of losing control of their appetite. Often the adolescent will maintain a picture of herself as overweight even when she is cachectic. Anorectic patients eat alone, are extremely obsessive, and demonstrate bizarre behavior around food. Although they eat alone they enjoy cooking for and serving the family. There is a lack of normal response to hunger or fatigue. They engage in excessive, rigid exercise programs. Although active and successful, they are loners. They have little or no interest in the opposite sex. In a society where almost 1 of every 2 marriages is ending in divorce it is striking that the families of anorectics have low divorce rates. The family fails to recognize dysfunctional interaction patterns when they exist. They often state that the only significant problem in family interaction is how to cope with their anorectic child.

The search continues for specific physiologic etiologies. The endocrine manifestations such as delayed release of TSH, prepubertal secretory pattern of FSH and LH, low T_4 for the low, normal level of TSH, normal to increased cortisol secretion, and increased cholesterol have all been observed in starvation states not due to anorexia.

The accompanying amenorrhea can precede, coincide with or occur after significant weight loss. Reduced gonadal function and a prepubertal secretion pattern of LH (absence of nocturnal secretory spikes) are the hallmarks of a patient with anorexia. In spite of low gonadotropin levels, the responses of LH and FSH to administration of gonadotropin-releasing hormone are often normal. In some patients, the LH response may be delayed or blunted while the FSH response is better preserved or even increased. Frisch and McArthur have proposed that each woman must attain a certain critical weight before cyclic gonadotropin secretion can occur. In addition, it has been estimated that the degree of fatness, i.e. 17% of body weight as fat rather than the absolute body weight, may be the critical determinant in timing of menarche. Most anorectic patients do, in fact, restore normal pituitary responsiveness and LHRH secretion after weight gain to 85 to 90% or above of ideal body weight and normalization of psychosocial function. However, as high as 30% of patients may have prolonged amenorrhea in the face of weight stabilization and psychosocial recovery. These patients may then seek medical care for infertility, lack of normal vaginal lubrication or small breasts.

The etiology of anorexia nervosa is a combination of biopsychosocial factors. Unknown genetic determinants may create a biologic vulnerability. Early life experiences and family interaction patterns may create intrapsychic conflicts that add a psychologic predisposition. Social and cultural factors, such as an obsession with thinness or emphasis on eating behavior, may be additive to the biologic and psychologic predisposition. Puberty with its coincident biologic, psychologic and social stress may tip the uneasy balance and initiate the clinical symptoms. Such an explanation can also account for the variance in clinical severity from a mild form with spontaneous remission to a severe form with progression to chronic dehabilitating disease and on occasion death in spite of appropriate treatment. Minuchin formulated the following model of psychosomatic disease that explains how anorexia nervosa is defined by the interrelationship of all family members (Fig. 71.3). A vulnerable child, perhaps due to genetic factors, is played upon by extrafamilial stresses, family function and her own physiology to become a symptomatic child.

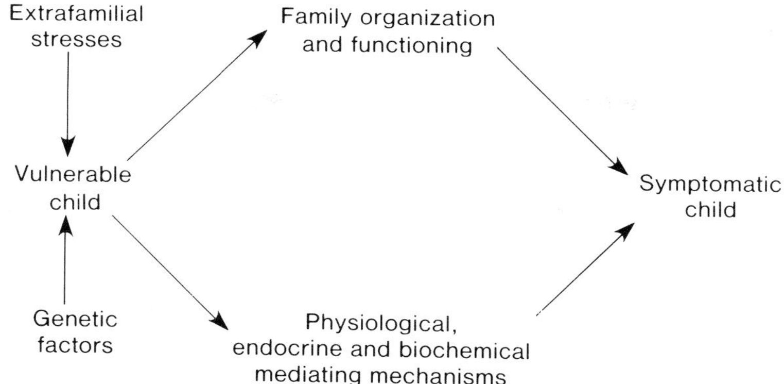

Figure 71.3 Scheme for interaction of psychosocial and biologic predisposing factors in anorexia nervosa to produce a symptomatic patient.

CLINICAL MANIFESTATION

These patients may come to the emergency department with several complaints. Often they are brought in by parents with the symptoms of vomiting secondary to stomach pain. The initial contact may be for guidance for altering the adolescent's bizarre eating habits. For example, an anorectic patient may go on a lettuce diet and eat only lettuce for weeks. She may be so concerned about fat in the food that she attempts to separate out any fat from the meat by combing through it with a fork. Cutting food into tiny portions and eating exactly one half or one fourth of the usual portion is another common behavior pattern. Eating alone, hiding food rather than eating it, or vomiting after eating are common presenting complaints. In addition to the unusual eating habits, parents will complain that the patient is obsessed with dieting, abuses laxatives, is irritable, moody and withdrawn. All teenage girls diet, but beware the teenager who is successful at rigid dieting while her companions who started to diet with her have discarded their weight-losing efforts.

The physical examination is distinctive—a severely emaciated, cachectic girl who denies she is ill. There is a decrease of muscle mass along with decreased subcutaneous tissue. The hands and feet are ice cold and may show bluish mottling. Bradycardia, usually 45 to 50, hyporeflexia, hypothermia and orthostatic hypotension may be seen. Associated laboratory findings include hypokalemia, metabolic alkalosis, hypoglycemia, and ketonuria.

It is important to realize that anorexia nervosa is a spectrum of disease from mild to severe. Although a greater than 25% weight loss is necessary to fulfill criteria for diagnosis, treatment is indicated when the clinical description noted is present, regardless of percentage weight loss. In addition, some anorectic patients will present as apparent psychogenic vomiters, vomiting consistently after food intake. Presence or absence of distorted body image should be a key differentiating factor. Another presentation is that of the patient who cannot eat because of abdominal pain. Again, it is important to look for the associated historical features already described as well as distorted body image.

MANAGEMENT

The first step in management is to complete the initial evaluation including a general medical, social and family history with special emphasis on the factors noted above. A complete physical examination is indicated with Tanner staging and a good examination of external genitalia. Pelvic and rectal examination should be performed as indicated for amenorrhea or other medical indications. The physician may need to explain the reason for the examination in order to gain the patient's cooperation.

A differential diagnosis should be considered including brain tumor or other malignancy, infectious process such as tuberculosis, inflammatory disease such as a rheumatic disease or inflammatory bowel disease, endocrine disorders such as diabetes, hypothyroidism, hyperthyroidism or adrenal insufficiency, anatomic abnormality of gastrointestinal tract such as superior mesenteric artery syndrome, psychogenic vomiting, depression, and schizophrenia.

The final evaluation step involves laboratory studies including CBC, sedimentation rate, electrolytes, blood sugar, BUN, creatinine, urinalysis, skull film with lateral view of sella, 24-hour urinary free cortisol (or a.m. and p.m. cortisol), chest x-ray, T_4, T_3, TSH, PPD, FSH, LH, and prolactin. Additional laboratory studies should be carried out as indicated by historical information or physical findings. If, for example, the patient complains of severe headaches a CAT scan might be considered. If there is a history of persistent stomach pain along with vomiting or diarrhea, gastrointestinal GI x-rays should be done even though gastrointestinal somatization is common. All of these studies do not need to be done in every anorectic but are appropriate for the anorectic patient who is failing treatment, who is hospitalized, or whose diagnosis is being questioned. An elevated ESR or hypochromic, microcytic anemia are uncommon in anorectics and may prompt diagnostic studies.

Once the diagnosis is made the patient and family should be referred promptly for psychiatric treatment with a therapist who has had experience treating anorectic patients. Various combinations of family therapy, individual therapy and group therapy are being used today in the successful treatment of this disease. In general, any patient still living at home should be treated with the family, while individual psychotherapy is appropriate for patients who have separated from the parental home. Most therapists use a combination of individual and family visits in the course of therapy. Antidepressants and tranquilizers may be used in conjunction with psychotherapy but should not be used in place of therapy and should be prescribed by the psychotherapist.

Indications for medical hospitalization include greater than 40% weight loss, orthostatic hypotension, electrolyte imbalance (usually a hypokalemic alkalosis), dehydration, hypoglycemia, severe or unremitting weight loss, intercurrent infection in a severely cachectic anorectic, or marked family disturbance (massive denial or inability to engage in outpatient therapy). An absence of ketonuria in the presence of severe starvation may be ominous as it suggests that all adipose stores have been depleted. Since some anorectic patients are severely depressed, the patient must be cleared as a suicide risk for continued outpatient management. Bruising and pedal edema are additional indications of severe malnutrition that may indicate admission.

The anorectic patient is a difficult but gratifying patient to treat. They have good potential and, in general, favored socioeconomic status. Their personality characteristics are those revered by society. When treated, they usually channel their energies to productive endeavors by society's standards.

RUNAWAYS

BACKGROUND

Most adolescent runaways who are referred to runaway treatment centers are referred by police, a school or a parent. They are not usually referred by medical centers. Emergency rooms, however, may become involved in the case of runaways because of injuries from abuse perpetuated by a family member or a street incident in the course of a runaway episode. They may also present to the emergency department for treatment of an acute medical complaint, often a gynecologic or drug use or abuse problem. In all such situations, it is important that the emergency room staff, in addition to providing necessary medical care, be prepared to obtain a detailed social history and that family relationships be assessed.

Runaways in the National Statistical Survey were almost equally divided between males (53%) and females (47%). The national statistical survey on runaway youth (1976) stated that 733,000 youths aged 10 to 17 ran away at least overnight during that year. Eighty percent were 15 to 17 years. The largest proportion (31%) were 16 years of age, 24% were 17, 25% were 15. Runaways are most likely to come from low income families, their rate being 40% higher than average. The lowest rate of running away comes from the middle income range. Social differences are slight. White collar and blue collar families have identical runaway rates. Cities and towns have higher rates than do suburbs and rural areas. Cumulative data in the National Statistical Survey showed that 8.4% of families had experienced a runaway event at some time. Based on the survey data it is estimated that 1 child in 8 will run away before his or her 18th birthday.

When viewed in a historical perspective, children from poor families often run away to escape the effects of poverty. For many adolescents, running away is a response to an unhealthy family or work situation and at times it is attempted as a problem-solving behavior. Since early colonial days, running away has been synonymous with adventure, romance, fortune seeking and independence. Periods of social or economic upheaval have always resulted in increased runaway behavior.

With 1 million runaways in 1972 it is clear that runaways are not a passing fad. Even though runaways now tend to stay in closer proximity to their home town as compared to runaways in the late 1960s, the problem of runaways will continue to be a major concern. Currently, our society often labels runaway children as psychopathological or delinquent, yet a historical review reveals evidence to the contrary. Running away to America was part of the founding of this nation, and there is a lot of evidence to suggest that the runaway child has played an important part in the growth of the country as far back as 1648. The Commonwealth of Massachusetts passed the first law that specifically prohibited runaway behavior in its attempt to control indentured servants or apprentices.

Industrialization followed by urbanization created a different system of child labor. The apprentice system was gradually replaced with factory work. Poor and immigrant children flocked to the cities. Growing poverty, idleness and crime rates followed. There was a prevalence of uncontrolled and unproductive youth, and society became increasingly alarmed about adolescents who left home prematurely. In the last half of the 19th century, police and social workers frequently interceded on behalf of runaways and street children, and some children were placed in alternative living situations. Contemporary programs of delinquency control can be traced back to this time.

The juvenile justice system was inaugurated at the beginning of the 1900s. Young delinquent children were not sent to special institutions for youthful offenders. With the advent of the Great Depression, the runaway youth problem was greatly exacerbated. Special services that included lodgings, education, vocational training and recreation and work programs were developed. In the late 1960s, with the development of the countercultural youth movement, for the first time a majority of runaway youths adopted a simple life-style with little interest in succeeding in the existing social order. The first runaway programs were established in large cities with a large influx of young people. In 1974 the Runaway Youth Act first provided federal legislation specifically for young people who had run away from home.

DYNAMICS

Three general types of runaways have been characterized by a review of the research literature:

1. First, there are those for whom the positive elements are dominant. These include an opportunity to meet new people, see new places, have new experiences. They are not leaving a bad situation but running to a more exciting world.
2. Second, there are those who are unhappy about one or more major components of their lives. This usually includes elements of conflict with and alienation from parents, truancy from school, feelings of rejection by teachers combined with rejection of school, poor academic performance, and poor peer relationships. Often they are incorporated into delinquent peer groups, and may already have been in trouble with police and courts. Their major motive is to leave a place and relationships about which they have negative feelings.

3. Third, there are those youths who, although they are characterized runaways, are actually abandoned or expelled from home. Displaced families sometimes disown sons or daughters or tell a youth not to return. In other instances, youth are so belittled and degraded that it becomes clear that the parents would prefer it if the adolescent would leave.

In summary, perspectives on the etiology of running away have shifted from an earlier focus on deviant personality of the teenager who runs away to a focus on relationships of the teenager with the family, school and peer group. Brennan et al. (*The Social Psychology of Runaways,* 1978) state that if youths are involved in satisfying roles, feel they are viewed positively by societal groups, have high self-esteem, feel positive about school and community, and feel they have control over their lives, they are less likely to run away.

Another theoretical perspective is the problem behavior proneness theory of Jessor and Jessor (1977) which looks to the individual for conventional attitudes and values versus tolerant attitudes toward deviance and values attained through deviant behavior. In addition, in the social environment, they look for the level of support and controls favorable to conventional behavior versus approval and models for deviant behavior. Neither of these perspectives can account for the youth who runs away from a good environment nor for those with multiple personality, family and school problems who do not run away. Both perspectives probably contribute to an understanding of the broad spectrum of runaway youth.

CLINICAL MANIFESTATIONS

When runaways present themselves to the emergency room special attention needs to be paid to their medical problems. Runaways are at special risk for physical, sexual, and drug abuse so the history and physical examination should be directed toward a search for abuse-related findings. Risk-taking behavior that may have resulted in physical injury needs to be assessed in terms of suicidal intent. Venereal disease such as gonorrhea, herpes, syphilis, and diseases such as scabies or pubic or head lice must be considered. Hepatitis is a common problem among drug-using street population and should be considered in the medical evaluation. The runaway's mental health status needs formal evaluation to rule out depression or suicidal ideation. Finally, runaways often have ongoing uncorrected medical problems that need to be referred for evaluation and treatment. Most commonly these include visual or hearing problems, or developmental lags that have interfered with school performance.

The runaway may be brought by the police or an interested friend or on occasion a parent to the emergency room. Sometimes they are brought in for a medical check after returning home. Commonly, they may be seeking care only for an acute injury or medical complaint, but the opportunity must be seized to do a complete assessment.

MANAGEMENT

A complete history and physical examination including genitalia and a pelvic for the female is indicated. A sexual history, including questions to elicit a history of sexual abuse, is essential. The physical examination should include a search for the signs of primary or secondary syphilis such as a chancre or generalized maculopapular rash. Even in the absence of positive findings a VDRL should be obtained. Pap smear and cervical culture for gonorrhea should be obtained. A drug use history should be obtained and attention paid to veins for puncture marks or burns about the nose or chest, a tip-off to cocaine snorting. Even in the absence of a positive drug history a toxic screen should be sent on blood and urine for determination of common street drugs, such as PCP, THC, amphetamine, barbituates, and narcotics. Careful attention must be paid to menstrual history in females with a view to ruling out pregnancy. A pregnancy test might be indicated. Skin conditions such as scabies, pubic or hair lice should be ruled out on physical examinations.

The runaway should be interviewed by a social service worker for information about family circumstances, peer group and school relationships. The circumstances of the run should be investigated and the youth's future plans evaluated. With this assessment a decision can be made as to the need for involvement acutely of a mental health professional or not. In any event a mental evaluation is indicated. When this medical, psychosocial assessment is completed, the next issue is one of disposition. Since the Juvenile Justice and Delinquency Prevention Act of 1974 (JJDPA) mandated the de-institutionalization of status offenders and decriminalized running away from home, services for runaways have been extremely variable from state to state. Although the elimination of police apprehension and detention of runaways is an advantage on the one hand, on the other it may mean that a given community will not provide assistance or shelter for them.

Disposition should be negotiated with representatives of agencies dealing with runaway youth locally, legal agencies if involved, and the family. Relinquishment of the runaway youth to a juvenile detention center should be avoided if possible in order to protect the youth's record for the future and to avoid the stigmatization.

CHRONIC ORGANIC COMPLAINTS

BACKGROUND

Every doctor who has worked in an emergency room is familiar with the semihysterical teenager who arrives complaining of severe pain, accompanied by a highly anxious, somewhat hostile family. The physical examination is negative and screening laboratory tests are normal. Often there is a history of prior episodes notable for a negative evaluation. The symptoms have frequently caused significant time loss from school and a disruption of the teen's and the family's life. The pain often has a history of waxing and waning independent of obvious life stress. It is not sufficient for the emergency room physician to tell the patient that there is no evidence of a significant medical problem. The patient and family correctly know that there is a problem and will simply return (or doctor shop) each time there is a crisis of symptoms. Similarly it is important that a diagnosis of conversion or psychosomatic symptoms be supported by positive criteria rather than the mere absence of physical and laboratory findings.

DYNAMICS

In psychogenic pain the pain seems to represent a misperception of an emotional state. An emotional conflict can produce somatic symptoms, usually pain, or can be converted into a functional impairment involving voluntary muscles or organs of special senses. In the extreme, fear or some other unacceptable feeling can be converted into actual paralysis. A history of the pain may demonstrate that there are marked variations in intensity based upon mental influences such as attitude, emotional state and life experiences. The attitude of "la belle indifference" or lack of concern about the symptoms is common because insofar as the symptoms reduce conflict they lessen anxiety.

The teenager usually complains about the limitations due to his symptoms although he may be deriving considerable secondary gain, as well as primary gain. The secondary gain occurs because concerned parents or friends may become very focused on the ill teenager and offer attentions that were not forthcoming when the teenager was asymptomatic. This situation may meet the psychological needs of the parents as well, and thus the original symptoms get reinforced. Both parents and teenager can become dependent upon the existence of the conversion symptoms.

The type of symptoms experienced by an individual patient is dependent upon the teenager's memory of symptoms experienced by himself or more often perception of symptoms experienced by relatives, family members or close friends. Additional discussion of this problem may be found in Chapter 70, in the sections on "School Refusal" and "Depression."

CLINICAL MANIFESTATIONS

The conversion symptoms may closely mimic physical disease, yet most adolescents cannot describe their symptoms so that they are fully consistent with the pertinent anatomical structures and physiological processes. The past medical history often reveals unexplained somatic symptoms especially abdominal pain or headaches and frequent absenteeism from school. The presence of the criteria listed in Table 71.9 helps to establish a diagnosis of conversion symptoms.

Recurrent pain in adolescents is usually in the abdomen, head, limbs or chest. Oster's 8-year longitudinal study on an unselected population of Danish school children, 6 to 19 years old, revealed a prevalence of 14.4% for abdominal pain, 20.6% for headaches and 15.5% for limb pain (Table 71.10). The pains were noted to peak in severity at 9 to 12 years and then progressively decrease throughout adolescence. These painful conditions have been noted to occur monosymptomatically and in various combinations. Apley suggested that these pains be grouped together as an expression of a reactive pattern which is usually associated with emotional disturbance and is often part of a familial pattern. In general, it is pain proneness as opposed to a more specific bodily localization that shows a familial tendency. As years go on varying sites of pain may be alternated.

Table 71.9
Chronic Organic Complaints

1. Symptoms often have symbolic meaning
2. Usually a model among family or acquaintances for the symptoms
3. More common in individuals with a hysterical personality
4. Frequent use of health issues and symptoms in family communication
5. Apparent lack of concern about symptoms
6. Symptoms reduce anxiety (primary gain)
7. Symptoms help adolescent cope with the environment (secondary gain)
8. Parents often overprotective, rigid and deny family problems
9. Manifest poor problem solving within the family
10. Family members are overinvolved with one another and normal boundaries between individuals tend to be lost

MANAGEMENT

It is important to take a precise history attempting to elicit an exact description of the symptom. Do not supply the patient with cue words to suggest sensations he has not experienced. Symptoms that were initially diffuse sometimes get molded into classic disease patterns after repeated history taking. A complete physical examination should be performed and not one that is directed only to the area of complaints. This is important in order to convince the referring doctor, patient, and parents that a physical cause has not been overlooked. Appropriate screening laboratory tests should be performed if they are rational and answer a voiced concern of the patient or parent. The interaction of the patient and family members should be observed during the course of the evaluation. Overly anxious, infantilizing, overly involved parental behavior should be noted. When parents are extremely upset as the patient gives a history of pain but does not appear to be in pain, it is suggestive of a psychosomatic complaint. The family is often anxious, defensive and hostile if they have made multiple visits to medical services for the same complaints without being given a diagnosis.

The most important role of the physician in the emergency department is to rule out an existing medical emergency, provide symptomatic relief, and to arrange the appropriate long-term medical care. The patient and family need to be told that the patient has symptoms that require treatment because they are interfering with function, but that there is no evidence of a specific underlying disease. An explanation that emphasizes the interrelationship of the

Table 71.10
Adolescent Pain

Pain	9 to 12 Years		16 to 17 Years	
	Male	Female	Male	Female
Recurrent abdominal pain (%)	21.0	30.0	5	5
Recurrent headache (%)	23.0	27	12	20
Limb pain (%)	20	30	4	13–14

mind and body and points out how various mind states produce physical symptoms is important. Diabetes, migraine and asthma are good examples of how mental states can specifically induce organic symptoms.

Further assessment is best done by a simultaneous pediatric, psychiatric evaluation and a family interview. If symptoms have been ongoing and the family has not been able to accept a diagnosis of psychosomatic pain, a planned stay on an adolescent inpatient unit can be helpful. It permits 24-hour observation of the pain and a determination of the presence or absence of environmentally related causes. Furthermore, it removes the aura of crisis from an episode of pain and permits better evaluation since the complicating factor of acute parental concern is temporarily removed. Finally, it is easier to implement simultaneous medical and psychiatric evaluation in an inpatient setting without any attached stigma.

Most published studies indicate that complete disappearance of symptoms frequently is not achieved. However, the physician's role is to assist the adolescent to cope with them and function in spite of them so that his dependency on the secondary gain is decreased. If the adolescent continues to be disabled by symptoms, psychiatric evaluation and treatment is indicated. In a review of psychogenic pain, Friedman found that a substantial proportion of the patients were reported as improved after several years, whether treated or not. Thus it is likely that many of these psychogenic symptoms of adolescence are related to environmental stress or a developmental crisis.

The following sections will cover the management of specific complaints or syndromes.

Hyperventilation Syndrome

Breathing in excess of physiologic requirements causes a decreased CO_2 in alveolar gas and in capillary blood. The resulting alkalosis and decreased CO_2 alter the excitability of the peripheral as well as central nervous system. The biochemical processes that produce the various symptoms are largely unknown. Subjectively the patient experiences breathlessness, chest pain, paraesthesias, dizziness, blurred vision, headache, trembling, fatigue, difficulty in thinking clearly, nervousness and anxiety without any cause. A persistent aching pain can occur over the left precordia, probably due to muscle fatigue from the abnormal breathing pattern in which the lower chest muscles and diaphragm are relatively fixed while the upper chest is overexerted. Brief, sharp pains have been described over the precordia or rib margin, possibly due to the accompanying aerophagia. Finally, intercostal muscle spasm from electrolyte changes can produce a constrictive type pain. Typically, the patient is totally unaware of the hyperventilation. Sighing usually accompanies an attack, but is more noticeable to observers than to the patient. Hyperventilation is also described in Chapter 72. Treatment includes tranquilizers, such as diazepam 2.5 to 5 mg, chlordiazepoxide 500 mg, or rebreathing into a paper bag.

Aerophagia

Aerophagia is a common psychophysiologic, gastrointestinal syndrome which, by producing stomach distention and an upward deflection of the left diaphragm, produces pain above and below the left rib margin but may occasionally be precordial. This condition is produced by frequent swallowing, bolting food and gulping liquids. Aerophagia is suggested by a history of borborygmi and belching with relief from passing flatus. Treatment includes instructing the patient to eat leisurely, chew thoroughly, drink by sipping instead of gulping and to discontinue gum chewing and drinking carbonated fluids.

Psychogenic Chest Pain

Psychogenic chest pain is also commonly referred to as irritable heart, neurocirculatory asthenia, or effort syndrome. The symptoms are similar to those of hyperventilation syndrome, namely chest pain, palpitation, heart consciousness, shortness of breath, fatigue, and insomnia. Pain is of two types, a dull aching pain not well localized or a sharp stabbing pain in the area of the cardiac apex.

Cardiospasm

Cardiospasm is caused by spasm of the sphincter at the lower end of the esophagus and can cause pain identical to angina pectoris. The pain can be retrosternal, boring pain or it may radiate between the scapulae or into the neck. It may be spastic with a waxing and waning quality.

Although angina pectoris is almost nonexistent in the otherwise healthy adolescent age group, it is an uppermost worry in the minds of parents and adolescents who present with psychogenic or psychophysiologic heart pain. Therefore, in order to convince the patient of the true diagnosis it is important to go through the diagnostic process of excluding angina. The treatment of patients with functional chest pain begins with a meticulous history and physical examination. History is the most important objective evidence, since neither laboratory tests nor physical examination are likely to reveal positive findings. Anginal pain is more often substernal or symmetrical while functional pain is away from midline and unilateral, most often in the area of the cardiac apex. Spontaneous pain without exertion is uncommon in angina but common in functional pain. Functional pain rarely occurs with intercourse. Furthermore, description of organic pain is likely to be more specific than that of functional pain. Life stress can precipitate both types of pain and is not useful in differentiation. Similarly, nitroglycerin can give relief of pain in both situations since it relieves smooth muscle spasm which often causes functional chest pain. The doctor's attitude must be accepting and not hostile, and it is important to explain how emotional stress can cause real pain. It is essential to convey that the doctor appreciates that the symptoms are real even though there may be no disease present. An example can be given of other disorders of severe pain brought on by emotional tension such as irritable bowel, migraine, or tension headaches. A chest x-ray and ECG will need to be on record but other tests should not be routinely performed without specific indications. Extensive and obscure studies will reinforce the patient's symptoms and convince the patient that if enough studies are done the answer will be found.

Irritable Bowel Syndrome

One of the commonest of the psychosomatic abdominal pain syndromes is that of spastic colon or irritable bowel syndrome. It is defined by a chronic episodic disturbance of bowel habit (constipation or diarrhea) and recurrent bouts of abdominal pain. The definition assumes a normal sigmoidoscopic examination, normal barium enema and upper gastrointestinal series, absence of ova and parasites or pathogenic bacteria on stool examination and culture, and a negative history of lactose intolerance. The history will usually reveal a relationship between life stress and abdominal pain. Not infrequently patients with irritable bowel syndrome will present during a period of rest or relaxation after a stressful period.

When silver-tipped electrodes are attached to the mucosa of the sigmoid colon in normal fasting individuals with an empty rectum, two types of basal electric rhythm (BER) can be recorded, 3 cycle/min and 6 cycle/min. Patients with irritable bowel syndrome have been noted to have increased their 3 cycle/min BER to approximately 45% of their total BER activity. The exact link between this increased percentage of 3 cycle/min BER and emotional stress, food intake and rectal distention has not been demonstrated. The pain is periodic. The patient may have pain all day for 2 to 3 days, then have a 2-day pain-free interval or pain over a longer period of time such as 2 weeks. The quality of pain is variable, like a gas pain but from sharp to dull. It is unusual for the pain to awaken a patient from sleep, and this symptom, if present, should point to a consideration of peptic ulcer or gallbladder disease. The relationship of the pain to food intake is also variable. A common bowel pattern is a loose stool accompanied by a rush of mucus. The location of the pain differs according to the physiologic aberration. If aerophagia is present, dilatation of hepatic and splenic flexures will occur. If there is only spasm of a segment of the colon it will manifest itself as right lower quadrant or left lower quandrant pain. If the patient has aerophagia, the physical examination of the abdomen will reveal hyperresonance. If there is significant spasm, that part of the colon will be tender to palpation. Other important considerations in the adolescent with abdominal pain include inflammatory bowel disease, peptic ulcer disease, gastroenteritis, lactose intolerance, gallbladder disease, pelvic inflammatory disease, ovarian cysts or tumors, and endometriosis.

The mainstay of treatment of the irritable bowel syndrome has been dietary manipulation, anticholinergics to decrease spasm, and tranquilizers or sedatives. A high fiber diet with increased bulk may provide some symptomatic relief. In addition, attention to eating slowly and at three regular times of the day decrease aerophagia. Anticholinergics such as clidinium or belladonna alone or in combination with tranquilizers such as chlordiazepoxide or Butisol are often used for symptomatic relief. Librax (clidinium and chlordiazepoxide), 1 tablet before meals. Clidinium has been shown to decrease 3 cycle/min BER and colonic motility when given with a meal. Lomotil (diphenoxylate with atropine) 1 tablet every 4 hours, or Metamucil, 1 teaspoon 1 to 3 times a day, has also been used to control the symptoms with varying success. Some attempt should also be made to counsel the symptomatic individual to evaluate their life-style and address such issues as overcommitment and daily stress.

References

General

Hofmann A, Becker RD, Gabriel HP: *The Hospitalized Adolescent; A Guide to Managing the Ill and Injured Youth.* Macmillan, New York, 1976.

Drug Abuse

Abramowicz M (ed.): Diagnosis and management of reactions to drug abuse. *Med Lett* 19: 13–16 (Feb. 11) 1977.

Barton CH, et al.: Phencyclidine intoxication; clinical experience in 27 cases confirmed by urine assay. *Ann Emerg Med* 10: 243–246, 1981.

Bernstein JG: Marijuana—new potential, new problems. *Drug Ther* pp. 38–47, December 1980.

Bettinger J: Cocaine intoxication; massive oral overdose. *Ann Emerg Med* 9: 429–430, 1980.

Burks JS, et al.: Tricyclic antidepressant poisoning; reversal of coma, choreoathetosis, and myoclonus by physostigmine. *JAMA* 230: 1405–1407, 1974.

Donovan JE, Jessor R: Adolescent problem drinking; psychosocial correlates in a national sample study. *J Stud Alcohol* 39: 1506–1523, 1978.

Goodman LS, Gilman AG (eds.): *The Pharmacological Basis of Therapeutics*, Ed. 6. Macmillan, New York, 1980.

Granacher RP: The central anticholinergic syndrome; management with physostigmine. *J Ky Med Assoc* 73: 147, 1975.

Haddad LM: Management of hallucinogen abuse. *Acad Fam Pract* 14: 83–87, 1976.

Harford TC: Teenage alcohol abuse. *Postgrad Med* 60: 73–76, 1976.

Jessor R, Jessor SL: *Problem Behavior and Psychosocial Development; A Longitudinal Study of Youth.* Academic Press, New York, 1977.

Jessor R, Chase JA, Donovan JE: Psychosocial correlates of marijuana use and problem drinking in a national sample of adolescents. *Am J Public Health* 70: 604, 1980.

Johnston LD, Bachman JD, O'Malley PM: *Drug Use Among American High School Students 1975–77.* DHEW Publication ADM 78-619, National Institute of Drug Abuse, Washington, D.C., 1977.

McCarron M, et al.: Acute phencyclidine intoxication; incidence of clinical findings in 1,000 cases. *Ann Emerg Med* 10: 237–242, 1981.

Pascale R, Hurd M, Primavera LH: The effects of chronic marijuana use. *J Soc Psychol* 110: 273–283, 1980.

Patel R, et al.: Myoglobinuric acute renal failure in phencyclidine overdose; report of observations in eight cases. *Ann Emerg Med* 9: 549–553, 1980.

Rappolt RT, et al.: NAGD regimen for the coma of drug related overdose. *Ann Emerg Med* 9: 357–363, 1980.

Siomopoules V: Amphetamine psychosis; overview and a hypothesis. *Dis Nerv Syst* 35: 336, 1975.

Snyder S: Phencyclidine. *Nature* 285: 355–356, 1980.

Weller R, Halikas J: Objective criteria for the diagnosis of marijuana abuse. *J Nerv Ment Dis* 168: 98–103, 1980.

Anorexia Nervosa

Bruch H: *Eating Disorders: Obesity and Anorexia Nervosa, & the Person Within.* Basic Books, New York, 1973.

Crisp AH, Palmer RL, Kalucy RS: How common is anorexia nervosa? A prevalence study. *Br J Psychiatry* 128: 549–554, 1976.

Frisch RD, McArthur JW: Menstrual cycles: Fatness a determinant of minimum weight necessary for their maintenance or onset. *Science* 185: 949, 1974.

Hodas G, Liebman R, Collins M: Pediatric hospitalization in the treatment of anorexia nervosa. In *The Psychiatric Hospital and the Family,* edited by H Harbin, 1981.

Hsu JKG: Outcome of anorexia nervosa; a review of the literature (1954–1978). *Arch Gen Psychiatry* 37: 1041–1046, 1980.

Hsu LKG, Crisp AH, Harding B: Outcome of anorexia nervosa. *Lancet* 1: 62–65, 1976.

Lucas A: Toward the understanding of anorexia nervosa as a disease entity. *Mayo Clin Proc* 56: 254–264, 1981.

Minuchin S, Rosman B, Baker L: *Psychosomatic Families: Anorexia Nervosa in Context.* Harvard University Press, Cambridge, Mass., 1978.

Runaways

Nye FC, Edelbrock C: The runaway in America. *J Fam Issues* 1: 147–215, 1980.

Organic Complaints

Almy TP: Wrestling with the irritable colon. *Med Clin North Am* 62: 203, 1978.

Apley J: A common denominator in the recurrent pains of childhood. *Proc R Soc Med* 51: 1023–1024, 1958.

Brown RT: Costochondritis in adolescents. *J Adolesc Health Care* 1: 198–201, 1981.

Compernolle T, et al.: Diagnosis and treatment of the hyperventilation syndome. *Psychosomatics* 20: 612–625, 1979.

Epstein S, et al.: Chest wall syndrome; a common cause of unexplained chest pain. *JAMA* 241: 2793–2797, 1979.

Friedman S: Conversion symptoms in adolescents. *Pediatr Clin North Am* 20: 873–882, 1973.

Oster J: Recurrent abdominal pain, headache and limb pains in children and adolescents. *Pediatrics* 50: 429–436, 1972.

Rapp CE: Irritable bowel syndrome in the college population; pathophysiology, differential diagnosis and treatment (personal communication), 1982.

CHAPTER **72**

Behavioral Problems

FRED M. HENRETIG, M.D., AND DAVID JAFFE, M.D.

INTRODUCTION

This chapter reviews several conditions with prominent behavioral as well as somatic symptoms which may require emergency department management. The emergency physician needs to understand the interaction between the psychosocial and physiologic manifestations of these problems. The following disorders are discussed: (1) hyperventilation syndrome, (2) rumination syndrome, (3) tics, (4) breathholding attacks, and (5) sleep disorders.

The diagnosis of these disorders in the emergency department requires a certain index of suspicion. The behavior problems present with somatic symptoms and signs that may mimic serious medical emergencies; the sleep disorders may mimic far more serious neurologic disturbances. Nevertheless, the clinical picture in each of the above syndromes is generally so characteristic that the correct diagnosis can be strongly considered after a careful history and physical examination. Further exploration of psychosocial issues, and evaluation of family dynamics (see p. 1080 in Chapter 70) will usually strengthen the diagnosis of the behavioral disorders. The more common of the sleep disorders are physiologic in etiology, but also require reassurance and counsel as management, hence their inclusion here. Additional discussion of sleep disturbances in infancy can be found in Chapter 13. The more serious disorders of excess sleep, such as narcolepsy and sleep apnea, are also discussed briefly here.

Although the management of these disorders usually requires referral to a physician with a continuing relationship with the child and his or her family, their recognition by the emergency department practitioner is crucial in order to exercise the maxim: *primum non nocere*. The emergency physician can avoid harm by the avoidance of unnecessary diagnostic testing or medical therapy and by trying to lessen the patient's and family's anxiety.

HYPERVENTILATION SYNDROME

BACKGROUND

Hyperventilation has been defined by Missri and Alexander as "ventilation in excess of that required to maintain normal blood PaO_2 and $PaCO_2$. It may be produced either by an increase in frequency or depth of respiration." The hyperventilation syndrome may present with symptoms related to diverse organs including the heart, lungs, brain, abdomen and skeletal systems. The syndrome is common in adults but has received little attention in pediatric literature. It can nonetheless be a disabling clinical pediatric problem that is often misdiagnosed and improperly treated.

PATHOPHYSIOLOGY AND DYNAMICS

The pathophysiology of the hyperventilation syndrome contains two components: (1) the physiologic derangement produced by hyperventilation and (2) underlying psychiatric disturbance, most often including anxiety. A single deep breath can reduce

$PaCO_2$ by 7 to 16 mm, and the $PaCO_2$ can drop to half of normal after only 30 sec of hyperventilation. Thereafter, only an occasional deep breath superimposed on normal breathing is required to maintain low $PaCO_2$. After a prolonged period of hyperventilation renal compensatory mechanisms occur, resulting in the $PaCO_2$ remaining low while the alkalotic pH tends to normalize. Tissue oxygenation may be lowered by the Bohr effect, which is the shift of the oxyhemoglobin curve to the left in response to acute respiratory alkalosis. Thus, at any given oxygen tension, oxygen becomes more tightly bound to hemoglobin and less available to the tissues.

Lowered $PaCO_2$ also produces important changes in the cardiovascular system, including cerebrovascular constriction, causing decreased blood flow to the brain. Since the Bohr effect also reduces tissue oxygenation in the brain, cerebral hypoxia may be related to many of the CNS symptoms associated with hyperventilation. Electrocardiographic changes such as ST segment depression, and flattening and inversion of T-waves, both in resting and exercise ECG, have been reported in adults who hyperventilate. However, unlike ischemic ECG changes, these changes occur early during exercise and disappear as exercise continues.

When normal subjects voluntarily hyperventilate, the only metabolic derangement that occurs in addition to alkalosis and lowered $PaCO_2$ is lowered serum inorganic phosphorus. Other serum electrolytes remain normal. Voluntary hyperventilators experience relatively few and mild symptoms as compared to the exaggerated complaints observed in the clinical hyperventilation syndrome.

In addition to the physiologic effects described above, there are psychological disturbances to account for the apparent severity and variety of symptoms that patients with hyperventilation syndrome report. Several studies have shown that children with hyperventilation syndrome have received psychiatric or psychological diagnoses of anxiety, conversion reaction or hysterical personality, depression, irritability, sleep disturbance, or excessive worry about schoolwork.

CLINICAL MANIFESTATIONS

The typical clinical picture of hyperventilation syndrome includes noticeably rapid respirations, tetany, and paresthesia. However, patients rarely present with this triad of symptoms and signs. Enzer and Walker found that only 43% of 44 children with hyperventilation syndrome had chief complaints in any way related to respiration.

Patients almost always report that their symptoms occur in "spells" or "attacks." The symptoms that occur during these attacks include various combinations of chest pain, palpitations, coldness of extremities, breathlessness, air hunger, numbness, tingling, loss of consciousness, dizziness, abdominal bloating, abdominal pain, tremors, muscle pain or stiffness. It is not surprising that children who experience attacks of such potentially alarming symptoms come to the emergency department for evaluation.

DIFFERENTIAL DIAGNOSIS

The manifestations of hyperventilation syndrome are variable and can initially seem worrisome. There are relatively few organic disorders that require serious consideration in the differential diagnosis. These include pain, metabolic acidosis, drug intoxication (including salicylism), hypercapnea, cirrhosis, organic CNS disorders, fever, and the response to severe pain. A few paroxysmal disorders such as hypotensive syncope, Stokes-Adams attacks, epilepsy, migraine, and asthma must also be ruled out.

Many of these diagnoses can be excluded on the basis of careful history and physical examination. Elements of history that suggest the diagnosis of hyperventilation syndrome include: chronicity of the complaint, unrelatedness of symptoms, references to breathlessness, and expressions of anxiety. Sources of environmental stress should be investigated. Physical examination may reveal obvious hyperventilation, or, more commonly, the patient may be observed to take periodic deep, sighing respirations. It is often helpful to assess whether voluntary hyperventilation reproduces the patient's symptoms.

Extensive laboratory evaluation is rarely required. For example, a patient whose chief complaint is chest pain and whose history and physical examination suggest hyperventilation syndrome, would require chest x-ray and ECG examination only if there is a history of previous heart disease, or if an abnormality such as arrhythmia or heart murmur is discovered on physical examination, or if the pain seems extraordinarily severe or persistent.

Diabetic ketoacidosis, the most common cause of metabolic acidosis, can be excluded by urinalysis. Other causes of metabolic acidosis are uncommon, and can be detected by electrolyte and/or blood gas determination. These should be performed if acidosis is suspected, but it is not necessary to obtain an arterial blood gas simply to document the alkalosis and lowered $PaCO_2$ associated with the hyperventilation syndrome.

Epilepsy rarely presents as syncope alone, and the tetany and paresthesia associated with hyperventilation syndrome should be easily differentiated from most of the common movement disorders associated with seizures.

As in many clinical situations that result in a diagnosis with psychological or psychiatric implications, the emergency physician may elect to order laboratory data to support the diagnosis. The specific tests obtained should be determined by the patient's symptoms, but will usually be selected from among chest x-ray, ECG, and the electrolytes and blood gas determinations. The purpose and extent of investigation should be explained clearly to the patient's family at the onset so that there will be mutual agreement that a careful, thorough evaluation has been performed.

TREATMENT

The classic remedy for hyperventilation is breathing into a paper bag. The patient rebreathes his own expired air and thus inhales air enriched with CO_2. Although we have found no published data discussing the efficacy of this technique, the authors have found it to be frequently useful.

Most experts recommend that the patient understand the mechanism by which the symptoms are produced. For adolescents in particular, it is important to emphasize that the patient has control over the production of symptoms. This is often accomplished by voluntary overbreathing and careful educational effort by the emergency physician. It is not helpful to tell the patient that there is "nothing wrong." Counseling and supportive therapy are usually necessary to discover the sources of psychologic disturbance experienced by the child. These efforts should start in the emergency department, but psychiatric consultation and/or referral may be required.

Propranolol has been used successfully in children with chronic refractory hyperventilation in a study by Joorabchi. At present its use should be limited to patients who fail to respond to educational and counseling therapy.

INFANT RUMINATION SYNDROME

BACKGROUND

Infant rumination syndrome is a rare, but potentially fatal, chronic psychiatric disorder of infancy manifested by voluntary, recurrent, self-stimulatory regurgitation. Children with this disorder may appear in the emergency department with complaints of vomiting and failure to thrive. Careful observational efforts have led to the conclusion that rumination syndrome is primarily a response to a disordered relationship between parents and the infant. The prevalence of infant rumination has declined considerably since the early decades of the 20th century, possibly because of improvements in overall socieconomic conditions and in child care.

Fleisher has reviewed several characteristics of the rumination syndrome. Symptoms begin in early infancy (between the ages of 3 and 8 months), and the babies develop progressive inanition which does not respond to any conventional dietary or mechanical intervention. The behavior pattern of rumination is characteristic. Babies ruminate only when awake, and when not otherwise occupied with people or objects. They begin by contracting the pharynx, tongue and abdominal muscles until they regurgitate stomach contents, which are then rechewed and swallowed. The infants appear to enjoy the entire process, and they experience no distress.

Parenting is always deficient. While mothers may exhibit a range of styles from neglectful to overattentive, they all have difficulty establishing a comfortable closeness with their infants. Often, these parents have marital and other interpersonal problems.

CLINICAL MANIFESTATIONS

The baby with infant rumination syndrome is most likely to present to the emergency department with a history of chronic vomiting and/or failure to thrive. Careful history will often reveal difficulties in the parent-child interaction. If the syndrome has been longstanding, the child may appear quite cachetic. No abnormalities on abdominal or rectal examination will be found. Surreptitious observation may show the characteristic behavior pattern described above. Hiatus hernia, chalasia, gastroesophageal reflux, indolent pyloric stenosis, and other delayed gastric emptying syndromes must be considered in the differential diagnosis. Laboratory evaluation should always include electrolyte determination to evaluate the nature of fluid losses and to assess the need for intravenous fluid, electrolyte and acid/base repair. X-ray and contrast studies need not necessarily be performed, especially if the history and observational evaluations are characteristic of rumination. However, if the diagnosis is in doubt, barium swallow and upper gastrointestinal examination may help to rule out organic esophageal or gastric pathology.

MANAGEMENT

Infants with the rumination syndrome must almost always be hospitalized for the special intensive nursing required to restore a sensitive and responsive environment. The parents should receive psychotherapy concurrent with the infant's hospitalization; but, even if the family's psychopathology persists, successfully treated rumination rarely recurs. Emergently abnormal electrolytes and severe inanition may require a short period of intravenous therapy.

TICS

Tics are a common movement disorder in school-aged children thought to be related to underlying tension and anxiety. They consist of stereotyped, usually rotatory movements involving face, head, neck and shoulders. Common tics are eye blinking, lip smacking, tongue thrusting, neck twisting and shrugging of the shoulders. The movements are rapid, generally lasting less than 1 sec, and, though repetitive, occur at irregular intervals. Tics are not noted when the child is asleep, and they increase in frequency with obvious emotional stress.

Tics may begin as purposeful movements, but seem to become unintentional in time. Several clinical features serve to distinguish tics from other important movement disorders such as myoclonic seizures or Sydenham's chorea: the ability to exercise at least some voluntary inhibition over the tic, the stereotyped nature of the movement, the usual limitation of involved muscle groups to those of the head and neck supplied by the cranial motor nerves, the lack of associated change in level of consciousness or amnesia, and the frequent accompanying evidence of emotional disturbance.

Treatment of tics consists of parental guidance and reassurance. Most tics disappear in time, especially if efforts are made to decrease significant sources of emotional and environmental stress. Some families may need referral for counseling, but in many cases the tic will resolve if parents will consciously ignore it. Constant scolding of the affected child tends to increase the frequency of occurrence. Tics may occur in association with coprolalia in the severe psychiatric disorder, Gilles de la Tourette's syndrome. If this disorder is suspected, a referral to a psychiatrist is indicated for more definitive diagnosis and treatment.

BREATHHOLDING ATTACKS

BACKGROUND

Breathholding attacks are common in young children and, when first encountered, a source of great anxiety to parents. The attacks have been recognized since antiquity, and the description by Hippocrates (cited by Illingworth) has been little improved upon in the last 2000 years: "The onset may be from some mysterious terror or a fright from somebody shouting, or in the midst of crying the child is not able quickly to recover his breath, as often happens to children; but when any of these things happens to him, at once the body is chilled, he becomes speechless, does not draw his breath, the breathing fails, the brain stiffens, the blood is at a standstill."

PATHOPHYSIOLOGY

As Hippocrates observed, the precipitating factor for breathholding spells is usually a sudden insult such as pain, fright or anger. Lombroso and Lerman studied 225 children who were breathholders and found that two main patterns occurred. Most commonly, the child in response to being angered or frustrated, held his breath in expiration until cyanosis, followed by loss of consciousness, occurred. In severe attacks, the unconsciousness was associated with limpness, or the child became opisthotonic, and then exhibited several beats of clonus. Such "cyanotic" spells were distinguished from "pallid" syncope, in which children, usually in response to a sudden painful stimulus, seem to cry only 1 or 2 gasps, turn pale and then fall limp without the occurrence of significant cyanosis. These two patterns of breathholding attacks are believed to further represent different pathophysiologic bases. In cyanotic attacks, the vigorous crying is thought to cause cerebral ischemia via cerebral vasoconstriction due to decreased $PaCO_2$, apnea-induced hypoxemia, and prolonged Valsalva effect in decreasing cardiac output. Anemia may also be a contributing factor (and if found and treated, the attacks often abate). In the pallid form of the attacks, there appears to be an overactive vagal response to unexpected pain, especially that of minor head trauma, with subsequent cerebral ischemia due to prolonged asystole.

CLINICAL MANIFESTATIONS

Breathholding is a common pediatric occurrence. In Lombroso and Lerman's prospective study of nearly 5000 children, 4.6% developed breathholding attacks leading to loss of consciousness and collapse. Many such children had a positive family history for breathholding. The age of onset varied from as early as the first week of life to as late as 3 years, but the majority began between 6 and 18 months. The spells ended by age 6 years in 90% of patients.

Precipitating factors, as alluded to above, tend to separate into two categories. The children prone to cyanotic spells usually begin crying when angered by being restrained or punished, or if a playmate grabs away a toy. Those with pallid syncope more often are triggered by a sudden pain or fright, such as from hitting the head after a minor fall when learning to walk and climb stairs.

Electroencephalogram (EEG) findings during breathholding attacks were also studied by Lombroso and Lerner. The EEG changes correspond exactly to the degree of cerebral ischemia encountered during the attacks, and are typical of those found with hypoxia of any cause. Enhanced background activity is followed by theta (θ), then delta (δ) activity; as cerebral anoxia persists beyond 10 sec, electrical silence supervenes. Return to baseline occurs rapidly with resumption of normal cardiorespiratory action.

The most important differential diagnosis of breathholding, with its accompanying loss of postural tone and consciousness, and with its limpness or tonic stiffening followed by one to several beats of clonus, is obviously epilepsy. Many children are mistakenly diagnosed as having seizure disorders, and unfortunately are therapeutically tried on many anticonvulsant drugs without benefit. The distinction is made more difficult because physicians rarely witness the attacks, and history must be obtained from parents who were terrified at the site of their cyanotic, unresponsive and often jerking children. Nevertheless, a carefully taken history is critical. Thus, after a thorough examination in the family's presence, and reassurances to them that the child has fully recovered, meticulous reiteration of the order of events is the most valuable method of distinguishing breathholding attacks from grand mal seizures. Again, breathholding attacks are precipitated by sudden pain, fright or anger. Such events do not usually influence the onset of seizures. In a seizure, although there is occasionally a single cry, loss of consciousness is almost immediate, followed by a short tonic phase and then prolonged clonus. Cyanosis, if it occurs at all, occurs late. A seizure generally lasts at least 1 min, and at its conclusion, there is a postictal state of altered consciousness which usually lasts at least several minutes. By contrast, in addition to the precipitating event, significant loud crying precedes loss of consciousness and limpness in breathholding attacks. If the attacks are severe and unconsciousness prolonged, there may then ensue a few beats of clonus, or opisthotonus followed by clonus. Cyanosis or pallor occurs early, preceding the loss of consciousness; parents, when calm, often recall this striking change in complexion before the child's fall. The period of unconsciousness is rarely greater than 1 min in breathholding, and, aside from a degree of tiredness, there is no significant postictal state.

In addition to the actual description of the attacks, other features of breathholders may help to distinguish them from children with seizures. Breathholders more commonly have a history of onset in infancy and a positive family history for breathholding. While seizures can occur in sleep, breathholding attacks never do, since the latter are precipitated by a perceived noxious stimulus. The EEG between attacks in breathholders is usually normal, while that in epileptics is often abnormal. In some cases, therefore, an EEG may help in diagnosis when the history of the attacks is not precise. Last, children with syncope due to structural cardiac disease should have obvious persistent abnormalities on examination. Conceivably, syncope due to cardiac arrhythmias may also cause diagnostic confusion, although the stereotyped history of breathholding attacks should distinguish them from both types of cardiac syncope. The physical examination should be normal in breathholders. In cases where the history is not definitive, an ECG may be advised (see Chapter 36, "Syncope").

MANAGEMENT

The prognosis for breathholders is excellent. As noted above, attacks usually cease when children reach school age. There is no subsequent increased incidence of epilepsy or mental retardation in former breathholders, although some apparently are prone to vasovagal syncope as adults.

Treatment consists of reassurance and patience, with counsel to minimize precipitating factors to the degree possible. Drug therapy is generally considered to be of little value. For children with frequent attacks of severe nature, referral to a pediatric neurologist for re-evaluation is recommended.

SLEEP DISTURBANCES

BACKGROUND

Oh sleep! It is a gentle thing,
Beloved from pole to pole!
To Mary Queen, thy praise be given
She sent the gentle sleep from heaven
That slid into my soul.

The Rime of the Ancient Mariner
(Coleridge)

Childhood sleep disturbances are common. Most reflect the particular stresses of certain developmental stages in infants and toddlers. Such problems are chronic and, although annoying to parents, will rarely present to the emergency department. Such developmental sleep disorders include resistance to being put down for the night and frequent nighttime awakenings in infancy, and nightmares in the toddler. Anticipatory guidance on the part of the family physician or pediatrician can minimize the degree of such disturbances and their impact on the family. The management of such problems if they do become chronic requires repeated, patient listening, and counsel (see also Chapter 70).

Some sleep disorders, however, are based on disturbed sleep physiology and may present with dramatic, often paroxysmal clinical features which are very likely to present in the emergency department (Table 72.1). The differential diagnosis and management of these disorders will be discussed more fully. Prior to such discussion, however, it may be helpful to briefly review current knowledge of sleep physiology.

PHYSIOLOGIC CONSIDERATIONS

For centuries men have viewed sleep rather simply as the opposite of alert wake-

Table 72.1
Sleep-related Disorders

- *I. Disorders Primarily Related to Normal Developmental Stages*
  - A. Chronic resistance to sleep
  - B. Frequent nighttime awakening
  - C. Nightmares
  - D. Body rocking and head banging
- *II. Disorders of Sleep Physiology*
  - A. Non-REM dyssomnias
    1. Pavor nocturnus
    2. Somnambulism and somniloguy
    3. Primary nocturnal enuresis
  - B. Disorders of excess sleep
    1. Narcolepsy
    2. Sleep-apnea syndromes
    3. Post-traumatic, post-encephalitic syndromes
    4. Kleine-Levin syndrome
  - C. Drug-induced disorders
    1. Insomnia
    2. Excess sleep
  - D. Adolescent depression
    1. Insomnia
    2. Excess sleep
  - E. Sudden infant death syndrome (?)

fulness, a period of physiologic restitution during which all vegetative and higher cortical functions were switched to lowest levels of activity. In recent years, however, researchers have established that sleep is not a unitary physiologic state but rather two states of vastly different physiologic characteristics alternating in an orderly cycle. In the first such state, there are periods of active sleep characterized by facial and body movements and the occurrence of bilateral synchronous rapid eye movements (REM sleep). Such states alternate with periods of quiet sleep, during which body and eye movements are absent (non-REM sleep). These states can be further subdivided by EEG patterns. Stage 1 is reflected by low voltage fast activity and is comparable to an awake pattern during visual imaging. This pattern is seen during active-REM sleep, and during the lightest stage of non-REM sleep. As a subject descends into deeper stages of non-REM sleep, the EEG activity becomes progressively slower and higher in voltage. During non-REM sleep, the pulse and respiratory rates are slow and regular; there is presence of some baseline muscle tone with minimal body or eye movements. Mentation is slight during non-REM sleep, and imagery is not vivid or easily recalled by a subject awakened from it.

REM sleep conversely represents a period of heightened CNS activity, although arousal threshold (that stimulus necessary to awaken the subject) during REM periods is comparable to the deeper non-REM stages.

Dreaming occurs during REM sleep. Heart and respiratory rates are faster and more irregular than in non-REM sleep, while resting muscle tone is suppressed. Adults usually begin their night with descent from stage 1 non-REM through the deeper non-REM levels, and then emerge to a REM period; such cycles may occur 4 to 6 times in a typical night.

The sleep cycles in infants differ from the adult pattern in that the distinct EEG stages are not as sharply organized. Young infants usually begin their cycle with a brief REM period, and their cycles are shorter. EEG patterns mature rapidly and, by 3 months of age, quiet sleep can be subdivided into four non-REM stages.

CLINICAL MANIFESTATIONS AND MANAGEMENT

The most common disorders of sleep physiology in children include (1) pavor nocturnus (night terrors), (2) somnambulism and somniloquy, and (3) nocturnal enuresis. These can be classified by their observed relationships to the REM/non-REM sleep cycle. They all tend to occur in the transition from deep non-REM to light non-REM sleep, and are thus considered disorders of arousal. The arousal disorders all share common features: the various disorders may occur at different times in the same child; there is frequently a positive family history; males outnumber females; and they are paroxysmal, associated with automatism, unresponsiveness to the environment and retrograde amnesia for the episodes. Much less common are the disorders of excess sleep including narcolepsy, sleep apnea syndrome and drug related, posttraumatic or post-encephalitic dyssomnias.

Pavor nocturnus is usually seen in the preschool-aged children. The child will awaken 15 to 90 min after sleep onset. Striking features include extreme anxiety, many autonomic phenomena (sweating, hyperpnea, tachycardia) and the appearance of staring at an imaginary site. The child may be inconsolable for 10 to 15 min, and show little evidence of awakening, but then suddenly relax and fall back to quiet sleep. There is generally no dream recall nor remembrance of the attack the next morning. Night terrors usually occur so infrequently that treatment is not necessary. In contrast to night terrors, nightmares are bad dreams (REM-sleep) from which the child is usually quite awake and responsive by the time the parents arrive, and for which there can be substantial recall.

Somnambulism and *somniloquy* (sleepwalking and sleeptalking) present in the school-age child, occurring at least once in some 15% of all children. The child sits up suddenly with eyes glassy and staring, and may then arise and walk around clumsily. Episodes last from 15 sec to 30 min and are not remembered the next morning. As opposed to adult sleepwalkers, significant psychopathology is not commonly present in school-aged somnambulists. Temporal lobe epilepsy may be difficult to distinguish from somnambulism, but can usually be differentiated by adequate sleep EEG studies. Sleepwalkers can hurt themselves, and "sleepproofing" the home is an important part of management. In childhood, drug therapy of sleepwalking is rarely necessary. Parents can be reassured that most children will outgrow sleepwalking over a period of several years.

Primary nocturnal enuresis is defined as occurring in a child over age 3 years, who is otherwise well, and who has never been dry at night but who can stay dry all day. It is the most common non-REM disorder, with incidence estimates ranging from 5 to 17% of all children between 3 and 15 years of age. The enuretic episode usually occurs, as in the above conditions, with the transition from deep non-REM sleep to lighter non-REM sleep and the first REM period of the night. The episode is characterized by tachycardia, tachypnea, penile erection in males, increased intravesical pressure and spontaneous bladder contraction. The differential diagnosis includes other organic problems such as diabetes mellitus, diabetes insipidus and urinary tract infection, though these would be rare if the above definition were strictly adhered to. Treatment choices range from conditioning modalties to medications (such as imipramine) which have both anticholinergic effects on the bladder and stimulant effects on sleep stage patterns. Drug therapy of enuresis is considered a last resort to be prescribed only in severe cases and should be instituted under a pediatrician's guidance.

Disorders of excess sleep in children are much less common than the non-REM dyssomnias. *Narcolepsy* in its complete syndrome includes excess daytime somnolence (often first noted at school) with attacks of daytime sleep (which are usually bursts of stage 1-non-REM sleep). Patients may also experience cataplexy (sudden loss of muscle tone with preservation of consciousness), sleep paralysis and hypnagogic hallucination (experience of paralysis and vivid imagery just as one is falling asleep) and disturbed nighttime sleep. Most patients manifest only excess daytime sleep and cataplexy. The onset of symptoms may occur in the school-age child but diagnosis is rarely made prior to adolescence or early adulthood. When studied in a sleep physiology laboratory, these patients generally have an initial REM period at sleep onset, similar to the pattern in normal neonates. Management includes stimulant drugs such as methylphenidate hydrochloride for the daytime sleepiness and, if necessary, imipramine for severe cataplexy, sleep paralysis or hypnagogic hallucinations.

The term *"sleep-apnea syndrome"* refers to another condition, seen in children with various types of upper airway obstruction, disordered sleep stages (increased stages 1 and 2 and decreased stages 3 and 4 of non-REM sleep) and frequent apneic spells during sleep. There may be secondary cardiovascular effects including hypertension and cor pulmonale. Children present with loud snoring, excess daytime somnolence, morning headaches, hypertension and poor school performance. The occurrence of this syndrome probably implies both CNS and upper airway defects. Management involves otolaryngologic consultation for thorough airway evaluation and appropriate measures to relieve obstruction. Children in whom this diagnosis is entertained require emergency hospitalization.

Other pediatric causes of disordered sleep physiology include adolescent substance abuse and depression (see Chapters 70 and 71), post-traumatic and post-encephalitic syndromes, and the Kleine-Levin syndrome seen in boys with attacks of excess sleep punctuated by enormous increase of appetite and overeating binges. Last, major research efforts are currently being directed toward a population of babies including those diagnosed as "near-miss" sudden infant death syndrome (infants found apneic and cyanotic in their cribs who were successfully resuscitated at home by their parents) and siblings of victims. A hypothesis common to these studies is that in such children, although the causes may be multifactorial, the final common pathway involves disordered respiratory control during sleep.

References

Hyperventilation

Enzer NB, Walker PA: Hyperventilation syndrome in childhood. *J Pediatr* 70: 521, 1967.

Joorabchi B: Expressions of the hyperventilation syndrome in childhood. *Clin Pediatr* 16: 1110, 1977.

Missri JC, Alexander S: Hyperventilation syndrome; a brief review. *JAMA* 240: 2093, 1978.

Rice RL: Symptom patterns of the hyperventilation syndrome. *Am J Med* 8: 691, 1950.

Saltzman HA, Hegman A, Sieber HO: Correlation of clinical and physiologic manifestations of sustained hyperventilation. *N Engl J Med* 288: 1431, 1963.

Rumination

Fleisher DR: Infant rumination syndrome. *Am J Dis Child* 133: 266, 1979.

Richmond JB, Eddy E, Green M: Rumination; a psychosomatic syndrome of infancy. *Pediatrics* 22: 49, 1958.

Tics

Illingworth RS: *The Normal Child*, Ed. 5. Churchill Livingstone, Edinburgh, 1973.

Lockman LA: Movement disorders. In *The Practice of Pediatric Neurology*, pp. 218–257. C. V. Mosby, St. Louis, 1975.

Menkes JH: *Textbook of Child Neurology*. Lea & Febiger, Philadelphia, 1974.

Breathholding Attacks

Illingworth RS: *The Normal Child*, Ed. 5. Churchill Livingstone, Edinburgh, 1973.

Lombroso CT, Lerman P: Breathholding spells (cyanotic and pallid infantile syncope). *Pediatrics* 39: 563, 1967.

Sleep Disorders

Anders TF, Guilleminault C: The pathophysiology of sleep disorders in pediatrics. *Adv Pediatr* 22: 137, 1976.

Kales A, Kales JD: Sleep disorders; recent findings in the diagnosis and treatment of disturbed sleep. *N Engl J Med* 290: 487, 1974.

SECTION **VI**

Administration of the Emergency Department

CHAPTER **73**

Organization/Staffing

STEPHEN LUDWIG, M.D., AND GARY R. FLEISHER, M.D.

INTRODUCTION

Emergency medicine has been evolving as a specialty for more than two decades. Prior to 1960, physician coverage of hospital emergency departments was spotty. The medical staff generally were not present in the facility around the clock and were not required to have special competence in the care of the critically ill patient.

In 1961, two systems began to develop independently, improving the coverage for the emergency departments of their local hospitals. A group of physicians in Virginia formed the first full-time group to practice emergency medicine (Alexandria Plan) and, at a hospital in Michigan, 60 attending physicians agreed to provide continuous coverage at their institution but maintained their own practices (Pontiac Plan).

In 1968, the first national organization for emergency physicians was formed to be known as the American College of Emergency Physicians (ACEP), and, in 1979, the American Board of Medical Specialists accepted Emergency Medicine as the 23rd approved medical specialty. Shortly thereafter, the American Board of Emergency

Medicine administered its first certification examination. More than 10,000 physicians now belong to ACEP, and there are 60 residency programs training physicians in this specialty.

Rapid increases in the usage of emergency facilities provided a major stimulus for the development of improved emergency care services. Since the end of World War II, the number of emergency visits in the United States has increased more than 600%. More than 80 million individuals received treatment in an emergency department in this country during 1981. A survey of health care in Cook County, Illinois, in 1970, by Gibson and colleagues found that 5% of all patient visits to physicians took place in the emergency departments.

Simultaneous with the spiraling demand for emergency care, the government showed increasing interest in such services. In 1967, the National Academy of Sciences published a report documenting the large annual morbidy and mortality from accidents. Because of these tragic statistics, Congress passed the National Highway Traffic Safety Act in 1967. This legislation required states to develop safety programs in accordance with uniform standards. Then, in 1973, Congress adopted the Emergency Medical Services Systems Act which authorized funds to assist the states in upgrading their emergency services. Extensions to this act were passed in both 1976 and 1979.

Only in the last few years has Pediatric Emergency Medicine evolved as a subspecialty of pediatrics. Embryonic programs appeared initially at several pediatric hospitals in the United States in the latter half of the 1970's. Then, following several years of organizational meetings, the American Academy of Pediatrics (AAP) created a Section of Pediatric Emergency Medicine in 1981.

The section convened for the first time in October 1981, and already lists nearly 100 members. Although no mechanism for certification has been formalized, a fellowship in pediatric emergency medicine is currently offered by at least one institution.

The arrival of the new specialty of pediatric emergency medicine provided a focus for the careful evaluation of the current organization and staffing of the emergency departments serving children. Certainly, such facilities must adhere to the standards promulgated by the Joint Commission for the Accreditation of Hospitals (JCAH). However, experience tells us that standards established primarily to regulate services for adults will not be satisfactory for the care of children. It is the area beyond the requirements of the present JCAH regulations that this chapter will address.

ORGANIZATION

As with any professional endeavor, there are many intangibles that are important to the successful organization and operation of the emergency department. Perhaps the key to any organizational arrangement is having the members of the organization feel committed to the purposes of the group. When workers, either professional or nonprofessional, assume a sense of pride in their work, the organizational structure will be a good one. If the emergency department becomes just another place to earn a salary, even the best organizational scheme will fail. The intangibles of departmental function are hard to translate into practical suggestions. Nonetheless, there are some specific organizational recommendations which are important, especially for new emergency department groups.

Leadership

In the past, many hospital emergency departments have been supervised by a senior resident physician. This is an inadequate arrangement; although a senior resident physician may be extremely competent in many aspects of medical decision making and technical skill, he or she is unable to provide the continuity necessary to properly administer departmental affairs. The leadership of the emergency department must come from a full time attending physician with a long-term career commitment to the department. For pediatric emergency care, the director should be trained both in pediatrics and emergency care. The position should not be filled by either a physician-in-training or a physician looking for a temporary position until a different situation comes along. The director of the department must have overall responsibility for the provision of medical care. To do this, the director needs the support of the hospital staff and administration, and in the case of a teaching hospital the support of the academic departmental chairman and faculty. Jenkins and Van de Leuv describe the inefficiency of some emergency departments because of the existence of three separate and distinct lines of authority in the medical, nursing and administrative staff. At some point these lines of authority must intertwine in order to provide departmental leadership. The medical director requires a broad range of authority. Mackenzie and colleagues have enumerated the qualifications and responsibilities of a director in a teaching hospital setting (Table 73.1).

In addition to a medical director, the department must have a nursing supervisor, administrator, and a cadre of staff physicians with similar dedication. This leadership group must be of sufficient size that one of its members is always available to direct the functioning of the department. The group will also be aided by establishing a set of written policies and procedures. Many of these guidelines are required by state and hospital association accrediting bodies such as the JCAH. In addition to formulating the required policies, the emergency department leadership group can formalize its authority by establishing other important protocols.

Financial Management

Emergency department physician groups may enter into a number of different financial relationships with hospitals.

The members of the physician group, the hospital's executive officer, and, in the case of an academic center, the departmental chairman and medical school dean must be in agreement about the form of the financial arrangement. The hospital and academic authorities must be prepared to support the financial goals of the emergency department, since it may take a number of years to achieve financial independence. There must be clear expectations about the level and longevity of support which can be offered.

It is important that the relationships between the emergency department staff, the hospital and the academic department be detailed in a written contract. Contracting is essential, as it serves as a point of anchorage for all parties. Contracting forces individuals to establish priorities and to be held accountable. Details of contracting and other aspects of financial management are covered in Chapter 74.

Staff Development

Another important organizational consideration is staff development. This refers to the development of the group of people who will serve as the professional staff as well as the education of the individuals in their professional roles.

The size of the staff depends on several factors including (1) presence and number of house officers, (2) hours of coverage needed, and (3) number and severity of illness of patients. If the department serves a significant number of critically ill children it is important to have staff level coverage 24 hours a day. In less busy departments which are not large referral centers 16 hours per day coverage may be adequate.

Development of *special interests* by the staff is encouraged. If each staff member assumes an area of expertise, both the department and the physician benefit. Emergency physicians may wish to concentrate interest in special areas; for example, toxicology, cardiopulmonary resuscitation, or epidemiology. Specialization has advantages for the department, such as raising the level of patient care, providing a source for in-service education, opening avenues for research, and providing more independence for the staff (less reliance on consultants). For the emergency physician, special interest areas provide a higher level of job interest, positive feelings of competence or expertise, and opportunities for teaching and clinical research. Having a special interest area may be helpful in reducing the occupational "burnout" which is caused by working in the highly stressful emergency department environment.

Staff should also be given the opportu-

Table 73.1
The Emergency Department Director[a]

I. Qualifications
- A. Physician—licensed to practice medicine in state or province of appointment
- B. Specialized knowledge in the broad field of emergency medicine and/or certificate of competence in some aspect of emergency medicine from a recognized residency program

II. Appointment
- A. Hospital—by the board of governors on the recommendation of the medical advisory committee to the active staff and to the department of emergency medicine as chairman
- B. University—by the dean of medicine on behalf of the senate to the appropriate academic department and to the major scientific educational and research committees of the university. Rank—associate professor or higher
- C. Community—by the regional health council or other recognized community health body to the emergency care advisory committee of the region as the coordinator of education and research programs in emergency medicine; or as a representative where more than one university is involved

III. Remuneration
- A. By the university for research and educational endeavors
- B. By the hospital for patient care and administration

IV. Terms of Reference
- A. Define emergency department policies, standards and functions with the aid of the emergency department committee
- B. Plan, organize and manage space, facilities, equipment and personnel for the functions defined for the emergency department. This includes the right to hire and fire all emergency department personnel and to define and manage the emergency department budget (in consultation with the appropriate hospital or university department)
- C. Direct educational, scientific and research endeavors in emergency medicine
- D. Coordinate emergency medicine functions within other areas in the hospital, university or community
- E. Represent the hospital and university in emergency medicine affairs to outside bodies
- F. Continue to review and update knowledge of emergency medicine and to audit patient care

[a] From J. R. Mackenzie et al.: *JACEP, 5:* 364–376, 1976.

nity to pursue continuing education. Periodic refresher courses help both the individual and the department. Continuing education is particularly important in pediatric emergency care as it is a newly evolving specialty. Many changes in the practice of pediatric emergency care are likely to occur in the coming years. Beyond voluntary continuing education, there are required areas of education and certification which the emergency physician must acquire. Certification in basic and advanced life support and in advanced trauma life support should be mandatory for all staff emergency physicians.

Another aspect of staff development which should be encouraged is membership in relevant professional organizations. Currently such organizations include American Academy of Pediatrics—Emergency Medicine Section, American College of Emergency Physicians, University Association of Emergency Medicine and Society of Teachers of Emergency Medicine. Many urban areas have local and regional emergency medicine societies or conclaves which are an excellent source of professional contacts, emergency medical education, and political action.

Space and Facilities

The details of a child oriented emergency department design are covered in Chapter 76. In the organization of the department there must be careful consideration of the available space and facilities. The emergency care group should clearly define space and equipment needs. The fulfillment of the needs can be negotiated as part of the financial contract between the emergency department group and the hospital. Environmental considerations are extremely important. The failure to fully alleviate space and facility needs can severely limit staff and program development and can interfere with the proper performance of many tasks.

Intra-Hospital Relationships

The emergency department must have organized relationships with other parts of the hospital, such as surgical and medical specialty, ancillary services, the medical staff committees, and hospital administration.

Perhaps the most important hospital ties are those which must be formed with consultant services. There must be clear definitions as to (1) when to consult a surgical or medical specialist, (2) how to reach the consultant, and (3) what can be expected in response to a consultation. If a consultant feels he is being inappropriately called and fails to adequately respond, the emergency physician and the patient are left feeling frustrated. This kind of situation is common in emergency departments and results in poor patient care, increased malpractice liability, and professional resentment. The emergency department director must establish guidelines and procedures with each of the specialty service consultants.

In addition to the relationships with surgical and medical consultants, there must be clearly established protocols for interaction with the clinical laboratory, respiratory therapy, social work, pharmacy, admissions office, and radiology services. With clearly defined expectations, each service can be held accountable for what it has agreed to provide. Periodic renegotiation of expectations is always needed to accommodate to changes in the needs of the emergency department and the ability of the ancillary service to respond. Without this aspect of organization, the staff will experience conflict and frustration.

Most hospital medical staffs are organized into a number of working committees. It is important for emergency department representatives to be part of hospital structure. In particular, committees such as Patient Care, Audit/Quality Assurance, Disaster Planning, Pharmacy and Therapeutic Standards, and Medical Records will benefit from an emergency department perspective. Committee work is another way to strengthen intra-hospital relationships. The hospital medical staff should also appoint an Emergency Services Committee. This committee, headed by the department director, provides an opportunity for other departments to contribute to the policy making and operations of the emergency department. The committee should include representatives from the nursing service, hospital administration, surgery and social work as a working core. Additional members may be added, depending on the policies to be discussed and the particulars of the hospital's departmental structure.

The emergency department must also organize relationships to various members of the hospital administration. In particular, there should be good communication between the emergency department director and the hospital legal counsel or risk management representative (see Chapter 77). There must also be working agreements between the business office and the emergency department. It is also important for the Emergency Director to keep the hospital's public relations department informed of issues which are newsworthy, whether they relate to a patient or to a new departmental program. All levels of hospital administration (including the hospital's board of directors) should be kept informed about departmental progress and problems.

Extra-Hospital Relationships

Good organizational practice dictates that the emergency department staff form relationships outside the hospital. Organizational ties to other emergency physicians have been noted previously. There must also be contacts with local providers of prehospital medical care such as police, firemen and paramedics from public or private auspices. The department will further benefit from relationships with other emergency departments and specialty hospitals. Maintaining communication with primary care physicians will increase the number and quality of referrals.

Program Development

Once the basic departmental organization is working well, there are many new avenues available for program development. The pediatric emergency care service can quite naturally become the home for one or more new programs such as a (1) Poison Control Center, (2) Inter-hospital Transport Service, (3) Child Abuse or Sexual Abuse Center, (4) Resuscitation Team, or (5) Trauma Center. Many other specialized services may be initiated in the emergency department. Any specialized program will take time, staff, and financial resources. The benefits of any new program development must be weighed against the cost; they must never jeopardize the ongoing functioning of the department.

Research in the emergency department is another aspect of program expansion. The emergency department is an ideal location for clinical research. There is a constant source of new research questions for the physician with an inquiring mind, and a large patient population is also available. Research creates an academic atmosphere for the staff and may provide an opportunity for activity which will compliment responsibilities for direct patient care. Many research projects may be carried out with minimal expenditures, while other projects may be a source of funds which can be used to support staff or purchase equipment. Initially, the nursing staff and residents may show resistance to the introduction of research protocols in the emergency department. However, if the staff is committed to the value of this form of program development, most obstacles can be overcome. Clinical research which seeks to answer questions perplexing to the departmental staff will be best accepted.

Another area of program growth is in the realm of educational programs. Emergency department staff can participate in medical educational programs on the medical school, residency, fellowship, and postgraduate levels. Fellowships in pediatric emergency care can provide indepth training and will be offered more widely in the future. Educational events may also be offered to other professionals, for example, nurses and social workers, and to the general public. Public education may cover many specific topics (e. g. avoiding frostbite) or focus on the use of the emergency department as a community resource.

STAFFING

Medical Staff

Role

Every emergency department must have a group of attending physicians who assume responsibility for the department. This group of physicians will be concerned principally with two areas: administration of the emergency department and patient care.

Although the medical group as a whole accepts certain responsibilities, each individual staff physician may divide his or her time in a different fashion. Thus, a single director may oversee the operation of the emergency department or several may share the administrative tasks. The functions of the director are discussed in this chapter on p. 1154.

The ultimate responsibility for the care of every patient in the emergency department lies with the attending medical staff, both from an ethical and a legal point of view. In many cases, the staff physician will provide complete care for the patient, thereby directly discharging his or her responsibilities.

Other patients will receive part or all of their care from other personnel in the emergency department, including consultants, residents, nurses, or physician's assistants. If the attending physician requests a consultation, he should remain involved with the management of that patient until satisfied that the treatment or disposition has been appropriate. Any areas of disagreement need to be resolved by the emergency department physician and the consultant before the patient leaves the facility, since both physicians are now responsible for the care.

The staff emergency department physician is directly accountable for the care provided by emergency department personnel other than consultants and must supervise these encounters. Ideally, the staff emergency physician should have direct involvement with the care of every patient, particularly those classified as actual emergencies. At a minimum, a staff physician should be available around-the-clock in the emergency department and should review the record of every patient.

Qualifications

Pediatric Emergency Care is a new field and there are not yet established standards for practitioners, certified training programs, or qualifying examinations. Although such criteria are being or will be developed, some minimal qualifications are self-evident for the physician who will be responsible for children in the emergency department of a pediatric institution. Obviously, a physician in this setting must be knowledgeable in two different fields, pediatrics and emergency medicine. To acquire competence in both these areas requires residency training in one of the disciplines and postgraduate experience in the other. The pediatrician who pursued a career in the emergency care of children must be certified by the American Heart Association in Advanced Cardiac Life Support. Additionally, he or she must seek experience beyond that provided during residency in the management of medical emergencies, trauma and other surgical emergencies, anesthesia, and the legal aspects of emergency care. The physician completing a residency in emergency medicine has learned the many surgical and critical care skills but lacks the experience in applying this knowledge to children. In addition, he or she must become familiar with the full range of less emergent pediatric problems that often prompt a visit to the emergency department.

Schedules

Certain considerations affect the requirements for staff physicians, although the exact details will vary from center to center. Among these are the following: the number of children seen daily, the ratio of emergent and nonemergent cases, the duration of attending coverage, the distribution of night call, and the amount of ancillary help.

At a minimum, there should be one attending physician on duty in the emergency department at all times. If the attending staff are to remain participants in the daytime activities of the institution, eight physicians are needed. Assuming that one is usually on vacation, each of the other seven would cover the department one night weekly and have the succeeding day free. Alternatively, the staff may see their only goal as coverage of the emergency department, foregoing most of the usual conferences, daily teaching activities, and research. Such an arrangement allows some physicians to cover exclusively nights or weekends for a given period of time. If each member of the department were to take direct patient care responsibilities for approximately 40 hours weekly, six physicians would be required.

When the case load exceeds a certain limit, additional physicians must be constantly available to treat the patients. Particularly if the percentage of critically ill children is high, two or more physicians should be available at all times. Usually, residents will provide most of the additional manpower.

At The Children's Hospital of Philadelphia, approximately 200 children visit the Emergency Department daily. One fifth of these are judged to have conditions that require emergency care (i.e. cardiopulmonary arrest, respiratory distress, lacerations, fractures, meningitis, epiglottitis), while the remainder have less urgent problems. Most emergencies will occur during the daytime (8 a.m. to 4 p.m.) and evening (4 p.m. to midnight) shift. At The Children's Hospital of Philadelphia the patients are distributed as follows: days 61%, evening 32%, night 7%. On week days between 9:00 a.m. and 5:30 a.m., there are two attending physicians and five to seven residents; from 5:30 until 12:00 a.m. one attending and five residents are present; after 12:00 a.m., one attending and two residents are on duty.

Professional Considerations

The emergency care of children requires unique knowledge and skills, as do other subspecialties of pediatrics. Thus, physicians responsible for the treatment of children in the emergency department must demonstrate a commitment to developing and/or maintaining expertise in this field. If the physicians expect to remain competent in the diagnosis and management of the various types of emergency problems and to achieve personal satisfaction, the schedule must set aside time for continuing education. Within most teaching hospitals, additional opportunity for clinical or basic research should be available.

Nursing Staff

Role

The nursing service is involved with all aspects of patient care in the emergency department. Since the medical staff bears the ultimate responsibility for the outcome of the emergency department visit, they must play a role in helping to establish nursing policies and procedures and monitoring the quality of the care delivered. The physicians will not usually handle the day-to-day problems in the management of nursing personnel but should be familiar with the functions of the service.

The responsibilities of the nursing service will vary among departments but will always include a basic core of assignments. Through the head nurse and the appropriate committees, the staff must develop a set of policies and procedures to guide patient care. The initial evaluation of the sick child will often be performed by the nursing staff, so they must be capable of rapidly assessing the ill patient, especially with regard to the cardiovascular status. The nurses will also assist the medical staff in the diagnosis and treatment of the patients. Particularly in dealing with children, who are often uncooperative, such assistance is frequently necessary. The nursing staff should assume responsibility for the coordination of the activities of the emergency department with other departments and inpatient units. Properly trained nurses can appropriately perform triage of children coming to the department. The registered nurse may choose to delegate certain responsibilities to other personnel including licensed practical nurses or aides.

Qualifications

The backbone of the nursing staff should consist of registered nurses, supplemented by an appropriate number of licensed practical nurses and aides. Since the emergency department environment places great demands on the nurses, they should have at least a year of experience working as a nurse with children. Prior employment in an intensive care unit is particularly helpful.

All registered nurses in the department initially should achieve certification in basic life support and eventually in advanced cardiac life support. The delivery of effective cardiopulmonary resuscitation requires a thorough knowledge of the procedures, drugs, and equipment by the nurses.

Triage of incoming patients is a difficult task that demands clinical competence, a familiarity with the legal statutes in the field, and a sensitivity for the relationship of the hospital to the community. Nurses who perform triage must learn the established guidelines of the department and undergo a supervised trial.

Scheduling

The same consideration that figures into the determination of the number of medical staff will also play a role in the size of the nursing staff. The head nurse should assume responsibility for scheduling nurses and assigning responsibilities on each shift. Should problems in staffing become apparent to the medical director of the emergency department, he or she must resolve them with the head nurse.

Social Work Staff

Role

As the spectrum of services provided by the emergency department widens, the need for support from the social service department becomes more urgent. Physicians working in the pediatric emergency facility will care for children who have run away from home, ingested drugs, or become pregnant. Parents, relatives, or the police will bring victims of child abuse and rape, expecting not just medical treatment but a comprehensive approach to these multifaceted problems. Working alone, the physician cannot find the solutions. The social worker forms an essential part of the multidisciplinary team needed for these situations.

The social worker can assist the physician in obtaining background information on the family and the environment. Often, this type of interview requires more time than that which is available to the physician and demands inquiry into aspects of the history with which most practitioners are not familiar. As a team, the physicians, social workers, and nurses can then formulate a plan for further management. In many cases, governmental agencies, including the police and welfare departments, or private organizations, such as Women Organized Against Rape, will enter into the care of the child at this time. The experienced social worker provides an invaluable liaison with these agencies.

Qualifications

The social workers interacting with the staff of the emergency department should meet the same standards established for their counterparts in other hospital departments. They must have, or be committed to, acquiring knowledge of the specialized needs of children.

Scheduling

A social worker must be available to the emergency department around-the-clock. If the service is sufficiently busy, a single individual should be delegated to coordinate all the social work activities in the emergency department. Colleagues who have primarily inpatient responsibilities can share coverage for nights and weekends. The case load will determine the need for additional full-time personnel.

Clerical Staff

From both a medical and a legal viewpoint, the proper registration of patients and the maintenance of adequate records requires a large clerical staff. The clerks will have the responsibility for greeting the patients and their families, directing them to the nurse for triage, eliciting information for registration, and obtaining consent for diagnosis and treatment. Individuals in this position need secretarial skills as well as an awareness of their important role as public representatives of the physicians and the hospital administration.

Additional Personnel

Certain tasks may become so burdensome for the personnel described heretofore that they will dictate the creation of new positions. Once again, the individual characteristics of the emergency department will determine which positions and how many staff are needed.

As the group of physicians expands, their needs often surpass those provided by the secretarial and clerical staff. Financial affairs and personnel management may consume an unacceptably large portion of the director's time or that of his or her assistants. When this happens, the physicians may want to retain the services of an administrator for their group, distinct from the person appointed by the hospital to oversee the department.

Technological advances have produced a continuous increase in the type and amount of equipment needed for diagnosis and treatment, particularly for the critically ill child. A busy emergency department will need to maintain two or more areas set up for resuscitation of the patient who has sustained multiple trauma or a cardiopulmonary arrest. The maintenance and updating of the equipment will eventually require a full-time member to assume this responsibility. The individual who takes this position would need a background in nursing or biomedical engineering.

Every department will serve a unique population and will be subjected to the demands of its own hospital and regional governing bodies. As new demands arise, the medical staff must guard against overburdening themselves or other personnel in the department. Rather, consideration should be given to creating new positions to meet these developing needs.

References

Beck LC: *The Physician's Office*. Excerpta Medica, Princeton, N. J. 1977.

Gibson G, Bugbee G, Anderson OW: *Emergency Medical Services in the Chicago Area*. Center for Health Administration Studies, University of Chicago, Chicago, 1970.

Jenkins AL, Van de Leuv JH (Eds.): *Emergency Department Organization and Management*, Ed. 2. C. V. Mosby, St. Louis, 1972.

Mackenzie JR, Jelenko C, James P, Frey C: A guide for the organization of an emergency department in the university setting. *JACEP* 5: 364–376, 1976.

Riggs LM: A vigorous new specialty. *N Engl J Med* 304: 480–483, 1981.

CHAPTER 74

Financial Management

LEO C. LEFEBVRE, JR., AND GEORGE J. PECKHAM, M.D.

BACKGROUND

Financial Management: What Is It?

Financial management can be described as the art of economically obtaining needed funds and of making the best use of those funds once obtained. Financial management can be viewed as a decision-making process. Like all decision-making processes, factual information, financial tools and techniques are needed in order for it to function accurately and efficiently. Financial management is commonly thought to be synonymous with accounting practices; often these terms are used interchangeably. Financial management and accounting are not the same, but are related. Accounting can be defined as "the art of collecting, summarizing, analyzing, reporting, and interpreting monetary information about a business enterprise." This is an important function, but it is not as broad a function as financial management (Berman and Weeks). Financial management provides the means for effective decision making; the accounting system provides the data needed for accurate analysis. In the health care field today the political, economic and management environments are forcing improvements in operations. Financial management is an important and responsive tool to be used in meeting these challenges.

Objectives of Financial Management

As stated by Berman and Weeks, "Primarily, financial management tools and techniques can aid management in providing the community with quality services at least cost by furnishing the data which are necessary for making intelligent capital investment decisions, by guiding the operations of certain hospital subsystems, and by providing the systems and data needed to monitor and control operations." Figure 74.1 illustrates the value and usefulness of financial management from the hospital's vantage point.

From the physician's standpoint, a basic objective in financial management is to develop as efficient a routine as possible in order to allow the physician to practice medicine rather than devote a large portion of time to financial matters. The emergency physician, however, cannot totally divorce himself from financial matters. Some time and attention must be invested in financial matters in order to adequately control one's practice.

Growth of the Emergency Group Practices

Historically, hospitals have had the total responsibility for financial management of the emergency department. But, as the number of emergency department visits began to grow, the financial management of the emergency department, as well as its medical liability, became more uncontrollable. The American Hospital Association reported that "Hospital emergency department traffic has increased markedly during the past two decades. The American Hos-

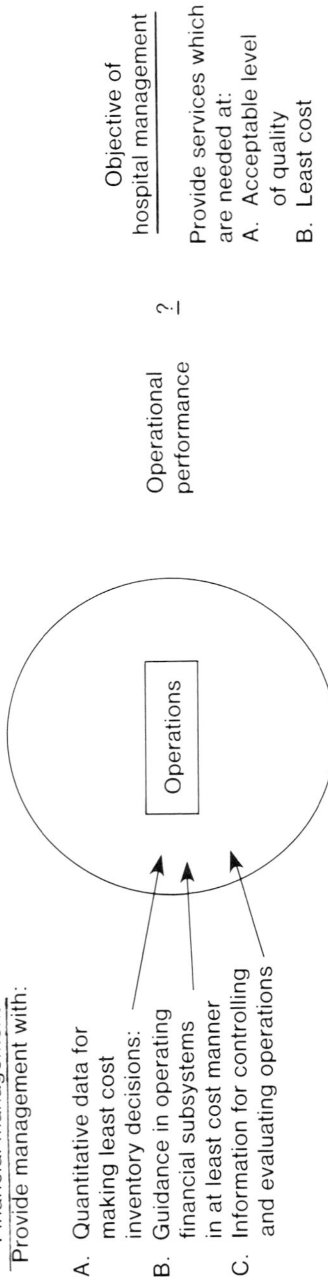

Figure 74.1 Financial management provides data and management which can assist management in guiding operational performance in order to meet the hospital's and physicians' objective.

pital Association annual survey of registered hospitals showed a 308% increase in the number of visits to the emergency departments of community (non-federal general short-term) hospitals from 1954 to 1970. From 1965 to 1970, the number of such visits rose from 28.7 million to 42.7 million, a gain of more than 14 million. Since the 1970s, the numbers of visits have continued to increase although at a much less dramatic rate.

At the Children's Hospital of Philadelphia, the figures confirm that there indeed has been a significant increase in emergency department activity. Table 74.1 shows that statistics from 1978 through 1981, and these numbers suggest a 17% increase in activity.

Because of the stresses noted above, many hospitals have contracted with a physician group for the provision of emergency services on a full-time basis. Although a relatively new concept, the contract group is gaining widespread acceptance in many hospitals. Hospitals are discovering that physician contracting is a viable method to insure efficient top quality patient care in the emergency department without fully assuming medical-legal or physician-administrative responsibilities.

The advantage of a group practice option of this type to the physicians is that there are financial incentives without sacrifice of the quality of care delivered. Emergency departments are a vital and necessary part of any community resource and as such should be operated for the benefit of the community. The primary objective of any physician group contracted by a hospital is to provide the community with the needed services at high quality levels and at the most economical costs. Physician contracting of emergency departments by hospitals appears to be a model that satisfies most of the requirements of both the hospital and the physicians.

For the future, "Rational planning for improved medical services requires that inclusion of hospital emergency departments be viewed as part of a broad spectrum of necessary ambulatory care services and facilities. Solutions to the problem of overu-

Table 74.1
The Children's Hospital of Philadelphia Emergency Department

	1978	1979	1980	1981
Acute care:	47,837	48,094	48,839	49,182
Emergency care:	15,957	16,056	20,179	25,446
Total	63,874	64,150	69,018	74,628
% Increase	—	—	7.6	8.1
% Increase	1978–1981 = 17%			

tilization of emergency departments will be found only by attacking the root causes of the overloading. A key cause of this problem is the lack of alternative sources of medical care for large segments of the population who use the emergency department for primary care. Alternative sources for primary care have been developed in the form of ambulatory care centers, primary care centers, neighborhood health centers, drop-in clinics adjacent to emergency departments, and outpatient departments that stay open evenings and weekends. The future development of these health care sources will bring additional changes to the emergency department group practice operation, and financial management.

ORGANIZATION

A Financial Plan

It may be well to point out that there is no need to reinvent the wheel when it comes to financial planning. Guidelines for a group practice state, "Financial planning normally begins with the development of fiscal policies addressing such issues as: establishing the accounting period, pooling of assets, developing wage and salary schedules and payroll procedures, developing accounting and information systems, adopting a chart of accounts, preparing balance sheets and income statements, creating books of account, determining credit and collection policies, establishing budgets, preparing for audits and developing a system of cash management. These considerations are somewhat technical in nature so that a newly forming group is well advised to acquire the assistance of a competent accountant, management consultation, or attorney—preferably one well versed in financial planning for physicians and medical groups."

Application of generally accepted financial principles from the business world is advisable, and a detailed annual budget is mandatory. The budget should include income and expenditures, capital requirements, equipment and one-time start-up costs as well as any other identified expense items. Some authorities estimate that only 2% of the private medical practices in this country prepare a budget of projected income and expenses. Virtually every commercial venture depends upon budget procedures for financial control.

A budget enables one to identify objectives as to income generation and expenditures. It defines the amount of required effort needed to achieve the groups stated goals. Budgets also provide methods of measuring progress toward those goals. Some expenditures to consider in establishing a budget are: staff salaries and fringe rates; trainees' salaries and fringe rates; secretaries' salaries and fringe rates; overhead expenses; operating expenses; billing and collecting expenses; capital equipment expenses; renovation expenses and any other defined one-time or on-going expenses.

Once a budget is established and agreed upon, adequate reports must be generated in a timely manner so that controls can be established and maintained throughout the year. Monthly financial reports should include a cash flow statement, an income statement and a balance sheet. A comparison of monthly and year-to-date actual figures as compared against budget figures is one objective way to measure performance. It is imperative that this information be provided in time so that corrective measures can have their maximum impact. There is nothing more frustrating than to be able to identify a correctable problem after it is too late to correct it. Monthly billing information is also useful in order to keep track of the collection rates.

Establishing Policies

In a 1974 study conducted by the Center for Research in Ambulatory Health Care Administration, seven policy areas were identified as being the most critical to the development of a new (emergency department practice) group. In order of priority they are:

1. Policies on organizational form and governance
2. Policies on physician compensation
3. Policies governing the addition or reduction of professional staff
4. Policies of medical service fees
5. Financial policies
6. Accounting policies
7. Policies governing growth of the group.

Business Systems

Wasserman and Miller have stated that, "A group cannot be viable unless the business system can handle the volume and diversity of transactions which the group generates. Such transactions include charge recording, receipts, adjustments, preparation of statements, insurance forms, as well as the general bookkeeping functions of the business. The latter include the preparation and maintenance of accounting records, payroll and the various quarterly financial reports required by the state and federal governments."

With the introduction of microcomputers and the proliferation of software programs, basic business systems, previously available to groups, are fast becoming obsolete. New programs for operational and work load data, accounting data, data base maintenance, and custom report generation will serve as powerful tools to effectively control and manage the business of the emergency department. Real time reports which are custom configured to organize and reorganize data into meaningful reports are now a reality. Only minimum personnel, expense, and time commitments are required to make a small computer system operational in a relatively short period of time. The director of any emergency group should decide what is required to maintain adequate control of the financial plan and should obtain the proper business system to meet that goal.

CONTRACTING

After considerable discussion and analysis at the Children's Hospital of Philadelphia, it was decided to form an emergency department physicians' group practice. The Pediatric Emergency Care Associates (PECA) was organized to fit within the already established structure and procedures within Medical Associates, Inc., which is the existing billing and collection arm of the staff physicians. Academically, PECA resides within the Department of Pediatrics. A three-party multiyear contract was written between the PECA group, the Department of Pediatrics and the Hospital. In general, a multiyear contract provides several advantages in this type of arrangement. First, there is the need to guarantee the financing of the operation for the first year in order to allow time to build up the accounts receivables into an ongoing self-supporting entity. Second, the contract specifically identifies and spells out the "arms length" relationship between the group and the Hospital. It establishes responsibilities: the physicians for the care of the patients and the Hospital for the support personnel and proper facilities. Third, other specific financial points such as revenue, expense budgets and profit sharing must be spelled out in as much detail as required for agreement by all parties. A long-term contract is highly recommended but needs to be flexible enough to be renogotiable each year.

ACCOUNTS RECEIVABLE

The control and management of accounts receivable is a complex problem, and begins when the patient first enters the emergency department and continues until the account is paid or a decision is made to write-off the account as uncollectable. In order to carefully control the size of group's assets, actual operating costs must be minimized while the quantity of working capital is optimized. Accounts receivable costs include: (1) carrying costs, (2) routine collections and credit costs, and (3) delinquency costs. Carrying costs are those sums of money committed to accounts receivable that could be utilized for some other investment opportunities. Hospitals, or entities within hospitals (such as the emergency department group), usually do not charge patients for the credit which is made available to them. If costs are to be minimized, accounts receivable and the granting of credit should be kept to an absolute minimum.

The Effect of the Payment Cycle

The main key in the control of the costs associated with accounts receivable is to minimize the time or the length of the payment cycle. There is a certain point at which the cost of carrying the accounts receivable is greater than the value of the accounts receivable. A realistic view of the emergency department accounts receivable would encourage collection at the time services are rendered because of the fact that billing self-pay patients or third party payers is one of limited control. Ideally, it should be the patient's responsibility to obtain reimbursements from third party payers and not the billing function's responsibility.

It is not realistic to think that any practice group can exercise control over a Blue Cross/Blue Shield plan or over the goverment (Medical Assistance) to either reduce the amount of required paperwork for billing or increase the frequency of their payment cycles. The only practical improvement that can be made to the accounts receivable is to streamline the inhouse paperwork processing procedures so that they are accelerated to the point where the rate of bill submissions is optimized. To minimize the internal processing time, a system must be designed to ensure that not only all requests for services are properly registered, but also that all services rendered are promptly and accurately charged to the proper patient's account. If extra time needs to be taken to try and identify ser vices or other information not properly recorded, or if incorrect charges are entered and must be corrected in a patient's account, internal processing time increases and costs increase. The length of the payment cycle can also be reduced by developing a systematic credit granting and follow-up procedure. Table 74.2 is a partial listing, adapted from the American Hospital Association, *Internal Control and Internal Auditing for Hospitals* that may help the streamlining of this process.

The Effect of Third Party Payers

Third party payers substantially affect the financial status of an emergency department. Today, third party payers are the major source of revenue and can usually be depended upon to pay within a defined payment system and within a reasonably predictable time frame. Berman and Weeks have noted that, "The major purchasers of hospital care today, Blue Cross and the Federal Goverment (principally Medicare and Medicaid), usually pay on a 'cost' or 'cost-plus' basis because they say they are wholesale buyers of care. The remainder of the purchasers of hospital care pay at rates higher than the 'cost' or 'cost-plus' reimbursement formulas. Some of these higher charges are partially covered by commercial insurance policies which pay certain indemnities for specified services. Any balance beyond the stated indemnities should be charged directly to the patient." Many physicians are reluctant to bill patients for this balance resulting in a loss of revenue that could be as high as 20% of the total amount billed.

Medical Assistance is a program that helps the medically indigent obtain medical services in which the federal goverment and the state share the expense. Medical Assistance applications and claims are processed through State Health Departments. Bills for services rendered are usually sent directly to the state agency and the charges for Medical Assistance patients are cost-based and negotiated between the State Health Department and the provider. Med-

Table 74.2
Accounts Receivable—Internal Control Checklist[a]

1. Are all charges made in accordance with the rate schedule?
2. Is a ledger account established for each patient admitted, and is it checked against the admission register?
3. Are satisfactory procedures followed in service departments to ensure the prompt reporting of ALL services involving charges?
4. Are charges for services checked for accurary of:
   a. Period covered?
   b. Type of services?
   c. Rates used?
   d. Extensions?
5. Are control totals developed from the charge media and balanced against the accounts receivable posting?
6. If statistical data are maintained, are they correlated with recorded revenues?
7. Is a reconciliation of the total of the individual accounts in the accounts receivable ledgers with the general ledger control:
   a. Prepared periodically?
   b. Reviewed by a responsible person?
8. Are statements of all accounts receivable mailed regularly?
9. Are aging schedules:
   a. Prepared periodically?
   b. Reviewed and tested periodically by a responsible person?
10. Are the following functions handled independently:
    a. Posting?
    b. Credit?
    c. Development of control totals?
    d. Cash receipts?
    e. Allowance approval?
11. Do persons independent of accounts receivable personnel and credit department personnel confirm accounts by mail and by:
    a. Checking patients' statements with accounts?
    b. Keeping statements under control to assure mailing?
    c. Receiving reported differences directly?
    d. Investigating reported differences

[a] Partial listing adapted from the American Hospital Association: *Internal Control and Internal Auditing for Hospitals*. American Hospital Association, Chicago, 1960.

ical Assistance helps reduce the bad debts and costs which have also plagued the emergency department. By paying a portion of the hospital bills of the medically indigent through negotiated rates, the Medical Assistance program was designed to make some contribution toward financial solvency for institutions providing free care.

Generation of Accounts Receivable

When a patient enters the emergency department, hospital personnel initiate an emergency department record where all the appropriate patient information is recorded. The record should indicate one of the four types of medical coverage that the patient will utilize (Blue Cross/Blue Shield, self-pay, private insurance, Medical Assistance). It is very important at this stage of the process to ensure that all the required data are properly entered correctly onto the record form. Any missing information or incorrect information will cause frustrating and costly delays at a time later in the process. The physician examines and treats the patient and should then fill out a billing form (Fig. 74.2) by coding the services rendered. In many states, if the patient has

PEDIATRIC EMERGENCY CARE

DOCTOR CODE ____________

BLUE SHIELD ☐ SELF PAY ☐

INSURANCE ☐ M.A. ☐

DATE ____/____/____

CODE	VISITS	AMOUNT	CODE	SERVICE	AMOUNT
HVOA	visit, accident related			**SURGICAL**	
HVOE	visit, emergency medical		12000	sim repair 2.5, trunk, arms, legs, neck, sca.p,	
90570	visit, prolonged detention			genitalia	
90540	visit, clinic		12020	sim rep. 2.5, face, lip, muc. membrane	
	SERVICE		12100	sim rep. 2.5-6.3, trunk, arms, legs	
	CPR		12120	sim rep. 2.5-6.3 scalp, neck, hands, feet	
31500	endotracheal intubation		12140	sim rep. 2.5-6.3, face, lip, muc. membrane	
36425	venipuncture-cutdown		12220	sim rep. 6.3-12.7, scalp, neck, hands, feet	
96020	cardioversion, external		12240	sim rep. 6.3-12.7, face, lip, muc. membrane	
DEFIB	defibrillation, external		12300	sim rep. over 12.7	
36480	CVP catherization		12400	dogbite-puncture wound	
36620	arterial cath. (MA94700)		10100	paronychia	
	OBTAIN CULTURES		10060	incision drainage-abscess or hematoma	
63200	lumbar puncture		11730	avulation-nail (MA11730)	
10160	aspiration abscess		13900	suture removal	
20600	arthrocentesis, small joint		16015	burn treatment	
20605	arthrocentesis, med. joint		11042	debridement simple	
20610	artrocentesis, large joint		10120	foreign body-simple	
51000	suprapubic aspiration		10121	foreign body-complicated	
51730	catherization bladder		64450	peripheral nerve block	
69420	myringotomy				
	ENT				
30905	nasal packing				
30901	nasal cauterization			**LAB. PROCEDURES**	
69200	otoscopy-removal for. body		36600	arterial puncture	
			83800	blood gas interpretation	
	EYE		81000	urinalysis	
65205	foreign body-conjunctiva		93005	EKG-tracing only	
			85055	hematocrit (MA85011)	
	ORTHO		85650	sed rate	
23505	clavicular fracture		89120	occult blood feces	
25565	dislocation radial head				
26700	dislocation finger				
26720	phalanx, fracture			**MISC.**	
	ASP./LAVAGE		59410	vaginal delivery	
89130	gastric lavage		36510	umbilical vein cath.	
32000	thoracentesis		36660	umbilical art. cath.	
49080	peritinocentesis		36431	transfusion	
33040	pericardiocentesis				
61000	subdural tap				
57456	culdocentesis				

AGNOSIS/RDA CODE

Amount Paid $ ☐ Check ☐ Cash

Total Charges $

Figure 74.2 Billing checklist used to itemize emergency department charges.

Medical Assistance coverage, it is imperative to obtain the authorized person's signature as it is required in order to request payment of benefits for physician services rendered. A copy of the emergency department record and the physician's billing form are forwarded to the billing and collection office where the physician's services are properly coded (ICDA) and charged out. We use a computerized billing system.

The patients who lack third party coverage ("self-pay") are billed automatically by the service bureau's computerized billing on a cycle billing scheme. This minimizes the time delay in presenting a bill to the patient for services rendered by the physician. Three monthly bills are usually generated to the patient. The last two have messages printed on them encouraging the patient to promptly remit their payment (Fig. 74.3). As payments are received, they are credited to the proper account via the same procedure as the patient entry data inputs.

The patients with coverage by Blue Cross/Blue Shield are entered into the system properly coded and a Doctor's Service Report form is completed and sent for payment to the appropriate regional office. An appropriate bill similar to the self-pay bill is sent to the patient, detailing any payments applied against the incurred charges as well as any remaining balance to be paid. Patients with private insurance are entered into the system properly coded and a Health Insurance Claim Group or Individual Standard Form is generated and sent to the carrier for payment. An appropriate bill is sent to the patient detailing any payments applied against the incurred charges as well as any remaining balance to be paid.

If a claim is rejected, for example because of an incorrect Medical Assistance Number, a postcard is sent out to the patient request-

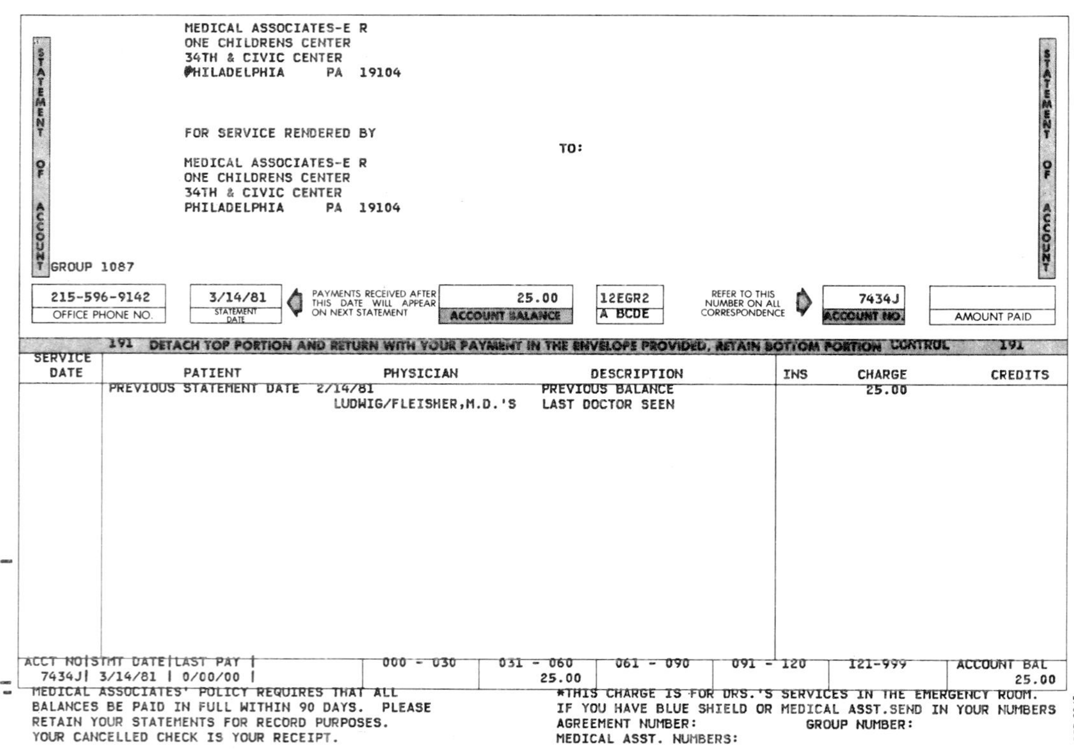

STATEMENT OF ACCOUNT

MEDICAL ASSOCIATES-E R
ONE CHILDRENS CENTER
34TH & CIVIC CENTER
PHILADELPHIA PA 19104

FOR SERVICE RENDERED BY

MEDICAL ASSOCIATES-E R
ONE CHILDRENS CENTER
34TH & CIVIC CENTER
PHILADELPHIA PA 19104

TO:

GROUP 1087

OFFICE PHONE NO.	STATEMENT DATE		ACCOUNT BALANCE			ACCOUNT NO.	AMOUNT PAID
215-596-9142	3/14/81	PAYMENTS RECEIVED AFTER THIS DATE WILL APPEAR ON NEXT STATEMENT	25.00	12EGR2 A BCDE	REFER TO THIS NUMBER ON ALL CORRESPONDENCE	7434J	

191 DETACH TOP PORTION AND RETURN WITH YOUR PAYMENT IN THE ENVELOPE PROVIDED, RETAIN BOTTOM PORTION CONTROL 191

SERVICE DATE	PATIENT	PHYSICIAN	DESCRIPTION	INS	CHARGE	CREDITS
	PREVIOUS STATEMENT DATE	2/14/81	PREVIOUS BALANCE		25.00	
		LUDWIG/FLEISHER,M.D.'S	LAST DOCTOR SEEN			

ACCT NO	STMT DATE	LAST PAY	000 - 030	031 - 060	061 - 090	091 - 120	121-999	ACCOUNT BAL
7434J	3/14/81	0/00/00		25.00				25.00

MEDICAL ASSOCIATES' POLICY REQUIRES THAT ALL BALANCES BE PAID IN FULL WITHIN 90 DAYS. PLEASE RETAIN YOUR STATEMENTS FOR RECORD PURPOSES. YOUR CANCELLED CHECK IS YOUR RECEIPT.

*THIS CHARGE IS FOR DRS.'S SERVICES IN THE EMERGENCY ROOM. IF YOU HAVE BLUE SHIELD OR MEDICAL ASST.SEND IN YOUR NUMBERS
AGREEMENT NUMBER: GROUP NUMBER:
MEDICAL ASST. NUMBERS:

OPR 8045

Figure 74.3 Typical patient bill.

Table 74.3
Service Bureau Summary Reports

Weekly
- Batch summary of payments, charges, adjustments
- Credit balance
- Zero balance
- Cycle billing recap
- Patient history eligibility
- Patient history exception
- Insurance claim register

Monthly
- Patient cross reference
- Accounts receivable
- Group procedure analysis
- Insurance company listing
- Physician coding listing
- Procedure adjustment register
- Physician procedure analysis
- Physician revenue allocation by physician, by patient
- Physician revenue allocation by total
- Year end statement recap (used for delinquent accounts)
- Statement selection audit report (microfiche only)

ing a correct number. If the claim is rejected for wrong information or coding errors, a new claim form is initiated correcting the errors and resubmitted. All pending claims are held and reviewed with each new payment received from the State Health Department, or the insurance company of the patient until a final disposition is made.

Uncollected Accounts

In the financial management of the emergency department, it is apparent that a considerable amount of physician care rendered and billed will not be recovered. It is necessary for the physicians to examine this issue and decide on how to set limits in this regard. The group must then define possible approaches to ensure that these limits will not be exceeded. Each year for a number of reasons a higher and higher percentage of billed physician services are uncollected. It has become a heavy burden for an emergency department group practice or a hospital to carry. Alternatives must be aggressively pursued in order to relieve this growing problem. Support for free medical care, for those who qualify, must become the burden of those in the geographical community being served. Industries, foundations and other community agencies must begin to be supportive. Hospitals must also actively solicit for this type of support, even though it may not be a traditional appeal for fund raising.

Monitoring Accounts Receivable

The computer service bureau issues a series of weekly and monthly reports analyzing the status of the accounts. Table 74.3 lists the reports available to help in the group's control of the financial management of the accounts receivable.

SUMMARY

Financial management is a decision-making process both for obtaining needed funds and for expending those funds in the most beneficial way. In the United States, changes in use of health care facilities have resulted in new styles of physician practice. The development of the emergency department group practice has been advantagous to both the hospitals and physicians.

Organization of an emergency department requires the formulation of a financial plan. A budget and a set of administrative policies are also key elements of the organization. The group must establish business systems to handle the volume and diversity of transactions. Microcomputers and software programs have added new dimensions to financial management.

The careful management of accounts receivable is the key to financial management. The length of the payment cycles and the policies established by third party payers are important influences on accounts receivable. The emergency department group practice must carefully analyze and control the generation of accounts receivable in order to maximize assets and minimize uncollected accounts.

In the future, changes in the patterns of health care, the available business, technology, and the economy will all influence the financial management of the emergency department.

References

Berman HT, Weeks LE: *The Financial Management of Hospitals*, Ed. 3. Health Administration Press, Ann Arbor, 1976.

Emergency Services—The Hospital Emergency Department in an Emergency Care System, Ch. 7, p. 6. American Hospital Association, 840 N. Lake Shore Dr., Chicago, IL 60611, copyright 1972.

Group Practice Guidelines to Forming or Joining a Medical Group, Section 3, p. 14. Published by Center for Research in Ambulatory Health Administration, prepared by representatives from: American Group Practice Association, AMA and the Medical Group Management Association, 1978.

The Physician's Office, Excerpta Medica, Nassau Bldg., 288 Alesander St., Princeton, NJ 08540, 1977.

Wasserman FW, Miller MC: *Building a group practice.* Charles C Thomas, Springfield, Ill., 1975.

CHAPTER **75**

Record Keeping and Information Systems

JANE B. KUNIEWICZ, B.S.N.

INTRODUCTION

Data systems (computerization), health care marketing (industrialization), standards for reimbursement (regulation), and the malpractice crisis (litigation) have been the key elements responsible for elevating the hospital medical record to its current state of notoriety. The resulting scrutiny of records is responsible for converting record keeping content and maintenance guidelines from a chore to a challenge. The purpose of this chapter is to review the elements of good record keeping and to apply them to a pediatric emergency system.

Medical records are communication systems. The essential role of any medical communication system is to accurately record pertinent and significant observable signs, symptoms and behaviors of the patient and to document the treatment given by the health care staff. A variety of health information systems exist, ranging from simple traditional systems to ones with rather complex capabilities. There are manual, mechanical and computerized systems that record and document patient findings. The tool most commonly used in hospitals is the familiar hospital chart, a document housing a complete compilation of medical observations on an individual from the time of his first admission to the events surrounding his last discharge.

With the advent of the industrialization of health care, the chart has come under the purview not only of the health care staff who create it, but other professionals who gain access to the document through multiple health related activities. Among the 6 million professionals and allied health care personnel in the United States who use patient charts are: researchers, reviewers of risk, quality of care and utilization, and auditors. These persons are usually internal to the organization. There are a number of non-health care professionals for whom the patient's chart provides information. Among these are commercial representatives, state and federal regulators, foundations and grant reviewers, and health insurance agents. In litigation, both defense and plantiff's attorneys depend on the accuracy of the record. Each such reviewer attempts to determine the quality of care when requesting information from and about the chart.

Proponents of good patient care argue that a corollary exists between care rendered and its documentation. The adage "good record keeping equals good patient care" is an ideal which may be obtainable. The physician who wonders if the level of care in his emergency department matches this goal might benefit from establishing minimal charting criteria and subsequently surveying records. In departments where the staff is technically competent and academically proficient, one would hope to routinely find records which are thorough and complete.

Emergency department record keeping is particularly difficult because of the rapidity with which events happen. The staff needs to be constantly reminded of their responsibility with respect to charting. It is difficult to record a quickly moving sequence of events. Within seconds, multiple patient problems can develop and be treated. An immediate notation alleviates later doubt and uncertainty about the chain of events. Many members of the team compete for access to the chart. A systematic plan for use and flow of the chart needs to be an integral part of the planning process in each emergency department. Quite often, in adult situations, the family waits outside the emergency department until the crisis is over. However, in a pediatric environment, it is not uncommon for parents to witness the care given their child. It is not surprising that the parent or witness may remember the sequence of treatment more readily than the physician who may have treated many children with similar problems. Thus, the volume of patients treated, the immediacy of the situation, the relationship of the parent to the physician, and the necessity to accurately record facts, make important immediate, sequential charting of all relevant information. The pediatric emergency department record is an indication of the quality of patient care. This chapter will discuss the general aspects of charting and emphasize aspects unique to pediatric emergency care.

ELEMENTS OF THE MEDICAL RECORD

Because the chart serves so many purposes, guidelines for documentation have been developed and prevail for charting in a pediatric emergency department and in an adult health care facility.

Guidelines

In over 7,000 hospitals in the United States, charting protocol includes the following generally accepted rules: (1) the patient's name must appear on every record page; (2) entries must be timed and dated using the 24-hour clock; (3) all entries should be signed, including the professional title (e.g. M.D., R.N., E.M.T., etc.); (4) entries must be typed or written in ink; and (5) entries should be objective, specific, comprehensive, and reflective of the recorder's evaluation. The record format is flexible. Methods such as SOAP (subjective, objective, assessment, plan), however, guide the recorder into a routine which guarantees consistency. Emphasis on the particulars of charting removes doubt about providers' intentions and proves to be a worthwhile exercise in the face of litigation.

Common Errors

Careless record keeping includes such commonly found errors as: (1) illegible writing; (2) use of unacceptable abbreviations; (3) obliterating inaccuracies with felt-tip markers or "white-out"; (4) skipping dates, times, and lines on a record; and (5) absence of countersignatures when indicated.

Corrections

Corrections in a record may be made according to a standard procedure: (1) draw a single line through the error, (2) date and initial the error, (3) enter corrections in chronological order, (4) indicate which entry correction is replacing which error, and (5) in a questionable situation, have the corrected notation witnessed by a colleague. To minimize the need for corrections, some hospitals provide an emergency department transcription service.

REGULATION OF RECORDS

Specifications on the content of patient's records are clearly delineated by medical staff, quality assurance committees, regulatory associations, and state and federal laws. If all these sources were consulted, over 120 screening criteria could be identified. Using even the most rigorous compliance with regulations and resolute determination, one may still appear deficient in creating the perfect record. Donabedian has commented that, "as standards of care are raised, perfection seems to become even more difficult to achieve."

Medical Staff

Within each hospital, the Executive Committee of the Medical Staff exercises the ultimate authority over who may make entries in a chart. Permission for staff and selected health care workers (e.g., student nurses, visiting practitioners, or teaching personnel) to write in the chart must be approved by the Executive Committee. In most hospitals, a Medical Records Committee serves as a standing committee of the Medical Staff. The Medical Records Committee approves chart forms and determines which forms should be retained as a part of the permanent record. The emergency department Director must monitor the permanency, precision, clarity, and content with which specific patient information is documented within the Department.

Quality Review Committee

The purpose of such committees is to monitor the care being given in a hospital and to recognize and correct deficiencies. Unfortunately the formulation of such a committee can build a false sense of security in practitioners who then take a "wait and see" attitude rather than correcting deficiencies on their own. Others think of audit as quality assurance and presume that the committee's existence serves as a standardbearer of excellence. Whatever the attitudes about quality review might be, the greatest hurdle in accomplishing a satisfactory review is the choice of an appropriate model to use in assessing a problem or issue. Educators and managers illustrate how difficult it is to accurately measure levels of care, because their assessment tools are either influenced by unexamined variables or by abstractors who rely on individual judgment to determine intended results (e.g. the questionable diagnosis). In his writings about variables, Donabedian says, "Each study of quality can be categorized in so many ways and the clusterings of attributes are so indistinct that it has been impossible to devise a satisfactory simple classification." Donabedian has developed a useful classification system of "criteria-mapping" which employs factors developed to avoid pitfalls of quality assurance programs "by linking strategies with careful clinical trials which will prove the bedrock of quality assessment, upon which all clinical medicine must ultimately rest." An example of the difficulties in abstracting medical records is documented in an Emergency Medical Services (EMS) study undertaken by Herrman to develop an index of injury/illness severity which would effectively summarize a patient's condition. The conclusion of the study states, "a more structured format would improve the quality of abstracted data."

Another report by Jhaveri further illustrates that there may be extraneous circumstances unrelated to audit format or abstractor's dilemmas that influence the error rate in a pediatric emergency department: (1) the change of interns brings about an increase in frequency of errors at the beginning of the academic year (July-October) and at the beginning of each month and (2) significantly more errors were found at the first year level than the second, emphasizing the need for attending level supervision for interns.

Association Regulations

Uniform compliance in establishing goals of safe, efficient patient care has been the objective of regulatory associations particularly, the Joint Commission on Hospital Accreditation (JCHA). Founded 65 years ago, the Commission has elicited the voluntary cooperation of hospitals in the United States who are interested in authenticating the quality and achieving acceptable standards and levels of care. The rapid growth of the health care industry and in particular the nearly explosive rate at which emergency departments are being used, warrants the type of guardianship offered by a surveyor. Emergency visits have increased at a faster rate than either hospital inpatient admissions or outpatient visits. Between 1962 and 1976 the number of patient visits to the emergency departments in the United States increased by 57 million, almost quadrupling. Under the pressures of this rapid growth, the fundamentals of care can become obscured. JCAH brings practitioners back to basics when it suggests the integration of at least

11 points around which a well executed emergency medical record can be developed.

1. Patient identification. When not available, the reason shall be entered into the records
2. Time and means of arrival
3. Pertinent history of the illness or injury and physical findings including the patient's vital signs
4. Emergency care given to the patient prior to arrival
5. Diagnostic and therapeutic orders
6. Clinical observations, including results of treatment
7. Reports of procedures, tests, and results
8. Diagnostic impression
9. Conclusion at the termination of evaluation/treatment, including a final disposition, the patient's condition on discharge or transfer, and any instructions given to the patient and/or family for follow-up care
10. Documentation of a patient's leaving against medical advice
11. The signature of the responsible practitioner.

State/Municipal Laws

Surveillance continues beyond the confines of the emergency department and the hospital. A separate hierarchy of officials on a local, state, and national level both control and assess standards of care. Two major areas of involvement are (1) regulations on the retention of records and (2) requirements to be informed of "reportable" diagnoses.

Record retention is a matter that might easily be overlooked by emergency department directors and staff. Compounding the problem is a lack of uniformity in the retention period assigned to the various elements of patient charts, summaries, and control registers. Pennsylvania provides a good example for the lack of uniformity. For example an instrument log book documenting safety testing of patient care equipment (which might be used in the emergency department) must be retained for the life of the equipment, while the emergency department patient log must be retained for only 3 years. The regulations for both the emergency department log and instrument care log are promulgated by the State Department of Health.

State and municipal reporting requirements for reportable diagnoses vary. Generally, reports include diagnoses such as sexual abuse, child abuse and neglect, gunshot and stab wounds, animal bites, communicable disease, and patients dead on arrival to the hospital. The reporting requirements include a wide range of communicable diseases. It is not sufficient to refer a patient for treatment. A copy of the referral must be attached to the chart or a notation made, stating to whom the reportable diagnosis was made. Weapon injuries are usually reported to the local police. A report is made to the coroner or medical examiner's officer in the event of a death in the emergency department. Venereal disease is reported to the local and then the state health department.

ADJUNCTS TO THE MEDICAL RECORD

The medical record may assume new dimensions by the addition of adjuncts. Adjunctive records can document special diagnostic and treatment circumstances. In the fast moving environment of the emergency department these addenda can record events which might otherwise be lost. If adjunctive documents are designed to save time, they can help the emergency department staff overcome the main deterrent to good record keeping. Several examples of medical record adjuncts are cited.

Pre-Hospital Care Records

In the pediatric emergency situation, the emergency medical technician (E.M.T.) or paramedic is often the first health care worker to meet the patient. The pre-hospital care record should include the patient's name, condition in which he was found, vital signs and a description of the services performed by the E.M.T., such as CPR, application of antishock trousers, and drug therapy. The time of the incident or injury as well as the time or arrival at the hospital can be significant predictors of the patient's outcome, and thus, important to the emergency department and physician. A signed copy of the E.M.T. record should be presented to the emergency department, and this should be retained as part of the hospital medical record.

Triage Forms

Triage systems are designed to make a brief but accurate determination about the immediacy of the problem and level of care required for the patient. Since the inception of the triage concept in 1963 at Yale New Haven Hospital, the sorting process has passed through many developmental stages. Although initially triage officers were physicians, now emergency medical technicians and emergency department nurses perform this important function.

Initial assessments and treatments made in triage should become a part of the medical record. Figure 75.1 shows the form used at the Children's Hospital of Philadelphia for this purpose. Since studies show that from 55 to 75% of the pediatric emergency department population does not require life-saving immediate emergency services, triage is now accepted as the preferred method of initial assessment.

Scoring and Screening Indices

Scoring and screening indices are used in an attempt to make patient assessment more objective and quantitative. They may be used in the triage process or to monitor the patient's progress through diagnosis and treatment. Examples of scoring indices include the Nelson severity index, the Children's Hospital of Philadelphia clinical asthma score, and the Glasgow coma score.

Nelson's "severity index" (Table 75.1) provides a tool for assessing the severity of illness. The author specifically suggests its use for triage of patients in pediatric emergency departments. It is a superb tool for the triage "novice," in that it predicts severity with a high incidence of reliability. Compared with a complete physician assessment, the "severity index" score had a 94.7% sensitivity for mild or moderate illness. Compared with the final diagnosis, the index had a predictive accuracy of 98.7% for diagnosing nonsevere illness. In predicting major illness the index had a prediction accuracy of 84.2%.

The clinical asthma score is a system for estimating the severity of an asthma attack and for predicting the risk of respiratory failure (Fig. 75.2) and has been in use at the Children's Hospital for several years. Developed by Wood and Downes, the score attempts to evaluate oxygenation, gas exchange, work of breathing, airway obstruction and cerebral function as affected by fatigue, hypoxia or carbon dioxide narcosis. This score was developed because clinical criteria of respiratory failure are sometimes difficult to analyze, interpret, and communicate to others. Our experience has shown that scoring compatibility is more easily achieved when one staff member assumes responsibility for the scoring process on an individual patient.

The Glasgow coma scale (GCS)(Table 75.2) is an assessment tool to describe level of consciousness. This scale was developed in 1974 at the University of Glasgow to standardize observations of levels of consciousness, particularly in patients with head injury. Familiarity with the scale facilitates rapid communication about a patient among staff members. The GCS is valuable in monitoring a patient as coma progresses or lightens or as a patient moves from one treatment area to another, for example, emergency department to radiology department to intensive care unit.

Algorithms

Some emergency departments prefer using algorithms as adjuncts to the medical record. Slay and Riskin's emergency department algorithms are used with a 96% accuracy rate. The concept can be appropriately applied to a pediatric emergency problem to make diagnosis and/or treatment uniform. Appropriate algorithms for a variety of signs and symptoms are presented in Chapters 5 through 42.

Checklists

Checklists are chart adjuncts which help the staff accomplish difficult multistep procedures. Two examples of checklists used in pediatrics are presented: (1) the sexual abuse checklist and (2) the death protocol. Both of these problems require that the

THE CHILDREN'S HOSPITAL OF PHILADELPHIA

EMERGENCY DEPARTMENT

TRIAGE INFORMATION

ROOM ASSIGNMENT

CHART #: ______

NAME: ______ AGE: ______ DATE: ______ TIME: ______ a.m. p.m.

CHIEF COMPLAINT: ______

______

ALLERGIES: Yes ☐ No ☐ LIST: ______

ASSESSMENT:

Temp. : ______ ______

Pulse : ______ ______

Resp. : ______ ______

B.P. : ______ ______

PROCEDURES IN TRIAGE: ______

______

______

SPECIAL REQUEST FOR M.D.: ______

TRIAGED TO: Circle one Acute E.R. E.R.

SOURCE OF REFERRAL and/or SOURCE OF ROUTINE HEALTH CARE:

NAME: ______

ADDRESS: ______

SIGNATURE (M.D., R.N., CCT, SNA): ______

2/4/81
#CH110

Figure 75.1 Triage information form.

physician pay attention to medical, social and legal concerns. The checklist allows the staff to work with the patient and family free of other concerns and ensures compliance with all procedural requirements.

The record for sexual assault (Fig. 75.3) was developed by the "Code R" team (a multidisciplinary team summoned to manage alleged sexual assault). It is intended to assist the emergency department in unrav-

Table 75.1
Scoring System for Severity Index[a]

Variable	Point Value		
	0	1	2
Respiratory effort	Labored or absent	Some distress	No distress
Color	Cyanotic	Pale, flushed, mottled	Normal
Activity	Delirium, stupor, coma	Lethargy	Normal
Temperature	<97.4 or >104°F (<36 or >40°C)	101.1–104°F (38–40°C)	97.4–101°F (36–38°C)
Play	Refuses to play	Decreased	Normal

[a] From K. G. Nelson: *American Journal of Public Health*, *70:* 804–807, 1980.

eling events surrounding an assault, with rapidity and sensitivity. The form serves as a reminder to the physician to record important and relevant facts. Sexual assault and incest complaints for children 12 years of age and under are treated in the Children's Hospital of Philadelphia Emergency Department. A more detailed discussion is covered in Chapter 68.

The death protocol checklist (Table 75.3) also reminds the staff of all the important things to do when a child dies in the emergency department. Knowing that all these details have been worked out in advance allows the staff to support the grieving family. The management of death and catastrophic illness is discussed in Chapter 69.

Special Purpose Records

A cardiopulmonary arrest record is an example of a special purpose record. The use of this adjunct form eliminates recopying records which the staff make during an emergency because: (1) the chart has not been "made up" or (2) the chart is being used by another member of the team. In a pediatric emergency department some critical factors to be included in this document are: (1) the age and weight of the child, (2) the rate and total volume of infused fluids, and (3) medication dosages. Recording the actions of the resuscitation team is equivalent to being at the finish line when each race is run simultaneously and all the horses are winners. Multiple events should happen at about the same time (depending on the expertise of the team) and all require documentation.

MECHANIZED INFORMATION SYSTEMS

Electronic Clipboard

Ornato and colleagues developed a mechanized system for accurately recording events during a cardiac arrest. The electronic clipboard device sends a timing signal into the electromagnetic tape recorder so that events recorded on the translucent flow sheet can be correlated with sections of the tape recording the ECG. In such a way, the entire cardiac arrest, including ECG can be reconstructed retrospectively. Comparing 18 patients whose CPR was recorded electronically with 18 patients whose records were conventionally recorded, Ornato reported "superiority of the newer technique with more total events recorded." Advantages of using the flow sheet are: (1) its usefulness in reconstructing events for scientific analysis, (2) legal documentation, and (3) education. The most outstanding feature of the clipboard is its ability to concomitantly record the ECG.

The Telescriber

The Telautograph (Telautograph Corp., Los Angeles) (Fig. 75.4) is a mechanized transcription device available for commercial use. It is valued in the emergency department because of the expediency it affords physicians and nurses in obtaining laboratory results. Instead of phoning "stat" clinical laboratory reports to the emergency department, the Telautograph provides a minitranscription service. At the

STAMP

THE CHILDREN'S HOSPITAL OF PHILADELPHIA

CLINICAL ASTHMA SCORE

DATE ____________

	0	1	2
PaO_2 mmHg	70-100 in air	70 in air	70 in 40% O_2
Cyanosis	None	in air	in 40% O_2
Inspiratory Breath Sounds	Normal	Unequal	Decreased to absent
Accessory Muscles	None	Moderate	Maximal
Expiratory Wheezing	None	Moderate	Marked
Cerebral Function	Normal	Depressed or agitated	Coma

(1) A score of 5 or more indicates impending respiratory failure - obtain blood-gases, notify anesthesia.
(2) A score of 6 may require transfer to I.C.U.
(3) A score of 7 or more with a $PaCO_2$ of 65 mmHg indicates existing respiratory failure.

Time	PaO_2	Inspiratory Sounds	Accessory Muscles	Expiratory Wheezing	Cerebral Function	Total Score	Blood Gases	Vital signs, Comments & Medications

Figure 75.2 Clinical asthma scoring record. (From D. W. Wood, J. J. Downes, and H. Lecks: *American Journal of Diseases of Children, 123:* 227, 1972.)

Children's Hospital of Philadelphia, urinalysis and hematology and chemistry reports are transcribed via the system. Other information on the report includes patient's name, hospital number, location, date, and time and signature of the technican recording the results. The machine beeps to alert personnel of an impending report. The physician frequently transcribes the values to the emergency department record, but the telescribed report may be approved for inclusion in the chart. Devices such as the Telautograph help significantly in the absence of a full service, on-line computer.

Table 75.2
Glasgow Coma Scale[a]

Eyes	Open	Spontaneously	4
		To verbal command	3
		To pain	2
	No response		1
Best motor response	To verbal command	Obeys	6
	To painful stimulus[b]	Localizes pain	5
		Flexion-withdrawal	4
		Flexion-abnormal (decorticate rigidity)	3
		Extension (decerebrate rigidity)	2
		No response	1
Best verbal response[c]		Oriented and converses	5
		Disoriented and converses	4
		Inappropriate words	3
		Incomprehensible sounds	2
		No response	1
Total			3–15

[a] The Glasgow coma scale, based upon eye opening, verbal, and motor responses, is a practical means of monitoring changes in level of consciousness. If response on the scale is given a number, the responsiveness of the patient can be expressed by summation of the figures. Lowest score is 3; highest is 15.
[b] Apply knuckles to sternum; observe arms.
[c] Arouse patient with painful stimulus if necessary.

COMPUTERIZED INFORMATION SYSTEMS

In *The Administrators Guide to Evaluating Records and the Medical Records Department*, Fox states:

> If it takes the medical record clerk or the medical record administrator more than five minutes to retrieve each chart, the effectiveness of the system and the person using the system should both be queried.

If such effectiveness existed in all medical records departments, one would have little need for integrating hospital information systems. Efficient data retrieval, however, continues to be a persistent problem, particularly in the delivery of pediatric emergency health care, since children cannot provide a reliable past medical history, especially if unaccompanied by a parent.

The frustration associated with securing known patient information can be partially averted through the use of a computer. Selection of an unsuitable patient information system, however, can introduce considerable anxiety. The key to a successful computerized operation lies in the system design, which is the critical factor in determining the success or failure of a conversion. In every situation, it is necessary to adapt program features to departmental needs. To do this, it is important to know well in advance of the system selection

The Children's Hospital of Philadelphia

PHYSICIAN'S SEXUAL ASSAULT CHECKLIST

Patient's Name ______________________ (last) (first)

Birthday ______________________

Current Telephone ______________________

Brought in by ______________________

Date, Time of Assault ______________________

CHOP Social Worker ______________________

Police Officer ______________________

CY47 filed? ______________________

History of Assault

____

COMPLETE THIS SECTION:

During assault, did any of these occur? coitus sodomy cunnilingus fellatio hand-genital contact

Did assailant ejaculate? ____________ Did patient lose consciousness? ____________

Since the assault, has patient eaten or rinsed mouth? ____________
bathed? ____________
douched? ____________
urinated or defecated? ____________

Patient's age at menarche ____________ LMP ____________ Cycle length ____________

Contraception? ____________ Method used ____________

Past Medical History ______________________

Other Problems ______________________

A

Physician's Signature ______________________ Date ____________

Figure 75.3 (*A–C*) Sexual assault checklist. (Courtesy of D. J. Paradise.)

exactly what it is the department hopes to accomplish by installing an automated system.

First, an investigative team should be assembled to examine: (1) *within the institution*: how the emergency department runs (i.e., functional components responsible for tying together the pieces in the delivery of pediatric emergency care) and (2) *within the data processing field*: the advantages, disadvantages, cost and capabilities of computer systems on the market.

Patient's Name________________________ Page 2

PHYSICAL EXAMINATION Temp______ P______ RR______ BP______ Wt______

General (include emotional state, condition of clothing)

Body Surface (include history of how bruises, lacerations, etc., occurred)

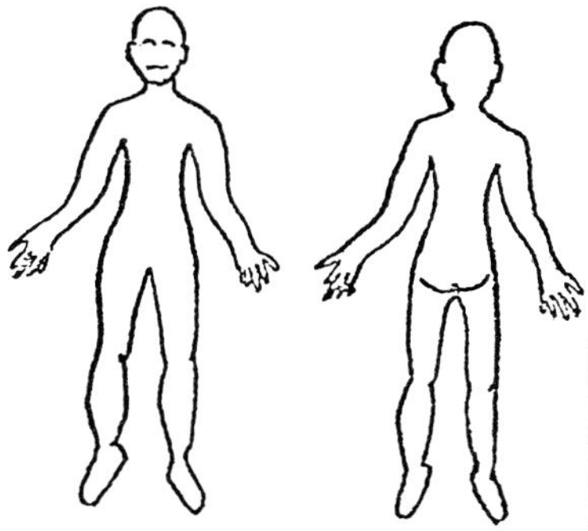

PE:	NORMAL	AB-NORMAL
(1) General		
(2) Head		
(3) Ears		
(4) Eyes		
(5) Nose		
(6) Throat		
(7) Neck		
(8) Chest		
(9) Heart		
(10) Abdomen		
(11) Genitalia		
(12) Extremities		
(13) Skin		
(14) Neuro		
(15) Psych		

Genital or Pelvic Examination

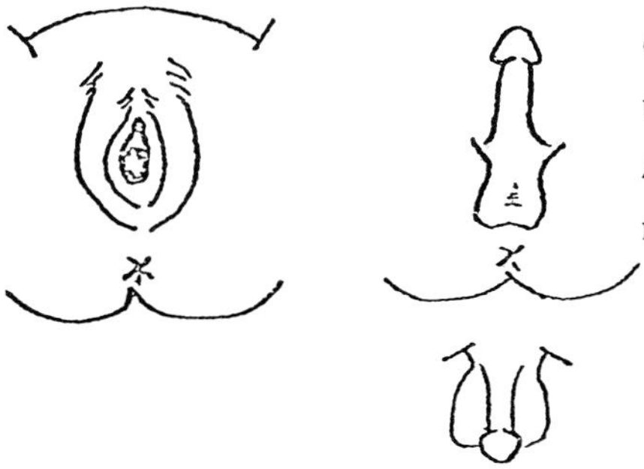

Vagina______________

Cervix______________

Uterus______________

Adnexa______________

Rectal______________

B

Physician's Signature________________________ Date__________

Fig. 75.3*B*

Investigative Team

Intrinsic to the effectiveness, popularity and ultimate utilization of a computerized system is the core of medical/management personnel who share a commitment to the idea of electronicization. The group should, ideally, be composed of the hospital's Chief Executive Officer, the Pediatric Emergency Department Director, Department Administrator, and the Data Processing Coordinator. It is inadvisable to proceed with the

Patient's Name________________________ Page 3

LABORATORY (check if done)

☐ Throat culture (GC)	☐ Pap smear	Other:
☐ Vaginal/cervical culture (GC)	☐ Urine pregnancy test	________
☐ Urethral culture (GC)	☐ Serum pregnancy test	________
☐ Rectal culture (GC)	☐ Urinalysis	________
☐ RPR	☐ Stool hematest	________

EVIDENTIARY MATERIAL (check if obtained)

Air-dried slides for sperm and acid phosphatase from:

☐ labia
☐ vagina/cervix
☐ rectum

Moist swab in 0.5 cc saline from:

☐ labia
☐ vagina/cervix
☐ rectum

☐ clothing (list)________________
☐ pubic hair and standards

Specimens given to:
____
Date, time________________

IMPRESSION:

THERAPY:

GC prophylaxis? DES? Anti-emetic?

FOLLOW-UP:

Pediatrics:

Social Work:

Gynecology:

Other:

C

Physician's Signature________________________Date__________

Fig. 75.3*C*

intent to convert from a manual system without a unified team whose intention it is to collaborate on the issues described. The value of forming such a group manifests itself (1) in the unity it represents to practitioners whose divergent needs tend to obscure the purpose of the change, (2) in its capacity to represent the clinical and managerial needs to the outside (sales and marketing representatives), and (3) in its ability to assess whether the application of a "total package" is both practical and efficient for use in a short-term pediatric critical care setting.

Table 75.3
Emergency Room Checklist for Sudden Death of Dead on Arrival (DOA)

1. Essential family members in the emergency room
2. Baptism performed or clergy requested, if indicated
3. Family provided private area to express grief; individual needs responded to by staff
4. Family permitted to "view" the child's body
5. Autopsy required explained to the family
6. Family is given information from whom to obtain the results of the autopsy
7. Social service contacted or consultation form completed and placed in social service folder
8. Emergency room chart completed
9. Forms completed for DOA or death in emergency room:
   a. Certificate of Death—two copies
   b. Medical Examiner's Notice and Pronouncement of Death—one copy
   c. Death Record—one copy
10. Completed emergency room chart and completed forms (9a, b, c) sent to hospital's pathology department or Medical Examiner's office with body
11. The Medical Examiner's office or hospital's pathology department notified
12. Private physician notified

Although its original designation is that of a "search committee," the investigative team should remain intact beyond the signing of any contractual agreement. Members must be encouraged to serve on a standing committee whose charge is to monitor long-range goals and eventually develop plans for expanded or revised system capabilities. Also, of practical importance is the team's ability to sustain a viable communication network among members of the committee and among prospective users of the system.

System Priorities

Once departmental information needs have been established, the investigative team should consider the advantages and disadvantages of each computer company's offer and the hospital's own financial resources. The advantages and disadvantages of the system designed for the Children's Hospital of Philadelphia Emergency Department will be discussed in some detail to help clarify this issue.

Advantages

The Emergency Department of the Children's Hospital of Philadelphia derives many benefits from its computerized outpatient system. The system design is appropriate, fast and manageable. The available information serves as a reliable reference point. It is responsible for forms production, daily statistics and demand bills. The system provides an audit trail from the point of registration to generation of the final bill.

Registration

The prospective patient enters the hospital and immediately approaches "triage," where a determination of the level of care required for the child's illness is made. The patient/parent takes a handwritten assessment of the patient's condition to the registrar. The registrar "pulls-up" the unit number on an "old" patient or the system designates a "new" number assignment for a "new" patient. The registrar then verifies information in the system and/or enters new demographic information. Payment for the visit is made or arranged between client and cashier. The chart then arrives from medical records, the request having been generated by the registration process.

The actual registration process should take less than a minute. Completion of the registration by securing consent signatures adds to the sign-in time. Having access to stored data makes the registration process less tedious to an already stressed parent or guardian. The system often supplies needed patient information on the child brought in by the police or a neighbor.

Other Applications

While waiting for the chart, the physician may obtain access to a *brief patient history*

THE CHILDREN'S HOSPITAL OF PHILADELPHIA

CLINICAL LABORATORIES

EMERGENCY REPORT FORM

PATIENT'S NAME			HOSPITAL NUMBER
LOCATION ER PICA IICU		DATE	TIME AM PM
GLUCOSE mg/dl	BUN mg/dl	CALCIUM mg/dl	CREATININE mg/dl
CHLORIDE meq/L	SODIUM meq/L	POTASSIUM meq/L	CO2 meq/L
BILIRUBIN (SPECTRO) mg/dl	BILIRUBIN (TOTAL) mg/dl	CSF GLUCOSE mg/dl	CSF PROTEIN mg/dl

CHEMISTRY

HBG	HCT	RBC	WBC
McV	McH	McHc	SEGS
BANDS	LYMPHS	ATYPICAL LYMPH	MONO
EOS	BASO	RBC RESULTS·	

HEMATOLOGY

1801

PLATELETS	FIBRINOGEN	PT SEC	CONTROL SEC	PTT SEC	NORMAL RANGE SEC

URINALYSIS		CSF CELL COUNT	CSF SMEAR
SPGR	PH	SEGS (CSF)	MONO (CSF)
SUGAR	CLINITEST	MICROSCOPIC	
PROTEIN	KETONES		
OCCULT BLOOD	BILIRUBIN	SIGNED	

URINALYSIS

MICROBIOLOGY

010
REV 1

315462

ENCIRCLED VALUES INDICATES ABNORMAL RESULT

Figure 75.4 Telautograph laboratory report form.

from the "update-file" of the computer. Such information as the date of the last Children's Hospital visit and final ICDA-9 diagnosis are available. A specific number of chronic conditions are stored in the system (e.g., glucose 6-phosphate dehydrogenase deficiency, diabetes, sickle cell anemia, hemophilia and allergies) as well as the immunization update on each child.

Should the physician want information about *bed availability* for a patient's possible admission, the computer can indicate the type and location of the vacancy. The system *requests charts* by a correct, verifiable unit number, making the margin of error in record retrieval minimal. When ancillary studies are ordered and/or chargeable items used, the appropriate billing is made through the computer.

Disposition

At the time of the patient's final disposition, a diagnosis is entered in the system by the emergency department clerk/registrar. If the patient is admitted, the admission process automatically transfers the emergency department bill to the inpatient invoice. The admission can be completed in the emergency department or in the Admitting Office.

Scheduling

A valuable feature of the system at the Children's Hospital of Philadelphia is the capability the system has to *schedule a follow-up appointment* for the patient. Initial appointments can also be made to specialty clinics by the registrars with the approval of the attending physician.

Disadvantages

Period of Adjustment

The transition from a manual to a computerized system requires a period of adjustment by the professional and clerical staff. Literally, months of conditioning must precede the actual conversion. The "hands-on" orientation to the system should closely parallel its installation and run until the system is on-line. Some employees cannot make the final adjustment to the system, and no amount of endurance on the part of the supervisor and/or employee will facilitate acceptance. The usual period of discomfort with the keyboard and CRT ranges from 3 weeks to 3 months. Many newcomers to the idea of computerization inherently anticipate failure, either for the system or for themselves. By the end of 3 months, however, staff confidence is at an acceptable level, at least until the system actually does "fail" for the first time.

Dependence

After 6 months, the staff becomes dependent on the computer. The manual system, which the staff tenaciously guarded and reluctantly discarded at the time of conversion, is the cause of much dread and aggravation when reimplemented. The realization that an inordinate amount of waiting accompanied the "old-way" finally dawns on the registrars and the staff, who then become forever wedded to technology. Living through this process, however, is decidedly a disadvantage.

Downtime/Manual Backup

The computer may not be available for several hours each day. Usually the downtime is scheduled after midnight, and the night shift must revert to the use of a manual plan. Problems may also occur when the system is down during the day for maintenance. It is important to anticipate a "failure" and have a backup manual system sufficiently developed so that chaos does not ensue.

Surveillance

Computer printouts require close scrutiny on a daily basis to counter errors which may be unconsciously but consistently made. When registering, scheduling or entering a diagnosis, a clerk may make a mistake. Because much of the computer information is coded, daily review of computer reports is needed.

Cost

The price of a system corresponds directly to the features suggested by the company. Often there is a fixed price for installation which may not include such items as hardware (CRT), physical plant reconstruction, cable outlets, etc. In addition, a monthly service charge, by department, must be considered. Pin-fed forms are expensive; depending on the emergency department census—$8,000 to $10,000 can be spent annually.

SUMMARY

Medical records are communication systems. The test of any system, basic or computerized, is whether or not it packages and distributes accurate information in an efficient way. In providing pediatric emergency care, the emergency department staff must relate to both the patient and the patient's family. The patient may be pre-verbal or unable to fully articulate his medical condition. The family is often distressed by the child's illness. As with most emergency department encounters, a pre-existing relationship with the staff does not exist. Thus, the importance and complexity of the medical record are increased. Not only will good patient care be reflected in complete medical records but meticulous record keeping will lead to improved care.

References

Accreditation Manual for Hospitals, 1981, Emergency Services, Standard VII, p. 33.

Barnell GA, Zielstroff RD: Data systems can enhance or hinder medical nursing activities. *Hospitals* 51: October 1977.

Donabedian A: The quality of medical care. *Science* 200: 856–863, 1978.

Fox L, Stearns G, Imbiorski W: *The Administrators Guide to Evaluating Records and Medical Record Department.* Cave Communications, Inc., Chicago, 1979.

Gluck J: Computerized medical record system, meeting a challenge for nursing. *J Nurs Adm* 9: 17–24 (Dec.), 1979.

Halperin R, et al.: Utilization of pediatric emergency room services, a critical review. *Pediatr Clin North Am* 4: 747–757, 1979.

Health Resource Statistics: U.S. Department of Health, Education and Welfare, Public Health Service, Office of Health Research, Statistics and Technology, p. 400. National Center for Health Statistics, Hyattsville, Md., Ed. 1976–77.

Herrman N, et al.: Interobserver and intraobserver reliability in the collection of emergency medical services data. *Health Serv Res* 15: Summer 1980.

Jhaveri RC, et al.: Analysis of medical records in a pediatric emergency room. *J Natl Med Assoc* 71: 569–71, 1979.

Jones C: Glasgow coma scale. *Am J Nurs* 79: 1551–1553, 1979.

Nelson KG: An index of severity for acute pediatric illness. *Am J Public Health* 70: 804–807, 1980.

Ornato JP, et al.: The electronic clipboard; an automated system for accurately recording events during a cardiac arrest. *Ann Emerg Med* 10: 27–30 (Mar.) 1981.

Slay LE, Riskin WG: Algorithm—directed triage in an emergency room. *JACEP* 5: 869–876, 1976.

Wood DW, et al.: A clinical scoring system for the diagnosis of respiratory failure. *Am J Dis Child* 123: 227–228, 1972.

CHAPTER 76

Child-oriented Emergency Department Design

ARON GOLDMAN, M.ARCH., M.D.

No matter how well architects and planners plan, or how carefully they design, they cannot by themselves create environments that have the variety and order we are after. An organic mixture can only be made by the action of a community, in which everyone helps to shape the parts of the environment that he knows best ... Participation is inherently good; it brings people together and involves them in their world; it creates feeling between people

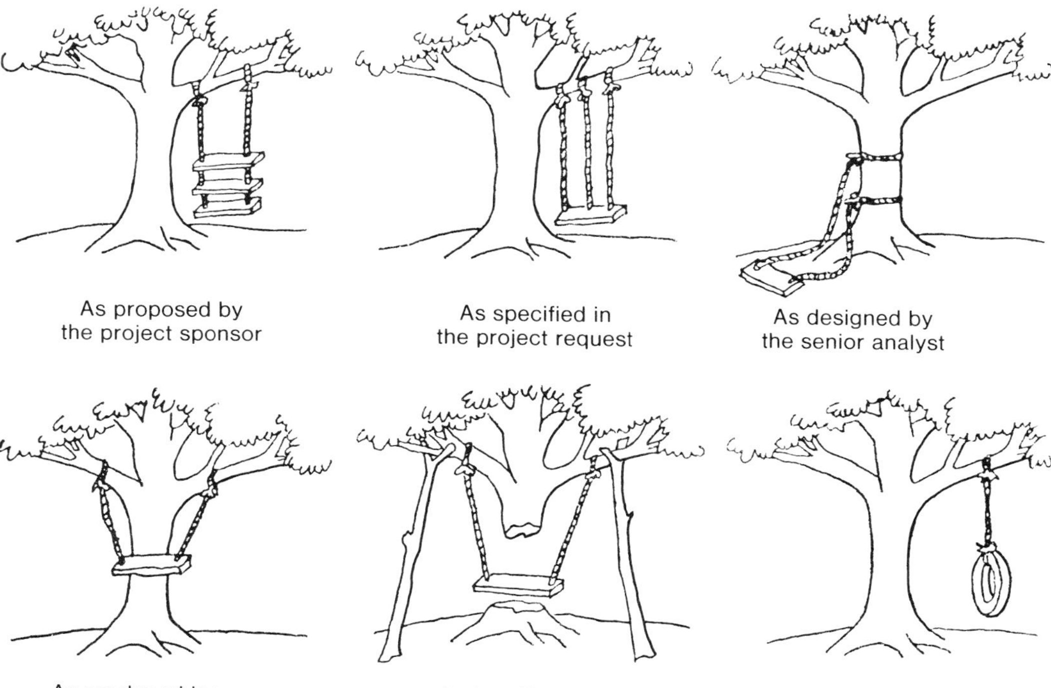

As proposed by the project sponsor

As specified in the project request

As designed by the senior analyst

As produced by the programmers

As installed at the user's site

What the user wanted

Figure 76.1

and the world around them, because it is a world which they have helped to make. The daily users of buildings know more about their needs than anyone else; so the process of participation tends to create places which are better adapted to human functions than those created by a centrally administered planning process.

—Christopher Alexander
The Oregon Experiment

INTRODUCTION

Architecture is created out of oppositions. These oppositions mold the built form by defining problems or conflicts inherent in the given circumstances. For example, "I need a quiet place to work" vs. "I like to have some informal contact with my fellow co-workers during the work day." This is the beginning of a statement of an architectural design problem. Another example, "I like to have a view from my office window" vs. "I often see patients in my office who need privacy," further delineates how this office or its windows may be designed. The more conflicts presented to the architect at the design stage, the better his solution will fit the problem. A poorly stated problem can only produce an unsatisfactory solution. In suggesting any procedure for approaching the design of the emergency department, one cannot underestimate developing a list of verbal criteria to describe the spaces.

The best design criteria are these that explain the space; irrational copying or duplication of emergency departments that seem to work well can lead to problems. For example, "The Emergency Department of Hospital X works well. It has a charting station at the center and patient rooms encircling it." It is more important to state specifically and nonspatially what process is going on that makes that particular emergency department work well, e.g., "It is important to have the charting station located so that all patients can be easily seen from it," or "It is desirable to keep the staff walking around the department to a minimum. The doctors frequently move between rooms x, y, and z. The nurses frequently move between rooms w, x, and y." In this way a more satisfactory architectural solution can be found without becoming locked into any particular spatial form. Function and spatial flow diagrams are helpful, and should be presented and discussed between the architects and staff (Fig. 76.2).

To get a satisfactory design, both hospital staff and architects must have good communication. As many members of the staff as possible should be consulted: administrators, nurses, doctors, security, social workers, maintenance people, and ambulance operators. A good ultimate design will have spaces that work well from the medical point of view, as well as an entryway that has good access, floors that are easily maintained, and so on. In particular, a pediatric hospital must consider the specific problems of a child's environment: a good design solution will take into account the problems of children and their parents in a hospital setting. Once the criteria have been developed, it is important to review the design as early as possible in its stages of development. Reviewing the early designs will allow for changes and may suggest other criteria that have been missed.

In the following pages I will provide some verbal sketches concerning some of the components of an emergency department and some of the criteria. Since each hospital will require a department that suits its size and needs, not all the elements suggested will be important. Each hospital staff should evaluate its current and future needs. The cost of constructing an emergency department is another factor which will influence the scope of any design. Of course, all of these needs must eventually be as specifically stated to the architect.

It is my hope that some of the ideas presented in this chapter will provide the beginnings of a discussion between the architect and the emergency room staff, when considering the design or remodeling of the emergency department space.

ACCESS

The drive and entryway to the emergency department should be easily visible from the street. Signs should be provided to direct incoming traffic clearly from the

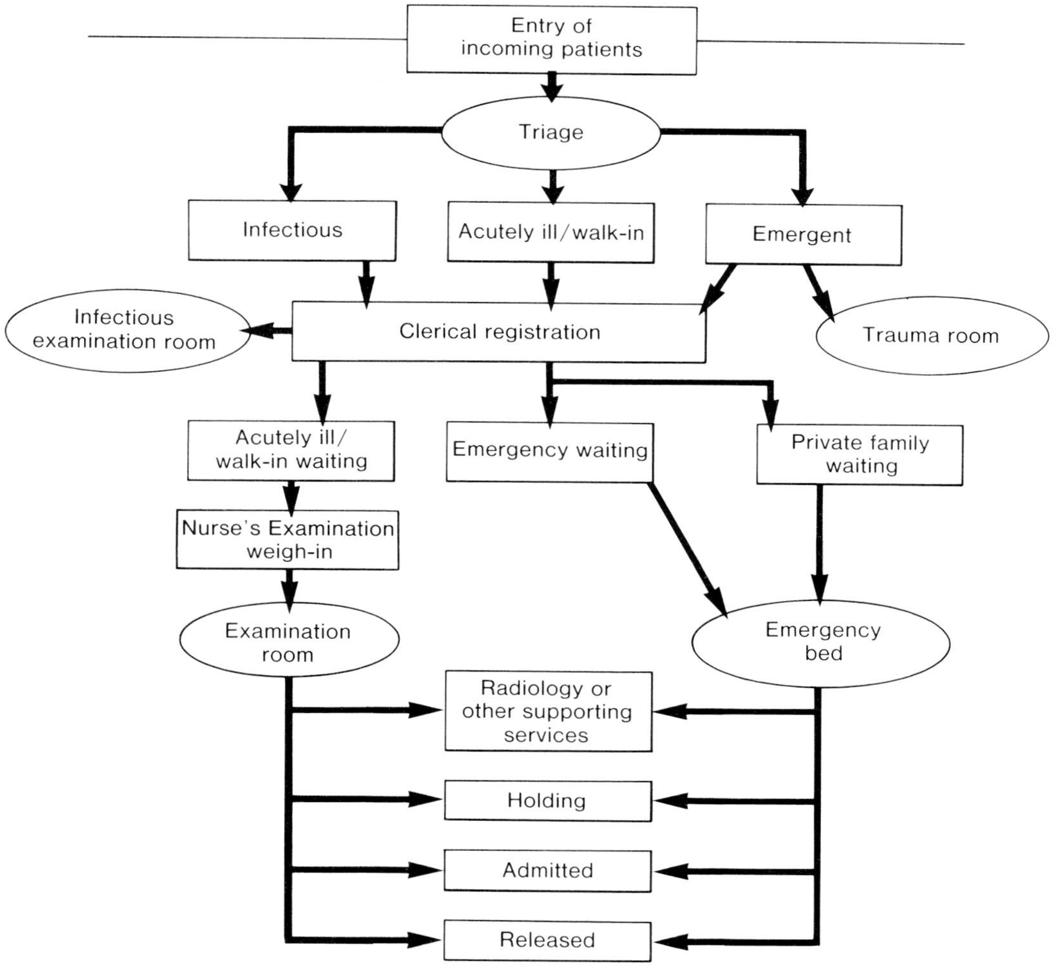

Figure 76.2

road, the sidewalk, and nearby public transportation stations.

Parking is a major problem at almost all hospitals, especially for the emergency patient brought by the private automobile. Facilities must be provided nearby for both patients and staff. If parking is a long distance away, an attendant should be provided to park the car for the parents driving. This is especially true in a pediatric hospital since it will be uncomfortable to separate the parent and child on arrival at the emergency room. The number of parking spaces provided varies with the patient population. In urban areas where most patients will not arrive in their own vehicle, the needs will not be the same as where almost every patient's family and staff member arrives in their own car. For the latter situation, the parking lot should have enough spaces for the maximum number of patients at any one time, plus staff parking (if provided in the same area) plus 10 extra spaces.

For the family who arrives at the entrance and needs assistance from the car, there should be some means of summoning aid. This could be done by bell or phone. Wheelchairs and stretchers should be stored at the entrance for immediate use, and there should be a radiation or chemical decontamination area that is weather pro-

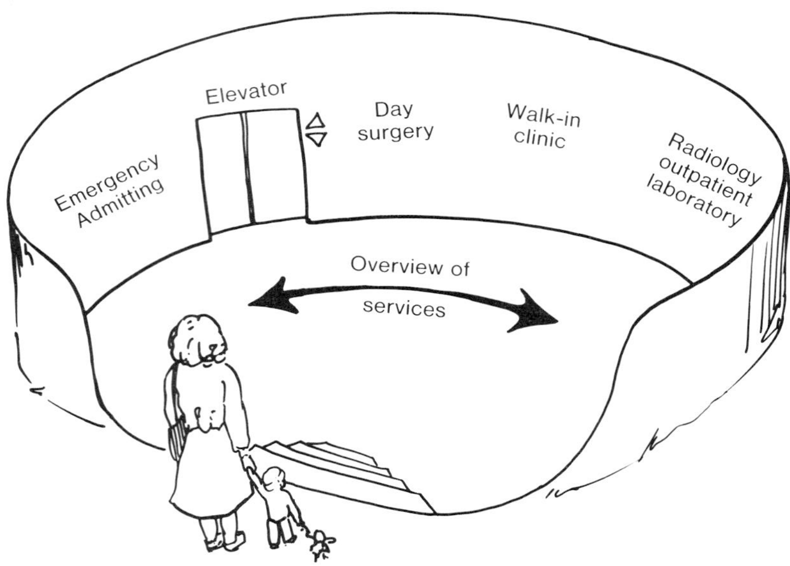

Figure 76.3

tected and is usable by stretcher and ambulatory patients.

The hospital security system must originate at the entrance to the emergency department. A uniformed guard must be present 24 hours a day to provide security and to control patient and family traffic flow. The emergency department entrance should not be the only 24-hour entrance to the hospital, and the general traffic flow of visitors and staff must be separated from the emergency department. Access to the rest of the hospital's service areas (surgery, radiology, laboratories, intensive care, etc.) from the emergency department has to be preserved (Fig. 76.3). Provisions must be made for emergencies generated within the hospital as well as emergencies generated within the community. There also should be an easy access way for life-threatening emergencies: "stats."

In a large-scale disaster, there must be a plan that allows a large volume of patients to arrive *en masse* without denying access to non-disaster patients. This plan must also provide for overflow of patients into contiguous service areas when the capacity of the emergency department is exceeded.

TRIAGE

The triage officer should be the first person whom the ambulatory patient and his relatives encounter when they enter the department. The officer is a medical person who will assess the priority of patient entry into the treatment area by the parameters of history and vital signs. If there is a separate ambulatory clinic area, this medically trained person can decide if this is the more important area for treatment. After this assessment has been made, the child and the relatives should be turned over to the clerical personnel. Ambulance patients bypass the triage officer and will be taken directly into the treatment area and be immediately evaluated by a nurse or a physician.

The triage interview area needs to have as much privacy as possible, which can be achieved by proper soundproofing and screening. There should be enough room in the triage area for the parent to sit down since they often arrive carrying children. Stretchers and wheelchairs should be stored nearby. Space should be provided for the child and his family waiting to be interviewed. The interview area should be contiguous with the waiting area to ensure that waiting patients are always under medical observation. In many cases, the triage officer will be the first to know that the patient who has just arrived needs resuscitation, and will need to alert the rest of the department, perhaps by using a bell or telephone system. The triage officer may also need to coordinate communications with clinics, radiology, and laboratories. One might also consider providing some space and equipment to do simple procedures such as splinting. In this area, the security system is also very important because of possible conflicts between patients' families and hospital staff.

WAITING

Whatever people are waiting for—an airplane, a business appointment or the doctor—has built-in uncertainties, which make it inevitable that they will spend some time doing nothing. They usually cannot enjoy this time since they never know exactly when their turn may come. They cannot even take a stroll or sit outside. They must stay in the narrow confines of the waiting room, and it can be an extremely demoralizing situation. Failure to provide reasonable waiting accommodations is not only inhuman, but not optimal from a utilitarian standpoint: the disposition of many pediatric patients is facilitated by his or her interactions and experiences immediately before he is seen by the staff. A noisy, crowded and uncomfortable waiting area may begin to deteriorate the relationship between the child, his family and the staff. The fundamental problem, then, is to get waiting people to spend their time enjoying the minutes or hours they are waiting almost as fully as the other hours of their day and still be on hand when they are ready to be seen.

Ideally, this is done best when the waiting is combined with some other activity that draws in the people who are waiting but is sufficiently engaging that one might want to be there regardless of the wait. This could be done by providing a cafe, pool tables, a reading room, where the activities and the seats around them are within an earshot of the signal that the staff is ready to see them. The Pediatrics Clinic at San Francisco General Hospital built a small playground beside the entrance to serve as a waiting area for children and a play area for the neighborhood. In another example, a horseshoe pit was built alongside a terrace where people came to wait for appointments. The people waiting inevitably started pitching horseshoes, others joined in, people left as their appointments came up. There was a flow between the activity area and the offices.

Waiting time could become a valuable resource for the education of the child and his family. The waiting room might be divided into smaller pocketed areas where the families and children could view videocasettes. Some of these could provide medical information, others could be pure entertainment for the children. A small video library could be available where parents and children would choose what they could watch. It might also be possible to develop an active play program for the waiting child and his siblings. This program could have its own budget and director, and might be supplemented by voluntary manpower. This central play area could become an important laboratory for observation of play by medical students and parents, in addition to making the wait time more meaningful for the child. Space for play is also important. Since children reduce anxiety by playing, they also need space to be mobile.

Waiting may also be a time when the parent and child wish to be quiet and still. The right atmosphere for being contemplative, or quiet enough to allow a sleeping infant to remain so, will come naturally if the waiting area provides some places that are quiet and protected. Some physical examples might be a seating arrangement facing a window or the street or a garden, or a private seat by a fish tank.

In the emergency department, one might want to separate the waiting areas for truly emergent and nonemergent patients. Both would be spatially between the process of triage and preparation for examination and treatment. Alternate spaces may be provided for children waiting for test results and follow-up appointment scheduling. These spaces should accommodate ambulatory, wheelchair, and stretcher patients, where appropriate. All spaces should be located so that there is easy observation and contact with the nursing staff. These spaces should be located so that the work of the staff is sufficiently shielded from possible interruption by waiting families. It may be desirable to separate the waiting families from the view of incoming patients. Often the arrival of an emergency case brought in by ambulance or police is trafficked directly through the main waiting area. This can frighten both the waiting children and families as well as the arriving patient. One might also consider a third, more private, waiting space for the family of a critically ill child in the resuscitation area.

To avoid continuous overflowing, one should try to estimate the number of waiting seats that will be required by the emergency department. This is the product of the average number of persons who accompany a child to the hospital, the maximum number of registrants per hour, and the average patient turnaround time. For example, an emergency department that has a peak registration of 20 children in 1 hour, a patient turnaround time of 1½ hours, and 1 person accompanying the child, would require 60 seats.

In summary, the people who are waiting should be given some freedom to do what they want. If they want to sit outside the interviewer's door, take a short stroll, play a game of pool, get a coffee or a hamburger, they can. If they want to sit quietly, they can. And they can do all this without fear of losing their place in line.

EXAMINING AND TREATMENT AREAS

In the design of an emergency facility, one must make an early decision concerning the degree of separation of the emergent and the nonemergent areas. Should there be separate examination rooms and a shared waiting area and nursing control, or should there be a complete separation (waiting areas, etc.) from the point of triage? If there are shared facilities these will determine where these activities will occur, i.e. at the border between the emergent and nonemergent areas (Figs. 76.4–76.10)

After the children have gone through triage and registration, they and their fam-

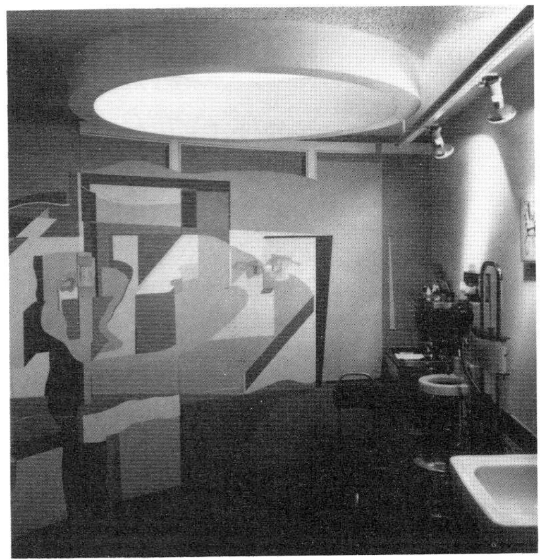

Figure 76.4. Examining room.

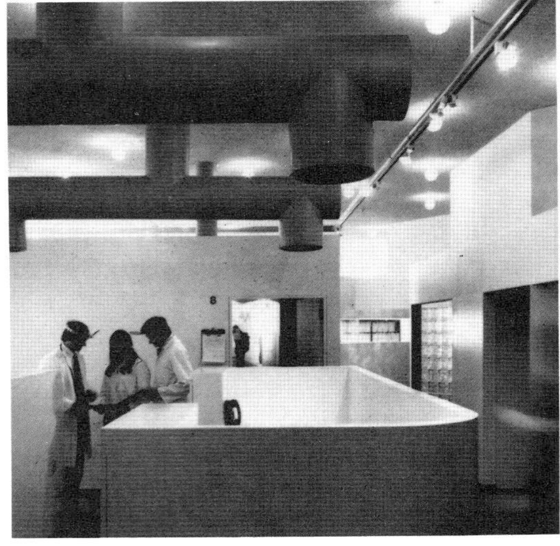

Figure 76.5. Nurses' station.

ilies must wait to be seen by the nursing staff for the preliminary work-up, vital signs and weigh-in. Adequate space for these functions should be provided close to the

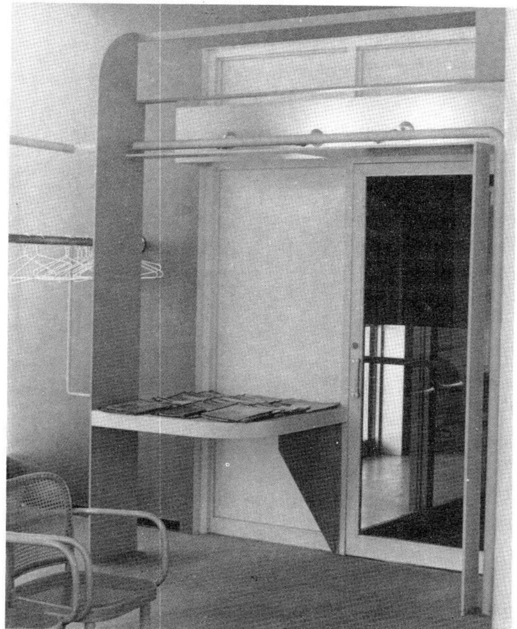

Figure 76.6. Details showing how "functional" events are transformed into an architecture that animates the wall.

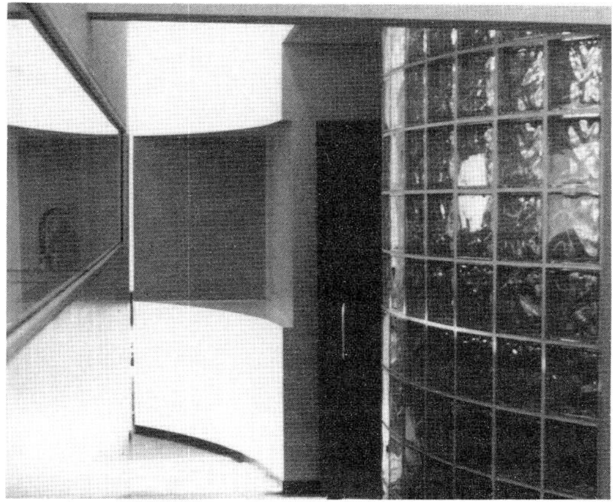

Figure 76.7. Varied materials, shapes and thicknesses of walls elucidate the individual spatial character and functions of the rooms they enclose.

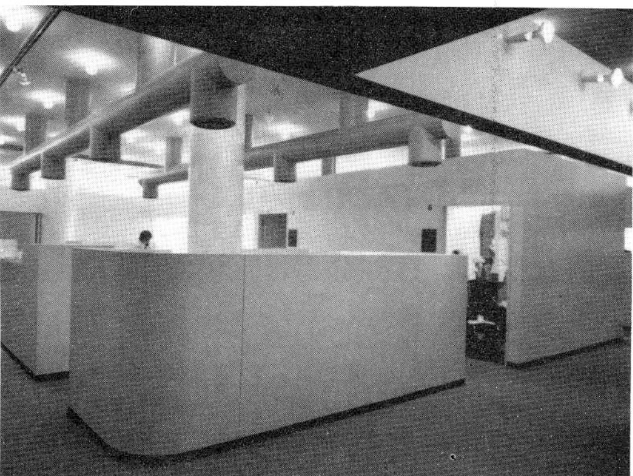

Figure 76.8. Ceiling height. This view of the nursing station shows how different ceiling heights and lighting patterns create qualitative differences among spaces that open into each other.

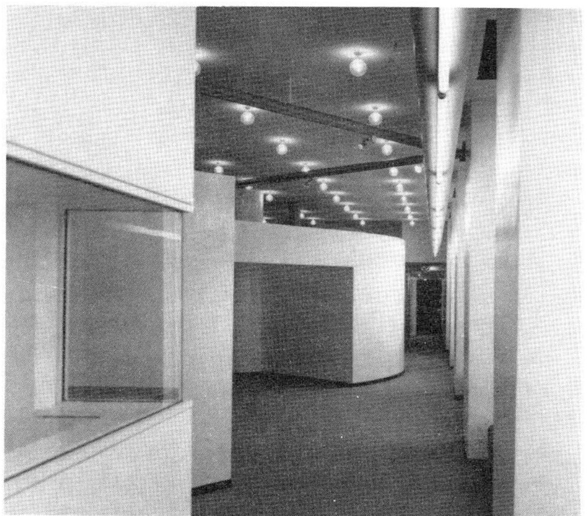

Figure 76.9. Example (see also Fig. 76.10) of corridors animated by the different characteristics of rooms along the way. Here the repetitive linear elements on the right are contrasted with the geometry of unique rooms on the left of the corridor. Note how this theme is reflected in the lighting pattern.

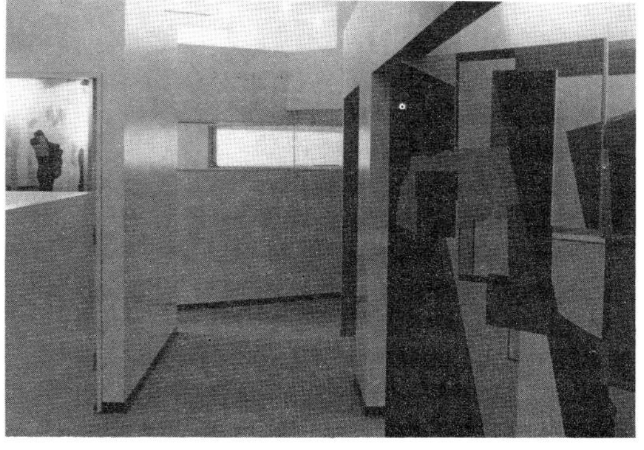

Figure 76.10. Events in the corridor include a mural by Michael Graves as well as a view of his mural inside an adjacent room, seen through a window into the corridor.

waiting and examination room areas. The "weigh-in area" should have adequate space for handling two children at one time, adequate privacy (the child may be partially unclothed), room for a scale, a sink, and areas for taking vital signs. One might also consider including a sink that is large enough for a sponge-bath for those children who require such treatment.

After the weigh-in the children are ready to be put in separate examining rooms. The number of examining cubicles needed is a function of the number of physicians on duty. There is some belief that in an ideal system, which incorporates sufficient paramedical and nursing personnel and rapid processing of laboratory and radiology results, each physician can efficiently use a maximum of six rooms. In departments where nurse scribes and physicians' assistants are used, the number of rooms per physician may be much greater. The average will probably be three rooms. In academic institutions where teaching is an important service, the number of examination cubicles may drop as low as one cubicle per physician. If the capacity exceeds six rooms per physician, there may be underutilization of the facility: the patients are merely being stored in the cubicles.

The smallest cubicle size is 8 by 9 feet, assuming a single doorway that opens inward. If any examination room has more than one doorway, the swing of the door will subtract from the usable area within the room, and additional area should be allowed to compensate for it. It is a good idea to include several examination rooms that are slightly larger (8 by 12). These larger examination rooms could be used for patients who come with both parents, or where the mother must bring siblings into the examination room. The larger rooms could also be used with a teaching case, where several staff members or students will be in the examination room at the same time. It is important to avoid hazardous location of equipment.

In hospitals with large volumes, or where similar facilities are not provided nearby within the hospital, specialized examination rooms may be necessary. One might wish to include an ENT-dental room, an infectious disease room, and a gynecological examination room.

The infectious room should be located away from the general examination room and waiting areas, and ideally very close to the entryway to the department. This will avoid trafficking these patients through large areas of the department.

The ENT-dental room will have the appropriate chair and equipment for those examinations. Having such a room in the department can avoid sending numbers of patients travelling around the hospital, and can be quite useful for the department if there is enough demand (Fig. 76.4).

The gynecological examination room should have the appropriate table and a small adjacent changing room and bathroom. It should be positioned within the department so that the adolescent or child will sense privacy.

If there is a central charting area, it should be conveniently located to the rooms and should allow the staff sufficient privacy so that charts can be written without disturbance. It may be convenient to have some writing areas in the corridors positioned so that some notes can be written while standing. Once again, there should be enough linear writing space for all members of the department to work comfortably.

TRAUMA RESUSCITATION ROOM

In the design of an emergency department, one important consideration is a trauma room. Should there be a special trauma room? If so, where should it be located and how large should it be?

Patients who require a trauma room (e.g. accident victims) are best off with the least amount of transport. For this reason, and because such patients may have a dramatic and disturbing appearance to other patients within the department, the trauma treatment area should be located close to the main entryway.

A two-bedded room would require approximately 16 by 15 feet of space. It may be useful to have equipment for taking x-rays within the area. This could be done with a portable x-ray unit or a unit suspended from the ceiling of the trauma room. There must be enough space for carts, and easily accessible shelves for storage. One might want to keep an area equipped for a thoracotomy, with surgical type lights, insulation, etc. One bed per 100 patients per day is a rough estimate of need.

MAJOR SURGICAL AREA

In most hospitals, it is be wrong to attempt to perform serious operations in an emergency department. Because of this, there must be easy access (elevators, etc.) between the emergency department and the operating area.

A large emergency department, however, may decide to make use of such a surgical suite. This room could be used for general anesthesia cases that do not need to be admitted (especially if used in conjunction with a nearby holding area) or for the patient who needs immediate surgery but cannot tolerate transport to the regular surgical suite.

In any case, the decision to include a surgical suite in the emergency department should be an early consideration. If not, appropriate access to the operating suite must be provided.

ACUTE CARE AREAS

The staff of the department must decide how many acute care beds it will need, in addition to those in the trauma room. All such areas should have suction, oxygen and a sink and should be electrically grounded and shielded for ECG use. In general, each bed and surrounding area will require approximately 8 by 15 feet of floor space. The acute area beds may surround a central nursing area without any intervening walls: in this case, some enclosure is provided by curtains. According to some staffs, this provides the greatest possible observation from a central nursing area. It also provides for less separation and privacy and an increase in the amount of noise within the area. As a compromise between enclosure and observation, one could provide areas that are separated by walls with glass above the waist level.

AUXILIARY FACILITIES

Laboratory

Whether or not to use the central laboratory or have a laboratory in the emergency department is up to the individual hospital. All emergency departments should have a space to do their own urinalyses, hematocrits, cultures and Gram stains.

It might also be a good idea to include a laboratory for the medical students in the context of a teaching hospital. This could be a counterspace 10 feet long, with a sink, and adequate cabinets for storage of culture media, staining materials, microscope, etc.

Radiology

The need for radiology facilities within the department depends on the volume and type of patients seen. If the ambulatory clinic is nearby, it can share facilities. If x-ray equipment is not located within the emergency department, it should be in close proximity and with a portable unit available. There should be adequate x-ray view boxes here and elsewhere in the department.

Nurse's Work Area

The nurse's work area (used for reporting, charting, etc., by all members of the medical staff) should have visual access to all patient care areas in the acute care facility. There always seems to be a critical shortage of writing and work space. To estimate the amount that might be needed, one should take the maximum number of staff members that would use the area at one time and give each approximately 5 linear feet of writing space, i.e., if there are 6 staff members working at the busiest times, there should be 30 feet of charting space. For good visual access, this charting area should be at the center of the acute care area, with the beds arranged circumferentially around the observation area (sometimes this is executed in a literal circle of beds around a circular area, but this may not be the most efficient space, and it is usually unnecessary and space wasting) (Fig. 76.5).

There should be a drug area with a lockbox, sink refrigerator, and counterspace on which to prepare drugs. In the equipment work area will be the autoclave, sink and so on. Sterile supplies can come from central supply if it is open 24 hours a day. If not, facilities for sterilization must be available. There should be a storage area for crutches and linen.

Holding Ward

The need for a holding ward, or an observation care unit, is a function of the work load of a department. It can be used for suspected head injuries, asthmatics, drug ingestion cases and patients waiting admission. The observation care unit usually requires a nursing staff whose sole responsibility is the unit. It should be an open room with good visual access. Space for 5 to 10 children could be included, and patients could be discharged or admitted if there is a need for more beds. Several criteria have been suggested for estimating the number of beds. One bed for every 100 inpatient beds has been suggested. Another criterion is one bed for every patient admitted from the emergency department. The limit of the patient stay will determine the complexity of the unit. If the patient's stay is more than 12 hours, toilet and dietary facilities need to be provided.

If one decided to include a holding area within the emergency department, it might be a good idea to locate it adjacent to the acute care beds area. If the holding area was not being utilized and there was a sudden need for acute care beds beyond the normal capacity, one would be able to put acute care patients in the adjacent holding ward beds. The opposite could also be provided for, if the holding area is in demand.

Conference Rooms

Architects have worked out some of the "science" of meetings, especially as it relates to spatial requirements. The upper range for a full casual voice is about 8 feet; a person with 20/20 vision can see details of facial expression up to 12 feet; two people whose heads are about 8 to 9 feet apart can pass an object if they both stretch; clear vision includes 12° horizontally and 3° vertically—which included one face, but not two, at distances up to about 10 feet.

Some architects believe that a small group discussion will function best if the members of the group are arranged in a rough circle, with a maximum diameter of about 8 feet. At this diameter, the circumference of the circle will be 25 feet. Since people require about 27 inches for their seats, there is room for 12 people. Investigators find that when meetings are held in rooms that are too large and half empty, people tend to sit back, and speakers face rows of empty seats.

If the meeting rooms are to foster contact and communication between co-workers, the locations of meeting rooms with respect to private offices must also be considered. Investigators find that meeting rooms work best when they are fairly near the participants' offices. Then discussions which begin in the meeting rooms are able to continue in the office or laboratory. When meeting rooms are a long walk from offices, the chances of this kind of informal business are drastically reduced.

The architect should also consider the spatial character of the meeting room. Will it need audiovisual aids or blackboards? Should there be a window with an interesting view; i.e., should it be located on an outside wall?

Teaching Areas

In a teaching hospital, it is often important to have spaces within the department where students can be grouped and brought aside to discuss work within the department without interfering with department activities and with due respect to patient privacy. If it is possible, one of the conference rooms can serve as a teaching area.

In the ambulatory area, one of the larger examination rooms can provide the setting for physical examinations where the room will be occupied by a greater than normal number of staff (students, interns, attendings) as well as the child and his accompanying family.

Offices

The staff should decide who will need to have offices within or adjacent to the emergency department. One should consider space for social workers, fellows, nurses, visiting staff, secretaries and attending doctors. The location of these offices within the department should be picked so that the normal department traffic pattern will not interfere with the work in offices.

Architects have tried to study the nature of work in a private or semi-private office space. They have developed numerous suggestions which can be considered in designing an office, listed below.

1. You feel more comfortable working in a space where there is a wall behind you. If your back is exposed, you may feel vulnerable.
2. You feel more comfortable in a workspace where there is a wall to one side. This is probably due to the fact that while it is possible to be vaguely aware of everything that is going on around you for 180°, to control vision of such a wide angle you must move your head all the time. If you have one wall at your side, you have a 90° angle, which is much easier to overview.
3. There should be no blank wall closer than 8 feet in front of you. When you look up, it should be possible to focus on something farther away than the desk.
4. Workspace where you spend most of the day should be at least 60 square feet.
5. Each workspace should be enclosed (50 to 75%) by walls or windows. Every workspace should have a view on life—outside or into an interior courtyard with visual interest and activity.
6. No other person should work closer than 8 feet from your space. In this way it is possible to have conversations on the phone that are private.
7. You should not be able to hear many noises that are different from the ones you make while working.
8. No one should be sitting directly opposite you or facing you.
9. Workspaces should allow an amount of visual and verbal communication when it is desired; you should be able to see two or three other persons while working, and able to talk to at least one from your space.

On-Call Rooms

Special rooms should be provided in a quiet area in the department for staff that must remain on-call during the night. It might be possible to use some offices which are empty at night to double as on-call rooms.

Staff Lounge, Lockers and Changing Areas

The emergency room is a stressful work situation. For this reason, a staff area may be provided adjacent to the emergency department. In this area, staff members may eat, smoke, rest, read, change clothes, shower, etc. If lockers are provided, this area should be in a secure place to prevent patients or outsiders from wandering in.

Bathrooms

Bathrooms should be provided near the waiting areas and adequately throughout the department to prevent dozens of pilgrimages across work areas. One may provide showers in bathrooms for the staff. Facilities for the wheelchair user should also be provided.

Family Waiting Area and Consultation Room

A number of emergency departments have realized the need for a room where a single family could stay for meetings with the staff. Ideally, this would be a quiet room near the reception area. It could be used for the families of a truly emergent case, where the parents are distressed by the condition of their child. It also could be used to inform relatives of a sudden death within the department without exposing their grief to the public gaze.

The room should be comfortable and "loungelike," holding 6 to 8 people. It should be near the patients' waiting area and nursing station. Physicians can use this room to discuss any private matter with the child's family. Psychiatrists and chaplains may also use this area.

Police and Ambulance Room

A police room is an essential area because of the mandatory reports following automobile accidents and personal violence. The room must be separate from the general waiting space and away from patient care areas. Ambulance personnel also could use this room.

DETAILING THE DESIGN

The Walls

Once the plan has been drawn with some accuracy, and many of the large-scale functional requirements of the spaces have been met, the details must be determined. These details will make a functional scheme provide more for its users. There are small spaces or "events" in the architecture which can relate to the user—especially the pediatric user. Niches, built-in seats, counters, closets and shelves should be added to the walls (Figs. 76.6 and 76.7).

Buildings with smooth, flat walls may appear impersonal or dead. Some of the walls should be made deep—containing shelves, cabinets, displays, special lights, special surfaces, deep window reveals, individual niches, built-in seats, and nooks. Items contained in these built-in walls can be built with the child in mind. There can be windows, mirrors and seats high enough only for a child. There can be walls with built-in seats for parents and children of different ages. There can be varying chair heights for children of different ages.

Built-in seats are sometimes too hard, too narrow and too stiff-backed. Make the side as wide as a comfortable chair (18 inches for adults) with a back that slopes gently, and put cushions on it to make it comfortable. Whenever possible, place the seat so that the occupant has a good view.

If possible, try to make the building interact with the child. For example, children love to be in tiny, cavelike places. In their play children often seek out cave-spaces to get into and under—old crates, tables, tents. In some part of the design, it may be possible to include such a cave—each child takes up approximately 5 square feet. One might want to make caves for one, three or five children at a time. Such a cave might be built in the left-over space under a stairwell. This is one of numerous ways that can create relationships between a child and the architecture he uses.

Ceiling Height

In a general way, low ceilings make for intimacy, high ceilings for formality. In buildings which are governed by standard components, it is very hard to make the ceiling height vary from room to room, and the psychological effects of varying heights tends to be forgotten.

If possible, the architect should try to vary the ceiling heights, for varying functions, especially in rooms that open into each other, so that the relative intimacy of different spaces can be felt. Rooms which are meant for large gatherings or are public should have high ceilings (greater than 10 feet), for smaller gatherings rooms should have ceilings which are lower (7 to 9 feet) and very low in rooms or alcoves for one or two people (6 to 7 feet). For children, it might be interesting to build in some spaces that are scaled down to their size (5 to 6 feet). Having some rooms with lowered ceilings may serve to overcome some of the feeling of being overwhelmed when entering a large building, such as a hospital (Fig. 76.8).

Color

The grays and greens often used in hospitals are often depressing and cold. A variety of wall and floor materials, generous amounts of sunlight, and a careful use of bright colors can make a great deal of difference between a monotonous environment and one that is active and engaging. While the use of bright color can be offensive, if it is carefully offset by ample neutral and white tones, it can create interest. If used in a more practical way, color can create a legibility in the building by giving a certain "color character" to its various parts. Places can be described as behind the blue door, down the yellow-tiled corridor, or at the red counter.

In the architecture of Michael Graves, murals and colors are used to demonstrate various "meanings" of rooms and spaces. It might be possible in the design of the emergency room to use colors and wall paintings that demonstrate to the users—child, parent, staff—how the building works, what it means, etc. (Figs. 76.4 and 76.10).

One could say that children especially require a bright, warm, and well-lit environment. However, adults also often find such an environment pleasing.

Corridors

In a building where a number of rooms must share a circulation path, it is common practice to string the rooms along a straight corridor. This often seems to be an efficient solution, since it minimizes the circulation space and reduces the construction costs of turning corners. However, people often dislike long corridors feeling they represent monotony and bureaucracy. In addition, one study of long corridors in mental hospitals by psychologists have shown that there are some disturbing perceptual distortions. Long passageways obscure the perception of human figure and face, and distort distance perception. There are disturbed visual cues with illusions involving room size, distance, walking speed, and time.

One architect has suggested a limit on the length of a corridor, based on some perceptual investigations. It is known that when a person sees 4 or 5 regularly spaced objects of some kind, he perceives them as a unit. He can judge their number without counting them. When the number of objects goes above 5 or 6, he can no longer estimate their number in one glance, he must count them. This means that a corridor tends to become perceptually less manageable when it has 5 or more doors down one side. While such studies are still speculative, it seems safe to say that very long uninterrupted corridors should be avoided whenever possible.

If one must make a longer corridor, it may be wise to break it down in some way. For example, a long corridor that is lit in patches from one side at short intervals can be pleasant; one has a chance to pause and glance out. The same effect can be produced by making hallways open into wider rooms every now and then (Fig. 76.9). Interior windows from the rooms opening off the corridor help animate the hall (Fig. 76.10). They establish a flow between the rooms and the passage, support a more informal style of communication, and give a person moving down the hall a taste of life inside the rooms. Even in an office, this contact can work provided the work space is protected by a partial wall or distance.

Another way to create a lively passage is to create events in the walls en route. If one provides special places with built-in seats, displays in the walls, small tables and places to lean, the corridor becomes a room in itself, rather than a purely functional conduit.

Windows

In a building with a large floor area and volume, only a limited number of spaces will have access to the outside wall. Therefore, a very careful consideration should be given to rooms that may require windows and rooms that do not.

One study showed that 81% of office workers chose to sit by a window. In general, people prefer windows with meaningful views—views of city life, nature. Windows need not face the exterior. In buildings with large well-lit courtyards, where there is some interest in seeing the courtyard, or even facing an interior corridor, windows can be positioned so that the person occupying the room could glimpse out into some interesting public space. Sills for windows could be positioned so that their height corresponds to a child's proportions.

Flexibility

The idea of a building's built-in ability to respond to change is one that has vexed architects for decades. At the present time, there is no single building design or construction method that provides a sweeping solution to the problem. Since the hospital is a mixture of stable and changing elements, each with distinct characteristics, and since different parts of the hospital will change at different rates, no single solution will satisfy every demand placed on it. As a solution to the inevitable problem of change, architects have proposed designing buildings or their parts to be convertible, reusable, expansible, contractible, or mobile. Each provides only a mediocre solution.

Convertibility can be achieved by technical means or by remodeling. Sometimes, moveable partitions are proposed. The client who requests such a flexible plan often has a poor idea of how his hospital may change; throwing in a few moveable walls is a poor solution. Moveable partitions have several problems:

1. If partitions are easy to move, they become lightweight and provide inadequate acoustic insulation. Those partitions that are easy to move and are well insulated acoustically are usually very expensive.
2. The actual cost of moving a partition, as well as a psychological inertia, is so high that even in highly flexible systems, the partitions are rarely moved. It is the nature of occupying a space that creates certain informal, semipermanent arrangements, e.g., furnishings, "ownership" of special spaces or windows. This makes occupants resistant to change.

Since program needs are constantly changing, it is not surprising that hospitals quickly become obsolete. But a building designed primarily to permit change will inevitably be characterized by a sense of indecisiveness. Hospital environments should be as complete as possible in any point of time; it is unsatisfactory to inhabit surroundings that are permanently temporary or incomplete.

Hospitals and other building types that undergo constant change in function must learn to live with remodeling. The minimal requirement for flexibility is that structural columns be adequately spaced so that subsequent nonstructural walls can be built in a relatively free open space and that mechanical facilities (electricity, water, air, etc.) be somewhat uniformly provided.

Acknowledgments. I would like to thank Michael Graves, architect, and Balthazar Korub, photographer, for permission to use photographs of the clinic in Fort Wayne, Indiana. The author feels that the level of design in this clinic is exemplary. I would also like to thank Christopher Alexander for permission to use the cartoon which appeared in *The Oregon Experiment.*

References

Alexander C, et al.: *A Pattern Language which Generates Multiservice Centers.* The Center for Environmental Structure, Berkeley, Calif., 1968.

Alexander C, et al.: *The Oregon Experiment.* The Center for Environmental Structure, Berkeley, Calif., 1975.

Alexander C, et al.: *A Pattern Language.* Oxford University Press, New York, 1977.

Goldsmith S: *Designing for the Handicapped.* RIBA Publications Ltd., London, 1976.

Kriedberg, M: *Problems of Pediatric Hospital Design.* U. S. Public Health Service, Tufts-New England Medical Center, Boston, 1965.

Rosenfeld I: *Hospitals—Integrated Design.* Reinhold Publishing, New York, 1951.

Editorials

A study of waiting time in an emergency department: *Can Med Assoc J* 109: 373–376, 1973.

An approach to studying emergency department utilization. *Va Med Month* 101: June 1974.

Checklist for a children's trauma room. *J Trauma* 16: 763–765, 1976.

Every emergency department should have one—an interview room. *Br Med J* January 10, 1976.

Forward looking architecture; flexibility with change in mind. *Hospitals* 52: 113, 1978.

Spatial design provides efficiency emergency-outpatient department. *Hospitals* 47: 36, 1973.

CHAPTER 77

Legal Aspects of Emergency Department Pediatrics

CHRISTOPHER C. BERGEN

INTRODUCTION

The risk of being sued is inherent in the practice of medicine. For a number of reasons, this risk is greater with respect to emergency department pediatrics than with respect to many other types of practice. There is generally no ongoing physician-patient-parent relationship outside of the emergency department encounter, and various conditions of many emergency departments make it difficult to establish such a relationship during the encounter. The medical problems which confront the emergency department physician treating a child are complex, and the patient's condition can change rapidly. The patients are frequently very young, unable to communicate, and incapable of caring for or making decisions for themselves. The parents upon whom the physician must rely to provide information, make decisions, and carry out instructions sometimes are no more than adolescents themselves or are too upset to be objective.

If treatment does result in an undesirable outcome, whether attributable to malpractice or not, parents may be persuaded relatively easily to protect and defend their children's interests or to attempt to punish anyone they think has violated them. Even if the parents do not find fault with the care, the child may, many years later. Each state has its own statute of limitations which sets a certain time period within which a person may bring suit for an alleged injury. When this period has passed, the suit may no longer be brought, regardless of its merits. These statutes apply to adults, whether suing on their own behalf or on behalf of their minor children. Because children are unable to initiate legal action, however, in almost all jurisdictions this time period does not begin for an injured child until he or she has reached the age of majority. Thus, either the parents, within the normal statute of limitations, or the child, within the same statute extended by the years it takes for him or her to reach majority, may bring suit against the physician treating pediatric patients.

With this in mind, the purpose of this chapter is to provide an overview of both the legal risks involved in emergency department pediatrics and the methods by which these risks can be managed. It is not the purpose of this chapter to give legal advice. Each jurisdiction has its own case law, statutes, rules and regulations, and only an attorney familiar with them can give sound legal advice.

THE LEGAL RISKS

Civil

Creative attorneys and sympathetic, precedent setting courts, which reflect the norms of modern society, make it impossible to compile a comprehensive list of allegations that might be made by plaintiffs in suits involving physicians. The most frequent allegation in such suits, however, is negligence or malpractice. Generally, the person alleging injury in a malpractice suit is the patient, but it is not uncommon for a physician to be held liable for damages suffered by persons other than the patient.

As examples, physicians may be held liable for losses suffered by the patient's family due to any incapacity suffered by the patient. If a physician fails to report suspected child abuse or a communicable disease to the proper authorities, and a third party (e.g. a sibling) is injured or contracts the disease as the direct result of that failure, the physician may be held liable. Failure to warn persons who the physician knows, or should know, are directly exposed to injury or illness as a result of a patient's condition may also lead to liability. Thus, liability may result from failure to warn parents of the contagious nature of a child's disease if other children in the family contract the disease when timely and reasonable precautions would have prevented its spread.

A physician may also be held liable for the consequences of not only his or her own actions but also the actions of certain other persons. Under the doctrine of *respondeat superior*, a physician may be held liable for the consequences of the actions of any of his or her agents or employees. Nurses, technicians and aides are generally hospital employees, but when working under the direct supervision of a physician, or following his or her specific instructions, they may become the physician's agents.

Other allegations commonly made by plaintiffs in suits involving physicians include battery, breach of contract and invasion of privacy. Battery is the unlawful touching of another's person. Such an allegation may be made as a result of treatment without consent or unreasonable contact in an attempt to restrain a patient. Breach of contract occurs when a physician fails to produce an outcome or deliver a service in accordance with a guarantee or promise. Invasion of privacy consists of a breach of the confidentiality of the physician-patient relationship. The information obtained by a physician in treating a patient is confidential and can be released only in accordance with the patient's consent, a court order or statute (e.g. child abuse and communicable disease reporting laws, laws governing release of medical record information, etc.). In the absence of one of these protections, private facts known to the physician only because of the physician-patient relationship may not be divulged privately for other than professional purposes if the patient is identified. Such facts may not be published or discussed publicly even for professional purposes if the patient is identified. Because information concerning parents or other family members may be obtained in treating a child, liability for such a breach of confidentiality may extend beyond the patient to third parties.

Criminal

Aside from the risk of being named in civil suits, a physician is exposed to the risk of criminal prosecution. In cases of death as a result of an extreme or outrageous breach of a physician's duty to a patient, the state may charge the physician with manslaughter. Such a charge may be made if the death is attributable to what the courts generally refer to as a physician's reckless or wanton conduct. According to *Black's Law Dictionary*, for conduct to be reckless "it must be such as to evince disregard of, or indifference to, consequences, under circumstances involving danger to the life or safety of others, although no harm was intended." *Black's* defines wanton as "recklessly disregardful of the rights or safety of others or of consequences."

In cases of failure to report suspected child abuse, drug abuse, certain types of wounds (e.g. gunshot and knife), venereal disease, or specified other communicable diseases in accordance with state statute, the physician may be charged with a misdemeanor. It should be noted that such reports, if made in good faith, will not expose a physician to a libel action in most jurisdictions.

MALPRACTICE—THE LEGAL PROCESS

Discovery

People turn to attorneys to discuss medical malpractice because they are angry. They perceive, correctly or incorrectly, that something has been done improperly during the course of diagnosis or treatment, and the physician has not responded adequately to their concerns. The attorney listens to the story and, if warranted, obtains and reviews the medical records, using consultant physicians if necessary.

At this point, if the attorney decides to pursue the case, the suit is started and the "discovery" phase of the legal process is begun. It is during this phase that attorneys use the power of subpoena to compel production of any document or physical evidence that might be relevant to their case, including: physician's personal records or notes, personnel files, policy and procedure manuals, maintenance records, budgets, formularies, incident reports, etc. The only documents not generally discoverable are the results of the hospital's peer review or quality assurance activities, defense counsel's work product, as protected by law. It should be noted that the attorney-client privilege prevents an attorney from disclosing information obtained in confidential communication with a client.

Once the attorney has reviewed and integrated all of this information, he or she may submit written interrogatories or requests for admission to the defendant, who must respond under oath and in writing within a specified number of days. Interrogatories are questions concerning anything that might lead to evidence relevant to the case. Requests for admission are statements of alleged fact pertaining to the case which must be admitted or denied. A fact that is admitted will be treated by the court as established and need not be proved at trial. Finally, the attorney may take the deposition of witnesses. A deposition is a formal interview, under oath, with counsel for all parties invited to attend. It usually takes place in an attorney's office and is transcribed by a reporter.

While the plaintiff's counsel is undertaking these activities, defense counsel is pursuing a similar course and making his or her own evaluation of the case. He or she will determine, along with the insurance carrier and, if the policy permits, the insured, whether to enter into settlement negotiations with plaintiff's counsel.

Trial

Most cases—approximately 90%—are settled or dropped. If the case goes to trial, however, the burden is on the plaintiff to demonstrate to the jury by a preponderance of the evidence the basic elements of a malpractice action: duty, breach of duty, injury and causal connection between the breach of duty and the injury. The plaintiff's injury and the causal connection between the alleged breach and the injury are often relatively easy to demonstrate. Thus, the outcome of a malpractice case usually depends upon the ability of plaintiff's counsel to demonstrate the extent of the physician's duty to the plaintiff and the breach of that duty.

The physician's duty to a patient arises out of the fiduciary or contractual nature of the physician-patient relationship. Because of the dependence of the patient on the physician or because of a contract implied by the consent of the patient to be treated and the physician to treat, the physician is duty bound to possess certain knowledge and skill and to apply them properly and with sound judgment and due care to the diagnosis and treatment of the patient's condition.

The standard of care required in carrying out this duty is an objective one. The physician must possess the knowledge and skill of a reasonable physician with similar training and must apply them with the judgment and care of that reasonable physician under similar circumstances (location, available equipment and personnel, emergency, etc.). Thus, the non-pediatrician confronted with a pediatric emergency is not judged by the same standard as the pediatrician, and the physician performing a procedure to save a life in an office is not judged by the same standard as the physician performing the same procedure in an emergency department. It should be noted that the standard is not that of an exceptionally well educated or highly skilled physician and that it does not require the physician to perform flawlessly at all times. Honest errors or mistakes in judgment are sometimes made by reasonable physicians in cases in which there are reasonable alternatives with respect to diagnosis or treatment, and performance of a procedure with a reasonable degree of skill may result in an error in a certain percentage of cases or under certain conditions. The standard is the reasonable physician, and he or she is not expected to be perfect.

Finally, with respect to the jury in a malpractice case, it is important to keep in mind that a physician will generally not be tried by a jury of his or her peers. The jury selection process is such that the jurors are usually not well educated or "professional" people. In addition, although in theory the cases are tried on the facts, sympathy and the ability to bear the financial burden frequently play a large part in the jury's decision.

RISK MANAGEMENT

Physician-Patient-Parent Relationship

There are two primary goals of risk management: to prevent suits and to minimize the cost of any suit which is not prevented. Prevention is, of course, the preferred method of management, and it is the method over which the physician has the greatest amount of control. As stated previously, people go to attorneys because they are angry. Cartwright reported that in the words of one plaintiff's attorney:

> In almost every case that comes into my office, particularly those involving the medical profession, the client is more angry about the doctor's lack of courtesy and consideration than about the injury or any other harm that took place. They complain that the doctor was short, uncommunicative, unfriendly, kept them waiting unmercifully and/or failed or refused to explain properly and communicate what was happening to them.

With this in mind, it is particularly important in an emergency department setting in which the wait is likely to be long, the processing through the system impersonal, and physician-patient-parent contact brief and without prior or subsequent history, to work very hard at establishing good physician-patient-parent relations. This aspect of a physician's emergency department practice cannot be overemphasized. Maximizing the time spent with patients and their parents will minimize the time spent with claims adjusters and attorneys.

Record Keeping to Prevent Suits

Equally as important as the physician-patient-parent relationship in preventing lawsuits is the quality of the medical record. Because it is the first document reviewed by parents, attorneys and their consulting physicians, its content and appearance could mean the difference between being sued or not in those cases in which there is an incorrect perception of improper treatment.

The medical record should be maintained as if it were a public document. The recorded information should be accurate and factual. All notes should be concise but complete. For efficiency, special forms, checklists and preprinted instruction sheets are encouraged. If instruction sheets are used, they should be written in the simplest language possible. Their use should be documented, and parents should be asked to sign a statement indicating that they received them and that they understand them.

The physician's notes should be consistent with the nurse's notes and the notes of any other discipline that appear in the chart. No extraneous comments should be made, and intramural battles should not be fought in the record. Comments about the difficulty of getting an x-ray performed or locating necessary personnel should not be made. Detailed and specific notes should be made with respect to the information given to parents about home care, danger signs and follow-up appointments. Unauthorized abbreviations should not be used, and insensitive observations should not be made (e.g. "FLK" or "funny looking kid").

Notes should always be dated and timed. Because so much activity is compressed within such a short span of time in an emergency situation, the exact time at which procedures are performed, or orders given or carried out, is frequently of crucial significance in determining the outcome of a malpractice case. The minutes and hours in the emergency department are the equivalent of days in an inpatient unit with respect to record keeping, and they should be treated accordingly.

In addition, it is extremely important that a chart never be altered. Whenever a change is made it should be initialed and dated, and the information being replaced should be struck out with one single line that does not destroy its legibility. It is very damaging to have even the appearance of a cover-up.

Statutes, Rules and Regulations, Policies and Procedures

Another means of preventing suits is to be familiar with and to practice in accordance with the various statutes, rules, regulations, policies and procedures that apply to practice in a particular hospital's emergency department. These include federal and state regulations on confidentiality; state laws governing treatment of minors, informed consent and the reporting of communicable disease, child abuse and specific types of injury; medical staff bylaws, rules and regulations; patient bill of rights; emergency department policy and procedure manual and formulary.

With respect to such policies, procedures, rules and regulations developed by the hospital and the medical staff, it is important to recognize that they establish a standard. If the standard cannot or will not be met, it should be changed or eliminated. It is better to have no standard at all than to have one which is not met.

Other Aspects of Suit Prevention

In addition to these general risk management guidelines for preventing suits, there are a number of more specific steps that should be taken. They are as follows.

1. Participate in quality assurance studies (mandated by the Joint Commission on the Accreditation of Hospitals (JCAH) for the purpose of discovering and correcting patient care problems)
2. Perform chart review with pre-established legal and medical criteria
3. Review and analyze personal and departmental incident statistics
4. Review and discuss records with all parents who want to see them; try to dissuade parents from looking at records alone
5. Be careful about statements made in public or in areas where conversations may be overheard
6. Encourage and attend hospital in-service programs on the legal aspects of medicine
7. Know how to contact both an administrator and an attorney 24 hours a day, 7 days a week
8. Know how to obtain a court order 24 hours a day, 7 days a week, or what to do if an order cannot be obtained.

Record Keeping to Minimize the Cost of Suits

To minimize the cost of any suit the quality of the medical record is again of primary importance. It is the most reliable source of information concerning the patient's treatment and in some cases may be the physician's only source. The parents who bring the suit will have had few, if any, similar encounters with an emergency department physician, and their recall will be excellent. The physician may subsequently have seen hundreds of patients under similar circumstances with similar symptoms and may remember nothing at all about this particular patient. The record may have to serve as a substitute for the physician's memory and should be maintained accordingly. In addition, the appearance of the record is very important. It should demonstrate a professional, competent and concerned approach to the patient. A record which demonstrates such an approach may do little or nothing to defend against an allegation of malpractice, but it gives plaintiff's counsel one less bit of evidence and may affect the degree of negligence perceived by the jury and, therefore, the size of the award.

Incident Reporting

Equally as important as the quality of the medical record in minimizing the cost of any suit is incident reporting. An "incident" is any unexpected occurrence that injures or has the potential to injure a patient or his/her family and should be reported immediately. Unfortunately, physicians have traditionally avoided reporting incidents. They have long held the view that if an incident is reported the chances of it resulting in a suit are increased. This may have been true 10 years ago, but with the coming of age of the consumer movement, the patient's increased expectation of cure, the publicity given malpractice cases, the increased litigiousness of society in general, and the physician's loss of stature in the eyes of the public, it is difficult to support this view today.

With all the players—attorneys, patients and their families, expert witnesses—looking so hard to discover malpractice, not reporting an incident would appear not to affect significantly the chance that it will result in a suit. It does, however, affect significantly the chance of being able to defend against a suit.

The reason for reporting incidents is to enable an insurance company to gather facts while they are still fresh in people's minds. It may be years before a suit arising out of a particular incident is filed. It is too late at that time to gather all of the factual information related to the event. It simply will not be recalled or will be recalled differently by different people. The plaintiff's almost total and sometimes self-serving recall will be difficult to rebut without all of the facts and without consistent explanations from all persons with knowledge of the incident. Thus, the resident's remark, reflecting a widely held belief, that "every time you file an incident report it costs the hospital $500" is simply not true. Because the cost of incident investigation is built into insurance premiums, it costs the hospital nothing and, indeed, may be saving the hospital and the physician thousands of dollars.

As stated previously, an incident report is discoverable. Consequently, as with the medical record, it should be treated as a public document. It should contain only very brief statements of fact. It should not contain opinions and should never describe an injury or condition as "iatrogenic." It should not be used to fight intramural battles or to reprimand other staff or employees for poor job performance. Because an incident report is discoverable, however, does not mean that it should be advertised. Copies should not be made; it should not be put on the chart, and a note that an incident report has been filed should not be made in the chart. If an incident occurs, the medical record need only include information that is necessary for the care of the child.

Once an incident report is received by the appropriate person, it is reviewed with respect to actual and potential consequences, and a detailed investigation is conducted if necessary. Depending upon state law and the manner in which the investigation is conducted, its results may or may not be discoverable. Keep in mind that incident investigation procedures are established in consultation with attorneys. If a damaging story is uncovered during the investigation, new discoverable documents do not have to be prepared. It may be quite desirable to prepare discoverable documents, however, when the investigation of an incident reveals no malpractice and offers a reasonable alternative explanation for an incident. Such a discoverable report may also be helpful in a situation in which malpractice is obvious (e.g. a child falling from an examining table and fracturing his or her skull) but in which there may have been mitigating circumstances or contributory negligence on the part of the parent (such as he or she offering to watch the child or stating after the fact that the child is hyperactive and has always been difficult to control).

INFORMED CONSENT

Because of the fiduciary or dependent nature of the physician-patient relationship and the right of an individual to self-determination, physicians are required to obtain informed consent from patients or, in the case of minors, their parents or guardians, prior to undertaking diagnostic or therapeutic procedures. For purposes of consent a guardian is a person or agency appointed by the court or a person designated by the parents on a temporary basis in their absence such as a teacher or relative. Guardians designated by parents must be adults and the designation must be written and signed.

The physician who actually performs the procedure should obtain the consent. Not only will this help promote a good relationship between the physician and the patient or parent, it will also assure that the information upon which the consent is based is accurate. The information should be conveyed in terms that the patient or parent can understand, and all questions should be answered. Written consent forms should be used, but it cannot be overemphasized that such forms do not represent informed consent in and of themselves. They are merely evidence that an informed consent has been obtained. Like all evidence, they may be refuted, and their validity is subject to determination of the jury.

To be informed, the consent must be given with an understanding as to the following aspects of the procedure under consideration.

1. Nature, scope and benefits of the procedure
2. Risks associated with the procedure
3. Risks associated with not undergoing the procedure
4. Risks and benefits of alternative procedures.

The extent of the disclosure required by the physician in order to enable a patient or parent to make an informed decision, particularly with respect to the risks associated with a procedure, is the most difficult area of the informed consent doctrine for both physicians and the courts. Legislation has been passed in over half of the states in an attempt to ease the difficulty. These statutes, along with the common law developed by the courts in the other states, establish two standards which may be used to determine the adequacy of the physician's disclosure in obtaining consent.

Disclosure Standards

The first disclosure standard is a professional one. The physician must disclose that which is ordinarily disclosed by a reasonable physician in similar circumstances. The second disclosure standard, and the one being recognized in more and more jurisdictions, is a material risk standard which requires the physician to disclose all of the information that an individual needs in order to make a decision. Some courts use a subjective test for materiality, determining it from the specific plaintiff's point of view, but most courts use an objective test which attempts to determine that information which would be material for the reasonable patient called upon to make the decision in question. For the most part, these standards are exclusive of one another, but some jurisdictions do apply them both.

Regardless of the standard used, the adequacy of the physician's disclosure is determined by the jury. The members of the jury consider expert testimony in determining whether the professional standard has been met, and they consider the severity and incidence of the risk under consideration in determining whether the material risk standard has been met. With respect to the latter, the jury's actual determination in various cases has been as follows:

1. 1/100 chance of a loss of hearing: disclosure required
2. 3/100 chance of death or paralysis: disclosure required
3. 3/200 chance of the loss of an eye: disclosure not required
4. 1/800,000 chance of developing aplastic anemia: disclosure not required
5. 1/250 to 1/500 chance of perforating the esophagus: disclosure not required.

These are just examples of decisions that have been made by juries, and it must be kept in mind that each situation will be reviewed on its own merits. For example, it seems reasonable that more complete disclosure of risks would be necessary when a reasonable alternative to the proposed procedure exists, and less complete disclosure of risks would be necessary if no alternative exists and failure to submit to the procedure would be dangerous for the patient.

Exceptions to the Disclosure Rule

There are, of course, exceptions to the requirement that the physician disclose information in accordance with either a professional or material risk standard when obtaining consent. Disclosure is not required when the risk is common knowledge or is already known to the patient. It is not required when the risk is not recognized by the medical profession or is one that exists only if the procedure is performed negligently. It is not required if the patient requests not to be informed, although this should never be encouraged by the physician, and if such a request is made it should be documented in the chart. Disclosure is also not required in situations where it would be detrimental to the physical or psychological health of the patient.

This last exception is commonly referred to as "therapeutic privilege," and it is a privilege which must be exercised with caution. Our legal system gives parents the right to make decisions with respect to the medical treatment of their children, and any infringement upon that right will be examined very closely by the courts. One situation in which therapeutic privilege might be exercised in the care of children in an emergency department is the discussion of the risk of paralysis as a result of a lumbar puncture. Given the severity of the risk, it might be one which would ordinarily be disclosed or which would be considered material despite its low incidence of occurrence. The risk of undetected meningitis, however, might be significant enough to justify withholding mention of the paralysis risk. An attorney should be consulted before establishing any policy concerning this issue.

Exceptions to the Parental Consent Rule

There are also exceptions to the requirement that a parent or guardian consent to treatment of a minor. All states have statutory or case law which defines emancipated minors and gives them the right to consent, to medical treatment. Other general exceptions to the requirement of parental consent, as described below, include life threatening emergencies, mature minors, and the unavailability of parents. In addition, some states allow treatment of minors without parental consent for venereal disease or other contagious disease.

The emancipated minor is generally one who has been married, graduated from high school or otherwise achieved independence from parental care, custody and control. Depending upon the jurisdiction, pregnant minors may or may not be considered emancipated and, if they are, may or may not revert to minority status following termination of the pregnancy. Over half of the states allow a minor to seek pregnancy care without the consent of a parent.

Each jurisdiction's legislation and case law determine the definition of "emergency." In general, however, emergencies are those situations in which there is an immediate threat to the child's life or permanent health. Mature minors are generally required to be at least 15 years of age and to be intellectually and emotionally capable of understanding their medical condition and the implications of their decisions with respect to their health. The unavailability of parents will justify the lack of consent only if their unavailability affects the timeliness of the treatment and if the treatment is necessary, even though not of an emergency nature. In such a situation, when alternative treatments with significantly different risks are available, the institution of treatment without consent should be delayed as long as is reasonable.

With the exception of the emancipated minor and, depending upon state law or physician judgment, pregnancy care or treatment for venereal disease or other communicable diseases, reasonable attempts should be made to contact the parents in all of these cases, and such attempts should be documented in the chart. Even after the treatment, reasonable attempts should be made to contact the parents in order to explain what was done and to answer any questions. This is not a legal requirement, but it is important with respect to the physician-patient-parent relationship.

When Consent Is Refused

If consent to a procedure or treatment cannot be obtained, this fact should be documented in the chart. This will help shift the responsibility to the parents in the event of an adverse outcome and will be helpful if they deny having rejected the recommended procedure or treatment. A specific example of this is the procedure for signing out against medical advice (AMA). Such a procedure should be used whenever a patient leaves the emergency department without being released by a physician. It is important, when signing out a child, that the parents understand the possible consequences of their action. The issue is essentially one of informed consent, and the appropriate information, if known by the physician, must be made available to the parents when they are making the decision to remove their child.

If a child's life is endangered by his or her parents' refusal to give consent to treatment, it may be necessary to obtain a court order to treat the child. It should be kept in mind that courts generally will not issue orders in violation of parental wishes if the situation is not life threatening. The right of parents to determine the medical treatment to be rendered their children is well established in the law and will generally not be infringed upon by the courts except in very limited circumstances involving life and death. The courtroom, for example, is not the place to bring a disagreement with parents over the method to be used in closing a laceration. The physician must abide by the parents' wishes in such a case.

In special circumstances, many states permit treatment of minors against the wishes of parents without a court order. Generally, in cases of suspected child abuse in these states, if the physician has reasonable cause to suspect that the child is in danger and if there is not sufficient time to obtain a court order, the child may be taken into protective custody (by the hospital or child protective services agency) and treated appropriately. Such custody is limited in time and a court order must be obtained as soon as possible.

SUMMARY

The major legal risk for any physician is malpractice, the failure to meet the standard of care set by the reasonable physician under a given set of conditions. Emergency department physicians treating children are no exception, and, indeed, for various reasons the risk is greater for them than for many other physicians. In general, suits alleging malpractice can be prevented or their cost can be minimized by developing good physician-patient-parent relationships, by maintaining medical records as if they were public documents, by reporting incidents, and by being familiar with and practicing in accordance with all relevant statutes, policies, procedures, rules and regulations.

References

Brown R, Truitt R: *The Right of Minors to Medical Treatment*, 28 *DePaul L. Rev.* 289, 1979.

Cartwright R: How to Protect the Professional From Consumerism. In *National Medicolegal Symposium*, pp. 84–85, San Francisco, March 17–20, 1977.

George J: *Law and Emergency Care.* C. V. Mosby, St. Louis, 1980.

Ludlum J: *Informed Consent.* American Hospital Assoc. 1978.

Miller L: Informed consent: I. *JAMA* 244: 2100, 1980.

Miller L: Informed consent: II. *JAMA* 244: 2347, 1980.

Miller L: Informed consent: III. *JAMA* 244: 2556, 1980.

Miller L: Informed consent: IV *JAMA* 244: 2661, 1980.

Wecht C: Physician's liability to non-patient third parties. *Trial*, p. 34, July 1979.

SECTION **VII**

Procedures

Illustrated Techniques of Pediatric Emergency Procedures

A. Michael Broennle, M.D., Michael H. Gewitz, M.D., Steven D. Handler, M.D., Charles G. Howell, M.D., David Jaffe, M.D., Robert G. Kettrick, M.D., William P. Potsic, M.D., Richard Ruddy, M.D., John M. Templeton, Jr., M.D., AND Josephine J. Templeton, M.D.

INTRODUCTION

This section, "Illustrated Techniques of Pediatric Emergency Procedures," provides a compendium of procedures often necessary in the emergency department. It includes methods for preparing and restraining the child, diagnostic techniques, and urgent therapeutic procedures.

Although they are not performed only by emergency physicians, the procedures in this section are often necessary for the care of children in the emergency department. Depending on the experience of the emergency physician, he or she may perform these procedures alone or with the collaboration of other specialists.

This section first describes general principles in patient preparation and restraint. Next, blood sampling and techniques for achieving vascular access are reviewed. Finally, we discuss the procedures pertinent to each region of the body (i.e., chest, abdomen, etc.).

The indications and potential complications for each procedure are listed, but the reader should refer to the appropriate chapters in the text for a more complete discussion on the clinical application of these techniques and the use of alternative approaches.

1.0. PREPARATION OF THE CHILD

The preparation of the child and family is a most important task to perform diagnostic and therapeutic procedures on children effectively in the emergency department. Many of the demonstrated procedures are time-consuming to the emergency physician, ancillary staff, patient, and family. Prepare the ancillary staff to assist in the procedure's performance to minimize delay. Have the appropriate assistance and necessary equipment available in the emergency department. Consider whether the emergency department is the appropriate location and environment in which the consequences and complications of a procedure can be cared for. Delay in care for other potentially ill children must be minimized.

Except when the procedure is immediately necessary for a life-threatening emergency, prepare the child and parents beforehand to obtain approval and support for the procedure. During the advanced life support of a resuscitation or other life-threatening situation, the emergency department staff should provide a professional person to privately prepare the family for the ensuing problems. In all cases, permission from the parent or guardian is mandatory, and should also be sought from the child, except when it seriously delays care. An informative, but efficient discussion of risks and benefits of the procedure for a particular child almost always reassures the parents of the need for the procedure. Assess the child's developmental maturity and use it to determine how capable the child is of understanding and cooperating in the performance of the procedure. There are substantial variations in developmental age which affect the fears of children.

Specifically, the parents need to understand the necessity of the procedure and of proper restraint or sedation of their child to minimize discomfort and maximize efficiency. Warn the parents of possible complications. Make them aware of the effects of sedation and of equipment that will be attached to their child, and of any discomfort subsequent to the procedure. The assurance that restraint may minimize repeated discomfort cannot be overemphasized. Last, prepare oneself to do the procedure. It is of no help to be upset, or angry, at having to perform a task on a child.

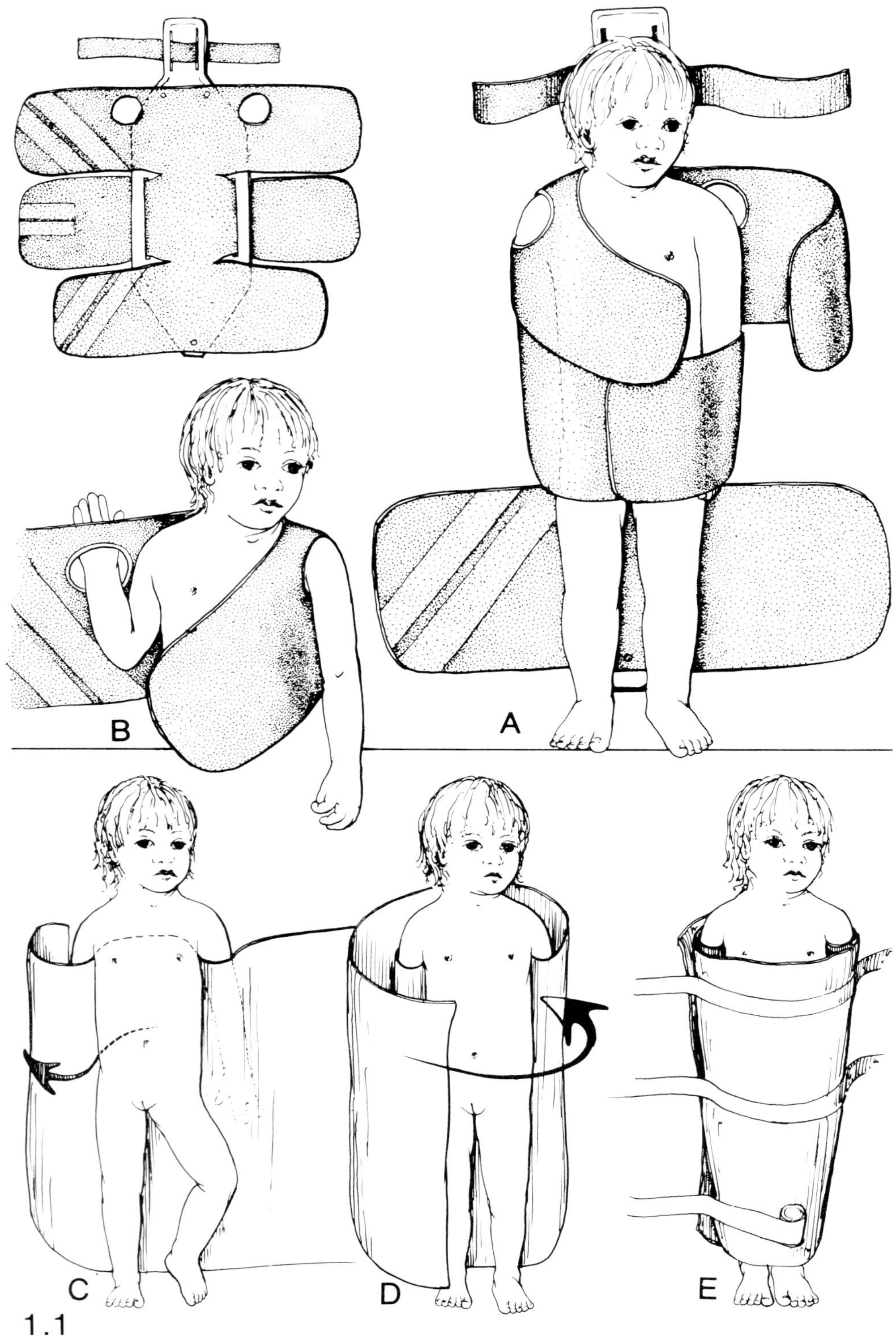

1.1

1.1. RESTRAINTS

INDICATIONS

Restraint should be used in performance of all procedures in which the child may be unmanageable, where it is possible they may directly hurt themselves, or indirectly delay treatment. Physical restraints are usually more effective than human restraints and are necessary in most infants, toddlers and preschool children.

COMPLICATIONS

1. Bruising, edema.
2. Vascular compromise (too tight a restraint or for excessive time).
3. Mistrust (if not discussed truthfully).

PROCEDURES

Papoose. Figure 1.1*A* represents the example of the papoose which is commonly used for restraint during repair of lacerations and other wounds. It is used to expose the head and extremities with minimal risk to the child.

After explaining the procedure to the family, open the papoose across the emergency department stretcher. Place the child supine on the papoose and expose the body area necessary for treatment. Beginning with the midabdominal restraints, cover the child across the midline with the Velcro-lined sides (Fig. 1.1*A*). Better exposure of the extremities, such as the hand, is obtained by flexion of the area under the harness (Fig. 1.1*B*). Before starting a wound repair or other procedure, reassess the immobility of the child and correct it if not adequate.

Mummy. The mummy is an alternative restraint to use while treating emergency problems of the head, especially trauma. By slight variation it also provides access to the distal extremities.

Prepare the patient and family for the procedures. Fold a bed sheet so the width measures from the axilla to the heel of the child. Stand the child on the bed, and place the bed sheet behind his back, under the axilla, and in front of his arms as in Figure 1.1*C*, with the short end of the sheet extending behind one arm. With the child standing, bring the long end of the sheet on the child's other side around the back to the front and across the trunk again to behind the child, as in Figure 1.1*D*. Lay the child supine or prone to best expose the injury to be treated. Extend several lengths of 2- or 3-inch width adhesive tape across the patient attaching it to the sides of the stretcher to firmly hold the trunk in place (Fig. 1.1*E*). Flexion of arm or shortening of the sheet width on the leg can usually suffice to expose the distal extremities to the operator.

Physical Restraint

There are many physical methods to restrain children for emergency procedures. Frequently a single assistant can grasp and immobilize a child. The specific positioning for several different procedures are shown with individual procedures. The assistant must be firm enough to prevent movement that would make the procedure more difficult to perform or more likely to induce complications. However, care should be taken not to use excessive force causing injury. In conjunction with restraint, sedation and local anesthetic may be indicated.

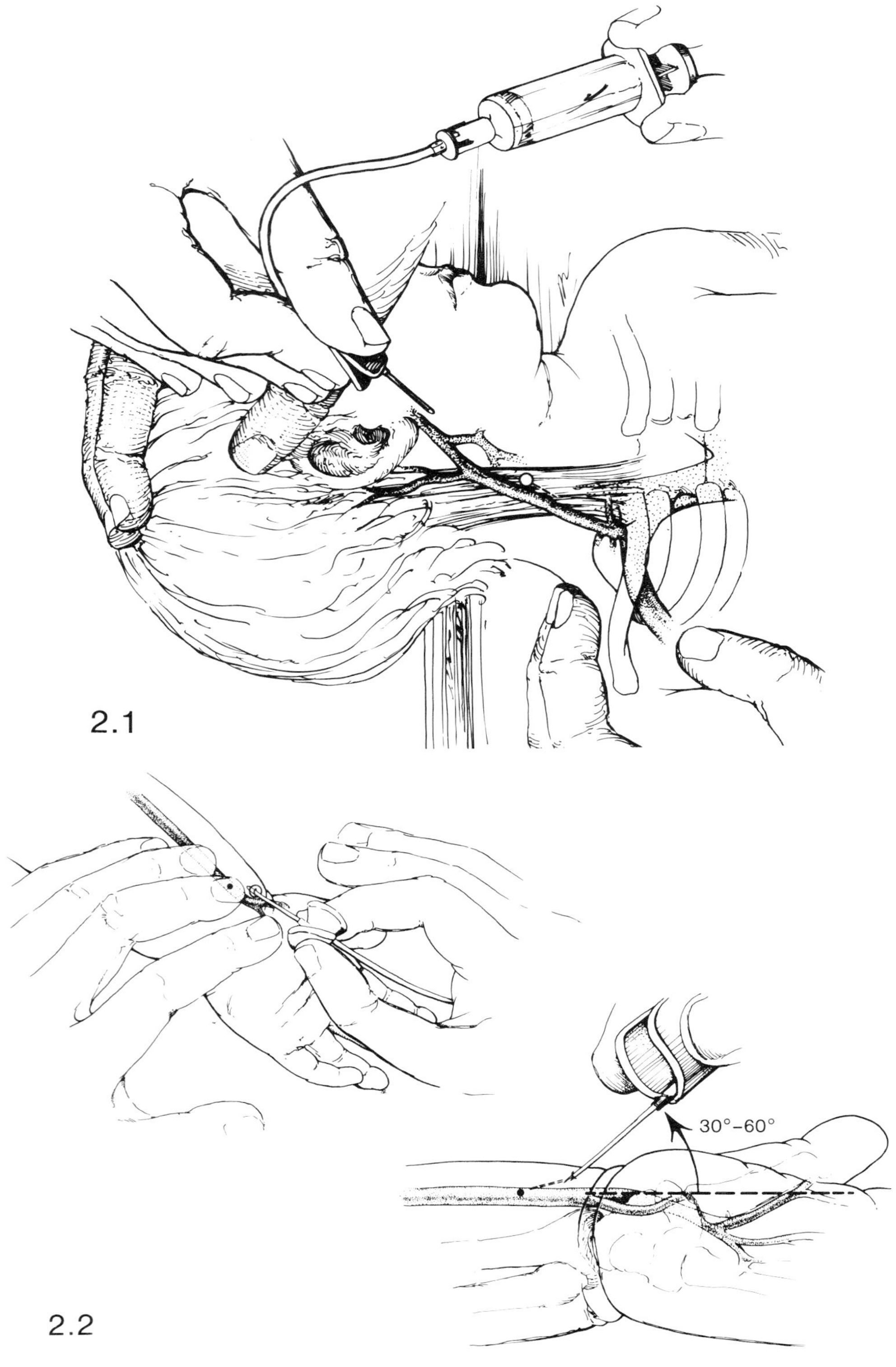
2.1
2.2
30°–60°

2.1 EXTERNAL JUGULAR VENIPUNCTURE

INDICATIONS

Venous blood sampling in infants less than 1 to 2 years of age with inadequate peripheral veins.

COMPLICATIONS

1. Hematoma.
2. Pneumothorax (apical)
3. Infection.

PROCEDURE

Place the infant on the examining table in the supine position with the infant's shoulders 7 to 10 cm from the end of the table. The assistant then holds the shoulder ipsilateral to the external jugular to be punctured with one hand and places the other hand over the zygoma and forehead, turning the head toward the contralateral shoulder and dropping it 15 to 20° over the table top. Have the assistant lean over the patient to stabilize the trunk.

The skin overlying the vein is cleansed with povidone-iodine solution circumferentially several times; wipe the area with 70% alcohol followed by dry sterile gauze. Attach a 21 or 23 gauge butterfly needle, 3 cm long, to a 5- to 10-ml syringe and check for patency. Stimulate the infant to cry to improve filling of the vessel. Align the butterfly needle parallel to the vessel as shown in Figure 2.1 and pierce the skin overlying or just next to the vein approximately ½ to ⅔ of the distance between the angle of the jaw and the shoulder. The puncture will often improve venous engorgement by stimulating the infant to cry. Then with constant suction on the syringe, advance the needle to enter the external jugular vein, keeping the needle steady with the heel of the hand on the infant's neck. After withdrawing an adequate blood sample, suction is relieved on the syringe and the needle withdrawn. Apply sterile dry gauze immediately. The assistant should bring the infant to the upright position and compress the venipuncture site for 5 min.

2.2 RADIAL ARTERIAL PUNCTURE

INDICATIONS

Procurement of blood samples, especially for arterial blood gas analysis.

COMPLICATIONS

1. Arterial occlusion by thrombosis/hematoma.
2. Infection—thrombophlebitis.
3. Ischemia (especially if the ulnar collateral circulation is insufficient).

PROCEDURE

Prepare the equipment—a 22 to 25 gauge, 3-cm butterfly needle on a 1- to 3-ml syringe. The syringe should be flushed with a small amount of sodium heparin (1000 units/ml) and then emptied.

The assistant must firmly restrain the infant or child, holding the arm just proximal to the wrist in supination, hyperextending the hand approximately 20 to 30°. Assess the adequacy of both radial and ulnar arterial flow by palpation before the puncture.

Cleanse the skin overlying the radial artery with povidone-iodine solution followed by 70% alcohol and then dry with sterile gauze. Using gentle pressure with the palpating fingers locate the vessel. Hold the needle as shown in Fig. 2.2 and pierce the skin between index and middle finger of the palpating hand, directing the needle at 30 to 60° from the horizontal plane. When the needle enters the radial artery, blood begins to flow into the tubing. It will freely flow into a glass syringe, but suction is needed to fill plastic syringes. If the initial thrust is unsuccessful, attempt to enter the artery from a different angle, either medially or laterally as determined by careful palpation. Because the blood gas analysis more reliably reflects the respiratory status of the child who is not agitated, every effort should be made to minimize the number of punctures.

After obtaining the specimen, quickly remove the needle and apply pressure to the puncture site for 5 min. Any air bubbles must be immediately removed from the sample to maintain accurate results.

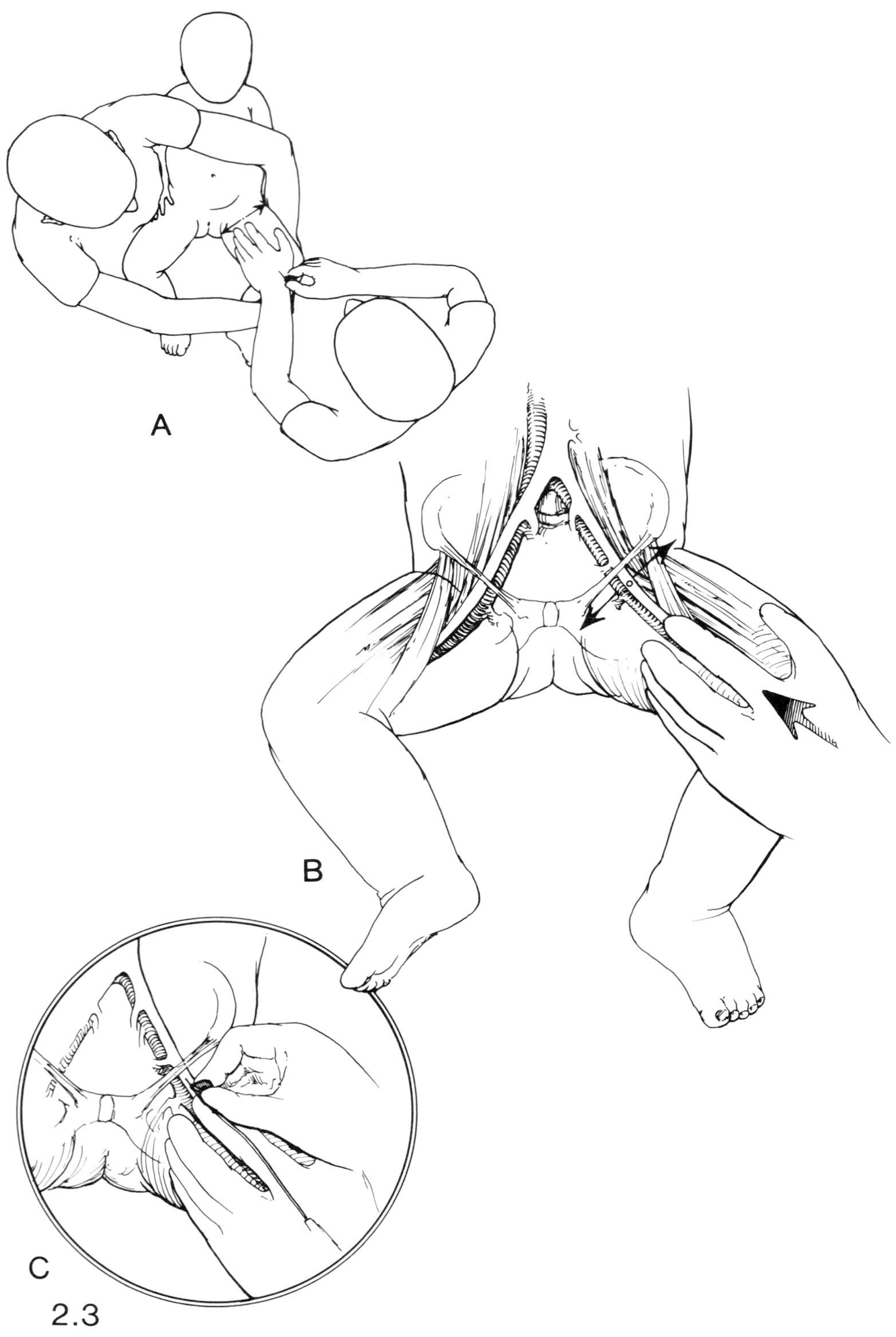
A
B
C
2.3

2.3 FEMORAL ARTERY/VEIN PUNCTURE

INDICATIONS

1. Arterial or venous blood sampling during acute resuscitations.
2. Venous blood sampling in infants with poor peripheral veins.

CONTRAINDICATIONS

Avoid it in children who have hypocoagulable and hypercoagulable states or cardiac shunts.

COMPLICATIONS

1. Hematoma of femoral triangle, including femoral nerve.
2. Thrombosis—femoral artery or vein.
3. Abscess.
4. Osteomyelitis/arthritis—proximal femur, hip joint.
5. Bladder or bowel puncture.

PROCEDURE

Prepare the necessary equipment—21 or 23 gauge, 3-cm butterfly needle, 5- to 10-ml syringe, povidone-iodine solution, 70% alcohol, sterile gauze, and blood sample containers.

Have the assistant restrain the infant. Two illustrated methods include the one in Figure 2.3*A*, where the trunk and contralateral leg are restrained by the assistant, and the ipsilateral leg by the operator. The other is diagrammed with the illustration for suprapubic bladder aspiration (see Fig. 11.2), where the assistant leans over the infant with arms pressing on the infant's arms above, and holding the distal thighs below in the frog leg position.

Gently flex the knee and externally rotate the hip to identify the landmarks of the femoral triangle. Locate the inguinal ligament, and gently palpate midway between the anterior superior iliac spine and pubic symphysis, for the femoral artery and vein (Fig. 2.3*B*). The empty space between flexor and extensor muscles of the medial thigh will also reveal the location of the vessels.

Cleanse the femoral triangle circumferentially with povidone-iodine several times, then wipe it off with 70% alcohol and dry with sterile gauze. With the palpating index finger, relocate the femoral artery approximately 2 cm below the inguinal ligament. Use the palm of this hand to control the movement of the child's leg. Minimize the infant's crying, as this will make the abdominal musculature taut and the transmitted pulse difficult to palpate.

Direct the butterfly needle 60 to 75° from the horizontal, just proximal to the palpating finger, as shown in Figure 2.3*C*. Then puncture the skin over the pulsatile femoral artery or 0.5 cm medially depending on desire for arterial or venous blood. Apply constant suction to the syringe as the needle is advanced into the thigh to assure that blood is obtained on entering the vessel. Avoid uncontrolled leg movements by the infant as this easily makes it possible to lose alignment of the needle and vessels. It is acceptable to withdraw the needle to just below skin surface and reattempt vessel puncture after shifting the medial or lateral alignment of the needle tip. After obtaining the sample, stop suction on the syringe. Concomitant with needle withdrawal, the assistant should provide constant pressure on the puncture site for longer than 5 min with a sterile gauze.

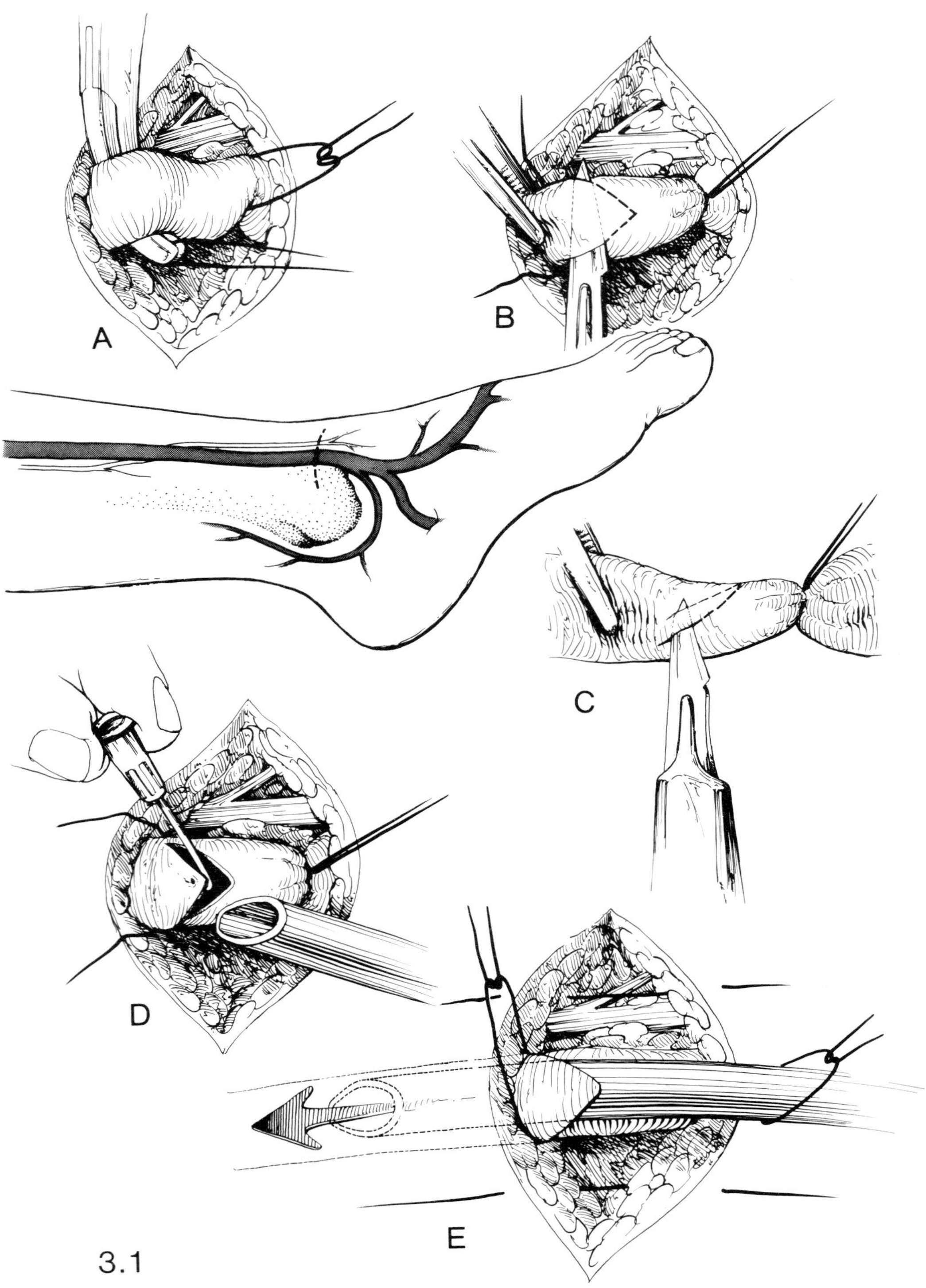

3.1

3.1 GREATER SAPHENOUS VEIN CUTDOWN

INDICATIONS

Emergency intravenous access if percutaneous attempts are unsuccessful. It is especially useful because of its consistent location when venous access is necessary during cardiopulmonary resuscitation.

COMPLICATIONS

1. Bleeding.
2. Infection/phlebitis.
3. Laceration of sensory nerves.
4. Catheter loss into the vein.

PROCEDURE

Prepare the child and the equipment needed for the procedure. Place the patient supine and externally rotate the leg and ankle. Restrain the patient's foot while allowing proper exposure of the area.

Palpate the medial malleolus of the tibia and anterior tibial tendon between which the saphenous vein lies. Cleanse the ankle with povidone-iodine solution followed by 70% alcohol and dry with sterile gauze. Wearing sterile gloves, drape the area with sterile towels leaving a rectangular 5- by 8-cm field exposed over the ankle. Inject 1% lidocaine to achieve local anesthesia at the incision site.

After relocating the landmarks, make a 2-cm transverse incision with a No. 15 scalpel blade just proximal and anterior to the bony prominence as shown by the dotted lines (Fig. 3.1). Do not use a proximal tourniquet as it may increase capillary bleeding and obscure the field.

With a curved hemostat, spread the subcutaneous tissue proximal from distal along the course of the vein. One can locate the vein by lifting up the tissue directly on top of the fascia. Just anterior to the vein there is a sensory nerve, which will be spared if the vein is well separated from the surrounding tissue. Isolate the vein and pass two 3-0 or 4-0 silk ties underneath it. Tie the distal suture, as is shown in Figure 3.1*A*, and hold it with a clamp distally. Then loosely knot the proximal tie.

As shown in Figure 3.1*B*, incise the vein after applying traction to it by exerting tension on the distal ligature. Use a No. 11 scalpel blade and insert its sharp point at 45° from the horizontal to produce a vein wall flap half way through the vein. Figure 3.1*C* shows the procedure in small veins where grasping the vein on either side flattens it out. This exposes the lateral vein surface and makes it easier to incise the 45° flap.

It is helpful to make a hook to hold the proximal vein flap. Use a hemostat to bend the tip of a 22 gauge needle into a curved hook. Lift the top of the vein flap with it to expose the venostomy opening.

Prepare the catheter for passage into the vein by attaching it distally to a stopcock and 10-ml syringe. Fill the catheter system with routine flushing solution. If it is a small vein, a beveled catheter end can be passed more easily. To prepare it, cut the catheter at a 30 to 45° angle. Then trim the edges to prevent a sharp edge from lacerating the vein.

Next, as in Figure 3.1*D*, hold the vein flap open with the curved hook and insert the beveled catheter through the vein opening and up the leg. Figure 3.1*E* shows the technique for advancing the catheter once patency is confirmed. Running intravenous fluids, while simultaneously advancing the catheter, dilates the vein and facilitates passage of 15 cm of catheter. At this point, secure the proximal tie around both the vein and indwelling catheter, and distal to the cutdown site, suture the catheter to the skin. The incision may be closed with several sutures. Apply a sterile dressing.

Rather than making an incision in the vein, the emergency physician may choose to insert an "over-the-needle" catheter into the vessel once it has been exposed. The technique is similar to that of percutaneous venipuncture except the vein is under direct visualization. After the catheter has been advanced and patency confirmed, secure it and close the incision as described above.

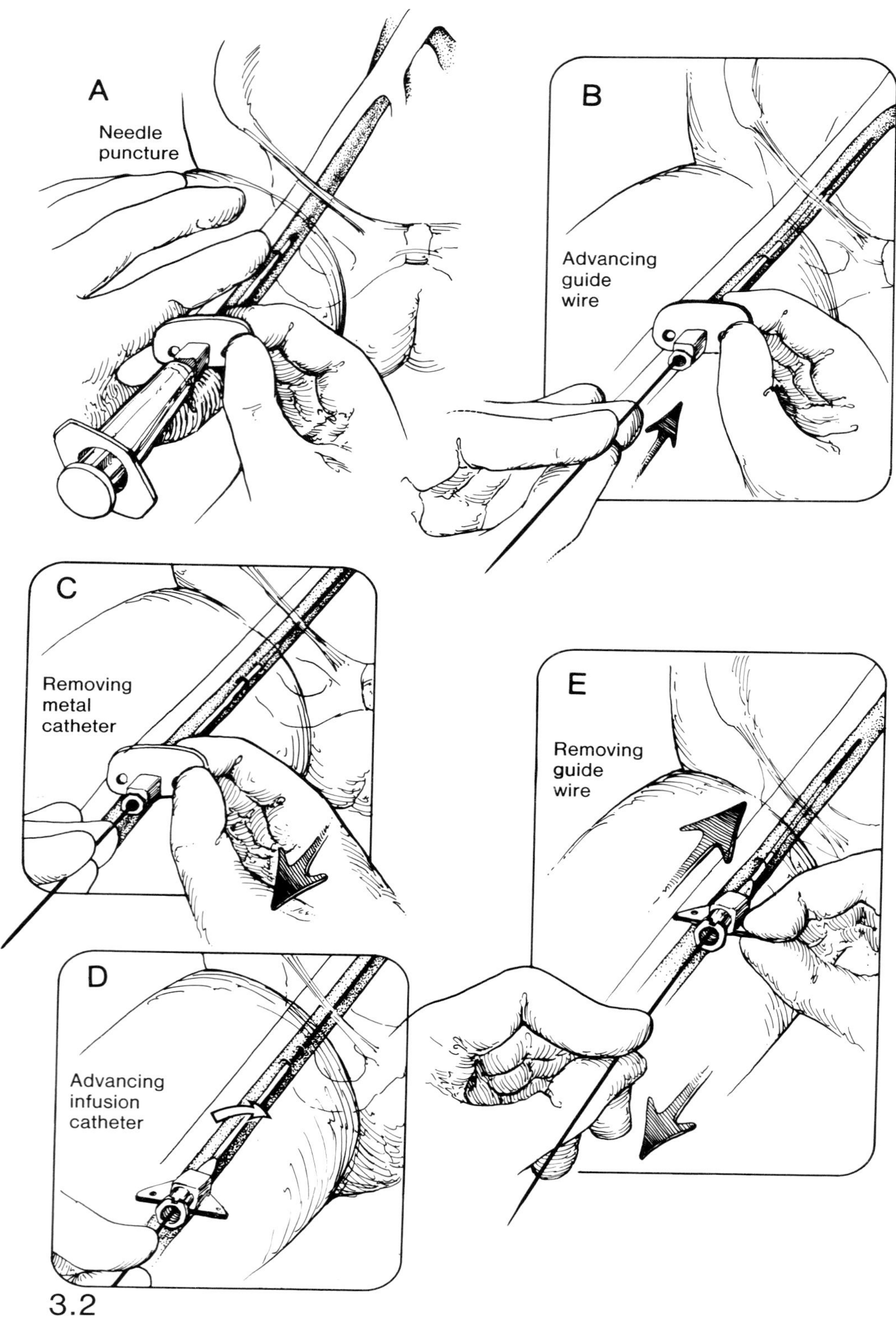
A
Needle puncture
B
Advancing guide wire
C
Removing metal catheter
D
Advancing infusion catheter
E
Removing guide wire

3.2

3.2. CENTRAL VENOUS CATHETER: PERCUTANEOUS SELDINGER TECHNIQUE

INDICATIONS

Emergency access to the central venous circulation. The femoral vein is more accessible than the external jugular vein during cardiopulmonary resuscitation but should be avoided when there is possible interruption of the inferior vena cava.

COMPLICATIONS

1. Arterial or venous laceration; 2. Infection; 3. Catheter fragment in circulation.

EQUIPMENT

Cook catheter (metal catheter, guide wire, No. 10 or 11 infusion catheter), sterile drapes and gloves, 5-10 ml syringe, T-connector, 3-way stop cock, infusion fluid, povidone-iodine solution, 70% alcohol, sterile gauze pads.

PROCEDURE

Femoral Approach

Restrain the lower extremities and trunk of the child. Externally rotate the hips to facilitate palpation of the femoral triangle. Palpate the femoral artery 1.5 cm below the inguinal ligament, half way between the anterior superior iliac spine and symphysis pubis. The femoral vein lies 0.5 cm medially.

Cleanse the site with povidine-iodine solution and 70% alcohol. Dry with gauze. Wearing sterile gloves, drape the area. Check all equipment, and attach a 5 ml syringe to the metal catheter.

Repalpate the femoral artery. Hold the metal catheter parallel to the blood vessel and 30° above the horizontal (Fig. 3.2*A*). Stabilize it with the heel of the lateral aspect of the hand against the child's leg.

Puncture the skin ½ cm medially to the arterial pulsation. Apply suction to the syringe while advancing the needle. When there is venous blood return, advance the metal catheter 1–2 mm and recheck for flow. Stabilize it against the thigh, and detach the syringe. Place a gloved thumb over the catheter to decrease bleeding.

Using the free hand, grasp the guide wire near the end that has a soft tip. Insert the wire through the metal catheter (Fig. 3.2*B*). Pass the end several centimeters past the catheter tip cephalad into the vein. If it does not pass easily, the metal catheter is usually not in the lumen of the vein. If so, remove the wire and reposition the catheter to establish blood flow again. Then replace the wire.

Stabilize the wire (against the thigh distally) with the hand which inserted it (Fig. 3.2*C*). Withdraw the metal catheter from the vein along the wire. Move the hand stabilizing the guide wire proximally once the wire is exposed at the puncture site. Support the wire and pull the metal catheter off the guide wire. Pick up the infusion catheter at the proximal end and advance it over the wire to the skin entry site. Twist it at the skin entry site (Fig. 3.2*D*) and advance it over the wire in a cephalad direction while stabilizing the wire distally. This rotary motion is helpful to enlarge the cutaneous puncture site.

Lastly, as in Figure 3.2*E*, withdraw the wire while holding the catheter in place; blood flows immediately if the vein has been cannulated. Attach the infusion system to the catheter; tape or suture it in place. Larger catheters can be placed by reinserting the wire, and increasing the size of the skin entry site.

External Jugular Vein (not illustrated)

Use the same technique as described above to cannulate the external jugular vein. After ensuring a patent airway and neck stabilization, use the landmarks and puncture site described in Procedure 2.1. Then follow the technique as described above for the femoral puncture. It may be helpful to use a guide wire which has a flexible, curved end to help make the turn towards the right atrium on entering the subclavian vein.

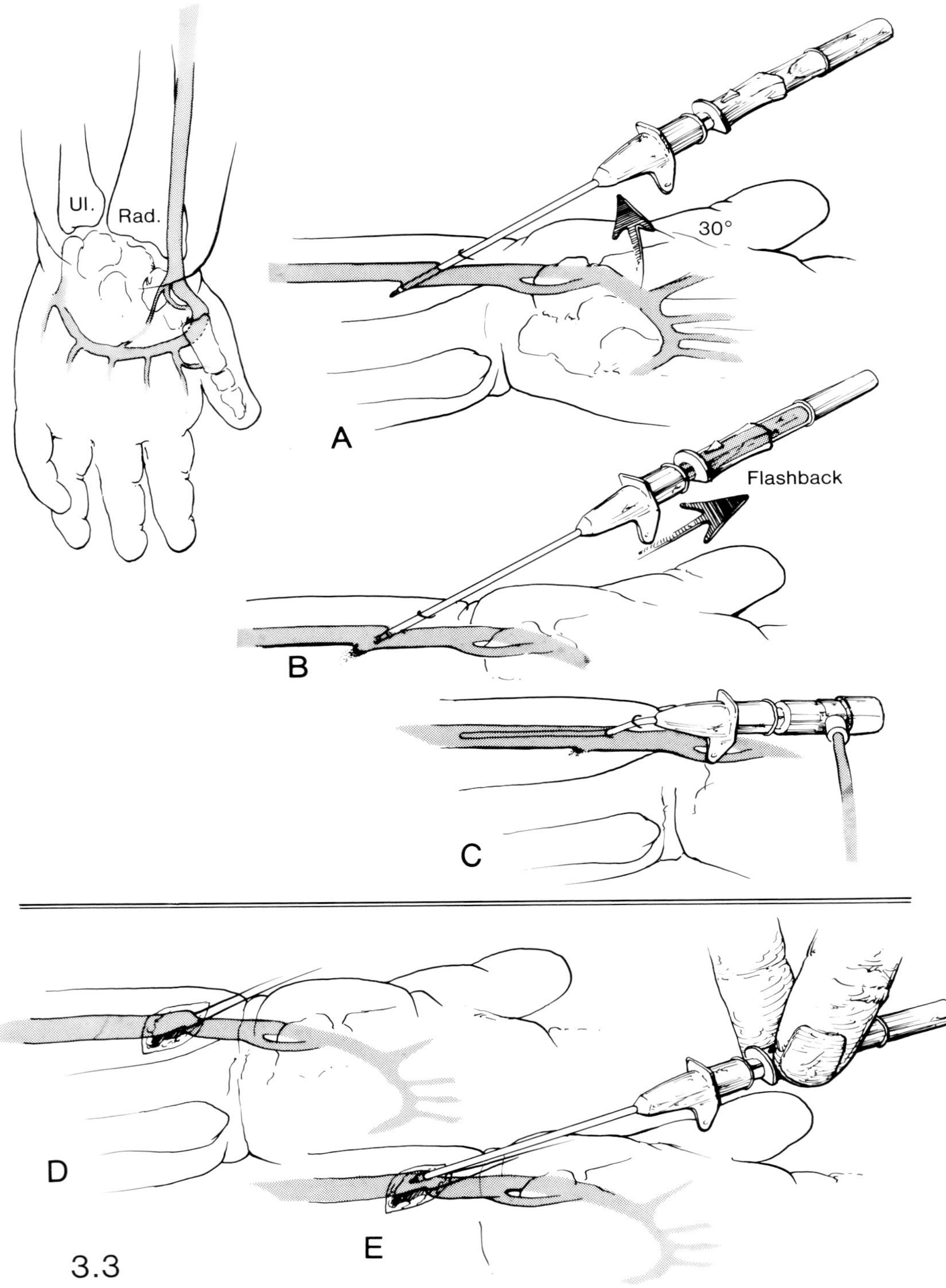
Ul.
Rad.
30°
A
Flashback
B
C
D
E
3.3

3.3. RADIAL ARTERY CATHETERIZATION

Percutaneous and Cutdown Techniques

INDICATIONS

Percutaneous

1. Frequent blood gas determinations
2. Continuous blood pressure monitoring in cardiovascular collapse/shock syndromes and major surgical procedures.

Cutdown

1. Infants weighing less than 5 kg.
2. Emergency arterial access if percutaneous attempts are unsuccessful.

COMPLICATIONS

1. Hemorrhage
2. Embolization or thrombosis
3. Ischemia and/or infarction of hand.
4. Infection.

Caution. No medications or hyperosmolar solutions should be administered through peripheral arterial catheters.

EQUIPMENT

Arm board, 1- and 2-inch tape, 1% lidocaine solution in a 3-ml syringe with a 25 gauge needle, 18 or 19 gauge sterile needle, povidone-iodine solution, 70% alcohol, gauze pads, catheter (20 or 22 gauge Angiocath® or Medicut®), T-connector, 5- or 10-ml syringe with heparin flush solution (10 units heparin/ml), *Cutdown tray*—drapes, scalpel blade, 4-0 silk ties, hemostats.

PROCEDURE

Percutaneous

Prepare the patient and the necessary equipment. Secure the child's hand and forearm to an arm board with the wrist in moderate extension using a gauze roll under the wrist. Cleanse the wrist with povidone-iodine several times followed by 70% alcohol and dry with sterile gauze. Locate the radial artery by palpation distally over the distal volar forearm as shown in Figure 3.3. Then, assess collateral circulation by palpation of the ulnar pulse. After infiltration with lidocaine make a puncture wound of the skin over the radial artery 0.5 to 1.0 cm proximal to the distal wrist crease.

Remove the syringe from the "over-the-needle" catheter system. Again, palpate the radial artery proximally to the previous puncture site while simultaneously advancing the catheter through the site. After puncturing the artery and obtaining blood flow, advance the needle 1 to 2 mm further; then hold the needle steady and slowly advance the catheter into the vessel.

If blood flow never occurs or stops spontaneously, the needle tip may have penetrated to posterior wall of the vessel as shown in Figure 3.3*A*. Remove the needle, holding the catheter steady, and begin pulling back the catheter a millimeter at a time until a sudden flash of arterial blood is identified (Fig. 3.3*B*). Then, advance the catheter forward into the artery. If no blood returns, make another attempt starting afresh as described above.

If blood flow is satisfactory in the position shown in Figure 3.3*C*, attach the connecting tubing to the catheter with a T-connector, stopcock and syringe and recheck arterial flow. The catheter should then be securely taped or sewn to the forearm to prevent dislodgment.

Cutdown (Fig. 3.3, *D* and *E*)

After preparing the equipment and the patient, the wrist is restrained, cleansed, and anesthetized as before. Wearing sterile gloves, drape the area. Make a 1-cm transverse skin incision proximal to the crease closest to the wrist joint. By carefully spreading the subcutaneous tissue along the incision line, visualize the artery with care to avoid cutting the adjacent veins.

The best approach is to directly puncture the exposed artery with the "over-the-needle" catheter setup, as shown in Figure 3.3*E*. A 4-0 silk tie is placed distal to the entry site and pulled to give back traction on the artery. This secures and accentuates it, usually enabling easy puncture and threading of the catheter. Attach the syringe and stopcock system and check for patency.

The system is secured by suturing the catheter to the skin distal to the incision. Closure of the incision should be accomplished with several 4-0 skin sutures and a dressing applied to stabilize and protect the system.

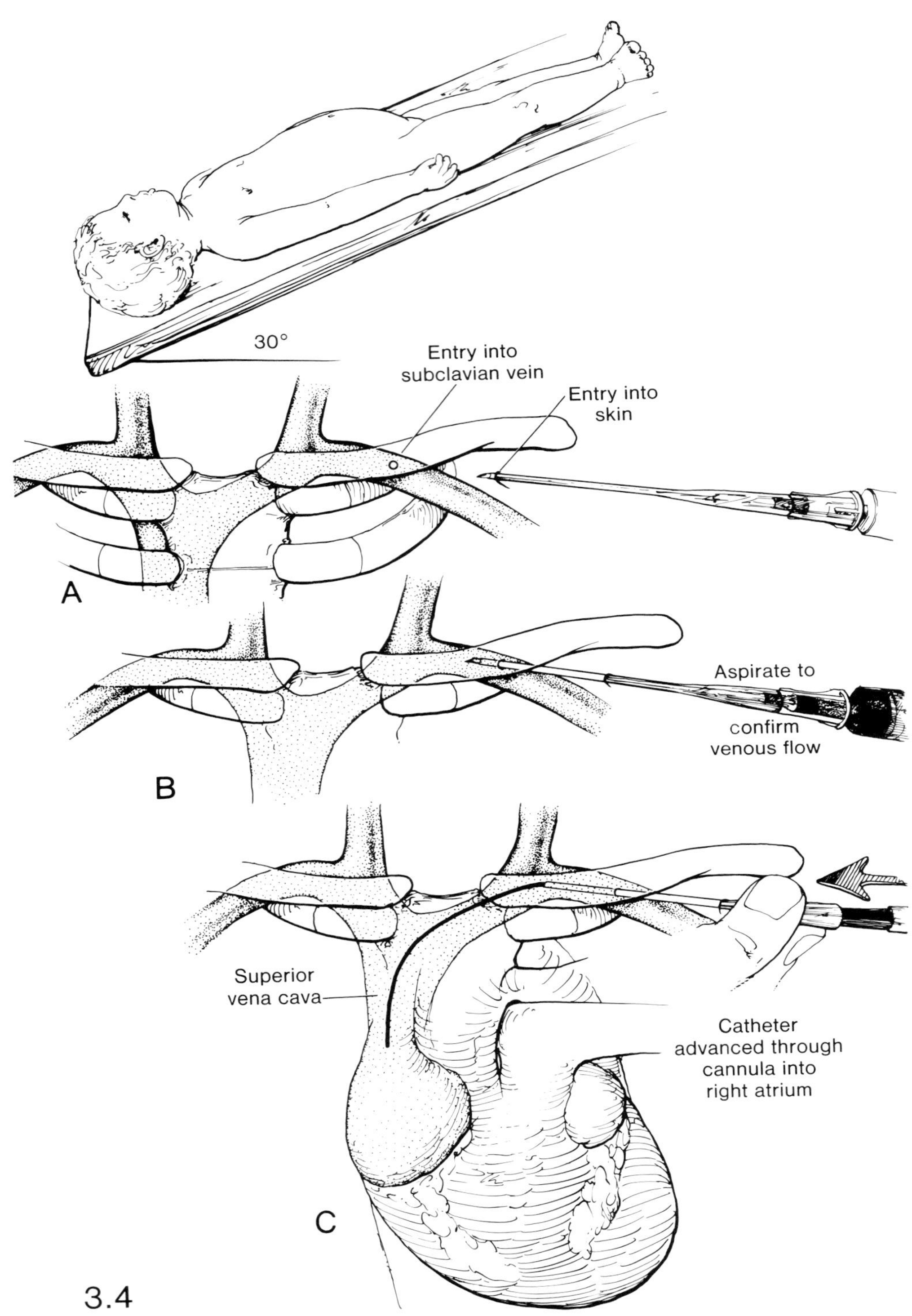
30°
Entry into subclavian vein
Entry into skin
A
Aspirate to
confirm venous flow
B
Superior vena cava
Catheter advanced through cannula into right atrium
C
3.4

3.4. TECHNIQUE OF SUBCLAVIAN VEIN PERCUTANEOUS CATHETERIZATION

INDICATIONS

Emergency access to the venous circulation in the absence of percutaneous peripheral, femoral, or external jugular access.

COMPLICATIONS

1. Pneumothorax, hemothorax or hydrothorax.
2. Infection, especially after prolonged maintenance following emergency placement.

PROCEDURE

Anesthesia. Except in premature infants or obtunded children, adequate restraint in the Trendelenburg position is difficult without heavy sedation or general anesthesia; this requirement precludes the insertion of a subclavian line in many situations. However, in children older than 6 years of age who are stable and cooperative, the procedure can be done, achieving local anesthesia with 1% lidocaine and/or sedation with intravenous diazepam (40 to 200 μg/kg) or a combination of morphine (0.1 mg/kg, to maximum 8 mg) and pentobarbital (4 mg/kg, to maximum 100 mg).

Technique. The technique of subclavian venous catheterization in children varies somewhat from the approach used in adults, but the positioning is similar. Place the child in the Trendelenburg position with a small towel roll under the thoracic spine to hyperextend the back. After preparation of the neck and upper chest on the side selected for catheterization with povidone-iodine, cover the area with a sterile aperture drape and towels. If the patient is awake but sedated, the intended tract of the subclavian line is anesthetized with 1% lidocaine, including the periosteum of the clavicle and adjacent first rib.

Make a small puncture at the intended entry site, a depression bordered by the deltoid and pectoralis major muscles, under the distal ⅓ of the clavicle, as shown in Figure 3.4*A*; use a No. 11 blade. This more lateral entry point maintains a greater distance between the skin surface and the entrance to the subclavian vein, decreasing the chance of infection. A more medial site is a less ideal, but an acceptable, alternative. Use a 20 gauge Argyle Intramedicut® cannula in newborns, an 18 gauge in young children, and a 14 gauge Centrasil® silastic catheter in patients over the age of 6 years.

Insert the needle through the puncture site as depicted in Figure 3.4*A* and direct it toward the junction of the first rib and clavicle. The needle is advanced underneath the clavicle at its midpoint while gentle steady aspiration is applied to the syringe. When the needle enters the vein, blood flows back briskly (Fig. 3.4*B*). Advancing the needle and catheter for several more millimeters assures that the catheter itself is in the vein.

Remove the needle leaving the Intramedicut cannula in the vein. If blood continues to return easily, insert the appropriate size catheter through the plastic cannula (Fig. 3.4*C*). If the blood return is not brisk, withdraw the plastic cannula back 1 mm at a time until the blood flows rapidly.

After the long catheter has been inserted, attach to it a 10-ml syringe and a T connector which have been filled with heparinized saline. After assessing for adequacy of blood return and infusion by alternately pushing and pulling on the plunger, secure the catheter temporarily while a chest x-ray is performed. This should confirm both the position of the catheter tip in the superior vena cava and the absence of a pneumothorax or a hemothorax. After the results of the chest x-ray are judged satisfactory, suture the catheter to the skin using 4-0 or 5-0 nylon and cover the area with sterile dressing.

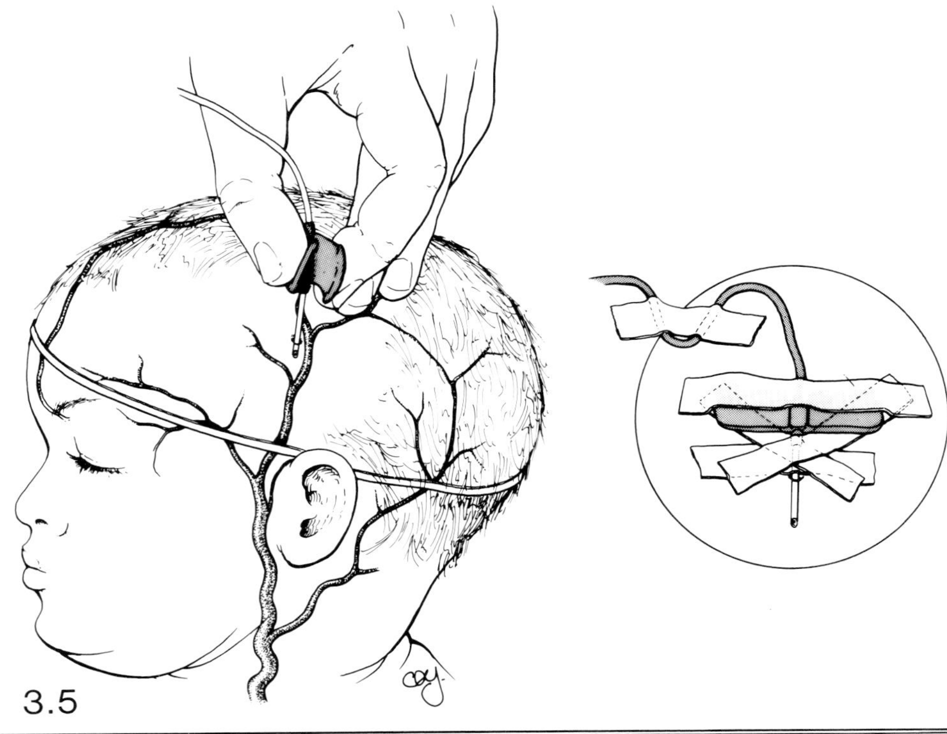

3.5

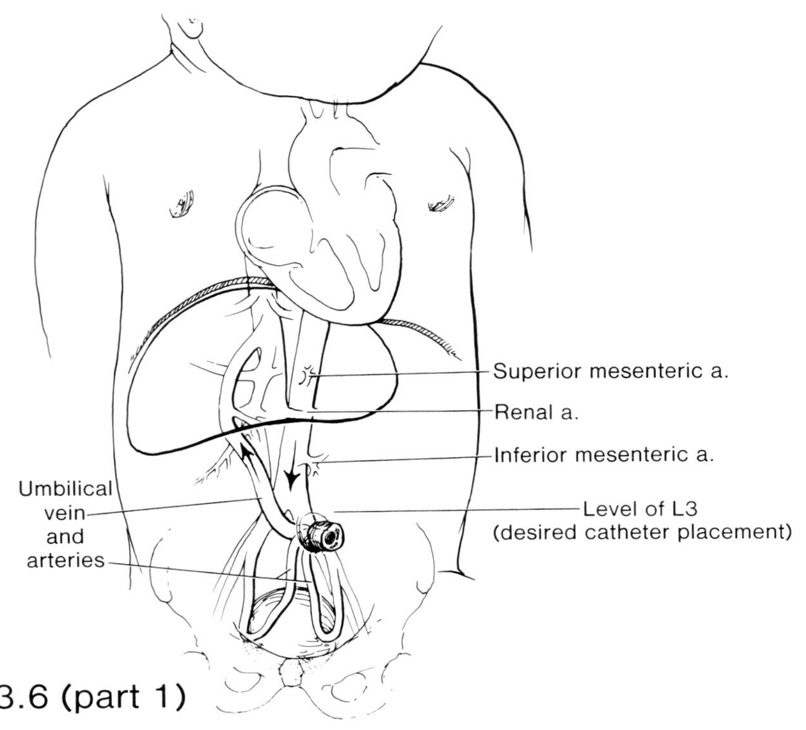
Superior mesenteric a.
Renal a.
Inferior mesenteric a.
Umbilical vein and arteries
Level of L3 (desired catheter placement)

3.6 (part 1)

3.5. SCALP VEIN CATHETERIZATION

INDICATIONS

To achieve intravenous access for delivering fluid and/or medication in an infant usually younger than 1 year, when peripheral extremity veins are unavailable.

COMPLICATIONS

1. Inadvertent arterial puncture.
2. Ecchymoses and hematoma of the scalp.
3. Antagonism of the parents. Care must be taken to explain the need for the use of these veins, and the absence of significant complications.

PROCEDURE

The infant under 1 year of age has several easily accessible scalp veins. These include the frontal, supraorbital, posterior facial, superficial temporal, and posterior auricular veins and their tributaries. Restrain the patient in a supine position and have an assistant stabilize the infant's head. Shave an area large enough to expose not only the desired veins but an area of surrounding scalp for adequate taping of the infusion needle. In this area, select a vein with a straight segment that is as long as the part of the needle that is to be inserted. Verify that the chosen vessel is a vein by palpating it to ensure that it does not pulsate.

Place a rubber band around the infant's head. Then, attach a small piece of tape to the rubber band to make it easier to lift and cut the rubber band after successful venipuncture.

Prepare the skin by cleansing with povidone-iodine solution followed by 70% alcohol. Grasp a No. 23, 25 or 27 "butterfly" scalp vein needle by the plastic tabs or "wings." Keep the needle and syringe unattached initially to facilitate evaluation of free blood return. Insert the needle in the direction of blood flow and pierce the skin approximately 0.5 cm proximal to the actual site where entry into the vein is anticipated. While applying mild traction on the skin of the scalp, slowly advance the needle through the skin toward the vein. Blood will enter the clear plastic tubing when successful venipuncture has occurred. Carefully cut the rubber band tourniquet, attach the syringe filled with saline flush solution, and slowly inject 0.5 ml of flush. If the needle is satisfactorily inserted into the lumen of the vein, the solution will flow easily. Appearance of a skin wheal indicates that the vein has not been satisfactorily cannulated, and another attempt must be made.

After successful venipuncture, carefully tape the scalp vein needle as shown in the diagram. Keep the infant restrained to prevent accidental removal or infiltration of the vein.

3.6. UMBILICAL ARTERY CATHETERIZATION

INDICATIONS

Respiratory failure or cardiovascular collapse in the newborn infant where percutaneous attempts for vascular access have failed.

COMPLICATIONS

1. Embolization or thrombosis—inferior mesenteric, renal, or lower extremity arteries.
2. Infection.
3. Ischemia/infarction.
4. Hemorrhage—from dislodgment of catheter or perforation of the vessel wall.
5. Arrhythmias—from direct cardiac stimulation if the catheter enters the heart.
6. Air embolization.

EQUIPMENT

1. 3-0 silk suture on straight or curved needle.
2. Antiseptic solution (povidone-iodine), sterile gauze pads, drapes and gloves.
3. Hemostats (4 pairs) and scissors.
4. Sterile scalpel and No. 11 or 15 blade.
5. 22 gauge needle.
6. 10-ml syringe filled with normal saline (T-connector (optional)) and 3-way stopcock.
7. Umbilical catheter—3½ Fr. (premature babies), or 5 Fr. (full term)
8. Infusion solution containing heparin (1 unit/ml)

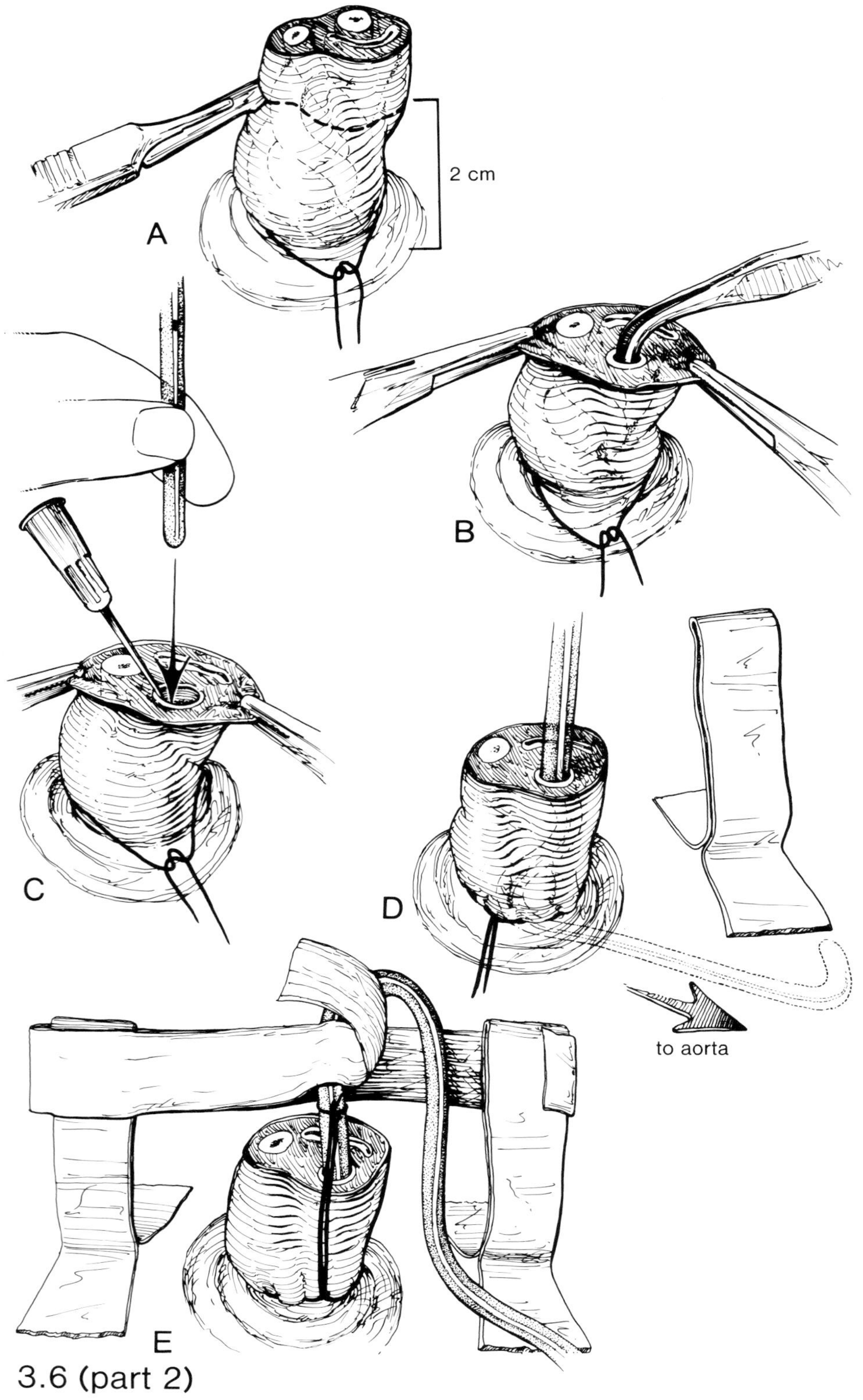

3.6 (part 2)

PROCEDURE

Initiate therapy for any cardiorespiratory disturbances prior to beginning procedure. During the catheterization monitor the cardiac rate, and keep the infant under a radiant heater to maintain euthermia. Figure 3.6 shows the anatomy of the area.

Place the infant supine in the frog leg position, and restrain him or her as necessary. Gauze pads may be wrapped around the ankles and wrists and either pinned or taped securely to the bed. Wearing mask, gown and gloves, hold the sterile umbilical catheter over the infant to measure the distance from the shoulder to the umbilicus. Advance the catheter into the artery 60% of this distance beginning at the skin surface so that its tip will reach the bifurcation of the aorta. Mark the catheter appropriately and attach it to the T-connector, stopcock and syringe. Flush it, leaving it full of fluid.

While lifting the umbilical cord with gauze in one hand, scrub the lower umbilical cord and the abdomen from the xiphoid process to the symphysis pubis. Drape the infant on both sides by folding two drapes into triangles or use an aperture drape; cover the area below the umbilicus with a third square drape.

At the base of the umbilical stump, suture a 3-0 or 4-0 silk tie around the cord to make a purse string, but leave the knot untied. While holding the gauze on the unsterile distal umbilicus, sever the cord 1.5 to 2 cm above the abdominal wall with the scalpel as shown in Figure 3.6*A*. Remove the cut umbilicus and gauze from the sterile area. Bleeding is usually minimal, stopping with gentle pressure or wiping; rarely, the purse string must be tightened.

Locate the umbilical vessels, usually two thick, white-walled arteries on one side, and a larger vein on the other. If the arteries in the stump are tortuous, cut it closer to the abdominal wall to facilitate cannulation.

Attach two clamps on opposite sides of the umbilicus, being careful to grasp a fibrous portion of the cord and not just Wharton's jelly or an artery. Evert the clamps to immobilize and expose the cord and use the small curved forceps, as in Figure 3.6*B*, to enter and then stretch the lumen of the artery. Gentle, repetitive stretching is most effective. Attempt at catheter placement should be undertaken when the artery remains dilated to a diameter which is greater than that of the catheter to a depth of 1 cm.

To insert the catheter, hold the distal end near the tip as in Figure 3.6*C* and place it in the arterial lumen between the prongs of the forceps that are holding the artery open. An alternative method, pictured in Figure 3.6*C*, shows the inner wall of the vessel held with a 22 gauge needle (bent with a a hemostat), allowing the vessel to be entered directly. Pass the catheter under gentle, constant tension in order to overcome the resistance that is encountered at the points where the artery turns. These locations are shown in Figure 3.6. Blood should flow readily after the second bend when the iliac artery is entered.

As shown in Figure 3.6*D*, advance the catheter as far as the mark made on it at the outset; confirm blood flow at the final point. Turn the handle of the stopcock toward the infant. Then, tighten and knot the purse string, leaving both ends of the suture long. Approximately 5 cm from the knot at the base of the cord, make a square knot and then loop and tie the suture around the catheter to help secure it in place as shown in Figure 3.6*E*. Place tape on the abdominal wall as shown also. Verify with an abdominal x-ray that the tip of the catheter lies below the level of third lumbar vertebral body, or withdraw it to this position manually.

Infuse solutions containing heparin (1 unit/ml) unless contraindicated for bleeding diathesis.

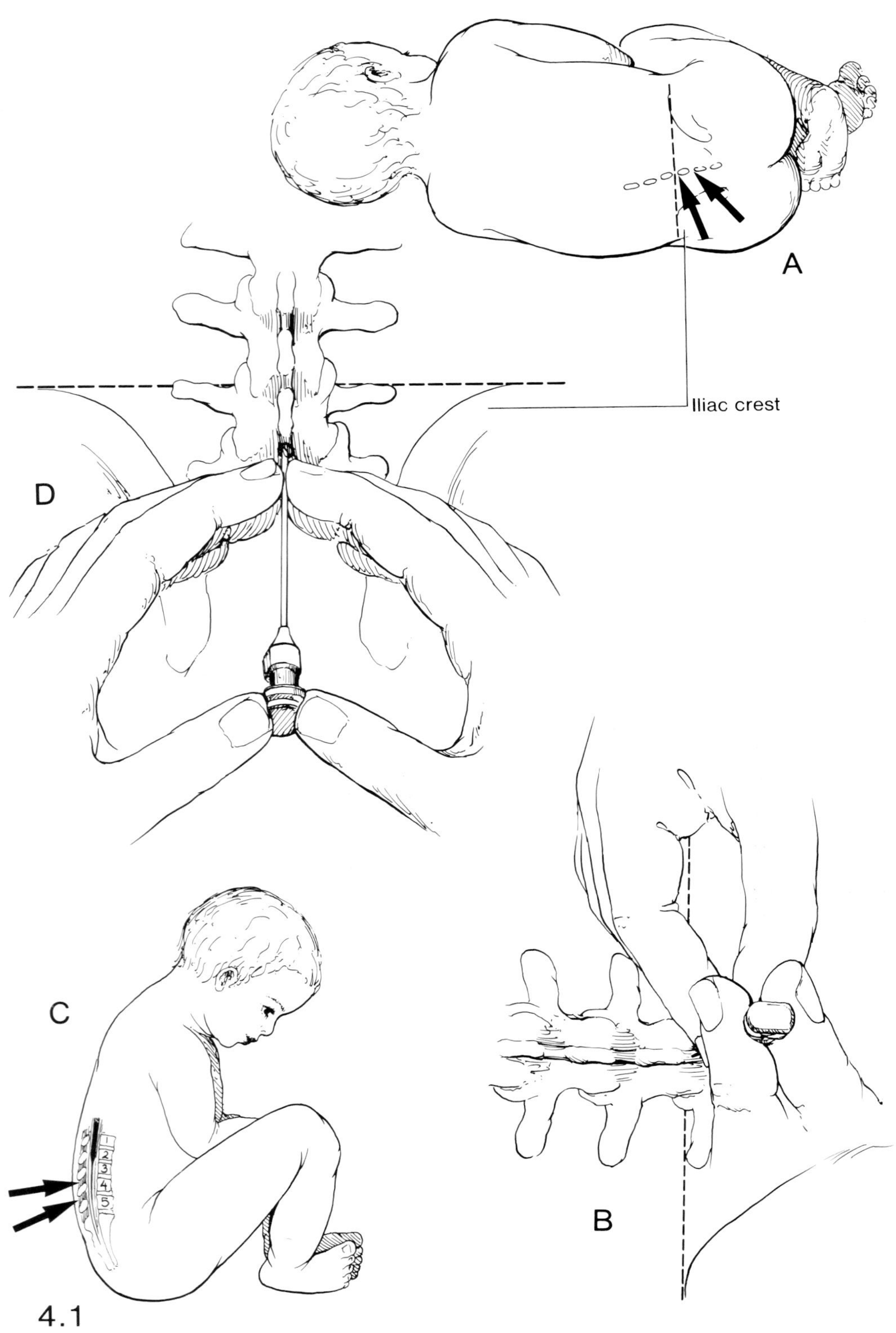
A
Iliac crest
D
C
1
2
3
4
5
B
4.1

4.1. LUMBAR PUNCTURE

INDICATIONS

To obtain cerebrospinal fluid (CSF) for the diagnosis of meningitis, meningoencephalitis, subarachnoid hemorrhage and other neurological syndromes.

COMPLICATIONS

Headache; local back pain—occasionally with short-lived referred limp; spinal cord bleeding—especially in the presence of bleeding diathesis; infection; subarachnoid epidermal cyst—secondary to foreign body reaction; ocular muscle palsy (transient); brainstem herniation—in the presence of symptomatic intracranial hypertension.

PROCEDURE

Lateral Decubitus Position

Restrain the patient firmly in the lateral decubitus position. Maximally flex the spine without compromising the upper airway.

The spinal cord ends at approximately the level of the L1 and L2 vertebral bodies. Caudal to L2, only the filum terminale is present. The desired sites for lumbar puncture are the interspaces between the posterior elements of L3 and L4 or L4 and L5. Locate these spaces by palpating the iliac crest (Fig. 4.1, A and D). Follow an imaginary "plumb line" from the iliac crest to the spine. The interspace encountered is L4-L5. Use it or the one cephalad to it.

Use sterile technique for the lumbar puncture (LP). Commercial LP trays and disposable manometers are available. Cleanse the skin with povidone-iodine solution after donning sterile gloves. Using sponges, begin at the intended puncture site and sponge in widening circles until an area of 10 cm diameter has been cleaned. Repeat this three times. Drape the child beneath his or her flank and over the back with the spine accessible to view.

Use local anesthesia in children older than 1 year of age. Anesthetize the site by injecting 1% lidocaine intradermally to raise a wheal, then advance the needle into desired interspace injecting anesthetic, being careful not to inject it into a blood vessel or spinal canal.

Select an appropriate length 22 gauge spinal needle as follows: less than 1 year, 3.75 cm (1.5 inch); 1 year to middle childhood 6.25 cm (2.5 inch); large children and adolescents, 8.75 cm (3.5 inch).

Check the spinal needle and make sure the stylet is secure. Grasp the spinal needle firmly with the bevel facing "up" toward the ceiling, making the bevel parallel to the direction of the fibers of the ligamentum flavum. Recheck the patient's position to ensure that the needle's trajectory is midsagittal to their back. Insert the needle into the skin over the selected interspace in the midline sagittal plane. Two methods of stabilizing and guiding the needle are shown. (Fig. 4.1, B and D). Insert the needle slowly, aiming slightly cephalad toward the umbilicus. When the ligamentum flavum and then the dura are punctured, a "pop" and decreased resistance are felt. Remove the stylet and check for flow of spinal fluid. If no fluid is obtained, reinsert the stylet, advance the needle slowly, and check frequently for the appearance to CSF.

When CSF flows, attach the manometer to the needle's hub to obtain an opening pressure reading. Collect 1 ml of CSF in each of the 3 sterile tubes. Send it for routine culture, glucose and protein determination, and cell count. Collect additional tubes as indicated. After collecting CSF, a closing pressure can be obtained. Reinsert the stylet and remove the spinal needle with one quick motion. Cleanse the back and cover the puncture site.

Sitting position

Restrain the child in the seated position with maximal spinal flexion (Figure 4.1C). Have the assistant hold the infant's hands between his or her flexed legs with one hand and flex the infant's head with the other hand.

Place drapes underneath the child's buttocks and on the shoulders with an opening near the intended spinal puncture site. Choose the interspace as noted earlier and follow the procedure as outlined for the lateral position. Insert the needle so it runs parallel to the spinal cord (Fig. 4.1D).

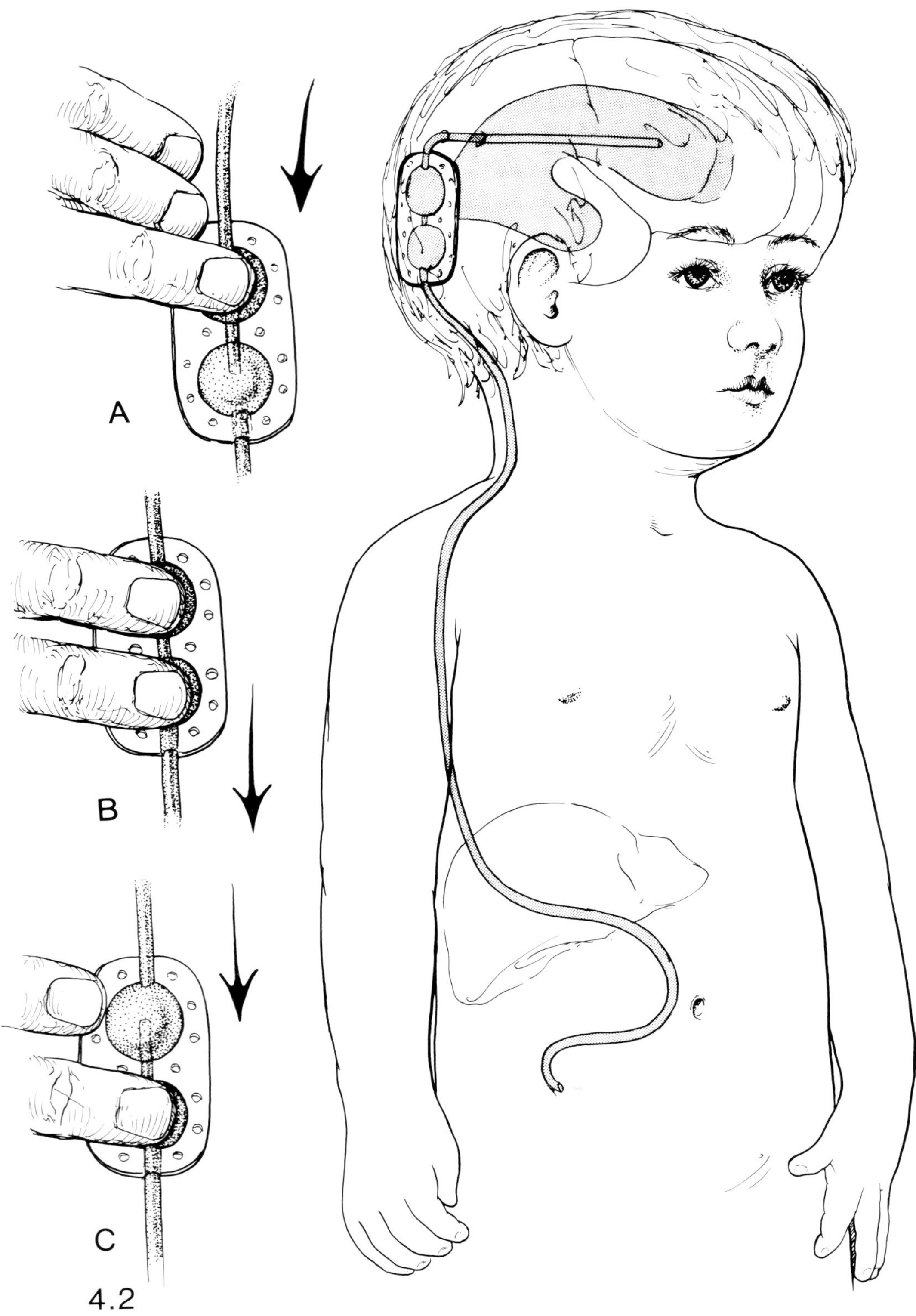

4.2

4.2. EVALUATION OF VENTRICULOPERITONEAL SHUNT

INDICATIONS

To evaluate any signs or symptoms of shunt malfunction including: vomiting, drowsiness, headache, seizures, bradycardia, coma, focal neurological findings, or swelling around the shunt site.

COMPLICATIONS

1. Proximal shunt dysfunction—rarely, repetitive pumping causes blockage of the proximal shunt with tissue from the choroid plexus or blood from irritation of the ventricular wall.
2. Cerebrospinal fluid leakage—if a complete blockage occurs distally, some patients develop a cerebrospinal fluid collection in the subgaleal space that may be exacerbated by vigorous pumping.

PROCEDURE

Figures 4.2 and 4.3 show two types of common permanent ventricular drainage systems.

Figure 4.2 is the standard Ames design "double-bubble" ventriculoperitoneal shunt. Its distal end, located in the abdominal cavity, has a 1-way valve. The shunt tubing travels from the lateral ventricle, through the skull, to the subcutaneous space of the scalp where a right angle is made. At this point, it connects to a "double-bubble" rubber reservoir that lies posterior and superior to the ear in the parietooccipital area of the skull. Finally, it continues subcutaneously, as shown, to the abdominal cavity, where the cerebrospinal fluid drains, if the system functions properly, and is absorbed by the peritoneum.

To check the function and patency of the system, place the child in a comfortable position during the physical examination. Locate the tubing and trace its entire course to look for disconnections, fluid accumulations, or insufficient length of the distal tubing. This should not cause pain, as it involves only mild pressure on skin surface.

In Figure 4.2, three maneuvers to assess patency are shown. First, compress the proximal bubble as in Figure 4.2*A*. This assures filling of the distal bubble for the next step, and empties the chamber to test proximal blockage later. While still compressing proximally, place a finger over the distal bubble and compress it as in Figure 4.2*B*. Normally there is no resistance to emptying of fluid through the valve into the abdominal cavity. Undue pressure suggests a distal tube blockage, disconnection, or insufficient length due to the growth of the child. Finally, release the proximal bubble as in Figure 4.2*C*. Now the negative pressure in this bubble should suck fluid into it from the ventricular cavity, and usually within 1 sec. A delay in filling of any longer often suggests a proximal blockage; however, if the shunt has been pumped several times in the previous hours, it may fill slowly because the proximal tip is sitting against the choroid plexus. Since there is no proximal valve, when the distal bubble is compressed, the proximal bubble can be repeatedly depressed to measure resistance to filling of the proximal shunt without draining excessive fluid from above.

Figure 4.3 displays a single reservoir, single pump Holter shunt. The circular chamber perpendicular to the shunt entering the skull is reservoir for obtaining specimens. More distally, there is a compressible rubber pump connected by tight purse strings on each end to plastic tubing. To pump this type, compress and release the distal soft tube. Each compression will test distal patency, while the release verifies proximal patency. Generally, the release is immediate in this shunt, so most any delay of filling suggests blockage or choroid collapse. Because the connections of the pump to the shunt tubing are purse strings on either end, this system can disconnect and leak cerebrospinal fluid subcutaneously.

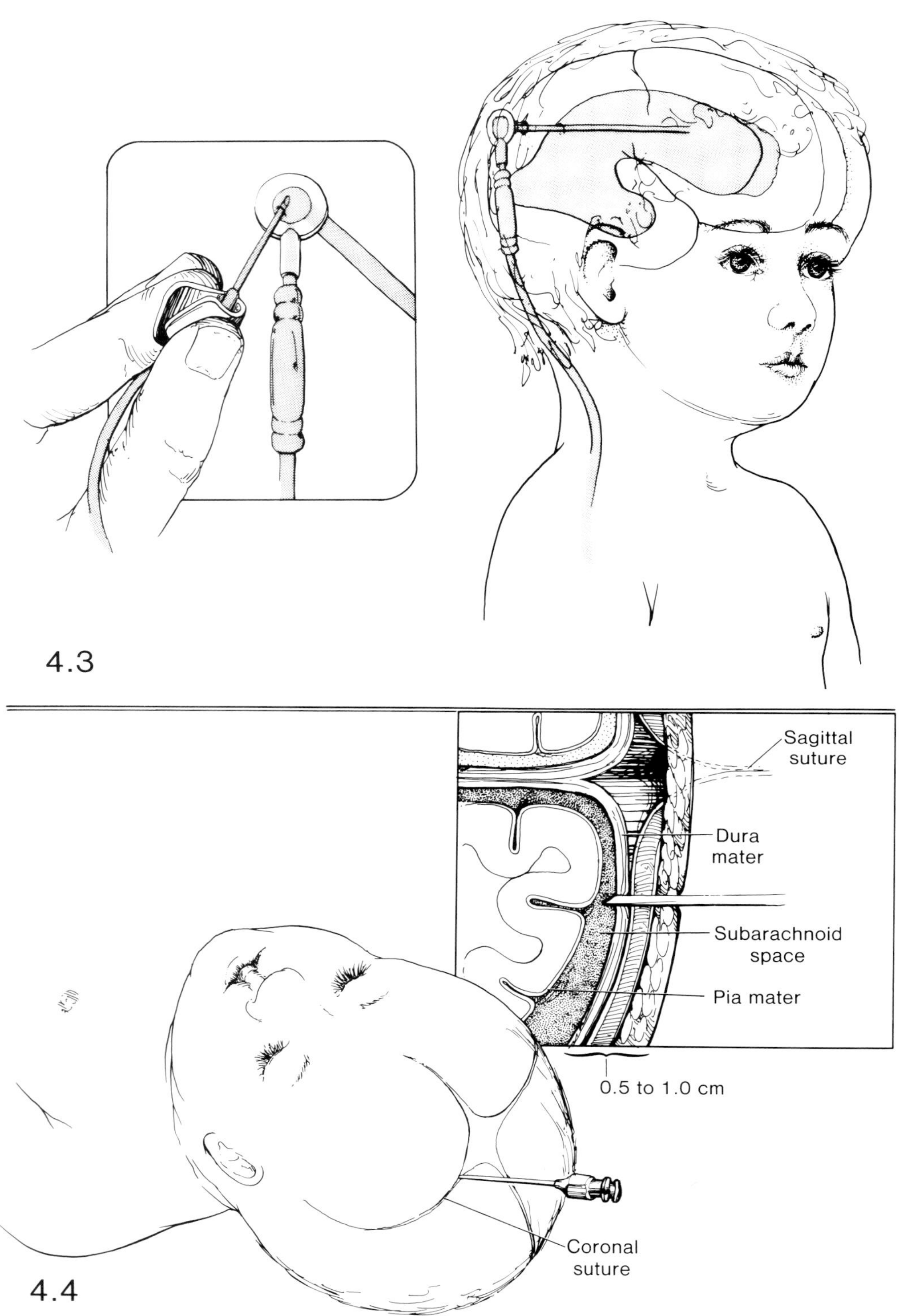
4.3
Sagittal suture
Dura mater
Subarachnoid space
Pia mater
0.5 to 1.0 cm
Coronal suture
4.4

4.3. DIAGNOSTIC TAP OF VENTRICULOPERITONEAL SHUNT

INDICATIONS

1. Reduction of intracranial pressure in a child with acute symptomatic hydrocephalus from shunt obstruction.
2. Diagnostic evaluation of possible ventricular or shunt infection.

COMPLICATIONS

1. Infection.
2. Cerebrospinal fluid leakage from use of a large bore needle or repeated taps.
3. Bleeding from trauma to vessels overlying the reservoir.

PROCEDURE

Locate the reservoir and pump(s), and assess the function of the shunt if the symptoms are suggestive of blockage. Restrain the patient in the supine position with the face turned toward the shoulder and the shunt reservoir facing up; shave the hair directly around the reservoir. Wash the site several times with povidone-iodine solution in a circumferential fashion; clean it off with 70% alcohol and dry the area with sterile gauze. Don sterile gloves. Prepare a 23 or 25 gauge butterfly infusion set and a 5- or 10-ml syringe, sample collection tubes, and sterile gauze on a sterile towel. A standard manometer can be used if pressure measurements are desired. Palpate the reservoir with one gloved finger. Puncture the skin and quickly enter the reservoir. If there is distal obstruction, the fluid will be under considerable pressure and will flow readily. Attach the manometer immediately and standardize the zero mark on it at the level of the cerebral ventricles. Samples of cerebrospinal fluid are collected aseptically into sterile tubes. Use slight negative pressure on the syringe to enhance flow if there is proximal obstruction or viscous infected fluid. If there is normal proximal function, refrain from appreciative suction on the syringe to minimize the chance of brain tissue entering the shunt.

Figure 4.3 shows the "single-bubble" system being tapped. In general, on the double-bubble setup, puncture either bubble in a similar fashion as described.

4.4. SUBDURAL TAP

INDICATIONS

Evacuation of subdural blood or fluid in young infants, when such collections cause symptoms (i.e., seizures, unilateral paresis) from increased intracranial pressure.

COMPLICATIONS

1. Intracranial hemorrhage
2. Contusion of the cerebral cortex.
3. Subgaleal collection of fluid or blood.
4. Infection.

PROCEDURE

Prepare the infant for the procedure in the supine position after performing the appropriate measures for resuscitation and stabilization. Have an assistant restrain the patient in a mummy wrap or by leaning over the infant with his or her arms firmly pinned at the side. The head should be face up. Continuous monitoring of the cardiac status is essential.

Shave the scalp widely in an area around the lateral boundaries of the anterior fontanel (the anterior two thirds of the head). Prep the site(s) with povidone-iodine solution and 70% alcohol and then dry with sterile gauze. Wearing sterile gloves, palpate the superior edge of the coronal suture at the lateral aspect of the anterior fontanel. If the fontanel is very small, move several millimeters further laterally in the coronal suture. Local anesthetic (i.e., 1% lidocaine) should be injected in the conscious child.

Grasp a 19 or 20 gauge subdural or spinal needle by the hub and check its patency. Hold it between the thumb and index finger and rest the heel of the hand against the infant's scalp. Puncture the skin at a right angle to surface, stretching it just slightly subcutaneously to obtain a Z-track. Advance the needle through the puncture site between the edges of the coronal suture until the feeling of resistance lessens. Then, remove the stylet to allow fluid or blood to drain; 10 to 15 ml can be safely evacuated from each side. Normally, the needle need be advanced no more than 5 to 8 mm below the scalp's surface. Some infants may require bilateral taps.

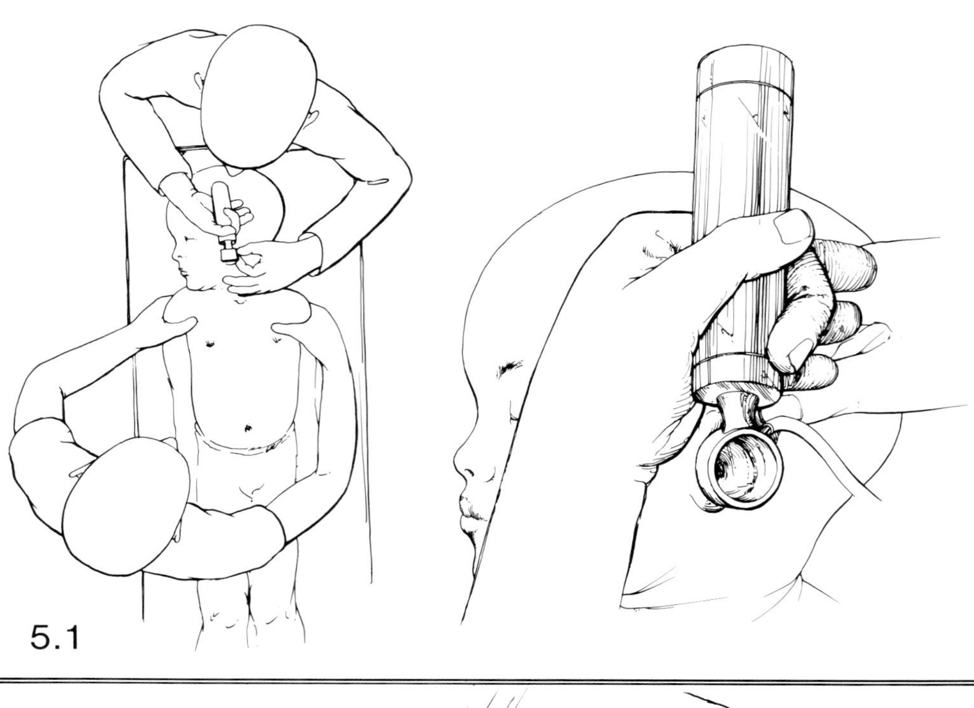

5.1

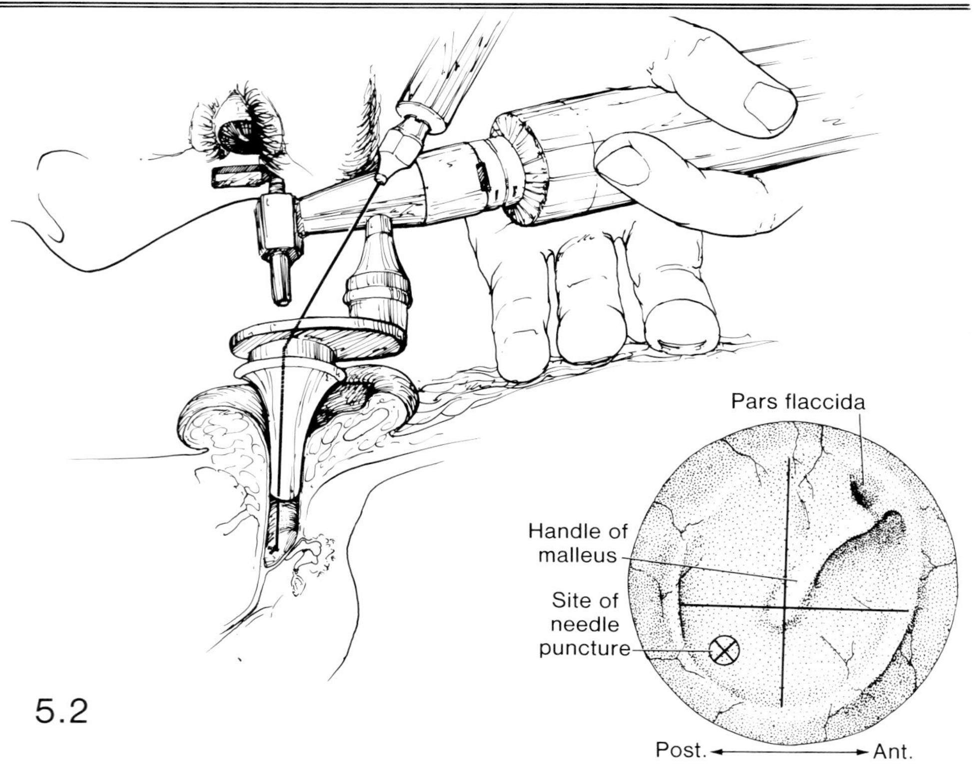
Pars flaccida
Handle of malleus
Site of needle puncture
Post.
Ant.

5.2

5.1. PNEUMATIC OTOSCOPIC EXAMINATION

INDICATIONS

Evaluation of middle ear.

COMPLICATIONS

Pain or contusion of the external canal.

PROCEDURE

To safely and accurately evaluate the middle ear structures in infants, restraint is extremely important; many young children fear the approach of a physician, particularly to examine their ears. Usually a parent can provide adequate immobilization. Place the infant supine, and ask a parent to hold the arms firmly next to the head, grasping them just above the elbow. Hold the otoscope as shown in Figure 5.1 grasping it between the thumb and index finger of the dominant hand. The heel of the hand should rest against the anterior portion of the infant's head to maintain constant, firm pressure against the temporal skull while bringing the infant's head horizontal to the table.

Once the infant is restrained, the nondominant hand should be used to grasp the upper portion of the helix, stretching it superiorly and posteriorly in the child to straighten the external canal. However, in young infants, pull the helix inferiorly and posteriorly to visualize the tympanic membrane. Simultaneously, observe the entrance to the auditory canal through the otoscope and flex the thumb to direct the speculum down the canal entrance. Then, straightening of the external canal is performed under direct visualization. The removal of cerumen obscuring the field may be necessary (see Procedure 5.3). Observe the tympanic membrane for color, contour, and presence of the bony and vascular landmarks. (See "Otitis Media" in Chapter 45.)

For evaluation of the compliance of the tympanic membrane, a tight seal is required between the auditory canal and the speculum. If the diameter of the speculum is found to be less than that of the canal, replace it with one of a larger size. Reenter the canal to ⅓ to ½ of its depth, establish a seal, and lightly squeeze the bulb while observing the tympanic membrane.

5.2. TYMPANOCENTESIS

INDICATIONS

1. Otitis media unresponsive to conventional therapy.
2. Otitis media in the neonate.
3. Otitis media in the immunosuppressed child (steroids or other chemotherapy).
4. Complicated otitis media (with meningitis or brain abscess).
5. Rarely for relief of severe pain due to otitis media or to rupture the bullae of bullous myringitis.

COMPLICATIONS

1. Bleeding (usually minor unless the jugular bulb is entered).
2. Disarticulation of the ossicular chain.
3. Laceration of the tympanic membrane.
4. Contamination of middle ear by bacteria in the external canal.

PROCEDURE

After explaining the procedure to the child and family, restrain the child securely in a supine position. Use the mummy papoose or ask an assistant to restrain the trunk. Have the child's head held in the horizontal plane by an assistant. Visualize the external canal and clean any wax or debris from it. Sterilize the ear canal by filling it with 70% alcohol or povidone-iodine solution for 60 sec, and then drain out excess solution by placing the ear down. Again restrain the child's head in the horizontal plane, and visualize the tympanic membrane with an otoscope fitted with an operating head. Insert the aspiration set (a 22 gauge, 8- to 10-cm spinal needle bent 30° 4 to 5 cm from the tip and attached to a 1-ml tuberculin syringe) into the otoscope, through the speculum as shown in Figure 5.2. Pierce the eardrum as shown in the inferoposterior quadrant. After entering the middle ear, aspirate with the syringe. Care should be taken not to contaminate the needle by touching the ear canal or otoscopic speculum. To send the small amount of fluid for culture, flush the spinal needle with nonbacteriostatic normal saline.

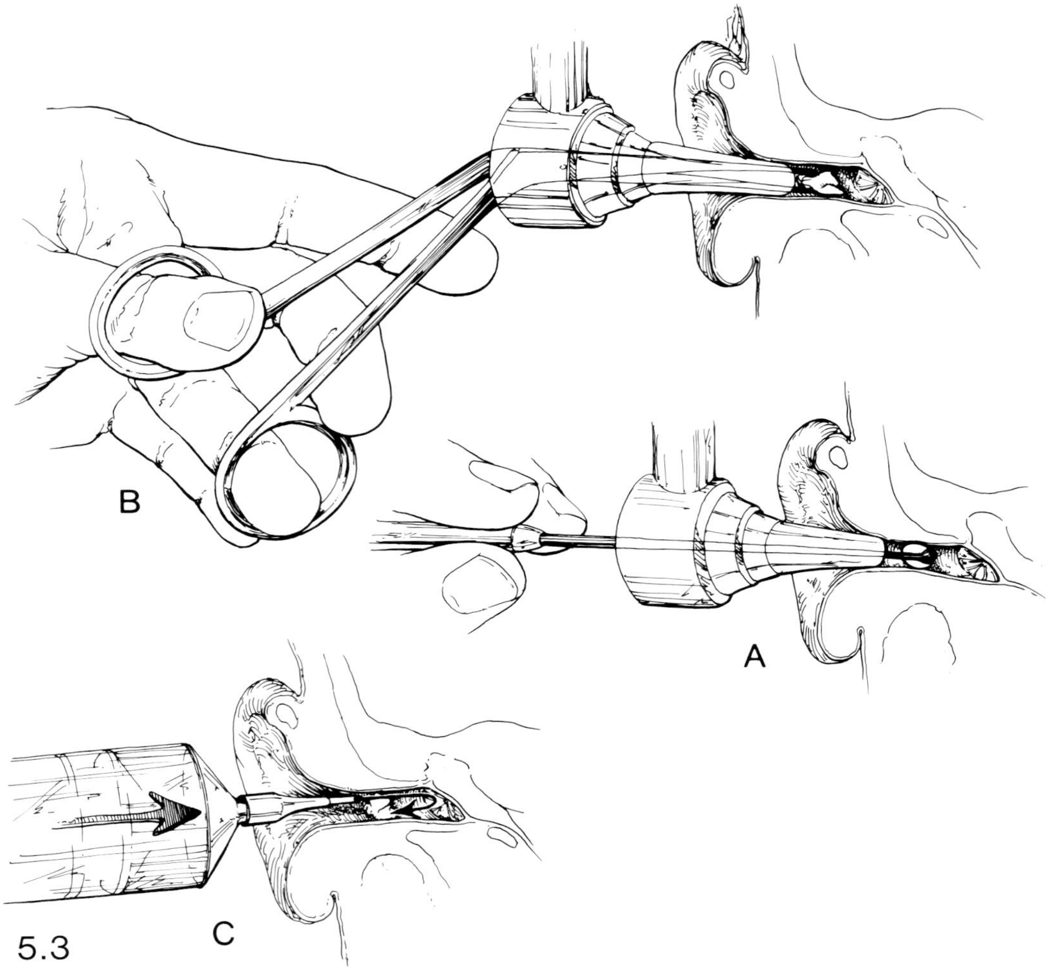

B

A

C

5.3

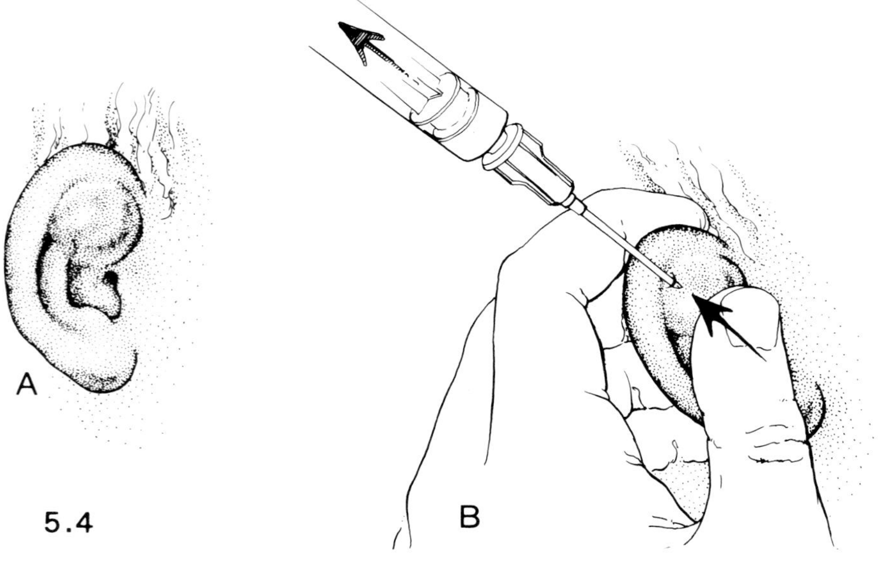

5.3. REMOVAL OF A FOREIGN BODY FROM THE EAR

INDICATIONS

Complete obstruction of the external canal by cerumen or foreign material which causes a conductive hearing deficit, severe pain or prevents visualization of the tympanic membrane of a febrile child.

COMPLICATIONS

1. Laceration of the wall of the external canal.
2. Perforation of the tympanic membrane.
3. Ossicular disruption.

PROCEDURE

Three methods are available for removal of a foreign body, all requiring cooperation or restraint of the child. Because a minor laceration of the ear canal is often unavoidable, the parents should be aware of this complication before the physician undertakes the use of a currette or forceps. After removal by any method, it is important to visualize the ear drum and document its condition.

A. Curette (Fig. 5.3*A*)

Visualize the foreign body with a speculum, preferably using an operating head otoscope. Then, very slowly advance the curette just beyond the foreign body as shown. While applying pressure to the foreign body, slowly withdraw the curette until the foreign body is removed.

B. Forceps (Fig. 5.3*B*)

Visualize the foreign body with a speculum and look for a protruding edge of the foreign material. Carefully guide the forceps under direct visualization through the speculum in the closed position. Just a few millimeters from the edge of the foreign body open the forceps and grasp the edge gently. Withdraw the forceps, visualizing the foreign body to minimize the chance of a complication.

C. Irrigation (Fig. 5.3*C*)

Straighten the ear canal and visualize the foreign body directly with a speculum, making sure the tympanic membrane is intact. If the foreign body is sponge, Styrofoam or expansile when wet, this method should be avoided. Remove the speculum and irrigate the ear canal by injecting a constant stream of water at body temperature. Use a 20- to 50-ml syringe attached to a flexible intravenous catheter tip (i.e., a cut section of tubing from a "butterfly" needle). Repeated irrigation may be necessary to provide complete emptying.

5.4. ASPIRATION OF AURICULAR HEMATOMA

INDICATIONS

Traumatic auricular hematoma or seroma.

COMPLICATIONS

1. Recurrent hematoma or seroma.
2. Infection in the hematoma or seroma (abscess).

PROCEDURE

Restrain the child in a standard method. Palpate the hematoma to find the most fluctuant portion. Then, cleanse the skin over the hematoma with povidone-iodine solution and dry with sterile gauze. Topical anesthesia may be provided with ethyl chloride sprayed directly on the hematoma. Use a 10- or 20-ml syringe with an 18 gauge straight needle.

While stabilizing the needle against the scalp with the nondominant hand, puncture the most fluctuant portion of the hematoma with the needle. Maintain negative pressure on the syringe with one hand, while "milking" the hematoma with the thumb and index finger of the other. Withdraw the needle after emptying the hematoma, but continue to maintain pressure on the auricle between the thumb and finger to tamponade any ongoing bleeding for several minutes. With wet cotton pledgets, reestablish the normal ear contours and apply a pressure dressing. In 12 to 24 hours, unwrap the dressing, check the ear and redress again.

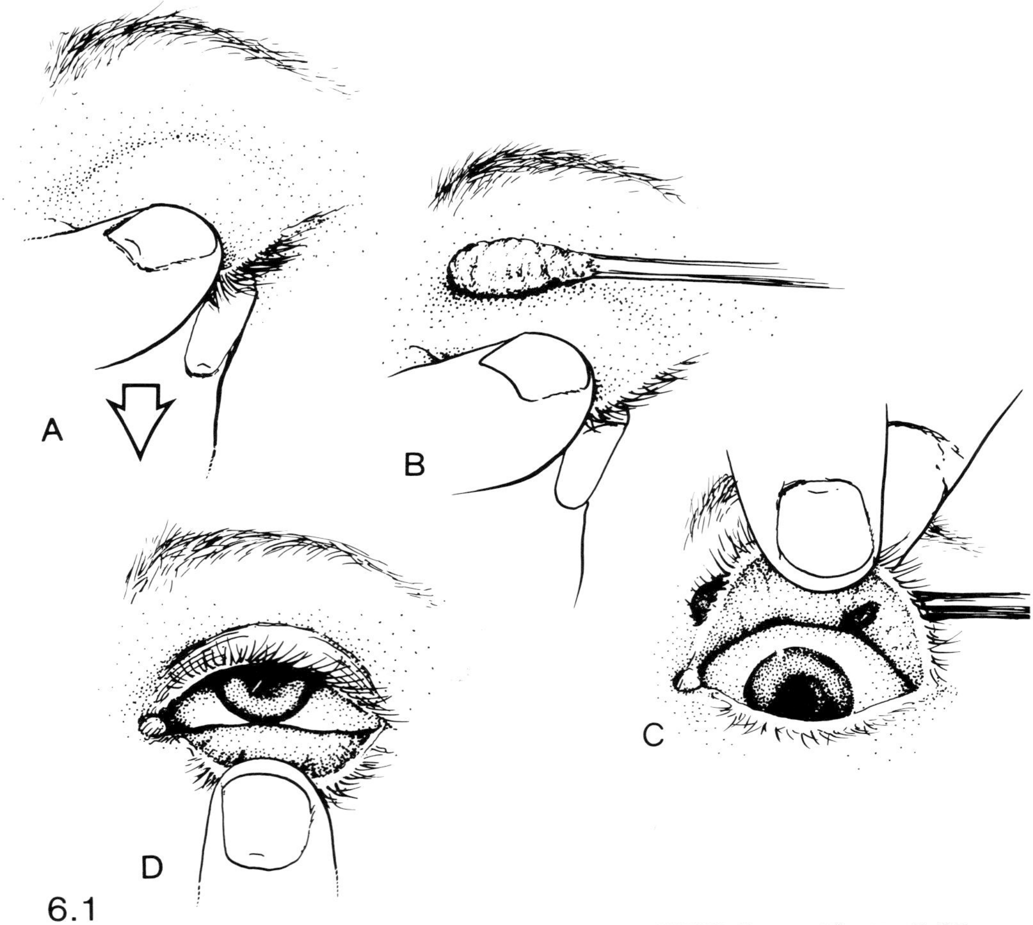

A

B

C

D

6.1

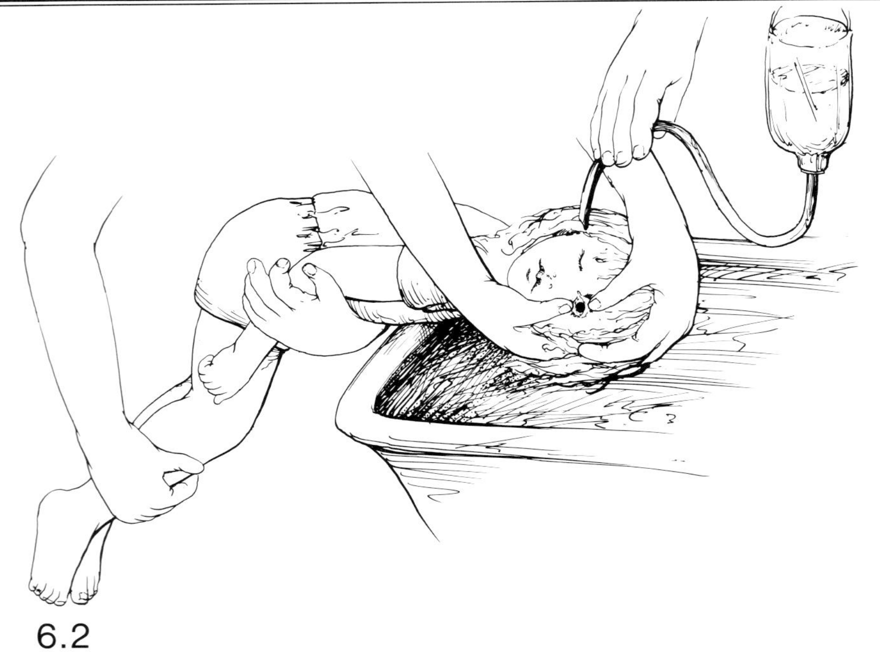

6.2

6.1. EVERSION OF THE EYELIDS

INDICATIONS

1. Identification of a foreign body or infection.
2. Instillation of medications to the conjunctiva.
3. Removal of a foreign body.

COMPLICATIONS

Mild contusion or ecchymoses (rarely).

PROCEDURE

Upper Lid

Upper lid eversion is the more difficult, normally requiring both cooperation or restraint, because the examiner needs to use both hands. After restraint, grasp the eyelash and distal upper lid between the index finger and thumb. Ask the child to look down at the floor if he or she will cooperate. Draw the eyelid downward as shown in Figure 6.1*A*. Place a clean, cotton swab across the superior tarsal margin as shown in Figure 6.1*B*. In one motion, move the swab slightly downward and pull the eyelid slightly upward. This maneuver should bend the eyelid slightly upward. This maneuver should bend the eyelid backward and expose the palpebral surface as shown in Figure 6.1*C*. To restore the lid to its usual position lift the swab slightly while maintaining pressure along the upper lid margin and turn the thumb and index finger downward.

Lower Lid

Have an assistant restrain the infant on the examining table in the supine position with the arms wrapped around the head. Alternatively, small infants can sit on the lap of a parent who then holds the infant's head still.

Place a thumb or finger at the base of the lower lid and gently retract it in a caudal and posterior direction while the child looks upward (Fig. 6.1*D*). While the eyelid is everted, removal of a foreign body can be accomplished. Use a clean cotton swab and apply it to the foreign body to flick it from the conjunctival surface.

6.2. IRRIGATION OF CONJUNCTIVA

INDICATIONS

Presence of a foreign body or caustic substance on the cornea or conjunctiva.

COMPLICATIONS

1. Subconjunctival hemorrhage or corneal abrasion (rare) in a child who is not adequately restrained.
2. Conjunctival erythema from overzealous irrigation.

PROCEDURE

Place the child supine over a large sink or pail. To restrain an uncooperative child, two assistants are necessary. The person holding the head should wear a gown and may use gauze under each thumb to help keep the eyelids open. Allow bacteriostatic normal saline solution (between room and body temperature) to flow through a set of intravenous tubing. Drip the fluid rapidly into the conjunctival sac. Irrigate for a minimum of 5 min for acid using at least 1 liter. Irrigate for 20 min for alkali or unknown substances. Tap water at room temperature is an acceptable alternative for irrigation fluid, especially if it can be done immediately.

After irrigation, the eye should be carefully examined for corneal and conjunctival integrity, including staining with fluorescein dye.

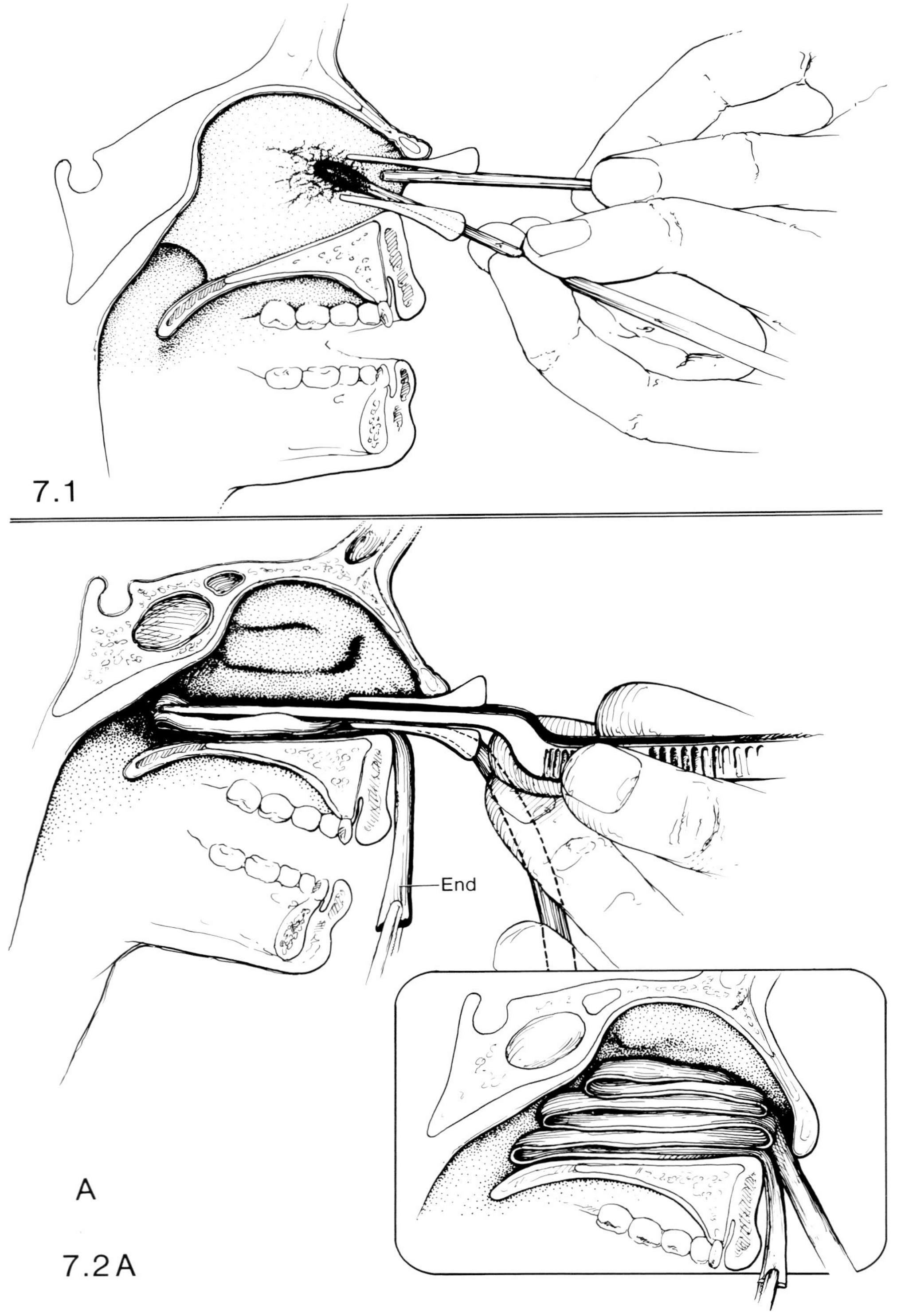
7.1
End
A
7.2A

7.1. NASAL CAUTERIZATION

INDICATIONS

Uncontrolled epistaxis.

CONTRAINDICATIONS

Bleeding diathesis (i.e., hemophilia, thrombocytopenia, etc.).

COMPLICATIONS

1. Secondary bacterial infection of the cauterized area.
2. Septal perforation.

PROCEDURE

The patient should be sitting or lying down and restrained, if necessary; sedation may be useful for the anxious child. Place cotton pledgets soaked with topical vasoconstricting and anesthetic agents (see Table 7.1) in the nostrils. This will shrink the nasal mucosa to allow better visualization of the interior of the nose and may slow or even stop the bleeding. Additionally, the topical anesthetic permits instrumentation of the nose without discomfort to the child. Insert the nasal speculum into the nose and open the blades widely, using a head light or directed light source (i.e., flashlight) to illuminate the interior of the nose. Since most epistaxis originates from Little's area (the anterior septum) this area should be examined first. Suction any clots or fresh blood gently with a Frazier suction tip on low pressure wall suction to expose the source of hemorrhage. Once the site of bleeding is located, apply the tip of a silver nitrate stick to it and roll it over the bleeding area (Fig. 7.1). Two or three sticks are often required to control an episode of epistaxis. Once the bleeding has stopped, put Vaseline or oxycel gauze (Surgicel®) on the septum to stabilize the clot and protect the area from further trauma.

If electrocautery is available, it can be used in place of the silver nitrate sticks, but certain precautions must be taken. While local anesthetics are usually unnecessary for the application of silver nitrate sticks, they are required prior to use of electric current to stop bleeding. Also, the electrocautery must be properly grounded and have manual setting so low voltage can be used.

With either method of cauterization, refrain from cauterizing both sides of the nasal septum at the same time. Vigorous bilateral cauterization may deprive the underlying septal cartilage of its blood supply and lead to a septal perforation.

TABLE 7.1
Equipment—Otorhinolaryngologic Procedures

Directed light source (headlight, flashlight, etc.)
Frazier suction tip
Nasal speculum
Bayonet forceps
Topical vasoconstrictor [phenylephrine (0.25%, 0.5%), epinephrine (1:1000), cocaine (3 to 5% solution)]
Topical anesthetics [cocaine (3 to 5% solution), lidocaine (4%) ethyl chloride]
Oxycel gauze (Surgicel)®
Silver nitrate sticks
Vaseline gauze (½ by 72 inch)
Gauze (4 × 4) to make posterior pack
Suture (0 silk) 18 inches length
Foley catheter (12 or 14 gauge with 30-ml balloon)
Red rubber catheters
Cuff (made of 1-inch length of suction tubing)
Syringe (30 ml)
Sterile saline solution
Hoffman clamp (for Foley catheter)
Scalpel blade, No. 15
Alligator forceps

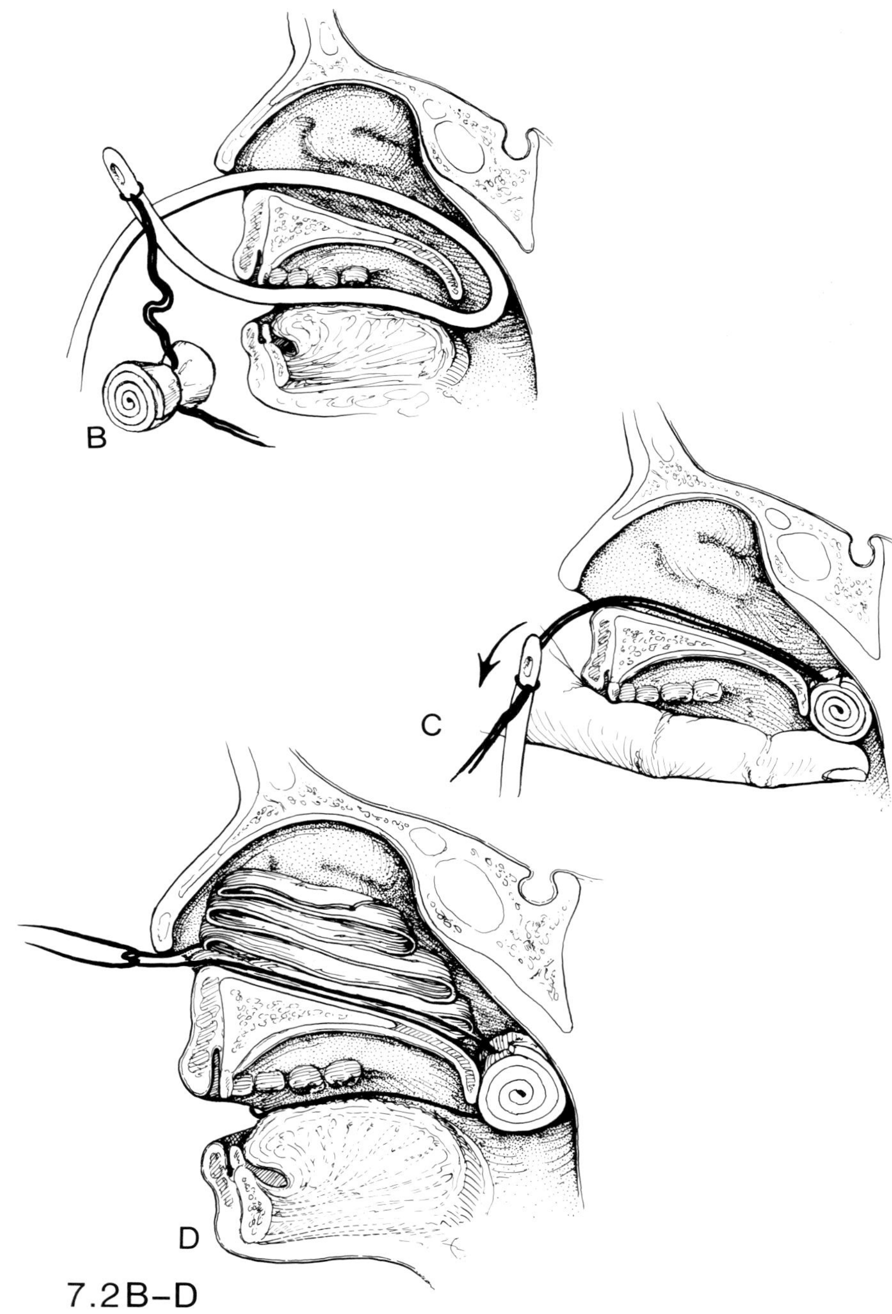

7.2B–D

7.2. NASAL PACKING—ANTERIOR AND POSTERIOR

INDICATIONS

Uncontrolled epistaxis.

COMPLICATIONS

1. Bacterial rhinosinusitis.
2. Nasal alar necrosis.
3. Septal ulceration or perforation.
4. Respiratory distress from sedation and nasal airway obstruction.

PROCEDURE

Anterior Pack (Fig. 7.2*A*)

Prepare the patient in the same manner as for cauterization. Using a bayonet forceps, grasp a length of Vaseline-impregnated gauze approximately 4 to 5 cm from its end, and insert it straight back along the floor of the nose, for 3 to 4 cm, not up along the bridge. The end of the gauze should protrude from the nostril by 2 to 3 cm to prevent it from falling into the nasopharynx and causing the child to gag. Withdraw the bayonet forceps and grasp the gauze again approximately 7 cm from where it is now exiting from the nose. This portion of the gauze should then be placed into the nose on top of the material that has already been placed. Repeat the process until the nasal cavity is filled with layers of gauze from bottom to top. A small piece of tape can be used to cover the nostril and prevent the child from disturbing the pack. Since the nasal pack causes stasis of the nasal secretions, oral antimicrobial drugs may be considered to prevent the occurrence of sinusitis.

Posterior Pack

If an anterior pack is not sufficient to stop an episode of epistaxis, a posterior pack may be required. Since the placement of posterior packs is very uncomfortable, sedation is strongly recommended.

Posterior packs can be made from either of two materials: 4 × 4 gauze or a Foley catheter. To make the gauze pack, roll up a 4 × 4 gauze sponge until it is approximately 2 to 5 cm long and 2 cm in diameter; three No. 0 silk sutures (50 cm length) are knotted around the middle of this roll. Next, thread a red rubber catheter into the nose and bring the end out the mouth by grasping it with a hemostat when it appears in the posterior oropharynx. Tie two of the silk sutures to the end of the catheter, as shown in Figure 7.2*B*, but hold the third with a hemostat. As the catheter is withdrawn from the nose, guide the pack into the mouth and then up into the nasopharynx (Fig. 7.2*C*). The pack is held in position by the two silk sutures which pull the pack up against the vomer (posterior nasal septum). Tie these sutures together after placing an anterior gauze pack as previously described. The third silk suture, which is protruding from the child's mouth, is taped to the cheek to prevent aspiration of the pack if the nasal ties should loosen.

An alternative is to use two red rubber catheters and insert one through each nares. On completion, there will be sutures on each side which can be loosely tied in front of the septum. An anterior pack is still used on the side of bleeding.

To place a posterior pack utilizing a Foley catheter, make a plastic cuff by cutting a 2- to 3-cm length of clear plastic tubing (such as suction tubing) and pass it over a 12 or 14 gauge Foley catheter that has a 30 ml balloon. The cuff serves to hold the catheter in place outside the nose. Slide the cuff up to the bifurcation of the catheter; the distal tip of the Foley catheter beyond the balloon should be cut off. Test the inflation of the balloon by injecting saline. Place the catheter into the nose and advance the end into the pharynx. After injecting 10 to 15 ml of saline into the balloon, pull the catheter back until the balloon is pressed tightly against the vomer (Fig. 7.2*E*). A standard anterior gauze pack is then placed in the nose. Slide the cuff of suction tubing down to contact the anterior gauze pack, making certain that the tubing is inside the nostril and not placing pressure on the nasal ala. A Hoffman clamp (or hemostat, in an emergency) is then used to clamp the Foley catheter just distal to the cuff of tubing to keep the catheter from slipping posteriorly

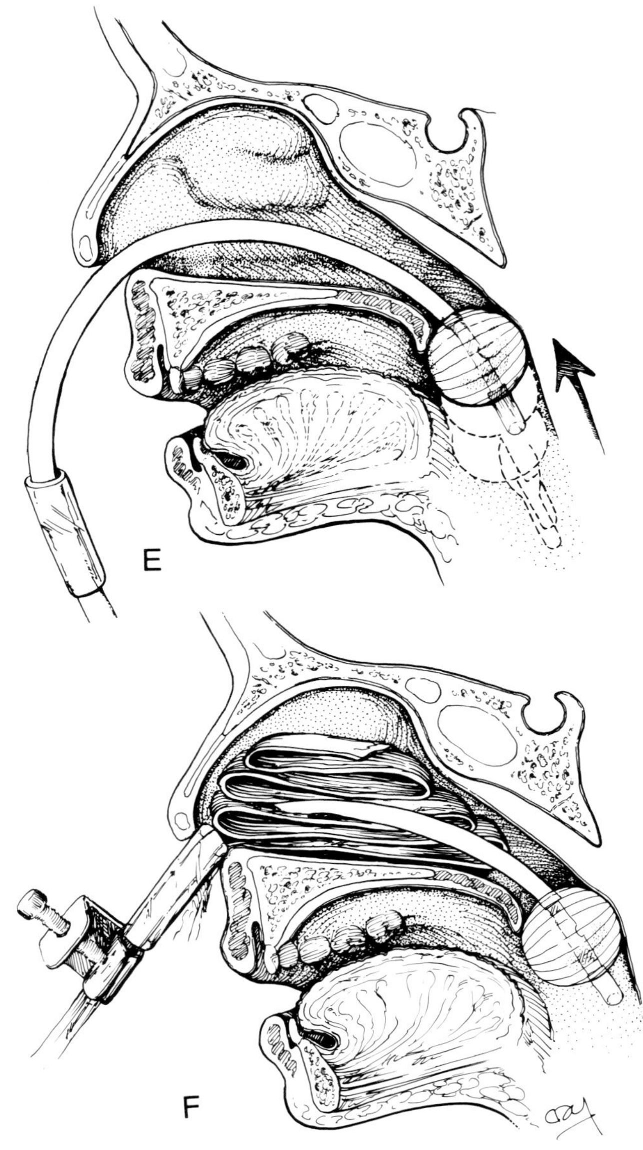

7.2 E–F

into the pharynx (Fig. 7.2*F*). Antimicrobial agents may be given to these children in an effort to prevent the occurrence of sinusitis.

Important Note. The placement of a posterior nasal pack may cause hypoxia and hypercapnia. Additionally, the sedation often required in these patients may decrease respiratory efforts and lead to significant respiratory embarrassment. For these reasons, any child with a posterior pack should be admitted to the hospital and observed in the intensive care unit.

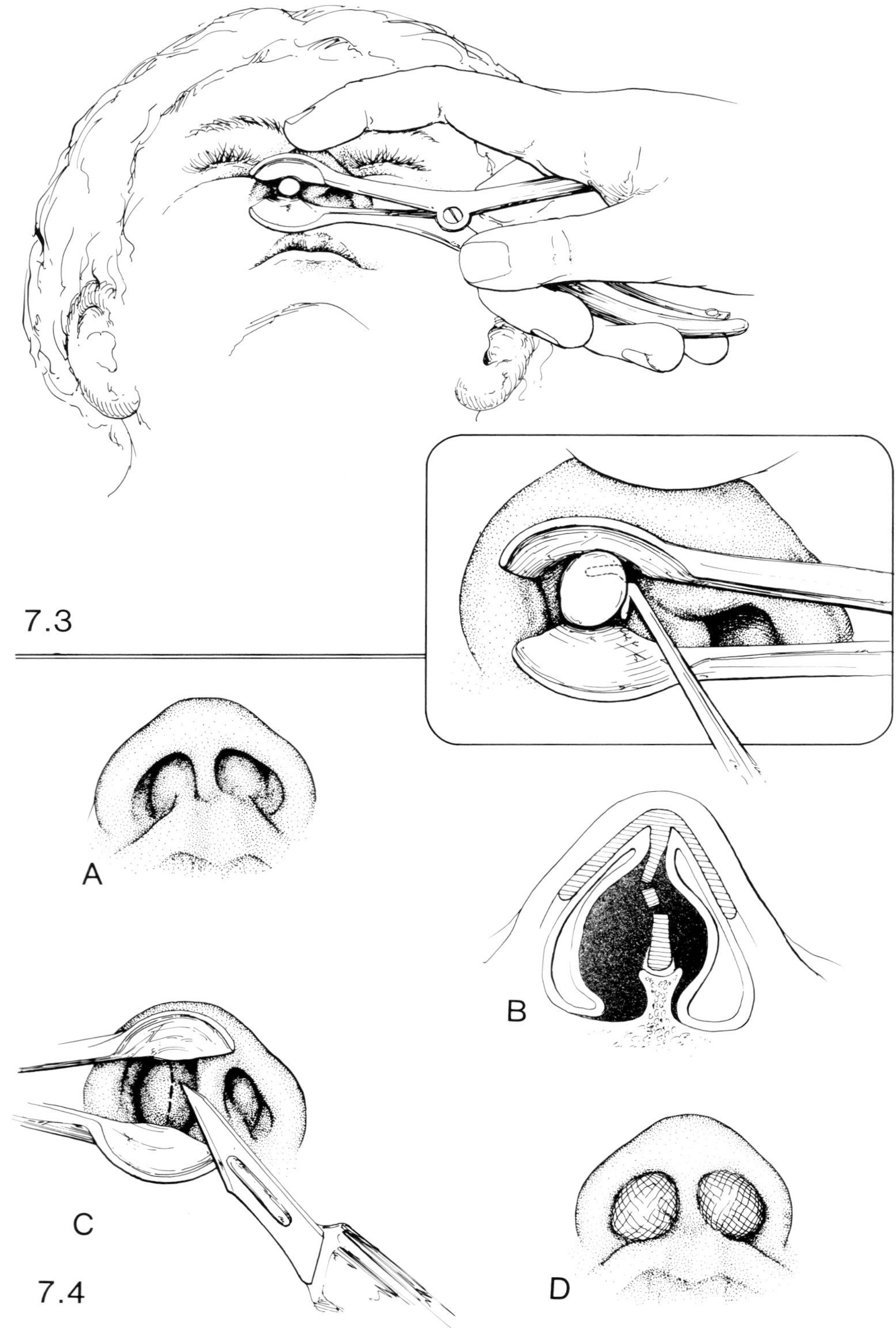
7.3
A
B
C
7.4
D

7.3. REMOVAL OF A NASAL FOREIGN BODY

INDICATION

Presence of a nasal foreign body.

COMPLICATIONS

1. Rhinosinusitis.
2. Mucosal laceration.
3. Epistaxis.
4. Aspiration.
5. Incomplete removal of the foreign body.

PROCEDURE

The child should be lying down and restrained. The patient must be kept still during instrumentation of the nose in order to prevent injury to the internal nasal structures. After applying a topical vasoconstrictor-anesthetic agent to shrink the nasal membranes, visualize the interior of the nose with a nasal speculum and a headlight or directed light. Purulent secretions should be gently removed with Frazier suction tip until the foreign body is clearly seen. Attempt to extract the object with either suction, a hook, or alligator forceps as determined by the size, nature and position of the object. Do not push the foreign body into the posterior nasopharynx as it may be aspirated by the struggling child. The use of irrigation is not recommended because the foreign body may slip posteriorly and be aspirated or hygroscopic foreign bodies (i.e., sponges) may swell and become lodged in the nose. After the foreign body has been removed, oral antimicrobials agents may be used in an effort to prevent an infection in the traumatized area.

7.4. DRAINAGE OF SEPTAL HEMATOMA/ABSCESS

INDICATION

Presence of a nasal septal hematoma or abscess.

COMPLICATIONS

1. Perichondritis.
2. Septal abscess.
3. Septal perforation.
4. Saddle nose deformity.

PROCEDURE

Figure 7.4, *A* and *B*, show the external appearance and anatomy of a septal hematoma. Since the drainage of a nasal septal hematoma/abscess is quite painful, this procedure is usually performed on a child in the operating room under a general anesthetic. If drainage is to be performed in the emergency department, the child requires adequate sedation and restraint.

After visualization of the hematoma or abscess with a headlight or directed light and a nasal speculum, anesthetize the membrane with topical 3 to 5% cocaine or injectable 1% lidocaine. Sterile gloves should be worn. Incise the bulging membrane on the affected side (or sides, if a bilateral abscess is present) of the nasal septum with a No. 15 scalpel blade as shown in Figure 7.4*C*. The material in the hematoma or abscess should be expressed manually and sent for culture. Then a *loose* anterior nasal pack should be placed to tamponade the nasal membranes against the septum (Fig. 7.4*D*). The child should receive oral antibiotic therapy after the procedure, and the pack changed in 12 to 24 hours.

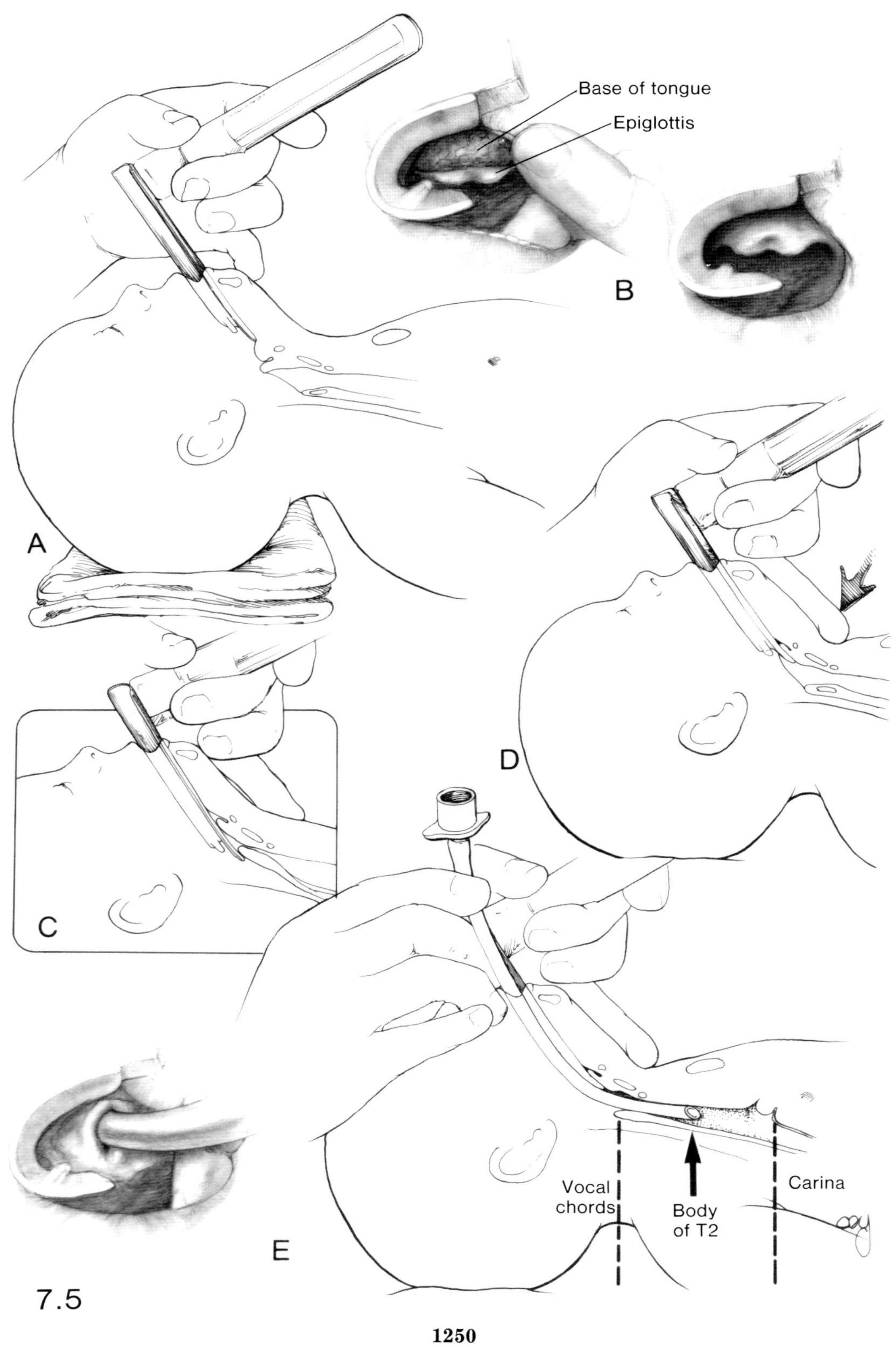

Base of tongue
Epiglottis
B
A
D
C
Vocal chords
Body of T2
Carina
E
7.5

7.5. OROTRACHEAL INTUBATION

INDICATIONS

1. Cardiopulmonary resuscitation.
2. Respiratory failure with hypoxemia or hypercarbia.
3. Absent pharyngeal reflexes: coma, brainstem dysfunction, and myopathy.
4. Unstable airway from facial trauma or an airway abnormality.

CAUTIONS

Caution should be exercised in the intubation of the child with a full stomach (see Chapters 1, 3, and 44), with temporomandibular ankylosis or a hypoplastic mandible (Chapter 3), or with a defect in blood coagulation.

COMPLICATIONS

1. Hypoxemia or cardiac arrest.
2. Bronchial intubation with secondary contralateal atelectasis or ipsilateral pneumothorax.
3. Vomiting and/or aspiration secondary to a full stomach.
4. Dislodgment of teeth.
5. Laceration of the lips and gums.
6. Laryngeal trauma.
7. Esophageal intubation.

EQUIPMENT

1. Resuscitator with mask and oxygen source.
2. Oropharyngeal airways (Guedel 00, 0, 1, 2, 3, 4).
3. Uncuffed orotracheal tubes 2.5- to 8.0-mm inner diameter (I.D.), cuffed tubes 6.0 to 8.0 mm I.D. (all with 15-mm male connector) (see Table 7.5*A*).
4. Laryngoscope handle and several blades (see Table 7.5*B*), extra batteries and bulbs.
5. Stylet: infant, adult teflon coated.
6. Magill forceps: child, adult sizes.
7. Suction equipment:
   a. Central or portable suction source
   b. Yankauer tonsil aspirator (replace tip by thick walled rubber tubing).
   c. Disposable sterile plastic suction catheters (French sizes 5, 8, 10, 14).

Table 7.5A
Endotracheal Tube Sizes

Age	Size (Inner Diameter, mm)
Premature	2.5
Term to 3 months	3.0
3 to 7 months	3.5
7 to 15 months	4.0
15 to 24 months	4.5
2 to 15 years	
Internal diameter (I.D.) = [16 + age (years)]/4	
(Round to the nearest 0.5 mm)	

Table 7.5B
Laryngoscope Blades

Age	Name and Size
Premature	Miller 0
Term to 1 year	Wis-Hipple 1 or Miller 1
1 to 1.5 years	Wis-Hipple 1½
1.5 to 12 years	Miller or Flagg 2
13 years +	Macintosh 3

PROCEDURE

Intubation is performed following preoxygenation: administer 100% O_2 at relatively high flows, i.e., up to 10 liters/min in pediatric patients by a T-piece system or high oxygen concentration self-inflating bag/mask for 3 min to a spontaneously ventilating patient. During resuscitations or in patients with inadequate ventilation, use assisted or controlled positive pressure ventilation by bag/mask before intubation for a least one minute or until cyanosis clears.

Prepare the awake patient with an appropriate anesthetic (see Chapters 1 and 3), and use proper restraint for any patient it is deemed should not receive temporary neuromuscular blockade. Then, with the patient supine and the head on a firm pad in the "sniffing" position (Fig. 7.5*A*), the operator opens the mouth with the right thumb and index finger by pulling the mandible open and forward. Insert the laryngoscope blade in the right corner of the mouth, then pull the blade to the center, depressing the tongue and clearing the lower lip from between the teeth and blade

(Fig. 7.5*B*). Advance the blade under direct visualization into the hypopharynx (Fig. 7.5*C*). Elevate the mandibular tissue block by exerting force along the axis of the laryngoscope handle to expose the posterior pharyngeal wall and the proximal esophagus. Avoid any direct pressure of the laryngoscope blade on the dentoalveolar ridge. Slowly withdraw the blade with an assistant applying simultaneous cricoid pressure (Fig. 7.5*D*); the larynx will ascend into view. If the epiglottis (Fig. 7.5*B*) obscures the glottic chink further elevation of the blade usually reestablishes a good view. Advance the endotracheal tube from the right side of the oropharynx to avoid blocking the view during tube passage. Pass it an appropriate distance (usually 2 to 3 cm) into the trachea (Fig. 7.5*E*).

Ventilate the patient using the T-piece system or self-inflating bag; determine tube position above the carina by auscultation of equal breath sounds in both axilla.

Use an oropharyngeal airway to protect the teeth and prevent biting of the orotracheal tube. Pick the airway that approximates the distance from the mouth to the angle of the jaw. Pass it into the pharynx curved downward maintaining the mouth open with a tongue depressor. Secure it with tape to the orotracheal tube and child's skin.

Confirm proper position of the tip of the tube by portable anteroposterior chest radiograph in order to help avoid accidental extubation or endobronchial intubation. Aim for the tip to be superimposed over the body of the second thoracic vertebrae, corresponding to a distance of at least 2 cm above the carina (Fig. 7.5*E*).

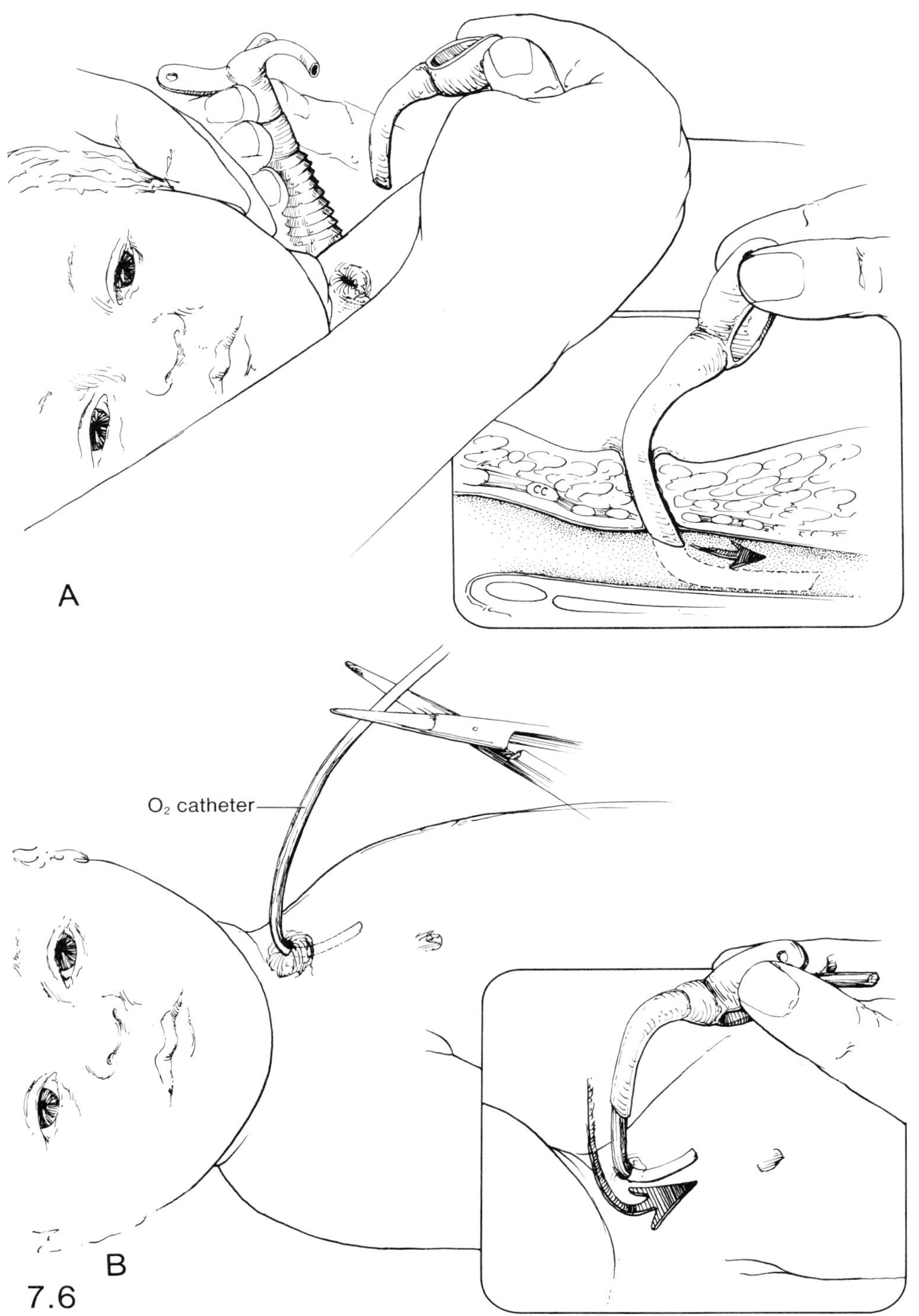
CC
A
O_2 catheter
B
7.6

7.6. REPLACEMENT OF A TRACHEOSTOMY CANNULA

INDICATIONS

1. Relief of obstruction of a tracheostomy tube (i.e., secretions, mucous plug, or foreign body).
2. Accidental decannulation.

COMPLICATIONS

1. Respiratory distress—hypoxemia and hypercarbia.
2. Creation of a false tracheal passage leading to pneumomediastinum and pneumothorax.

PROCEDURE

1. Replacement of an Obstructed Tracheostomy Cannula

The child with a tracheostomy who develops tachypnea, cyanosis, decreased breath sounds or severe retractions should be assumed to have a mechanical obstruction of his or her cannula until proven otherwise. Have an assistant obtain a scissors, a new cannula (often available from the parents), or an endotracheal tube of the same diameter or one size smaller than the obstructed tube. Ventilate the child with 100% oxygen. Place a small, folded towel under the child's shoulder and extend the head and neck. This maneuver exposes the tracheostomy site and eliminates redundancy or flaccidity of those tissues, which lie between the trachea and the anterior surface of the neck. The trachea is thereby forced closer to the plane of the skin. An attempt should be made to pass a suction catheter. If the catheter passes, apply suction at 80 to 120 cm of water and withdraw over a period of 3 to 5 sec. Immediately reventilate with 100% oxygen and continue suctioning. If the suction catheter will not pass through the tracheal cannula, the cannula must be changed immediately. Carefully cut the strings which secure the cannula with a bandage scissors so as not to lacerate the child's neck. Remove the tube. Observe the tract of the tracheocutaneous fistula and introduce the new cannula so that the tip follows the course of the tracheocutaneous fistula (see Fig. 7.6*A*). Press the flanges of the tracheostomy tube against the child's neck and attach a swivel connector and resuscitator to the system. Ventilate the child and check for symmetrical breath sounds by auscultation. Insert a hemostat through a flange hole and pull the tracheostomy twill (cloth tape) through so that you are left with two lengths of twill which are sufficiently long to go around the neck to knot through the opposite flange hole. Prior to securing the knot, apply adhesive-backed foam, if available, to the string crossing the back of the neck. With the neck flexed, tie the string snugly. If properly secured an index finger should fit snugly under the strings while the head is flexed. Obtain a chest x-ray to assure proper placement and to assess for pulmonary parenchymal change.

If a tracheostomy cannula is not immediately available, a standard endotracheal tube can be used instead. Care must be taken so as not to advance these beyond the carina. The chest should be auscultated for equal breath sounds bilaterally and, in addition, position of the distal tip should be confirmed by a chest roentgenogram.

2. Replacement of a Dislodged Cannula

When a tracheal cannula is dislodged from the stoma of a child totally dependent on that cannula, it must be replaced immediately. Time may not allow for acquisition of a clean tube. Cut the strings, and replace the cannula. Hold it firmly in place until it can be secured or until a clean cannula is made available. Occasionally the tracheocutaneous stomal tract will constrict so that the cannula cannot be replaced. Several actions can be considered. First, place a smaller tracheal cannula or endotracheal tube to allow oxygenation and ventilation. Then electively dilate the stoma and replace the appropriate size tube. Alternatively, as in Figure 7.6*B*, pass a smaller oxygen catheter (Fr. 10, 14). If the child is cyanotic, connect the catheter to an oxygen hose and run oxygen at a flow rate between 250 and 500 ml/min. If the child is not cyanotic move directly toward passing a tracheostomy cannula over the oxygen catheter into the stoma. The oxygen catheter will serve as a stylet and guideline to keep the tracheostomy cannula from being forced into a false passage. If the cannula cannot be advanced it may be necessary to oxygenate and ventilate the child with a resuscitator and mask through the upper airway while an assistant covers the stoma with a gloved finger. If the upper airway is obstructed, place a small endotracheal tube (size 3.5 to 4.5) through the stoma, hold it in place and use it to oxygenate while efforts are made toward mobilizing more direct surgical intervention.

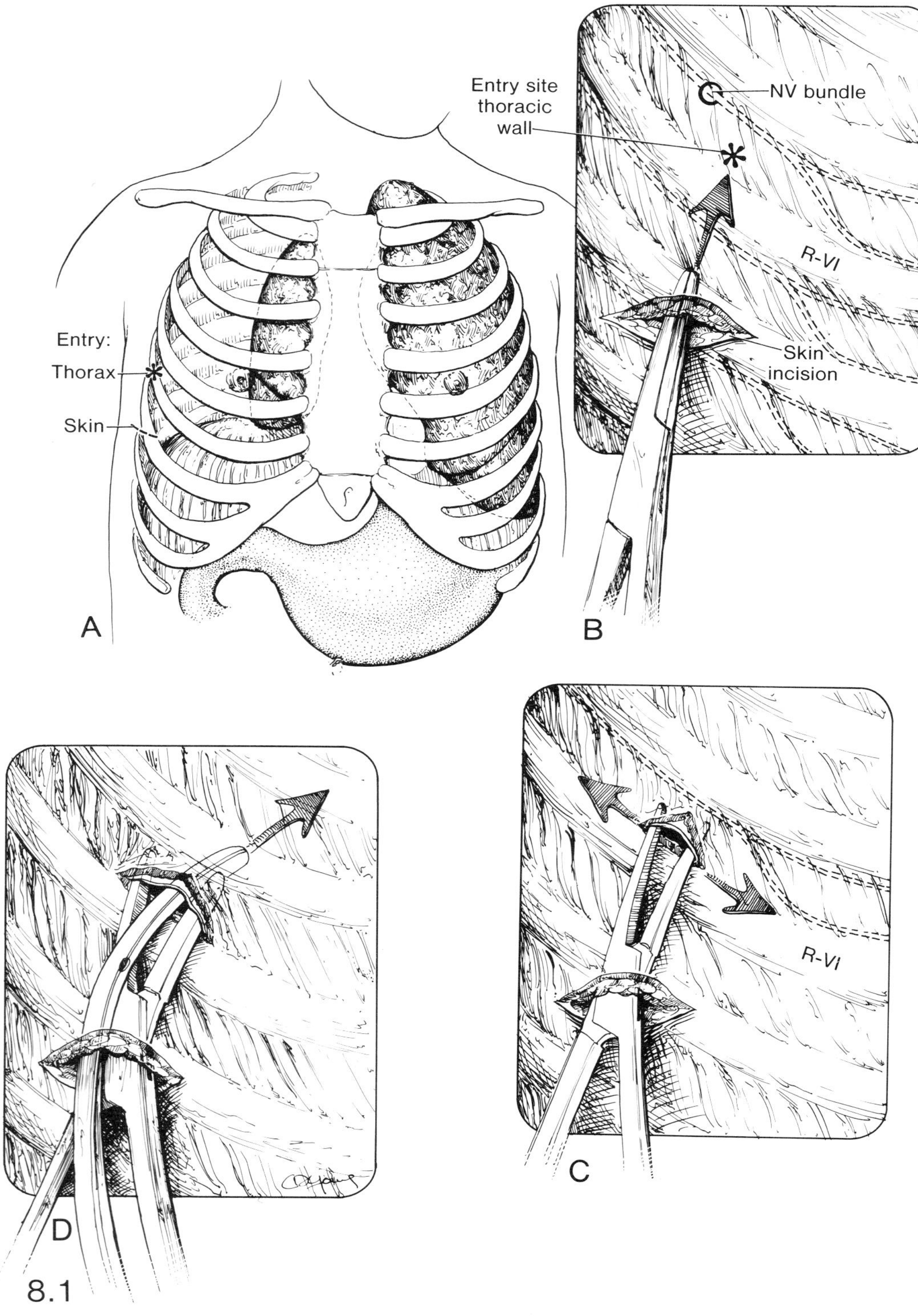
Entry site
thoracic
wall
NV bundle
R-VI
Skin
incision
Entry:
Thorax
Skin
A
B
C
R-VI
D
8.1

8.1. INSERTION OF CHEST TUBE

INDICATIONS

1. Evacuation of a pneumothorax.
2. Drainage of a hemothorax, symptomatic empyema, or large pleural effusion.

COMPLICATIONS

1. Bleeding—local.
2. Pulmonary contusion or laceration.
3. Pneumothorax or hemothorax.
4. Infection.
5. Bronchopleural fistula or pleural-cutaneous air leak.
6. Diaphragmatic, splenic, or liver puncture.

PROCEDURE

Identify the side(s) with the hemothorax or pneumothorax by physical examination and chest x-ray. Initiate treatment of cardiorespiratory disturbances prior to beginning the procedure. If abdominal distension is present, especially from a dilated stomach, pass a large bore nasogastric tube to reduce diaphragmatic elevation.

Figure 8.1*A* shows the anatomy of a child with a right-sided pneumothorax, from an anterior view, and the preferred sight of entry into the thorax between the anterior axillary and midaxillary lines at the level of the nipple (5th intercostal space).

Restrain the child if necessary; minimize any respiratory compromise. Generally, a young or seriously ill child should be supine, but the older cooperative patient may sit. Locate the landmarks and cleanse the site with povidone-iodine solution. Wearing sterile gloves, use a local anesthetic (1% lidocaine) to infiltrate the skin, subcutaneous tissue, and periosteum of the upper rib border. Make the skin incision at least one intercostal space below the rib over which the catheter will pass. This provides an oblique trajectory for the chest tube which helps maintain a seal when the tube is in position and after its removal.

Figure 8.1*B* shows a 1.5- to 2.0-cm transverse skin incision made with a No. 15 scalpel blade. Using a curved hemostat or Kelly clamp, bluntly dissect through the muscle and fascial layers to the upper surface of the chosen rib. Determine this by palpation with the tip of the instrument. Then, slide it over the superior rib margin, puncturing the intercostal muscles and pleura well below the neurovascular bundle of the adjacent cephalad rib, as shown in Figure 8.1*C*. The instrument should be controlled so that the tip does not enter more than 1 cm into the thoracic cavity. Open the instrument widely to provide an opening through the intercostal muscles and pleura that is at least 1.5 to 2 cm in diameter. At this point, any fluid or air under pressure in the pleural space may surge out.

As shown in Figure 8.1*D*, grasp the chest tube between the tips of the curved hemostat or clamp. In general, the smaller thoracic cavity in children as compared to adults makes the use of a trochar more dangerous. Then advance the instrument through the incision and up the previously dissected tract to the pleural space. When the tube tip has entered this cavity, open the hemostat and advance the catheter until it meets some resistance. The tip will most likely be at the apex of the hemithorax. Approximate the incision with several nylon sutures, some of which should encircle the tube to secure it in place. Sterile ointment and a sterile occlusive dressing should be applied to the wound. Further taping will help prevent dislodgment. After the tube has been attached to a drainage set (such as a Pleurovac®), obtain an upright or decubitus chest film immediately.

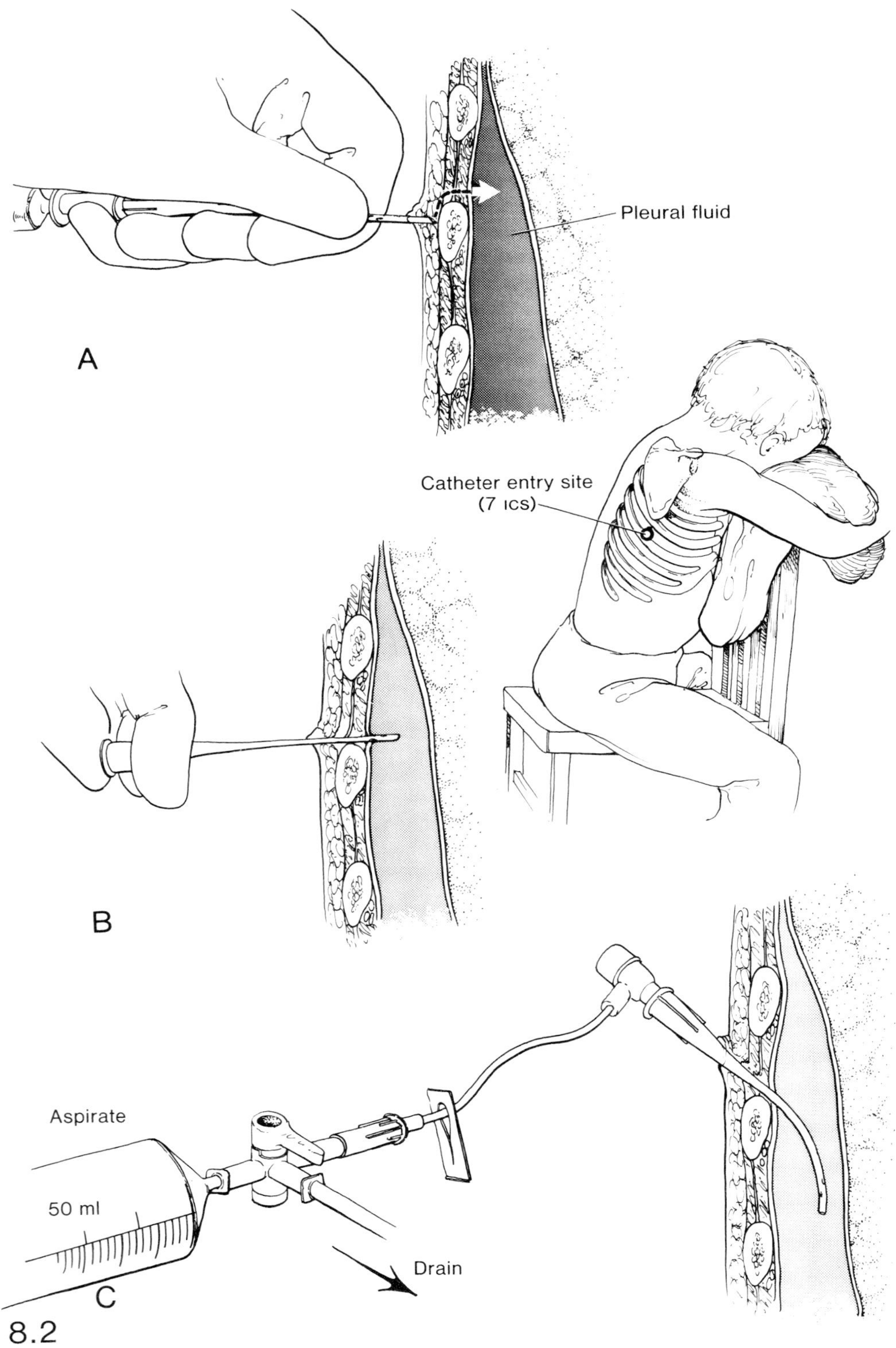
Pleural fluid
A
Catheter entry site
(7 ICS)
B
Aspirate
50 ml
Drain
C
8.2

8.2. THORACENTESIS

INDICATIONS

Diagnostic or therapeutic drainage of a pleural effusion or empyema.

COMPLICATIONS

1. Pneumothorax.
2. Pulmonary contusion.
3. Bleeding.

EQUIPMENT

1. Povidone-iodine solution, sterile gauze.
2. 5-ml syringe, 22 gauge needle, 1% lidocaine.
3. "Over the needle catheter," No. 16–20 Medicut® with extra holes cut in the catheter or large bore Argyle Intramedicut® catheter.
4. Stopcock, T-connector, 20- to 50-ml syringe.

PROCEDURE

To confirm the presence of a free pleural effusion and the side involved, obtain erect and decubitus chest radiographs prior to the procedure. Prepare the equipment and patient. Some children may do better with mild sedation, if they are not having respiratory distress, since restraint is difficult. Figure 8.2 shows the position useful in most toddlers and older children. Place the child in the sitting position with the arms and head supported on a pillow. With the arm on the involved side elevated, the lower tip of the scapula lies just above the 7th intercostal space in the posterior axillary line. Significant amounts of free fluid in the thoracic cavity will usually be present at this point. After donning sterile gloves, scrub the area of the intended puncture with povidone-iodine. Then anesthetize the site with 1% lidocaine from the skin to the periosteum of the rib. Figure 8.2*A* shows utilization of an "over the needle" catheter device. Advance the needle through the skin at a right angle to the chest wall at the point marked in Figure 8.2. Direct the needle against the upper rib surface of the rib then draw it back slightly. Next, lift up the catheter system gently and slowly advance it so that the needle slides over the top surface of the rib. Maintain continuous suction on the syringe while entering the pleural cavity; a decrease in the resistance to advancement of the needle and flow of fluid signals penetration of the parietal pleura. Advance the catheter slightly further, holding the needle steady.

As shown in Figure 8.2*B*, remove the syringe and needle and cover the hub of the catheter with the thumb. Since the catheter is soft, it can be advanced further into the thoracic cavity with little risk of puncturing lung. Aim caudally to achieve an optimal position for the evacuation of fluid.

As shown in Figure 8.2*C*, quickly attach a syringe (20 to 50 ml), stopcock, and T-connector to the catheter tip to minimize any leakage of air into the thorax. Increments of up to 50 ml can be removed for diagnostic studies or to provide symptomatic relief. If suction becomes difficult, reposition the catheter to maximize drainage. If insufficient fluid is obtained using a large bore Medicut®, insert a longer "through-the-needle" catheter deeper into the thorax to improve emptying. At the end of the procedure, quickly remove the catheter and apply a sterile occlusive dressing. An upright chest film should be obtained afterward to look for the presence of an iatrogenic pneumothorax.

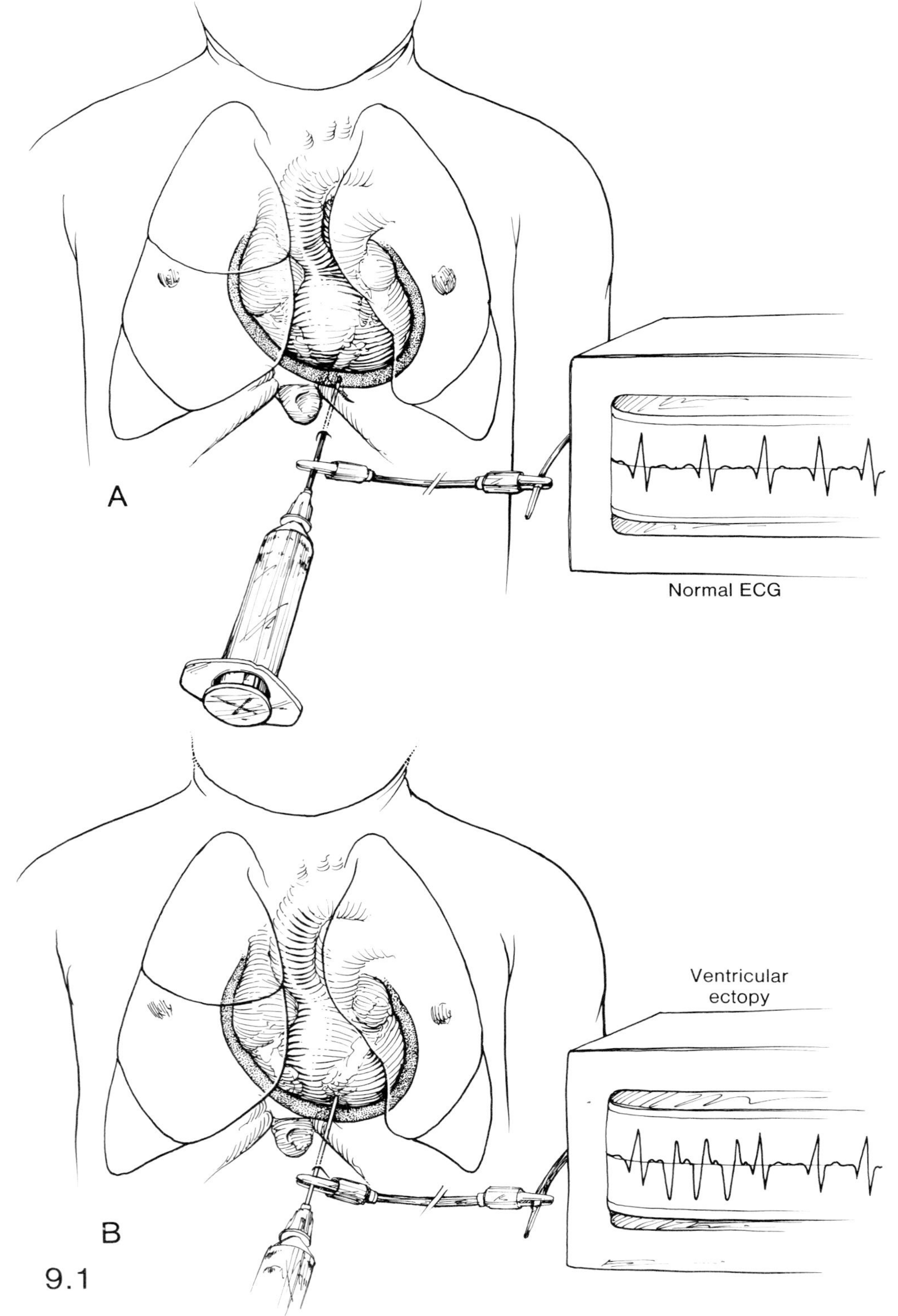
A
Normal ECG
Ventricular ectopy
B
9.1

9.1. PERICARDIOCENTESIS

INDICATIONS

1. Emergency removal of intrapericardial fluid in the treatment of pericardial tamponade.
2. Elective removal of pericardial fluid in the presence of a chronic or recurrent pericardial accumulation leading to an impairment of cardiac output.
3. As a diagnostic procedure for direct analysis of pericardial fluid.

COMPLICATIONS

A. During the procedure, one must observe for the following complications:
   1. Myocardial penetration or puncture of a cardiac chamber.
   2. Cardiac arrhythmias.
   3. Development of a hemorrhagic pericardial effusion (hemopericardium).
   4. Pneumothorax.

B. After the procedure, monitor the patient for the following:
   1. Continued pericardial leakage with the development of a cutaneous fistula.
   2. "Hidden" pericardial-peritoneal fistula.
   3. Slowly developing pneumothorax.
   4. Pneumopericardium.
   5. Infection at the puncture wound site.
   6. Slowly accumulating hemorrhagic pericardial effusion leading to pericardial tamponade.

PROCEDURES

Position the child supine at a 30 to 45° angle to the horizontal plane. Sedation usually is required and may necessitate capable airway management and ventilation to ensure the safety of the child. Attach the limb leads of an ECG monitor. Clean and sterilize the precordium with povidone-iodine solution and drape the area with sterile towels after donning sterile gloves. Infiltrate the area just below the xiphoid process with 1% lidocaine; penetrate through the muscle layer to achieve satisfactory local anesthesia.

Use a large bore (20 gauge) needle attached to a stopcock and a 20- to 50-ml syringe for the pericardial tap. Connect the "V" lead of the electrocardiogram to the hub of the needle with a sterile clip (alligator type) after checking that the lead is grounded. Turn ECG recorder on to "V" lead position.

Prior to the insertion of the needle, make a 2-mm incision just below the xiphoid to facilitate penetration of the skin. Holding the needle perpendicular to the skin, advance it through this incision; point the tip slightly cephalad and to the left of the midthoracic spine. Once below the skin, angle the needle at approximately 60 to 70° from the horizontal of the abdomen and slowly advance it, maintaining slight negative pressure on the syringe.

Capable medical personnel should monitor the ECG during this procedure. If an oscilloscope is not available, run a paper tracing continuously during the needle insertion. Close observation for a change in the ECG serves as a guide to the depth of the needle penetration. The appearance of a "ventricular" ECG complex or a "current of injury" pattern (ST segment changes and T-wave inversion) indicates penetration beyond the pericardium and into the myocardium. Should this occur, as shown in Figure 9.1*B*, withdraw the needle and observe closely for the return of the baseline pattern of the ECG (Fig. 9.1*A*).

Once in the pericardial space, the syringe fills with the pericardial fluid and the physician notes some spontaneous relief of the negative pressure being applied to the plunger. If drainage of a large volume of fluid is anticipated, introduce a flexible wire through the indwelling needle, followed by an end-hole catheter passed over the wire into the pericardial space.

After the procedure is completed, remove the needle (or catheter) and cover the puncture site with a sterile dressing. The patient should be observed very closely with frequent vital signs, until stable, in the intensive care unit. Obtain a chest x-ray to look for complications or a reaccumulation of pericardial fluid.

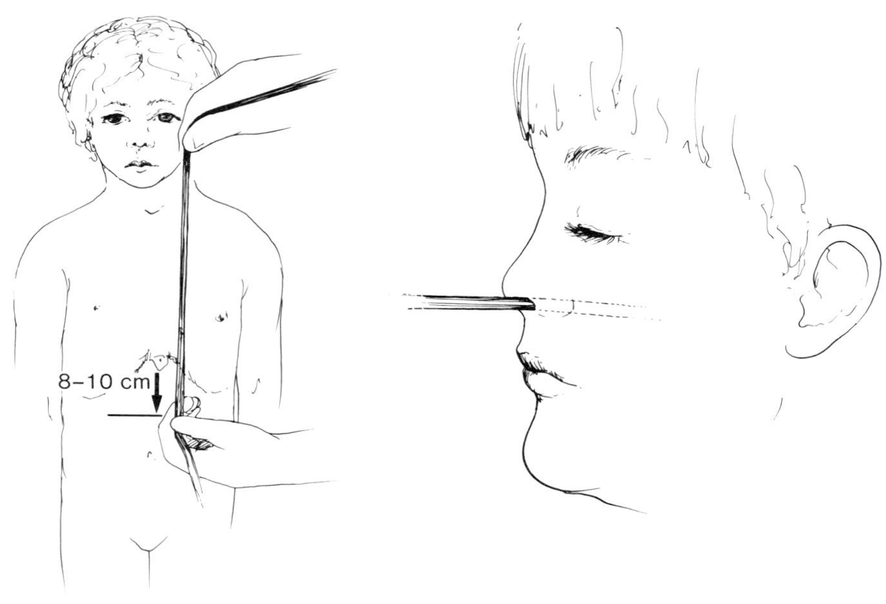

10.1

10.1. NASOGASTRIC TUBE PLACEMENT

INDICATIONS

1. Decompression of the stomach and proximal bowel for obstruction or trauma.
2. Gastric lavage in the child with upper gastrointestinal bleeding, or an ingestion.
3. Administration of medication.

COMPLICATIONS

1. Tracheal intubation.
2. Nasal or pharyngeal trauma or laceration.
3. Vomiting, leading to aspiration.

PROCEDURE

Choose the largest size tube feasible to perform the indicated task, without causing undue discomfort to the child. In general, choose an 8 Fr. tube in the newborn, around a 12 Fr. by a year. A teenager will usually tolerate an 18 Fr. In between, pick the size accordingly. It is advisable to cut extra side holes if gastric lavage or decompression is necessary. Estimate the length of tubing to be passed by adding 8 to 10 cm to the distance from the nares to the xiphoid process.

Prepare the child by explaining the procedure as fully as possible; sedation is rarely required. Older children, who are alert, can remain sitting. Infants and obtunded children require the supine position with their head turned to the side.

Straighten the curved tube out and check its patency with a syringe. If it is too pliable, stiffen it by immersion in ice water. Apply lubricant to facilitate atraumatic nasal passage. Grasp the tube 5 to 6 cm from the distal end and advance it posteriorly along the floor of the nose. If it is incorrectly directed up the nose, it may lacerate the inferior turbinate. Insert it with the natural curve of the tube pointing downward in order to pass the bend the posterior pharynx makes. One may ask the cooperative child to flex his or her head slightly and swallow some water to assist in glottic closure and easy passage into the esophagus; an assistant should flex the infant's neck. If the child coughs and gags persistently or the tube emerges from the mouth, temporarily discontinue the procedure.

When the tube is successfully passed to the measured length, check its position. Attach a syringe filled with air to the proximal end and, while depressing the plunger rapidly, listen with a stethoscope for gurgling over the stomach. Tape the tube securely to the nose, using tincture of benzoin on the skin in the uncooperative or diaphoretic child.

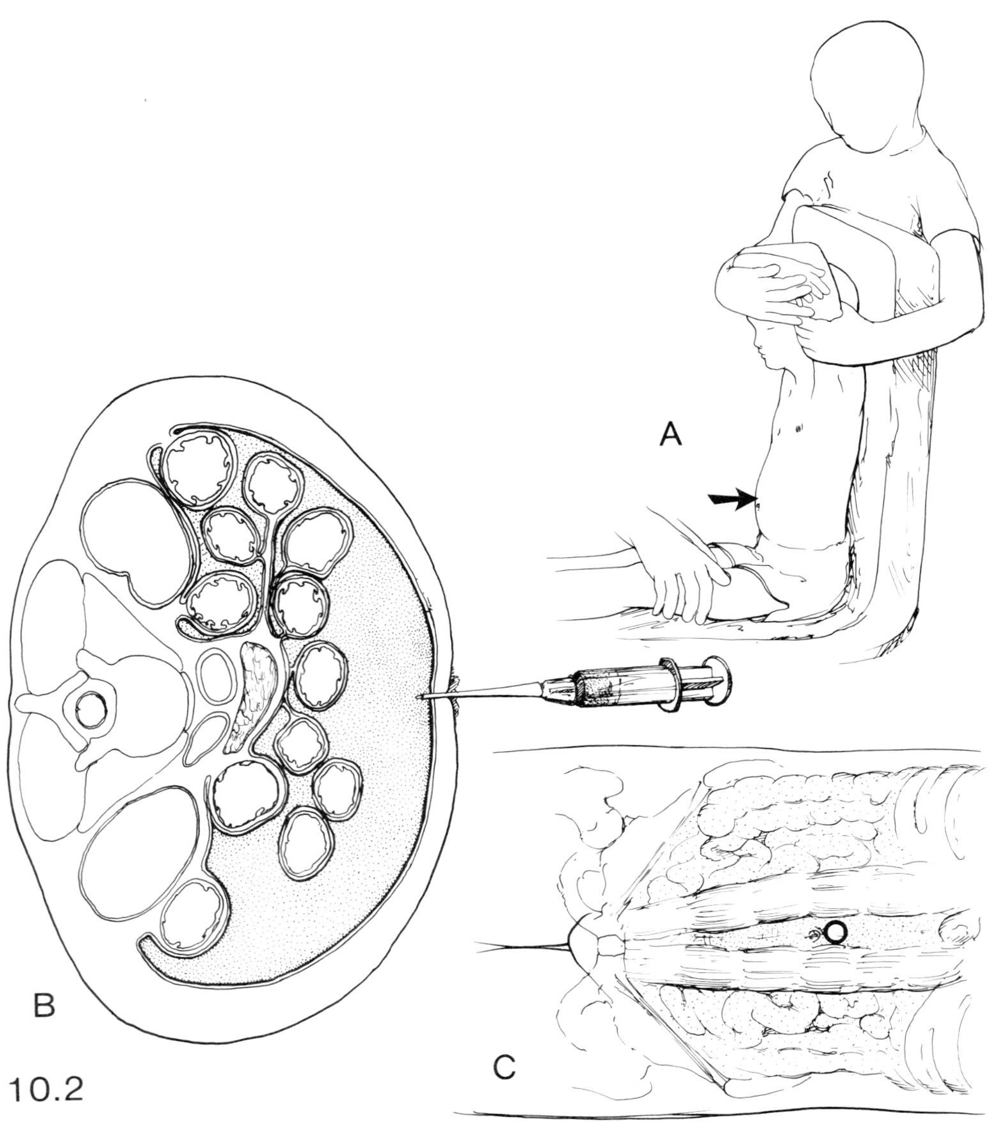
A
B
C
10.2

10.2 PERITONEAL TAP

INDICATION

1. To obtain peritoneal fluid for diagnostic purposes.
2. Relief of respiratory distress secondary to a large peritoneal collection of fluid.

COMPLICATIONS

1. Perforation of abdominal viscera.
2. Hemorrhage.
3. Peritonitis.

PROCEDURE

The child undergoing a diagnostic peritoneal aspiration may require sedation to permit safe access to the peritoneal cavity. If there is a large collection of intra-abdominal fluid, it may elevate the diaphragm, causing respiratory compromise. This serves as a relative contraindication to the use of general anesthetic for sedation.

Before attempting this procedure, carefully evaluate the abdominal anatomy. Verify the presence of ascites by percussion, being certain to note shifting dullness after the child is turned. Place the patient in the position in which the procedure is to be done, either sitting (Fig. 10.2*A*) or lateral decubitus (Fig. 10.2*C*) with an adequate amount of restraint. If there is a large amount of fluid, the child will have less respiratory embarrassment if allowed to sit.

For a diagnostic tap, use an 18, 20, or 22 gauge "over the needle" catheter (Medicut®). If a large amount of fluid must be evacuated, the plastic catheter, in contrast to a metal needle, allows for repositioning in the patient, and decreases the risk of bowel perforation during a prolonged procedure.

As shown in Figure 10.2*A*, a midline supraumbilical approach is probably the safest, either in the sitting or decubitus position. Cleanse a large area around the planned site with povidone-iodine solution. Then drape the patient with towels under and over the back, if in the decubitus position; drape towels on the lap, if in the sitting position. Wearing sterile gloves, inject the skin with 1% lidocaine.

After local anesthesia is achieved, take the needle and catheter in hand. Stabilize the tip of the needle with the thumb and index finger, placing the heel of this hand against the abdominal wall. With the other hand, direct the needle perpendicular to the abdominal wall. Puncture the skin, and then move the needle parallel to the midline for a short distance to a make a Z-track. Advance the needle with support until a "popping sensation" or decreased resistance is appreciated. Immediately verify penetration through the peritoneum by drawing fluid into the syringe. As shown schematically in Figure 10.2*B*, the abdominal viscera lie slightly away from the peritoneum if there is a moderate amount of fluid.

Slowly advance the needle several millimeters while continuing to aspirate fluid with the syringe. Then remove the needle and syringe from the catheter and cover the opening with the thumb. After attaching a larger syringe and T-connector, observe for a brisk flow of fluid. The catheter tip can be repositioned once the needle has been removed, and the patient safely turned to facilitate the collection of fluid. When completed, quickly pull the catheter straight out and firmly apply first a sterile gauze and then a pressure dressing to the puncture wound.

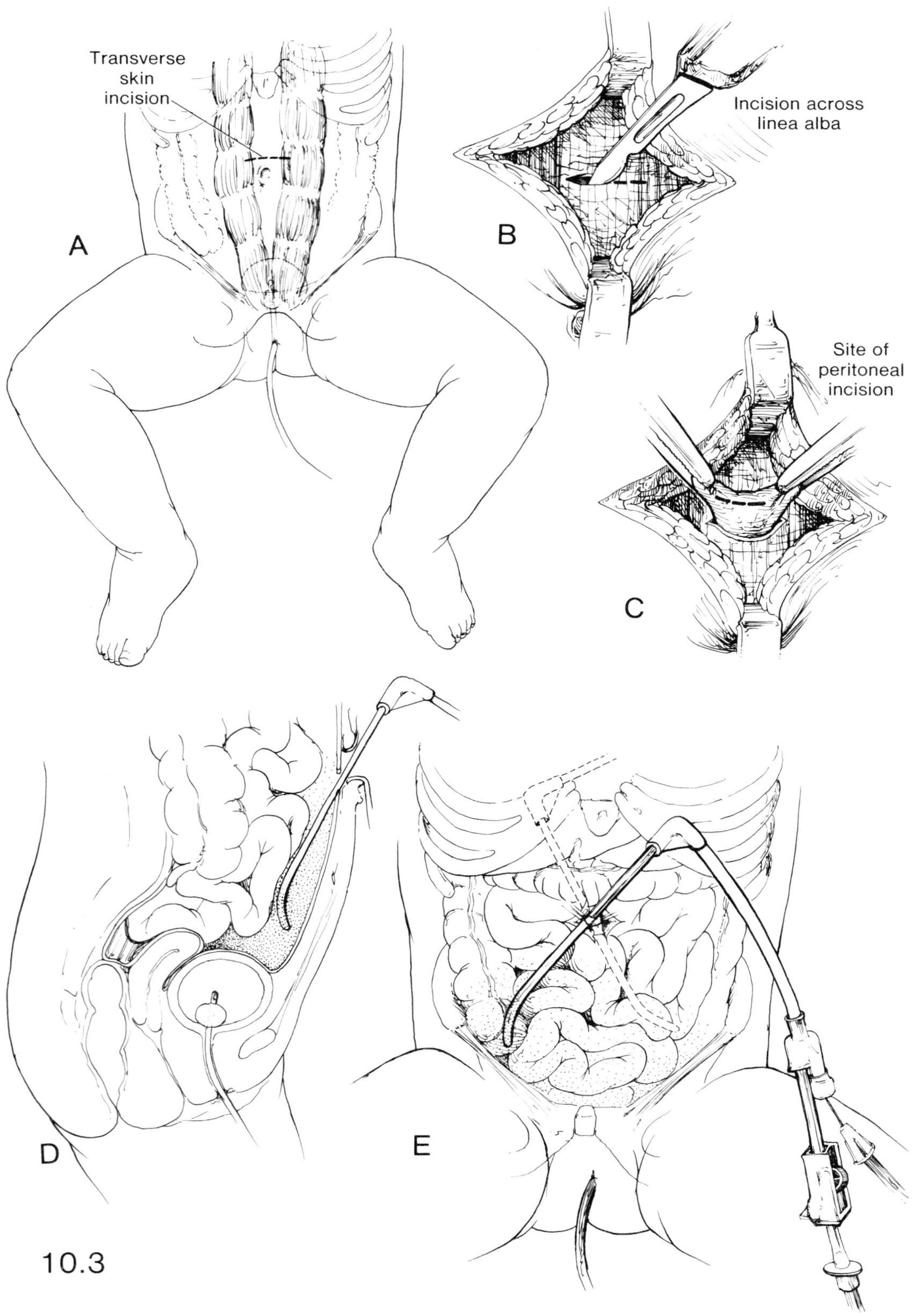
Transverse
skin
incision
A
Incision across
linea alba
B
Site of
peritoneal
incision
C
D
E

10.3

10.3. PERITONEAL LAVAGE

INDICATIONS

Multiple trauma in the child with coma, cardiovascular instability, or a falling hemoglobin.

COMPLICATIONS

1. Falsely positive test due to bleeding from the incision or blunt trauma to the bowel by the catheter.
2. Perforation of abdominal viscera by catheter (enhanced by prior abdominal adhesions).
3. Hemorrhage.
4. Peritonitis.

PROCEDURE

The child should receive an overall assessment, an intravenous infusion of saline through a large bore catheter, and the appropriate laboratory and radiographic evaluation. Correction of any cardiorespiratory disturbances is essential for the procedure to be safely performed.

Pass a nasogastric tube with extra side holes to decompress the stomach and a urinary catheter to empty the bladder. Select a site for the incision, either supraumbilical or infraumbilical, in the midline. A supraumbilical location is preferable in younger children whose bladder extends into the abdomen (Fig. 10.3*A*).

Prepare the anterior abdominal wall with povidone-iodine, wearing sterile gloves. Inject 1% lidocaine with epinephrine (to lessen bleeding) into the skin and subcutaneous tissue for local anesthesia. As shown in Figure 10.3*A*, make a 1.5- to 2-cm transverse incision in the skin with a No. 15 scalpel blade 1 to 2 cm above the umbilicus.

The subcutaneous tissue should be divided and the linea alba exposed by blunt dissection. Make a transverse or vertical incision through the linea alba as shown in Figure 10.3*B*, with care not to penetrate deeper than this fascial plane.

Using two hemostats, grasp the peritoneum at the center of the fascial opening, as shown in Figure 10.3*C*. The field should be maintained free of blood to prevent a falsely positive result. Between the hemostats, make a small incision through the peritoneum with the scalpel to provide access to the abdominal cavity. An immediate return of frankly bloody material constitutes a positive result.

If frankly bloody fluid is not obtained on opening the peritoneum, gently introduce a peritoneal dialysis catheter, without the trochar, through the peritoneal opening. Pass it caudally just inside the peritoneal lining into the pelvis to minimize the chance of perforating a viscus, as shown in cross section in Figure 10.3*D*. If aspiration through the catheter yields frankly bloody fluid, significant intra-abdominal bleeding has occurred.

If no blood is obtained, quickly infuse 10 to 20 ml/kg of Ringer's lactate solution into the abdominal cavity through the dialysis catheter, as shown in Figure 10.3*E*. Once the fluid has been instilled, turn the patient from side to side in order to promote its distribution throughout the peritoneal cavity. Then allow the fluid to run back out under gravity into a sterile collecting bag connected to intravenous tubing. Samples of the fluid should be sent for determination of red blood cell count, white blood count, amylase level, Gram stain, and examination for stool or food particles. At the completion of the lavage, whether the result is positive or negative, carefully remove the catheter. Use chromic sutures to close the peritoneum, and 2-0 or 3-0 absorbable sutures for the fascia and subcutaneous tissue. Place Steri-strips across the skin.

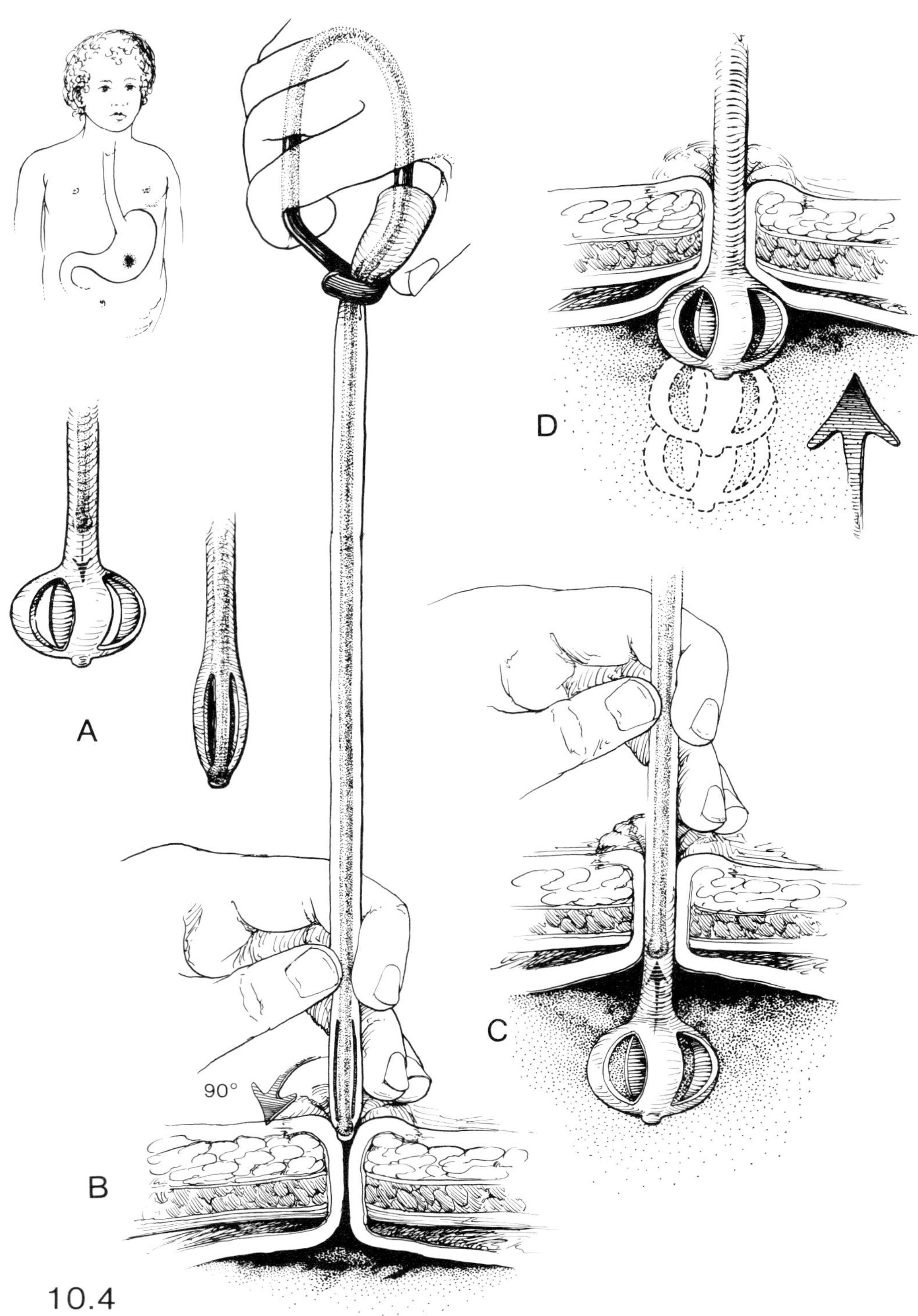
A
B
C
D
90°
10.4

10.4. REPLACEMENT OF A GASTROSTOMY TUBE

INDICATION

Obstruction or dislodgment of a gastrostomy tube.

COMPLICATIONS

1. Bleeding at the mucosal site.
2. Separation of the stomach from the abdominal wall.
3. Gastric outlet obstruction from an improperly positioned tube.

PROCEDURE

When a child with a gastrostomy appears in the emergency department following dislodgment of the tube, it should be replaced as soon as possible. The opening very quickly narrows, making passage of a replacement very difficult.

Perform a history and physical examination to be certain that there is not an intra-abdominal obstruction, and examine the gastrostomy site for bleeding or tears. The passage of a blunt tipped stylet through the opening allows the physician to assess the patency and direction of the tract.

Slide a Bard® or Mallincott® gastrostomy tube, of the same size as the one that is to be replaced, over a metal stylet, and as in Figure 10.4*A*, firmly stretch it to straighten out the mushroom or ball at the distal tip. An alternative is to use a Foley catheter of similar size. Hook the end of the tube and the handle of the stylet and generously apply lubricant to the distal portion.

Restrain the child in the supine position. Holding the system perpendicular to the abdominal wall, as in Figure 10.4*B*, aim it in the direction of the stoma tract as determined by the previous probing. Grasp the distal end of the tube between the index finger and thumb of one hand and stabilize it by placing the heel of this hand against the abdominal wall to prevent slippage. The other hand holds the handle of the stylet and the proximal portion of the tube.

Pass the tip of the catheter into the opening to the gastrostomy site and, with steady, firm pressure, push it down in the direction of the stomach, perpendicular to the abdominal wall. It may take 30 to 45 sec of this steady pressure to stretch the site enough to permit entry. Avoid sudden jerking of the tip, as this increases the chance of mucosal damage or separation.

When the stomach is entered, resistance suddenly lessens. As shown in Figure 10.4*C*, the tube must be inserted far enough so that the whole "mushroom" tip (balloon) is in the gastric cavity. After advancing several centimeters with little resistance, detach the handle of the stylet from the catheter and pass the catheter 4 to 5 cm further. The balloon will spontaneously open. Then fully withdraw the stylet and pull the tube gently out to appreciate the "clunk" on reaching the surface. If the tube is in the stomach, it will move freely and spontaneously drain gastric contents. Cover the distal end with clean gauze.

Occasionally the catheter may not be advanced far enough, leaving the balloon in the wall of the stomach. If this is the case, reinsert the stylet, stretch the tube, and with constant pressure, advance the catheter into the stomach. Similarly, if a child with a gastrostomy tube in place appears to be uncomfortable or have an obstructed tube, the tube may have been incorrectly placed or may have slipped out, so that the balloon is inflated in the gastric wall.

If the procedure causes mucosal trauma, the local application of lubricant gel or a neutralizing agent, such as an antacid, may decrease inflammation of the stoma.

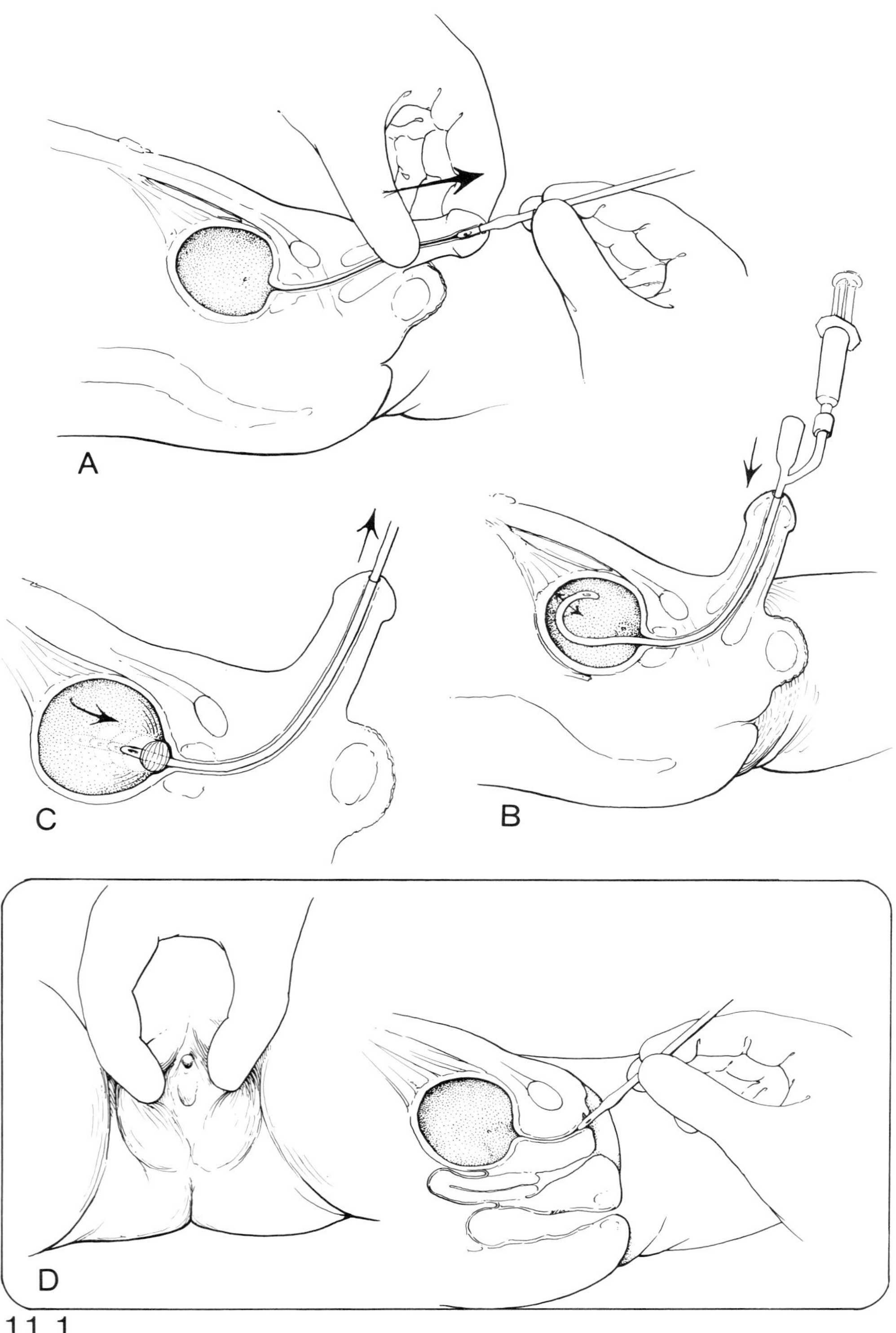

11.1

11.1. CATHETERIZATION OF THE BLADDER

INDICATIONS

1. Multiple trauma—especially for the evaluation of the urinary tract in the unconscious child.
2. Severe head trauma.
3. Shock.
4. Acute urinary retention.
5. To obtain a urine specimen for diagnosis.

CONTRAINDICATIONS

Urethral trauma.

COMPLICATIONS

1. Urethral trauma.
2. Vaginal catheterization.
3. Urinary tract infection.

PROCEDURE

Restrain the patient as necessary, using the method shown for suprapubic bladder aspiration in infants (see Fig. 11.2). The older child may require additional restraint if he or she is uncooperative. Prepare the urethral meatus and penis or the perineal area thoroughly by scrubbing with a povidone-iodine solution; select a Foley catheter of the appropriate size (size 8 Fr. in newborn, size 10 Fr. in most children and size 12 Fr. in older children). Inflate the balloon on the catheter with normal saline to test its competence. The catheter tip should be well lubricated with sterile lubricant to minimize local trauma.

Male

As shown in Figure 11.1*A* gently grasp and extend the penile shaft to straighten out the urethral pathway. Hold the catheter near the distal tip and advance it up the urethra unless resistance or an obstruction is encountered. If this occurs, select a smaller catheter. Generally, if an 8 Fr. is too large, a No. 8 feeding tube is a satisfactory alternative, but is more difficult to maintain in the bladder.

When the catheter reaches the junction of the penile shaft and the perineum, it may help to position the penis more vertically as shown in Figure 11.1*B*. The catheter should be passed into the bladder all the way to the Y- connection; this is important because urine may begin to flow while the catheter is in the proximal urethra, and inflation of the balloon in the urethra may lead to complications.

Figure 11.1*C* shows withdrawal of the catheter after inflation of the balloon. When the balloon strikes the wall, a "clunking" sensation is appreciated; this indicates that the balloon is resting on the trigone. Then tape the catheter to the child's leg, leaving a lax portion to prevent injury to the trigone if the catheter is accidently pulled.

Female

In the female, the principles of catheterization are similar to those in the male. Have an assistant carefully spread the labia, as shown in Figure 11.1*D*, if it is difficult to visualize the urethra. Then, introduce a well-lubricated, pretested Foley catheter into the bladder. Again, advance the catheter its entire length before inflating the balloon. A catheter that is passed in its entirety has not been inadvertently located in the small vagina of the young girl. After withdrawing the catheter until a clunking sensation is appreciated, secure it with tape.

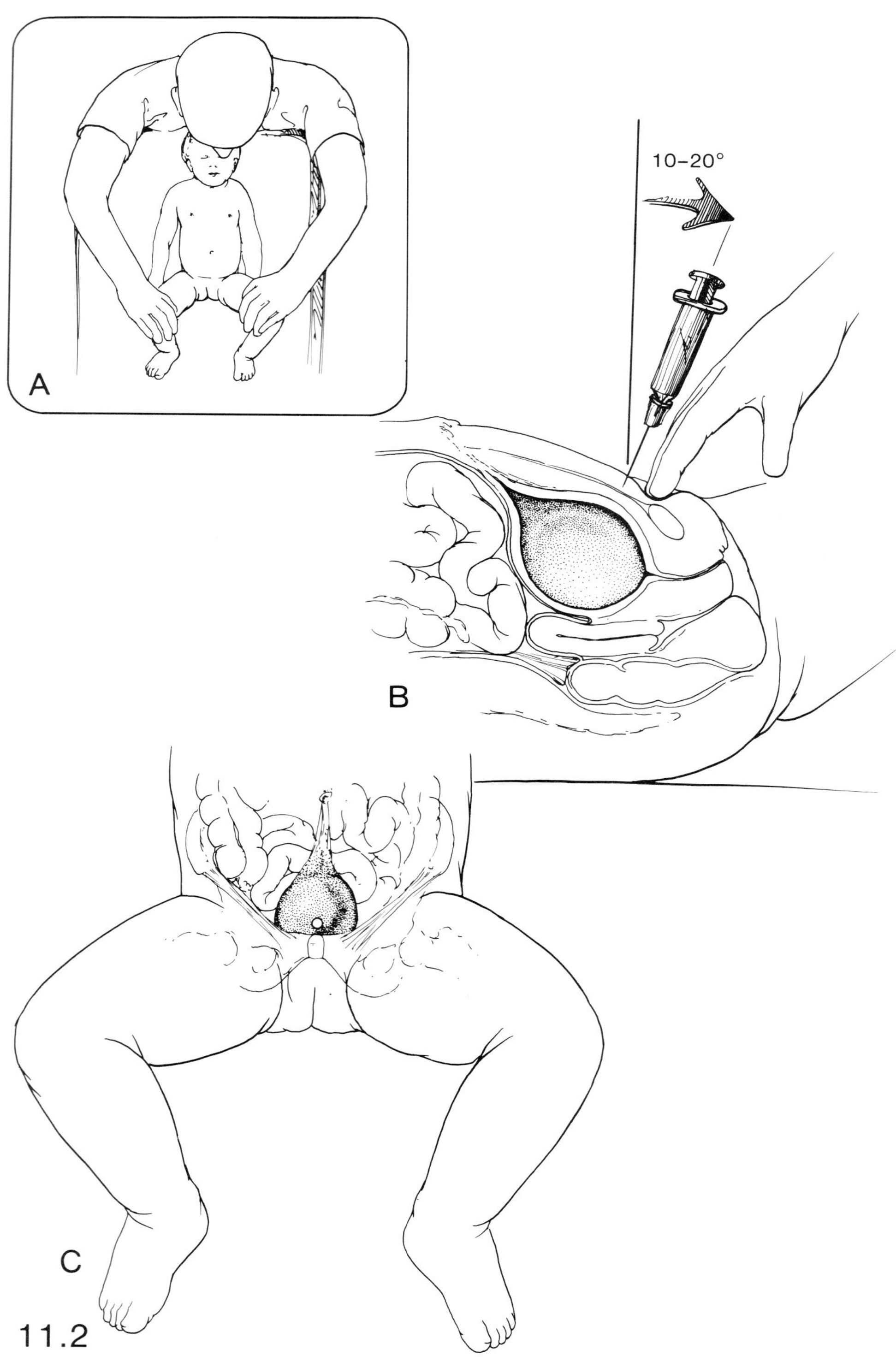

11.2

11.2. SUPRAPUBIC BLADDER ASPIRATION

INDICATIONS

To obtain a sterile urine specimen for culture in infants and children less than 2 years old. Above the age of 2, collect sterile urine by urethral catheterization.

COMPLICATIONS

1. Hematuria—microscopic hematuria virtually always occurs. Gross hematuria is uncommon.
2. Intestinal perforation.
3. Infection of the abdominal wall.

PROCEDURE

Position the infant supine. Holding the legs in the frog leg position as shown in Figure 11.2*A*, restrain the child firmly. Have an assistant occlude the penile urethra in a male infant to prevent urination while preparations are made. It is wise to wait at least 1 hour before doing this procedure if the infant has just voided.

Select a puncture site in the midline of the abdomen, approximately 1 to 2 cm cephalad to the superior edge of the pubic bone (Fig. 11.2, *B* and *C*). Prepare the skin by cleansing with povidone-iodine solution. After 3 applications of the antiseptic solution, wipe the area with 70% alcohol. Position a 22 gauge needle (with 3-ml syringe attached to it) at the planned puncture site perpendicular to the plane of the abdominal wall, which is generally 10–20° from the true vertical (Fig. 11.2*C*). Pierce the skin and then, with a second quick stabbing motion, enter the bladder. Withdraw the needle slowly while aspirating with the syringe simultaneously. If urine is not obtained, do not remove the needle from the abdomen completely. Instead, change the angle of the needle, and reinsert it as described above. Attempt the procedure at two different angles; first about 20° caudad to the perpendicular, and second about 20° cephalad to the perpendicular. If urine is not obtained after the third attempt, further trials are unlikely to be successful. Either perform urethral catheterization or wait 1 to 2 hours and try the suprapubic bladder tap again.

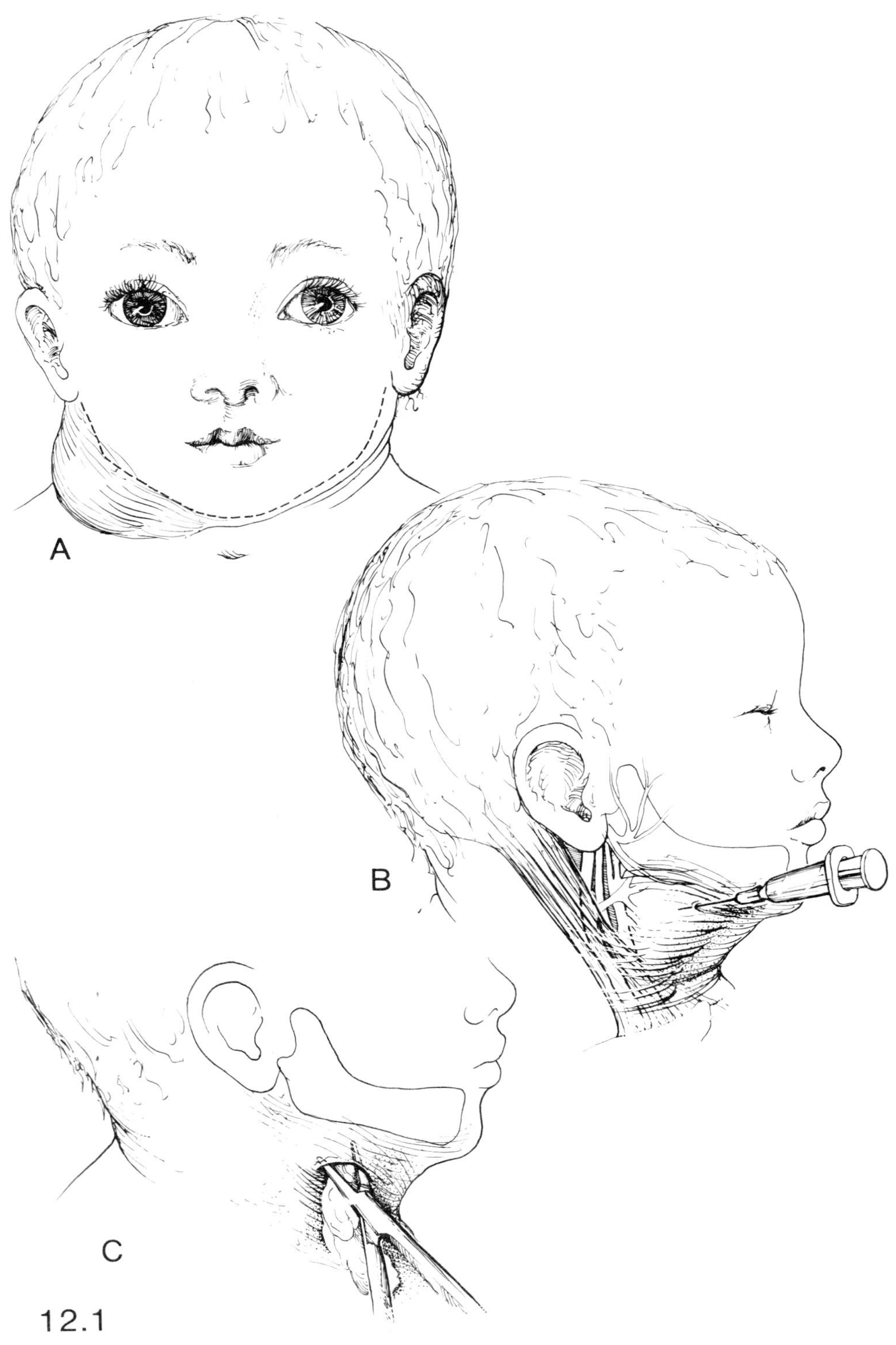
A
B
C
12.1

12.1. DRAINAGE OF AN ABSCESS

Aspiration, Incision and Drainage

INDICATIONS

Diagnostic and therapeutic drainage of fluctuant adenitis most commonly in the anterior cervical or submandibular region.

COMPLICATIONS

1. Scar formation (more common with incision and drainage).
2. Contusion or laceration of the carotid triangle structures, transverse cervical nerve or inferior branches of the facial nerve.
3. Fistula formation—usually only with myobacterial neck mass (scrofula).

PROCEDURE

Restrain the child supine with head turned 90° away from the midline to expose the neck. Have an assistant stabilize the head. In the child less than 2 years of age, one cannot expect cooperation during the procedure. Therefore, utilize a single puncture to drain the abscess without injecting a local anesthetic. First, spray ethyl chloride locally to minimize any discomfort. In the older child, a small amount of locally instilled 1% lidocaine or ethyl chloride sprayed over the intended puncture site provides adequate anesthesia for the patient during the actual aspiration.

Aspiration by Needle

Cleanse the area to be punctured with povidone-iodine solution and then anesthetize as described above. Use a simple large bore needle to aspirate the abscess for culture and drainage. Alternatively, use a large bore "over the needle" (i.e., Medicut®) catheter for drainage.

Direct the needle insertion parallel to the plane of the face to avoid injury to adjacent structures, as shown in Figure 12.1*B*. The needle and syringe should be held with one hand stabilized against the child's jaw to minimize movement of the needle if the child struggles. Puncture the abscess and advance the needle into the center of the abscess cavity. Apply suction and drain as much purulent material as possible. Remove the needle when complete and apply pressure with a sterile dressing. Repeated aspirations may be necessary, in addition to systemic antibiotics.

If using the Medicut® system, cut extra holes in the catheter and, as described above, puncture the abscess. Stabilize the catheter in the abscess and remove the needle, attaching a 10-ml syringe. To the system, now apply suction to withdraw fluid. With a plastic catheter one can move the system about without fear of unnecessary injury to the nearby structures of the neck. Moreover, manual pressure can be applied to the abscess while aspirating on the indwelling plastic catheter.

Incision and Drainage

When a formal incision and drainage is required, cleanse the skin with povidone-iodine solution and anesthetize it as previously described. With a No. 15 scalpel blade, incise the skin over the abscess parallel to the natural creases of the neck to the depth of the superficial fascia. Then, bluntly open the abscess with a hemostat for at least 1 cm as shown in the Figure 12.1*C*. Insert a gloved little finger into the abscess to break up any septae. Pack the wound lightly with iodoform gauze to provide hemostasis, but not so tightly as to impede drainage. Remove the packing in 1 to 2 days.

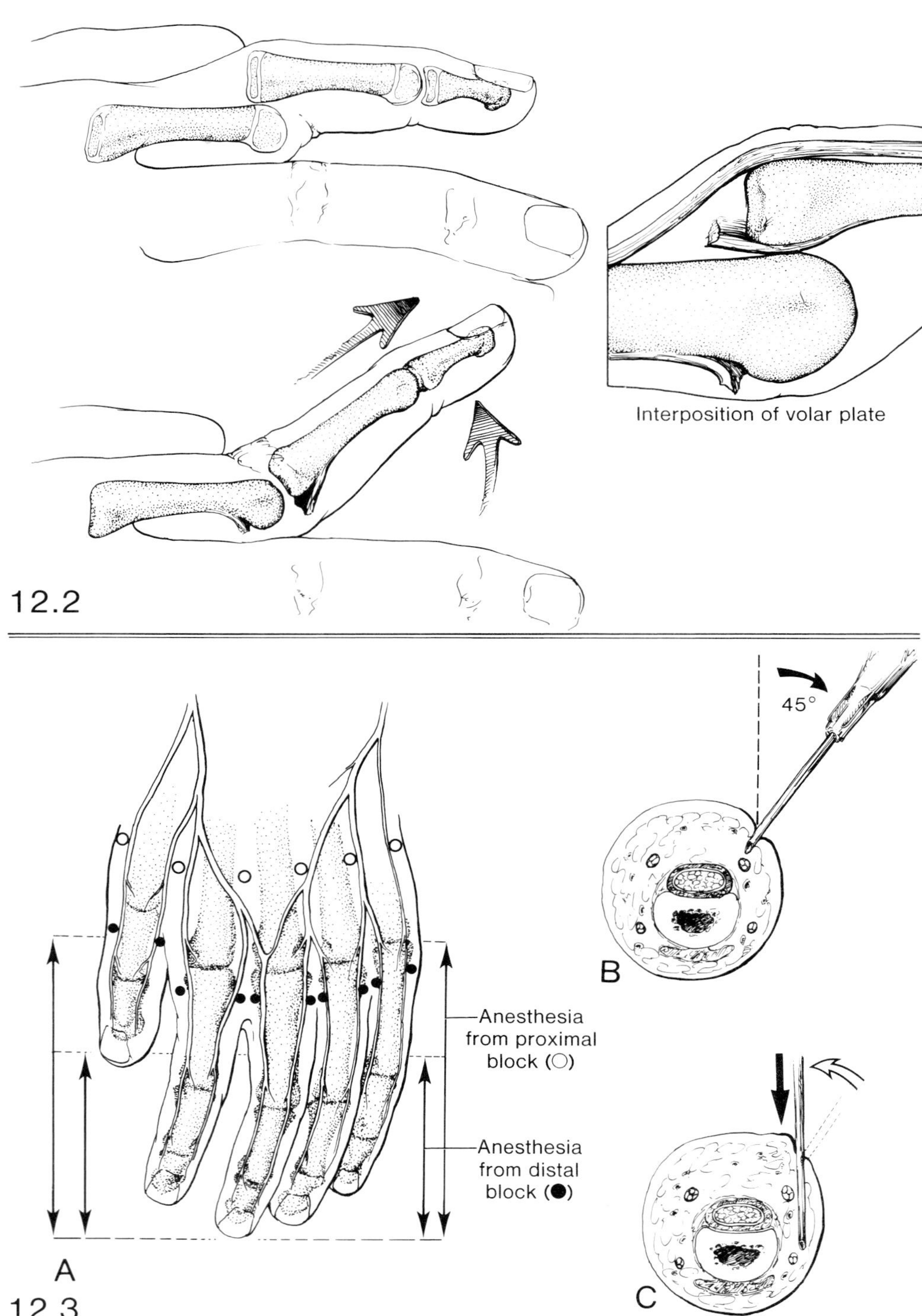
Interposition of volar plate
12.2
45°
B
Anesthesia
from proximal
block (○)
Anesthesia
from distal
block (●)
C
A
12.3

12.2. CLOSED REDUCTION OF A FINGER DISLOCATION

INDICATIONS

Interphalangeal and metacarpal-phalangeal dislocations.

COMPLICATIONS

Fractures secondary to attempted reduction.

CAUTION

Closed reduction of a dislocation may not be possible when there is dorsal dislocation with interposition of the volar plate or entrapment of the metacarpal head (see Fig. 12.2).

PROCEDURE

Splint the deformed finger for comfort. Check the integrity of the neurovascular supply in the distal finger. Have radiographs of at least two views taken to ascertain the presence of obvious fractures or interposition of the volar plate of the distal phalanx.

If necessary, have an assistant restrain the child. Grasp the hand proximal to the dislocation and also near the tip of the distal phalanx. Assert traction longitudinally along the distal aspect of the finger. The joint will usually slide into proper position.

If this method is unsuccessful, apply pressure distally to increase the deformity a few degrees while applying traction to the finger longitudinally along the distal phalanx.

Immobilize the joint for three weeks afterwards and refer for a reassessment of the joint and instruction in range of motion exercises. If there is a small avulsion of the volar lip of the distal phalanx, apply a dorsal splint to prevent hyperextension of the affected joint.

In cases where the reduction is unsuccessful, the volar plate is interposed, or the second metacarpal bone is trapped, consult an orthopedic surgeon to assess the need of open reduction.

12.3. DIGITAL NERVE BLOCK

INDICATIONS

Anesthesia of fingers and toes for surgical procedures (i.e., drainage of a felon or paronychia, removal of a foreign body, or laceration repair).

COMPLICATIONS

1. Infection.
2. Bleeding.

CAUTION

Do not use vasoconstrictor such as epinephrine with the anesthetic agent.

PROCEDURE

Identify the area requiring anesthetic carefully. If it includes more than the distal two thirds to three fourths of the finger or toes, alternate procedures need to be performed to achieve adequate anesthesia. Check the digit for blood supply, sensation and motor nerve function before injecting the anesthetic agent. The site of puncture on the digits is shown in Figure 12.3*A*.

Restrain the child. A "mummy" restraint is good in the young child leaving exposed the extremity to be anesthetized. Have an assistant grasp the extremity proximal to the digit to prevent movement.

The digital nerves, as shown in Figure 12.3*B*, are both dorsal and volar in the body of the digit, and anesthesia must be injected at both levels.

Scrub thoroughly the planned puncture sites, on the medial and lateral aspect(s) of the finger, with povidone-iodine solution. Dry with sterile gauze and don gloves. Use a 22 gauge needle attached to a 5-ml syringe and 1% lidocaine (without epinephrine). Inject the site at a 45° angle from vertical until the needle hits the periosteum. Release the tension on the needle and gently rotate the syringe to the vertical as shown in Figure 12.3*C*. Then advance the needle to the volar surface while injecting anesthetic until at least three quarters through the digit. Remove the needle from the tissue and then repeat the procedure on the other side of the digit in a similar manner. The digit should be anesthetized after several minutes.

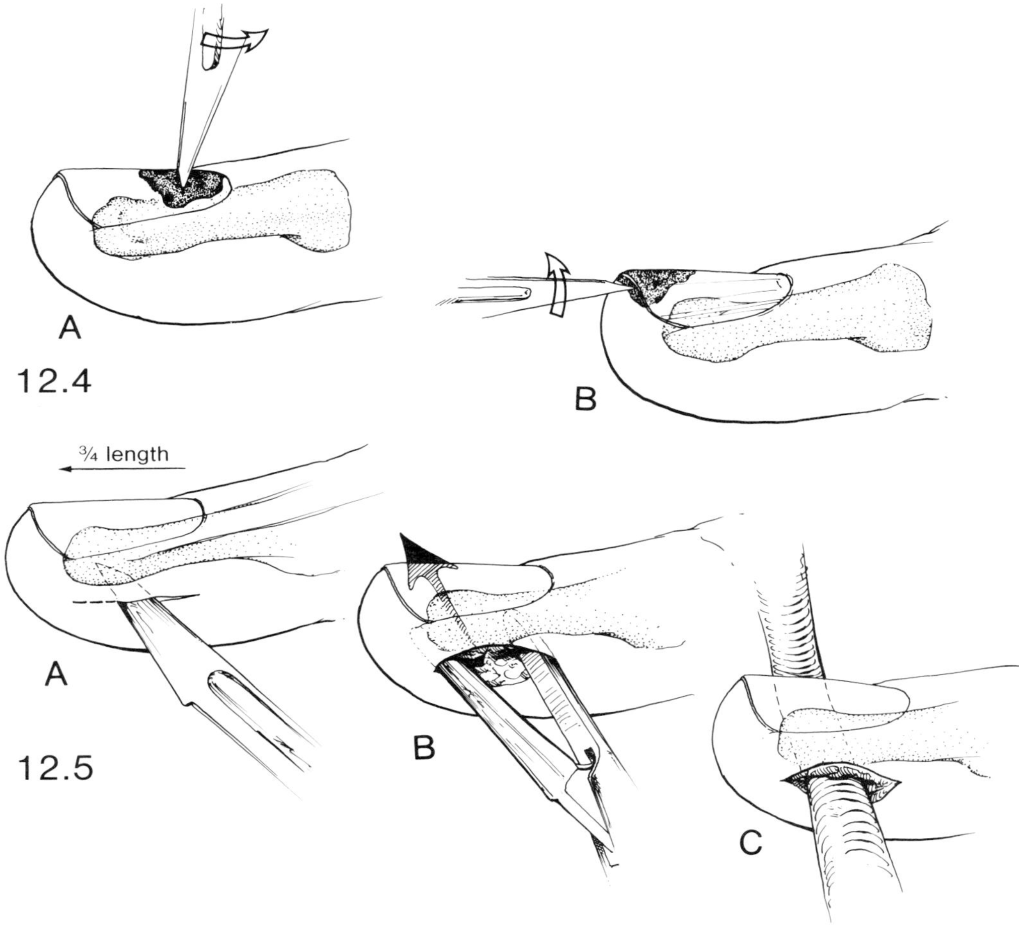
A
12.4
B
¾ length
A
12.5
B
C

12.4. DRAINAGE OF A SUBUNGUAL HEMATOMA

INDICATION

Blood under pressure beneath a nail bed, either proximally or distally.

COMPLICATIONS

1. Bleeding.
2. Infection.

PROCEDURE

Subungual hematomas occur from trauma in the proximal or distal nail bed as shown in Figure 12.4. Generally the hematoma causes pain that is immediately relieved with drainage. A digital nerve block may be used for anesthesia but is usually not necessary.

A hematoma of the proximal nail bed is relieved by making a hole in the nail. Restrain the child and digit on a table. Soak the fingertip in povidone-iodine solution for several minutes. Hold a scalpel with No. 11 blade perpendicular to the nail in the center of the hematoma. Puncture the nail by simultaneously applying downward and rotary pressure as shown in Figure 12.4*A*. Apply pressure sterile gauze to drain the blood for several minutes, and then cover with a sterile dressing.

Alternatively, a heated metal wire (Thermolance®) can be used to puncture the nail. If available this technique is more rapid and less painful than making a hole with a scalpel.

A distal hematoma is shown in Figure 12.4*B*. Restrain the child and finger on a firm surface. Clean the nail with povidone-iodine solution. Take a scalpel with No. 11 blade and lance the hematoma by inserting the blade directly under the nail parallel to its course. Keep the blade against the under surface of the nail. Cover with a sterile gauze while blood is draining and apply a sterile dressing.

12.5. INCISION AND DRAINAGE OF FELON

INDICATION

A felon, or digital pulp space abscess, requires drainage to relieve severe pain and to decrease the spread of infection.

COMPLICATIONS

1. Scar formation.
2. Bleeding.

PROCEDURE

Restrain the child sitting in a chair or supine in a papoose. Have the assistant hold the hand supinated on a hard table top. Locate the felon in the pulp space between the volar soft tissues and the periosteum of the distal phalanx. Be sure to distinguish it from a paronychia, a more superficial abscess of the tissues beneath the nail.

Anesthetize the distal finger with a digital nerve block as described in Procedure 12.3. After obtaining anesthesia, scrub the fingertip with povidone-iodine solution for several minutes. Don sterile gloves.

Align the cutting edge of a No. 11 blade perpendicular to the long axis of the finger at its distal medial aspect. Incise the digit, as in Figure 12.5*A*, half of the distance to the volar surface beginning at the proximal end of the nail bed and extending for about three fourths of the length of the nail distally. Extend the incision all the way through from the medial to lateral surface of the fingertip. With a small, straight hemostat, spread the incised septa to promote drainage of purulent material in the pulp of the finger as shown in Figure 12.5*B*.

After sufficient spreading of the tissues, prepare a drain 8 to 10 cm in length. Place the drain in one side of the incision and pull it through the tunnel, leaving exposed ends on both sides of the finger (Fig. 12.5*C*). Make a bulky dressing using sterile gauze to protect the wound. In 2 to 24 hours remove the dressing, and inspect the wound. Systemic antibiotics are recommended.

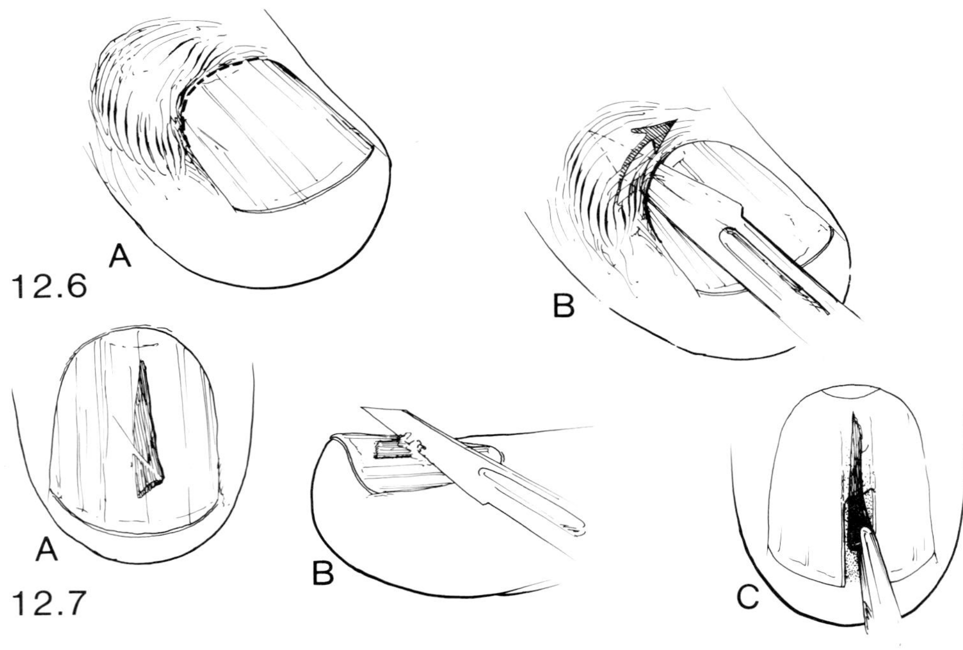
A
12.6
B
A
12.7
B
C

12.6. INCISION AND DRAINAGE OF A PARONYCHIA

INDICATION

Failure of this infection of the soft tissue along the edges of the nail to respond to medical treatment.

COMPLICATIONS

1. Bleeding.
2. Scar formation.

PROCEDURE

Restrain the child appropriately for age. Prepare the site for the surgical procedure with povidone-iodine solution and cover with sterile disposable drapes. Inject 1% lidocaine for a digital block as in Procedure 12.3, or spray the skin locally with ethyl chloride for anesthesia. Using a No. 11 surgical blade, incise the skin at its junction with the nail. As indicated in Figure 12.6*B* extend the incision along the base of the nail to permit adequate drainage. If the paronychia is only on one side of the nail bed, make the incision along the lateral margin of the nail bed distal to the cuticle. Dress the wound and instruct the patient to use warm compresses.

12.7. REMOVAL OF A SUBUNGUAL SPLINTER

INDICATIONS

1. Painful subungual splinter.
2. To prevent infection or a foreign body reaction to a splinter in the nail bed.

COMPLICATIONS

Bleeding.

PROCEDURE

Restrain the child's hand with the fingers extended. Use a No. 11 blade to scrape the nail down to the nail bed. Hold the blade perpendicular to the direction of the splinter and at 90° from the horizontal as in Figure 12.7*B*. Scrape the nail off in a proximal to distal fashion, applying pressure gently to minimize discomfort from squeezing the nail onto the splinter. The shape of the nail removed is similar to that of a "U." With a small tweezers or forceps, grasp the splinter once it is exposed and tug it gently to remove it from the nailbed. Soak the finger in a warm povidone-iodine and water solution several times per day to decrease the chance of infection.

Large splinters or those embedded deeply under the nail require prolonged scraping and are best removed by excision of a large portion of nail after digital block.

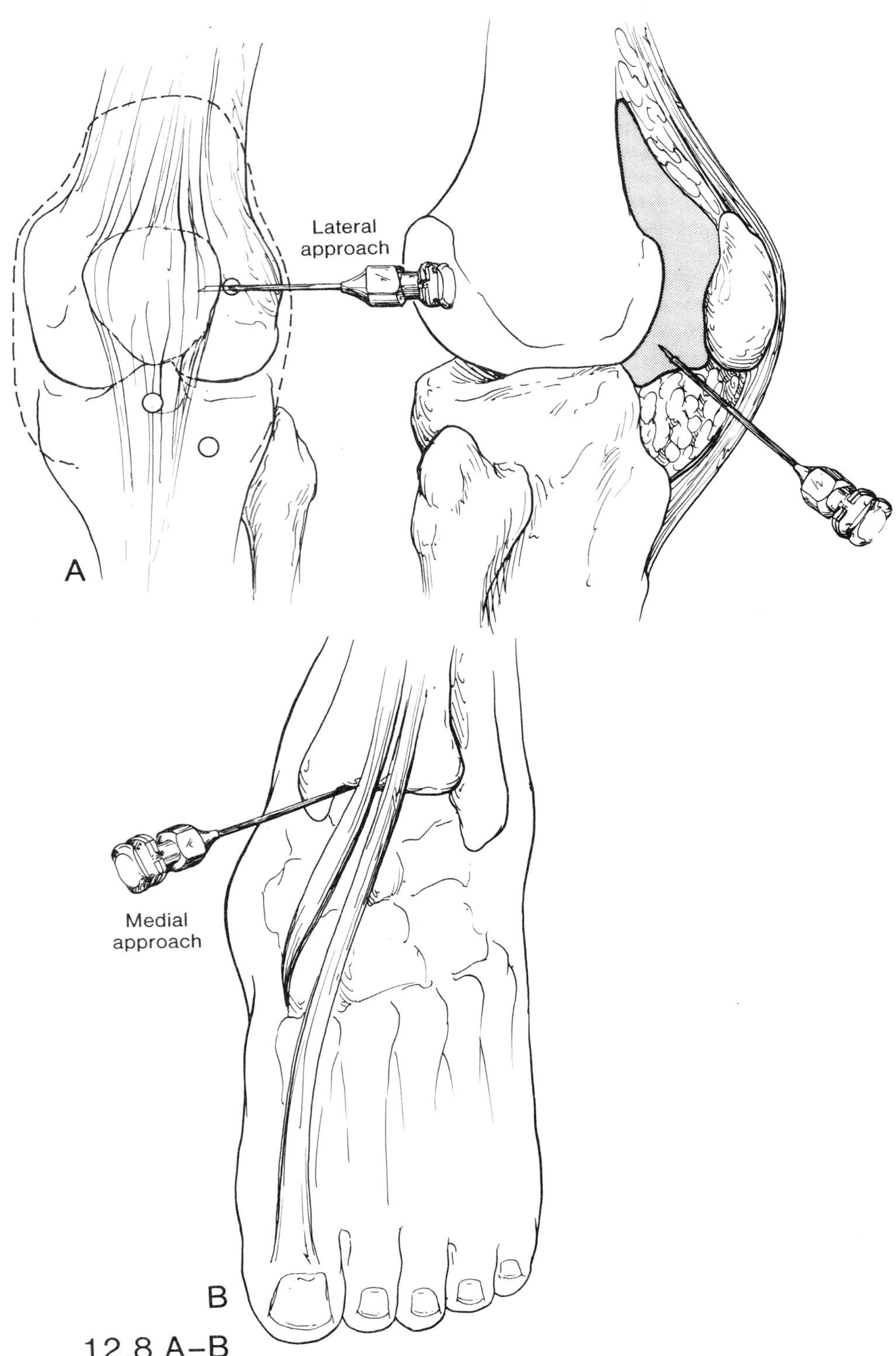

12.8 A–B

12.8. ARTHROCENTESIS—GENERAL CONSIDERATIONS

INDICATIONS

1. Removal of a joint effusion causing severe pain and distension that limits function.
2. Suspected septic arthritis.
3. To obtain joint fluid for the diagnosis of systemic illness (i.e., collagen disease).

COMPLICATIONS

1. Bleeding.
2. Infection—joint space or bone.

CONTRAINDICATIONS (RELATIVE)

1. Bleeding diathesis—patients with bleeding diatheses (i.e., hemophilia), as the cause of the joint effusion usually require only immobilization and replacement of coagulation factors.
2 Presence of a fracture around the joint space. Aspiration may increase the chance of infection when a fracture is present.

12.8*A*. THE KNEE JOINT

PROCEDURE

The knee is the commonest joint requiring aspiration in children, primarily to evaluate possible bacterial infection or to drain a large traumatic effusion. Radiographs should usually be obtained before tapping the joint.

Place the child supine on the examining table, with the knee actively extended as far as possible. Restrain the child as necessary. Have an assistant hold both the thigh and calf of the leg to be tapped.

The lateral approach to the knee is preferred because it avoids passage through the vastus medialus muscle. Pick a puncture point at the midpatellar level in the anteroposterior view (Fig. 12.8*A*) and at the posterior margin of the patella in the lateral view (Fig. 12.8*A*).

Cleanse the area to be punctured circumferentially with povidone-iodine solution. Use a 23 or 25 gauge needle attached to a 3-ml syringe to inject 1% lidocaine into the skin and subcutaneous tissues for anesthesia or, alternatively, spray ethyl chloride locally. Take care not to have bacteriostatic solutions enter the joint space if a bacterial infection is suspected, yet still undiagnosed.

Wearing sterile gloves, attach an 18 gauge needle to a 10-ml syringe. Hold the syringe in one hand, while palpating the lateral margin of the patella with the other. Puncture the skin with syringe 10 to 20° above the horizontal at the anesthetized site. Advance the needle, applying suction on the plunger of the syringe, until it passes into the joint space near the margin of the patella. When the joint space is entered, the syringe will fill with joint fluid. Stabilize the syringe against the patient's leg with the heel of the hand during the aspiration. Move the needle slightly in varied directions to effectively evacuate the joint, but take care not to injure the synovium.

At completion, remove the syringe and apply a sterile gauze pad over the puncture site. Send the aspirate for appropriate studies. Immobilize the knee joint with a supportive dressing.

12.8*B*. THE ANKLE JOINT

PROCEDURE

Restrain the patient in the supine position on the examining table. Have an assistant hold the foot in slight plantar flexion (approximately 110°). Place a soft brace under the plantar surface of the foot to provide further immobilization.

Identify two landmarks, the medial malleolus of the distal tibia and the thick halluces longus extensor tendon. The latter structure is found approximately 1 cm anterolateral to the medial malleolus as shown in Figure 12.8*B*.

Pick a puncture site between these landmarks. Cleanse it circumferentially with povidone-iodine solution. Wearing sterile gloves, inject 1% lidocaine or spray ethyl chloride locally to anesthetize the skin. Use either an 18 or 20 gauge plain or spinal needle attached to 10-ml syringe.

Puncture the skin aiming the needle slightly inferiorly toward the tibial-talar articulation as Figure 12.8*B* shows. Apply suction to the syringe. Aspirate the fluid from the joint and remove the needle when satisfied that an adequate specimen has been obtained (often only a small amount). Apply sterile gauze to the puncture site and immobilize the joint.

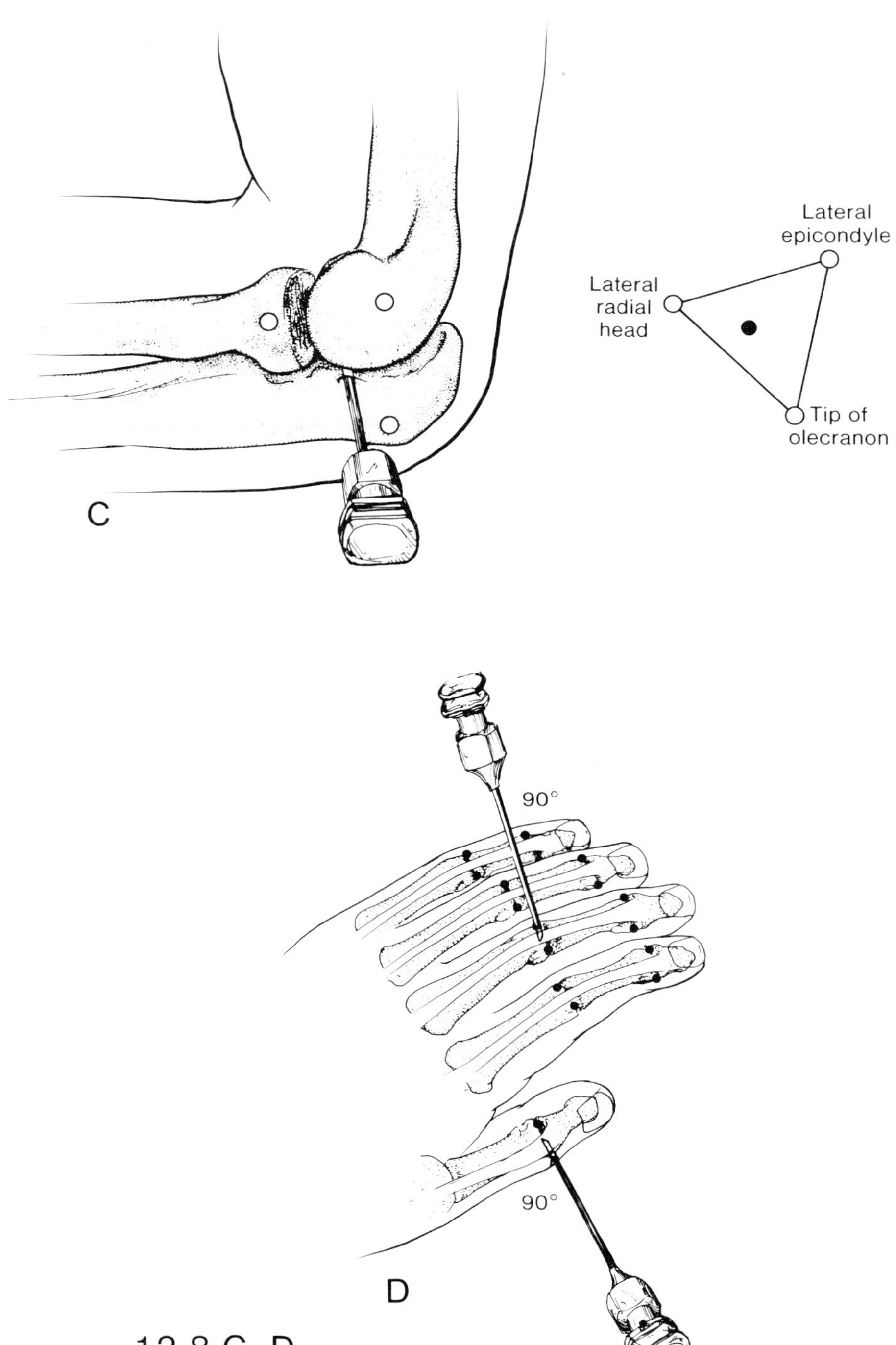
Lateral epicondyle
Lateral radial head
Tip of olecranon
C
90°
90°
D

12.8 C–D

12.8*C*. THE ELBOW JOINT

PROCEDURE

Rest the child prone or seated with his or her arm extended, and elbow flexed 90° to maximally open the joint space. Restrain the patient, maintaining the arm and forearm in this flexed position.

The needle puncture site should lie in the center of the triangle formed by the head of the radius, the lateral humeral epicondyle and the olecranon, as demonstrated in the Figure 12.8*C*.

Sterilize the site with povidone-iodine solution. Wearing sterile gloves, inject the skin with 1% lidocaine or spray with ethyl chloride for anesthesia. Use a large bore, 18 or 20 gauge needle on a 10-ml syringe.

Puncture the skin perpendicularly to the surface of the arm. Hold the syringe in one hand and guide the needle tip with the thumb and index finger of the other, leaning against the patient's arm. Advance the syringe while applying suction to the plunger, until the needle enters the elbow joint. If there is difficulty entering the joint space, pull the needle back and reassess the location of the landmarks. Readvance it in a new line. Continue to stabilize the syringe while aspirating fluid. Remove the needle and press sterile gauze over the puncture site. Immobilize the joint.

12.8*D*. THE INTERPHALANGEAL JOINT

PROCEDURE

Sit the child with the forearm extended over the examining table or place him or her prone with the arms extended over the head. Restrain if necessary. Have an assistant immobilize the finger proximally and distally. Locate the joint to be aspirated, using the radiograph as necessary. Choose a puncture site on the dorsal surface because the skin of the palm is tougher and because slight flexion opens the joint space, facilitating a dorsal approach.

Cleanse the surface with povidone-iodine solution and allow to dry. Using a 22 gauge needle attached to a 5-ml syringe, puncture the skin perpendicularly to the long axis of the finger and advance the needle to the joint space. Be sure to puncture the skin and joint in the middle of the finger to avoid the digital vessels which run peripherally. Aspirate fluid with suction on the syringe. Remove the needle and press sterile gauze over the puncture. Immobilize the joint.

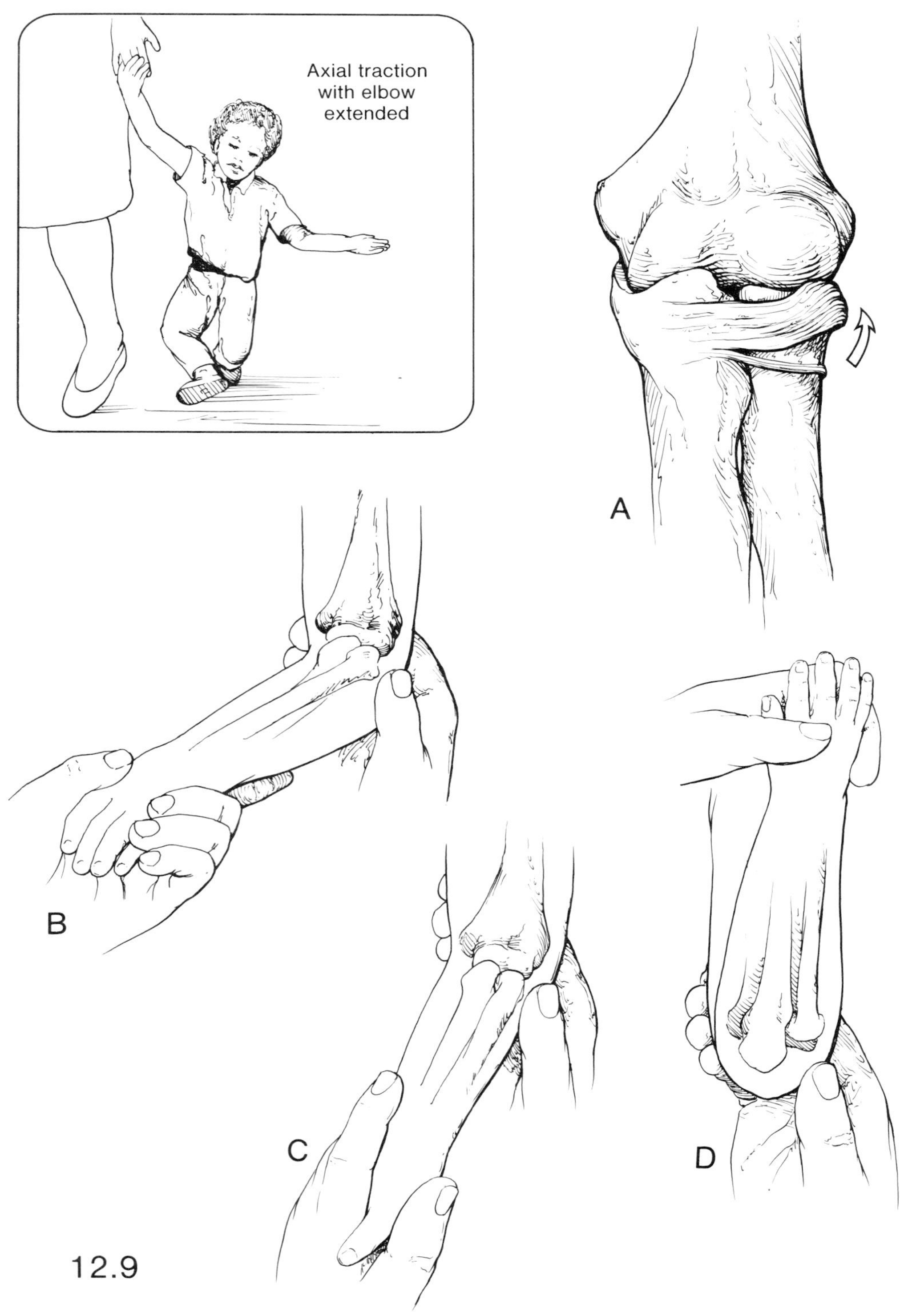

12.9

12.9. REDUCTION OF A NURSEMAID'S ELBOW

INDICATIONS

Perform this maneuver when a radial head dislocation (nursemaid's elbow) is suspected in toddlers. This injury occurs when the child has had excessive axial traction placed across the elbow joint, most often during a fall while holding hands with an adult (see Fig. 12.9). The injury probably represents interposition of the annular ligament between the radial head and the capitellum (Fig. 12.9*A*).

COMPLICATIONS

Vascular or musculoskeletal damage if the maneuver is performed on a child with a fracture (i.e., supracondylar fracture of humerus).

PROCEDURE

Obtain a clear history and examine the toddler in the parent's arms. Gentle manipulation of the contralateral arm first may make examination of the injured arm easier. The affected arm is generally held at the child's side, slightly flexed at the elbow in pronation. Assess it for point tenderness along the length of the arm and shoulder, and after failing to observe any, instruct the parent of what is to be done.

Have a parent or assistant restrain the child in the sitting position. As shown in Figure 12.9*B*, grasp the palm of the child's hand as if to shake it. Encircle the elbow with the other hand with the thumb over the annular ligament of the radius. Gently supinate the palm of the hand (Fig. 12.9*C*), and in a continuous motion flex the elbow to the shoulder (Fig. 12.9*D*). During the flexion maneuver the physician feels a "pop" with the thumb that lies over the radial head.

Generally the child uses the arm normally within 10 to 15 min. Repeat the maneuver if unsatisfied with the child's use of the arm. An x-ray of the arm is helpful to be certain that there is no other injury. Rarely, when a prolonged period has elapsed before reduction, it will take somewhat longer for the child to regain normal function after the maneuver is performed.

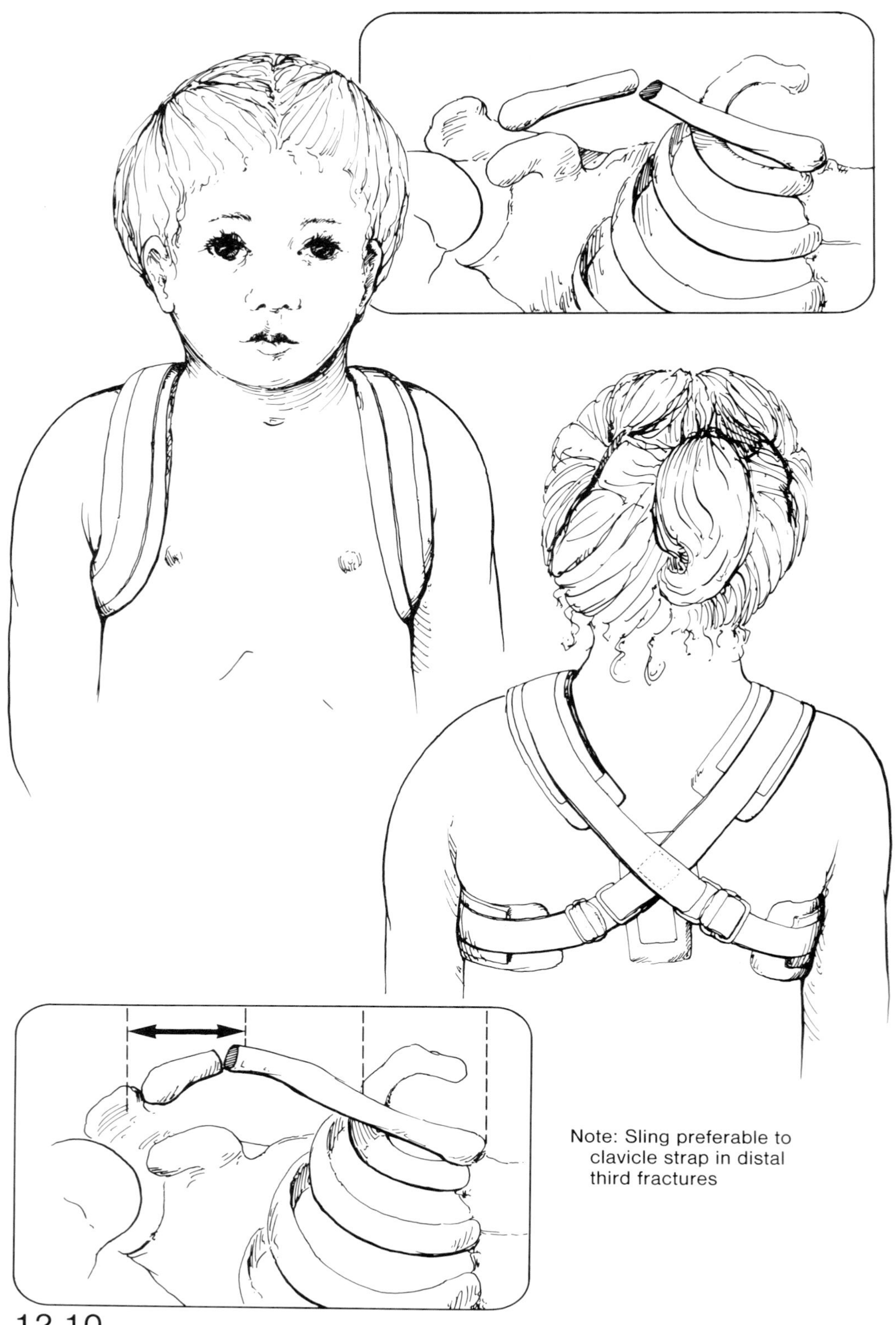
Note: Sling preferable to clavicle strap in distal third fractures

12.10

12.10. APPLICATION OF FIGURE-OF-EIGHT HARNESS

INDICATION

To immobilize midshaft clavicular fractures for comfort during healing.

COMPLICATIONS

1. Pressure sores (tight application).
2. Pain (loose application).

PROCEDURE

Obtain radiographs in two views to confirm the presence and location of the fracture. Then choose a figure of eight dressing by measuring the child's chest circumference and picking the closest available size (Table 12.10).

Stand the child up and loosely drape the harness over his or her shoulders to assess how much to tighten the straps. Remove the harness and manually adjust the straps by sliding the cloth through the metal clips. Make it slightly tighter than estimated during the fitting to pull the shoulders slightly back from their usual forward, rounded position.

Reapply the harness around the shoulders from the front to the back with the soft padding against the skin of the axillae. Approximate the buckles in the midline of the back and clip them. The harness should fit snugly, and the shoulders should be straight. Tighten the straps as necessary.

Have the patient wear the harness except during bathing for 3 weeks. The parent should demonstrate the successful reapplication of the harness before leaving the emergency department.

It is appropriate to manage distal clavicular fractures with a shoulder sling rather than a figure-of-eight dressing.

Table 12.10
Figure-of-Eight Harness Sizes

Size	Chest Circumference (cm)
Extra extra small	<20
Extra small	20–25
Small	25–30
Medium	30–35
Medium long	33–39

APPENDIX A

The Children's Hospital of Philadelphia Resuscitation Equipment

1. *Resuscitation Cart*
   1.1. 3-Drawer Craftsman Cart (Sears Roebuck) with side shelf
   1.2. Cardiac arrest board with hooks for storage on side of cart
   1.3. Defibrillator
   1.4. ECG with 1 extra roll of paper, ECG paste, ECG leads
   1.5. Monitor screen with ECG interconnection cable
   1.6. E-Cylinder rack
   1.7. Sphygmomanometer Aneroid
   1.8. STAT worksheet—on clipboard affixed by hook to side of cart
   1.9. E-Cylinder
   1.10. O_2 flow meter (Bordon type)
   1.11. O_2 tubing
   1.12. Cylinder key
2. *Airway Box (Inventory Card Inside Lid)*
   2.1. Laryngoscope handle with knurled finish
   2.2. Laryngoscope blades:
      2.2.1 Miller 0, 1, 2, 3
      2.2.2. Wis-Hipple 1.5
      2.2.3. MacIntosh 2,3
   2.3. Extra "C" batteries (2)
   2.4. Endotracheal tubes
      2.4.1. Uncuffed sizes 2.5–8.5 (two of each)
      2.4.2. Cuffed sizes 7–9 (two of each)
   2.5. Stylets
      2.5.1. Infant (1)
      2.5.2. Adult (1)
   2.6. Magill forceps (1)
   2.7. Nasopharyngeal airways—12, 16, 20, 24, 28, 30 Fr. (one of each)
   2.8. Oropharyngeal airways—0–5 (one of each)
3. *Resuscitation Bag—(Heavy Transparent Plastic Bag to Hang from Side of Cart)*
   3.1. Self-inflating resuscitator—adult
   3.2. Self-inflating resuscitator—infant
4. *Drawer 1*
   4.1. Tongue blades (5)
   4.2. Yankauer suction tip (1)
   4.3. Tracheal catheters: 6, 8, 10 Fr. (two of each)
   4.4. Oxygen catheters: 10, 14 Fr. (two of each)

5. *Drawer 2*
    5.1. Salem sump nasogastric tube: size 10, 16 (2 of each)
    5.2. Feeding tubes: size 3½–8 Fr. (2 of each)
    5.3. K-Y jelly (4)
    5.4. ½ inch waterproof tape
6. *Drawer 3*
    6.1. Unit dose prepackage drugs: (2 of each)
        6.1.1. Epinephrine 1:10,000—10 ml
        6.1.2. Atropine 0.4 mg/0.5 ml
        6.1.3. Bicarbonate full strength 7.5%—50 ml
        6.1.4. Bicarbonate ½ strength 4.2%—10 ml
        6.1.5. Calcium gluceptate 4.5 meq/5 ml
        6.1.6. Calcium chloride 10%—10 ml
        6.1.7. Lidocaine 1%—10 ml
        6.1.8. Dextrose 25%—10 ml
        6.1.9. Syringes: 1 to 50 ml (five of each)
        6.1.10. Needles: 21, 23, 25 (five of each)
        6.1.11. Blood gas kit
        6.1.12. Sterile saline 1-L bottle with 4 × 4 attached
        6.1.13. Masks: graduated sizes infant to adult (0, 1, 2, 3, 4, 5)
        6.1.14. Mapelson D system:
            1–500 ml bag
            1–1.0 L bag
            1–2.0 L bag
7. *Resuscitation Stretcher*
    7.1. Masks (graduated sizes infant through adult to be arrayed at head of bed): Size 0, 1, 2, 3, 4 (one of each)
    7.2. Cardiac board
    7.3. Mapelson D system with 1.0 liter bag connected to O_2 flow meter
8. *Additional Resuscitation Equipment*
    8.1. Sealed emergency drug box
    8.2. Blood pressure cuffs: infant, small child, large child, adult
    8.3. I.V. solutions and equipment (room A–i.v. cabinet)
        8.3.1. Albumin–5%, 25%
        8.3.2. 500 ml 5% dextrose in normal saline
        8.3.3. 500 ml normal saline solution (NSS)
        8.3.4. 500 ml Ringer's lactate
        8.3.5. 500 ml mannitol 20%
        8.3.6. Solusets Administration Sets
        8.3.7. Venosets Administration Sets
    8.4. STAT i.v. tray
        8.4.1. CVP #10 kit (2)
        8.4.2. CVP #11 kit (2)
        8.4.3. Medicuts—22, 20, 18, 16 (2 of each)
        8.4.4. Butterflys—25, 23, 21, 18 (4 of each)
        8.4.5. Intracaths 8 inch, small, medium, large (2 of each)
        8.4.6. Tourniquets (3)
        8.4.7. 4 × 4 sponges
        8.4.8. Betadine swabs (10)
        8.4.9. Alcohol swabs (10)
        8.4.10. Tape
            Waterproof ½, 1, 2 inch (1 roll of each)
            Clear ½, 1 inch (1 roll of each)

8.4.11. Stopcocks (2)
8.4.12. T-connectors (2)
8.4.13. Venatubes 30 inches (2)
8.4.14. Armboards (2 of each size)
8.4.15. Tincture benzoin (individual applicators)
8.4.16. 1 bottle prep solution povidone
8.4.17. Betadine ointment (2 packs)
8.4.18. Eye drape (2)
8.4.19. Band Aids—Effodine

8.5. STAT Trays
8.5.1. Cutdown trays (2)
Scalpel blades sizes #10, 11, 15
Sterile gloves
Size 7 (2 of each)
Size 8 (2 of each)
Suture material (3-0 straight) 2 packs
8.5.2. Umbilical tray (1)
8.5.3. Catheterization tray(2)
Foley catheters (two of each size)
8.5.4. Tracheostomy tray with all size trach tubes
8.5.5. Chest (Thoracotomy) tray with all sizes chest tubes
Extra clamps—hemostats (Kellys)
8.5.6. Peritoneal lavage tray
8.5.7. Minor procedure tray

8.6. MAST Trousers
Pediatric
Adult

APPENDIX B

Emergency Drug Compendium*

KATHLEEN R. ROSENBERRY, PHARM.D.

RESUSCITATION DRUG LIST

Drug: ATROPINE

Route of Administration: Intravenous, intratracheal

Dose: Initial — 0.01 mg/kg or a minimum dose 0.2 mg

Subsequent — The initial dose may be repeated every 5–10 min to a maximum total dose of 2.0 mg

Precautions: Because paradoxical bradycardia occurs with low doses, a minimum of 0.2 mg should be administered

Adverse Effects: Tachycardia, myocardial ischemia

Available: Injection: 0.4 mg/0.5 ml, 0.4 mg/ml, prefilled syringe, 1 mg/ml, 1 ml vial, 0.4 mg/ml, 20 ml vial

Drug: BRETYLIUM (BRETYLOL)

Route of Administration: Intravenous

Dose: Initial — 5 mg/kg given rapidly followed by defibrillation

Subsequent — If defibrillation is unsuccessful, give 10 mg/kg

Precautions: Bretylium should not be given with digitalis products. Because hypotension may be seen with bretylium, the patient should be placed in a Trendelenberg position and the physician should be prepared to support the blood pressure with administration of fluid

Adverse Effects: Hypotension, vomiting

Available: Injection: 50 mg/ml, 10 ml ampule

Drug: CALCIUM (CALCIUM CHLORIDE OR CALCIUM GLUCONATE)

Route of Administration: Intravenous

Dose: Initial — Calcium chloride: 10 mg/kg

Calcium gluconate: 30 mg/kg

Subsequent — The initial dose may be repeated once

Precautions: Calcium chloride should be given only through a central i.v.; calcium gluconate may be given through a peripheral i.v. Calcium in any form should be infused slowly while the patient is being observed by a cardiac monitor for appearance of bradycardia

Adverse Effects: Hypercalcemia, cardiac arrest

* *EDITORS NOTE:* This compendium is not meant to be a complete listing. We have compiled only a limited number of drugs, and provided dosages for the more common indications.

Available: Calcium chloride: Injection: 10% (13.5 meq calcium per gram), 10 ml ampules or prefilled syringes.
Calcium gluconate: Injection: 10% (4.8 meq of calcium per gram), 10 ml ampule

Drug: DOPAMINE (INTROPIN)

Route of Administration: Intravenous

Dose: Initial 2–20 μg/kg/min

Subsequent Titrate to desired cardiovascular effect

Precautions: Dopamine is unstable in alkaline solutions (pH greater than 6.85). Solutions containing sodium bicarbonate or aminophylline should not be used concurrently with dopamine. A standard infusion may be made by mixing 60 mg of dopamine with 100 ml of 5% dextrose in water (D5W). Infuse this solution initially at a rate of 1 ml/kg/hr. This will deliver 10 μg/kg/min

Adverse Effects: Hypertension and tachycardia may be seen with rapid infusion

Available: Injection: 200 mg/5 ml, 5 ml ampule

Drug: EPINEPHRINE

Route of Administration: Intravenous, intratracheal

Dose: Initial 10 μg/kg (0.1 ml of 1:10,000 solution)

Subsequent 20 μg/kg i.v., then 40 μg/kg if still no response

Precautions: Epinephrine solution for infusion should be prepared by adding 6 mg of epinephrine (1:1,000) to 100 ml of D5W which produces a solution containing 60 μg/ml. This solution should be infused at 1 ml/kg/hr which allows a dose of 1 μg/kg/min. Do not mix bicarbonate with epinephrine for the epinephrine will be inactivated. Cardiac injection of epinephrine should be avoided for this route is associated with greater risk

Adverse Effects: Hypotension

Available: Injection: 100 μg/ml (1:10,000), 10 ml and 3 ml prefilled syringe; 1000 μg/ml (1:1,000), 1 ml ampule

Drug: FUROSEMIDE (LASIX)

Route of Administration: Oral, intravenous

Dose: Initial 1 mg/kg

Subsequent If no response in 20–30 min, a repeat dose of 1–2 mg/kg may be given

Precautions: Hypokalemia in a patient on digoxin may result in the development of life-threatening arrhythmias. Furosemide should be administered at a rate of no more than 4 mg/min to avoid vasodilation of the pulmonary vasculature

Adverse Effects: Hypokalemia, hyperosmolarity, metabolic alkalosis, and worsening of hypotension

Available: Injection: 10 mg/ml, 2 ml ampule and 10 mg/ml prefilled syringes; elixir: 10 mg/ml; tablets: 20 mg, 40 mg, 80 mg

Drug: GLUCOSE

Route of Administration: Intravenous

Dose: Initial 1 g/kg infused as a 25% solution

Subsequent Subsequent doses should be based on the serum glucose level

Precautions: None

Adverse Effects: Hyperglycemia, hyperosmolarity

Available: Injection: 25 g/100 ml, 50 ml vials; 25 g/100 mg, 10 ml, prefilled syringe

Drug: ISOPROTERENOL (ISUPREL)

Route of Administration: Intravenous

Dose: 0.1–1 μg/kg/min. A standard infusion may be prepared by adding 0.6 mg of isoproterenol to 100 ml of D5W. Infuse this solution at a rate of 1 ml/kg/hr to deliver 1 μg/kg/min

Precautions: Isoproterenol should be used with extreme caution in children on digitalis products. In the dehydrated or hypovolemic patient, isoproterenol may produce or aggravate existing hypotension; thus, the physician must be prepared to support a decrease in blood pressure. Isoproterenol should not be mixed with any drugs

Adverse Effects: Tachyarrhythmias, myocardial ischemia, hypertension

Available: Injection: 200 μg, 1 ml ampule

Drug: LIDOCAINE (XYLOCAINE)

Route of Administration: Intravenous, intratracheal

Dose: Initial 1 mg/kg

Subsequent The initial dose may be repeated up to 3 times at 5-min intervals. Once the initial bolus has been given, an infusion of lidocaine 10–20 μg/kg/min should be initiated

Precautions: Dosage must be modified in children with congestive heart failure or liver disease

Adverse Effects: Nausea, vomiting, lethargy, paresthesias, disorientation, and seizures are seen early. Later, symptoms of cardiac toxicity including depression of the myocardium and ventricular irritability may occur. Heart block and drug-induced asystole may also occur

Available: Injection: 100 mg/ml and 500 mg/ml, multidose vials; prefilled syringe 10 mg/ml, 10 ml

Drug: METHYLPREDNISOLONE (SOLU-MEDROL)

Route of Administration: Intravenous

Dose: Initial 30 mg/kg/i.v. or dexamethasone 1 ml/kg/i.v.

Subsequent Repeat in 2–4 hr

Precautions: None

Adverse Effects: No known adverse effects from short-term use

Available: Injections: 40 mg, 125 mg and 1 g vials

Drug: NALOXONE (NARCAN)

Route of Administration: Intravenous

Dose: Initial 0.01 mg/kg

Subsequent The initial dose may be repeated every 3–5 min up to a maximum of 5 doses

Precautions: None

Adverse Effects: Narcotic withdrawal symptoms may occur when naloxone is administered too rapidly or too often to reverse narcotic effect; otherwise very safe

Available: Injection: 400 μg/ml, 1 ml ampule and 20 μg/ml, 2 ml ampule

Drug: OXYGEN

Route of Administration: Delivered by breathing mask or ventilation

Dose: 100% until circulation is restored

Precautions: Use with self inflating bag valve mask *with* attached reservoir

Available: Pressurized cylinders

Drug: SODIUM BICARBONATE

Route of Administration: Intravenous

Dose: Initial 1 meq/kg full strength (1 meq/ml) for children more than 6 mo old, use half-strength (0.5 meq/ml) for children less than 6 mo old

Subsequent — Determined by calculating the base deficit from the measured arterial pH and pCO_2: meq of bicarbonate (HCO_3) = (base deficit × wt (kg) × 0.4)/2

Precautions: Bicarbonate should be given by direct i.v. administration and followed by saline flush to avoid precipitation in the i.v. line with other drugs such as calcium. Bicarbonate is irritating to the airways and destroys lung parenchyma; thus, it should not be given by the intratracheal route

Adverse Effects: Hypernatremia (11.9 meq of sodium per 1 g) alkalosis, and hyperosmolarity may be produced. Bicarbonate should always be used in conjunction with an airway when corrrecting respiratory acidosis

Available: Injection: 1 meq/ml, 50 ml prefilled syringe

GENERAL DRUG LIST

Drug: ACETAMINOPHEN
Route of Administration: Oral, rectal
Dose: 60–90 mg/kg/day in 6 divided doses (maximum daily dose 3.6 gm)
Precautions: Use cautiously in patients with liver disease
Available: Tablets: 80 mg (chewable) and 325 mg; elixir, 160 mg/5 ml and 100 mg/ml; suppositories, 120 mg and 650 mg

Drug: ACETYLSALICYLIC ACID (ASPIRIN)
Route of Administration: Oral, rectal
Dose: Antipyretic dose, 60 mg/kg/day in 4–6 divided doses. Acute rheumatoid arthritis dose, 80–90 mg/kg/day in 4 divided doses (maximum daily dose 3.6 gm)
Precautions: Enhances the activity of methotrexate and warfarin and decreases the activity of probenicid. Use with caution in bleeding disorders
Adverse Effects: Gastrointestinal upset, tinnitus
Available: Tablets: 80 mg, 325 mg; suppositories: 325 mg

Drug: ALBUTEROL (PROVENTIL, VENTOLIN)
Route of Administration: Inhalation
Dose: 1–2 puffs every 4–6 hr (each puff delivers 90 μg)
Precautions: Beta(β)-blockers inhibit the activity of albuterol and should not be used concomitantly. If used too frequently, paradoxical bronchospasm may occur. Use with caution in patients with cardiac disease, thyroid disease and diabetes mellitus
Adverse Effects: Palpitation, tremor, nausea, nervousness, hypertension, headache and drying or irritation of the oropharynx
Available: Inhaler unit supplied with oral adapter

Drug: ϵ-AMINOCAPROIC ACID (AMICAR)
Route of Administration: Oral, intravenous
Dose: Oral or slow intravenous 100 mg/kg/dose initially followed by ⅓ of initial dose hourly to achieve plasma level of 130 μg/ml for inhibition of systemic hyperfibrinolysis (maximum daily dose 30 g)
Precautions: To be used for mouth bleeding but not for urinary tract bleeding associated with hemophilia
Available: Injection: 250 mg/ml, 20 ml vial; tablets: 500 mg; syrup: 1.25 g/ 5 ml

AMINOPHYLLINE—**see THEOPHYLLINE (p. 1310)**

Drug: AMITRIPTYLINE (ELAVIL)
Route of Administration: Oral

Dose: <12 yr: 5 mg/kg/24 hr; >12 yr: 25 mg daily at bedtime, increasing by 25 mg every 3 days to a total of 150 mg/day
Adverse Effects: Drowsiness, dry mouth, blurred vision, diplopia
Available: Tablets: 10 mg, 25 mg, 50 mg, 75 mg, 100 mg, 150 mg

Drug: AMOXICILLIN (AMOXIL, POLYMOX)
Route of Administration: Oral
Dose: <10 kg 125 mg t.i.d.; >10 kg, 250 mg t.i.d.
Adverse Effects: Diarrhea, maculopapular rash
Available: Capsules: 250 mg and 500 mg; oral suspension: 125 mg/5 ml and 250 mg/5 ml

Drug: d-AMPHETAMINE (DEXEDRINE)
Route of Administration: Oral
Dose: 2.5–5 mg once daily, gradually increasing to a maximum of 20 mg/day
Precautions: Tolerance may develop requiring adjustment of the dosage
Adverse Effects: Insomnia, nervousness, loss of appetite, irritability, tachycardia
Available: Tablets: 5 mg, 10 mg; spansules: 10 mg, 15 mg; elixir: 5 mg/5 ml

Drug: AMPICILLIN (GENERIC)
Route of Administration: Oral, intramuscular, intravenous
Dose: 0–7 days of age: 50–100 mg/kg/day in 2 divided doses.
7 days to 1 month of age: 100 to 200 mg/kg/day in 4–6 divided doses
>1 month of age: oral: 50–100 mg/kg/day in 4 divided doses; parenteral: 150–400 mg/kg/day in 4–6 divided doses
Precautions: When given orally, ampicillin should be administered on an empty stomach
Available: Injection: 125 mg, 250 mg, 500 mg and 1 g vials; suspension: 125 mg/5 ml, 100 and 200 ml, 250 mg/5 ml, 100 ml and 200 ml; capsules: 250 and 500 mg

Drug: AZATHIOPRINE (IMURAN)
Route of Administration: Oral, intravenous
Dose: Antirheumatic dose, 1–2 mg/kg/day in 1–2 divided doses
Precautions: Reduce dose to 25–30% when allopurinol is also being administered
Adverse Effects: Leukopenia, thrombocytopenia, macrocytic anemia, nausea and vomiting
Available: Injection: 100 mg/20 ml vial, tablets: 25 mg, 50 mg

Drug: BECLOMETHASONE (BECLOVENT)
Route of Administration: Inhalation
Dose: 1–2 puffs 3–4 times daily; maximum not to exceed 10 puffs per day (each puff delivers 42 μg)
Precautions: Caution should be used in converting asthmatic patients from oral steroids to inhaled steroids. Withdrawal symptoms include muscle and joint pain, malaise, anorexia, nausea, headache and depression
Adverse Effects: Hoarseness, dry mouth (rarely), bronchospasm (rarely)
Available: Inhaler supplied with oral adapter

Drug: BENZTROPINE (CONGENTIN)
Route of Administration: Oral, intramuscular
Dose: 1–2 mg/day, once or twice daily
Adverse Effects: Atropine-like symptoms
Available: Tablets: 500 μg, 1 mg, 2 mg; injection: 1 mg/ml

Drug: CARBAMAZEPINE (TEGRETOL)
Route of Administration: Oral
Dose: 20–30 mg/kg/day in 3 divided doses

Adverse Effects: Sedation, transient leukopenia, vertigo, dizziness, diplopia, ataxia, nystagmus, hepatotoxicity; may interact when used with clonazepam, theophylline, phenobarbital, phenytoin and valproic acid
Available: Tablets: 200 mg, 100 mg (chewable)

Drug: CARBENICILLIN (GEOCILLIN)
Route of Administration: Oral, intravenous
Dose: Oral: 40–100 mg/kg/day in 4 divided doses; intravenous: 0–7 days, 100 mg/kg/day in 2 divided doses: 7 days but <2000 g; 300 mg/kg/day in 3 divided doses; >7 days and >2000 g 400–600 mg/kg/day in 4–6 divided doses (maximum intravenous daily dose is 40 g)
Precautions: Each gram of carbenicillin contains 4.8 meq of sodium
Adverse Effects: May cause hypernatremia or hypokalemia when large doses are given
Available: Injection: 2, 5, and 10 g vial; tablets: 382 mg

Drug: CEFACLOR (CECLOR)
Route of Administration: Oral
Dose: 20–60 mg/kg/day in 3–4 divided doses (maximum daily dose of 2–3 g)
Adverse Effects: Serum sickness
Available: Capsules: 250 mg, 500 mg; suspension: 125 mg/5 ml, 250 mg/5 ml

Drug: CEFAZOLIN (ANCEF)
Route of Administration: Intramuscular, intravenous
Dose: 100 mg/kg/day in 3 divided doses
Precautions: May have cross-sensitivity with penicillin
Available: Injection: 1 g and 5 g vials

Drug: CEPHALEXIN (KEFLEX)
Route of Administration: Oral
Dose: 50–100 mg/kg/day (maximum daily dose 4 g) given in 4 divided doses
Precautions: The drug should be given on an empty stomach
Adverse Effects: Nausea, vomiting and diarrhea; possible cross-sensitivity in patients who are allergic to penicillin
Available: Capsules: 125 mg, 250 mg, 500 mg; suspension: 125 mg/5 ml, 250 mg/5 ml

Drug: CHLORAL HYDRATE (NOCTEC)
Route of Administration: Oral, rectal
Dose: 30 mg/kg/dose, may be repeated once at ½ the initial dose
Adverse Effects: Sedation, drowsiness, somnolence
Available: Capsules: 500 mg; syrup: 50 mg/5 ml; suppositories: 300 mg and 600 mg

Drug: CHLORAMPHENICOL (CHLOROMYCETIN)
Route of Administration: Oral, intravenous
Dose: Full term newborns in the first week, 25 mg/kg/day in 2 divided doses; infants 1–4 wk of age, 50 mg/kg/day in 2 divided doses; older children, 50–100 mg/kg/day in 4 divided doses (maximum daily dose 4–6 g)
Precautions: If given with a bactericidal agent (i.e., penicillin), chloramphenicol should be given 1 hr following bactericidal drug. Concurrent administration may increase the blood level of phenytoin
Adverse Effects: Gray baby syndrome, usually seen in newborn infants of low birth weight started on the drug in the first 48 hr of life
Available: Injection: 100 mg/ml after reconstitution; capsules: 50 mg, 100 mg, 250 mg; suspension: 150 mg/5 ml

Drug: CHLOROTHIAZIDE (DIURIL)
Route of Administration: Oral, intravenous
Dose: <6 mo, 20–30 mg/kg/day in 2 divided doses; >6 mo, 20 mg/kg/day in 2 divided doses (maximum daily dose 2 g/y)
Precautions: Use with caution in liver and severe renal disease
Adverse Effects: Hyperbilirubinemia, hypokalemia and hyperglycemia
Available: Injection: 500 mg/20 ml; tablets: 250 mg, 500 mg

Drug: CHLORPHENIRAMINE MALEATE (CHLOR-TRIMETON)
Route of Administration: Oral, intramuscular, subcutaneous
Dose: 0.35 mg/kg/day in 3 or 4 divided doses or: <6 yr, 12 mg/24 hr; 6–12 yr, 24 mg/24 hr; >12 yr, 36 mg/24 hr
Precautions: With repeated use, patients may develop tolerance to drowsiness and to therapeutic effect. May lower seizure threshhold. Use with caution in patients with asthma
Adverse Effects: Drowsiness, dry mouth
Available: Injection: 10 mg/ml, 100 mg/ml; syrup: 2 mg/5 ml; tablets: 4 mg; sustained-release tablets and capsules: 8 mg, 12 mg

Drug: CHLORPROMAZINE (THORAZINE)
Route of Administration: Oral, intramuscular
Dose: 2 mg/kg/day in 4–6 divided doses, titrate in emergencies
Precautions: Use cautiously in patients with liver, pulmonary, and cardiovascular disease
Adverse Effects: Hypotension, extrapyramidal reactions, dystonias, drowsiness, jaundice, agranulocytosis
Available: Injection: 25 mg/ml, 1 ml and 2 ml ampule; 25 mg/ml, 10 ml vial; tablets: 10 mg, 25 mg, 50 mg; syrup: 10 mg/5 ml

Drug: CLOTRIMAZOLE (GYNE-LOTRIMIN, MYCELEX-G)
Route of Administration: Topical
Dose: 1 tablet/day inserted vaginally for 7 days; apply cream locally
Adverse Effects: May cause erythema, blistering or urticaria where applied
Available: Vaginal tablet: 100 mg; cream: 1%; solution: 1%

Drug: COCAINE HCl
Route of Administration: Topical
Dose: Topical administration in each nostril
Available: 1%, 5%, 10% solutions

Drug: CROMOLYN SODIUM (INTAL, AARANE)
Route of Administration: Inhalation
Dose: 1 capsule inserted in Spinhaler and inhaled every 6 hr (each capsule contains 20 mg)
Precautions: When used for exercise-induced bronchospasm, cromolyn should be administered 30 min prior to exercise
Adverse Effects: Hoarseness, oropharyngeal irritation, dry mouth, chest tightness or bronchospasm, nasal congestion, nausea and urticaria
Available: Capsules: 20 mg

Drug: CYCLOPHOSPHAMIDE (CYTOXAN)
Route of Administration: Oral, intravenous
Dose: Antirheumatic dose 0.5–2.5 mg/kg/day in 1–2 divided doses
Precautions: The rate of metabolism and hence the leukopenic activity of cyclophosphamide is increased by phenobarbital. Good hydration is recommended to reduce incidence of hemorrhagic cystitis. Should be

used with caution in patients with impaired hepatic or renal function

Adverse Effects: Leukopenia, thrombocytopenia, anemia, anorexia, nausea, vomiting, hemorrhagic cystitis, gonadal suppression, alopecia, interstitial pulmonary fibrosis

Available: Injection: 100 mg, 200 mg, 500 mg/vial; tablets: 25 mg, 50 mg

Drug: CYPROHEPTADINE HYDROCHLORIDE (PERIACTIN)

Route of Administration: Oral

Dose: <14 yr, 0.25 mg/kg/day in 4 divided doses; >14 yr, 0.5 mg/kg/day in 4 divided doses

Precautions: Use with caution in asthma

Adverse Effects: Atropine-like efffects

Available: Tablets: 4 mg; syrup: 2 mg/5 ml

Drug: DEXAMETHASONE (DECADRON, HEXADROL)

Route of Administration: Oral, intramuscular, intravenous, inhalation

Dose: Oral, intramuscular, intravenous: 0.5–1 mg/day (for acute increased intracranial pressure); maintenance dose: 0.25–0.5 mg/kg/day in 4 divided doses

Precautions: Every other day therapy is advised once dosage is established to minimize growth retardation

Adverse Effects: Sodium and water retention, growth retardation

Available: Injection: 4 mg/ml, 10 mg/ml, 24 mg/ml; tablets: 0.5 mg, 0.75 mg, 1.5 mg, 4 mg; oral liquid: 0.5 mg/5 ml; nasal insufflation (each spray delivers 100 μg)

Drug: DIAZEPAM (VALIUM)

Route of Administration: Oral, intravenous

Dose: Intravenous: 0.1–0.3 mg/kg to maximum of 10 mg infused at 1 mg/min; oral, 1–2.5 mg/dose, 3–4 times daily

Precautions: Given intravenously to interrrupt status epilepticus, diazepam has a very short duration of action requiring repeat doses or administration of another anticonvulsant. Diazepam may cause prolonged sedation

Adverse Effects: Sedation, cardiorespiratory depression, hypotension

Available: Injection: 5 mg/ml; tablets: 2 mg, 5 mg, 10 mg

Drug: DIAZOXIDE (HYPERSTAT)

Route of Administration: Intravenous

Dose: 5 mg/kg/dose; may be repeated in 30 min if necessary. Daily maximum dose 10–15 g/kg; should be administered rapidly as an i.v. push

Precautions: Patients should remain recumbent for 30 min following the dose. Intravenous furosemide is customarily given to prevent fluid retention

Adverse Effects: Tachycardia and salt and water retention

Available: Injection: 300 mg/20 ml ampule

Drug: DIGOXIN (see text, p. 296)

Drug: DIPHENHYDRAMINE (BENADRYL)

Route of Administration: Oral, intramuscular, intravenous

Dose: 5 mg/kg/day in 4 divided doses (maximum daily dose 300 mg)

Precautions: Should be avoided in neonates

Adverse Effects: Drowsiness, sedation, dry mouth

Available: Injection: 50 mg/ml; capsules: 25 mg, 50 mg; dye-free elixir: 12.5 mg/5 ml

Drug: ERYTHROMYCIN (E-MYCIN, EES, PEDIAMYCIN)

Route of Administration: Oral, intravenous

Dose: Oral: erythromycin estolate salt, 20–50 mg/kg/day in 2–4 divided doses to a maximum of 2–3 g; erythromycin ethylsuccinate, 50 mg/kg/day in 4 divided doses (maximum daily dose 2–3 g). Intravenous: erythromycin base for injection 20 mg/kg/day in 4 divided doses to a maximum of 2–4 g/day

Precautions: Erythromycin is metabolized by the liver and should be used with caution in liver failure. There is a possibility of jaundice occurring with the estolate salt; however; this rarely occurs among children 12 yr of age or younger. For intravenous use, the drug should be diluted properly and infused over 30–60 min since the drug may cause phlebitis. Orally, both salts of erythromycin can be taken with food

Available: Injection: various concentrations. Chewable tablets: 200 mg and 400 mg; capsules: 125 mg and 250 mg; suspension: 125 mg/5 ml, 250 mg/5 ml

Drug: ESTROGEN, CONJUGATED (PREMARIN)

Route of Administration: Intravenous, topical

Dose: Topical: apply at bedtime for 2–4 wk; intravenous: 10 mg to 25 mg once

Precautions: Inject slowly

Available: Injection: 25 mg; vaginal cream

Drug: ETHACRYNIC ACID (EDECRIN)

Route of Administration: Oral, intravenous

Dose: Oral: 1 mg/kg once or twice daily; intravenous: 0.4–0.6 mg/kg/dose given once or twice daily

Precautions: When given with aminoglycoside antibiotics, the potential for ototoxicity is increased

Adverse Effects: Ototoxicity, electrolyte imbalance

Available: Injection: 50 mg vial (as sodium ethacrynate); tablets: 25 mg, 50 mg

Drug: FERROUS SULFATE (FER-IN-SOL, VARIOUS GENERICS)

Route of Administration: Oral, intramuscular, intravenous

Dose: 4–6 mg/kg/day of elemental iron given in 3 divided doses orally (Fer-in-sol solution contains 25 mg elemental iron per ml)

Precautions: When administered i.v., infusion should be given slowly over 2 hr following a test dose. If ferrous sulfate (20% elemental iron) is not tolerable, ferrous gluconate (12% elemental iron) may be tried since side effects are directly related to amount of elemental iron consumed

Adverse Effects: Epigastric distress, nausea, constipation (p.o.); hypotension, bradycardia, myalgias, headache, lymphadenopathy and urticaria (i.v.); pain at injection site and brown discoloration of skin (i.m.)

Available: Liquid: Fer-in-sol, 125 mg/5 ml (25 mg elemental iron/ml); Feosol, 220 mg/5 ml (45 mg elemental iron/5 ml). Tablets: 325 mg (60 mg elemental iron). Injection: 50 mg/ampule

Drug: FLUPHENAZINE (PROLIXIN)

Route of Administration: Oral, intramuscular

Dose: Recommended for adolescents only, 1–20 mg/day

Precautions: Similar to thioridazine

Adverse Effects: Similar to thioridazine

Available Injection: 2.5 mg/ml, 10 ml vial; tablets: 1 mg, 2.5 mg, 5 mg, 10 mg; elixir: 0.5 mg/ml

Drug: FOLIC ACID (FOLVITE)

Route of Administration: Oral, intramuscular, intravenous

Dose: 1 mg/day

Available: Injection: 5 mg/ml; tablets: 1 mg

Drug: FUROSEMIDE (LASIX)
Route of Administration: Oral, intramuscular, intravenous
Dose: Oral, 1–4 mg/kg/day in a single dose; intravenous, 0.5–1 mg/kg/dose (increments may be made according to clinical response)
Precautions: May reduce arterial responsiveness to pressors and enhance the affect of tubocurarine. If used with antihypertensive drugs, their dose should be reduced. Electrolyte abnormalities are more prone to occur with furosemide than with other diuretics. Furosemide therapy may also be accompanied by metabolic alkalosis. Hypokalemia induced by furosemide may render a digitalized patient more prone to digitalis toxicity. The i.v. injection should be given at a rate not faster than 4 mg/min because of the vasodilating effect of furosemide on the pulmonary vasculature
Adverse Effect: Electrolyte abnormalities, ototoxicity
Available: Injection: 10 mg/ml in 2 ml, 4 ml, 8 ml, 10 ml units; tablets: 20 mg, 40 mg and 80 mg; oral solution: 10 mg/ml

Drug: GENTAMICIN (GARAMYCIN)
Route of Administration: Intravenous, intramuscular, intrathrecal
Dose: Parenteral: 1–7 days and <1500 gm, 2.5 mg/kg every 24 hr; 1500–2000 g, 2.5 mg/kg every 18 hr; 2000 g, 2.5 mg/kg every 12 hr. 7–21 days and <1500 gm, 2.5 mg/kg every 12 hr; >1500 gm, 2.5 mg/kg every 8 hr. After day 21 and all weights, 2.5 mg/kg every 8 hr (maximum daily dose 300 mg)
Precautions: Reduce dose with renal insufficiency
Adverse Effects: Ototoxicity and renal toxicity
Available: Injection: various concentrations; ophthalmic preparation

Drug: HALOPERIDOL (HALDOL)
Route of Administration: Oral, intramuscular
Dose: 0.025–0.05 mg/kg/day initially, increasing to 0.1–0.3 mg/kg/day
Adverse Effects: Sedation, hypotension, extrapyramidal reactions
Available: Injection: 5 mg/ml; tablets: 0.5, 1, 2, 5, 10 mg; solution: 2 mg/ml

Drug: HEPARIN
Route of Administration: Subcutaneous, intravenous
Dose: 50–100 units/kg as a bolus every 4 hr *or* 12.5–25 units/kg/hr by continuous i.v. infusion after bolus injection of 50–100 units/kg
Precautions: Use PTT of 1–1½ × normal as therapeutic index. With continuous infusion use a control device to prevent overheparinization
Adverse Effects: Hemorrhage
Available: Injection; various concentration

Drug: HYDRALAZINE (APRESOLINE)
Route of Administration: Oral, intramuscular, intravenous
Dose: I.V.: 0.1–0.2 mg/kg given as an infusion over 15–30 min, repeated every 4–6 hr to a daily maximum of 1–2 mg/kg or maximum total daily dose of 100 mg. Oral dosage: 0.75–1 mg/kg/day given every 4–6 hr
Precautions: When given intravenously, hydralazine should be infused slowly and blood pressure monitored
Adverse Effects: Tachycardia, flushing, headache, vomiting, and salt and water retention
Available: Injection: 20 mg/ml, 1 ml ampule; tablets: 10 mg, 25 mg and 50 mg

Drug: HYDROCHLOROTHIAZIDE (HYDRODIURIL)
Route of Administration: Oral
Dose: 2–3 mg/kg/day in 2 divided doses
Precautions: Use with caution in liver and severe renal disease
Adverse Effects: Hyperbilirubinemia, hypokalemia, and hyperglycemia
Available: Tablets: 25 mg, 50 mg, 100 mg

Drug: HYDROCORTISONE (SOLU-CORTEF)
Route of Administration: Oral, intramuscular, intravenous
Dose: Gram-negative shock (sodium succinate): initial dose 50 mg/kg i.v.; subsequent dose 50–75 mg/kg/day in 4 divided doses. Status asthmaticus: 4 mg/kg/dose every 2 hr for 5–6 doses, then 10 mg/kg/day in 4 divided doses
Precautions: Every other day therapy is advised once dosage and therapy is established to minimize growth retardation
Adverse Effects: Sodium and water retention, growth retardation
Available: Injection: 100 mg/2 ml; tablets: 10 mg, 20 mg; oral suspension: 10 mg/5 ml

Drug: HYDROXYCHLOROQUINE (PLAQUENIL)
Route of Administration: Oral
Dose: Antirheumatic dose, 3–6 mg/kg/day in a single daily dose (maximum 400 mg/day)
Precautions: This drug should be given with extreme caution in children and in all patients with G6PD deficiency
Adverse Effects: Headache, vertigo, tinnitus, nystagmus, seizures, ataxia, emotional changes, skeletal muscle weakness, corneal deposits, retinopathy (may be irreversible), rashes, bleaching of hair, alopecia, blood dyscrasias, gastrointestinal upset, lassitude
Available: Tablets: 200 mg

Drug: HYDROXYZINE (ATARAX, VISTARIL)
Route of Administration: Oral, intramuscular
Dose: Oral: 2 mg/kg/day in 4 divided doses; intramuscular: 0.5–1.0 mg/kg/dose given every 4 hr
Precautions: May potentiate barbiturates or meperidine
Adverse Effects: Drowsiness, dry mouth
Available: Injection (Vistaril): 50 mg/ml; tablets (hydrochloride—Atarax): 10 mg, 25 mg; capsules (pamoate—Vistaril): 25 mg, 50 mg; syrup (Atarax): 25 mg/5 ml

Drug: IBUPROFEN (MOTRIN)
Route of Administration: Oral
Dose: 300–400 mg/dose in 4–6 divided doses
Precautions: The lowest effective dose should be utilized. Ibuprofen should be avoided in patients with bronchospastic reactivity to aspirin and used with caution in patients with underlying cardiac and renal disease
Adverse Effects: Common: nausea, epigastric pain, heartburn, indigestion, dizziness, rash. Less common: bleeding, photoallergic skin reactions, headache, nervousness, tinnitus, decreased appetite, edema, fluid retention
Available: Tablets: 300 mg, 400 mg, 600 mg

Drug: IMIPRAMINE (TOFRANIL)
Route of Administration: Oral
Dose: Enuresis: 25–75 mg at bedtime
Adverse Effects: Drowsiness, dry mouth, blurred vision, diplopia
Available: Tablets: 10 mg, 25 mg, 50 mg

Drug: INDOMETHACIN (INDOCIN)
Route of Administration: Oral
Dose: 0.5–2.5 mg/kg/day in 2 or 3 divided doses (maximum daily dose 100 mg)
Precautions: Indomethacin should be used with caution in children with coagulation defects and renal disease
Adverse Effects: Common: nausea, vomiting, indigestion, diarrhea, abdominal distress, headache, dizziness. Less common: constipation somnolence, listlessness, visual problems, edema, hematologic abnormalities, dyspnea, angioedema and vaginal bleeding
Available: Capsules: 25 mg, 50 mg

Drug: LITHIUM CARBONATE (ESKALITH, LITHONATE, AND OTHERS)
Route of Administration: Oral
Dose: 300–900 mg/day (serum lithium levels must be maintained between 0.6 and 1.2 meq/L)
Precautions: Serum lithium levels must be monitored carefully and frequently since toxicity is directly related to the serum level. Patients should be instructed to discontinue lithium therapy if diarrhea, vomiting, tremor, mild ataxia, drowsiness or muscle weakness develop. Haloperidol should be avoided in patients receiving lithium
Adverse Effects: Mild thirst at initiation of therapy, transient and mild nausea during first few days of therapy. Other severe CNS toxicities are dose related (see "Precautions")
Available: Capsules: 300 mg; tablets: 300 mg

Drug: MEDROXYPROGESTERONE ACETATE (PROVERA)
Route of Administration: Oral
Dose: 10–20 mg/day
Precautions: Should be avoided during pregnancy, in patients with history of thromboembolic or liver disease, breast malignancy, migraine, undiagnosed vaginal bleeding or depression
Adverse Effects: Breast tenderness, sensitivity reactions, edema, fluid retention, acne, thrombophlebitis, menstrual abnormalities, cholestatic jaundice, headache, dizziness, alopecia, pruritus
Available: Tablets: 2.5 mg, 10 mg

Drug: MEPERIDINE (DEMEROL)
Route of Administration: Oral, intramuscular, intravenous
Dose: 1.5–2.0 mg/kg/dose i.m. or p.o. every 4–6 hrs
Precautions: Monitor respirations, blood pressure and heart rate following parenteral meperidine. Use with caution in renal failure. May potentiate other CNS depressants
Adverse Effects: Drowsiness, sedation, apathy, orthostatic hypotension, nausea, vomiting, urinary retention, respiratory depression
Available: Injection: 25 mg/ml, 50 mg/ml, 75 mg/ml, 100 mg/ml; tablets: 50 mg, 100 mg; syrup: 50 mg/5 ml

Drug: METAPROTERENOL (ALUPENT, METAPREL)
Route of Administration: Oral, inhalation
Dose: Oral: $<$30 kg, 10 mg qid or 1.5 mg/kg/day in 3–4 divided doses; $>$30 kg, 20 mg qid in 3–4 divided doses. Inhalation: 2 puffs every 4 hr not to exceed 5 doses per day (each puff delivers 0.65 mg metaproterenol sulfate)
Precautions: Patients should be carefully instructed in the proper use of the inhaler
Adverse Effects: Nausea, headache, tremor, nervousness, tachycardia, palpitations, dizziness, flushing

Available: Tablets: 10 mg, 20 mg; syrup: 10 mg/5 ml; aerosol: 0.65 mg/inhalation

Drug: METHENAMINE (MANDELAMINE)
Route of Administration: Oral
Dose: Initial: 100 mg/kg/day in 4 divided doses; maintenance: 50 mg/kg/day in 4 divided doses (maximum daily dose 3 g)
Precautions: Should not be used in newborns or with renal insufficiency. Ascorbic acid should be given with each dose to acidify the urine
Adverse Effects: Dysuria
Available: Tablets: 250 mg, 500 mg, 1000 mg; suspension: 250 mg/5 ml, 500 mg/5 ml

Drug: METHYLENE BLUE
Route of Administration: Intravenous
Dose: 1–2 mg/kg/dose
Available: 1% solution

Drug: METHYLPHENIDATE (RITALIN)
Route of Administration: Oral
Dose: 0.3–1.0 mg/kg/day in 2–3 divided doses
Precautions: Tolerance may develop requiring dosage adjustment
Adverse Effects: Insomnia, nervousness, loss of appetite, irritability, possible growth suppression, tachycardia
Available: Tablets: 5 mg, 10 mg, 20 mg

Drug: METRONIDAZOLE (FLAGYL)
Route of Administration: Oral
Dose: For amebiasis: 35–50 mg/kg/day in 3 divided doses for 10 days; for giardiasis: 15 mg/day for 5 days; for trichomonas: 15 mg/kg/day for 7 days or a single dose of 2 g
Precautions: Avoid taking metronidazole with alcohol
Adverse Effects: Metallic taste, gastrointestinal distress, CNS toxicity
Available: Tablets: 250 mg

Drug: MICONAZOLE (MONISTAT)
Route of Administration: Topical
Dose: Cream or lotion: applied b.i.d. for 2–4 weeks; vaginal cream: 1 applicator full daily for 7 days
Available: Cream 2%, lotion 2%, vaginal cream 2%

Drug: MORPHINE SULFATE (GENERIC)
Route of Administration: Oral, intramuscular, intravenous, subcutaneous
Dose: 0.1–0.2 mg/kg every 4– 6 hr (maximum dose 15 mg)
Precautions: Morphine intravenous should be administered slowly (4–5 min) while monitoring respirations, blood pressure and heart rate. May potentiate other CNS depressants
Adverse Effects: Drowsiness, sedation, hypotension, nausea, vomiting, urinary retention, apnea
Available: Injection: 8 mg/ml, 10 mg/ml, 15 mg/ml; tablets: 10 mg, 15 mg

Drug: NAPROXEN (NAPROSYN)
Route of Administration: Oral
Dose: Dysmenorrhea: 500 mg once, followed by 250 mg qid; juvenile rheumatoid arthritis: 10 mg/kg/day in 2 divided doses
Precautions: Should be used with caution in patients with underlying renal, cardiac, or peptic ulcer disease
Adverse Effects: Common: constipation, heartburn, abdominal pain, nausea, headache, dizziness, drowsiness, pruritus, skin erruptions, ecchymosis, tinnitus, edema, dyspnea. Less common: thirst, palpitations, vomiting, ne-

phrotic syndrome, abnormal liver function tests, hematuria, blood dyscrasias, weakness, alopecia, depression, malaise

Available: Tablets: 250 mg, 375 mg

Drug: NITROFURANTOIN (MACRODANTIN)

Route of Administration: Oral

Dose: For acute infections: 5–7 mg/kg/day in 4 divided doses; for prophylaxis or chronic therapy: 2–3 mg/kg/day in 1 or 2 divided doses

Precautions: Medication should be administered with food to minimize gastrointestinal distress. Impaired renal function requires reduction of drug dosage

Adverse Effects: Gastrointestinal distress including nausea, vomiting, abdominal pain, anorexia; infrequently, interstitial pneumonitis and peripheral neuritis

Available: Capsules and tablets: 25 mg, 50 mg, 100 mg; suspension: 25 mg/5 ml

Drug: NITROPRUSSIDE, SODIUM (NIPRIDE)

Route of Administration: Intravenous

Dose: Slow infusion at 0.5–8 μg/kg/min

Precautions: The onset of action is instantaneous. Nitroprusside should be infused in D5W; the solution should be protected from light and changed every 4 hr because of the instability of the drug. A discolored solution should be discarded. Careful and frequent monitoring of arterial pressure, pulmonary wedge pressure and cardiac output is crucial. If possible, nitroprusside should be administered by infusion pump

Adverse Effects: Anxiety, apprehension, confusion, muscle twitching, hyperreflexia, sweating, increased cardiac output, lowered blood pressure, accumulation of thiocyanate (in the presence of severe liver or renal impairment or prolonged infusion). Symptoms of cyanide intoxication include fatigue, anorexia, acidosis, weakness, tinnitus, confusion and seizures. These symptoms occur at levels greater than 12 mg/100 ml

Available: Injection: 50 mg ampule

Drug: NORETHINDRONE ACETATE (NORLUTATE)

Route of Administration: Oral

Dose: 10–20 mg/day

Precautions: Use cautiously in patients with renal or cardiac disease

Adverse Effects: Fluid retention

Available: Tablets: 5 mg

Drug: NYSTATIN (MYCOSTATIN, NILSTAT)

Route of Administration: Oral, topical

Dose: <28 days: 200,000–400,000 units/day in 4 divided doses; >28 days: 400,000–2,000,000 units/day in 4 divided doses

Adverse Effects: Gastrointestinal upset

Available: Topical cream, ointment and powder; tablets: 500,000 units; oral suspension: 100,000 units/ml

Drug: OXACILLIN (PROSTAPHLIN, BACTOCIL)

Route of Administration: Oral, intramuscular, intravenous

Dose: <1 week of age and <2000 g: 50 mg/kg/day given in 2 divided doses; >1 week of age and <2000 g: 100 mg/kg/day given in 2 divided doses. Children: 150 mg/kg/day given in 4 divided doses (maximum daily dose 12 g)

Precautions: Each gram of oxacillin contains 3.1 meq of sodium. Dosage of oxacillin may need to be modified in liver failure

Adverse Effects: May cross-react with penicillin, hematuria and nephritis

Available: Injection: 4 g and 10 g vial; capsules: 250 mg, 500 mg; oral solution: 250 mg/5 ml

Drug: PARALDEHYDE

Route of Administration: Oral, intramuscular, intravenous, rectal
Dose: 0.1–0.15 mg/kg (mix 4 ml in 100 ml of normal saline)
Precautions: Give only in a glass syringe and protect from light
Available: Injection: 2 ml and 5 ml ampules

Drug: PEMOLINE (CYLERT)

Route of Administration: Oral
Dose: 37.5 mg to start; increase at weekly intervals to achieve the desired clinical response or a maximal daily dose of 112.5 mg; usual dose range is 56.25–75 mg/day
Precautions: Same as methylphenidate, D-amphetamine
Adverse Effects: Same as methylphenidate, D-amphetamine
Available: Tablets: 18.75 mg, 37.5 mg (chewable), 75 mg

Drug: D-PENICILLAMINE (DEPEN, CUPRIMINE)

Route of Administration: Oral
Dose: 5–10 mg/kg/day given as a single dose (maximum 500 mg/day)
Precautions: Should be given with food or flavored food substance to improve palatibility
Adverse Effects: Anorexia, nausea, vomiting, diarrhea, bitter taste, stomatitis, blood dyscrasias, proteinuria, glomerulonephritis, pruritus, dermatitis, cross-sensitivity with penicillins
Available: Capsules: 125 mg, 250 mg

Drug: PENICILLIN G, BENZATHINE (BICILLIN, BIBENZYL PENICILLIN)

Route of Administration: Intramuscular
Dose: 0.2–1.2 million units per dose (1 mg is equivalent to 1600 units)
Precautions: Same as penicillin G, potassium
Adverse Effects: Same as penicillin G, potassium
Available: Injection: 300,000 units/ml, vial; 600,000 units/ml, Tubex

Drug: PENICILLIN G, POTASSIUM (PLAIN PENICILLIN)

Route of Administration: Oral, intramuscular, intravenous
Dose: Intravenous or intramuscular: <7 days of age: 50,000–100,000 units/kg/day in 2 divided doses; 7–28 days of age: 250,000 units/kg/day in 4 divided doses; children (i.v. or i.m.): 100,000–800,000 units/kg/day in 4–6 divided doses. Oral: 60,000 units/kg/day in 4 divided doses (maximum daily dose 20,000,000 units)
Precautions: Each 1,000,000 units contains 3 meq of potassium
Adverse Effects: Allergic reactions, seizures (high doses only)
Available: Injection: 1,000,000 units, 5,000,000 units and 20,000,000 units/vial; sodium penicillin G is available in vials of 1,000,000 and 5,000,000 units; tablets: 200,000 units, 400,000 units; liquid: 200,000 units and 400,000 units/5 ml

Drug: PENICILLIN G, PROCAINE

Route of Administration: Intramuscular
Dose: 50,000 units/kg/day in 2 divided doses; gonorrhea dose: 100,000 units/kg once preceded by oral probeneid (maximum dose 4.8 million units)
Available: Injection: 300,000 units, 600,000 units and 1,200,000 units, Tubex; 600,000 units/1.2 ml, 10 ml vial

Drug: PENICILLIN V, POTASSIUM (PEN VK, V-CILLIN K)

Route of Administration: Oral
Dose: 25,000–50,000 units/kg/day or 40 mg/kg/day in 4 divided doses; rheumatic fever prophylaxis: 400,000 units twice daily
Precautions: Same as penicillin G, potassium

Adverse Effects: Same as penicillin G, potassium
Available: Tablets: 200,000 units, 400,000 units; oral solution: 200,000 units/5 ml, 400,000 units/5 ml

Drug: PHENOBARBITAL (LUMINAL)
Route of Administration: Oral, intramuscular, intravenous
Dose: Initial 10 mg/kg; may be repeated once
Subsequent 3–6 mg/kg/day in 2 divided doses in children; 1–2 mg/kg/day in 2 divided doses in adolescents
Precautions: Due to slower availability, intramuscular phenobarbital should not be used for the actively convulsing child. Drug interactions may occur when phenobarbital is combined with valproic acid, phenytoin, oral anticoagulants and theophylline
Adverse Effects: Sedation, somnolence, ataxia, paradoxical excitation or hyperexcitability, hypotension, cardiorespiratory depression (especially when administered with diazepam to control status epilepticus)
Available: Injection: 65 mg/ml, 1 ml vial; tablets: 15 mg, 30 mg, 60 mg, 100 mg; elixir: 20 mg/5 ml

Drug: PHENYLEPHRINE HYDROCHLORIDE (NEO-SYNEPHRINE)
Route of Administration: Oral, intramuscular, intravenous, intranasal, subcutaneous
Dose: Hypotension: 0.1 mg/kg/dose every 1–2 hr as needed. (To prepare infusion, mix 10 ml per 100 ml saline, adjust dosage rate to desired effect.) Intranasal: 2–3 drops topically in each nostril of a 0.25% solution. Oral (decongestant): 1 mg/kg/day in 4 divided doses
Precautions: Use cautiously in the presence of hypertension, arrhythmias, hyperthyroidism, or hyperglycemia
Available: Injection: 10 mg/ml, 1 ml ampule; nasal solution: 0.25, 0.5 and 1%; elixir: 5 mg/5 ml

Drug: PHENYTOIN (DILANTIN, VARIOUS GENERICS)
Route of Administration: Oral, intravenous
Dose: Initial 10 mg/kg, may be repeated once
Subsequent <20 kg: 5–10 mg/kg/day in 2 divided doses, 20–40 kg: 5–7 mg/kg/day in 2 divided doses; >40 kg: 5 mg/kg/day in 2 divided doses
Precautions: Intravenous phenytoin should be administered directly into a vein or intravenous tubing. If dilution is unavoidable, normal saline is required since other solutions will result in crystallization of phenytoin. The dose should be administered slowly over 10 min with cardiac monitoring. Intramuscular phenytoin should be avoided due to erratic and incomplete absorption
Adverse Effects: Sedation, somnolence, nystagmus, ataxia, gingival hyperplasia, rare rashes and Stevens-Johnson syndrome, nausea, hepatotoxicity, vitamin deficiency. Drug interactions may occur when phenytoin is combined with phenobarbital, chloramphenicol, isoniazid, salicylates, oral anticoagulants and corticosteroids
Available: Injection: 100 mg/2 ml, 250 mg/5 ml; capsules 30 mg, 100 mg; chewable tablets: 50 mg; elixir: 20 mg/5 ml

Drug: POLYSTYRENE SULFONATE SODIUM (KAYEXALATE)
Route of Administration: Oral, rectal
Dose: 1 g/kg; orally the drug may be administered with food or beverage or by nasogastric tube; rectally it may be administered by making an enema with 10% glucose and water, 1 g in 4 ml
Precautions: The enema must be retained for at least 30 min. Kayexalate may bind other drugs
Available: Powder

Drug: PREDNISONE (DELTASONE)
Route of Administration: Oral
Dose: Antirheumatic dose: 1–2 mg/kg/day in 1–4 divided doses; nephrotic syndome: 2 mg/kg/day
Precautions: Every other day therapy is advised once dosage is established to minimize growth retardation
Adverse Effects: Sodium and water retention, growth retardation
Available: Tablets: 1 mg, 2.5 mg, 5 mg, 10 mg, 50 mg

Drug: PROCAINAMIDE (PRONESTYL)
Route of Administration: Oral, intramuscular, intravenous
Dose: Oral: 15–50 mg/kg/day given in 4 divided doses. Intravenous: 2 mg/kg/dose (maximum 100 mg) diluted and given slowly over 15–30 min. May be repeated every 30 min. Maximum total daily dose is 2–4 g oral or i.m. or 1–2 g i.v.
Precautions: Dosage adjustment is recommended for patients with reduced renal function due to prolonged excretion; procainamide should not be given in patients with myasthenia gravis or complete heart block
Adverse Effects: Hypertension, myocardial depression, conduction block and arrhythmias, lupus-like syndrome, nausea and vomiting. A prolonged QRS interval sec suggests toxicity
Available: Injection: 100 mg/ml; capsules: 250 mg, 375 mg, 500 mg

Drug: PROPRANOLOL (INDERAL)
Route of Administration: Oral, intravenous
Dose: Acute antiarrhythmic dose: Intravenous: 0.01 mg/kg/dose given slowly; may repeat every 6–8 hr as needed; Oral: 1.0 mg/kg/day in 4 divided doses (maximum oral daily dose 60 mg)
Precautions: i.v. injection should be given over 10 min. Propranolol should be used with extreme caution in patients with asthma, diabetes or congestive heart failure. Should be discontinued 48 hr prior to cardiac surgery
Adverse Effects: Hypoglycemia, hypotension, nausea and vomiting
Available: Injection: 1 mg/ml, 1 ml ampule; tablets: 10 mg, 20 mg, 40 mg, 80 mg

Drug: QUINIDINE SULFATE (VARIOUS GENERICS)
Route of Administration: Oral, intramuscular, intravenous
Dose: Test dose of 2 mg/kg orally. Sulfate: 3–6 mg/kg/dose repeated every 2–3 hr for up to 5 times per day. Gluconate: 2–10 mg/kg/dose repeated every 3–6 hr
Precautions: Intravenous use of quinidine is only recommended when a cardiologist is in attendance. Absorption from the i.m. site is erratic and unreliable. Oral quinidine may be taken with food
Adverse Effects: Cinchonism is a sign of quinidine toxicity and is characterized by tinnitus, headache, nausea and disturbed vision
Available: Gluconate injection: 80 mg/ml; quinidine sulfate capsules: 200 mg, 300 mg; quinidine gluconate tablets: 324 mg

Drug: RESERPINE (RAU-SED, SANDRIL, SERPASIL)
Route of Administration: Oral, intramuscular
Dose: Oral: 10–20 μg/kg/day; intramuscular: 0.15 mg/kg/day in 2 divided doses
Precautions: Intramuscular route is to be used only for acute hypertension. Use with caution in patients with peptic ulcer
Adverse Effects: Nasal stuffiness and lethargy
Available: Injection: 2.5 mg/ml, 2 ml ampule; tablets: 100 μg, 250 μg, 1 mg; elixir: 250 μg/5 ml

Drug: SPECTINOMYCIN (TROBICIN)

Route of Administration: Intramuscular
Dose: 40 mg/kg/dose intramuscularly (maximum 2 g)
Precautions: Not effective for syphilis
Available: Injection: 2 and 4 g vials

Drug: SPIRONOLACTONE (ALDACTONE)
Route of Administration: Oral
Dose: 1.5–3 mg/kg/daily in 1 or 2 divided doses (maximum daily dose 100 mg)
Precautions: Observe for hyperkalemia, hyponatremia, elevated BUN or mild acidosis; contraindicated in acute renal failure; may potentiate β-blocking agents and other hypotensive drugs
Available: Tablets: 25 mg

Drug: SULFISOXAZOLE (GANTRISIN)
Route of Administration: Oral, intramuscular, intravenous
Dose: 120 mg/kg/day (maximum daily dose 4–6 g). Initial loading dose is ½ the daily dose
Precautions: With oral Sulfisoxazole, fluid intake should be encouraged to enhance excretion of the metabolites. Use with caution in presence of renal or liver disease or G6PD deficiency
Adverse Effects: Gastrointestinal distress, rash, fever, allergic reaction
Available: Injection: 400 mg/ml, 5 ml ampules; tablets: 500 mg; pediatric suspension: 500 mg/5 ml; oral suspension: 1 g/5 ml (Lipo-Gantrisin)

Drug: TERBUTALINE (BRETHINE, BRICANYL)
Route of Administration: Oral, subcutaneous, inhalation
Dose: Not recommended for children less than 12 yr. Oral: 2.5–5 mg t.i.d.; subcutaneous: 0.25 mg/dose may repeat × 1 in 15–30 min
Adverse Effects: Nervousness, tremor, headache, nausea, and others as with all sympathomimetic agents
Available: Injection: 1 mg/ml; tablets: 2.5 mg, 5 mg

Drug: TETRACYCLINE (ACHROMYCIN)
Route of Administration: Oral and intravenous
Dose: Oral: 20–40 mg/kg/day given in 4 divided doses (maximum daily dose 2–3 g); i.v. 10–20 mg/kg/day given in 2 divided doses (maximum daily dose 2 g)
Precautions: Due to deposition of the drug in the enamel and dentin of teeth resulting in enamel hypoplasia and discoloration of permanent teeth, tetracycline is not recommended in children under 8 yr of age. Intravenous route of administration is not recommended because it carries a high risk of hepatotoxicity due to fatty infiltration. Concomitant use of any products that contain calcium (milk), iron or antacids should be avoided, for tetracycline chelates with divalent ions, producing lowered serum levels. Absorption of the drug is reduced in an alkaline medium
Adverse Effects: Gastrointestinal distress, hepatotoxicity, superinfection and photosensitivity
Available: Injection: 100 mg, 250 mg, 500 mg vials; capsules: 100 mg, 250 mg, 500 mg; syrup: 125mg/5 ml

Drug: THEOPHYLLINE (ELIXIOPHYLLIN, THEOPHYL, THEODUR, SLO-PHYLLIN)
Route of Administration: Oral, intravenous, rectal
Dose: Initial — *Status asthmaticus.* Children: 6 mg/kg over 20–30 min i.v.
Subsequent — 0.9–1.1 mg/kg/hr. *Chronic asthma.* Oral: 4–6 mg/kg/dose given every 6 hr. Sustained-released preparations are given every 8 or 12 hr. Levels should be used to monitor therapy. *Neonatal apnea. Initial:* 6 mg/kg

infused over 20–30 min. *Subsequent:* 3–4 mg/kg/dose either orally or intravenously every 8 hrs (monitor level)

Precautions: Rectal suppositories are erratically absorbed and should not be administered to children. Use with caution in cardiac, renal, hepatic and ulcer disease and glaucoma

Adverse Effects: CNS irritability, nervousness and insomnia, seizures (associated with levels >40 μg/ml), hypotension, tachyarrhythmias, nausea, vomiting, abdominal cramping

Available: Injection: aminophylline 250 mg/10 ml; tablets and capsules: 100 mg, 125 mg, 200 mg, 250 mg; sustained-released tablets and capsules: 60 mg, 100 mg, 125 mg, 200 mg, 250 mg, 300 mg; elixir and syrup: 80 mg/15 ml

Drug: THIORIDAZINE (MELLARIL)

Route of Administration: Oral

Dose: 10 mg b.i.d. initially; increase weekly to 50–800 mg/day

Precautions: Similar to chlorpromazine

Adverse Effects: Similar to chlorpromazine. In addition, ocular disturbances may occur

Available: Tablets: 10 mg, 25 mg, 50 mg, 100 mg, 150 mg and 200 mg; syrup: 30 mg/5 ml, 100 mg/5 ml

Drug: TOLMETIN (TOLECTIN)

Route of Administration: Oral

Dose: Start at 15 mg/kg/day, increase gradually as tolerated to 30 mg/kg (maximum daily dose 1800 mg). Daily dose should be given in 3 divided doses

Precautions: Cross-sensitivity with aspirin may occur in patients receiving tolmetin. Concomitant aspirin may lower tolmetin peak level

Adverse Effects: Headache, dizziness, drowsiness, vertigo, dyspepsia, abdominal pain, nausea and vomiting, prolonged bleeding time, possible hepatotoxicity

Available: Tablets: 200 mg

Drug: TRIFLUOPERAZINE (STELAZINE)

Route of Administration: Oral, intramuscular

Dose: Recommended for adolescents only, 5–30 mg/day

Precautions: Similar to chlorpromazine

Adverse Effects: Similar to chlorpromazine

Available: Injection: 2 mg/ml, 10 ml vials; tablets: 5 mg, 10 mg

Drug: TRIMETHOPRIM SULFAMETHOXAZOLE (BACTRIM, SEPTRA)

Route of Administration: Oral, intravenous

Dose: Minor infections: 8 mg/kg/day of trimethoprim (TMP) and 40 mg/kg of sulfamethoxazole (SMZ) given in 2 divided doses; for pneumocystis: 20 mg/kg of TMP and 100 mg/kg/day of SMZ in 4 divided doses. Intravenous: 15–20 mg/kg/day (based on the TMP component) given in 4 divided doses

Precautions: Rapid infusion must be avoided. The parenteral preparation should not be given intramuscularly

Adverse Effects: Bone marrow suppression and occasional gastrointestinal disturbances

Available: Injection: 80 mg trimethoprim and 400 mg sulfamethoxazole per 5 ml ampule. Tablets: trimethoprim 80 mg, sulfamethoxazole 400 mg; double strength tablets—trimethoprim 160 mg, sulfamethoxazole 800 mg. Suspension: trimethoprim 40 mg and sulfamethoxazole 200 mg/5 ml

Drug: VANCOMYCIN (VANCOCIN)

Route of Administration: Intravenous

Dose: <1 month of age and full term: 45 mg/kg/day in 3 divided doses; <1

month of age and low birth weight: 30 mg/kg/day in two divided doses. Children: 40 mg/kg/day in 4 divided doses (maximum daily dose 2–4 g)

Precautions: Administer slowly over 30–60 min to reduce incidence of thrombophlebitis. Major dosage modification is required in renal disease

Available: Injection: 50 mg/ml, 10 ml vial

Drug: VITAMIN B_{12}

Route of Administration: Oral, intramuscular, intravenous

Dose: 10–30 μg once or twice weekly

Adverse Effects: Possible allergic reactions

Available: Injection: 100 μg/ml, 1000 μg/ml; oral: vitamin B complex tablets

Index